VOLUME 2

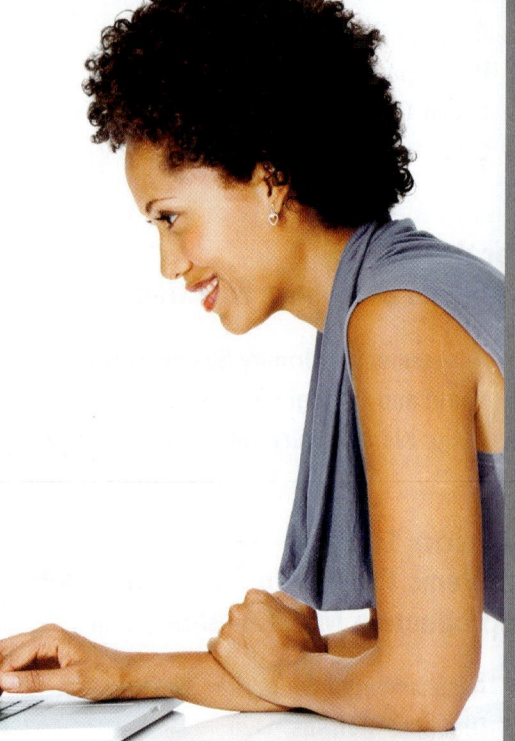

10th Edition

MEDICAL-SURGICAL NURSING

Assessment and Management of Clinical Problems

Volume 2

Sharon L. Lewis, RN, PhD, FAAN

Professor Emerita, University of New Mexico, Albuquerque, New Mexico
Former Castella Distinguished Professor, School of Nursing, University of Texas Health Science Center at San Antonio, San Antonio, Texas
Developer and Consultant, Stress-Busting Program for Family Caregivers

Linda Bucher, RN, PhD, CEN, CNE

Emerita Professor, School of Nursing, University of Delaware, Newark, Delaware
Per Diem Staff Nurse, Emergency Department, Virtua Memorial Hospital, Mt. Holly, New Jersey

Margaret McLean Heitkemper, RN, PhD, FAAN

Professor and Chairperson, Biobehavioral Nursing and Health Systems, Elizabeth Sterling Soule Endowed Chair in Nursing, School of Nursing
Adjunct Professor, Division of Gastroenterology, School of Medicine, University of Washington, Seattle, Washington

Mariann M. Harding, RN, PhD, CNE

Associate Professor of Nursing, Kent State University at Tuscarawas, New Philadelphia, Ohio

Section Editors

Jeffrey Kwong, DNP, MPH, ANP-BC, FAANP
Associate Professor of Nursing at CUMC
Program Director, Adult-Gerontology Nurse Practitioner Program
Program Director, HIV Sub-Specialty
Program Director, Elder LGBT Interprofessional Collaborative Care Program (ELINC)
Program Director, Collaborative Access for LGBT Adults (CALA)
Columbia University School of Nursing
New York, New York

Dottie Roberts, RN, EdD, MSN, MACI, OCNS-C, CMSRN, CNE
Executive Director,
Orthopaedic Nurses Certification Board,
Chicago, Illinois;
Editor, "MEDSURG Nursing,"
Official Journal of the Academy
of Medical-Surgical Nurses
Pitman, New Jersey

ELSEVIER

ELSEVIER

3251 Riverport Lane
St. Louis, Missouri 63043

MEDICAL-SURGICAL NURSING; ASSESSMENT AND MANAGEMENT
OF CLINICAL PROBLEMS, 10TH EDITION

ISBN (two-volume set): 978-0-323-35593-3
ISBN (Volume 2): 978-0-323-49758-9

Notices

Knowledge and best practice in this field are constantly changing. As new research and experience broaden our understanding, changes in research methods, professional practices, or medical treatment may become necessary.

Practitioners and researchers must always rely on their own experience and knowledge in evaluating and using any information, methods, compounds, or experiments described herein. In using such information or methods they should be mindful of their own safety and the safety of others, including parties for whom they have a professional responsibility.

With respect to any drug or pharmaceutical products identified, readers are advised to check the most current information provided (i) on procedures featured or (ii) by the manufacturer of each product to be administered, to verify the recommended dose or formula, the method and duration of administration, and contraindications. It is the responsibility of practitioners, relying on their own experience and knowledge of their patients, to make diagnoses, to determine dosages and the best treatment for each individual patient, and to take all appropriate safety precautions.

To the fullest extent of the law, neither the Publisher nor the authors, contributors, or editors, assume any liability for any injury and/or damage to persons or property as a matter of products liability, negligence or otherwise, or from any use or operation of any methods, products, instructions, or ideas contained in the material herein.

Herdman, T.H. & Kamitsuru, S. (Eds.). (2014). *NANDA International Nursing Diagnoses: Definitions & Classification, 2015-2017*. Oxford: Wiley Blackwell.

Previous editions copyrighted 2014, 2011, 2007, 2004, 2000, 1996, 1992, 1987, and 1983 by Mosby, Inc., an affiliate of Elsevier Inc.

Library of Congress Cataloging-in-Publication Data

Names: Lewis, Sharon Mantik, author.
Title: Medical-surgical nursing : assessment and management of clinical problems / Sharon L. Lewis
  [and five others].
Description: Tenth edition. | St. Louis, Missouri : Elsevier, Inc, [2017] | Includes bibliographical references and
  index.
Identifiers: LCCN 2016018182| ISBN 9780323328524 (v. 1 : hardcover : alk. paper) | ISBN 9780323355933
  (v. 2 : hardcover : alk. paper)
Subjects: | MESH: Nursing Care | Nursing Assessment | Perioperative Nursing
Classification: LCC RT41 | NLM WY 100 | DDC 617/.0231—dc23 LC record available at
  https://lccn.loc.gov/2016018182

Senior Content Strategist: Jamie Blum
Content Development Manager: Jean Sims Fornango
Content Development Specialist: Jennifer Hermes, Melissa Rawe
Publishing Services Manager: Julie Eddy
Senior Project Manager: Mary G. Stueck
Design Direction: Ashley Miner, Renée Duenow

Printed in the United States of America

Last digit is the print number: 9 8 7 6 5 4 3 2 1

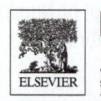

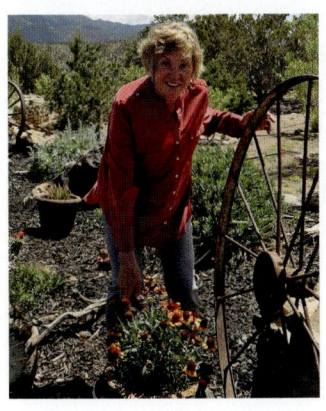

SHARON L. LEWIS, RN, PhD, FAAN

Sharon Lewis received her Bachelor of Science in nursing from the University of Wisconsin–Madison, Master of Science in nursing with a minor in biological sciences from the University of Colorado–Denver, and PhD in immunology from the Department of Pathology at the University of New Mexico School of Medicine. She had a 2-year postdoctoral fellowship from the National Kidney Foundation. Her more than 45 years of teaching experience include inservice education and teaching in associate degree, baccalaureate, master's degree, and doctoral programs in Maryland, Illinois, Wisconsin, New Mexico, and Texas. Favorite teaching areas are pathophysiology, immunology, and family caregiving. She has been actively involved in clinical research for the past 35 years, investigating altered immune responses in various disorders and developing a stress management program for family caregivers. Her current primary professional responsibility is disseminating the Stress-Busting for Family Caregivers Program that she developed. Her free time is spent biking, landscaping, gardening, and being a grandmother.

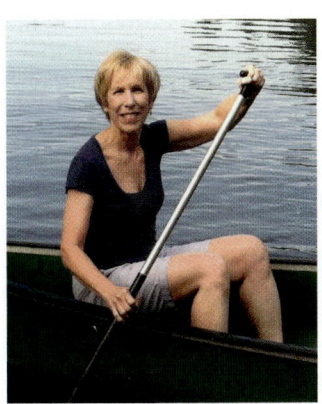

LINDA BUCHER, RN, PhD, CEN, CNE

Linda Bucher is an Emerita Professor in the School of Nursing at the University of Delaware in Newark, Delaware. She received her Bachelor of Science in nursing from Thomas Jefferson University in Philadelphia, her Master of Science in adult health and illness from the University of Pennsylvania in Philadelphia, and her doctorate in nursing from Widener University in Chester, Pennsylvania. Her 40 years of nursing experience have spanned staff and patient education, acute and critical care nursing, and teaching in associate, baccalaureate, and graduate nursing programs in New Jersey, Pennsylvania, and Delaware. Her preferred teaching areas include emergency and cardiac nursing and evidence-based practice. She maintains her clinical practice by working as an emergency nurse, actively participates in the American Association of Critical Care Nurses, and volunteers as a postoperative nurse for Operation Smile. In her free time, she enjoys traveling and skiing with her family.

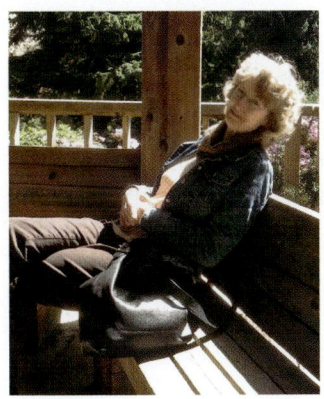

MARGARET MCLEAN HEITKEMPER, RN, PhD, FAAN

Margaret Heitkemper is Professor and Chairperson, Department of Biobehavioral Nursing and Health Systems at the School of Nursing, and Adjunct Professor, Division of Gastroenterology at the School of Medicine at the University of Washington. She is also Director of the National Institutes of Health-National Institute for Nursing Research–funded Center for Research on Management of Sleep Disturbances at the University of Washington. In the fall of 2006, Dr. Heitkemper was appointed the Elizabeth Sterling Soule Endowed Chair in Nursing. Dr. Heitkemper received her Bachelor of Science in nursing from Seattle University, a Master of Nursing in gerontologic nursing from the University of Washington, and a doctorate in Physiology and Biophysics from the University of Illinois–Chicago. She has been on faculty at the University of Washington since 1981 and has been the recipient of three School of Nursing Excellence in Teaching awards and the University of Washington Distinguished Teaching Award. In addition, in 2002 she received the Distinguished Nutrition Support Nurse Award from the American Society for Parenteral and Enteral Nutrition (ASPEN), in 2003 the American Gastroenterological Association and Janssen Award for Clinical Research in Gastroenterology, and in 2005 she was the first recipient of the Pfizer and Friends of the National Institutes for Nursing Research Award for Research in Women's Health.

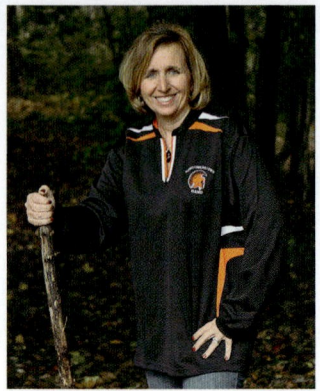

MARIANN M. HARDING, RN, PhD, CNE

Mariann Harding is an Associate Professor of Nursing at Kent State University Tuscarawas, New Philadelphia, Ohio, where she has been on the faculty since 2005. She received her diploma in nursing from Mt. Carmel School of Nursing in Columbus, Ohio, her Bachelor of Science in nursing from Ohio University in Athens, Ohio, her Master of Science in Nursing as an adult nurse practitioner from the Catholic University of America in Washington D.C., and her doctorate in nursing from West Virginia University in Morgantown, West Virginia. Her 29 years of nursing experience has primarily been in critical care nursing, and teaching in licensed practical, associate, and baccalaureate nursing programs. She currently teaches medical-surgical nursing, health care policy, and evidence-based practice. Her research has focused on promoting student success and health promotion among individuals with gout and facing cancer. Free time is spent with her family or traveling, walking, and reading.

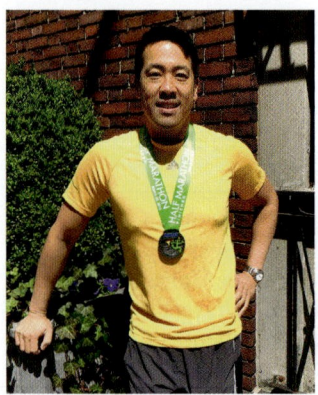

JEFFREY KWONG, DNP, MPH, ANP-BC, FAANP

Jeffrey Kwong is an Associate Professor of Nursing at Columbia University School of Nursing where he also serves as Director of the Adult-Gerontology Nurse Practitioner Program. He has worked in the area of adult primary care with a special focus on HIV for over 20 years. He received his undergraduate degree from the University of California–Berkeley, his nurse practitioner degree from the University of California–San Francisco, and completed his doctoral training at the University of Colorado–Denver. He also has a Master's Degree in Public Health with a focus on Health Education and Behavioral Sciences from the University of California–Los Angeles and was appointed a Hartford Geriatric Interprofessional Scholar while completing his gerontology education at NYU. In addition to teaching, Dr. Kwong maintains a clinical practice at Gotham Medical Group in New York City. In 2015 he was inducted as a Fellow in the American Association of Nurse Practitioners.

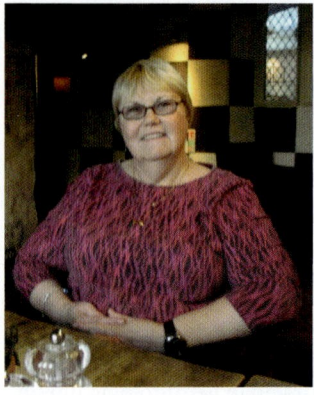

DOTTIE ROBERTS, RN, EdD, MSN, MACI, OCNS-C, CMSRN, CNE

Dottie Roberts received her Bachelor of Science in nursing from Beth-El College of Nursing, Colorado Springs, Colorado, Master of Science in adult health nursing from Beth-El College of Nursing and Health Sciences, Master of Arts in curriculum and instruction from Colorado Christian University, Colorado Springs, Colorado, and EdD in healthcare education from Nova Southeastern University, Ft. Lauderdale, Florida. She has over 25 years of experience in medical-surgical and orthopaedic nursing, and holds certifications in both specialties. She has also taught in two baccalaureate programs in the Southeast and is certified as a nurse educator. For her dissertation, Dottie completed a phenomenological study on facilitation of critical-thinking skills by clinical faculty in a baccalaureate nursing program. She has been Executive Director of the Orthopaedic Nurses Certification Board since 2005 and editor of "MEDSURG Nursing," the official journal of the Academy of Medical-Surgical Nurses, since 2003. Her free time is spent traveling, reading, and cross-stitching.

Richard B. Arbour, RN, MSN, CCRN, CNRN, CCNS, FAAN
Clinical Faculty
School of Nursing
LaSalle University
Philadelphia, Pennsylvania

Adena Bargad, RN, PhD, CNM
Assistant Professor, Columbia University Medical Center
Director, Sub-Specialty Program in Women's Health
Columbia University School of Nursing
New York, New York

Diana Taibi Buchanan, RN, PhD
Associate Professor
Biobehavioral Nursing and Health Systems
University of Washington
Seattle, Washington

Darcy Burbage, RN, MSN, AOCN, CBCN
Survivorship Nurse Navigator
Helen F. Graham Cancer Center and Research Institute
Newark, Delaware

Kim K. Choma, RN, DNP, WHNP
Women's Health Nurse Practitioner–Training Consultant
NY/NJ AIDS Education and Training Centers (AETC)
New York, New York

Susan Collazo, MSN, APN-CNP
Thoracic Surgery
Northwestern Memorial Hospital
Chicago, Illinois

Paula P. Cox-North, PhD, ARNP
Clinical Assistant Professor
School of Nursing
University of Washington School of Nursing
Seattle, Washington

Hazel A. Dennison, RN, DNP, APNc, CPHQ, CNE
Director of Education Services
American Nephrology Nurses Association
Anthony J. Jannetti, Pub.
Pitman, New Jersey

Jane K. Dickinson, RN, PhD, CDE
Program Coordinator/Faculty
Diabetes Education and Management
Teachers College
Columbia University
New York, New York

Rose Ann DiMaria-Ghalili, RN, PhD, CNSC
Associate Professor of Nursing
College of Nursing and Health Professions
Drexel University
Philadelphia, Pennsylvania

Mechele Fillman, RN, MSN
Nursing Practitioner
Pain Management
Stanford Healthcare
Palo Alto, California

Diana L. Gallagher, RN, MS, CWOCN, CFCN
Clinical Nursing and Education
HealthMatters Consulting
Fayetteville, Arkansas

Sherry A. Greenberg, RN, PhD, GNP-BC
Coordinator, Advanced Practice Nursing: Geriatrics Program
Hartford Institute for Geriatric Nursing
New York University College of Nursing
New York, New York

Angela DiSabatino Herman, RN, MS
Manager, Cardiovascular Clinical Trials
Christiana Care Health Services
Newark, Delaware

Christine R. Hoch, RN, MSN
Nursing Instructor
University of Delaware
Newark, Delaware

David M. Horner, CRNA, MS, APN
CRNA Anesthesia
Marlton Hospital
Marlton, New Jersey

Melissa L. Hutchinson, RN, MN, CCNS, CCRN
Clinical Nurse Specialist
MICU/CCU
VA Puget Sound Health Care System
Seattle, Washington

Katherine A. Kelly, RN, DNP, FNP-C, CEN
Assistant Professor of Nursing
California State University
Sacramento, California

Judy Knighton, RN, MScN
Clinical Nurse Specialist—Burns
Ross Tilley Burn Centre
Sunnybrook Health Sciences Centre
Toronto, Ontario, Canada

Nancy Kupper, RN, MSN
Associate Professor of Nursing
Tarrant County College
Fort Worth, Texas

Janet Lenart, RN, MN, MPH
Senior Lecturer and Director for Online Education
University of Washington School of Nursing
Seattle, Washington

Linda Littlejohns, RN, MSN, CNRN, FAAN
Neuroscience Clinical Nursing Consultant
San Juan Capistrano, California

Amy McKeever, PhD, CRNP, WHNP-BC
Assistant Professor
College of Nursing
Villanova University
Villanova, Pennsylvania

De Ann F. Mitchell, RN, PhD
Director of Nursing
Tarrant County College
Fort Worth, Texas

Carolyn Moffa, RN, MSN, FNP-C, CHFN
Clinical Leader, Heart Failure Program
Christiana Care Health System
Newark, Delaware

Eugene E. Mondor, RN, MN, CNCC(C)
Clinical Nurse Educator—Adult Critical Care
Royal Alexandra Hospital
Edmonton, Alberta, Canada

Janice A. Neil, RN, PhD
Associate Professor and Chair
Undergraduate Nursing Science Junior Division
College of Nursing
East Carolina University
Greenville, North Carolina

Suzanne Teresa Parsell, MSN, ANP-BC, CUNP
Division of Endourology
University of Michigan
Ann Arbor, Michigan

Madona Dawn Plueger, RN, MSN, ACNS-BC, CNRN
Neuroscience Clinical Nurse Specialist
Barrow Neurological Institute
St. Joseph's Hospital and Medical Center
Phoenix, Arizona

Carolee Polek, RN, PhD, AOCNS, BMTCN
Associate Professor
School of Nursing
University of Delaware
Newark, Delaware

Rosemary C. Polomano, RN, PhD, FAAN
Professor of Pain Practice
Department of Biobehavioral Health Sciences
University of Pennsylvania School of Nursing;
Professor of Anesthesiology and Critical Care (Secondary)
University of Pennsylvania Perelman School of Medicine
Philadelphia, Pennsylvania

Matthew C. Price, RN, MS, CNP, ONP-C, RNFA
Manager, Orthopedic Advanced Practice Providers
Orthopedics
Riverside Methodist Hospital
Columbus, Ohio

Susanne A. Quallich, RN, MSN, ANP-BC, NP-C, CUNP
Andrology Nurse Practitioner
Urology
University of Michigan Health System
Ann Arbor, Michigan

Kathleen A. Rich, RN, PhD, CCNS, CCRN-CSC, CNN
Cardiovascular Clinical Specialist
Patient Care Services
IU Health La Porte Hospital
La Porte, Indiana

Sandra Irene Rome, RN, MN, AOCN, CNS
Clinical Nurse Specialist
Blood and Marrow Transplant Program
Cedars-Sinai Medical Center
Los Angeles, California

Jennifer Saylor, RN, PhD, ACNS-BC
Assistant Professor
School of Nursing
University of Delaware
Newark, Delaware

Maureen A. Seckel, RN, MSN, APN, ACNS-BC, CCNS, CCRN
Clinical Nurse Specialist
Medical Pulmonary Critical Care
Christiana Care Health System
Newark, Delaware

Rose Shaffer, RN, MSN, ACNP-CS, CCRN
Cardiology Nurse Practitioner
Thomas Jefferson University Hospital
Philadelphia, Pennsylvania

Anita Jo Shoup, RN, MSN, CNOR
Perioperative Clinical Nurse Specialist
Swedish Edmonds
Edmonds, Washington

Cindy M. Sullivan, MN, ANP-C, CNRN
Nurse Practitioner
Neurosurgery
Barrow Neurological Institute
Phoenix, Arizona

Linda A. L. Upchurch, DNP, ANP-BC
Assistant Professor
School of Nursing
Georgia Southern University
Statesboro, Georgia

Deidre D. Wipke-Tevis, RN, PhD
Associate Professor
PhD Program Director
MU Sinclair School of Nursing
University of Missouri
Columbia, Missouri

Mary K. Wollan, RN, BAN, ONC
Orthopaedic Nurse Educator
Excelen
Minneapolis, Minnesota

Kathy H. Wu, MSN, ANP-BC
Nurse Practitioner
Liver Transplant Center
New York Columbia Presbyterian Hospital
New York, New York

Meg Zomorodi, RN, PhD, CNL
Clinical Associate Professor
School of Nursing
University of North Carolina at Chapel Hill
Chapel Hill, North Carolina

Michael E. Zychowicz, RN, DNP, ANP, ONP, FAAN, FAANP
Associate Professor and Director, MSN Program
School of Nursing
Duke University
Durham, North Carolina

Karen S. Abate, PhD, FNP-BC
Trenton, New Jersey

Marian Altman, RN, MS, CNS-BC, ANP
Richmond, Virginia

Carol Annesser, RN, MSN, BC, CNE
Toledo, Ohio

Tara Back, RN, MSN
St. Louis, Missouri

Carolyn Baird, DNP, MBA, RN-BC, CARN-AP, CCDPD, FIAAN
Canonsburg, Pennsylvania

Adena Bargad, PhD, CNM
New York, New York

Janica Barnett, JD, AGPCNP-BC
New York, New York

Margaret Barton-Burke, RN, PhD, FAAN
St. Louis, Missouri

Vera Barton-Caro, RN, PhD, FNP-BC, CHFN
Wheeling, West Virginia

Cecilia M. Bidigare, RN, MSN, CNS-BC, CNE
Dayton, Ohio

Sonya H. Blevins, RN, DNP, CMSRN, CNE
Greenville, South Carolina

Donna C. Bond, RN, DNP, CCNS, AE-C, CTTS
Roanoke, Virginia

Marilyn Borkgren, APN, MS, CCNS
Elk Grove Village, Illinois

Elisabeth G. Bradley, MS, APN, ACNS-BC, AGPCNP-BC
Newark, Delaware

Marylee Bressie, RN, DNP, CCRN, CCNS, CEN
Minneapolis, Minnesota

Barbara Brunow, RN, MSN, MEd, CNS, CNE
Sandusky, Ohio

Diana Taibi Buchanan, RN, PhD
Seattle, Washington

Geraldine M. Budd, RN, PhD, FNP-BC, FAANP
Harrisburg, Pennsylvania

Darcy Burbage, RN, MSN, AOCN, CBCN
Newark, Delaware

Patricia Gable Burke, RN, BSN, CWOCN
Cincinnati, Ohio

Hope Bussenius, DNP, APRN, FNP-BC
Atlanta, Georgia

Judy Carlyle, RN, MNSc
Nashville, Arkansas

Kim K. Choma, RN, DNP, WHNP
New York, New York

Kim Clevenger, RN, EdD, BC
Morehead, Kentucky

Deborah Cline, RN, MS
Reno, Nevada

Susan Collazo, MSN, APN-CNP
Chicago, Illinois

Janie Corbitt, RN, MLS
Milledgeville, Georgia

Hazel A. Dennison, RN, DNP, APNc, CPHQ, CNE
Pitman, New Jersey

Jane K. Dickinson, RN, PhD, CDE
New York, New York

Vickie Lee Doscher, MSN, FNP-C, APRN
Chesapeake, Virginia

Deborah Ehlers, RN, MSN
Yakima, Washington

Susan J. Eisel, RN, MSEd
Toledo, Ohio

Rowena W. Elliott, RN, PhD, CNN, CNE, AGNP-C, FAAN
Hattiesburg, Mississippi

Dana R. Epstein, RN, PhD
Tempe, Arizona

Deborah Erickson, RN, PhD
Peoria, Illinois

Christine Espina, RN, DNP
Seattle, Washington

Cora Espina, RN, MN, ARNP, CWN
Seattle, Washington

Abimbola Farinde, PharmD, MS
Orange Beach, Alabama

Brian J. Fasolka, RN, MSN, CEN
Philadelphia, Pennsylvania

Marianne Ferrin, MSN, ACNP-BC
Philadelphia, Pennyslvania

Diana L. Gallagher, RN, MS, CWOCN, CFCN
Fayetteville, Arkansas

Karen Gilbert, RN, MSN, CNSC, CRNP
Riverton, New Jersey

Nelda S. Godfrey, RN, PhD, ACNS-BC, FAAN
Kansas City, Kansas

Roberta Goff, MSN Ed, RN-BC, ACNS-BC, ONC
Traverse City, Michigan

Regina Gonzalez-Lama, RN, MS
Staten Island, New York

Debra B. Gordon, RN-BC, DNP, ACNS-BC, FAAN
Seattle, Washington

Shari Gould, RN, MSN
Victoria, Texas

Sherry A. Greenberg, RN, PhD, GNP-BC
New York, New York

Kelly S. Grimshaw, RN, MSN, APRN, CCRN, CCTN
New Haven, Connecticut

Sharon Haas, RN, MSN, CDN
Milwaukee, Wisconsin

Debra Hagler, RN, PhD, ACNS-BC, CNE, CHSE, ANEF, FAAN
Phoenix, Arizona

Cynthia Hambach, RN, MSN, CCRN
Philadelphia, Pennsylvania

Janet L. Hannah, RN, CGRN
Leesburg, Virginia

Carla V. Hannon, MS, APRN, CCRN, CCNS
New Haven, Connecticut

Helene Harris, RN, MSN
Temple, Texas

Misty Hobart, RN, MSN, CNE
Spokane, Washington

Deena Hollingsworth, MSN, FNP-BC, CORLN
Arlington, Virginia

Michele M. Hughes, RN, MSN, ACNP, ONP-C
Mechanicsville, Virginia

Melissa Hutchinson, RN, MN, CCNS, CCRN
Seattle, Washington

Stephanie Jackson, RN, MSN, AOCNS
Los Angeles, California

Suzanne Jed, MSN, FNP-BC
Pretoria, South Africa

Monica L. Johnson, RN, MSN, MBA-HCM, CMSRN, ONC, LNC
New Orleans, Louisiana

Jane Kaufman, MS, CRNP, ANP-BC
Philadelphia, Pennsylvania

Christina D. Keller, RN, MSN-Ed
Radford, Virginia

Lauren Kemph, RN, DNP, AGPCNP
New York, New York

Tracy H. Knoll, RN, MSN
St. Louis, Missouri

Regina Kukulski, RN, MSN, ACNS, BC, CNE
Trenton, New Jersey

Jane E. Lacovara, RN, MSN, CMSRN
Tucson, Arizona

Katherine A. Ladetto, RN, MSN, APRN, ANP-BC, GNP-BC
Peabody, Massachusetts

Susan C. Landis, RN, MN
Seattle, Washington

Marci Langenkamp, RN, MS
Piqua, Ohio

Patricia Lea, RN, DNP, CCRN
Galveston, Texas

Judith M. Lewis, DNP, APRN, CRNA
Akron, Ohio

Linda R. Lewis, MSN, RN-BC
Scranton, Pennsylvania

Rebecca Liebert, RN, MSN, FNP-C, ONP-C
Tomah, Wisconsin

Linda Littlejohns, RN, MSN, CNRN, FAAN
San Juan Capistrano, California

Anthony R. Lutz, RN, MSN, A-GNP-C
Charlotte, North Carolina

Carolyn Lyon, RN, MSN
Roanoke, Virginia

Angela M. Martinelli, RN, PhD, CNOR
Fairfield, Connecticut

Donna E. McCabe, DNP, APRN-BC, GNP
New York, New York

Molly McClelland, RN, PhD, ACNS-BC, CMSRN
Detroit, Michigan

Tara McMillan-Queen, RN, MSN, ANP, GNP
Charlotte, North Carolina

Molly McNett, RN, PhD, CNRN
Cleveland, Ohio

Karen Meneses, RN, PhD, FAAN
Birmingham, Alabama

Eugene E. Mondor, RN, MN, CNCC(C)
Edmonton, Alberta, Canada

Heidi E. Monroe, MSN, RN-BC, CPAN, CAPA
Green Bay, Wisconsin

Anna P. Moore, RN, MS
Richmond, Virginia

Kathy Morrison, RN, MSN, CNRN, SCRN
Hershey, Pennsylvania

Pamela K. Newland, RN, PhD, CMSRN
St. Louis, Missouri

Lorraine Nowakowski-Grier, MSN, APRN-BC, CDE
Newark, Delaware

Ellen Odell, DNP, ACNS-BC, CNE, APRN
Siloam Springs, Arkansas

Suzanne Teresa Parsell, MSN, ANP-BC, CUNP
Ann Arbor, Michigan

Jessica Pastor, MSN, DNP(c), ACNP-BC, SANE-A, TNCC
Detroit and Troy, Michigan

Rebecca Personett, RN, PhD, NEA-BC
Gainesville and Dallas, Texas

Madona Dawn Plueger, RN, MSN, ACNS-BC, CNRN
Phoenix, Arizona

Carolee Polek, RN, PhD, AOCNS, BMTCN
Newark, Delaware

Julia R. Popp, RN, MSN
Toledo, Ohio

Sarah Byram Poppe, MSN, ANP-BC
Olympia, Washington

Matthew C. Price, RN, MS, CNP, ONP-C, RNFA
Columbus, Ohio

Susanne A. Quallich, RN, MSN, ANP-BC, NP-C, CUNP
Ann Arbor, Michigan

Margaret R. Rateau, RN, PhD, CNE
East Liverpool, Ohio

Patricia S. Regojo, RN, MSN
Philadelphia, Pennsylvania

Courtney Reinisch, RN, DNP, APN-BC, DCC
Newark, New Jersey

Janet M. Riggs, RN, DrNP
Philadelphia, Pennsylvania

Julie Rogan, RN, MSN, ACCNS-AG, AOCNS, CCRN
Philadelphia, Pennsylvania

Diane Marie Rudolphi, RN, MS
Newark, Delaware

Diane Ryzner, MSN, APN, CNS, OCNS-C
Arlington Heights, Illinois

Susan A. Sandstrom, RN, MSN, BC, CNE
Omaha, Nebraska

Christine L. Savage, RN, PhD, CARN, FAAN
Baltimore, Maryland

Jennifer Saylor, RN, PhD, ACNS-BC
Newark, Delaware

Mary Scheid, RN, MSN, OCN, CBCN
Greeley, Colorado

Teresa J. Seright, RN, PhD, CCRN
Bozeman, Montana

Crystal Sheaves, RN, MSN, APRN, FNP-BC
Charleston, West Virginia

Crystal R. Sherman, DNP, CNP, FNP-BC, APHN-BC
Portsmouth, Ohio

Michelle Smeltzer, RN, MSN, DNPc, CEN
East Norriton, Pennsylvania

Matthew Soos, RN, BSN, BA, EMT
Atlantic City, New Jersey

Lisa Spruce, DNP, ACNS, ACNP, ANP, CNOR, CNS-CP
Denver, Colorado

Whitney Starr, MSN, FNP-BC
Denver, Colorado

Cynthia M. Steinwedel, RN, PhD, CNE
Peoria, Illinois

Laura A. Stokowski, RNC, MS
Falls Church, Virginia

Beth D. Strauss, RN, DNP, ACNS-BC
Madison, Wisconsin

Cindy M. Sullivan, MN, ANP-C, CNRN
Phoenix, Arizona

Joseph Tariman, RN, PhD, ANP-BC
Chicago, Illinois

Allison J. Terry, RN, PhD
Montgomery, Alabama

Tamekia L. Thomas, MSN, APN, PCCN, ACNS-BC
Newark, Delaware

Andrea H. Thurler, RN, DNP, FNP-BC
Boston, Massachusetts

Bonnie Tong, MSN, ACNP-BC
New York, New York

Mary Ellen Tresgallo, DNP, MPH, FNP-BC
New York, New York

Kathryn J. Trotter, DNP, CNM, FNP-C
Durham, North Carolina

Linda A. L. Upchurch, DNP, ANP-BC
Statesboro, Georgia

Olga Van Dyke, RN, MSN, CAGS
Boston, Massachusetts

Dawn M. Vanderhoef, PhD, DNP, PMHNP/CS-BC
Nashville, Tennessee

Deborah Kirk Walker, DNP, FNP-BC, NP-C, AOCN
Birmingham, Alabama

Colleen R. Walsh, RN, DNP, ONC, ONP-C, CNS, ACNP-BC
Evansville, Indiana

Daryle Wane, PhD, ARNP, FNP-BC
New Port Richey, Florida

Robert M. Welch, RN, MSN, FNP, CRNO
Reno, Nevada

Laura C. Williams, RN, MSN, CNS, ONC, CCNS
Orlando, Florida

Daniel Worrall, MSN, ANP-BC
Boston, Massachusetts

Kathy H. Wu, MSN, ANP-BC
New York, New York

Elsa Wuhrman, DNP, RN-BC, FNP, BC, DCC
New York, New York

Kenneth Wysocki, PhD, FNP-BC, FAANP
Scottsdale, Arizona

Linda H. Yoder, RN, PhD, AOCN, FAAN
Austin, Texas

Meg Zomorodi, RN, PhD, CNL
Chapel Hill, North Carolina

**To the Profession of Nursing
and to the Important People in Our Lives**

Sharon
*My husband Peter and our grandchildren
Malia, Halle, Aidan, Cian, Layla, Ryker, and Archer*

Linda
*My nieces, Stefany and Jayme,
who so admirably reflect the ideals of the nursing profession
and my godchild, Liz, for her love of written words.*

Margaret
*My husband David, our daughters Elizabeth and Ellen,
and our grandsons Jaxon James and Axel*

Mariann
My husband Jeff and our daughters Kate and Sarah

Jeff
*To my mother, Virginia, whose dedication to the field of nursing
led me on this wonderful journey.*

Dottie
*My husband Steve and my children Megan, E.J., Jessica, and Matthew,
who have supported me through four college degrees and countless writing projects,
and to our grandsons Oscar and Stephen.*

The tenth edition of *Medical-Surgical Nursing: Assessment and Management of Clinical Problems* has been thoroughly revised to incorporate the most current medical-surgical nursing information in an easy-to-use format. More than just a textbook, this is a comprehensive resource containing essential information that students need to prepare for lectures, classroom activities, examinations, clinical assignments, and the safe, comprehensive care of patients. In addition to the readable writing style and full-color illustrations, the text and accompanying resources include many special features to help students learn key medical-surgical nursing content, including patient and caregiver teaching, gerontology, interprofessional care, cultural and ethnic considerations, patient safety, genetics, nutrition and drug therapy, evidence-based practice, and much more.

The comprehensive and timely content, special features, attractive layout, and student-friendly writing style combine to make this the number one medical-surgical nursing textbook used in more nursing schools than any other medical-surgical nursing textbook.

The strengths of the first nine editions have been retained, including the use of the nursing process as an organizational theme for nursing management. Numerous new features have been added to address some of the rapid changes in practice. Contributors have been selected for their expertise in specific content areas; one or more specialists in the subject area have thoroughly reviewed each chapter to increase accuracy. The editors have undertaken final rewriting and editing to achieve internal consistency. All efforts have been directed toward building on the strengths of the previous edition while preparing an even more effective new edition.

ORGANIZATION

Content is organized into two major divisions. The first division, Section 1 (Chapters 1 through 10), discusses general concepts related to adult patients. The second division, Sections 2 through 12 (Chapters 11 through 68), presents nursing assessment and nursing management of medical-surgical problems.

The various body systems are grouped to reflect their interrelated functions. Each section is organized around two central themes: assessment and management. Chapters dealing with assessment of a body system include a discussion of the following:

1. A brief review of anatomy and physiology, focusing on information that will promote understanding of nursing care
2. Health history and noninvasive physical assessment skills to expand the knowledge base on which treatment decisions are made
3. Common diagnostic studies, expected results, and related nursing responsibilities to provide easily accessible information

Management chapters focus on the pathophysiology, clinical manifestations, diagnostic studies, interprofessional care, and nursing management of various diseases and disorders. The nursing management sections are organized into assessment, nursing diagnoses, planning, implementation, and evaluation. To emphasize the importance of patient care in various clinical settings, nursing implementation of all major health problems is organized by the following levels of care:

1. Health Promotion
2. Acute Care
3. Ambulatory Care

CLASSIC FEATURES

- **Nursing management** is presented in a consistent and comprehensive format, with headings for Health Promotion, Acute Care, and Ambulatory Care. Over 60 nursing care plans on the Evolve website incorporate Nursing Interventions Classification (NIC) and Nursing Outcomes Classification (NOC) in a way that clearly shows the linkages among NIC, NOC, and nursing diagnoses, and applies them to nursing practice.

- **Cultural and ethnic health disparities** content and boxes in the text highlight risk factors and important issues related to the nursing care of various ethnic groups. A special Culturally Competent Care heading denotes cultural and ethnic content related to diseases and disorders. Chapter 2: Health Disparities and Culturally Competent Care discusses health status differences among groups of people related to access to care, economic aspects of health care, gender and cultural issues, and disease risk.

- **Interprofessional care** is highlighted in special Interprofessional Care sections in all management chapters and Interprofessional Care tables throughout the text.

- **Coverage on delegation and prioritization** includes the following:
  - Teamwork & Collaboration boxes highlight the nurse's role in working with members of the interprofessional team and also cover specific topics and skills related to delegation
  - Delegation and prioritization questions in case studies and Bridge to NCLEX Examination Questions
  - Nursing interventions throughout the text are listed in order of priority
  - Nursing diagnoses in the nursing care plans are listed in order of priority

- **Focused Assessment boxes** in all assessment chapters provide brief checklists that help students do a more practical "assessment on the run" or bedside approach to assessment. They can be used to evaluate the status of previously identified health problems and monitor for signs of new problems.

- **Safety Alert boxes** highlight important patient safety issues and focus on the National Patient Safety Goals.

- **Pathophysiology Maps** outline complex concepts related to diseases in flowchart format, making them easier to understand.

- **Patient and caregiver teaching** is an ongoing theme throughout the text. Chapter 4: Patient and Caregiver Teaching emphasizes the increasing importance and prevalence of patient management of chronic illnesses and conditions and the role of the caregiver in patient care.

- **Gerontology and chronic illness** are discussed in Chapter 5: Chronic Illness and Older Adults, and included throughout the text under Gerontologic Considerations headings and in Gerontologic Differences in Assessment tables.

- **Nutrition** is highlighted throughout the book. Nutritional Therapy tables summarize nutritional interventions and promote healthy lifestyles in patients with various health problems.
- *Healthy People* boxes present health care goals as they relate to specific disorders such as diabetes and cancer.
- **Extensive drug therapy** content includes Drug Therapy tables and concise Drug Alerts highlighting important safety considerations for key drugs.
- **Genetics content** includes:
  - Genetics in Clinical Practice boxes that summarize the genetic basis, genetic testing, and clinical implications for genetic disorders that affect adults
  - A genetics chapter that focuses on practical application of nursing care as it relates to this important topic
  - Genetic Risk Alerts in the assessment chapters call attention to important genetic risks
  - Genetic Link headings in the management chapters highlight the specific genetic bases of many disorders
- **Gender Differences** boxes discuss how women and men are affected differently by conditions such as pain and hypertension.
- **Complementary & Alternative Therapies boxes** expand on this information and summarize what nurses need to know about therapies such as herbal remedies, acupuncture, and biofeedback.
- **Ethical/Legal Dilemmas boxes** promote critical thinking for timely and sensitive issues that nursing students may deal with in clinical practice—topics such as informed consent, advance directives, and confidentiality.
- **Emergency Management tables** outline the emergency treatment of health problems most likely to require emergency intervention.
- **Assessment Abnormalities tables** in assessment chapters alert the nurse to frequently encountered abnormalities and their possible etiologies.
- **Nursing Assessment tables** summarize the key subjective and objective data related to common diseases. Subjective data are organized by functional health patterns.
- **Health History tables** in assessment chapters present key questions to ask patients related to a specific disease or disorder.
- **Evidence-based practice** is covered throughout the book in Applying the Evidence boxes, Translating Research Into Practice boxes, and evidence-based practice-focused questions in the case studies.
- **Student-friendly pedagogy** includes the following:
  - Learning Outcomes and Key Terms at the beginning of each chapter help students identify the key content for that chapter.
  - Evolve website boxes at the end of each chapter alert students to supplemental online content and exercises, making it easy for students to facilitate online learning.
  - Bridge to NCLEX® Examination Questions at the end of each chapter are matched to the learning outcomes and help students learn the important points in the chapter. Answers are provided just below the questions for immediate feedback, and rationales are provided on the Evolve website.

- Case Studies with photos bring patients to life. Management chapters have case studies at the end of the chapters. These cases help students learn how to prioritize care and manage patients in the clinical setting. Unfolding case studies are included in each assessment chapter and case studies that focus on managing care of multiple patients are included at the end of each section. Discussion questions with a focus on prioritization, delegation, and evidence-based practice are included in all case studies. Answer guidelines are provided on the Evolve website.
- A **glossary** of key terms and definitions is provided at the back of the text. An expanded version of the glossary with audio pronunciations is included on the Evolve website.

NEW FEATURES

- **Check Your Practice boxes** challenge students to think critically, analyze patient assessment data, and implement the appropriate intervention. Scenarios and discussion questions are provided to promote active learning.
- **Becoming a Nurse Leader boxes** introduce students to concepts related to being a responsible team member and leader. They cover topics such as how nurses can build supportive relationships in the work environment, how to manage a team when providing care, dealing with a changing environment, and more.
- **Informatics boxes and content** in the Patient and Caregiver Teaching chapter reflect the current use and importance of technology as it relates to patient self-management.
- **Increased focus on developing critical thinking skills** is apparent in the Evidence-Based Practice boxes where students are engaged in discussing the implications of EBP findings for nursing practice. The unfolding case studies in assessment chapters also include additional discussion questions to facilitate critical thinking.
- **Increased focus on ambulatory and chronic care** addresses the increasing management of patients on an outpatient basis.
- **QSEN competencies** are highlighted in the core content, case studies, and nursing care plans.

LEARNING SUPPLEMENTS FOR STUDENTS

- The handy **Clinical Companion** presents approximately 200 common medical-surgical conditions and procedures in a concise, alphabetical format for quick clinical reference. Designed for portability, this popular reference includes the essential, need-to-know information for treatments and procedures in which nurses play a major role. An attractive and functional four-color design highlights key information for quick, easy reference.
- An exceptionally thorough **Study Guide** contains over 500 pages of review material that reflect the content found in the book. It features a wide variety of clinically relevant exercises and activities, including NCLEX-format multiple choice and alternate format questions, case studies, anatomy review, critical thinking activities, and much more. It features an attractive four-color design and many alternate-item format questions to better prepare students for the NCLEX examination. An answer key is included to provide students with immediate feedback as they study.

- The **Evolve Student Resources** are available online at http://evolve.elsevier.com/Lewis/medsurg and include the following valuable learning aids organized by chapter:
  - Printable **Key Points** summaries for each chapter
  - 1000 NCLEX Examination **Review Questions**
  - **Answer Guidelines** to the case studies in the textbook
  - **Rationales for the Bridge to NCLEX® Examination Questions** in the textbook
  - 55 **Interactive Case Studies** with state-of-the-art animations and a variety of learning activities, which provide students with immediate feedback. Ten of the case studies are enhanced with photos and narration of the clinical scenarios.
  - Customizable **Nursing Care Plans**
  - **Conceptual Care Map Creator** and conceptual care maps for selected case studies in the textbook
  - **Audio glossary** of key terms, available as comprehensive alphabetical glossary and organized by chapter
  - **Stress-Busting Kit**
  - **Supporting Media**, including animations and audio clips
  - **Fluids and Electrolytes Tutorial**
  - **Content Updates**
- **Virtual Clinical Excursions (VCE)** is an exciting learning tool that brings learning to life in a "virtual" hospital setting. VCE simulates a realistic, yet safe, nursing environment where the routine and rigors of the average clinical rotation abound. Students can conduct a complete assessment of a patient and set priorities for care, collect data, analyze and interpret data, prepare and administer medications, and reach conclusions about complex problems. Each lesson has a textbook reading assignment and online activities based on "visiting" patients in the hospital. Instructors receive an implementation manual with directions for using VCE as a teaching tool.
- More than just words on a screen, **Elsevier eBooks** come with a wealth of built-in study tools and interactive functionality to help students better connect with the course material and their instructors. Plus, with the ability to fit an entire library of books on one portable device, students have the ability to study when, where, and how they want.

TEACHING SUPPLEMENTS FOR INSTRUCTORS

- The **Evolve Instructor Resources** (available online at http://evolve.elsevier.com/Lewis/medsurg) remain the most comprehensive set of instructor's materials available, containing the following:
  - **TEACH for Nurses Lesson Plans** with electronic resources organized by chapter to help instructors develop and manage the course curriculum. This exciting resource includes:
    - Objectives
    - Teaching focus
    - Key terms
    - Nursing curriculum standards
    - Student and instructor chapter resource listings
    - Teaching strategies with learning activities and assessment methods tied to learning outcomes
    - **Case studies** with answer guidelines
  - The **Test Bank** features over 2000 NCLEX Examination test questions with text page references and answers coded for NCLEX Client Needs category, nursing process, and cognitive level. The test bank includes hundreds of prioritization, delegation, and multiple patient questions. All alternate item format questions are included. The ExamView software allows instructors to create new tests; edit, add, and delete test questions; sort questions by NCLEX category, cognitive level, nursing process step, and question type; and administer and grade online tests.
  - The **Image Collection** contains more than 800 full-color images from the text for use in lectures.
  - An extensive collection of **PowerPoint Presentations** includes over 125 different presentations focused on the most common diseases and disorders. The presentations have been thoroughly revised to include helpful instructor notes/teaching tips, unfolding case studies, new illustrations and photos not found in the book, new animations, and updated audience response questions for use with iClicker and other audience response systems.
  - Course management system.
  - Access to all student resources listed above.
- The **Simulation Learning System (SLS)** is an online toolkit that helps instructors and facilitators effectively incorporate medium- to high-fidelity simulation into their nursing curriculum. Detailed patient scenarios promote and enhance the clinical decision-making skills of students at all levels. The SLS provides detailed instructions for preparation and implementation of the simulation experience, debriefing questions that encourage critical thinking, and learning resources to reinforce student comprehension. Each scenario in the SLS complements the textbook content and helps bridge the gap between lecture and clinical. The SLS provides the perfect environment for students to practice what they are learning in the text for a true-to-life, hands-on learning experience.

ACKNOWLEDGMENTS

The editors are especially grateful to many people at Elsevier who assisted with this major revision effort. In particular, we wish to thank the team of Jamie Blum, Jennifer Hermes, Mary Stueck, Julie Eddy, and Ashley Miner. In addition, we want to thank Becky Ramsaroop in marketing.

Special thanks and appreciation go to Peter Bonner who assisted with many details of manuscript preparation and review and photography for the book and interactive case studies.

We are particularly indebted to the faculty, nurses, and student nurses who have put their faith in our book to assist them on their path to excellence. The increasing use of this book throughout the United States, Canada, Australia, and other parts of the world has been gratifying. We appreciate the many users who have shared their comments and suggestions on the previous editions. All feedback is welcome.

We also wish to thank our contributors and reviewers for their assistance with the revision process. We sincerely hope that this book will assist both students and clinicians in practicing truly professional nursing.

Sharon L. Lewis
Linda Bucher
Margaret McLean Heitkemper
Mariann M. Harding
Jeffrey Kwong
Dottie Roberts

AUTHORS OF TEACHING AND LEARNING RESOURCES

TEST BANK

Debra Hagler, RN, PhD, ACNS-BC, CNE, CHSE, ANEF, FAAN
Clinical Professor
College of Nursing and Healthcare Innovation
Arizona State University
Phoenix, Arizona

CASE STUDIES

Interactive and Managing Care of Multiple Patients Case Studies

Katherine A. Kelly, RN, DNP, FNP-C, CEN
Assistant Professor of Nursing
California State University
Sacramento, California

Sarah Barnes, RN, DNP
Assistant Professor of Nursing
California State University
Sacramento, California

POWERPOINT PRESENTATIONS

Jane E. Oehme, RN, MS
Associate Professor of Nursing
Pennsylvania College of Technology
Williamsport, Pennsylvania

Michele A. Walczak, RN, MSN
Associate Professor of Nursing
Pennsylvania College of Technology
Williamsport, Pennsylvania

TEACH FOR NURSES

Margaret R. Rateau, RN, PhD, CNE
Associate Professor of Nursing
Kent State University–Columbiana at East Liverpool
East Liverpool, Ohio

AUDIENCE RESPONSE QUESTIONS

Jane E. Oehme, RN, MS
Associate Professor of Nursing
Pennsylvania College of Technology
Williamsport, Pennsylvania

Michele A. Walczak, RN, MSN
Associate Professor of Nursing
Pennsylvania College of Technology
Williamsport, Pennsylvania

NCLEX EXAMINATION REVIEW QUESTIONS

Mary Boyce, RN, MSN, CCRN, CNE
Mesa Community College
Mesa, Arizona

Sarah Barnes, RN, DNP
Assistant Professor of Nursing
California State University
Sacramento, California

Leigh W. Moore, RN, MSN, CNOR, CNE
Associate Professor of Nursing–ADN
Southside Virginia Community College
Alberta, Virginia

STUDY GUIDE

Susan A. Sandstrom, RN, MSN, BC, CNE
Associate Professor in Nursing, Retired
College of Saint Mary
Omaha, Nebraska

CLINICAL COMPANION

Debra Hagler, RN, PhD, ACNS-BC, CNE, CHSE, ANEF, FAAN
Clinical Professor
College of Nursing and Healthcare Innovation
Arizona State University
Phoenix, Arizona

ETHICAL/LEGAL DILEMMAS BOXES

Katherine K. Anselmi, JD, PhD, WHNP-BC
Associate Clinical Professor
Assistant Dean of Accreditation/Regulatory Affairs and Online Innovation
College of Nursing and Health Professions
Drexel University
Philadelphia, Pennsylvania

Vicki D. Lachman, RN, PhD, APRN, FAAN, NEA-BC
President
V.L. Associates
Avalon, New Jersey

EVIDENCE-BASED PRACTICE BOXES

Shannon Ruff Dirksen, RN, PhD, FAAN
Associate Professor
College of Nursing and Health Innovation
Arizona State University
Phoenix, Arizona

NURSING CARE PLANS

Collin Bowman-Woodall, RN, MS
Assistant Professor
Samuel Merritt University
San Francisco Peninsula Learning Center
San Mateo, California

BECOMING A NURSE LEADER BOXES

Donna Jean Middaugh, RN, PhD
Associate Dean for Academic Programs
College of Nursing
University of Arkansas for Medical Sciences
Little Rock, Arkansas

GLOSSARY

Cory Retherford, MSOM
Former Research Assistant
University of Texas Health Science Center at San Antonio
San Antonio, Texas

SPECIAL PROJECTS

Peter Bonner, MS
Former Professor and Research Statistician
New Mexico Highlands University
Las Vegas, New Mexico;
DSI
Placitas, New Mexico

CONTENTS

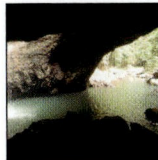
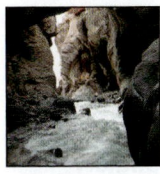
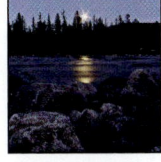
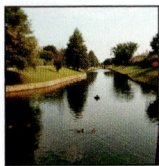
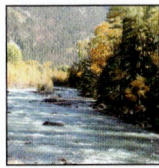
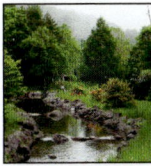
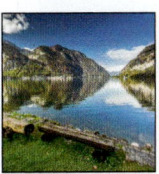

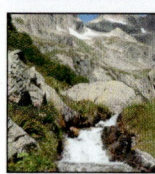
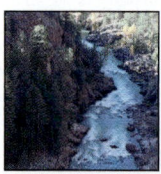
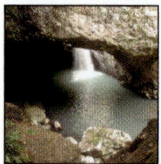
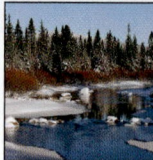
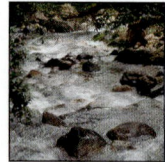

SPECIAL FEATURES

EMERGENCY MANAGEMENT TABLES

ETHICAL/LEGAL DILEMMAS BOXES

EVIDENCE-BASED PRACTICE BOXES

Applying the Evidence Boxes

Translating Research Into Practice Boxes

FOCUSED ASSESSMENT BOXES

GENDER DIFFERENCES BOXES

GENETICS IN CLINICAL PRACTICE BOXES

GERONTOLOGIC ASSESSMENT DIFFERENCES TABLES

HEALTH HISTORY TABLES

HEALTHY PEOPLE BOXES

INFORMATICS IN PRACTICE BOXES

INTERPROFESSIONAL CARE TABLES

NURSING ASSESSMENT TABLES

NURSING MANAGEMENT TABLES

NUTRITIONAL THERAPY TABLES

PATIENT & CAREGIVER TEACHING TABLES

TEAMWORK & COLLABORATION BOXES

MEDICAL-SURGICAL NURSING

Assessment and Management of Clinical Problems

Problems of Ingestion, Digestion, Absorption, and Elimination

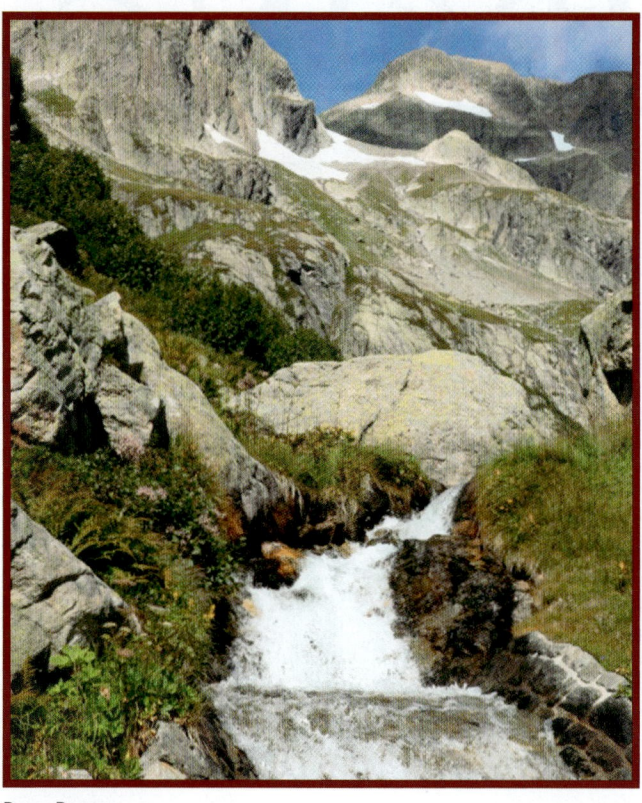

Peter Bonner

Let the mountains talk, let the river run. Once more, and forever.

David Brower

Assessment of Gastrointestinal System

Paula Cox-North

Nothing compares to the stomach ache you get from laughing with your best friends.

Unknown author

http://evolve.elsevier.com/Lewis/medsurg/

LEARNING OUTCOMES

1. Describe the structures and functions of the organs of the gastrointestinal tract.
2. Describe the structures and functions of the liver, gallbladder, biliary tract, and pancreas.
3. Differentiate the processes of ingestion, digestion, absorption, and elimination.
4. Explain the processes of biliary metabolism, bile production, and bile excretion.
5. Link the age-related changes of the gastrointestinal system to the differences in assessment findings.
6. Obtain significant subjective and objective assessment data related to the gastrointestinal system from a patient.
7. Perform a physical assessment of the gastrointestinal system using appropriate techniques.
8. Differentiate normal from abnormal findings of a physical assessment of the gastrointestinal system.
9. Describe the purpose, significance of results, and nursing responsibilities related to diagnostic studies of the gastrointestinal system.

KEY TERMS

absorption, p. 835
bilirubin, p. 837
borborygmi, Table 38-10, p. 847
cheilosis, Table 38-10, p. 846
deglutition, p. 834

digestion, p. 835
endoscopy, p. 851
hematemesis, Table 38-10, p. 846
Kupffer cells, p. 837
melena, Table 38-10, p. 847

pyorrhea, Table 38-10, p. 846
pyrosis, Table 38-10, p. 846
steatorrhea, Table 38-10, p. 847
tenesmus, Table 38-10, p. 847
Valsalva maneuver, p. 836

The gastrointestinal (GI) system, also called the *digestive system*, consists of the GI tract and its associated organs and glands. Included in the GI tract are the mouth, esophagus, stomach, small intestine, large intestine, rectum, and anus. The associated organs are the liver, pancreas, and gallbladder (Fig. 38-1).

STRUCTURES AND FUNCTIONS OF GASTROINTESTINAL SYSTEM

The GI tract extends approximately 30 ft (9 m) from the mouth to the anus. The GI tract is essentially a tube composed of four layers. From the inside to the outside, these layers are (1) mucosa lining; (2) submucosa connective tissue, which contains glands, blood vessels, and lymph nodes; (3) muscle; and (4) serosa (Fig. 38-1). The muscular coat has two layers: circular (inner) layer and longitudinal (outer) layer.

Parasympathetic and sympathetic branches of the autonomic nervous system (ANS) innervate the GI tract. The parasympathetic (cholinergic) system is mainly excitatory. The sympathetic (adrenergic) system is mainly inhibitory. For example, parasympathetic stimulation increases peristalsis and sympathetic stimulation decreases it. Both sympathetic and parasympathetic afferent fibers relay sensory information.

The GI tract has its own nervous system: the enteric nervous system (ENS) or intrinsic nervous system. The ENS system regulates motility and secretion along the entire GI tract. The ENS is composed of two networks: (1) Meissner plexus in the submucosa and (2) Auerbach (myenteric) plexus between the muscle layers. The submucosal plexus controls secretion and is involved in many sensory functions. The myenteric plexus is the major nerve supply to the GI tract and controls GI movements. Although the ENS receives innervation from the ANS, it operates independently of the brain and spinal cord.

Circulation in the GI system is unique in that venous blood draining the GI tract organs empties into the portal vein, which then perfuses the liver. This allows the liver to clean the blood of bacteria and toxins from the GI tract. The celiac artery, superior mesenteric artery (SMA), and the inferior mesenteric artery (IMA) supply arterial blood to the GI tract. The stomach and duodenum receive their blood supply from the celiac axis. The distal small intestine to mid large intestine receives its blood supply from branches of the hepatic and SMA. The distal large

Reviewed by Barbara Brunow, RN, MSN, MEd, CNS, CNE, Assistant Director, Firelands Regional Medical Center, School of Nursing, Sandusky, Ohio; and Christina D. Keller, RN, MSN-Ed, Instructor, Radford University, Radford, Virginia.

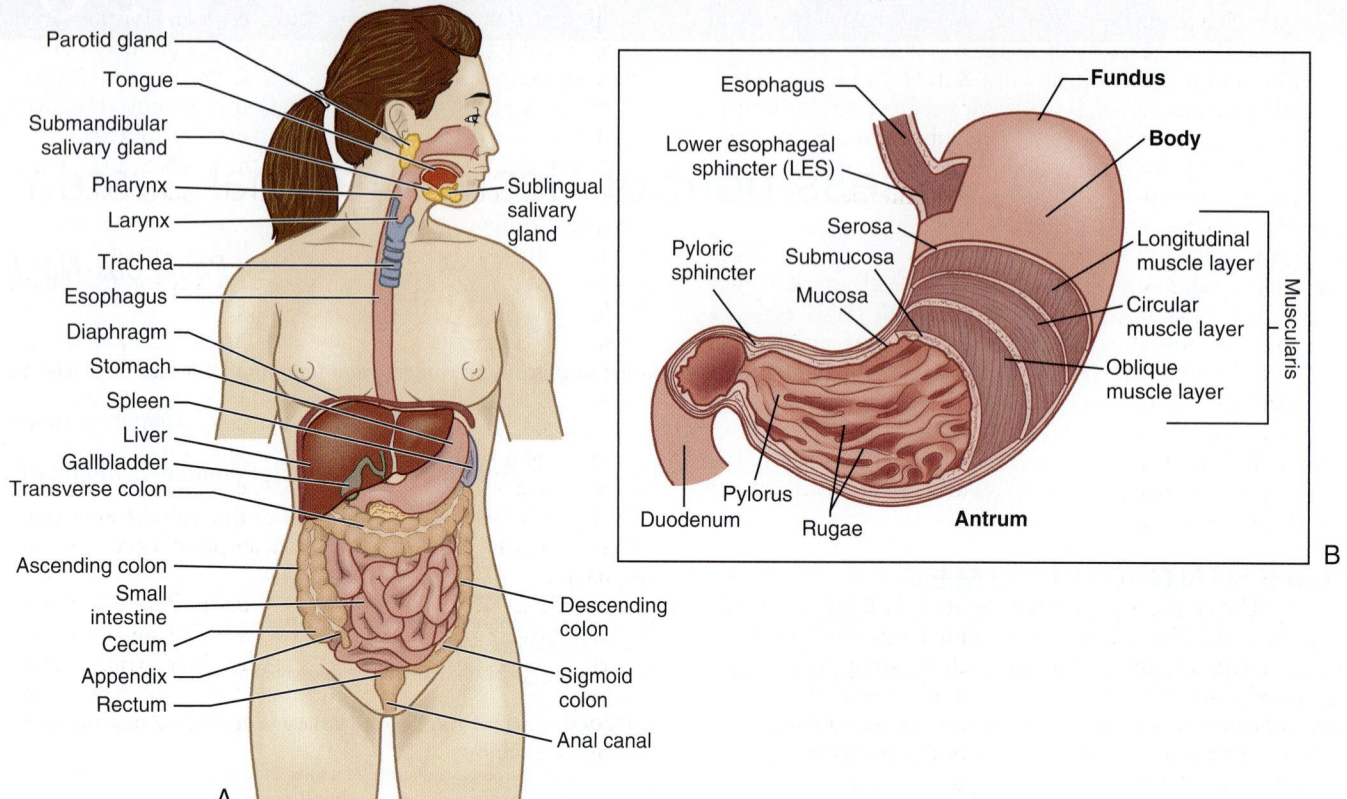

FIG. 38-1 A, Location of organs of the gastrointestinal system. **B,** Parts of the stomach.

intestine through the anus receives its blood supply from the IMA. The GI tract and accessory organs receive approximately 25% to 30% of the cardiac output at rest and 35% or more after eating. Because such a large percentage of the cardiac output perfuses these organs, the GI tract is a major source from which to divert blood flow during exercise, stress, or injury.

The peritoneum almost completely covers the abdominal organs. The two layers of the peritoneum are the *parietal layer,* which lines the abdominal cavity wall, and the *visceral layer,* which covers the abdominal organs. The peritoneal cavity is the potential space between the parietal and visceral layers. The two folds of the peritoneum are the mesentery and omentum. The mesentery attaches the small intestine and part of the large intestine to the posterior abdominal wall and contains blood and lymph vessels. The omentum hangs like an apron from the stomach to the intestines and contains fat and lymph nodes.

The main function of the GI system is to supply nutrients to body cells. This is accomplished through the processes of (1) *ingestion* (taking in food), (2) *digestion* (breaking down food), and (3) *absorption* (transferring food products into circulation). *Elimination* is the process of excreting the waste products of digestion.

Ingestion

Ingestion is the intake of food. *Appetite,* the desire to ingest food, influences how much food a person eats. An appetite center is located in the hypothalamus. A number of factors, including hypoglycemia, an empty stomach, and a decrease in body temperature, stimulate appetite. The hormone *ghrelin* released from the stomach mucosa plays a role in appetite stimulation. Another hormone, *leptin,* is involved in appetite suppression.

(See Chapter 40 for a discussion of ghrelin and leptin.) The sight, smell, and taste of food frequently stimulate appetite. Stomach distention, illness (especially accompanied by fever), hyperglycemia, nausea and vomiting, and certain drugs (e.g., amphetamines) inhibit appetite.

Deglutition, or swallowing, is the mechanical component of ingestion. The organs involved in the deglutition of food are the mouth, pharynx, and esophagus.

Mouth. The mouth consists of the lips and oral (buccal) cavity. The lips surround the opening of the mouth and function in speech. The hard and soft palates form the roof of the oral cavity. The oral cavity contains the teeth, used in *mastication* (chewing), and the tongue. The tongue is a solid muscle mass and assists in chewing and moving food to the back of the throat for swallowing. The taste receptors (taste buds) are on the sides and tip of the tongue. The tongue is also important in speech.

Within the oral cavity are three pairs of salivary glands: parotid, submaxillary, and sublingual glands. These glands produce saliva, which consists of water, protein, mucin, inorganic salts, and salivary amylase.

Pharynx. The pharynx is a muscular tube lined with mucous membrane. It has three divisions: nasopharynx, oropharynx, and laryngeal pharynx. The mucous membrane is continuous with the nasal cavity, mouth, auditory tubes, and larynx. During ingestion, the oropharynx provides a route for food from the mouth to the esophagus. Food or liquid stimulates receptors in the oropharynx, initiating the swallowing reflex. During swallowing, the epiglottis closes over the opening to the larynx and prevents food from entering the respiratory tract. The tonsils and adenoids, composed of lymphoid tissue, assist the body in preventing infection.

Esophagus. The esophagus is a hollow, muscular tube that receives food from the pharynx and moves it to the stomach. It is 7 to 10 in (18 to 25 cm) long and 0.8 in (2 cm) in diameter. The esophagus is located in the thoracic cavity. It is structurally composed of four layers: inner mucosa, submucosa, muscularis propria, and outermost adventitia. The upper third of the esophagus is composed of striated skeletal muscle. The distal two thirds are composed of smooth muscle.

Between swallows, the esophagus remains collapsed and the *upper esophageal sphincter* (UES) closed. With swallowing, the UES relaxes and a peristaltic wave moves the bolus into the esophagus. The muscular layers contract *(peristalsis)* and propel the food to the stomach. The *lower esophageal sphincter* (LES) at the distal end of the esophagus controls the opening of the esophagus into the stomach. It remains contracted except during swallowing, belching, or vomiting. The LES is an important barrier that normally prevents reflux of acidic gastric contents into the esophagus.

Digestion and Absorption

Stomach. The stomach's functions are to store food, mix food with gastric secretions, and empty contents in small boluses into the small intestine. The stomach absorbs only small amounts of water, alcohol, electrolytes, and certain drugs.

The stomach is usually J shaped and lies obliquely in the epigastric, umbilical, and left hypochondriac regions of the abdomen (Fig. 38-5 later in the chapter). It always contains gastric fluid and mucus. The three main parts of the stomach are the fundus (cardia), body, and antrum (Fig. 38-1). The pylorus is a small portion of the antrum proximal to the pyloric sphincter. The LES and pyloric sphincter guard the entrance to and exit from the stomach.

The stomach wall has four layers. The serous (outer) layer of the stomach is continuous with the peritoneum. The muscular layer consists of the longitudinal (outer) layer, circular (middle) layer, and oblique (inner) layer. The mucosal layer forms folds called *rugae* that contain many small glands. In the fundus the glands contain (1) chief cells, which secrete pepsinogen and (2) parietal cells, which secrete hydrochloric (HCl) acid, water, and intrinsic factor. The secretion of HCl acid makes gastric juice acidic. This acidic pH aids in the protection against ingested organisms. Intrinsic factor promotes cobalamin (vitamin B_{12}) absorption in the small intestine.

Small Intestine. The two primary functions of the small intestine are digestion and absorption, the uptake of nutrients from the gut lumen to the bloodstream. The small intestine is a coiled tube approximately 23 ft (7 m) in length and 1 to 1.1 in (2.5 to 2.8 cm) in diameter. It extends from the pylorus to the ileocecal valve. The small intestine is composed of the duodenum, jejunum, and ileum. The ileocecal valve prevents reflux of large intestine contents into the small intestine.

The mucosa of the small intestine is thick, vascular, and glandular. The functional units of the small intestine are *villi*, which are minute, fingerlike projections in the mucous membrane. Villi contain epithelial cells that produce the intestinal digestive enzymes. The epithelial cells on the villi also have *microvilli*. The circular folds in the mucous and submucous layers, along with the villi and microvilli, increase the surface area for digestion and absorption.

The digestive enzymes on the brush border of the microvilli chemically break down nutrients for absorption. Between the bases of the villi lie the crypts of Lieberkühn, which contain the

multipotent stem cells that are the precursors for the other epithelial cell types. Brunner's glands in the submucosa of the duodenum secrete an alkaline fluid containing bicarbonate that neutralizes acidic fluids and protects the mucosa. Intestinal goblet cells secrete mucus that also protects the mucosa.

Physiology of Digestion. Digestion is the physical and chemical breakdown of food into absorbable substances. The timely movement of food through the GI tract and the secretion of specific enzymes facilitate digestion. These enzymes break down foodstuffs to particles of appropriate size for absorption (Table 38-1).

The process of digestion begins in the mouth, where food is chewed, mechanically broken down, and mixed with saliva. Saliva facilitates swallowing by lubricating food. Saliva contains amylase, which breaks down starches to maltose. Chewing and the sight, smell, thought, and taste of food stimulate the release of saliva. A person produces about 1 L of saliva each day. After swallowing, food moves through the esophagus to the stomach. No digestion or absorption occurs in the esophagus.

Both GI secretion and motility are under neural and hormonal control. Food entering the stomach and small intestine triggers the release of hormones into the bloodstream (Tables 38-2 and 38-3). These hormones play important roles in the control of HCl acid secretion, production and release of digestive enzymes, and motility.

TABLE 38-1 Gastrointestinal Secretions

Daily Amount (mL)	Secretions, Enzymes	Action
Salivary Glands		
1000-1500	Salivary amylase	Initiation of starch digestion
Stomach		
2500	Pepsinogen	Protein digestion
	HCl acid	Activation of pepsinogen to pepsin
	Lipase	Fat digestion
	Intrinsic factor	Essential for cobalamin absorption in ileum
Small Intestine		
3000	Enterokinase	Activation of trypsinogen to trypsin
	Amylase	Carbohydrate digestion
	Peptidases	Protein digestion
	Aminopeptidases	Protein digestion
	Maltase	Maltose to two glucose molecules
	Sucrase	Sucrose to glucose and fructose
	Lactase	Lactose to glucose and galactose
	Lipase	Fat digestion
Pancreas		
700	Trypsinogen	Protein digestion
	Chymotrypsin	Protein digestion
	Amylase	Starch to disaccharides
	Lipase	Fat digestion
Liver and Gallbladder		
1000	Bile	Emulsification of fats and aid in absorption of fatty acids and fat-soluble vitamins (A, D, E, K)

In the stomach, muscle action mixes the food with gastric secretions to form *chyme*, which is now ready for absorption. Protein digestion begins with the release of pepsinogen from chief cells. The stomach's acidic environment results in the conversion of pepsinogen to its active form, pepsin. Pepsin begins the breakdown of proteins. There is minimal digestion of starches and fats. The stomach also serves as a reservoir for food, releasing it slowly into the small intestine. The length of time that food remains in the stomach depends on the composition of the food. The average meal remains in the stomach for 3 to 4 hours.

In the small intestine, the physical presence and chemical nature of chyme stimulates motility and secretion. Secretions involved in digestion include enzymes from the pancreas, bile from the liver, and enzymes from the small intestine (Table 38-1). Carbohydrates are broken down to monosaccharides, fats to glycerol and fatty acids, and proteins to amino acids. Enzymes on the brush border of the microvilli complete the digestion process. These enzymes break down disaccharides to monosaccharides and peptides to amino acids for absorption.

The absorption of most of the end products of digestion occurs in the small intestine. The movement of the villi enables these end products to come in contact with the absorbing membrane. Monosaccharides, fatty acids, amino acids, water, electrolytes, vitamins, and minerals are absorbed.

Elimination

Large Intestine. The large intestine is a hollow, muscular tube approximately 5 to 6 ft (1.5 to 1.8 m) long and 2 in (5 cm) in diameter. The four parts of the large intestine are shown in Fig. 38-2.

The most important function of the large intestine is the absorption of water and electrolytes. The large intestine also forms feces and serves as a reservoir for the fecal mass until defecation occurs. Feces are composed of water (75%), bacteria, unabsorbed minerals, undigested foodstuffs, bile pigments, and desquamated (shed) epithelial cells. The large intestine secretes mucus, which acts as a lubricant and protects the mucosa.

Microorganisms in the colon contribute to digestion by (1) producing vitamin K and some B vitamins and (2) breaking down proteins that are not digested or absorbed in the small intestine into amino acids. Bacteria deaminate the amino acids, resulting in ammonia. Ammonia is carried to the liver, where it is converted to urea, which is excreted by the kidneys. Bacteria produce gas that escapes the colon through the anus, a phenomenon called *flatulence* or *flatus*. If an infection or antibiotics alter the normal microbiome, an overgrowth of pathogenic bacteria can occur and cause disease.

The movements of the large intestine are usually slow. However, propulsive (mass movements) peristalsis also occurs. Food entering the stomach and duodenum triggers gastrocolic and duodenocolic reflexes, resulting in peristalsis in the colon. These reflexes are more active after the first daily meal and frequently result in bowel evacuation.

Defecation is a reflex action involving voluntary and involuntary control. Feces in the rectum stimulate sensory nerve endings that produce the desire to defecate. The reflex center for defecation is in the parasympathetic nerve fibers in the sacral portion of the spinal cord. These fibers produce contraction of the rectum and relaxation of the internal anal sphincter. When a person feels the desire to defecate, he or she can voluntarily relax the external anal sphincter. An acceptable environment for defecation is usually necessary, or the urge to defecate will be ignored. If defecation is suppressed over long periods, problems can occur, such as constipation or fecal impaction.

The Valsalva maneuver, often referred to as "bearing down," can facilitate defecation. During this maneuver, the person inspires deeply and holds the breath, closing the airway, while contracting abdominal muscles and bearing down. This increases both intraabdominal and intrathoracic pressures and reduces venous return to the heart. The heart rate temporarily decreases along with a decrease in cardiac output. This results in a transient drop in BP. When the patient relaxes, thoracic pressure falls, resulting in a sudden flow of blood into the heart, increased heart rate, and an immediate rise in BP. The Valsalva maneuver may be contraindicated in the patient with a head injury, eye surgery, cardiac problems,

---

TABLE 38-2 Phases of Gastric Secretion

Stimulus to Secretion	Secretion
Cephalic (nervous) Sight, smell, taste of food (before food enters stomach). Initiated in the CNS and mediated by the vagus nerve.	HCl acid, pepsinogen, mucus
Gastric (hormonal and nervous) Food in antrum of stomach, vagal stimulation.	Release of gastrin from antrum into circulation to stimulate gastric secretions and motility
Intestinal (hormonal) Presence of chyme in small intestine.	Acidic chyme (pH <2): Release of secretin, gastric inhibitory polypeptide, cholecystokinin into circulation to decrease HCl acid secretion Chyme (pH >3): Release of gastrin from duodenum to increase acid secretion

---

TABLE 38-3 Hormones Controlling GI Secretion and Motility

Hormone	Source	Activating Stimuli	Function
Gastrin	Gastric and duodenal mucosa	Stomach distention, partially digested proteins in pylorus	Stimulates gastric acid secretion and motility. Maintains lower esophageal sphincter tone.
Secretin	Duodenal mucosa	Acid entering small intestine	Inhibits gastric motility and acid secretion. Stimulates pancreatic bicarbonate secretion.
Cholecystokinin	Duodenal mucosa	Fatty acids and amino acids in small intestine	Contracts gallbladder and relaxes sphincter of Oddi. Allows increased flow of bile into duodenum. Release of pancreatic digestive enzymes.
Gastric inhibitory peptide	Duodenal mucosa	Fatty acids and lipids in small intestine	Inhibits gastric acid secretion and motility.

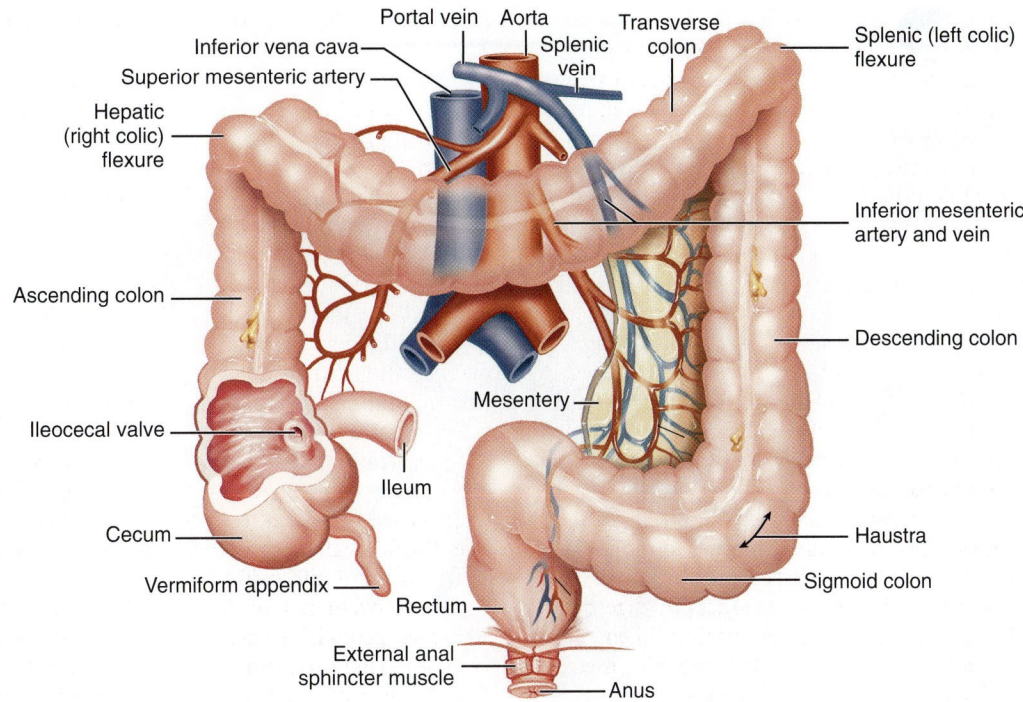

FIG. 38-2 Anatomic locations of the large intestine. (From Patton KT, Thibodeau GA: *Anatomy and physiology*, ed 8, St Louis, 2013, Mosby.)

hemorrhoids, abdominal surgery, or liver cirrhosis with portal hypertension.

Liver, Biliary Tract, and Pancreas

Liver. The liver is the largest internal organ in the body, weighing approximately 3 lb (1.36 kg). It lies in the right epigastric region (Fig. 38-5 later in the chapter). Most of the liver is enclosed in peritoneum. It has a fibrous capsule that divides it into right and left lobes (Fig. 38-3).

The functional units of the liver are lobules. A lobule consists of rows of hepatic cells *(hepatocytes)* arranged in cords that radiate out from a central vein. Capillaries called *sinusoids* are located between the rows of hepatocytes. Sinusoids are lined with **Kupffer cells**, which carry out phagocytic activity, removing bacteria and toxins from the blood. The hepatic cells secrete bile into tiny canals called *canaliculi*. These merge with other canals to form larger, interlobular bile ducts, which unite into the two main left and right hepatic ducts.

The liver has a rich blood supply. The portal circulatory system brings blood to the liver from the stomach, intestines, spleen, and pancreas. About one fourth of the blood supply comes from the hepatic artery, a branch of the celiac artery. Three fourths comes from the portal vein. The portal vein carries absorbed products of digestion directly to the liver. Once in the liver, the portal vein branches and comes in contact with each lobule.

The liver performs numerous functions and is essential for life. It has metabolic, secretory, vascular, and storage functions (Table 38-4). The hepatic cells constantly make bile. Bile consists of water, cholesterol, bile salts, electrolytes, fatty acids, and bilirubin. It provides the alkaline medium needed for the action of pancreatic lipase. Bile salts are needed for fat emulsification and digestion.

Bilirubin Metabolism. **Bilirubin,** a pigment derived from the breakdown of hemoglobin, is constantly produced (Fig. 38-4). When released into the bloodstream, it binds to albumin. This

TABLE 38-4	Functions of Liver
Function	**Description**
Metabolic Functions	
Carbohydrate metabolism	Performs glycogenesis (conversion of glucose to glycogen), glycogenolysis (process of breaking down glycogen to glucose), gluconeogenesis (formation of glucose from amino acids and fatty acids).
Protein metabolism	Synthesis of nonessential amino acids, synthesis of plasma proteins (except gamma globulin), synthesis of clotting factors, urea formation (NH_4) from ammonia (NH_3). NH_3 formed from deamination of amino acids by action of bacteria in colon.
Fat metabolism	Synthesis of lipoproteins, breakdown of triglycerides into fatty acids and glycerol, formation of ketone bodies, synthesis of fatty acids from amino acids and glucose, synthesis and breakdown of cholesterol.
Detoxification	Inactivation of drugs and harmful substances and excretion of their breakdown products.
Blood clotting	Synthesis of prothrombin (factor I), fibrinogen (factor II) and factors V, VII, IX, and X.
Secretory Functions	
Bile production	Formation of bile, containing bile salts, bile pigments (mainly bilirubin), and cholesterol.
Bilirubin	Conjugation and secretion of bilirubin.
Vascular Functions	
Blood filtration	Breakdown of old RBCs, WBCs, bacteria, and other particles. Breakdown of hemoglobin from old RBCs to bilirubin and biliverdin.
Blood reservoir	Serves as temporary storage for blood within general circulation.
Storage Functions	
Storage	Stores glucose in form of glycogen; vitamins, including fat-soluble (A, D, E, K) and water-soluble (B_1, B_2, cobalamin, folic acid); fatty acids; minerals (iron, copper); and amino acids in form of albumin and beta-globulins.

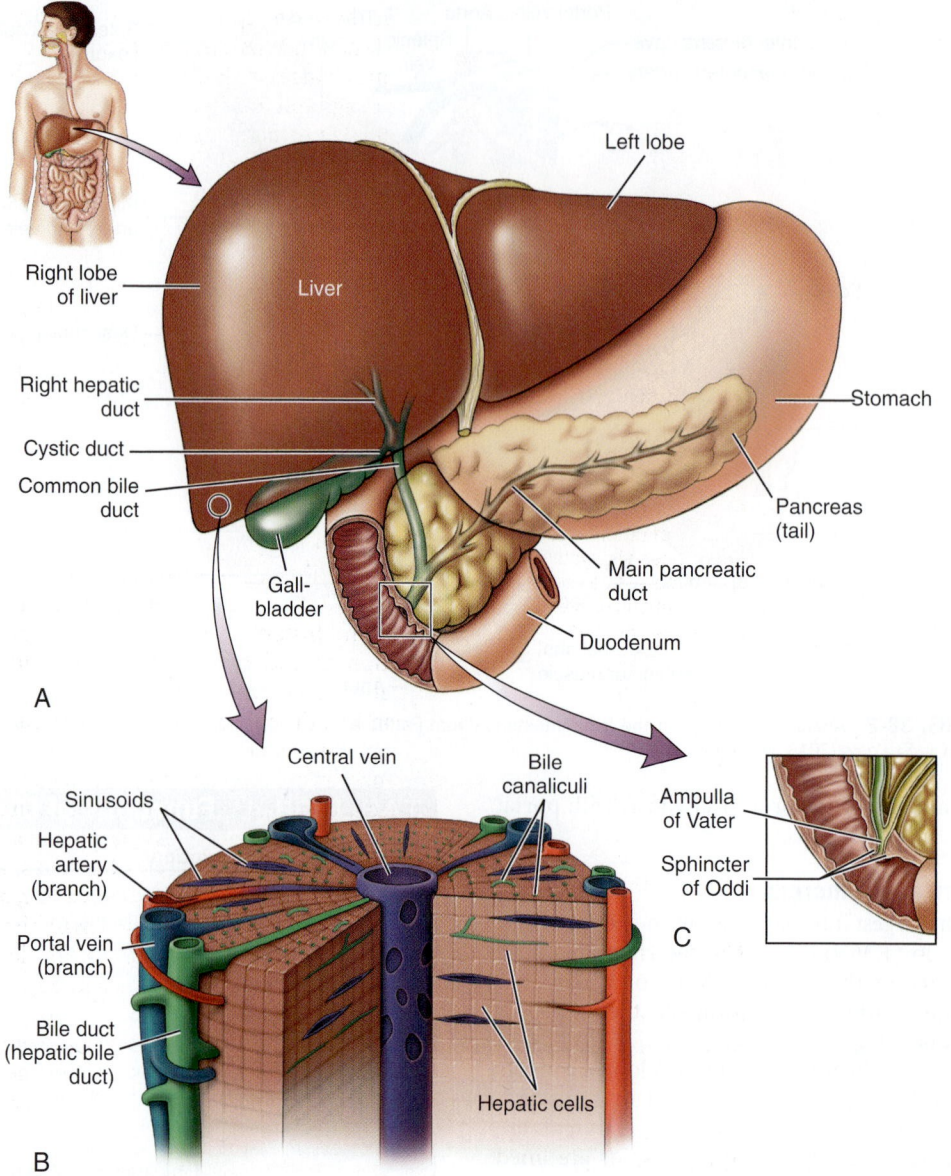

FIG. 38-3 **A,** Gross structure of the liver, gallbladder, pancreas, and duct system. **B,** Liver lobule. **C,** Entrance of the common bile duct into the duodenum.

form of bilirubin is referred to as *unconjugated*. It is insoluble in water and transported to the liver. In the liver, unconjugated bilirubin is conjugated with glucuronic acid and is excreted in bile into the intestine. *Conjugated* bilirubin is soluble in water. In the intestines, bacterial action reduces bilirubin to stercobilinogen and urobilinogen. Stercobilinogen accounts for the brown color of stool. A small amount of urobilinogen is reabsorbed into the blood, where it is returned to the liver through the portal circulation. There, it is excreted again in the bile or entered into circulation and excreted by the kidneys.

Biliary Tract. The biliary tract consists of the gallbladder and ducts that connect the liver, gallbladder, and duodenum. The gallbladder is a pear-shaped sac located below the liver. The gallbladder's function is to concentrate and store bile. It holds approximately 45 mL of bile. The presence of fat in the upper duodenum triggers the release of cholecystokinin, which causes the gallbladder to contract and release bile.

The hepatic ducts receive bile from the canaliculi in the liver lobules. The left and right hepatic ducts merge with the cystic duct from the gallbladder to form the common bile duct. Bile moves down the common bile duct to enter the duodenum at the ampulla of Vater (Fig. 38-3). The pancreatic duct also enters the duodenum at this point.

Pancreas. The pancreas is a long, slender gland lying behind the stomach and in front of the first and second lumbar vertebrae. It consists of a head, body, and tail. The peritoneum covers the anterior surface of the pancreas. The pancreas contains lobes and lobules. The pancreatic duct extends along the gland and enters the duodenum through the common bile duct at the ampulla of Vater (Fig. 38-3).

The pancreas has both exocrine and endocrine functions. The exocrine function contributes to digestion through the production and release of enzymes (Table 38-1). The endocrine function occurs in the islets of Langerhans, whose β cells secrete

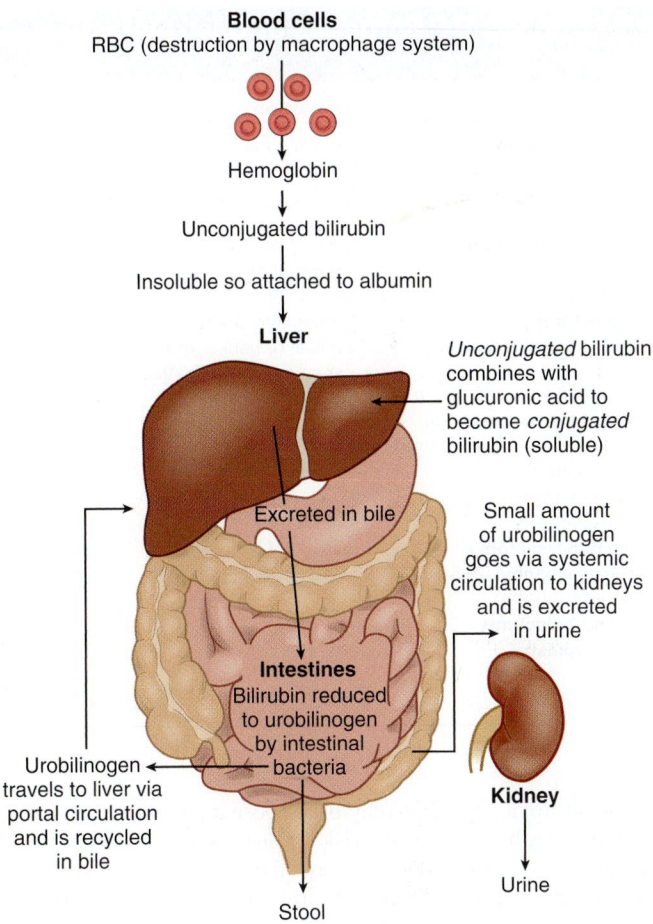

Blood cells
RBC (destruction by macrophage system)

Hemoglobin

Unconjugated bilirubin

Insoluble so attached to albumin

Liver

Excreted in bile

Unconjugated bilirubin combines with glucuronic acid to become *conjugated* bilirubin (soluble)

Intestines
Bilirubin reduced to urobilinogen by intestinal bacteria

Small amount of urobilinogen goes via systemic circulation to kidneys and is excreted in urine

Urobilinogen travels to liver via portal circulation and is recycled in bile

Kidney

Urine

Stool

FIG. 38-4 Bilirubin metabolism and conjugation.

insulin and amylin; α cells secrete glucagon; δ cells secrete somatostatin; and F cells secrete pancreatic polypeptide.

Gerontologic Considerations: Effects of Aging on Gastrointestinal System

The process of aging changes the functional ability of the GI system. Diet, alcohol intake, and obesity affect organs of the GI system, making it a challenge to separate the sole effects of aging from lifestyle. Many factors can lead to a decrease in appetite and make eating less pleasurable. Caries and periodontal disease can lead to loss of teeth. Taste buds decline in number and the sense of smell lessens, leading to decreased ability to taste. With less saliva, a very dry mouth *(xerostomia)* is common.

Age-related changes in the esophagus include delayed emptying, resulting from smooth muscle weakness, reduced UES opening, and an incompetent LES.[1] Although motility of the GI system decreases with age, secretion and absorption are affected to a lesser extent. The older patient often has a decrease in HCl acid secretion *(hypochlorhydria)* and a reduction in the secretion of intrinsic factor.

The prevalence of constipation in adults over age 60 is about 34%.[2] Factors that may increase the risk for constipation include slower peristalsis, anorectal dysfunction, inactivity, decreased dietary fiber, inadequate fluid intake, constipating medications, and laxative abuse. Neurologic, cognitive, and metabolic disorders may also play a role.[3] (See Chapter 42 for a detailed discussion of constipation.)

The liver size decreases after 50 years of age, but results of liver function tests remain within normal ranges. Age-related enzyme changes in the liver decrease the liver's ability to metabolize drugs and hormones.

The size of the pancreas is unaffected by aging, but it does undergo structural changes, such as fibrosis, fatty acid deposits, and atrophy. Gallbladder diseases increase with age.[4]

Older adults, especially those over 85, are at risk for decreased food intake. The economic inability to purchase food supplies affects nutritional intake, especially in the older adult. Economic constraints may reduce the number of fresh fruits and vegetables consumed and thus the amount of fiber. Immobility limits the ability to obtain and prepare meals. Age-related changes in the GI system and differences in assessment findings are presented in Table 38-5.

ASSESSMENT OF GASTROINTESTINAL SYSTEM

Subjective Data

Important Health Information

Past Health History. Obtain information from the patient about the history or existence of the problems related to GI functioning and fully explore any symptoms. Inquire about any abdominal pain, nausea, vomiting, diarrhea, constipation, abdominal distention, jaundice, heartburn, dyspepsia, changes in appetite, hematemesis, indigestion, excessive gas, bloating, melena, trouble swallowing, or rectal bleeding. Document related conditions such as food intolerance or allergies, lactose intolerance, and anemia. Ask the patient about a history or existence of diseases such as reflux, gastritis, hepatitis, colitis, gallstones, hemorrhoids, peptic ulcer, cancer, diverticuli, or hernias.

Question the patient about weight history. Explore in detail any unexplained or unplanned weight loss or gain within the past 6 to 12 months. Document a history of chronic dieting and repeated weight loss and gain.

Medications. Assess the patient's past and current use of medications. Ask about the reason for taking the medication, its name, the dose and frequency, length of time taken, its effect, and any

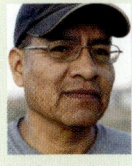

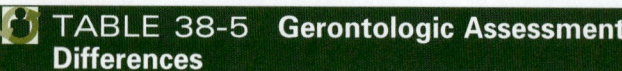

TABLE 38-5 Gerontologic Assessment Differences

Gastrointestinal System

Expected Aging Changes	Differences in Assessment Findings
Mouth	
Gingival retraction	Loss of teeth, dental implants, dentures, difficulty chewing
Decreased taste buds, decreased sense of smell	Diminished sense of taste (especially salty and sweet)
Decreased volume of saliva	Dry oral mucosa
Atrophy of gingival tissue	Poor-fitting dentures
Esophagus	
Lower esophageal sphincter pressure decreased, motility decreased	Epigastric distress, dysphagia, potential for hiatal hernia and aspiration
Abdominal Wall	
Thinner and less taut	More visible peristalsis, easier palpation of organs
Decreased number and sensitivity of sensory receptors	Less sensitivity to surface pain
Stomach	
Atrophy of gastric mucosa, decreased blood flow	Food intolerances, signs of anemia as result of cobalamin malabsorption, slower gastric emptying
Small Intestines	
Slightly decreased motility and secretion of most digestive enzymes	Complaints of indigestion, slowed intestinal transit, delayed absorption of fat-soluble vitamins
Liver	
Decreased size and lowered position	Easier palpation because of lower border extending past costal margin
Decreased protein synthesis, ability to regenerate decreased	Decreased drug and hormone metabolism
Large Intestine, Anus, Rectum	
Decreased anal sphincter tone and nerve supply to rectal area	Fecal incontinence
Decreased muscular tone, decreased motility	Flatulence, abdominal distention, relaxed perineal musculature
Increased transit time, decreased sensation to defecation	Constipation, fecal impaction
Pancreas	
Pancreatic ducts distended, lipase production decreased, pancreatic reserve impaired	Impaired fat absorption, decreased glucose tolerance

TABLE 38-6 Surgeries of Gastrointestinal System

Procedure	Description
Appendectomy	Removal of appendix
Cholecystectomy	Removal of gallbladder
Choledochojejunostomy	Opening between common bile duct and jejunum
Choledocholithotomy	Opening into common bile duct for removal of stones
Colectomy	Removal of colon
Colostomy	Opening into colon
Esophagoenterostomy	Removal of portion of esophagus with segment of colon attached to remaining portion
Esophagogastrostomy	Removal of esophagus and anastomosis of remaining portion to stomach
Gastrectomy	Removal of stomach
Gastrostomy	Opening into stomach
Glossectomy	Removal of tongue
Hemiglossectomy	Removal of half of tongue
Herniorrhaphy	Repair of a hernia
Ileostomy	Opening into ileum
Mandibulectomy	Removal of mandible
Pyloroplasty	Enlargement and repair of pyloric sphincter area
Vagotomy	Resection of branch of vagus nerve

side effects. Include information about over-the-counter (OTC) medications, prescription drugs, herbal products, vitamins, probiotics, and nutritional supplements. This is a critical aspect of history taking. Many medications not only affect the GI system, but they are also affected by abnormalities of the GI system.

Many chemicals and drugs are potentially hepatotoxic (see *livertox.nih.gov*) and result in significant harm unless monitored closely. For example, chronic high doses of acetaminophen and nonsteroidal antiinflammatory drugs (NSAIDs) may be hepatotoxic. NSAIDs may predispose a patient to upper GI bleeding, with an increasing risk as the person ages. Other medications, such as antibiotics, may change the normal bacterial composition in the GI tract, resulting in diarrhea. Antacids and laxatives may affect the absorption of certain medications. Ask the patient about laxative or antacid use, including the kind and frequency.

Surgery or Other Treatments. Obtain information about hospitalizations for any problems related to the GI system. Document data related to any abdominal or rectal surgery, including the year, reason for surgery, postoperative course, and possible blood transfusions. Terms related to surgery of the GI system are listed in Table 38-6.

Functional Health Patterns. Key questions to ask a patient with a GI problem are presented in Table 38-7.

Health Perception–Health Management Pattern. Ask about the patient's health practices related to the GI system, such as maintenance of normal body weight, proper dental care, adequate nutrition, and effective elimination habits.

Query the patient about recent foreign travel with possible exposure to hepatitis or parasitic infestation. Ask about risk behaviors for hepatitis exposure. Document whether the patient has received hepatitis A and B vaccination.

Assess the patient for habits that directly affect GI functioning. The intake of alcohol in large quantities or for long periods has detrimental effects on the stomach mucosa. Chronic alcohol exposure causes fatty infiltration of the liver and can cause damage, leading to cirrhosis and hepatocellular carcinoma. Obtain a history of cigarette smoking. Nicotine is irritating to the GI tract mucosa. Cigarette smoking is related to GI cancers (especially mouth and esophageal cancers), esophagitis, and ulcers. Smoking delays the healing of ulcers.

Family history is an important component of this health pattern. About one third of cases of colorectal cancer occur in patients with a family history. Because of the relationship

TABLE 38-7   Health History

Gastrointestinal System

Health Perception–Health Management
- Describe any measures used to treat GI symptoms such as diarrhea or constipation.
- Do you smoke?* Do you drink alcohol?*
- Are you exposed to any chemicals on a regular basis?* Have you been exposed in the past?*
- Have you recently traveled outside the United States?*

Nutritional-Metabolic
- Describe your usual daily food and fluid intake.
- Do you take any supplemental vitamins or minerals?*
- Have you experienced any changes in appetite or food tolerance?*
- Has there been a weight change in the past 6-12 mo?*
- Are you allergic to any foods?*

Elimination
- Describe the frequency and time of day you have bowel movements. What is the consistency of the bowel movement?
- Do you use laxatives or enemas?* If so, how often?
- Have there been any recent changes in your bowel pattern?*
- Do you have any pain with bowel movements or pain relieved by bowel movements?
- Describe any skin problems caused by GI problems.
- Do you need any assistive equipment, such as ostomy equipment, raised toilet seat, commode?

Activity-Exercise
- Do you have limitations in mobility that make it difficult for you to obtain and prepare food?*

Sleep-Rest
- Do you experience any difficulty sleeping because of a GI problem?*
- Are you awakened by symptoms such as gas, abdominal pain, diarrhea, or heartburn?*

Cognitive-Perceptual
- Have you experienced any change in taste or smell that has affected your appetite?*
- Do you have any heat or cold sensitivity that affects eating?*
- Does pain interfere with food preparation, appetite, or chewing?*
- Do pain medications cause constipation, diarrhea, or appetite suppression?*

Self-Perception–Self-Concept
- Describe any changes in your weight that have affected how you feel about yourself.
- Have you had any changes in normal elimination that have affected how you feel about yourself?*
- Have any symptoms of GI disease caused physical changes that are a problem for you?*

Role-Relationship
- Describe the impact of any GI problem on your usual roles and relationships.
- Have any changes in elimination affected your relationships?*
- Do you live alone? Describe how your family or others assist you with your GI problems.

Sexuality-Reproductive
- Describe the effect of your GI problem on your sexual activity.

Coping–Stress Tolerance
- Do you experience GI symptoms in response to stressful or emotional situations?
- Describe how you deal with any GI symptoms that result.

Value-Belief
- Describe any culturally specific health beliefs regarding food and food preparation that may influence the treatment of your GI problem.

*If yes, describe.

GENETIC RISK ALERT

Colorectal Cancer

- Colorectal cancer may run in families if first-degree relatives (parents, siblings) or many other family members (grandparents, aunts, uncles) have had colorectal cancer. This is especially true when family members are diagnosed with colorectal cancer before age 50.
- Genetic conditions associated with an increased risk of colorectal cancer include:
  - Hereditary nonpolyposis colorectal cancer (HNPCC), which is caused by mutations in several different genes.
  - Familial adenomatous polyposis (FAP), which is characterized by multiple polyps that are noncancerous at first but eventually develop into cancer if not treated. Most cases of FAP are due to mutations of the adenomatous polyposis coli (APC) gene.

GENETIC RISK ALERT

Inflammatory Bowel Disease (IBD)

- People with IBD have a genetic predisposition or susceptibility to the disease.
- First-degree relatives have a 5- to 20-fold increased risk of developing IBD.

between colorectal and breast cancer, inquire about a history of either type of cancer in the family.

Nutritional-Metabolic Pattern. A thorough nutritional assessment is essential. Take a diet history and inquire about both content and amount or portion size. Food preferences and preparation may vary by culture. Open-ended questions allow the patient to express beliefs and feelings about the diet. For example, you can say, "Please tell me about your food and beverage intake over the past 24 hours." A 24-hour dietary recall can be used to analyze the adequacy of the diet. Assist the patient in recalling the preceding day's food intake, including early morning and nighttime intake, snacks, liquids, and vitamin supplements. You can then evaluate the diet in relation to recommended servings for dietary intake using a guide such as MyPlate (www.choosemyplate.gov). A 1-week recall may provide additional information on usual dietary patterns. Compare weekday and weekend dietary intake patterns in relation to both the quality and quantity of food.

Ask the patient about the use of sugar and salt substitutes, use of caffeine, and amount of fluid and fiber intake. Note any changes in appetite, food tolerance, and weight. Anorexia and weight loss may indicate cancer or inflammation. Decreased food intake can also be the consequence of economic problems or depression.

Ask about food allergies and dietary intolerances, including lactose and gluten. Have the patient describe the allergic response and any GI symptoms.

Elimination Pattern. Elicit a detailed account of the patient's bowel elimination pattern. Note the frequency, time of day, and usual stool consistency. Ask about the presence of pain with bowel movements or if bowel movements relieve pain. Document the use of laxatives and enemas, including type, frequency, and results. Investigate any recent change in bowel patterns.

Document the amount and type of fluid and fiber intake because these influence the frequency and consistency of stools. Inadequate fiber intake can be associated with constipation. Investigate the possible association between a skin problem and a GI problem. Food allergies can cause skin lesions, pruritus, and edema. Diarrhea can result in redness, irritation, and pain in the perianal area. External drainage systems, such as an ileostomy or ileal conduit, may cause local skin irritation.

Activity-Exercise Pattern. Activity and exercise affect GI motility. Immobility is a risk factor for constipation. Assess ambulatory status to determine if the patient is capable of securing and preparing food. If the patient is unable to do these tasks, determine if a family member or an outside agency is meeting this need.

Note any limitation in the ability to feed oneself. Assess for access to a toilet. Identify the use of and access to supplies such as a commode or ostomy supplies.

Sleep-Rest Pattern. GI symptoms can interfere with the quality of sleep. Nausea, vomiting, diarrhea, indigestion, and bloating can produce sleep problems. Ask the patient if GI symptoms affect sleep or rest. For example, a patient with gastroesophageal reflux disease (GERD) may wake with burning, epigastric pain.

A patient may have a bedtime ritual that involves a particular food or beverage. Herbal teas may be sleep inducing. Document individual routines and comply with these whenever possible to avoid sleeplessness. Hunger can prevent sleep and a light, easily digested snack may be helpful.

Cognitive-Perceptual Pattern. Sensory alterations can result in problems related to the acquisition, preparation, and ingestion of food. Changes in taste or smell can affect appetite and eating pleasure. Vertigo can make shopping and standing at a stove difficult and dangerous. Heat or cold sensitivity can make certain foods painful to eat. Problems in expressive communication limit the patient's ability to state personal dietary preferences. If a patient has a GI disorder, ask questions to determine his or her understanding of the illness and its treatment.

Both acute and chronic pain influence dietary intake. Behaviors associated with pain include avoiding activity, fatigue, and disrupted eating patterns. For patients receiving opioid medications, assess for constipation, nausea, sedation, and appetite suppression.

Self-Perception–Self-Concept Pattern. Many GI and nutritional problems affect the patient's self-perception. Overweight and underweight persons may have problems related to self-esteem and body image. Repeated attempts to achieve a personally acceptable weight can be discouraging and depressing for some people. The way a person recounts a weight history can alert you to potential problems in this area.

The need for external devices to manage elimination, such as a colostomy or an ileostomy, may be challenging for some patients. The patient's willingness to engage in self-care and to discuss this situation provides you with valuable information related to body image and self-esteem.

The altered physical changes often associated with advanced liver disease can be disturbing for the patient. Jaundice and ascites cause significant changes in external appearance. Assess the patient's attitude about these changes.

Role-Relationship Pattern. Problems related to the GI system such as cirrhosis, hepatitis, ostomies, obesity, and carcinoma may alter the patient's ability to maintain usual roles and relationships. A chronic illness may necessitate leaving a job or reducing work hours. Changes in body image and self-esteem can affect relationships.

Sexuality-Reproductive Pattern. Changes related to sexuality and reproductive status can result from problems of the GI system. For example, obesity, jaundice, anorexia, and ascites could decrease the acceptance of a potential sexual partner. An ostomy could affect the patient's confidence related to sexual activity. Your sensitive questioning can identify potential problems.

Anorexia can affect the reproductive status of a female patient. Obesity leads to reduced fertility and increased miscarriage rates in women.

Coping–Stress Tolerance Pattern. Determine what is stressful for the patient and what coping mechanisms the patient uses. Factors outside the GI tract can influence its functioning. Both psychologic and emotional factors, such as stress and anxiety, influence GI functioning in many people. Stress can manifest as anorexia, nausea, epigastric and abdominal pain, or diarrhea. It can also aggravate some diseases of the GI system, such as peptic ulcer disease, irritable bowel syndrome, and IBD. However, never attribute GI symptoms solely to psychologic factors.

Value-Belief Pattern. Assess the patient's spiritual and cultural beliefs regarding food and food preparation. Whenever possible, respect these preferences. Determine if any value or belief could interfere with planned interventions. For example, if the patient with anemia is a vegetarian, you will need to consider how to increase dietary intake of iron-rich foods other than meat. Thoughtful assessment and consideration of the patient's beliefs and values usually increase adherence and satisfaction.

Objective Data
Physical Examination
Mouth

Inspection. Inspect the mouth for symmetry, color, and size. Observe for abnormalities such as pallor or cyanosis, cracking, ulcers, or fissures. The dorsum (top) of the tongue should have a thin white coating. The undersurface should be smooth. Observe for any lesions. Using a tongue blade, inspect the buccal mucosa and note the color, any areas of pigmentation, and any lesions. Dark-skinned individuals normally have patchy areas of pigmentation. In assessing the teeth and gums, look for caries; loose teeth; abnormal shape and position of teeth; and swelling, bleeding, discoloration, or gingival inflammation. Note any distinctive breath odor.

Inspect the pharynx by tilting the patient's head back and depressing the tongue with a tongue blade. Observe the tonsils, uvula, soft palate, and anterior and posterior pillars. Instruct the patient to say "ah." The uvula and soft palate should rise and remain in the midline.

Palpation. Palpate any suspicious areas in the mouth. Note ulcers, nodules, indurations, and areas of tenderness. The mouth of the older adult requires careful assessment. Give particular attention to dentures (e.g., fit, condition), ability to swallow, the tongue, and lesions. Ask the patient with dentures to remove them during an oral examination to allow for good visualization and palpation of the area.

Abdomen. Two systems are used to anatomically describe the surface of the abdomen. One system divides the abdomen into four quadrants by a perpendicular line from the sternum to the pubic bone and a horizontal line across the abdomen at the umbilicus (Fig. 38-5, *A*, and Table 38-8). The other system divides the abdomen into nine regions (Fig. 38-5, *B*). Only the epigastric, umbilical, and suprapubic or hypogastric regions are commonly assessed.

For the abdominal examination, good lighting should shine across the abdomen. The patient should be in the supine position and as relaxed as possible. To help relax the abdominal muscles, have the patient slightly flex the knees and raise the head of the bed slightly. The patient should have an empty bladder. Use warm hands when doing the abdominal examination to avoid eliciting muscle guarding. Ask the patient to breathe slowly through the mouth.

The standard approach for examining the abdomen is appropriate for an older adult. The abdomen may be thinner and more lax unless the patient is obese.

Inspection. Assess the abdomen for skin changes (color, texture, scars, striae, dilated veins, rashes, lesions), umbilicus (location and contour), symmetry, contour (flat, rounded [convex], concave, protuberant, distended), observable hernias or masses, and movement (pulsations and peristalsis). A normal aortic pulsation may be seen in the epigastric area. Look across the abdomen tangentially (across the abdomen in a line) for peristalsis. Peristalsis is not normally visible in an adult but may be visible in a thin person.

Auscultation. When you examine the abdomen, auscultate before percussion and palpation because these latter procedures may alter the bowel sounds. Use the diaphragm of the stethoscope to auscultate bowel sounds because they are relatively high pitched. Use the bell of the stethoscope to detect lower-pitched sounds. Warm the stethoscope in your hands before auscultating to help prevent abdominal muscle contraction. Listen in the epigastrium and in all four quadrants. Start in the right lower quadrant because bowel sounds are normally present there. Listen for bowel sounds for at least 2 minutes. Do not count bowel sounds. Determine if they are normal, hypoactive, or hyperactive.

The frequency and intensity of bowel sounds vary depending on the phase of digestion. Normal sounds are relatively high pitched and gurgling. Stomach growling or loud gurgles

CASE STUDY

Subjective Data

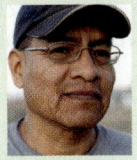
(©iStockphoto/ Thinkstock)

A focused subjective assessment of L.C. revealed the following information:
- **PMH:** Negative history for medical or surgical problems.
- **Medications:** None.
- **Health Perception–Health Management:** L.C. states he has not been feeling well for the past several weeks. He feels weak and is easily fatigued. Denies exposure to chemicals. No recent travel outside of the United States. Smokes approximately 1 pack of cigarettes/day for 20 yr. Drinks beer on a daily basis, typically 3 or 4 bottles per day.
- **Nutritional-Metabolic:** L.C. is 5 ft, 9 in tall and weighs 140 lb (BMI: 20.7 kg/m²). States has been losing weight over the past several months and does not have an appetite. No food allergies.
- **Elimination:** States has had alternating episodes of constipation and diarrhea. He noticed some bright red blood in stools. Has not had a bowel movement for 4 days.
- **Cognitive-Perceptual:** Rates pain as a 9 on a scale of 0 to 10. States pain comes and goes in waves. Prefers to lie still with knees flexed and drawn into his abdomen.

Discussion Questions

1. Which subjective assessment findings are of most concern to you?
2. Based on these subjective assessment findings, what should be included in the physical assessment? What would you be looking for?
3. What would be your priority assessment?
   You will learn more about physical examination of the gastrointestinal system in the next section.
   (See p. 845 for more information on L.C.)

Answers available at *http://evolve.elsevier.com/Lewis/medsurg.*

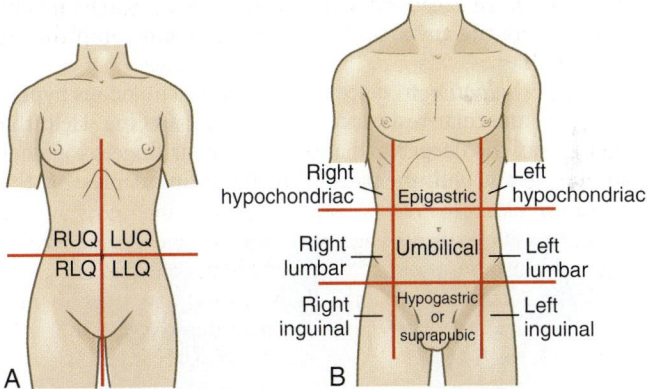

FIG. 38-5 A, Abdominal quadrants. **B,** Abdominal regions. *LLQ,* Left lower quadrant; *LUQ,* left upper quadrant; *RLQ,* right lower quadrant; *RUQ,* right upper quadrant.

TABLE 38-8 Structures Located in Abdominal Regions

Right Upper Quadrant	Left Upper Quadrant	Right Lower Quadrant	Left Lower Quadrant
• Liver and gallbladder	• Left lobe of liver	• Lower pole of right kidney	• Lower pole of left kidney
• Pylorus	• Spleen	• Cecum and appendix	• Sigmoid flexure
• Duodenum	• Stomach	• Portion of ascending colon	• Portion of descending colon
• Head of pancreas	• Body of pancreas	• Bladder (if distended)	• Bladder (if distended)
• Right adrenal gland	• Left adrenal gland	• Right ovary and salpinx	• Left ovary and salpinx
• Portion of right kidney	• Portion of left kidney	• Uterus (if enlarged)	• Uterus (if enlarged)
• Hepatic flexure of colon	• Splenic flexure of colon	• Right spermatic cord	• Left spermatic cord
• Portion of ascending and transverse colon	• Portion of transverse and descending colon	• Right ureter	• Left ureter

(borborygmi) indicate hyperperistalsis. The bowel sounds are more high pitched (rushes and tinkling) when the intestines are under tension, as in intestinal obstruction. Listen for decreased or absent bowel sounds. A perfectly "silent abdomen" is uncommon.[5] If you are patient and listen for several minutes, you will frequently find the bowel sounds are not absent but are hypoactive. If you do not hear bowel sounds, note the amount of time you listened in each quadrant without hearing bowel sounds.

Listen for vascular sounds. A *bruit,* best heard with the bell of the stethoscope, is a swishing or buzzing sound and indicates turbulent blood flow. Normally you should not hear aortic bruits.

Percussion. The purpose of percussing the abdomen is to estimate the size of the liver and determine the presence of fluid, distention, and masses. Sound waves vary according to the density of underlying tissues. Air produces a higher-pitched, hollow sound termed *tympany.* Fluid or masses produce a short, high-pitched sound with little resonance termed *dullness.* Lightly percuss all four quadrants of the abdomen and assess the distribution of tympany and dullness (Fig. 38-6). Tympany is the predominant percussion sound of the abdomen.

To percuss the liver, start below the umbilicus in the right midclavicular line and percuss lightly upward until you hear dullness, thus determining the lower border of the liver. Next, start at the nipple line in the right midclavicular line and percuss downward between ribs to the area of dullness indicating the upper border of the liver. Measure the height or vertical space between the two borders to determine the size of the liver. The normal range of liver height in the right midclavicular line is 2.4 to 5 in (6 to 12.7 cm).

Palpation. Use palpation to assess the abdominal organs and detect any tenderness, distension, masses, or fluid. Palpation is important because it may reveal a tumor. Begin with light palpation. Palpate any areas in which the patient complains of tenderness last.

Use *light palpation* to detect tenderness or cutaneous hypersensitivity, muscular resistance, masses, and swelling. Help the patient relax for deeper palpation. Keep your fingers together and press gently with the pads of the fingertips, depressing the abdominal wall about 0.4 in (1 cm). Use smooth movements and palpate all quadrants (Fig. 38-7, *A*).

Use *deep palpation* to delineate abdominal organs and masses (Fig. 38-7, *B*). Use the palmar surfaces of your fingers to press more deeply. Again, palpate all quadrants and note the location, size, and shape of masses, as well as the presence of tenderness. During these maneuvers, observe the patient's facial expression because it will provide nonverbal cues of discomfort or pain.

An alternative method for deep abdominal palpation is the two-hand method. Place one hand on top of the other and apply pressure to the bottom hand with the fingers of the top hand. With the fingers of the bottom hand, feel for organs and masses. Practice both methods of palpation to determine which one is most effective.

Check a problem area on the abdomen for rebound tenderness by pressing in slowly and firmly over the painful site. Withdraw the palpating fingers quickly. Pain on withdrawal of the fingers indicates peritoneal inflammation. Because assessing for rebound tenderness may produce pain and severe muscle spasm, it should be done at the end of the examination and only by an experienced practitioner.

To palpate the liver, place your left hand behind the patient to support the right eleventh and twelfth ribs (Fig. 38-8). The patient may relax on your hand. Press the left hand forward and place the right hand on the patient's right abdomen lateral to the rectus muscle. The fingertips should be below the lower border of liver dullness and pointed toward the right costal margin. Gently press in and up. The patient should take a deep breath with the abdomen so that the liver drops and is in a better position for palpation. Try to feel the liver edge as it comes down to the fingertips. During inspiration, the liver edge should feel firm, sharp, and smooth. Describe the surface and contour and any tenderness. If the patient has chronic obstructive pulmonary disease, large lungs, or a low diaphragm, the liver may be palpated 0.4 to 0.8 in (1 to 2 cm) below the right costal margin.

To palpate the spleen, move to the patient's left side. Place your right hand under the patient, and support and press the patient's left lower rib cage forward. Place your left hand below the left costal margin, and press it in toward the spleen. Ask the patient to breathe deeply. The fingertips can feel the tip or edge of an enlarged spleen. The spleen is normally not palpable. If it is palpable, do not continue because manual compression of an enlarged spleen may cause it to rupture.

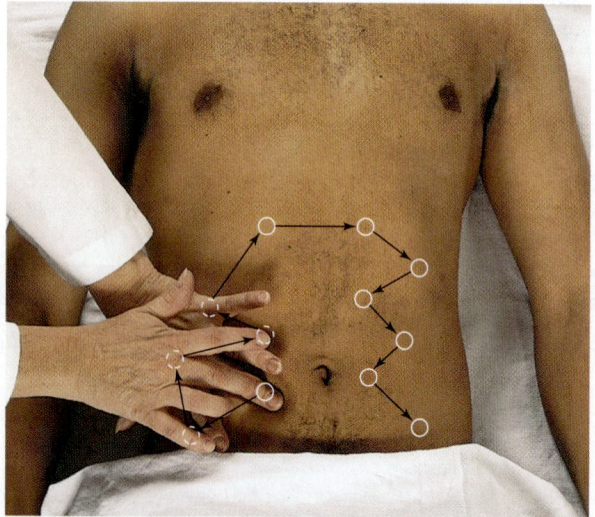

FIG. 38-6   Technique for percussion of the abdomen. Moving clockwise, percuss lightly in all four quadrants. (From Jarvis C: *Physical examination and health assessment,* ed 6, St Louis, 2012, Saunders.)

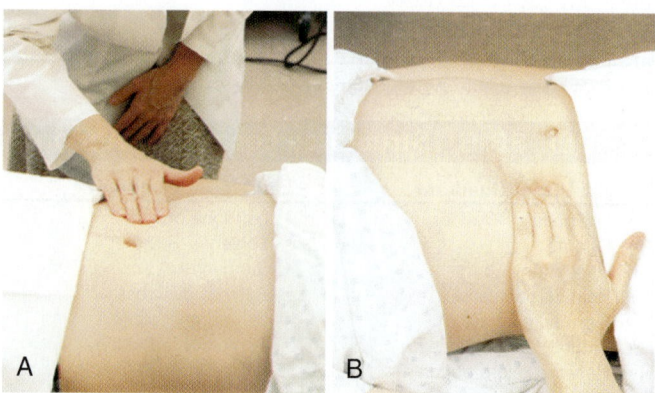

FIG. 38-7   **A,** Technique for light palpation of the abdomen. **B,** Technique for deep palpation.

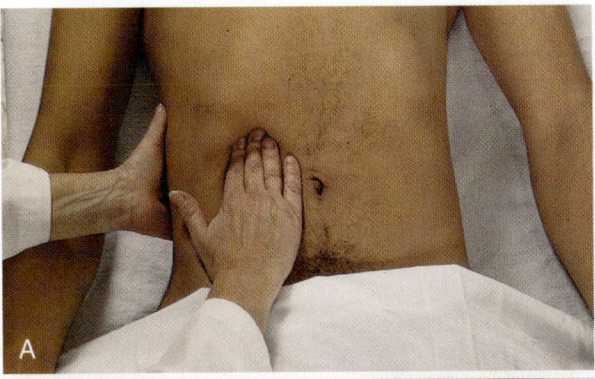

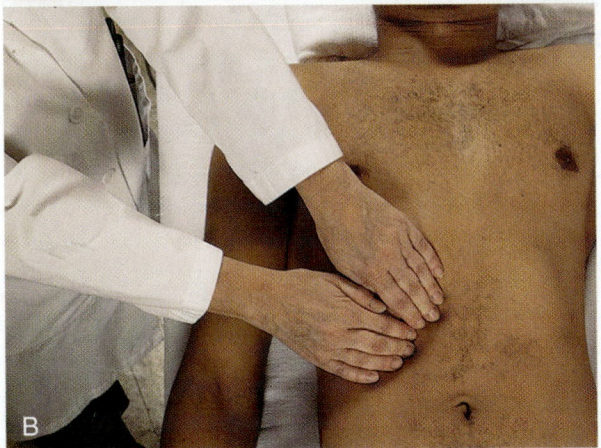

FIG. 38-8 A, Technique for liver palpation. **B,** Alternative technique to palpate liver with fingers hooked over the costal region. (From Jarvis C: *Physical examination and health assessment,* ed 6, St Louis, 2012, Saunders.)

Rectum and Anus. Inspect perianal and anal areas for color, texture, masses, rashes, scars, erythema, fissures, and external hemorrhoids. Palpate any masses or unusual areas with a gloved hand.

For the digital examination of the rectum, place a gloved, lubricated index finger against the anus while having the patient gently bear down (Valsalva maneuver). Then, as the sphincter relaxes, insert the finger. Point the finger toward the umbilicus. Try to get the patient to relax. Insert the finger into the rectum as far as possible, and palpate all surfaces. Assess any nodules, tenderness, or irregularities. Use the gloved finger to remove a stool sample and check it for occult blood. However, a single guaiac-based fecal occult blood test has limited sensitivity in detecting colorectal cancer.

Findings of a normal physical assessment of the GI system are given in Table 38-9. Table 38-10 outlines assessment abnormalities. Gerontologic differences in the GI system and differences in assessment findings are described in Table 38-5. A *focused assessment* is used to evaluate the status of previously identified GI problems and to monitor for signs of new problems. A focused assessment of the GI system is presented on p. 846.

DIAGNOSTIC STUDIES OF GASTROINTESTINAL SYSTEM

Table 38-11 presents common diagnostic studies of the GI system. Selected diagnostic studies are described in more detail below.

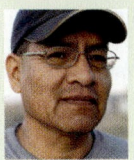
For most diagnostic studies, make sure a signed consent form for the procedure has been completed and is in the medical record. The HCP doing the procedure is responsible for explaining the procedure and obtaining written consent. You play an important role in teaching patients about the procedures. When preparing the patient, it is important to ask about any known allergies to drugs, iodine, shellfish, or contrast media.

Many GI system diagnostic procedures require (1) measures to cleanse the GI tract and (2) ingestion or injection of a contrast medium or a radiopaque tracer. Often the patient has a series of GI diagnostic tests done. Monitor the patient closely to ensure adequate hydration and nutrition during the testing period.

Some diagnostic studies are especially difficult and uncomfortable for the older adult. Adjustments may be needed during the preparation to avoid dehydration or worsening renal function. Make sure to consider any physical limitations when positioning the older patient during testing. Close monitoring is needed to avoid problems such as dehydration from prolonged fluid restriction and diarrhea from bowel-cleansing procedures.

Radiologic Studies

Upper Gastrointestinal Series. An upper GI series with small bowel follow-through provides visualization of the oropharyngeal area, esophagus, stomach, and small intestine. The procedure consists of the patient swallowing contrast medium (a thick barium solution or gastrograffin) and then assuming different positions on the x-ray table. The movement of the contrast medium is observed with fluoroscopy and a series of x-rays are taken. An upper GI series is useful in identifying esophageal strictures, polyps, tumors, hiatal hernias, foreign bodies, and ulcers.

Lower Gastrointestinal Series. The purpose of a lower GI series, or a barium enema, is to observe (using fluoroscopy) the colon filling with contrast medium and to observe (by x-ray) the filled colon. It consists of administering an enema of contrast medium to the patient. This procedure identifies polyps, tumors, and other lesions in the colon. Adding air contrast after

Text continued on p. 851

TABLE 38-9 Normal Physical Assessment of Gastrointestinal System

Mouth

- Moist and pink lips
- Pink and moist buccal mucosa and gingivae without plaques or lesions
- Teeth in good repair
- Protrusion of tongue in midline without deviation or fasciculations
- Pink uvula (in midline), soft palate, tonsils, and posterior pharynx
- Swallows smoothly without coughing or gagging

Abdomen

- Flat without masses or scars. No bruises
- Bowel sounds in all quadrants
- No abdominal tenderness; nonpalpable liver and spleen
- Liver 10 cm in right midclavicular line
- Generalized tympany

Anus

- Absence of lesions, fissures, and hemorrhoids
- Good sphincter tone
- Rectal walls smooth and soft
- No masses
- Stool soft, brown, and heme negative

FOCUSED ASSESSMENT
Gastrointestinal System

Use this checklist to make sure the key assessment steps have been done.

Subjective
Ask the patient about any of the following and note responses.

Loss of appetite	Y	N
Abdominal pain	Y	N
Changes in stools (e.g., color, blood, consistency, frequency, pain)	Y	N
Nausea, vomiting	Y	N
Painful swallowing	Y	N

Objective: Diagnostic
Check the following results for critical values.

Endoscopy: colonoscopy, sigmoidoscopy, esophagogastroduodenoscopy	✓
CT scan	✓
Radiologic series: upper GI, lower GI	✓
Stool for occult blood or ova and parasites	✓
Liver function tests	✓

Objective: Physical Examination
Inspect

Skin for color, lesions, scars, petechiae, etc.	✓
Abdominal contour for symmetry and distention	✓
Perianal area for intact skin, hemorrhoids	✓

Auscultate*

Bowel sounds	✓

Palpate

Abdominal quadrants using light touch	✓
Abdominal quadrants using a deep technique	✓

*NOTE: Do auscultation before palpation.

TABLE 38-10 Assessment Abnormalities
Gastrointestinal System

Finding	Description	Possible Etiology and Significance
Mouth		
Ulcer, plaque on lips or in mouth	Sore or lesion	Carcinoma, viral infections
Cheilosis	Softening, fissuring, and cracking of lips at angles of mouth	Riboflavin deficiency
Cheilitis	Inflammation of lips (usually lower) with fissuring, scaling, crusting	Often unknown
Geographic tongue	Scattered red, smooth (loss of papillae) areas on dorsum of tongue	Unknown
Smooth tongue	Red, slick appearance	Cobalamin deficiency
Leukoplakia	Thickened white patches	Premalignant lesion
Pyorrhea	Recessed gingivae, purulent pockets	Periodontitis
Herpes simplex	Benign vesicular lesion	Herpesvirus
Candidiasis	White, curdlike lesions surrounded by erythematous mucosa	*Candida albicans*
Glossitis	Reddened, ulcerated, swollen tongue	Exposure to streptococci, irritation, injury, vitamin B deficiencies, anemia
Acute marginal gingivitis	Friable, edematous, painful, bleeding gingivae	Irritation from ill-fitting dentures or orthodontic appliances, calcium deposits on teeth, food impaction
Esophagus and Stomach		
Dysphagia	Difficulty swallowing, sensation of food sticking in esophagus	Esophageal problems, cancer of esophagus
Hematemesis	Vomiting of blood	Esophageal varices, bleeding peptic ulcer
Pyrosis	Heartburn, burning in epigastric or substernal area	Hiatal hernia, esophagitis, incompetent lower esophageal sphincter
Dyspepsia	Burning or indigestion	Peptic ulcer disease, gallbladder disease
Odynophagia	Painful swallowing	Cancer of esophagus, esophagitis
Eructation	Belching	Gallbladder disease
Nausea and vomiting	Feeling of impending vomiting, expulsion of gastric contents through mouth	GI infections, common manifestation of many GI diseases; stress, fear, and pathologic conditions

TABLE 38-10 Assessment Abnormalities

Gastrointestinal System—cont'd

Finding	Description	Possible Etiology and Significance
Abdomen		
Distention	Excessive gas accumulation, enlarged abdomen, generalized tympany	Obstruction, paralytic ileus
Ascites	Accumulated fluid within abdominal cavity, eversion of umbilicus (usually)	Peritoneal inflammation, heart failure, metastatic carcinoma, cirrhosis
Bruit	Humming or swishing sound heard through stethoscope over vessel	Partial arterial obstruction (narrowing of vessel), turbulent flow (aneurysm)
Hyperresonance	Loud, tinkling rushes	Intestinal obstruction
Borborygmi	Waves of loud, gurgling sounds	Hyperactive bowel as result of eating
Absent bowel sounds	No bowel sounds on auscultation	Peritonitis, paralytic ileus, obstruction
Absence of liver dullness	Tympany on percussion	Air from viscus (e.g., perforated ulcer)
Masses	Lump on palpation	Tumors, cysts
Rebound tenderness	Sudden pain when fingers withdrawn quickly	Peritoneal inflammation, appendicitis
Nodular liver	Enlarged, hard liver with irregular edge or surface	Cirrhosis, carcinoma
Hepatomegaly	Enlargement of liver, liver edge >1-2 cm below costal margin	Metastatic carcinoma, hepatitis, venous congestion
Splenomegaly	Enlarged spleen	Chronic leukemia, hemolytic states, portal hypertension, some infections
Hernia	Bulge or nodule in abdomen, usually appearing on straining	Inguinal (in inguinal canal), femoral (in femoral canal), umbilical (herniation of umbilicus), or incisional (defect in muscles after surgery)
Rectum and Anus		
Hemorrhoids	Thrombosed veins in rectum and anus (internal or external)	Portal hypertension, chronic constipation, prolonged sitting or standing, pregnancy
Mass	Firm, nodular edge	Tumor, carcinoma
Pilonidal cyst	Opening of sinus tract, cyst in midline just above coccyx	Probably congenital
Fissure	Ulceration in anal canal	Straining, irritation
Melena	Abnormal, black, tarry stool containing digested blood	Cancer, bleeding in upper GI tract from ulcers, varices
Tenesmus	Painful and ineffective straining at stool. Sense of incomplete evacuation	Inflammatory bowel disease, irritable bowel syndrome, diarrhea secondary to GI infection (e.g., food poisoning)
Steatorrhea	Fatty, frothy, foul-smelling stool	Chronic pancreatitis, biliary obstruction, malabsorption problems

TABLE 38-11 Diagnostic Studies

Gastrointestinal System

Study	Description and Purpose	Nursing Responsibility
Radiology		
Upper gastrointestinal (GI) or barium swallow	Fluoroscopic x-ray study using contrast medium. Used to diagnose structural abnormalities of esophagus, stomach, and duodenum.	*Before:* Explain procedure including the need to drink contrast medium and assume various positions on x-ray table. Keep patient NPO for at least 8 hr. Tell patient to avoid smoking after midnight. *After:* Take measures to prevent contrast medium impaction (fluids, laxatives). Tell patient that stool may be white for up to 72 hr.
Small bowel series	Contrast medium is ingested and films taken every 30 min until medium reaches terminal ileum.	Same as for upper GI.
Lower GI or barium enema	Fluoroscopic x-ray examination of colon using contrast medium, which is administered rectally (enema) (Fig. 38-9). Double-contrast or air-contrast barium enema is test of choice. Air is infused after the barium flows through transverse colon. Used to detect the presence of tumors, diverticula, and polyps.	*Before:* Administer laxatives and enemas until colon is clear of stool evening before procedure. Administer clear liquid diet evening before procedure. Keep patient NPO for 8 hr before test. Instruct patient about barium being given by enema. Explain that cramping and urge to defecate may occur during procedure and patient may be placed in various positions on tilt table. *After:* Give fluids, laxatives, or suppositories to assist in expelling barium. Observe stool for passage of contrast medium. Tell patient that stool may be white for up to 72 hr.

Continued

TABLE 38-11 Diagnostic Studies
Gastrointestinal System—cont'd

Study	Description and Purpose	Nursing Responsibility
Radiology—cont'd **Cholangiography**		
• Percutaneous transhepatic (PTC)	Under local anesthesia and monitored anesthesia care, a long needle is passed into liver (under fluoroscopy) and into bile duct. Bile is removed and radiopaque contrast medium directly injected into biliary system. Used to determine filling of hepatic and biliary ducts.	*Before:* Assess patient's medications for possible contraindications, precautions, or complications with use of contrast medium. Keep patient NPO for 8-12 hr before test. Initiate prophylactic IV antibiotics 1 hr prior. *After:* Observe patient for signs of hemorrhage, bile leakage, and infection. Observe safety precautions until sedation wears off. Maintain bed rest for 6 hr.
• Surgical cholangiogram	Contrast medium is injected into common bile duct during surgery on biliary structures.	*Before:* Explain that anesthetic will be used. Assess patient's medications for possible contraindications, precautions, or complications with use of contrast medium.
• Magnetic resonance cholangiopancreatography (MRCP)	Use of MRI technology to obtain images of biliary and pancreatic ducts.	*Before:* Explain procedure to patient. Assess for contraindications, including pregnancy and presence of metal implants (e.g., pacemaker).
Ultrasound	Noninvasive procedure using high-frequency ultrasound waves, which are passed into body structures and recorded as they are reflected. Used to show size and configuration of an organ.	
• Abdominal ultrasound	A conductive gel is applied to skin and a transducer is placed on the area. Detects abdominal masses (tumors, cysts), gallstones, biliary and liver disease.	*Before:* Instruct patient to be NPO for 8-12 hr. Air or gas can reduce quality of images. Food intake can cause gallbladder contraction, resulting in suboptimal study.
• Endoscopic ultrasound (EUS)	Small ultrasound transducer is installed on tip of endoscope. Because EUS transducer gets close to the organ(s) being examined, images obtained are more accurate and detailed than those provided by traditional ultrasound. Detects and stages esophageal, gastric, rectal, biliary, and pancreatic tumors and abnormalities.	Same as esophagogastroduodenoscopy (EGD).
• Ultrasound elastography (Fibroscan)	Transient elastography uses an ultrasound transducer to assess level of liver fibrosis. Used to monitor patients with chronic liver disease.	*Before:* Explain the need to lie in dorsal decubitus position with right arm in extreme abduction.
Nuclear imaging scans (scintigraphy)	Tracer doses of a radioactive isotope are injected IV and a scanning device picks up radioactive emission, which is recorded on paper. Shows size, shape, and position of organ. Functional disorders and structural defects may be identified.	*Before:* Tell patient that the substance used contains only traces of radioactivity and poses little to no danger. Schedule no more than one radionuclide test a day. Explain to patient need to lie flat during scanning.
• Gastric emptying studies	Radionuclide study (scintigraphy) is used to assess ability of stomach to empty solids. Patient eats cooked egg containing Tc-99m and toast with water. Images are obtained at 0, 1, 2, and 4 hr later. Study is used in patients with gastric emptying disorders caused by ulcers, ulcer surgery, diabetes, gastric malignancies, or functional disorders.	Same as above.
• Hepatobiliary scintigraphy (HIDA)	Patient is given IV injection of Tc-99m and positioned under camera to record distribution of tracer dose in liver, biliary tree, gallbladder, and proximal small intestine. Used to identify obstructions of bile ducts (gallstones, tumors), diseases of gallbladder, and bile leaks.	Same as above.
• Scintigraphy of GI bleeding	Tc-99m–labeled sulfur colloid or Tc-99m labeling of the patient's own RBCs to determine the site of active GI blood loss. Sulfur colloid or patient's RBCs are injected, and images of abdomen are obtained at intermittent intervals.	Same as above.
Gastric emptying breath test (GEBT)	Noninvasive test that measures CO_2 in a patient's breath. Used to diagnose delayed gastric emptying (gastroparesis). Baseline breath test done and then patient eats a special test meal that includes a scrambled egg–mix and *Spirulina platensis*, a type of protein that has been enriched with carbon-13, which can be measured in breath samples. Both carbon-12 and a very small amount of carbon-13 are normally found in exhaled CO_2. By adding carbon-13 to the test meal, the GEBT can determine how fast the stomach empties the meal by measuring the ratio of carbon-13 to carbon-12 collected in breath samples at multiple time points after the meal is consumed compared to baseline.	*Before:* Instruct patient to be NPO after midnight and that the test takes 4 hr. *During:* Can be done in any clinical setting since it does not require the special training or special precautions related to radiation (as does scintigraphy).

TABLE 38-11 Diagnostic Studies

Gastrointestinal System—cont'd

Study	Description and Purpose	Nursing Responsibility
Computed tomography (CT) scan	Noninvasive radiologic examination allows for exposures at different depths. Using oral and IV contrast medium accentuates density differences. Detects biliary tract, liver, and pancreatic disorders.	*Before:* Explain procedure. Determine sensitivity to iodine or shellfish if contrast material used.
Magnetic resonance imaging (MRI)	Noninvasive procedure using radiofrequency waves and a magnetic field. IV contrast medium (gadolinium) may be used. Used to detect hepatobiliary disease, hepatic lesions, and sources of GI bleeding and stage colorectal cancer.	*Before:* Explain procedure to patient. Assess for contraindications, including pregnancy and presence of metal implants (e.g., pacemaker).
Virtual colonoscopy	Combines CT scanning or MRI with computer virtual reality software. Air is introduced via a tube placed in rectum to enlarge colon to enhance visualization. Images obtained while patient is on back and abdomen. Computer combines images to form 2-D and 3-D pictures that are viewed on monitor. Detects intestine and colon diseases, including polyps, cancer, diverticulosis, and lower GI bleeding.	*Before:* Bowel preparation similar to colonoscopy (see Colonoscopy).
Defecography	Uses fluoroscopy or MRI to assess the shape and position of the rectum during defecation. Using a lubricated small plastic tip, fill rectum and anus with barium. Oral barium allows small bowel to be visualized. The person then sits on a toilet-like seat attached to the x-ray table, and is asked to push and empty the rectum. Images are taken while person is sitting at rest, straining, squeezing, and during defecation. Detects pelvic floor abnormalities.	*Before:* Keep patient NPO for 2 hr. Two enemas are given 2 hr before, 15 minutes apart. Oral barium is given 1 hr before.
Endoscopy Esophagogastroduodenoscopy (EGD)	Directly visualizes mucosal lining of esophagus, stomach, and duodenum with flexible endoscope. Test may use video imaging to visualize stomach motility. Detects inflammation, ulcerations, tumors, varices, or Mallory-Weiss tears. Biopsies may be taken. Varices can be treated with band ligation or sclerotherapy.	*Before:* Keep patient NPO for 8 hr. Make sure signed consent is on chart. Give preoperative medication if ordered. Explain to patient that local anesthesia may be sprayed on throat before insertion of scope and that patient will be sedated during procedure. *After:* Keep patient NPO until gag reflex returns. Gently tickle back of throat to determine reflex. Use warm saline gargles for relief of sore throat. Check temperature q15-30min for 1-2 hr (sudden temperature spike is sign of perforation).
Colonoscopy	Directly visualizes entire colon up to ileocecal valve with flexible fiberoptic scope. Patient's position is changed frequently during procedure to assist with advancement of scope to cecum. Used to diagnose or detect inflammatory bowel disease, polyps, tumors, and diverticulosis and dilate strictures. Procedure allows for biopsy and removal of polyps without laparotomy.	*Before:* Bowel preparation prior varies depending on HCP. For example, patient follows either a low-residue or full liquid diet the day before until bowel cleansing begins. Bowel cleansing follows a split-dose regimen. The evening before the procedure the patient drinks 2 L of oral polyethylene glycol (PEG) lavage solution. The second 2 L dose begins 4-6 hr before procedure. Explain to patient that a flexible scope will be inserted while patient in side-lying position and sedation will be given. *After:* Patient may experience abdominal cramps caused by stimulation of peristalsis because the bowel is constantly inflated with air during procedure. Observe for rectal bleeding and manifestations of perforation (e.g., malaise, abdominal distention, tenesmus). Check vital signs.
Video capsule endoscopy (VCE)	Patient swallows a vitamin-sized capsule with camera, which provides endoscopic visualization of GI tract (Fig. 38-11). Camera takes >50,000 images during 8-hr examination, relaying images to monitoring device that patient wears on belt. Afterwards, images are downloaded to a workstation. Used to visualize small intestine and diagnose diseases such as Crohn's disease, small bowel tumors, small bowel injury due to NSAIDs, celiac disease, and malabsorption syndrome and to identify sources of possible GI bleeding in areas not accessible by upper endoscopy or colonoscopy.	*Before:* Instruct patient to fast overnight. May have bowel preparation similar to colonoscopy. Video capsule is swallowed, and clear liquids resumed after 2 hr and food and medications after 4 hr. *During:* 8 hr after swallowing the capsule, the patient returns to have the monitoring device removed. A patency capsule may be used first in patients assessed to be high risk for capsule retention due to strictures. *After:* Peristalsis causes passage of the disposable capsule with a bowel movement.

Continued

TABLE 38-11 **Diagnostic Studies**

Gastrointestinal System—cont'd

Study	Description and Purpose	Nursing Responsibility
Endoscopy—cont'd		
Sigmoidoscopy	Directly visualizes rectum and sigmoid colon with lighted flexible endoscope. Sometimes a special table is used to tilt patient into knee-chest position. Used to detect tumors, polyps, inflammatory and infectious diseases, fissures, hemorrhoids.	*Before:* Bowel preparation similar to colonoscopy (see Colonoscopy). Explain to patient knee-chest position (unless patient is older or very ill), need to take deep breaths during insertion of scope, and possible urge to defecate as scope is passed. Encourage patient to relax and let abdomen go limp. *After:* Observe for rectal bleeding after polypectomy or biopsy.
Endoscopic retrograde cholangiopancreatography (ERCP)	Fiberoptic endoscope (using fluoroscopy) is orally inserted into descending duodenum. Then common bile and pancreatic ducts are cannulated. Contrast medium is injected into ducts and allows for direct visualization of structures. Can be used to retrieve a gallstone from distal common bile duct, dilate strictures, biopsy, and diagnose pseudocysts.	*Before:* Explain procedure. Keep patient NPO 8 hr before. Ensure consent form signed. Administer sedation immediately before and during procedure. Administer antibiotics if ordered. *After:* Check vital signs. Check for signs of perforation or infection. Be aware that pancreatitis is most common complication. Check for return of gag reflex.
Laparoscopy (peritoneoscopy)	Visualize peritoneal cavity and contents with laparoscope. Double-puncture peritoneoscopy permits better visualization of abdominal cavity, especially liver. Done in operating room. Can obtain biopsy specimen.	*Before:* Make sure signed consent is on chart. Keep patient NPO 8 hr. Administer preoperative sedative medication. Ensure bladder and bowels are emptied. *After:* Observe for possible complications of bleeding and bowel perforation after the procedure.
Blood Studies		
Amylase	Enzyme secreted by pancreas. Important in diagnosing acute pancreatitis. Level of amylase peaks in 24 hr and then drops to normal in 48-72 hr. Depending on method, *reference interval* is 30-122 U/L (0.51-2.07 µkat/L).	*Before:* Explain procedure to patient.
Lipase	Enzyme secreted by pancreas. Important in diagnosing pancreatitis. Level stays elevated longer than serum amylase in acute pancreatitis. *Reference interval:* 31-186 U/L (0.5-3.2 µkat/L).	*Before:* Explain procedure to patient.
Gastrin	Hormone secreted by cells of the antrum of the stomach, the duodenum, and the pancreatic islets of Langerhans. *Reference interval:* 25-100 pg/mL when fasting.	*Before:* Explain procedure to patient.
Liver Biopsy	Percutaneous procedure uses needle inserted between 6th and 7th or 8th and 9th intercostal spaces on the right side to obtain specimen of hepatic tissue. Often done with ultrasound or CT guidance	*Before:* Check patient's coagulation status (prothrombin time, clotting or bleeding time). Ensure patient's blood is typed and crossmatched. Take baseline vital signs. Explain need to hold breath after expiration when needle is inserted. Ensure informed consent has been signed. *After:* Check vital signs to detect internal bleeding q15min × 2, q30min × 4, q1hr × 4. Keep patient lying on right side for minimum of 2 hr to splint puncture site. Keep patient in bed in flat position for 12-14 hr. Assess patient for complications such as bile peritonitis, shock, pneumothorax.
Fecal Tests		
Fecal analysis	Form, consistency, and color are noted. Specimen examined for mucus, blood, pus, parasites, and fat content. May test for occult blood (guaiac test, Hemoccult, Hemoccult II, Hemoccult-SENSA, Hematest) and DNA testing (PreGen-Plus, Cologuard) to detect colorectal cancer	*Before:* Keep diet free of red meat for 24-48 hr before occult blood test. *During:* Observe patient's stools. Collect stool specimens. Check stools for blood.
Stool culture	Tests for the presence of bacteria, including *Clostridium difficile*	*During:* Collect stool specimen.

the barium provides better visualization (Fig. 38-9). Because it requires the patient to retain the barium, an older or immobile patient may not tolerate it very well.

Virtual Colonoscopy. *Virtual colonoscopy* combines CT scanning or MRI with computer software to produce images of the colon and rectum. The test is less invasive than a conventional colonoscopy and the patient does not need sedation. It does require radiation and prior cleansing of the colon.

Compared to conventional colonoscopy, virtual colonoscopy provides a better view inside the colon that is narrow from inflammation or a growth.[6] There are a few disadvantages of virtual colonoscopy. If a polyp is found, it will have to be biopsied or removed by conventional colonoscopy. Virtual colonoscopy may be less sensitive in obtaining information on the details and color of the mucosa and in detecting small (less than 10 mm) or flat polyps.

Endoscopy

Endoscopy refers to the direct visualization of a body structure through an endoscope. An endoscope is a fiberoptic instrument with a light and camera attached, allowing the ability to take video and still pictures (Fig. 38-10). Some endoscopes contain a channel through which to pass instruments, such as biopsy forceps and cytology brushes.

GI structures that can be examined by endoscopy include the esophagus, stomach, duodenum, and colon. An *endoscopic retrograde cholangiopancreatography* (ERCP) is used to visualize the pancreatic, hepatic, and common bile ducts. Endoscopy is often combined with diagnostic procedures, including biopsy and cytologic studies and invasive and therapeutic procedures. Examples include polypectomy, sclerosis or banding of varices, laser treatment, cauterization of bleeding sites, papillotomy, common bile duct stone removal, and balloon dilation.

The major complication of GI endoscopy is perforation through the structure being scoped. Many endoscopic procedures require short-acting IV sedation. All endoscopic procedures require informed, written consent. Specific endoscopy procedures are discussed in Table 38-11.

Capsule endoscopy is a noninvasive approach to visualize the GI tract (Fig. 38-11). Colon capsule endoscopy may be useful in monitoring inflammation in patients with inflammatory bowel disease. Its sensitivity in detecting small lesions, colonic polyps, and colorectal cancer is under investigation.[7]

Liver Biopsy

The purpose of a liver biopsy is to obtain hepatic tissue to use in establishing a diagnosis of cancer or assessing and staging fibrosis. It may also be useful for following the progress of liver disease, such as chronic hepatitis.

The two types of liver biopsy are open and closed. The *open method* involves making an incision and removing a wedge of tissue. It is done in the operating room with the patient under general anesthesia, often concurrently with another surgical procedure. The *closed,* or *needle, biopsy* is a percutaneous procedure. The site is infiltrated with a local anesthetic and a needle

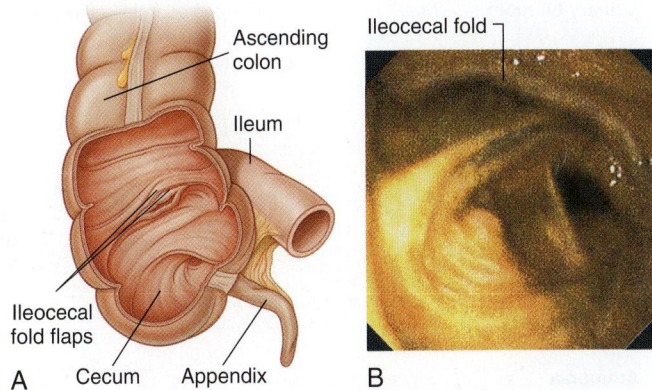

FIG. 38-10 A, Illustration showing the ileocecal junction and the ileocecal fold. **B,** Endoscopic image of the ileocecal fold. (From Drake RL, Vogl W, Mitchell AWM: *Gray's anatomy for students,* ed 3, Edinburgh, 2015, Churchill Livingstone.)

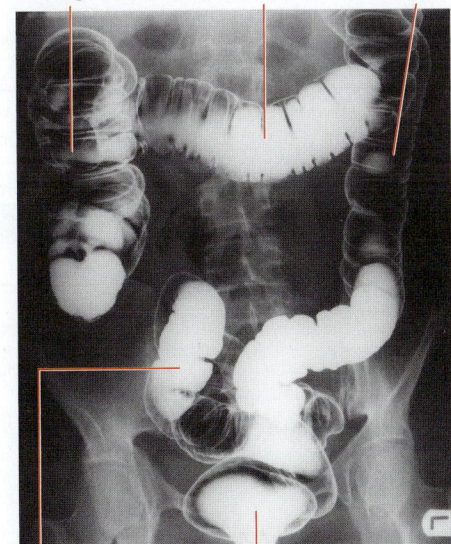

FIG. 38-9 Barium enema x-ray showing the large intestine. (From Drake RL, Vogl W, Mitchell AWM: *Gray's anatomy for students,* ed 3, Edinburgh, 2014, Churchill Livingstone.)

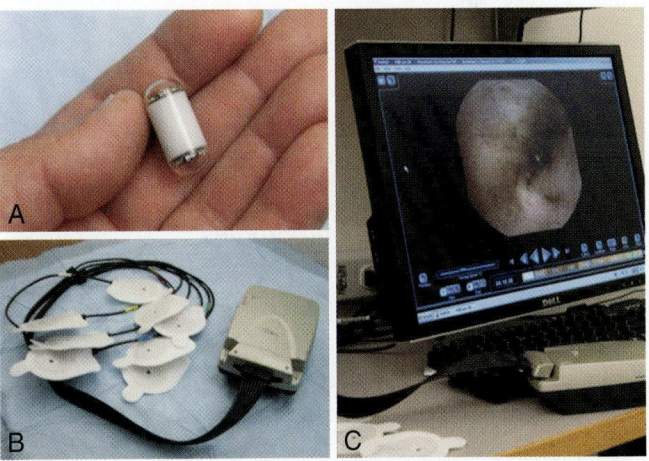

FIG. 38-11 Capsule endoscopy. **A,** The pill-sized video capsule has its own camera and light source. **B,** As it travels through the GI tract, it sends messages through sensing electrodes placed on the chest and abdomen to a data recorder worn on a waist belt. **C,** After the test, the images are viewed on a computer. (From Dye CE, Gaffney RR, Dykes TM, et al: Endoscopic and radiographic evaluation of the small bowel in 2012, *Am J Med* 125:1228e1, 2012.)

inserted between the sixth and seventh or eighth and ninth intercostal spaces on the right side. The patient lies supine with the right arm over the head. Instruct the patient to expire fully and not breathe when the needle is inserted.

Liver Function Studies

Liver function tests (LFTs) are laboratory (blood) studies that reflect hepatic disease. Table 38-12 describes the most common LFTs.

TABLE 38-12 Diagnostic Studies

Liver Function Tests

Test	Description and Purpose
Bile Formation and Excretion	
Serum bilirubin	Measurement of liver's ability to conjugate and excrete bilirubin, allowing differentiation between unconjugated (indirect) and conjugated (direct) bilirubin in plasma
• Total	Measurement of direct and indirect total bilirubin *Reference interval:* 0.2-1.2 mg/dL (3-21 μmol/L)
• Direct	Measurement of conjugated bilirubin. Elevated in obstructive jaundice *Reference interval:* 0.1-0.3 mg/dL (1.7-5.1 μmol/L)
• Indirect	Measurement of unconjugated bilirubin. Elevated in hepatocellular and hemolytic conditions *Reference interval:* 0.1-1.0 mg/dL (1.7-17 μmol/L)
Urinary bilirubin	Measurement of urinary excretion of conjugated bilirubin *Reference interval:* 0 or negative
Protein Metabolism	
Protein (serum)	Measurement of serum proteins made by liver • Albumin, *reference interval:* 3.5-5.0 g/dL (35-50 g/L) • Globulin, *reference interval:* 2.0-3.5 g/dL (20-35 g/L) • Total protein, *reference interval:* 6.4-8.3 g/dL (64-83 g/L) • A/G ratio, *reference interval:* 1.5:1-2.5:1
α-Fetoprotein	Indication of hepatocellular cancer *Reference interval:* <10 ng/mL (<10 mcg/L)
Ammonia	Conversion of ammonia to urea normally occurs in liver. Increase can result in hepatic encephalopathy secondary to liver cirrhosis. *Reference interval:* 15-45 mcg N/dL (11-32 μmol N/L)

Test	Description and Purpose
Hemostatic Function	
Prothrombin time (PT)	Determination of prothrombin activity *Reference interval:* 11-16 sec
International normalized ratio (INR)	Standardized system of reporting PT based on a reference calibration model and calculated by comparing the patient's PT with a control value *Reference interval:* In general, 2-3 is the desired therapeutic level with warfarin (Coumadin), depending on laboratory.
Vitamin K	Essential cofactor for many clotting factors *Reference interval:* 0.1-2.2 ng/mL (0.22-4.88 nmol/L)
Serum Enzymes	
Alkaline phosphatase (ALP)	Originates from bone and liver. Serum levels rise when excretion is impaired because of obstruction in biliary tract. *Reference interval:* 38-126 U/L (0.65-2.14 μkat/L), depending on method and age
Aspartate aminotransferase (AST)	Elevated in liver damage and inflammation *Reference interval:* 10-30 U/L (0.17-0.51 μkat/L)
Alanine aminotransferase (ALT)	Elevated in liver damage and inflammation *Reference interval:* 10-40 U/L (0.17-0.68 μkat/L)
γ-Glutamyl transpeptidase (GGT)	Present in biliary tract (not in skeletal or cardiac muscle). Increase in hepatitis and alcoholic liver disease. More sensitive for liver dysfunction than ALP *Reference interval:* 0-30 U/L (0-0.5 μkat/L)
Lipid Metabolism	
Cholesterol (serum)	Synthesis and excretion by liver. Increase in biliary obstruction. Decrease in cirrhosis and malnutrition *Reference interval:* <200 mg/dL (<5.2 mmol/L), varying with age

A/G, Albumin/globulin.

CASE STUDY

Objective Data: Diagnostic Studies

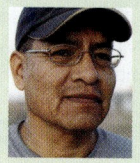

(©iStockphoto/Thinkstock)

The ED physician performs a rectal examination and finds a palpable mass. The following diagnostic tests are ordered:
• CBC
• Electrolytes
• Liver function tests
• Urinalysis
• CT scan of the abdomen
• Colonoscopy

The CBC reveals an Hgb of 6.8 g/dL and Hct of 20%. The WBC count is normal. The electrolytes, liver function tests, and urinalysis are within normal limits. The CT scan reveals pockets of gas and fluid in the ascending colon and two medium-sized tumors in the transverse colon.

Discussion Questions
1. Which diagnostic study results are of most concern to you?
2. With this information, what additional diagnostic studies would you anticipate being ordered for L.C.?
3. What are the interprofessional team's priorities for L.C. at this time? Case study continued in Chapter 42 on p. 971.

Answers available at *http://evolve.elsevier.com/Lewis/medsurg.*

BRIDGE TO NCLEX EXAMINATION

The number of the question corresponds to the same-numbered outcome at the beginning of the chapter.

1. A patient is admitted to the hospital with a diagnosis of diarrhea with dehydration. The nurse recognizes that increased peristalsis resulting in diarrhea can be related to
   a. sympathetic inhibition.
   b. mixing and propulsion.
   c. sympathetic stimulation.
   d. parasympathetic stimulation.

2. A patient has an elevated blood level of indirect (unconjugated) bilirubin. One cause of this finding is that
   a. the gallbladder is unable to contract to release stored bile.
   b. bilirubin is not being conjugated and excreted into the bile by the liver.
   c. the Kupffer cells in the liver are unable to remove bilirubin from the blood.
   d. there is an obstruction in the biliary tract preventing flow of bile into the small intestine.

3. As gastric contents move into the small intestine, the bowel is normally protected from the acidity of gastric contents by the
   a. inhibition of secretin release.
   b. release of bicarbonate by the pancreas.
   c. release of pancreatic digestive enzymes.
   d. release of gastrin by the duodenal mucosa.

4. A patient is jaundiced and her stools are clay colored (gray). This is *most* likely related to
   a. decreased bile flow into the intestine.
   b. increased production of urobilinogen.
   c. increased bile and bilirubin in the blood.
   d. increased production of cholecystokinin.

5. An 80-year-old man states that, although he adds a lot of salt to his food, it still does not have much taste. The nurse's response is based on the knowledge that the older adult
   a. should not experience changes in taste.
   b. has a loss of taste buds, especially for sweet and salt.
   c. has some loss of taste but no difficulty chewing food.
   d. loses the sense of taste because the ability to smell is decreased.

6. When the nurse is assessing the health perception–health maintenance pattern as related to GI function, an appropriate question to ask is
   a. "What is your usual bowel elimination pattern?"
   b. "What percentage of your income is spent on food?"
   c. "Have you traveled to a foreign country in the last year?"
   d. "Do you have diarrhea when you are under a lot of stress?"

7. During an examination of the abdomen the nurse should
   a. position the patient in the supine position with the bed flat and knees straight.
   b. listen for bowel sounds in the epigastrium and all four quadrants for 2 minutes.
   c. describe bowel sounds as absent if no sound is heard in a quadrant after 2 minutes.
   d. use the following order of techniques: inspection, palpation, percussion, auscultation.

8. Normal physical assessment findings of the GI system are (*select all that apply*)
   a. nonpalpable liver and spleen.
   b. borborygmi in upper right quadrant.
   c. tympany on percussion of the abdomen.
   d. liver edge 2 to 4 cm below the costal margin.
   e. finding of a firm, nodular edge on the rectal examination.

9. In preparing a patient for a colonoscopy, the nurse explains that
   a. a signed permit is not necessary.
   b. sedation will be used during the procedure.
   c. one cleansing enema is necessary for preparation.
   d. light meals should be eaten for 3 days before the procedure.

1. d, 2. b, 3. b, 4. a, 5. b, 6. c, 7. b, 8. a, c, 9. b

For rationales to these answers and even more NCLEX review questions, visit *http://evolve.elsevier.com/Lewis/medsurg*.

EVOLVE WEBSITE

http://evolve.elsevier.com/Lewis/medsurg
Review Questions (Online Only)
Key Points
Answer Keys for Questions
• Rationales for Bridge to NCLEX Examination Questions
• Answer Guidelines for Case Studies on pp. 839, 843, 845, and 852
Conceptual Care Map Creator
Audio Glossary
Supporting Media
• Animation
  • Rectal Examination
Content Updates

REFERENCES

1. Omari T, Kritas S, Fraser R, et al: Swallowing dysfunction in healthy older people using pharyngeal pressure-flow analysis, *Neurogastroenterol Motil* 26:59, 2014.
*2. Bharucha A, Pemberton J, Locke G: American Gastroenterological Association technical review on constipation, *J Gastro* 144:218, 2013.
3. Bailes B, Reeve K: Constipation in older adults, *Nurs Pract* 38:21, 2013.
4. McArthur T, Planz V, Fineberg N, et al: The common duct dilates after cholecystectomy and with advancing age: reality or myth? *J Ultrasound Med* 32:8, 2013.
5. Jarvis C: *Physical examination and health assessment*, ed 6, St Louis, 2012, Saunders.
6. National Digestive Diseases Information Clearinghouse: virtual colonoscopy. Retrieved from *www.niddk.nih.gov/health-information/health-topics/diagnostic-tests/virtual-colonoscopy/Pages/diagnostic-test.aspx*.
7. Tal A, Vermehren J, Albert J: Colon capsule endoscopy: current status and future directions, *World J Gastroenterol* 20:44, 2014.

*Evidence-based information for clinical practice.

39

Nutritional Problems

Rose Ann DiMaria-Ghalili

Let thy food be thy medicine and thy medicine be thy food.

Hippocrates

ⓔ http://evolve.elsevier.com/Lewis/medsurg/

LEARNING OUTCOMES

1. Relate the essential components of a well-balanced diet to their impact on health outcomes.
2. Describe the common etiologic factors, clinical manifestations, and management of malnutrition.
3. Describe the components of a nutritional assessment.
4. Explain the indications, complications, and nursing management principles related to the use of enteral nutrition.
5. Explain the indications, complications, and nursing management related to the use of parenteral nutrition.
6. Compare the etiologic factors, clinical manifestations, and nursing management of eating disorders.

KEY TERMS

This chapter focuses on problems related to nutrition. A review of normal nutrition provides a basis for evaluating nutritional status. Malnutrition and types of supplemental nutrition, including enteral and parenteral nutrition, are discussed.

NUTRITIONAL PROBLEMS

Nutrition is the sum of processes by which one takes in and uses nutrients.[1] Nutritional status can be viewed on a continuum from undernutrition to normal nutrition to overnutrition. Any alteration in the process of nutrient intake or use can cause nutritional problems. Nutritional problems occur in all ages, cultures, ethnic groups, socioeconomic classes, and across all educational levels.

Many factors influence nutritional status. A person establishes attitudes towards food and eating habits early. Dietary intake frequently reflects cultural or religious preferences. The financial status of a person or family influences the type and amount of nutritionally sound food that can be purchased.[2]

NORMAL NUTRITION

Nutrition is important for energy, growth, and maintaining and repairing body tissues. Optimal nutrition (in the absence of any underlying disease process) results from eating a balanced diet. The major components of the basic food groups are macronutrients (carbohydrates, fats, proteins), micronutrients (vitamins, minerals, electrolytes), and water. Optimal nutrition and daily physical activity are essential for a healthy lifestyle.

Body type, age, gender, medications, physical activity, and the presence or absence of disease influence a person's daily caloric requirements. Adjustments in caloric intake are necessary depending on changes in health status and daily activity level. There are several ways to estimate caloric need. The Mifflin–St. Jeor equation calculates daily adult energy (calorie) requirements based on resting metabolic rate[3] (Table 39-1). A simpler way to estimate daily calories needed is by kilocalories per kilogram (kcal/kg). An average adult should consume 20 to 25 cal/kg body weight to lose weight, 25 to 30 cal/kg to maintain body weight, and 30 to 35 cal/kg to gain weight.[4] Energy needs may be greater during illness.

Carbohydrates, the body's primary source of energy, yield approximately 4 cal/g. They are classified as either simple or complex, depending on the number of sugars they contain. Simple carbohydrates come in two forms: monosaccharides (e.g., glucose, fructose), which are found in fruits and honey, and disaccharides (e.g., sucrose, maltose, lactose), which are found in foods such as table sugar, malted cereal, and milk,

Reviewed by Karen Gilbert, RN, MSN, CNSC, CRNP, Nutrition Support Clinical Nurse Specialist, Thomas Jefferson University Hospital, Riverton, New Jersey; and Allison J. Terry, RN, PhD, Associate Professor of Nursing, Assistant Dean of Clinical Practice, School of Nursing, Auburn University Montgomery, Montgomery, Alabama.

TABLE 39-1 Estimating Daily Energy (Calorie) Requirements

Mifflin–St. Jeor Equation

For each gender, use the formula below to calculate energy expenditure:

Men: 10 × weight (kg) + 6.25 × height (cm) − 5 × age (yr) + 5
Women: 10 × weight (kg) + 6.25 × height (cm) − 5 × age (yr) − 161

To determine total daily calorie needs, the energy expenditure has to be multiplied by the appropriate activity factor, as follows:

1.200 = sedentary (little or no exercise)
1.375 = lightly active (light exercise/sports 1-3 days/wk)
1.550 = moderately active (moderate exercise/sports 3-5 days/wk)
1.725 = very active (hard exercise/sports 6-7 days a wk)
1.900 = extra active (very hard exercise/sports and physical job)

Example

Man: Weight 180 lb (82 kg), height 5 ft 10 in (178 cm), age 50, very active
Energy expenditure = 10 (82) + 6.25 (178) − 5 (50) + 5 × 1.725 = 2911

Woman: Weight 150 lb (68 kg), height 5 ft 6 in (168 cm), age 60, lightly active
Energy expenditure = 10 (68) + 6.25 (168) − 5 (60) −161 × 1.375 = 1745

TABLE 39-2 Nutritional Therapy
Foods High in Protein

Complete Proteins	Incomplete Proteins
• Milk and milk products (e.g., cheese) • Eggs • Fish • Meats • Poultry	• Grains (e.g., corn) • Legumes (e.g., navy beans, soybeans, peas) • Nuts (e.g., peanuts) • Seeds (e.g., sesame seeds, sunflower seeds)

respectively. Complex carbohydrates or polysaccharides include starches, such as cereal grains, potatoes, and legumes.

Carbohydrates are the chief protein-sparing ingredient in a nutritionally sound diet. The Dietary Reference Intake (DRI) recommendations are that 45% to 65% of total calories should come from carbohydrates.[4] A person should take approximately 14 g of dietary fiber per 1000 calories eaten per day from fruits, vegetables, and whole grains. This equates to roughly 28 to 30 g for a typical 2000-calorie diet. Individuals should choose food and beverages with little added sugar or caloric sweeteners.

Fats are a major source of energy for the body. One gram of fat yields 9 calories. Fats are stored in adipose tissue and the abdominal cavity. They act as carriers of essential fatty acids and fat-soluble vitamins. Fats provide a feeling of satiety after eating. Fat intake should be no more than 20% to 35% of total calories.[4]

Fats can be divided into (1) potentially harmful (saturated fat and *trans* fat) and (2) healthier dietary fat (monounsaturated and polyunsaturated fat). One type of polyunsaturated fat, omega-3 fatty acids, may be especially beneficial to your heart. Omega-3 fatty acids (found in some types of fatty fish) appear to decrease the risk of coronary artery disease.

Diets high in excess calories, usually in the form of fats, contribute to the development of obesity. Individuals should consume less than 10% of calories from saturated fatty acids (approximately 20 g of saturated fat per day in a 2000-calorie diet and choose foods with no *trans*-fatty acids.

Proteins are an essential component of a well-balanced diet. They are required for tissue growth, repair, and maintenance; body regulatory functions; and energy production. Ideally, 10% to 35% of daily caloric needs should come from protein.[4] The recommended daily protein intake is 0.8 to 1 g/kg of body weight. One gram of protein yields 4 calories. Amino acids are the fundamental units of protein structure. The 22 amino acids are classified as essential and nonessential. The body can synthesize nonessential amino acids if an adequate supply of protein is available. The body cannot synthesize the 9 essential amino acids. Their availability depends totally on dietary sources. We obtain them from both animal and plant sources. *Complete proteins* contain all the essential amino acids. Proteins that lack one or more of the essential amino acids are *incomplete proteins*. Table 39-2 lists foods high in protein.

Vitamins are organic compounds required in small amounts for normal metabolism. Vitamins function primarily in enzyme reactions that facilitate amino acid, fat, and carbohydrate metabolism. A diet consisting of foods from the five basic food groups is essential for obtaining the recommended dietary allowances of essential vitamins. Vitamins are divided into two categories: *water-soluble* vitamins (vitamin C and the B-complex vitamins) and *fat-soluble* vitamins (vitamins A, D, E, and K). Since the body stores excess fat-soluble vitamins, consuming too much can result in toxicity. Upper limits have been established for vitamins A, D, and E.

❤ HEALTHY PEOPLE
Health Impact of a Well-Balanced Diet

- Reduces incidence of anemia
- Maintains normal body weight and prevents obesity
- Maintains good bone health and reduces risk of osteoporosis
- Lowers the risk of developing elevated cholesterol and type 2 diabetes mellitus
- Decreases the risk of heart disease, hypertension, and certain types of cancers

Mineral salts (e.g., magnesium, iron, calcium) make up approximately 4% of the total body weight. Minerals are necessary for the body to build and repair tissues, regulate body fluids, and assist in various functions. Minerals required in amounts greater than 100 mg/day are called *major minerals*. Minerals present in minute amounts are *trace elements*. Table 39-3 lists the major minerals and trace elements. Some minerals are stored and can be toxic if taken in excess amounts. The amount of minerals needed daily varies greatly, from a few micrograms of trace minerals to 1 g or more of the major minerals, such as calcium, phosphorus, and sodium. A well-balanced diet usually meets the daily requirements of minerals. However, deficiency and excess states can occur.

VEGETARIAN DIET

The common element among all vegetarians is the exclusion of red meat from the diet. There are many types of vegetarians and no strict definition of the word "vegetarian." Many vegetarians are *vegans,* who are pure or total vegetarians and eat only plants, and *lacto-ovo-vegetarians,* who eat plants, dairy products, and eggs.

TABLE 39-3   Major Minerals and Trace Elements

Major Minerals	Trace Elements
• Calcium	• Chromium
• Chloride	• Copper
• Magnesium	• Fluoride
• Phosphorus	• Iodine
• Potassium	• Iron
• Sodium	• Manganese
• Sulfur	• Molybdenum
	• Selenium
	• Zinc

TABLE 39-4   Nutritional Therapy

Foods High in Iron

These foods provide 25%-39% of the Dietary Reference Intake (DRI) of iron.

Food	Selected Serving Size
Breads, Cereals, and Grain Products	
Farina, regular or quick cooked (enriched)	⅔ cup
Oatmeal, instant, fortified, prepared (enriched)	⅔ cup
Ready-to-eat cereals, fortified (enriched)	1 oz
Meat, Poultry, Fish, and Alternatives	
Beef liver, braised	3 oz
Pork liver, braised	3 oz
Chicken or turkey liver, braised	½ cup diced
Clams: steamed, boiled, or canned (drained)	3 oz
Oysters: baked, broiled, steamed, or canned (undrained)	3 oz
Soybeans, cooked	½ cup

Without a well-planned diet, vegetarians can have vitamin or protein deficiencies. Plant protein, although a lesser quality than animal protein, fulfills most of the protein requirements. Combinations of vegetable protein foods (e.g., cornmeal, kidney beans) can increase the nutritional value. Milk made from soybeans or almonds is an excellent protein source and should be calcium fortified. Other deficiencies that may be present in a vegan diet include calcium, zinc, and vitamins A and D.

The primary deficiency for a strict vegan is lack of cobalamin (vitamin B_{12}). Cobalamin is only obtained from animal protein, special supplements, or foods fortified with the vitamin. Vegans not using cobalamin supplements are susceptible to the development of megaloblastic anemia and the neurologic signs of cobalamin deficiency.

Strict vegetarians and lacto-ovo-vegetarians are at risk for iron deficiency. Table 39-4 lists examples of foods high in iron.

Culturally Competent Care: Nutrition

People have unique cultural heritages that may affect eating customs and nutritional status. Each culture has its own beliefs and behaviors related to food and the role that food plays in the etiology and treatment of disease. In addition, culture and religion can influence what food is considered edible, how it is prepared, when it is eaten, and how and who prepares it. For example, some religions, such as Judaism and Islam, have specific laws regarding food. Assess the extent to which Jewish or Muslim patients adhere to Kosher or Halal dietary practices to ensure that appropriate meals are served. The websites for

Kosher Quest (*www.kosherquest.org*) and the Islamic Food and Nutrition Council of America (*www.ifanca.org*) provide detailed information.

Assess the patient's diet history and implement necessary dietary changes. Avoid *cultural stereotyping* by not making assumptions or generalizations about diet based on a person's cultural background. Dietary habits differ considerably within and among ethnic groups. Acculturation (extent to which immigrants adopt attributes of a new culture) can also affect dietary practices.[5]

It is important to know whether the patient eats "traditional foods" associated with the culture. Assess the impact of eating traditional foods on health. For example, many traditional foods eaten by some African Americans tend to be high in fat, cholesterol, and sodium. Traditional foods eaten by some Asian Americans may be high in fiber and low in fat and cholesterol. The diet may be low in calcium because of limited dairy product intake.

Considering cultural beliefs is important when planning and monitoring acceptance of dietary changes. Culture can also influence perception of body weight and size. Ask the patient or family about how culture affects dietary choices and weight maintenance. For example, in some cultures obesity does not carry the stigma that it does in Western cultures. This may make teaching regarding weight reduction more challenging. A Jewish patient who eats only Kosher food may be comforted in knowing that an enteral nutrition formula is Kosher. Another example of culturally sensitive planning is adjusting meal plans for the Muslim patient observing Ramadan (the Islamic month of *fasting*, in which Muslims refrain from eating and drinking during daylight hours).

MALNUTRITION

Malnutrition is a deficit, excess, or imbalance of essential nutrients. It may occur with or without inflammation. Malnutrition affects body composition and functional status.[6] Other terms used to describe malnutrition include *undernutrition* and *overnutrition*.

Undernutrition describes a state of poor nourishment because of inadequate diet or diseases that interfere with normal appetite and assimilation of ingested food. *Overnutrition* refers to the ingestion of more food than is required for body needs, as in obesity.

Malnutrition is a problem in both developing and developed countries across the care continuum (community, hospital, long-term care). Prevalence rates for malnutrition in the hospital setting range from 30% to 50%.[7] The prevalence of malnutrition in older adults based on the Mini Nutritional Assessment (MNA) ranges from approximately 6% (community-dwelling older adults) to 50% (rehabilitation settings).[8]

Etiology of Malnutrition

Several terms describe the types and causes of adult malnutrition. Older terms still used in some settings include *primary* or *secondary protein-calorie malnutrition* (PCM), *marasmus,* and *kwashiorkor.* Marasmus and kwashiorkor describe forms of malnutrition seen in children in developing countries. These terms should not be used to describe malnutrition in adults.

The following etiology-based terms are the preferred ones to use in clinical practice settings, since they indicate the interaction and importance of inflammation on nutritional status.[6]

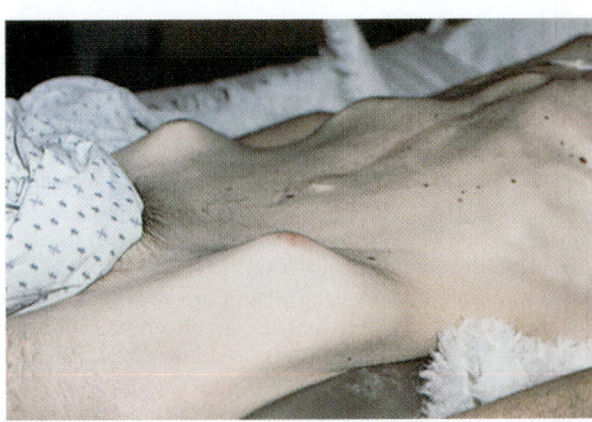

FIG. 39-1 Patient with malnutrition. (From Morgan SL, Weinsier RL: *Fundamentals of clinical nutrition*, ed 2, St Louis, 1998, Mosby.)

TABLE 39-5   Conditions That Increase the Risk for Malnutrition

- Dementia
- Depression
- Chronic alcoholism
- Excessive dieting to lose weight
- Swallowing disorders (e.g., head and neck cancer)
- Decreased mobility that limits access to food or its preparation
- Nutrient losses from malabsorption, dialysis, diarrhea, or wounds
- Drugs with antinutrient or catabolic properties such as corticosteroids and oral antibiotics
- Extreme need for nutrients because of hypermetabolism or stresses such as infection, burns, trauma, or fever
- No oral intake and/or receiving standard IV solutions (5% dextrose) for 10 days (adults) or for 5 days (older adults)

- *Starvation-related malnutrition,* or primary PCM, occurs when nutritional needs are not met (Fig. 39-1). In primary PCM, there is chronic starvation without inflammation (e.g., anorexia nervosa).
- *Chronic disease–related malnutrition,* or secondary PCM, is associated with conditions that have sustained mild to moderate inflammation. This occurs when dietary intake does not meet tissue needs, although it would under normal conditions. Examples of conditions associated with this type of malnutrition include organ failure, cancer, rheumatoid arthritis, obesity, and metabolic syndrome.
- *Acute disease– or injury-related malnutrition* is associated with acute disease or injury states with marked inflammatory response (e.g., major infection, burns, trauma, surgery).

Contributing Factors to Malnutrition

Many factors contribute to the development of malnutrition, including socioeconomic factors, physical illnesses, incomplete diets, and drug-nutrient interactions. Table 39-5 lists conditions that increase the risk for malnutrition.

Socioeconomic Factors. Persons or families with limited financial resources may have *food insecurity* (inadequate access).[2] Food insecurity is a major public health problem. It affects the overall quality of food that is available in both quantity and nutritional value. Those with food insecurity usually choose less expensive "filling" foods, which are more energy dense (high fat) and lack nutritional value. This type of diet increases the risk of nutrient deficiencies.

To help obtain food, people may use "safety net programs." These include food assistance programs; housing and energy subsidies; and in-kind contributions from relatives, friends, food pantries, or charitable organizations. Consult with social workers to help patients gain access to government and local programs such as Meals on Wheels that deliver nutritious meals to homebound people.

The "heat or eat" phenomenon is problematic, as those with limited economic resources struggle to pay household utility bills or put food on the table. Older adults on a fixed income have an added burden of deciding on whether to pay for medications or food. You and the dietitian can assist patients in making food choices that meet nutritional requirements while staying within their limited resources.

Physical Illnesses. Malnutrition is a common consequence of illness, surgery, injury, or hospitalization. The hospitalized patient, especially the older adult, is at risk of becoming malnourished. Prolonged illness, major surgery, sepsis, draining wounds, burns, hemorrhage, fractures, and immobilization can all contribute to malnutrition. Undernutrition can aggravate a pathologic condition. An existing deficiency state is likely to become more severe during illness.

Anorexia, nausea, vomiting, diarrhea, abdominal distention, and abdominal cramping may accompany GI disease. Any combination of these symptoms interferes with normal food consumption and metabolism. In addition, a patient may restrict intake to a few foods or fluids that may not be nutritionally sound out of fear of aggravating an existing GI problem.

Malabsorption syndrome is the impaired absorption of nutrients from the GI tract. Decreases in digestive enzymes or in bowel surface area can quickly lead to a deficiency state. Many drugs have undesirable GI side effects and alter normal digestive and absorptive processes. For example, antibiotics change the normal flora of the intestines, decreasing the body's ability to synthesize biotin.

Fever accompanies many illnesses, injuries, and infections, with a concomitant increase in the body's basal metabolic rate (BMR) and nitrogen loss. Each degree of temperature increase on the Fahrenheit scale raises the BMR by about 7%. Without an increase in caloric intake, the body uses protein stores to supply calories, and protein depletion develops. After the body temperature returns to normal, the rate of protein breakdown and resynthesis may be increased for several weeks.

Consider the nutritional requirements of a patient who is not overtly ill but is undergoing diagnostic studies. This patient may be nutritionally fit on entering the hospital but can become malnourished because of the dietary restrictions imposed by multiple diagnostic studies.

Incomplete Diets. Vitamin deficiencies are rare in most developed countries. When vitamin imbalances do occur, they usually involve several vitamins, rather than a single one. This may happen with persons with a pattern of alcohol and drug abuse, those who are chronically ill, and those who follow poor dietary practices. Persons who had surgery on the GI tract may be at risk for vitamin deficiencies. For example, resection of the terminal ileum poses a risk for deficiencies of fat-soluble vitamins. After a gastrectomy, patients require cobalamin supplementation because intrinsic factor (normally made in the stomach) is not available to bind with cobalamin so that this vitamin can be absorbed in the ileum. Followers of fad diets or poorly planned vegetarian diets are also at risk.

TABLE 39-6 Recommended Daily Vitamin Intake and Manifestations of Deficiencies

Vitamin	Dietary Reference Intake	Manifestations of Deficiencies
A (retinol)	Men: 900 mcg/retinol equivalents* Women: 700 mcg/ retinol equivalents	Dry, scaly skin. Increased susceptibility to infection, night blindness, anorexia, eye irritation, keratinization of respiratory and GI mucosa, bladder stones, anemia, retarded growth
D	Adults ages 19-70: 600 IU Adults age >70: 800 IU	Muscular weakness, excessive sweating, diarrhea and other GI disturbances, bone pain, active or healed rickets, osteomalacia
E	Adults: 15 mg	Neurologic deficits
K	Men: 120 mcg Women: 90 mcg	Defective blood coagulation
B₁ (thiamine)	Men: 1.2 mg Women: 1.1 mg	Anorexia, fatigue, nervous irritability, constipation, paresthesias, insomnia
B₆ (pyridoxine)	Men ages 19-50: 1.3-1.7 mg Men age >51: 1.7 mg Women ages 19-50: 1.3-1.5 mg Women age >51: 1.5 mg	Seizures, dermatitis, anemia, neuropathy with motor weakness, anorexia
B₁₂ (cobalamin)	Adults: 2.4 mcg	Megaloblastic anemia, anorexia, glossitis, sore mouth and tongue, pallor, neurologic problems such as depression and dizziness, weight loss, nausea, constipation
C	Men: 90 mg Women: 75 mg	Bleeding gums, loose teeth, easy bruising, poor wound healing, scurvy, dry, itchy skin
Folate (folic acid)	Adults: 400 mcg	Impaired cell division and protein synthesis, megaloblastic anemia, anorexia, fatigue, sore tongue, diarrhea, forgetfulness

*1 retinol equivalent = 10 international units vitamin A activity from β-carotene or 3.33 international units vitamin A activity from retinol.

Clinical manifestations of vitamin imbalances range from skin conditions to neurologic signs. The recommended dietary allowances for essential vitamins and manifestations of imbalances are presented in Table 39-6.

Drug-Nutrient Interactions. A *drug-nutrient interaction* occurs when a drug affects the use of nutrients in the body. Many drug and food or beverage interactions may occur. Potential adverse interactions include incompatibilities, altered drug effectiveness, and impaired nutritional status. For example, many drugs produce side effects such as changes in taste, appetite, and nausea. Grapefruit juice can increase the absorption of some drugs, enhancing their effect. Drug-nutrient interactions can also occur with the use of herbs and dietary supplements. Monitor and prevent these potential interactions for patients in the hospital and at home.

Pathophysiology of Starvation

Knowing the pathophysiology of the starvation process will help you understand the physiologic changes that occur in malnutrition. Initially, the body selectively uses carbohydrates (glycogen) rather than fat and protein to meet metabolic needs. These carbohydrate stores, found in the liver and muscles, are minimal. They may be totally depleted within 18 hours. During the early phase of starvation, protein is used only in its normal participation in cellular metabolism.

However, once carbohydrate stores are depleted, the body converts skeletal protein to glucose for energy. Alanine and glutamine are the first amino acids used in *gluconeogenesis*, the process by which the liver forms glucose. The resulting plasma glucose allows metabolic processes to continue. When these amino acids are used as energy sources, the person may be in negative nitrogen balance (nitrogen excretion exceeds nitrogen intake).

Within 5 to 9 days, the body mobilizes fat to supply much of the needed energy. In prolonged starvation, fat provides up to 97% of calories, conserving protein. Depletion of fat stores depends on the amount available. Fat stores are generally used up in 4 to 6 weeks. Once fat stores are gone, the body uses visceral and body proteins, including those in internal organs and plasma. They rapidly decrease because they are the only remaining body source of energy available.

If a malnourished patient has surgery, experiences physical trauma, or has an infection, the stress response is superimposed on the starvation response. The body uses protein stores for energy to meet the increased metabolic energy expenditure.

As protein depletion continues, liver function becomes impaired, and protein synthesis decreases. The decrease in protein synthesis lowers plasma oncotic pressure. A major function of plasma proteins, primarily albumin, is to maintain the osmotic pressure of blood. When the oncotic pressure decreases, body fluids shift from the vascular space into the interstitial compartment. Eventually albumin leaks into the interstitial space along with the fluid. Edema becomes clinically observable. Often edema in the patient's face and legs masks the underlying muscle wasting.

As the total blood volume decreases, the skin appears dry and wrinkled. As fluids shift to the interstitial space, ions also move. Sodium (a predominant extracellular ion) increases in amount within the cell. Potassium (a predominant intracellular ion) and magnesium shift to the extracellular space. The sodium-potassium exchange pump has high-energy needs, using 20% to 50% of all calories ingested. When the diet is extremely deficient in calories and essential proteins, the pump will fail. This leaves sodium inside the cell (along with water), and the cell expands.

The liver is the body organ that loses the most mass during protein deprivation. Fat gradually infiltrates the liver due to decreased synthesis of lipoproteins. If dietary protein and other necessary nutrients are not given, death will rapidly ensue.

Impact of Inflammation. Inflammation affects nutrient metabolism and is an important component of nutritional status. During the starvation process, there is a decreased BMR, sparing of skeletal muscle, and decreased protein breakdown. However, in inflammatory states, there are alterations in the expression of proinflammatory (e.g., interleukin-6) and antiinflammatory cytokines (e.g., interleukin-10). These cytokine changes result in increased protein and skeletal muscle breakdown, increased BMR, increased glucose turnover, decreased negative acute

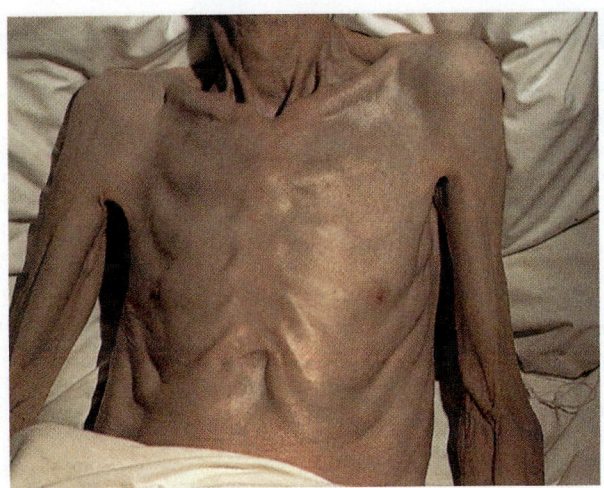

FIG. 39-2 Severe malnutrition that results in wasting and extensive loss of adipose tissue. (From Kamal A, Brockelhurst JC: *Color atlas of geriatric medicine,* ed 2, St Louis, 1991, Mosby.)

phase protein (albumin, prealbumin) production, and increased positive acute phase protein (e.g., C-reactive protein [CRP]) production.[6,7,9]

Clinical Manifestations

The clinical manifestations of malnutrition range from mild to emaciation and death (Fig. 39-2). The most obvious signs on physical examination are apparent in the skin (dry and scaly skin, brittle nails, rashes, hair loss), mouth (crusting and ulceration, changes in tongue), muscles (decreased mass and weakness), and CNS (mental changes such as confusion, irritability). The speed at which malnutrition develops depends on the quantity and quality of the protein intake, caloric value, illness, and the person's age.

The manifestations of malnutrition result from numerous interactions at the cellular level. As protein intake declines, the muscles (which are the largest store of protein in the body) become wasted and flabby. This leads to weakness and fatigability. Decreased protein is available for tissue repair, causing delayed wound healing. The person is more susceptible to infections. Both humoral and cell-mediated immunity are deficient. Leukocytes decrease in the peripheral blood. Impaired phagocytosis occurs because of the lack of energy needed to drive the process. Many malnourished persons are anemic, generally because of nutritional deficiencies in iron and folic acid (necessary building blocks for red blood cells [RBC]).

Diagnostic Studies

History and Physical Examination. The diagnosis of malnutrition is best determined by body composition, including a thorough history of weight loss, nutrient intake, and measures of functional status. A dietary history of foods eaten over the past week reveals a great deal about the patient's diet habits and knowledge of good nutrition. In addition to height, weight, and vital signs, assess and document the patient's physical state and each body system. Table 39-7 summarizes the assessment and findings of the patient with malnutrition.

Laboratory Studies. Serum albumin has a half-life of approximately 20 to 22 days. In the absence of marked fluid loss (e.g., from hemorrhage or burns), the serum albumin value lags behind actual protein changes by more than 2 weeks. This makes albumin a poor indicator of acute changes in nutritional status. Prealbumin, a protein synthesized by the liver, has a half-life of 2 days. It is a better indicator of recent or current nutritional status. However, the extent to which visceral proteins, including albumin and prealbumin, are true markers of malnutrition is questionable.

Albumin and prealbumin are *negative acute phase proteins.* This means that during an inflammatory response, the liver decreases synthesis of these proteins. So low or below normal levels of these negative acute phase proteins may indicate an inflammatory state rather than accurately depicting nutritional status. One way to determine if low albumin and prealbumin levels are due to malnutrition is to measure CRP, a *positive acute phase protein.* CRP is typically elevated during inflammation. A high CRP and low albumin or prealbumin suggests that inflammation is driving the change in albumin and prealbumin levels.[9]

Serum electrolyte levels reflect changes taking place between the intracellular and extracellular spaces. The serum potassium level is often elevated. The RBC count and hemoglobin level indicate the presence and degree of anemia. The total lymphocyte count decreases with malnutrition. Calculate it by multiplying the percent of lymphocytes times the total white blood cell (WBC) count. Liver enzyme levels may be elevated during malnutrition. Serum levels of both fat-soluble and water-soluble vitamins are usually decreased. Low serum levels of fat-soluble vitamins correlate with the clinical signs of *steatorrhea* (fatty stools).

Anthropometric Measurements. Anthropometric measurements are gross measures of fat and muscle contents. They consist of measures of skinfold thickness at various sites (indicators of subcutaneous fat stores) and midarm muscle circumference (indicator of protein stores). The sites most reflective of body fat are those over the biceps and triceps, below the scapula, above the iliac crest, and over the upper thigh. The measures obtained are compared with standards for healthy persons of the same age and gender.

Anthropometric measurements are most beneficial when done serially and by persons trained in anthropometry. They evaluate the long-term effects of malnutrition or responses to nutritional interventions. Both skinfold thickness and midarm circumference decrease in malnutrition. Shifts in hydration status influence these measurements. The exact relationship of the midarm circumference measure to morbidity and mortality remains to be established.

Waist circumference and hip-to-waist ratio are commonly used to reflect nutritional status. These measures are discussed in Chapter 40.

Functional Measurements. Functional assessment focuses on performance of activities of daily living (ADL) tools.[10] The most frequently used tools are the Katz Index and Lawton Scale.[11] Measuring muscle strength can assess physical functional status, an important outcome of nutrition status. Handgrip strength is measured with a hand dynamometer. Timed gait and chair stands are markers of lower extremity strength.[10]

❖ NURSING AND INTERPROFESSIONAL MANAGEMENT: MALNUTRITION

◆ Nursing Assessment

As a nurse, you are responsible for nutritional screening across care settings. Nutritional screening identifies those who are

TABLE 39-7   Nursing Assessment
Malnutrition

Subjective Data
Important Health Information

Past health history: Severe burns, major trauma, hemorrhage, draining wounds, bone fractures with prolonged immobility, chronic renal or liver disease, cancer, malabsorption syndromes, GI obstruction, infectious diseases, acute (e.g., trauma, sepsis) or chronic inflammatory condition (e.g., rheumatoid arthritis)

Medications: Corticosteroids, chemotherapy, diet pills, dietary supplements, herbs

Surgery or other treatments: Recent surgery, radiation

Functional Health Patterns

Health perception–health management: Alcohol or drug abuse. Malaise, apathy

Nutritional-metabolic: Increase or decrease in weight, weight problems. Increase or decrease in appetite, typical dietary intake, food preferences and aversions, food allergies or intolerance. Ill-fitting or absent dentures. Dry mouth, difficulty in chewing or swallowing, bloating, or gas. ↑ sensitivity to cold, delayed wound healing

Elimination: Constipation, diarrhea, nocturia, decreased urine output

Activity-exercise: Increase or decrease in activity patterns. Weakness, fatigue, decreased endurance

Cognitive-perceptual: Pain in mouth. Paresthesias, loss of position and vibratory sense

Role-relationship: Change in family (e.g., loss of a spouse), financial resources

Sexual-reproductive: Amenorrhea, impotence, decreased libido

Objective Data
General

Listless, cachectic, underweight for height

Eyes

Pale or red conjunctivae, gray keratinized epithelium on conjunctiva (Bitot's spots). Dryness and dull appearance of conjunctivae and cornea, soft cornea. Blood vessel growth in cornea. Redness and fissuring of eyelid corners

Integumentary

Dry, brittle, sparse hair with color changes and lack of luster, alopecia. Dry, scaly lips. Fever blisters, angular crusts and lesions at corners of mouth (cheilosis). Brittle, ridged nails. Decreased tone and elasticity of skin. Cool, rough, dry, scaly skin with brown-gray pigment changes. Reddened, scaly dermatitis, scrotal dermatitis. Slight cyanosis, peripheral edema

Respiratory

Decreased respiratory rate, ↓ vital capacity, crackles, weak cough

Cardiovascular

Increased or decreased heart rate, ↓ BP, dysrhythmias

Gastrointestinal

Swollen, smooth, raw, beefy red tongue (glossitis), hypertrophic or atrophic papillae. Dental cavities, absent or loose teeth, discolored tooth enamel. Spongy, pale, receded gums with a tendency to bleed easily, periodontal disease. Ulcerations, white patches or plaques. Redness, swelling of oral mucosa. Distended, tympanic abdomen. Ascites, hepatomegaly, decreased bowel sounds, steatorrhea

Neurologic

Decreased or loss of reflexes, tremor; irritability, confusion, syncope, peripheral neuropathy

Musculoskeletal

Decreased muscle mass with poor tone, "wasted" appearance, bowlegs, knock-knees, beaded ribs, chest deformity, prominent bony structures

Possible Diagnostic Findings

↓ Hemoglobin and hematocrit, ↓ MCV (mean corpuscular volume), MCH (mean corpuscular hemoglobin), or MCHC (mean corpuscular hemoglobin concentration). Altered serum electrolyte levels, especially hyperkalemia. ↓ BUN and creatinine, ↓ serum albumin, transferrin, and prealbumin. ↑ CRP, ↓ lymphocytes, ↑ liver enzymes, ↓ serum vitamin levels

---

malnourished or at risk for malnutrition. The Joint Commission requires nutritional screening for all patients within 24 hours of admission, with a detailed nutrition assessment if a patient is at risk. Following a standard approach to nutritional screening, using valid and reliable tools, will accurately identify those at risk. Many nutritional screening and assessment tools are available. Hospital-specific screening tools review common admission assessment data, including history of weight loss, intake before admission, use of nutritional support, chewing or swallowing issues, and skin breakdown.[12]

The Mini Nutritional Assessment (MNA) assesses nutrition status in older adults. In long-term care, the Minimum Data Set (MDS) form is used to obtain nutrition information.[13] In home care settings, the Outcome and Assessment Information Set (OASIS) is used to collect information on diet, oral intake, dental health, swallowing difficulties, and any need for meal assistance.[13]

If screening identifies a person at nutritional risk, perform a full nutritional assessment. A nutritional assessment is a comprehensive approach that includes medical, nutritional, and medication histories; physical examination; anthropometric measurements; and laboratory data (Table 39-8). Nutritional assessment provides the basis for nutritional intervention.

Across all care settings, be aware of the patient's nutritional status. Obtaining an accurate measure of body weight and height and recording this information are critical components of this assessment. When assessing weight, obtain a detailed weight history, noting weight loss. Ask whether the weight loss was intentional or unintentional and the period over which it took place. A loss of more than 5% of usual body weight over 6 months (whether intentional or unintentional) is a critical indicator for further assessment, especially in the older adult.[13] If an involuntary weight loss exceeds 10% of the usual weight, determine the reason. Unintentional weight loss is important to consider in the obese person. Latent malnutrition may be present despite excess body weight. Determine the patient's current weight in relation to ideal body weight.

When possible, measure the patient's actual height rather than using the patient's self-report. Alternatives to standing height (stature) measurements include arm demi-span and knee-height measurements. The *arm demi-span* is the distance from a point on the midline at the suprasternal notch to the

TABLE 39-8   Components of Nutritional Assessment

Anthropometric Measurements
- Height and weight
- Body mass index (BMI)
- Rate of weight change
- Amount of weight loss

Physical Examination
- Physical appearance
- Muscle mass and strength
- Dental and oral health

Health History
- Personal and family history
- Acute or chronic illnesses
- Current medications, herbs, supplements
- Cognitive status, depression

Diet History
- Chewing and swallowing ability
- Changes in appetite or taste
- Food and nutrient intake
- Availability of food

Laboratory Data
- Glucose
- Electrolytes
- Lipid profile
- Blood urea nitrogen (BUN)
- Albumin, prealbumin, CRP

Functional Status
- Ability to perform basic and instrumental activities of daily living
- Handgrip strength
- Performance tests (e.g., timed walk tests)

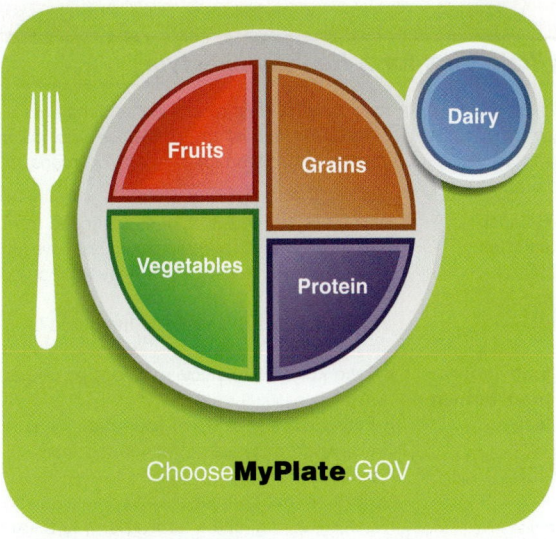

FIG. 39-3   MyPlate is the primary food group symbol that serves as a reminder to make healthy food choices and to build a healthy plate at mealtimes. It is a visual cue that identifies the five basic food groups from which to select healthy foods. The plate is divided into four slightly different-sized quadrants, with fruits and vegetables taking up half the space and grains and protein making up the other half. The vegetables and grains portions are the largest of the four. Next to the plate is a blue circle for dairy, which could be a glass of milk or a food such as cheese or yogurt. For more information, see *www.choosemyplate.gov*. (US Department of Agriculture, Center for Nutrition Policy and Promotion: Guidance on Use of USDA's MyPlate and Statements about Amounts of Food Groups Contributed by Foods on Food Product Labels, Washington, DC.)

web between the middle and ring fingers with the arm horizontally outstretched. For persons confined to bed, using a Luft ruler is an alternative to standing height.

Body mass index (BMI) is a measure of weight for height (see Fig. 40-2). A BMI of less than 18.5 kg/m^2 is considered underweight, normal weight is a BMI between 18.5 and 24.9 kg/m^2, and overweight is a BMI between 25 and 29.9 kg/m^2. A BMI of 30 kg/m^2 or greater is obese. BMIs outside the normal weight range are associated with increased morbidity and mortality.

Obtain a complete diet history from the patient or caregiver. Often the patient's nutritional state is not the reason for seeking medical care. However, it may be a contributing factor to the disease and have an impact on management and recovery.

◆ Nursing Diagnoses

Nursing diagnoses for the patient with malnutrition include, but are not limited to, the following:

- Imbalanced nutrition: less than body requirements *related to* decreased access, ingestion, digestion, or absorption of food or *related to* anorexia, dysphagia, or increased metabolic needs
- Feeding self-care deficit *related to* decreased strength and endurance, fatigue, and apathy
- Deficient fluid volume *related to* factors affecting access to or absorption of fluids
- Risk for impaired skin integrity *related to* poor nutritional state
- Noncompliance *related to* alteration in perception, lack of motivation, or incompatibility of regimen with lifestyle or resources

◆ Planning

The overall goals are that the patient with malnutrition will (1) achieve an appropriate weight, (2) consume a specified number of calories per day on an individualized diet; and (3) have no adverse consequences related to malnutrition or nutritional therapies.

◆ Nursing Implementation

◆ Health Promotion.   It is part of your role to teach and reinforce healthy eating habits. Use MyPlate, Dietary Guidelines for Americans 2015, and Nutrition Facts food labels to promote healthy nutrition. The MyPlate approach provides a visual guide for sensible meal planning. It helps Americans eat healthfully and make good food choices. MyPlate focuses on the proportions of five food groups (grains, protein, fruits, vegetables, and dairy) that you should eat at each meal (Fig. 39-3, Table 39-9). At the health professionals' link at *www.choosemyplate.gov*, you can download daily food plans, sample menus, and tips for how to be physically active. These materials are valuable to use in patient teaching. MyPlate materials for older adults are available at *www.nutrition.tufts.edu/research/myplate-older-adults*.

There are many resources to help people eat a nutritious diet and maintain a healthy weight. Electronic and print sources are available for determining nutritional information in commonly consumed foods. Many food products have Nutrition Facts labels (Fig. 39-4). Consumer and health professional education materials on Nutrition Facts labels are available on the U.S. Food and Drug Administration (FDA) website (*www.fda.gov/ Food/IngredientsPackagingLabeling/LabelingNutrition*).

Interactive web-based programs and mobile device applications are available to track physical activity, calories, nutrients, and foods eaten. Mobile device applications assist with making healthy eating choices easier. Some use built-in barcode scanners to scan foods quickly and give individual food items' nutrition facts. Users can compare items for their nutrition benefit and cost. Other applications give information on portion sizes and adjustments needed to reduce calories, sodium, or fat in the diet based on the user's height, weight, and activity level.

TABLE 39-9   Nutritional Therapy

MyPlate Tips for a Healthy Lifestyle

Making food choices for a healthy lifestyle can be as simple as using these 10 tips. Use the ideas in this list to (1) balance your calories, (2) choose foods to eat more often, and (3) cut back on foods to eat less often.

1. **Balance calories**	• Find out how many calories you need for a day as a first step in managing your weight. Go to www.choosemyplate.gov to find your calorie level. • Being physically active also helps you balance calories.
2. **Enjoy your food, but eat less**	• Take the time to enjoy your food as you eat it. • Eating too fast or when your attention is elsewhere may lead to eating too many calories. • Pay attention to hunger and fullness cues before, during, and after meals. Use them to recognize when to eat and when you have had enough.
3. **Avoid oversized portions**	• Use a smaller plate, bowl, and glass. • Portion out foods before you eat. • When eating out, choose a smaller size option, share a dish, or take home part of your meal.
4. **Foods to eat more often**	• Eat more vegetables, fruits, whole grains, and fat-free or 1% milk and dairy products. • These foods have the nutrients you need for health, including potassium, calcium, vitamin D, and fiber. • Make them the basis for meals and snacks.
5. **Make half your plate fruits and vegetables**	• Choose red, orange, and dark-green vegetables such as tomatoes, sweet potatoes, and broccoli, along with other vegetables, for your meals. • Add fruit to meals as part of main or side dishes or as dessert.
6. **Switch to fat-free or low-fat (1%) milk**	• They have the same amount of calcium and other essential nutrients as whole milk. • They have fewer calories and less saturated fat.
7. **Make half your grains whole grains**	• To eat more whole grains, substitute a whole-grain product for a refined product. • For example, eat whole-wheat bread instead of white bread, or brown rice instead of white rice.
8. **Foods to eat less often**	• Cut back on foods high in solid fats, added sugars, and salt. • They include cakes, cookies, ice cream, candies, sweetened drinks, pizza, and fatty meats like ribs, sausages, bacon, and hot dogs. • Use these foods as occasional treats, not everyday foods.
9. **Compare sodium in foods**	• Use the Nutrition Facts label (Fig. 39-4) to choose lower sodium versions of foods such as soup, bread, and frozen meals. • Select foods labeled "low sodium," "reduced sodium," or "no salt added."
10. **Drink water instead of sugary drinks**	• Cut calories by drinking water or unsweetened beverages. • Soda, energy drinks, and sports drinks are a major source of added sugar and calories in American diets.

Source: US Department of Agriculture Center for Nutrition Policy and Promotion: Nutrition education series, DG Tips Sheet No 1, June 2011. Retrieved from www.choosemyplate.gov and www.health.gov/dietaryguidelines.

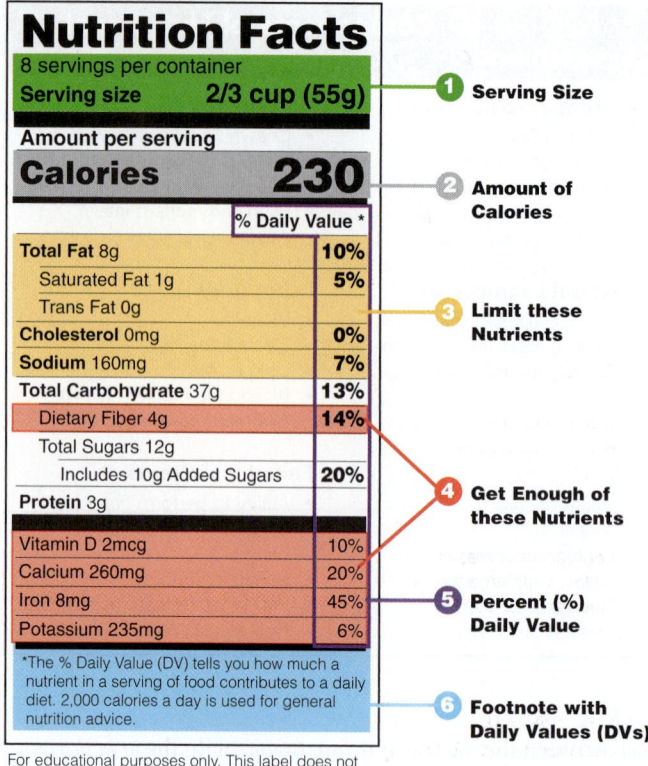

For educational purposes only. This label does not meet the labeling requirements described in 21 CFR 101.9.

FIG. 39-4   Sample of a Nutrition Facts label. (US Department of Health and Human Services, Nutrition Facts Label, Silver Spring, Md.)

◆ **Acute Care.** Collaborate with the HCP and dietitian to identify malnutrition and implement appropriate interventions to meet the patient's nutritional needs. Assess the patient's nutritional state during your assessment of the patient's other physical problems. Identify risk factors for malnutrition and why they exist. With increased stress, such as surgery, severe trauma, and sepsis, the patient needs more calories and protein. Wound healing requires increased protein synthesis. The patient undergoing major surgery who is malnourished or is at risk for malnutrition needs several weeks of increased protein and calorie intake preoperatively to promote healing postoperatively.

Teach the patient and caregiver the importance of good nutrition and the rationale for recording the daily weight, intake, and output. Measure weight and height on admission, and routinely assess and document the person's weight. Daily weights give an ongoing record of body weight gain or loss. Rapid gains and losses are usually the result of shifts in fluid balance. In conjunction with accurate recording of food and fluid intake, the body weight provides a clearer picture of the patient's fluid and nutritional state.

If the patient is able to take food by mouth, obtain a daily calorie count and diet diary to give an accurate record of food intake. You and the dietitian can assist the patient and family in selecting high-calorie and high-protein foods (unless medically contraindicated). Table 39-10 gives examples of high-calorie, high-protein foods. Offering foods preferred by the patient enhances intake. Encourage the family to bring the patient's favorite foods from home.

Make sure the environment is conducive to eating. Provide a quiet environment. Offer oral hygiene and provide hand

TABLE 39-10 Nutritional Therapy

High-Calorie, High-Protein Diet

Suggestions for high-calorie, high-protein foods include the following.

Breads and Cereals
- Hot cereals (oatmeal, cream of wheat) prepared with milk, added fat (butter or margarine), and sugar
- Potatoes prepared with added fat (butter and whole milk)
- Granola and other cereals with dried fruit
- Croissants, buttermilk biscuits, muffins, banana bread, zucchini bread

Vegetables
- Vegetables prepared with added fat (margarine, butter)
- Fried vegetables

Fruits
- Canned fruit in heavy syrup
- Dried fruit

Meat
- Fried meats
- Meats covered in cream sauces or gravy
- Casseroles

Milk and Milk Products
- Milkshakes
- Whole milk and milk products (yogurt, ice cream, cheese)
- Whipping cream or heavy cream
- Whole milk with added nutritional supplements

hygiene. Assist the patient to a comfortable position and place the bedside table at the appropriate height. Clear the bedside table of clutter. Place urinals, bedpans, and emesis basins out of sight. If needed, open cartons and packages. Protect mealtime from unnecessary interruptions by performing non-urgent care before or after mealtime.

The undernourished patient usually needs to have between-meal supplements. These may consist of items prepared in the dietary department or commercially prepared products. Eating these items provides extra calories, proteins, fluids, and nutrients. If the patient is unable to consume enough nutrition with a high-calorie, high-protein diet, consider adding oral liquid nutritional supplements.

Some patients may benefit from appetite stimulants such as megestrol acetate (Megace) or dronabinol (Marinol) to improve nutritional intake. If the patient is still unable to take in enough calories, enteral feedings may be considered (Fig. 39-5). Contraindications for enteral nutrition include GI obstruction, prolonged ileus, severe diarrhea or vomiting, and enterocutaneous fistula. If enteral feedings are not feasible, consider initiating parenteral nutrition (PN).

Ambulatory Care. Many patients are discharged on a therapeutic diet. Discharge preparation for both the patient and caregiver is essential. Teach them about the cause of the undernourished state and ways to avoid the problem in the future. They need to be aware that undernourishment, whatever the cause, can recur and that adhering to a diet high in protein and calories for a few weeks cannot fully restore a normal nutritional state. It may take many months to reach this goal.

Assess their ability to comply with the dietary instructions in light of past eating habits, religious and ethnic preferences, age, income, other resources, and state of health. Emphasize the need for continual follow-up care to accomplish and maintain rehabilitation. In the discharge planning, ensure proper follow-up such as visits by the home health nurse and outpatient dietitian referrals.

Determine the need for nutritious meals and snacks after discharge from the hospital. Access to a dietitian may be limited

and you may be the primary source of nutritional information. In your assessment, consider the availability and acceptability of community resources that provide meals such as Meals on Wheels, senior congregate feeding sites, and the Supplemental Nutrition Assistance Program (SNAP, formerly known as Food Stamps). Help the patient identify reliable Internet sources that provide evidence-based food and nutrition recommendations.

Keeping a diet diary for 3 days at a time is one way to analyze and reinforce healthful eating patterns. These records are also helpful to the interprofessional care team in the follow-up care. Encourage self-assessment of progress by having the patient weigh himself or herself once or twice a week and keep a weight record.

◆ Evaluation

The expected outcomes are that the patient who is malnourished will
- Achieve and maintain optimal body weight
- Consume a well-balanced diet
- Experience no adverse outcomes related to malnutrition
- Maintain optimal physical functioning

Gerontologic Considerations: Malnutrition

Nutrition affects quality of life, functional status, and health in older adults. They are particularly vulnerable to malnutrition across care settings. You play an important role in assessing the physiologic, functional, environmental, dietary, psychologic, and social factors related to nutritional risk in older adults.[10] Older hospitalized adults with malnutrition are more likely to have poor wound healing, pressure ulcers, infections, decreased muscle strength, postoperative complications, and increased morbidity and mortality risks. They are less able to regain body weight after periods of undernutrition due to illness or surgery.

Older adults may report little or no appetite, problems with eating or swallowing, inadequate servings of nutrients, and fewer than two meals per day. Limited incomes may cause them to restrict the number of meals or the dietary quality of meals eaten. Social isolation is a problem in older adults. Those who live alone may lose their desire to cook and report decreased appetite. Functional limitations may affect the ability to feed oneself, purchase food, or cook and prepare meals.[10] Some may lack transportation to buy food.

Chronic illnesses associated with aging can also affect nutritional status. For example, depression and dysphagia (secondary to stroke) can affect intake. Poor oral health from cavities, gum disease (gingivitis), and missing teeth, as well as *xerostomia* (dry mouth), can impair the older adult's ability to lubricate, masticate, and swallow food. Medications can cause dry mouth, alter the taste of food, or decrease appetite.

Physiologic changes associated with aging include a decrease in lean body mass and redistribution of fat around internal organs, which can decrease caloric requirements. Sarcopenia (loss of lean body mass with aging) affects muscle strength and function.[14] Older adults on bed rest or prolonged inactivity lose more lean body mass than younger adults.[15] Changes in odor and taste perception (from medications, nutrient deficiencies, or taste-bud atrophy) can alter nutritional status.

Daily requirements for healthy older adults for maintaining weight include 30 cal/kg of body weight and 0.8 to 1 g/kg of protein per day, with no more than 30% of calories from fat. Requirements may differ depending on the degree of malnutrition and physiologic stress. To prevent loss of muscle mass and

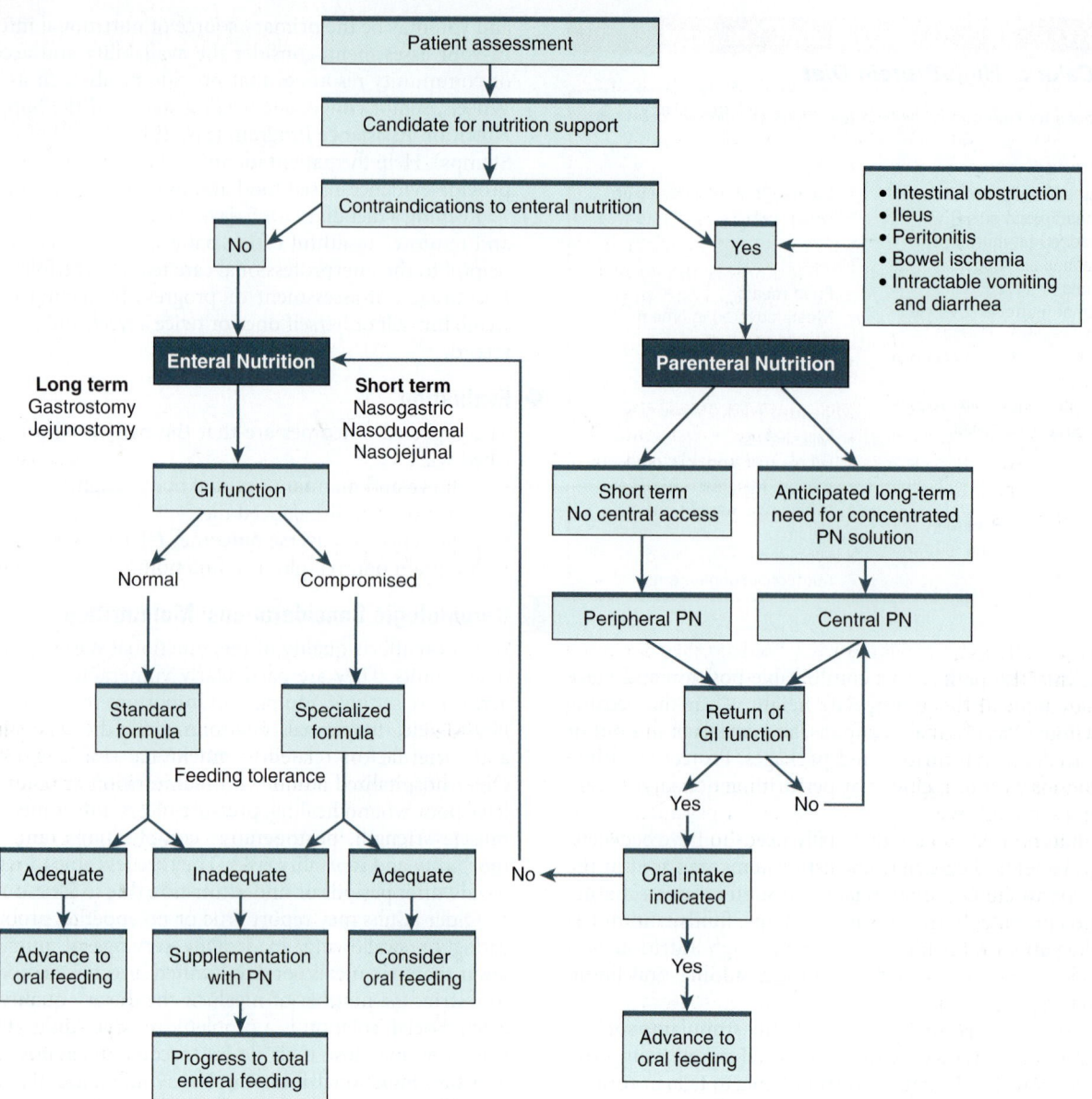

FIG. 39-5 Nutritional support algorithm. (Adapted from Ukleja A, Freeman KL, Gilbert K, and the ASPEN Board of Directors: Standards for nutrition support: adult hospitalized patients, *Nutr Clin Pract* 25:403, 2010.)

maintain function, older adults should consume a moderate amount of high-quality protein at each meal.[14] Daily vitamin D requirements are higher for older adults (Table 39-6).

Focus your initial care strategies on improving oral intake and providing a stimulating environment for meals. Special strategies, such as use of adaptive devices (e.g., such as large-handled eating utensils often are helpful in increasing the patient's dietary intake).

Oral liquid supplements have a role in improving the nutritional status of older adults. Do not use supplements as meal substitutes, rather use them as snacks between meals. In long-term care, using these beverages instead of water for oral medication administration increases caloric intake. Some older adults may require nutritional support therapies until their strength and general health improve. Before starting any nutritional support therapy (e.g., enteral or parenteral nutrition) for an older patient unable to give consent, review his or her

advance directives regarding the use of artificial nutrition and hydration.

Malnourished or nutritionally at-risk older adults are vulnerable when discharged from the hospital to the home. Older adults may not be able to shop for or prepare foods during the initial recovery period.[10] Consult with the social worker and dietitian to ensure the older adult has access to food on discharge. Home-delivered meals or senior congregate feeding programs are an appropriate referral. Many community nutritional programs are available to the older person to make mealtime a pleasant, social event. Improving the social setting of a meal frequently improves dietary intake. SNAP is another alternative that allows low-income households, regardless of age, to buy more food of a greater variety.

Older adults with dementia or a stroke present unique nursing challenges with regard to eating and feeding. (Dementia is discussed in Chapter 59; strokes are discussed in Chapter 57.)

SPECIALIZED NUTRITIONAL SUPPORT

If patients are unable to maintain or achieve adequate nutritional status, nutritional support may be necessary. For a decision-making plan related to nutritional support, see Fig. 39-5.

Some institutions have nutritional support teams composed of a physician, nurse, dietitian, and pharmacist. The team's function is to oversee the nutritional support of select inpatients and outpatients. The nutritional support nurse on that team is a key resource for issues regarding patients' nutrition and nutritional access.

Oral Feeding

Oral supplements are used as an adjunct to meals and fluid intake in the patient whose nutritional intake is deficient. They provide advanced nutrition and calories and are relatively inexpensive. These include milkshakes, puddings, or commercially available products (e.g., Carnation Instant Breakfast, Ensure, Boost).

Enteral Nutrition

Enteral nutrition (EN), also known as tube feeding, is nutrition (e.g., a nutritionally balanced liquefied food or formula) delivered into the GI tract distal to the oral cavity via a tube, catheter, or stoma. EN is used with the patient who has a functioning GI tract but is unable to take any or enough oral nourishment, or when it is unsafe to do so.

Indications for EN include persons with anorexia, orofacial fractures, head and neck cancer, neurologic or psychiatric conditions that prevent oral intake, extensive burns, or critical illness (especially if mechanical ventilation is required), and those receiving chemotherapy or radiation therapy. EN is easily administered, safer, more physiologically efficient, and less expensive than parenteral nutrition (PN).

There is a wide variety of enteral formulas. Their concentration, flavor, osmolality, and amounts of protein, sodium, and fat vary. There are special formulas for patients with diabetes and liver, kidney, or lung disease. Most are lactose free. Concentrations range from 1 to 2 cal/mL. Most standard formulas provide between 1 and 1.5 cal/mL. The more calorically dense the formula, the less water it contains. The number and size of particles in the formula determines its osmolality. The more hydrolyzed or broken down the nutrients, the greater the osmolality.

A formula with a high sodium content is contraindicated in the patient with cardiovascular problems, such as heart failure. Those with short bowel syndrome or ileocecal resection should not receive one with a high fat content because of impaired fat absorption. Patients receiving feedings with a protein content greater than 16% require supplemental fluids through the feeding tube or by mouth (if permitted) to avoid dehydration.

Common delivery options are continuous infusion or cyclic feedings by infusion pump, intermittent infusion by gravity, and intermittent bolus by syringe. Critically ill patients often receive EN by continuous infusion. Intermittent feeding may be preferred as the patient improves or is receiving EN at home.[16]

Nasally and orally placed tubes (orogastric, nasogastric [NG], nasoduodenal, or nasojejunal) are appropriate for short-term feeding (less than 4 weeks). Nasoduodenal and nasojejunal tubes are transpyloric tubes. They are used when pathophysiologic conditions such as risk of aspiration warrant feeding the patient below the pyloric sphincter. If feedings are necessary for an

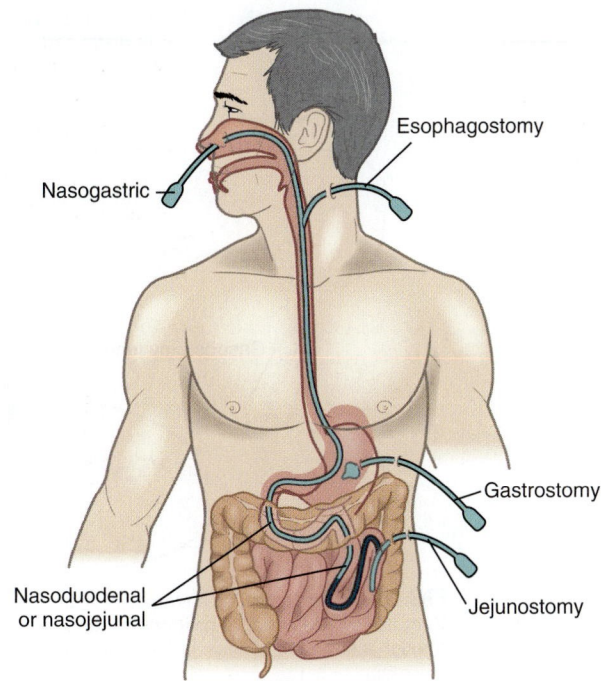

FIG. 39-6 Common enteral feeding tube placement locations.

extended time, tubes are placed in the stomach or small bowel by surgical, endoscopic, or fluoroscopic procedures. Fig. 39-6 shows the locations of commonly used enteral feeding tubes.

Orogastric, Nasogastric, and Nasointestinal Tubes. Polyurethane or silicone feeding tubes are long, small in diameter, soft, and flexible. This design decreases the risk of mucosal damage from prolonged placement. These tubes are radiopaque, making their position readily identified by x-ray. Placement into the small intestine decreases the chance of regurgitating gastric contents into the esophagus and subsequent aspiration.[16] However, the patient can still aspirate gastric secretions if the stomach is not emptying properly. A stylet is used for tube placement in a comatose patient because the ability to swallow is not essential during insertion. A complication that can result from using a stylet is increased risk for perforation.

Although smaller feeding tubes have many advantages over wider-lumen tubes, such as the standard decompression NG tube, there are some disadvantages. Because of the small diameter, these tubes clog easily when feedings are thick. They are more difficult to use for checking residual volumes. They are particularly prone to obstruction if you do not thoroughly crush and dissolve oral drugs before administration. Failure to flush the tubing before and after both drug administration and residual volume determination can result in tube clogging. Vomiting or coughing can dislodge the tubes. They can become knotted or kinked. Problems with a tube may necessitate removal and insertion of a new tube, which adds to cost and patient discomfort.

Gastrostomy and Jejunostomy Tubes. A gastrostomy tube may be used when a patient requires EN for an extended time (Fig. 39-6). Gastrostomy tubes can be placed surgically, radiologically, or endoscopically. The patient must have an intact, unobstructed GI tract. The esophageal lumen must be wide enough to pass the endoscope for percutaneous endoscopic gastrostomy (PEG) tube placement (Fig. 39-7). PEG tube and radiologically placed gastrostomy tube procedures have fewer risks than

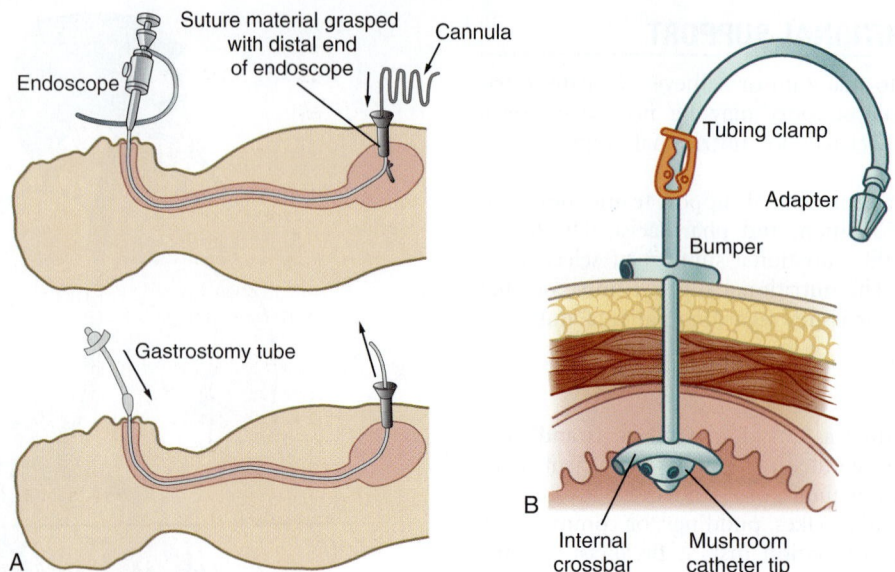

FIG. 39-7   Percutaneous endoscopic gastrostomy. **A,** Gastrostomy tube placement via percutaneous endoscopy. With use of endoscopy, a gastrostomy tube is inserted through the esophagus into the stomach and then pulled through a stab wound made in the abdominal wall. **B,** A retention disk and bumper secure the tube.

surgical placement. The procedure requires IV sedation and local anesthesia. IV antibiotics are given before the procedure.

For the patient with chronic reflux, feeding through a jejunostomy (J-tube) may be necessary to reduce the risk of aspiration. Jejunostomy tubes are placed either endoscopically or with open or laparoscopic surgery. Combination gastrojejunostomy (G-J) tubes allow for simultaneous gastric decompression and small bowel feeding. When a patient has a G-J tube, it is important to know which port is the gastric and which is the jejunal.

Enteral feedings can start within 24 to 48 hours after a surgically placed gastrostomy or jejunostomy tube without waiting for flatus or a bowel movement. Most PEG tube feeding can start within 2 hours of insertion, although the institution's policies may vary.[17] The feeding tube is either premarked or marked at the skin insertion site.

Tube Feedings and Safety.   You have a critical role in ensuring that tube feedings are administered safely. Aspiration and dislodged tubes are two important safety concerns. Nursing management of tube feedings is addressed in Table 39-11.

Accidental tube removal can result in delayed feedings and potential discomfort with tube replacement. The management of common problems in patients receiving tube feedings is presented in Table 39-12. A nursing care plan for the patient receiving enteral nutrition (eNCP 39-1) is available on the website for this chapter.

Specific care and teaching related to feeding tubes and enteral nutrition are summarized in the following section. Remember that is important to teach the patient and caregiver how to care for the feeding tube and properly administer enteral nutrition.

Patient Position.   Proper patient positioning decreases the risk of aspiration. To prevent aspiration, elevate the head of bed to a minimum of 30 degrees, but preferably 45 degrees. If the patient does not tolerate a backrest elevation, use a reverse Trendelenburg position to elevate the head of the bed, unless contraindicated. If you need to lower the head of the bed for a procedure, return the patient to an elevated position as soon as possible. Follow the institution's policy for suspending feeding

TABLE 39-11   **Nursing Management of Tube Feedings**
1. Check tube placement before feeding and before each drug administration.
2. Assess for bowel sounds before feeding.
3. Use liquid medications rather than pills.   • Dilute viscous liquid medications.   • Do not add medications to enteral feeding formula.
4. If using tablets, crush drugs to a fine powder and dissolve in water to avoid clogging feeding tubes.
5. Follow measures to decrease aspiration risk: • Keep head of bed elevated to 30- to 45-degree angle.   • Check for residual volumes per facility policy.
6. Assess regularly for complications (e.g., aspiration, diarrhea, abdominal distention, hyperglycemia, constipation, and fecal impaction).

while the patient is supine. If intermittent delivery is used, the head should remain elevated for 30 to 60 minutes after feeding.

Aspiration Risk.   Evaluate all enterally fed patients for risk of aspiration. Before starting tube feedings, ensure the tube is in the proper position. Maintain head-of-bed elevation as described above. Checking gastric residual volumes is important when giving feedings into the stomach. An increased residual volume increases the risk for aspiration of the formula into the lungs.[16]

Check gastric residual volumes every 4 hours during the first 48 hours for gastrically fed patients. After attaining the enteral feeding rate goal, decrease gastric residual monitoring to every 6 to 8 hours in non–critically ill patients or continue every 4 hours in critically ill patients. Promotility drugs such as erythromycin or metoclopramide improve gastric emptying and may reduce aspiration risk. Feeding tubes may need to be advanced below the ligament of Treitz (jejunostomy) if gastric residual volumes consistently measure more than 500 mL. Do not obtain residual volumes for EN delivered through a jejunostomy tube.

TABLE 39-12 Management of Tube Feeding Problems

Problems and Causes	Management
Vomiting	
Improper placement of tube	• Replace tube in proper position. • Check tube position before beginning feeding and every 4 hr if continuous feedings.
Delayed gastric emptying, increased residual volume	• If gastric residual volume is ≥250 mL after second gastric residual check, consider a promotility drug. • If gastric residual volume is >500 mL, hold feeding and reassess patient tolerance. • Advance tube below the ligament of Treitz if gastric residual volume consistently remains >500 mL.
Dehydration	
Excessive diarrhea, vomiting	• Decrease rate or change formula. • Check drugs that patient is receiving, especially antibiotics. • Avoid bacterial contamination of formula and equipment.
Poor fluid intake	• Increase intake and check amount and number of feedings. • Increase amount of fluid intake if appropriate.
High-protein formula	• Change formula to one with less protein.
Hyperosmotic diuresis	• Check blood glucose levels frequently. • Change formula to one with less glucose.
Diarrhea	
Feeding too fast	• Dilute or decrease rate of feeding. • Change to continuous drip feedings. • Discontinue excess water boluses.
Infection	• Obtain stool culture for fecal leukocyte determination, *C. difficile*, and/or toxin assay.
Medications	• Check for drugs that may cause diarrhea (e.g., sorbitol in liquid medications, antibiotics).
Low-fiber formula	• Change to formula with more fiber.
Tube moving distally	• Properly secure tube before beginning feeding. • Check placement before each feeding or at least every 24 hr if continuous feedings.

Contaminated formula	• Refrigerate unused formula and record date opened.
	• Discard outdated formula.
	• Discard formula left standing for longer than manufacturer's guidelines.
	  • 8 hr for ready-to-feed formulas (cans)
	  • 4 hr for reconstituted formula
	  • 24-48 hr for closed-system enteral formulas
	• Use closed system to prevent contamination.

Constipation	
Formula components	• Change formula to one with more fiber content. • Give as-needed laxative.
Poor fluid intake	• Increase fluid intake if not contraindicated. • Give total fluid intake of 30 mL/kg body weight.
Drugs	• Check for drugs that may be constipating.
Impaction	• Perform rectal examinations and manually remove feces if present.
Inactivity	• Encourage ambulation unless contraindicated. • Collaborate with physical therapy to promote activity.

TEAMWORK & COLLABORATION

Nasogastric and Gastric Tubes and Enteral Feedings

Role of Nursing Personnel

Registered Nurse (RN)
- Insert nasogastric (NG) tube for unstable patient.
- Irrigate NG or gastrostomy tube for unstable patient.
- Insert nasointestinal tube.
- Give bolus or continuous enteral feeding for unstable patient.
- Give medications through the NG or gastrostomy tube to unstable patient.
- Evaluate nutritional status of patient receiving enteral feedings.
- Monitor for complications related to tubes and enteral feedings.
- Develop plan for gastrostomy or jejunostomy tube care.
- Teach patient and caregiver about home enteral feeding and gastrostomy or jejunostomy tube care.
- Evaluate for therapeutic effect of NG tube connected to suction (e.g., decreased nausea or distention).

Licensed Practical/Vocational Nurse (LPN/LVN)
- Insert NG tube for stable patient.
- Irrigate NG and gastrostomy tubes.
- Give bolus or continuous enteral feeding for stable patient.
- Remove NG tube.
- Give medications through NG or gastrostomy tube to stable patient.
- Provide skin care around gastrostomy or jejunostomy tubes.

Unlicensed Assistive Personnel (UAP)
- Provide oral care to patient with NG, gastrostomy, or jejunostomy tube.
- Weigh patient who is receiving enteral feeding.
- Position and maintain patient receiving enteral feeding with the head of bed elevated.
- Notify RN or LPN about patient symptoms (e.g., nausea, diarrhea) that may indicate problems with enteral feedings.
- Alert RN or LPN about enteral feeding infusion pump alarms.
- Empty drainage devices and measure output.

Role of Other Team Members

Dietitian
- Evaluate nutritional status of patient receiving enteral feedings.
- Select appropriate enteral feeding formula.
- Monitor for and manage complications related to enteral feedings.
- Teach patient and caregiver about home enteral feedings.

Tube Position. Obtain x-ray confirmation of newly inserted nasal or orogastric tubes (small bore or large bore) to confirm proper position in the GI tract before administering feedings or medications. Smaller feeding tubes can pass directly into the bronchus on insertion without any obvious respiratory manifestations. Do not rely on the auscultation method to differentiate between gastric and respiratory or gastric and small bowel placement. Placing a tube under electromagnetic guidance is associated with reduced tube misplacement.[18] Capnography, a direct monitor of breath-to-breath CO_2 level, can determine tube placement in the respiratory tract. However, it still requires x-ray confirmation to verify location before feeding.[16]

Maintain proper placement of the tube after starting feedings. A small bowel tube may dislocate upward into the stomach or the tube's tip can dislocate upward into the esophagus. To determine if a feeding tube is still in the proper position, mark the exit site of the feeding tube at the time of the initial x-ray and check the tube external length at regular intervals.

Observe for negative pressure when attempting to withdraw fluid from the feeding tube.[17] You are more likely to feel negative pressure during attempts to aspirate fluid from a small bowel than from a gastric tube. Observe for unexpected changes in residual volume. An increase in gastric residual volume may indicate displacement of a small intestine tube into the stomach.[17] If you see a significant increase in the external length, use other bedside tests to help determine whether the tube has become dislocated. These measures include assessing aspirate color and pH. Because each of these measures has limitations, confirm placement with more than one test. Consider applying a nasal bridle in patients who attempt to pull out a tube or for whom taping the nose is difficult.

Site Care. Skin care around gastrostomy and jejunostomy tube sites is important because the action of digestive juices irritates the skin. Daily assess the skin around the feeding tube for signs of redness and maceration. Monitor bumper tension and routinely check for pressure injury.

 BECOMING A NURSE LEADER

Practicing Safe Delegation

Situation

It is the beginning of a hectic shift on a medical-surgical unit. You are a new RN and have a full patient care assignment. You observe Janet, a fellow RN, whispering something to Tony, the unlicensed assistive personnel (UAP). Immediately thereafter, you see Tony going into Mr. Jade's room with his enteral feeding and a medication cup. You carefully watch from the hallway as you see Tony inserting the medication and enteral feeding into Mr. Jade's NG tube. Although you realize that all of you are very busy, Tony is not qualified to administer medications or enteral feedings.

Points for Consideration

- The RN may delegate components of care but certain nursing functions cannot be delegated or assigned to UAP.[1]
- The RN uses critical thinking and professional judgment when following the Five Rights of Delegation (see Table 1-7) to be sure that the delegation or assignment is:
  - The right task
  - Under the right circumstances
  - To the right person
  - With the right directions and communication
  - Under the right supervision and evaluation
- RNs decide what patient care interventions are necessary and how, when, and by whom these interventions need to be provided.
- Effective delegation is based on one's state nurse practice act and an understanding of the concepts of responsibility, authority, and accountability.
- Each person involved in the delegation process is accountable for his or her own actions or inaction and is potentially liable if competent and safe care is not provided.[2]

Discussion Questions

1. Why is it inappropriate to delegate the administrations of medication or enteral feedings via an NG tube to Tony?
2. Who could be liable in this situation? Why?
3. What action should you take after you witnessed what Tony did?

References

1. American Nurses Association (ANA) and the National Council of State Boards of Nursing (NCSBN). Retrieved from *www.ncsbn.org/ Delegation_joint_statement_NCSBN-ANA.pdf*.
2. Anderson L: General guidelines to effective delegation in nursing. Retrieved from *www.nursetogether.com/guidelines-to-effective -nursing-delegation*.

To keep the skin clean and dry, initially rinse it with sterile water and dry it. Apply a dressing until the site is healed. After that, wash with mild soap and water. A protective ointment (zinc oxide, petroleum gauze) or a skin barrier (Karaya, Stoma-hesive) may be used on the skin around the tube. If the skin is irritated, consider using other types of drain or tube pouches. A wound, ostomy, and continence nurse (WOCN) can provide assistance if issues arise.

Tube Patency. All enteral feedings require routine flushing. Flush feedings tubes in adults with 30 mL of warm tap water every 4 hours during continuous feedings or before and after each intermittent feeding. Use sterile water in immunocom-promised and critically ill patients. Always flush tubes between each medication and after all medications are given. Try to only use liquid medications and do not mix medications.[17] Flush clogged tubes with warm water, using a back-and-forth motion.

Misconnection. An *enteral feeding misconnection* is an inad-vertent connection between an enteral feeding system and a non-enteral system such as an IV line, a peritoneal dialysis catheter, or a tracheostomy tube cuff. With an enteral feeding misconnection, nutritional formula intended for the GI tract is given IV or into the respiratory tract. Severe patient injury and death can result from tubing misconnection. Table 39-13 provides tips to decrease the risk of enteral feeding misconnections.

 Gerontologic Considerations: Enteral Nutrition

EN feeding strategies are used in the older patient to improve nutritional status. Because of physiologic changes associated with aging, the older adult is more vulnerable to complications associated with nutritional interventions, especially fluid and

TABLE 39-13 Decreasing Enteral Feeding Misconnections

The following are tips to help you decrease your risk of making an enteral tube feeding misconnection.

1. Teach visitors, LPN/LVNs, and UAP to notify nurse if an enteral feeding line becomes disconnected and not to reconnect any line.
2. Do not modify or adapt IV or feeding devices, because you may compromise the safety features incorporated into their design.
3. Do not use an IV pump or IV tubing to deliver an enteral feeding.
4. When making a reconnection or connecting any new device or infusion, trace lines back to their origins and ensure connections are secure.
5. When patient arrives on a new unit or setting or during shift handoff, recheck connections and trace all tubes.
6. Route tubes and catheters that have different purposes in unique and standardized directions (e.g., route IV lines toward the patient's head and enteral lines toward the feet).
7. Package together all parts needed for enteral feeding and reduce the availability of additional adapters and connectors. This will minimize the availability of dissimilar tubes or catheters that could be improperly connected.
8. Label or color-code feeding tubes and connectors. Teach staff about the labeling or color-coding process in the institution's enteral feeding system.
9. When there are several access points and/or several bags hanging, place proximal and distal labels on all tubings.
10. Check the patient's vital signs after making any connection.
11. Identify and confirm a solution's label, since a three-in-one parenteral nutrition solution can appear similar to an enteral nutrition formulation bag. Label the bags with large, bold statements such as "WARNING! For Enteral Use Only—NOT for IV Use."
12. Make all connections under proper lighting conditions.

TABLE 39-14 Common Indications for Parenteral Nutrition

- Chronic severe diarrhea and vomiting
- Complicated surgery or trauma
- GI obstruction
- Intractable diarrhea
- Severe anorexia nervosa
- Severe malabsorption
- Short bowel syndrome
- GI tract anomalies and fistulae

electrolyte imbalances. Complications such as diarrhea can leave the patient dehydrated. Decreased thirst perception or impaired cognitive function decreases the patient's ability to seek additional fluids.

With aging, there is an increased risk of glucose intolerance. As a result, the older patient may be more susceptible to hyperglycemia in response to the high carbohydrate load of some EN formulas. The older adult with compromised cardiovascular function (e.g., heart failure) will have a decreased ability to handle large volumes of formula. If this happens, the patient may need a more concentrated formula (2.0 cal/mL). The older adult has an increased risk for aspiration caused by gastroesophageal reflux disease (GERD), delayed gastric emptying, hiatal hernia, or diminished gag reflex. Physical mobility, fine motor movement, and visual system changes associated with aging may contribute to difficulties in managing EN in the home setting.

Parenteral Nutrition

Parenteral nutrition (PN) is the administration of nutrients directly into the bloodstream. PN is used when the GI tract cannot be used for the ingestion, digestion, and absorption of essential nutrients. Table 39-14 lists common indications for the use of PN. PN is a relatively safe method of providing complete nutritional support.

Composition. PN is customized to meet the needs of each patient. The composition is reformulated as the patient's condition changes. This requires you to collaborate with the interprofessional team in delivering PN to the patient.

Commercially prepared PN base solutions are available. These base solutions contain dextrose and protein in the form of amino acids. The pharmacy adds prescribed electrolytes (e.g., sodium, potassium, chloride, calcium, magnesium, and phosphate), vitamins, and trace elements (e.g., zinc, copper, chromium, and manganese) to meet the patient's needs. A three-in-one or total nutrient admixture containing an IV fat emulsion, dextrose, and amino acids is widely used. Premixed PN solutions are relatively new and require manipulation of the dextrose and amino acid chambers prior to use. Standard electrolytes are available in some premixed solutions; multivitamins are added prior to use.[19]

Calories. Calories in PN are supplied primarily by carbohydrates in the form of dextrose and by fat in the form of fat emulsion. The administration of 100 to 150 g of dextrose daily (1 g provides approximately 3.4 calories, as opposed to oral carbohydrates, which provide 4 calories) has a protein-sparing effect. Providing adequate nonprotein calories in the form of glucose and fat allows the use of amino acids for wound healing and not for energy. However, overfeeding can lead to metabolic complications. To minimize these problems, the recommended energy intake is 25 to 35 cal/kg/day in a nonobese patient.

Fat-emulsion solutions of 10%, 20%, and 30% are available. Fat emulsions provide approximately 1 cal/mL (10% solution) or 2 cal/mL (20% solution). Fat emulsions primarily contain soybean or safflower triglycerides with egg phospholipids added as an emulsifier. They provide a large number of calories in a relatively small amount of fluid. This is beneficial when the patient is at risk for fluid overload.

IV fat emulsions should provide up to 20% to 30% of total calories of PN. Most stable patients receive 1 g/kg/day. The maximum daily lipid dose is 2.5 g/kg/day. Critically ill patients may not tolerate this dose and may receive less than 1 g/kg/day. Serum triglyceride levels are done at the beginning of PN and then closely monitored. Give IV fat emulsions administered separately over 8 to 10 hours. The infusion rate should not exceed 0.11 g/kg/hr.[19]

Nausea, vomiting, and elevated temperature may occur, especially when lipids are infused quickly. Fat emulsions are contraindicated in the patient with a disturbance in fat metabolism such as hyperlipidemia. They are used cautiously in the patient at risk for fat embolism (e.g., fractured femur) and the patient with an allergy to eggs or soybeans.

Protein. The normal healthy person of average body size needs approximately 45 to 65 g of protein daily. Protein is provided at the rate of 1 to 1.5 g/kg/day depending on the patient's needs. In a nutritionally depleted patient who is under the stress of illness or surgery, protein requirements can exceed 150 g/day (1.5 to 2 g/kg/day) to ensure a positive nitrogen balance. Burn patients, who are often on PN, EN, and oral food, may need upward of 2 g/kg protein. Protein needs may be lower than 1 g/kg and restricted in those with end-stage renal disease who are not on dialysis.

Electrolytes. The exact amount of electrolytes needed depends on the patient's health problem and on serum electrolyte levels. Assess individual requirements daily at the beginning of therapy and then several times a week as the treatment progresses. The following are ranges for average daily electrolyte requirements for adult patients without renal or liver impairment:[19]

- Sodium: 1 to 2 mEq/kg
- Potassium: 1 to 2 mEq/kg
- Chloride: as needed to maintain acid-base balance
- Magnesium: 8 to 20 mEq
- Calcium: 10 to 15 mEq
- Phosphate: 20 to 40 mmol

Trace Elements and Vitamins. Zinc, copper, chromium, manganese, selenium, molybdenum, and iodine supplements may be added according to the patient's condition and needs. Monitor levels of these elements. The HCP may order additional amounts added to the PN. The daily addition of a multivitamin preparation to the PN generally meets the vitamin requirements.

Methods of Administration. PN is administered as central PN or peripheral parenteral nutrition (PPN). Central PN and PPN differ in nutrient content and tonicity, which is measured in milliosmoles (mOsm; the concentration of particles in a fluid).

Central Parenteral Nutrition. *Central PN* is indicated when long-term support is necessary or when the patient has high protein and caloric requirements. Central PN is administered through a central venous catheter or a peripherally inserted central catheter (PICC) whose tip lies in the superior vena cava (see Chapter 16). Central PN solutions are hypertonic, measuring at least 1600 mOsm/L. The high glucose content ranges from 20% to 50%. Central PN must be infused in a large central vein so that rapid dilution can occur. The use of a peripheral vein for hypertonic, central PN solutions would cause irritation and thrombophlebitis.

Peripheral Parenteral Nutrition. PPN is administered through a peripherally inserted catheter or vascular access device into a large vein. PPN is used when (1) nutritional support is needed for only a short time, (2) protein and caloric requirements are not high, (3) the risk of a central catheter is too great, or (4) PN is used to supplement inadequate oral intake.

Compared with central PN, PPN contains fewer nutrients. Although this makes PPN less hypertonic, it still has an osmolality of up to 800 mOsm/L. This increases the risk of phlebitis. Another potential complication is fluid overload. PPN requires large volumes of fluid, which many patients cannot tolerate.

❖ NURSING MANAGEMENT: PARENTERAL NUTRITION

Nursing management of patients receiving PN is presented in Table 39-15 and eNursing Care Plan 39-2 (available on the website for this chapter).

◆ Complications

Complications associated with PN are related either to the catheter or to the PN infusion itself (Table 39-16).

Refeeding syndrome is characterized by fluid retention and electrolyte imbalances (hypophosphatemia, hypokalemia,

---

TABLE 39-15 Management of Parenteral Nutrition Infusions

Preparation of Parenteral Nutrition (PN) Solutions

- All PN solutions must be prepared by a pharmacist or a trained technician using strict aseptic techniques under a laminar flow hood.
- Add nothing to PN solutions after they are prepared in the pharmacy. Danger of drug incompatibilities and contamination is high.
- Limit number of personnel involved in preparing and administering PN to reduce risk of infection.
- PN solutions are ordered daily to adjust to the patient's current needs.
- PN solution label indicates the nutrient content, all additives, time mixed, and date and time of expiration. In general, solutions are good for 24 hr and must be refrigerated until 30 min before use.

Maintaining PN Infusions

- Follow proper aseptic techniques to reduce infection risk.
- Use a 0.22-micron Millipore filter with parenteral solutions not containing fat emulsion and a 1.2-micron filter with solutions containing fat emulsion.
- Change filters and IV tubing q24 hr if giving PN with lipids and q72 hr for PN with amino acids and dextrose.
- Label tubing and filter with date and time they are put into use.
- If a multilumen catheter is present, use a dedicated line for PN.
- Control the infusion rate. Give PN using an infusion pump.
- Set an alarm to alert for tubing obstruction.
- Periodically check the volume infused because pump malfunctions can alter the rate.

Catheter Site Care

- Change dressings covering catheter site according to the institution's protocol.
- Carefully observe the catheter site for signs of inflammation and infection. Phlebitis can readily occur in the vein because of the hypertonic infusion, and the area can become infected.
- After the catheter is removed, change dressing daily and assess for wound healing.
- If an infection is suspected during a dressing change, send a culture specimen of the site and drainage and notify the HCP immediately.

Ensuring Patient Safety

- Before starting PN, check label and ingredients in solution to make sure they match what the HCP ordered.
- Examine the solution for leaks, color changes, particulate matter, clarity, and fat emulsions cracking (separating into layers). If present, promptly return it to the pharmacy for replacement.
- Discontinue a PN solution and replace it with a new solution if bag is not empty at the end of 24 hr. At room temperature, the solution (especially when containing fat emulsion) is a good medium for microorganism growth.
- If fat emulsions are infused separately from the PN solution, the preferred delivery method is a continuous low volume, such as 20% lipids delivered over 12 hr.
- Monitor for adverse reactions, including allergic manifestations, dyspnea, cyanosis, fever, flushing, phlebitis, chest and back pain, and pain at IV site.

Hypoglycemia

- If a PN formula bag should empty before the next solution is available, a 10% or 20% dextrose solution (based on the amount of dextrose in the central PN solution) or 5% dextrose solution (based on the amount of dextrose in the peripheral PN solution) can be given to prevent hypoglycemia.

Hyperglycemia

- Check glucose blood levels at bedside q4-6hr with glucose-testing meter.
- Maintain a glucose range of 110-150 mg/dL. Give sliding scale doses of insulin to keep the glucose level in normal range.
- Insulin can be added to the PN admixture, but the dosage will not be able to be changed for 24 hr.

Catheter-Related Infections

- Catheter-related infection and septicemia can occur. Local manifestations: erythema, tenderness, and exudate at the catheter insertion site. Systemic manifestations: fever, chills, nausea, vomiting, and malaise.
- If no other causes can be identified, a catheter-related infection is suspected. Blood cultures are drawn. A chest x-ray is taken to detect changes in pulmonary status.
- Immunosuppressed patients are at high-risk for infection. Note subtle signs in patients receiving chemotherapy, corticosteroids, or antibiotics, which can mask signs of infection.
- To reduce the risk of infection, catheters with antibiotic or antiseptic surfaces may be used. Follow institutional central line infection prevention measures (see Chapter 16).
- Antibiotics may be prescribed. A new central line may or may not be placed depending on the patient's condition.

Transitioning to Oral Nutrition

- Encourage oral nourishment and maintain a careful record of intake. A general rule is that 60% of caloric needs should be met orally before discontinuation of PN.
- Begin with clear liquids and advance as tolerated to a soft diet.
- Limit full liquids because of an increased risk of lactose deficiency resulting in nausea, diarrhea, and bloating.

Assessing Effectiveness

- Monitor initial vital signs q4-8hr in the patient receiving PN.
- Weigh patient daily as a measure of the patient's hydration status.
- Maintain an accurate intake and output record.
- Determine the cause of any weight changes (e.g., fluid gained from edema, actual increase or decrease in tissue weight).
- Assess blood levels of glucose, electrolytes, and urea nitrogen.
- Complete blood count and hepatic enzyme studies are followed a minimum of three times per week until stable and then weekly as the patient's condition warrants.

TABLE 39-16   Complications of Parenteral Nutrition

Metabolic Problems	Catheter-Related Problems
• Refeeding syndrome	• Air embolus
• Hyperglycemia, hypoglycemia	• Pneumothorax, hemothorax, and hydrothorax
• Altered renal function	• Hemorrhage
• Essential fatty acid deficiency	• Dislodgment
• Liver dysfunction	• Thrombosis of vein
• Hyperlipidemia	• Phlebitis
	• Catheter-related sepsis
	• Occlusion

hypomagnesemia). Hypophosphatemia is the hallmark of refeeding syndrome and is associated with serious outcomes, including cardiac dysrhythmias, respiratory arrest, and neurologic disturbances (e.g., paresthesias). Conditions that predispose patients to refeeding syndrome include long-standing malnutrition states, such as chronic alcoholism, vomiting and diarrhea, chemotherapy, and major surgery. Refeeding syndrome can occur any time a malnourished patient starts aggressive nutritional support.

◆ Home Nutritional Support

Home PN or EN is an accepted mode of nutritional therapy for the person who does not require hospitalization but needs continued nutritional support. Some patients successfully receive home therapy for many months, even years. It is important for you to teach the patient and caregiver about catheter or tube care, proper technique in mixing and handling of the solutions and tubing, and side effects and complications.

Home nutritional therapies are expensive. Specific criteria must be met for expenses to be reimbursed. The discharge planning team must be involved early to help plan for such issues. Home nutritional support may be a burden for the patient and caregivers and affect quality of life. Tell the family about support groups such as the Oley Foundation (www.oley.org) that provide peer support and advocacy.

EATING DISORDERS

Eating disorders are psychiatric conditions associated with physiologic alterations and risk for death. The manifestations of eating disorders vary across gender, age, socioeconomic status, and race and ethnicity.[20] Patients with eating disorders may be hospitalized for fluid and electrolyte alterations; cardiac dysrhythmias; and nutritional, endocrine, and metabolic disorders.[20]

Menstrual problems may be reported in women of childbearing age. A number of nutritional problems associated with these disorders require you to implement a nutritional plan of care.

The three most common types of eating disorders are anorexia nervosa, bulimia nervosa, and binge-eating disorder. *Binge-eating disorder* is less severe than bulimia nervosa and anorexia nervosa. Those with binge-eating disorder do not have a distorted body image and are often overweight or obese.

Eating disorders also occur in some who are health conscious. For example, men with *bigorexia* or muscle dysmorphia (an extreme concern with becoming more muscular) may use steroids or other drugs to increase muscle mass. They may also use supplements and protein shakes to increase their body weight and mass.

The *female athlete triad* is a syndrome in which eating disorders, amenorrhea, and osteoporosis are present.[21] The triad is seen in females participating in sports that emphasize leanness and low body weight.

Anorexia Nervosa

Anorexia nervosa is characterized by self-starvation, an intense fear of being fat, and disrupted self-image.[20] Anorexia nervosa clinically manifests as extreme thinness, unwillingness to maintain a healthy weight, intense fear of gaining weight, distorted body image, *lanugo* (soft, downy hair covering the body except the palms and soles), refusal to eat, continuous dieting, hair loss, sensitivity to cold, compulsive exercise, dry and yellowish skin, constipation, and absent or irregular menstruation in women of childbearing age.[20] Signs of malnutrition are noted during the physical examination.

Diagnostic studies often show osteopenia or osteoporosis, iron-deficiency anemia, an elevated blood urea nitrogen level from marked intravascular volume depletion, and abnormal renal function. A lack of dietary potassium and potassium loss in the urine lead to potassium deficiency. Manifestations of potassium deficiency include muscle weakness, cardiac dysrhythmias, and renal failure. Leukopenia, hypoglycemia, hyponatremia, hypomagnesemia, and hypophosphatemia may be present.

Interprofessional treatment must involve a combination of nutritional support and psychiatric care. Nutritional care

EVIDENCE-BASED PRACTICE
Translating Research Into Practice

What Is the Effect of Internet-Based Interventions on Eating Disorders?

Clinical Question

In persons with eating disorders (P), are Internet-based interventions (I) effective in the treatment of eating-disorder behaviors (O)?

Synthesis of Best Available Evidence

• Systematic review of randomized controlled trials (RCTs) and nonrandomized controlled studies
• 8 studies of persons (n = 609) diagnosed with bulimia nervosa, binge eating, or more than one eating disorder. Participants were mainly females (97%) with average age of 24 to 45 years old. In most studies, cognitive behavioral therapy (CBT) with a guided self-help component was the basis of the intervention. Planned contact between coach and participant averaged once per week. Outcomes were symptoms of eating disorder–behaviors (e.g., binge eating and purging), anxiety, depression, and quality of life.
• Significant reductions were noted in binge eating and purging. Improvements in depressive symptoms, anxiety, and quality of life were also reported.

Conclusions

• Internet-based interventions using CBT have positive effects on reducing bulimia nervosa and binge eating.

Implications for Nursing Practice

• Why is it important for health care providers to facilitate alternative methods of treatment delivery other than face-to-face?
• How would you help a patient with an eating disorder who resides in a rural area who regularly misses clinic appointments because of transportation problems?

Reference for Evidence

Dolemeyer R, Tietjen A, Kersting A, et al: Internet-based interventions for eating disorders in adults: a systematic review, *BMC Psychiatry* 13:207, 2013.

P, Patient population of interest; *I,* intervention or area of interest; *C,* comparison of interest or comparison group; *O,* outcomes of interest; *T,* timing (see p. 15).

focuses on reaching and maintaining a healthy weight, normal eating patterns, and perception of hunger and satiety. Hospitalization may be necessary if the patient has medical complications that cannot be managed in an outpatient therapy program. Nutritional repletion must be closely supervised to ensure consistent and ongoing weight gains. Refeeding syndrome is a rare but serious complication of refeeding programs. The use of EN or PN may be necessary.

Improved nutrition, however, is not a cure for anorexia nervosa. The underlying psychiatric problem must be addressed by identifying disturbed patterns of personal and family interactions, followed by personal and family counseling.

Bulimia Nervosa

Bulimia nervosa is a disorder characterized by episodes of binge eating, inappropriate behaviors to avoid weight gain (vomiting, laxative abuse, over exercise), and a persistent concern with body image.[20] Those with bulimia nervosa may have normal weight for height or their weight may fluctuate with bingeing and purging. They may abuse laxatives, diuretics, exercise, or diet drugs. They may have signs of frequent vomiting, such as macerated knuckles, swollen salivary glands, broken blood vessels in the eyes, and dental problems. The person with bulimia nervosa goes to great lengths to conceal abnormal eating habits. Abnormal laboratory parameters, including hypokalemia, metabolic alkalosis, and elevated serum amylase, may occur with frequent vomiting.[20]

The cause of bulimia remains unclear. It is thought to be similar to that of anorexia nervosa. Substance abuse, anxiety, affective disorders, and personality disturbances have been reported among persons with bulimia. Over time, problems associated with bulimia become increasingly hard to deal with effectively. A treatment combination of psychologic counseling (i.e., cognitive behavioral therapy) and nutritional counseling is essential.

Fluoxetine (Prozac) is the only FDA-approved antidepressant for treating bulimia nervosa. It may not be appropriate in all patients with bulimia. Education and emotional support for the patient and family are vital. Support groups such as the National Association of Anorexia Nervosa and Associated Disorders (ANAD) (www.anad.org) are helpful to those affected by these disorders.

CASE STUDY

Undernutrition

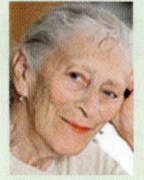

(©iStockphoto/ Thinkstock)

Patient Profile

M.S. is a 70-yr-old white woman who is 5 ft 4 in tall and weighs 100 lb. She was recently admitted to the inpatient medical unit.

Subjective Data

- Reports 30-lb weight loss in past 2 mo
- Recently had a thrombotic stroke with hemiparesis and dysphagia
- Has a history of rheumatoid arthritis
- Has had nothing by mouth for the past 24 hr and just started enteral nutrition via PEG tube
- Lives with her daughter, who is at her bedside

Objective Data

Physical Examination

- Has left-sided weakness
- BP is 150/90 mm Hg
- A PEG tube was recently placed

Laboratory Results

- Serum albumin 2.9 g/dL
- Prealbumin 11.0 mg/dL
- C-reactive protein 0.9 mg/L

Discussion Questions

1. What are M.S.'s risk factors for malnutrition?
2. What is her BMI?
3. What are contributing factors to her developing dysphagia and malnutrition?
4. What should you include in a successful weight gain program for M.S.?
5. For which possible complications of enteral nutrition could M.S. be at risk?
6. **Priority Decision:** What is the priority of the nursing care for M.S.?
7. **Priority Decision:** Based on the assessment data presented, write one or more appropriate nursing diagnoses. Are there any collaborative problems?
8. **Teamwork and Collaboration:** How would you use unlicensed assistive personnel (UAP) to care for M.S.?
9. **Evidence-Based Practice:** M.S.'s daughter tells you that her mother's abdomen appears bloated and she wonders if she should massage it.
10. **Teamwork and Collaboration:** What is the interprofessional team's top priority at this time for M.S.?
11. **Safety:** To ensure M.S.'s safety, what nursing interventions are necessary considering M.S.'s recent weight loss?

Answers available at *http://evolve.elsevier.com/Lewis/medsurg*.

BRIDGE TO NCLEX EXAMINATION

The number of the question corresponds to the same-numbered outcome at the beginning of the chapter.

1. The percentage of daily calories for a healthy person consists of
   a. 50% carbohydrates, 25% protein, 25% fat, and <10% of fat from saturated fatty acids.
   b. 65% carbohydrates, 25% protein, 25% fat, and >10% of fat from saturated fatty acids.
   c. 50% carbohydrates, 40% protein, 10% fat, and <10% of fat from saturated fatty acids.
   d. 40% carbohydrates, 30% protein, 30% fat, and >10% of fat from saturated fatty acids.

2. Place in order the substrates the body uses for energy during starvation, beginning with 1 for the first component and ending with 4 for the last component.
   ___ a. skeletal protein.
   ___ b. glycogen.
   ___ c. visceral protein.
   ___ d. fat stores.

3. A complete nutritional assessment including anthropometric measurements is *most* important for the patient who
   a. has a BMI of 25.5 kg/m².
   b. complains of frequent nocturia.
   c. reports a 5-year history of constipation.
   d. reports an unintentional weight loss of 10 lb in 2 months.

4. Which method is *best* to use when confirming initial placement of a blindly inserted small-bore NG feeding tube?
   a. x-ray.
   b. air insufflation.
   c. observing patient for coughing.
   d. pH measurement of gastric aspirate.

5. A patient is receiving peripheral parenteral nutrition. The parenteral nutrition solution is completed before the new solution arrives on the unit. The nurse gives
   a. 20% intralipids.
   b. 5% dextrose solution.
   c. 0.45% normal saline solution.
   d. 5% lactated Ringer's solution.

6. A patient with anorexia nervosa shows signs of malnutrition. During initial refeeding, the nurse carefully assesses the patient for
   a. hyperkalemia.
   b. hypoglycemia.
   c. hypercalcemia.
   d. hypophosphatemia.

1a, 2, b, a, d, 3, d, c, 5, b, a, 4, 5, b, d, 6, d

For rationales to these answers and even more NCLEX review questions, visit *http://evolve.elsevier.com/Lewis/medsurg*.

EVOLVE WEBSITE

http://evolve.elsevier.com/Lewis/medsurg
Review Questions (Online Only)
Key Points
Answer Keys for Questions
- Rationales for Bridge to NCLEX Examination Questions
- Answer Guidelines for Case Study on p. 872
Nursing Care Plans
- eNursing Care Plan 39-1: Patient Receiving Enteral Nutrition
- eNursing Care Plan 39-2: Patient Receiving Parenteral Nutrition
Conceptual Care Map Creator
Audio Glossary
Content Updates

REFERENCES

1. American Society for Parenteral and Enteral Nutrition (A.S.P.E.N.) Board of Directors and Clinical Practice Committee: Definition of terms, style, and conventions used in A.S.P.E.N. Retrieved from *www.nutritioncare.org/uploadedFiles/Home/Guidelines_and_Clinical _Practice/DefinitionsStyleConventions.pdf*.
2. United States Department of Agriculture: Scientific report of the 2015 Dietary Guidelines Advisory Committee. Retrieved from *www.health.gov/dietaryguidelines/2015-scientific-report*.
3. Mifflin MD, St. Jeor ST, Hill LA, et al: A new predictive equation for resting energy expenditure in healthy individuals, *Am J Clin Nutr* 51:242, 1990. (Classic)
4. U.S. Department of Health and Human Services and U.S. Department of Agriculture: *2015-2020 Dietary Guidelines for Americans,* ed 8. Retrieved from *www.health.gov/dietaryguidelines/2015-scientific-report*.
5. Colby SE: Multicultural food perspectives: Strategies for health care providers, *Am J Lifestyle Med* 7:13, 2013.
6. White JV, Guenter P, Jensen G, et al: Consensus statement of the Academy of Nutrition and Dietetics/American Society for Parenteral and Enteral Nutrition: Characteristics recommended for the identification and documentation of adult malnutrition, *J Acad Nutr Diet* 112:730, 2012. (Classic)
7. Jensen GL: Malnutrition and inflammation—"Burning Down the House" inflammation as an adaptive physiologic response versus self-destruction, *J Parenter Enteral Nut* 39:56, 2015.
8. Kaiser MJ, Bauer JM, Ramsch C, et al: Frequency of malnutrition in older adults: A multinational perspective using the Mini Nutritional Assessment, *J Am Geriatr Soc* 58:1734, 2010. (Classic)
9. Jensen GL, Hsiao PY, Wheeler D: Adult nutrition assessment tutorial, *J Parenter Enteral Nutr* 36:267, 2012. (Classic)
10. DiMaria-Ghalili RA: Integrating nutrition in the comprehensive geriatric assessment, *Nutr Clin Pract* 29:420, 2014.
11. Russell MK: Functional assessment of nutrition status, *Nutr Clin Pract* 30:211, 2015.
*12. Guenter P, DiMaria-Ghalli RA: Survey of nurses' nutrition screening and assessment practices in hospitalized patients, *MedSurg Matters* 22:10, 2013.
13. Bales C, Locher J, Slatzman E: *Handbook of clinical nutrition and aging,* New York, 2015, Springer Publishing.
14. Litchford MD: Counteracting the trajectory of frailty and sarcopenia in older adults, *Nutr Clin Pract* 29:428, 2014.
*15. Deutz NE, Pereira SL, Hays NP, et al: Effect of β-hydroxy-β-methylbutyrate (HMB) on lean body mass during 10 days of bed rest in older adults, *Clin Nutr* 32:704, 2013.
16. Enteral Nutrition Practice Recommendations Task Force: Enteral nutrition practice recommendations, *J Parenter Enteral Nutr* 33:122, 2009. (Classic)
17. Boullata J, Carney LN, Guenter P: *A.S.P.E.N. enteral nutrition handbook,* Silver Springs, Md, 2010, ASPEN. (Classic)
18. Taylor S, Allen K, McWilliam H, et al: Confirming nasogastric tube position with electromagnetic tracking versus pH or x-ray and tube radio-opacity, *Br J Nurs* 23:352, 2014.
19. Ayers P, Guenter P, Holcombe B, et al: *A.S.P.E.N. parenteral nutrition handbook,* ed 2, Silver Spring, Md, 2014, ASPEN.
20. Dickstein LP, Franco KN, Rome ES, et al: Recognizing, managing medical consequences of eating disorders in primary care, *Cleve Clin J Med* 81:255, 2014.
21. De Souza MJ, Nattiv A, Joy E, et al: 2014 Female Athlete Triad Coalition consensus statement on treatment and return to play of the female athlete triad, *Br J Sports Med* 48:289, 2014.

*Evidence-based information for clinical practice.

40

Obesity

Sharon L. Lewis

Our greatest weakness lies in giving up. The most certain way to succeed is always to try just one more time.

Thomas A. Edison

http://evolve.elsevier.com/Lewis/medsurg/

LEARNING OUTCOMES

1. Discuss the epidemiology and etiology of obesity.
2. Compare the classification systems for determining a person's body size.
3. Explain the health risks associated with obesity.
4. Discuss nutritional therapy and exercise plans for the obese patient.
5. Differentiate among the bariatric surgical procedures used to treat obesity.
6. Describe the nursing and interprofessional management related to conservative and surgical therapies for obesity.
7. Describe the etiology, clinical manifestations, and nursing and interprofessional management of metabolic syndrome.

KEY TERMS

bariatric surgery, p. 885
body mass index (BMI), p. 874
extreme obesity, p. 874

lipectomy, p. 890
metabolic syndrome, p. 890
obese, p. 874

obesity, p. 874
overweight, p. 874
waist-to-hip ratio (WHR), p. 875

OBESITY

Obesity is an excessively high amount of body fat or adipose tissue (Fig. 40-1). Obesity is a major health problem because it increases the risk of many other diseases such as diabetes and cancer.[1] Whether obesity should be labeled as a disease has been controversial. In 2008 the Obesity Society announced their support for calling obesity a disease. In 2013 the American Medical Association designated obesity as a disease.[2]

Attitudes about obesity can create biases and discrimination against people who are obese. Obesity must be viewed and treated as a chronic disease similar to other chronic diseases, such as diabetes and hypertension.

Classifications of Body Weight and Obesity

An important part of your patient assessment is to determine and classify a patient's body weight. A number of assessment methods are available, including body mass index (BMI), waist circumference, waist-to-hip ratio (WHR), and body shape. The most widely used and endorsed measures are BMI and waist circumference. These measures are cost-effective, reliable, and easily used in all practice settings.

Body Mass Index. The most common measure of obesity is the **body mass index (BMI)**. BMI is calculated by dividing a person's weight (in kilograms) by the square of the height in meters (Fig. 40-2). Individuals with a BMI less than 18.5 kg/m² are considered underweight, whereas those with a BMI between 18.5 and 24.9 kg/m² reflect a normal body weight. A BMI of 25 to 29.9 kg/m² is classified as being **overweight,** and those with values at 30 kg/m² or above are considered **obese**. The term **extreme obesity** (*morbid* or *severe obesity*) is used for those with a BMI greater than 40 kg/m².

Table 40-1 shows the classification of overweight and obesity by BMI. The BMI, which provides an overall assessment of fat mass, must be considered in relation to the patient's age, gender, and body build. For example, a body builder may have a BMI associated with obesity, but because of a high muscle mass, the BMI would not be an accurate assessment. In contrast, in individuals who have lost body mass (e.g., older adults), the BMI would underestimate the degree of obesity. For this reason, other measures must be combined with the BMI for an accurate evaluation of a person's weight.

Waist Circumference. *Waist circumference* is another way to assess and classify a person's weight (Table 40-1). The average waist size has increased by more than 1 inch (from 37.6 inches to 38.8 inches) in the past decade. Health risks increase if the waist circumference is greater than 40 inches in men and greater than 35 inches in women.[3] People who have visceral

Reviewed by Geraldine M. Budd, RN, PhD, FNP-BC, FAANP, Assistant Dean and Professor, Widener University School of Nursing, Harrisburg, Pennsylvania; Lorraine Nowakowski-Grier, MSN, APRN, BC, CDE, Diabetes Nurse Practitioner, Christiana Care Health Services, Nursing Development & Education, Newark, Delaware; Sarah Byram Poppe, MSN, ANP-BC, Nurse Practitioner, Gastroenterology Associates, Olympia, Washington; and Daryle Wane, PhD, ARNP, FNP-BC, RN to BSN Coordinator, Professor of Nursing, Department of Health Occupations, Pasco-Hernando Community College, New Port Richey, Florida.

TABLE 40-1	**Classification of Overweight and Obesity**			
			DISEASE RISK* RELATIVE TO NORMAL WEIGHT AND WAIST CIRCUMFERENCE	
	BMI (kg/m²)	Obesity Class	Men ≤40 in (102 cm) Women ≤35 in (89 cm)	Men >40 in (102 cm) Women >35 in (89 cm)
Underweight	<18.5	—	—	—
Normal†	18.5-24.9	—	—	—
Overweight	25.0-29.9	—	Increased	High
Obesity	30.0-34.9	Class I	High	Very high
	35.0-39.9	Class II	Very high	Very high
Extreme obesity	≥40.0	Class III	Extremely high	Extremely high

Source: National Heart, Lung, and Blood Institute: Classification of overweight and obesity by BMI, waist circumference, and associated disease risks. Retrieved from *www.nhlbi.nih.gov/health/public/heart/obesity/lose_wt/bmi_dis.htm.*
BMI, Body mass index.
*Disease risk for type 2 diabetes, hypertension, and cardiovascular disease.
†Increased waist circumference can also be a marker for increased risk in persons of normal weight.

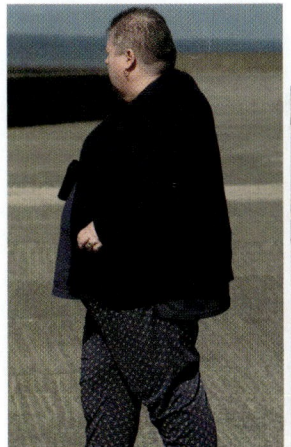
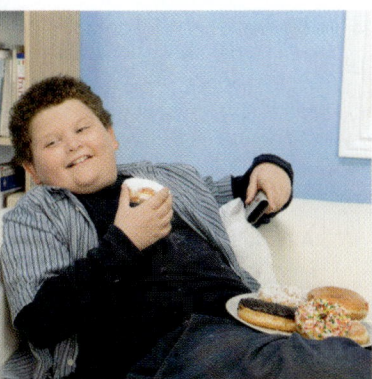

A B

FIG. 40-1 The obesity epidemic has taken its toll on both adults **(A)** and children **(B)** in the United States. (Source: *A,* Marilyn Barbone/Hemera/Thinkstock; *B,* IPGGutenbergUKLtd/iStock/Thinkstock.)

$$BMI\ (kg/m2) = \frac{Weight\ (pounds) \times 703}{Height\ (inches)^2}$$

FIG. 40-2 Body mass index (BMI) chart. Healthy weight: BMI 18 to 24.9 kg/m²; overweight: BMI 25 to 29.9 kg/m²; obesity: BMI 30 kg/m². BMI = weight (kg)/height (m²).

fat with truncal obesity are at an increased risk for cardiovascular disease and metabolic syndrome (discussed later in this chapter).

Waist-to-Hip Ratio. The waist-to-hip ratio (WHR) is another method used to assess obesity. This ratio is a method of describing the distribution of both subcutaneous and visceral adipose tissue. The ratio is calculated by using the waist measurement divided by the hip measurement. A WHR less than 0.8 is optimal. A WHR greater than 0.8 indicates more truncal fat, which puts the individual at a greater risk for health complications.

Body Shape. *Body shape* is another method of identifying those who are at a higher risk for health problems (Table 40-2). Individuals with fat located primarily in the abdominal area, an *apple-shaped body,* have *android obesity.* Those with fat distribution in the upper legs, a *pear-shaped body,* have *gynoid obesity.* Genetics has an important role in determining a person's body shape and weight.[4]

Epidemiology of Obesity

The magnitude of the obesity problem is a public health crisis. After decades of rising obesity rates among adults, the rate of increase is beginning to slow, but rates remain far too high. Currently, about 34% of adults in the United States are obese. Women have a slightly higher incidence of obesity than men.[1]

Significant geographic, racial and ethnic, and income disparities exist. Obesity rates are highest in the South (Fig. 40-3) and among African Americans, Hispanics, and lower-income, less-educated Americans[1] (Fig. 40-4).

Obesity in adulthood is often a problem that begins in childhood or adolescence. One in ten children becomes obese as early as age 2 to 5.[1] Reversing the childhood obesity crisis is key to addressing the overall obesity epidemic.

Etiology and Pathophysiology

Obesity is an increase in body weight beyond the body's physical requirements. This results in an abnormal increase and

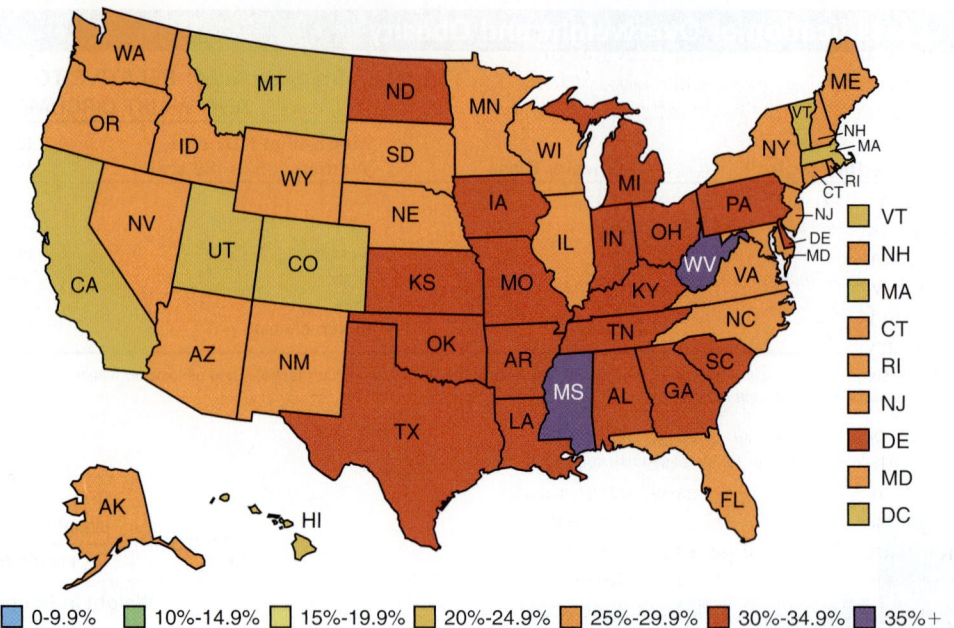

FIG. 40-3 Percent of obese adults (BMI >30 kg/m²) in the United States. Mississippi and West Virginia have the highest rates of obesity at 35.1%, whereas Colorado has the lowest rate at 21.3%. Twenty states have rates at or above 30%, 43 states have rates of at least 25%, and every state is above 20%. (Source: Trust for America's Health, Robert Wood Johnson Foundation. The state of obesity. 2014. Retrieved from *http://stateofobesity.org*.)

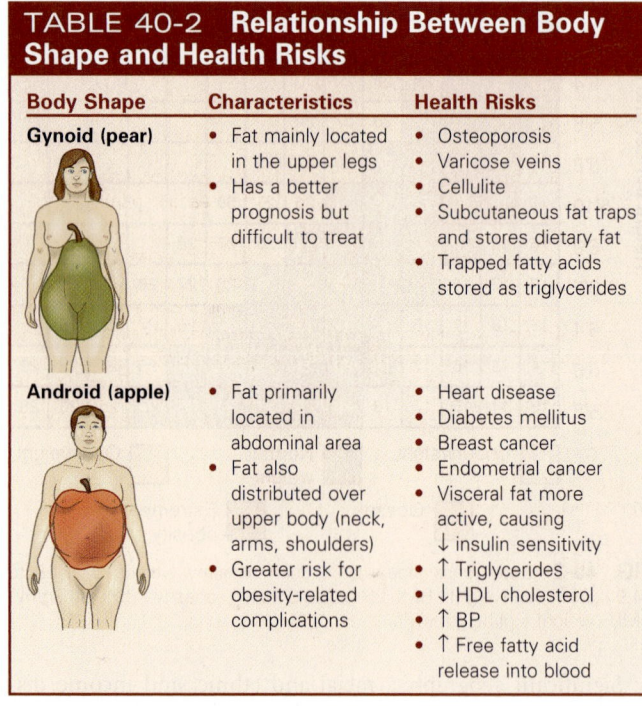

TABLE 40-2 Relationship Between Body Shape and Health Risks

Body Shape	Characteristics	Health Risks
Gynoid (pear)	• Fat mainly located in the upper legs • Has a better prognosis but difficult to treat	• Osteoporosis • Varicose veins • Cellulite • Subcutaneous fat traps and stores dietary fat • Trapped fatty acids stored as triglycerides
Android (apple)	• Fat primarily located in abdominal area • Fat also distributed over upper body (neck, arms, shoulders) • Greater risk for obesity-related complications	• Heart disease • Diabetes mellitus • Breast cancer • Endometrial cancer • Visceral fat more active, causing ↓ insulin sensitivity • ↑ Triglycerides • ↓ HDL cholesterol • ↑ BP • ↑ Free fatty acid release into blood

HDL, High-density lipoprotein.

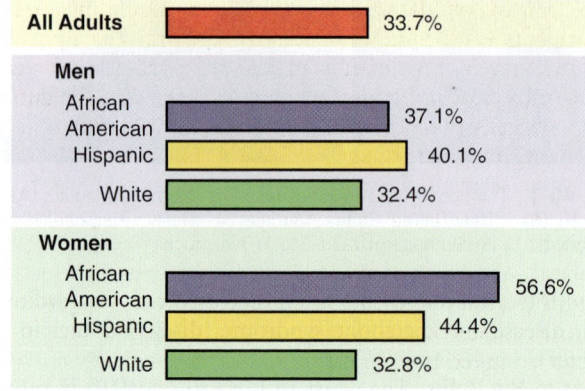

FIG. 40-4 Obesity affects some groups disproportionately. Among U.S. adults, African American and Hispanic populations have substantially higher rates of obesity than do white populations. This is true among both men and women. (Source: Trust for America's Health, Robert Wood Johnson Foundation. The state of obesity. 2014. Retrieved from *http://stateofobesity.org*.)

accumulation of fat cells. However, the processes leading to and sustaining the obese state are complex and still undergoing investigation.

In obesity, there is an increase in the number of adipocytes *(hyperplasia)* and an increase in their size *(hypertrophy)*. Adipocyte *hypertrophy* is a process by which adipocytes can increase their volume several thousand–fold to accommodate large increases in lipid storage. In addition, preadipocytes are trig-gered to become adipocytes once storage of existing fat cells is exceeded. This process occurs primarily in the visceral (intraabdominal) and subcutaneous tissues. The process of *hyperplasia* (increase in numbers) of adipocytes is greatest from infancy through adolescence.

The majority of obese persons have *primary obesity,* which is excess calorie intake over energy expenditure for the body's metabolic demands. Others have *secondary obesity,* which can result from various congenital anomalies, chromosomal anomalies, metabolic problems, central nervous system lesions and disorders, or drugs (e.g., corticosteroids, antipsychotics).

The cause of obesity involves significant genetic and biologic factors that are highly influenced by environmental and psychosocial factors. Each of these factors can and should be considered individually, but in reality they are interrelated.

Genetic Link

Studies of twins suggest the existence of genetic factors in obesity.[5] However, genetic factors do not totally account for the etiology of obesity. Estimates of obesity as an inherited problem are more than 50%.[6]

A number of genes have been identified as being linked to obesity. Genes actually may influence how calories are stored and energy released. "Energy-thrifty" genes, once protective against long periods when food was not available, are now maladaptive in societies in which food availability is no longer a primary issue. Genes may be responsible for why two individuals living in the same environment can vary considerably in body size.

A strong link exists between a gene known as *FTO* (fat mass and obesity-associated gene) and BMI. Variants of this gene may explain why some people become overweight, whereas others do not. People with two copies of a certain allele at the *FTO* gene weigh 7 to 8 lb more and have a greater risk of obesity than those who do not have the risk allele.[7] More research is needed to better understand the role of genes in obesity.

Physiologic Regulatory Mechanisms in Obesity. Research has focused on the physiologic regulatory processes that control eating behavior, energy metabolism, and body fat metabolism. Knowing how appetite is triggered and energy is expended provides important information for understanding obesity and specific targets for the development of drugs.

The hypothalamus, gut, and adipose tissue synthesize hormones and peptides that stimulate or inhibit the appetite (Fig. 40-5). The hypothalamus is a major site for regulating appetite. Neuropeptide Y, produced in the hypothalamus, is a powerful appetite stimulant. When it is imbalanced, it leads to overeating and obesity. Hormones and peptides produced in the gut and adipocyte cells affect the hypothalamus and have a critical role in appetite and energy balance (Table 40-3).

Leptin, secreted from adipocytes when they fill with fat, acts in the hypothalamus to suppress appetite and increase fat metabolism. A genetic deficiency of leptin causes extreme obesity. In obesity the level of leptin is actually increased, which has raised the question of whether obese people are insensitive to leptin. Possible causes of obesity include failure to produce enough leptin receptors or production of receptors that are faulty.

TABLE 40-3 Hormones and Peptides in Obesity

Where Produced	Normal Function	Alteration in Obesity
Anorexins (Suppress Appetite)		
Leptin		
Adipocytes	Suppresses appetite and hunger Regulates eating behavior	Obesity is associated with high levels. Leptin resistance develops; thus obese people may lose the effect of appetite suppression.
Insulin		
Pancreas	Decreases appetite	Increased insulin secretion which stimulates ↑ liver synthesis of triglycerides and ↓ HDL production
Peptide YY		
Colon	Inhibits appetite by slowing GI motility and gastric emptying	Circulating levels are decreased. ↓ Release after eating
Cholecystokinin		
Small intestine	Inhibits gastric emptying Sends satiety signals to hypothalamus	Unknown role
Glucagon-Like Peptide-1 (GLP-1)		
Small intestine	Stimulates insulin secretion from pancreas Increases satiety (mediated by GLP-1 receptors in brain)	Unknown role
Orexins (Stimulate Appetite)		
Neuropeptide Y		
Hypothalamus	Stimulates appetite	Imbalance causes increased appetite
Ghrelin		
Stomach (primarily)	Stimulates appetite ↑ After food deprivation ↓ In response to food in the stomach	Normal postprandial decline does not occur, which can lead to increased appetite and overeating

HDL, High-density lipoprotein.

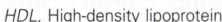

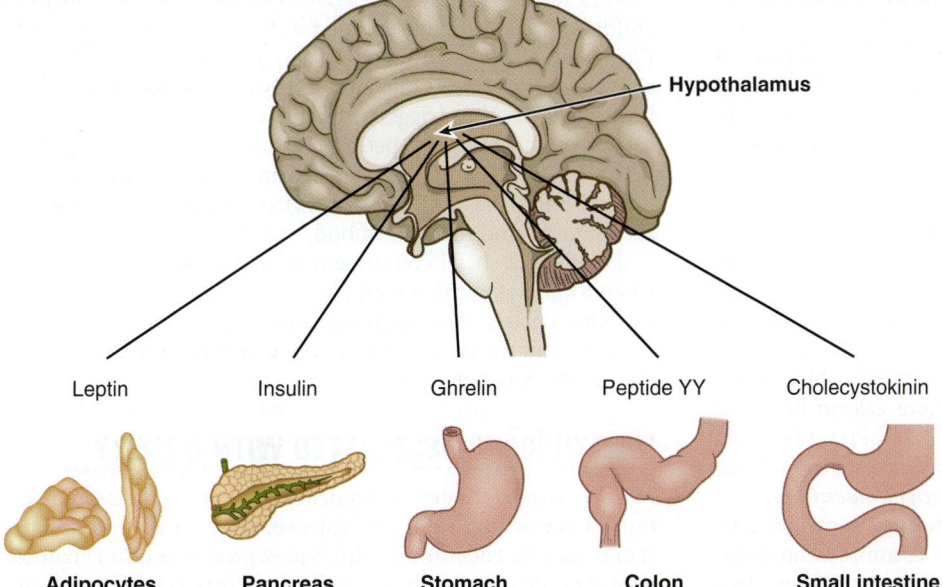

FIG. 40-5 Some of the common hormones and peptides that interact with the hypothalamus to control and influence eating patterns, metabolic activities, and digestion. Obesity disrupts this balance (Table 40-3).

TABLE 40-4   Portion Sizes: 30 Years Ago vs. Today

	30 Yr Ago	Today
Turkey sandwich	320 cal	820 cal
Bagel	3-in diameter, 140 cal	6-in diameter, 350 cal
Cheeseburger	333 cal	590 cal
Soda	6½ oz, 85 cal	20 oz, 250 cal

Ghrelin, a gut hormone, regulates appetite through inhibition of leptin. In a fasting state, ghrelin is increased. Ghrelin acts in the hypothalamus by working on the reward system that triggers overeating. Ghrelin is thought to play a part in compulsive eating. In gastric bypass surgery, ghrelin is decreased significantly, which helps suppress appetite.[8]

The two major consequences of obesity are due to the sheer increase in fat mass and production of adipokines produced by fat cells. Adipocytes produce at least 100 different proteins. These proteins, secreted as enzymes, adipokines, growth factors, and hormones, contribute to the development of insulin resistance and atherosclerosis.

An increased release of cytokines from fat cells may disrupt immune factors, thus predisposing the person to certain cancers. Because visceral fat accumulation is associated with more alterations of these adipokines, people with abdominal obesity have more complications of obesity.[8]

Environmental Factors. Environmental factors play an important role in obesity. In today's culture, people have greater access to food (particularly prepackaged and fast foods) and soft drinks, which have poor nutritional quality. In addition, eating outside of the home interferes with the ability to control the quality and quantity of food.

Portion size of meals has increased dramatically (Table 40-4). Underestimating portion sizes and therefore caloric intake is common. The Centers for Disease Control and Prevention has developed visual programs that demonstrate how portions have increased over time (*www.cdc.gov/healthyweight/index.html*).

Lack of physical exercise is another factor that contributes to weight gain and obesity. With increases in the use of technology, labor-saving devices, and cars, Americans are expending less energy in their everyday lives. Elimination of physical education programs in schools, along with increased time spent playing video games and watching TV, has contributed to the increase in sedentary habits.

Socioeconomic status is a known risk factor for obesity in a variety of ways.[1] People with low incomes may attempt to stretch their food dollars by purchasing less expensive foods that often have poor nutritional quality with a greater caloric content. For example, people with low incomes are more likely to purchase pasta, bread, and canned fruit packed with sugar rather than chicken and fresh fruits and vegetables. Low-income residents may also live in environments that do not accommodate outdoor activities (e.g., safe playgrounds, walking tracks, tennis, swimming pools).

Psychosocial Factors. People use food for many reasons besides its nutritional value. Associations with food begin in childhood, such as the use of food for comfort or rewards. Furthermore, when overeating develops at an early age and continues into adulthood, one's ability to sense fullness *(satiety)* is altered. Whether triggered by specific foods or by the wide variety of choices, some people consume more food than their bodies need. The lack of hunger that drives eating has been termed "mindless eating" and leads to consumption of unnecessary calories and increase in body weight.

Finally, the social component of eating begins early in life when food is associated with pleasure and fun at such events as birthday parties, Thanksgiving, and religious holidays. All of these factors must be included when considering the etiology and treatment of obesity.

HEALTH RISKS ASSOCIATED WITH OBESITY

Hippocrates wrote that "corpulence is not only a disease itself, but the harbinger of others," thus recognizing that obesity has major adverse effects on health. Many problems occur in obese people at higher rates than people of normal weight (Fig. 40-6).

Mortality rates rise as obesity increases, especially when obesity is associated with visceral fat.[9] In addition to these problems, obese patients have a reduced quality of life. Fortunately, most of these conditions can improve if an individual loses weight.

Cardiovascular Problems

Obesity is a significant risk factor for cardiovascular disease in both men and women. Android obesity is the best predictor of these risks and is linked with increased low-density lipoproteins (LDLs), high triglycerides, and decreased high-density lipoproteins (HDLs).[10] Obesity is also associated with hypertension, which can occur because of increased circulating blood volume, abnormal vasoconstriction, increased inflammation (damaging blood vessels), and increased risk of sleep apnea (raises BP). Altered lipid metabolism and hypertension can increase the long-term risk of heart disease and stroke. Excess body fat can also lead to chronic inflammation throughout the body, especially in blood vessels, thus increasing the risk of heart disease.

Diabetes Mellitus

Obesity is a major risk factor for the development of type 2 diabetes.[11] Hyperinsulinemia and insulin resistance, common features of type 2 diabetes, are also found in obesity. The term *diabesity* reflects the combined effects of diabetes and obesity.

Excess weight decreases the effectiveness of insulin. When insulin does not work effectively, too much glucose stays in the bloodstream. Thus more insulin is made to compensate. Pancreatic β cells (cells that make insulin) may get overworked and become worn out. Over time, the pancreas is no longer able to keep blood glucose in normal range. Adiponectin, a peptide that increases insulin sensitivity, is decreased in obese people.

Obesity complicates the management of type 2 diabetes by increasing insulin resistance and glucose intolerance. These factors make drug treatment for diabetes less effective.

Gastrointestinal and Liver Problems

Gastroesophageal reflux disease (GERD) and gallstones are more prevalent in obese people. Gallstones occur due to supersaturation of the bile with cholesterol. Nonalcoholic steatohepatitis (NASH) is a condition in which lipids are deposited in the liver, resulting in a fatty liver. NASH is associated with elevated hepatic glucose production. NASH can eventually progress to cirrhosis and can be fatal. Weight loss can improve NASH.

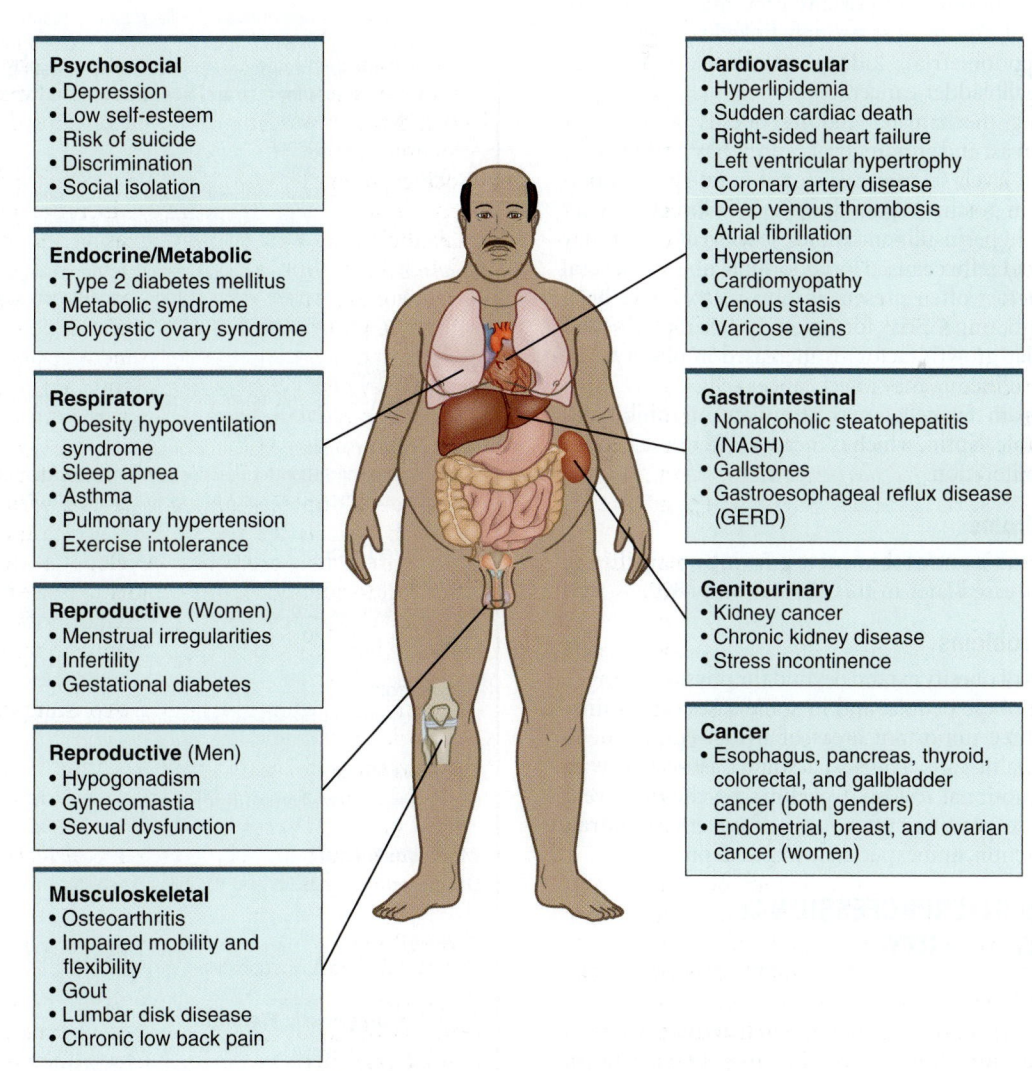

Psychosocial
• Depression
• Low self-esteem
• Risk of suicide
• Discrimination
• Social isolation

Endocrine/Metabolic
• Type 2 diabetes mellitus
• Metabolic syndrome
• Polycystic ovary syndrome

Respiratory
• Obesity hypoventilation syndrome
• Sleep apnea
• Asthma
• Pulmonary hypertension
• Exercise intolerance

Reproductive (Women)
• Menstrual irregularities
• Infertility
• Gestational diabetes

Reproductive (Men)
• Hypogonadism
• Gynecomastia
• Sexual dysfunction

Musculoskeletal
• Osteoarthritis
• Impaired mobility and flexibility
• Gout
• Lumbar disk disease
• Chronic low back pain

Cardiovascular
• Hyperlipidemia
• Sudden cardiac death
• Right-sided heart failure
• Left ventricular hypertrophy
• Coronary artery disease
• Deep venous thrombosis
• Atrial fibrillation
• Hypertension
• Cardiomyopathy
• Venous stasis
• Varicose veins

Gastrointestinal
• Nonalcoholic steatohepatitis (NASH)
• Gallstones
• Gastroesophageal reflux disease (GERD)

Genitourinary
• Kidney cancer
• Chronic kidney disease
• Stress incontinence

Cancer
• Esophagus, pancreas, thyroid, colorectal, and gallbladder cancer (both genders)
• Endometrial, breast, and ovarian cancer (women)

FIG. 40-6 Health risks associated with obesity.

Respiratory and Sleep Problems

The increased fat mass associated with obesity may lead to sleep apnea and obesity hypoventilation syndrome. The increased distribution of fat around the diaphragm causes a reduced chest wall compliance, increased work of breathing, and decreased total lung capacity. Sleep apnea results from increased fat around the neck, leading to snoring and hypoventilation while sleeping. Weight loss can improve lung function.

Poor sleep and sleep deprivation may increase appetite. Sleep deprivation has been associated with obesity. Building up a sleep debt over a matter of days can impair metabolism and disrupt hormone levels. The level of leptin falls in people who are sleep deprived, thus promoting appetite.

Musculoskeletal Problems

Obesity is associated with an increased incidence of osteoarthritis because of the stress put on weight-bearing joints, especially the knees and hips. Increased body fat also triggers inflammatory mediators and contributes to deterioration of cartilage. Hyperuricemia and gout are often found in people who are obese and in those who have metabolic syndrome (discussed later in this chapter).

Cancer

Obesity is one of the most important preventable causes of cancer. The types of cancer most strongly linked to excess body fat are breast, endometrial, kidney, colorectal, pancreatic, esophageal, and gallbladder cancer.[12]

The underlying mechanisms linking obesity and cancer remain unclear. Breast and endometrial cancer may be due to the increased estrogen levels (estrogen is stored in fat cells) associated with obesity in postmenopausal women. Colorectal cancer has been linked to hyperinsulinemia, and esophageal cancer may be secondary to acid reflux caused by abdominal obesity. Several hormones and factors often present in obese states have been identified as potentiating the risk for cancer. For example, insulin (a powerful cellular growth factor) is increased in obesity. The resulting hyperinsulinemia may affect cancer cells.

Adipokines (from fat cells) may stimulate or inhibit cell growth. For example, leptin, which is increased in obese people, promotes cell proliferation.

Metabolic Syndrome

Metabolic syndrome is one of the fastest-growing obesity health concerns. It is discussed later in this chapter on p. 890.

Psychosocial Problems

The consequences of obesity extend beyond the physical changes. Stigmatization of obese people, and in some cases discrimination, occurs in three important areas of living: employment, education, and health care. The social stigma associated with obesity has an emotional toll on a person's psychologic well-being. Many obese persons suffer low self-esteem, withdraw from social interaction, and experience major depression.[13]

❖ NURSING AND INTERPROFESSIONAL MANAGEMENT: OBESITY

◆ Nursing Assessment

The first step in the treatment of obesity is to determine whether any physical conditions are present that may be causing or contributing to obesity. This requires a thorough history and physical examination.

Table 40-5 lists information that can assist you in understanding an obese patient and provides a basis for intervention. When assessing an individual who is overweight or obese, be sensitive and nonjudgmental in asking specific and leading questions about weight, diet, and exercise (Table 40-6). In doing so, you can often obtain information that the patient may have withheld out of embarrassment or shyness. Patients need to understand the rationale for questions asked about weight or dietary habits, and you must be ready to respond to their concerns.

TABLE 40-5   Nursing Assessment

Obese Patient

Subjective Data

Important Health Information

Past health history: Time of obesity onset; diseases related to metabolism and obesity, such as hypertension, cardiovascular problems, stroke, cancer, chronic joint pain, respiratory problems, diabetes mellitus, cholelithiasis, metabolic syndrome

Medications: Thyroid preparations, diet pills, herbal products

Surgery or other treatments: Prior weight-reduction procedures (bariatric surgery)

Functional Health Patterns

Health perception–health management: Family history of obesity; perception of problem; methods of weight loss attempted

Nutritional-metabolic: Amount and frequency of eating; overeating in response to boredom, stress, specific times, or activities; history of weight gain and loss

Elimination: Constipation

Activity-exercise: Typical physical activity; drowsiness, somnolence; dyspnea on exertion, orthopnea, paroxysmal nocturnal dyspnea

Sleep-rest: Sleep apnea, use of continuous positive airway pressure (CPAP)

Cognitive-perceptual: Feelings of rejection, depression, isolation, guilt, or shame; meaning or value of food; adherence to prescribed reducing diets, degree of long-term commitment to a weight loss program

Role-relationship: Change in financial status or family relationships; personal, social, and financial resources to support a reducing diet

Sexuality-reproductive: Menstrual irregularity, heavy menstrual flow in women, birth control practices, infertility; effect of obesity on sexual activity and attractiveness to significant other

Objective Data

General

Body mass index ≥ 30 kg/m^2; waist circumference: woman >35 in (89 cm), man >40 in (102 cm)

Respiratory

Increased work of breathing; wheezing; rapid, shallow breathing

Cardiovascular

Hypertension, tachycardia, dysrhythmias

Musculoskeletal

Decreased joint mobility and flexibility; knee, hip, and low back pain

Reproductive

Gynecomastia and hypogonadism in men

Possible Diagnostic Findings

Elevated serum glucose, cholesterol, triglycerides; chest x-ray demonstrating enlarged heart; electrocardiogram showing dysrhythmia; abnormal liver function tests

TABLE 40-6   Assessing Patients With Obesity

When assessing patients with obesity and before selecting a weight loss strategy, ask the following questions.

- What is your history with weight gain and weight loss?
- Are other family members overweight?
- How has your health been affected by your body weight?
- What do you think contributes to your weight?
- What does food mean to you? How do you use food (e.g., to relieve stress, provide comfort)?
- What is your motivation for losing weight?
- What have you already tried to lose weight? Was it successful? If not, why not?
- Would you like to manage your weight differently? If so, how?
- What sort of barriers do you think impede your weight loss efforts?
- Are there any major stresses that will make it difficult to focus on weight control?
- How much time can you devote to exercise on a daily or weekly basis?
- What type of support do you have from family and/or friends for losing weight?

? CHECK YOUR PRACTICE

You are working in the hypertension clinic, and the attending physician has asked you to do an assessment on a 54-yr-old man for possible referral to a weight loss program. He is 5'9" and weighs 242 pounds. His BP has been difficult to control with drugs and diet. While trying to do an assessment (using the questions in Table 40-6), he interrupts you and asks you if he can leave. He angrily tells you, "I do not want to give up my favorite foods, quit drinking, or exercise. Do you understand that?"

- How would you respond to him?

Assess a patient's willingness to change and potential for change. If people are not ready for change, offer them the opportunity to return for further discussion when they are ready to discuss their weight again and make lifestyle changes.

When obtaining the history, explore genetic and endocrine factors such as hypothyroidism, hypothalamic tumors, Cushing syndrome, hypogonadism in men, and polycystic ovary syndrome in women. Laboratory tests of liver function and thyroid function, a fasting glucose level, and a lipid panel (triglyceride level, LDL and HDL cholesterol levels) assist in evaluating the cause and effects of obesity. When no organic cause (e.g., hypothyroidism) is associated with obesity, the disorder should be considered a chronic, complex disease.

As part of the initial nursing history and physical examination, examine each body system with particular attention to the organ system in which the patient has expressed a problem or concern. Measurements used with the obese person may include height (without shoes), weight (obtain in a private location and in a gown if possible), waist circumference, and BMI. Have the right equipment to take these measurements. Provide special chairs, examination tables, and scales that can accommodate an obese person.

Also assess for any co-morbid diseases associated with obesity (e.g., hypertension, sleep apnea). These obesity-related complications require special treatment.

◆ **Planning**

The overall goals are that the obese patient will (1) modify eating patterns, (2) participate in a regular physical activity program, (3) achieve and maintain weight loss to a specified level, and (4) minimize or prevent health problems related to obesity.

◆ **Nursing Implementation**

Obesity is one of the most challenging health problems. For the majority of patients who are obese, successful weight management will be a difficult, lifelong project. Obesity treatment begins with patients understanding their weight history and deciding on a plan that is best for them.

Together with other members of the interprofessional care team, you have a major role in planning for and managing the care of an obese patient. First, examine your own personal beliefs and any potential biases related to obesity. If you associate obesity with a lack of willpower and overindulgence, your attitude may be conveyed to patients. They may experience shame in a setting that claims to be a caring one.

You are in a pivotal position to help overweight and obese individuals. Interventions include (1) helping obese patients explore and deal with their negative experiences and (2) teaching other health professionals about stigma and biases experienced by obese patients.

Although health care for obese people has greater demands, HCPs often fail to address these needs. In addition, obese people underutilize health care opportunities available to them. HCPs are often reluctant to counsel patients about obesity for a variety of reasons, including (1) time constraints during appointments make it difficult, (2) weight management may be viewed as professionally unrewarding, (3) reimbursement for weight management services is difficult to obtain, and (4) many HCPs do not feel knowledgeable about giving weight loss advice.

Despite the known benefits of weight loss, it is a difficult process for most individuals. Achieving an "ideal" BMI is not necessary and may not be a realistic goal. Modest weight loss of even 3% to 5% of starting weight can have clinical benefits, and greater weight losses produce greater benefits.[14] In general, the average weight loss program (except for bariatric surgery) results in a 10% reduction of body weight. This average reduction should not be considered a failure, since it is associated with significant health benefits.[15]

Exploring an individual's motivation for weight loss is essential for overall success. Using principles from motivational interviewing (discussed in Chapter 4 on p. 47), you can help patients understand their desire to lose weight and gain confidence in achieving weight loss.

Focusing on the reasons for wanting to lose weight may help patients develop strategies for a weight loss program. Any supervised plan of care must be directed at two different processes: (1) successful weight loss, which requires a short-term energy deficit, and (2) successful weight control, which requires long-term behavior changes.

A multicomponent approach for weight loss must be used that includes nutritional therapy, exercise, behavior modification, and for some, drugs or surgical intervention (Table 40-7). Focusing on more than one aspect provides for more effective weight loss and weight control efforts. While teaching patients, stress healthy eating habits and adequate physical activity as lifestyle patterns to develop and maintain.

◆ **Nutritional Therapy.** There are no "magic" diets for weight loss. No one diet is superior for weight loss. All diets can work if they achieve a reduced caloric intake relative to expenditure.[14]

Restricting dietary intake so that it is below energy requirements is a cornerstone for any weight loss or maintenance program. A good weight loss plan should contain foods from

TABLE 40-7   Interprofessional Care

Obesity

Diagnostic Assessment
- History and physical examination
- Family history
- BMI, waist circumference, waist-to-hip ratio
- Assessment of health risks and co-morbidities

Management
- Management of co-morbidities
- Lifestyle interventions
  - Participation in weight loss program
  - Support groups
  - Behavior modification
- Nutritional therapy
- Exercise
- Behavior modification
- Support groups
- Drug therapy (Table 40-9)
- Surgical therapy (Table 40-10)

BMI, Body mass index.

TABLE 40-8   Nutritional Therapy

1200-Calorie–Restricted Weight-Reduction Diet*

General Principles
1. Eat regularly. Do not skip meals.
2. Measure foods to determine the correct portion size.
3. Avoid concentrated sweets, such as sugar, candy, honey, pies, cakes, cookies, and regular sodas.
4. Reduce fat intake by baking, broiling, or steaming foods.
5. Maintain a regular exercise program for successful weight loss.

Meal	Exchanges	Menu Plan
Breakfast	1 meat	1 hard-boiled egg
	2 bread	1 slice toast
		¾ cup dry cereal (unsweetened)
	1 fruit	½ small banana
	1 fat	1 tsp margarine
	1 dairy†	1 cup low-fat milk
	Beverage	Coffee
Lunch	2 meat	Cheese enchiladas (made with 2 oz
	2 bread	cheese, two corn tortillas, lettuce,
	Vegetable	chili sauce)
	1 fruit	Fresh grapes (12)
	Beverage	Diet soda
Dinner	2 meat	2 oz baked chicken
	1 bread	Corn on the cob with 1 tsp margarine
	Vegetable	Tossed salad and 1 Tbsp salad dressing
	1 fruit	¾ cup strawberries
	1 milk	1 cup low-fat milk

*For 1000 cal, omit 1 fruit exchange and change low-fat milk to skim milk. For 1500 cal, add 1 meat exchange, 1 fruit exchange, and 2 fat exchanges; change low-fat milk to whole milk. For 1800 cal, add 2 bread exchanges, 3 meat exchanges, 3 fat exchanges, and 1 fruit exchange; change low-fat milk to whole milk.
†One extra fat exchange allowed for each cup of 2% low-fat milk; 2 extra fat exchanges allowed for each cup of skim milk.

EVIDENCE-BASED PRACTICE

Translating Research Into Practice

What Types of Diet Programs Result in Weight Loss?

Clinical Question

For adults who are overweight or obese (P), what is the effect of low-fat and low-carbohydrate diet programs (I) versus control group (C) on weight loss at 6 and 12 months (T)?

Synthesis of Best Available Evidence
- Meta-analysis of randomized controlled trials (RCTs)
- 48 RCTs (n = 7286) of overweight or obese adults (BMI ≥25 kg/m^2). Interventions were popular branded diet programs (e.g., Atkins low-carbohydrate diet, Ornish low-fat diet) with and without exercise and/or behavioral support such as counseling. Control groups included wait-listed controls, no specific diet, or competing dietary programs. Outcomes were weight loss measurements at 6 and 12 months.
- At 6-month follow-up, all diet programs resulted in some weight loss with low-carbohydrate and low-fat diets having the greatest weight loss.
- At 12-month follow-up, weight loss for all diets was about 1 to 2 kg less than after 6-month follow-up. Low-carbohydrate and low-fat diets had strongest effect on weight loss.
- Exercise and behavioral support were related to increased weight loss.

Conclusions
- Low-carbohydrate and low-fat diets are associated with significant weight loss.
- Differences in weight loss among types of low-carbohydrate and low-fat diets were small.

Implications for Nursing Practice
- What factors are important to discuss with a patient who asks what diet will help the most in losing weight?
- How will you assist the patient on a diet incorporate exercise into his or her lifestyle?
- What strategies will you use to help patients maintain weight loss after 6 months?

Reference for Evidence

Johnston BC, Kanters S, Bandayrel K, et al: Comparison of weight loss among named diet programs in overweight and obese adults: a meta-analysis, *JAMA* 312: 923, 2014.

P, Patient population of interest; *I,* intervention or area of interest; *C,* comparison of interest or comparison group; *O,* outcomes of interest; *T,* timing (see p. 15).

C requirements. Lean meat, fish, and eggs provide sufficient protein and the B-complex vitamins.

It is rare to find an obese person who has not at some time attempted to lose weight. Some people have met with limited and temporary success, and others have met only with failure. Many individuals attempt weight loss by trying one of the many fad diets that offer the enticement of quick weight loss with little effort. Often these quick weight-reduction diets (found in the popular media) advocate the elimination of one category of foods (e.g., carbohydrates). Therefore these should be discouraged. Low-carbohydrate diets do produce a rapid weight loss but reduce the opportunity to get adequate amounts of fiber, vitamins, and minerals. These restrictive diets are difficult to maintain on a long-term basis. The more restrictive the regimen, the greater the demand for intense discipline in the face of an intense desire to eat foods not allowed on the diet.

It is best to recommend a dietary approach in which calorie restriction includes all food groups (e.g., MyPlate). Patients will

the basic food groups (MyPlate is presented in Fig. 39-1 and Table 39-1). (Table 40-8 presents an example of a 1200-calorie diet.)

A supervised diet plan may be prescribed that limits calories to a total of 800 or less per day (very-low-calorie diet), but this is not sustainable on a long-term basis. These diets should be provided only by trained professionals in a medical care setting. Persons on very-low-calorie diets need frequent professional monitoring, because the severe energy restriction places them at risk for multiple health complications.[14]

In general, it is best to recommend a diet that includes adequate amounts of fruits and vegetables, provides enough bulk to prevent constipation, and meets daily vitamin A and vitamin

find it easier to incorporate such a change into their lifestyle and not become as bored with their food options. However, the ability to adhere to a diet and degree of weight loss strongly depends on the patient's motivation.

The degree of success of any diet depends in part on the amount of weight to be lost. A moderately obese person will obviously attain his or her goal more easily than a person with extreme obesity. Because men have a higher percentage of lean body mass, they are often able to lose weight more quickly than women. Women have a higher percentage of body fat, which is metabolically less active than muscle tissue. Postmenopausal women are particularly prone to weight gain, especially increased abdominal fat.

The obese patient must recognize the advantages of weight loss and weight control. You can assist by helping the patient track eating patterns with a diet diary. Through a frank discussion of eating patterns, the patient often realizes that eating is "mindless" and the result of bad habits picked up over time. These eating behaviors must be changed, or any weight loss will only be temporary.

Setting a realistic and healthy goal, such as losing 1 to 2 lb/wk, should be mutually agreed on at the beginning of a weight loss program. Trying to lose too much too fast usually results in a sense of frustration and failure for the patient. You can help patients understand that losing large amounts of weight in a short period causes skin and underlying tissue to lose elasticity and tone. Slower weight loss offers better cosmetic results.

Inevitably, the patient reaches plateau periods during which no weight is lost. These plateaus may last from several days to several weeks. Remind the patient that plateaus are normal occurrences during weight reduction. A weekly check of body weight is a good method of monitoring progress. Daily weighing is not recommended because of the frequent fluctuations resulting from retained water (including urine) and elimination of feces. Instruct the patient to record the weight at the same time of the day, wearing the same type of clothing.

There is no clear consensus on the number of meals to be eaten when a person is on a diet. Some nutritionists advocate several small meals per day because the body's metabolic rate is temporarily increased immediately after eating. However, when eating several small meals a day, patients may consume more calories unless they carefully adhere to portion sizes and total daily calorie allotment.

When a person first starts a weight loss program, food portion sizes must be carefully determined to stay within the dietary guidelines. Portion sizes over the past 30 years have increased considerably (Table 40-4). Food portions can be weighed using a scale, or everyday objects can be used as a visual cue to determine portion sizes. The size of a woman's fist or a baseball is equivalent to a serving of vegetables or fruit. A serving of meat is about the size of a person's palm or a deck of cards. A serving of cheese is about the size of a thumb or six dice. A portion size quiz is available at *www.nhlbi.nih.gov/health/educational/wecan/eat-right/distortion.htm*.

Another aspect of the American diet that must be considered is which foods contribute the most calories—animal sources, fruits, grains, or vegetables. Two thirds or more of an individual's diet should be plant-source foods, and the other one third or less should be from animal protein. Being aware of personal consumption habits and striving for the two-thirds to one-third ratio is a simple goal that can be achieved without weighing and measuring foods at every meal. Once this ratio has been adopted

into the patient's meal planning, portions can gradually be reduced as activity levels are gradually increased to achieve healthy weight loss. The recommended portion size of animal protein is 3 oz. The standard size for chopped vegetables is ½ cup, according to MyPlate guidelines (Table 39-1).

A list of healthy or low-calorie foods serves as a good reference and permits an occasional meal to be eaten at a restaurant. Furthermore, the patient who carefully follows the prescribed diet may not need to take vitamin supplements.

Encourage the appropriate fluid intake in the form of water. Alcoholic and sugary beverages should be limited or avoided, since they increase caloric intake and are low in nutritional value.

◆ **Exercise.** Exercise is an essential part of a weight loss program. Patients should exercise daily, preferably 30 minutes to an hour. There is no evidence that increased activity promotes an increase in appetite or leads to dietary excess. In fact, exercise frequently has the opposite effect. The addition of exercise produces more weight loss than does dieting alone and has a favorable effect on body fat distribution. With regular exercise, WHR is reduced. Finally, exercise is especially important in maintaining weight loss.

When large muscles are involved in the exercise program, a primary benefit is cardiovascular conditioning. Exercise is of benefit to overweight and obese persons even if it does not make them lean. Many psychologic benefits can be derived from an increased physical activity program. Exercise decreases tension and stress, promotes better-quality sleep and rest, increases stamina and energy, improves self-concept and self-confidence, improves attitudes, and increases optimism about the future.[16]

Explore with patients possible ways to incorporate exercise in daily routines. It may be as simple as parking farther from their place of employment or taking the stairs versus an elevator. Encourage individuals to wear a pedometer to track their activity with a goal of 10,000 steps a day. However, success may be walking one third of the recommended steps with incremental increases over time. Although joining a health club can be one way of getting exercise, it is not necessary. Patients can walk, swim, and cycle, all of which have long-term benefits. Stress to patients that engaging in weekend exercise only or in spurts of strenuous activity is not advantageous and can actually be dangerous.

◆ **Behavior Modification.** The assumption behind behavior modification is twofold: (1) obesity is a learned disorder caused by overeating and (2) often the critical difference between an obese person and a person of normal weight is the cues that regulate eating behavior. Therefore most behavior-modification programs deemphasize the diet and focus on how and when to eat. Ideally, behavior intervention should begin with counseling sessions with a trained interventionist.[14]

Teach people to restrict their eating to designated meals and to increase the amount of physical activity in their lives. Persons who participate in a behavioral therapy program are more successful in maintaining their losses over an extended time than those who do not participate in such training.

Various behavioral techniques for patients engaged in a weight loss program include (1) self-monitoring, (2) stimulus control, and (3) rewards. *Self-monitoring* may involve keeping a record of the type and time food was consumed and how the person was feeling when eating. *Stimulus control* is aimed at separating events that trigger eating from the act of eating. *Rewards* may be used as incentives for weight loss. Short- and long-term goals are useful benchmarks for earning rewards. It is important that the reward for a specified weight loss not be associated with food, such as dinner out or a favorite treat. Reward items do not have to have a monetary component. For example, time for a hot bath or an hour of pleasure reading would be an enjoyable reward for many people.

Praise your patient's successes, even small ones, at every opportunity. Changing existing behaviors is difficult.

◆ **Support Groups.** People who are on a weight management plan are often encouraged to join a group in which others are also trying to modify their eating habits. Many self-help groups are available that offer support and information on dieting tips. For example, Take Off Pounds Sensibly (TOPS) (*www.tops.org*) is the oldest nonprofit organization of this type. Behavior modification is an integral part of the program, along with nutrition education. Weight Watchers International, Inc. (*www.weightwatchers.com*), Jenny Craig (*www.jennycraig.com*), and Nutrisystems (*www.nutrisystem.com*) are probably the most successful commercial weight-loss programs.[17] Weight Watchers offers a food plan that is nutritionally balanced and practical to follow. Group leaders, all of whom have successfully lost weight with Weight Watchers, teach members various behavior-modification techniques.

Commercial weight-reduction centers have proliferated across the nation. Many of these programs are staffed by nurses and dietitians. These weight-reduction centers are cost prohibitive for those with limited financial resources. Many of these programs also offer special prepackaged foods and supplements that must be purchased as part of the weight-reduction plan. Only these prescribed foods and drinks are to be consumed until an agreed-on amount of weight is lost. The patient is encouraged to buy the same type of foods for the maintenance phase of the program, lasting from 6 months to 1 year. Behavior-modification training is incorporated in these programs as well. Individuals must learn how to adjust their diet once they are no longer using the commercial products. This can be challenging for many, and the weight lost may be regained once the restricted food program is completed.[18]

In recent years, a number of employers have begun weight loss programs at the workplace. The rationale for such programs is that better health repays the cost of the programs through improved work performance, decreased absenteeism, less hospitalization, and lower insurance costs. Such programs have been well accepted by both employees and employers.

◆ Drug Therapy

Drugs should never be used alone. Rather, they should be part of a comprehensive weight loss program that includes reduced-calorie diet, exercise, and behavior modification.[19-21] Drugs should be reserved for adults with a BMI of 30 kg/m² or greater (obese), or adults with a BMI of 27 kg/m² or greater (overweight) who have at least one weight-related condition, such as hypertension, type 2 diabetes, or dyslipidemia. The drugs currently approved by the U.S. Food and Drug Administration (FDA) for obesity are presented in Table 40-9.

◆ **Appetite-Suppressing Drugs.** The sympathomimetic amines suppress appetite by increasing the availability of norepinephrine in the brain, thus stimulating the central nervous system. The sympathomimetics fall into two groups: amphetamines and nonamphetamines. The amphetamines have a much higher abuse potential than the nonamphetamines. Amphetamines are not recommended, nor are they approved by the FDA for either short- or long-term weight loss.

Drug	Mechanism of Action	Nursing Considerations
orlistat (Xenical, Alli [low-dose form available over the counter])	• Blocks fat breakdown and absorption in intestine • Inhibits the action of intestinal lipases, resulting in undigested fat excreted in feces	• Associated with leakage of stool, flatulence, diarrhea, and abdominal bloating, especially if a high-fat diet is consumed • Severe liver injury may occur. • Fat-soluble vitamin levels may have to be supplemented.
lorcaserin (Belviq)	• Selective serotonin (5-HT) agonist • Suppresses appetite and creates a sense of satiety	• Common side effects are headache, dizziness, fatigue, nausea, dry mouth, and constipation.
bupropion/ naltrexone (Contrave)	*bupropion:* antidepressant *naltrexone:* opioid antagonist	• Common side effects are nausea, constipation, headache, vomiting, dizziness, insomnia, dry mouth, and diarrhea. • Suicidal thoughts and behaviors and neuropsychiatric reactions can occur. • Can increase BP and heart rate and should not be used in patients with uncontrolled hypertension • Can cause seizures and must not be used in patients who have seizure disorder
phentermine/ topiramate (Qsymia)	*phentermine:* sympathomimetic anorectic *topiramate:* antiseizure drug that induces satiety	• Common side effects are paresthesias, dizziness, insomnia, constipation, dry mouth. • Must not be used in patients with glaucoma or hyperthyroidism • Can increase heart rate, and should not be used in patients with uncontrolled hypertension or heart disease
liraglutide (Saxenda)	• Glucagon-like peptide 1 (GLP-1) agonist • Induces satiety	• Used to treat type 2 diabetes • Must be injected • Side effects include thyroid tumors and pancreatitis.

Nonamphetamines are not usually recommended for weight loss because of the potential for abuse. If used, these drugs should only be used short term (for 3 months or less).

Nonamphetamines include phentermine (Adipex-P, Fastin, Ionamin), diethylpropion (Tenuate), phendimetrazine (Bontril), and benzphetamine (Didrex). Adverse effects of these drugs include palpitations, tachycardia, overstimulation, restlessness, dizziness, insomnia, weakness, and fatigue.

◆ **Nursing Interventions Related to Drug Therapy.** Drugs will not cure obesity, and individuals must understand that without substantial changes in food intake and increased physical activity, they will gain weight when drug therapy is stopped.

As with any drug treatment, there are side effects (Table 40-9). Careful evaluation for other medical conditions can help determine which drugs, if any, would be advisable for a given patient. Many insurance companies do not cover the cost of weight loss drugs.

Your role related to drug therapy is to teach the patient about proper administration, side effects, and how the drugs fit into the overall weight loss plan. The modification of dosage without consultation with the HCP can have detrimental effects. Emphasize that diet and exercise regimens are the cornerstones of permanent weight loss. Finally, discourage the purchase of over-the-counter diet aids except for Allī.

BARIATRIC SURGICAL THERAPY

Bariatric surgery, surgery on the stomach and/or intestines to help a person with extreme obesity lose weight, has become a viable option for treating obesity. Surgery is currently the only treatment that has been found to have a successful and lasting impact for sustained weight loss for individuals with extreme obesity.[14]

Criteria guidelines for bariatric surgery include having a BMI of 40 kg/m^2 or more or a BMI of 35 kg/m^2 or more with other significant co-morbidities (e.g., hypertension, type 2 diabetes mellitus, heart failure, sleep apnea).

The majority of people who undergo bariatric surgery successfully improve their overall quality of life. In addition to losing weight, patients often experience resolution of co-morbidities such as diabetes. Although overall mortality is very low, a number of complications can arise from surgery. Therefore the option to have surgery must be carefully considered.[22]

Many insurance carriers do not cover the cost of bariatric surgery. If they do consider reimbursing for the surgery, most of them require documentation of a medically supervised weight loss program for approximately 6 months.

Before being considered candidates for surgery, patients must be screened for psychologic, physical, and behavioral conditions that have been associated with poor surgical outcomes. These include untreated depression, binge eating disorders, and drug and alcohol abuse that may interfere with a commitment to lifelong behavioral changes. Other contraindications to surgery include illnesses that are known to reduce life expectancy and are not likely to be improved with weight reduction. These conditions include advanced cancer; end-stage kidney, liver, and cardiopulmonary disease; severe coagulopathy; or inability to comply with nutritional recommendations.

Bariatric surgeries fall into one of three broad categories: restrictive, malabsorptive, or a combination of malabsorptive and restrictive (Table 40-10 and Fig. 40-7). In restrictive procedures the stomach is reduced in size (less food eaten), and in malabsorptive procedures the small intestine is shortened or bypassed (less food absorbed). The majority of procedures are performed laparoscopically, thus decreasing postoperative recuperation as compared to an open procedure. With laparoscopy, patients have fewer wound infections, shorter hospital stays, and a faster recovery period.

Restrictive Surgeries

Restrictive bariatric surgery reduces either the size of the stomach, which causes the patient to feel full more quickly, or the amount allowed to enter the stomach. In these surgeries, digestion is not altered, so the risk of anemia or cobalamin deficiency is low. The most common restrictive surgeries include adjustable gastric banding and sleeve gastrectomy.

Adjustable Gastric Banding. Laparoscopic adjustable gastric banding (AGB), the most common restrictive procedure done, involves limiting the stomach size with an inflatable band placed around the fundus of the stomach (Fig. 40-7, A). This restrictive procedure can be done using a Lap-Band or Realize Band system. The band is connected to a subcutaneous port and can be inflated or deflated (by fluid injection in the HCP's office) to change the stoma size to meet the patient's needs as weight is lost. The restrictive effect of the band creates a sense of fullness as the upper portion of the stomach now accommodates less than the average stomach. The band then causes a delay in stomach emptying, providing patients with further satiety.

The procedure can be either modified or reversed at a later date if necessary. AGB is the preferred option for patients who are surgical risks, because it is a less invasive approach.

Sleeve Gastrectomy (Gastric Sleeve). In the sleeve gastrectomy (gastric sleeve), about 75% of the stomach is removed, leaving a sleeve-shaped stomach (Fig. 40-7, B). Although the stomach is drastically reduced in size, its function is preserved. The removal of the majority of the stomach also results in the elimination of hormones produced in the stomach that stimulate hunger, such as ghrelin.

Research is ongoing on a procedure called endoscopic sleeve gastroplasty. It involves using an endoscope rather than making a surgical incision. When the endoscope reaches the stomach, the surgeon places sutures in the stomach, making it smaller and changing its shape.

Gastric Plication. Gastric plication is a minimally invasive weight-loss surgery that reduces the size of the stomach. It is done by folding the stomach wall inward, and then sutures are placed to secure the folded stomach wall. This reduces the stomach volume by as much as 70%.

Intragastric Balloons. Intragastric balloons involve a weight-loss system (Orbera, ReShape) that uses a gastric balloon that occupies space in the stomach. The balloon is placed into the stomach through the mouth, using a minimally invasive endoscopic procedure, while the patient is under mild sedation. Once in place, the balloon is filled with saline so that it expands. The balloon can be filled with different amounts of saline (from 400 to 700 mL). When it is time to remove the balloon, it is first deflated and then removed using another endoscopic procedure.

The intragastric balloon does not change or alter the stomach's natural anatomy. It is designed to help patients feel more full, curb the appetite, and reduce food intake. Patients are advised to follow a diet and exercise plan to assist with their weight loss efforts.

The balloons are less invasive than having gastric bypass surgery. This device should not be used in patients who have had previous gastrointestinal or bariatric surgery or who have been diagnosed with inflammatory bowel disease, large hiatal hernia, symptoms of delayed gastric emptying, or active Helicobacter pylori infection.

Once the device is placed in the stomach, patients may experience vomiting, nausea, abdominal pain, and feelings of indigestion. Other potential risks are gastric ulcers and balloon deflation.

Combination of Restrictive and Malabsorptive Surgery

Roux-en-Y Gastric Bypass. The Roux-en-Y gastric bypass (RYGB) procedure is a combination of restrictive and

TABLE 40-10 Surgical Therapy for Obesity*

Description	Advantages	Disadvantages
Restrictive Surgery		
Adjustable Gastric Banding (AGB) (Lap-Band, Realize Band)		
• Inflatable band encircles stomach • Creation of gastric pouch with about 30 mL (1 oz) capacity • Later stretches to 60-90 mL (2-3 oz) • Upper gastric pouch connected by very narrow channel to lower section of stomach	• Food digestion occurs through normal process • Band can be adjusted to ↑ or ↓ restriction • Surgery can be reversed • Absence of dumping syndrome • Lack of malabsorption • Low complication rate	• Some nausea and vomiting initially (eating too much too quickly) • Problems with adjustment device • Band may slip or erode into stomach wall • Gastric perforation • Weight loss may be more limited than with other types of surgery
Sleeve Gastrectomy (Gastric Sleeve)		
• About 75% of stomach removed • Creation of sleeve-shaped stomach with 60-150 mL (2-5 oz) capacity	• Function of stomach preserved • No bypass of intestine • Avoids complications of obstruction, anemia, vitamin deficiencies	• Weight loss may be more limited than with other types of surgery • Leakage related to stapling • Irreversible
Gastric Plication		
• Adapted version of sleeve gastrectomy (gastric sleeve) • Sleeve created by suturing rather than removing stomach	• Minimal surgery compared to sleeve gastrectomy • No rerouting of intestines • Natural nutrient absorption capabilities maintained	• Requires hospital stay of 24-48 hr • Nausea common after procedure • Risks include stomach leakage from sutured areas, blockage of stomach from swelling or fold too tight
Intragastric Balloon		
• Involves placing a deflated balloon into stomach using an endoscope • Balloon then filled with saline and occupies space in stomach	• Does not require invasive surgery • Done as outpatient procedure	• Can only be left in place for 6 months • Once device in stomach, patients may experience nausea, vomiting, abdominal pain, indigestion, and gastric ulcers
Malabsorptive Surgery		
Biliopancreatic Diversion (BPD) With or Without Duodenal Switch		
• 70% of the stomach removed horizontally • Anastomosis between stomach and intestine • Decreases the amount of small intestine available for nutrient absorption • Duodenal switch cuts the stomach vertically and is shaped like a tube	• Able to eat larger meals than with gastric bypass or banding procedures • Less food intolerance • Rapid weight loss • Greater long-term weight loss	• Abdominal bloating, diarrhea, and foul-smelling gas (steatorrhea) • Three or four loose bowel movements a day • Malabsorption of fat-soluble vitamins • Iron deficiency • Protein-calorie malnutrition • Dumping syndrome • Most complicated of weight loss surgeries
Combination of Restrictive and Malabsorptive Surgery		
Roux-en-Y Gastric Bypass (RYGB)		
• Surgery on stomach to create a pouch (restrictive) • Small gastric pouch connected to jejunum • Remaining stomach and first segment of small intestine are bypassed (malabsorptive)	• Better weight loss results than with restrictive procedures • Lower incidence of malnutrition and diarrhea • Rapid improvement of weight-related co-morbidities • Good long-term results	• Leak at site of anastomosis • Anemia: iron deficiency, cobalamin deficiency, folic acid deficiency • Calcium deficiency • Dumping syndrome • Irreversible
Implanted Gastric Stimulation Device		
Maestro Rechargeable System (Fig. 40-8)		
• Device implanted into abdomen • Works like pacemaker to deliver electrical impulses to vagus nerve, which tells brain when stomach is full.	• Least invasive of weight loss surgeries • Procedure done on outpatient basis	• Device must be charged 1-2 times/week • If battery completely drained, device needs to be reprogrammed • Side effects include nausea, vomiting, heartburn, belching, swallowing problems

*Fig. 40-7.

malabsorptive surgery. This surgical procedure is the most common bariatric procedure performed in the United States. It is considered the gold standard among bariatric procedures.[14]

This procedure involves creating a small gastric pouch and attaching it directly to the small intestine using a Y-shaped limb of the small bowel (Fig. 40-7, D). After the procedure, food bypasses 90% of the stomach, the duodenum, and a small segment of jejunum.

Overall, it has low complication rates, has excellent patient tolerance, and sustains long-term weight loss. Outcomes include improved glucose control with improvement or reversal of dia-

betes, normalization of BP, decreased total cholesterol and triglycerides, decreased GERD, and decreased sleep apnea.

A complication of the RYGB is *dumping syndrome*, in which gastric contents empty too rapidly into the small intestine, overwhelming its ability to digest nutrients. Symptoms can include vomiting, nausea, weakness, sweating, faintness, and, on occasion, diarrhea. Patients are discouraged from eating sugary foods after surgery to avoid dumping syndrome. Because sections of the small intestine are bypassed, poor absorption of iron can cause iron-deficiency anemia. Patients need to take a multivitamin with iron and calcium supplements. Chronic anemia caused

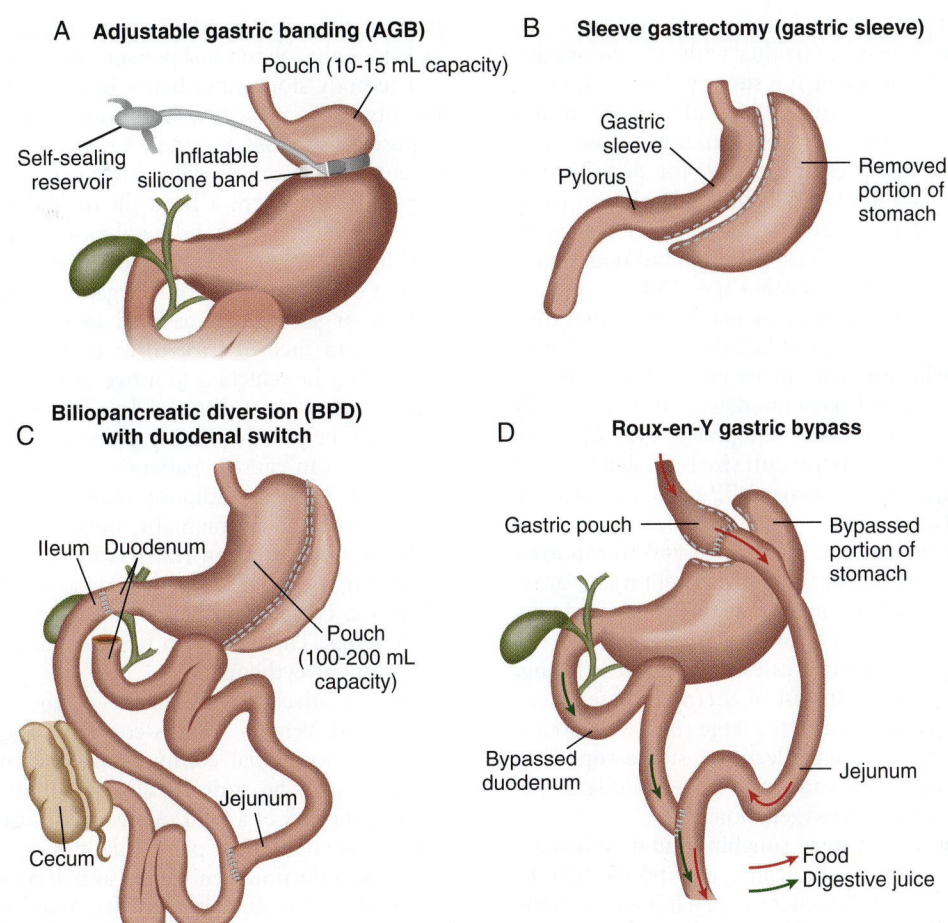

FIG. 40-7 Bariatric surgical procedures. **A,** Adjustable gastric banding (AGB) uses a band to create a gastric pouch. **B,** Sleeve gastrectomy involves creating a sleeve-shaped stomach by removing about 75% of the stomach. **C,** Biliopancreatic diversion (BPD) with duodenal switch procedure creates an anastomosis between the stomach and intestine. **D,** Roux-en-Y gastric bypass procedure involves constructing a gastric pouch whose outlet is a Y-shaped limb of small intestine.

by cobalamin deficiency may also occur. This problem can usually be managed with parenteral or intranasal cobalamin.

Implantable Gastric Stimulation

An implantable gastric stimulation device (e.g., Maestro Rechargeable System) consists of a pacemaker-like electrical pulse generator, wire leads, and electrodes that are implanted in the abdomen (Fig. 40-8). The Maestro System works by sending intermittent electrical pulses to the vagus nerve, which is involved in regulating stomach emptying and signaling to the brain that the stomach feels empty or full. External controllers allow the patient to charge the device and allow HCPs to adjust the device's settings in order to provide optimal therapy.

❖ NURSING MANAGEMENT: PERIOPERATIVE CARE OF THE OBESE PATIENT

◆ Nursing Implementation

This section discusses general nursing considerations for the care of the obese patient who is having surgery. Special nursing considerations are described for the patient who is having bariatric surgery. (Care of the surgical patient is discussed in Chapters 17 to 19.)

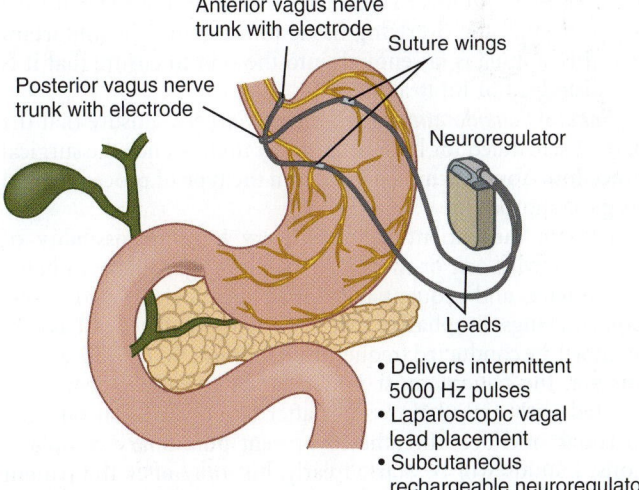

FIG. 40-8 The Maestro Rechargeable System is an electrical stimulator that is surgically implanted into the abdomen. It works by sending intermittent electrical pulses to the vagus nerve, which is involved in regulating stomach emptying and signaling to the brain that the stomach feels empty or full.

◆ **Preoperative Care.** Special considerations are necessary for the obese patient, especially the individual with extreme obesity, who is admitted to the hospital for surgery. Before surgery, interview the patient to identify past and current health information and any assistive devices currently in use (e.g., continuous positive airway pressure [CPAP] for sleep apnea). Co-morbidities secondary to obesity increase the risk for complications in the perioperative period. It may be necessary to coordinate care with the patient's cardiologist, pulmonologist, gynecologist, gastroenterologist, or other specialists.

Have a plan in place before the patients arrive so that they receive optimal care and do not feel like they are a burden to the nursing staff. Nursing units must have available appropriate size hospital gowns, beds that accommodate an increased body size, and necessary patient transfer equipment.[23] To correctly measure BP in obese people, a larger cuff size is needed to avoid artifactual errors. Ensure that oversized BP cuffs are available and placed in the patient's room.

Consider how the patient will be weighed and transported throughout the hospital. A wheelchair with removable arms that is large enough to safely accommodate the patient and pass easily through doorways should be available.

Preoperative and postoperative assessment of heart, lung, and bowel sounds may require the use of alternative assessment techniques. For example, because of the large chest wall, breath and heart sounds are often distant. Electronic stethoscopes can be used to amplify lung, heart, and bowel sounds. Pulse oximetry may also be used to assess oxygenation status.

Instruct the patient in the proper coughing and deep breathing techniques and methods of turning and positioning to prevent pulmonary complications after surgery. If possible, demonstrate the use of a spirometer before surgery. Use of the spirometer helps prevent and treat postoperative lung congestion. Practicing these strategies preoperatively can help the patient perform them correctly postoperatively. Furthermore, if the patient uses CPAP at home for sleep apnea, make arrangements for the use of a machine while the patient is hospitalized.

Obtaining venous access may be complicated by excess adipose tissue. A longer IV catheter is helpful (longer than 1 in) to go through the overlying tissue to the vein. It is important that the cannula is far enough into the vein to ensure that it is not dislodged or infiltrated.

◆ *Special Considerations for Bariatric Surgery.* Ensure that the patient scheduled for bariatric surgery understands the surgical procedure. Your teaching depends on the type of procedure and surgical approach.[24]

Prepare the patient before surgery for the possibility of returning with one or more of the following: urinary catheter, IV catheter, and sequential compression device or compression stockings. Emphasize that vital signs and a general assessment will be conducted frequently to monitor for complications. Further, the patient must understand that he or she will be assisted with ambulation soon after surgery and encouraged to cough and deep breathe to prevent pulmonary complications. Liquids will be started early, but only after the patient is fully awake and there is no evidence of any anastomosis leaks.

◆ **Postoperative Care.** The initial postoperative care focuses on careful assessment and immediate intervention for cardiopulmonary complications, thrombus formation, anastomosis leaks, and electrolyte imbalances. The transfer from surgery may require many trained staff members. During the transfer, the patient's airway should remain stabilized and attention given to managing the patient's pain. Maintain the patient's head at a 35- to 40-degree angle to reduce abdominal pressure and increase lung expansion.

The body stores anesthetics in adipose tissue, thus placing patients with excess adipose tissue at risk for re-sedation. As adipose cells release anesthetics back into the bloodstream, the patient may become sedated after surgery. If this happens, be prepared to perform a head-tilt or jaw-thrust maneuver and keep the patient's oral and nasal airways open.

Diligence in turning and ambulation postoperatively will prevent complications from surgery. Tell the patient that typically he or she will be assisted in walking the evening after surgery and then at least three or four times each day. The patient may be reluctant to move or may not have the stamina to walk even a short distance. In either situation, you will need additional help in facilitating movement in an obese patient.

Obesity can cause a patient's breathing to become shallow and rapid. The extra adipose tissue in the chest and abdomen compresses the diaphragmatic, thoracic, and abdominal structures. This compression restricts the chest's ability to expand, preventing the lungs from working as efficiently as they would otherwise. The patient retains more CO_2 with less O_2 delivered to the lungs. This results in hypoxemia, pulmonary hypertension, and polycythemia.

Postoperatively the risk for deep venous thrombosis (DVT) is increased. Venous stasis is common due to the pressure on the veins. Sequential compression stockings or compression stockings may be ordered along with low-dose heparin to decrease the risk of a DVT. Active and passive range-of-motion exercises are a frequent part of daily care.

Wound infection, dehiscence, and delayed healing are potential problems for all obese patients. Assess the patient's skin for any complications related to wound healing. Keep skinfolds clean and dry to prevent dermatitis and secondary bacterial or fungal infections.

◆ *Special Considerations for Bariatric Surgery.* Patients experience considerable abdominal pain after bariatric surgery. Give pain medications as necessary during the immediate postoperative period (first 24 hours). Be aware that pain could be from an anastomosis leak rather than typical surgical pain.

Abdominal wounds require frequent observation for the amount and type of drainage, condition of the incision, and signs of infection. Protect the incision against undue straining that accompanies turning and coughing. Monitor vital signs to assist in identifying problems such as infection.

During the immediate postoperative period water and sugar-free clear liquids are given (30 mL every 2 hours while awake). Before discharge, instruct patients on a measured amount of a high-protein liquid diet. The patient is taught to eat slowly, stop eating when feeling full, and not consume liquids with solid food. Vomiting is a common complication during this time. A dietitian is usually part of the bariatric team and assists the patient with the transition to the new diet.

◆ **Ambulatory and Home Care**

◆ *Special Considerations for Bariatric Surgery.* The patient who has undergone major surgical treatment for obesity has not been successful in the past in following or maintaining a prescribed diet. Now the patient is forced to reduce oral intake because of the anatomic changes from the surgical procedure. The patient's adherence to a reduced intake is necessary because of the concern for abdominal distention, cramping abdominal pain, and perhaps diarrhea.

Weight loss is considerable during the first 6 to 12 months. During this time the patient must learn to adjust intake sufficiently to maintain a stable weight. Although behavior modification is not necessarily an intended outcome with these surgical procedures, it becomes an unexpected secondary gain. For example, a person who has had bariatric surgery cannot overeat or binge eat without consequences.

The diet generally prescribed should be high in protein and low in carbohydrates, fat, and roughage and consist of six small feedings daily. Fluids should not be ingested with the meal, and in some cases, fluids should be restricted to less than 1000 mL/day. Fluids and foods high in carbohydrate tend to promote diarrhea and symptoms of the dumping syndrome. Generally, calorically dense foods (foods high in fat) should be avoided to permit more nutritionally sound food to be consumed.[25]

The patient must clearly understand the proper diet. Late complications can be anticipated after bariatric surgery, including anemia, vitamin deficiencies, diarrhea, and psychologic problems. Failure to lose weight or loss of too much weight may be caused by the surgical formation of too large a stomach pouch or of an outlet that is much too small, respectively. Peptic ulcer formation, dumping syndrome, and small bowel obstruction may be seen late in the recovery and rehabilitation stage.

Emphasize the importance of long-term follow-up care, in part because of potential complications late in the recovery period. Encourage patients to adhere strictly to the prescribed diet and to inform the HCP of any changes in their physical or emotional condition. Some patients have been known to overeat when they return home and gain rather than lose weight.

INFORMATICS IN PRACTICE

Use of Cell Phone for Weight Loss

- Cell phone apps (e.g., My Fitness Pal) are available to help track calories, weight, exercise, and eating patterns.
- Apps are popular for accountability, reflection, and motivation.
- Tracking systems may provide immediate access to nutritional information for better dietary decision making.
- Some apps (e.g., Foodmeter) can be used to scan the barcode of foods in the grocery store and give nutritional information.
- Calorie tracker apps can be used to monitor daily calorie intake and keep a record of weight loss progress.
- With text messaging, a phone "buddy" can be used to provide support when a person's will power is lacking.
- Share progress with friends and family. Some weight loss apps for cell phones sync with social media accounts so that a person can share milestones by adding them to Twitter and Facebook.

CHECK YOUR PRACTICE

You are working in the bariatric surgery outpatient clinic. When you walk into the clinic room where a 36-yr-old woman is waiting for her follow-up visit, you find her distraught and crying. You ask her what is wrong. She responds, "I am a total failure. I have been fat all my life and I had to have this horrible surgery to help me. Why couldn't I do it on my own?"
- What is an effective way for you to handle this situation?

Several potential psychologic problems may arise after surgery. Some patients express guilty feelings that weight loss was achieved by surgical interventions rather than by the "sheer willpower" of reduced dietary intake and exercise. Be ready to provide support and assist the patient in moving away from such negative feelings.

By 6 to 8 months after surgery, considerable weight loss has usually occurred, and patients are able to see how much their appearance has changed. Discussion of this possible

EVIDENCE-BASED PRACTICE
Applying the Evidence

Obesity Interventions in Faith-Based Organizations

J.W. is a 39-year-old African American woman who is 5 ft 6 in tall and weighs 196 lb. You work in the outpatient clinic that she visits for health care. Your clinic is referring patients who would benefit from losing weight to weight loss programs. She tells you she has been trying to lose weight by "watching what she eats" and that she is "not sure what else she can do." In further conversations with her, you learn she is an active member of her neighborhood church.

Making Clinical Decisions

Best Available Evidence. Faith-based organizations are places where effective programs have helped obese individuals improve weight-related behaviors and lose weight.

Clinician Expertise. You know it is important for J.W. to engage in a weight loss program that will assist her in adopting healthy behaviors. You also know churches can play a major role in providing health promotion programs in African American communities.

Patient Preferences and Values. J.W. indicates she is interested in learning about a weight loss program at her church.

Implications for Nursing Practice

1. Why is it important to discuss with J.W. her motivation for attending the program at her church?
2. How will you help J.W. to set realistic short- and long-term goals related to weight loss? How may these goals differ?
3. At each clinic visit, how will you support J.W.'s efforts to lose weight?

Reference for Evidence

Lancaster K, Carter-Edwards L, Grilo S, et al: Obesity interventions in African American faith-based organizations: a systematic review, *Obes Rev* 15:159, 2014.

outcome with the patient before surgery and again during the rehabilitation phase facilitates the patient's adjustment to a new body image. Do not hesitate to encourage counseling for unresolved psychologic issues.

Massive weight loss often leaves the patient with large quantities of flabby skin that can result in problems related to altered body image (Fig. 40-9). Cosmetic surgery may alleviate this situation.

Often one result of bariatric surgery is the return of fertility in women. Pregnancy complications can result from anemia and nutritional deficiencies. Furthermore, depending on the type of surgery, intestinal obstructions and hernias are commonly experienced in pregnancy. Women must carefully consider the risk of pregnancy after bariatric surgery. In general, encourage women to postpone pregnancy for 12 to 18 months after bariatric surgery.

◆ Evaluation

The expected outcomes are that the obese patient will
- Experience long-term weight loss
- Have improvement in obesity-related co-morbidities
- Integrate healthy practices into daily routines
- Monitor for adverse side effects of surgical therapy
- Have an improved self-image

Gerontologic Considerations: Obesity in Older Adults

The prevalence of obesity is increasing in all age groups, including older people. The number of obese older persons has markedly risen because of increases in both the total number of older persons and the percentage of the older adults who are obese. Obesity is more common in older women than in older men.

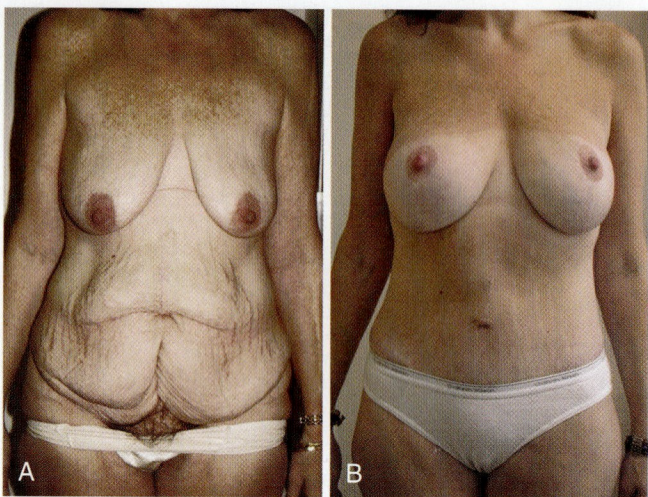

FIG. 40-9 A, Preoperative view of a 37-year-old woman with massive weight loss who had gastric bypass surgery. **B,** Postoperative view 2½ years after abdominoplasty. She also underwent breast surgery, thighlift, backlift with excision of excess skin of the lower back and upper buttocks, and upper arm surgery. (From Shermak MA: Contouring the epigastrium, *Aesthet Surg J* 25:506, 2005.)

TABLE 40-11	Criteria for Metabolic Syndrome*
Measure	**Criteria**
Waist circumference	≥40 in (102 cm) in men
	≥35 in (89 cm) in women
Triglycerides	>150 mg/dL (1.7 mmol/L)
	OR
	Drug treatment for elevated triglycerides
High-density lipoprotein (HDL) cholesterol	<40 mg/dL (0.9 mmol/L) in men
	<50 mg/dL (1.1 mmol/L) in women
	OR
	Drug treatment for elevated cholesterol
BP	≥130 mm Hg systolic BP
	OR
	≥85 mm Hg diastolic BP
	OR
	Drug treatment for hypertension
Fasting blood glucose	≥110 mg/dL
	OR
	Drug treatment for elevated glucose

Source: National Heart, Lung, and Blood Institute: How is metabolic syndrome diagnosed? Retrieved from *www.nhlbi.nih.gov/health/dci/Diseases/ms/ms_diagnosis.html.*
*Any three of the five measures are needed for a diagnosis of metabolic syndrome.

A decrease in energy expenditure is an important contributor to a gradual increase in body fat with age.

Obesity in older adults can exacerbate age-related declines in physical function and lead to frailty and disability. Obesity is associated with decreased survival. Individuals who are obese live 6 to 7 years less than people of normal weight.

Many of the changes associated with aging are exacerbated by obesity. Excess body weight places more demands on arthritic joints. The mechanical strain on weight-bearing joints can lead to premature immobility. Excess weight also affects other body systems. Older adults may find that excess intraabdominal weight causes problems with urinary incontinence. In addition, excess weight may contribute to hypoventilation and sleep apnea.

Obesity affects the quality of life for older adults. Weight loss can improve physical functioning and obesity-related health complications. The same therapeutic approaches for obesity as were discussed earlier also apply to the older adult.

COSMETIC SURGICAL THERAPY

Lipectomy

Lipectomy (adipectomy) is performed to remove unsightly flabby folds of adipose tissue (Fig. 40-9). There is no evidence that a regeneration of adipose tissue occurs at the surgical sites. However, emphasize to the patient that surgical removal does not prevent obesity from recurring, especially if lifetime eating habits remain the same. Although body image and self-esteem may be enhanced by such procedures, these operations are not without complications. The dangerous effects of anesthesia and the potential for poor wound healing in the obese patient cannot be overemphasized.

Liposuction

Another cosmetic surgical procedure is liposuction, or suction-assisted lipectomy. It is used for cosmetic purposes and not for weight reduction. This surgical intervention helps improve facial appearance or body contours. A good candidate for this type of surgery is a person who has achieved weight reduction

but who has excess fat under the chin, along the jaw line, in the nasolabial folds, over the abdomen, or around the waist and upper thighs. A long, hollow, stainless steel cannula is inserted through a small incision over the fatty tissue to be suctioned. This surgical procedure is not usually recommended for the older person because the skin is less elastic and will not accommodate the new underlying shape.

METABOLIC SYNDROME

Metabolic syndrome is a group of metabolic risk factors that increase an individual's chance of developing cardiovascular disease, stroke, and diabetes mellitus. About one in three adults have metabolic syndrome. The syndrome is more prevalent in those 60 years of age and older.[26]

Metabolic syndrome is characterized by a cluster of health problems, including obesity, hypertension, abnormal lipid levels, and high blood glucose. Metabolic syndrome is diagnosed if an individual has three or more of the conditions listed in Table 40-11.

Currently health professionals are debating whether metabolic syndrome should be viewed as a distinct condition. Since there is not one standard treatment for the syndrome itself, interventions are focused on each risk factor.

Etiology and Pathophysiology

The main underlying risk factor for metabolic syndrome is insulin resistance related to excessive visceral fat (Fig. 40-10). Insulin resistance is the body's cells diminished ability to respond to the action of insulin. The pancreas compensates by secreting more insulin, resulting in hyperinsulinemia.

Other characteristics of metabolic syndrome include hypertension, increased risk for clotting, and abnormalities in cholesterol levels. The net effect of these conditions is an increased prevalence of coronary artery disease.

Clinical Manifestations and Diagnostic Studies

The signs of metabolic syndrome are impaired fasting blood glucose, hypertension, abnormal cholesterol levels, and obesity.

PATHOPHYSIOLOGY MAP

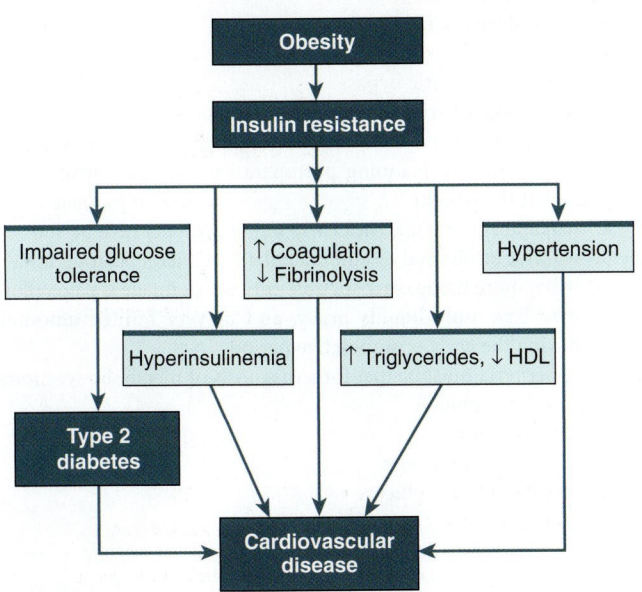

FIG. 40-10   Relationship among insulin resistance, obesity, diabetes mellitus, and cardiovascular disease. *HDL,* High-density lipoprotein.

Medical problems develop over time if the condition remains unaddressed. Patients with this syndrome are at a higher risk of heart disease, stroke, diabetes, renal disease, and polycystic ovary syndrome. Patients who have metabolic syndrome and smoke are at an even higher risk.

❖ NURSING AND INTERPROFESSIONAL MANAGEMENT: METABOLIC SYNDROME

Lifestyle modifications are the first-line interventions to reduce the risk factors for metabolic syndrome. Management or reversal of metabolic syndrome can be achieved by reducing the major risk factors of cardiovascular disease: reducing LDL cholesterol, stopping smoking, lowering BP, and reducing glucose levels. For long-term risk reduction, weight should be decreased, physical activity increased, and healthy dietary habits established.

There is no specific management of metabolic syndrome. You can assist patients by providing information on healthy diets, exercise, and positive lifestyle changes. The diet, which should be low in saturated fats, should promote weight loss. Weight reduction and maintenance of a lower weight should be the first priority in those with abdominal obesity and metabolic syndrome.

Because sedentary lifestyles contribute to metabolic syndrome, increasing regular physical activity will lower a patient's risk factors. In addition to assisting in weight reduction, regular exercise has been found to decrease the triglyceride level and increase the HDL cholesterol level in patients with metabolic syndrome.[26]

Patients unable to lower risk factors with lifestyle therapies alone or those at high risk for a coronary event or diabetes may be considered for drug therapy. Although there is no specific medication for metabolic syndrome, cholesterol-lowering and antihypertensive drugs can be used. Metformin (Glucophage) has also been used to prevent diabetes by lowering glucose levels and enhancing the cells' sensitivity to insulin.

CASE STUDY

Obesity

Patient Profile

S.R. is a 48-yr-old white woman who comes to the clinic with complaints of hip pain.

(©Thinkstock)

Subjective Data

- States that it is "getting hard to get around"
- Reports gradual weight gain of 40 lb over past 40 yr
- Lives in a rural community with no sidewalks
- Spends most of her free time watching television
- Reports health problems related to type 2 diabetes mellitus, shortness of breath, hypertension, and osteoarthritis
- Had knee replacement surgery at age 46 for osteoarthritis
- Has tried orlistat (Xenical) but hated the side effects

Objective Data

Physical Examination

- 5 ft 6 in tall; weighs 230 lb; BMI 37 kg/m², waist circumference of 40 in
- Has obese, nontender, soft round, abdomen
- BP 160/100 mm Hg

Laboratory Results

- Fasting blood glucose 250 mg/dL (13.9 mmol/L)
- Total cholesterol 205 mg/dL (5.3 mmol/L)
- Triglyceride 298 mg/dL (3.36 mmol/L)
- HDL cholesterol 31 mg/dL (0.8 mmol/L)
- LDL cholesterol 114 mg/dL

Interprofessional Care

- Referral to a community weight loss program
- Consultation with bariatric surgeon

Discussion Questions

1. What are S.R.'s risk factors for obesity?
2. Of the possible complications of obesity, which ones does S.R. have? Why did she develop them?
3. *Patient-Centered Care:* How would you assist S.R. in designing a successful weight loss and weight management program?
4. *Teamwork and Collaboration:* How could a comprehensive community weight loss program be beneficial to S.R.?
5. What are S.R.'s risk factors for metabolic syndrome?
6. Is S.R. a candidate for bariatric surgery? Why or why not?
7. *Evidence-Based Practice:* S.R. tells you that she is not sure surgery will work for her. She asks you, "What is the best surgery for me?"

Answers available at *http://evolve.elsevier.com/Lewis/medsurg.*

BRIDGE TO NCLEX EXAMINATION

The number of the question corresponds to the same-numbered outcome at the beginning of the chapter.

1. Which statement *best* describes the etiology of obesity?
   a. Obesity primarily results from a genetic predisposition.
   b. Psychosocial factors can override the effects of genetics in the etiology of obesity.
   c. Obesity is the result of complex interactions between genetic and environmental factors.
   d. Genetic factors are more important than environmental factors in the etiology of obesity.

2. The obesity classification that is *most* often associated with cardiovascular health problems is
   a. primary obesity.
   b. secondary obesity.
   c. gynoid fat distribution.
   d. android fat distribution.

3. Health risks associated with obesity include (*select all that apply*)
   a. colorectal cancer.
   b. rheumatoid arthritis.
   c. polycystic ovary syndrome.
   d. nonalcoholic steatohepatitis.
   e. systemic lupus erythematosus.

4. The *best* nutritional therapy plan for a person who is obese is
   a. the Zone diet.
   b. the Atkins diet.
   c. Sugar Busters.
   d. foods from the basic food groups.

5. This bariatric surgical procedure involves creating a gastric pouch that is reversible and no malabsorption occurs. What surgical procedure is this?
   a. Vertical gastric banding
   b. Biliopancreatic diversion
   c. Roux-en-Y gastric bypass
   d. Adjustable gastric banding

6. A patient with extreme obesity has undergone Roux-en-Y gastric bypass surgery. In planning postoperative care, the nurse anticipates that the patient
   a. may have severe diarrhea early in the postoperative period.
   b. will not be allowed to ambulate for 1 to 2 days postoperatively.
   c. will require nasogastric suction until the drainage is pale yellow.
   d. may have only liquids orally, and in very limited amounts, during the early postoperative period.

7. Which criteria must be met for a diagnosis of metabolic syndrome (*select all that apply*)?
   a. Hypertension
   b. Elevated triglycerides
   c. Elevated plasma glucose
   d. Increased waist circumference
   e. Decreased low-density lipoproteins

1.c, 2.d, 3.a,c,d, 4.d, 5.d, 6.d, 7.a,b,c,d

For rationales to these answers and even more NCLEX review questions, visit *http://evolve.elsever.com/Lewis/medsurg*.

ⓔ EVOLVE WEBSITE

http://evolve.elsevier.com/Lewis/medsurg

Review Questions (Online Only)
Key Points
Answer Keys for Questions
· Rationales for Bridge to NCLEX Examination Questions
· Answer Guidelines for Case Study on p. 891
Student Case Study
· Patient With Obesity and Osteoarthritis
Conceptual Care Map Creator
Audio Glossary
Content Updates

REFERENCES

1. Trust for America's Health, Robert Wood Johnson Foundation. The state of obesity. 2014. Retrieved from *http://stateofobesity.org*.
2. Breymaier SOB: AMA adopts new policies on second day of voting at annual meeting. 2013. Retrieved from *www.ama-assn.org/ama/pub/news/news/2013/2013-06-18-new-ama-policies-annual-meeting.page*.
*3. Ford ES, Maynard LM, Li C: Trends in mean waist circumference and abdominal obesity among US adults, 1999-2012, *JAMA* 312(11):1151, 2014.
4. Modern Genetics: Genetics of body shape: apple or pear? Retrieved from *http://sirens-space.blogspot.com/2012/03/genetics-of-body-shape-apple-or-pear.html*.
*5. Naukkarinen J, Rissanen A, Kaprio J, et al: Causes and consequences of obesity: the contribution of recent twin studies, *Int J Obes (Lond)* 36(8):1017, 2012.
6. Malis C, Rasmussen EL, Foulsen P, et al: Total and regional fat distribution is strongly influenced by genetic factors in young and elderly twins, *Obesity Res* 13:2139, 2005. (Classic)
7. Tung YC, Yeo GS, O'Rahilly S, et al: Obesity and FTO: changing focus at a complex locus, *Cell Metab* 20(5):710, 2014.
8. Troke RC, Tan TM, Bloom SR: The future role of gut hormones in the treatment of obesity, *Ther Adv Chronic Dis* 5(1):4, 2014.
*9. Flegal KM, Kit BK, Orpana H, et al: Association of all-cause mortality with overweight and obesity using standard body mass index categories: a systematic review and meta-analysis, *JAMA* 309(1):71, 2013.
10. Lavie CJ, McAuley PA, Church TS, et al: Obesity and cardiovascular diseases: implications regarding fitness, fatness, and severity in the obesity paradox, *J Am Coll Cardiol* 63(14):1345, 2014.
11. Gregg EW, Zhuo X, Cheng YJ, et al: Trends in lifetime risk and years of life lost due to diabetes in the USA, 1985-2011: a modelling study, *Lancet Diabetes Endocrinol* 2(11):867, 2014.
12. Gallagher EJ, LeRoith D: Obesity and diabetes: the increased risk of cancer and cancer-related mortality, *Physiol Rev* 95(3):727, 2015.
13. Budd GM, Peterson JA: The obesity epidemic, Part 1: Understanding the origins, *AJN* 114:40, 2014.
*14. Jensen MD, Ryan DH, Donato KA, et al: Guidelines (2013) for managing overweight and obesity in adults, *Obesity* 22(S2):S1, 2014.
15. The National Weight Control Registry. NWCR facts. Retrieved from *www.nwcr.ws/Research/default.htm*.
16. Budd GM, Peterson JA: The obesity epidemic, Part 2: Nursing assessment and intervention, *AJN* 115:38, 2015.
17. Gudzune KA, Doshi RS, Mehta AK, et al. Efficacy of commercial weight-loss programs: an updated systematic review, *Ann Intern Med* 162(7):501, 2015.
18. Wee CC: The role of commercial weight-loss programs, *Ann Intern Med* 162(7):522, 2015.
19. Schumacher D: Pharmacological management of the obese patient, *Am J Lifestyle Med* 9(2):137, 2015.
*20. Apovian CM, Aronne LJ, Bessesen DH, et al: Pharmacological management of obesity: an Endocrine Society Clinical Practice Guideline, *J Clin Endocrinol Metab* 100(2):342, 2015.
21. Pucci A, Finer N: New medications for treatment of obesity: metabolic and cardiovascular effects, *Can J Cardiol* 31(2):142, 2015.
22. Dunham M: Caring for patients undergoing bariatric surgery, *Nursing* 43:43, 2013.
23. Gardner LA: Caring for Class III obese patients, *AJN* 113:66, 2013.
24. Idzik S, Troeleman N, Mielke A: Be prepared for bariatric patients in the OR, *OR Nurse J* 7:13, 2013.
25. Dietary Guidelines After Bariatric Surgery. Retrieved from *www.ucsfhealth.org/education/dietary_guidelines_after_gastric_bypass*.
26. National Heart, Lung, and Blood Institute. What is metabolic syndrome? Retrieved from *www.nhlbi.nih.gov/health/health-topics/topics/ms*.

*Evidence-based information for clinical practice.

41

Upper Gastrointestinal Problems

Paula P. Cox-North

As with stomachs, we should pity minds that do not eat.

Victor Hugo

http://evolve.elsevier.com/Lewis/medsurg/

LEARNING OUTCOMES

1. Describe the etiology, complications, interprofessional care, and nursing management of nausea and vomiting.
2. Describe the etiology, clinical manifestations, and treatment of common oral inflammations and infections.
3. Describe the etiology, clinical manifestations, complications, interprofessional care, and nursing management of oral cancer.
4. Explain the types, pathophysiology, clinical manifestations, complications, and interprofessional care (including surgical therapy and nursing management) of gastroesophageal reflux disease (GERD) and hiatal hernia.
5. Describe the pathophysiology, clinical manifestations, complications, and interprofessional care of esophageal cancer, diverticula, achalasia, and esophageal strictures.
6. Differentiate between acute and chronic gastritis, including the etiology, pathophysiology, interprofessional care, and nursing management.
7. Compare and contrast gastric and duodenal ulcers, including the etiology, pathophysiology, clinical manifestations, complications, interprofessional care, and nursing management.
8. Describe the clinical manifestations, interprofessional care, and nursing management of stomach cancer.
9. Explain the common etiologies, clinical manifestations, interprofessional care, and nursing management of upper gastrointestinal bleeding.
10. Identify common types of foodborne illnesses and nursing responsibilities related to food poisoning.

KEY TERMS

achalasia, p. 908
Barrett's esophagus, p. 901
dysphagia, p. 898
esophageal cancer, p. 905
esophageal diverticula, p. 907

esophagitis, p. 901
gastritis, p. 909
gastroesophageal reflux disease (GERD), p. 900
hiatal hernia, p. 904
Mallory-Weiss tear, p. 894

nausea, p. 893
peptic ulcer disease (PUD), p. 910
stomach (gastric) cancer, p. 919
stress-related mucosal disease (SRMD), p. 922
vomiting, p. 893

NAUSEA AND VOMITING

Nausea and vomiting are the most common manifestations of gastrointestinal (GI) disease. Although nausea and vomiting can occur independently, they are closely related and usually treated as one problem. **Nausea** is a feeling of discomfort in the epigastrium with a conscious desire to vomit. **Vomiting** is the forceful ejection of partially digested food and secretions *(emesis)* from the upper GI tract.

Etiology and Pathophysiology

Nausea and vomiting occur in a wide variety of GI disorders and in many conditions unrelated to GI disease. These include pregnancy; infection; central nervous system (CNS) disorders (e.g., meningitis, tumor); cardiovascular problems (e.g., myocardial infarction, heart failure); metabolic disorders (e.g., diabetes mellitus, Addison's disease, renal failure); postoperatively after general anesthesia; side effects of drugs (e.g.,

chemotherapy, opioids); psychologic factors (e.g., stress, fear); and conditions in which the GI tract becomes overly irritated, excited, or distended. Women are more likely to have nausea and vomiting associated with anesthesia and motion sickness.[1]

A vomiting center in the medulla coordinates the multiple components involved in vomiting. This center receives input from various stimuli. Neural impulses reach the vomiting center via afferent pathways through branches of the autonomic nervous system. Receptors for these afferent fibers are located in the GI tract, kidneys, heart, and uterus. When stimulated, these receptors relay information to the vomiting center, which then initiates the vomiting reflex (Fig. 41-1).

Vomiting is a complex act. It requires the coordinated activity of several structures: closure of the glottis, deep inspiration with contraction of the diaphragm in the inspiratory position, closure of the pylorus, relaxation of the stomach and lower esophageal sphincter (LES), and contraction of the abdominal muscles with increasing intraabdominal pressure. These

Reviewed by Susan C. Landis, RN, MN, Senior Lecturer, University of Washington School of Nursing, Seattle, Washington; Heidi E. Monroe, MSN, RN-BC, CPAN, CAPA, Assistant Professor of Nursing, Bellin College and Bellin Hospital, Green Bay, Wisconsin; Sarah Byram Poppe, MSN, ANP-BC, Nurse Practitioner, Gastroenterology Associates, Olympia, Washington; and Andrea H. Thurler, RN, DNP, FNP-BC, Nurse Practitioner, Massachusetts General Hospital, Harvard University, Massachusetts General Institute of Health Professions, Boston, Massachusetts.

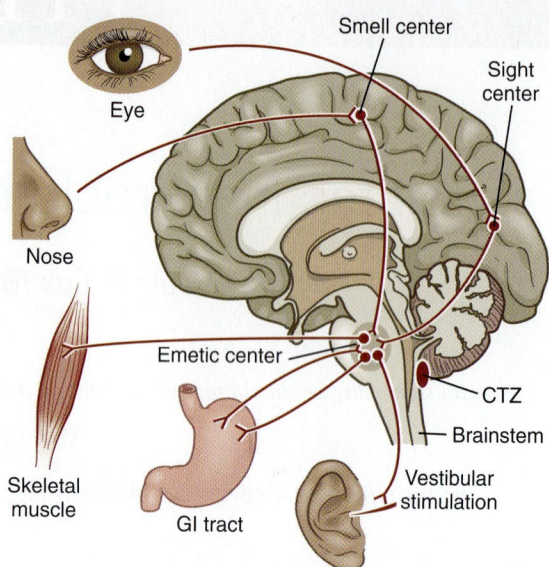

Eye

Smell center

Sight center

Nose

Emetic center

CTZ

Brainstem

Vestibular stimulation

Skeletal muscle

GI tract

FIG. 41-1 Stimuli involved in the act of vomiting. *CTZ*, Chemoreceptor trigger zone. (Modified from McKenry L, Tessier E, Hogan M: *Mosby's pharmacology in nursing*, ed 22, St Louis, 2006, Mosby.)

simultaneous activities force the stomach contents up through the esophagus, into the pharynx, and out the mouth.

The *chemoreceptor trigger zone* (CTZ) located in the brainstem responds to chemical stimuli from drugs, toxins, and labyrinthine stimulation (e.g., motion sickness). Once stimulated, the CTZ transmits impulses directly to the vomiting center. This action activates the autonomic nervous system, resulting in both parasympathetic and sympathetic stimulation. Sympathetic activation produces tachycardia, tachypnea, and diaphoresis. Parasympathetic stimulation causes relaxation of the LES, an increase in gastric motility, and a pronounced increase in salivation.

Clinical Manifestations

Nausea is a subjective complaint. *Anorexia* (lack of appetite) usually accompanies nausea. When nausea and vomiting occur over a long period, dehydration can develop rapidly. Water and essential electrolytes (e.g., potassium, sodium, chloride, hydrogen) are lost. As vomiting persists, the patient may have severe electrolyte imbalances, extracellular fluid volume loss, decreased plasma volume, and eventually circulatory failure.

Metabolic alkalosis can result from loss of gastric hydrochloric (HCl) acid. When contents of the small intestine are vomited, metabolic acidosis can occur. However, metabolic acidosis is less common than metabolic alkalosis. Weight loss resulting from fluid loss can occur in a short time with severe vomiting.

Interprofessional Care

The goals of interprofessional care are to determine and treat the underlying cause of the nausea and vomiting and provide symptomatic relief. Assess the patient for precipitating factors, and describe the contents of the emesis.

It is important to differentiate among vomiting, regurgitation, and projectile vomiting. *Regurgitation* is an effortless process in which partially digested food slowly comes up from the stomach. Retching or vomiting rarely occurs before it. *Projectile vomiting* is a forceful expulsion of stomach contents

without nausea. It is characteristic of CNS (brain and spinal cord) tumors.

Emesis containing partially digested food several hours after a meal indicates gastric outlet obstruction or delayed gastric emptying. The presence of fecal odor and bile after prolonged vomiting suggests intestinal obstruction below the level of the pylorus. Bile in the emesis suggests obstruction below the ampulla of Vater.

The color of the emesis aids in identifying the presence and source of any bleeding. Bright red blood indicates active bleeding. This could be due to a **Mallory-Weiss tear** (disruption of the mucosal lining near the esophagogastric junction), esophageal varices, gastric or duodenal ulcer, or cancer. Vomitus with a "coffee-ground" appearance is related to gastric bleeding. The blood changes to dark brown because of its interaction with HCl acid.

The timing of nausea and vomiting can help determine its cause. Early morning vomiting is common in pregnancy. Emotional stressors with no evident pathologic disorder may elicit vomiting during or immediately after eating. Those with *cyclic vomiting syndrome* have recurring episodes of nausea, vomiting, and fatigue that last from a few hours up to 10 days.

Drug Therapy. The use of drugs to treat nausea and vomiting depends on the cause of the problem (Table 41-1). Many antiemetic drugs act in the CNS via the CTZ to block the neurochemicals that trigger nausea and vomiting. Because the cause cannot always be readily determined, use drugs with caution. Using antiemetics before determining the cause can mask the underlying disease process and delay diagnosis and treatment.

> **DRUG ALERT**   **Promethazine Injection**
> - Do not administer into an artery or under the skin because of the risk of severe tissue injury, including gangrene.
> - When given IV, it can leach out of the vein and cause serious damage to surrounding tissue.
> - Deep muscle injection is the preferred route of injection administration.

> **DRUG ALERT**   **Metoclopramide (Reglan)**
> - Chronic use or high doses carry the risk of tardive dyskinesia.
> - Tardive dyskinesia is a neurologic condition characterized by involuntary and repetitive movements of the body (e.g., extremity movements, lip smacking).
> - Tardive dyskinesia may persist after discontinuing the drug.

Serotonin (5-HT$_3$) receptor antagonists are effective in reducing chemotherapy-induced vomiting caused by delayed gastric emptying and nausea and vomiting related to migraine headache, anesthesia, and anxiety.[2] They are effective in preventing and treating postoperative nausea and vomiting. Dexamethasone is given in combination with other antiemetics to manage acute and delayed chemotherapy-induced vomiting. Aprepitant (Emend) and rolapitant (Varubi), neurokinin-1 receptor antagonists (NK$_1$RA), are used to prevent chemotherapy-induced and postoperative nausea and vomiting.

Dronabinol (Marinol) is an orally active cannabinoid. It is used alone or in combination with other antiemetics for preventing chemotherapy-induced vomiting. Because of the potential for abuse as well as drowsiness and sedation, it is used only when other therapies are not effective.

Nutritional Therapy. The patient with severe vomiting requires IV fluid therapy with electrolyte and glucose replacement until able to tolerate oral intake. Some patients may need a nasogastric (NG) tube and suction to decompress the stomach. Start oral nutrition beginning with clear liquids once symptoms

TABLE 41-1   Drug Therapy
Nausea and Vomiting

Drug	Mechanism of Action	Side Effects
Serotonin (5-HT₃) Antagonists dolasetron (Anzemet) granisetron ondansetron (Zofran) palonosetron (Aloxi)	Block action of serotonin (causes nausea and vomiting)	Constipation, diarrhea, headache, fatigue, malaise, elevated liver function tests
Phenothiazines chlorpromazine perphenazine prochlorperazine trifluoperazine promethazine	Act in the CNS level of the chemoreceptor trigger zone (CTZ) Block dopamine receptors that trigger nausea and vomiting	Dry mouth, hypotension, sedative effects, rashes, constipation
Antihistamines meclizine (Antivert) dimenhydrinate (Dramamine) hydroxyzine (Vistaril) diphenhydramine	Block histamine receptors that trigger nausea and vomiting	Dry mouth, hypotension, sedative effects, rashes, constipation
Prokinetic Agents metoclopramide (Reglan)	Inhibit action of dopamine ↑ Gastric motility and emptying	CNS side effects ranging from anxiety to hallucinations Extrapyramidal side effects, including tremor and dyskinesias (similar to Parkinson's disease)
Anticholinergic (Antimuscarinic) scopolamine transdermal trimethobenzamide (Tigan)	Block cholinergic pathways to vomiting center	Xerostomia, somnolence
Butyrophenone droperidol	Block neurochemicals that trigger nausea and vomiting	Dry mouth, hypotension, sedative effects, rashes, constipation
Neurokinin-1 Receptor Antagonist aprepitant (Emend) netupitant and palonosetron (Akynzeo) rolapitant (Varubi)	Block interaction of Substance P at NK-1 receptor preventing nausea and vomiting	Headache, hiccups, fatigue, constipation, diarrhea, anorexia
Corticosteroids dexamethasone	Not well understood how it prevents nausea and vomiting	Hyperglycemia, insomnia, euphoria
Cannabinoids dronabinol (Marinol) nabilone (Cesamet)	Inhibit vomiting control mechanism in the medulla oblongata	Xerostomia, amnesia, ataxia, confusion, coordination problems, dizziness, and somnolence

have subsided. Water is the initial fluid of choice for oral rehydration. Have the patient sip small amounts of fluid (5 to 15 mL) every 15 to 20 minutes. Other options include carbonated beverages with the carbonation removed at room temperature and warm tea. Extremely hot or cold liquids are often difficult to tolerate. Broth and sports drinks (e.g., Gatorade) are high in sodium, so give them with caution. Dry toast or crackers may be helpful.

As the patient's condition improves, provide a diet high in carbohydrates and low in fat. Items such as a baked potato, plain gelatin, rice, and cereal are ideal. Many patients do not tolerate coffee, spicy foods, highly acidic foods, and those with strong odors. Tell the patient to eat food slowly and in small amounts to prevent overdistending the stomach. Liquids taken between meals rather than with meals also reduce overdistention. Consult a dietitian about nutritious foods that are well tolerated by the patient.

Nondrug Therapy. For some patients, acupressure or acupuncture at specific points is effective in reducing postoperative nausea and vomiting.[3] Some patients use herbs such as ginger and peppermint oil. Relaxation breathing exercises, changes in body position, or exercise may help some patients.

🌿 COMPLEMENTARY & ALTERNATIVE THERAPIES
Ginger

Scientific Evidence
- May be effective for nausea and vomiting of pregnancy when used at recommended doses for short periods
- If taken 1 hr before surgery, may reduce nausea and vomiting for up to 24 hr

Nursing Implications
- Few adverse effects reported with short-term use
- May inhibit platelet aggregation and increase risk of bleeding
- Possibly lowers blood glucose levels

Source: Based on a systematic review of scientific literature. Retrieved from www.nlm.nih.gov/medlineplus/druginfo/natural/961.html.

❖ NURSING MANAGEMENT: NAUSEA AND VOMITING
◆ Nursing Assessment

Each patient with a history of prolonged and persistent nausea or vomiting requires a thorough nursing assessment before you

TABLE 41-2   Nursing Assessment
Nausea and Vomiting

Subjective Data
Important Health Information
Past health history: GI disorders, chronic indigestion, food allergies, pregnancy, infection, CNS disorders, recent travel, eating disorders, metabolic disorders, cancer, cardiovascular disease, renal disease
Medications: Antiemetics, digitalis, opioids, ferrous sulfate, aspirin, aminophylline, alcohol, antibiotics, chemotherapy. General anesthesia.
Surgery or other treatments: Recent surgery

Functional Health Patterns
Nutritional-metabolic: Amount, frequency, character, and color of vomitus. Dry heaves. Anorexia, weight loss
Activity-exercise: Weakness, fatigue
Cognitive-perceptual: Abdominal tenderness or pain
Coping–stress tolerance: Stress, fear

Objective Data
General
Lethargy, sunken eyeballs

Integumentary
Pallor, dry mucous membranes, poor skin turgor

Gastrointestinal
Amount, frequency, character (e.g., projectile), content (undigested food, blood, bile, feces), and color of vomitus (red, "coffee ground," green-yellow)

Urinary
Decreased output, concentrated urine

Possible Diagnostic Findings
Altered serum electrolytes (especially hypokalemia), metabolic alkalosis, abnormal upper GI findings on endoscopy or abdominal x-rays

develop a specific plan of care. Although many conditions are associated with nausea and vomiting, you should have a basic understanding of the common conditions and be able to identify the patient who is at high risk. Knowing the physiologic mechanisms involved in nausea and vomiting is important in the assessment process. Table 41-2 presents subjective and objective data to obtain from a patient with nausea and vomiting.

◆ Nursing Diagnoses
Nursing diagnoses for the patient with nausea and vomiting may include, but are not limited to, the following:
- Nausea *related to* multiple etiologies
- Deficient fluid volume *related to* prolonged vomiting
- Imbalanced nutrition: less than body requirements *related to* nausea and vomiting

Additional information on nursing diagnoses is presented in eNursing Care Plan 41-1 (available on the website for this chapter).

◆ Planning
The overall goals are that the patient with nausea and vomiting will (1) experience minimal or no nausea and vomiting, (2) have normal electrolyte levels and hydration status, and

(3) return to a normal pattern of fluid balance and nutrient intake.

◆ Nursing Implementation
◆ Acute Care.
Most people with nausea and vomiting remain at home. When nausea and vomiting persist, hospitalization may be necessary for diagnosis of the underlying problem. Until a diagnosis is confirmed, the patient is on nothing-by-mouth (NPO) status and given IV fluids. The patient with persistent vomiting, a possible bowel obstruction, or paralytic ileus may need an NG connected to suction. Secure the NG tube to prevent its movement in the nose and back of the throat, because this can stimulate nausea and vomiting.

With prolonged vomiting, there is a chance of dehydration and acid-base and electrolyte imbalances. Record intake and output, monitor vital signs, and assess for signs of dehydration. Provide physical and emotional support. Maintain a quiet, odor-free environment. Observe for changes in the patient's physical comfort and mentation. The risk of pulmonary aspiration is a concern when vomiting occurs in older or unconscious patients or in patients with conditions that impair the gag reflex. To prevent aspiration, put the patient who cannot adequately manage self-care in a semi-Fowler's or side-lying position.

? CHECK YOUR PRACTICE

You are caring for a newly admitted 76-yr-old man who reports vomiting for the past 3 days. He says, "I cannot keep anything down, not even water."
- What assessment findings do you need to monitor in this man?
- What findings would indicate that he is experiencing dehydration?
- What are your priority nursing interventions for him?

◆ Ambulatory Care.
Teach the patient and caregiver (1) how to manage the unpleasant sensation of nausea, (2) methods to prevent nausea and vomiting, and (3) strategies to maintain fluid and nutritional intake. Tell them to keep the immediate environment quiet, free of noxious odors, and well ventilated. Avoiding sudden changes of position and unnecessary activity are helpful. Encourage the use of relaxation techniques, frequent rest periods, effective pain management strategies, and diversional tactics. Cleansing the face and hands with a cool washcloth and providing mouth care between episodes increase the person's comfort level. When symptoms occur, stop all foods and drugs until the acute phase is over.

If you suspect a medication is the cause, notify the HCP immediately. The HCP can change the drug dose or prescribe a new drug. Advise the patient that stopping the drug without consulting the HCP may have detrimental effects on the person's health. The patient should take an antiemetic drug only if prescribed by the HCP. Taking over-the-counter (OTC) drugs to relieve symptoms may make the problem worse.

When food is the precipitating cause of nausea and vomiting, help the patient identify the specific food. Determine when it was eaten, prior history with the food, and whether anyone else who ate the food is sick. A patient may be reluctant to resume fluid intake because of fear of symptoms recurring. Suggest that he or she begin with clear liquids or cola beverages, sports drinks (e.g., Gatorade), tea or broth, dry crackers or toast, and plain gelatin. Bland foods, such as cereal, rice, baked potato, and cooked chicken, are generally tolerated in small amounts.

◆ Evaluation

The expected outcomes are that the patient with nausea and vomiting will
- Be comfortable with minimal or no nausea and vomiting
- Have electrolyte levels within normal range
- Be able to maintain adequate intake of fluids and nutrients

Gerontologic Considerations: Nausea and Vomiting

The older adult experiencing nausea and vomiting requires careful assessment and monitoring, particularly during periods of fluid loss and subsequent rehydration therapy. Older patients are more likely to have cardiac or renal insufficiency that places them at greater risk for life-threatening fluid and electrolyte imbalances. Excessive fluid and electrolytes replacement may result in adverse consequences for a person with heart failure or renal disease. The older adult with a decreased level of consciousness is at high risk for aspirating vomitus. Close monitoring of the patient's physical status and level of consciousness during episodes of vomiting is important.

Older adults are particularly susceptible to the CNS side effects of antiemetic drugs. These drugs may produce confusion and increase their risk for falls. Dosages should be reduced and efficacy closely evaluated. Use safety precautions for these patients (e.g., removing rugs that may cause slipping).

ORAL INFLAMMATION AND INFECTIONS

Oral inflammation and infections may be due to specific mouth diseases or secondary to systemic disorders such as leukemia or vitamin deficiency. Common inflammations and infections of the oral cavity are presented in Table 41-3. The patient who is immunosuppressed (e.g., receiving chemotherapy for cancer) or using corticosteroid inhalant treatment for asthma is at risk for oral infections (e.g., candidiasis). Oral infections may predispose the patient to infections in other body organs. For example, the oral cavity is a potential reservoir for respiratory pathogens. Oral pathogens have been associated with diabetes and heart disease.[4]

Managing these conditions focuses on identifying the cause, eliminating infection, providing comfort measures, and maintaining nutritional intake. Oral inflammation and infections can severely impair oral ingestion. Regular and good oral and dental hygiene reduces oral infections and inflammation.

TABLE 41-3 Infections and Inflammation of the Mouth

Infection or Inflammation	Etiology	Manifestations	Treatment
Gingivitis	• Neglected oral hygiene, malocclusion, missing or irregular teeth, faulty dentistry • Eating of soft rather than fibrous foods	• Inflamed gingivae and interdental papillae • Bleeding during tooth brushing • Development of pus, formation of abscess with loosening of teeth (periodontitis)	• Prevention through health teaching, dental care, gingival massage, professional cleaning of teeth • Eat fibrous foods • Conscientious brushing habits with flossing
Vincent's infection (acute necrotizing ulcerative gingivitis, trench mouth)	• Fusiform bacteria, Vincent spirochetes • Predisposing factors of stress, excessive fatigue, poor oral hygiene • Nutritional deficiencies (B and C vitamins)	• Painful, bleeding gingivae • Eroding necrotic lesions of interdental papillae • Ulcerations that bleed • Increased saliva with metallic taste, fetid mouth odor • Anorexia, fever, general malaise	• Rest (physical and mental) • Avoidance of smoking and alcohol • Soft, nutritious diet • Correct oral hygiene habits • Topical applications of antibiotics • Mouth irrigations with chlorhexidine (Hibiclens) and saline solutions
Oral candidiasis (moniliasis or thrush)	• *Candida albicans* (a yeastlike fungus) • Debilitation • Prolonged high-dose antibiotic or corticosteroid therapy	• Pearly, bluish white "milk-curd" membranous lesions on mucosa of mouth and larynx • Sore mouth, yeasty halitosis	• Miconazole buccal tablets (Oravig) • Nystatin or amphotericin B as oral suspension or buccal tablets • Good oral hygiene
Herpes simplex (cold sore, fever blister) (see Table 23-6)	• Herpes simplex virus (type 1 or 2) • Predisposing factors of upper respiratory tract infections, excessive exposure to sunlight, food allergies, emotional tension, onset of menstruation	• Lip lesions, mouth lesions, vesicle formation (single or clustered) • Shallow, painful ulcers	• Spirits of camphor, corticosteroid cream, mild antiseptic mouthwash, viscous lidocaine • Removal or control of predisposing factors • Antiviral agents (e.g., acyclovir [Zovirax], famciclovir [Famvir], valacyclovir [Valtrex])
Aphthous stomatitis (canker sore)	• Recurrent and chronic form of infection • Secondary to systemic disease, trauma, stress, or unknown causes	• Ulcers of mouth and lips, causing extreme pain • Ulcers surrounded by erythematous base	• Corticosteroids (topical or systemic) • Tetracycline oral suspension
Parotitis (inflammation of parotid gland, surgical mumps)	• *Staphylococcus* species usually • *Streptococcus* species occasionally • Debilitation and dehydration with poor oral hygiene • Extended NPO status	• Pain in area of gland and ear • Absence of salivation • Purulent exudate from gland, erythema, ulcers	• Antibiotics, mouthwashes, warm compresses • Preventive measures such as chewing gum, sucking on hard candy (lemon drops) • Adequate fluid intake
Stomatitis (inflammation of mouth)	• Trauma, pathogens, irritants (tobacco, alcohol) • Renal, liver, and hematologic diseases • Side effect of chemotherapy and radiation	• Excessive salivation • Halitosis • Sore mouth	• Removal or treatment of cause • Oral hygiene with soothing solutions, topical medications • Soft, bland diet

ORAL CANCER

There are two types of oral cancer: *oral cavity cancer,* which starts in the mouth, and *oropharyngeal cancer,* which develops in the part of the throat just behind the mouth (the oropharynx). *Head and neck squamous cell carcinoma* (HNSCC) is a broad term used for cancers of the oral cavity, pharynx, and larynx, which account for 90% of malignant oral tumors. Annually 42,440 Americans are diagnosed with oral cancer. An estimated 8,390 people die from the disease.[5]

Oral cancer is more prevalent in African American men, and their survival rate is lower than that of white men. Oral cancer is more common after age 35. The average age at diagnosis is 65 years. It is two times more common in men than in women. The 5-year survival rate is 83% for localized cancer and 61% for all stages of cancer of the oral cavity and pharynx combined.[5]

Most oral cancer lesions occur on the lower lip. Other common sites are the lateral border and undersurface of the tongue, labial commissure, and buccal mucosa. Lip cancer has the most favorable prognosis of any of the oral tumors. The visibility of lip lesions usually leads to an earlier diagnosis.

Etiology and Pathophysiology

Although the definitive cause of oral cancer is unknown, it has a number of predisposing factors (Table 41-4). Of those with

CULTURAL & ETHNIC HEALTH DISPARITIES
Oral, Pharyngeal, and Esophageal Problems

Nausea and Vomiting
- Asian Americans, Middle Easterners, and African Americans are more likely to experience nausea and vomiting than whites.

Cancers of Oral Cavity and Pharynx
- Incidence and mortality rates are higher in African American men than in whites.
- Death rates from oral cancer are decreasing in whites but increasing in nonwhites.

Esophageal Cancer
- Highest incidence is in non-Hispanic white men.
- Higher incidence occurs in Alaska Natives than in whites.

Stomach Cancer
- Asian Americans and Pacific Islanders, Hispanics, and African Americans have higher rates of stomach cancer than non-Hispanic whites.
- Asian Americans show significantly higher survival rates than other ethnic groups.

oral cancer, 75% to 90% report either using tobacco or a history of frequent alcohol consumption. More than 30% of patients with cancer of the lip have outdoor occupations, indicating that prolonged exposure to sunlight is a risk factor. Irritation from the pipe stem resting on the lip is a factor in pipe smokers. Human papillomavirus (HPV) contributes to 25% of oral cancer cases.[5] HPV-associated oropharyngeal cancer is associated with multiple sexual partners, especially multiple oral sex partners.[6]

Clinical Manifestations

The common manifestations of oral cancer are shown in Table 41-4. Patients may report nonspecific symptoms such as chronic sore throat, sore mouth, and voice changes. *Leukoplakia,* called "smoker's patch," is a white patch on the mouth mucosa or tongue. It is a precancerous lesion, although less than 15% actually transform into cancer cells. The patch becomes *keratinized* (hard and leathery) and is sometimes described as hyperkeratosis. Leukoplakia is the result of chronic irritation, especially from smoking. *Erythroplasia* (erythroplakia), which is a red velvety patch on the mouth or tongue, is another precancerous lesion. More than 50% of cases of erythroplakia progress to squamous cell carcinoma. About 30% of patients with oral cancer have an asymptomatic neck mass.

Cancer of the lip usually appears as an indurated, painless ulcer on the lip. The first sign of cancer of the tongue is an ulcer or area of thickening. Soreness or pain of the tongue may occur, especially when eating hot or highly seasoned foods. Lesions are most likely to develop in the proximal half of the tongue. Some patients have limited tongue movement. Later symptoms of cancer of the tongue include increased salivation, slurred speech, dysphagia (difficulty swallowing), toothache, and earache.

Diagnostic Studies

Diagnostic tests are done to identify oral dysplasias, which are precursors to oral cancer (Table 41-5). Oral exfoliative cytologic

TABLE 41-5   Interprofessional Care
Oral Cancer

Diagnostic Assessment	Management

• History and physical examination
• Biopsy
• Oral exfoliative cytology
• Toluidine blue test
• CT, MRI, PET
	• Surgical therapy
	  • Surgical excision of the tumor
	  • Radical neck dissection
	• Radiation (internal or external) therapy
	• Combined surgical and radiation therapy
	• Chemotherapy

TABLE 41-4   Types and Characteristics of Oral Cancer

Location	Predisposing Factors	Clinical Manifestations	Treatment
Lip	Constant overexposure to sun, ruddy and fair complexion, recurrent herpetic lesions, irritation from pipe stem, syphilis, immunosuppression	Indurated, painless ulcer	Surgical excision, radiation
Tongue	Tobacco, alcohol, chronic irritation, syphilis	Ulcer or area of thickening, soreness or pain Increased salivation, slurred speech, dysphagia, toothache, earache (later signs)	Surgery (hemiglossectomy or glossectomy), radiation
Oral cavity	Poor oral hygiene, tobacco usage (pipe and cigar smoking, snuff, chewing tobacco), chronic alcohol intake, chronic irritation (jagged tooth, ill-fitting prosthesis, chemical or mechanical irritants), human papillomavirus (HPV)	Leukoplakia, erythroplakia, ulcerations, sore spot, rough area, pain, dysphagia, a lump or thickening in the cheek A sore throat or a feeling that something is stuck Difficulty chewing and speaking (later signs)	Surgery (mandibulectomy, radical neck dissection, resection of buccal mucosa), internal and external radiation

study involves scraping the suspicious lesion and spreading the scraping on a slide for microscopic examination. The toluidine blue test is a screening test for oral cancer. When toluidine blue is applied topically to stain an area, cancer cells preferentially take up the dye. A negative cytologic smear or negative toluidine blue test does not necessarily rule out a malignant condition. Once cancer is diagnosed, CT scan, MRI, and positron emission tomography (PET) are used for staging of the cancer.[7]

Interprofessional Care

Management of the patient with oral cancer usually consists of surgery, radiation, chemotherapy, or a combination of these. The curative treatments are usually surgery and radiation.

Surgical Therapy. Surgery remains the most effective treatment, especially for early-stage disease. The procedure done depends on the location and extent of the tumor. Some patients with small tumors in the mouth and throat are candidates for minimally invasive robotic-assisted surgery. However, many of the operations are radical procedures involving extensive resections. Some examples are partial *mandibulectomy* (removal of the mandible), *hemiglossectomy* (removal of half of the tongue), *glossectomy* (removal of the tongue), resections of the buccal mucosa and floor of the mouth, and radical neck dissection.

Radical neck dissection includes wide excision of the primary lesion with removal of the regional lymph nodes, the deep cervical lymph nodes, and their lymphatic channels. The following structures are removed or transected depending on the extent of the primary lesion: sternocleidomastoid muscle and other closely associated muscles, internal jugular vein, mandible, submaxillary gland, part of the thyroid and parathyroid glands, and spinal accessory nerve. The patient usually has a tracheostomy. Drainage tubes are inserted into the surgical area and connected to suction to remove fluid and blood. (Head and neck surgery is described in more detail in Chapter 26.)

Nonsurgical Therapy. Radiation therapy may be used alone to treat small cancers or when lesions cannot be removed. Patients usually do not have radiation before surgery because it is difficult to remove radiated tissue. The tissue becomes fibrotic and heals slower.[8] Most patients begin radiation about 6 weeks after surgery.

Chemotherapy can shrink lesions before surgery, decrease metastasis, sensitize cancer cells to radiation, or treat distant metastases. Chemotherapy drugs include 5-fluorouracil (5-FU), methotrexate, cisplatin, carboplatin, paclitaxel, docetaxel, ifosfamide (Ifex), and bleomycin. A commonly used combination is cisplatin and 5-FU. This combination is more effective than either drug alone. (Chemotherapy is discussed in Chapter 15.)

Palliative treatment is the best management when the prognosis is poor, the cancer is inoperable, or the patient decides against surgery. Palliation aims to treat the symptoms and make the patient more comfortable. If it becomes difficult for the patient to swallow, placing a gastrostomy tube will allow for adequate nutritional intake. Give analgesic medications freely. Frequent suctioning of the oral cavity is necessary when swallowing becomes difficult. (Other palliative and end-of-life nursing measures are discussed in Chapter 9.)

Nutritional Therapy. Many patients are malnourished before surgery. They may require placement of a percutaneous endoscopic gastrostomy (PEG) and enteral nutrition before radiation treatment or surgery. After radical neck surgery, the patient may be unable to ingest nutrients orally because of mucositis, swelling, location of sutures, or difficulty swallowing. Parenteral fluids are given for the first 24 to 48 hours. After that time, enteral nutrition is given via NG, gastrostomy, or jejunostomy. (See Chapter 39 for information on PEG and parenteral and enteral feedings.) Cervical esophagostomy and pharyngostomy are options for some patients.

Observe for feeding tolerance and adjust the amount, time, and formula if nausea, vomiting, diarrhea, or distention occurs. Give small amounts of water when the patient can swallow. Observe for choking. Suctioning may be necessary to prevent aspiration.

❖ NURSING MANAGEMENT: ORAL CANCER

◆ Nursing Assessment

Subjective and objective data to obtain from a patient with oral cancer are presented in Table 41-6.

◆ Nursing Diagnoses

Nursing diagnoses for the patient with oral cancer may include, but are not limited to, the following:

- Imbalanced nutrition: less than body requirements *related to* oral pain, difficulty chewing and swallowing, surgical resection, and radiation treatment
- Chronic pain *related to* the tumor, surgery, or radiation
- Anxiety *related to* diagnosis of cancer, uncertain future, potential for disfiguring surgery, and prognosis

◆ Planning

The overall goals are that the patient with cancer of the oral cavity will (1) have a patent airway, (2) be able to communicate, (3) have adequate nutritional intake to promote wound healing, and (4) have relief of pain and discomfort.

TABLE 41-6 Nursing Assessment

Oral Cancer

Subjective Data

Important Health Information

Past health history: Recurrent oral herpetic lesions, human papillomavirus (HPV) infection or vaccination, syphilis, exposure to sunlight
Medications: Immunosuppressants
Surgery or other treatments: Removal of prior tumors or lesions

Functional Health Patterns

Health perception–health management: Use of alcohol and tobacco, pipe smoking. Poor oral hygiene
Nutritional-metabolic: Reductions in oral intake, weight loss, difficulty chewing food, increased salivation, intolerance to certain foods or temperatures of food
Cognitive-perceptual: Mouth or tongue soreness or pain, toothache, earache, neck stiffness, dysphagia, difficulty speaking

Objective Data

Integumentary

Indurated, painless ulcer on lip. Painless neck mass

Gastrointestinal

Areas of thickening or roughness, ulcers, leukoplakia, or erythroplakia on the tongue or oral mucosa. Limited movement of the tongue. Increased salivation, drooling. Slurred speech. Foul breath odor

Possible Diagnostic Findings

Positive exfoliative smear cytology (microscopic examination of cells removed by scraping), positive biopsy

◆ **Nursing Implementation**

You have a significant role in early detection and treatment of oral cancer. Identify patients at risk (Table 41-4) and provide information about predisposing factors. Inform the patient who smokes about smoking cessation programs available in the community. Warn adolescents and teenagers about the danger of using snuff or chewing tobacco. (Smoking cessation is discussed in Chapter 10 and Tables 10-3 to 10-6.)

Because early detection of oral cancer is important, teach the patient to report unexplained pain or soreness of the mouth, unusual bleeding, dysphagia, sore throat, voice changes, or swelling or lump in the neck. Refer any person with an ulcerative lesion that does not heal within 2 to 3 weeks to the HCP.

Preoperative care for the patient who will have a radical neck dissection must consider the patient's physical and psychosocial needs. Physical preparation is the same as that for any major surgery, with special emphasis on oral hygiene. Explanations and emotional support should include information on postoperative communication and feeding. Explain the surgical procedure, and ensure that the patient understands the information. (See Chapter 26 and eNursing Care Plan 26-2 for more information about the nursing management of a patient undergoing a radical neck dissection).

◆ **Evaluation**

The expected outcomes are that the patient with oral cancer will
- Have no respiratory complications
- Be able to communicate
- Maintain an adequate nutritional intake to promote wound healing
- Experience minimal pain and discomfort with eating, drinking, and talking

ESOPHAGEAL DISORDERS

GASTROESOPHAGEAL REFLUX DISEASE

Gastroesophageal reflux disease (GERD) is a chronic symptom of mucosal damage caused by reflux of stomach acid into the lower esophagus. GERD is not a disease but a syndrome. GERD is the most common upper GI problem. Approximately 10% to 20% of the U.S. population experience GERD symptoms (heartburn or regurgitation) at least once a week.[9]

Etiology and Pathophysiology

GERD has no one single cause (Fig. 41-2). GERD results when the reflux of acidic gastric contents into the esophagus overwhelms the esophageal defenses. Gastric HCl acid and pepsin secretions in reflux cause esophageal irritation and inflammation (esophagitis). If the reflux contains intestinal

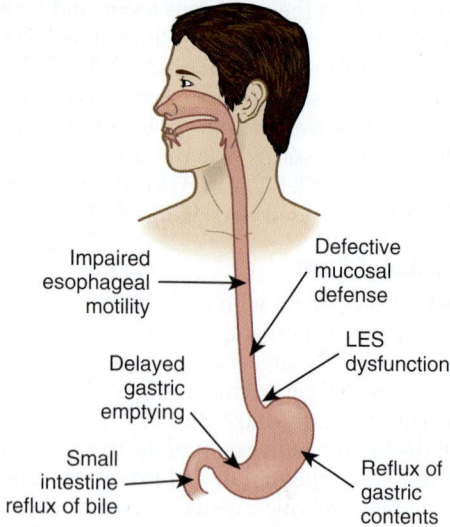

FIG. 41-2 Factors involved in the pathogenesis of gastroesophageal reflux disease (GERD). *LES,* Lower esophageal sphincter.

TABLE 41-7	**Factors Affecting Lower Esophageal Sphincter Pressure**
Increase Pressure	• Tea, coffee (caffeine)
• bethanechol (Urecholine)	• Drugs
• metoclopramide (Reglan)	• Anticholinergics
	• β-Adrenergic blockers
Decrease Pressure	• Calcium channel blockers
• Alcohol	• Diazepam (Valium)
• Chocolate (theobromine)	• Morphine sulfate
• Fatty foods	• Nitrates
• Nicotine	• Progesterone
• Peppermint, spearmint	• Theophylline

proteolytic enzymes (e.g., trypsin) and bile, this further irritates the esophageal mucosa. The degree of inflammation depends on the amount and composition of the gastric reflux and on the esophagus's mucosal defense mechanisms.

One of the primary etiologic factors in GERD is an incompetent LES. Under normal conditions, the LES acts as an antireflux barrier. An incompetent LES lets gastric contents move from the stomach to the esophagus when the patient is supine or has an increase in intraabdominal pressure.

Decreased LES pressure can be due to certain foods and drugs (Table 41-7). Obesity is a risk factor for GERD.[10] In an obese person the intraabdominal pressure is increased, which can exacerbate GERD. Cigarette and cigar smoking can contribute to GERD. Hiatal hernia, discussed in the next section, commonly causes GERD.

Clinical Manifestations

The symptoms of GERD vary from person to person. The persistence of mild symptoms (i.e., more than twice a week) or moderate to severe symptoms once a week is considered GERD.

Heartburn *(pyrosis)* is the most common manifestation. Heartburn is a burning, tight sensation felt intermittently beneath the lower sternum and spreading upward to the throat or jaw. It may occur after ingesting food or drugs that decrease the LES pressure or directly irritate the esophageal mucosa. An HCP should evaluate heartburn that occurs more than twice a week, is severe, is associated with dysphagia, or occurs at night and wakes a person from sleep. Older adults who complain of recent onset of heartburn should receive medical evaluation.

Patients may complain of dyspepsia or regurgitation. *Dyspepsia* is pain or discomfort centered in the upper abdomen (mainly in or around the midline as opposed to the right or left hypochondrium). Regurgitation is often described as hot, bitter, or sour liquid coming into the throat or mouth.

A person with GERD may report respiratory symptoms, including wheezing, coughing, and dyspnea. Nocturnal discomfort and coughing can awaken the person, resulting in disturbed sleep patterns. Otolaryngologic symptoms include hoarseness, sore throat, a *globus sensation* (sense of a lump in the throat), hypersalivation, and choking.

GERD-related chest pain can mimic angina. It is described as burning; squeezing; or radiating to the back, neck, jaw, or arms. Complaints of chest pain are more common in older adults with GERD. Unlike angina, GERD-related chest pain is relieved with antacids.

Complications

Complications of GERD are due to the direct local effects of gastric acid on the esophageal mucosa. **Esophagitis** (inflammation of the esophagus) is a common complication of GERD. Esophagitis with esophageal ulcerations is shown in Fig. 41-3. Repeated esophagitis may lead to scar tissue formation, stricture, and dysphagia.

Another complication of chronic GERD is **Barrett's esophagus** (esophageal metaplasia). *Metaplasia* is the reversible change from one type of cell to another type because of an abnormal stimulus. In Barrett's esophagus, the flat epithelial cells in the distal esophagus change into columnar epithelial cells. These cell changes are primarily due to GERD. However, some people with no history of GERD develop Barrett's esophagus.

Barrett's esophagus is a precancerous lesion that increases the patient's risk for esophageal adenocarcinoma. About 5% to 20% of people with chronic GERD have Barrett's esophagus.[11] Compared with whites, African Americans and Asians are at lower risk for Barrett's esophagus. Because of the risk for esophageal cancer, a surveillance endoscopy every 2 to 3 years or radiofrequency ablation is recommended.[11]

Respiratory complications of GERD include cough, bronchospasm, laryngospasm, and cricopharyngeal spasm. These complications are due to gastric secretions irritating the upper airway. Asthma, chronic bronchitis, and pneumonia may develop from aspiration into the respiratory system. Dental erosion, especially in the posterior teeth, may result from acid reflux into the mouth.[12]

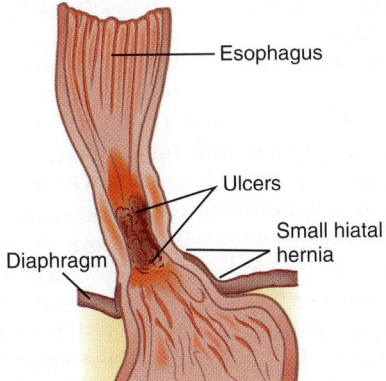

FIG. 41-3 Esophagitis with esophageal ulcerations.

Diagnostic Studies

GERD is usually diagnosed based on symptoms and the patient's response to behavioral and drug therapies. Diagnostic tests are done when usual therapy is ineffective or when complications are suspected. Diagnostic studies done to determine the cause of the GERD are shown in Table 41-8.

Endoscopy is useful in assessing the LES competence and the degree of inflammation (if present), potential scarring, and strictures. Biopsy and cytologic specimens can be used to distinguish stomach or esophageal cancer from Barrett's esophagus. In addition, the degree of dysplasia (low grade versus high grade) is determined. Manometric studies measure pressure in the esophagus and LES and esophageal motility function. Ambulatory esophageal pH monitoring may be done for patients with refractory symptoms and no evidence of mucosal inflammation. Radionuclide tests can detect reflux of gastric contents and the rate of esophageal clearance.

Interprofessional Care

Most patients with GERD can successfully manage the condition through lifestyle modifications and drug therapy. These approaches require patient teaching and adherence to therapies. When these therapies are ineffective, surgery is an option (Table 41-8).

Lifestyle Modifications. Teach the patient with GERD to avoid factors that trigger symptoms. Give particular attention to food and drugs that may affect the LES, acid secretion, or gastric emptying. Recommend weight reduction if the patient is overweight. A patient and caregiver teaching guide is provided in Table 41-9.

Encourage patients who smoke to stop. If needed, refer the patient to community resources for assistance in stopping smoking. (See Chapter 10 for more information related to smoking cessation.) If stress seems to cause symptoms, discuss measures to cope with stress. (See Chapter 6 for stress management techniques.)

TABLE 41-8 Interprofessional Care

Gastroesophageal Reflux Disease (GERD) and Hiatal Hernia

Diagnostic Assessment	Drug Therapy (Table 41-10)
• History and physical examination	• Proton pump inhibitors
• Upper GI endoscopy with biopsy and cytologic analysis	• H₂-receptor blockers
	• Prokinetic drug therapy
• Esophagram (barium swallow)	• Cholinergic drugs
• Motility (manometry) studies	• Antacids
• pH monitoring (laboratory or 24 hr ambulatory)	
• Radionuclide studies	*Surgical Therapy*
	• Nissen fundoplication
	• Toupet fundoplication
Management	
Conservative	*Endoscopic Therapy*
• Elevate head of bed on 4- to 6-in blocks	• Intraluminal valvuloplasty
• Avoid reflux-inducing foods (fatty foods, chocolate, peppermint)	• Radiofrequency therapy
• Avoid alcohol	
• Reduce or avoid acidic pH beverages (colas, red wine, orange juice)	

TABLE 41-9   Patient & Caregiver Teaching
Gastroesophageal Reflux Disease (GERD)

Include the following instructions when teaching the patient and caregiver about management of GERD.

1. Explain the reason for a low-fat diet.
2. Encourage the patient to eat small, frequent meals to prevent gastric distention.
3. Explain the reason for avoiding alcohol, smoking (causes an almost immediate, marked decrease in lower esophageal sphincter pressure), and beverages that contain caffeine.
4. Advise the patient to not lie down for 2-3 hr after eating, wear tight clothing around the waist, or bend over (especially after eating).
5. Have the patient avoid eating within 3 hr of bedtime.
6. Encourage the patient to sleep with head of bed elevated on 4- to 6-in blocks (gravity fosters esophageal emptying).
7. Provide information about drugs, including reason for their use and common side effects.
8. Discuss strategies for weight reduction if appropriate.
9. Encourage patient and caregiver to share concerns about lifestyle changes and living with a chronic problem.

Nutritional Therapy. Diet does not cause GERD, but food can aggravate symptoms. No specific diet is necessary. Some patients may need to avoid foods that decrease LES pressure, such as chocolate, peppermint, fatty foods, coffee, and tea (Table 41-7), which predispose them to reflux. Certain foods (e.g., tomato-based products, orange juice, cola, red wine) may irritate the esophagus. Tell the patient to avoid late evening meals, nocturnal snacking, and milk, especially at bedtime, since it increases gastric acid secretion. Small, frequent meals and drinking fluids between meals help prevent overdistention of the stomach. Increased saliva production by chewing gum and oral lozenges may help with mild symptoms.

Drug Therapy. Drug therapy for GERD focuses on decreasing the volume and acidity of reflux, improving LES function, increasing esophageal clearance, and protecting the esophageal mucosa[13] (Table 41-10). Proton pump inhibitors (PPIs) and histamine (H_2)-receptor blockers are the most common and effective treatments for symptomatic GERD. The goal of HCl acid suppression treatment is to reduce the acidity of the gastric refluxate. Patients who are symptomatic with GERD but do not have evidence of esophagitis (*nonerosive GERD*) achieve symptom relief with PPIs and H_2-receptor blockers.

PPIs are more effective in healing esophagitis than H_2-receptor blockers. PPIs are also beneficial in decreasing the incidence of esophageal strictures, a complication of chronic GERD. PPIs are available in prescription or OTC preparations. Therapy should start with once a day dosing, before the first meal of the day. Long-term use of PPIs has been associated with decreased bone density, chronic hypochlorhydria, and increased risk of pneumonia.[14]

 DRUG ALERT   Proton Pump Inhibitors (PPIs)

- Long-term use or high doses may increase the risk of fractures of hip, wrist, and spine.
- Patients should take the lowest dose for the shortest duration needed to treat their condition.
- Use is associated with an increased risk of new and recurrent *Clostridium difficile* infection in hospitalized patients.[15]

H_2-receptor blockers reduce symptoms and promote esophageal healing in 50% of patients. These drugs are available in OTC and prescription formulations. Some formulations include an H_2-receptor blocker plus antacid combination. For example,

EVIDENCE-BASED PRACTICE
Translating Research Into Practice

Do Proton Pump Inhibitors Increase Gastric Cancer Risk?
In adults with acid-related gastric problems (P), what is the effect of taking proton pump inhibitors (I) for at least 6 months (T) versus endoscopy or no treatment (C) and the risk of developing gastric cancer (O)?

Synthesis of Best Available Evidence
- Systematic review of randomized controlled trials (RCTs)
- Seven RCTs of patients (*n* = 1789) taking proton pump inhibitors (PPIs) for at least 6 months and without gastric cancer at start of trial. Intervention was taking PPIs for an acid-related gastric disorder. Comparison groups received no treatment or surgery/endoscopic treatment only. Outcome was to examine development and progression of gastric precancerous lesions.
- PPIs are commonly prescribed worldwide and are the most effective drugs to reduce gastric acid secretion.
- PPIs did not increase risk of atrophy or metaplasia of gastric mucosa.
- Higher incidence of developing focal cell hyperplasia (thickening of stomach lining) with PPIs
- No participants had dysplastic or neoplastic gastric mucosa changes.

Conclusions
- Taking PPIs for ≥6 months does not appear to promote development of precancerous gastric lesions.

Implications for Nursing Practice
1. How would you counsel a patient who is concerned about the long-term effects of taking a PPI?
2. What information would you provide to a patient who due to reported adverse effects with PPIs is self-treating frequent heartburn with OTC medications that are not effective?

Reference for Evidence
Song H, Zhu J, Lu D: Long-term proton pump inhibitor (PPI) use and the development of gastric pre-malignant lesions, *Cochrane Database Syst Rev* 12: CD010623, 2014.

P, Patient population of interest; *I*, intervention or area of interest; *C*, comparison of interest or comparison group; *O*, outcomes of interest; *T*, timing (see p. 15).

Pepcid Complete includes famotidine, calcium carbonate, and magnesium hydroxide.

Cholinergic drugs (e.g., bethanechol [Urecholine]) increase LES pressure, improve esophageal emptying in the supine position, and increase gastric emptying. However, cholinergic drugs increase HCl acid secretion. Prokinetic (motility-enhancing) drugs (metoclopramide [Reglan]) promote gastric emptying and reduce the risk of gastric acid reflux but are not a primary therapy for GERD.

Antacids produce quick but short-lived relief of heartburn. They are most effective taken 1 to 3 hours after meals and at bedtime. Antacids with or without alginic acid (e.g., Gaviscon) may be useful in patients with mild, intermittent heartburn. However, in patients with moderate to severe or frequent symptoms or patients with documented esophagitis, antacids are not effective in relieving symptoms or healing lesions.

Surgical Therapy. Surgical therapy (*antireflux* surgery) is reserved for patients with complications, including esophagitis, medication intolerance, stricture, Barrett's esophagus, and persistent severe symptoms. The goal of surgical therapy is to reduce reflux by enhancing the integrity of the LES. Most surgical procedures are done laparoscopically. The fundus of the

TABLE 41-10   Drug Therapy
Gastroesophageal Reflux Disease (GERD) and Peptic Ulcer Disease (PUD)

Drug	Mechanism of Action	Side Effects
Proton Pump Inhibitors (PPIs) dexlansoprazole (Dexilant) esomeprazole (Nexium) lansoprazole (Prevacid) omeprazole (Prilosec) pantoprazole (Protonix) rabeprazole (Aciphex) omeprazole and sodium bicarbonate (Zegerid)	↓ HCl acid secretion by inhibiting the proton pump (H⁺-K⁺-ATPase) responsible for the secretion of H⁺ ↓ Irritation of the esophageal and gastric mucosa	Headache, abdominal pain, nausea, diarrhea, vomiting, flatulence
Histamine (H₂)-Receptor Blockers cimetidine famotidine (Pepcid) nizatidine (Axid) ranitidine (Zantac)	Block the action of histamine on the H₂ receptors to ↓ HCl acid secretion ↓ Conversion of pepsinogen to pepsin ↓ Irritation of the esophageal and gastric mucosa	Headache, abdominal pain, constipation, diarrhea
Prokinetic Agents metoclopramide (Reglan)	Block effect of dopamine ↑ Gastric motility and emptying Reduce reflux	CNS side effects ranging from anxiety to hallucinations Extrapyramidal side effects (tremor and dyskinesias similar to Parkinson's disease)
Antiulcer, Protectants sucralfate (Carafate)	Act to form a protective layer and serve as a barrier against acid, bile salts, and enzymes in the stomach	Constipation
Cholinergic bethanechol (Urecholine)	↑ Lower esophageal sphincter pressure, improve esophageal emptying, increase gastric emptying	Lightheadedness, syncope, flushing, diarrhea, stomach cramps, dizziness
Antacids, Acid Neutralizers ***Single Substance*** aluminum hydroxide calcium carbonate (Tums, Titralac) magnesium oxide (MagOx) sodium bicarbonate (Alka-Seltzer) sodium citrate (Bicitra) ***Aluminum and Magnesium*** Gelusil, Maalox, Mylanta aluminum/magnesium trisilicate (Gaviscon)	Neutralize HCl acid Taken 1-3 hr after meals and at bedtime	*Aluminum hydroxide:* Constipation, phosphorus depletion with chronic use *Calcium carbonate:* Constipation or diarrhea, hypercalcemia, milk-alkali syndrome, renal calculi *Magnesium preparations:* Diarrhea, hypermagnesemia *Sodium preparations:* Milk-alkali syndrome if used with large amounts of calcium. Use with caution in patients on sodium restrictions
Prostaglandin (Synthetic) misoprostol (Cytotec)	Protect lining of stomach *Cytoprotective:* Increase production of gastric mucus and mucosal secretion of bicarbonate *Antisecretory:* ↓ HCl acid secretion	Abdominal pain, diarrhea, GI bleeding, uterine rupture if pregnant

stomach is wrapped around the lower portion of the esophagus to reinforce and repair the defective barrier. Nissen and Toupet fundoplications are common laparoscopic antireflux surgeries (Fig. 41-4).

A LINX Reflux Management System is an option for patients who have symptoms despite maximum medical management. A LINX system is a ring of small, flexible magnets enclosed in titanium beads and connected by titanium wires. Once implanted laparoscopically into the LES, the ring provides strength to a weakened LES. Under resting (nonswallowing) conditions, the magnetic attraction between the beads helps keep a weak LES closed to prevent reflux. When the person swallows, the force of pressure associated with the movement of fluids or foods overwhelms the magnetic forces and the fluid or food passes to the stomach. Adverse events with the system include difficulty swallowing, vomiting, nausea, chest pain, and

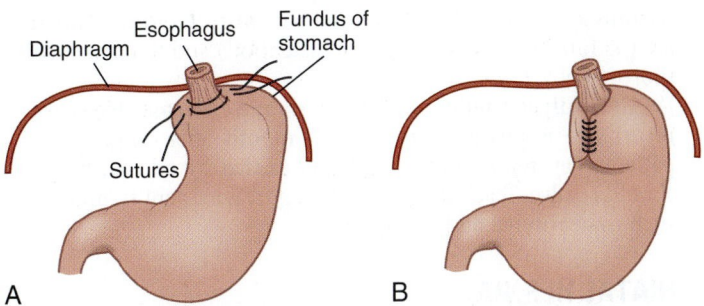

FIG. 41-4 Nissen fundoplication for repair of hiatal hernia. **A,** Fundus of stomach is wrapped around distal esophagus. **B,** The fundus is then sutured to itself. (Modified from Doughty DB, Jackson DB: *Mosby's clinical nursing series: gastrointestinal disorders,* St Louis, 1993, Mosby.)

pain when swallowing food. Tell patients who have a LINX system not to have an MRI as it could cause serious harm.
Endoscopic Therapy. Alternatives to surgical therapy include endoscopic mucosal resection (EMR), photodynamic therapy, cryotherapy, and radiofrequency ablation (image-guided technique that kills cells through heating). For patients with high-grade dysplasia, EMR can be used as a diagnostic test to obtain biopsy samples. The results of the biopsy can determine whether cancer is present.

❖ NURSING MANAGEMENT: GASTROESOPHAGEAL REFLUX DISEASE

Nursing care for the patient with acute symptoms of GERD consists of encouraging the patient to follow the necessary regimen. The head of the bed is elevated to approximately 30 degrees. This can be done using pillows or with 4- to 6-in blocks under the bed. The patient should not be supine for 2 to 3 hours after a meal. Teach the patient to avoid food and activities that cause reflux (e.g., late night eating). Have patients contact the HCP if symptoms persist.

The patient on a PPI needs to take the medication before the first meal of the day. Teach the patient about possible medication side effects. Tell the patient on a prescription H_2-receptor agent to take the medication as prescribed and not to stop without checking with the HCP.

Postoperative care focuses on preventing respiratory complications, maintaining fluid and electrolyte balance, and preventing infection. Laparoscopic fundoplication is often an outpatient procedure. However, patients at risk for complications, including those with prior upper abdominal surgeries or co-morbidities (e.g., cardiac disease, obesity), may be hospitalized after the procedure. A small percentage of patients experience complications, including gastric or esophageal injury, splenic injury, pneumothorax, perforation, bleeding, infection, and pneumonia.

Since most procedures are done laparoscopically, the risk of respiratory complications is reduced. If an open high abdominal incision is used, respiratory complications can occur. Respiratory assessment includes respiratory rate and rhythm, pulse rate and rhythm, and signs of pneumothorax (e.g., dyspnea, chest pain, cyanosis). Have the patient cough and deep breathe to expand the lungs. Patients may require medications to prevent nausea and vomiting and to control pain. Measure and record the intake and output. When peristalsis returns, only give fluids initially. Solids are added gradually with the goal of resuming a normal diet. Teach the patient to avoid foods that are gas forming (prevents gastric distention) and to chew food thoroughly.

After surgery, reflux symptoms should decrease. However, recurrence is possible. In the first month after surgery, the patient may report mild dysphagia caused by edema, but it should resolve. Teach the patient to report persistent symptoms such as heartburn and regurgitation.

HIATAL HERNIA

Hiatal hernia is herniation of a portion of the stomach into the esophagus through an opening, or hiatus, in the diaphragm. It is also referred to as *diaphragmatic hernia* and *esophageal hernia*. Hiatal hernias are the most common abnormality found on x-ray examination of the upper GI tract. They are common in older adults and occur more often in women.

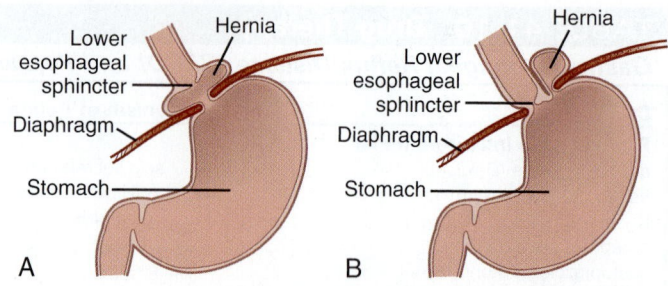

FIG. 41-5 **A**, Sliding hiatal hernia. **B**, Rolling or paraesophageal hernia.

There are two types of hiatal hernias (Fig. 41-5):
1. *Sliding:* The junction of the stomach and esophagus is above the diaphragm, and a part of the stomach slides through the hiatal opening in the diaphragm. This occurs when the patient is supine. The hernia usually goes back into the abdominal cavity when the patient is standing upright. This is the most common type of hiatal hernia.
2. *Paraesophageal* or *rolling:* The fundus and greater curvature of the stomach roll up through the diaphragm, forming a pocket alongside the esophagus. The esophagogastric junction remains in the normal position. Acute paraesophageal hernia is a medical emergency.

Etiology and Pathophysiology

Many factors contribute to the development of a hiatal hernia. Structural changes (weakening of the muscles in the diaphragm around the esophagogastric opening) occur with aging. Factors that increase intraabdominal pressure may predispose patients to developing a hiatal hernia. These include obesity, pregnancy, ascites, tumors, intense physical exertion, and heavy lifting on a continual basis.

Clinical Manifestations and Complications

Some people with hiatal hernia are asymptomatic. When present, manifestations of hiatal hernia are similar to those described for GERD on pp. 900-901.

Complications that may occur with hiatal hernia include GERD, esophagitis, hemorrhage from erosion, stenosis (narrowing of the esophagus), ulcerations of the herniated portion of the stomach, strangulation of the hernia, and regurgitation with tracheal aspiration.

Diagnostic Studies

An esophagram (barium swallow) may show the protrusion of gastric mucosa through the esophageal hiatus. Endoscopic visualization of the lower esophagus provides information on the degree of mucosal inflammation or other abnormalities. Other tests done are the same as those for GERD (Table 41-8).

❖ NURSING AND INTERPROFESSIONAL MANAGEMENT: HIATAL HERNIA

Conservative therapy of hiatal hernia is similar to that described for GERD (pp. 901-904). Teach the patient to reduce intraabdominal pressure by eliminating constricting garments and avoiding lifting and straining.

Surgical approaches to hiatal hernias can include reduction of the herniated stomach into the abdomen, *herniotomy* (excision of the hernia sac), *herniorrhaphy* (closure of the hiatal defect), an antireflux procedure, and *gastropexy* (attachment of the stomach subdiaphragmatically to prevent rehemiation). The goals are to reduce the hernia, provide an acceptable LES pressure, and prevent movement of the gastroesophageal junction. Surgery to repair hiatal hernia is often done laparoscopically by either Nissen or Toupet techniques (Fig. 41-4). The approach used (thoracic or abdominal) depends on the patient.

Gerontologic Considerations: GERD and Hiatal Hernia

The incidence of hiatal hernia and GERD increases with age. Hiatal hernia is associated with weakening of the diaphragm, obesity, kyphosis, or other factors (e.g., wearing girdles) that increase intraabdominal pressure. Older patients may take medications known to decrease LES pressure (e.g., nitrates, calcium channel blockers, antidepressants). Other agents such as nonsteroidal antiinflammatory drugs (NSAIDs) and potassium can irritate the esophageal mucosa (*medication-induced esophagitis*).

Some older adults with hiatal hernia and GERD are asymptomatic or have less severe symptoms. The first indication may be a serious problem such as esophageal bleeding secondary to esophagitis or respiratory complications (e.g., aspiration pneumonia) related to aspiration of gastric contents.

The clinical course and management of GERD and hiatal hernia in the older adult are similar to those for the younger adult. Changes in lifestyle, including eliminating dietary factors (such as caffeine-containing beverages and chocolate) and elevating the head of the bed on blocks may be challenging for the older adult.

Laparoscopic procedures reduce the risk associated with surgical repair. An older patient with cardiovascular and pulmonary problems may not be a good candidate for surgical intervention.

ESOPHAGEAL CANCER

Esophageal cancer is not common. However, the rates are increasing. In the United States, approximately 16,980 new cases are diagnosed and 15,590 deaths occur from esophageal cancer each year.[5] The 5-year survival rate is 37% for localized cancer and 18% for regional cancer.

Most esophageal cancers are adenocarcinomas. The others are squamous cell tumors. Adenocarcinomas arise from the glands lining the esophagus and resemble cancers of the stomach and small intestine. The incidence of esophageal cancer increases with age. Those between 70 and 84 are at greatest risk. There is a higher incidence in non-Hispanic white men and Alaska Natives compared with other ethnic groups. The incidence is higher in men than in women.

Etiology and Pathophysiology

The cause of esophageal cancer is unknown. Several important risk factors include Barrett's esophagus, smoking, excessive alcohol intake, and obesity. For example, current smoking or a history of smoking is associated with a twofold higher risk of esophageal cancer. Those with injury to the esophageal mucosa (e.g., from occupational exposure to asbestos and cement dust) are at greater risk. *Achalasia,* a condition marked by delayed emptying of the lower esophagus, is associated with squamous cell cancer.

Most esophageal tumors are located in the middle and lower portions of the esophagus. The tumor usually appears as an ulcerated lesion. It may penetrate the muscular layer and extend outside the wall of the esophagus. The majority of patients have advanced disease at the time of diagnosis. The cancer spreads via the lymph system, with the liver and lung being common sites of metastasis.

Clinical Manifestations and Complications

By the time the patient experiences symptoms, the tumor is often advanced. Progressive dysphagia is the most common symptom. It may be described as a substernal feeling that food is not passing. Initially the dysphagia occurs only with meat, then with soft foods, and eventually with liquids.

Pain develops late. It occurs in the substernal, epigastric, or back areas and usually increases with swallowing. The pain may radiate to the neck, jaw, ears, and shoulders. If the tumor is in the upper third of the esophagus, symptoms such as sore throat, choking, and hoarseness may occur. Most patients lose weight. When esophageal stenosis (narrowing) is severe, regurgitation of blood-flecked esophageal contents is common.

Hemorrhage occurs if the cancer erodes through the esophagus and into the aorta. Esophageal perforation with fistula formation into the lung or trachea sometimes develops. The tumor may enlarge enough to cause esophageal obstruction, particularly in the later stages.

Diagnostic Studies

Endoscopic biopsy is necessary to make a definitive diagnosis of esophageal cancer. Endoscopic ultrasonography (EUS) is an important tool used to stage esophageal cancer. Esophagram (barium swallow) may show narrowing of the esophagus at the tumor site (Table 41-11).

Interprofessional Care

The treatment of esophageal cancer depends on the tumor's location and whether invasion or metastasis is present. Esophageal cancer usually has a poor prognosis because it is often not diagnosed until the disease is advanced. The best results are obtained with a multimodal approach, including surgery, endoscopic ablation, chemotherapy, and radiation therapy. Depending on the location and cancer spread, only chemotherapy and radiation may be used. Palliative therapy consists of restoring swallowing function and maintaining nutrition and hydration.

Surgical Therapy. The types of surgical procedures done are (1) removal of part or all of the esophagus (*esophagectomy*) with use of a Dacron graft to replace the resected part, (2) resection of a portion of the esophagus and anastomosis of the remaining

TABLE 41-11 Interprofessional Care

Esophageal Cancer

Diagnostic Assessment	Management
• History and physical examination	• Surgical therapy
	• Esophagectomy
• Endoscopy of esophagus with biopsy	• Esophagogastrostomy
	• Esophagoenterostomy
• Endoscopic ultrasonography	• Endoscopic therapy
• Esophagram (barium swallow)	• Photodynamic therapy
• Bronchoscopy	• Endoscopic mucosal resection
• CT, MRI	• Radiofrequency ablation
	• Laser therapy
	• Dilation
	• Stent or prosthesis placement
	• Radiation therapy
	• Chemotherapy

portion to the stomach (*esophagogastrostomy),* and (3) resection of a portion of the esophagus and anastomosis of a segment of colon to the remaining portion (*esophagoenterostomy).* The surgical approaches may be open (thoracic, abdominal incision) or laparoscopic.

Minimally invasive esophagectomy (e.g., laparoscopic vagal nerve–sparing surgery) is being done more frequently. It has the advantage of using smaller incisions, decreasing intensive care unit (ICU) and hospital stays, and producing fewer pulmonary complications.

Endoscopic Therapy. Endoscopic therapy includes photodynamic therapy, endoscopic mucosal resection (EMR), and radiofrequency ablation. In photodynamic therapy, the patient receives an IV injection of porfimer sodium (Photofrin), which is a photosensitizer. Although most tissues absorb porfimer, cancer tissue absorbs it to a greater degree. The HCP directs light towards the cancerous area using a fiber passed through an endoscope. The light reacts with porfimer, starting a reaction that destroys the cancer cells. Warn patients to avoid direct sunlight for up to 4 weeks after the procedure.

Endoscopic mucosal resection (EMR) is an option for some small, very early stage cancers. It involves the removal of malignant tissue using an endoscope. Radiofrequency ablation is used to kill cancer cells using electric current.

Dilation, stent placement, or both can relieve obstruction. Dilation increases the lumen of the esophagus. It often relieves dysphagia and allows for improved nutrition. There are various types of dilators. Placement of stents or expandable stents may help when dilation is no longer effective.[16] Stents allow food and liquid to pass through the stenotic area of the esophagus. Self-expandable metal stents are available with features to prevent stent migration and tumor ingrowth. Stents may be placed before surgery to improve the patient's nutritional status.

Endoscopic laser therapy may be used in combination with dilation. Laser therapy can be repeated if obstruction recurs as the tumor grows. Sometimes these procedures are combined with radiation therapy.

Radiation Therapy. Depending on the type and stage of esophageal cancer, chemotherapy with or without radiation therapy may be given. Concurrent radiation and chemotherapy are given for palliation of symptoms, especially dysphagia, and to increase survival. Some patients receive radiation therapy before surgery.

Chemotherapy. Many different chemotherapy drugs can be used to treat esophageal cancer. Common combination regimens are carboplatin and paclitaxel, cisplatin and 5-fluorouracil (5-FU), ECF (epirubicin [Ellence], cisplatin, and 5-FU), DCF (docetaxel, cisplatin, and 5-FU), cisplatin with capecitabine (Xeloda), and oxaliplatin with either 5-FU or capecitabine. Other chemotherapy drugs that have been used include bleomycin, mitomycin, methotrexate, vinorelbine (Navelbine), topotecan, and irinotecan (Camptosar). (Chemotherapy is discussed in Chapter 15.)

Targeted Therapy. Some esophageal cancers have too much HER-2 protein on their cell surfaces, which helps cancer cells to grow. Trastuzumab (Herceptin) is a drug that targets the HER-2 protein and kills the cancer cells.

Ramucirumab (Cyramza), an angiogenesis inhibitor, binds to the receptor for *vascular endothelial growth factor* (VEGF), a compound that stimulates blood vessel growth. Thus ramucirumab prevents VEGF from binding to the receptor and signaling the body to make more blood vessels. This can help slow or stop the growth and spread of cancer. Ramucirumab is used to treat advanced cancers that start at the gastroesophageal (GE) junction. (Targeted therapies are discussed in Chapter 15.)

Nutritional Therapy. After esophageal surgery parenteral fluids are given. A jejunostomy, gastrostomy, or esophagostomy feeding tube may be placed to feed the patient depending on the type of surgery (e.g., esophagogastrectomy) performed. A swallowing study is often done before allowing the patient to have oral fluids. When starting fluids, give water (30 to 60 mL) hourly and gradually progress to small, frequent, bland meals. Place the patient in an upright position to prevent regurgitation. With tube feeding, observe the patient for signs of intolerance to the feeding or leakage of the feeding into the mediastinum. Symptoms that indicate leakage are pain, increased temperature, and dyspnea. (Enteral nutrition is discussed in Chapter 39.)

❖ NURSING MANAGEMENT: ESOPHAGEAL CANCER

◆ Nursing Assessment

Ask the patient about a history of GERD, hiatal hernia, achalasia, Barrett's esophagus, and tobacco and alcohol use. Assess the patient for progressive dysphagia and *odynophagia* (burning, squeezing pain while swallowing). Ask about the type of substances (e.g., meats, soft foods, liquids) that cause dysphagia. Assess the patient for pain (substernal, epigastric, or back areas), choking, heartburn, hoarseness, cough, anorexia, weight loss, and regurgitation.

◆ Nursing Diagnoses

Nursing diagnoses for the patient with esophageal cancer include, but are not limited to, the following:

- Chronic pain *related to* the compression of tumor on surrounding tissues, esophageal stenosis
- Imbalanced nutrition: less than body requirements *related to* dysphagia, odynophagia, weakness, chemotherapy, and radiation therapy
- Risk for aspiration *related to* difficulty swallowing, choking, and regurgitation
- Anxiety and grieving *related to* diagnosis of cancer, uncertain future, and prognosis

◆ Planning

The overall goals are that the patient with esophageal cancer will (1) have relief of symptoms, including pain and dysphagia; (2) achieve optimal nutritional intake; and (3) experience a quality of life appropriate to stage of disease and prognosis.

◆ Nursing Implementation

◆ Health Promotion. Counsel the patient with GERD, Barrett's esophagus, or hiatal hernia about the importance of regular follow-up evaluation. Health counseling should focus on elimination of smoking and excessive alcohol intake, as well as other risk factors for GERD (Table 41-7). Maintaining good oral hygiene and dietary habits (e.g., intake of fresh fruits and vegetables) is important. Encourage patients to seek medical attention for any esophageal problems, especially dysphagia.

◆ Acute Care

◆ *Preoperative Care.* The patient and caregiver usually react with shock, disbelief, and depression when they are told about a diagnosis of esophageal cancer. Provide emotional and physical support, provide information, clarify test results, and maintain a positive attitude with respect to the patient's immediate recovery and long-term survival.

In addition to general preoperative teaching and preparation, pay particular attention to the patient's nutritional needs. Many patients are poorly nourished because of the inability to ingest adequate amounts of food and fluids. A high-calorie, high-protein diet is recommended. Some patients require a liquid form of this diet. Others may need IV fluid replacement or parenteral nutrition. Teach the patient and caregiver how to keep an intake and output record and assess for signs of fluid and electrolyte imbalance. Some treatment protocols require preoperative radiation and chemotherapy.

Meticulous oral care is essential. Cleanse the mouth thoroughly, including the tongue, gingivae, and teeth or dentures. It may be necessary to use swabs or a gauze pad and to scrub the mouth, including the tongue. Milk of magnesia with mineral oil helps remove crust formation.

Teaching should include information about chest tubes (if an open thoracic approach is used), IV lines, NG tubes, pain management, gastrostomy or jejunostomy feeding, turning, coughing, and deep breathing. (General preoperative care is discussed in Chapter 17.)

Postoperative Care. The patient usually has an NG tube in place and may have bloody drainage for 8 to 12 hours. The drainage gradually changes to greenish yellow. Assessing the drainage, maintaining the tube, and providing oral and nasal care are nursing responsibilities. Do not reposition the NG tube or reinsert it without consulting the surgeon.

Because of the location of the surgery and the patient's general condition, emphasize preventing respiratory complications. Have the patient turn, cough, and deep breathe, and use an incentive spirometer every 2 hours.

Cardiac dysrhythmias may result from the proximity of the pericardium to the surgical site. Other complications that can occur after esophagectomy include esophageal anastomotic leaks, fistula formation, interstitial pulmonary edema, and acute respiratory distress related to the disruption of the mediastinal lymph nodes.

Position the patient in a semi-Fowler's or Fowler's position to prevent reflux and aspiration of gastric secretions. When the patient can drink fluids or eat, maintain the upright position for at least 2 hours after eating to assist with gastric emptying.

Ambulatory Care. Many patients require long-term follow-up care after surgery for esophageal cancer. The patient may undergo chemotherapy and radiation treatment after surgery. Encourage and assist the patient in maintaining adequate nutrition. A permanent feeding gastrostomy may be required. The patient usually has fears and anxieties about a diagnosis of cancer. Know what the HCP has told the patient about the prognosis and provide appropriate counseling.

Referral to a palliative care or home health nurse may be needed. (See Chapter 15 for the care of the cancer patient and Chapter 9 for a discussion of palliative and end-of-life care.)

◆ **Evaluation**

The expected outcomes are that the patient with esophageal cancer will
- Maintain a patent airway
- Have relief of pain
- Be able to swallow comfortably and consume adequate nutritional intake
- Experience a quality of life appropriate to stage of disease and prognosis

OTHER ESOPHAGEAL DISORDERS

Eosinophilic Esophagitis

Eosinophilic esophagitis (EoE) is characterized by swelling of the esophagus from an infiltration of *eosinophils*. People with EoE frequently have a personal or family history of other allergic diseases. The most common food triggers are milk, egg, wheat, rye, and beef. Environmental allergens, such as pollens, molds, cat, dog, and dust mite allergens, may be involved in the development of EoE.

Clinical manifestations include severe heartburn, difficulty swallowing, food impaction in the esophagus, nausea, vomiting, and weight loss. The diagnosis is based on symptoms and biopsy findings of eosinophils infiltrating esophageal tissue obtained from endoscopy.

Allergy skin testing helps to determine the person's allergens. A trial of avoidance of the foods to which the person has positive allergy tests is the initial form of treatment. Other common treatments include the use of PPIs (Table 41-10) and corticosteroids. Corticosteroids are frequently used to treat EoE when avoiding allergic triggers does not relieve symptoms.

Corticosteroids may be used orally (prednisone) or as a topical therapy with inhaled corticosteroids (e.g., fluticasone [Flovent]). The patient takes a puff of fluticasone, and rather than inhaling it, swallows the medication. This directly delivers the drug to the esophagus. The most common side effect is a yeast infection of the throat (esophageal candidiasis).

Esophageal Diverticula

Esophageal diverticula are saclike outpouchings of one or more layers of the esophagus. They occur in three main areas: (1) above the upper esophageal sphincter (*Zenker's diverticulum*), which is the most common location; (2) near the esophageal midpoint (traction diverticulum); and (3) above the LES (epiphrenic diverticulum) (Fig. 41-6). Pharyngeal pouches (Zenker's diverticula) occur commonly in people over 60 years.

Typical symptoms include dysphagia, regurgitation, chronic cough, aspiration, and weight loss. Food becomes trapped in the outpouches. This causes tasting sour food and smelling a foul odor. Complications include malnutrition, aspiration, and perforation. Endoscopy or barium studies can easily establish a diagnosis.

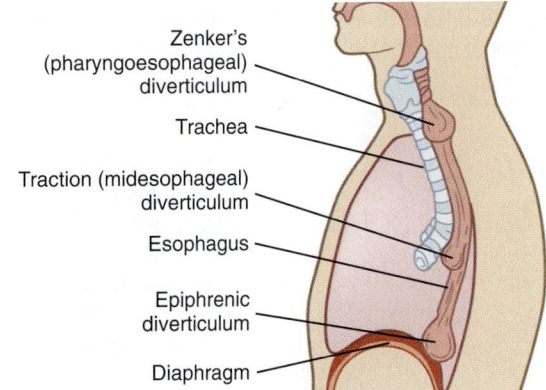

FIG. 41-6 Possible sites for esophageal diverticula. These hollow outpouchings may occur just above the upper esophageal sphincter (Zenker's, the most common type of pulsion diverticulum), near the midpoint of the esophagus (traction), and just above the lower esophageal sphincter (epiphrenic). (Modified from Price SA, Wilson LM: *Pathophysiology: clinical concepts of disease processes*, ed 6, St Louis, 2003, Mosby.)

There is no specific treatment for esophageal diverticula. Some patients find that they can empty the pocket of food that collects by applying pressure at a point on the neck. The diet may have to be limited to foods that pass more readily (e.g., blenderized foods). Surgical treatment may be necessary if nutrition is disrupted. Treatment by endoscopic stapling diverticulotomy or diverticulostomy is associated with decreased complications compared with the open approaches. The most serious surgical complication is esophageal perforation.

Esophageal Strictures

The most common cause of *esophageal strictures* (or narrowing) is chronic GERD. The ingestion of strong acids or alkalis, external beam radiation, and surgical anastomosis can also create strictures. Trauma such as throat lacerations and gunshot wounds can lead to strictures because of scar formation. Strictures can result in dysphagia, regurgitation, and ultimately weight loss.

Strictures can be dilated using mechanical *bougies* (dilating instruments) or balloons. Dilation may be done with or without endoscopy, or with fluoroscopy. Surgical excision with anastomosis is sometimes necessary. The patient may have a temporary or permanent gastrostomy.

Achalasia

In achalasia, peristalsis of the lower two thirds (smooth muscle) of the esophagus is absent. Achalasia is a rare, chronic disorder. The exact cause is unknown. With achalasia, the pressure in the LES increases along with incomplete relaxation. Esophageal obstruction at or near the diaphragm occurs. Food and fluid accumulate in the lower esophagus. The result is dilation of the esophagus proximal to (above) the tapering affected segment of the lower esophagus (Fig. 41-7). There is a selective loss of inhibitory neurons, resulting in unopposed contraction of the LES.

The onset of achalasia is usually insidious. Dysphagia is the most common symptom and occurs with both liquids and solids. Patients may report a globus sensation and/or substernal chest pain (similar to angina pain) during or immediately after a meal. About a third of the patients experience nocturnal regurgitation. *Halitosis* (foul-smelling breath) and the inability to eructate (belch) are other symptoms. Patients with achalasia may report symptoms of GERD and regurgitation of sour-tasting food and liquids, especially when they are lying down. Weight loss is typical.

Diagnosis is made with esophagram (barium swallow), manometric evaluation (high-resolution manometry), and/or endoscopic evaluation. Treatment focuses on symptom management. The goals of treatment are to relieve dysphagia and regurgitation, improve esophageal emptying by disrupting the LES, and prevent the development of megaesophagus (enlargement of the lower esophagus).

Endoscopic pneumatic dilation involves dilating the LES muscle using balloons of progressively larger diameter (3.0, 3.5, and 4.0 cm) (Fig. 41-8). It is an outpatient procedure. If this is ineffective, the next option is a Heller myotomy, done laparoscopically. In this procedure, the surgeon cuts through the muscles of the LES, allowing food to pass. Because GERD with esophagitis and stricture is a common complication, the patient often has antireflux surgery at the same time. The patient typically returns to usual activities 1 to 2 weeks afterwards.

Medical therapy is less effective than invasive procedures. The injection of botulinum toxin endoscopically into the LES gives short-term relief of symptoms and improves esophageal emptying. It works by promoting relaxation of the smooth muscle. This treatment is used for older patients for whom surgery and pneumatic dilation may not be appropriate due to other chronic illnesses.

Smooth muscle relaxants, such as nitrates (isosorbide dinitrate [Isordil]) and calcium channel blockers (e.g., nifedipine [Procardia]), taken sublingually 30 to 45 minutes before meals may improve dysphagia. Side effects (e.g., headache), drug tolerance, and short duration of action limit their use. Symptomatic treatment consists of eating a semisoft diet, eating slowly and drinking fluid with meals, and sleeping with the head elevated.

Esophageal Varices

Esophageal varices are dilated, tortuous veins occurring in the lower portion of the esophagus because of portal hypertension. Esophageal varices are a common complication of liver cirrhosis. They are discussed in Chapter 43.

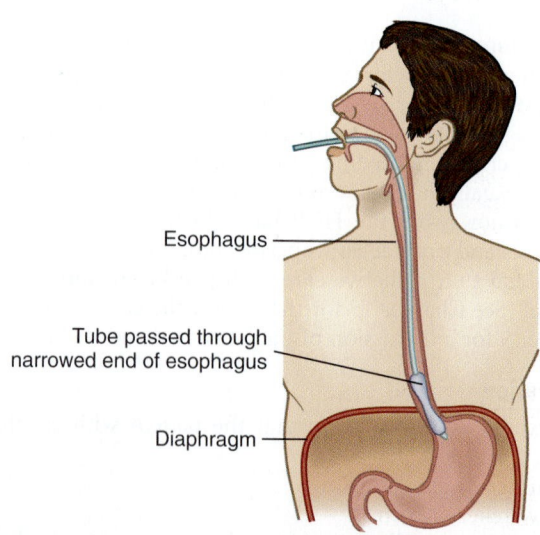

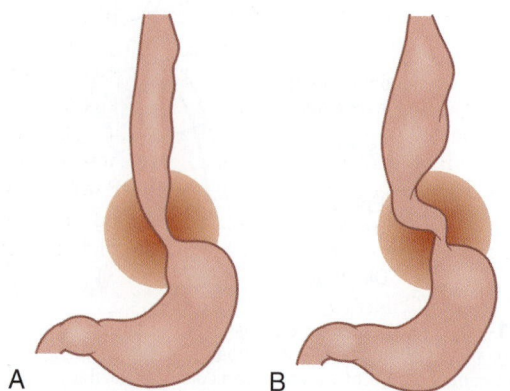

FIG. 41-7 Esophageal achalasia. **A,** Early stage, showing tapering of lower esophagus. **B,** Advanced stage, showing dilated, tortuous esophagus.

FIG. 41-8 Pneumatic dilation attempts to treat achalasia by maintaining an adequate lumen and decreasing lower esophageal sphincter (LES) tone. (Modified from Price SA, Wilson LM: *Pathophysiology: clinical concepts of disease processes,* ed 6, St Louis, 2003, Mosby.)

DISORDERS OF THE STOMACH AND UPPER SMALL INTESTINE

GASTRITIS

Gastritis, an inflammation of the gastric mucosa, is one of the most common problems affecting the stomach. Gastritis may be acute or chronic and diffuse or localized.

Etiology and Pathophysiology

Gastritis occurs as the result of a breakdown in the normal gastric mucosal barrier. This mucosal barrier normally protects the stomach tissue from the corrosive action of HCl acid and pepsin. When the barrier is broken, HCl acid and pepsin can diffuse back into the mucosa. This back diffusion results in tissue edema, disruption of capillary walls with loss of plasma into the gastric lumen, and possible hemorrhage.

Risk Factors. Risk factors and causes of gastritis are listed in Table 41-12. Some of the risk factors are discussed in this section.

Drug-Related Gastritis. Drugs contribute to the development of acute and chronic gastritis. NSAIDs, including aspirin, and corticosteroids inhibit the synthesis of prostaglandins that are protective to the gastric mucosa. This makes the mucosa more susceptible to injury. NSAID-related gastritis is associated with many drugs, including piroxicam (Feldene), naproxen (Naprosyn), indomethacin, diclofenac (Voltaren), and ibuprofen.[17]

Risk factors for NSAID-induced gastritis include being female; being over age 60; having a history of ulcer disease; taking anticoagulants, other NSAIDs (including low-dose aspirin), or other ulcerogenic drugs (including corticosteroids); and having a chronic debilitating disorder such as cardiovascular disease. Some drugs such as digitalis (digoxin) and alendronate (Fosamax) have direct irritating effects on the gastric mucosa.

Diet. Dietary indiscretions can result in acute gastritis. After an alcoholic drinking binge, acute damage to the gastric mucosa can range from localized injury of superficial epithelial cells to destruction of the mucosa with mucosal congestion, edema, and hemorrhage. Prolonged damage induced by repeated alcohol abuse results in chronic gastritis. Eating large quantities of spicy, irritating foods can cause acute gastritis.

Helicobacter pylori. An important cause of chronic gastritis is *Helicobacter pylori* infection. *H. pylori* infection causes acute gastritis in most infected persons. In some patients, chronic gastritis develops. Prolonged inflammation leads to functional changes in the stomach and in some cases, stomach cancer. *H. pylori* is discussed later in this chapter on p. 911.

Other Risk Factors. Although not as common as *H. pylori*, other bacterial, viral, and fungal infections are associated with chronic gastritis. Gastritis can occur from reflux of bile salts from the duodenum into the stomach because of anatomic changes following surgical procedures (e.g., gastroduodenostomy, gastrojejunostomy). Prolonged vomiting may cause reflux of bile salts. Intense emotional responses and CNS lesions may produce inflammation of the mucosal lining from hypersecretion of HCl acid.

Autoimmune Gastritis. Autoimmune metaplastic atrophic gastritis (also called *autoimmune atrophic gastritis*) is an inherited condition in which there is an immune response directed against parietal cells. It most commonly affects women of northern European descent. Patients often have other autoimmune disorders. The loss of parietal cells leads to low chloride levels, inadequate production of intrinsic factor, cobalamin (vitamin B_{12}) malabsorption, and pernicious anemia. It is associated with an increased risk of stomach cancer.

Clinical Manifestations

The symptoms of *acute gastritis* include anorexia, nausea and vomiting, epigastric tenderness, and a feeling of fullness. Hemorrhage is commonly associated with alcohol abuse and at times is the only symptom. Acute gastritis is self-limiting, lasting from a few hours to a few days. Complete healing of the mucosa is expected.

The manifestations of *chronic gastritis* are similar to those of acute gastritis. Some patients are asymptomatic. However, when parietal cells are lost because of atrophy, the source of intrinsic factor is also lost. *Intrinsic factor* is essential for the absorption of cobalamin in the terminal ileum. Once the body's cobalamin stores in the liver are depleted, a state of cobalamin deficiency exists. Because it is essential for the growth and maturation of red blood cells (RBCs), the lack of cobalamin results in pernicious anemia and neurologic complications. (Cobalamin deficiency anemia is discussed in Chapter 30.)

Diagnostic Studies

Acute gastritis is usually diagnosed based on the patient's symptoms and a history of drug or alcohol use. Occasionally, an endoscopic examination with biopsy is necessary to provide a definitive diagnosis. Breath, urine, serum, stool, and gastric tissue biopsy tests are available to assess for *H. pylori* infection. A complete blood count (CBC) may show anemia from blood loss or lack of intrinsic factor. Stools are tested for occult blood. Serum tests for antibodies to parietal cells and intrinsic factor may be done. A tissue biopsy can rule out gastric cancer.

❖ NURSING AND INTERPROFESSIONAL MANAGEMENT: GASTRITIS

◆ Acute Gastritis

Eliminating the cause and preventing or avoiding it in the future are generally all that is needed to treat acute gastritis. The

TABLE 41-12	Causes of Gastritis
Drugs	**Environmental Factors**
• Aspirin	• Radiation
• Bisphosphonates	• Smoking
• Corticosteroids	
• Iron supplements	**Diseases/Disorders**
• Nonsteroidal antiinflammatory drugs (NSAIDs)	• Burns
	• Large hiatal hernia
Diet	• Physiologic stress
• Alcohol	• Crohn's disease
• Large quantities of spicy, irritating foods	• Reflux of bile and pancreatic secretions
	• Renal failure
	• Sepsis
Microorganisms	• Shock
• *Helicobacter pylori*	
• Mycobacterium species	**Other Factors**
• Salmonella organisms	• Endoscopy procedures
• Staphylococcus organisms	• Nasogastric tube
• Cytomegalovirus	• Psychologic stress
• Syphilis	

TABLE 41-13   Drug Therapy

Helicobacter pylori *Infection*

Treatment	Duration	Eradication Rate
Triple-drug therapy proton pump inhibitor (PPI) amoxicillin clarithromycin (Biaxin)	7-14 days	70%-85%
Quadruple therapy PPI bismuth tetracycline metronidazole (Flagyl)	10-14 days	85%

plan of care is supportive and similar to that described for nausea and vomiting. If vomiting accompanies acute gastritis, rest, NPO status, and IV fluids may be prescribed. Antiemetics are given (Table 41-1). Monitor for dehydration. It can occur rapidly in acute gastritis with vomiting.

In severe cases of acute gastritis, an NG tube may be used to (1) monitor for bleeding, (2) lavage the precipitating agent from the stomach, or (3) keep the stomach empty and free of noxious stimuli. Clear liquids are resumed when symptoms have subsided. Reintroduce solids gradually.

If the patient is at risk for hemorrhage, frequently check vital signs and test the vomitus for blood. All of the management strategies discussed in the section on upper GI bleeding apply to the patient with severe gastritis (see pp. 923-925).

Drug therapy focuses on reducing irritation of the gastric mucosa and providing symptomatic relief. H_2-receptor blockers (e.g., ranitidine, cimetidine) or PPIs (e.g., omeprazole, lansoprazole) reduce gastric HCl acid secretion (Table 41-10). Teach the patient about the therapeutic effects of PPIs and H_2-receptor blockers.

◆ Chronic Gastritis

The treatment of chronic gastritis focuses on evaluating and eliminating the specific cause (e.g., cessation of alcohol intake, abstinence from drugs, *H. pylori* eradication). Antibiotic combinations are used to eradicate *H. pylori* (Table 41-13). The patient with pernicious anemia needs lifelong cobalamin therapy (see Chapter 30).

The patient undergoing treatment for chronic gastritis may have to adapt to lifestyle changes and strictly adhere to a drug regimen. Some patients find a nonirritating diet consisting of six small feedings a day helpful. Smoking is contraindicated in all forms of gastritis. An interprofessional team approach in which the HCP, nurse, dietitian, and pharmacist provide consistent information and support will increase the patient's success in making these changes.

PEPTIC ULCER DISEASE

Peptic ulcer disease (PUD) is a condition characterized by erosion of the GI mucosa from the digestive action of HCl acid and pepsin. Any portion of the GI tract that is in contact with gastric secretions is susceptible to ulcer development. This includes the lower esophagus, stomach, duodenum, and margin of a gastrojejunal anastomosis after surgical procedures. About 25 million people in the United States are affected by PUD in their lifetime.[18]

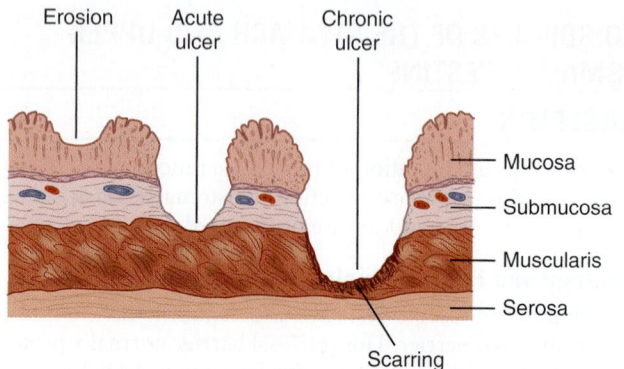

FIG. 41-9 Peptic ulcers, including an erosion, an acute ulcer, and a chronic ulcer. Both the acute ulcer and the chronic ulcer may penetrate the entire wall of the stomach. (Modified from Price SA, Wilson LM: *Pathophysiology: clinical concepts of disease processes,* ed 6, St Louis, 2003, Mosby.)

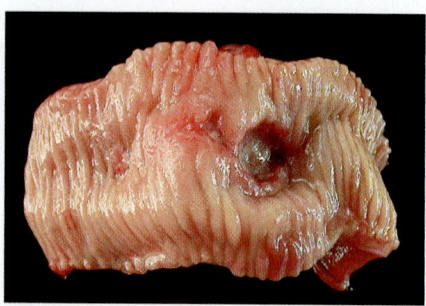

FIG. 41-10 Peptic ulcer of the duodenum. (From Kumar V, Abbas AK, Aster JC, Fausto N: *Robbins and Cotran pathologic basis of disease,* ed 8, Philadelphia, 2010, Saunders.)

Types

Peptic ulcers are classified as acute or chronic, depending on the degree and duration of mucosal involvement, and gastric or duodenal, according to the location. The *acute ulcer* (Fig. 41-9) is associated with superficial erosion and minimal inflammation. It is of short duration and resolves quickly when the cause is identified and removed. A chronic ulcer (Fig. 41-10) is one of long duration, eroding through the muscular wall with the formation of fibrous tissue. It is present continuously for many months or intermittently throughout the person's lifetime. Chronic ulcers are more common than acute erosions.

Although gastric and duodenal ulcers are both considered PUD, they are different in their incidence and presentation (Table 41-14). Generally, the treatment of all types of ulcers is similar.

Etiology and Pathophysiology

Peptic ulcers develop only in an acid environment. However, an excess of HCl acid may not be necessary for ulcer development. Pepsinogen, the precursor of pepsin, changes to pepsin in the presence of HCl acid and a pH of 2 to 3. When food or antacids neutralize the stomach acid level or drugs block acid secretion, the pH increases to 3.5 or more. At a pH of 3.5 or more, pepsin has little or no proteolytic activity.

The pathophysiology of ulcer development is outlined in Fig. 41-11. The back diffusion of HCl acid into the gastric mucosa results in cellular destruction and inflammation. Histamine is released from the damaged mucosa, resulting in vasodilation and increased capillary permeability and further secretion of acid and pepsin. Fig. 41-12 depicts the interrelationship between

TABLE 41-14 Comparison of Gastric and Duodenal Ulcers

Gastric Ulcers	Duodenal Ulcers
Lesion	
Superficial, smooth margins. Round, oval, or cone shaped	Penetrating (associated with deformity of duodenal bulb from healing of recurrent ulcers)
Location of Lesion	
Predominantly antrum, also in body and fundus of stomach	First 1-2 cm of duodenum
Gastric Secretion	
Normal to decreased	Increased
Incidence	
Greater in women	Greater in men, but increasing in women (especially postmenopausal)
Peak age 50-60 yr	Peak age 35-45 yr
Increased cancer risk	No increase in cancer risk
H. pylori infection in 80%	*H. pylori* infection in 90%
↑ With incompetent pyloric sphincter and bile reflux	Associated with other diseases (e.g., chronic obstructive pulmonary disease, pancreatic disease, hyperparathyroidism, Zollinger-Ellison syndrome, chronic renal failure)
Clinical Manifestations	
Burning or gaseous pressure in epigastrium	Burning, cramping, pressure-like pain across midepigastrium and upper abdomen. Back pain with posterior ulcers
Pain 1-2 hr after meals. If penetrating ulcer, aggravation of discomfort with food	Pain 2-5 hr after meals and midmorning, midafternoon, middle of night. Periodic and episodic. Pain relief with antacids and food
Recurrence Rate	
High	High

the mucosal blood flow and disruption of the gastric mucosal barrier. As described in the section on gastritis, a number of factors damage the mucosal barrier.

Helicobacter pylori. *H. pylori* is associated with PUD. About 70% of people in developing countries and 40% in the U.S. and industrialized countries are infected with *H. pylori*.[18] Infection likely occurs during childhood with transmission from family members to the child, possibly through a fecal-oral or oral-oral route. In the United States, those more likely to be infected are people born before 1940 and those of low socioeconomic status.

In the stomach, the bacteria can survive a long time by colonizing the gastric epithelial cells within the mucosal layer. The bacteria produce urease, which metabolizes urea-producing ammonium chloride and other damaging chemicals. Urease activates the immune response with both antibody production and the release of inflammatory cytokines. This leads to increased gastric secretion and produces tissue damage, leading to PUD.

Although most people with *H. pylori* never develop ulcers, it appears that those infected with *CagA*-positive strains are more likely to have PUD. Other factors influencing risk for PUD include genetics, smoking, NSAID use, and diet. It is thought that the higher risk of PUD among persons of lower socioeconomic status is due to their having a higher prevalence of *H. pylori* infection.

PATHOPHYSIOLOGY MAP

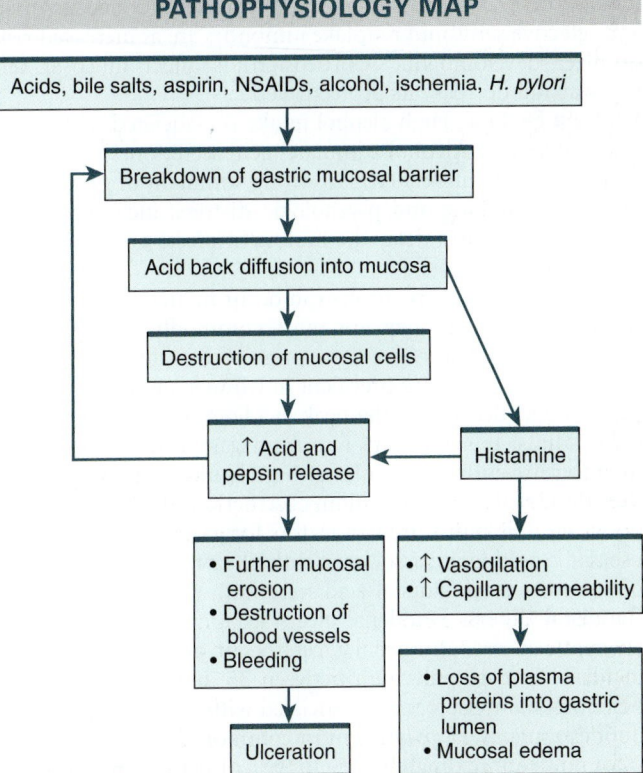

FIG. 41-11 Disruption of gastric mucosa and pathophysiologic consequences of back diffusion of acids.

PATHOPHYSIOLOGY MAP

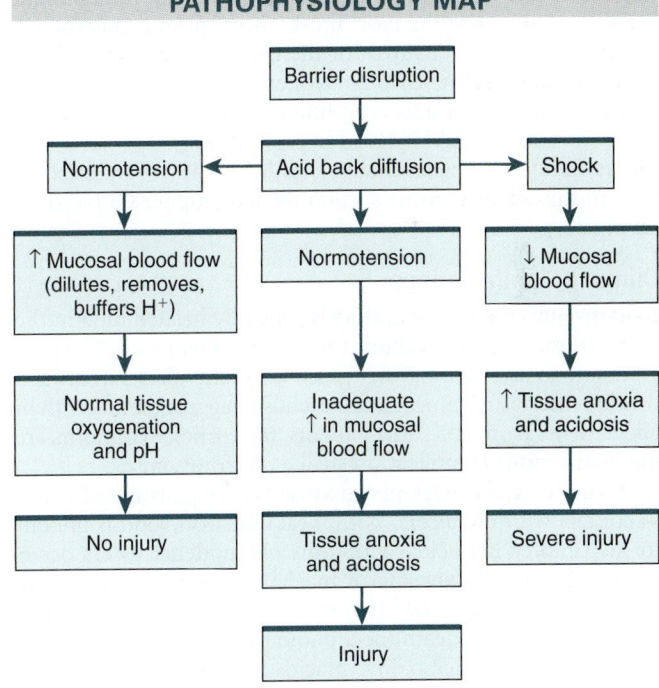

FIG. 41-12 Relationship between mucosal blood flow and disruption of the gastric mucosal barrier.

Medication-Induced Injury. Ulcerogenic drugs, such as aspirin and NSAIDs, inhibit prostaglandin synthesis, increase gastric acid secretion, and reduce the integrity of the mucosal barrier. The use of NSAIDs is responsible for the majority of non–*H. pylori* peptic ulcers. NSAIDs in the presence of *H. pylori* increase the risk of PUD.[17] Patients on corticosteroids, anticoagulants, and selective serotonin reuptake inhibitors are at increased risk of ulcer development.[19] Corticosteroids affect mucosal cell renewal and decrease its protective effects.

Lifestyle Factors. High alcohol intake is associated with acute mucosal lesions. Alcohol stimulates acid secretion. Coffee (caffeinated and decaffeinated) is a strong stimulant of gastric acid secretion. Smoking and psychologic distress, including stress and depression, can delay the healing of ulcers once they have developed.

Gastric Ulcers. Gastric ulcers can occur in any portion of the stomach. However, they are most commonly found in the antrum. Gastric ulcers are less common than duodenal ulcers. Gastric ulcers are more prevalent in women and those over 50 years of age. Because of the peak incidence of gastric ulcers in older adults, the mortality rate from gastric ulcers is greater than that from duodenal ulcers. Gastric ulcers are more likely than duodenal ulcers to result in obstruction. *H. pylori*, medications, and bile reflux are risk factors for gastric ulcers. Alcohol use and smoking are associated with ulcer formation. They are both known stimulants of acid secretion.

Duodenal Ulcers. Duodenal ulcers account for about 80% of all peptic ulcers. Duodenal ulcers occur at any age, but the incidence is especially high between 35 and 45 years of age. Although many factors are associated with the development of duodenal ulcers, *H. pylori* is most common. *H. pylori* infection is found in approximately 90% to 95% of patients with duodenal ulcers.

The development of duodenal ulcers is often associated with a high HCl acid secretion. Alcohol ingestion and smoking are also associated with duodenal ulcer formation. Several patient groups at high risk include those with chronic obstructive pulmonary disease, cirrhosis of the liver, chronic pancreatitis, hyperparathyroidism, chronic kidney disease, and *Zollinger-Ellison syndrome* (a rare condition characterized by severe peptic ulceration and HCl acid hypersecretion).

Stress-Related Mucosal Disease (SRMD). SRMD is described later in this chapter in the section on acute upper GI bleeding on p. 922.

Clinical Manifestations

In gastric ulcers, the discomfort is generally located high in the epigastrium and occurs about 1 to 2 hours after meals. The pain is described as "burning" or "gaseous." If the ulcer has eroded through the gastric mucosa, food tends to aggravate rather than alleviate the pain. For some patients, the earliest symptoms are due to a serious complication such as perforation.

In duodenal ulcers, symptoms occur when gastric acid comes in contact with the ulcers. With meal ingestion, food is present to help buffer the acid. Symptoms of duodenal ulcers occur generally 2 to 5 hours after a meal. The pain is described as "burning" or "cramplike." It is most often located in the mid-epigastric region beneath the xiphoid process. Duodenal ulcers can also produce back pain. Antacids alone or in combination with an H_2-receptor blocker, as well as food, neutralize the acid to provide relief. A characteristic of duodenal ulcer is its tendency to occur continuously for a few weeks or months and then disappear for a time, only to recur some months later.

Some patients experience bloating, nausea, vomiting, and early feelings of fullness. Not all patients with ulcers experience pain or discomfort. *Silent* peptic ulcers are more likely to occur in older adults and those taking NSAIDs. The presence or absence of symptoms is not directly related to the size of the ulcer or the degree of healing.

Complications

The three major complications of chronic PUD are hemorrhage, perforation, and gastric outlet obstruction. All these complications are considered emergency situations and may require surgical intervention.

Hemorrhage. Hemorrhage is the most common complication of PUD. Duodenal ulcers account for a greater percentage of upper GI bleeding episodes than gastric ulcers.

Perforation. Perforation is considered the most lethal complication of PUD. Perforation is commonly seen in large penetrating duodenal ulcers (Fig. 41-13). Even though duodenal ulcers are more prevalent and perforate more often, mortality rates associated with perforation of gastric ulcers are higher. The patient with gastric ulcers is older and often has concurrent medical problems, which accounts for the higher mortality rate.

With perforation, the ulcer penetrates the serosal surface with spillage of either gastric or duodenal contents into the peritoneal cavity. Larger perforations require immediate surgical closure. Small perforations may spontaneously seal themselves and symptoms cease. Spontaneous sealing occurs because of fibrin production in response to the perforation. This can lead to fibrinous fusion of the duodenum or gastric curvature to adjacent tissue (mainly the liver) and strictures that can obstruct the flow of intestinal contents and the passage of stool.

The clinical manifestations of perforation are sudden and dramatic in onset. During the initial phase (0 to 2 hours after perforation), the patient has sudden, severe upper abdominal pain that quickly spreads throughout the abdomen. The pain radiates to the back and shoulders. Food or antacids do not relieve the pain. The abdomen appears rigid and boardlike as the abdominal muscles attempt to protect from further injury. The patient's respirations become shallow and rapid. The heart rate is elevated (tachycardia), and the pulse is weak. Bowel sounds are usually absent. Nausea and vomiting may occur.

The contents entering the peritoneal cavity from the stomach or duodenum may contain air, saliva, food particles, HCl acid, pepsin, bacteria, bile, and pancreatic fluid and enzymes. If the condition is untreated, bacterial peritonitis may occur within 6 to 12 hours. The intensity of peritonitis is proportional to the amount and duration of the spillage through the perforation. It is difficult to determine from the symptoms alone whether a

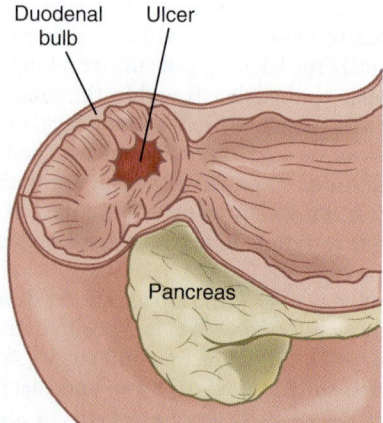

FIG. 41-13 Duodenal ulcer of the posterior wall penetrating into the head of the pancreas, resulting in walled-off perforation.

gastric or duodenal ulcer has perforated, because the manifestations of peritonitis are the same (see Chapter 42).

Gastric Outlet Obstruction. Both acute and chronic PUD can result in gastric outlet obstruction. Obstruction in the distal stomach and duodenum is the result of edema, inflammation, or pylorospasm and fibrous scar tissue formation. With obstruction the patient reports discomfort or pain that is worse toward the end of the day as the stomach fills and dilates. Belching or self-induced vomiting may provide some relief. Vomiting is common and often projectile. The vomitus may contain food particles that were ingested hours or days before. Constipation occurs because of dehydration and decreased diet intake secondary to anorexia. Over time dilation of the stomach and visible swelling in the upper abdomen may occur.

Diagnostic Studies

The diagnostic tests used to determine the presence and location of an ulcer are similar to those used for acute upper GI bleeding. Endoscopy is the most accurate diagnostic procedure. Endoscopy allows for direct viewing of the gastric and duodenal mucosa (Fig. 41-14). During endoscopy, tissue specimens are obtained to determine if *H. pylori* is present and rule out stomach cancer. Endoscopy can also be used to determine the degree of ulcer healing after treatment.

Several noninvasive and invasive tests are available to confirm *H. pylori* infection. The gold standard for diagnosing *H. pylori* infection is a biopsy of the antral mucosa with testing for urease (rapid urease testing). Noninvasive tests include serology, stool, and breath testing. The urea breath test can identify active infection. Urea is a by-product of the metabolism of *H. pylori* bacteria. Stool antigen tests are not as accurate as the urea breath test. Serum or whole blood antibody tests, particularly immunoglobulin G (IgG), do not distinguish between past and current infection.

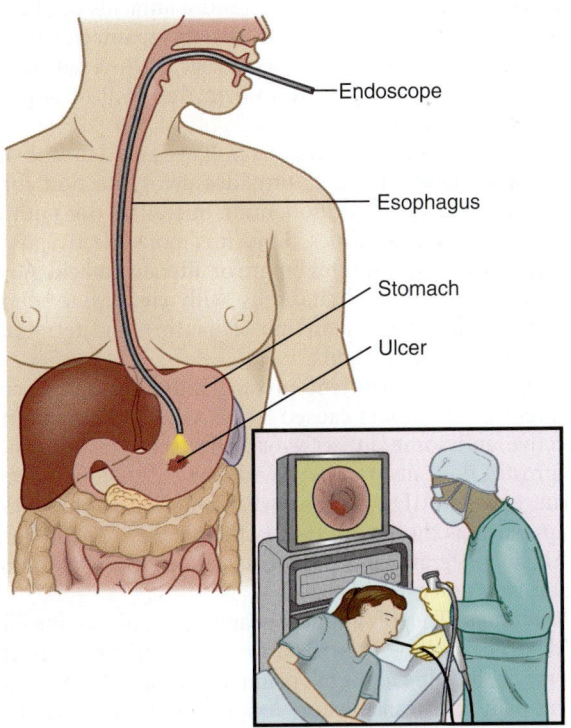

FIG. 41-14 Esophagogastroduodenoscopy (EGD) directly visualizes the mucosal lining of the stomach with a flexible endoscope. Ulcers or tumors can be directly visualized and biopsies taken.

A barium contrast study may be used to diagnose gastric outlet obstruction or for ulcer detection in those who cannot undergo endoscopy. Elevated fasting serum gastrin levels may indicate the presence of a possible gastrinoma (Zollinger-Ellison syndrome). A secretin stimulation test can discern patients with gastrinomas from those with other causes of hypergastrinemia.

Laboratory tests, including a CBC, liver enzyme studies, serum amylase, and stool examination, should be done. A CBC may indicate anemia secondary to ulcer bleeding. Liver enzyme studies help detect any liver problems (e.g., cirrhosis) that may complicate ulcer treatment. Stools are tested for blood. A serum amylase evaluates pancreatic function when posterior duodenal ulcer penetration of the pancreas is suspected.

Interprofessional Care: Conservative Therapy

A treatment regimen begins after diagnostic studies confirm the presence of PUD (Table 41-15). The regimen consists of adequate rest, drug therapy, smoking cessation, dietary modifications (if needed), and long-term follow-up care. The aim of treatment is to decrease gastric acidity and enhance mucosal defense mechanisms.

Patients are generally treated in ambulatory care clinics. Pain disappears after 3 to 6 days, but ulcer healing is much slower. Complete healing may take 3 to 9 weeks, depending on ulcer size, treatment regimen, and patient adherence. Endoscopic examination is the most accurate method to monitor ulcer healing. The usual follow-up endoscopic evaluation is done 3 to 6 months after diagnosis and treatment.

Aspirin and nonselective NSAIDs are discontinued for 4 to 6 weeks. When aspirin must be continued, co-administration with a PPI, H_2-receptor blocker, or misoprostol (Cytotec) may be prescribed. Patients receiving low-dose aspirin for cardiovascular and stroke risk who have a history of ulcer disease or complications may need to receive long-term treatment with a PPI.[20] Enteric-coated aspirin decreases localized irritation but has not been proved to reduce the overall risk for GI bleeding.

Smoking has an irritating effect on the mucosa and delays mucosal healing. The patient should either stop or severely reduce smoking. (See Chapter 10 for ways to enhance patient smoking cessation.) Adequate rest, both physical and emotional, is important for ulcer healing and may require some modifications in the patient's daily routine. Avoiding or restricting alcohol intake will enhance healing.

Drug Therapy. Drugs are a vital part of therapy (Table 41-10). Drug therapy focuses on reducing gastric acid secretion and, if needed, eliminating *H. pylori* infection. Patients with *H. pylori* infection need treatment with antibiotics and a PPI. After the ulcer has healed, many patients can stop H_2-receptor blocker and PPI therapy. Some may need to continue low-dose maintenance therapy.

Because ulcers frequently recur, interrupting or discontinuing therapy can have harmful results. Strict adherence to the prescribed drug regimen is important. Encourage the patient to adhere to therapy and continue with follow-up care as prescribed. Teach the patient and caregiver about each drug prescribed, why it is ordered, and the expected benefits. Review what to do if pain and discomfort recur or there is blood in vomitus or stools.

Antibiotic Therapy. Eradicating *H. pylori* is the most important part of treating PUD in patients positive for *H. pylori*. Antibiotic therapy is prescribed concurrently with a PPI for 7

TABLE 41-15 Interprofessional Care
Peptic Ulcer Disease

Diagnostic Assessment
- History and physical examination
- Upper GI endoscopy with biopsy
- Endoscopic ultrasound
- *Helicobacter pylori* testing of breath, urine, blood, tissue
- Complete blood cell count
- Liver enzymes
- Serum amylase
- Stool testing for blood

Management
Conservative Therapy
- Adequate rest
- Smoking and alcohol cessation
- Stress management (see Chapter 6)

Drug Therapy (Tables 41-10 and 41-13)
- Antibiotics for *H. pylori*
- Proton pump inhibitors
- H_2-receptor blockers
- Cytoprotective drugs
- Antacids

Acute Exacerbation Without Complications
- NPO
- NG suction
- Adequate rest
- IV fluid replacement

Drug Therapy
- Proton pump inhibitors
- H_2-receptor blockers
- Antacids
- Sedatives

Acute Exacerbation With Complications (Hemorrhage, Perforation, Obstruction)
- NPO
- NG suction
- IV proton pump inhibitor
- Bed rest
- IV fluid replacement (lactated Ringer's solution)
- Blood transfusions
- Stomach lavage (possible)

Surgical Therapy
- *Perforation:* Simple closure with omentum graft
- Gastric outlet obstruction: Pyloroplasty and vagotomy
- Ulcer removal or reduction
  - Billroth I and II
  - Vagotomy and pyloroplasty

to 14 days (Table 41-13). If the patient has a penicillin allergy, metronidazole is used instead of amoxicillin in the triple-drug regimen. Bismuth can be given alone or as part of a combination capsule (Pylera) containing bismuth, tetracycline, and metronidazole. Because of the existence of antibiotic-resistant organisms, a growing number of patients do not have *H. pylori* eradicated with a single round of therapy.

Proton Pump Inhibitors. PPIs are more effective than H_2-receptor blockers in reducing gastric acid secretion and promoting ulcer healing. PPIs are used in combination with antibiotics to treat ulcers caused by *H. pylori*. Several PPIs are available as both prescription and OTC preparations.

Histamine (H$_2$)-Receptor Blockers. H_2-receptor blockers promote ulcer healing. The onset of action of H_2-receptor blockers is 1 hour. Depending on the specific drug, therapeutic effects last up to 12 hours. Several H_2 receptor blockers are available as both prescription and OTC preparations. Famotidine, ranitidine, and cimetidine can be given orally or IV. Nizatidine is only available orally.

Antacids. Antacids are sometimes used as adjunct therapy for PUD. They increase gastric pH by neutralizing the HCl acid. As a result, they reduce the acid content of chyme reaching the duodenum. In addition, some antacids (e.g., aluminum hydroxide) can bind to bile salts, thus decreasing the damaging effects of bile on the gastric mucosa.

Common antacids consist of magnesium hydroxide or aluminum hydroxide as single preparations or in various combinations (Table 41-10). The neutralizing effects of antacids taken on an empty stomach last only 20 to 30 minutes. When antacids are taken after meals, the effects may last as long as 3 to 4 hours. After an acute phase of bleeding, antacids may be given hourly, either orally or through the NG tube. If an NG tube is in place, the stomach contents should be aspirated and tested periodically for pH level. If pH is less than 5, intermittent suction may be used, or the frequency or dosage of the antacid or antisecretory agent increased.

The type and dosage of antacid given depend on side effects and potential drug interactions. Antacids high in sodium (e.g., sodium citrate [Bicitra]) are used cautiously in older adults and patients with liver cirrhosis, hypertension, heart failure, and renal disease. Patients with renal failure should not take magnesium preparations because of the risk of magnesium toxicity. An antacid combination of aluminum and magnesium seems to decrease the side effects of both.

Antacids can interact unfavorably with many drugs. They can enhance the absorption of drugs such as dicumarol and amphetamines. Calcium and magnesium antacids can potentiate the effects of digitalis. In some instances, antacids decrease the absorption rates of prescribed drugs, such as tetracycline. Before antacid therapy begins, inform the HCP of any drugs that a patient is taking.

Cytoprotective Drug Therapy. Sucralfate is used for the short-term treatment of ulcers. It provides cytoprotection for the esophagus, stomach, and duodenum. Sucralfate does not have acid-neutralizing capabilities. Since it is most effective at a low pH, give it at least 60 minutes before or after an antacid. Adverse side effects are minimal. It binds with cimetidine, digoxin, warfarin (Coumadin), phenytoin (Dilantin), and tetracycline, reducing their bioavailability.

Misoprostol is a synthetic prostaglandin analog prescribed to prevent gastric ulcers caused by NSAIDs and aspirin. It has protective and some antisecretory effects on gastric mucosa. Misoprostol does not interfere with the therapeutic effects of aspirin and NSAIDs. People who require chronic NSAID therapy, such as those with osteoarthritis, may benefit from its use. Since it is teratogenic, it is used with caution in women of childbearing potential.

Other Drugs. Tricyclic antidepressants (e.g., imipramine [Tofranil], doxepin) may be prescribed for some patients. Antidepressants may contribute to overall pain relief through their effects on afferent pain fiber transmission. In addition, tricyclic antidepressants have varying degrees of anticholinergic properties, which result in reduced acid secretion.

Anticholinergic drugs are occasionally used for PUD treatment. Anticholinergics are associated with a number of side effects, such as dry mouth, warm skin, flushing, thirst, tachycardia, dilated pupils, blurred vision, and urine retention.

Nutritional Therapy. There is no specific recommended dietary modification for PUD. Patients should eat and drink foods and fluids that do not cause any distressing symptoms. Foods that commonly cause gastric irritation include pepper, carbonated beverages, broth (meat extract), and hot, spicy foods. Caffeine-containing beverages and foods can increase symptoms in some patients. Teach the patient to avoid alcohol use because it can delay healing.

Therapy Related to Complications of Peptic Ulcer Disease

Acute Exacerbation. Patients with an acute exacerbation frequently experience bleeding, increased pain and discomfort, and nausea and vomiting. Management is similar to that described for upper GI bleeding later in this chapter (see pp. 923-925).

Perforation. The immediate focus of managing a patient with a perforation is to stop the spillage of gastric or duodenal contents into the peritoneal cavity and restore blood volume. An NG tube can provide continuous aspiration and gastric decompression to stop spillage through the perforation. For duodenal aspiration, the tube is placed as near to the perforation site as possible to facilitate decompression.

Circulating blood volume is replaced with lactated Ringer's and albumin solutions. These solutions substitute for the fluids lost from the vascular and interstitial space as peritonitis develops. Blood replacement in the form of packed RBCs may be necessary. A central venous pressure line and an indwelling urinary catheter may be inserted and monitored hourly. The patient with a history of cardiac disease requires electrocardiographic (ECG) monitoring or placement of a pulmonary artery catheter for accurate assessment of left ventricular function. Broad-spectrum antibiotic therapy is started immediately to treat bacterial peritonitis.

Either open or laparoscopic procedures are used for perforation repair depending on the location of the ulcer and surgeon preference. The procedure involving the least risk to the patient is simple oversewing of the perforation and reinforcement of the area with a graft of omentum. Excess gastric contents are suctioned from the peritoneal cavity during the surgical procedure.

Gastric Outlet Obstruction. The aim of therapy for obstruction is to decompress the stomach, correct any existing fluid and electrolyte imbalances, and improve the patient's general state of health. An NG tube is used as described previously. With continuous decompression for several days, the ulcer can begin healing, and the inflammation and edema will subside. Pain relief results from the decompression.

IV fluids and electrolytes are replaced according to the degree of dehydration, vomiting, and electrolyte imbalance indicated by laboratory studies. A PPI or H_2-receptor blocker is used if the obstruction is due to an active ulcer as determined by endoscopy. Pyloric obstruction may be treated endoscopically by balloon dilations. Surgical intervention may be needed to remove scar tissue.

❖ NURSING MANAGEMENT: PEPTIC ULCER DISEASE

◆ Nursing Assessment

Subjective and objective data to obtain from a patient with PUD are presented in Table 41-16.

◆ Nursing Diagnoses

Nursing diagnoses related to PUD may include, but are not limited to, the following:

TABLE 41-16 Nursing Assessment

Peptic Ulcer Disease

Subjective Data

Important Health Information

Past health history: Chronic kidney disease, pancreatic disease, chronic obstructive pulmonary disease, serious illness or trauma, hyperparathyroidism, cirrhosis of the liver, Zollinger-Ellison syndrome

Medications: Aspirin, corticosteroids, nonsteroidal antiinflammatory drugs

Surgery or other treatments: Complicated or prolonged surgery

Functional Health Patterns

Health perception–health management: Chronic alcohol abuse, smoking, caffeine use. Family history of peptic ulcer disease

Nutritional-metabolic: Weight loss, anorexia, nausea and vomiting, hematemesis, dyspepsia, heartburn, belching

Elimination: Black, tarry stools

Cognitive-perceptual
- *Duodenal ulcers:* Burning, midepigastric or back pain occurring 2-5 hr after meals and relieved by food; nocturnal pain common
- *Gastric ulcers:* High epigastric pain occurring 1-2 hr after meals. Pain may be precipitated or aggravated by food.

Coping–stress tolerance: Acute or chronic stress

Objective Data

General

Anxiety, irritability

Gastrointestinal

Epigastric tenderness

Possible Diagnostic Findings

Anemia. Guaiac-positive stools. Positive blood, urine, breath, or stool tests for *Helicobacter pylori*. Abnormal upper gastrointestinal endoscopic and barium studies.

- Acute pain *related to* increased gastric secretions
- Ineffective health management *related to* lack of knowledge of long-term management of PUD
- Nausea *related to* acute exacerbation of disease process

Additional information on nursing diagnoses for the patient with PUD is presented in eNursing Care Plan 41-2 available on the website for this chapter.

◆ Planning

The overall goals are that the patient with PUD will (1) adhere to the prescribed therapeutic regimen, (2) experience a reduction in or absence of discomfort, (3) exhibit no signs of GI complications, (4) have complete healing of the peptic ulcer, and (5) make appropriate lifestyle changes to prevent recurrence.

◆ Nursing Implementation

Health Promotion. You play an important role in identifying patients at risk for PUD. Early detection and effective treatment of ulcers are important aspects of reducing morbidity risks associated with PUD. Patients who are taking ulcerogenic drugs (e.g., aspirin, NSAIDs) are at risk for PUD. Encourage patients to take these drugs with food. Teach patients to report symptoms related to gastric irritation, including epigastric pain, to their HCP.

Acute Care. During an acute exacerbation, the patient often complains of increased pain, nausea, and vomiting. Some may have evidence of bleeding. Initially many patients attempt to cope with the symptoms at home before seeking medical assistance.

During the acute phase, the patient may be NPO for a few days, have an NG tube inserted and connected to intermittent suction, and have IV fluid replacement. Explain to the patient and caregiver the reasons for these therapies so they understand that the advantages far outweigh any temporary discomfort. Regular mouth care alleviates the dry mouth. Cleaning and lubricating the nares facilitate breathing and decrease soreness. Analysis of gastric contents may include pH testing and analysis for blood, bile, or other substances. When the stomach is empty of gastric secretions, pain diminishes and ulcer healing begins.

The volume of fluid lost, the patient's signs and symptoms, and laboratory test results (hemoglobin, hematocrit, and electrolytes) determine the type and amount of IV fluids administered. Take vital signs initially and then at least hourly to detect and treat shock. Give IV fluids as ordered and record intake and output.

Physical and emotional rest is helpful to ulcer healing. The patient's environment should be quiet and restful. Give pain medications as ordered. A mild sedative or tranquilizer has beneficial effects when the patient is anxious and apprehensive. Use good judgment before sedating a person who is becoming increasingly restless because the drug could mask the signs of shock secondary to upper GI bleeding.

◆ *Hemorrhage.* Changes in vital signs and an increase in the amount and redness of aspirate often signal massive upper GI bleeding. With bleeding, the patient's pain often decreases because the blood helps neutralize the acidic gastric contents. It is important to maintain the patency of the NG tube so that blood clots do not obstruct the tube. If the tube becomes blocked, the patient can develop abdominal distention. Use interventions similar to those described for upper GI bleeding on pp. 923-925.

◆ *Perforation.* With perforation, the patient complains of sudden, severe upper abdominal pain that quickly becomes generalized throughout the abdomen. Other manifestations include a rigid, boardlike abdomen; severe back and shoulder pain; shallow respirations; and a weak, rapid heart rate. Bowel sounds that may have been previously normal or hyperactive may diminish and become absent. When the patient with an ulcer demonstrates these changes, suspect perforation and notify the HCP immediately.

Take vital signs promptly and record them every 15 to 30 minutes. Temporarily stop all oral or NG drugs and feedings. If perforation exists, anything taken orally can add to the spillage into the peritoneal cavity and increase discomfort. If you are giving IV fluid, maintain the rate or increase it per institutional protocol to replace the depleted plasma volume. Giving pain medications provides comfort.

Those with confirmed perforation start on antibiotic therapy. If the perforation fails to seal spontaneously, surgical closure is necessary. Since surgery is done as soon as possible, there may not be time to adequately prepare the patient and family.

◆ *Gastric Outlet Obstruction.* Gastric outlet obstruction can happen at any time. It is most likely to occur in the patient whose ulcer is located close to the pylorus. The onset of symptoms is usually gradual. Constant NG aspiration of stomach contents can help relieve symptoms. This allows edema and inflammation to subside and permits normal flow of gastric contents through the pylorus.

Regularly irrigate the NG tube with a normal saline solution per institutional policy to assist proper functioning. It may be helpful to reposition the patient from side to side so that the tube tip is not constantly lying against the mucosal surface. It is important to maintain accurate intake and output records, especially of the gastric aspirate.

To check for ongoing obstruction, clamp the NG tube intermittently and measure the gastric residual volume. The frequency and amount of time the tube remains clamped are related to the amount of aspirate obtained and the patient's comfort level. A method commonly followed is to clamp the tube overnight (approximately 8 to 12 hours) and measure the gastric residual volume in the morning. When the aspirate falls below 200 mL, it is within a normal range and the patient can begin oral intake of clear liquids. Oral fluids begin at 30 mL/hr and then gradually increase in amount. As the amount of gastric residual decreases, solid foods are added and the tube removed.

If the patient has resumed oral feedings and you note symptoms of obstruction, promptly inform the HCP. Generally, all that is necessary to treat the problem is to resume gastric aspiration so that the edema and inflammation resulting from the acute episode resolve. IV fluids with electrolyte replacement keep the patient hydrated during this period. If conservative treatment is not successful, surgery is done after the acute phase has passed.

◆ **Ambulatory Care.** Patients with PUD have specific needs to prevent recurrence and complications. Teaching should cover aspects of the disease process, drugs, possible changes in lifestyle (alcohol intake, smoking), and regular follow-up care. Table 41-17 provides a patient and caregiver teaching guide for PUD.

Knowing the etiology and pathophysiology of PUD may motivate the patient to become involved in care and improve adherence to therapy. Work with the dietitian to elicit a dietary history and plan ways to incorporate any needed dietary modifications into the patient's home and work setting.

Teach the patient about prescribed drugs, including their actions, side effects, and dangers if omitted for any reason.

TABLE 41-17 Patient & Caregiver Teaching

Peptic Ulcer Disease (PUD)

Include the following instructions when teaching the patient and caregiver about management of PUD.

1. Follow dietary modifications, including avoiding foods that may cause epigastric distress such as acidic foods.
2. Avoid cigarettes. In addition to promoting ulcer development, smoking delays ulcer healing.
3. Reduce or eliminate alcohol intake.
4. Avoid OTC drugs unless approved by the HCP. Many preparations contain ingredients, such as aspirin, that should not be taken unless approved by the HCP. Check with the HCP about the use of nonsteroidal antiinflammatory drugs.
5. Do not interchange brands of antacids, H_2-receptor blockers, and proton pump inhibitors that can be purchased OTC without checking with the HCP. This can lead to harmful side effects.
6. Take all medications as prescribed. This includes both antisecretory and antibiotic drugs. Failing to take medications as prescribed can result in relapse.
7. It is important to report any of the following:
   • Increased nausea or vomiting
   • Increased epigastric pain
   • Bloody emesis or tarry stools
8. Stress can be related to signs and symptoms of PUD. Learn and use stress management strategies (see Chapter 6).
9. Share concerns about lifestyle changes and living with a chronic illness.

Make sure the patient knows not to take OTC drugs (e.g., aspirin, NSAIDs) unless approved by the HCP.[20] Because you can buy several H$_2$-receptor blockers and PPIs without a prescription, tell the patient that substituting prescription with OTC preparations without checking with the HCP can lead to harmful side effects.

Try to obtain information about the patient's psychosocial status. Knowledge of lifestyle, occupation, and coping behaviors can be helpful in planning care. The patient may be reluctant to talk about personal subjects, the stress experienced at home or on the job, the usual methods of coping, or dependence on drugs or alcohol.

The patient may not be honest about habitual use of alcohol or cigarettes. Provide information about the negative effects of alcohol and cigarettes on PUD and ulcer healing. Changes, such as smoking cessation and alcohol abstinence, are difficult for many people. The patient may do better in reducing, rather than totally eliminating, use of these substances. However, the goal should always be total cessation.

PUD is often a chronic, recurring disorder. Inform patients with chronic PUD about potential complications, the clinical manifestations indicating their presence, and what to do until they see the HCP. Emphasize the need for long-term follow-up care. Encourage the patient to seek immediate intervention if symptoms return. The patient may be frustrated, especially if the patient followed prescribed therapy and it failed to prevent a recurrence.

Some patients do not adhere to the plan of care and experience repeated exacerbations. Patients quickly learn that they often experience no discomfort when they omit prescribed drugs, smoke, or drink alcohol. Consequently, they make no or little alterations in their lifestyle. After an acute exacerbation, the patient is likely to be more amenable to following the plan of care and open to suggestions for changes in lifestyle.

◆ Evaluation

Expected outcomes are that the patient with PUD will
- Have pain controlled without the use of analgesics
- Verbalize an understanding of the treatment regimen
- Commit to self-care and management of the disease
- Have no complications (hemorrhage, perforation)

Additional information on expected outcomes for the patient with PUD is presented in eNursing Care Plan 41-2 (available on the website for this chapter).

Interprofessional Care: Surgical Therapy for Peptic Ulcer Disease

With the use of drug therapy and endoscopic therapy to treat PUD, surgery is used less frequently. Surgery is done on patients with complications that are unresponsive to medical management or concerns about stomach cancer.

Surgical procedures include partial gastrectomy, vagotomy, and pyloroplasty. Partial gastrectomy with removal of the distal two thirds of the stomach and anastomosis of the gastric stump to the duodenum is called a *gastroduodenostomy* or *Billroth I* operation (Fig. 41-15, *A*). If the gastric stump is anastomosed to the jejunum, the surgery is a *gastrojejunostomy* or *Billroth II* operation (Fig. 41-15, *B*).

Vagotomy is the severing of the vagus nerve, either totally (*truncal*) or selectively (*highly selective vagotomy*). These procedures decrease gastric acid secretion. *Pyloroplasty* consists of surgical enlargement of the pyloric sphincter to facilitate the

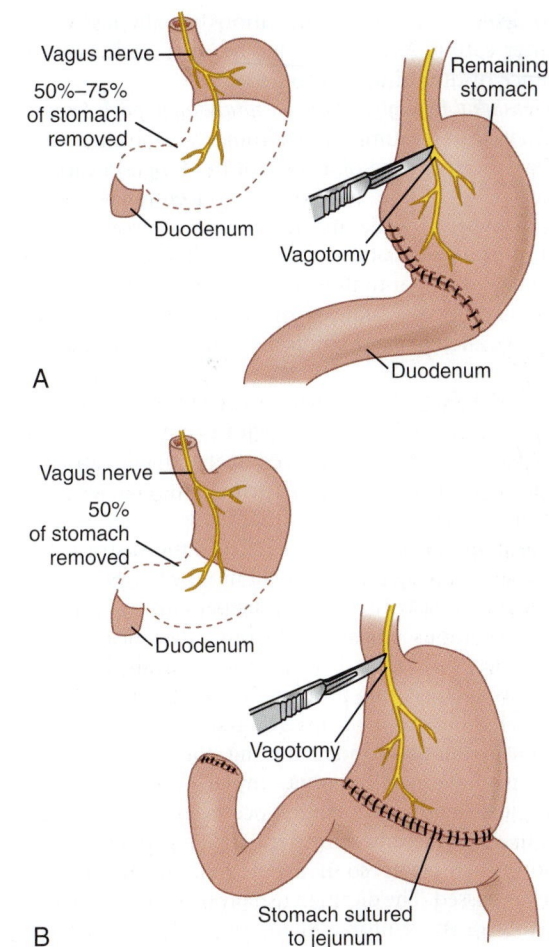

FIG. 41-15 **A,** Billroth I procedure (subtotal gastric resection with gastroduodenostomy anastomosis). **B,** Billroth II procedure (subtotal gastric resection with gastrojejunostomy anastomosis).

easy passage of contents from the stomach. It is commonly done after vagotomy or to enlarge an opening that is constricted from scar tissue.

Postoperative Complications. As with all surgeries, acute postoperative bleeding at the surgical site can occur. Monitoring of patients is similar to that described under acute upper GI bleeding. The most common long-term postoperative complications from PUD surgery are (1) dumping syndrome, (2) postprandial hypoglycemia, and (3) bile reflux gastritis.

Dumping Syndrome. Dumping syndrome is the direct result of surgical removal of a large portion of the stomach and pyloric sphincter. Approximately 20% of patients experience dumping syndrome after PUD surgery.

Normally, gastric chyme enters the small intestine in small amounts. After surgery, the stomach no longer has control over the amount of gastric chyme entering the small intestine. Therefore a large bolus of hypertonic fluid enters the intestine and causes fluid to be drawn into the bowel lumen. This creates a decrease in plasma volume, distention of the bowel lumen, and rapid intestinal transit.

Symptoms begin within 15 to 30 minutes after eating. The patient usually describes feelings of generalized weakness, sweating, palpitations, and dizziness. These symptoms are due to the sudden decrease in plasma volume. The patient complains of abdominal cramps, *borborygmi* (audible abdominal sounds produced by hyperactive intestinal peristalsis), and the urge to defecate. These manifestations usually last less than 1 hour after eating. A short rest period after each meal reduces the chance of dumping syndrome.

Postprandial Hypoglycemia. *Postprandial hypoglycemia* is considered a variant of dumping syndrome. It is the result of uncontrolled gastric emptying of a bolus of fluid high in carbohydrate into the small intestine. The bolus of concentrated carbohydrate results in hyperglycemia and the release of excess amounts of insulin into the circulation. This results in reflex hypoglycemia. Symptoms are similar to those of any hypoglycemic reaction and include sweating, weakness, mental confusion, palpitations, tachycardia, and anxiety. Symptoms generally occur 2 hours after eating.

Bile Reflux Gastritis. Gastric surgery that involves either reconstruction or removal of the pylorus can result in reflux of bile into the stomach. Prolonged contact with bile causes damage to the gastric mucosa, chronic gastritis, and recurrence of PUD.

The main symptom is continuous epigastric distress that increases after meals. Vomiting relieves the distress, but only temporarily. Although only a small number of patients experience bile reflux gastritis, caution the patient to notify the HCP of any continuous epigastric distress after meals. Cholestyramine (Questran), given before or with meals, has been used successfully to treat this problem. Cholestyramine binds with the bile salts that are the source of gastric irritation.

Nutritional Therapy. Understanding the surgery performed and the patient's resulting anatomy are important. Nutrition interventions help minimize the occurrence of expected complications and maximize nutrient intake (Table 41-18). Start nutrition teaching as soon as the immediate postoperative period has passed. The dietitian usually provides dietary instructions. You must reinforce them. Reassure the patient that unpleasant symptoms are usually of short duration. Following dietary measures will decrease symptoms within a few months and is essential to long-term adherence.

Because gastric resection decreases the stomach's reservoir, patients must reduce their meal size accordingly. Teach the patient to limit drinking fluids with meals. Initially, dry foods

---

with a low carbohydrate content and moderate protein and fat content are better tolerated. To avoid hypoglycemic episodes, teach the patient to limit the amount of sugar consumed with each meal and eat small, frequent meals with moderate amounts of protein and fat. The immediate ingestion of sugared fluids or candy relieves hypoglycemic symptoms.

❖ NURSING MANAGEMENT: SURGICAL THERAPY FOR PEPTIC ULCER DISEASE

◆ Preoperative Care

Surgery can involve either laparoscopic or open surgery techniques. The surgeon will provide the necessary information about the procedure and expected outcomes so that the patient can make an informed decision. Help the patient and caregiver by clarifying and interpreting their questions. Teach them what to expect after surgery, including comfort measures, pain relief, coughing and breathing exercises, use of an NG tube, and IV fluid administration (see Chapter 17).

◆ Postoperative Care

Care of the patient after major abdominal surgery is similar to the postoperative care after abdominal laparotomy (see Chapter 42). An NG tube is used to decompress the remaining portion of the stomach. This decreases pressure on the suture line and allows edema and inflammation resulting from surgical trauma to resolve.

Observe the gastric aspirate for color, amount, and odor. The aspirate is usually bright red at first, with a gradual darkening within the first 24 hours after surgery. Normally the color changes to yellow-green within 36 to 48 hours. If the tube becomes clogged, the HCP may order periodic gentle irrigations with normal saline solution. It is essential that the NG suction is working and that the tube remains patent so that accumulated gastric secretions do not put a strain on the anastomosis. This can lead to distention of the remaining portion of the stomach and result in (1) rupture of the sutures, (2) leakage of gastric contents into the peritoneal cavity, (3) hemorrhage, and (4) possible abscess formation. If the tube must be replaced or repositioned, call the HCP to perform this task because of the danger of perforating the gastric mucosa or disrupting the suture line.

Observe the patient for signs of decreased peristalsis, including abdominal distention and lower abdominal discomfort, which may indicate intestinal obstruction. Monitor and record accurate intake and output every 4 hours.

Keep the patient comfortable and free of pain by giving analgesics and frequently changing position. In an open surgical approach, the incision is relatively high in the epigastrium and may interfere with deep breathing and coughing. Splinting the area with a pillow while encouraging the patient to deep breathe helps prevent pulmonary complications. Splinting also protects the abdominal suture line from rupturing during coughing. Observe the dressing for signs of bleeding or odor and drainage indicative of an infection. Encourage early ambulation.

While the NG tube is connected to suction, maintain IV therapy. Administer potassium and vitamin supplements as ordered until oral feedings are resumed. Before the NG tube is removed, the patient begins clear liquids to determine the tolerance level. The stomach may be aspirated within 1 or 2 hours to assess the amount remaining and its color and consistency. When fluids are well tolerated, the NG tube is removed. Fluids

---

🫛 TABLE 41-18   Nutritional Therapy

Postgastrectomy Dumping Syndrome

Purposes
- To slow the rapid passage of food into the intestine
- To control symptoms of dumping syndrome (dizziness, sense of fullness, diarrhea, tachycardia), which sometimes occurs after a partial or total gastrectomy

Diet Principles
- Divide meals into six small feedings to avoid overloading the stomach and intestine at mealtimes.
- Do not take fluids with meals but at least 30-45 min before or after meals. This helps prevent distention or a feeling of fullness.
- Avoid concentrated sweets (e.g., honey, sugar, jelly, jam, candies, sweet pastries, sweetened fruit) because they sometimes cause dizziness, diarrhea, and a sense of fullness.
- Increase protein and fats to promote rebuilding of body tissues and to meet energy needs. Meat, cheese, and eggs are specific foods to increase in the diet.
- Amount of time these restrictions should be followed varies. The HCP decides the proper amount of time to remain on this prescribed diet according to the patient's clinical condition and progress.

are increased in frequency, with a slow progression to regular foods. The patient begins a regimen of six small meals a day.

Pernicious anemia is a long-term complication of total gastrectomy and may occur after partial gastrectomy. Pernicious anemia is due to the loss of intrinsic factor, which is produced by the parietal cells. The patient will require cobalamin replacement therapy (see Chapter 30). PUD is a chronic problem, and ulcers can recur, especially at the site of the anastomosis.

Gerontologic Considerations: Peptic Ulcer Disease

The morbidity and mortality rates associated with PUD in older adults are higher than for younger adults because of concurrent health problems and a decreased ability to withstand hypovolemia. Monitor older adults who use NSAIDs for osteoarthritis for signs and symptoms of PUD. In older patients, pain may not be the first symptom associated with an ulcer. For some patients the first manifestation is frank gastric bleeding or a decrease in hematocrit.

The treatment and management of PUD in older adults are similar to those in younger adults. An emphasis is placed on preventing gastritis and PUD. This includes teaching the patient to take NSAIDs and other gastric-irritating drugs with food, milk, or antacids. Teach the patient to avoid irritating substances, adhere to the PPI or H$_2$-receptor blocker therapy as prescribed, and report abdominal pain or discomfort to the HCP.

STOMACH CANCER

Stomach (gastric) cancer is an adenocarcinoma of the stomach wall (Fig. 41-16). It accounts for more than 24,590 new cancer cases and 10,720 deaths annually.[5] The rate of stomach (particularly distal) cancer has been steadily declining in the United States. However, cancer in the proximal gastric and gastroesophageal junction is increasing.

Asian Americans, Pacific Islanders, Hispanics, and African Americans have higher rates of stomach cancer than non-Hispanic whites. In the U.S., the incidence is higher in men than in women by a 2:1 ratio. Stomach cancer mostly affects older people. The average age of people when they are diagnosed is 69.

At the time of diagnosis, only 10% to 20% of patients have disease confined to the stomach. More than 50% have advanced metastatic disease. The 5-year survival rate is 71% in persons with early stage disease (confined to the stomach). The overall 5-year survival rate of all people with stomach cancer is about 29%.[5]

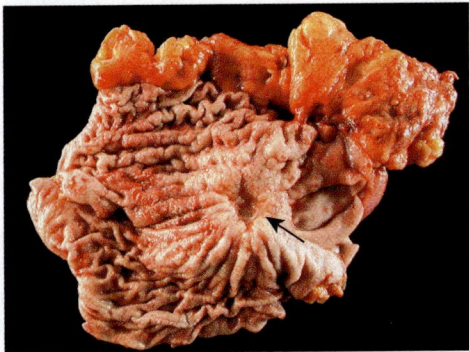

FIG. 41-16 Stomach cancer. Gross photograph showing an ill-defined, excavated central ulcer surrounded by irregular, heaped-up borders. (From Kumar V, Abbas AK, Aster JC, Fausto N: *Robbins and Cotran pathologic basis of disease*, ed 8, Philadelphia, 2010, Saunders.)

Etiology and Pathophysiology

While many factors are implicated in the development of stomach cancer, no single causative agent has been identified. Stomach cancer probably begins with a nonspecific mucosal injury because of infection (*H. pylori*), autoimmune-related inflammation, or repeated exposure to irritants such as bile, antiinflammatory agents, and tobacco use.

Stomach cancer has been associated with diets containing smoked foods, salted fish and meat, and pickled vegetables. Whole grains and fresh fruits and vegetables are associated with reduced rates of stomach cancer. Infection with *H. pylori*, especially at an early age, is a risk factor for stomach cancer. It is possible that *H. pylori* and resulting cell changes can induce a sequence of transitions from dysplasia to cancer. People with lymphoma of the stomach (mucosa-associated lymphoid tissue [MALT]) are at higher risk of stomach cancer.

Other predisposing factors include atrophic gastritis, pernicious anemia, adenomatous polyps, hyperplastic polyps, and achlorhydria. Smoking and obesity both increase the risk of stomach cancer. Although first-degree relatives of patients with stomach cancer are at increased risk, only 8% to 10% of stomach cancers have an inherited component.[21]

Stomach cancer spreads by direct extension and typically infiltrates rapidly to the surrounding tissue and liver. Seeding of tumor cells into the peritoneal cavity occurs late in the course of the disease.

Clinical Manifestations

Stomach cancers often spread to adjacent organs before any distressing symptoms occur. Clinical manifestations include unexplained weight loss, indigestion, abdominal discomfort or pain, and signs and symptoms of anemia. The patient may report *early satiety,* or a sense of being full sooner than usual. Anemia is common. It is caused by chronic blood loss as the lesion erodes through the mucosa or from pernicious anemia (caused by loss of intrinsic factor). The person appears pale and weak and complains of fatigue, weakness, dizziness, and, in extreme cases, shortness of breath. The stool may be positive for occult blood. Supraclavicular lymph nodes that are hard and enlarged suggest metastasis via the thoracic duct. The presence of ascites is a poor prognostic sign.

Diagnostic Studies

The diagnostic studies for stomach cancer are presented in Table 41-19. Upper GI endoscopy is the best diagnostic tool. The stomach can be distended with air during the procedure, stretching the mucosal folds. Tissue biopsy and subsequent histologic examination are important in diagnosing stomach cancer.

Endoscopic ultrasound, CT, and PET scanning can be used to stage the disease. Barium studies do not always detect small lesions of the cardia and fundus. Laparoscopy is done to determine peritoneal spread.

Blood studies detect anemia and determine its severity. Elevations in liver enzymes and serum amylase levels may indicate liver and pancreatic involvement. Stool examination provides evidence of occult or gross bleeding. The presence of tumor markers can help diagnose cancer.

Interprofessional Care

The treatment of choice for stomach cancer is surgical removal of the tumor. Preoperative management focuses on correcting nutritional deficits and treating anemia. Transfusions of packed

TABLE 41-19 Interprofessional Care

Stomach Cancer

Diagnostic Assessment	Management

• History and physical examination
• Endoscopy and biopsy
• CT and PET scans
• Upper GI barium study
• Exfoliative cytologic study
• Endoscopic ultrasonography
• Complete blood count
• Urinalysis
• Stool examination
• Liver enzymes
• Serum amylase
• Tumor markers
• Carcinoembryonic antigen (CEA)
• Carbohydrate antigen (CA)–19-9, CA-125, CA 72-4
• α-Fetoprotein
	• Surgical therapy
	  • Subtotal gastrectomy (Billroth I or II procedure)
	  • Total gastrectomy with esophagojejunostomy
	• Radiation therapy
	• Chemotherapy
	• Targeted therapy

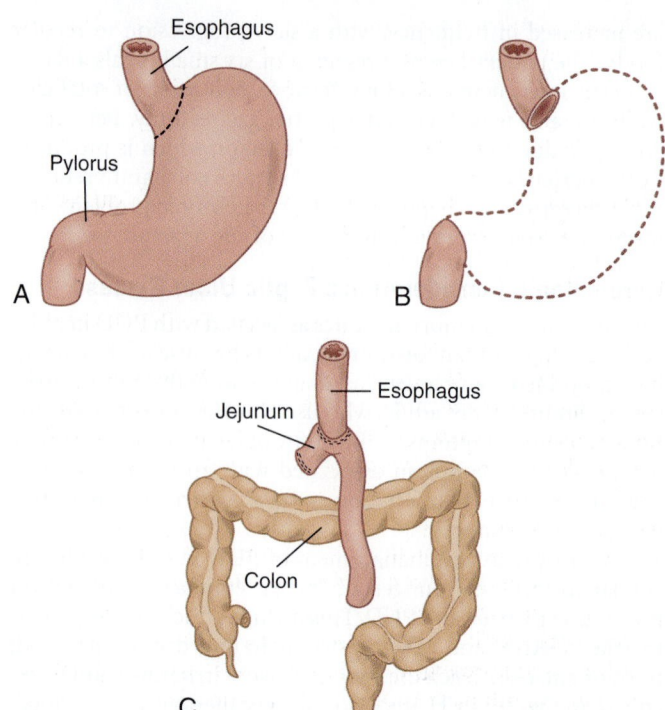

FIG. 41-17 Total gastrectomy for stomach cancer. **A,** Normal anatomic structure of the stomach. **B,** Removal of the stomach (total gastrectomy). **C,** Anastomosis of the esophagus with the jejunum (esophagojejunostomy).

RBCs correct the anemia. If gastric outlet obstruction occurs, gastric decompression may be necessary before surgery.

Surgical Therapy. The surgical interventions used in the treatment of stomach cancer are the same procedures used for PUD. The location and extent of the lesion, the patient's physical condition, and the surgeon's preference determine the specific surgery used (e.g., open versus laparoscopic).

The surgical aim is to remove as much of the stomach as necessary to remove the tumor and a margin of normal tissue. Lesions located in the antrum or pyloric region are generally treated by either a Billroth I or II procedure (Fig. 41-15). When the lesion is located in the fundus, a total gastrectomy with esophagojejunostomy is performed (Fig. 41-17). When metastasis has occurred to adjacent organs, such as the spleen, ovaries, or bowel, the surgical procedure is extended as necessary. If the tumor extends into the transverse colon, partial colon resection is required.

Chemotherapy and Radiation Therapy. A number of chemotherapy drugs can be used to treat stomach cancer. These include 5-FU (fluorouracil) (often given with leucovorin [folinic acid]), capecitabine (Xeloda), carboplatin, cisplatin, docetaxel (Taxotere), epirubicin (Ellence), irinotecan (Camptosar), oxaliplatin (Eloxatin), and paclitaxel. Combination therapies are commonly used as the drugs affect different phases of the cell cycle. Examples of combination therapy include ECF (epirubicin, cisplatin, and 5-FU) and DCF (docetaxel, cisplatin, and 5-FU). Intraperitoneal administration of chemotherapy agents may also be used to treat metastatic disease. (Chemotherapy is discussed in Chapter 15.)

Radiation therapy may be used together with chemotherapy to reduce the recurrence or as a palliative measure to decrease tumor mass and provide temporary relief of obstruction.

Targeted Therapy. Trastuzumab (Herceptin) and ramucirumab (Cyramza) are targeted therapies used to treat stomach cancer. About 20% of patients with stomach cancer have too much HER-2 (growth-promoting protein) on the surface of the cancer cells. Trastuzumab (Herceptin) targets the HER-2 protein and kills the cancer cells.[22] Ramucirumab (Cyramza) binds to the receptor for VEGF and prevents VEGF from binding to the receptor, thus preventing the growth and spread of cancer. These drugs are also used for esophageal cancer as discussed on p. 906. (Targeted therapies are discussed in Chapter 15.)

❖ NURSING MANAGEMENT: STOMACH CANCER

◆ Nursing Assessment

The assessment of a person with possible stomach cancer is similar to that for PUD (Table 41-16). Important data to obtain from the patient and caregiver include a nutritional assessment, a psychosocial history, the patient's perceptions of the health problem and need for care, and a physical examination.

The nutritional assessment obtains information about appetite and changes in eating patterns over the previous 6 months. Determine the patient's normal weight and any recent changes in it. Unexplained weight loss is common. Evaluate the patient's nutritional status. Cachexia may be evident if oral intake has been reduced for an extended period. A malnourished patient does not respond well to chemotherapy or radiation therapy and is a poor surgical risk. The patient may report a history of vague abdominal symptoms, including dyspepsia and intestinal gas discomfort or pain. If the patient reports pain, explore where and when it occurs and how it is relieved.

Determine the patient's personal perception of the health problem and method of coping with hospitalization, diagnostic tests, and procedures. The possibility of a diagnosis of cancer and a treatment regimen that may include surgery, chemotherapy, or radiation treatment is stressful. Support the patient, caregiver, and family. If surgery is planned, assess the patient's expectations regarding surgery (cure or palliation) and how the patient has responded to previous surgical procedures.

◆ Nursing Diagnoses

Nursing diagnoses for the patient with stomach cancer include, but are not limited to, the following:

• Imbalanced nutrition: less than body requirements *related to* inability to ingest, digest, or absorb nutrients

- Acute pain *related to* underlying disease process and side effects of surgery, chemotherapy, or radiation therapy
- Anxiety and grieving *related to* diagnosis of cancer, uncertain future, and prognosis

◆ Planning

The overall goals are that the patient with stomach cancer will (1) experience minimal discomfort, (2) achieve optimal nutritional status, and (3) maintain a degree of spiritual and psychologic well-being appropriate to the disease stage.

◆ Nursing Implementation

◆ **Health Promotion.** Your role in the early detection of stomach cancer focuses on identifying the patient at risk because of specific disorders such as *H. pylori* infection, pernicious anemia, and achlorhydria. Be aware of symptoms associated with stomach cancer and the significant findings on physical examination. Symptoms often occur late and mimic other conditions, such as PUD. Poor appetite, weight loss, fatigue, and persistent stomach distress are symptoms of stomach cancer. Encourage patients with a positive family history of stomach cancer to undergo diagnostic evaluation if anemia, PUD, or vague epigastric distress are present. It is important that you recognize the possibility of stomach cancer in a patient who is treated for PUD and fails to have relief with prescribed therapy.

◆ **Acute Care**

◆ *Preoperative Care.* When diagnostic tests confirm cancer, the patient and family generally react with shock, disbelief, and depression. Provide emotional and physical support, provide information, clarify test results, and maintain a positive attitude with respect to the patient's immediate recovery and long-term survival.

Because of changes in appetite and early satiety, the patient's current nutritional status may be poor. Surgery may be delayed until the patient is more physically able to withstand it. A positive nutritional state enhances wound healing and the ability to deal with infection and other possible postoperative complications. The patient may better tolerate several small meals a day than three regular meals. It may be challenging to persuade the patient to eat when he or she has no appetite and is depressed. Getting the patient's caregiver to assist with meals and encourage intake may be beneficial. The diet may be supplemented by a variety of commercial liquid supplements and vitamins. If the patient is unable to ingest oral feedings, the HCP may prescribe enteral (tube feeding) or parenteral nutrition (see Chapter 39).

If needed, packed RBCs and fluid volume restoration may be given during the preoperative period. Closely observe for transfusion reactions. Monitor hemoglobin and hematocrit levels.

The preoperative teaching plan before stomach cancer surgery is similar to that for PUD (see the section on surgical therapy for PUD on pp. 918).

◆ *Postoperative Care.* Postoperative care is similar to that following a procedure for PUD (see the section on surgical therapy for PUD earlier in this chapter). If the patient had a Billroth I or II procedure, the postoperative care is similar to that of the patient having this procedure for PUD. When the surgical intervention involves a total gastrectomy, the plan of care is somewhat different. A total gastrectomy requires resection of the lower esophagus, removal of the entire stomach, and anastomosis of the esophagus to the jejunum. If the chest cavity is entered,

postoperative drainage is accomplished by the insertion of chest tubes. (Chest surgery and drainage tubes are discussed in Chapter 27.)

After total gastrectomy, the NG tube does not drain a large quantity of secretions because removal of the stomach has eliminated the reservoir capacity. The NG tube is removed when intestinal peristalsis has resumed. Small amounts of clear fluid are then started. Closely observe the patient for signs of fluid leakage at the anastomosis site as evidenced by an elevation in the temperature and increasing dyspnea. When the patient tolerates fluids without distress, fluid intake is increased and some solid foods added.

After a total gastrectomy, the patient experiences symptoms of dumping syndrome. Weight loss often occurs. Postoperative wound healing may be impaired because of poor nutritional intake. This necessitates IV or oral replacement of vitamins C, D, and K; the B-complex vitamins; and cobalamin. These vitamins (with the exception of cobalamin) must be replaced because they are normally absorbed in the duodenum.

Radiation therapy or chemotherapy is used as an adjuvant to surgery or for palliation. Your role is to provide detailed instructions, reassure the patient, and ensure completion of the designated number of treatments. Start by assessing the patient's knowledge of these therapies. Teach the patient about skin care, need for nutrition and fluid intake during therapy, and appropriate use of antiemetic drugs. (Specific care of the patient receiving chemotherapy and radiation therapy is discussed in Chapter 15.)

◆ **Ambulatory Care.** Most dietary measures useful after PUD surgery are applicable after stomach cancer surgery. Make plans for pain relief, including comfort measures and the judicious use of analgesics. Teach wound care (if needed) to the primary caregiver in the home setting. Dressings, special equipment, or special services may be required. Provide the patient with a list of community agencies (e.g., American Cancer Society) that are available for assistance before the patient goes home.

When chemotherapy or radiation treatment is continuing after discharge, a referral to home health care may be beneficial. The home health nurse can assist with recovery, determine the degree of patient adherence, and provide consultation to the patient and caregiver. Encourage the patient to adhere to the prescribed therapies, keep appointments for chemotherapy administration or radiation treatments, and keep the HCP informed of changes in physical condition. (Long-term management of the cancer patient is discussed in Chapter 15.)

◆ Evaluation

Expected outcomes are that the patient with stomach cancer will

- Experience no or minimal discomfort, pain, or nausea
- Achieve optimal nutritional status
- Maintain a degree of psychologic well-being appropriate to the disease stage

UPPER GASTROINTESTINAL BLEEDING

In the United States approximately 300,000 hospital admissions occur each year for upper GI bleeding. Approximately 60% of these are adults over age 65. Despite advances in drug management of predisposing conditions and identification of risk factors, the mortality rate for upper GI bleeding has remained at approximately 6% to 13% for the past 45 years.[23]

Etiology and Pathophysiology

Although the most serious loss of blood from the upper GI tract is characterized by a sudden onset, insidious occult bleeding can be a major problem. The severity of bleeding depends on whether the origin is venous, capillary, or arterial. Types of upper GI bleeding are presented in Table 41-20. Bleeding from an arterial source is profuse, and the blood is bright red, indicating it has not been in contact with gastric HCl acid secretion. In contrast, "coffee-ground" vomitus indicates that the blood has been in the stomach for some time. *Melena* (black, tarry stools) indicates slow bleeding from an upper GI source. The longer the passage of blood through the intestines, the darker the stool color because of the breakdown of hemoglobin and release of iron.

Discovering the cause of the bleeding is not always easy. A variety of areas in the GI tract may be involved. Table 41-21 lists the common causes of upper GI bleeding.

Stomach and Duodenal Origin. Bleeding peptic ulcers account for 40% of the cases of upper GI bleeding. Drugs are a major cause of upper GI bleeding. Aspirin, NSAIDs, and corticosteroids can cause irritation and disruption of the gastroduodenal mucosa. About 25% of people on chronic NSAIDs (e.g., ibuprofen) develop ulcer disease; of these, 2% to 4% will bleed. Even low-dose aspirin is associated with a risk for GI bleeding. Many OTC preparations contain aspirin. A careful history of all commonly used drugs is necessary whenever upper GI bleeding is suspected.

Stress-related mucosal disease (SRMD), also called *physiologic stress ulcers,* is a continuum of conditions ranging from stress-related injury (superficial mucosal damage) to stress ulcers (focal deep mucosal damage). SRMD is most commonly seen in critically ill patients who have had severe burns, trauma, or major surgery. Patients with coagulopathy and those who experience respiratory failure resulting in mechanical ventilation for more than 48 hours are at highest risk for SRMD.[24]

Esophageal Origin. Bleeding from the esophagus is most likely due to chronic esophagitis, Mallory-Weiss tear, or esophageal varices. Chronic esophagitis can be caused by GERD, smoking, alcohol use, and the ingestion of drugs irritating to the mucosa. Esophageal varices most often occur from cirrhosis of the liver. (Esophageal varices are discussed in Chapter 43.)

Diagnostic Studies

Endoscopy is the primary tool for diagnosing the source (e.g., esophageal or gastric varices, gastritis) of upper GI bleeding. Angiography is used when endoscopy cannot be done or when bleeding persists after endoscopic therapy. Angiography is a procedure requiring preparation and setup time and may not be appropriate for a high-risk, unstable patient. In this procedure, a catheter is inserted into the femoral artery and advanced to the left gastric or superior mesenteric artery until the site of bleeding is found.

Laboratory studies include CBC, blood urea nitrogen (BUN), serum electrolytes, prothrombin time, partial thromboplastin time, liver enzymes, arterial blood gases (ABGs), and a type and crossmatch for possible blood transfusions. All vomitus and stools are tested for gross and occult blood.

Monitor the patient's laboratory studies to estimate the effectiveness of therapy. The hemoglobin and hematocrit values are not of immediate help in estimating the degree of blood loss, but they provide a baseline for guiding further treatment. The initial hematocrit may be normal and may not reflect the loss until 4 to 6 hours after fluid replacement, since initially the loss of plasma and RBCs is equal.

Assess the patient's BUN level. During a significant hemorrhage, GI tract bacteria break down proteins, resulting in elevated BUN levels. An elevated BUN level may also indicate renal hypoperfusion or renal disease.

Interprofessional Care

A massive upper GI hemorrhage is a loss of more than 1500 mL of blood or 25% of intravascular blood volume. Although 80% to 85% of patients with massive hemorrhage spontaneously stop bleeding, the cause must be identified and treatment started immediately.

Emergency Assessment and Management. A complete history of events leading to the bleeding episode is deferred until emergency care has been started. To facilitate early intervention, focus your physical examination on identifying signs and symptoms of shock, such as tachycardia, weak pulse, hypotension, cool extremities, prolonged capillary refill, and apprehension. (Shock is discussed in Chapter 66.)

Urine output is one of the best measures of vital organ perfusion. An indwelling urinary catheter is inserted so that hourly output can be accurately assessed. Hemodynamic monitoring provides an accurate and quick assessment of blood flow and pressure in the cardiovascular system (see Chapter 65). A central venous pressure line may be used for fluid volume status assessment. If the patient has a history of valvular heart disease, coronary artery disease, or heart failure, a pulmonary artery catheter may be necessary. Administer supplemental O_2 to increase blood O_2 saturation.

The patient is at risk for perforation and peritonitis. Do a thorough abdominal examination. Note the presence of a tense,

---

TABLE 41-20 Types of Upper Gastrointestinal Bleeding

Type	Manifestations
Obvious bleeding	
• Hematemesis	Bloody vomitus appearing as fresh, bright red blood or "coffee-ground" appearance (dark, grainy digested blood).
• Melena	Black, tarry stools (often foul smelling) caused by digestion of blood in the GI tract. Black appearance is from the presence of iron.
Occult bleeding	Small amounts of blood in gastric secretions, vomitus, or stools not apparent by appearance. Detectable by guaiac test

---

TABLE 41-21 Causes of Upper Gastrointestinal Bleeding

Stomach and Duodenum
- Stomach cancer
- Erosive gastritis
- Peptic ulcer disease
- Polyps
- Stress-related mucosal disease
- Drug-induced
  - Corticosteroids
  - Nonsteroidal antiinflammatory drugs (NSAIDs)
  - Salicylates

Esophagus
- Esophageal varices
- Esophagitis
- Mallory-Weiss tear

Systemic Diseases
- Blood dyscrasias (e.g., leukemia, aplastic anemia)
- Renal failure

rigid, boardlike abdomen and the presence or absence of bowel sounds.

The type and amount of fluids infused are based on physical and laboratory findings. Generally, an isotonic crystalloid solution (e.g., lactated Ringer's solution) is started. Whole blood, packed RBCs, and fresh frozen plasma may be used for volume replacement in massive hemorrhage. When upper GI bleeding is less profuse, infusion of isotonic saline solution followed by packed RBCs restores the hematocrit more quickly and does not create complications related to fluid volume overload. (The use of blood transfusions and volume expanders is discussed in Chapter 30.)

Endoscopic Therapy. The first-line management of upper GI bleeding is endoscopy. Endoscopy performed within the first 24 hours of bleeding is important for diagnosis, determining the need for surgical intervention, and providing treatment.

The goal of endoscopic hemostasis is to coagulate or thrombose the bleeding vessel. Several techniques are used including (1) thermal (heat) probe, (2) multipolar and bipolar electrocoagulation probe, (3) argon plasma coagulation (APC), (4) neodymium:yttrium-aluminum-garnet (Nd:YAG) laser, and (5) mechanical therapy with endoscopic clips or bands. Multipolar electrocoagulation and thermal probe are the two most commonly used procedures. The heat probe coagulates tissue by directly applying a heating element to the bleeding site. The APC is a noncontact coagulation that delivers monopolar current to tissue. Endoscopic clips and bands directly compress the bleeding vessel. For variceal bleeding, other strategies include variceal ligation, injection sclerotherapy, and balloon tamponade (see Chapter 43).

Surgical Therapy. Surgical intervention is indicated when bleeding continues regardless of the therapy provided and when the site of the bleeding has been identified. Surgical therapy may be necessary when the patient continues to bleed after rapid transfusion of up to 2000 mL of whole blood or remains in shock after 24 hours. The site of the hemorrhage determines the choice of surgery. Mortality rates increase considerably in older patients.

Drug Therapy. During the acute phase of upper GI bleeding, drugs are used to decrease bleeding, decrease HCl acid secretion, and neutralize the HCl acid that is present. Empiric PPI therapy with high-dose IV bolus and subsequent infusion to decrease acid secretion is often started before endoscopy (Table 41-10). Efforts are made to reduce acid secretion because the acidic environment can alter platelet function and interfere with clot stabilization. This may decrease the amount of bleeding and need for endoscopic therapy.

Injection therapy with epinephrine (1:10,000 dilution) during endoscopy is effective for acute hemostasis. Epinephrine produces tissue edema and, ultimately, pressure on the source of bleeding (Table 41-22). Octreotide (Sandostatin) or vasopressin may be given when upper GI bleeding is from esophageal or gastric varices (Chapter 43).

❖ NURSING MANAGEMENT: UPPER GASTROINTESTINAL BLEEDING

◆ Nursing Assessment

A thorough and accurate nursing assessment is an essential first step as you begin care of the patient admitted with upper GI bleeding. The patient may not be able to provide specific information about the cause of the bleeding until immediate

---

TABLE 41-22   Nursing Assessment
Upper Gastrointestinal Bleeding
Subjective Data
Important Health Information
Past health history: Precipitating events before bleeding episode, previous bleeding episodes and treatment, peptic ulcer disease, esophageal varices, esophagitis, acute and chronic gastritis, stress-related mucosal disease
Medications: Aspirin, nonsteroidal antiinflammatory drugs, corticosteroids, anticoagulants
Functional Health Patterns
Health perception–health management: Family history of bleeding, smoking, alcohol use
Nutritional-metabolic: Nausea, vomiting, weight loss, thirst
Elimination: Diarrhea. Black, tarry stools. Decreased urine output. Sweating
Activity-exercise: Weakness, dizziness, fainting
Cognitive-perceptual: Epigastric pain, abdominal cramps
Coping–stress tolerance: Acute or chronic stress
Objective Data
General
Fever
Integumentary
Clammy, cool, pale skin. Pale mucous membranes, nail beds, and conjunctivae. Spider angiomas, jaundice, peripheral edema
Respiratory
Rapid, shallow respirations
Cardiovascular
Tachycardia, weak pulse, orthostatic hypotension, slow capillary refill
Gastrointestinal
Red or "coffee-ground" vomitus. Tense, rigid abdomen, ascites. Hypoactive or hyperactive bowel sounds. Black, tarry stools
Urinary
Decreased urine output, concentrated urine
Neurologic
Agitation, restlessness. Decreasing level of consciousness
Possible Diagnostic Findings
↓ Hematocrit and hemoglobin, hematuria. Guaiac-positive stools, emesis, or gastric aspirate. ↓ Levels of clotting factors, ↑ liver enzymes, abnormal endoscopy results

physical needs are met. Perform an immediate nursing assessment while you are getting the patient ready for initial treatment. The assessment includes the patient's level of consciousness, vital signs, skin color, and capillary refill. Check the abdomen for distention, guarding, and peristalsis. Immediate determination of vital signs indicates whether the patient is in shock from blood loss and provides a baseline BP and pulse for monitoring the progress of treatment. Signs and symptoms of shock include low BP; rapid, weak pulse; increased thirst; cold, clammy skin; and restlessness. Monitor the patient's vital signs every 15 to 30 minutes. Inform the HCP of any significant changes.

Once the immediate interventions have begun, the patient or caregiver should answer the following questions: Is there a history of previous bleeding episodes? Has the patient received blood transfusions in the past? Were there any transfusion reactions? Are there any other illnesses (e.g., liver disease, cirrhosis) or medications that may contribute to bleeding or interfere with treatment? Does the patient have a religious preference that prohibits the use of blood or blood products?

Subjective and objective data to obtain from the patient or caregiver are presented in Table 41-22.

◆ Nursing Diagnoses

Nursing diagnoses for the patient with upper GI bleeding include, but are not limited to, the following:

- Risk for decreased cardiac output *related to* loss of blood
- Deficient fluid volume *related to* acute loss of blood and gastric secretions
- Ineffective peripheral tissue perfusion *related to* loss of circulatory volume
- Anxiety *related to* upper GI bleeding, hospitalization, uncertain outcome, source of bleeding

◆ Planning

The overall goals are that the patient with upper GI bleeding will (1) have no further GI bleeding, (2) have the cause of the bleeding identified and treated, (3) experience a return to a normal hemodynamic state, and (4) experience minimal or no symptoms of pain or anxiety.

◆ Nursing Implementation

◆ **Health Promotion.** Although not all cases of upper GI bleeding can be prevented, you have an important role in identifying patients at high risk. Always consider the patient with a history of chronic gastritis, cirrhosis, or PUD at high risk. The patient who has had a previous upper GI bleeding episode is more likely to have another bleed. Patients on daily low-dose aspirin to reduce cardiovascular disease risk are at risk for upper GI bleeding, especially those over 60 years old with a history of PUD.

Teach the at-risk patient to avoid known gastric irritants such as alcohol and smoking and to take only prescribed medications. OTC drugs can be harmful because they may contain ingredients (e.g., aspirin) that increase the risk of bleeding. Review how to test vomitus or stools for occult blood. Teach them to report positive results promptly to the HCP. Stress the importance of treating an upper respiratory tract infection promptly. Severe coughing or sneezing can increase pressure on the already fragile varices and may result in massive hemorrhage (see Chapter 43).

The patient who requires regular doses of drugs that produce gastroduodenal toxicity (peptic ulcer formation, bleeding), such as aspirin, corticosteroids, or NSAIDs, needs to be taught about the potential for GI bleeding. Taking these drugs with meals or snacks lessens their direct irritation. Patients receiving low-dose aspirin who have a history of ulcer disease or complications may need to receive long-term treatment with a PPI, H_2-receptor blocker, or misoprostol (Cytotec).[20]

Patients with blood dyscrasias (e.g., aplastic anemia), liver dysfunction, or those who are taking chemotherapy drugs are at risk due to a decrease in clotting factors and platelets. Teach patients about their disease process, drugs, and increased risk of GI bleeding.

◆ **Acute Care.** Emergency management of acute GI bleeding is presented in Table 41-23. Place IV lines, preferably two, with a 16- or 18-gauge needle for fluid and blood replacement. Administer fluid or blood replacement as ordered. An accurate intake and output record is essential so that the patient's hydration status can be assessed. Measure the urine output hourly. If the patient has a central venous pressure line or pulmonary artery

---

✚ TABLE 41-23 Emergency Management
Acute Gastrointestinal Bleeding

Assessment Findings	Interventions
Abdominal and GI Findings • Hematemesis • Melena • Nausea • Abdominal pain • Abdominal rigidity **Hypovolemic Shock** • ↓ BP • ↓ Pulse pressure • Tachycardia • Cool, clammy skin • ↓ Level of consciousness • ↓ Urine output (<0.5 mL/kg/hr) • Slow capillary refill	**Initial** • If unresponsive, assess circulation, airway, and breathing. • If responsive, monitor airway, breathing, and circulation. • Establish IV access with large-bore catheter and start fluid replacement therapy. Insert additional large-bore catheter if shock present. • Give O₂ via nasal cannula or non-rebreather mask. • Initiate ECG monitoring. • Obtain blood for CBC, clotting studies, and type and crossmatch as appropriate. • Insert NG tube as needed. • Insert indwelling urinary catheter. • Give IV proton pump inhibitor (PPI) therapy to decrease acid secretion. **Ongoing Monitoring** • Monitor vital signs, level of consciousness, O₂ saturation, ECG, bowel sounds, and intake/output. • Assess amount and character of emesis. • Keep patient NPO. • Provide reassurance and emotional support to patient and caregiver.

👤 CHECK YOUR PRACTICE

You are admitting a 71-yr-old man to the clinical unit from the emergency department. He has a diagnosis of upper GI bleeding. He complains of heartburn and pain (6 on a scale of 10) in the upper epigastric region and has just had a 250 mL coffee-ground emesis.
- What assessment data do you need to obtain?
- What are the priority nursing interventions for this man?

---

catheter in place, record these readings every 1 to 2 hours. Use ECG monitoring to evaluate cardiac function. Close monitoring of vital signs, especially in the patient with cardiovascular disease, is important because dysrhythmias may occur.

Observe the older adult or the patient with a history of cardiovascular problems closely for signs of fluid overload. However, volume overload and pulmonary edema are concerns in all patients who are receiving large amounts of IV fluids within a short time. Auscultate breath sounds and closely observe the respiratory effort. Keep the head of the bed elevated to provide comfort and prevent aspiration.

When an NG tube is present, pay special attention to keeping it in proper position and observe the aspirate for blood. Although gastric lavage (room temperature, cool, or iced) is used in some institutions, its effectiveness as a treatment for upper GI bleeding is questionable. When lavage is used, approximately 50 to 100 mL of fluid is instilled at a time into the stomach. The lavage fluid may be aspirated from the stomach or drained by gravity. When aspiration is the method used, it is important not to aspirate if you feel resistance. The tip of the NG tube may be up against the gastric mucosal lining. When resistance is a factor, use the gravity method.

Approach the patient in a calm manner to help decrease the level of anxiety. Use caution when administering sedatives for restlessness because it is one of the warning signs of shock and may be masked by the drugs.

Assess the stools for blood (hematochezia, black-tarry, bright red). Black, tarry stools are not usually associated with a brisk hemorrhage but are indicative of prolonged bleeding. Determine if menses or bleeding are possible sources of blood in the stools. When vomitus contains blood but the stool contains no gross or occult blood, the hemorrhage is considered to be of short duration.

When beginning oral nourishment, observe the patient for symptoms of nausea and vomiting and a recurrence of bleeding. Feedings initially consist of clear fluids. They are given hourly until tolerance is determined. Gradually introduce foods if the patient exhibits no signs of discomfort.

When hemorrhage is the result of chronic alcohol abuse, closely observe the patient for delirium tremens as alcohol withdrawal takes place. Symptoms indicating the onset of delirium tremens are agitation, uncontrolled shaking, sweating, and vivid hallucinations. (Alcohol withdrawal is discussed in Chapter 10.)

◆ **Ambulatory Care.** Teach the patient and caregiver how to avoid future bleeding episodes. Ulcer disease, drug or alcohol use, and liver and respiratory diseases can all result in upper GI bleeding. Help the patient and caregiver to be aware of the consequences of not adhering to drug therapy.

Emphasize not to take any drugs (especially aspirin, NSAIDs) other than those prescribed by the HCP. Support the patient in smoking and alcohol cessation because they are sources of irritation and interfere with tissue repair. Long-term follow-up care may be necessary because of possible recurrence. Teach the patient and caregiver what to do if an acute hemorrhage occurs in the future.

◆ **Evaluation**

The expected outcomes are that the patient with upper GI bleeding will
- Have no upper GI bleeding
- Maintain normal fluid volume
- Experience a return to a normal hemodynamic state
- Understand potential etiologic factors and make appropriate lifestyle modifications

FOODBORNE ILLNESS

Foodborne illness (food poisoning) is a nonspecific term that describes acute GI symptoms such as nausea, vomiting, diarrhea, and cramping abdominal pain caused by the intake of contaminated food or liquids.[25] There are 31 known foodborne pathogens. Each year one out of six Americans, approximately 48 million, experiences a foodborne illness. Of these, 128,000 are hospitalized and approximately 3000 die.[26]

Bacteria account for most foodborne illnesses. The most common source is raw foods that become contaminated during growing, harvesting, processing, storing, shipping, or final preparation. When food is uncooked and left out for more than 2 hours at room temperature, bacteria can multiply quickly. One example is prepackaged cookie dough. The most common bacterial food poisonings are presented in Table 41-24.

Focus interventions on preventing infection. Teaching includes correct food preparation and cleanliness, adequate cooking, and refrigeration (Table 41-25). For the hospitalized patient, emphasize correcting fluid and electrolyte imbalances from diarrhea and vomiting. With botulism, additional assessment and care relative to neurologic symptoms are indicated (see Chapter 60).

Escherichia coli O157:H7 Poisoning

Escherichia coli O157:H7 causes hemorrhagic colitis and kidney failure. In the very young and older adults, *E. coli* O157:H7 can be life threatening. *E. coli* O157:H7 is found primarily in undercooked meats, particularly poultry and hamburger.[26] *E. coli* outbreaks have been observed with contaminated leafy vegetables, fruits, and nuts. Infection can occur after drinking raw milk, unpasteurized juice, or contaminated fruit juices and after swimming in or drinking sewage-contaminated water.

TABLE 41-24	**Bacterial Food Poisoning**		
Type and Cause	**Sources**	**Manifestations**	**Treatment and Prevention**
Staphylococcal Toxin from *Staphylococcus aureus*	Meat, bakery products, cream fillings, salad dressings, milk. Skin and respiratory tract of food handlers	Onset: 30 min to 7 hr Vomiting, nausea, abdominal cramping, diarrhea	*Treat:* Symptomatic, fluid and electrolyte replacement, antiemetics *Prevent:* Immediate refrigeration of foods, monitoring of food handlers
Clostridial *Clostridium perfringens*	Meat or poultry dishes cooked at lower temperature (stew, pot pie), rewarmed meat dishes, gravies, improperly canned vegetables	Onset: 8-24 hr Diarrhea, nausea, abdominal cramps, vomiting (rare), midepigastric pain	*Treat:* Symptomatic, fluid replacement *Prevent:* Correct preparation of meat dishes. Serving food immediately after cooking or rapid cooling of food
Salmonella *Salmonella typhimurium* (grows in gut)	Improperly cooked poultry, pork, beef, lamb, and eggs	Onset: 8 hr to several days Nausea and vomiting, diarrhea, abdominal cramps, fever and chills	*Treat:* Symptomatic, fluid and electrolyte replacement *Prevent:* Correct preparation of food
Botulism Toxin from *Clostridium botulinum*; ingested toxin absorbed from gut and blocks acetylcholine at neuromuscular junction	Improperly canned or preserved food, home-preserved vegetables (most common), preserved fruits and fish, canned commercial products	Onset: 12-36 hr *GI:* Nausea, vomiting, abdominal pain, constipation, distention *Central nervous system:* Headache, dizziness, muscular incoordination, weakness, inability to talk or swallow, diplopia, breathing difficulties, paralysis, delirium, coma	*Treat:* Maintenance of ventilation, polyvalent antitoxin, guanidine hydrochloric acid (enhances acetylcholine release) *Prevent:* Correct processing of canned foods, boiling of suspected canned foods for 15 min before serving
Escherichia coli *E. coli* O157:H7	Contaminated beef, pork, milk, cheese, fish, cookie dough	Onset: 8 hr to 1 wk (varies by strain) Bloody stools, hemolytic uremic syndrome, abdominal cramping, profuse diarrhea	*Treat:* Symptomatic, fluid and electrolyte replacement *Prevent:* Correct preparation of food

TABLE 41-25 Patient & Caregiver Teaching

Prevention of Food Poisoning

Include the following instructions when teaching the patient and caregiver how to prevent food poisoning.

1. Cook all ground beef and hamburger thoroughly.
   - Use a digital instant-read meat thermometer to ensure thorough cooking (ground beef can turn brown before disease-causing bacteria are killed).
   - Cook ground beef until a thermometer inserted into several parts of the patty, including the thickest part, reads at least 160° F.
   - People who cook ground beef without using a thermometer can decrease their risk of illness by not eating ground beef patties that are still pink in the middle.
2. If you are served an undercooked hamburger or other ground beef product in a restaurant, send it back for further cooking. Also ask for a new bun and a clean plate.
3. Avoid spreading harmful bacteria. Keep raw meat separate from ready-to-eat foods. Wash hands, counters, and utensils with hot soapy water after they touch raw meat. Never place cooked hamburgers or ground beef on the unwashed plate that held raw patties. Wash meat thermometers in between tests of patties that require further cooking.
4. Drink only pasteurized milk, juice, or cider. Commercial juice with an extended shelf-life that is sold at room temperature (e.g., juice in cardboard boxes, vacuum-sealed juice in glass containers) has been pasteurized. Juice concentrates are heated sufficiently to kill pathogens.
5. Wash fruits and vegetables thoroughly, especially those that will not be cooked.
6. Do not eat raw food products that are supposed to be cooked. Follow package directions for cooking at proper temperatures.
7. People who are immunocompromised should avoid eating alfalfa sprouts until the safety of the sprouts can be ensured.

Person-to-person contact in families, nursing homes, and child-care centers is an important mode of transmission.

Most strains of *E. coli* are harmless and live in the intestines of healthy humans and animals. *E. coli* O157:H7 produces a powerful toxin and can cause severe illness. The manifestations of *E. coli* O157:H7 include diarrhea (often bloody) and abdominal cramping pain for 2 to 8 days (average 3 to 4 days) after swallowing the organism. The diarrhea is variable, ranging from mild to bloody. It may start out as watery but may progress to bloody. Systemic complications, including hemolytic uremia and thrombocytopenic purpura, and even death can occur.

Infection with *E. coli* O157:H7 is diagnosed by detecting the bacteria in the stool. All people who suddenly have diarrhea with blood should have a stool culture for *E. coli* O157:H7.

Treatment involves supportive care to maintain blood volume. Antibiotic therapy remains controversial. Most people recover without antibiotics or other specific treatment. There is no evidence that antibiotics improve the course of disease. It is thought that treatment with some antibiotics may precipitate kidney complications. Patients should avoid antidiarrheal agents, such as loperamide (Imodium). Other therapies may include dialysis and plasmapheresis.

In a small percentage of infections, particularly in young children and older adults, hemolytic uremic syndrome (HUS) occurs. With HUS, the RBCs are destroyed and the kidneys fail. It is a life-threatening condition usually treated in an ICU. Blood transfusions and kidney dialysis are often required. Approximately 3% to 5% of patients with HUS die. About one third of people with HUS have abnormal kidney function for years after. A few require long-term dialysis. Additional long-term complications of HUS include hypertension, seizures, blindness, and paralysis.

CASE STUDY

Peptic Ulcer Disease

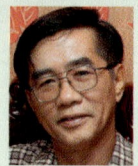
(©iStockphoto/Thinkstock)

Patient Profile
F.H., a 40-yr-old male immigrant from Vietnam, has a 1-yr history of epigastric distress. Increasingly, it is not relieved by over-the-counter omeprazole (Prilosec). He is scheduled for an upper endoscopy this morning.

Subjective Data
- Reports increasing substernal pain, especially 2 to 3 hr after eating
- Currently avoids alcohol and is taking an over-the-counter PPI
- Smoking history of 1 pack of cigarettes per day for 20 yr
- Complains of increasing fatigue with exercise
- Reports occasional black bowel movement
- Takes Chinese medicine for frequent back pain

Objective Data
Physical Examination
- Height 5 ft, 5 in tall and weight 140 lb

Diagnostic Studies
- Endoscopy reveals a duodenal ulcer
- Hgb 10.2 g/dL; Hct 30%
- Histology of biopsied tissue reveals *Helicobacter pylori* infection

Interprofessional Care
- omeprazole 20 mg bid × 10 days
- clarithromycin 500 mg bid × 10 days
- amoxicillin 1 gram bid × 10 days

Discussion Questions
1. Explain the pathophysiology of peptic ulcer disease.
2. What are the risk factors for duodenal ulcers? Which of these did F.H. have?
3. What is the pathophysiology of *H. pylori*?
4. **Priority Decision:** Based on the assessment data provided, what are the priority nursing diagnoses? Are there any collaborative problems?
5. **Patient-Centered Care:** How will you consider F.H.'s cultural preferences in planning care?
6. **Priority Decision:** What are the priority nursing interventions for F.H.?
7. **Teamwork and Collaboration:** For the interventions that you identified in question 6, which of the following personnel could be responsible for implementing them: registered nurse (RN), licensed practical nurse (LPN), unlicensed assistive personnel (UAP)?
8. What lifestyle interventions would you recommend for F.H.?
9. **Evidence-Based Decision:** F.H. asks you if the treatment will work and this will be the end of his problems. How will you respond?
10. **Teamwork and Collaboration:** What referrals may be indicated?

Answers available at *http://evolve.elsevier.com/Lewis/medsurg*.

BRIDGE TO NCLEX EXAMINATION

The number of the question corresponds to the same-numbered outcome at the beginning of the chapter.

1. M.J. calls the clinic and tells the nurse that her 85-year-old mother has been nauseated all day and has vomited twice. Before the nurse hangs up and calls the HCP, she should tell M.J. to
   a. administer antiemetic drugs and observe skin turgor.
   b. give her mother sips of water and elevate the head of her bed to prevent aspiration.
   c. offer her mother a high-protein liquid supplement to drink to maintain her nutritional needs.
   d. offer her mother large quantities of Gatorade to decrease the risk of sodium depletion.

2. The nurse explains to the patient with Vincent's infection that treatment will include
   a. tetanus vaccinations.
   b. viscous lidocaine rinses.
   c. amphotericin B suspension.
   d. topical application of antibiotics.

3. The nurse teaching young adults about behaviors that put them at risk for oral cancer includes
   a. discouraging use of chewing gum.
   b. avoiding use of perfumed lip gloss.
   c. avoiding use of smokeless tobacco.
   d. discouraging drinking of carbonated beverages.

4. Which instructions would the nurse include in a teaching plan for a patient with mild gastroesophageal reflux disease (GERD)?
   a. "The best time to take an as-needed antacid is 1 to 3 hours after meals."
   b. "A glass of warm milk at bedtime will decrease your discomfort at night."
   c. "Do not chew gum; the excess saliva will cause you to secrete more acid."
   d. "Limit your intake of foods high in protein because they take longer to digest."

5. A patient who has undergone an esophagectomy for esophageal cancer develops increasing pain, fever, and dyspnea when a full liquid diet is started postoperatively. The nurse recognizes that these symptoms are *most* indicative of
   a. an intolerance to the feedings.
   b. extension of the tumor into the aorta.
   c. leakage of fluids into the mediastinum.
   d. esophageal perforation with fistula formation into the lung.

6. The pernicious anemia that may accompany gastritis is due to
   a. chronic autoimmune destruction of cobalamin stores in the body.
   b. progressive gastric atrophy from chronic breakage in the mucosal barrier and blood loss.
   c. a lack of intrinsic factor normally produced by acid-secreting cells of the gastric mucosa.
   d. hyperchlorhydria from an increase in acid-secreting parietal cells and degradation of RBCs.

7. The nurse is teaching the patient and family that peptic ulcers are
   a. caused by a stressful lifestyle and other acid-producing factors such as *H. pylori*.
   b. inherited within families and reinforced by bacterial spread of *Staphylococcus aureus* in childhood.
   c. promoted by factors that tend to cause oversecretion of acid, such as excess dietary fats, smoking, and *H. pylori*.
   d. promoted by a combination of factors that may result in erosion of the gastric mucosa, including certain drugs and alcohol.

8. An optimal teaching plan for an outpatient with stomach cancer receiving radiation therapy should include information about
   a. cancer support groups, alopecia, and stomatitis.
   b. nutrition supplements, ostomy care, and support groups.
   c. prosthetic devices, wound and skin care, and grief counseling.
   d. wound and skin care, nutrition, drugs, and community resources.

9. The teaching plan for the patient being discharged after an acute episode of upper GI bleeding includes information concerning the importance of *(select all that apply)*
   a. limiting alcohol intake to one serving per day.
   b. only taking aspirin with milk or bread products.
   c. avoiding taking aspirin and drugs containing aspirin.
   d. only taking drugs prescribed by the health care provider.
   e. taking all drugs 1 hour before mealtime to prevent further bleeding.

10. Several patients are seen at an urgent care center with symptoms of nausea, vomiting, and diarrhea that began 2 hours ago while attending a large family reunion potluck dinner. You question the patients specifically about foods they ingested containing
    a. beef.
    b. meat and milk.
    c. poultry and eggs.
    d. home-preserved vegetables.

1, b, 2, d, 3, c, 4, a, 5, c, 6, c, 7, d, 8, d, 9, c, d, 10, b

For rationales to these answers and even more NCLEX review questions, visit *http://evolve.elsevier.com/Lewis/medsurg*.

ⓔ EVOLVE WEBSITE

http://evolve.elsevier.com/Lewis/medsurg
Review Questions (Online Only)
Key Points
Answer Keys for Questions
• Rationales for Bridge to NCLEX Examination Questions
• Answer Guidelines for Case Study on p. 926
Student Case Studies
• Patient With Oral Cancer
• Patient With Peptic Ulcer Disease

Nursing Care Plans
• eNursing Care Plan 41-1: Patient With Nausea and Vomiting
• eNursing Care Plan 41-2: Patient With Peptic Ulcer Disease
Conceptual Care Map Creator
Audio Glossary
Content Updates

REFERENCES

*1. Gang TJ, Diemunsch P, Habib AS, et al: Consensus guidelines for the management of postoperative nausea and vomiting, *Anesthes Analg* 118:85, 2014.

2. National Comprehensive Cancer Network (NCCN): NCCN Clinical practice guidelines in oncology. Retrieved from *www.nccn.org/professionals/physician_gls/f_guidelines.asp*.

*3. Song HJ, Seo HJ, Lee H, et al: Effect of self-acupressure for symptom management: a systematic review, *Complement Ther Med* 23:68, 2015.

*4. Linden GJ, Lyons A, Scannapieco FA: Periodontal systemic associations: review of the evidence, *J Periodontol* 84:S8, 2013.

5. National Cancer Institute: SEER stat fact sheets. Retrieved from *http://seer.cancer.gov/statfacts/html*.

6. Chai RC, Lambie D, Verma M, et al: Current trends in the etiology and diagnosis of HPV-related head and neck cancers, *Cancer Med* 4:596, 2015.

7. Fedele S: Diagnostic aids in the screening of oral cancer, *Head Neck Oncol* 1:5, 2009. (Classic)

*8. Omura K: Current status of oral cancer treatment strategies, *Int J Clin Oncol* 19:423, 2014.

9. Badillo R, Francis D: Diagnosis and treatment of gastroesophageal reflux disease, *World J Gastrointest Pharmacol Ther* 5:105, 2014.

10. Chang P, Friedenberg F: Obesity and GERD, *Gastroenterol Clin North Am* 43:795, 2014.

*11. Spechler SJ, Sharma P, Souza RF, et al: American Gastroenterological Association medical position statement on the management of Barrett's esophagus, *Gastroenterol* 140:1084, 2011. (Classic)

*12. Kosalram K, Whittle T, Byth K, et al: An investigation of risk factors associated with tooth surface loss: A pilot study, *J Oral Rehabil* 41:675, 2014.

*13. Katz PO, Gersen LB, Vela MF: American College of Gastroenterology: Diagnosis and management of gastroesophageal reflux disease, *Am J Gastroenterol* 108:308, 2013.

*14. Leontiadis GI, Moayyedi P: Proton pump inhibitors and risk of bone fractures, *Curr Treat Options Gastroenterol* 12:414, 2014.

*15. Deshpande A, Pasupuleti V, Thota P, et al: Risk factors for recurrent *Clostridium difficile* infection: A systematic review and meta-analysis, *Infect Control Hosp Epidemiol* 36:452, 2015.

*16. Dai Y, Li C, Xie Y, et al: Interventions for dysphagia in esophageal cancer, *Cochrane Database Syst Rev* (10):CD005048, 2014.

17. Goldstein JL, Cryer B: Gastrointestinal injury associated with NSAID use: a case study and review of risk factors and preventative strategies, *Drug Healthcare Patient Saf* 7:31, 2015.

18. Centers for Disease Control and Prevention: *Helicobacter pylori* and peptic ulcer disease: the key to cure. Retrieved from *www.cdc.gov/ulcer/keytocure.htm*.

*19. Jiang HY, Chen HZ, Hu XJ, et al: Use of selective serotonin reuptake inhibitors and risk of upper gastrointestinal bleeding: a systematic review and meta-analysis, *Clin Gastroenterol Hepatol* 13:42, 2015.

20. Yasuda H, Matsuo Y, Sato Y: Treatment and prevention of gastrointestinal bleeding in patients receiving antiplatelet therapy, *World J Crit Care Med* 4:40, 2015.

21. Oliveira C, Pinheiro H, Figueiredo J, et al: Familial gastric cancer: Genetic susceptibility, pathology, and implications for management, *Lancet Oncol* 16:e60, 2015.

22. Lordick F, Lorenzen S, Yamada Y: Optimal chemotherapy for advanced gastric cancer: is there a global consensus? *Gastric Cancer* 17:213, 2014.

*23. Lu Y, Loffroy R, Lau JY: Multidisciplinary management strategies for acute non-variceal upper gastrointestinal bleeding, *Br J Surg* 10:e34, 2014.

24. Bardou M, Quenot JP, Barkun A: Stress-related mucosal disease in the critically ill patient, *Nat Rev Gastroenterol Hepatol* 12:98, 2015.

25. National Digestive Diseases Information Clearinghouse: Bacteria and foodborne illness. Retrieved from *www.niddk.nih.gov/health-information/health-topics/digestive-diseases/foodborne-illnesses/Pages/facts.aspx*.

26. Centers for Disease Control and Prevention: *Escherichia coli* O157:H7. Retrieved from *www.cdc.gov/Features/EcoliInfection*.

*Evidence-based information for clinical practice.

42

Lower Gastrointestinal Problems

Diana L. Gallagher, Mariann M. Harding

In this life we cannot do great things. We can only do small things with great love.

Mother Teresa

ⓔ http://evolve.elsevier.com/Lewis/medsurg/

LEARNING OUTCOMES

1. Explain the common etiologies, interprofessional care, and nursing management of diarrhea, fecal incontinence, and constipation.
2. Describe common causes of acute abdominal pain and nursing management of the patient after an exploratory laparotomy.
3. Describe the interprofessional care and nursing management of acute appendicitis, peritonitis, and gastroenteritis.
4. Compare and contrast the inflammatory bowel diseases of ulcerative colitis and Crohn's disease, including pathophysiology, clinical manifestations, complications, interprofessional care, and nursing management.
5. Differentiate among mechanical and nonmechanical bowel obstructions, including causes, interprofessional care, and nursing management.
6. Describe the clinical manifestations and interprofessional care of colorectal cancer.
7. Explain the anatomic and physiologic changes and nursing management of the patient with a fistula and a fecal diversion.
8. Differentiate between diverticulosis and diverticulitis, including clinical manifestations, interprofessional care, and nursing management.
9. Compare and contrast the types of hernias, including etiology and surgical and nursing management.
10. Describe the types of malabsorption syndromes and interprofessional care of celiac disease, lactase deficiency, and short bowel syndrome.
11. Describe the types, clinical manifestations, interprofessional care, and nursing management of anorectal conditions.

KEY TERMS

anal fistula, p. 970
appendicitis, p. 942
celiac disease, p. 966
constipation, p. 934
Crohn's disease, p. 944
diarrhea, p. 929
diverticulitis, p. 963
fecal incontinence, p. 933

fistula, p. 962
gastroenteritis, p. 944
hemorrhoids, p. 968
hernia, p. 964
inflammatory bowel disease (IBD), p. 944
intestinal obstruction, p. 950
irritable bowel syndrome (IBS), p. 940
lactase deficiency, p. 967

ostomy, p. 958
paralytic ileus, p. 950
peritonitis, p. 943
short bowel syndrome (SBS), p. 967
steatorrhea, p. 965
stoma, p. 958
ulcerative colitis, p. 944

The wide variety of intestinal problems presented in this chapter include the disorders of diarrhea, constipation, and fecal incontinence; inflammatory and infectious bowel disorders; bowel trauma; bowel obstructions; colorectal cancer; abdominal and bowel surgery (including ostomy formation); and malabsorption disorders.

DIARRHEA

Diarrhea is the passage of at least three loose or liquid stools per day. It may be acute, lasting 14 days or less, or persistent, lasting greater than 14 days. Chronic diarrhea lasts 30 days or longer.[1]

Etiology and Pathophysiology

The primary cause of acute diarrhea is ingesting infectious organisms (Table 42-1). Viruses cause most cases of infectious diarrhea in the United States. While some viral infections can be deadly, most are mild and last less than 24 hours. Therefore most patients rarely seek treatment.

Bacterial infection with *Escherichia coli* O157:H7, a type of enterohemorrhagic *E. coli,* is the most common cause of bloody diarrhea in the United States. It is transmitted by undercooked beef or chicken contaminated with the bacteria or in fruits and vegetables exposed to contaminated manure. Other pathologic *E. coli* strains are endemic in developing countries and commonly cause traveler's diarrhea. *Giardia lamblia* is the most

Reviewed by Janica Barnett, JD, AGPCNP-BC, Adult Gerontology Nurse Practitioner, Mt. Sinai Hospital, New York, New York; Janet L. Hannah, RN, CGRN, Staff Nurse, Inova Loudoun ASC, Leesburg, Virginia; Susan C. Landis, RN, MN, Senior Lecturer, University of Washington School of Nursing, Seattle, Washington; Sarah Byram Poppe, MSN, ANP-BC, Nurse Practitioner, Gastroenterology Associates, Olympia, Washington; Andrea H. Thurler, RN, DNP, FNP-BC, Nurse Practitioner, Massachusetts General Hospital, Harvard University, Massachusetts General Institute of Health Professions, Boston, Massachusetts; and Daryle Wane, PhD, ARNP, FNP-BC, RN to BSN Coordinator, Professor of Nursing, Department of Health Occupations, Pasco-Hernando State College, New Port Richey, Florida.

TABLE 42-1	Causes and Manifestations of Acute Infectious Diarrhea	
Type of Organism	**Manifestations**	**Source of Infection/Susceptibility**
Viral		
Rotavirus	• Fever, vomiting, and profuse watery diarrhea • Lasts 3 to 8 days	• Highly contagious • Transmitted mainly by fecal-oral route
Norovirus (also called *Norwalk-like virus*)	• Nausea, vomiting, diarrhea, stomach cramping • Rapid onset. Lasts 1-2 days	• Very contagious • Virus is present in stool and emesis
Bacterial		
Enterotoxigenic *Escherichia coli*	• Watery or bloody diarrhea, abdominal cramps • Nausea, vomiting, and fever may be present • Mean duration >60 hr	• Most common cause of traveler's diarrhea • Transmitted in water or food contaminated with infected feces
Enterohemorrhagic *E. coli* (e.g., *E. coli* O157:H7)	• Severe abdominal cramping, bloody diarrhea, and vomiting • Low-grade fever • Usually lasts 5-7 days	• Can cause serious illness, especially in older adults • May progress to life-threatening renal failure • Transmitted in water or food contaminated with infected feces
Shigella	• Diarrhea (sometimes bloody), fever, and stomach cramps • Usually lasts 5-7 days • Postinfection arthritis may occur	• Transmitted via fecal-oral route or in food or water contaminated with infected feces • Can contaminate recreational water
Salmonella	• Diarrhea, fever, and abdominal cramps • Lasts 4-7 days	• Reservoir is poultry, reptiles, and other animals (especially turtles, lizards, snakes, chicks, and young birds) • Can be transmitted by handling animals • Found in undercooked poultry, meat, and foods prepared with raw eggs
Staphylococcus	• Nausea, vomiting, abdominal cramps, and diarrhea • Usually mild • May cause illness in as little as 30 min • Lasts 1-3 days	• 25%-50% of people are carriers in mucous membranes, skin, or hair • Transmitted in food contaminated by food workers who are carriers or through contaminated milk and cheese
Campylobacter jejuni	• Diarrhea, abdominal cramps, and fever. Sometimes nausea and vomiting • Lasts about 7 days	• Undercooked poultry and unpasteurized milk • Most frequent in summer months
Clostridium perfringens	• Diarrhea, abdominal cramps, nausea, and vomiting • Occurs 6-24 hr after eating contaminated food and lasts approximately 24 hr	• Associated with meats, gravies, and stews. Commonly associated with dried or pre-cooked foods • Can cause serious illness in anyone, especially older adults
Clostridium difficile	• Watery diarrhea, fever, anorexia, nausea, abdominal pain	• Prolonged use of antibiotics followed by exposure to feces-contaminated surfaces • Spores on hands and environmental surfaces are extremely difficult to kill
Parasitic		
Giardia lamblia	• Abdominal cramps, nausea, diarrhea • May interfere with nutrient absorption	• Highly contagious • Transmitted via fecal-oral route • Found in fresh lakes and rivers. Has been transmitted in swimming pools, water parks, and hot tubs
Entamoeba histolytica	• Diarrhea, abdominal cramping • Only 10%-20% are ill, and symptoms are usually mild	• Fecally contaminated food, water, or hands • Most common in developing countries • In the United States, high-risk groups include travelers, recent immigrants, and homosexual men
Cryptosporidium	• Watery diarrhea • Lasts about 2 wk • May have abdominal cramps, nausea, vomiting, fever, dehydration, weight loss • May be fatal in those who are immunocompromised (e.g., AIDS)	• Lives in human intestines and is transmitted in stool of infected human or animal • Outer shell allows it to live for long periods outside of body and makes it resistant to chlorine • Common cause of waterborne disease (swimming pools, lakes, drinking water, food contaminated with feces)

common intestinal parasite that causes diarrhea in the United States.

Infectious organisms attack the intestines in different ways. Some organisms (e.g., *Rotavirus A, Norovirus, G. lamblia*) alter secretion and/or absorption of the enterocytes of the small intestine without causing inflammation. Other organisms (e.g., *Clostridium difficile*) impair absorption by destroying cells, cause inflammation in the colon, and produce toxins that cause damage.

Secretory diarrhea is a common result of bacterial or viral infections. It occurs when ingested pathogens survive in the GI tract long enough to absorb into the enterocytes. The resulting chain reaction changes cell permeability and results in the oversecretion of water and sodium and chloride ions into the bowel.

Organisms enter the body in contaminated food (e.g., *Salmonella* in undercooked eggs and chicken) or contaminated drinking water (*G. lamblia* in contaminated lakes or pools). Travelers often get diarrhea, especially if they travel to countries with poorer sanitation than their own. Infection can spread from one person to another via the fecal-oral route. For example, adult day care workers can transmit infection from one resident to another if they do not wash their hands thoroughly after changing soiled diapers and linens.

A person's age, gastric acidity, intestinal microflora, and immune status influence susceptibility to pathogenic organisms. Older adults are most likely to suffer life-threatening diarrhea. Since stomach acid kills ingested pathogens, taking medications designed to decrease stomach acid (e.g., proton pump inhibitors and histamine [H_2]-receptor blockers) increases the likelihood that pathogens will survive.[2]

The healthy human colon contains short-chain fatty acids and bacteria such as *E. coli*. These organisms aid in fermentation and provide a microbial barrier against pathogenic bacteria. Antibiotics kill off the normal flora, making the person more susceptible to pathogenic organisms. For example, patients receiving broad-spectrum antibiotics (e.g., clindamycin [Cleocin], cephalosporins, fluoroquinolones) are susceptible to pathogenic strains of *C. difficile*. *C. difficile* infection (CDI) causes the most serious antibiotic-associated diarrhea and is the most common cause of hospital-related GI illness in the United States.[2] Probiotics such as *Saccharomyces boulardii* and *Lactobacillus* may be helpful in preventing antibiotic-induced diarrhea in some patients.

People who are immunocompromised because of disease (e.g., human immunodeficiency virus [HIV]) or immunosuppressive medications are susceptible to gastrointestinal (GI) tract infection. Immunocompromised patients receiving jejunal enteral nutrition are especially prone to CDI and other foodborne infections. Jejunostomy and nasointestinal feedings, which bypass the stomach's acid environment, do not contain the poorly digestible fiber that is necessary for the survival of normal colonic bacteria.

Diarrhea is not always due to infection. Drugs and specific food intolerances can cause diarrhea. Large amounts of undigested carbohydrate in the bowel, lactose intolerance, and certain laxatives (e.g., lactulose, sodium phosphate, magnesium citrate) produce osmotic diarrhea. *Osmotic diarrhea* results from rapid GI transit that prevents absorption of fluid and electrolytes. Bile salts and undigested fats lead to excessive fluid secretion into the GI tract. Diarrhea from celiac disease and short bowel syndrome results from malabsorption in the small intestine.

Clinical Manifestations

Infections that attack the upper GI tract (e.g., *Norovirus*, *G. lamblia*) usually produce large-volume, watery stools, cramping, and periumbilical pain (Table 42-1). Patients have either a low-grade or no fever and often experience nausea and vomiting before the diarrhea begins. Infections of the colon and distal small bowel (e.g., *Shigella*, *Salmonella*, *C. difficile*) produce fever and frequent bloody diarrhea with a small volume.

Leukocytes, blood, and mucus may be present in the stool, depending on the causative agent. Severe diarrhea produces life-threatening dehydration, electrolyte disturbances (e.g., hypokalemia), and acid-base imbalances (metabolic acidosis). CDI can progress to fulminant colitis and intestinal perforation.

Diagnostic Studies

Since most cases of diarrhea resolve quickly, stool cultures are done only in patients who are very ill, have a high fever, or have had diarrhea longer than 3 days. Stools are examined for blood, mucus, white blood cells (WBCs), and parasites. Cultures reliably identify infectious organisms. Multiple-pathogen tests can concurrently detect common viral, parasitic, and bacterial organisms from a single stool sample. Toxins produced by *C. difficile* can usually be detected in a stool sample.

Testing for ova and parasites is reserved for people who have had diarrhea more than 2 weeks. The WBC count may be elevated. People with long-standing diarrhea can develop anemia from iron and folate deficiencies. Increased hematocrit, blood urea nitrogen (BUN), and creatinine levels are signs of fluid deficit.

In patients with chronic diarrhea, measuring stool electrolytes, pH, and osmolality helps determine whether the diarrhea is from decreased fluid absorption or increased fluid secretion. Measuring stool fat and undigested muscle fibers may indicate fat and protein malabsorption conditions, including pancreatic insufficiency. Some patients with secretory diarrhea have elevated serum levels of GI hormones such as vasoactive intestinal polypeptide and gastrin.

Interprofessional Care

Treatment of diarrhea depends on the cause. Acute infectious diarrhea is usually self-limiting. The major concerns are preventing transmission, replacing fluid and electrolytes, and protecting the skin. Patients usually tolerate oral fluids. Solutions containing glucose and electrolytes (e.g., Pedialyte) may be sufficient to replace losses from mild diarrhea. If losses are severe, parenteral administration of fluids, electrolytes, vitamins, and nutrition is necessary. Teach the patient to avoid foods and drugs that cause diarrhea. Insoluble fiber (psyllium) may be helpful in thickening the stool.

Antidiarrheal agents are sometimes used short term. They coat and protect mucous membranes, absorb irritating substances, inhibit intestinal transit, decrease intestinal secretions, or decrease central nervous system stimulation of the GI tract (Table 42-2). Antidiarrheal agents are contraindicated in treating some infectious diarrheas because they potentially prolong exposure to the organism. They are used cautiously in

TABLE 42-2 **Drug Therapy**	
Antidiarrheal Drugs	
Drug	**Mechanism of Action**
bismuth subsalicylate (Pepto-Bismol)	Decreases secretions and has weak antibacterial activity. Used to prevent traveler's diarrhea
calcium polycarbophil (Mitrolan)	Bulk-forming agent that absorbs excessive fluid from diarrhea to form a gel. Used when intestinal mucosa cannot absorb fluid
loperamide (Imodium, Pepto Diarrhea Control)	Inhibits peristalsis, delays transit, increases absorption of fluid from stools
diphenoxylate with atropine (Lomotil)	Opioid and anticholinergic. Decreases peristalsis and intestinal motility
paregoric (camphorated tincture of opium)	Opioid. Decreases peristalsis and intestinal motility
Donnagel-PG (combination of kaolin, pectin, and paregoric)	Decreases peristalsis and intestinal motility
octreotide acetate (Sandostatin)	Suppresses serotonin secretion, stimulates fluid absorption from GI tract, decreases intestinal motility

inflammatory bowel disease (IBD) because of the danger of causing *toxic megacolon* (colonic dilation greater than 5 cm).

Antibiotics are rarely used to treat acute diarrhea. They are used for certain infections or when the infected person is severely ill or immunosuppressed. For example, a nonabsorbable antibiotic, rifaximin (Xifaxan), is used to treat traveler's diarrhea caused by *E. coli.*[1]

Clostridium difficile Infection. CDI is a particularly hazardous health care–associated infection (HAI). The risk for contracting CDI is highest in patients receiving antimicrobial, chemotherapy, or immunosuppressive agents. Additional risk factors include an ICU stay, a prolonged hospital stay, having surgery, and receiving drugs that suppress gastric acid.[2] *C. difficile* spores can survive for up to 70 days on objects, including commodes, telephones, thermometers, bedside tables, and floors. Health care workers who do not adhere to strict infection control precautions can transmit *C. difficile* from patient to patient. Meticulous hand washing with soap and water and frequently changing gloves are extremely important in limiting the spread of *C. difficile.*

CDI is treated with either metronidazole (Flagyl) or vancomycin (Vancocin).[2] Metronidazole is the first line of treatment of mild to moderate CDI. Vancomycin is used for severe CDI or in patients who do not respond to metronidazole therapy within 5 to 7 days. Vancomycin is given orally or by enema. All nonessential antibiotics, stool softeners, laxatives, and antidiarrheal agents should be stopped. Patients who are at risk for relapse from certain strains of *C. difficile* or have recurrent CDI may receive the antibiotic fidaxomicin (Dificid).

Recurrent CDI occurs in about 20% of patients. The risk increases with the use of additional antibiotics and subsequent CDI recurrences.[2] *Fecal microbiota transplantation* (FMT) is emerging as the most effective treatment for recurrent CDI.[3] FMT reestablishes healthy intestinal flora by infusing fecal bacteria obtained from healthy donor stool into the patient's colon. To perform an FMT, feces obtained from the donor is pureed into a liquid, slurry consistency using saline, water, or pasteurized cow's milk. The donor stool is then placed in the GI tract via an enema, nasoenteral tube, or during colonoscopy. The major concern with FMT is the potential for transmitting infectious agents in the donor stool. Using feces from donors who have intimate physical contact with the recipient and careful screening minimize this risk. Most patients have diarrhea immediately after the procedure.

❖ **NURSING MANAGEMENT:
ACUTE INFECTIOUS DIARRHEA**

◆ **Nursing Assessment**

Begin the nursing assessment with a thorough history and physical examination (Table 42-3). Ask the patient to describe his or her stool pattern and associated symptoms. Focus on the duration, frequency, character, and consistency of stool, and the relationship to other symptoms such as pain and vomiting. Inquire about medical conditions that may cause diarrhea and whether the person is taking medications such as antibiotics and laxatives that are known to cause diarrhea, decrease stomach acidity, or cause immunosuppression. Determine whether the patient has traveled to a foreign country, been at a day care facility recently, and if other family members are ill. Ask about food preparation practices, food intolerances (e.g., milk), and changes in diet and appetite.

TABLE 42-3 **Nursing Assessment**
Diarrhea
Subjective Data
Important Health Information
Past health history: Recent travel, hospitalization, infections, stress. Diverticulitis or malabsorption, metabolic disorders, inflammatory bowel disease, irritable bowel syndrome
Medications: Laxatives or enemas, magnesium-containing antacids, sorbitol-containing suspensions or elixirs, antibiotics, methyldopa, digitalis, colchicine; OTC antidiarrheal medications
Surgery or other treatments: Stomach or bowel surgery, radiation
Functional Health Patterns
Health perception–health management: Chronic laxative abuse, malaise
Nutritional-metabolic: Ingestion of fatty and spicy foods, food intolerances. Anorexia, nausea, vomiting, weight loss. Thirst
Elimination: Increased stool frequency, volume, and looseness. Change in color and character of stools. Steatorrhea, abdominal bloating. Decreased urine output
Cognitive-perceptual: Abdominal tenderness, abdominal pain and cramping, tenesmus
Objective Data
General
Lethargy, sunken eyeballs, fever, malnutrition
Integumentary
Pallor, dry mucous membranes, poor skin turgor, perianal irritation
Gastrointestinal
Frequent soft to liquid stools that may alternate with constipation, altered stool color. Abdominal distention, hyperactive bowel sounds. Pus, blood, mucus, or fat in stools. Fecal impaction
Urinary
Decreased output, concentrated urine
Possible Diagnostic Findings
Abnormal serum electrolyte levels. Anemia, leukocytosis, eosinophilia, hypoalbuminemia. Positive stool cultures. Ova, parasites, leukocytes, blood, or fat in stool. Abnormal sigmoidoscopy or colonoscopy findings. Abnormal lower GI series

Assess for fever and signs of dehydration (dry skin, low-grade fever, orthostatic changes in pulse and BP, decreased and concentrated urine). Assess the abdomen for distention, pain, and guarding. Inspect the perineal skin for signs of redness and breakdown from the diarrhea.

◆ **Nursing Diagnoses**

Nursing diagnoses for the patient with acute infectious diarrhea may include, but are not limited to, the following:

• Diarrhea *related to* acute infectious process
• Deficient fluid volume *related to* excessive fluid loss and decreased fluid intake

For additional information on nursing diagnoses for diarrhea, see eNursing Care Plan 42-1 on the website for this chapter.

◆ **Planning**

The overall goals are that the patient with diarrhea will have (1) no transmission of the microorganism causing the infectious diarrhea; (2) cessation of diarrhea and resumption of normal bowel patterns; (3) normal fluid, electrolyte, and acid-base balance; (4) normal nutritional status; and (5) no perianal/perineal skin breakdown.

◆ Nursing Implementation

Consider all cases of acute diarrhea as infectious until the cause is known. Strict infection control precautions are necessary to prevent the illness from spreading to others. Wash your hands before and after contact with each patient and when handling body fluids of any kind. Flush vomitus and stool in the toilet. Teach the patient and caregiver to wash contaminated clothing immediately with soap and water. Teach them the principles of hygiene, infection control precautions, and the potential dangers of an illness that is infectious to themselves and others. Discuss proper food handling, cooking, and storage with the patient and caregiver (see Tables 41-24 and 41-25).

Viruses and *C. difficile* spores are extremely difficult to kill. Alcohol-based hand cleaners and ammonia-based disinfectants are ineffective, and even vigorous cleaning with soap and water does not kill everything. Immediately put patients with CDI in isolation, and ensure that visitors and health care providers wear gloves and gowns. Give infected patients their own disposable stethoscopes and thermometers. Consider all objects in the room contaminated. Ensure surfaces and equipment are disinfected with a 10% bleach solution or a disinfectant labeled as *C. difficile* sporicidal.[2]

FECAL INCONTINENCE

Etiology and Pathophysiology

Fecal incontinence is the involuntary passage of stool. It occurs when the normal structures that maintain continence are damaged or disrupted. Defecation is a voluntary action when the neuromuscular system is intact (see Chapter 38). Problems with motor function (contraction of sphincters and rectal floor muscles) and/or sensory function (ability to perceive the presence of stool or to experience the urge to defecate) can result in fecal incontinence. Contributing factors include weakness or disruption of the internal or external anal sphincter, damage to the pudendal nerve or other nerves that innervate the anorectum, damage to the anal tissue, and trauma to the puborectalis muscle (Table 42-4).

For women, obstetric trauma is the most common cause of sphincter disruption. Childbirth, aging, and menopause contribute to the development of fecal incontinence. With diarrhea, the likelihood is increased that stool will be accidentally discharged. Chronic constipation can lead to *fecal impaction,* a collection of hardened feces in the rectum or sigmoid colon that a person cannot expel. Incontinence occurs as liquid stool seeps around the hardened feces. Fecal impaction is a common problem in older adults with limited mobility. Constipated individuals tend to strain during defecation. Straining contributes to incontinence because it weakens the pelvic floor muscles.

Anorectal surgery can damage the sphincters and pudendal nerves. Radiation for prostate cancer decreases rectal compliance. Neurologic conditions, including stroke, spinal cord injury, and multiple sclerosis, interfere with defecation. Even people with normally functioning defecation experience incontinence if immobility prevents timely access to a toilet.

Diagnostic Studies and Interprofessional Care

The diagnosis and effective management of fecal incontinence require a thorough health history and physical examination.

TABLE 42-4	Causes of Fecal Incontinence	

Traumatic
- Anorectal surgery for hemorrhoids, fistula, and fissures
- Childbirth injury (episiotomy is a risk factor)
- Perineal trauma or pelvic fracture

Inflammatory
- Infection
- Inflammatory bowel disease
- Radiation

Pelvic Floor Dysfunction
- Medications
- Rectal prolapse

Functional
- Physical or mobility impairments affecting toileting ability (e.g., frail older person who cannot get to the bathroom in time)

Neurologic
- Brain tumor
- Cauda equina nerve injury
- Congenital abnormalities (e.g., spina bifida, myelomeningocele)
- Dementia
- Diabetes mellitus (secondary to neuropathy)
- Multiple sclerosis
- Rectal surgery
- Spinal cord injuries
- Stroke

Other
- Chronic constipation
- Denervation of pelvic muscles from chronic excessive straining
- Fecal impaction
- Loss of rectal elasticity
- Rapid transit of large diarrheal stools

Ask the patient about the number of incontinent episodes per week, stool consistency and volume, and the degree that incontinence interferes with work and social activities. A rectal examination can reveal reduced anal canal muscle tone and contraction strength of the external sphincter, as well as detect internal prolapse, rectocele, hemorrhoids, fecal impaction, and masses. If the impaction is higher in the colon, an abdominal x-ray or a CT scan may be helpful. Other tests include anorectal manometry, anorectal ultrasonography, and defecography. Sigmoidoscopy or colonoscopy can identify inflammation, tumors, fissures, and other pathologic conditions.

Treatment of incontinence depends on the underlying cause. Fecal incontinence from fecal impaction usually resolves after manual removal of the hard feces and cleansing enemas. To prevent recurrence, maintaining normal stool consistency and a bowel management program are important. This includes regular defecation, a high-fiber diet, and increased intake of caffeine free fluids. Patients with dehydration will need fluid replacement therapy.

Dietary fiber supplements or bulk-forming laxatives such as psyllium (Metamucil, Konsyl) increase stool bulk, firm consistency, and promote the sensation of rectal filling. Patients may need to reduce or eliminate foods that cause diarrhea and rectal irritation. Common food triggers include coffee, dried fruit, onions, mushrooms, green vegetables, fruit with peels, spicy foods, and foods with monosodium glutamate. Antidiarrheal agents (e.g., loperamide [Imodium]) are useful in slowing intestinal transit.

Kegel exercises (see Table 45-18) can strengthen and coordinate the pelvic floor muscles to improve continence. Biofeedback therapy can improve awareness of rectal sensation, coordinate internal and external anal sphincters, and increase the strength of external sphincter contraction. Biofeedback training requires intact sensory and motor nerves and motivation to learn. It is a safe, painless, and effective treatment.[4]

Mild electrical stimulation of the sacral nerves targets communication problems between the brain and nerves that control the pelvic floor muscles and sphincters. Electrical stimulation can improve quality of life, and some patients may achieve complete continence.[4]

For patients who do not respond to conservative treatment, treatment with dextranomer/hyaluronic acid gel (Solesta) may be used. In this treatment, the gel is injected into the deep submucosa of the patient's anal canal. It works by building up tissue in the anal area, narrowing the anal canal and allowing muscles to more adequately close. No anesthesia is required. Postinjection pain and bleeding may occur.

Surgery (e.g., sphincter repair procedures) is an option when other conservative treatments fail, the patient has a full-thickness prolapse, or the anal sphincter needs repair. A colostomy is sometimes necessary.

❖ NURSING MANAGEMENT: FECAL INCONTINENCE

◆ Nursing Assessment

Fecal incontinence is embarrassing, uncomfortable, and irritating to the skin. Its unpredictable nature makes it difficult to maintain school and work activities and hampers social or intimate contact. Be sensitive to the patient's feelings when discussing incontinence. Ask about daily activities (mealtimes and work), diet, and family and social activities.

If the underlying cause cannot be corrected, help the patient reestablish a predictable pattern of defecation. Ask about bowel patterns before the incontinence developed; current bowel habits; stool consistency and frequency; and symptoms, including pain during defecation and a feeling of incomplete evacuation (*tenesmus*). Assess whether the patient has a sensation of urgency to evacuate the bowel or sensation of passing flatus and leaking stool. Check the perineal area for irritation or breakdown. The Bristol Stool Scale is helpful to assess stool consistency (*www.poopreport.com/Poll/bristol_scale.html*).

Patients who have fecal incontinence are at risk for *incontinence-associated dermatitis* (IAD).[5] IAD results from chemical irritants in the feces causing skin damage. It is characterized by location, redness, skin loss, and rash. The location of IAD is usually the perianal or perineal area, buttocks, or upper thighs. Fungal infection is common and frequently seen as a dark red center surrounded by satellite lesions. Your assessment is important in differentiating IAD from pressure ulcer development.

◆ Nursing Implementation

Regardless of the cause of fecal incontinence, bowel training is an effective strategy for many patients. Bowel elimination occurs at regular intervals in most people. Knowing the patient's usual bowel pattern can assist you in planning a bowel program that will achieve optimal stool consistency and predictable bowel elimination patterns. For the hospitalized patient, placement on a bedpan, assistance to a bedside commode, or walks to the bathroom at a regular time daily help to establish regular defecation. A good time to schedule elimination is within 30 minutes after breakfast.

If these techniques are ineffective in reestablishing bowel regularity, administer bisacodyl (Dulcolax), a glycerin suppository, or a small phosphate enema 15 to 30 minutes before the usual evacuation time. These preparations stimulate the anorectal reflex. Since stimulation will not occur unless the suppository or enema touches the rectal wall, first check for stool in the rectum and digitally remove it before inserting the laxative. Once a regular pattern is established, discontinue these drugs. Digital stimulation is another method for stimulating the

anorectal reflex and is commonly included in bowel programs for people with neurogenic bowels (e.g., from spinal cord injury). Irrigating the rectum and colon (usually with tap water) at regular intervals is another way to achieve continence in patients with neurogenic bowel.

Maintaining perineal skin integrity is of utmost importance, especially in the bedridden patient. Feces can contaminate wounds, damage skin, cause bladder infections, and spread infections such as *C. difficile*. Containment of the feces is essential. One option to contain stool is a fecal management system (e.g., Flexi-Seal, DignaCare, Actiflo, Instaflo). A fecal management system funnels liquid stool from the rectum into a containment system. Common features include a retention cuff that sits above the anal sphincter and soft tubing that extends from this cuff to a secure hub that allows a person to change the containment canister when it is full. A system can remain in place for weeks. Fecal management systems may decrease the risk of CDI, skin damage from exposure to stool, IAD, and pressure ulcer development.[6] Avoid the use of rectal tubes or urinary catheters. They can reduce the responsiveness of the rectal sphincter and potentially irritate or ulcerate the rectal mucosa.

Perform frequent skin assessments when absorbent products are used. Incontinence briefs may help minimize risk of developing IAD, but only if changed promptly after each episode of incontinence. Use absorbent products in combination with a defined skin care program. This includes prompt cleansing, moisturizing, and skin protection. Soap is not an ideal product since it can be drying. Cleanse the perineal skin gently with tap water or a pH-balanced cleanser to remove feces. Apply a moisture barrier and, if needed, a skin barrier cream for more protection. For patients unable to care for themselves at home, you should teach caregivers how to maintain skin integrity.

Fecal incontinence is an overwhelming burden for most patients. Be sensitive to their fears. Teach strategies to help patients reduce incontinent episodes and better cope with them when they do occur. Help patients identify food triggers that may worsen symptoms. Encourage them to avoid those foods and exercise after meals. Tell them to try to use bathrooms when they are available. Patients may be more confident when they use discreet, disposable briefs or pads. Have them wear dark-colored clothing that they can quickly remove for toileting. Ready access to a spare set of clothing and cleansing cloths is important.

CONSTIPATION

Constipation is a syndrome defined by difficult or infrequent stools; hard, dry stools that are difficult to pass; or a feeling of incomplete evacuation.[7] Because people vary, it is important to compare the current symptoms with the patient's normal pattern of elimination.

Etiology and Pathophysiology

Common causes of constipation include taking in insufficient dietary fiber or fluids, decreasing physical activity, and ignoring the defecation urge (Table 42-5). Many drugs, especially opioids, cause constipation. Constipation occurs with diseases that slow GI transit and hamper neurologic function such as diabetes mellitus, Parkinson's disease, and multiple sclerosis. Emotions, including anxiety, depression, and stress, affect the GI tract and can contribute to constipation.

Some people believe that they are constipated if they do not have a daily bowel movement. This can result in chronic laxative

TABLE 42-5   Causes of Constipation

Colonic Disorders
- Diverticular disease
- Inflammation-induced strictures
- Intussusception
- Irritable bowel syndrome
- Luminal or extraluminal obstructing lesions
- Rectocele
- Volvulus

Drug-Induced Causes
- Antacids (calcium and aluminum)
- Anticholinergics
- Antidepressants
- Antihypertensives
- Antipsychotics
- Barium sulfate
- Bismuth
- Calcium supplements
- Iron supplements
- Laxative abuse
- Opioids

Systemic Disorders
Metabolic/Endocrine
- Celiac disease
- Diabetes mellitus
- Hypercalcemia/hyperparathyroidism
- Hypokalemia
- Hypothyroidism
- Pheochromocytoma
- Pregnancy

Collagen Vascular Disease
- Amyloidosis
- Systemic sclerosis (scleroderma)

Neurologic Disorders
- Autonomic neuropathy (resulting from diabetes mellitus)
- Hirschsprung's megacolon
- Multiple sclerosis
- Neurofibromatosis
- Parkinson's disease
- Spinal cord lesions or injury
- Stroke

EVIDENCE-BASED PRACTICE
Applying the Evidence

Probiotics and Constipation

L.R. is an 82-yr-old female patient with decreased mobility after a recent hip fracture. During a check-up visit at the orthopedic clinic, L.R. mentions she is experiencing discomfort due to constipation. She tells you she is following her discharge instructions and is drinking "lots of water all day and trying to increase fiber in her diet."

Making Clinical Decisions

Best Available Evidence. In adults with constipation, there is an association between the use of probiotics, especially products containing *Bifidobacterium lactis,* and significant improvements in gut transit time, stool frequency, and stool consistency. Quality of life diminishes with increased severity in constipation symptoms.

Clinician Expertise. You recently read about the potential benefit of probiotics in relieving constipation. You also understand that diet can play a major role in treating and preventing constipation.

Patient Preferences and Values. L.R. asks if you know of anything else she can do as she does not want to take any more of those "constipation" drugs.

Implications for Nursing Practice

1. What information would you share with L.R. related to probiotics and constipation?
2. What additional data would you obtain from L.R. related to her diet, mobility, and fluid intake?
3. Why is it important for you to know about alternative therapies? What is your role in supporting patients who desire alternatives to drug therapy?

Reference for Evidence

Dimidi E, Christodoulides S, Fragkos K, et al: The effect of probiotics on functional constipation in adults: a systematic review and meta-analysis of randomized controlled trials, *Am J Clin Nutr* 100:1075, 2014.

use and subsequent *cathartic colon syndrome,* a condition in which the colon becomes dilated and atonic (lacking muscle tone). Ultimately, the person cannot defecate without a laxative.

Ignoring the urge to defecate for a prolonged period can cause the muscles and mucosa of the rectum to become insensitive to the presence of feces. In addition, the prolonged retention of feces results in drying of stool due to water absorption. The harder and drier the feces, the more difficult it is to expel.

Clinical Manifestations

The clinical presentation of constipation may vary from a mild discomfort to a more severe event mimicking an "acute abdomen." Stools are absent or hard, dry, and difficult to pass. Abdominal distention, bloating, increased flatulence, and increased rectal pressure may be present.

Hemorrhoids are the most common complication of chronic constipation. They result from venous engorgement caused by repeated *Valsalva maneuvers* (straining) and venous compression from hard, impacted stool. Valsalva maneuver may have serious outcomes for patients with heart failure, cerebral edema, hypertension, and coronary artery disease. During straining, the patient inspires deeply and holds the breath while contracting abdominal muscles and bearing down. This increases both intraabdominal and intrathoracic pressures and reduces venous return to the heart. The heart rate temporarily decreases along with a decrease in cardiac output. This results in a transient drop in arterial pressure. When the patient relaxes, thoracic pressure falls, resulting in a sudden flow of blood into the heart, increased heart rate, and an immediate rise in arterial pressure. These changes may be fatal for the patient who cannot compensate for the sudden increased blood flow returning to the heart.

In the presence of *obstipation* (severe constipation with no passage of gas or stool) or fecal impaction secondary to constipation, colonic perforation may occur. Perforation, which is life threatening, causes abdominal pain, nausea, vomiting, fever,

and an elevated WBC count. Rectal mucosal ulcers and fissures may occur from stool stasis or straining. Diverticulosis is another potential complication of chronic constipation. These complications are most common in older patients.

Diagnostic Studies and Interprofessional Care

Perform a thorough history and physical examination to identify the underlying cause of constipation. Ask the patient about usual defecation patterns and habits, diet, exercise, laxative use, and past history such as obstetric injuries that could contribute to difficulties with defecation. Diagnostic testing may include abdominal x-rays, barium enema, colonoscopy, sigmoidoscopy, rectal balloon expulsion test, anorectal manometry, defecography with barium or fluoroscopy, and colonic transit tests.

Increasing dietary fiber, maintaining adequate fluid intake, and exercise can prevent many cases of constipation. Laxatives (Table 42-6) and enemas are an option in treating acute constipation. They are used cautiously because overuse leads to chronic constipation. The choice of laxative or enema depends on the severity of the constipation and the patient's health. Daily bulk-forming laxatives (psyllium) can prevent constipation because they work like dietary fiber and do not cause dependence. Bisacodyl tablets and suppositories, milk of magnesia, and lactulose act more rapidly but are more likely to cause dependence. Enemas are fast acting and beneficial for immediate treatment of constipation but must be used cautiously. Soapsuds enemas produce inflammation of colon mucosa, tap water enemas can potentially lead to water intoxication, and

TABLE 42-6 Drug Therapy

Constipation

Mechanism of Action	Example	Comments
Bulk Forming Absorbs water. Increases bulk, thereby stimulating peristalsis *Action:* Usually within 24 hr	methylcellulose (Citrucel) psyllium (Metamucil, Perdiem, Konsyl, Hydrocil, Fiberall)	Contraindicated in patients with abdominal pain, nausea, and vomiting and in patients suspected of having appendicitis, biliary tract obstruction, or acute hepatitis. Must be taken with fluids (≥8 oz). Best choice for initial treatment of constipation
Stool Softeners and Lubricants Lubricate intestinal tract and soften feces, making hard stools easier to pass. Do not affect peristalsis *Action:* Softeners in 72 hr, lubricants in 8 hr	*Softeners:* docusate (Colace, Surfak, Peri-Colace) *Lubricants:* mineral oil (Fleet's Oil Retention Enema, Kondremul Plain)	Can block absorption of fat-soluble vitamins such as vitamin K, which may increase risk of bleeding in patients on anticoagulants
Saline and Osmotic Solutions Cause retention of fluid in intestinal lumen caused by osmotic effect *Action:* Within 15 min-3 hr	Magnesium salts (magnesium citrate, Milk of Magnesia) Sodium phosphates (Fleet Enema, Phospho-soda) lactulose (Constulose) polyethylene glycol (MiraLAX, GoLYTELY, CoLyte)	Magnesium-containing products may cause hypermagnesemia in patients with renal insufficiency
Stimulants Increase peristalsis by irritating colon wall and stimulating enteric nerves *Action:* Usually within 12 hr	cascara sagrada, senna (Senokot) phenolphthalein: sennosides (Ex-Lax), bisacodyl (Correctol, Feen-a-Mint, Dulcolax), docusate/phenolphthalein (Doxidan)	Cause melanosis coli (brown or black pigmentation of colon). Are most widely abused laxatives. Should not be used in patients with impaction or obstipation
Selective Chloride Channel Activator Increases intestinal fluid secretion and motility *Action:* Usually within 24 hr	lubiprostone (Amitiza)	Used in the treatment of idiopathic constipation and irritable bowel syndrome with constipation (women only). Contraindicated in patients with history of mechanical GI obstruction
Intestinal Secretagogue Increases fluid secretion and accelerates intestinal transit *Action:* Usually within 24 hr	linaclotide (Linzess)	Used in the treatment of idiopathic constipation and irritable bowel syndrome with constipation

sodium phosphate (e.g., Fleet) enemas may cause electrolyte imbalances in patients with cardiac and renal problems.

Intestinal secretagogues, lubiprostone (Amitiza) and linaclotide (Linzess), increase intestinal chloride and water secretion, accelerating transit and easing evacuation. They are useful in treating chronic idiopathic constipation.[7]

Newer medications include methylnaltrexone (Relistor) and naloxegol (Movantik), peripherally acting opioid receptor antagonists that decrease constipation caused by opioid use. These drugs do not block the analgesic effects of opioids.

Other therapies target specific patient needs. Biofeedback therapy may benefit patients who have constipation because of *anismus* (uncoordinated contraction of the anal sphincter during straining).

A patient with severe constipation related to bowel motility or mechanical disorders may require more intense treatment. Diagnostic studies include anorectal manometry, GI tract transit studies, and sigmoidoscopic rectal biopsies. A patient with unrelenting constipation may need a colostomy, ileostomy, or continent fecal diversion. (These procedures are discussed later in this chapter.)

Nutritional Therapy. Diet is an important factor in preventing and treating constipation. Many patients experience improved symptoms when they increase their dietary fiber intake. Dietary fiber is found in fruits, vegetables, and grains (Table 42-7). Wheat bran and prunes are especially effective for preventing and treating constipation. Whole wheat and bran are high in insoluble fiber.

Dietary fiber adds to the stool bulk directly by attracting water. Therefore adequate fluid intake (2 L/day) is essential. Large, bulky stools move through the colon much more quickly than small stools. However, the recommended fluid intake may be contraindicated in a patient with cardiac disease or renal failure. Tell the patient that increasing fiber intake may initially increase gas production because of fermentation in the colon, but this effect decreases over several days.

❖ NURSING MANAGEMENT: CONSTIPATION

◆ Nursing Assessment

Table 42-8 outlines the subjective and objective data you should obtain from a patient with constipation.

◆ Nursing Implementation

Tailor the nursing management of constipation to your assessment of the patient's symptoms. Teach the patient about the importance of diet, fluids, and activity in the prevention and treatment of constipation (Table 42-9). Emphasize the importance of a high-fiber diet, adequate fluid intake, and regular exercise. Teach the patient to establish a regular time to defecate and not to suppress the urge to defecate. Discourage the use of laxatives and enemas to achieve fecal elimination.

Defecation is easiest when the person is sitting on a commode with the knees higher than the hips. The sitting position allows gravity to aid defecation, and flexing the hips straightens the angle between the anal canal and rectum so that stool flows out

TABLE 42-7 Nutritional Therapy

High-Fiber Foods

High-fiber foods are recommended for patients with diverticulosis, irritable bowel syndrome, constipation, hemorrhoids, atherosclerosis, hyperlipidemia, and diabetes mellitus.

	Fiber/Serving (g)	Serving Size	Calories/Serving
Vegetables			
Asparagus	3.5	½ cup	18
Beans			
• Navy	8.4	½ cup	80
• Kidney	9.7	½ cup	94
• Lima	8.3	½ cup	63
• Pinto	8.9	½ cup	78
• String	2.1	½ cup	18
Broccoli	3.5	½ cup	18
Carrots, raw	1.8	½ cup	15
Corn	2.6	½ medium ear	72
Peas, canned	6.7	½ cup	63
Potatoes			
• Baked	1.9	½ medium	72
• Sweet	2.1	½ medium	79
Squash, acorn	7.0	1 cup	82
Tomato, raw	1.5	1 small	18
Fruits			
Apple	2.0	½ large	42
Blackberries	6.7	¾ cup	40
Orange	1.6	1 small	35
Peach	2.3	1 medium	38
Pear	2.0	½ medium	44
Raspberries	9.2	1 cup	42
Strawberries	3.1	1 cup	45
Grain Products			
Bread, whole wheat	1.3	1 slice	59
Cereal			
• All Bran (100%)	8.4	⅓ cup	70
• Corn Flakes	2.6	¾ cup	70
• Shredded Wheat	2.8	1 biscuit	70
Popcorn	3.0	3 cups	62

TABLE 42-8 Nursing Assessment

Constipation

Subjective Data

Important Health Information

Past health history: Colorectal disease, neurologic dysfunction, bowel obstruction, environmental changes, cancer, irritable bowel syndrome, diabetes mellitus

Medications: Aluminum and calcium antacids, anticholinergics, antidepressants, antihistamines, antipsychotics, diuretics, opioids, iron, laxatives, enemas

Functional Health Patterns

Health perception–health management: Chronic laxative or enema abuse. Rigid beliefs regarding bowel function. Malaise

Nutritional-metabolic: Changes in diet or mealtime. Inadequate fiber and fluid intake. Anorexia, nausea

Elimination: Change in usual elimination patterns. Hard, difficult-to-pass stool, decrease in frequency and amount of stools. Flatus, abdominal distention. Tenesmus, rectal pressure. Fecal incontinence (if impacted)

Activity-exercise: Change in daily activity routines. Immobility, sedentary lifestyle

Cognitive-perceptual: Dizziness, headache, anorectal pain. Abdominal pain on defecation

Coping–stress tolerance: Acute or chronic stress

Objective Data

General

Lethargy

Integumentary

Anorectal fissures, hemorrhoids, abscesses

Gastrointestinal

Abdominal distention. Hypoactive or absent bowel sounds. Palpable abdominal mass. Fecal impaction. Small, hard, dry stool. Stool with blood

Possible Diagnostic Findings

Guaiac-positive stools. Abdominal x-ray demonstrating stool in lower colon

TABLE 42-9 Patient & Caregiver Teaching

Constipation

Include the following instructions when teaching the patient and caregiver about management of constipation.

1. Eat Dietary Fiber

Eat 20 to 30 g of fiber per day. Gradually increase the amount of fiber eaten over 1 to 2 wk. Fiber softens hard stool and adds bulk to stool, promoting evacuation.
• Foods high in fiber: raw vegetables and fruits, beans, breakfast cereals (All Bran, oatmeal)
• Fiber supplements: Metamucil, Citrucel, FiberCon
Eat prunes or drink prune juice daily. Prunes stimulate defecation.

2. Drink Fluids

Fluid softens hard stools. Drink 2 L per day. Drink water or fruit juices. Avoid caffeinated coffee, tea, and cola. Caffeine stimulates fluid loss through urination.

3. Exercise Regularly

Walk, swim, or bike at least three times per wk. Contract and relax abdominal muscles when standing or by doing sit-ups to strengthen muscles and prevent straining. Exercise stimulates bowel motility and moves stool through the colon.

4. Establish a Regular Time to Defecate

First thing in the morning or after the first meal of the day is a good time because people often have the urge to defecate at this time.

5. Do Not Delay Defecation

Respond to the urge to have a bowel movement as soon as possible. Delaying defecation results in hard stools and a decreased "urge" to defecate. Water is absorbed from stool by the intestine over time. The colon becomes less sensitive to the presence of stool in the rectum.

6. Record Your Bowel Elimination Pattern

Develop a habit of recording when you have a bowel movement on your calendar. Regular monitoring of bowel movement will assist in early identification of a problem.

7. Avoid Laxatives and Enemas

Do not overuse laxatives and enemas because they cause dependence. People who overuse them are unable to have a bowel movement without them.

more easily. Place a footstool in front of the toilet to promote flexion of the thighs. It is challenging to defecate while sitting on a bedpan. For a patient in bed, elevate the head of the bed as high as the patient can tolerate.

The sights, odors, and sounds of defecation embarrass most people. Provide as much privacy as possible and use an odor eliminator. Encourage patients to maintain abdominal muscle tone. Prompt patients to contract abdominal muscles several times a day. Sit-ups and straight-leg raises can help improve abdominal muscle tone.

For the patient whose perceived constipation is related to rigid beliefs regarding bowel function, initiate a discussion about these concerns. Give appropriate information on normal bowel function and discuss the adverse consequences of excessive use of laxatives and enemas.

ACUTE ABDOMINAL PAIN

Etiology and Pathophysiology

Acute abdominal pain is pain of recent onset. It may signal a life-threatening problem and therefore requires immediate attention. Causes include damage to organs in the abdomen and pelvis, which leads to inflammation, infection, obstruction, bleeding, and perforation (Fig. 42-1). Perforation of the GI tract results in irritation of the *peritoneum* (serous membrane lining the abdominal cavity) and peritonitis. Hypovolemic shock occurs from bleeding or obstruction and peritonitis causing large amounts of fluid to move from the vascular space into the abdomen.

Clinical Manifestations

Pain is the most common symptom of an acute abdominal problem. The patient may have nausea, vomiting, diarrhea, constipation, flatulence, fatigue, fever, rebound tenderness, and bloating.

Diagnostic Studies and Interprofessional Care

Diagnosis begins with a complete history and physical examination. Description of the pain (frequency, timing, duration, location), accompanying symptoms, and sequence of symptoms (e.g., pain before or after vomiting) provide vital clues about the origin of the problem. Note the patient's position. The fetal posture is common with peritoneal irritation (e.g., appendicitis), a supine posture with outstretched legs with visceral pain, and restlessness with a seated posture with bowel obstructions or obstructions from kidney stones and gallstones.

Physical examination includes examination of the abdomen, rectum, and pelvis. A complete blood count (CBC), urinalysis, abdominal x-ray, and electrocardiogram are done, along with an ultrasound or CT scan. Women of childbearing age may need a pregnancy test to rule out an ectopic pregnancy.

Emergency management of the patient with acute abdominal pain is presented in Table 42-10. The goal of management is to identify and treat the cause, and monitor and treat complications, especially shock. Careful use of pain medications (e.g., morphine) provides pain relief without interfering with diagnostic accuracy when patients have nontraumatic acute abdominal pain.

In patients with acute abdominal pain, an immediate surgical consult is needed. The surgeon may perform a diagnostic

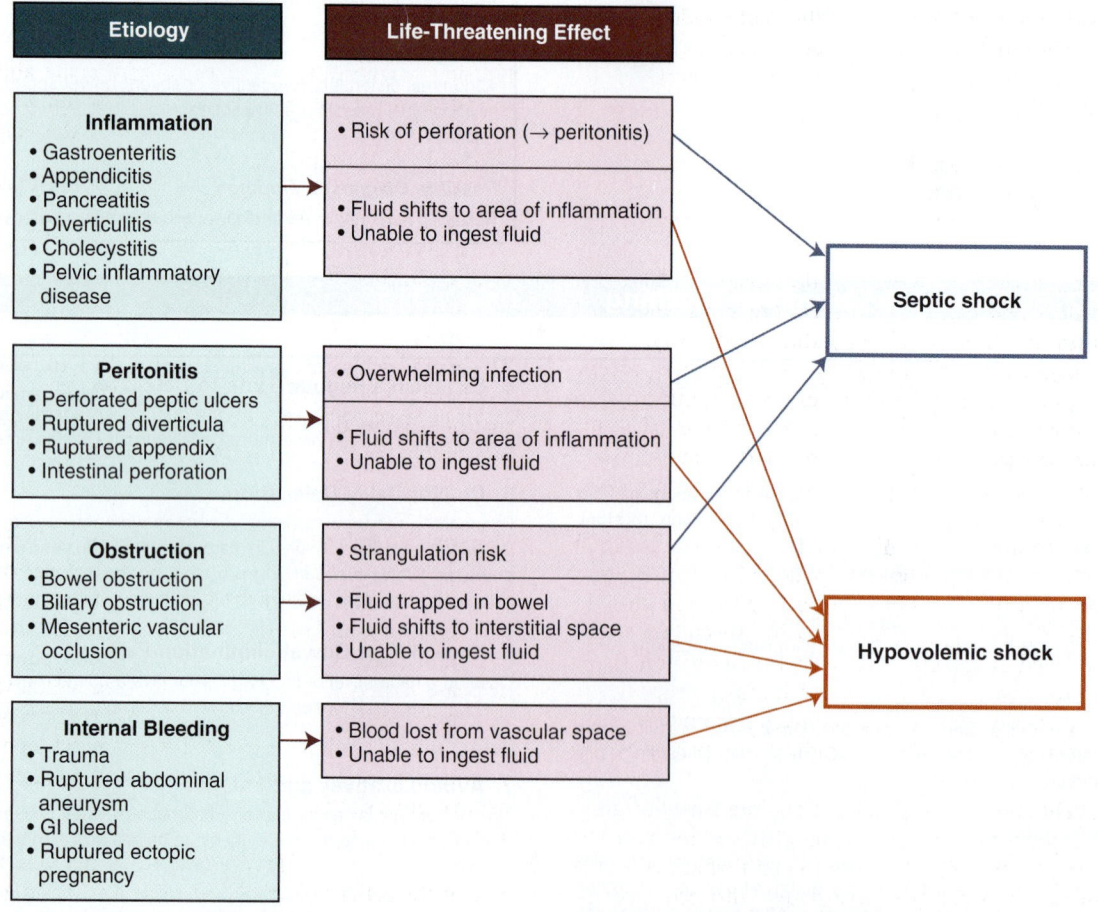

FIG. 42-1 Etiology of acute abdominal pain and pathophysiologic sequelae.

✚ TABLE 42-10 Emergency Management

Acute Abdominal Pain

Etiology	Assessment Findings	Interventions
Inflammation	**Abdominal and GI Findings**	**Initial**
• Appendicitis	• Diffuse, localized, dull, burning, or sharp abdominal pain or tenderness	• Ensure patent airway.
• Cholecystitis	• Rebound tenderness	• Administer O_2 via nasal cannula or non-rebreather mask.
• Crohn's disease	• Abdominal distention	• Establish IV access with large-bore catheter and infuse warm normal saline or lactated Ringer's solution. Insert additional large-bore catheter if shock present.
• Gastritis	• Abdominal rigidity	
• Pancreatitis	• Nausea and vomiting	
• Pyelonephritis	• Diarrhea	• Obtain blood for CBC and electrolyte levels.
• Ulcerative colitis	• Hematemesis	• Anticipate order for amylase level, pregnancy tests, clotting studies, and type and crossmatch as appropriate.
Vascular Problems	• Melena	
• Ruptured aortic aneurysm	**Hypovolemic Shock**	• Insert indwelling urinary catheter.
• Mesenteric vascular occlusion	• ↓ BP	• Obtain urinalysis.
Gynecologic Problems	• ↓ Pulse pressure	• Insert NG tube as needed.
• Pelvic inflammatory disease	• Tachycardia	**Ongoing Monitoring**
• Ruptured ectopic pregnancy	• Cool, clammy skin	• Monitor vital signs, level of consciousness, O_2 saturation, and intake/output.
• Ruptured ovarian cyst	• ↓ Level of consciousness	• Assess quality and amount of pain.
Infectious Disease	• ↓ Urine output (<0.5 mL/kg/hr)	• Assess amount and character of emesis.
• *Escherichia coli* O157:H7		• Anticipate surgical intervention.
• *Giardia*		• Keep patient NPO.
• *Salmonella*		
Other		
• Obstruction or perforation of abdominal organ		
• Gastrointestinal bleeding or ischemia		
• Trauma		

laparoscopy to inspect the surface of abdominal organs, obtain biopsy specimens, perform laparoscopic ultrasounds, and remove organs. A laparotomy is used when laparoscopic techniques are inadequate. If the cause of the acute abdomen can be surgically removed (e.g., inflamed appendix) or surgically repaired (e.g., ruptured abdominal aneurysm), surgery is considered definitive therapy.

❖ NURSING MANAGEMENT: ACUTE ABDOMINAL PAIN

◆ Nursing Assessment

For the patient complaining of acute abdominal pain, take vital signs immediately and again at frequent intervals. Increased pulse and decreasing BP indicate impending shock. An elevated temperature suggests an inflammatory or infectious process. Intake and output measurement provides essential information about the adequacy of vascular volume. Altered mental status indicates poor cerebral perfusion. Skin color, skin temperature, and peripheral pulse strength provide information about perfusion.

Inspect the abdomen for distention, masses, abnormal pulsation, symmetry, hernias, rashes, scars, and pigmentation changes. Apply light pressure when inspecting the abdomen to help determine the level of a patient's pain. Auscultate bowel sounds. Diminished or absent bowel sounds in a quadrant may indicate a bowel obstruction, acute peritonitis, or paralytic ileus. Perform palpation gently. Determine pain from peritoneal irritation by asking the person to cough, gently palpating the abdomen, or shaking the bed.

Ask the patient about the onset, location, intensity, duration, frequency, and character of pain. Note whether the pain has spread or moved to new sites (quadrants) and what makes the pain worse or better. Is the pain associated with other symptoms, such as nausea, vomiting, changes in bowel and bladder habits, or vaginal discharge in women? Assessment of vomiting includes the amount, color, consistency, and odor of the emesis. Ask about usual and changes in bowel patterns and habits.

◆ Nursing Diagnoses

Nursing diagnoses for the patient with acute abdominal pain include, but are not limited to, the following:
- Acute pain *related to* inflammation of the peritoneum and abdominal distention
- Risk for deficient fluid volume *related to* collection of fluid in peritoneal cavity secondary to inflammation or infection
- Anxiety *related to* pain and uncertainty of cause or outcome of condition

◆ Planning

The overall goals are that the patient with acute abdominal pain will have (1) relief of abdominal pain, (2) resolution of inflammation, (3) freedom from complications (especially hypovolemic shock), and (4) normal nutritional status.

◆ Nursing Implementation

General care for the patient with acute abdominal pain involves management of fluid and electrolyte imbalances, pain, and anxiety. Assess the quality and intensity of pain at regular intervals, and provide medication and other comfort measures. Maintain a calm environment and provide information to help decrease anxiety. A nasogastric (NG) tube with low suction may decrease vomiting and relieve discomfort from gastric distention. Conduct ongoing assessments of vital signs, intake and output, and level of consciousness, which are key indicators of hypovolemic shock.

◆ Acute Care

◆ *Preoperative Care.* Preoperative care includes the emergency care of the patient described in Table 42-10 and general care of the preoperative patient (see Chapter 17).

◆ *Postoperative Care.* Postoperative care depends on the type of surgical procedure performed. See eNursing Care Plan 19-1, a general plan for the postoperative patient, on the website for Chapter 19.

Postoperatively some patients will have an NG tube with low suction to empty the stomach and prevent gastric dilation. If the upper GI tract was entered, drainage from the NG tube may be dark brown to dark red for the first 12 hours. Later it should be light yellowish brown, or it may have a greenish tinge because of bile. If a dark red color continues or you observe bright red blood, notify the surgeon because of the possibility of hemorrhage. "Coffee-ground" granules in the drainage indicate blood that has been changed by acidic gastric secretions.

Nausea and vomiting are common after a laparotomy and result from the surgery, decreased peristalsis, or pain medications. Antiemetics such as ondansetron (Zofran), promethazine (Phenergan), and prochlorperazine (Compazine) may be ordered. Monitor fluid and electrolyte status along with BP, heart rate, and respirations. (See Chapter 41 for further discussion of managing nausea and vomiting.)

Swallowed air and reduced peristalsis from decreased mobility, manipulation of the abdominal organs during surgery, and anesthesia can result in abdominal distention and gas pains. Early ambulation helps restore peristalsis, expel flatus, and reduce gas pain. Gradually, as intestinal activity increases, distention and gas pain disappear.

◆ **Ambulatory Care.** Preparation for discharge begins soon after surgery. Teach the patient and caregiver about any modifications in activity, care of the incision, diet, and drug therapy. Initially the patient starts on clear liquids after surgery and then, if tolerated, progresses to a regular diet.

Early ambulation speeds recovery, but normal activities are resumed gradually, with planned rest periods. Patients generally have restrictions not to lift anything heavier than a few pounds. The patient and caregiver should be aware of possible complications after surgery. Teach them to notify the surgeon immediately if fever greater than 101° F (38.6° C), vomiting, pain, weight loss, incisional drainage, or changes in bowel function occur.

◆ **Evaluation**

The expected outcomes are that the patient with acute abdominal pain will have

- Resolution of the cause of the acute abdominal pain
- Relief of abdominal pain and discomfort
- Freedom from complications, especially hypovolemic shock and septicemia
- Normal fluid, electrolyte, and nutritional status

CHRONIC ABDOMINAL PAIN

Chronic abdominal pain may originate from abdominal structures or be referred from a site with the same or a similar nerve supply. The pain is often described as dull, aching, or diffuse. Common causes of chronic abdominal pain include irritable bowel syndrome (IBS), peptic ulcer disease, chronic pancreatitis, hepatitis, pelvic inflammatory disease, adhesions, and vascular insufficiency.

Diagnosing the cause of chronic abdominal pain begins with a thorough history and description of specific pain characteristics, including severity, location, frequency, duration, and onset. The assessment includes factors that increase or decrease the pain, such as eating, defecation, and activities.

Endoscopy, CT scan, MRI, laparoscopy, and barium studies may be done. Treatment for chronic abdominal pain depends on the underlying cause.

IRRITABLE BOWEL SYNDROME

Irritable bowel syndrome (IBS) is a disorder characterized by chronic abdominal pain or discomfort and alteration of bowel patterns. Diarrhea or constipation may predominate, or they may alternate. As a functional GI disorder, IBS has no known organic cause.

The manifestations of IBS are intermittent and may occur for years. Patients often report a history of GI infections and food intolerances. However, the role of food allergies in IBS is unclear. Other dietary factors that may contribute to symptoms include fermentable oligo-, di-, and monosaccharides and polyols (FODMAPs). Examples include fructans (found in wheat, rye, onions, garlic, and legumes), galactans, lactose (found in milk and yogurt), fructose (found in honey, apples, pears, and high-fructose corn syrup), sorbitol, and xylitol. Psychologic stressors (e.g., depression, anxiety, sexual abuse, posttraumatic stress disorder) are associated with development and exacerbation of IBS.

IBS is diagnosed solely on symptoms. The Rome III criteria for diagnosing IBS require the presence of abdominal pain and/or discomfort at least 3 months that is associated with two or more of the following: improvement with defecation, change in stool frequency at onset, or change in the stool appearance at onset.[8] Depending on the stool patterns, IBS is categorized as IBS with constipation, IBS with diarrhea, IBS mixed, and IBS unsubtyped. Other common symptoms include abdominal distention, nausea, flatulence, bloating, urgency, mucus in the stool, and sensation of incomplete evacuation. Non-GI symptoms may include fatigue, headache, and sleep disturbances.

GENDER DIFFERENCES
Irritable Bowel Syndrome (IBS)

Men	Women
• More likely to have IBS with diarrhea	• Affects women 2 to 2.5 times more often than men
• Less likely to admit to symptoms or seek help for them	• More likely to have IBS with constipation
• Experience more interpersonal difficulties	• Report more extraintestinal co-morbidities (e.g., migraine headache, insomnia, fibromyalgia)

The key to accurate diagnosis is a thorough history and physical examination. Ask patients to describe symptoms, past health history (including psychosocial factors such as stress and anxiety), family history, and drug and diet history. Determine if and how IBS symptoms interfere with school, work, or recreational activities. Diagnostic tests are selectively used to rule out other disorders such as colorectal cancer, IBD, endometriosis, and malabsorption disorders (lactose intolerance, celiac disease).

No single therapy is effective for all patients with IBS. Treatment may include dealing with psychologic factors, dietary changes, and drugs to regulate stool output and reduce discomfort. Patients may benefit from keeping a diary of symptoms, diet, and episodes of stress to help identify any factors that trigger the IBS symptoms. Cognitive behavior therapy and stress management techniques may help a patient cope. Participating in regular exercise reduces bloating and constipation as well as reduces symptoms of anxiety and depression. Acupuncture and hypnosis can also be used.

Review with the patient foods that are high in FODMAPs and teach them to follow a low FODMAP diet.[9] Advise the patient whose primary symptoms are abdominal distention and flatulence to avoid common gas-producing foods such as broccoli and cabbage. If dairy products tend to cause symptoms, yogurt may be the best option because of the lactobacillus bacteria it contains. Some patients benefit from certain probiotic combinations. For those with constipation, encourage an intake of enough dietary fiber to produce soft, painless bowel movements.

Drug therapy is individualized. Antispasmodic medications (hyoscyamine, dicyclomine [Bentyl]) decrease GI motility and smooth muscle spasms, reducing pain and diarrhea. An option for women with severe pain and diarrhea is alosetron (Lotronex). Because of serious side effects (e.g., severe constipation, ischemic colitis), it is available only in a restricted access program for those who have not responded to other IBS therapies.

 DRUG ALERT Alosetron (Lotronex)
- Patients taking this drug may experience severe constipation and ischemic colitis (reduced blood flow to intestines).
- Teach the patient to discontinue the drug and contact the HCP if constipation, rectal bleeding, bloody diarrhea, or abdominal pain occurs.

Loperamide (Imodium), a synthetic opioid that slows intestinal transit, is another option for those with diarrhea. Eluxadoline (Viberzi) is used to treat the symptoms of diarrhea and abdominal pain.

Women with IBS with constipation may benefit from lubiprostone (Amitiza). Men or women with constipation symptoms can take linaclotide (Linzess). It is contraindicated in patients with a history of mechanical obstruction or prior bowel surgery. Low doses of tricyclic antidepressants and selective serotonin reuptake inhibitors (SSRIs) may reduce symptoms.[8]

ABDOMINAL TRAUMA

Etiology and Pathophysiology

Injuries to the abdominal area usually are a result of blunt trauma or penetrating injuries. Common injuries of the abdomen include lacerated liver, ruptured spleen, mesenteric artery tears, diaphragm rupture, urinary bladder rupture, great vessel tears, renal or pancreas injury, and stomach or intestine rupture.

Blunt trauma commonly occurs with motor vehicle accidents, direct blows, and falls and may not be obvious because it does not leave an open wound. Both compression injuries (e.g., direct blow to the abdomen) and shearing injuries (e.g., rapid deceleration in a motor vehicle crash allowing some tissue to move forward while other tissues stay stationary) occur with blunt trauma. *Penetrating injuries* occur when a gunshot or stabbing produces an obvious, open wound into the abdomen.

When solid organs (liver, spleen) are injured, bleeding can be profuse, resulting in hypovolemic shock. When contents from hollow organs (e.g., bladder, stomach, intestines) spill into the peritoneal cavity, the patient is at risk for peritonitis. In addition, abdominal compartment syndrome can develop.

Abdominal compartment syndrome, or abdominal hypertension, is excessively high pressure in the abdomen. Anything that increases the volume in the abdominal cavity (e.g., edematous organs, bleeding) increases abdominal pressure. High abdominal pressure restricts ventilation, potentially leading to respiratory failure. The high pressure decreases cardiac output, venous return, and arterial perfusion of organs. Decreased perfusion to the kidneys can lead to renal failure.

Clinical Manifestations

Careful assessment provides important clues to the type and severity of injury. Intraabdominal injuries are often associated with rib fractures, fractured pelvis, spinal injury, and thoracic injury. If the patient was in an automobile accident, a contusion or abrasion across the lower abdomen may indicate internal organ trauma due to seat belt use. Seat belts can produce blunt trauma to abdominal organs by pressing the intestine and pancreas into the spinal column.

Classic manifestations of abdominal trauma are (1) guarding and splinting of the abdominal wall (indicating peritonitis); (2) a hard, distended abdomen (indicating intraabdominal bleeding); (3) decreased or absent bowel sounds; (4) abrasions or bruising over the abdomen; (5) abdominal pain; (6) hematemesis or hematuria; and (7) signs of hypovolemic shock (Table 42-11). Ecchymosis around the umbilicus (*Cullen's sign*) or flanks (*Grey Turner's sign*) may indicate retroperitoneal hemorrhage. Loss of bowel sounds occurs with peritonitis. If the diaphragm ruptures, you can hear bowel sounds (if present) in the chest. Auscultation of bruits is indicative of arterial damage.

Diagnostic Studies

Laboratory tests include a baseline CBC and urinalysis. Even when bleeding, the patient will have normal hemoglobin and hematocrit because fluids are lost at the same rate as the red blood cells. Deficiencies are evident after fluid resuscitation begins. Blood in the urine may be a sign of kidney or bladder damage. Additional laboratory work includes arterial blood gases, prothrombin time, electrolytes, BUN and creatinine, and type and crossmatch (in anticipation of possible blood transfusions). An abdominal CT scan and focused abdominal ultrasound are the most common diagnostic methods, but the patient must be stable before going for CT.

Diagnostic peritoneal lavage can be used to detect blood, bile, intestinal contents, and urine in the peritoneal cavity. It is generally used only for unstable patients to identify blood in the peritoneum.

❖ NURSING AND INTERPROFESSIONAL MANAGEMENT: ABDOMINAL TRAUMA

Emergency management of abdominal trauma is presented in Table 42-11. IV access is established, and volume expanders or blood given if the patient is hypotensive. An NG tube with low suction will decompress the stomach and prevent aspiration. Frequent ongoing assessment is necessary to monitor fluid status, detect deterioration in condition, and determine the necessity for surgery. Do not remove an impaled object until skilled care is available. Removal may cause further injury and bleeding. The decision about whether to do surgery depends on clinical findings, diagnostic test results, and the patient's response to conservative management.

✚ TABLE 42-11   Emergency Management

Abdominal Trauma

Etiology	Assessment Findings	Interventions
Blunt	**Hypovolemic Shock**	**Initial**
• Falls	• ↓ Level of consciousness	• If unresponsive, assess circulation, airway, and breathing.
• Motor vehicle collisions	• Tachypnea	• If responsive, monitor airway, breathing, and circulation.
• Pedestrian event	• Tachycardia	• Administer appropriate O_2 therapy.
• Assault with blunt object	• ↓ BP	• Control external bleeding with direct pressure or sterile pressure
• Crush injuries	• ↓ Pulse pressure	dressing.
• Explosions		• Establish IV access with two large-bore catheters and infuse normal
	Surface Findings	saline or lactated Ringer's solution.
Penetrating	• Abrasions or ecchymoses on abdominal	• Obtain blood for type and crossmatch and CBC.
• Knife	wall, flank, or peritoneum	• Remove clothing.
• Gunshot wounds	• Open wounds: lacerations, eviscerations,	• Stabilize impaled objects with bulky dressing—*do not remove.*
• Impalement	puncture wounds, gunshot wounds	• Cover protruding organs or tissue with sterile saline dressing.
• Other missiles	• Impaled object	• Insert indwelling urinary catheter if there is no blood at the meatus,
		pelvic fracture, or boggy prostate.
	Abdominal and GI Findings	• Obtain urine for urinalysis.
	• Nausea and vomiting	• Insert NG tube if no evidence of facial trauma.
	• Hematemesis	• Anticipate diagnostic peritoneal lavage.
	• Absent or decreased bowel sounds	
	• Hematuria	**Ongoing Monitoring**
	• Abdominal distention	• Monitor vital signs, level of consciousness, O_2 saturation, and urine
	• Abdominal rigidity	output.
	• Abdominal pain with palpation	• Maintain patient warmth using blankets, warm IV fluids, or warm
	• Rebound tenderness	humidified O_2.

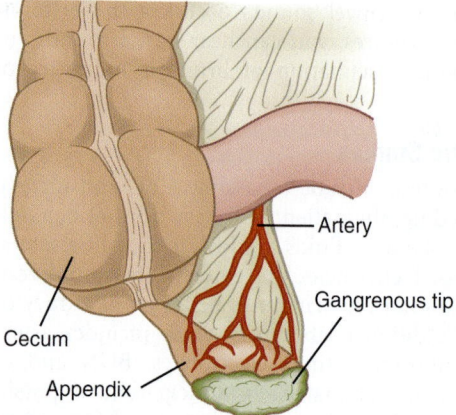

FIG. 42-2 In appendicitis the blood supply of the appendix is impaired by inflammation and bacterial infection, which may result in gangrene.

(labels: Artery, Gangrenous tip, Cecum, Appendix)

INFLAMMATORY DISORDERS

APPENDICITIS

Appendicitis is inflammation of the appendix, a narrow blind tube that extends from the inferior part of the cecum (Fig. 42-2). It is the most common reason for emergency abdominal surgery.

Etiology and Pathophysiology

About 7% of people will develop appendicitis sometime during their lifetime.[10] It is most common in individuals 10 to 30 years of age. A common cause of appendicitis is obstruction of the lumen by a fecalith (accumulated feces). Obstruction results in distention; venous engorgement; and the accumulation of mucus and bacteria, which can lead to gangrene, perforation, and peritonitis.

Clinical Manifestations

Diagnosis can be difficult because many patients do not have classic symptoms. Appendicitis typically begins with dull periumbilical pain, followed by anorexia, nausea, and vomiting. The pain is persistent and continuous, eventually shifting to the right lower quadrant and localizing at *McBurney's point* (halfway between the umbilicus and right iliac crest). A low-grade fever may develop. Further assessment reveals localized tenderness, rigidity, rebound tenderness, and muscle guarding. Coughing, sneezing, and deep inhalation worsen pain. The patient usually prefers to lie still, often with the right leg flexed. The older adult may report less severe pain, slight fever, and discomfort in the right iliac fossa.

Diagnostic Studies and Interprofessional Care

Patient examination includes a complete history, physical examination, and a differential WBC count. Most patients have a mildly to moderately elevated WBC count. A urinalysis is done to rule out genitourinary conditions that mimic appendicitis. CT scan is the preferred diagnostic procedure. However, ultrasound and MRI are also used.

If there is a delay in diagnosis and treatment, the appendix can rupture and the resulting peritonitis can be fatal. The treatment of appendicitis is an immediate *appendectomy* (surgical removal of appendix). If the inflammation is localized, surgery should be done as soon as the diagnosis is made. Antibiotics and fluid resuscitation are started before surgery.

If the appendix has ruptured and there is evidence of peritonitis or an abscess, giving parenteral fluids and antibiotic therapy for 6 to 8 hours before the appendectomy helps prevent dehydration and sepsis.

❖ NURSING MANAGEMENT: APPENDICITIS

Managing the patient presenting with manifestations of appendicitis focuses on preventing fluid volume deficit, relieving pain, and preventing complications. To ensure the stomach is empty in case surgery is needed, keep the patient on nothing-by-mouth (NPO) status until the HCP evaluates the patient. Monitor vital signs and perform ongoing assessment to detect any deterioration in condition. Administer IV fluids, analgesics, and antiemetics as ordered. Provide comfort measures.

Postoperative care for the patient who had an appendectomy is similar to the patient after a laparotomy. Patients are usually discharged within 24 hours following an uncomplicated laparoscopic appendectomy. Ambulation begins a few hours after surgery and the diet advanced as tolerated. Most patients resume normal activities 2 to 3 weeks after surgery.

> ### ⓘ CHECK YOUR PRACTICE
>
> A 28-yr-old female patient comes to the emergency department with acute abdominal pain.
> - What manifestations would make you suspect appendicitis is the cause of the patient's abdominal pain rather than other causes of abdominal pain?

PERITONITIS

Etiology and Pathophysiology

Peritonitis results from a localized or generalized inflammatory process of the peritoneum. Causes of peritonitis are listed in Table 42-12. Primary peritonitis occurs when blood-borne organisms enter the peritoneal cavity. For example, the ascites that occurs with cirrhosis of the liver provides an excellent liquid environment for bacteria to flourish. Organisms can enter the peritoneum during peritoneal dialysis. (Peritoneal dialysis is described in Chapter 46.)

Secondary peritonitis is much more common. It occurs when abdominal organs perforate or rupture and release their contents (bile, enzymes, and bacteria) into the peritoneal cavity. Common causes include a ruptured appendix, perforated gastric or duodenal ulcer, severely inflamed gallbladder, and trauma from gunshot or knife wounds.

Intestinal contents and bacteria irritate the normally sterile peritoneum and produce an initial chemical peritonitis. Bacterial peritonitis develops a few hours later. The resulting inflammatory response leads to massive fluid shifts (peritoneal edema) and adhesions as the body attempts to wall off the infection.

Clinical Manifestations

Abdominal pain is the most common symptom of peritonitis. A universal sign is tenderness over the involved area. Rebound tenderness, muscular rigidity, and spasm are other signs of peritoneal irritation. Patients may lie still and take only shallow breaths because movement worsens the pain. Abdominal distention, fever, tachycardia, tachypnea, nausea, vomiting, and altered bowel habits may be present. These manifestations vary, depending on the severity and acuteness of the underlying condition. Complications of peritonitis include hypovolemic shock,

sepsis, intraabdominal abscess formation, paralytic ileus, and acute respiratory distress syndrome. Peritonitis can be fatal if treatment is delayed.

Diagnostic Studies and Interprofessional Care

A CBC is done to determine elevations in WBC count and hemoconcentration from fluid shifts (Table 42-13). Peritoneal aspiration may be performed and the fluid analyzed for blood, bile, pus, bacteria, fungus, and amylase content. An abdominal x-ray may show dilated loops of bowel consistent with paralytic ileus, free air if perforation has occurred, or air and fluid levels if an obstruction is present. Ultrasound and CT scans may be useful in identifying ascites and abscesses. Peritoneoscopy may be helpful in the patient without ascites. It allows for direct examination of the peritoneum and the ability to obtain biopsy specimens for diagnosis.

Patients with milder cases of peritonitis or those who are poor surgical risks receive conservative care. Treatment consists of antibiotics, NG suction, analgesics, and IV fluid administration. Surgery is indicated to locate the cause of the inflammation, drain purulent fluid, and repair any damage (e.g., perforated organs).

❖ NURSING MANAGEMENT: PERITONITIS

◆ Nursing Assessment

Assessment of the patient's pain, including the location, is important and may help to determine the cause of peritonitis.

TABLE 42-12 Causes of Peritonitis

Primary	Secondary
• Blood-borne organisms	• Appendicitis with rupture
• Genital tract organisms	• Blunt or penetrating trauma to abdominal organs
• Cirrhosis with ascites	• Diverticulitis with rupture
	• Ischemic bowel disorders
	• Pancreatitis
	• Perforated intestine
	• Perforated peptic ulcer
	• Peritoneal dialysis
	• Postoperative (breakage of anastomosis)

TABLE 42-13 Interprofessional Care

Peritonitis

Diagnostic Assessment
- History and physical examination
- CBC, including WBC differential
- Serum electrolytes
- Abdominal x-ray
- Abdominal paracentesis and culture of fluid
- CT scan or ultrasound
- Peritoneoscopy

Management
Preoperative or Nonoperative
- NPO status
- IV fluid replacement
- NG to low-intermittent suction
- O₂ PRN
- Parenteral nutrition as needed

Drug Therapy
- Antibiotic therapy
- Analgesics (e.g., morphine)
- Antiemetics as needed

Postoperative
- NPO status
- NG to low-intermittent suction
- Semi-Fowler's position
- IV fluids with electrolyte replacement
- Parenteral nutrition as needed
- Blood transfusions as needed

Drug Therapy
- Antibiotic therapy
- Sedatives and opioids
- Antiemetics as needed

Assess the patient for the presence and quality of bowel sounds, increasing abdominal distention, abdominal guarding, nausea, fever, and manifestations of hypovolemic shock.

◆ Nursing Diagnoses

Nursing diagnoses for the patient with peritonitis include, but are not limited to, the following:

- Acute pain *related to* inflammation of the peritoneum and abdominal distention
- Risk for deficient fluid volume *related to* fluid shifts into the peritoneal cavity secondary to trauma, infection, or ischemia
- Anxiety *related to* uncertainty of cause or outcome of the condition and pain

◆ Planning

The overall goals are that the patient with peritonitis will have (1) resolution of inflammation, (2) relief of abdominal pain, (3) freedom from complications (especially sepsis and hypovolemic shock), and (4) normal nutritional status.

◆ Nursing Implementation

The patient with peritonitis is extremely ill and needs skilled supportive care. Establish IV access so that you can administer replacement fluids lost to the peritoneal cavity and have access for antibiotic therapy. Monitor the patient for pain and response to analgesics. You may position the patient with knees flexed to increase comfort. Sedatives may be given to relieve anxiety.

Accurate monitoring of fluid intake and output and electrolyte status is necessary to determine replacement therapy. Frequently monitor vital signs. Administer antiemetics to decrease nausea and vomiting and prevent further fluid and electrolyte losses. Place the patient on NPO status. The patient may need an NG tube to decrease gastric distention and further leakage of bowel contents into the peritoneum. Administer low-flow oxygen therapy as needed.

If the patient had an open surgical procedure, drains are inserted to remove purulent drainage and excess fluid. Postoperative care is similar to that of the patient who had a laparotomy.

GASTROENTERITIS

Gastroenteritis is an inflammation of the mucosa of the stomach and small intestine. Features of *acute gastroenteritis* are sudden diarrhea accompanied by nausea, vomiting, fever, and abdominal cramping. Viruses are the most common cause of gastroenteritis (Table 42-1).

Norovirus is a leading cause of foodborne outbreaks of acute gastroenteritis. Laboratory testing to identify norovirus is useful when a number of people have simultaneously contracted gastroenteritis and there is a clear avenue for virus transmission, such as a shared location or food.

Most cases of gastroenteritis are self-limiting. Encourage oral fluids containing glucose and electrolytes (e.g., Pedialyte) to prevent and treat dehydration. Older adults and chronically ill patients may be unable to consume enough fluids to compensate for fluid loss. If dehydration occurs, IV fluid replacement may be necessary. Nursing management of the patient with gastroenteritis is the same as for the patient with acute diarrhea (see pp. 932-933).

INFLAMMATORY BOWEL DISEASE

Inflammatory bowel disease (IBD) is a chronic inflammation of the GI tract characterized by periods of remission interspersed with periods of exacerbation. The exact cause is unknown, and there is no cure. IBD is classified as either Crohn's disease or ulcerative colitis based on clinical manifestations (Table 42-14). As the name suggests, ulcerative colitis is usually limited to the colon. Crohn's disease can involve any segment of the GI tract from the mouth to the anus.

Both ulcerative colitis and Crohn's disease commonly occur during the teenage years and early adulthood, and both have a second peak in the sixth decade. IBD occurs more commonly in people of white and Ashkenazic Jewish origin than in other racial and ethnic groups. Many people with IBD have a family member with the disorder.

Etiology and Pathophysiology

IBD is an autoimmune disease involving an immune reaction to a person's own intestinal tract. Some agent or a combination of agents triggers an overactive, inappropriate, sustained immune response. The resulting inflammation causes widespread tissue destruction.

IBD is caused by a combination of factors, including environmental factors, genetic predisposition, and alterations in immune function. Environmental factors such as diet, exposure to air pollution, stress, and smoking increase susceptibility by influencing the environment of the GI microbial flora and the immune system. IBD is more prevalent in industrialized countries. Dietary factors unique to these countries contribute to the development of IBD. High dietary intake of total fats, polyunsaturated fatty acid (PUFA), omega-6 fatty acids, and meat is associated with an increased risk of IBD. High fiber and fruit intake is associated with a decreased risk of Crohn's disease, whereas a high vegetable intake is associated with a decreased risk of ulcerative colitis.[11] Oral contraceptives and nonsteroidal antiinflammatory drugs (NSAIDs) exacerbate Crohn's disease.

Genetic Link

IBD occurs more frequently in family members of people with IBD, especially monozygotic twins. Numerous genome-wide association studies have confirmed a genetic predisposition. Certain genetic mutations are associated with Crohn's disease, others are associated with ulcerative colitis, and many are associated with both. IBD is more likely to occur in those with other genetic syndromes, including cystic fibrosis. An increased prevalence occurs in the presence of other inflammatory disorders with genetic susceptibility, such as psoriasis and multiple sclerosis.[12]

The recent identification of the first gene associated with Crohn's disease, the *NOD2* gene, was a major breakthrough. *NOD2* gene changes are associated with a form of Crohn's disease that affects the ileum in persons of northern European descent. Changes in the *NOD2* gene trigger an abnormal immune response that allows bacteria to grow unchecked and invade intestinal cells, causing chronic inflammation and digestive problems.[13]

The discovery of numerous gene variations suggests that IBD is a group of diseases that produce similar types of mucosal destruction. A genetically susceptible person who is not exposed to a triggering agent will not become ill, and a person who is not genetically susceptible will not develop IBD even if exposed to a triggering agent. The pathway from genetic mutation to

TABLE 42-14 Comparison of Ulcerative Colitis and Crohn's Disease

Characteristic	Ulcerative Colitis	Crohn's Disease
Clinical		
Usual age at onset	Teens to mid-30s. After 60	Teens to mid-30s. After 60
Diarrhea	Common	Common
Abdominal pain	Common, severe constant	Common, cramping
Fever (intermittent)	During acute attacks	Common
Weight loss	Rare	Common, may be severe
Rectal bleeding	Common	Sometimes
Tenesmus	Common	Rare
Malabsorption and nutritional deficiencies	Minimal incidence	Common
Pathologic		
Location	Usually starts in rectum and spreads in a continuous pattern up the colon	Occurs anywhere along GI tract. Most frequent site is distal ileum.
Small bowel involvement	Minimal	Common
Distribution	Continuous areas of inflammation	Healthy tissue interspersed with areas of inflammation (skip lesions)
Depth of involvement	Mucosa	Entire thickness of bowel wall (transmural)
Cobblestoning of mucosa	Rare	Common
Pseudopolyps	Common	Rare
Complications		
Perianal abscess and fistulas	Rare	Common
Strictures	Occasional	Common
C. difficile infection	Increased incidence and severity	Increased incidence and severity
Perforation	Common (because of toxic megacolon)	Common (because inflammation involves entire bowel wall)
Toxic megacolon	More common	Rare
Carcinoma	Increased incidence of colorectal cancer after 10 yr of disease	Increased incidence of small intestinal cancer Increased incidence of colorectal cancer but not as much as with ulcerative colitis

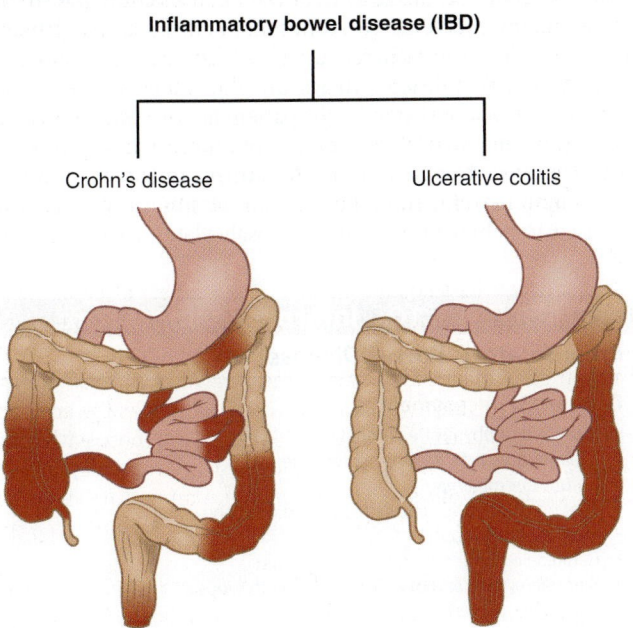

FIG. 42-3 Comparison of distribution patterns of Crohn's disease and ulcerative colitis.

abnormal immune responses varies depending on which gene or genes are affected. This genetic variation may explain differences in patient responses to various drug therapies for IBD.
Pattern of Inflammation in Ulcerative Colitis vs. Crohn's Disease. The pattern of inflammation differs between Crohn's disease and ulcerative colitis (Fig. 42-3). Crohn's disease can occur anywhere in the GI tract from the mouth to the anus but most commonly involves the distal ileum and proximal colon.

Segments of normal bowel can occur between diseased portions, so-called "skip" lesions (Table 42-14). The inflammation in Crohn's disease involves all layers of the bowel wall. Typically, ulcerations are deep and longitudinal and penetrate between islands of inflamed edematous mucosa, causing the classic cobblestone appearance. Strictures at the areas of inflammation can cause bowel obstruction. Since the inflammation goes through the entire wall, microscopic leaks can allow bowel contents to enter the peritoneal cavity and form abscesses or produce peritonitis. In active Crohn's disease, fistulas are common.

Ulcerative colitis usually starts in the rectum and moves in a continual fashion toward the cecum. Although mild inflammation may occur in the terminal ileum, ulcerative colitis is a disease of the colon and rectum. The inflammation and ulcerations occur in the mucosal layer, the innermost layer of the bowel wall. Fistulas and abscesses are rare since inflammation does not extend through all bowel wall layers. Because water and electrolytes are not absorbed through inflamed mucosa, diarrhea with large fluid and electrolyte losses is common. Breakdown of cells results in protein loss through the stool. Areas of inflamed mucosa form *pseudopolyps*, tongue-like projections into the bowel lumen.

Clinical Manifestations

Both forms of IBD are chronic disorders with mild to severe acute exacerbations that occur at unpredictable intervals over many years. Although the manifestations of Crohn's disease and ulcerative colitis are similar (diarrhea, weight loss, abdominal pain, fever, and fatigue), there are differences (Table 42-14).

In Crohn's disease, diarrhea and cramping abdominal pain are common symptoms. If the small intestine is involved, weight loss occurs from inflammation of the small intestine causing malabsorption. Rectal bleeding sometimes occurs with Crohn's disease, although not as often as with ulcerative colitis.

In ulcerative colitis, the primary manifestations are bloody diarrhea and abdominal pain. Pain may vary from the mild lower abdominal cramping associated with diarrhea to severe, constant pain associated with acute perforations. With *mild disease,* diarrhea may consist of no more than four semi-formed stools daily that contain small amounts of blood. The patient may have no other manifestations. In *moderate disease,* the patient has increased stool output (up to 10 stools/day), increased bleeding, and systemic symptoms (fever, malaise, mild anemia, anorexia). In *severe disease,* diarrhea is bloody, contains mucus, and occurs 10 to 20 times a day. In addition, fever, rapid weight loss greater than 10% of total body weight, anemia, tachycardia, and dehydration are present.

Complications

Patients with IBD experience both local (confined to the GI tract) and systemic (extraintestinal) complications (Table 42-15). GI tract complications include hemorrhage, strictures, perforation (with possible peritonitis), abscesses, fistulas, CDI, and colonic dilation (toxic megacolon). Patients with toxic megacolon are at risk of perforation and may need an emergency colectomy. Toxic megacolon is more common with ulcerative colitis. Perineal abscess and fistulas occur in up to a third of patients with Crohn's disease. CDI increases in frequency and severity in patients with IBD.[14]

Hemorrhage may lead to anemia. Blood transfusions and iron supplements are used to treat the anemia. Nutritional problems are especially common in Crohn's disease when the terminal ileum is involved. Bile salts and cobalamin are exclusively absorbed in the terminal ileum. Thus disease in the terminal ileum can result in fat malabsorption and anemia.

Patients with a history of IBD have an increased risk for colorectal cancer. Those with Crohn's disease are at increased risk for small intestinal cancer. Cancer screening at regular intervals is important in persons with IBD.

Some people with IBD suffer from systemic complications, including joint, eye, mouth, kidney, bone, vascular, and skin problems (Table 42-15). Circulating factors such as cytokines trigger inflammation in these areas. Routine liver function tests are important because primary sclerosing cholangitis, a complication of IBD, can lead to liver failure.

Diagnostic Studies

The diagnosis of IBD includes ruling out other diseases with similar symptoms and then determining whether the patient has Crohn's disease or ulcerative colitis. The symptoms of early Crohn's disease are similar to those of IBS. Diagnostic studies provide information about disease severity and complications. A CBC typically shows iron-deficiency anemia from blood loss. An elevated WBC count may be an indication of toxic megacolon or perforation. Decreased serum sodium, potassium, chloride, bicarbonate, and magnesium levels occur due to fluid and electrolyte losses from diarrhea and vomiting. Hypoalbuminemia is present with severe disease because of poor nutrition or protein loss. Elevated erythrocyte sedimentation rate, C-reactive protein, and WBCs reflect inflammation. The stool is examined for blood, pus, and mucus. Stool cultures can determine if infection is present.

Imaging studies such as double-contrast barium enema, small bowel series (small bowel follow through), transabdominal ultrasound, CT, and MRI are useful for diagnosing IBD. Colonoscopy allows for examination of the entire large intestine lumen and sometimes the most distal ileum. The extent of inflammation, ulcerations, pseudopolyps, and strictures is determined, and biopsy specimens taken for a definitive diagnosis. Since a colonoscope can enter only the distal ileum, capsule endoscopy (see Chapter 38) may be used to diagnose Crohn's disease in the small intestine.

Interprofessional Care

The goals of treatment of IBD are to (1) rest the bowel, (2) control the inflammation, (3) combat infection, (4) correct malnutrition, (5) alleviate stress, (6) provide symptomatic relief, and (7) improve quality of life. Since the cause is unknown, treatment relies on drugs to treat the inflammation and maintain remission (Table 42-16). A number of drugs are available to treat IBD. Since the recurrence rate is high after surgical treatment of Crohn's disease, drugs are the preferred treatment. Hospitalization is indicated if the patient fails to respond to drug therapy, the disease is severe, or complications are suspected.

Drug Therapy. The goal of drug treatment in IBD is to induce and maintain remission. Five major classes of medications are used to achieve this goal: aminosalicylates, antimicrobials,

---

TABLE 42-15 Extraintestinal Complications of IBD

Joints
- Peripheral arthritis (colitic)
- Ankylosing spondylitis
- Sacroiliitis
- Finger clubbing

Skin
- Erythema nodosum
- Pyoderma gangrenosum

Mouth
- Aphthous ulcers

Eye
- Conjunctivitis
- Uveitis
- Episcleritis

Other
- Gallstones
- Kidney stones
- Liver disease: primary sclerosing cholangitis
- Osteoporosis
- Thromboembolism

TABLE 42-16 Interprofessional Care

Inflammatory Bowel Disease

Diagnostic Assessment
- History and physical examination
- CBC, erythrocyte sedimentation rate
- Serum chemistries
- Testing of stool for occult blood and infection
- Capsule endoscopy
- Radiologic studies with barium contrast
- Sigmoidoscopy and/or colonoscopy with biopsy

Management
- High-calorie, high-vitamin, high-protein, low-residue, lactose-free (if lactase deficiency) diet
- Elemental diet or parenteral nutrition
- Drug therapy (Table 42-17)
  - Aminosalicylates
  - Antimicrobials
  - Corticosteroids
  - Immunosuppressants
  - Biologic and targeted therapy (immunomodulators)
- Physical and emotional rest
- Referral for counseling or support group
- Surgical therapy (Table 42-18)

TABLE 42-17   Drug Therapy
Inflammatory Bowel Disease

Class	Action	Examples
5-Aminosalicylates (5-ASA)	Decrease inflammation by suppressing proinflammatory cytokines and other inflammatory mediators	*Systemic:* sulfasalazine (Azulfidine), mesalamine (Asacol, Pentasa), olsalazine (Dipentum), balsalazide (Colazal)
Antimicrobials	Prevent or treat secondary infection	*Topical:* 5-ASA enema (Rowasa), mesalamine suppositories (Canasa) metronidazole (Flagyl), ciprofloxacin (Cipro), clarithromycin (Biaxin)
Corticosteroids	Decrease inflammation	*Systemic:* corticosteroids (prednisone, budesonide [Uceris]) (oral); hydrocortisone or methylprednisolone (IV for severe IBD)
		Topical: hydrocortisone suppository or foam (Cortifoam) or enema (Cortenema)
Immunosuppressants	Suppress immune response	azathioprine (Imuran), 6-mercaptopurine (6-MP), methotrexate, cyclosporine
Biologic and targeted therapy (immunomodulators)	Inhibit the cytokine tumor necrosis factor (TNF)	infliximab (Remicade), adalimumab (Humira), certolizumab pegol (Cimzia), golimumab (Simponi)
	Prevent migration of leukocytes from bloodstream to inflamed tissue	natalizumab (Tysabri), vedolizumab (Entyvio)

corticosteroids, immunosuppressants, and biologic and targeted therapy (Table 42-17). Drug selection depends on the location and severity of inflammation. Patients are treated with either a "step-up" or a "step-down" approach. With the step-up approach, the patient begins with less toxic therapies (e.g., aminosalicylates and antimicrobials) and is started on more toxic medications (e.g., biologic and targeted therapy) when initial therapies do not work. The step-down approach uses biologic and targeted therapy first.

Medications containing 5-aminosalicylic acid (5-ASA) remain a mainstay in achieving and maintaining remission and preventing flare-ups of IBD. They include sulfasalazine (Azulfidine) and the new generation of sulfa-free drugs (olsalazine [Dipentum], mesalamine [Pentasa]). Aminosalicylates are more effective for ulcerative colitis. However, they are first-line therapies for mild to moderate Crohn's disease, especially when the colon is involved.

The exact mechanism of action of 5-ASA is unknown, but topical application to the intestinal mucosa suppresses proinflammatory cytokines and other inflammatory mediators. The benefits of these drugs usually depend on the dose: the larger the dose, the more likely patients will improve during the acute phase and remain in remission. However, many people cannot tolerate the side effects of sulfasalazine. Headaches, nausea, and fatigue occur at the higher doses. In men, long-term sulfasalazine treatment may cause abnormal sperm production, leading to infertility. These effects are reversible if sulfasalazine is discontinued.

DRUG ALERT   Sulfasalazine (Azulfidine)
- May cause yellowish orange discoloration of skin and urine
- Avoid exposure to sunlight and ultraviolet light until photosensitivity is determined.

The sulfa-free drugs are as effective as sulfasalazine and better tolerated when administered orally. Topical 5-ASA preparations include rectal suppositories and enemas. Topical treatment offers the advantage of delivering the 5-ASA directly to the affected tissue and minimizing systemic effects. The combination of oral and rectal therapy is better than oral or rectal therapy alone.

Corticosteroids are used to achieve remission in IBD. They are given for the shortest possible time because of side effects associated with long-term use. Patients with disease in the left colon, sigmoid, and rectum benefit from suppositories, enemas, and foams because they deliver the corticosteroid directly to the inflamed tissue with minimal systemic effects. Oral prednisone

is given to patients with mild to moderate disease who did not respond to either 5-ASA or topical corticosteroids. Those with severe inflammation may require a short course of IV corticosteroids. Corticosteroids must be tapered to very low levels when surgery is planned to prevent postoperative complications (e.g., infection, delayed wound healing, fistula formation).

Immunosuppressants (6-mercaptopurine, azathioprine [Imuran]) are given to maintain remission after corticosteroid induction therapy. These drugs require regular CBC monitoring because they can suppress the bone marrow and lead to inflammation of the pancreas or liver. They have a delayed onset of action and are therefore not useful for acute flare-ups.

Methotrexate is most useful in patients with Crohn's disease who cannot stop corticosteroid use without a flare-up or in whom other medications have been ineffective. Many patients have flu-like symptoms with use, and some develop bone marrow depression and liver dysfunction. Correct dosing is critical to minimize the risk of toxicity. Careful monitoring of the CBC and liver enzymes is essential. Advise women of childbearing age to avoid pregnancy because use causes birth defects and fetal death.

Currently there are six biologic and targeted medications.[15] Four are antitumor necrosis factor (TNF) agents: infliximab (Remicade), adalimumab (Humira), certolizumab pegol (Cimzia) and golimumab (Simponi). Infliximab is a monoclonal antibody to TNF (proinflammatory cytokine). This drug is given IV to induce and maintain remission in patients with Crohn's disease and in patients with draining fistulas who do not respond to conventional drug therapy. The other TNF agents are given subcutaneously and have effects similar to those of infliximab.

The anti-TNF agents have similar side effects. The most common adverse effects are upper respiratory and urinary tract infections, headaches, nausea, joint pain, and abdominal pain. More serious effects include reactivation of hepatitis and tuberculosis (TB); opportunistic infections; and malignancies, especially lymphoma. Patients need to know the risks before starting therapy. They are tested for TB and hepatitis before treatment begins and cannot receive live virus immunizations. Teaching includes how to prevent infection and recognize early signs and symptoms (e.g., fever, cough, malaise, dyspnea).

Two biologic and targeted medications are integrin receptor antagonists: natalizumab (Tysabri) and vedolizumab (Entyvio). They inhibit leukocyte adhesion by blocking α_4-integrin, an adhesion molecule. The use of integrin receptor antagonists is limited to those who have not had an adequate response with other therapies (corticosteroids, immunosuppressants, or TNF agents). Both are given by IV infusion. Their use is associated

TABLE 42-18	Indications for Surgical Therapy for IBD
• Drainage of abdominal abscess • Failure to respond to conservative therapy • Fistulas • Inability to decrease corticosteroids	• Intestinal obstruction • Massive hemorrhage • Perforation • Severe anorectal disease • Suspicion of carcinoma

with increased risk of infection, hepatotoxicity, and hypersensitivity reactions. Because of the risk of progressive multifocal leukoencephalopathy, natalizumab is available only through a restricted program.

The biologic and targeted agents do not work for everyone. They are costly and may produce allergic reactions. They are immunogenic, meaning that patients receiving them frequently produce antibodies against them. Immunogenicity leads to acute infusion reactions and delayed hypersensitivity-type reactions. The drugs are most effective when given at regular intervals. Infusion reactions are more likely if a drug is stopped and then restarted.

Surgical Therapy

Ulcerative Colitis. Indications for surgery for ulcerative colitis are presented in Table 42-18. Since ulcerative colitis affects only the colon, a total proctocolectomy is curative. Surgical procedures used to treat ulcerative colitis include (1) total proctocolectomy with ileal pouch/anal anastomosis and (2) total proctocolectomy with permanent ileostomy. These procedures can be performed laparoscopically.

Total proctocolectomy with ileal pouch/anal anastomosis (IPAA). The most commonly used surgical procedure for ulcerative colitis is a total proctocolectomy with ileal pouch/anal anastomosis (IPAA). In this procedure, a diverting ileostomy is performed, and an ileal pouch is created and anastomosed directly to the anus (Fig. 42-4). It requires two surgical procedures performed approximately 8 to 12 weeks apart. The first procedure includes colectomy, rectal mucosectomy, ileal pouch (reservoir) construction, ileoanal anastomosis, and temporary ileostomy. The second surgery involves closure of the ileostomy to direct stool toward the new pouch. Initially, patients may have 4 to 6 stools or more daily, but adaptation over the next 3 to 6 months will result in a decreased number of bowel movements. The patient is able to control defecation at the anal sphincter. The major complication of this procedure is acute or chronic pouchitis. A permanent ileostomy may be done if pouchitis does not resolve.

Total proctocolectomy with permanent ileostomy. A proctocolectomy with a permanent ileostomy is a one-stage surgery involving the removal of the colon, rectum, and anus with closure of the anal opening. The end of the terminal ileum is brought out through the abdominal wall to form a stoma (ostomy). The stoma is usually placed in the right lower quadrant below the belt line. With a permanent ileostomy, continence is not possible.

Crohn's Disease. Surgery for Crohn's disease is usually performed for complications such as strictures, obstructions, bleeding, and fistula (Table 42-18). Most patients with Crohn's disease eventually require surgery. The most common surgery involves resection of the diseased segments with reanastomosis of the remaining intestine. Unfortunately, the disease often recurs at the anastomosis site. Repeated removal of sections of small intestine can lead to short bowel syndrome. *Short bowel*

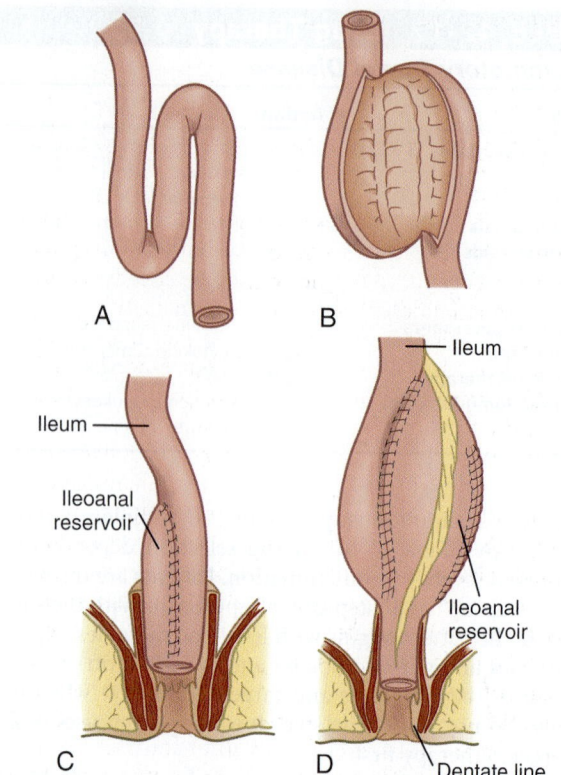

FIG. 42-4 Ileoanal pouch (reservoir). **A,** Formation of a pouch. **B,** Posterior suture lines completed. **C,** J-shaped configuration for ileoanal pouch (J-pouch). **D,** S-shaped configuration for ileoanal pouch (S-pouch).

syndrome (SBS) occurs when either surgery or disease leaves too little small intestine surface area to maintain normal nutrition and hydration. Lifetime fluid boluses and parenteral nutrition may be needed. For more detail, see the discussion on short bowel syndrome later in this chapter on p. 967.

The other common surgery for Crohn's disease is a strictureplasty, which opens up narrowed areas obstructing the bowel. Since the intestine remains intact, it reduces the risk of developing short-bowel syndrome and its associated complications. Recurrences at the site of the strictureplasty are uncommon.

Postoperative Care. Postoperative care after surgical procedures for IBD is similar to that described in the general nursing care plan for the postoperative patient (see eNursing Care Plan 19-1 on the website for Chapter 19). If an ileostomy is formed, monitor stoma viability, the mucocutaneous juncture (the area where the mucous membrane of the bowel interfaces with the skin), and peristomal skin integrity. Your patient should return from surgery with a clear ileostomy pouch in place. Replace pouches if feces leak onto the skin. (See the later discussion on ileostomy care on pp. 961-962.)

Immediately after surgery, ileostomy output initially may be as high as 1500 to 1800 mL/24 hr. Observe the patient for signs of fluid and electrolyte imbalance, hemorrhage, abdominal abscess, small bowel obstruction, dehydration, and other related complications. If an NG tube is used, remove it when bowel function returns. Over a period of days to weeks, the proximal small bowel adapts and increases fluid absorption. Then, feces will thicken to a paste-like consistency and the volume decrease. Patients, especially those with Crohn's disease, are at risk for developing a bowel obstruction during the first 30 days postoperatively.

Transient incontinence of mucus is a result of intraoperative manipulation of the anal canal. Initial drainage through the ileoanal anastomosis will be liquid. Have the patient start Kegel exercises about 4 weeks after surgery to strengthen the pelvic floor and sphincter muscles (see Table 45-18). Perianal skin care is important to protect the epidermis from mucous drainage and maceration. Instruct the patient to gently clean the skin with a mild cleanser, rinse well, and dry thoroughly. A moisture barrier ointment and a perineal pad may be used.

Nutritional Therapy. An individualized diet is an important component in the treatment of IBD. It is essential that people with IBD eat a balanced, healthy diet with sufficient calories, protein, and nutrients. Consult a dietitian regarding dietary recommendations. The goals of diet management are to (1) provide adequate nutrition without exacerbating symptoms, (2) correct and prevent malnutrition, (3) replace fluid and electrolyte losses, and (4) prevent weight loss.

Nutritional deficiencies are due to decreased oral intake, blood loss, and, depending on the location of the inflammation, malabsorption of nutrients. Patients may reduce food intake in an effort to reduce diarrhea. Inflammatory mediators reduce appetite. Bloody diarrhea leads to iron-deficiency anemia, which may require treatment with supplemental iron (ferrous sulfate or ferrous gluconate). Parenteral or IV iron may be needed for patients who cannot tolerate oral iron or if anemia is severe.

Disease of the terminal ileum reduces absorption of cobalamin and bile acids. Reduced cobalamin contributes to anemia, and bile salts are important for fat absorption and contribute to osmotic diarrhea. Those who develop anemia should receive cobalamin injections. Cholestyramine, an ion-exchange resin that binds unabsorbed bile salts, helps control diarrhea. Zinc deficiency can result from severe or chronic diarrhea, and supplementation may be necessary.

Medications can contribute to nutritional problems. Patients receiving sulfasalazine should receive folate (folic acid) daily. Those receiving corticosteroids are prone to osteoporosis and need calcium supplements. Potassium supplements may be necessary with corticosteroids. Vitamin D deficiency requiring supplementation is common. This may be due to malabsorption due to inflammation, surgical resection of intestine, reduced sunlight exposure, and decreased dietary intake.[16]

During an acute exacerbation, patients with IBD may not be able to tolerate a regular diet. Liquid enteral feedings are preferred over parenteral nutrition because atrophy of the gut and bacterial overgrowth occur when the GI tract is not used. (Enteral and parenteral nutrition are discussed in Chapter 39.) Enteral nutrition is high in calories and nutrients, lactose free, and easily absorbed. Enteral feedings help achieve remission and improve nutritional status. Restarting regular foods gradually will help identify food intolerances or sensitivities.

There are no universal food triggers for IBD, but some may find that certain foods cause diarrhea. A food diary helps to identify problem foods to avoid. Because many patients with IBD are lactose intolerant, avoiding milk and milk products improves symptoms. Lactose-intolerant patients can use yogurt as a substitute. High-fat foods, cold foods, and high-fiber foods (cereal with bran, nuts, raw fruits with peels) may trigger diarrhea.

❖ NURSING MANAGEMENT: INFLAMMATORY BOWEL DISEASE

◆ Nursing Assessment

Table 42-19 outlines the subjective and objective data you should obtain from a patient with IBD.

TABLE 42-19 Nursing Assessment

Inflammatory Bowel Disease

Subjective Data
Important Health Information
Past health history: Infection, autoimmune disorders
Medications: Antidiarrheal medications

Functional Health Patterns
Health perception–health management: Family history of ulcerative colitis or Crohn's disease. Fatigue, malaise
Nutritional-metabolic: Nausea, vomiting; anorexia. Weight loss
Elimination: Diarrhea. Blood, mucus, or pus in stools
Cognitive-perceptual: Lower abdominal pain (worse before defecation), cramping, tenesmus

Objective Data
General
Intermittent fever, emaciated appearance, fatigue

Integumentary
Pale skin with poor turgor, dry mucous membranes. Skin lesions, anorectal irritation, skin tags, cutaneous fistulas

Gastrointestinal
Abdominal distention, hyperactive bowel sounds, abdominal cramps

Cardiovascular
Tachycardia, hypotension

Possible Diagnostic Findings
Anemia, leukocytosis. Electrolyte imbalance, hypoalbuminemia, vitamin and trace metal deficiencies. Guaiac-positive stool. Abnormal sigmoidoscopic, colonoscopic, and/or barium enema findings

---

◆ Nursing Diagnoses

Nursing diagnoses for the patient with IBD include, but are not limited to, the following:

- Diarrhea *related to* bowel inflammation and intestinal hyperactivity
- Imbalanced nutrition: less than body requirements *related to* decreased absorption and increased nutrient loss through diarrhea
- Ineffective coping *related to* chronic disease, lifestyle changes, inadequate confidence in ability to cope

For additional information on nursing diagnoses on IBD, see eNursing Care Plan 42-2 on the website for this chapter.

◆ Planning

The overall goals are that the patient with IBD will (1) have fewer and less severe acute exacerbations, (2) maintain normal fluid and electrolyte balance, (3) be free from pain or discomfort, (4) adhere to medical regimens, (5) maintain nutritional balance, and (6) have an improved quality of life.

◆ Nursing Implementation

During the acute phase, focus your attention on hemodynamic stability, pain control, fluid and electrolyte balance, and nutritional support. Maintain accurate intake and output records, and monitor the number and appearance of stools. Assess for the presence of blood in stools and emesis. Administer IV fluids, electrolytes, analgesics, and antiinflammatory medications as ordered. Monitor serum electrolytes, CBC, and vital signs, being alert for any changes related to diarrhea and dehydration. If the patient experiences orthostatic hypotension, teach the patient to change position slowly and use safety precautions.

Until diarrhea is controlled, help the patient stay clean, dry, and free of odor. Place a deodorizer in the room. Meticulous perianal skin care using plain water (no harsh soap) together with a moisturizing skin barrier cream prevents skin breakdown. Dibucaine (Nupercainal), witch hazel, sitz baths, and other soothing compresses or ointments may reduce irritation and discomfort of the anus.

Calculate the adequacy of the daily calorie intake. Obtain a daily weight. Assess the abdomen, including bowel sounds, as needed. Consult with a dietitian regarding diet modifications and the need for nutritional supplements.

IBD is a chronic illness. Assist the patient in accepting the chronicity of IBD and learning strategies to cope with its recurrent, unpredictable nature. Teaching includes (1) the importance of rest and diet management, (2) perianal care, (3) drug action and side effects, (4) symptoms of recurrence of disease, (5) when to seek medical care, and (6) ways to reduce stress. Excellent teaching resources, written in easily comprehensible language are available from the Crohn's and Colitis Foundation of America (www.ccfa.org).

It is important to establish rapport and encourage the patient to talk about self-care strategies. Ask patients what you can do to facilitate their self-care. An explanation of all procedures and treatments helps to build trust, decrease apprehension, and increase self-control. Once you have established a therapeutic relationship, talk with smokers who have Crohn's disease about quitting since smoking is associated with more severe disease.[17]

The patient and caregiver may need your help setting realistic short- and long-term goals. Patients may suffer severe fatigue, which limits their energy for physical activity. Rest is important. Patients may lose sleep because of frequent episodes of diarrhea and abdominal pain. Nutritional deficiencies and anemia leave the patient feeling weak and listless. Teach them to schedule activities around rest periods.

Many patients experience intermittent exacerbations and remissions of symptoms. Given the chronicity and uncertainty related to the frequency and severity of flares, the patient may experience frustration, depression, and anxiety. Psychotherapy and behavioral therapies may help patients deal with their feelings about the disease and help to manage their symptoms. Because of the relationship between emotions and the GI tract, teach the patient strategies for managing stress (see Chapter 6). Suggest that your patient seek support through a local or online support group from the Crohn's and Colitis Foundation of America.

◆ Evaluation

The expected outcomes are that the patient with IBD will
- Experience a decrease in the number of diarrhea stools
- Maintain body weight within a normal range
- Be free from pain and discomfort
- Demonstrate the use of effective coping strategies

For additional information on expected outcomes for IBD, see eNursing Care Plan 42-2 on the website for this chapter.

 ### Gerontologic Considerations:
Inflammatory Bowel Disease

A second peak in occurrence of IBD is in the sixth decade. The etiology, natural history, and clinical course of IBD are similar to those observed in younger patients. However, in the older patient, proctitis and left-sided ulcerative colitis are more common. Diagnosis is sometimes difficult in older adults, since IBD can be confused with CDI and the colitis associated with diverticulosis or NSAID ingestion.

For the healthy older adult, the interprofessional care of IBD is similar to that of the younger patient. For the frail older patient with IBD, the usual treatments may increase the risk of adverse events, hospitalization, or mortality.[18] Older adults are more prone to adverse events from corticosteroids. Immunosuppressants and biologic therapy have a higher risk of infection and malignancy in older patients. Those with diminished renal and cardiovascular function are more vulnerable to the consequences of volume depletion from diarrhea. Those with physical limitations may have difficulty handling fecal urgency and multiple trips to the bathroom without assistance.

In addition to Crohn's disease and ulcerative colitis, older adults are vulnerable to inflammation of the colon (colitis) from drug use and systemic vascular disease. Drugs such as NSAIDs, digitalis, sumatriptan (Imitrex), vasopressin, estrogen, and allopurinol (Zyloprim) have been associated with the development of colitis in the older patient. Colitis may also be secondary to ischemic bowel disease related to atherosclerosis and heart failure.

INTESTINAL OBSTRUCTION

Intestinal obstruction occurs when intestinal contents cannot pass through the GI tract. The obstruction may occur in the small intestine or colon and can be partial or complete, simple or strangulated. Partial obstructions do not completely occlude the intestinal lumen, allowing for some fluid and gas to pass through. They usually resolve with conservative treatment. A complete obstruction totally occludes the lumen and usually requires surgery. A simple obstruction has an intact blood supply; a strangulated one does not.

Types of Intestinal Obstruction

The causes of intestinal obstruction are classified as mechanical or nonmechanical.

Mechanical. In *mechanical obstruction*, there is a physical obstruction of the intestinal lumen. Most intestinal obstructions occur in the small intestine.[19] Surgical adhesions are the most common cause of small bowel obstructions and can occur within days of surgery or several years later (Fig. 42-5). Other causes of small bowel obstruction are hernia, strictures from Crohn's disease, and intussusception after bariatric abdominal surgery. The most common cause of colon obstruction is colorectal cancer (malignant obstruction) followed by diverticular disease and sigmoid volvulus. A *volvulus* is an intestinal obstruction that occurs by the bowel twisting on itself.

Nonmechanical. A *nonmechanical obstruction* occurs with reduced or absent peristalsis due to altered neuromuscular transmission of the parasympathetic innervation to the bowel.[19] It may result from a neuromuscular or vascular disorder. **Paralytic ileus** (lack of intestinal peristalsis and bowel sounds) is the most common form of nonmechanical obstruction. It occurs to some degree after any abdominal surgery. It can be difficult to know whether postoperative obstruction is due to paralytic ileus or adhesions. One clue is that bowel sounds usually return before postoperative adhesions develop. Other causes of paralytic ileus include peritonitis, inflammatory responses (e.g., acute pancreatitis, acute appendicitis), electrolyte abnormalities

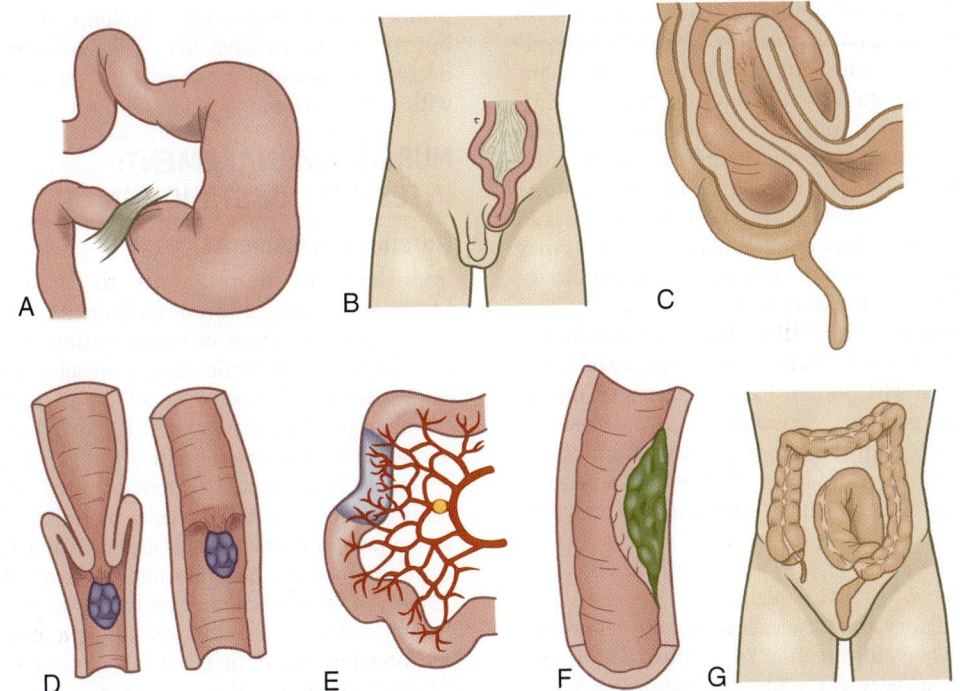

FIG. 42-5 Bowel obstructions. **A,** Adhesions. **B,** Strangulated inguinal hernia. **C,** Ileocecal intussusception. **D,** Intussusception from polyps. **E,** Mesenteric occlusion. **F,** Neoplasm. **G,** Volvulus of the sigmoid colon.

(especially hypokalemia), and thoracic or lumbar spinal fractures.

Pseudo-obstruction is a mechanical obstruction of the intestine without any cause found on radiologic imaging. There are several conditions that are associated with a pseudo-obstruction. These include myocardial infarction, renal failure, Parkinson's disease, trauma, recent major orthopedic surgery, opiate use, and metabolic disturbances (e.g., hypokalemia).[19]

Vascular obstructions are rare and are the result of an interference with the blood supply to a portion of the intestines. The most common causes are emboli and atherosclerosis of the mesenteric arteries. Emboli may originate from thrombi in patients who have chronic atrial fibrillation, diseased heart valves, and prosthetic valves. Venous thrombosis may occur in conditions of low blood flow, such as heart failure and shock.

Etiology and Pathophysiology

About 6 to 8 L of fluid enter the small intestine daily. Most of the fluid is absorbed before it reaches the colon. Approximately 75% of intestinal gas is swallowed air. When an obstruction occurs, fluid, gas, and intestinal contents accumulate proximal to the obstruction. Distention reduces fluid absorption and initially stimulates intestinal secretions. Distal to the obstruction, the bowel empties and then collapses. As distention increases in the proximal bowel, intraluminal bowel pressure rises. The increased pressure leads to an increase in capillary permeability and extravasation of fluids and electrolytes into the peritoneal cavity. Eventually the intestinal muscle becomes fatigued, and peristalsis stops. Retention of fluids in the intestine and peritoneal cavity leads to a severe reduction in circulating blood volume. This leads to hypotension and hypovolemic shock.

If blood flow is inadequate, bowel tissue becomes ischemic, then necrotic, and the bowel may perforate. In the most dangerous situation the bowel becomes so distended that the blood flow stops, causing edema, cyanosis, and gangrene of a bowel segment. This is called *intestinal strangulation* or *intestinal infarction*. If

TABLE 42-20 Manifestations of Small and Large Intestinal Obstructions

Manifestation	SMALL INTESTINE		Large Intestine
	Proximal	Distal	
Onset	Rapid	Rapid	Gradual
Vomiting	Frequent and copious	Less frequent	Late or absent
Pain	Colicky, cramping, occurs at frequent intervals	Colicky, occurs more intermittently	Persistent, cramping
Bowel movement	Feces for a short time	Gradual constipation	Absolute constipation
Abdominal distention	Minimal	Increased	Increased

not quickly corrected, the bowel will become necrotic and rupture, leading to infection, septic shock, and death.

The location of the obstruction determines the extent of fluid, electrolyte, and acid-base imbalances. If the obstruction is high (e.g., upper duodenum), metabolic alkalosis may result from the loss of gastric hydrochloric (HCl) acid through vomiting or NG intubation and suction. When the obstruction is located in the small intestine, dehydration occurs rapidly. Dehydration and electrolyte imbalances do not occur early in large bowel obstruction. If the obstruction is below the proximal colon, solid fecal material accumulates until symptoms of discomfort appear.

Clinical Manifestations

The four hallmark clinical manifestations of an obstruction are abdominal pain, vomiting, distention, and constipation. The order and degree these appear vary by the location and type of the obstruction (Table 42-20). Colicky abdominal pain is usually the first manifestation of an obstruction. In small bowel obstruction, the pain is often of sudden onset. It occurs at 4- to 5-minute intervals for proximal obstructions and less frequently for distal obstructions. The nature of the vomiting gives a clue to the level of obstruction. In a proximal obstruction, patients rapidly develop nausea and vomiting. It may be projective and contain bile. Vomiting usually provides temporary relief from abdominal pain in higher obstructions. Vomiting from a more distal small bowel obstruction is more gradual in onset and more fecal and foul smelling. Auscultation of bowel sounds may reveal high-pitched sounds above the area of obstruction. Bowel sounds are usually absent with paralytic ileus.

Signs of colonic obstruction include abdominal distention, either absolute constipation or a marked change in bowel function, and lack of flatus. The patient has persistent, cramping abdominal pain. Bowel sounds are usually present and become progressively hypoactive. Vomiting is rare. Strangulation causes severe, constant pain that is rapid in onset. Abdominal tenderness and rigidity occur and the patient's temperature may rise above 100° F (37.8° C).

Diagnostic Studies

Perform a thorough history and physical examination. Imaging can identify the presence and location of an obstruction and guide decisions about surgery. CT scans and abdominal x-rays are ordered. Sigmoidoscopy or colonoscopy may provide direct visualization of an obstruction in the colon.

Blood tests include a CBC and blood chemistries. An elevated WBC count may indicate strangulation or perforation. Elevated hematocrit values may reflect hemoconcentration. Decreased hemoglobin and hematocrit values may indicate bleeding from a neoplasm or strangulation with necrosis. Serum electrolytes, BUN, and creatinine are monitored frequently to assess the degree of dehydration. Metabolic alkalosis can develop from vomiting.

Interprofessional Care

Treatment of a bowel obstruction depends on the cause. If a strangulated obstruction or perforation is present, the patient will require emergency surgery to relieve the obstruction and survive. In some, especially those due to surgical adhesions, an obstruction may resolve without surgery.

The initial medical treatment includes placing the patient on NPO status, inserting an NG tube for decompression, providing IV fluid therapy with either normal saline or lactated Ringer's solution (since fluid losses from the GI tract are isotonic), adding potassium to IV fluids after verifying renal function, and administering analgesics for pain control. Some patients require parenteral nutrition to allow bowel rest and improve nutritional status before surgery.

Surgery may involve simply resecting the obstructed segment of bowel and anastomosing the remaining healthy bowel back together. Partial or total colectomy, colostomy, or ileostomy may be required when extensive obstruction or necrosis is present. Occasionally, an obstruction can be removed nonsurgically. Colonoscopy offers a means to remove polyps, dilate strictures, and remove and destroy tumors with a laser.

The treatment goal for a patient with a malignant bowel obstruction is to regain patency and resolve the obstruction. Stents can be placed via endoscopic or fluoroscopic procedures. They are used for palliative purposes or as "a bridge to surgery," allowing a patient to avoid emergency surgery. This gives the interprofessional care team time to correct fluid volume problems and treat other problems, thus improving surgical outcomes. Corticosteroids with antiemetic properties that decrease edema and inflammation may be used in combination with stent placement.

❖ NURSING MANAGEMENT: INTESTINAL OBSTRUCTION

◆ Nursing Assessment

Intestinal obstruction is a potentially life-threatening condition. Major concerns are preventing fluid and electrolyte deficiencies and early recognition of deterioration in the patient's condition (e.g., hypovolemic shock, bowel strangulation). Nursing assessment begins with a detailed patient history and physical examination. Determine the location, duration, intensity, and frequency of abdominal pain.

Record the onset, frequency, color, odor, and amount of vomitus. Assess bowel function, including the passage of flatus. Auscultate for bowel sounds and document their character and location. Inspect the abdomen for scars, visible masses, and distention. Assess whether abdominal tenderness or rigidity is present. Measure the abdominal girth, and check for signs of peritoneal irritation (e.g., muscle guarding, rebound pain, pain if bed is shaken). If the surgeon decides to wait and see if the obstruction resolves on its own, assess the patient regularly and notify the surgeon of changes in vital signs, changes in bowel sounds, decreased urine output, increased abdominal distention, and pain.

Maintain a strict intake and output record, including emesis and tube drainage. A urinary catheter allows for hourly monitoring of urine output. Immediately report if the urine output is less than 0.5 mL/kg of body weight per hour, because this indicates inadequate vascular volume and the potential for acute kidney injury. Rising serum creatinine and BUN levels are additional indicators of acute kidney injury.

◆ Nursing Diagnoses

Nursing diagnoses for the patient with intestinal obstructions include, but are not limited to, the following:
- Acute pain *related to* abdominal distention and increased peristalsis
- Deficient fluid volume *related to* a decrease in intestinal fluid absorption, third space fluid shifts into the bowel lumen and peritoneal cavity, NG suction, and vomiting

◆ Planning

The overall goals are that the patient with an intestinal obstruction will have (1) relief of the obstruction and return to normal bowel function, (2) minimal to no discomfort, and (3) normal fluid and electrolyte and acid-base status.

◆ Nursing Implementation

Monitor the patient closely for signs of dehydration and electrolyte imbalances. Administer IV fluids as ordered. Watch for signs and symptoms of fluid overload, since some patients, especially older adults, may not tolerate rapid fluid replacement. Monitor serum electrolyte levels closely. A patient with a high intestinal obstruction is more likely to have metabolic alkalosis. A patient with a low obstruction is at greater risk for metabolic acidosis. The patient is often restless and constantly changes position to relieve the pain. Provide comfort measures and promote a restful environment. Nursing care of the patient after surgery for an intestinal obstruction is similar to care of the patient after a laparotomy (see p. 940).

With an NG tube in place, oral care is extremely important. Vomiting leaves an unpleasant taste in the patient's mouth, and fecal odor may be present. The patient breathes through the mouth, drying the mouth and lips. Encourage and help the patient to brush the teeth frequently. Mouthwash and water for rinsing the mouth and water-soluble lubricant for the lips should be readily available to the patient. Check the nose for signs of irritation from the NG tube. Clean and dry this area daily, apply water-soluble lubricant, and retape the tube. Check the NG tube every 4 hours for patency.

POLYPS OF LARGE INTESTINE

Colonic polyps arise from the mucosal surface of the colon and project into the lumen. They may be *sessile* (flat, broad based, and attached directly to the intestinal wall) or *pedunculated* (attached to the intestinal wall by a thin stalk). Polyps tend to be sessile when small and become pedunculated as they enlarge (Fig. 42-6). They may be found anywhere in the large intestine. As patients age, polyps are increasingly present in the proximal colon. Rectal bleeding and occult blood in the stool are the most common signs, but most patients with polyps are asymptomatic.

Types of Polyps

The most common types of polyps are hyperplastic and adenomatous. *Hyperplastic polyps* are non-neoplastic growths. They rarely grow larger than 5 mm and never cause clinical symptoms. Other benign (nonneoplastic) polyps include inflammatory polyps, lipomas, and juvenile polyps.

Adenomatous polyps are neoplastic and closely linked to colorectal adenocarcinoma. There are three types of adenomatous polyps: tubular, tubulovillous, and villous. Large or villous adenomatous polyps are more likely to have cancers develop in them. Removing adenomatous polyps decreases the occurrence of colorectal cancer.

Genetic Link

Familial adenomatous polyposis (FAP) is the most common polyposis syndrome (see the Genetics in Clinical Practice box).

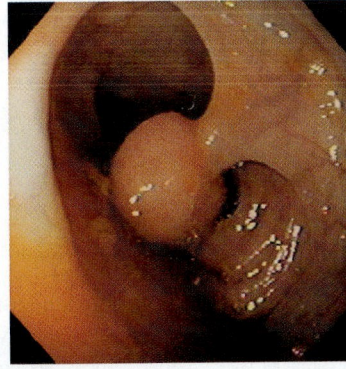

FIG. 42-6   Endoscopic image of pedunculated polyp in descending colon. (Courtesy David Bjorkman, MD, University of Utah School of Medicine, Department of Gastroenterology. In McCance KL, Huether SE: *Pathophysiology: the biologic basis for disease in adults and children*, ed 6, St Louis, 2010, Mosby.)

GENETICS IN CLINICAL PRACTICE
Familial Adenomatous Polyposis (FAP)

Genetic Basis
- Classic form of disease
  - Autosomal dominant disorder
  - Mutations in adenomatous polyposis coli *(APC)* gene
  - Normally this is a tumor suppressor gene involved in DNA repair.
  - Normally this gene produces a special substance (a protein) that keeps polyps from developing in the colon.
- Autosomal recessive FAP
  - Autosomal recessive disorder
  - Mutations in the *mutY* homolog *(MUTYH)* gene
  - Normally this gene is involved in DNA repair.

Incidence
- Affects 1 in 7000 to 22,000 people
- Equally affects men and women

Genetic Testing
- DNA testing is available.

Clinical Implications
- FAP accounts for about 1% of all colorectal cancers.
- Persons with classic FAP have hundreds to thousands of colorectal polyps.
- Polyps are not present at birth but appear during adolescence and early adulthood.
- Autosomal recessive FAP is characterized by fewer polyps, typically <100.
- If untreated, almost all persons with classic FAP will develop colorectal cancer before age 40.
- With classic FAP, there are other benign and malignant tumors sometimes present, especially in the small intestine, stomach, liver, thyroid, and other tissues.
- Many deaths related to FAP can be prevented with early and aggressive monitoring and treatment, including frequent colonoscopies and total colectomy.
- Individuals with a family history of FAP can benefit from genetic counseling.

FAP is a genetic disorder characterized by hundreds or sometimes thousands of polyps in the colon that eventually become cancerous, usually by age 40. Since it is autosomal dominant, 50% of the offspring of a patient with FAP carry the FAP gene. Anyone with a family history of FAP should undergo genetic testing during childhood. If the FAP gene is present, colorectal screening begins at puberty, and annual colonoscopy begins at age 16. Since cancer is inevitable, the colon and rectum are removed, usually by age 25, and proctocolectomy with an IPAA or an ileostomy is performed (see p. 948). Patients with FAP are at risk for cancers of the thyroid, small intestine, liver, and brain, so lifetime cancer surveillance is essential.

Diagnostic Studies and Interprofessional Care

Colonoscopy, sigmoidoscopy, barium enema, and virtual colonoscopy (CT or MRI colonography) are used to discover polyps. Colonoscopy is preferred because it allows evaluation of the total colon. All polyps are considered abnormal and should be removed. Polyps can be removed immediately *(polypectomy)* with colonoscopy or sigmoidoscopy. They cannot be removed during barium enema and virtual colonoscopy. After polypectomy, observe the patient for rectal bleeding, fever, severe abdominal pain, and abdominal distention, which may indicate hemorrhage or perforation.

COLORECTAL CANCER

Of cancers that affect both men and women, colorectal cancer (CRC) is the second leading cause of cancer-related deaths and is the third most common cancer in men and women. Annually about 136,800 people in the United States are diagnosed with CRC and 50,300 people die from CRC.[20]

CRC is more common in men than in women. Mortality rates are highest among African American men and women. The risk of CRC increases with age, with about 90% of new CRC cases detected in people older than 50. However, while the incidence of CRC in people over 50 years is decreasing due to increased screening efforts to detect precancerous lesions, the number of cases in people aged 20 to 49 years is rising and expected to continue to do so.

Etiology and Pathophysiology

Unlike some other cancers, no single risk factor accounts for most cases of CRC (Table 42-21). The risk is highest in those with first-degree relatives with CRC and people with IBD. About one third of cases of CRC occur in patients with a family history of CRC. Hereditary forms of CRC, including FAP and hereditary nonpolyposis colorectal cancer (HNPCC) syndrome (Lynch syndrome), account for 5% to 10% of those cases.

About 30% to 50% of people with CRC have an abnormal *KRAS* gene.[21] The *KRAS* gene, which is primarily involved in regulating cell division, belongs to a class of genes known as *oncogenes*. When mutated, oncogenes have the potential to cause normal cells to become cancerous.

Physical exercise and a diet with large amounts of fruits, vegetables, and grains may decrease the risk of CRC. Long-term use of NSAIDs (e.g., aspirin) is associated with reduced CRC risk.

Adenocarcinoma is the most common type of CRC. Approximately 85% of CRCs arise from adenomatous polyps. As the

TABLE 42-21 Risk Factors for Colorectal Cancer

- Family history of colorectal cancer (first-degree relative)
- Personal history of inflammatory bowel disease
- Personal history of colorectal cancer
- Family or personal history of familial adenomatous polyposis (FAP)
- Family or personal history of hereditary nonpolyposis colorectal cancer (HNPCC) syndrome
- Obesity (body mass index ≥30 kg/m²)
- Red meat (≥7 servings/wk)
- Cigarette smoking
- Alcohol (≥4 drinks/wk)
- Personal history of diabetes mellitus

tumor grows, the cancer invades and penetrates the muscularis mucosae (Fig. 42-7). Eventually tumor cells gain access to the regional lymph nodes and vascular system and spread to distant sites. Since venous blood leaving the colon and rectum flows through the portal vein and the inferior rectal vein, the liver is a common site of metastasis. The cancer spreads from the liver to other sites, including the lungs, bones, and brain. CRC can also spread directly into adjacent structures.

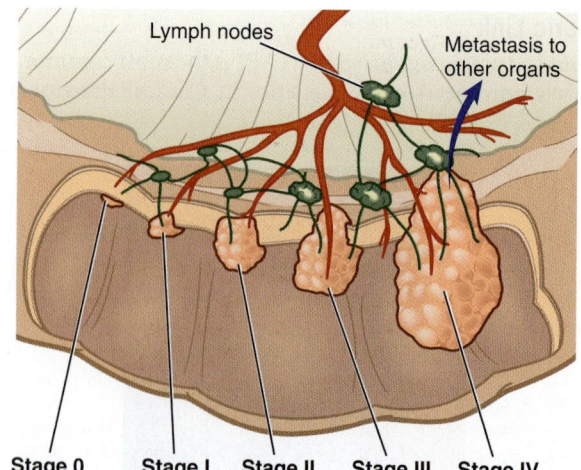

FIG. 42-7 The five stages of colorectal cancer. Stage 0 cancer has not grown beyond the mucosal layer. Stage I cancer has grown beyond the mucosa into the submucosa, but no lymph nodes are involved. Stage II cancer has grown beyond the submucosa into the muscle but there is no lymph node involvement or metastasis. Stage III cancer is any tumor with lymph node involvement but no metastasis. Stage IV cancer is any tumor with lymph node involvement and metastasis.

Clinical Manifestations

CRC has an insidious onset, and symptoms do not appear until the disease is advanced. Common clinical manifestations include iron-deficiency anemia, rectal bleeding, abdominal pain, change in bowel habits, and intestinal obstruction or perforation.

Physical findings may include the following:
- *Early disease:* Nonspecific findings (fatigue, weight loss) or none at all
- *More advanced disease:* Abdominal tenderness, palpable abdominal mass, hepatomegaly, ascites

Bleeding can occur with both right- and left-sided CRC. Bleeding on the right side, which is more common than the left side, is often unrecognized and an early manifestation is often anemia. Hematochezia (fresh blood in the stool) is more often caused by left-sided CRC than right-sided CRC.

Right-sided lesions are more likely to cause diarrhea, while left-sided tumors are usually detected later and could present with bowel obstruction (Fig. 42-8). Complications of CRC include obstruction, bleeding, perforation, peritonitis, and fistula formation.

Diagnostic Studies

Obtain a thorough history with close attention to family history (Table 42-22). Since symptoms of CRC do not become evident

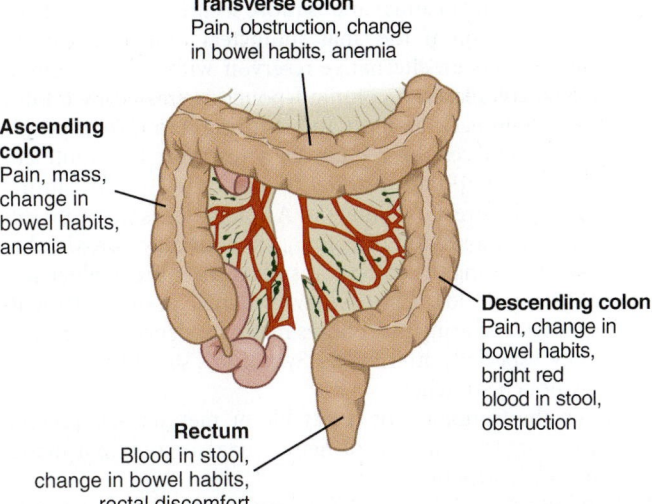

Transverse colon
Pain, obstruction, change in bowel habits, anemia

Ascending colon
Pain, mass, change in bowel habits, anemia

Descending colon
Pain, change in bowel habits, bright red blood in stool, obstruction

Rectum
Blood in stool, change in bowel habits, rectal discomfort

FIG. 42-8 Signs and symptoms of colorectal cancer by location of primary cancer. (Modified from McCance KL, Huether SE: *Pathophysiology: the biologic basis for disease in adults and children,* ed 6, St Louis, 2010, Mosby.)

TABLE 42-22 Interprofessional Care
Colorectal Cancer

Diagnostic Assessment	Management
• History and physical examination	• Surgery
• Digital rectal examination	• Right hemicolectomy
• Testing of stool for occult blood	• Left hemicolectomy
• CBC	• Abdominal-perineal resection
• Liver function tests	• Laparoscopic colectomy
• Barium enema	• Chemotherapy
• Sigmoidoscopy and/or colonoscopy with biopsy	• Targeted therapy
• Abdominal CT scan, ultrasound, or MRI	• Radiation therapy
• Carcinoembryonic antigen (CEA) test	

until the disease is advanced, there is an increased emphasis on screening. Beginning at age 50 and continuing until age 75, men and women at average risk for developing CRC should have screening tests to detect both polyps and cancer based on one of these testing schedules:
- Flexible sigmoidoscopy (every 5 years)
- Colonoscopy (every 10 years)
- Double-contrast barium enema (every 5 years)
- CT colonography (virtual colonoscopy) (every 5 years)
- Tests that primarily find cancer include the following:
  - High sensitivity fecal occult blood test (FOBT) (every year), or
  - Fecal immunochemical test (FIT) (every year)

Colonoscopy is the gold standard for CRC screening, because the entire colon is examined (only 50% of CRCs are detected by sigmoidoscopy), biopsies can be obtained, and polyps can be immediately removed and sent to the laboratory for examination. People at average risk of CRC should have a colonoscopy every 10 years beginning at age 50.

Persons at risk (Table 42-21) should begin screening earlier and have screening done more often. African Americans should have their first colonoscopy at age 45. Those who have a first-degree relative who developed CRC before age 60 or have two first-degree relatives with CRC should have a colonoscopy every 5 years beginning at age 40 or 10 years earlier than when the youngest relative developed cancer. Those who have one first-degree relative who had CRC after age 60 should have a colonoscopy every 10 years beginning at age 40.[22]

Less favorable, but acceptable, screening methods include stool testing for fecal blood. The FOBT and FIT look for blood in the stool. Stool tests must be done frequently, since tumor bleeding occurs at intervals and may easily be missed if a single test is done. In addition to testing for blood in human stool, new tests (PreGen-Plus, Cologuard) can detect DNA mutations that may indicate the presence of CRC.

Once tissue biopsies confirm the diagnosis of CRC, additional laboratory studies include a CBC to check for anemia and liver function tests. A CT scan or MRI of the abdomen may be helpful in detecting liver metastases, retroperitoneal and pelvic disease, and depth of penetration of tumor into the bowel wall. However, liver function tests may be normal even when metastasis has occurred.

Carcinoembryonic antigen (CEA) is a complex glycoprotein sometimes produced by CRC cells. It may be used to monitor for disease recurrence after surgery or chemotherapy but is not a good screening tool because of the large number of false positives. CEA levels may also be increased in non-colon carcinomas (e.g., gastric, pancreatic, lung carcinoma, breast, and thyroid carcinoma) as well as some non-neoplastic conditions, such as IBD, pancreatitis, cirrhosis, and COPD.

Interprofessional Care

The prognosis and treatment of CRC correlate with pathologic staging of the disease. The most commonly used staging system is the tumor, node, metastasis (TNM) staging (Table 42-23). As with other cancers, prognosis worsens with greater size and depth of tumor, lymph node involvement, and metastasis (Table 42-24).

Surgical Therapy. Goals of surgical therapy include (1) complete resection of the tumor, (2) a thorough exploration of the abdomen to determine if the cancer has spread, (3) removing all lymph nodes that drain the area where the cancer is located,

TABLE 42-23   TNM Classification of Colorectal Cancer

T	Primary Tumor
T_x	Primary tumor cannot be assessed because of incomplete information.
T_{is}	Carcinoma in situ. Cancer is in earliest stage and has not grown beyond mucosa layer.
T_1	Tumor has grown beyond mucosa into the submucosa.
T_2	Tumor has grown through submucosa into muscularis propria.
T_3	Tumor has grown through the muscularis propria into the subserosa but not to neighboring organs or tissues.
T_4	Tumor has spread completely through the colon or rectal wall and into nearby tissues or organs.
N	**Lymph Node Involvement**
N_x	Lymph nodes cannot be assessed.
N_0	No regional lymph node involvement is found.
N_1	Cancer is found in one to three nearby lymph nodes.
N_2	Cancer is found in four or more nearby lymph nodes.
M	**Metastasis**
M_x	Presence of distant metastasis cannot be assessed.
M_0	No distant metastasis is seen.
M_1	Distant metastasis is present.

TABLE 42-24   Classification System Used to Stage Colorectal Cancer

Stage*	TNM†	Duke's	5-Yr Survival Rate
0	$T_{is}\ N_0\ M_0$		>96%
I	$T_1\ N_0\ M_0$	A	>90%
	$T_2\ N_0\ M_0$	B_1	85%
II	$T_3\ N_0\ M_0$	B_2	70%-80%
III	Any T, $N_1\ M_0$	C	64%
IV	Any T, any N, M_1	D	8%

*Staging system is shown in Fig. 42-7.
†See Table 42-23.

(4) restoring bowel continuity so that normal bowel function will return, and (5) preventing surgical complications.

Some polyps can be removed during colonoscopy, whereas others require surgery. Polypectomy during colonoscopy can be used to resect CRC in situ and is considered successful when the resected margin of the polyp is free of cancer, the cancer is well differentiated, and there is no apparent lymphatic or blood vessel involvement.

The decision for surgical treatment of CRC depends on the staging and location of the cancer and ability to restore normal bowel function and continence. Surgical removal of stage I cancer includes removal of the tumor and at least 5 cm of intestine on either side of the tumor, plus removal of nearby lymph nodes. The remaining cancer-free ends are sewn back together (anastomosis). Laparoscopic surgery is sometimes used for stage I tumors, especially those in the left colon. Low-risk stage II tumors are treated with wide resection and reanastomosis, and chemotherapy is used in addition to surgery for high-risk stage II tumors. Stage III tumors are treated with surgery and chemotherapy. Radiation and chemotherapy may be done before surgery to reduce tumor size. Once the cancer has spread to distant sites (stage IV), any surgery is usually palliative, with chemotherapy and radiation used to control the spread and provide pain relief. Select patients with limited lung or liver metastases can achieve a cure after primary and metastatic tumor resection and chemotherapy.[23] A patient who has a perforation, peritonitis, or is hemodynamically unstable may need a temporary colostomy or ileostomy.

In rectal cancer, the location and size of the tumor determines the course of treatment. Local excision may be an option. If the tumor is in the distal rectum (1 to 2 cm from the anorectal junction) and the sphincters cannot be preserved, the patient will undergo an *abdominal-perineal resection (APR)*. An APR involves removing the entire rectum with the tumor, and the patient will have a permanent colostomy. The perineal wound may be closed around a drain or left open with packing to allow healing by granulation. Complications that can occur include delayed wound healing, hemorrhage, persistent perineal sinus tracts, infections, and urinary tract and sexual dysfunction.

If the tumor is in the mid or proximal rectum, it may be possible to preserve the sphincters. In this situation, a low anterior resection (LAR) can be done. A LAR involves removing the rectum and anastomosing the colon to the anal canal. A temporary ileostomy or colostomy may be done to divert stool and allow time for the anastomosis to heal, usually about 8 to 12 weeks. Then the ostomy can be "taken down," and the ends of the colon surgically reconnected. An LAR is increasingly common because of advancements in laparoscopy and stapling techniques. End-to-end anastomosis stapling involves less tissue (less than 5 cm from anus) and is more secure with less leakage.

Another option if the anal sphincters remain is for the surgeon to create an alternative reservoir with either a colonic J-pouch or coloplasty. A colonic J-pouch is created by folding the distal colon back on itself and suturing it to form a pouch. The pouch replaces the rectum as a reservoir for stool. The patient has a temporary ostomy to allow the J-pouch sutures time to heal before stool enters it. A coloplasty is made by slitting the side of a section of colon a short distance proximal to the anus, stretching the colon transversely to make it wider, and then suturing it closed in the new widened position. Patients with sphincter-sparing procedures may experience urgency and frequency, especially after meals. Symptoms should improve as the new pouch stretches.

When the tumor is not resectable or metastasis is present, palliative surgery can control hemorrhage or relieve a malignant bowel obstruction.

Chemotherapy and Targeted Therapy. Chemotherapy can be used to shrink the tumor before surgery, as an adjuvant therapy after colon resection, and as palliative treatment for nonresectable cancer. Adjuvant chemotherapy is recommended for patients with stage III tumors and high-risk stage II tumors. Current chemotherapy protocols include varying doses of 5-fluorouracil (5-FU) and folinic acid (leucovorin) alone or in combination with oxaliplatin (Eloxatin) or irinotecan (Camptosar). The preferred protocol includes oxaliplatin. It is omitted if patients have too many side effects. Oral fluoropyrimidines (e.g., capecitabine [Xeloda]) in combination with oxaliplatin are an alternative to 5-FU/folinic acid therapy.[24]

Several targeted therapies have a role in treating metastatic CRC. Angiogenesis inhibitors, which inhibit the blood supply to tumors, include aflibercept (Zaltrap), bevacizumab (Avastin), and ramucirumab (Cyramza). Bevacizumab is often added to a combination chemotherapy regimen (e.g., 5-FU and irinotecan or 5-FU, leucovorin, oxaliplatin) to treat metastatic CRC. Regorafenib (Stivarga) is a multikinase inhibitor that blocks several enzymes that promote cancer growth. Cetuximab (Erbitux) and panitumumab (Vectibix) block the epidermal growth factor receptor.

Lonsurf, which is a combination of trifluridine and tipiracil, is used in patients with metastatic CRC who are no longer responding to other therapies. Trifluridine impairs DNA function and angiogenesis. Tipiracil prevents the rapid metabolism of trifluridine, thus increasing its bioavailability.

Radiation Therapy. Some patients may receive radiation therapy as an adjuvant to surgery and chemotherapy or as a palliative measure for those with metastatic cancer. As a palliative measure, the primary objective is to reduce tumor size and provide symptomatic relief. Radiation therapy is described in Chapter 15.

❖ NURSING MANAGEMENT: COLORECTAL CANCER

◆ Nursing Assessment

Table 42-25 outlines the subjective and objective data you should obtain from a patient with CRC.

◆ Nursing Diagnoses

Nursing diagnoses for the patient with CRC include, but are not limited to, the following:

- Diarrhea or constipation *related to* altered bowel elimination patterns
- Fear and anxiety *related to* diagnosis of CRC, surgical or therapeutic interventions, and possible terminal illness
- Ineffective coping *related to* diagnosis of cancer and side effects of treatment

TABLE 42-25 Nursing Assessment
Colorectal Cancer

Subjective Data

Important Health Information

Past health history: Previous breast or ovarian cancer, familial polyposis, villous adenoma, adenomatous polyps, inflammatory bowel disease

Medications: Use of any medications affecting bowel function (e.g., laxatives, antidiarrheal drugs)

Functional Health Patterns

Health perception–health management: Family history of colorectal, breast, or ovarian cancer; weakness, fatigue

Nutritional-metabolic: High-calorie, high-fat, low-fiber diet. Anorexia, nausea and vomiting, weight loss

Elimination: Change in bowel habits, alternating diarrhea and constipation, defecation urgency. Rectal bleeding, mucoid stools. Black, tarry stools. Increased flatus, decrease in stool caliber. Feelings of incomplete evacuation

Cognitive-perceptual: Abdominal and low back pain, tenesmus

Objective Data

General

Pallor, cachexia, lymphadenopathy (later signs)

Gastrointestinal

Palpable abdominal mass, distention, ascites, and hepatomegaly (liver metastasis)

Possible Diagnostic Findings

Anemia. Guaiac-positive stools, palpable mass on digital rectal examination. Positive sigmoidoscopy, colonoscopy, barium enema, or CT scan. Positive biopsy

◆ Planning

The overall goals are that the patient with CRC will have (1) normal bowel elimination patterns, (2) quality of life appropriate to the disease progression, (3) relief of pain, and (4) feelings of comfort and well-being.

◆ Nursing Implementation

◆ **Health Promotion.** Encourage all persons over 50 to have regular CRC screening. Help identify those at high risk who need screening at an earlier age. Discuss with patients how participating in early cancer screening helps decrease mortality rates. Realize that barriers exist, including lack of accurate information and fear of diagnosis.

Endoscopic and radiographic procedures can only reveal polyps when the bowel has been adequately prepared to eliminate stool. Provide teaching about bowel cleansing for outpatient diagnostic procedures, and administer cleansing preparations to inpatients. The patient should follow either a low-residue or a full liquid diet the day before the procedure until bowel cleansing begins. Bowel cleansing should follow a split-dose regimen. The evening before the procedure, the patient should drink 2 L of oral polyethylene glycol (PEG) lavage solution. The second 2 L dose should begin 4 to 6 hours before the procedure. A split-dose regimen started early morning the day of a procedure provides better cleansing for patients scheduled in the afternoon. Because many people find the PEG lavage solution difficult to drink and experience nausea and bloating, manufacturers have modified the PEG solutions to improve taste and palatability. Magnesium citrate solution or bisacodyl tablets or suppositories are sometimes given before the PEG lavage to remove the bulk of stool so that only 2 L of solution are needed.[25] Encourage the patient to drink all of the solution. Stools will be clear or clear yellow liquid when the colon is clean.

◆ **Acute Care.** Depending on your practice setting and surgeon preference, you may see patients undergoing a preoperative bowel cleansing routine prior to elective bowel surgeries. In the past, many patients underwent a cleansing routine with polyethylene glycol solutions (e.g., MiraLAX, GoLYTELY), enemas, and/or laxatives to reduce bacterial counts. There is very little evidence that supports this practice. There is no difference in surgical outcome between those who underwent a preoperative cleansing routine and those who did not.[25]

Nursing care for the patient after a colon resection is similar to care of the patient after a laparotomy (see p. 940). If enough healthy bowel remained that the surgeon could reconnect the bowel ends, normal bowel function is maintained and routine postoperative care is appropriate. Patients with more extensive surgery (e.g., APR) may have an open wound and drains (e.g., Jackson-Pratt, Hemovac) and a permanent ostomy. Postoperative care includes sterile dressing changes, care of drains, and patient and caregiver teaching about the ostomy.

A patient who has open and packed wounds requires meticulous care. Reinforce dressings and change them frequently during the first several hours postoperatively when drainage is likely to be profuse. Carefully assess all drainage for amount, color, and consistency. The drainage is usually serosanguineous. Examine the wound regularly and record bleeding, excessive drainage, and unusual odor. Use aseptic technique with dressing changes. Some patients experience phantom rectal pain or still feel as if they need to have a bowel movement. This is normal and often subsides over time. Be astute in distinguishing phantom sensations from perineal abscess pain. Consult with a wound, ostomy, and continence nurse (WOCN) if available. Ostomy care is discussed in depth in the next section on pp. 960-962.

If the patient's wound is closed or partially closed, assess the incision for suture integrity and signs and symptoms of wound inflammation and infection. Examine the drainage for amount, color, and characteristics. Observe the skin around the drain for signs of inflammation, and keep the area around the drain clean and dry. Monitor for edema, erythema, and drainage around the suture line, as well as fever and an elevated WBC count.

Sexual dysfunction is a possible complication after APR. The likelihood of sexual dysfunction depends on the surgical technique used. The surgeon should discuss the possibility with the patient. Members of the interprofessional care team should be available to address the patient's questions and concerns. Erection, ejaculation, and orgasm involve different nerve pathways, and a dysfunction of one does not mean complete sexual dysfunction. The WOCN is an important source of information concerning sexual dysfunction resulting from an APR.

◆ **Ambulatory Care.** Psychologic support for the patient and caregiver dealing with the diagnosis of cancer is important. Discuss the patient's feelings about his or her prognosis and future screening. Patients need much emotional support because recurrent cancer is painful, debilitating, and demoralizing. The special needs of the cancer patient are discussed in Chapter 15. You may need to address issues surrounding palliative care, end-of-life issues, and hospice (see Chapter 9).

Patients with CRC need to know how to manage changes that are the result of the cancer and cancer treatment. Those who had sphincter-sparing surgery may experience diarrhea and incontinence of feces and gas. They may need antidiarrheal drugs or bulking agents to control the diarrhea, but overuse can result in constipation. A consult with a dietitian or WOCN may help patients and caregivers understand how to manage food and fluid options. Ostomy rehabilitation, including teaching and ongoing support, should be available for all ostomy patients. Patients with skin changes from incontinence and/or radiation therapy will need assistance in managing these conditions.

◆ **Evaluation**

The expected outcomes for the patient with CRC are that the patient will have
- Minimal alterations in bowel elimination patterns
- Optimal nutritional intake
- Quality of life appropriate to disease progression
- Feelings of comfort and well-being

OSTOMY SURGERY

Types

An ostomy is a surgically created opening on the abdomen that allows the discharge of body waste. The outermost portion that is visible is a stoma. The stoma is the result of the large or small bowel being brought to the outside of the abdomen and sutured in place. When a stoma is created as a fecal diversion, feces will drain through the stoma instead of the anus.

An ostomy is necessary when the normal elimination route is no longer possible. For example, if a person has Stage III CRC, the surgeon will remove the diseased portion of the colon along with a certain margin of healthy tissue. If the tumor involves the rectum and is large enough to necessitate the removal of the anal sphincters, the anus will be sutured shut and a permanent

ostomy created. Patients at high risk for CRC, such as those with FAP, and patients with ulcerative colitis may have a total colectomy and an ileostomy.

Ostomies are named according to their location and type (Fig. 42-9). An ostomy in the ileum is called an *ileostomy*. An ostomy in the colon is called a *colostomy*. The ostomy is further characterized by its anatomic site (e.g., ascending, transverse, or sigmoid colostomy). The more distal the ostomy, the more the functioning bowel remains and the more likely that the intestinal contents will resemble the feces that would have been eliminated from an intact colon and rectum. Ileostomy output will be a liquid to thin paste since it did not enter the colon. Patients have no control over ileostomy drainage; it is involuntary. An ileostomy drains frequently, and the patient must wear an ostomy appliance (pouch) to collect the drainage (effluent). In contrast, output from a sigmoid colostomy resembles normal formed stool. Some patients are able to regulate emptying time with colostomy irrigation and may not need to wear a pouch. See Table 42-26 for a comparison of colostomies and ileostomies.

Ostomies may be temporary or permanent. For example, the person with a draining fistula may need a temporary ostomy to prevent stool from reaching the diseased area. Patients who have trauma to the intestines (e.g., gunshot wound, stabbing) may need a temporary ostomy. Cancer involving the rectum requires a permanent ostomy if all bowel distal to the ostomy is removed.

Permanent ostomies may be continent or traditional. *Continent ileostomies* (e.g., Koch pouch, Barnett Continent Ileal Reservoir) use 40 to 45 cm of the terminal ileum to fashion an internal pouch, nipple valve, and abdominal stoma. The internal pouch can hold approximately 500 mL or more of material. Continent ostomies are an option for patients who have had a prior APR with ileostomy for ulcerative colitis or FAP. They are not normally done for Crohn's disease because of the risk of disease reoccurrence and the loss of a significant length of small bowel. Appropriate patients must be motivated and compliant. Patients must drain the pouch manually by inserting a catheter through the nipple valve. Initially, this is needed every 1 to 2 hours. As the pouch enlarges, the frequency decreases to four times daily and as needed. They must keep the stool consistency relatively fluid by following a low-residue diet.

The major types of traditional ostomies include end, double-barreled, and loop ostomy.

End Stoma. An end stoma is constructed by dividing the bowel and bringing out the proximal end as a single stoma, making a colostomy or ileostomy. The distal portion of the GI tract is either surgically removed or the distal segment is oversewn and left in the abdominal cavity with its mesentery intact. If the distal bowel is removed, the stoma is permanent. When the distal bowel is oversewn and not removed, the procedure is called a *Hartmann's pouch* (Fig. 42-10). With a Hartmann's pouch, the potential exists for the bowel to be reanastomosed and the stoma closed (referred to as a *takedown*).

Loop Stoma. A loop stoma is constructed by bringing a loop of bowel to the abdominal surface and then opening the anterior wall of the bowel to provide fecal diversion. This results in one stoma with a proximal opening for feces and a distal opening for mucus drainage from the distal colon. An intact posterior wall separates the two openings. A plastic rod holds the loop of bowel in place for 7 to 10 days after surgery to prevent it from slipping back into the abdominal cavity (Fig. 42-11). A loop stoma is usually temporary.

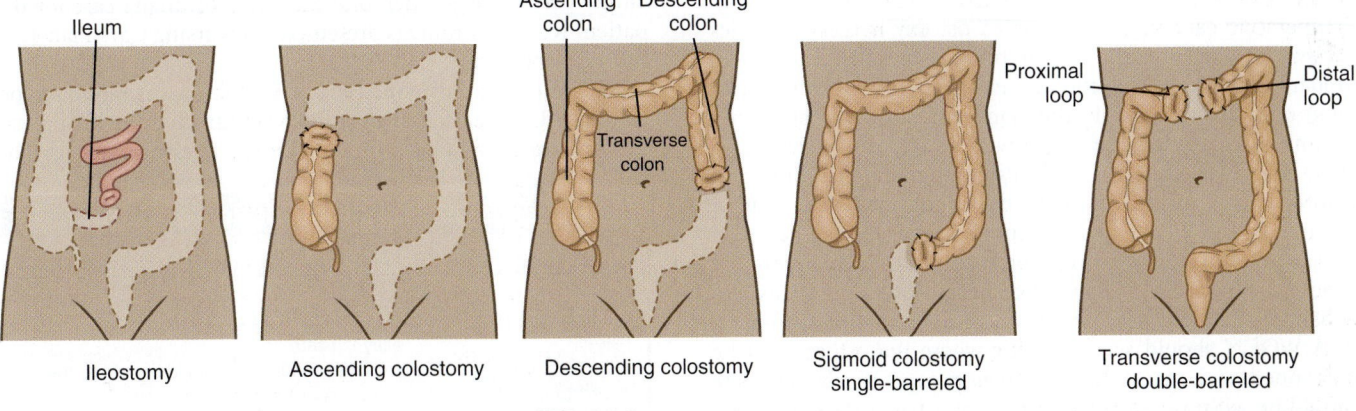

FIG. 42-9 Types of ostomies.

TABLE 42-26	**Comparison of Ileostomy and Colostomy**			
		COLOSTOMY		
Characteristic	**Ileostomy**	**Ascending**	**Transverse**	**Sigmoid**
Stool consistency	Liquid to semiliquid	Semiliquid	Semiliquid to semiformed	Formed
Fluid requirement	Increased	Increased	Possibly increased	No change
Bowel regulation	No	No	No	Yes (if there is a history of a regular bowel pattern)
Pouch and skin barriers	Yes	Yes	Yes	Dependent on regulation
Irrigation	No	No	No	Possibly every 24-48 hr (if patient meets criteria)
Indications for surgery	Ulcerative colitis, Crohn's disease, diseased or injured colon, familial polyposis, trauma, cancer	Perforating diverticulum in lower colon, trauma, rectovaginal fistula, inoperable tumors of colon, rectum, or pelvis	Same as for ascending	Cancer of the rectum or rectosigmoid area, perforating diverticulum, trauma

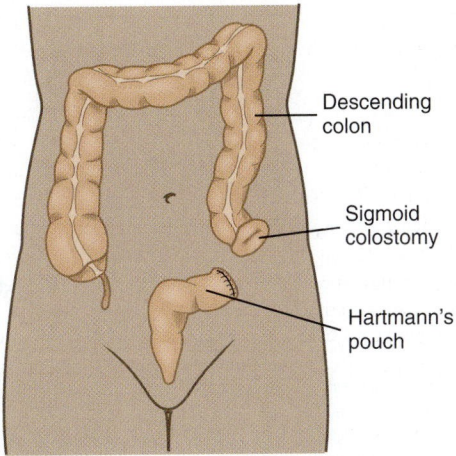

FIG. 42-10 Sigmoid colostomy. Distal bowel is oversewn and left in place to create Hartmann's pouch.

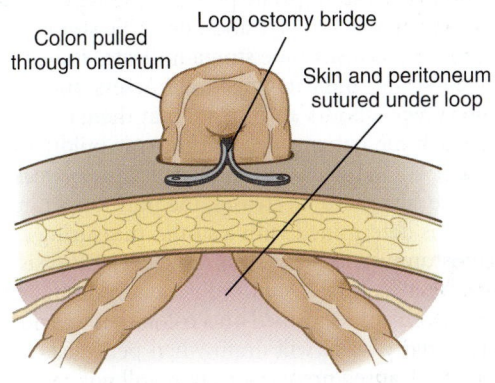

FIG. 42-11 Loop colostomy.

Double-Barreled Stoma. To create a double-barreled stoma, the surgeon divides the bowel and both the proximal and distal ends are brought through the abdominal wall as two separate stomas (Fig. 42-9). The proximal one is the functioning stoma. The distal, nonfunctioning stoma is referred to as the *mucus fistula*. The double-barreled stoma is usually temporary.

❖ NURSING MANAGEMENT: OSTOMY SURGERY

Two major aspects of nursing care for the patient with an ostomy are (1) emotional support as the patient copes with a radical change in body image and (2) patient and caregiver teaching about ostomy care. Accurate information, emotional support, and mastering basic skills will help patients learn to live a full life with an ostomy and accept the changes in body appearance and function. Without accurate information, fear and misconceptions can be overwhelming. People with ostomies lose control over flatus and feces and worry about odor and leakage. They question the patency of ostomy pouches and wonder how the ostomy will change their lives. With time and proper support, people learn to manage the stoma and resume work, social, and sexual activities. Adjusting to any major change in health status and personal appearance is highly individualized. People with new ostomies need time and support to adjust to the changes but should be reassured they can adjust and resume their previous lifestyle.

Preoperative Care

Preoperative care that is unique to ostomy surgery includes (1) psychologic preparation for the ostomy, (2) educational preparation, and (3) selection of an optimal site for the placement of the stoma. Ideally, the management of patients facing ostomy surgery begins preoperatively and continues throughout the postoperative period. Psychologic preparation and emotional support are particularly important as the person begins to cope with the change in body image, loss of control over elimination, and fear of odors. Provide the patient opportunities for verbalization of concerns and questions. This will enhance the patient's feelings of control and thus ability to cope.

A WOCN should select the site where the ostomy will be positioned and mark the abdomen preoperatively. The site should be within the rectus muscle, on a flat surface, and in a place that the patient is able to see. Stomas placed outside the rectus muscle may increase the chance of developing a hernia. A flat site makes it much easier to create a good seal and avoid leakage from the bag. Being able to see the stoma makes caring for it easier. Whenever possible, it should be discreetly hidden under clothing and appropriate for normal activities.

It is normal for the patient and caregiver to have questions concerning the procedures. If available, a WOCN should visit with the patient and caregiver to determine the patient's ability to perform self-care, identify support systems, and determine any modifications that could facilitate learning during rehabilitation. The patient and caregiver should understand the extent of surgery, the type of stoma planned, and basic stoma care.

Postoperative Care

Postoperative nursing care includes assessment of the stoma and provision of an appropriate pouching system that protects the skin and contains drainage and odor. The stoma should be rosy pink to red. A dusky blue stoma indicates ischemia, and a brown-black stoma indicates necrosis. Assess and document stoma color every 4 hours and ensure that there is no excessive bleeding. Teach the patient that the stoma is mildly to moderately swollen. Edema will resolve over the first 6 weeks (Table 42-27). As the stoma size decreases, the pouch opening will be smaller. This is determined with a stoma-measuring card.

The colostomy starts functioning when peristalsis returns. Record the volume, color, and consistency of the drainage. When a colostomy is performed on a colon that was not cleaned out before surgery, stool will drain when peristalsis returns. If the bowel was cleansed preoperatively, it will not begin producing stool until a few days after the patient is eating again. Excessive amounts of gas are common during the first 2 weeks. Because this can be distressing to patients, assure them this is temporary.

Colostomy Care

An appropriate pouching system is vital to protect the skin and provide dependable stool collection. Most pouching systems have an adhesive skin barrier and a pouch to collect the feces. Most skin barriers are made of pectin-based or karaya mediums with hydrocolloid properties. Adhesion occurs in two phases. First, the wafer's backing has adhesive material that forms an immediate bond with the skin. Second, the hydrocolloids interface with the moisture on the skin to form a tighter seal. If the abdominal stoma site has bends or creases, it is difficult to get a good seal and the skin barrier will pull away faster. Since excessive weight of collected stool pulls the wafer away from the skin,

empty ostomy bags when one-third full. (Nursing care for the patient with an ostomy is presented in eNursing Care Plan 42-3 on the website.)

Use a transparent pouch in the initial postoperative period so that you can easily assess stoma viability and pouch application by the patient. Each time the pouch is changed, assess the

TABLE 42-27	**Characteristics of Stoma**
Characteristic	**Description or Cause**
Color*	
Rose to brick-red	Viable stoma mucosa.
Pale	May indicate anemia.
Blanching, dark red to purple	Indicates inadequate blood supply to the stoma or bowel.
Edema†	
Mild to moderate edema	Normal in initial postoperative period. Trauma to the stoma.
Moderate to severe edema	Obstruction of the stoma, allergic reaction to food, gastroenteritis.
Bleeding	
Small amount	Oozing from stoma mucosa when touched is normal because of its high vascularity.
Moderate to large amount	Could indicate lower gastrointestinal bleeding, coagulation factor deficiency, stomal varices secondary to portal hypertension.

*Report sustained color changes to surgeon.
†Closely observe and report to the surgeon and adjust the stoma opening size in the pouch.

░ TEAMWORK & COLLABORATION

Ostomy Care

Although licensed practical/vocational nurses (LPN/LVNs) and unlicensed assistive personnel (UAP) provide much of the ostomy care for patients with established ostomies, patients with new ostomies have complex needs and require frequent assessment, planning, intervention, and evaluation by a registered nurse (RN).

Role of Nursing Personnel

Registered Nurse (RN)*

- Assess and document stoma appearance.
- For patient with a new ostomy, assess patient's psychologic preparation for ostomy care.
- Choose appropriate ostomy pouching system (skin barrier and bag or pouch) for patient.
- Place ostomy pouching system for a new ostomy.
- Develop plan of care for skin care around the ostomy.
- Teach ostomy care and skin care to patient and caregiver.
- Irrigate new colostomy.
- Teach colostomy irrigation to patient and caregiver.
- Teach patient and caregivers about appropriate dietary choices.

Licensed Practical/Vocational Nurse (LPN/LVN)

- Monitor the volume, color, and odor of the ostomy drainage.
- Monitor the skin around the ostomy for breakdown.
- Provide skin care around the ostomy.
- Irrigate colostomy in stable patient.

Unlicensed Assistive Personnel (UAP)

- Empty ostomy bag and measure liquid contents.
- Place the ostomy pouching system for an established ostomy.
- Assist stable patient with colostomy irrigation.

*In agencies where a wound, ostomy, and continence nurse (WOCN) is available, many of these roles will be assumed by that person.

skin for irritation. If the peristomal skin is irritated and raw, additional products may have to be applied. Do not allow feces to remain on the skin or irritation will quickly develop. If a pouch has failed, it must be changed immediately.

A colostomy in the ascending and transverse colon has semi-liquid stools. Have the patient use a drainable pouch. A drainable pouch may last up to 4 to 7 days.

A colostomy in the sigmoid or descending colon has semi-formed or formed stools. The patient can use a drainable pouch or choose a disposable, closed end pouch changed every day. Another option is irrigation. Patients who irrigate may not need a regular pouch as they may be able to regulate when the colon empties. Optional charcoal filters can deodorize and automatically release flatus. They are available for both drainable and nondrainable pouches.

With shorter hospital stays, patient teaching should focus on the critical aspects that patients need to master. Teaching must include (1) basic skills about managing the ostomy (e.g., emptying and changing the pouch), (2) food and fluid requirements, and (3) how to get help for problems. Additional teaching should include expanded information on these topics plus skin care, managing gas and odor, care of the stoma, potential complications, resuming activities of daily living, and sources for support and assistance.[26] Teach the patient when to seek health care. Home care and outpatient follow-up may be helpful, especially if there is access to a WOCN. Provide written information about the particular ostomy, instructions for pouch changes, basic supplies needed, where to purchase supplies (including retailers' names and phone numbers), any follow-up appointments, and contact information for the surgeon and WOCN. Patient and caregiver teaching is presented in Table 42-28.

Teach the patient about the importance of fluids and a healthy diet. A well-balanced diet and adequate fluid intake are important. The effect of food on stoma output is individual. Most patients with colostomies can eat anything they want. However, some choose to avoid certain foods because of possible increased gas, odor, or stoma output[27] (Table 42-29). Teach patients to chew their food very well to reduce the chance of blockage.

The patient can resume activities of daily living within 6 to 8 weeks but should avoid heavy lifting. The patient's physical condition determines when he or she can resume sports. Swimming with an ostomy pouch intact is not a problem. The patient can bathe and shower with or without the pouching system in place because water does not harm the stoma.

◆ **Colostomy Irrigations.** Colostomy irrigations may be used to stimulate emptying of the colon. Regularity is possible only when the stoma is in the distal colon. If the colon is irrigated and emptied on a regular basis, the bowel can be trained, and little or no spillage should occur between irrigations. The patient may need to wear only a pad or small pouch over the stoma. Irrigation requires manual dexterity and adequate vision. People who irrigate regularly should still have ostomy bags readily available in case they develop diarrhea from foods or illness.

◆ **Ileostomy Care**

Nursing care for a patient with an ileostomy is similar to that for a patient with a colostomy. Because the stool from an ileostomy is caustic to the skin, a secure pouching system is important. This is easier with stoma protrusion of at least 1 to 1.5 cm. When the stoma is flat, recessed, or in a crease, seepage occurs

TABLE 42-28	Patient & Caregiver Teaching

Ostomy Self-Care

Include the following instructions when teaching the patient and/or caregiver about self-care of an ostomy.

1. Explain what an ostomy is and how it functions.
2. Describe the underlying condition that resulted in the need for an ostomy.
3. Demonstrate and allow the patient and caregiver to practice the following activities:
   - Remove the old skin barrier, cleanse the skin, and correctly apply new skin barriers.
   - Apply, empty, clean, and remove the pouch.
   - Empty the pouch before it is one-third full to prevent leakage.
4. Irrigate the colostomy to regulate bowel elimination (optional).
5. Explain how to contact the wound, ostomy, and continence nurse with questions.
6. Describe how to obtain additional ostomy supplies.
7. Explain dietary and fluid management.
   - Identify a well-balanced diet and dietary supplements to prevent nutritional deficiencies.
   - Identify foods to avoid to reduce diarrhea or gas.
   - Promote fluid intake of least 3000 mL/day to prevent dehydration (unless contraindicated).
   - Increase fluid intake during hot weather, excessive perspiration, and diarrhea to replace losses and prevent dehydration.
   - Describe symptoms of fluid and electrolyte imbalance.
   - Explain how to contact the dietitian with questions.
   - Explain how to recognize problems (fluid and electrolyte deficits, fever, diarrhea, skin irritation, stomal problems) and how to contact the appropriate health care provider.
8. Describe community resources to assist with emotional and psychologic adjustment to the ostomy.
9. Explain the importance of follow-up care.
10. Describe the ostomy's potential effects on sexual activity, social life, work, and recreation and strategies to manage these changes.

TABLE 42-29	Nutritional Therapy

Effects of Food on Stoma Output

Odor Producing	Gas Forming	Diarrhea Causing
Eggs	Beans	Alcohol
Garlic	Cabbage family	Beer
Onions	Onions	Cabbage family
Fish	Beer	Spinach
Asparagus	Carbonated beverages	Green beans
Cabbage	Cheeses (strong)	Coffee
Broccoli	Sprouts	Spicy foods
Alcohol		Fruits (raw)

and results in altered skin integrity. The patient must wear a pouch at all times since regularity is not possible with an ileostomy. An open-ended, drainable pouch is needed so that drainage can be easily emptied. A drainable pouch usually lasts for 4 to 7 days before having to be changed. If leakage occurs, the pouch must be promptly removed, the skin cleansed, and a new pouch applied. The skin barrier should completely protect the skin from any exposure to stool. Caulking strips or "paste" around the stoma may help ensure a secure seal.

Observe the patient with an ileostomy for signs and symptoms of fluid and electrolyte imbalance, particularly potassium, sodium, and fluid deficits. In the first 24 to 48 hours after surgery, the amount of drainage from the stoma may be negligible. Patients with new ileostomies lose the absorptive functions provided by the colon and the delay provided by the ileocecal valve. As a result, they may experience a period of high-volume output of 1500 to 1800 mL/day when peristalsis returns. Later, as the proximal small bowel adapts, the average amount can be 500 mL/day. If the small bowel was been shortened by surgery, drainage from the ileostomy may be greater. Patients need to increase fluid intake to at least 2 to 3 L/day or more when there are excessive fluid losses from heat and sweating. They may also need to ingest additional sodium. Patients must learn signs and symptoms of fluid and electrolyte imbalance so that they can take appropriate action.

The ileostomy patient is susceptible to obstruction because the lumen is less than 1 inch in diameter. It may narrow further at the point where the bowel passes through the fascia/muscle layer of the abdomen. Foods such as nuts, raisins, popcorn, coconut, mushrooms, olives, stringy vegetables, foods with skins, dried fruits, and meats with casings must be chewed extremely well before swallowing.[27] If the terminal ileum was removed, the patient may need cobalamin treatment.

◆ Psychologic Adaptation to an Ostomy

The patient's response to a new ostomy is highly individualized. Some have minimal difficulty and view their ostomy positively. It may be curative if their presenting condition was ulcerative colitis or a step toward remission if the diagnosis was CRC. Other patients may experience a grief reaction from the loss of a body part and an alteration in body image. They may be angry, depressed, or resentful. Anxiety and fear are normal. Concerns about stool leaking, odor, sounds of flatus, pouch reliability, and changes in normal life style are all valid worries.

The patient's emotional state may limit his or her ability to participate in teaching and ostomy care. Emotional support, interventions from skillful WOCNs, and visits from people who have successfully learned to manage their ostomies will help patients learn to cope with and manage the new stoma.

Discuss with the patient the psychologic impact of the stoma and its effect on body image and self-esteem. Assist the patient in identifying ways of coping with depression and anxiety resulting from the illness, surgery, or postoperative problems. Support from the caregiver, family, and friends is vital and reassures the patient that he or she is still cherished and valued despite having the ostomy. Encourage patients to share their concerns and ask questions. Provide information in an easily understood manner and help patients develop confidence and competence in managing the stoma.

New ostomy patients will have questions on a variety of topics ranging from managing gas to intimacy to travel. Provide the names and contact information for support groups. The Wound Ostomy Continence Nurses Society (*www.wocn.org*), local support groups, and United Ostomy Associations of America (*www.ostomy.org*) provide practical information about living with an ostomy. Online support groups are also available. Ask the patient if he or she would like to meet with a person who has adjusted to an ostomy. Most hospitals have a visitor's program. Visitor's programs give the patient and caregiver an opportunity to talk with a person who has adjusted well to an ostomy and has experienced some of the same feelings and concerns they have.

◆ Sexual Function After Ostomy Surgery

Sexual function and sexuality concerns affect both men and women with an ostomy. The patient with a stoma may fear rejection by a partner or that others will not find him or her desirable. Incorporate a discussion of sexuality and sexual function in the plan of care. Help the patient realize that it takes time to adjust to the pouch and to body changes before feeling secure in his or her sexual functioning.

Help the patient understand if specific aspects of surgery and treatment have the potential for sexual dysfunction. Pelvic surgery can disrupt nerve and vascular supplies to the genitalia. Radiation therapy, chemotherapy, and medications can alter sexual function. The patient's overall physical health influences sexual desire. Generalized fatigue caused by illness can decrease desire. Understanding this information can help patients plan the timing of sexual activity.

For men, the main concern may be erection and ejaculation. Erection of the penis depends on intact parasympathetic and nonadrenergic noncholinergic nerves as well as adequate blood supply. Nerve-sparing surgical techniques are used when possible to preserve sexual function. Unfortunately, any pelvic surgery that removes the rectum has the potential of damaging the parasympathetic nerve plexus. Sympathetic nerve damage in the presacral area can disrupt the ability to ejaculate. This can occur with the APR procedure. Sexual dysfunction may be temporary and resolve in 3 to 12 months. Pelvic radiation can reduce blood flow to the pelvis by causing scarring in the small blood vessels.

For women, the main issues may be vaginal lubrication, clitoral congestion, and dyspareunia. Nerve damage can result in vaginal dryness and decreased sensation in the vagina and clitoris, making arousal and achieving orgasm more challenging. Experimenting with positions and using lubrication may help. A woman with an ostomy can still become pregnant.

Teach the patient to empty the pouch before sexual activities. Some may apply a smaller pouch during sexual activity. Women may consider wearing open panties, a short slip, or similar lingerie. Men may consider wearing a wrap or cummerbund around the midsection to secure the pouch. There are many types of pouch covers that patients can make or purchase.

FISTULAS

A **fistula** is an abnormal tract between two hollow organs or a hollow organ and the skin. Fistulas are named by the track that they take from one body part to another. For example, an enterocutaneous fistula is an opening between the small intestine and skin. An enterovaginal fistula is between the small intestine and vagina, allowing stool and gas to drain through the vagina.

A GI fistula occurs between the lumen of the GI tract and another organ. GI fistulas are a serious complication associated with increased morbidity and mortality, extended hospital stays, and increased costs. Most fistulas occur after surgery, or are associated with IBD, cancer, or adhesions. Fistulas can form in the presence of diverticulitis, pancreatitis, trauma, hypotension, sepsis, and corticosteroid use. Fistulas are classified as simple or complex and by the amount of output. A simple fistula has only one short, direct tract. A complex fistula is associated with an abscess, involves multiple organs, and may open into the base of a wound. High output fistulas drain more than 500 mL/day, moderate output fistulas drain 200 to 500 mL/day, and low output fistulas drain less than 200 mL/day.[28]

Fever and abdominal pain are early indicators of a fistula. Other manifestations vary depending on the type of fistula.

With an enterocutaneous fistula, there may be pus or intestinal contents draining through the skin opening. Patients with a colocutaneous (colon to skin) fistula may have stool or pus draining through the opening. If a colovesical (colon to urinary tract) fistula is present, manifestations include fecaluria (passing stool with urination), recurrent urinary tract infections, dysuria, and hematuria.

❖ NURSING AND INTERPROFESSIONAL MANAGEMENT: GASTROINTESTINAL FISTULAS

The development of a draining fistula can be disheartening for the patient and caregiver and a time-consuming challenge for HCPs. Managing a fistula requires (1) identifying the fistula tract, (2) maintaining fluid and electrolyte balance, (3) controlling infection, (4) protecting the surrounding skin, (5) managing output, and (6) providing nutritional support.[28] Most fistulas heal spontaneously. Surgery may be necessary to treat the complications.

Appropriate fluid and electrolyte replacement can be challenging, especially when the patient has a high output fistula. Monitor the volume of fistula output as this guides replacement therapies and nutritional support. Assess the character of the drainage, noting the color, consistency, and odor. Monitor laboratory values. Hypokalemia, hypomagnesemia, and hypophosphatemia from the loss of GI fluids are common. Administer IV fluids and electrolyte replacement as ordered. Keep an accurate intake and output record. To reduce intestinal output, many patients require NPO status and receive somatostatin or octreotide to decrease GI secretions. Measure vital signs frequently and be alert for signs of dehydration.

Malnutrition is a significant problem, particularly if the patient is on NPO status or has a small intestinal fistula. Consult a dietitian. High-calorie, high-protein parenteral or enteral nutrition is necessary for providing enough calories and protein to replace losses and support healing. Many patients require trace element (e.g., copper, zinc, magnesium) and vitamin supplements.

> ### ❓ CHECK YOUR PRACTICE
>
> A 51-yr-old female is 4 days postop following a proctocolectomy for ulcerative colitis. You note a 2.5 cm of erythema in the center of her incision with heavy, foul-smelling tan drainage pooling on her skin. Suspecting she is developing an enterocutaneous fistula, you notify the surgeon and WOCN.
> • What will you do to protect her skin?

Maintaining skin integrity and optimizing healing is essential. Consult a WOCN if available. Although low output fistulas may be managed with a simple absorbent dressing, a high-output enterocutaneous fistula often requires advanced techniques, including specialty pouches; barrier creams, powders, and sealants to protect the skin; and negative pressure wound therapy.

DIVERTICULOSIS AND DIVERTICULITIS

Diverticula are saccular dilations or outpouchings of the mucosa that develop in the colon (Fig. 42-12). Diverticulosis is the presence of multiple noninflamed diverticula. **Diverticulitis** is inflammation of one or more diverticula, resulting in perforation into the peritoneum. Clinically, diverticular disease covers

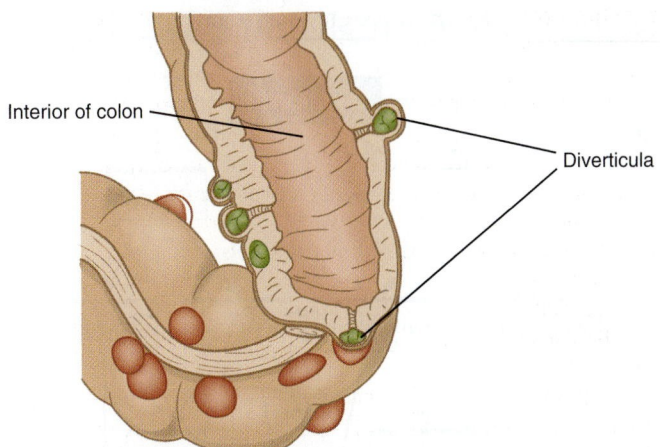

FIG. 42-12 Diverticula are outpouchings of the colon. When they become inflamed, the condition is diverticulitis. The inflammatory process can spread to the surrounding area in the intestine.

a spectrum from asymptomatic, uncomplicated diverticulosis to diverticulitis with complications such as perforation, abscess, fistula, and bleeding. Diverticula are common, especially in older adults, but most people never develop diverticulitis.[29]

Etiology and Pathophysiology

Diverticula may occur anywhere in the GI tract but are most common in the left (descending, sigmoid) colon. They seem to occur at weak points in the intestinal wall, such as where the blood vessels pass through the muscle layer. The main factor thought to contribute to the development of diverticulosis is a lack of dietary fiber intake. The disease is more prevalent in Western, industrialized populations, where people tend to consume diets low in fiber and high in refined carbohydrates. Inadequate dietary fiber slows transit time, allowing more water to be absorbed from the stool, making it more difficult to pass through the lumen. Decreased stool size increases intraluminal pressure. This places stress on the weakened areas and promotes diverticula formation. Diverticula are uncommon in vegetarians. Other risk factors for diverticula are obesity, inactivity, smoking, excessive alcohol use, and immunosuppression.

Clinical Manifestations and Complications

The majority of patients with diverticulosis have no symptoms. Those with symptoms typically have abdominal pain, bloating, flatulence, and changes in bowel habits. In more serious situations, the diverticula bleed or diverticulitis develops. The most common signs and symptoms of diverticulitis are acute pain in the left lower quadrant (location of sigmoid colon), a palpable abdominal mass, nausea, vomiting, and systemic symptoms of infection (fever, increased C-reactive protein, leukocytosis with a shift to the left). Older adults with diverticulitis may be afebrile, with a normal WBC count and little, if any, abdominal tenderness. Diverticulitis can cause erosion of the bowel wall and perforation into the peritoneum (Fig. 42-13). A localized abscess develops when the body is able to wall off the area of perforation. Peritonitis develops if it cannot be contained. Bleeding can be extensive but usually stops spontaneously.

Diagnostic Studies

Diverticular disease can be asymptomatic and is typically discovered during routine sigmoidoscopy or colonoscopy. Diagnosis of diverticulitis is based on the history and physical

PATHOPHYSIOLOGY MAP

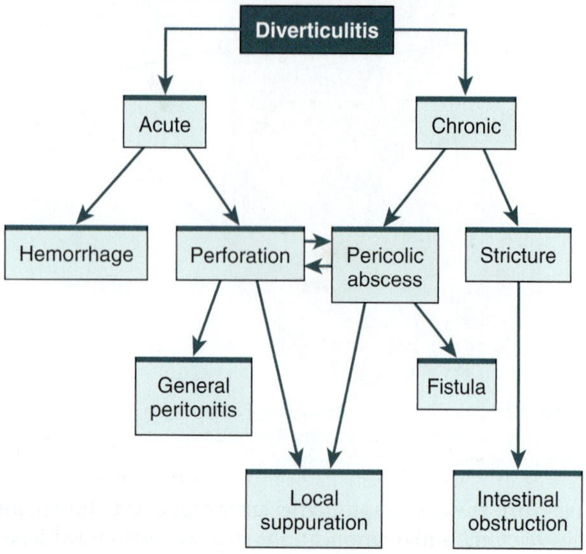

FIG. 42-13   Complications of diverticulitis.

examination (Table 42-30). The preferred diagnostic test is a CT scan with oral contrast. Abdominal and chest x-ray rule out other causes of acute abdominal pain.

❖ NURSING AND INTERPROFESSIONAL MANAGEMENT: DIVERTICULOSIS AND DIVERTICULITIS

A high-fiber diet, mainly from fruits and vegetables, with a decreased intake of fat and red meat is the best way to prevent diverticular disease. High levels of physical activity also seem to decrease the risk. Currently there is no evidence to support the theory that diverticulitis can be prevented by avoiding nuts and seeds.

In acute diverticulitis, the goal of treatment is to let the colon rest and the inflammation subside. Some patients can be managed at home with oral antibiotics and a clear liquid diet. Hospitalization is necessary if symptoms are severe, the patient is unable to tolerate oral fluids, there are systemic manifestations of infection (fever, significant leukocytosis), or the patient has co-morbid conditions (e.g., immunosuppression).

If hospitalized, the patient is kept on NPO status and IV fluids and antibiotics are given. Observe for signs of abscess, bleeding, and peritonitis, and monitor the WBC count. Administer analgesics as needed. When the acute attack subsides, give oral fluids first and then progress the diet to semisolids.

Patients with frequently reoccurring diverticulitis or complications, such as an abscess or obstruction, may need surgery. The usual surgical procedure involves resection of the involved colon with a primary anastomosis. If the surgeon is not able to anastomose the colon, then the patient will have a temporary diverting colostomy. After the colon heals, the temporary colostomy can be "taken down" and the ends of the colon reconnected.

Provide the patient with diverticular disease with a full explanation of the condition. Patients who understand the disease process well and adhere to the prescribed regimen are less likely to experience an exacerbation of the disease and complications. Teach them the importance of following a

---

TABLE 42-30   Interprofessional Care

Diverticulosis and Diverticulitis

Diagnostic Assessment
- History and physical examination
- Testing of stool for occult blood
- CBC
- Urinalysis
- Barium enema
- Sigmoidoscopy and/or colonoscopy with biopsy
- Blood culture
- CT scan with oral contrast
- Abdominal and/or chest x-ray

Management

Conservative Therapy
- High-fiber diet
- Dietary fiber supplements
- Stool softeners
- Anticholinergics
- Clear liquid diet
- Oral antibiotics
- Mineral oil
- Bulk laxatives
- Weight reduction (if overweight)

Acute Care: Diverticulitis
- Antibiotic therapy
- NPO status
- IV fluids
- NG suction
- Surgery
- Possible resection of involved colon
- Possible temporary colostomy

---

high-fiber diet (Table 42-7) and encourage a fluid intake of at least 2L/day.

Weight reduction is important for the obese person with diverticular disease. A patient with diverticular disease should avoid increased intraabdominal pressure because it may precipitate an attack. Factors that increase intraabdominal pressure are straining at stool, vomiting, bending, heavy lifting, and wearing tight, restrictive clothing.

HERNIAS

A **hernia** is a protrusion of the viscus (internal organ such as the intestine) through an abnormal opening or a weakened area in the wall of the cavity in which it is normally contained. A hernia may occur in any part of the body, but it usually occurs within the abdominal cavity. *Reducible* hernias easily return into the abdominal cavity. Reducing can be done manually or may occur spontaneously when the person lies supine. *Irreducible,* or *incarcerated,* hernias cannot be placed back into the abdominal cavity and have abdominal contents trapped in the opening. Strangulation occurs if the blood supply to the contents trapped in an irreducible hernia becomes compromised. The result is an acute intestinal obstruction. Gangrene and necrosis of the hernia contents are possible.

Types

The *inguinal hernia* is the most common type of hernia and occurs at the point of weakness in the abdominal wall where the spermatic cord (in men) or the round ligament (in women) emerges (Fig. 42-14, *C*).

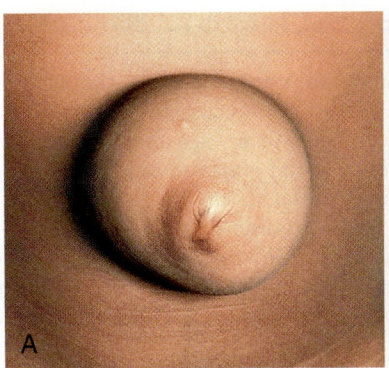 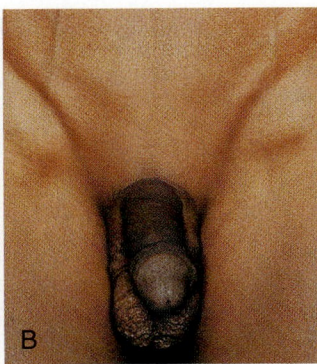 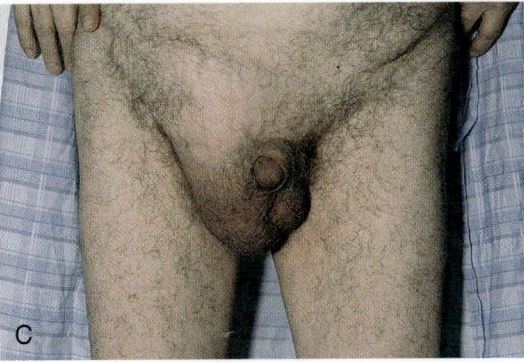

FIG. 42-14 **A,** Umbilical hernia. **B,** Femoral hernias (note swelling below the inguinal ligaments). **C,** Right inguinal hernia. (*A* and *B,* From Zitelli BJ, McIntire SC, Nowalk AJ: *Zitelli and Davis' atlas of pediatric physical diagnosis,* ed 6, Philadelphia, 2012, Saunders. *C,* From Swartz MH: *Textbook of physical diagnosis: history and examination,* ed 6, Philadelphia, 2010, Saunders.)

GENDER DIFFERENCES

Hernia

Men	Women
• Inguinal hernias are more common in men.	• Femoral hernias are more common in women, particularly older women.
• Men have a 25% lifetime risk of developing a groin hernia.	• Women have less than a 5% lifetime risk of developing a groin hernia.
• Men undergo 90% of the 750,000 groin hernia repairs done annually in the United States.	

An *umbilical hernia* occurs when the rectus muscle is weak (as with obesity) or the umbilical opening fails to close after birth (Fig. 42-14, *A*). A *femoral hernia* occurs when there is a protrusion through the femoral ring into the femoral canal. It appears as a bulge below the inguinal ligament. Femoral hernias easily strangulate (Fig. 42-14, *B*).

Ventral or *incisional hernias* are due to weakness of the abdominal wall at the site of a previous incision. They occur most commonly in patients who are obese, have had multiple surgical procedures in the same area, or have had inadequate wound healing because of poor nutrition or infection. Peristomal hernias are ventral hernias.

Clinical Manifestations

Pain is the classic symptom of a hernia. It may worsen with activities that increase intraabdominal pressure, such as lifting, coughing, and straining. A hernia may be readily visible, especially when the person tenses the abdominal muscles. If the hernia becomes strangulated, the patient will have severe pain and symptoms of a bowel obstruction such as vomiting, cramping abdominal pain, and distention.

❖ NURSING AND INTERPROFESSIONAL MANAGEMENT: HERNIAS

Diagnosis of a hernia is usually based on history and physical examination findings. Ultrasound, CT, and MRI can assist in identifying a hernia and determining the contents. Laparoscopic surgery is the treatment of choice. The surgical repair of a hernia, known as a *herniorrhaphy,* is usually an outpatient procedure. Reinforcing the weakened area with wire, fascia, or mesh is known as a *hernioplasty.* Emergency surgery is required for strangulated hernias or inflamed, irreducible hernias.

Surgery for strangulated hernias involves resecting the involved area with possible placement of a temporary colostomy.

After a hernia repair, the patient may have difficulty voiding. Measure intake and output and observe for a distended bladder. Scrotal edema is a painful complication after an inguinal hernia repair. A scrotal support with application of an ice bag and elevating the scrotum may help relieve pain and edema. Encourage deep breathing, but not coughing. Teach patients to splint the incision and keep their mouths open when coughing or sneezing is unavoidable. The patient may be restricted from heavy lifting (>10 lb) for 6 to 8 weeks.

MALABSORPTION SYNDROME

Malabsorption results from impaired absorption of fats, carbohydrates, proteins, minerals, and vitamins. The stomach, small intestine, liver, and pancreas regulate normal digestion and absorption. Digestive enzymes ordinarily break down nutrients so that absorption can take place. Malabsorption may occur if this process is interrupted at any point. Several problems can cause malabsorption (Table 42-31). Lactose intolerance is the most common malabsorption disorder, followed by IBD, celiac disease, tropical sprue, and cystic fibrosis.

The most common signs of malabsorption are weight loss, diarrhea, and steatorrhea (bulky, foul-smelling, yellow-gray, greasy stools with putty-like consistency) (Table 42-32). Steatorrhea does not occur with lactose intolerance.

Tests used to determine the cause of malabsorption include qualitative examination of stool for fat (e.g., Sudan III stain), a

TABLE 42-31	Causes of Malabsorption
Biochemical or Enzyme Deficiencies	**Bacterial Proliferation**
• Biliary tract obstruction	• Parasitic infection
• Chronic pancreatitis	• Tropical sprue
• Cystic fibrosis	
• Lactase deficiency	**Small Intestinal Mucosal Disruption**
• Pancreatic insufficiency	• Celiac disease
• Zollinger-Ellison syndrome	• Crohn's disease
	• Whipple's disease
Disturbed Lymphatic and Vascular Circulation	**Surface Area Loss**
• Heart failure	• Billroth II gastrectomy
• Ischemia	• Distal ileal resection, disease, or bypass
• Lymphangiectasia	• Short bowel syndrome
• Lymphoma	

TABLE 42-32   Manifestations of Malabsorption

Manifestations	Pathophysiology
Gastrointestinal	
Weight loss	Malabsorption of fat, carbohydrates, and protein leading to loss of calories. Marked reduction in caloric intake or increased use of calories.
Diarrhea	Impaired absorption of water, sodium, fatty acids, bile salts, and carbohydrates
Flatulence	Bacterial fermentation of unabsorbed carbohydrates
Steatorrhea	Undigested and unabsorbed fat
Glossitis, cheilosis, stomatitis	Deficiency of iron, riboflavin, cobalamin, folic acid, and other vitamins
Hematologic	
Anemia	Impaired absorption of iron, cobalamin, and folic acid
Hemorrhagic tendency	Vitamin C deficiency. Vitamin K deficiency inhibiting production of clotting factors II, VII, IX, and X
Musculoskeletal	
Bone pain	Osteoporosis from impaired calcium absorption. Osteomalacia secondary to hypocalcemia, hypophosphatemia, inadequate vitamin D
Tetany	Hypocalcemia, hypomagnesemia
Weakness, muscle cramps	Anemia, electrolyte depletion (especially potassium)
Muscle wasting	Protein malabsorption
Neurologic	
Altered mental status	Dehydration
Paresthesias	Cobalamin deficiency
Peripheral neuropathy	Cobalamin deficiency
Night blindness	Thiamine deficiency, vitamin A deficiency
Integumentary	
Bruising	Vitamin K deficiency
Dermatitis	Fatty acid deficiency, zinc deficiency, niacin and other vitamin deficiencies
Brittle nails	Iron deficiency
Hair thinning and loss	Protein deficiency
Cardiovascular	
Hypotension	Dehydration
Tachycardia	Hypovolemia, anemia
Peripheral edema	Protein malabsorption, protein loss in diarrhea

72-hour stool collection for quantitative measurement of fecal fat, serologic testing for celiac disease, and fecal elastase testing to determine if there is pancreatic insufficiency. Near-infrared reflectance analysis (NIRA) for fecal fat is available at some centers in the United States.

Other diagnostic studies include a CT scan and endoscopy to obtain a small bowel biopsy specimen. A small bowel barium enema can identify abnormal mucosal patterns. Capsule endoscopy is useful in assessing the small intestine for alterations in mucosal integrity and inflammation. Tests for carbohydrate malabsorption include the D-xylose test and the lactose tolerance test. Laboratory studies that are frequently ordered include a CBC, measurement of prothrombin time (to see if vitamin K absorption is adequate), serum vitamin A and carotene levels, serum electrolytes, cholesterol, and calcium. Treatment depends on the cause.

CELIAC DISEASE

Celiac disease is an autoimmune disease characterized by damage to the small intestinal mucosa from ingesting wheat, barley, and rye.[30] It can occur at any age and has a wide variety of symptoms. *Celiac sprue* and *gluten-sensitive enteropathy* are other names for celiac disease.

Celiac disease is not the same disease as *tropical sprue*, a chronic disorder occurring primarily in tropical areas. Tropical sprue causes progressive disruption of jejunal and ileal tissue, resulting in nutritional difficulties. It is treated with folic acid and tetracycline.

Celiac disease is most common in people of European ancestry and affects about 1% of the population of the United States.[30] High-risk groups include first- or second-degree relatives of someone with celiac disease and people with disorders associated with the disease such as migraine and myocarditis. It is slightly more common in women. Symptoms often begin in childhood.

Etiology and Pathophysiology

Three factors necessary for developing celiac disease are genetic predisposition, gluten ingestion, and an immune-mediated response.

Genetic Link

About 90% to 95% of patients with celiac disease have human leukocyte antigen (HLA) allele HLA-DQ2. The other 5% to 10% have HLA-DQ8. However, not everyone with these genetic markers develops celiac disease, and some people with celiac disease do not have these HLA alleles.

As with other autoimmune diseases, the tissue destruction that occurs with celiac disease is the result of chronic inflammation. Gluten contains specific peptides called *prolamines*. Partial digestion of gluten releases the prolamine peptides, which are absorbed into the intestinal submucosa. In genetically susceptible individuals, the peptides bind to HLA-DQ2 and/or HLA-DQ8 and activate an inflammatory response. Inflammation damages the microvilli and brush border of the small intestine, ultimately decreasing the amount of surface area available for nutrient absorption. Damage is most severe in the duodenum, probably because it has more exposure to gluten. The inflammation lasts as long as gluten ingestion continues.

Clinical Manifestations

Classic manifestations of celiac disease include foul-smelling diarrhea, steatorrhea, flatulence, abdominal distention, and malnutrition.[30] Some people have no obvious GI symptoms and may instead have atypical signs and symptoms such as decreased bone density and osteoporosis, dental enamel hypoplasia, iron and folate deficiencies, peripheral neuropathy, and reproductive problems. An intensely pruritic, vesicular skin lesion, called *dermatitis herpetiformis*, is sometimes present and occurs as a rash on the buttocks, scalp, face, elbows, and knees. Celiac disease is also associated with other autoimmune diseases, particularly rheumatoid arthritis, type 1 diabetes mellitus, and thyroid disease.

Protein, fat, and carbohydrate absorption is affected. Weight loss, muscle wasting, and other signs of malnutrition may be present. Abnormal serum folate, iron, and cobalamin levels can occur. Iron-deficiency anemia is common. Patients may exhibit lactose intolerance and need to refrain from lactose-containing products until the disease is under control. Inadequate calcium intake and vitamin D absorption can lead to decreased bone density and osteoporosis.

Diagnostic Studies and Interprofessional Care

Early diagnosis and treatment can prevent complications. Screening is recommended for close relatives of patients known to have the disease, young patients with decreased bone density, those with anemia once other causes are ruled out, and certain autoimmune diseases.

Celiac disease is confirmed by a combination of findings from the history and physical exam, serology testing, and histologic analysis of small intestine biopsies.[31] Have the patient complete diagnostic testing before starting a gluten-free diet, since the diet will alter the results. Serologic testing for immunoglobulin A (IgA) antitissue transglutaminase and IgA endomysial antibody provides good sensitivity and specificity. Histologic evidence remains the gold standard for confirming the diagnosis. Biopsies show flattened mucosa and noticeable losses of villi. Genotyping involves testing for HLA-DQ2 and/or HLA-DQ8 antigens.

A gluten-free diet (Table 42-33) is the only effective treatment for celiac disease. Most patients need to maintain on a gluten-free diet for the rest of their lives. If the disease is untreated, chronic inflammation and hyperplasia continue. Individuals with celiac disease have an increased risk of non-Hodgkin's lymphoma and GI cancers. Those with refractory disease who do not respond to a gluten-free diet alone may need corticosteroid therapy.

Refer all patients for a dietary consultation. You can work with a dietitian to teach the patient how to eat a nutritionally adequate diet while staying within a budget. Teach the patient to avoid wheat, barley, oats, and rye products. Although pure oats do not contain gluten, wheat, rye, and barley can contaminate oat products during the milling process. Teach the patient to read medication and food labels. Some medications and many food additives, preservatives, and stabilizers contain gluten. The patient needs to know where to purchase gluten-free products. Good sources are health food stores, many grocery stores, and through Internet sites.

Maintaining a gluten-free diet can be difficult, particularly when traveling or eating in restaurants. Many with celiac disease describe feeling embarrassed or like a burden when having to discuss gluten-free menu options with restaurant staff or when dining in other's homes. Mobile phone users will find apps listing gluten-free menu options at popular restaurants helpful. Many restaurants now indicate which food choices are gluten free. The Celiac Sprue Association website (*www.csaceliacs.info*) and the Celiac Disease Foundation (*www.celiac.org*) provide suggestions for maintaining a gluten-free diet and living with celiac disease.

LACTASE DEFICIENCY

Lactase deficiency is a condition in which the lactase enzyme is deficient or absent. Lactase is the enzyme that breaks down lactose into two simple sugars: glucose and galactose. Primary lactase insufficiency is most commonly a result of genetic factors. Certain ethnic or racial groups, especially those with Asian or African ancestry, develop low lactase levels in childhood. Less common causes include low lactase levels resulting from premature birth and congenital lactase deficiency, a rare genetic disorder. Lactose malabsorption can occur when conditions leading to bacterial overgrowth promote lactose fermentation in the small bowel or when intestinal mucosal damage interferes with absorption. The latter occurs with IBD and celiac disease.

Symptoms of lactose intolerance include bloating, flatulence, cramping abdominal pain, and diarrhea. Diarrhea results from the excess, undigested lactose in the small intestine attracting water molecules, which prevents them from being properly absorbed. Symptoms generally occur within 30 minutes to several hours after drinking a glass of milk or ingesting a milk product. Lactose intolerance is diagnosed with a lactose tolerance test, a lactose hydrogen breath test, or genetic testing.

Treatment consists of eliminating lactose from the diet by avoiding milk and milk products, and/or replacing lactase with commercially available preparations. A lactose-free diet generally results in prompt resolution of symptoms. Many lactose-intolerant persons are aware of their condition. They likely have been avoiding lactose-containing products and using lactose-free milk products. Lactase enzyme (Lactaid) is available as an over-the-counter product. It breaks down the lactose present in ingested milk. A number of milk products treated with lactase enzyme are readily available.

The diet may gradually advance to a low-lactose diet as tolerated by the patient. Many lactose-intolerant persons may not exhibit symptoms if they have lactose in small amounts. Cheese contains less lactose than milk and ice cream. Live culture yogurt has less lactose because the bacteria help digest the lactose. Teach the patient to read labels to detect any hidden sources of milk products. Some people tolerate lactose better if taken with meals. Teach the patient that adhering to the diet is important. Since avoiding milk and milk products can lead to calcium deficiency, supplements may be necessary to prevent osteoporosis.

SHORT BOWEL SYNDROME

Short bowel syndrome (SBS) is a condition in which the small intestine does not have adequate surface area to absorb enough nutrients. This leaves the person unable to meet energy, fluid, electrolyte, and nutritional needs to stay healthy on a normal diet. Causes of SBS include diseases that damage the intestinal

---

TABLE 42-33 Nutritional Therapy

Celiac Disease

Foods to Eat	Foods to Avoid
• Butter	• Baked goods, including muffins, cookies, cakes, pies
• Cheese, cottage cheese	• Barley
• Coffee, tea, and cocoa	• Bread, including wheat bread, white bread, "potato" bread
• Corn tortillas	• Flour
• Eggs	• Gluten stabilizers
• Flax, corn, and rice	• Oats
• Fresh fruits	• Pasta, pizza, bagels
• Gluten-free flour breads, crackers, pasta, and cereals	• Rye
• Meat, fish, poultry (not marinated or breaded)	• Wheat
• Peanut butter	
• Potatoes	
• Soy products	
• Tapioca	
• Unflavored milk	
• Yogurt	

mucosa, surgical removal of too much small intestine (primarily in patients with Crohn's disease), and congenital defects.

SBS is likely to develop in patients with a loss of two-thirds length of the small intestine. The length and area of the remaining small intestine and the presence of the colon affect the patient's outcome. If the terminal ileum and ileocecal valve remain intact, the remaining intestine undergoes adaptive changes that are most pronounced in the ileum. The villi and crypts increase in size, and the absorptive capacity of the remaining intestine increases. When the colon is present, fluid and electrolyte absorption increases. Those with an end jejunostomy often have little to no adaptation. Providing enteral nutrition and a normal diet after surgery stimulates the remaining intestine to adapt and function better.

Clinical Manifestations

The predominant manifestation of SBS is chronic diarrhea. Other manifestations include abdominal pain, flatulence, and steatorrhea. Signs of malnutrition as well as vitamin and mineral deficiencies include weight loss, cobalamin and zinc deficiency, and hypocalcemia. The patient may develop lactase deficiency and bacterial overgrowth. Oxalate kidney stones may form because of increased colonic absorption of oxalate.

Interprofessional Care

The treatment goals are that the patient will have fluid and electrolyte balance, normal nutritional status, and control of diarrhea. The main treatment is nutritional support involving parenteral nutrition, enteral nutrition, medications, and a tailored diet. In the immediate period after massive bowel resection, patients receive parenteral nutrition to replace fluid, electrolyte, and nutrient losses and to rest the bowel. Those with severe resections will require parenteral nutrition indefinitely. Enteral nutrition and a normal diet are gradually resumed to stimulate the remaining intestine to function better. Some can eventually discontinue parenteral nutrition.

Refer the patient to a dietitian. The optimal diet is high in protein and complex carbohydrates and low in fat and concentrated sweets. Oral supplements of calcium, zinc, and multivitamins may be required. Soluble fiber is encouraged if the colon is present. The patient should eat at least six small meals per day to increase the time of contact between food and the intestine. Oral intake may be supplemented with elemental nutrient formulas and tube feeding during the night. For patients with severe malabsorption, parenteral nutrition is necessary (see Chapter 39).

Patients often take multiple medications to help control fecal output. Excess fluid secretion is reduced with H_2 blockers, proton pump inhibitors, α-adrenergic receptor agonists (e.g., clonidine), or octreotide. Opioid antidiarrheal drugs are the most effective in decreasing intestinal motility (Table 42-2). For patients who have limited ileal resections, cholestyramine (Questran) reduces diarrhea resulting from unabsorbed bile acids by increasing their excretion in feces. Bile acids stimulate intestinal fluid secretion and reduce colonic fluid absorption. Antibiotic therapy is used if bacterial overgrowth is contributing to diarrhea.[32]

Three drugs have FDA approval for the treatment of SBS: somatropin (Zorbtive), glutamine, and teduglutide (Gattex). Somatropin enhances intestinal adaption and increases the flow of water, electrolytes, and nutrients into the bowel. Glutamine improves intestinal absorption. Teduglutide helps to increase the surface area of the intestine and improve intestinal absorption of fluids and nutrients.

Intestinal transplantation is a procedure performed at a few specialized transplant centers in the United States. It is considered the only long-term treatment option for patients with intestinal failure who have irreversible complications from parenteral nutrition. The leading cause of intestinal failure is SBS. Transplantation may include the intestine alone, liver and intestine, or multivisceral combinations (stomach, duodenum, jejunum, ileum, colon, and/or pancreas).

GASTROINTESTINAL STROMAL TUMORS

Gastrointestinal stromal tumors (GISTs) are a rare form of cancer that originates in cells found in the wall of the GI tract. These cells, known as *interstitial cells of Cajal,* help control the movement of food and liquid through the stomach and intestines. About 55% of GISTs are in the stomach; 35% are in the small intestine; and the rest are in the gallbladder, esophagus, colon, or peritoneum.[33] Most GISTs occur in people between the ages of 50 and 70. While the exact cause of GISTs is unknown, genetic mutations likely play a role. A few GISTs occur in people with familial mutations in either the KIT or platelet-derived growth factor receptor a (PDGFRa) oncogenes or occur in those with neurofibromatosis type 1.[33]

The manifestations of GISTs depend on the part of the GI tract affected. Early manifestations are often subtle, including early satiety, fatigue, bloating, nausea or vomiting, and a change in bowel habits. Because these manifestations are similar to those of many other GI problems, early detection of the cancer is difficult. Later manifestations may include GI bleeding and obstruction caused by growth of the tumor. GISTs are often found during imaging for other problems. Diagnosis is based on histologic examination of biopsied tissue. Endoscopic ultrasound, CT, or MRI are used to determine the extent of disease.

Patients initially undergo surgery to remove the tumor, but the GIST has often metastasized by the time of diagnosis or commonly recurs. GISTs are unresponsive to conventional chemotherapy. However, discovery of genetic mutations led to the development of tyrosine kinase inhibitor drugs (e.g., imatinib mesylate [Gleevec], regorafenib [Stivarga]) that are highly effective against certain GISTs.[33]

ANORECTAL PROBLEMS

HEMORRHOIDS

Hemorrhoids are dilated hemorrhoidal veins. They may be internal (occurring above the internal sphincter) or external (occurring outside the external sphincter) (Figs. 42-15 and 42-16). In affected persons, hemorrhoids appear periodically, depending on the amount of anorectal pressure.

Etiology and Pathophysiology

Hemorrhoids develop because of increased anal pressure and weakening of the connective tissue that supports the hemorrhoidal veins. Weakened supporting tissue allows for downward displacement of the hemorrhoidal veins, causing them to dilate. Blood flow through the veins of the hemorrhoidal plexus is impaired. An intravascular clot in the venule results in a thrombosed external hemorrhoid. Many factors increase the risk for hemorrhoids, including pregnancy, prolonged constipation,

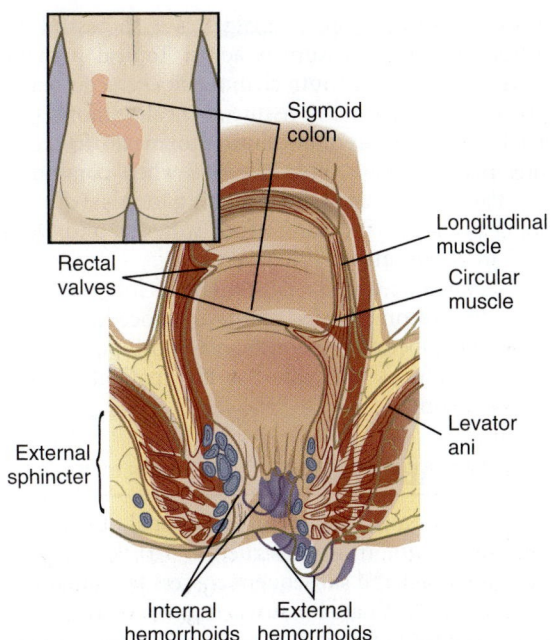

FIG. 42-15 Anatomic structures of the rectum and anus with external and internal hemorrhoids.

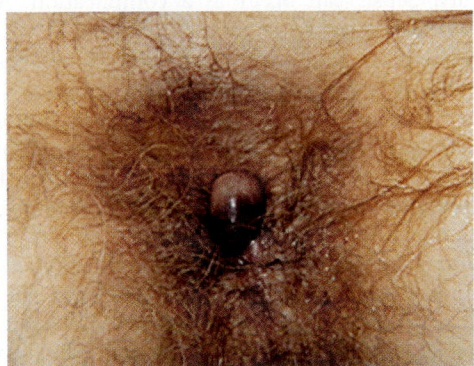

FIG. 42-16 Thrombosed external hemorrhoids. (From Townsend CM, Beauchamp RD, Evers BM, et al: *Sabiston textbook of surgery: the biological basis of modern surgical practice,* ed 19, Philadelphia, 2012, Saunders.)

straining in an effort to defecate, heavy lifting, prolonged standing and sitting, obesity, and portal hypertension.

Clinical Manifestations

Hemorrhoids are the most common reason for bleeding with defecation. Other manifestations include anal pruritus, prolapse, and pain. Internal hemorrhoids most often cause painless bright red bleeding with stools, on the toilet paper, or dripping into the toilet water. If internal hemorrhoids become constricted, the patient will report pain. Internal hemorrhoids can prolapse into the anal canal or externally. Symptoms of prolapse include pressure with defecation and a protruding mass.

External hemorrhoids are reddish blue and seldom bleed. There may be itching, burning, and edema. They usually do not cause pain unless thrombosis (blood clots) is present. Thrombosed hemorrhoids are a bluish purple tinge and palpable at the anal orifice. They usually cause pain and inflammation. The clot can erode through the overlying stretched skin, causing bleeding with defecation. Constipation or diarrhea can aggravate these symptoms.

Diagnostic Studies and Interprofessional Care

Internal hemorrhoids are diagnosed by digital examination, anoscopy, and sigmoidoscopy. External hemorrhoids are easily diagnosed by visual inspection and digital examination.

Therapy is based on the cause and the patient's symptoms. A high-fiber diet and increased fluid intake prevent constipation and reduce straining, which allows engorgement of the veins to subside. The resulting stool bulk may also decrease stool leakage and therefore itching. Ointments such as dibucaine; creams, suppositories, and impregnated pads that contain antiinflammatory agents (e.g., hydrocortisone); or astringents and anesthetics (e.g., witch hazel, benzocaine) may be used to shrink the mucous membranes and relieve discomfort. The use of topical corticosteroids should be limited to 1 week or less to prevent side effects such as contact dermatitis and mucosal atrophy. Stool softeners can keep the stools soft. Sitz baths help relieve pain.

External hemorrhoids are usually managed by conservative therapy unless they become thrombosed. For internal hemorrhoids, nonsurgical approaches (rubber band ligation, infrared coagulation, sclerotherapy, laser treatment) are options.[34] Rubber band ligation is the most widely used technique. The surgeon inserts an anoscope to identify the hemorrhoid and then ligates it with a rubber band. The rubber band around the hemorrhoid constricts circulation, and the tissue becomes necrotic, separates, and sloughs off. There is some local discomfort with this procedure, but no anesthetic is required.

A *hemorrhoidectomy* is the surgical excision of hemorrhoids. Surgery is indicated when there is marked prolapse, excessive pain or bleeding, or large or multiple thrombosed hemorrhoids. Surgical removal is done by cautery, clamp, or excision. After removing the hemorrhoids, the tissue is either sutured and the wound heals by primary intention or the area is left open and healing takes place by secondary intention.

❖ NURSING MANAGEMENT: HEMORRHOIDS

Conservative nursing management for the patient with hemorrhoids includes teaching measures to prevent constipation and to avoid prolonged standing or sitting, and proper use of OTC drugs for hemorrhoidal symptoms. Teach the patient to seek medical care for severe symptoms of hemorrhoids (e.g., excessive pain and bleeding, prolapsed hemorrhoids). Sitz baths (15 to 20 minutes, two or three times each day) may help to reduce discomfort and swelling associated with hemorrhoids.

Nursing care after a hemorrhoidectomy focuses on pain control and promoting wound healing. Be aware that although the procedure is minor, the pain is severe and feared by many. There are several analgesic regimens, using a combination of medications. Most patients initially receive an opioid and NSAID in conjunction with topical preparations that provide anesthesia or reduce internal sphincter spasms, such as glyceryl trinitrate (GTN), calcium channel blockers (e.g., nifedipine with lidocaine, diltiazem), or nitroglycerin preparations.

The patient usually dreads the first bowel movement and often resists the urge to defecate. Give pain medication before the bowel movement to reduce discomfort. Stool softeners (e.g., docusate [Colace]) and bulking agents help form a soft, bulky stool that is easier to pass. If the patient does not have a bowel movement within 2 or 3 days, an oil-retention enema is given.

Sitz baths are started 1 or 2 days after surgery and continued for 1 to 2 weeks. A warm sitz bath provides comfort and keeps the anal area clean. A sponge ring in the sitz bath helps relieve pressure on the area. Initially, do not leave the patient alone because of the possibility of weakness or fainting. Instruct the patient that pressure relief cushions are acceptable to ease discomfort when sitting. Tell the patient not to use a pressure relief ring or "doughnut" because they can reduce blood flow to the area.

The patient may have packing in the rectum to absorb drainage, with a T-binder to hold the dressing in place. Packing is usually removed on the first or second postoperative day. Assess for rectal bleeding, especially in patients taking clopidogrel or oral anticoagulants. The patient may be embarrassed when the dressing is changed. Provide as much privacy as possible.

Teach the patient the importance of diet, care of the anal area, symptoms of complications (especially bleeding), and avoidance of constipation and straining. Hemorrhoids may recur. Occasionally, anal strictures develop and dilation is necessary. Regular checkups are important to prevent any further problems.

ANAL FISSURE

An *anal fissure* is a skin ulcer or a crack in the lining of the anal wall. Many times the initiating factor is the passage of hard stools. Other fissures are related to trauma (anal intercourse, insertion of a foreign body such as endoscope), local infection (syphilis; tuberculosis; gonorrhea; or infection with *Chlamydia*, herpes simplex virus, or HIV), or inflammation (Fig. 42-17). An anal fissure is considered acute when it is of recent onset (less than 6 weeks), and chronic if it has been present for a longer period. Chronic fissures have a characteristic appearance that includes perianal skin tag and fibrotic edges.[35]

Anal tissue ulcerates because of ischemia caused by a combination of high pressure in the internal anal sphincter and poor blood supply to the area. The ischemic tissue may ulcerate spontaneously or when traumatized by factors such as hard stools that would not normally cause tissue breakdown. Ischemia must be corrected for a fissure to heal.

The hallmark of an anal fissure is severe anal pain. It tends to be worse with defecation and with direct pressure on the site (e.g., sitting). Acute fissures tend to bleed slightly, and patients may report red blood on the toilet paper. Constipation results because of fear of pain associated with bowel movements.

Anal fissures are easy to diagnose with a physical examination. Conservative care with fiber supplements, adequate fluid intake, sitz baths, and topical analgesics is successful in most cases, especially if the fissure is acute. Topical preparations, including nitrates and calcium channel blockers, decrease rectal anal pressure and allow the fissure to heal without sphincter damage. Local injections of botulinum toxin can decrease rectal anal pressure. They are most effective when combined with nitrates. Pain is managed by softening stools with a bulk-producing agent (psyllium) or stool softener, and warm sitz baths (15 to 20 minutes, 3 times per day).[35]

If conservative treatment fails, a lateral internal sphincterotomy is the recommended surgical procedure. It carries the risk of postoperative incontinence. Postoperative nursing care is the same as the care for the patient who had a hemorrhoidectomy.

ANORECTAL ABSCESS

An *anorectal abscess* is a collection of perianal pus (Fig. 42-17). The abscess results from obstruction of the anal glands, leading to infection and subsequent abscess formation. Abscess formation occurs with anal fissures, trauma, or IBD. The most common causative organisms are *E. coli*, staphylococci, and streptococci. Clinical manifestations include local severe pain and swelling, foul-smelling drainage, tenderness, and elevated temperature. Sepsis can occur as a complication. Anorectal abscesses are diagnosed by rectal examination.

Anorectal abscesses require surgical drainage. Larger abscesses require packing afterwards with impregnated gauze or placement of drains (e.g., Penrose) to promote drainage. The area then heals by granulation. Patients who have diabetes, cellulitis, or are immunocompromised (e.g., chemotherapy) may require antibiotic therapy. Nursing care includes warm, moist heat applications and changing packing daily. The patient is usually more comfortable lying on the abdomen or side. A low-fiber diet is given. The patient may leave the hospital with the wound still open. Teach the patient about wound care and the importance of sitz baths, thorough cleaning after urinating or bowel movements, and follow-up visits with the HCP.

ANAL FISTULA

An **anal fistula** is an abnormal tunnel leading from the anus or rectum. It may extend to the outside of the skin, vagina, or buttocks and often precedes an abscess. Anal fistulas are a complication of Crohn's disease and may resolve when drug treatment (i.e., with infliximab) achieves remission of the disease. About 50% of anal fistulas are due to anorectal abscess.

Feces may enter the fistula and cause an infection. There may be persistent, bloody, or purulent discharge, or stool leakage from the fistula. The patient may need to wear a pad to avoid staining clothes.

Surgical treatment of an anal fistula depends on the location and nature of the fistula. In a fistulotomy, the surgeon opens the fistula and healthy tissue is allowed to granulate in the wound. Care is the same as that after a hemorrhoidectomy. Options for complex fistulas include ligation of the intersphincteric fistula tract (LIFT), or the use of rectal flaps, setons, plugs, or fibrin glue injections to seal the fistula.

ANAL CANCER

Anal cancer is uncommon in the general population, but the incidence is increasing. In the United States approximately 7200

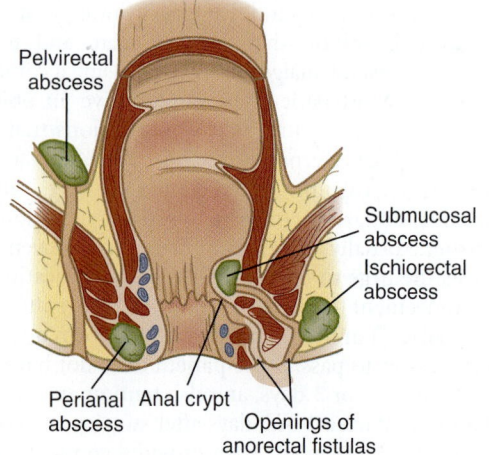

Pelvirectal abscess

Submucosal abscess

Ischiorectal abscess

Perianal abscess   Anal crypt

Openings of anorectal fistulas

FIG. 42-17 Common sites of anorectal abscesses and fistula formation.

people are diagnosed with anal cancer each year.[36] It mainly occurs in older adults, with the average age being in the early 60s. Human papillomavirus (HPV) is associated with about 80% of the cases of anal cancer. Those at high risk for anal cancer include smokers, men who have sex with men, women with cervical or vulvar cancer or precancerous lesions, and people who are immunocompromised (e.g., posttransplantation immunosuppression) or HIV-positive.[37]

The most frequent initial symptom is rectal bleeding. Other symptoms include rectal pain and sensation of a rectal mass. Some patients have no symptoms, which leads to delayed diagnosis and treatment.

It is especially important to screen high-risk individuals using DRE and anal Pap tests. In an anal Pap test, the anal lining is swabbed and the cells examined to identify any cell changes (e.g., dysplasia, neoplasia). High-resolution anoscopy allows for visualization of the mucosa and biopsy. An endoanal (endorectal) ultrasound may also be done.

Review with the patient behavior practices used to reduce the risk of sexually transmitted infections. Encourage the use of condoms, avoiding unprotected anal sex, and limiting sexual partners. Two HPV vaccines are available to help prevent cervical, vulvar, vaginal, and anal cancers and associated precancerous lesions. Both Gardasil and Gardasil 9 vaccines protect against HPV types 6, 11, 16, and 18. Gardasil 9 protects against 5 additional HPV types, 31, 33, 45, 52, and 58. After vaccination with HPV vaccine, patients at risk need to continue their recommended screening program.[37]

Treatment of anal cancer depends on the size and depth of the lesions. Topical therapy with bichloroacetic or trichloroacetic acid may be used to remove genital warts and kill the HPV virus. Options for precancerous lesions are surgical removal or treatment with topical imiquimod (Aldara) and 5-FU. Cancer therapy involves surgery or a combination of radiation and chemotherapy. Chemotherapy regimens include combinations of mitomycin, cisplatin, and 5-FU.

PILONIDAL SINUS

A *pilonidal sinus* is a small tract under the skin between the buttocks in the sacrococcygeal area. It is thought to be of congenital origin. It may have several openings and is lined with epithelium and hair, hence the name *pilonidal* ("a nest of hair"). The skin is moist, and movement of the buttocks causes the short, wiry hair to penetrate the skin. If the irritated skin becomes infected, it forms a pilonidal cyst or abscess. There are no symptoms with a pilonidal sinus unless there is an infection. Then the patient complains of pain and swelling at the base of the spine.

An abscess requires incision and drainage. The wound may be closed, or left open to heal by secondary intention. The wound is packed, and sitz baths are ordered. Nursing care includes warm, moist heat applications when an abscess is present. The patient is usually more comfortable lying on the abdomen or side. Teach the patient to avoid contaminating the dressing when urinating or defecating and to avoid straining whenever possible.

Colorectal Cancer

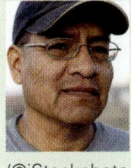

(©iStockphoto/ Thinkstock)

Patient Profile
L.C., a 58-yr-old Native American man, is from a Pueblo tribe in northern New Mexico. L.C.'s wife and family drove 50 miles to take him to the Indian Health Service hospital because of his deteriorating health (see the case study in Chapter 38 on p. 839).

Subjective Data
See the case study in Chapter 38 on p. 843.

Objective Data

Physical Examination
See the case study in Chapter 38 on p. 845.

Laboratory Tests
• CT scan and colonoscopy show two medium-sized tumors in the transverse colon.

Interprofessional Care

Surgical Procedure
• Transverse hemicolectomy performed and lymph node biopsies taken.
• Pathology results indicate that the adenocarcinoma tumor has invaded the muscle wall of colon and 2 out of 5 lymph nodes are positive for cancer.

Postoperative
• Feels like his life has ended and does not want to leave hospital.
• States that there is "no one" to take care of him at his home and he is far away from the hospital.

Follow-Up Treatment
Scheduled for outpatient chemotherapy

Discussion Questions
1. What signs and symptoms of colorectal cancer did L.C. manifest (see the case study in Chapter 38 on p. 852)?
2. What stage of CRC does L.C. probably have? What treatment is recommended for this stage of CRC?
3. How could you provide emotional support to L.C. and his family?
4. *Patient-Centered Care:* What is a culturally sensitive way for you to support L.C. and his family in making decisions about his continued health care?
5. *Priority Decision:* Based on the assessment data, what are the priority nursing diagnoses? Are there any collaborative problems?
6. *Priority Decision:* What are the priority nursing interventions for L.C. at this stage of his illness?
7. *Teamwork and Collaboration:* What referrals may be indicated at this time?
8. *Evidence-Based Practice:* L.C. had not had a previous colonoscopy. He is worried that other members of his family may have colon cancer. What can you tell him about the recommendations for colorectal cancer screening?
9. *Quality Improvement:* What outcomes would indicate nursing interventions were successful?

Answers available at *http://evolve.elsevier.com/Lewis/medsurg.*

BRIDGE TO NCLEX EXAMINATION

The number of the question corresponds to the same-numbered outcome at the beginning of the chapter.

1. The *most* appropriate therapy for a patient with acute diarrhea caused by a viral infection is to
   a. increase fluid intake.
   b. administer an antibiotic.
   c. administer an antimotility drug.
   d. quarantine the patient to prevent spread of the virus.

2. A 35-year-old female patient is admitted to the emergency department with acute abdominal pain. Which medical diagnoses should you consider as possible causes of her pain *(select all that apply)*?
   a. Gastroenteritis
   b. Ectopic pregnancy
   c. Gastrointestinal bleeding
   d. Irritable bowel syndrome
   e. Inflammatory bowel disease

3. Assessment findings suggestive of peritonitis include *(select all that apply)*
   a. rebound tenderness.
   b. a soft, distended abdomen.
   c. dull, intermittent abdominal pain.
   d. shallow respirations with bradypnea.
   e. observing that the patient is lying still.

4. In planning care for the patient with Crohn's disease, the nurse recognizes that a major difference between ulcerative colitis and Crohn's disease is that Crohn's disease
   a. frequently results in toxic megacolon.
   b. causes fewer nutritional deficiencies than ulcerative colitis.
   c. often recurs after surgery, whereas ulcerative colitis is curable with a colectomy.
   d. is manifested by rectal bleeding and anemia more often than is ulcerative colitis.

5. The nurse performs a detailed assessment of the abdomen of a patient with a possible bowel obstruction, knowing that manifestations of an obstruction in the large intestine are *(select all that apply)*
   a. persistent abdominal pain.
   b. marked abdominal distention.
   c. diarrhea that is loose or liquid.
   d. colicky, severe, intermittent pain.
   e. profuse vomiting that relieves abdominal pain.

6. A patient with stage I colorectal cancer is scheduled for surgery. Patient teaching for this patient would include an explanation that
   a. chemotherapy will begin after the patient recovers from the surgery.
   b. both chemotherapy and radiation can be used as palliative treatments.
   c. follow-up colonoscopies will be needed to ensure that the cancer does not recur.
   d. a wound, ostomy, and continence nurse will visit the patient to identify an abdominal site for the ostomy.

7. The nurse determines a patient undergoing ileostomy surgery understands the procedure when the patient states
   a. "I should only have to change the pouch every 4 to 7 days."
   b. "The drainage in the pouch will look like my normal stools."
   c. "I may not need to wear a drainage pouch if I irrigate it daily."
   d. "Limiting my fluid intake should decrease the amount of output."

8. In contrast to diverticulitis, the patient with diverticulosis
   a. has rectal bleeding.
   b. often has no symptoms.
   c. has localized cramping pain.
   d. frequently develops peritonitis.

9. A nursing intervention that is *most* appropriate to decrease postoperative edema and pain after an inguinal herniorrhaphy is
   a. applying a truss to the hernia site.
   b. allowing the patient to stand to void.
   c. supporting the incision during coughing.
   d. applying a scrotal support with an ice bag.

10. The nurse determines that the goals of dietary teaching have been met when the patient with celiac disease selects from the menu
    a. scrambled eggs and sausage.
    b. buckwheat pancakes with syrup.
    c. oatmeal, skim milk, and orange juice.
    d. yogurt, strawberries, and rye toast with butter.

11. What should a patient be taught after a hemorrhoidectomy?
    a. Take mineral oil before bedtime.
    b. Eat a low-fiber diet to rest the colon.
    c. Administer oil-retention enema to empty the colon.
    d. Use prescribed pain medication before a bowel movement.

1. a, 2. a, b, c, d, e, 3. a, e, 4. c, 5. a, b, d, 6. c, 7. a, 8. b, 9. d, 10. a, 11. d

For rationales to these answers and even more NCLEX review questions, visit *http://evolve.elsevier.com/Lewis/medsurg*.

EVOLVE WEBSITE

http://evolve.elsevier.com/Lewis/medsurg
Review Questions (Online Only)
Key Points
Answer Keys for Questions
• Rationales for Bridge to NCLEX Examination Questions
• Answer Guidelines for Case Study on p. 971
Student Case Study
• Patient With Ulcerative Colitis
Nursing Care Plans
• eNursing Care Plan 42-1: Patient With Acute Infectious Diarrhea
• eNursing Care Plan 42-2: Patient With Inflammatory Bowel Disease
• eNursing Care Plan 42-3: Patient With a Colostomy/Ileostomy
Conceptual Care Map Creator
Audio Glossary
Content Updates

REFERENCES

1. Hamilton AC, Moises A: Diarrhea, *Hosp Med Clin* 2:e227, 2013.
*2. Surawicz C, Brandt L, Zuckerbraun B, et al: Guidelines for diagnosis, treatment, and prevention of *Clostridium difficile* infections, *Am J Gastroenterol* 108:478, 2013.
3. Orenstein R, Griesbach CL, DiBaise JK: Moving fecal microbiota transplantation into the mainstream, *Nutr Clin Pract* 28:589, 2013.
*4. Whitehead W, Rao S, Hamilton F, et al: Treatment of fecal incontinence: state of the science summary for the National Institute of Diabetes and Digestive and Kidney Diseases workshop, *Am J Gastroenterol* 110:138, 2015.
*5. Kottner J, Blume-Peytavi U, Lohrmann C, et al: Associations between individual characteristics and incontinence-associated dermatitis, *Int J Nurs Stud* 51:1373, 2014.
6. Whiteley I, Sinclair G: Fecal management systems for disabling incontinence or wounds, *Br J Nurs* 23:881, 2014.

*7. Bharucha A, Pemberton J, Locke G: American Gastroenterological Association technical review on constipation, *Gastroenterol* 144:218, 2013.

8. Peyton L, Greene J: Irritable bowel syndrome: current and emerging treatment options, *P&T* 38:567, 2014.

*9. Anusha T, Eamonn MQ: Diet and irritable bowel syndrome, *Curr Opin Gastroenterol* 31:605, 2015.

10. Teixeira PG, Demetrios D: Appendicitis: changing perspectives, *Adv in Surg* 47:119, 2013.

*11. Hou JK, Lee D, Lewis J: Diet and inflammatory bowel disease: review of patient-targeted recommendations, *Clin Gastroenterol Hepatol* 12:1592, 2014.

12. Ek WE, D'Amato M, Halfvarson J: The history of genetics in inflammatory bowel disease, *Ann Gastroenterol* 27:294, 2014.

13. NOD2. Retrieved from *http://ghr.nlm.nih.gov/gene/NOD2*.

*14. Berg AM, Kelly CP, Farraye FA: Clostridium difficile infection in the inflammatory bowel disease patient, *Inflamm Bowel Dis* 19:194, 2013.

15. Park SC, Jeen YT: Current and emerging biologics for ulcerative colitis, *Gut and Liver* 9:18, 2015.

*16. Pappa H: Vitamin D deficiency and supplementation in patients with IBD, *Gastroenterol Hepatol* 10:127, 2014.

*17. Parkes GC: Smoking in inflammatory bowel disease: impact on disease course and insights into the etiology of its effect, *J Crohns* 8:717, 2014.

*18. Gisbert JP: Systematic review with meta-analysis: inflammatory bowel disease in the elderly, *Aliment Pharmacol Ther* 39:459, 2014.

19. Glancy DG: Intestinal obstruction, *Surgery* 32:204, 2014.

20. Colorectal cancer facts and figures. Retrieved from *www.cancer.org/ research/cancerfactsstatistics/colorectal-cancer-facts-figures*.

*21. Brenner H, Matthias K, Christian PP: Effect of screening sigmoidoscopy and colonoscopy on colorectal cancer incidence and mortality, *Lancet* 383:1490, 2014.

22. American Cancer Society recommendations for colorectal cancer early detection. Retrieved from *www.cancer.org/cancer/colonandrectumcancer/ moreinformation/colonandrectumcancerearlydetection/colorectal-cancer -early-detection-acs-recommendations*.

23. Brenner H, Kloor M, Pox C: Colorectal cancer, *Lancet* 383:1490, 2014.

24. Colon cancer treatment. Retrieved from *www.cancer.gov/cancertopics/ pdq/treatment/colon/HealthProfessional*.

25. Johnson D, Barkun A, Rex D, et al: Optimizing adequacy of bowel cleansing for colonoscopy: recommendations from the US multi-society task force on colorectal cancer, *Gastroenterol* 147:903, 2014.

26. Prinz A, Colwell J, Cross H, et al: Discharge planning for a patient with a new ostomy: best practice for clinicians, *J Wound Ostomy Continence Nurs* 42:79, 2015.

27. Willcutts K, Touger-Decker R: Nutritional management for ostomates, *Top Clin Nutr* 28:373, 2013.

28. Haack C, Galloway JR, Srinivasan S: Enterocutaneous fistulas: a look at causes and management, *Curr Surg Rep* 10:1, 2014.

29. Coyne PE, Kalbassi MR: Diverticular disease, *Surgery* 32:431, 2014.

30. Levy J, Bernstein L, Silber N: Celiac disease: an immune dysregulation syndrome, *Curr Probl Pediatr Adolesc Health Care* 44:324, 2014.

*31. Rubio-Tapia A, Hill ID, Kelly CP, et al: ACG clinical guidelines: diagnosis and management of celiac disease, *Am J Gastroenterol* 108:656, 2013.

32. Kumpf VJ: Pharmacologic management of diarrhea in patients with short bowel syndrome, *J Parenter Enteral Nutr* 38:38S, 2014.

33. Heikki J, Hohenberger P, Corless CL: Gastrointestinal stromal tumor, *Lancet* 382:973, 2013.

34. Rakinic J, Poola VP: Hemorrhoids and fistulas: new solutions to old problems, *Curr Prob Surg* 51:98, 2014.

35. Higuero T: Update on the management of anal fissure, *J Visceral Surg* 152:S37, 2015.

36. American Cancer Society: Anal cancer. Retrieved from *www.cancer.org/ cancer/analcancer/detailedguide/anal-cancer-what-is-key-statistics*.

*37. Shridhar R, Shibata D, Chan E, et al: Anal cancer: current standards in care and recent changes in practice, *CA Canc J for Clin* 65:139, 2015.

*Evidence-based information for clinical practice.

43

Liver, Pancreas, and Biliary Tract Problems

Kathy H. Wu

Neither should a ship rely on one small anchor, nor should life rest on a single hope.

Epictetus

e http://evolve.elsevier.com/Lewis/medsurg/

LEARNING OUTCOMES

1. Differentiate among the types of viral hepatitis, including etiology, pathophysiology, clinical manifestations, complications, and interprofessional care.
2. Describe the nursing management of the patient with viral hepatitis.
3. Describe the pathophysiology, clinical manifestations, complications, and interprofessional care of the patient with nonalcoholic fatty liver disease.
4. Explain the etiology, pathophysiology, clinical manifestations, complications, interprofessional care, and nursing management of the patient with cirrhosis of the liver.
5. Describe the clinical manifestations and management of liver cancer.
6. Differentiate between acute and chronic pancreatitis related to pathophysiology, clinical manifestations, complications, interprofessional care, and nursing management.
7. Explain the clinical manifestations, interprofessional care, and nursing management of the patient with pancreatic cancer.
8. Describe the pathophysiology, clinical manifestations, complications, and interprofessional care of gallbladder disorders.
9. Describe the nursing management of the patient undergoing surgical treatment of cholecystitis and cholelithiasis.

KEY TERMS

Nursing management of patients with liver, pancreatic, and gallbladder problems is the focus of this chapter. Viral hepatitis, cirrhosis, acute pancreatitis, cholecystitis, and cholelithiasis are described in detail.

DISORDERS OF THE LIVER

HEPATITIS

Hepatitis is inflammation of the liver. Hepatitis is most commonly caused by viruses. It can also be caused by substances (e.g., alcohol, medications, chemicals), autoimmune diseases, and metabolic abnormalities.

Viral Hepatitis

There are several types of viral hepatitis, and each type is designated by a letter (A, B, C, D, E). The different types of viral hepatitis have similar clinical manifestations, but their modes of transmission and disease course vary (Table 43-1). Some types of viral hepatitis infection can lead to chronic liver disease. Other less common viruses can also cause liver disease. These include cytomegalovirus (CMV), Epstein-Barr virus (EBV), herpesvirus, coxsackievirus, and rubella virus.

Hepatitis A Virus. Hepatitis A is a self-limiting infection that can cause a mild flu-like illness and jaundice. In more severe cases, it can cause acute liver failure. Hepatitis A virus (HAV) is a ribonucleic acid (RNA) virus that is transmitted primarily through the fecal-oral route. It frequently occurs in small outbreaks caused by fecal contamination of food or drinking water. Poor hygiene, improper handling of food, crowded situations, and poor sanitary conditions are contributing factors.

Transmission occurs between family members, institutionalized individuals, and children in day care centers. Foodborne hepatitis A outbreaks are usually due to food contaminated by

Reviewed by Marian Altman, RN, MS, CNS-BC, ANP, Patient Care Services Safety Manager, Virginia Commonwealth University Health System, Richmond, Virginia; Brian J. Fasolka, RN, MSN, CEN, Assistant Clinical Professor, College of Nursing and Health Professions, Drexel University, Philadelphia, Pennsylvania; Lauren Kemph, RN, DNP, AGPCNP, Nurse Practitioner, Center for Liver Disease and Transplantation at New York Presbyterian, New York, New York; Katherine A. Ladetto, RN, MSN, APRN, ANP-BC, GNP-BC, Nurse Practitioner, North Shore Physicians Group, Peabody, Massachusetts; and Heidi E. Monroe, MSN, RN-BC, CPAN, CAPA, Assistant Professor of Nursing, Bellin College and Bellin Hospital, Green Bay, Wisconsin.

TABLE 43-1 Characteristics of Hepatitis Viruses

Incubation Period and Mode of Transmission	Sources of Infection	Infectivity
Hepatitis A Virus (HAV) *Incubation:* 15-50 days (average 28) • Fecal-oral (primarily fecal contamination and oral ingestion)	• Crowded conditions (e.g., day care, nursing home) • Poor personal hygiene • Poor sanitation • Contaminated food, milk, water, shellfish • Persons with subclinical infections, infected food handlers, sexual contact, IV drug users	• Most infectious during 2 wk before onset of symptoms • Infectious until 1-2 wk after the start of symptoms
Hepatitis B Virus (HBV) *Incubation:* 45-180 days (average 56-96) • Percutaneous (parenteral) or permucosal exposure to blood or blood products • Sexual contact • Perinatal transmission	• Contaminated needles, syringes, and blood products • Sexual activity with infected partners. Asymptomatic carriers • Tattoos or body piercing with contaminated needles • HBV-infected mother (perinatal transmission)	• Before and after symptoms appear • Infectious for 4-6 mo • Carriers continue to be infectious for life
Hepatitis C Virus (HCV) *Incubation:* 14-180 days (average 56) • Percutaneous (parenteral) or mucosal exposure to blood or blood products • High-risk sexual contact • Perinatal contact	• Blood and blood products • Needles and syringes • Sexual activity with infected partners	• 1-2 wk before symptoms appear • Continues during clinical course • 75%-85% go on to develop chronic hepatitis C and remain infectious
Hepatitis D Virus (HDV) *Incubation:* 2-26 wk • HBV must precede HDV • Chronic carriers of HBV always at risk	• Same as HBV • Can cause infection only when HBV is present • Routes of transmission same as for HBV	• Blood infectious at all stages of HDV infection
Hepatitis E Virus (HEV) *Incubation:* 15-64 days (average 26-42 days) • Fecal-oral route • Outbreaks associated with contaminated water supply in developing countries	• Contaminated water, poor sanitation • Found in Asia, Africa, and Mexico • Not common in United States	• Not known • May be similar to HAV

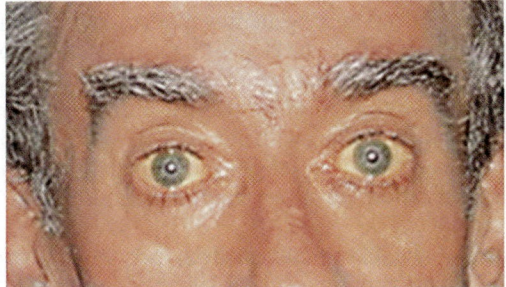

FIG. 43-1 Jaundiced patient. (From Butcher GP: *Gastroenterology: an illustrated colour text*, London, 2004, Churchill Livingstone.)

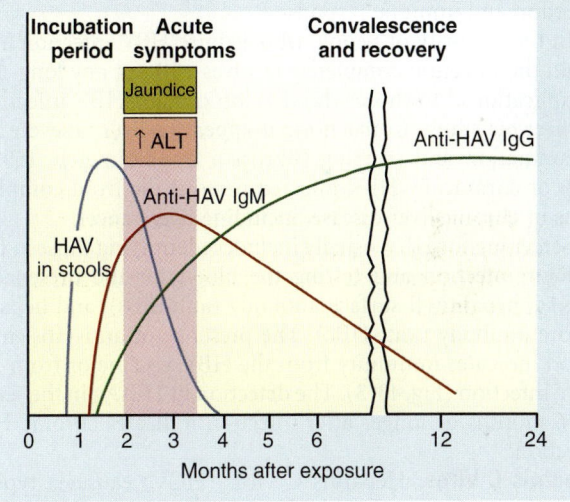

FIG. 43-2 Course of infection with hepatitis A virus *(HAV)*. *ALT,* Alanine aminotransferase. (From McCance KL, Huether SE: *Pathophysiology: the biologic basis for disease in adults and children,* ed 6, St Louis, 2010, Mosby.)

an infected food handler. Individuals at increased risk for hepatitis A infection include drug users (both injection and noninjection drugs), men who have sex with men (MSM), and persons traveling to developing countries.

The virus is present in feces during the incubation period. Therefore it can be carried and transmitted by persons who have undetectable, subclinical infections. The greatest risk of transmission occurs before clinical symptoms appear. HAV is found in feces 2 or more weeks before the onset of symptoms and up to 1 week after the onset of jaundice (Fig. 43-1). It is present only briefly in blood.

Anti-HAV (antibody to HAV) immunoglobulin (Ig) M appears in the serum as the stool becomes negative for the virus. Detection of hepatitis A IgM indicates acute hepatitis. Although not commonly tested clinically, hepatitis A IgG indicates past infection. IgG antibody provides lifelong immunity (Fig. 43-2). Hepatitis A vaccination and thorough hand washing are the best measures to prevent outbreaks. In the United States, the incidence of hepatitis A viral infection has declined since vaccination was recommended for at-risk persons and children (at the age of 1 year).[1]

Hepatitis B Virus. Hepatitis B virus (HBV) is a blood-borne pathogen that can cause either acute or chronic hepatitis. Since the 1990s, the incidence of HBV infection has decreased because of the widespread use of the HBV vaccine.[1]

Asians and Pacific Islanders have a high incidence of HBV hepatitis. Perinatal transmission is the most common mode of transmission in this population and often results in chronic HBV infection.

HBV is a deoxyribonucleic acid (DNA) virus. It can be transmitted several ways: (1) perinatally from mothers infected with HBV to their infants; (2) percutaneously (e.g., IV drug use, accidental needle-stick punctures); or (3) via small cuts on mucosal surfaces and exposure to infectious blood, blood products, or other body fluids (e.g., semen, vaginal secretions, saliva).

Sexual transmission is a common mode of HBV transmission. MSM (especially those practicing unprotected anal intercourse) are at an increased risk for HBV infection. It is generally believed that casual encounters such as hugging, kissing, and sharing utensils do not transmit the disease.

Other at-risk individuals include those who live with chronically HBV-infected persons, patients on hemodialysis, health care personnel, and public safety workers. HBV can live on a dry surface for at least 7 days, and it is 50 to 100 times more infectious than human immunodeficiency virus (HIV).[2]

HBV has been detected in almost every body fluid. Infected semen and saliva contain much lower concentrations of HBV than blood, but the virus can be transmitted via these secretions. If gastrointestinal (GI) bleeding occurs, feces can be contaminated with the virus from the blood. There is no evidence that urine, feces (without GI bleeding), breast milk, tears, and sweat are infectious. Organ and tissue transplantation is another potential source of infection. However, in some patients with acute hepatitis B, there is no readily identifiable risk factor.[1]

HBV is a complex structure with three distinct antigens: surface antigen (HBsAg), core antigen (HBcAg), and e antigen (HBeAg). Each antigen along with its corresponding antibody may appear or disappear in serum depending on the phase of infection and immune response.

In the majority of people who acquire HBV infection as an adult, the infection completely resolves without any long-term complications.[3] In those who develop chronic HBV infections, the liver may range from a normal-appearing liver to severe liver inflammation and scarring (fibrosis). Approximately 15% to 25% of chronically HBV-infected persons die from complications of chronic liver disease, including liver cancer.

Screening for HBV usually includes identifying those at high risk for infection and testing the blood for the presence of HBsAg, hepatitis B surface antibody (anti-HBs), and hepatitis B core antibody (anti-HBc). The presence of anti-HBs in the blood indicates immunity from the HBV vaccine or from past HBV infection (Fig. 43-3). The detection of HBsAg in the serum for 6 months or longer after infection indicates chronic HBV infection.

Hepatitis C Virus. Hepatitis C virus (HCV) causes a type of hepatitis that can result in both acute illness as well as chronic infection. Acute hepatitis C, which can be mild in presentation, can be difficult to detect unless a diagnosis is made with laboratory testing. The most common causes of acute hepatitis C outbreaks are among injection drug users and HIV-positive MSM.

HCV is an RNA virus that is primarily transmitted percutaneously. The most common mode of HCV transmission is the sharing of contaminated needles and equipment among injection drug users. High-risk sexual behavior (e.g., unprotected sex, multiple partners), especially among MSM, is associated with increased risk of transmission.

Approximately 10% of all cases of HCV infection in the United States are due to occupational exposure, hemodialysis,

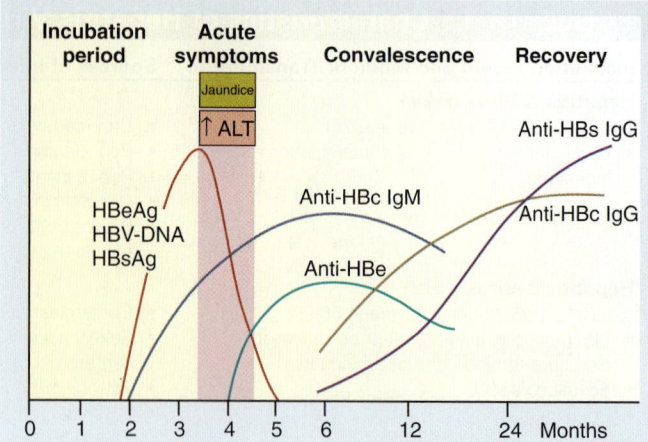

FIG. 43-3   Course of infection with hepatitis B virus *(HBV)*. *ALT,* Alanine aminotransferase; *anti-HBc,* antibody to hepatitis B core antigen; *anti-HBe,* antibody to HBeAg; *anti-HBs,* antibody to HBsAg; *HBeAg,* hepatitis B e antigen; *HBsAg,* hepatitis B surface antigen. (From McCance KL, Huether SE: *Pathophysiology: the biologic basis for disease in adults and children,* ed 6, St Louis, 2010, Mosby.)

and perinatal transmission.[2] The risk of perinatal HCV transmission is higher in women who are co-infected with both HIV and HCV. Persons who were given blood or blood products before 1992 (when blood product testing for HCV began) are at higher risk for chronic HCV infection and should be routinely tested.[4] Some patients with HCV infection cannot identify a source of infection.

The majority of patients who acquire hepatitis C usually develop chronic infection. However, because signs and symptoms of HCV infection are generally mild, most individuals are unaware of their infection. Hepatitis C is the most common cause of chronic liver disease and liver failure, with 20% to 30% of these patients developing cirrhosis and eventually liver failure and/or liver cancer.[4] Along with chronic HBV, HCV account for 80% of the cases of liver cancer.[5] HCV hepatitis is the most common indication for liver transplantation in the United States.[4]

Because of the 15- to 20-year delay between infection and the clinical manifestations of liver damage, long-term effects of HCV infection pose important health care challenges.

Persons at risk for HCV infection are also at risk for HBV and HIV infections. About 30% to 40% of HIV-infected patients also have HCV. This high rate of co-infection is primarily related to IV drug use. Co-infection with HIV and HCV places the patient at greater risk for progression to cirrhosis.

Screening for HCV infection should be conducted on those at increased risk. This includes individuals who engage in high-risk sexual practices, injection drug users, persons of the "baby boomer" generation born between 1945 and 1965, those who may have had blood or blood products prior to 1992, and/or those who have abnormal liver function tests. A positive antibody test for HCV (anti-HCV) is usually sufficient for a diagnosis.[4]

Hepatitis D Virus. Hepatitis D virus (HDV), also called *delta virus,* is uncommon in the United States. HDV is a defective single-stranded RNA virus that cannot survive on its own and requires hepatitis B to replicate. It can be acquired at the same time as HBV, or a person with HBV can be infected with HDV at a later time. HDV is also transmitted percutaneously, similar to HBV. It can cause a spectrum of illness ranging from an asymptomatic chronic carrier state to acute liver failure. There is no vaccine for HDV. However, vaccination against HBV reduces the risk of HDV co-infection.

Hepatitis E Virus. Hepatitis E virus (HEV) is an RNA virus transmitted by the fecal-oral route. The usual mode of transmission is drinking contaminated water. Hepatitis E infection occurs primarily in developing countries, with epidemics reported in India, Asia, Mexico, and Africa. Only a few cases of HEV have been reported in the United States, primarily in persons who recently traveled to an HEV-endemic area.

Pathophysiology

Liver. In viral hepatitis, hepatocytes become targets of the virus in one of two ways: through direct action of the virus (as in HCV infection) or through a cell-mediated immune response to the virus (as in HBV infection).[5,6]

During acute viral hepatitis, large numbers of infected hepatocytes are destroyed. The destruction of hepatocytes leads to a wide range of liver-related dysfunction. Bile production, coagulation, blood glucose, and protein metabolism can be affected. Detoxification and processing of drugs, hormones, and metabolites (e.g., ammonia from protein catabolism) may also be disrupted.

After resolution of an acute infection, liver cells can regenerate. If no complications occur, the liver can resume its normal appearance and function. In certain cases, the acute hepatitis can become so severe and irreversible that people experience liver failure or even death.

TABLE 43-2 Manifestations of Hepatitis	
Acute Hepatitis	**Chronic Hepatitis**
• Anorexia	• ALT, AST elevations (may be normal in some people)
• Dark urine	• Anemia
• Decreased sense of taste and smell	• Ascites and lower extremity edema
• Diarrhea or constipation	• Asterixis ("liver flap")
• Fatigue, lethargy, malaise	• Bleeding abnormalities (thrombocytopenia, easy bruising, prolonged clotting time)
• Flu-like symptoms (e.g., headache)	• Fatigue, malaise
• Hepatomegaly	• Hepatic encephalopathy: confusion, difficulty concentrating, easy agitation
• Jaundice	
• Clay-colored stools	• Hepatomegaly
• Low-grade fever	• Hyperbilirubinemia
• Lymphadenopathy	• Jaundice
• Myalgias and/or arthralgias	• Myalgias and/or arthralgias
• Nausea, vomiting	• Palmar erythema
• Pruritus	• Spider angiomas
• Right upper quadrant tenderness	
• Splenomegaly	
• Weight loss	

ALT, Alanine aminotransferase; *AST,* aspartate aminotransferase.

Chronic viral hepatitis can be insidious and silent, causing persistent and continual destruction of infected hepatocytes. Over time scar tissue can develop, which leads to fibrosis and compromised liver function. Fibrosis can lead to cirrhosis and liver failure. Cirrhosis is a generally irreversible condition that can increase one's risk for liver dysfunction, portal hypertension, and primary liver cancer. (Cirrhosis is discussed later in this chapter.)

Systemic Effects. In the early phases of hepatitis infection, antigen-antibody complexes between the virus and its corresponding antibody form circulating immune complexes. The circulating immune complexes activate the complement system (see Chapter 11). The clinical manifestations of this activation are rash, angioedema, arthritis, fever, and malaise. *Cryoglobulinemia* (abnormal proteins found in the blood), glomerulonephritis, and vasculitis can occur secondary to immune complex activation.

Clinical Manifestations and Complications

The clinical manifestations of the different viral hepatitis infections can be classified into acute hepatitis and chronic hepatitis (Table 43-2).

Acute Hepatitis. Many patients with acute hepatitis have no symptoms and may not even know they have been infected. However, others may have intermittent or ongoing anorexia, lethargy, nausea, vomiting, low-grade fever, skin rashes, diarrhea or constipation, malaise, fatigue, myalgias, arthralgias, other flu-like symptoms, and right upper quadrant tenderness (caused by liver inflammation).

Although the acute phase of viral hepatitis varies depending on the type of hepatitis, it usually lasts from 1 to 6 months. During this time, the patient may have a decreased sense of smell and find food repugnant. Smokers may have distaste for cigarettes. Physical examination often reveals hepatomegaly, lymphadenopathy, abdominal tenderness, and sometimes splenomegaly. The acute phase is the period of maximal infectivity.

A patient in the acute phase of hepatitis may be *icteric* (jaundiced) or anicteric. (Types of jaundice are presented in

TABLE 43-3 Classification of Jaundice

	Hemolytic Jaundice	Hepatocellular Jaundice	Obstructive Jaundice
Causes	• Blood transfusion reactions, sickle cell crisis, hemolytic anemia.	• Hepatitis, cirrhosis, hepatocellular carcinoma.	• Hepatitis, cirrhosis, hepatocellular carcinoma. • Common bile duct obstruction from stone(s), biliary strictures, sclerosing cholangitis, and pancreatic cancer.
Description	• Caused by increased breakdown of RBCs, which produces an increased amount of unconjugated bilirubin in blood. • Liver is unable to handle increased load.	• Results from liver's altered ability to take up bilirubin from blood or to conjugate or excrete it. • In hepatocellular disease, damaged hepatocytes leak bilirubin.	• Results from decreased or obstructed flow of bile through liver or biliary duct system. • Obstruction may occur in intrahepatic or extrahepatic bile ducts. • Intrahepatic obstructions are due to swelling or fibrosis of the liver's canaliculi and bile ducts.
Diagnostic Findings ***Serum Bilirubin***			
Unconjugated (indirect)	↑	↑	↑
Conjugated (direct)	Normal	↑ or ↓ (severe disease)	↑
Urine Bilirubin	Negative	↑	↑
Urobilinogen			
Stool	↑	Normal, ↓	↓
Urine	↑	Normal, ↑	↓

Table 43-3.) Jaundice, a yellowish discoloration of body tissues, results from an alteration in normal bilirubin metabolism or disruption of the flow of bile into the hepatic or biliary duct systems. (Normal bilirubin metabolism is presented in Fig. 38-4.)

The urine may appear darker because of excess bilirubin being excreted by the kidneys. If conjugated bilirubin cannot pass into the intestines from the liver because of obstruction or inflammation of the bile ducts, the stools will be light or clay colored.

Pruritus (intense generalized itching) sometimes accompanies jaundice. It occurs as a result of the accumulation of bile salts beneath the skin. The pruritus can be intolerable to the patient.

As jaundice fades, the convalescent phase begins. The convalescent phase can last for weeks to months, with an average of 2 to 4 months. During this period, patients typically experience malaise and easy fatigability. Hepatomegaly remains for several weeks, but splenomegaly (if present) subsides during this period.

Most patients with acute viral hepatitis recover completely. Almost all cases of acute hepatitis A resolve. However, some patients may have a relapse in the first 2 to 3 months after the infection. The disappearance of jaundice does not mean the patient has totally recovered. Some HBV infections and the majority of HCV infections result in chronic hepatitis.

The overall mortality rate for acute hepatitis is less than 1%. The mortality rate is higher in older adults and those with underlying debilitating illnesses (including chronic liver disease).

Complications that can result from acute hepatitis are acute liver failure, chronic hepatitis, cirrhosis of the liver, portal hypertension, and hepatocellular carcinoma.

Acute Liver Failure. Occasionally acute liver failure (fulminant hepatic failure) may occur, which is a serious condition with a poor prognosis. Manifestations include encephalopathy, gastrointestinal bleeding, disseminated intravascular coagulation, fever with leukocytosis, renal manifestations (oliguria, azotemia), ascites, edema, hypotension, respiratory failure, hypoglycemia, bacterial infections, thrombocytopenia, and coagulopathies. Liver transplantation is usually the cure for these patients. (Acute liver failure is discussed in this chapter on p. 996.)

Chronic Hepatitis. Manifestations of chronic hepatitis are presented in Table 43-2. Chronic HBV is more likely to develop in infants born to infected mothers and in those who acquire the infection before age 5 than in those who acquire the virus after age 5.[3]

Alterations in the patient's cellular immune response may be important in the development of the chronic HBsAg carrier state and the progression of acute HBV to chronic HBV. For example, persons with chronic kidney disease undergoing dialysis tend to have a depressed cellular immune response, which may explain why they are more at risk for developing chronic infection after acquiring the acute form of HBV.[6]

HCV infection is more likely than HBV to become chronic.[4] As previously mentioned, many patients with chronic HCV infection develop chronic liver disease, cirrhosis, portal hypertension, and liver cancer. Risk factors for progression to cirrhosis include male gender, alcohol consumption, concomitant fatty liver disease, and excess iron deposition in the liver. People with metabolic syndrome (obesity, elevated cholesterol or triglycerides, hypertension, and diabetes mellitus) are also at risk for progression of HCV to cirrhosis.[4] In some patients, co-infection with HIV may also cause complications or require modification of treatment. Manifestations of chronic hepatitis include anemia and coagulation problems (easy bruising and bleeding). The liver is responsible for producing clotting factors, so in persons with liver disease, clotting and bleeding times can be impaired or prolonged.

Skin manifestations may include spider angiomas, palmar erythema, and gynecomastia. Some patients have splenomegaly, hepatomegaly, or cervical lymph node enlargement.

In patients with severe liver damage, *hepatic encephalopathy* is a potentially life-threatening spectrum of neurologic, psychiatric, and motor disturbances. Hepatic encephalopathy results from the liver's inability to remove toxins (especially ammonia) from the blood. (Hepatic encephalopathy is discussed later in this chapter on p. 990.)

Ascites, a common manifestation of hepatitis (especially chronic hepatitis), is the accumulation of excess fluid in the peritoneal cavity. Fluid accumulates due to reduced protein levels in the blood, which reduces the plasma oncotic pressure. (Ascites is discussed later in this chapter on p. 988.)

TABLE 43-4 Diagnostic Studies

Viral Hepatitis

Virus	Tests	Significance
A	Anti-HAV immunoglobulin M (IgM)	Acute infection
	Anti-HAV immunoglobulin G (IgG)	Previous infection or immunization. Not routinely done in clinical practice
B	HBsAg (hepatitis B surface antigen)	Marker of infectivity
		Present in acute or chronic infection
		Positive in chronic carriers
	Anti-HBs (hepatitis B surface antibody)	Indicates previous infection with HBV or immunization
	HBeAg (hepatitis B e antigen)	Indicates high infectivity
		Used to determine the clinical management of patients with chronic hepatitis B
	Anti-HBe (hepatitis B e antibody)	Indicates previous infection
		In chronic hepatitis B, indicates a low viral load and low degree of infectivity
	Anti-HBc (antibody to hepatitis B core antigen) IgM	Indicates acute infection
		Does not appear after vaccination
	Anti-HBc IgG	Indicates previous infection or ongoing infection with hepatitis B
		Does not appear after vaccination
	HBV DNA quantitation	Indicates active ongoing viral replication
		Best indicator of viral replication and effectiveness of therapy in patient with chronic hepatitis B
	HBV genotyping	Indicates the genotype of HBV
C	Anti-HCV (antibody to HCV)	Marker for acute or chronic infection with HCV
	HCV RNA quantitation	Indicates active ongoing viral replication
	HCV genotyping	Indicates the genotype of HCV
D	Anti-HDV	Present in past or current infection with HDV
	HDV Ag (hepatitis D antigen)	Present within a few days after infection
E*	Anti-HEV IgM and IgG	Present 1 wk-2 mo after illness onset
	HEV RNA quantitation	Indicates active ongoing viral replication

A, Hepatitis A virus (HAV); *B*, hepatitis B virus (HBV); *C*, hepatitis C virus (HCV); *D*, hepatitis D virus (HDV); *E*, hepatitis E virus (HEV).
*Currently, no serologic tests to diagnose HEV infection are commercially available in the United States. However, diagnostic tests are available in research laboratories to detect IgM and IgG anti-HEV and HEV RNA levels.

Diagnostic Studies

The only definitive way to distinguish among the various types of viral hepatitis is by testing the patient's blood for the specific antigen or antibody. In some types of viral hepatitis, the blood can be tested for the viral load (viral level). Tests for the different types of viral hepatitis are presented in Table 43-4.

In viral hepatitis, many results of liver function tests show significant abnormalities such as those shown in Table 43-5.

Several tests are available to determine the presence of HCV. Initial testing for HCV infection includes HCV antibody testing. If the antibody test is positive, HCV RNA testing is done to assess for chronic infection; a positive result confirms chronic infection. A few patients may have a false-positive HCV antibody result with a negative HCV RNA test. If recent HCV infection is suspected, HCV RNA testing is usually done because it may take several weeks or longer for HCV antibodies to develop.

HCV RNA testing may used for immunocompromised patients (e.g., patient with HIV). Because of altered or delayed antibody response to HCV, these patients may not have detectable antibody levels even though they are infected with HCV.

Viral genotype testing is done in patients undergoing drug therapy for HBV or HCV infection. HBV has at least eight different genotypes (A to H). In some centers, HBV genotyping is performed before starting treatment. HBV genotype may be useful in predicting disease course and treatment outcomes.

HCV has six genotypes and more than 50 subtypes. In the United States, 75% of HCV infections are caused by HCV genotype 1. For patients who test positive for HCV, genotyping is obtained before drug therapy is started.[4] The genotype determines the choice and duration of therapy. It is also one of the strongest predictors of a patient's response to drug therapy.

TABLE 43-5 Diagnostic Findings in Acute Hepatitis

Test	Abnormal Finding	Etiology
Aminotransferases		
• Aspartate aminotransferase (AST)	Increased in acute phase	Liver cell injury
	Decreases as jaundice disappears	
• Alanine aminotransferase (ALT)	Increased in acute phase	Liver cell injury
	Decreases as jaundice disappears	
γ-Glutamyl transpeptidase (GGT)	Increased	Liver cell injury
Alkaline phosphatase	Moderately increased	Impaired excretory function of liver
Serum proteins		
• γ-Globulin	Normal or increased	Impaired clearance from liver
• Albumin	Normal or decreased	Liver cell injury
Serum bilirubin (total)	Increased to about 8-15 mg/dL (137-257 μmol/L)	Liver cell injury
Urinary bilirubin	Increased	Conjugated hyperbilirubinemia
Urinary urobilinogen	Increased 2-5 days before jaundice	Diminished reabsorption of urobilinogen
Prothrombin time	Prolonged	Decreased prothrombin production by liver

A liver biopsy is not indicated in acute hepatitis unless the diagnosis is in doubt. In chronic hepatitis, a liver biopsy may be done for histologic examination of liver cells and characterization of the degree of inflammation, fibrosis, or cirrhosis that may be present. A patient who has a bleeding disorder may not be an appropriate candidate for a percutaneous liver biopsy because of the risk of bleeding. In these patients, a transjugular biopsy may be an alternative. This type of biopsy consists of obtaining liver tissue through a rigid cannula introduced into one of the hepatic veins, typically using jugular venous access.

Techniques for noninvasive assessment of liver fibrosis may eventually replace the need for liver biopsy. Options include the use of ultrasound elastography (FibroScan), which uses an ultrasound transducer to determine the degree of liver fibrosis. FibroSure (FibroTest) is a biomarker that uses the results of serum tests (e.g., liver enzyme levels) to assess the extent of hepatic fibrosis.[7]

Interprofessional Care

There is no specific treatment for acute viral hepatitis. Most patients can be managed at home. Emphasis is on providing adequate nutrition and measures to rest the body and assist the liver to regenerate and repair (Table 43-6). Rest reduces the metabolic demands on the liver and promotes liver cell regeneration. The degree of rest depends on the severity of symptoms, but usually alternating periods of activity and rest are adequate. Counseling should include the importance of avoiding alcohol and notification of possible contacts for testing and prophylaxis, if indicated.

In patients with chronic viral hepatitis, care may involve hepatologists, infectious disease specialists, pharmacists,

---

TABLE 43-6 Interprofessional Care
Viral Hepatitis

Diagnostic Assessment
- History and physical examination
- Liver function tests
- Alanine aminotransferase (ALT)
- Aspartate aminotransferase (AST)
- Serum bilirubin
- Prothrombin time (PT) and INR
- Alkaline phosphatase
- γ-Glutamyl transpeptidase
- Hepatitis testing
  - *Hepatitis A:* Anti-HAV IgM
  - *Hepatitis B:* HBsAg, anti-HBs, HBeAg, anti-HBe, anti-HBc IgM and IgG, HBV DNA quantitation, HBV genotyping
  - *Hepatitis C:* Anti-HCV, HCV RNA quantitation, HCV genotyping
  - *Hepatitis D:* Anti-HDV, HDV Ag
- FibroScan
- FibroSure (FibroTest)

Management
Acute and Chronic
- Well-balanced diet
- Vitamin supplements
- Rest (degree of strictness varies)
- Avoidance of alcohol intake and drugs detoxified by liver

Chronic HBV and HCV
- Drug therapy (Table 43-7)

HAV, Hepatitis A virus; *HB,* hepatitis B; *HBeAg,* hepatitis B e antigen; *HBsAg,* hepatitis B surface antigen; *HBV,* hepatitis B virus; *HCV,* hepatitis C virus; *HDV Ag,* hepatitis D antigen; *HDV,* hepatitis D virus; *INR,* international normalized ratio.

---

dietitians, and mental health or substance abuse specialists. The role and extent of involvement of team members is based on the patient's specific needs.

Drug Therapy
Acute Hepatitis. There are no drug therapies for treating acute HAV infection. Treatment of acute HBV may be indicated only in patients with severe hepatitis and liver failure.

In acute hepatitis C, some patients may choose to be monitored for spontaneous clearance of the infection. For those patients who choose treatment, one of the direct-acting antivirals (DAAs) may be used. (DAAs are discussed later in the section on chronic hepatitis.)

Supportive drug therapy may include antihistamines for generalized itching and antiemetics for nausea. These drugs include promethazine (Phenergan) and ondansetron (Zofran).

🌿 COMPLEMENTARY & ALTERNATIVE THERAPIES
Milk Thistle (Silymarin)

Scientific Evidence
- Previous studies suggested that milk thistle may benefit the liver by protecting and promoting the growth of liver cells and inhibiting inflammation. These studies were small and not well designed.
- A meta-analysis found no real benefit from using milk thistle:
  - Silymarin was no better than placebo for chronic hepatitis C in people who had not responded to standard antiviral treatment.
  - Hepatitis C patients who used silymarin had fewer and milder symptoms of liver disease and somewhat better quality of life but no change in virus activity or liver inflammation.

Nursing Implications
- Appears to be well tolerated in recommended doses for up to 6 yr.
- May lower blood glucose.
- May interfere with the liver's cytochrome P450 enzyme system.

Source: National Center for Complementary and Alternative Therapy: Milk thistle. Retrieved from *https://nccih.nih.gov/health/milkthistle/ataglance.htm.*

Chronic Hepatitis B. Drug therapy for chronic HBV is focused on decreasing the hepatitis B viral load and liver enzymes, and in turn slowing the rate of disease progression. Long-term goals are preventing development of cirrhosis, portal hypertension, liver failure, and hepatocellular cancer. Current drug therapies for chronic HBV do not eradicate the virus but suppress viral replication and prevent complications of hepatitis B. First-line therapies now include primarily nucleoside and nucleotide analogs (Table 43-7) and occasionally interferon therapy.[8]

Nucleoside and nucleotide analogs. Nucleoside and nucleotide analogs inhibit viral DNA replication. HBV reproduces by making copies of its viral DNA nucleosides and nucleotides. The nucleoside and nucleotide analog drugs mimic normal building blocks for DNA, but are actually faulty viral DNA building blocks. Once they become incorporated into the viral DNA, they halt DNA synthesis.

Nucleoside and nucleotide analogs do not prevent all viral reproduction, but they can substantially lower the amount of virus in the body. These medications include lamivudine (Epivir), adefovir (Hepsera), entecavir (Baraclude), telbivudine (Tyzeka), and tenofovir (Viread). These oral medications are indicated in the treatment of chronic HBV when there is evidence of significant active viral replication and liver inflammation.[8]

Nucleoside and nucleotide analogs also reduce viral load, decrease liver damage, and decrease serum levels of liver

TABLE 43-7   Drug Therapy
Viral Hepatitis B and C

Drug Class	Examples	Mechanism of Action	Indication
Nucleoside and Nucleotide Analogs	adefovir dipivoxil (Hepsera) entecavir (Baraclude) lamivudine (Epivir HBV) telbivudine (Tyzeka) tenofovir (Viread) ribavirin* (Copegus, Rebetol, Ribasphere)	Inhibits HBV DNA polymerase enzyme by competing with natural substrates. Prevents viral replication	Chronic hepatitis B
Immune Modulator	pegylated interferon (PegIntron, Pegasys)	Has antiviral, antiproliferative, immune-regulating actions	Chronic hepatitis B and C†
Direct-Acting Antivirals ***NS3/4A Protease Inhibitors***	simeprevir (Olysio) grazoprevir‡ paritaprevir‡	Blocks viral protease enzyme. Prevents viral replication in genotype 1 HCV	Chronic hepatitis C
NS5B Polymerase Inhibitors	sofosbuvir (Sovaldi) dasabuvir‡	Nucleoside and nucleotide inhibitors of HCV polymerase. Prevent replication of RNA HCV	Chronic hepatitis C
NS5A Inhibitors	daclatasvir (Daklinza) ledipasvir‡ ombitasvir‡ elbasvir‡ velpatasvir‡	Blocks nonstructural protein 5A (NS5A) at early stage in RNA HCV replication	Chronic hepatitis C
Combination Therapy	sofosbuvir + ledipasvir (Harvoni) ombitasvir + paritaprevir + ritonavir§ + dasabuvir (Viekira Pak) ombitasvir + paritaprevir + ritonavir (Technivie) elbasvir + grazoprevir (Zepatier) sofosbuvir + velpatasvir (Epclusa)	More than one drug combined in single tablet. Drugs may be from the same or different classes.	Chronic hepatitis C

*Also used for chronic hepatitis C.
†Use of all oral or noninterferon therapies for chronic hepatitis C is preferred.
‡Used only in combination therapy.
§CYP3A inhibitor used to enhance the pharmacokinetics of the other agents.

enzymes. Most patients with HBV require long-term treatment with these medications. Frequently when these drugs are stopped, patients' (except those who have seroconverted) HBV DNA and liver enzyme levels return to pretreatment levels.

Severe exacerbations of hepatitis B can develop after discontinuation of treatment. If these drugs are discontinued for any reason, closely monitor liver function for several months.

Interferon. Interferon is a naturally occurring immune protein made by the body during an infection to recognize and respond to pathogens. It has antiviral, antiproliferative, and immune-modulating effects. (Interferon is discussed in Chapter 13 on p. 194.) Pegylated interferon (PegIntron, Pegasys) is given by subcutaneous injection.

The numerous side effects with interferon therapy, including flu-like symptoms (e.g., fever, malaise, fatigue), make adherence to therapy challenging for some patients. Currently the use of interferon is limited due to the availability of better tolerated and more effective oral treatments.

Patients receiving interferon should have blood counts and liver function tests performed every 4 to 6 weeks. Depression is a side effect of interferon. Patients must be screened for depression and other mood disorders before starting interferon treatment and monitored frequently while on therapy.[9]

Chronic Hepatitis C. Treatment of chronic hepatitis C is individualized and based on the genotype of the HCV, severity of liver disease, and presence of other health problems (e.g., HIV). Drug therapy is directed at eradicating the virus and preventing HCV-related complications.[10] Treatment for HCV primarily includes the use of direct-acting antivirals (DAAs) (Table 43-7), which block proteins needed for HCV replication.

With DAAs, patients complete treatment with oral drugs, typically with only 12 weeks of therapy. The majority of individuals who complete treatment with the DAAs are now able to cure their chronic HCV infection.

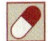 **DRUG ALERT   Ribavirin (Rebetol, Copegus, Ribasphere)**
- May cause severe birth defects. During treatment, pregnancy must be avoided both by women taking the drug and by women whose male partners are taking the drug.
- Monitor hemoglobin and hematocrit as it may cause anemia.

Many patients with HIV also have HCV. Patients who have stable HIV and relatively intact immune systems (CD4+ counts greater than 200/μL) are treated for HCV with the goal of eradicating HCV and reducing the risk of progression to cirrhosis. HCV treatment may reduce CD4+ counts and increase the patient's risk for anemia and leukopenia.

Patients with advanced fibrosis or cirrhosis can undergo drug therapy as long as liver decompensation (e.g., ascites, variceal rupture, jaundice, wasting, encephalopathy) is not present. **Nutritional Therapy.** No special diet is required in the treatment of viral hepatitis. Emphasis is placed on a well-balanced diet that the patient can tolerate. During acute viral hepatitis, adequate calories are important because the patient usually loses weight. If fat content is poorly tolerated because of decreased bile production, it should be reduced. Vitamin supplements, particularly B-complex vitamins and vitamin K, are frequently used. If anorexia, nausea, and vomiting are severe, IV solutions of glucose or supplemental enteral nutrition therapy may be used. Fluid and electrolyte balance must be maintained.

❖ NURSING MANAGEMENT: VIRAL HEPATITIS

◆ Nursing Assessment

Subjective and objective data that should be obtained from a person with hepatitis are presented in Table 43-8.

◆ Nursing Diagnoses

Nursing diagnoses for the patient with viral hepatitis may include, but are not limited to, the following:

- Imbalanced nutrition: less than body requirements *related to* anorexia and nausea
- Activity intolerance *related to* fatigue and weakness
- Risk for impaired liver function *related to* viral infection

---

TABLE 43-8 Nursing Assessment
*Hepatitis**

Subjective Data
Important Health Information

Past health history: Hemophilia, exposure to infected persons, ingestion of contaminated food or water. Exposure to benzene, carbon tetrachloride, or other hepatotoxic agents. Crowded, unsanitary living conditions. Exposure to contaminated needles. Recent travel, organ transplant recipient, exposure to new drug regimens, hemodialysis, transfusion of blood or blood products before 1992. HIV status (if known)
Medications: Use and misuse of acetaminophen, new prescription, over-the-counter, or herbal medications or supplements

Functional Health Patterns

Health perception–health management: IV drug and chronic alcohol use. Malaise, distaste for cigarettes (in smokers), high-risk sexual behaviors
Nutritional-metabolic: Weight loss, anorexia, nausea, vomiting. Feeling of fullness in right upper quadrant
Elimination: Dark urine, light-colored stools, constipation or diarrhea, skin rashes, hives
Activity-exercise: Fatigue, arthralgias, myalgias
Cognitive-perceptual: Right upper quadrant pain and liver tenderness, headache, pruritus
Role-relationship: Exposure as health care worker, resident in long-term care institution, incarceration, homelessness

Objective Data
General

Low-grade fever, lethargy, lymphadenopathy

Integumentary

Rash or other skin changes, jaundice, icteric sclera, injection sites

Gastrointestinal

Hepatomegaly, splenomegaly

Possible Diagnostic Findings

Elevated liver enzyme levels. ↑ serum total bilirubin, hypoalbuminemia, anemia, bilirubin in urine and increased urobilinogen, prolonged prothrombin time, positive tests for hepatitis, including anti-HAV IgM, HBsAg, anti-HBs, HBeAg, anti-HBe, anti-HBc IgM and IgG, HBV DNA quantitation, anti-HCV, HCV RNA quantitation, anti-HDV, HDV Ag. Abnormal liver scan, abnormal results on liver biopsy

HAV, Hepatitis A virus; *HBcAg,* hepatitis B core antigen; *HBeAg,* hepatitis B e antigen; *HBsAg,* hepatitis B surface antigen; *HBV,* hepatitis B virus; *HCV,* hepatitis C virus; *HDV Ag,* hepatitis D antigen; *HDV,* hepatitis D virus.
*Hepatitis includes both viral and nonviral causes. History questions should be tailored to the type of hepatitis.

Additional information on nursing diagnoses for the patient with hepatitis is presented in eNursing Care Plan 43-1 available on the website for this chapter.

◆ Planning

The overall goals are that the patient with viral hepatitis will (1) have relief of discomfort, (2) be able to resume normal activities, and (3) return to normal liver function without complications.

◆ Nursing Implementation

Health Promotion. Viral hepatitis is a public health problem. Your role is important in the prevention and control of this disease. It is helpful to understand the epidemiology of the different types of viral hepatitis before considering appropriate control measures. Preventive and control measures for hepatitis A, B, and C are summarized in Table 43-9.

◆ *Hepatitis A.* Outbreaks of viral hepatitis are usually due to HAV. Preventive measures include personal and environmental hygiene and health education to promote good sanitation. Hand washing is probably the most important precaution. Teach about careful hand washing after bowel movements and before eating.

Vaccination is the best protection against HAV. All children at 1 year of age should receive the vaccine. Adults at risk should also receive the vaccine. These include people who travel to areas with increased rates of hepatitis A, MSM, injecting and noninjecting drug users, persons with clotting factor disorders (e.g., hemophilia), and persons with chronic liver disease.

HAV vaccine is inactivated HAV. There are currently several forms of HAV vaccine: Havrix, Vaqta, and Avaxim. Primary immunization consists of a single dose administered IM in the deltoid muscle. A booster is recommended 6 to 12 months after the primary dose to ensure adequate antibody titers and long-term protection. The primary immunization provides immunity within 30 days after a single dose in more than 95% of those vaccinated.

Twinrix, a combined HAV and HBV vaccine, is available for people over 18 years of age. Immunization consists of three doses, given on a 0-, 1-, and 6-month schedule, the same schedule as that used for the single HBV vaccine. Twinrix may be given to high-risk individuals, including patients with chronic liver disease, users of illicit IV drugs, patients on hemodialysis, MSM, and people with clotting factor disorders who receive therapeutic blood products. The side effects of the vaccine are mild and usually limited to soreness and redness at the injection site.

Isolation is not required for HAV infection. For a patient with HAV infection, use infection control precautions. A private room is indicated if the patient is incontinent of stool or has poor personal hygiene.

Both hepatitis A vaccine and immune globulin (IG) are used for prevention of HAV infection after exposure to an infected person *(postexposure prophylaxis).* The vaccine is used for preexposure prophylaxis, and IG can be used either before or after exposure. IG provides temporary (1 to 2 months) passive immunity and is effective for preventing hepatitis A if given within 2 weeks after exposure. IG is recommended for persons who do not have anti-HAV antibodies and are exposed as a result of close (household, day care center) contact with persons who have HAV or foodborne exposure. Because patients with HAV are most infectious just before the onset of symptoms (the preicteric phase), those exposed through household contact or

TABLE 43-9 Preventive Measures for Viral Hepatitis*

Hepatitis A

General Measures
- Hand washing
- Proper personal hygiene
- Environmental sanitation
- Control and screening (signs, symptoms) of food handlers
- Serologic screening for those carrying virus
- Active immunization: HAV vaccine

Use of Immune Globulin
- Early administration (1-2 wk after exposure) to those exposed
- Prophylaxis for travelers to areas where hepatitis A is common if not vaccinated with HAV vaccine

Special Considerations for Health Care Personnel
- Wash hands after contact with a patient or removal of gloves
- Use infection control precautions

Hepatitis B and C

Percutaneous Transmission
- Screening of donated blood
- *HBV:* HBsAg
- *HCV:* Anti-HCV
- Use of disposable needles and syringes

Sexual Transmission
- Acute exposure: HBIG administration to sexual partner of HBsAg-positive person
- HBV vaccine series administered to uninfected sexual partners
- Condoms used for sexual intercourse

General Measures
- Hand washing
- Avoid sharing toothbrushes and razors
- HBIG administration for one-time exposure (needle stick, contact of mucous membranes with infectious material)
- Active immunization: HBV vaccine

Special Considerations for Health Care Personnel
- Use infection control precautions
- Reduce contact with blood or blood-containing secretions
- Handle the blood of patients as potentially infective
- Dispose of needles properly
- Use needleless IV access devices when available

HAV, Hepatitis A virus; *HBIG,* hepatitis B immune globulin; *HBsAg,* hepatitis B surface antigen; *HBV,* hepatitis B virus; *HCV,* hepatitis C virus.
*A suggested guideline for general practice to prevent you from contracting viral hepatitis from diagnosed and undiagnosed patients and carriers is for you to wear disposable gloves, goggles, and gowns (sometimes) when fecal or blood contamination is likely in handling (1) soiled bedpans, urinals, and catheters and (2) when the patient's bed linens are soiled by body excreta or secretions.

contracting HBV to reduce risks by maintaining good hygienic practices, including hand washing, and using gloves when expecting contact with blood. Patients should not share razors, toothbrushes, and other personal items. Teach patients to use a condom for sexual intercourse. In addition, the partner should be vaccinated.

The HBV vaccine is the best means of prevention. The HBV vaccines (Recombivax HB, Engerix-B) contain HBsAg, which promotes the synthesis of specific antibodies directed against HBV. The vaccine is given in a series of three IM injections in the deltoid muscle. The second dose is administered within 1 month of the first one, and the third one within 6 months of the first. The vaccine is more than 95% effective. Only minor adverse reactions have been reported with vaccination, including transient fever and soreness at the injection site. The vaccine is not contraindicated in pregnancy.

The first dose of hepatitis B vaccine should be given at birth, with the vaccine series completed by age 6 to 18 months. Older children and adolescents who did not previously receive the hepatitis B vaccine should also be vaccinated.[8] It is also important to vaccinate adults who are in the at-risk groups and are not immune. Household members of the patient with HBV should be tested and vaccinated if they are HBsAg and antibody negative. Hepatitis vaccination is recommended for patients with chronic kidney disease before they start dialysis. Dialysis patients should routinely have their antibody titer levels checked to determine the need for revaccination.

For postexposure prophylaxis, the HBV vaccine and hepatitis B immune globulin (HBIG) are used. HBIG contains antibodies to HBV and confers temporary passive immunity. HBIG is prepared from plasma of donors with a high titer of anti-HBs. HBIG is recommended for postexposure prophylaxis in cases of needle stick, mucous membrane contact, or sexual exposure and for infants born to mothers who are positive for HBsAg. Ideally HBIG should be given within 24 hours of exposure. The vaccine series should also be started.

The Centers for Disease Control and Prevention (CDC) recommends following standard precautions for the patient with HBV (see Table 14-9). This includes using disposable needles and syringes and disposing of them in puncture-resistant units without recapping, bending, or breaking.

◆ ***Hepatitis C.*** No vaccine is currently available for hepatitis C. Therefore it is important to identify individuals at high risk for contracting HCV and teach them how to reduce their risks. Primary measures to prevent HCV transmission include (1) screening of blood, organ, and tissue donors; (2) using infection control precautions; and (3) modifying high-risk behavior.

In the United States there are many people who have undiagnosed hepatitis C. Because of this, the Centers for Disease Control and Prevention (CDC) recommends universal screening for all persons born between 1945 and 1965.[11] The CDC does not recommend IG or antiviral agents (e.g., interferon) for postexposure prophylaxis for HCV infection (e.g., needle-stick exposure from an infected patient). After an acute exposure (e.g., needle stick), the person should have anti-HCV testing done. For the person exposed to HCV, baseline anti-HCV and ALT levels should be measured, with follow-up testing at 4 to 6 months. Testing for HCV RNA may be performed at 4 to 6 weeks.[11]

◆ **Acute Care.** In patients with hepatitis, assess for the presence and degree of jaundice. In light-skinned persons, jaundice is

foodborne outbreaks should receive IG. Although IG may not prevent infection in all persons, it may modify the illness to a subclinical infection. When hepatitis A occurs in a food handler, IG should be administered to all other food handlers at the establishment. Patrons may also need to be given IG.

Persons who are exposed to HAV who have received a dose of HAV vaccine more than 1 month previously or who have a history of laboratory-confirmed HAV infection do not require IG.

◆ ***Hepatitis B.*** The best way to reduce HBV infection is to identify those at risk, screen them for HBV, and vaccinate those who have not been infected. Teach individuals at high risk of

usually observed first in the sclera of the eyes and later in the skin. In dark-skinned persons, jaundice is observed in the hard palate of the mouth and inner canthus of the eyes. The urine may have a dark brown or brownish red color because of bilirubin excretion from the kidneys. Comfort measures to relieve pruritus (if present), headache, and arthralgias are helpful.

? CHECK YOUR PRACTICE

You are caring for a 32-yr-old man who has acute hepatitis A. He has been having severe nausea and vomiting. He is admitted to the hospital for IV hydration and monitoring. The patient says, "I'm so weak and I feel like I'm going to vomit all the time. Isn't there something you can do to help me?"
- How would handle this situation?
- What information and teaching will you provide him?

Ensuring that the patient receives adequate nutrition is not always easy. The anorexia and distaste for food may cause nutritional problems. Assess the patient's tolerance of specific foods and eating pattern. Small, frequent meals may be preferable to three large ones and may also help prevent nausea. Often a patient with hepatitis finds that anorexia is not as severe in the morning, so it is easier to eat a good breakfast than a large dinner. Measures to stimulate the appetite, such as mouth care, antiemetics, and attractively served meals in pleasant surroundings, should be included in your nursing care plan. Drinking carbonated beverages and avoiding very hot or very cold foods may help alleviate anorexia. Adequate fluid intake (2500 to 3000 mL/day) is also important.

Rest is a critical factor in promoting hepatocyte regeneration. Assess the patient's response to the rest and activity plan, and modify it accordingly. Liver function tests and symptoms are used as a guide to activity level.

Psychologic and emotional rest is as essential as physical rest. Limited activity may produce anxiety and extreme restlessness in some patients. Diversion activities, such as reading and hobbies, may help a patient cope with the plan of care and ensure adequate rest.

◆ **Ambulatory Care.** Most patients with viral hepatitis are cared for at home. Assess the patient's knowledge of nutrition and provide the necessary dietary teaching. Caution the patient about overexertion and the need to follow the HCP's advice about when to return to work. For patients who suffer from fatigue, tell them to plan activities after periods of rest when energy levels are highest. Teach the patient and caregiver how to prevent transmission to other family members. Also teach what symptoms should be reported to the HCP.

Assess the patient for any manifestations of complications. These include bleeding tendencies with increasing prothrombin time values, manifestations of encephalopathy, sudden increase in weight and abdominal girth (may indicate fluid retention and/or ascites), bloody or tarry stools, vomiting of blood, or elevated liver enzymes.

Instruct the patient to have regular follow-ups for at least 1 year after the diagnosis of hepatitis. Because relapses occur with hepatitis B and C, teach the patient the symptoms of recurrence and the need for follow-up evaluations. All patients with chronic HBV or HCV should avoid alcohol, since it can accelerate disease progression.

It should also be noted that patients who are positive for HBsAg (chronic carrier status) or HCV antibody cannot be blood donors.

◆ **Evaluation**

Expected outcomes are that the patient with hepatitis will
- Maintain food and fluid intake adequate to meet nutritional needs
- Avoid alcohol and other hepatotoxic agents
- Demonstrate gradual increase in activity tolerance
- Perform daily activities with scheduled rest periods

Additional information on expected outcomes for the patient with hepatitis is presented in eNursing Care Plan 43-1 available on the website for this chapter.

DRUG- AND CHEMICAL-INDUCED LIVER DISEASES

Alcohol consumption is the most frequent cause of both acute and chronic liver disease. It can cause injury and subsequent necrosis of liver tissue. Alcohol consumption can cause a spectrum of manifestations, ranging from mild elevation in liver enzymes (aspartate aminotransferase [AST] and alanine aminotransferase [ALT]) to acute alcoholic hepatitis. It may also cause advanced fibrosis and cirrhosis, which usually occurs after decades of excessive alcohol intake. Patients may also have serious liver disease caused by another chronic disease (e.g., chronic HCV infection) in combination with alcoholic liver disease, which can significantly compound the problem.

Acute alcoholic hepatitis is a syndrome of hepatomegaly, jaundice, elevation of liver enzyme tests (AST, ALT, alkaline phosphate), low-grade fever, and possibly ascites and prolonged prothrombin time. These manifestations may improve with cessation of alcohol intake.

Even at the end-stage of cirrhosis, abstinence can result in significant reversal in some patients. If liver function does not recover after abstaining from alcohol for 6 months or longer, liver transplantation may be considered.

Chemical hepatotoxicity is liver injury caused by exposure to certain compounds (e.g., carbon tetrachloride, gold compounds). Some agents can cause hepatotoxicity, while others may induce cholestasis, necrosis, or liver cancer. Fortunately because of the declining use of these agents, the incidence of chemically induced liver toxicity has diminished since the 1980s.

Drug-induced liver injury (DILI) is one of the more common causes of jaundice.[12] Many medications (prescription, over-the-counter [OTC], diet and herbal supplements) can cause an increase in liver enzymes and, in severe cases, jaundice and acute liver failure. The pattern of injury depends on the drug causing the reaction. The most common cause of DILI is acetaminophen. In patients with chemical hepatotoxicity or DILI, the agents that are identified as the cause of liver injury should be stopped or discontinued.

💊 DRUG ALERT   Acetaminophen (Tylenol)

- Drug is safe if taken at recommended levels. However, its prevalence in a variety of pain relievers, fever reducers, and cough medicines may mean that patients do not realize they are taking several drugs that all contain acetaminophen and overdose may occur.
- Acute liver failure can occur as a result of overdosing, either intentionally or unintentionally.
- The FDA has asked drug manufacturers to limit the strength of acetaminophen in prescription drug products to 325 mg per tablet, capsule, or other dosage unit, making these products safer.
- Combining the drug with alcoholic beverages increases the risk of liver damage.

AUTOIMMUNE, GENETIC, AND METABOLIC LIVER DISEASES

Autoimmune Hepatitis

Autoimmune hepatitis is a chronic inflammatory disorder of the liver in which the patient's own immune system attacks the liver. The cause of this condition is unknown. Autoimmune hepatitis is characterized by the presence of autoantibodies and high levels of serum immunoglobulins. It frequently occurs together with other autoimmune diseases.

The majority of patients with autoimmune hepatitis are women. Laboratory tests useful in the diagnosis include antinuclear antibody (ANA) and/or anti–smooth muscle antibody testing (ASMA). A liver biopsy is usually done to confirm the diagnosis and guide the treatment decision.[13]

Although autoimmune hepatitis can cause acute liver failure, the spectrum of disease is variable, with most patients developing chronic hepatitis. Untreated autoimmune hepatitis can progress to cirrhosis. Prednisone with or without azathioprine (Imuran) is the recommended treatment for active autoimmune hepatitis. Cyclosporine (Gengraf), tacrolimus (Prograf, FK506), budesonide (Entocort), methotrexate, and mycophenolate mofetil (CellCept) have also been used in patients who do not respond to prednisone and azathioprine.[13]

Wilson's Disease

Wilson's disease is an autosomal recessive disorder involving cellular copper transport. A defect in biliary excretion leads to accumulation of copper in the liver, causing progressive liver injury and cirrhosis. Approximately 1 in 40,000 people have Wilson's disease. It affects both men and women equally. Symptoms appear between ages 5 and 35.[14]

Once cirrhosis occurs, copper leaks into the plasma, leading to multiple complications including neurologic, hematologic, and renal disease. The hallmark of Wilson's disease is corneal Kayser-Fleischer rings. These are brownish red rings that can be seen in the cornea near the limbus on eye examination. Low serum ceruloplasmin levels and measurable copper concentrations from liver biopsy samples are also present. Diagnosis is based on clinical findings, including the corneal rings and neurologic symptoms. First-degree relatives of patients with Wilson's disease should be screened for the disease.

The recommended initial treatment of symptomatic patients or those with active disease is chelating agents such as D-penicillamine (Cuprimine) or trientine (Syprine), which promote the excretion of urinary copper. Zinc acetate (Galzin), which has also been used as therapy, interferes with the absorption of copper. Once the amount of copper in the body has been reduced, treatment focuses on preventing copper from building up again. When liver damage is severe, liver transplantation may be required.

Hemochromatosis

Hemochromatosis is a condition in which excessive amounts of iron accumulate in the body. Although it is primarily caused by a genetic defect *(hereditary hemochromatosis)*, it may also be caused by liver disease and chronic blood transfusions that are used to treat thalassemia and sickle cell disease. (Hemochromatosis is discussed in Chapter 30.)

Primary Biliary Cholangitis

Primary biliary cholangitis (PBC), formerly known as primary biliary cirrhosis, is a chronic disease of the small bile ducts of the liver. In PBC, there is a T cell–mediated attack of the small bile duct cells, resulting in loss of bile ducts and ultimately *cholestasis* (blockage of bile flow). Over time, this leads to liver fibrosis and cirrhosis.

Most patients diagnosed with PBC are women between ages 30 and 65.[15] The disease is associated with other autoimmune disorders such as rheumatoid arthritis, Sjögren's syndrome, and scleroderma. Elevated serum alkaline phosphatase levels, antimitochondrial antibodies (AMAs), ANAs, and serum lipid levels are seen in patients with PBC.

The goals of treatment are the suppression of ongoing liver damage, prevention of complications, and symptom management. Drugs for PBC include ursodeoxycholic acid (ursodiol [Actigall]), a bile acid, and obeticholic acid (Ocaliva), which decreases the bile in the liver. Management focuses on preventing or minimizing malabsorption, skin disorders such as pruritus and xanthomas (cholesterol deposits in the skin), hyperlipidemia, vitamin deficiencies, anemia, and fatigue. Cholestyramine is used to treat pruritus. Patients are monitored for progression to cirrhosis. Liver transplantation is a treatment option for end-stage liver disease in patients with PBC.

Primary Sclerosing Cholangitis

Primary sclerosing cholangitis (PSC) is a disease of unknown etiology characterized by chronic inflammation, fibrosis, and strictures (narrowing) of the medium and large bile ducts both inside and outside the liver. The majority of patients with PSC also have ulcerative colitis. Complications of PSC can include cholangitis, cholestasis with jaundice, cholangiocarcinoma (bile duct cancer), and cirrhosis.

Drug therapy is not beneficial. Treatment is directed at reducing the incidence of biliary complications and screening for bile duct and colorectal cancer, which is related to the high incidence of ulcerative colitis. Patients with advanced liver disease may require liver transplantation.

Nonalcoholic Fatty Liver Disease and Nonalcoholic Steatohepatitis

Nonalcoholic fatty liver disease (NAFLD) refers to a wide spectrum of liver diseases ranging from a fatty liver (steatosis) to nonalcoholic steatohepatitis (NASH) to cirrhosis. The term *nonalcoholic* is used because NAFLD and NASH occur in individuals who do not consume excessive amounts of alcohol. However, a pathologic analysis of liver cells in NAFLD is similar to that found in alcoholic liver disease.

The common characteristic of NAFLD is the accumulation of fatty infiltration in the hepatocytes. In NASH the fat accumulation is associated with varying degrees of inflammation and fibrosis of the liver. If NASH is left untreated, it can become a serious liver disease that can cause cirrhosis, hepatocellular cancer, and liver failure.

Currently, NAFLD affects about 10% to 20% of the U.S. population. This percentage is increasing because of the growing number of people who are obese. NAFLD should be considered in patients with risk factors such as obesity, diabetes, hyperlipidemia, and hypertension (also known as *metabolic syndrome*). NASH affects 2% to 5% of the U.S. population.[16]

Elevations in liver function tests (ALT, AST) are often the first sign of NAFLD. Ultrasound and CT scans can be used to diagnose NAFLD. Definitive diagnosis is by a liver biopsy.

There is no currently approved treatment for NAFLD. The goal of therapy is directed at reducing risk factors, which includes (1) reducing body weight, hyperlipidemia, and hypertension and (2) managing diabetes.

CIRRHOSIS

Cirrhosis is the end-stage of liver disease. Cirrhosis is characterized by extensive degeneration and destruction of the liver cells. This results in the replacement of liver tissue by fibrosis (scar tissue) and regenerative nodules that occur from the liver's attempt to repair itself (Fig. 43-4). The development of cirrhosis usually happens after decades of chronic liver disease. Cirrhosis (combined with chronic liver diseases) ranks as the eighth leading cause of death in the United States. It is twice as common in men as compared to women.

Etiology and Pathophysiology

Any chronic liver disease, including disease from excessive alcohol intake and NAFLD, can cause cirrhosis. The most common causes of cirrhosis in the United States are chronic hepatitis C infection and alcohol-induced liver disease. In patients with alcohol-induced liver disease, some controversy exists as to whether the cause is the alcohol or the malnutrition

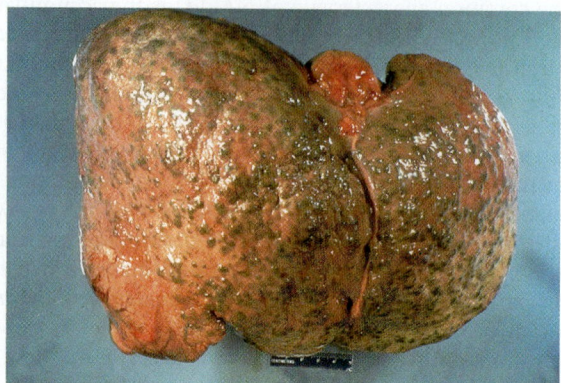

FIG. 43-4 Cirrhosis that developed secondary to alcoholism. The characteristic diffuse nodularity of the surface is due to the combination of regeneration and scarring of the liver. (From Kumar V, Abbas AK, Aster JC, Fausto N: *Robbins and Cotran pathologic basis of disease*, ed 8, Philadelphia, 2010, Saunders.)

that often coexists with alcoholism. Some cases of nutrition-related cirrhosis have resulted from extreme dieting, malabsorption, and obesity. Environmental factors and genetic predisposition may also lead to the development of cirrhosis, regardless of dietary or alcohol intake.

Approximately 20% of patients with chronic hepatitis C and 10% to 20% of those with chronic hepatitis B develop cirrhosis.[17] Chronic inflammation and cell necrosis from viral hepatitis can result in progressive fibrosis and, ultimately, cirrhosis. Chronic hepatitis combined with alcohol ingestion has a synergistic effect in accelerating liver damage.

Biliary causes of cirrhosis include primary biliary cholangitis (PBC) and primary sclerosing cholangitis (PSC). Both are described earlier in this chapter.

Cardiac cirrhosis includes a spectrum of hepatic derangements that result from long-standing, severe, right-sided heart failure. It causes hepatic venous congestion, parenchymal damage, necrosis of liver cells, and fibrosis over time. The treatment is aimed at managing the patient's underlying heart failure.

In cirrhosis, the liver cells attempt to regenerate, but the regenerative process is disorganized, resulting in abnormal blood vessel and bile duct architecture. The overgrowth of new and fibrous connective tissue distorts the liver's normal lobular structure, resulting in lobules of irregular size and shape with impeded blood flow. Eventually, irregular and disorganized liver regeneration, poor cellular nutrition, and hypoxia (from inadequate blood flow and scar tissue) result in decreased liver function.

Clinical Manifestations

Early Manifestations. Patients may be unaware of their liver condition because there are relatively few symptoms in early-stage disease. If an individual does have symptoms, it may include fatigue or an enlarged liver. Blood tests may show normal liver function (compensated cirrhosis). The diagnosis of cirrhosis is often made later when a patient manifests symptoms of more advanced liver disease.

Late Manifestations. Late manifestations result from liver failure and portal hypertension (Fig. 43-5). Jaundice, peripheral edema, and ascites develop gradually. Other late manifestations include skin lesions, hematologic disorders, endocrine disturbances, and peripheral neuropathies (Fig. 43-6). In the advanced stages, the liver becomes small and nodular. Liver function is dramatically diminished.

Jaundice. Jaundice results from decreased ability to conjugate and excrete bilirubin into the small intestines (Table 43-3). There is an overgrowth of connective tissue in the liver, which compresses the bile ducts and leads to an obstruction. This results in an increase in the bilirubin in the vascular system, and jaundice occurs. (Normal bilirubin metabolism is presented in Fig. 38-4.) The jaundice may be minimal or severe, depending on the degree of liver damage.

Skin Lesions. Various skin manifestations are commonly seen in cirrhosis. Spider angiomas (*telangiectasia* or *spider nevi*) are small, dilated blood vessels with a bright red center point and spiderlike branches. They occur on the nose, cheeks, upper trunk, neck, and shoulders. *Palmar erythema* (a red area that blanches with pressure) is located on the palms of the hands. Both of these lesions are due to an increase in circulating estrogen as a result of the damaged liver's inability to metabolize steroid hormones.

Hematologic Problems. Hematologic problems include thrombocytopenia, leukopenia, anemia, and coagulation disorders.

PATHOPHYSIOLOGY MAP

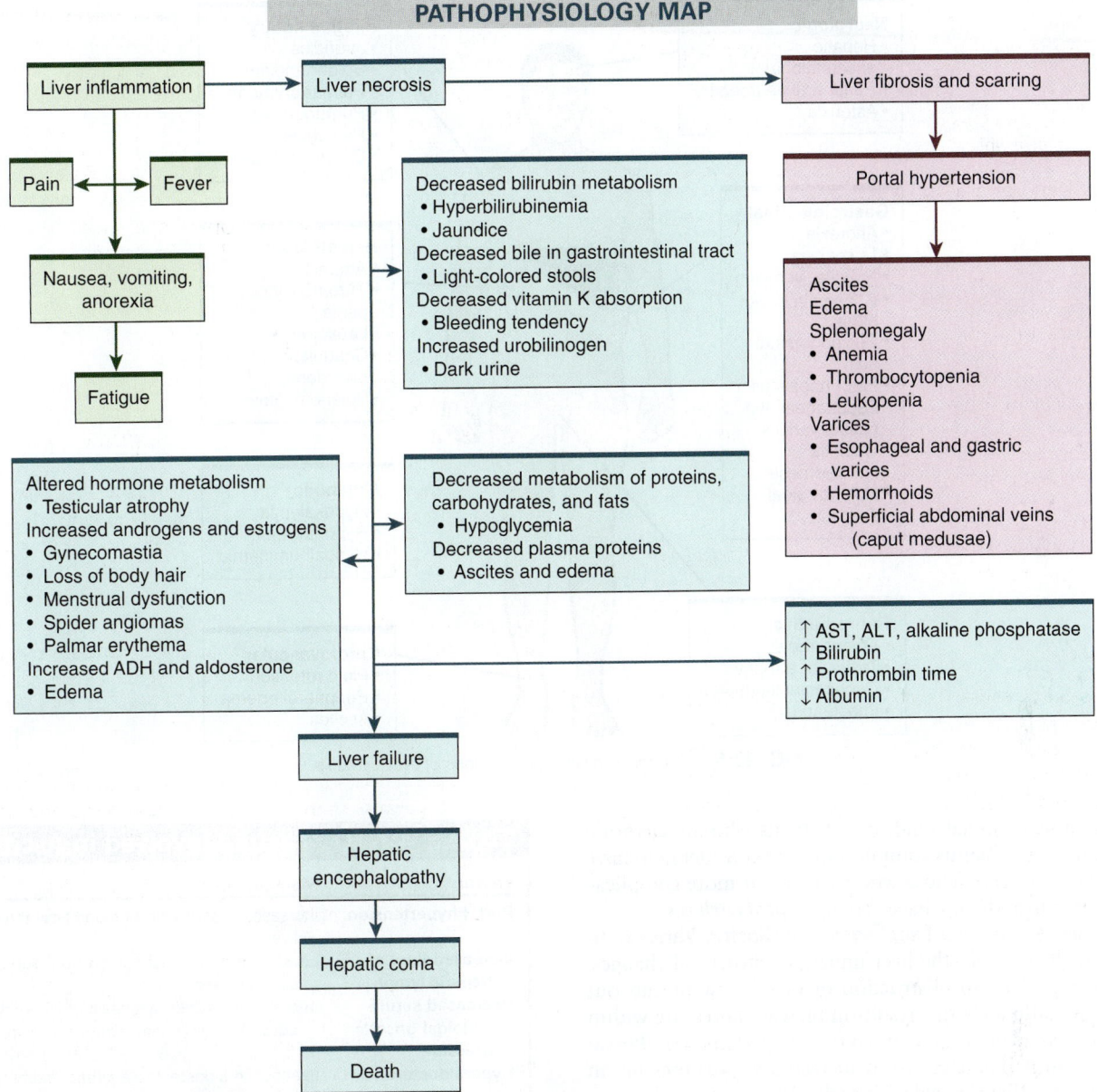

FIG. 43-5 Continuum of liver dysfunction in cirrhosis and resulting manifestations. *ADH,* Antidiuretic hormone; *ALT,* alanine aminotransferase; *AST,* aspartate aminotransferase. (Adapted from Huether SE, McCance KL: *Understanding pathophysiology,* ed 5, St Louis, 2012, Mosby.)

Thrombocytopenia, leukopenia, and anemia are thought to be caused by the splenomegaly that results from backup of blood from the portal vein into the spleen (portal hypertension). Overactivity of the enlarged spleen results in increased removal of blood cells from circulation. Anemia can result from inadequate red blood cell (RBC) production and survival, poor diet, poor absorption of folic acid, and bleeding from varices.

The coagulation problems result from the liver's inability to produce prothrombin and other factors essential for blood clotting. Manifestations of coagulation problems (bleeding tendencies) include epistaxis, purpura, petechiae, easy bruising, gingival bleeding, and heavy menstrual bleeding.

Endocrine Problems. The liver plays an important role in the metabolism of hormones, such as estrogen and testosterone. In men with cirrhosis, gynecomastia (benign growth of the glandular tissue of the male breast), loss of axillary and pubic hair, testicular atrophy, and impotence with loss of libido may

occur because of increased estrogen levels. Younger women with cirrhosis may develop amenorrhea, and older women may have vaginal bleeding. Aldosterone, an important hormone associated with fluid balance, can also be altered. If the liver fails to metabolize aldosterone adequately, it can lead to hyperaldosteronism with subsequent sodium and water retention and potassium loss.

Peripheral Neuropathy. Peripheral neuropathy is a common finding in alcoholic cirrhosis and is probably due to a dietary deficiency of thiamine, folic acid, and cobalamin. The neuropathy usually results in sensory and motor symptoms, but sensory symptoms may predominate.

Complications

Major complications of cirrhosis are portal hypertension, esophageal and gastric varices, peripheral edema, abdominal ascites, hepatic encephalopathy (mental status changes, including

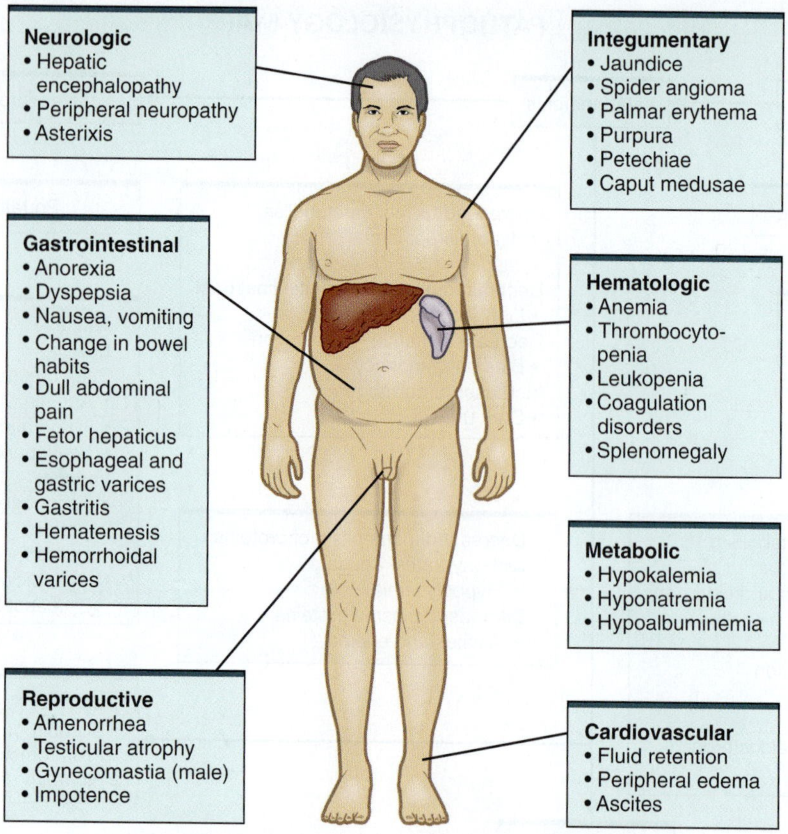

Neurologic
• Hepatic encephalopathy
• Peripheral neuropathy
• Asterixis

Integumentary
• Jaundice
• Spider angioma
• Palmar erythema
• Purpura
• Petechiae
• Caput medusae

Gastrointestinal
• Anorexia
• Dyspepsia
• Nausea, vomiting
• Change in bowel habits
• Dull abdominal pain
• Fetor hepaticus
• Esophageal and gastric varices
• Gastritis
• Hematemesis
• Hemorrhoidal varices

Hematologic
• Anemia
• Thrombocytopenia
• Leukopenia
• Coagulation disorders
• Splenomegaly

Metabolic
• Hypokalemia
• Hyponatremia
• Hypoalbuminemia

Reproductive
• Amenorrhea
• Testicular atrophy
• Gynecomastia (male)
• Impotence

Cardiovascular
• Fluid retention
• Peripheral edema
• Ascites

FIG. 43-6 Systemic clinical manifestations of liver cirrhosis.

coma), and hepatorenal syndrome. Patients who are cirrhotic but who have no obvious complications are considered to have *compensated cirrhosis.* Those who have one or more complications of their liver disease have *decompensated cirrhosis.*

Portal Hypertension and Esophageal and Gastric Varices. In patients with cirrhosis, the liver undergoes structural changes. These changes lead to obstruction of blood flow in and out of the liver. Ultimately this results in increased pressure within the liver's circulatory system (portal hypertension). Portal hypertension is characterized by increased venous pressure in the portal circulation, splenomegaly, large collateral veins, ascites, and gastric and esophageal varices.

As a way of reducing pressure, the body develops alternate circulatory pathways, referred to as *collateral circulation.*[18] The collateral channels commonly form in the lower esophagus, anterior abdominal wall, parietal peritoneum, and rectum. Varicosities (distended veins) develop in areas where the collateral and systemic circulations communicate, resulting in esophageal and gastric varices, *caput medusae* (ring of varices around the umbilicus), and hemorrhoids.

Esophageal varices are a complex of tortuous, enlarged veins at the lower end of the esophagus. Gastric varices are located in the upper portion of the stomach. These varices are fragile and do not tolerate high pressure, thus they can bleed easily. Large varices are more likely to bleed. Esophageal varices are responsible for approximately 80% of variceal hemorrhages.[19] The remaining 20% of variceal hemorrhages are due to gastric varices. The patient may present with melena or hematemesis. Ruptured esophageal varices are the most life-threatening complication of cirrhosis and considered a medical emergency.

TABLE 43-10	Factors Involved in Ascites
Factor	**Mechanism**
Portal hypertension	Increase in resistance of blood flow through liver.
Increased flow of hepatic lymph	Leaking of protein-rich lymph from surface of cirrhotic liver.
Decreased serum colloidal oncotic pressure	Impairment of liver synthesis of albumin. Loss of albumin into peritoneal cavity.
Hyperaldosteronism	Increase in aldosterone secretion stimulated by decreased renal blood flow. Decreased liver catabolism of circulating aldosterone.
Impaired water excretion	Increase in antidiuretic hormone (ADH) stimulated by decrease in renal blood flow.

Peripheral Edema and Ascites. Peripheral edema occurs in the lower extremities and presacral area. Peripheral edema can occur before, concurrently with, or after ascites development. Edema results from decreased colloidal oncotic pressure from impaired liver synthesis of albumin and increased portacaval pressure from portal hypertension.

Ascites is the accumulation of serous fluid in the peritoneal or abdominal cavity. It is a common manifestation of cirrhosis. Several mechanisms lead to ascites. One mechanism of ascites occurs with portal hypertension, which causes proteins to shift from the blood vessels into the lymph space (Fig. 43-7). When the lymphatic system is unable to carry off the excess proteins and water, they leak into the peritoneal cavity. The osmotic pressure of the proteins pulls additional fluid into the peritoneal cavity (Table 43-10).

PATHOPHYSIOLOGY MAP

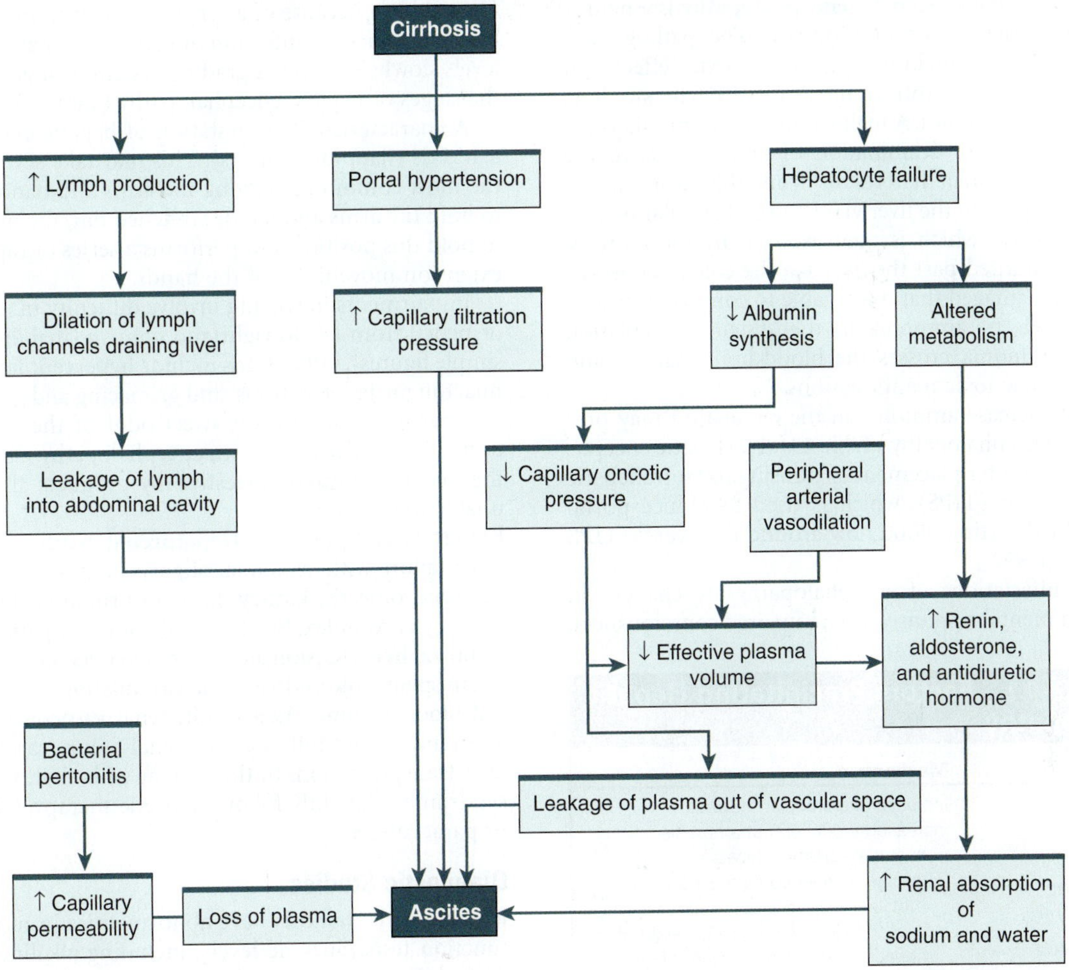

```
                              ┌──────────┐
                              │ Cirrhosis │
                              └──────────┘
          ┌────────────────────────┼──────────────────────────────┐
          ▼                        ▼                               ▼
  ┌──────────────┐        ┌──────────────────┐          ┌──────────────────┐
  │ ↑ Lymph      │        │ Portal           │          │ Hepatocyte       │
  │ production   │        │ hypertension     │          │ failure          │
  └──────────────┘        └──────────────────┘          └──────────────────┘
          │                        │                      ┌────────┴────────┐
          ▼                        ▼                      ▼                 ▼
  ┌──────────────┐        ┌──────────────────┐    ┌──────────────┐  ┌──────────────┐
  │ Dilation of  │        │ ↑ Capillary      │    │ ↓ Albumin    │  │ Altered      │
  │ lymph        │        │ filtration       │    │ synthesis    │  │ metabolism   │
  │ channels     │        │ pressure         │    └──────────────┘  └──────────────┘
  │ draining liver│       └──────────────────┘
  └──────────────┘                              ┌──────────────┐  ┌──────────────┐
          │                                     │ ↓ Capillary  │  │ Peripheral   │
          ▼                                     │ oncotic      │  │ arterial     │
  ┌──────────────┐                              │ pressure     │  │ vasodilation │
  │ Leakage of   │                              └──────────────┘  └──────────────┘
  │ lymph into   │
  │ abdominal    │                                    ┌──────────────┐  ┌──────────────────┐
  │ cavity       │                                    │ ↓ Effective  │  │ ↑ Renin,         │
  └──────────────┘                                    │ plasma       │→ │ aldosterone,     │
                                                      │ volume       │  │ and antidiuretic │
  ┌──────────────┐                                    └──────────────┘  │ hormone          │
  │ Bacterial    │                                                      └──────────────────┘
  │ peritonitis  │              ┌──────────────────────────────────┐
  └──────────────┘              │ Leakage of plasma out of          │
          │                     │ vascular space                    │
          ▼                     └──────────────────────────────────┘
  ┌──────────────┐  ┌──────────┐  ┌──────────┐  ┌──────────────────┐
  │ ↑ Capillary  │→ │ Loss of  │→ │ Ascites  │← │ ↑ Renal          │
  │ permeability │  │ plasma   │  │          │  │ absorption of    │
  └──────────────┘  └──────────┘  └──────────┘  │ sodium and water │
                                                 └──────────────────┘
```

FIG. 43-7 Mechanisms for development of ascites. (Adapted from Huether SE, McCance KL: *Understanding pathophysiology*, ed 5, St Louis, 2012, Mosby.)

A second mechanism of ascites formation is hypoalbuminemia resulting from the liver's decreased ability to synthesize albumin. The hypoalbuminemia results in decreased colloidal oncotic pressure.

A third mechanism of ascites is hyperaldosteronism, which occurs when the hormone aldosterone is metabolized by damaged hepatocytes. The increased level of aldosterone causes increased sodium reabsorption by the renal tubules. This retention of sodium, combined with an increase in antidiuretic hormone in blood, leads to additional water retention. Because of edema formation, there is decreased intravascular volume and, subsequently, decreased renal blood flow and glomerular filtration.

Ascites is manifested by abdominal distention with weight gain (Fig. 43-8). If the ascites is severe, the increase in abdominal pressure from the fluid accumulation may cause eversion of the umbilicus. Abdominal striae with distended abdominal wall veins may be present. Patients may show signs of dehydration (e.g., dry tongue and skin, sunken eyeballs, muscle weakness) and a decrease in urine output. Hypokalemia is common and is due to an excessive loss of potassium caused by hyperaldosteronism. Low potassium levels can also result from diuretic therapy used to treat the ascites.

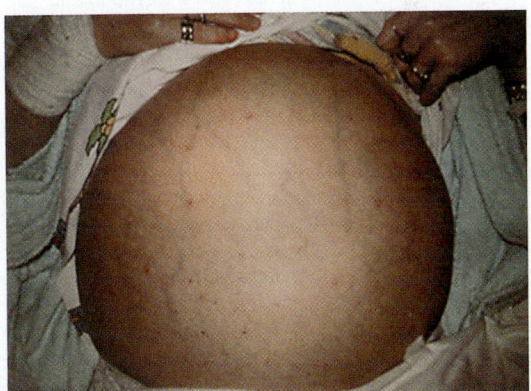

FIG. 43-8 Gross ascites. (From Butcher GP: *Gastroenterology: an illustrated colour text*, London, 2004, Churchill Livingstone.)

Because of alterations in immune function associated with cirrhosis, patients with ascites are at risk for *spontaneous bacterial peritonitis* (SBP). SBP is a bacterial infection of the ascitic fluid. In SBP, bacteria normally found in the intestines are translocated into the peritoneal space. The bacteria most frequently responsible for the infection are a gram-negative enteric pathogen such as *Escherichia coli*. SBP occurs in approximately

15% to 25% of hospitalized patients with cirrhosis and ascites. It is particularly common after variceal hemorrhage.[20]

Hepatic Encephalopathy. Hepatic encephalopathy is a neuropsychiatric manifestation of liver disease. The pathogenesis is multifactorial and includes the neurotoxic effects of ammonia, abnormal neurotransmission, astrocyte swelling, and inflammatory cytokines. A major source of ammonia is the bacterial and enzymatic deamination of amino acids in the intestines. The ammonia that results from this deamination process normally goes to the liver via the portal circulation and is converted to urea, which is then excreted by the kidneys. When blood is shunted past the liver via the collateral vessels or the liver is so damaged that it is unable to convert ammonia to urea, the levels of ammonia in the systemic circulation increase. The ammonia crosses the blood-brain barrier and produces neurologic toxic manifestations.

Factors that increase ammonia in the circulation may precipitate hepatic encephalopathy (Table 43-11). Hepatic encephalopathy can occur after placement of transjugular intrahepatic portosystemic shunt (TIPS), which is used to reduce portal hypertension by diverting blood flow around the liver.[21] (TIPS is discussed on p. 992.)

Clinical manifestations of encephalopathy are changes in neurologic and mental responsiveness; impaired consciousness; and inappropriate behavior, ranging from sleep disturbances to trouble concentrating to deep coma. Changes may occur (1) suddenly because of an increase in ammonia in response to bleeding varices or infection or (2) gradually as blood ammonia levels slowly increase. A grading system is often used to classify the stages of hepatic encephalopathy (Table 43-12).

A characteristic manifestation of hepatic encephalopathy is asterixis (flapping tremors). This may take several forms, with the most common involving the arms and hands. When asked to hold the arms and hands stretched out, the patient is unable to hold this position and performs a series of rapid flexion and extension movements of the hands.

Impairments in writing involve difficulty in moving the pen or pencil from left to right and *apraxia* (inability to construct simple figures). Other signs include hyperventilation, hypothermia, tongue fasciculations, and grimacing and grasping reflexes.

Fetor hepaticus (musty, sweet odor of the patient's breath) occurs in some patients with encephalopathy. This odor is from the accumulation of digestive by-products that the liver is unable to degrade.

Hepatorenal Syndrome. Hepatorenal syndrome is a type of renal failure with azotemia, oliguria, and intractable ascites. In this syndrome, the kidneys have no structural abnormality. The etiology is complex, but the final common pathway is likely to be portal hypertension along with liver decompensation, resulting in splanchnic and systemic vasodilation and decreased arterial blood volume. As a result, renal vasoconstriction occurs, and renal failure follows. This renal failure can be reversed by liver transplantation. In the patient with cirrhosis, hepatorenal syndrome frequently follows diuretic therapy, GI hemorrhage, or paracentesis.

Diagnostic Studies

Patients with cirrhosis have abnormalities in most of the liver function tests. Enzyme levels, including alkaline phosphatase, AST, ALT, and γ-glutamyl transpeptidase (GGT), are initially elevated because of their release from inflamed liver cells. However, in end-stage liver disease, AST and ALT levels may be normal due to the death and loss of hepatocytes. Patients with cirrhosis will also have decreased serum total protein and albumin, increased serum bilirubin (Table 43-3) and globulin levels, and prolonged prothrombin time. Alterations in fat metabolism are reflected by decreased cholesterol levels.

Although a liver ultrasound may be able to detect the presence of cirrhosis, it is not a reliable diagnostic test for cirrhosis. Ultrasound elastography (Fibroscan) is a noninvasive test that is used to quantify the degree of liver fibrosis. A liver biopsy, which may be done to identify liver cell changes, is the gold standard for a definitive diagnosis of cirrhosis.

TABLE 43-11 Factors Precipitating Hepatic Encephalopathy

Factor	Mechanism
GI hemorrhage	Increase in ammonia in GI tract.
Constipation	Increased production of ammonia from bacterial action on feces.
Hypokalemia	Potassium is needed by brain to metabolize ammonia.
Hypovolemia	Increase in blood ammonia because of hepatic hypoxia. Impairment of cerebral, hepatic, and renal function because of decreased blood flow.
Infection	Increase in metabolic rate and increase in cerebral sensitivity to toxins.
Cerebral depressants (e.g., opioids)	Decrease in metabolism by liver, causing higher drug levels and cerebral depression.
Metabolic alkalosis	Facilitation of transport of ammonia across blood-brain barrier. Increase in renal production of ammonia.
Paracentesis	Loss of sodium and potassium ions. Decrease in blood volume.
Dehydration	Potentiates ammonia toxicity.
Increased metabolism	Increase in workload of liver.
Uremia (renal failure)	Retention of nitrogenous metabolites.

TABLE 43-12 Grading Scale for Hepatic Encephalopathy

Grade	Level of Consciousness	Intellectual Function	Neurologic Findings
0	Normal to minimal change	Subtle to no change in personality, behavior, memory, concentration	Asterixis absent May have abnormal psychometric test
1	Lack of awareness, sleep disturbance	Short attention span, impaired computational skills, personality change, decrease in short-term memory, mild confusion, depression	Incoordination, asterixis may be absent
2	Lethargy, drowsiness	Disoriented to time, inappropriate behavior, deficits in executive function	Asterixis, abnormal reflexes
3	Somnolent, arousable	Disoriented to time, loss of meaningful conversation, marked confusion, incomprehensible speech	Asterixis, abnormal reflexes
4	Not arousable, comatose	Absent	Decerebrate May be responsive to painful stimuli

Interprofessional Care

The goal of treatment is to slow the progression of cirrhosis and to prevent and treat any complications. Interprofessional care measures are listed in Table 43-13. Management of specific problems associated with cirrhosis is described next.

Ascites. Management of ascites focuses on sodium restriction, diuretics, and fluid removal. Patients may be encouraged to limit sodium intake to 2 g/day.[22] Patients with severe ascites may need to restrict their sodium intake to 250 to 500 mg/day. Very low sodium intake can result in reduced nutritional intake and subsequent problems associated with malnutrition. The patient is usually not on restricted fluids unless severe ascites develops. When caring for patients with ascites, accurately assess and monitor fluid and electrolyte balance. Albumin infusion may be used to help maintain intravascular volume and adequate urine output by increasing plasma colloid oncotic pressure.

Diuretic therapy is an important part of management. Often a combination of drugs that work at multiple sites of the nephron is more effective than a single agent. Spironolactone (Aldactone) is an effective diuretic, even in patients with severe ascites. Spironolactone is also an antagonist of aldosterone and is potassium sparing. Other potassium-sparing diuretics include amiloride (Midamor) and triamterene (Dyrenium). A high-potency loop diuretic, such as furosemide (Lasix), is frequently used in combination with a potassium-sparing drug.

Tolvaptan (Samsca), a vasopressin-receptor antagonist, is used to correct hyponatremia, which is often seen in patients with cirrhosis. It causes an increase in water excretion, resulting in an increase in serum sodium concentration.

A paracentesis is a sterile procedure in which a catheter is used to withdraw fluid from the abdominal cavity. This procedure can be used to diagnose a medical condition or relieve pain, pressure, or difficulty breathing. In the patient with cirrhosis, this procedure is reserved for the person with impaired respiration or abdominal discomfort caused by severe ascites who does not respond to diuretic therapy. It is only a temporary measure of palliation because the fluid tends to reaccumulate rapidly.

TIPS (discussed later in this section) is used to alleviate ascites that does not respond to diuretics. Peritoneovenous shunt is a surgical procedure that provides continuous reinfusion of ascitic fluid into the venous system. Its use has almost been eliminated because of the high rate of complications.

Esophageal and Gastric Varices. The main therapeutic goal for esophageal and gastric varices is to prevent bleeding and variceal rupture by reducing portal pressure. The patient who has esophageal and/or gastric varices should avoid ingesting alcohol, aspirin, and nonsteroidal antiinflammatory drugs (NSAIDs).

All patients with cirrhosis should have an upper endoscopy (esophagogastroduodenoscopy [EGD]) to screen for varices. Patients with varices at risk of bleeding are generally started on a nonselective β-blocker (nadolol [Corgard] or propranolol [Inderal]) to reduce the incidence of hemorrhage. β-Blockers decrease high portal pressure, which decreases the risk for rupture.

When variceal bleeding occurs, the first step is to stabilize the patient and manage the airway. IV therapy is initiated and may include administration of blood products. Management that involves a combination of drug therapy and endoscopic therapy is more successful than either approach alone.

Drug therapy for bleeding varices may include the somatostatin analog octreotide (Sandostatin) or vasopressin. The main goal of drug therapy is first to stop the bleeding and identify the source and apply interventions to prevent further bleeding. IV administration of octreotide or vasopressin produces vasoconstriction of the splanchnic arterial bed, decreases portal blood flow, and decreases portal hypertension. Currently, octreotide is more widely used in this setting because of its limited side effect profile when compared with vasopressin.

At the time of endoscopy, band ligation or sclerotherapy of varices may be used to prevent rebleeding. Endoscopic variceal ligation (EVL, or "banding") is performed by placing a small rubber band (elastic O-ring) around the base of the *varix* (enlarged vein). Sclerotherapy involves injection of a sclerosing solution into the swollen veins through an injection needle that is placed through the endoscope.

Balloon tamponade may be used when acute esophageal or gastric variceal hemorrhage cannot be controlled on initial endoscopy. Balloon tamponade controls the hemorrhage by mechanical compression of the varices. Different types of tubes are available. The Sengstaken-Blakemore tube has two balloons,

---

TABLE 43-13 Interprofessional Care

Cirrhosis of the Liver

Diagnostic Assessment
- History and physical examination
- Liver function tests (ALT, AST, alkaline phosphatase, γ-glutamyl transpeptidase [GGT])
- Liver biopsy (percutaneous needle)
- Upper endoscopy (esophagogastroduodenoscopy)
- CT scan, MRI
- Liver ultrasound (e.g., FibroScan)
- Serum electrolytes
- Prothrombin time
- Total bilirubin
- Serum albumin
- Complete blood count

Management
Conservative Therapy
- Rest
- B-complex vitamins
- Avoidance of alcohol
- Minimization or avoidance of aspirin, acetaminophen, and NSAIDs

Ascites
- Low-sodium diet
- Diuretics
- Paracentesis (if indicated)

Esophageal and Gastric Varices
- Endoscopic band ligation or sclerotherapy
- Balloon tamponade
- Transjugular intrahepatic portosystemic shunt (TIPS)

Drug Therapy
- Nonselective β-blocker (e.g., propranolol [Inderal])
- octreotide (Sandostatin)
- vasopressin

Hepatic Encephalopathy
Drug Therapy
- Antibiotics (rifaximin [Xifaxan])
- lactulose

ALT, Alanine aminotransferase; *AST*, aspartate aminotransferase.

gastric and esophageal, with three lumens: one for the gastric balloon, one for the esophageal balloon, and one for gastric aspiration. Two other types of balloons are the Minnesota tube (a modified Sengstaken-Blakemore tube with an esophageal suction port above the esophageal balloon) and the Linton-Nachlas tube.

! **SAFETY ALERT** **Balloon Tamponade**
- Label each lumen to avoid confusion.
- Secure the tube to prevent movement of the tube that could result in occlusion of the airway.
- Deflate balloons for 5 min every 8-12 hr per institutional policy to prevent tissue necrosis.

Supportive measures during an acute variceal bleed include administration of fresh frozen plasma and packed RBCs, vitamin K, and proton pump inhibitors (e.g., pantoprazole [Protonix]). Lactulose and rifaximin (Xifaxan) may be administered to prevent hepatic encephalopathy from breakdown of blood and the release of ammonia in the intestine. Antibiotics are given to prevent bacterial infection.

Because of the high incidence of recurrent bleeding with each bleeding episode, continued therapy is necessary. Long-term management of patients who have had an episode of bleeding includes nonselective β-blockers, repeated band ligation of the varices, and portosystemic shunts in patients who develop recurrent bleeding.

Shunting Procedures. Nonsurgical and surgical methods of shunting blood away from the varices are available. Shunting procedures tend to be used more after a second major bleeding episode than during an initial bleeding episode. *Transjugular intrahepatic portosystemic shunt (TIPS)* is a nonsurgical procedure in which a tract (shunt) between the systemic and portal venous systems is created to redirect portal blood flow. A catheter is placed in the jugular vein and then threaded through the superior and inferior vena cava to the hepatic vein. The wall of the hepatic vein is punctured, and the catheter is directed to the portal vein. Stents are positioned along the passageway, overlapping in the liver tissue and extending into both veins.

This procedure reduces portal venous pressure and decompresses the varices, thus controlling bleeding. TIPS does not interfere with a future liver transplantation. Limitations of the procedure include the increased risk of hepatic encephalopathy (toxin-containing blood bypasses the liver) and stenosis of the stent. TIPS is contraindicated in patients with severe hepatic encephalopathy, hepatocellular carcinoma, severe hepatorenal syndrome, and portal vein thrombosis.

Various surgical shunting procedures may be used to decrease portal hypertension by diverting some of the portal blood flow while allowing adequate liver perfusion. Currently, the surgical shunts most commonly used are the portacaval shunt and the distal splenorenal shunt (Fig. 43-9).

Hepatic Encephalopathy. The goal of management of hepatic encephalopathy is the reduction of ammonia formation. Ammonia formation in the intestines is reduced with lactulose, a drug that traps ammonia in the gut. It can be given orally, as an enema, or through a nasogastric (NG) tube. The laxative effect of the drug expels the ammonia from the colon. Antibiotics such as rifaximin may also be given, particularly in patients who do not respond to lactulose. Constipation should be prevented, and regular and frequent bowel movements are necessary to minimize the ammonia buildup.

Control of hepatic encephalopathy also involves treatment of precipitating causes (Table 43-10). This includes lowering

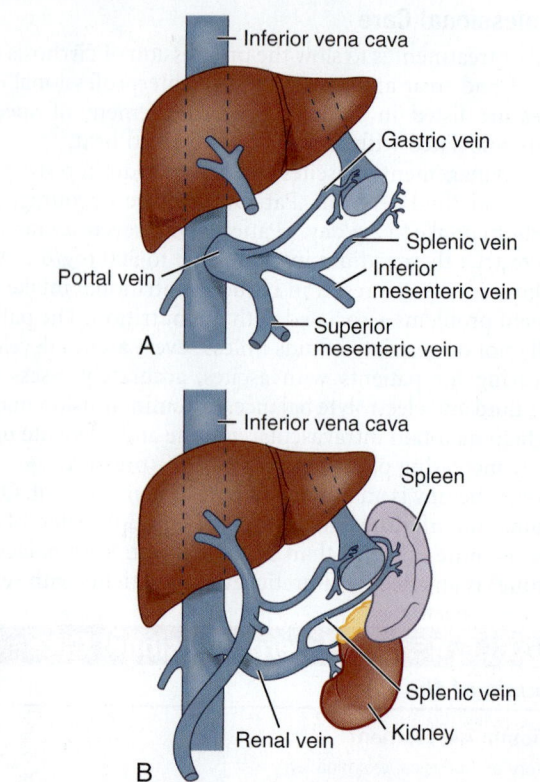

FIG. 43-9 Portosystemic shunts. **A,** Portacaval shunt. The portal vein is anastomosed to the inferior vena cava, diverting blood from the portal vein to the systemic circulation. **B,** Distal splenorenal shunt. The splenic vein is anastomosed to the renal vein. The portal venous flow remains intact while esophageal varices are selectively decompressed. (The short gastric veins are decompressed.) The spleen conducts blood from the high pressure of the esophageal and gastric varices to the low-pressure renal vein.

one's dietary protein intake, preventing and controlling GI bleeds, and in the event of a bleed, removing the blood promptly from the GI tract to decrease the protein accumulation in the gut.[23]

Drug Therapy. There is no specific drug therapy for cirrhosis. However, a number of drugs are used to treat symptoms and complications of advanced liver disease (Table 43-14).

Nutritional Therapy. The diet for the patient who has cirrhosis without complications is high in calories (3000 cal/day) with high carbohydrate content and moderate to low levels of fat. Protein restriction may be appropriate in some patients immediately after a severe flare of symptoms (i.e., episodic hepatic encephalopathy). However, protein restriction is rarely justified in patients with cirrhosis and persistent hepatic encephalopathy. For many patients, malnutrition is a more serious clinical problem than hepatic encephalopathy.[24]

A patient with alcoholic cirrhosis frequently has protein-calorie malnutrition. Oral nutritional supplements containing protein from branched-chain amino acids that are metabolized by the muscles may be recommended. These supplements provide protein that is more easily metabolized by the liver. Parenteral nutrition or enteral nutrition therapy may be required, although rarely used, and only reserved for severe cases of malnutrition.

The patient with ascites and edema is put on a low-sodium diet. The degree of sodium restriction depends on the patient's condition. Instruct the patient and caregiver about the degree of restriction. Table salt is a well-known source of sodium, but sodium is also present in baking soda and baking powder. Foods

TABLE 43-14 Drug Therapy
Cirrhosis

Drug	Mechanism of Action
octreotide (Sandostatin) vasopressin	Hemostasis and control of bleeding in esophageal and gastric varices, constriction of splanchnic arterial bed
propranolol (Inderal) nadolol (Corgard)	Reduction of portal venous pressure and esophageal variceal bleeding
lactulose	Acidification of feces in bowel and trapping of ammonia, causing its elimination in feces
rifaximin (Xifaxan) neomycin sulfate	Decrease bacterial flora, thus reducing formation of ammonia
magnesium sulfate	Magnesium replacement (hypomagnesemia possible with liver dysfunction)
Vitamin K	Correction of clotting abnormalities from decreased levels of this vitamin
Proton pump inhibitors (e.g., pantoprazole [Protonix])	Decrease in gastric acidity
Diuretics	
• spironolactone (Aldactone)	Blocks actions of aldosterone, potassium sparing
• furosemide (Lasix)	Acts on distal tubule and loop of Henle to decrease reabsorption of sodium and water

that are high in sodium content include canned soups and vegetables, many frozen foods, salted snacks (e.g., potato chips), nuts, smoked meats and fish, crackers, breads, olives, pickles, ketchup, and beer. Advise the patient to read labels for sodium content. Provide suggestions to the patient and caregiver about how to make the diet more palatable. Seasonings such as garlic, parsley, onion, lemon juice, and spices may make food more appetizing. Collaborate with a dietitian regarding dietary strategies.

❖ NURSING MANAGEMENT: CIRRHOSIS

◆ Nursing Assessment

Subjective and objective data that should be obtained from an individual with cirrhosis are presented in Table 43-15.

◆ Nursing Diagnoses

Nursing diagnoses for the patient with cirrhosis include, but are not limited to, the following:
- Imbalanced nutrition: less than body requirements *related to* anorexia, nausea, and impaired utilization and storage of nutrients
- Impaired skin integrity *related to* peripheral edema, ascites, and pruritus
- Excess fluid volume *related to* portal hypertension and hyperaldosteronism
- Ineffective health management *related to* ineffective coping and abuse of alcohol

Additional information on nursing diagnoses for the patient with cirrhosis is presented in eNursing Care Plan 43-2 available on the website for this chapter.

◆ Planning

The overall goals are that the patient with cirrhosis will (1) have relief of discomfort, (2) have minimal to no complications

TABLE 43-15 Nursing Assessment
Cirrhosis

Subjective Data
Important Health Information
Past health history: Previous viral, toxic, or idiopathic hepatitis. Alcohol intake, metabolic syndrome, chronic biliary obstruction and infection, severe right-sided heart failure
Medications: Adverse reaction to any medication. Use of anticoagulants, aspirin, NSAIDs, acetaminophen

Functional Health Patterns
Health perception–health management: Chronic alcohol abuse. Weakness, fatigue
Nutritional-metabolic: Anorexia, weight loss, dyspepsia, nausea and vomiting, gingival bleeding
Elimination: Dark urine, decreased urine output, light-colored or black stools, flatulence, change in bowel habits. Dry, yellow skin, bruising
Cognitive-perceptual: Dull, right upper quadrant or epigastric pain. Numbness, tingling of extremities. Pruritus
Sexuality-reproductive: Impotence, amenorrhea

Objective Data
General
Fever, cachexia, wasting of extremities

Integumentary
Icteric sclera, jaundice, petechiae, ecchymoses, spider angiomas, palmar erythema, alopecia, loss of axillary and pubic hair, peripheral edema

Respiratory
Shallow, rapid respirations. Epistaxis

Gastrointestinal
Abdominal distention, ascites, distended abdominal wall veins, palpable liver and spleen, foul breath. Hematemesis. Black, tarry stools. Hemorrhoids

Neurologic
Altered mentation, asterixis

Reproductive
Gynecomastia, testicular atrophy, and impotence (men); loss of libido (men and women); amenorrhea or heavy menstrual bleeding (women)

Possible Diagnostic Findings
Anemia, thrombocytopenia; leukopenia. ↓ serum albumin, potassium. Abnormal liver function studies. ↑ INR, ↓ platelets, ↑ ammonia, ↑ bilirubin levels. Abnormal abdominal ultrasound, CT, or MRI

INR, International normalized ratio.

(ascites, esophageal varices, hepatic encephalopathy), and (3) return to as normal a lifestyle as possible.

◆ Nursing Implementation

◆ **Health Promotion.** Common risk factors for cirrhosis include alcoholism, malnutrition, viral hepatitis, biliary obstruction, obesity, and right-sided heart failure. Prevention and early treatment of cirrhosis focus on reducing or eliminating these risk factors. Urge patients to abstain from alcohol, and encourage those with a chronic alcohol use history to enroll in Alcoholics Anonymous or other support groups. (The treatment of alcohol dependence is discussed in Chapter 10.)

Adequate nutrition, especially for the person who abuses alcohol and other individuals at risk for cirrhosis, is essential to promote normal liver regeneration. Identify and treat acute hepatitis early so that it does not progress to chronic hepatitis and cirrhosis. Bariatric surgery for morbidly obese individuals reduces the incidence of NAFLD.

◆ **Acute Care.** Nursing care for the patient with cirrhosis focuses on conserving the patient's strength while maintaining muscle strength and tone. When the patient requires complete bed rest, implement measures to prevent pneumonia, thromboembolic problems, and pressure ulcers. Modify the activity and rest schedule according to signs of clinical improvement (e.g., decreasing jaundice, improvement in liver function studies).

Anorexia, nausea and vomiting, pressure from ascites, and poor eating habits all interfere with adequate intake of nutrients. Oral hygiene before meals may improve the patient's taste sensation. Make between-meal snacks available so that the patient can eat them at times when food is best tolerated. Provide food preferences whenever possible. Explain the reason for any dietary restrictions to the patient and caregiver.

Nursing assessment and care should include the patient's physical status. Is jaundice present? Where is it observed— sclera, skin, hard palate? What is the progression of jaundice? If the jaundice is accompanied by pruritus, carry out measures to relieve itching. Cholestyramine or hydroxyzine (Atarax) may be ordered to help relieve the pruritus. Other measures to alleviate pruritus include baking soda or moisturizing bath oils (Alpha Keri), lotions containing calamine, antihistamines, soft or old linens, and control of the temperature (not too hot and not too cold). Keep the patient's nails short and clean. Teach patients to rub with their knuckles rather than scratch with their nails when they cannot resist scratching.

Note the color of urine and stools and assess for improvement or normalization of color. When jaundice is present, the urine is often dark brown and the stool is gray or tan.

Edema and ascites are frequent manifestations of cirrhosis and require nursing assessments and interventions. Accurate calculation and recording of intake and output, daily weights, and measurements of extremities and abdominal girth help in the ongoing assessment of the location and extent of the edema. Mark the abdomen with a permanent marker so that the girth is measured at the same location each time.

Immediately before a paracentesis have the patient void to prevent puncturing of the bladder during the procedure. When the paracentesis is completed, have the patient sit on the side of the bed or place him/her in high Fowler's position. Also monitor for hypovolemia and electrolyte imbalance. Check and monitor BP and heart rate following the procedure. Check the dressing for bleeding and/or leakage of ascitic fluid.

Dyspnea is a frequent problem for the patient with severe ascites and can lead to pleural effusions. A semi-Fowler's or Fowler's position allows for maximal respiratory efficiency. Use pillows to support the arms and chest to increase the patient's comfort and ability to breathe.

Meticulous skin care is essential because the edematous tissues are prone to breakdown. Use an alternating-air pressure mattress or other special mattress. A turning schedule (minimum of every 2 hours) must be adhered to rigidly. Support the abdomen with pillows. If the abdomen is taut, cleanse it gently. The patient will tend to avoid moving because of abdominal discomfort and dyspnea. Range-of-motion exercises are helpful. Implement measures such as coughing and deep breathing to prevent respiratory problems. The lower extremities may be elevated. If scrotal edema is present, a scrotal support provides some comfort.

When the patient is taking diuretics, monitor the serum levels of sodium, potassium, chloride, and bicarbonate. Monitor renal function (blood urea nitrogen [BUN], serum creatinine) routinely and with any change in the diuretic dosage. Observe for signs of fluid and electrolyte imbalance, especially hypokalemia. Hypokalemia may be manifested by cardiac dysrhythmias, hypotension, tachycardia, and generalized muscle weakness. Water excess (hyponatremia) is manifested by muscle cramping, weakness, lethargy, and confusion.

Observe for and provide nursing care for any hematologic problems. These include bleeding tendencies, anemia, and increased susceptibility to infection.

Assess the patient's response to altered body image resulting from jaundice, spider angiomas, palmar erythema, ascites, and gynecomastia. The patient may experience anxiety and embarrassment about these changes. Explain these phenomena and be a supportive listener. Provide nursing care with concern and encouragement to help the patient maintain his or her self-esteem.

❓ CHECK YOUR PRACTICE

You are caring for a 69-yr-old male patient with advanced cirrhosis who just underwent banding for esophageal varices. The unlicensed assistive personnel (UAP) tells you that the patient's BP is 80/60 mm Hg and he is difficult to arouse.
- What would you do?
- What are your nursing priorities?
- What are you concerned about?

◆ ***Bleeding Varices.*** If the patient has esophageal or gastric varices, observe for any signs of bleeding from the varices, such as hematemesis and melena. If hematemesis occurs, assess the patient for hemorrhage, call the HCP, and be ready to transfer the patient to the endoscopy suite and/or assist with equipment to control the bleeding. The patient's airway must be maintained. Patients with bleeding varices are usually admitted to the ICU.

Balloon tamponade may be used in patients who have bleeding that is unresponsive to band ligation or sclerotherapy. When balloon tamponade is used, explain to the patient and caregiver the use of the tube and how it will be inserted. Check the balloons for patency. It is usually the HCP's responsibility to insert the tube by either the nose or mouth. Then the gastric balloon is inflated with approximately 250 mL of air, and the tube is retracted until resistance (lower esophageal sphincter) is felt. The tube is secured by placement of a piece of sponge or foam rubber at the nostrils (nasal cuff). For continued bleeding, the esophageal balloon is then inflated. A sphygmomanometer is used to measure and maintain the desired pressure at 20 to 40 mm Hg. The position of the balloons is verified by x-ray.

Nursing care includes monitoring for complications of rupture or erosion of the esophagus, regurgitation and aspiration of gastric contents, and occlusion of the airway by the balloon. If the gastric balloon breaks or is deflated, the esophageal balloon will slip upward, obstructing the airway and causing asphyxiation. If this happens, cut the tube or deflate the esophageal balloon. Keep scissors at the bedside. Minimize regurgitation by oral and pharyngeal suctioning and by keeping the patient in a semi-Fowler's position.

The patient is unable to swallow saliva because of the inflated esophageal balloon occluding the esophagus. Encourage the patient to expectorate, and provide an emesis basin and tissues. Frequent oral and nasal care provides relief from the taste of blood and irritation from mouth breathing.

◆ *Hepatic Encephalopathy.* Nursing care of the patient with hepatic encephalopathy focuses on maintaining a safe environment, sustaining life, and assisting with measures to reduce the formation of ammonia. Patients with hepatic encephalopathy may exhibit confusion and be at risk for falls or other injuries. Assess the patient's (1) level of responsiveness (e.g., reflexes, pupillary reactions, orientation), (2) sensory and motor abnormalities (e.g., hyperreflexia, asterixis, motor coordination), (3) fluid and electrolyte imbalances, (4) acid-base imbalances, and (5) response to treatment measures.

Assess the neurologic status, including an exact description of the patient's behavior at least every 2 hours. Plan your care of the patient based on the severity of the encephalopathy.

Institute measures to prevent falls or injuries. In addition, measures to minimize constipation are important to reduce ammonia production. Give drugs, laxatives, and enemas as ordered. Encourage fluids, if not contraindicated. Any GI bleeding may worsen encephalopathy. Assess the patient taking lactulose for diarrhea and excessive fluid and electrolyte losses.

Control factors known to precipitate encephalopathy as much as possible, including anything that may cause constipation (e.g., dehydration, opioid medications). In patients with altered levels of consciousness or whose airway may become compromised, have safety measures and emergency equipment readily available.

◆ **Ambulatory Care.** The patient with cirrhosis may be faced with a prolonged course and the possibility of life-threatening problems and complications. The patient and caregiver need to understand the importance of continual health care and medical supervision. Supportive measures include proper diet, rest, avoidance of potentially hepatotoxic OTC drugs such as acetaminophen in high doses, and abstinence from alcohol. Abstinence from alcohol is important and results in improvement in most patients. However, some patients find abstinence extremely difficult and require a lot of emotional support. Explore your own attitude towards the patient whose cirrhosis is secondary to chronic alcohol use. Always provide care without being condescending or judgmental. Treat patients with respect and concern for their well-being (see Chapter 10).

Cirrhosis is a chronic disease and people can live many years with symptoms and complications secondary to cirrhosis. The patient is affected not only physically but also psychologically, socially, and economically. Major lifestyle changes may be required, especially if chronic alcohol use is the primary cause. Provide information regarding community support programs, such as Alcoholics Anonymous, for help with chronic alcohol use.

Teach the patient and caregiver about complications and when to seek medical attention (Table 43-16). Include instructions about adequate rest periods, how to detect early signs of complications, skin care, drug therapy side effects, observation for bleeding, and protection from infection.

Referral to a community or home health nurse may sometimes be necessary to ensure patient adherence to prescribed therapy. Home care for the patient with cirrhosis should focus on helping the patient with activities of daily living while maintaining the highest level of wellness possible.

◆ **Evaluation**

Expected outcomes are that the patient with cirrhosis will
- Maintain food and fluid intake adequate to meet nutritional needs
- Maintain skin integrity with relief of edema and pruritus
- Experience normalization of fluid balance as a result of medical and nursing interventions
- Acknowledge and get treatment for a substance use problem

ETHICAL/LEGAL DILEMMAS
Rationing

Situation

T.H., a 43-yr-old female patient with cirrhosis of the liver, is frequently admitted to the hospital. She has been told that her continued alcohol consumption will inevitably lead to her death. Now she has been admitted for GI bleeding and needs blood transfusions. She has a rare blood type that is difficult to match. Should you ask for an ethics consultation?

Ethical/Legal Points for Consideration

- *Rationing,* or the controlled distribution of scarce resources, is a difficult ethical problem. The needs of an individual patient or group of patients are weighed against the needs of many patients, who may have a greater chance of recovery, and the availability of the necessary resources.
- Health interests can supersede the interests or rights of an individual. For example, in anticipation of an anthrax attack, the government could confiscate all relevant antibiotics and restrict their use to treat the disease.
- Two individual rights that must be considered with regard to rationing are the (1) constitutional right to privacy and (2) right to consent to or refuse medical procedures and therapy.
- The competent adult is the only person who may consent to or refuse treatment for his or her health care problems.
- If T.H. consents to a blood transfusion, an intervening party may be permitted to refuse that treatment only given substantial intervening circumstances and not as a threat to compel compliant future behavior.
- If involved parties cannot reach an agreement, legal intervention by way of a court order may become necessary.

Discussion Questions

1. Do you think patients with diseases that have a behavioral component such as substance abuse, deserve aggressive treatment?
2. Would you request an ethics committee consultation in T.H.'s case?

TABLE 43-16 Patient & Caregiver Teaching
Cirrhosis

When teaching the patient and caregiver about management of cirrhosis, do the following.

1. Explain that cirrhosis is a chronic illness and requires continual health care.
2. Teach the symptoms of complications and when to seek medical attention to enable prompt treatment.
3. Teach the patient to avoid potentially hepatotoxic over-the-counter drugs, because the diseased liver is unable to metabolize them.
4. Encourage abstinence from alcohol because continued use increases the rate of liver disease progression and risk of liver complications.
5. Instruct the patient with esophageal or gastric varices to avoid aspirin and NSAIDs to prevent hemorrhage.
6. Teach the patient with portal hypertension and varices that straining at stool, coughing, sneezing, and retching and vomiting may increase the risk of variceal hemorrhage.

Additional information on expected outcomes for the patient with cirrhosis is presented in eNursing Care Plan 43-2 available on the website for this chapter.

ACUTE LIVER FAILURE

Acute liver failure, or *fulminant hepatic failure,* is a potentially life-threatening clinical syndrome. It is characterized by a rapid onset of severe liver dysfunction in someone with no prior history of liver disease. It is often accompanied by hepatic encephalopathy.

The most common cause of acute live failure is drugs, usually acetaminophen in combination with alcohol.[25] Other drugs that can cause acute liver failure include isoniazid, halothane, sulfa-containing drugs, and NSAIDs. Drugs can cause hepatocyte damage by disrupting essential intracellular processes or causing an accumulation of toxic metabolic products. Other causes can include viral hepatitis, in particular HBV. Hepatitis A is a less common cause. Although the disease can run its course over 8 weeks, it can last as long as 26 weeks. The survival rate is approximately 60%.[26]

Clinical Manifestations and Diagnostic Studies

Manifestations of acute liver failure include jaundice, coagulation abnormalities, and encephalopathy. In acute liver failure, changes in cognitive function are the first clinical sign. Patients are susceptible to a wide variety of complications, including cerebral edema, renal failure, hypoglycemia, metabolic acidosis, sepsis, and multiorgan failure.

Serum bilirubin is elevated, and the prothrombin time is prolonged. Liver enzyme levels (AST, ALT) are often markedly elevated. Additional laboratory tests include blood chemistries (especially glucose, since hypoglycemia may be present and require correction), complete blood count (CBC), acetaminophen level, screening for other drugs and toxins, viral hepatitis serology (especially HAV and HBV), serum ceruloplasmin (enzyme synthesized in liver) and α_1-antitrypsin levels, iron levels, and autoantibodies (antinuclear and anti–smooth muscle antibodies). Plasma ammonia levels may also be obtained.

CT or MRI is helpful in providing information about the liver size and contour, presence of ascites or tumors, and patency of the blood vessels.

❖ NURSING AND INTERPROFESSIONAL MANAGEMENT: ACUTE LIVER FAILURE

Since acute liver failure may progress rapidly, with hour-by-hour changes in consciousness, the patient is usually transferred to the ICU once the diagnosis is made. Planning for transfer to a transplant center should begin in patients with grade 1 or 2 encephalopathy because they may worsen rapidly. Early transfer is important because the risks involved with patient transport may increase or even preclude transfer once stage 3 or 4 encephalopathy develops (Table 43-12).

Renal failure is a frequent complication of liver failure and may be due to dehydration, hepatorenal syndrome, or acute tubular necrosis. The frequency of renal failure may be even greater with acetaminophen overdose or other toxins, with which direct renal toxicity occurs. Although few patients die of renal failure alone, it often increases the mortality risk and may worsen the prognosis. Protect renal function by maintaining adequate fluid balance, avoiding nephrotoxic agents (e.g., aminoglycosides, NSAIDs), and promptly identifying and treating infection.

Liver transplantation is the treatment of choice for and increases survival rates in patients with acute liver failure. Cerebral edema, cerebellar herniation, and brainstem compression are the most common causes of death. Treatment of cerebral edema is described in Chapter 56.

Monitoring and management of hemodynamic and renal function, as well as glucose, electrolytes, and acid-base status, are critical. Conduct frequent neurologic evaluations for signs of elevated intracranial pressure. Position the patient with the head elevated at 30 degrees. Avoid excessive patient stimulation. Maneuvers that cause straining or Valsalva-like movements may increase intracranial pressure (ICP). (ICP monitoring is discussed in Chapter 56.)

Assess the patient regularly for baseline level of consciousness and orientation and report any changes to the HCP. Avoid the use of any sedatives because of their effects on mental status and the effect of their use can be confused with worsening encephalopathy. Only minimal doses of benzodiazepines should be used due to their delayed metabolism by the failing liver. Additional measures include padding bedrails to avoid injury from possible seizures, closely observing the patient to prevent injuries, monitoring intake and output for renal function, and providing good skin and oral care to avoid breakdown and infection.

Alterations in level of consciousness may compromise nutritional intake and vitamin supplementation should be implemented. Factors such as coagulation problems may also influence whether enteral nutrition is initiated. An NG tube may be irritating to the nasal and esophageal mucosa, and cause bleeding.

LIVER CANCER

Primary liver cancer starts in the liver. The most common types of liver cancer are hepatocellular carcinoma [HCC] (75% of cases) and intrahepatic cholangiocarcinoma (bile duct cancer). Annually about 35,660 people in the United States are diagnosed with liver cancer and 24,550 die. Worldwide liver cancer is the fifth most common cancer and second most common cause of cancer death.[27]

Liver cancer is the most common cause of death in patients with cirrhosis. Cirrhosis caused by hepatitis C is the most common cause of HCC in the United States, followed by alcoholic cirrhosis.[27]

Liver cancer incidence rates are higher in men than women. The incidence of HCC is increasing in the United States because of the large number of patients infected with chronic hepatitis C.[27]

In primary liver cancer, lesions may be singular or numerous and nodular or diffusely spread over the entire liver. Some tumors infiltrate other organs such as the gallbladder or move into the peritoneum or the diaphragm. Primary liver cancer commonly metastasizes to the lung.

Metastatic carcinoma of the liver is more common than primary liver cancer (Fig. 43-10). The liver is a common site of metastatic growth because of its high rate of blood flow and extensive capillary network. Cancer cells in other parts of the body are commonly carried to the liver via the portal circulation.

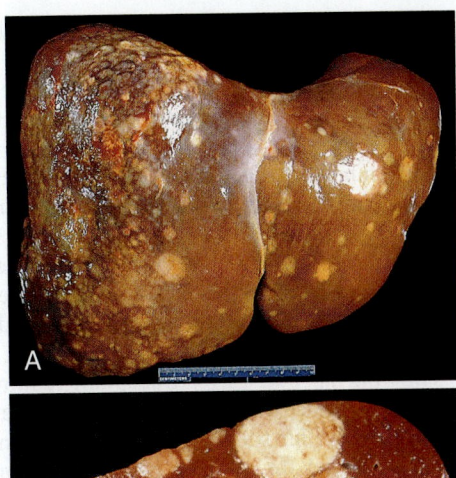

FIG. 43-10 Multiple hepatic metastases from a primary colon cancer. **A,** Gross specimen showing outside of liver. **B,** Liver section showing metastatic lesions. (*A,* From Kumar V, Abbas AK, Fausto N: *Robbins and Cotran pathologic basis of disease,* ed 7, Philadelphia, 2005, Saunders. *B,* From Kumar V, Abbas AK, Aster JC, Fausto N: *Robbins and Cotran pathologic basis of disease,* ed 8, Philadelphia, 2010, Saunders.)

Clinical Manifestations and Diagnostic Studies

The clinical manifestations of early liver cancer can be absent or subtle. They are often a result of the underlying cirrhosis rather than from the actual liver tumor(s). The patient may present with hepatomegaly, splenomegaly, fatigue, peripheral edema, ascites, and other complications from portal hypertension. In late stages, patients will commonly have manifestations of fever/chills, jaundice, anorexia, weight loss, palpable mass, and right upper quadrant pain.

Diagnostic and screening for liver cancer are ultrasound, CT, and MRI. Recent advancements in MRI scanning have allowed for accurate diagnosis of liver cancers without the need for a percutaneous biopsy.[28] Occasionally, a biopsy may be performed when the results of diagnostic imaging studies are inconclusive or tissue is needed to guide treatment. Risks of a biopsy include bleeding and potential tumor cell seeding along the needle tract. Therefore a biopsy is generally avoided unless a diagnosis cannot be made by CT or MRI and clinical presentation.

Serum α-fetoprotein (AFP) levels are elevated in approximately 60% of patients with HCC. The level of elevation may not correlate with the clinical features of HCC (e.g., stage or prognosis). (AFP is discussed in Chapter 15.)

❖ NURSING AND INTERPROFESSIONAL MANAGEMENT: LIVER CANCER

Prevention of liver cancer focuses on identifying and treating chronic hepatitis B and C viral infections. Treatment of chronic alcohol abuse may also lower the risk of liver cancer. Screening for at-risk patients (e.g., those with cirrhosis) usually involves a combination of serum AFP and either CT, MRI, or ultrasound imaging of the liver.

Treatment of liver cancer depends primarily on the stage of cancer: number, size, and location of tumors, involvement of any blood vessels, patient's age and overall health, and extent of underlying liver disease. Surgical liver resection (partial hepatectomy) offers the best chance for a cure. However, only about 15% of people have sufficient healthy liver tissue for this to be an option. The underlying cirrhosis and portal hypertension often compromises liver function and may cause liver failure postoperatively. Furthermore, many patients tend to be diagnosed at an advanced stage of liver cancer, when surgery is not an option. For those patients who have relatively early stage liver cancer and have impaired liver function, liver transplantation offers another option with good prognosis.

Nonsurgical therapies include percutaneous ablation, chemoembolization, radioembolization, and sorafenib (Nexavar) oral therapy.[29] In ablation, a thin needle is inserted into the core of the tumor. Then various substances can be injected (ethanol, acetic acid) and the temperature of the probe (radiofrequency, microwave, cryotherapy) can be altered for ultimate destruction of the tumor. This procedure can be done percutaneously, laparoscopically, or through an open incision. This method is typically limited by the number, size, and location of liver tumors. It is usually offered to patients with early stage liver cancer. Although complications are not common, they can include infection, bleeding, dysrhythmias, and skin burn.

In those patients with multinodular HCC or intermediate stage liver cancer, embolization of the tumors is another intervention. There are two options typically used: transarterial chemoembolization (TACE) or transarterial radioembolization (TARE). TACE and TARE are minimally invasive procedures performed by interventional radiologists. A catheter is placed via the femoral artery or radial artery and advanced to the arterial blood supply of the tumors in the liver. Either a chemotherapy drug (TACE) or radioactive beads (TARE) along with embolizing agents are then injected into the arteries of the tumor(s) region. TACE works by shutting off the blood supply to the tumors and exposing liver tumor cells to the chemotherapy agent. TARE destroys the tumor(s) by slowly releasing radioactive material directly to the site of the tumor. It can take up to 3 months for complete results.

In patients with advanced HCC, sorafenib (Nexavar) is typically the first-line treatment. It is a kinase inhibitor, a type of targeted therapy, that blocks certain proteins (kinases) that play a role in tumor growth and cancer progression (see Table 15-13). This drug has the potential to slow tumor progression and prolong life.

Nursing intervention for the patient with liver cancer focuses on keeping the patient as comfortable as possible. Since these patients manifest the same problems as any patient with advanced liver disease, the nursing interventions discussed for cirrhosis of the liver are used for these patients (see pp. 993-995.) (See Chapter 15 for care of the patient with cancer.)

Although the prognosis for patients with liver cancer is poor, it is improving with early screening and surveillance programs for those with chronic hepatitis and/or cirrhosis. The cancer progresses relatively rapidly, and patients often have complications both from the advancing cancer and declining liver function. Without treatment, death may occur within 6 to 12 months, most commonly as a result of hepatic encephalopathy or massive blood loss from GI bleeding.

LIVER TRANSPLANTATION

Liver transplantation has become a practical option for many people with end-stage liver disease or localized HCC. Liver disease related to chronic viral hepatitis is the leading indication for liver transplantation. Other indications include congenital biliary abnormalities (biliary atresia), inborn errors of metabolism, sclerosing cholangitis, acute liver failure, and chronic end-stage liver disease. Liver transplants are not recommended for the patient with widespread cancer. Currently about 17,000 people are waiting for liver transplants. However, only 6000 transplants are performed annually.[30]

Liver transplant candidates must go through a rigorous transplant evaluation prior to being listed on the transplant list. This is done to confirm the diagnosis of end-stage liver disease and to assess for other co-morbid conditions (e.g., cardiovascular disease, chronic kidney disease) that may affect the patient's surgical outcome. The evaluation includes physical examination, laboratory tests (CBC, liver function tests), cardiac and pulmonary evaluations, endoscopy, CT scan, and psychologic testing. Potential recipients receive counseling regarding cigarette smoking and alcohol abstinence. Contraindications for liver transplant include severe extrahepatic disease, advanced HCC or other cancer, ongoing drug or chronic alcohol use, and inability to comprehend or comply with the rigorous posttransplant care.

Liver transplantation is performed using both deceased (cadaver) and live donor livers. (See Chapter 13 for a general discussion of organ transplants.) The live donor liver transplant was developed initially for children whose parents wanted to serve as donors. Today, some liver transplant centers are performing live liver transplant procedures for adults. In this procedure, the living person donates a portion of his or her liver to another. However, live liver donation poses potential risks to the donor, including biliary problems, hepatic artery thrombosis, wound infection, postoperative ileus, and pneumothorax.

Because of the limited number of donor livers, when a liver becomes available for transplant it may be divided into two parts (split liver transplant) and implanted into two recipients. The decision to use a split donor liver is based on the donor's size and health. The recipients of the split liver generally are smaller than the donor. The success rate associated with split liver transplantation is somewhat lower than that associated with whole organ transplantation.

Postoperative complications of liver transplant include bleeding, infection, and rejection. However, the liver is subject to a less aggressive immunologic attack than other organs such as the kidneys. (Transplants and immunosuppressive therapy are discussed in Chapter 13.)

Immunosuppressive therapy generally involves a combination of corticosteroids (prednisone), a calcineurin inhibitor (cyclosporine or tacrolimus), and an antiproliferative agent (e.g., azathioprine). (Immunosuppressive therapy is presented in Table 13-16.) Tacrolimus appears to be superior to cyclosporine in liver transplantation. Standard immunosuppressive regimens often change during the course of a liver transplant recipient's life. In addition, corticosteroid withdrawal may be done and is relatively safe to do in liver transplant recipients.

About 80% of patients survive more than 5 years after liver transplant. Long-term survival depends on the cause of liver failure (e.g., localized HCC, chronic hepatitis B or C, biliary disease). Patients who have liver disease secondary to hepatitis B or C often experience reinfection of the transplanted liver. For patients with hepatitis B, treatment after surgery with IV HBIG and one of the nucleoside or nucleotide analogs (used to treat HBV infection) has reduced the rates of reinfection of the transplanted liver.

After a liver transplant, patients with HCV typically have lower survival rates than other patient groups. However, with the new direct-acting antivirals (DAAs) that can cure HCV infection, the need for liver transplant may decrease. For those patients with chronic hepatitis C who still need a transplant, the possibility of reinfection may still exist. Research is ongoing to determine if DAAs should be initiated before or after transplant.

The patient who has had a liver transplant requires highly skilled nursing care, either in an ICU or in some other specialized unit. Postoperative nursing care includes assessing neurologic status; monitoring for signs of hemorrhage; preventing pulmonary complications; monitoring drainage, electrolyte levels, and urine output; and monitoring for manifestations of infection and rejection. Common respiratory problems are pneumonia, atelectasis, and pleural effusions. To prevent these complications, encourage the patient to use measures such as coughing, deep breathing, incentive spirometry, and repositioning. Measure the drainage from the Jackson-Pratt drain, NG tube, and T tube, and note the color and consistency of the drainage at regular intervals.

The first 2 months after surgery are critical for monitoring for infection. Causes of infection can be viral, fungal, or bacterial. Fever may be the only sign of infection. Adherence to the medication regimen can be challenging, especially in the beginning. Emotional support and teaching for the patient and caregiver are essential to the success of the patient with a liver transplant.

 Gerontologic Considerations: Liver Disease in the Older Adult

The incidence of liver disease increases with age. With aging, the liver's size and metabolic breakdown of drugs decrease, and hepatobiliary function is altered. The liver has a decreased capacity to respond to injury. This especially applies to regeneration after injury.[31] Transplanted livers take longer to regenerate in the older adult compared with the younger adult.

Older adults are particularly vulnerable to drug-induced liver injury. This is due to several factors, including the increased use of multiple prescription and OTC drugs, which can lead to drug interactions and potential drug toxicity. Age-related decreases in liver function result in decreased drug metabolism. In addition, with aging the liver is less able to recover from drug-induced injury.

A growing number of older adults have chronic hepatitis C and the resulting cirrhosis. Antibodies to HCV and elevated liver enzymes may be found during a routine health assessment in asymptomatic patients.

Lifetime health behaviors may also influence the development of chronic liver disease in the older adult. Chronic alcohol use and obesity can contribute to cirrhosis, fatty liver inflammation (NASH), and subsequent liver failure and its complications. Because of many older adults' concomitant cardiovascular and pulmonary diseases and possible anticoagulant therapy, variceal bleeding can cause significant morbidity and mortality and needs immediate medical intervention. In the older adult with liver disease, hepatic encephalopathy can sometimes be misdiagnosed as dementia and often overlooked.

PATHOPHYSIOLOGY MAP

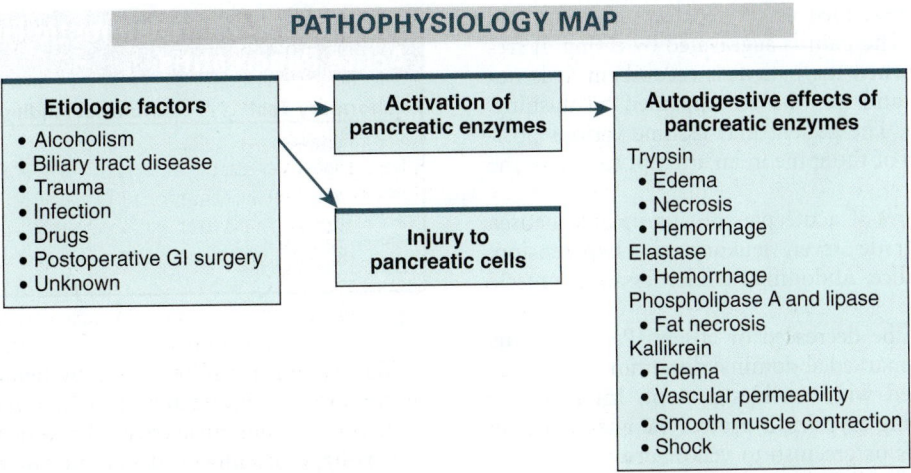

FIG. 43-11 Pathogenic process of acute pancreatitis.

Because older adults tend to have more co-morbid conditions, transplantation may have more risks for complications. Therefore older adults are not good candidates for liver transplants.

DISORDERS OF THE PANCREAS

ACUTE PANCREATITIS

Acute pancreatitis is an acute inflammation of the pancreas. Spillage of pancreatic enzymes into surrounding pancreatic tissue causes autodigestion and severe pain. The degree of inflammation varies from mild edema to severe hemorrhagic necrosis. Acute pancreatitis is most common in middle-aged men and women. It affects women and men equally. The rate of pancreatitis in African Americans is three times higher than in whites.

Etiology and Pathophysiology

Many factors can cause injury to the pancreas. In the United States, the most common cause is gallbladder disease (gallstones), which is more common in women. The second most common cause is chronic alcohol intake, which is more common in men.

Smoking is an independent risk factor for acute pancreatitis. Biliary sludge, or microlithiasis, which is a mixture of cholesterol crystals and calcium salts, is found in 20% to 40% of patients with acute pancreatitis.[32] The formation of biliary sludge is seen in patients with bile stasis.

Acute pancreatitis attacks are also associated with hypertriglyceridemia (serum levels over 1000 mg/dL). Other less common causes of acute pancreatitis include trauma (postoperative, postprocedure following an endoscopic retrograde cholangiopancreatography [ERCP]), viral infections (mumps, coxsackievirus B, HIV), penetrating duodenal ulcer, cysts, abscesses, cystic fibrosis, Kaposi sarcoma, certain drugs (corticosteroids, thiazide diuretics, oral contraceptives, sulfonamides, NSAIDs), metabolic disorders (hyperparathyroidism, renal failure), and vascular diseases.[32] In some cases the cause is unknown (idiopathic).

The most common pathogenic mechanism in acute pancreatitis is autodigestion of the pancreas (Fig. 43-11). The etiologic factors injure pancreatic cells or activate the pancreatic enzymes in the pancreas rather than in the intestine. This may be due to

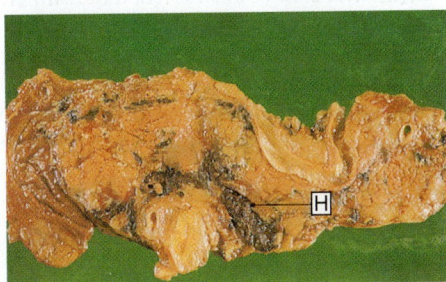

FIG. 43-12 In acute pancreatitis, the pancreas appears edematous and is commonly hemorrhagic *(H)*. (From Stevens A, Lowe J: *Pathology: illustrated review in colour,* ed 2, London, 2000, Mosby.)

reflux of bile acids into the pancreatic ducts through an open or distended sphincter of Oddi. This reflux may be caused by blockage created by gallstones. Obstruction of pancreatic ducts results in pancreatic ischemia.

Consuming alcohol is another cause of pancreatitis. The exact mechanism by which chronic alcohol intake predisposes a person to pancreatitis is not known. It is thought that alcohol increases the production of the digestive enzymes in the pancreas. Approximately 5% to 10% of chronic alcohol users develop pancreatitis. This suggests that certain environmental (high-fat diet, smoking) and genetic factors may also be contributing factors.

The pathophysiologic involvement of acute pancreatitis is classified as either *mild pancreatitis* (also known as *edematous* or *interstitial pancreatitis*) or *severe pancreatitis* (also called *necrotizing pancreatitis*) (Fig. 43-12). In severe pancreatitis, approximately half the patients have permanent decreases in pancreatic endocrine and exocrine function. Patients with severe pancreatitis are also at high risk of developing pancreatic necrosis, organ failure, and septic complications, resulting in a 25% mortality rate.[32]

Clinical Manifestations

Abdominal pain is the predominant manifestation of acute pancreatitis. The pain is due to distention of the pancreas, peritoneal irritation, and obstruction of the biliary tract. The pain is usually located in the left upper quadrant, but it may be mid-epigastric. It commonly radiates to the back because of the retroperitoneal location of the pancreas. The pain has a sudden onset and is described as severe, deep, piercing, and continuous or steady. The pain is aggravated by eating. It frequently has its onset when the patient is recumbent. It is not relieved by vomiting and may be accompanied by flushing, cyanosis, and dyspnea. The patient may assume various positions involving flexion of the spine in an attempt to relieve the severe pain.

Other manifestations of acute pancreatitis include nausea and vomiting, low-grade fever, leukocytosis, hypotension, tachycardia, and jaundice. Abdominal tenderness with muscle guarding is common.

Bowel sounds may be decreased or absent. Paralytic ileus may occur and causes marked abdominal distention. The lungs are frequently involved with crackles present. Intravascular damage from circulating trypsin (a proteolytic enzyme) may cause areas of cyanosis or greenish to yellow-brown discoloration of the abdominal wall. Other areas of ecchymoses are the flanks (*Grey Turner's spots* or *sign,* a bluish flank discoloration) and the periumbilical area (*Cullen's sign,* a bluish periumbilical discoloration). These result from seepage of bloodstained exudate from the pancreas and may occur in severe cases.

Shock may occur because of hemorrhage into the pancreas, toxemia from the activated pancreatic enzymes, or hypovolemia as a result of fluid shift into the retroperitoneal space (massive fluid shifts).

Complications

The severity of the acute pancreatitis depends on the extent of pancreatic destruction. Acute pancreatitis can be life threatening. Some patients recover completely, others have recurring attacks, and others develop chronic pancreatitis.

Two significant local complications of acute pancreatitis are pseudocyst and abscess. A *pancreatic pseudocyst* is an accumulation of fluid, pancreatic enzymes, tissue debris, and inflammatory exudates surrounded by a wall adjacent to the pancreas. Manifestations of pseudocyst are abdominal pain, palpable epigastric mass, nausea, vomiting, and anorexia. The serum amylase level frequently remains elevated. CT, MRI, and endoscopic ultrasound (EUS) may be used in the detection of a pseudocyst. The cysts usually resolve spontaneously within a few weeks but may perforate, causing peritonitis or rupture into the stomach or the duodenum. Treatment options include surgical drainage, percutaneous catheter placement and drainage, and endoscopic drainage.

When a pseudocyst gets infected, a *pancreatic abscess* results from extensive necrosis in the pancreas. It may rupture or perforate into adjacent organs. Manifestations of an abscess include upper abdominal pain, abdominal mass, high fever, and leukocytosis. Pancreatic abscesses require prompt surgical drainage to prevent sepsis.

The main systemic complications of acute pancreatitis are pulmonary (pleural effusion, atelectasis, pneumonia, and acute respiratory distress syndrome [ARDS]) and cardiovascular (hypotension). The pulmonary complications are likely due to the passage of exudate containing pancreatic enzymes from the peritoneal cavity through transdiaphragmatic lymph channels. Enzyme-induced inflammation of the diaphragm occurs with the result being atelectasis caused by reduced diaphragm movement. Trypsin can activate prothrombin and plasminogen, increasing the patient's risk for intravascular thrombi, pulmonary emboli, and disseminated intravascular coagulation (DIC).

TABLE 43-17	Diagnostic Findings in Acute Pancreatitis
Laboratory Test	**Abnormal Finding**
Serum amylase	↑
Serum lipase	↑
Urinary amylase	↑
Blood glucose	↑
Serum calcium	↓
Serum triglycerides	↑

Tetany, which can be caused by hypocalcemia, is a sign of severe disease. It is due in part to the combining of calcium and fatty acids during fat necrosis. The exact mechanisms of how or why hypocalcemia occurs are not well understood.

Patients with severe acute pancreatitis are at risk for abdominal compartment syndrome secondary to intraabdominal hypertension and edema. Abdominal compartment syndrome is discussed in Chapter 42.

Diagnostic Studies

The primary diagnostic tests for acute pancreatitis are serum amylase and lipase (Table 43-17). The serum amylase level is usually elevated early and remains elevated for 24 to 72 hours. Serum lipase level, which is also elevated in acute pancreatitis, is an important test because other disorders (e.g., mumps, cerebral trauma, renal transplantation) may increase serum amylase levels. Other serum findings include an increase in liver enzymes, triglycerides, glucose, and bilirubin and a decrease in calcium.

Diagnostic evaluation of acute pancreatitis is also directed at determining the cause. An abdominal ultrasound, x-ray, or contrast-enhanced CT scan can be used to identify pancreatic problems. CT scan is the best imaging test for pancreatitis and related complications such as pseudocysts and abscesses. ERCP is used (although ERCP can cause acute pancreatitis), along with EUS, magnetic resonance cholangiopancreatography (MRCP), and angiography. Chest x-rays may show pulmonary changes, including atelectasis and pleural effusions.

Interprofessional Care

Goals of interprofessional care for acute pancreatitis include (1) relief of pain; (2) prevention or alleviation of shock; (3) reduction of pancreatic secretions; (4) correction of fluid and electrolyte imbalances; (5) prevention or treatment of infections; and (6) removal of the precipitating cause, if possible (Table 43-18).

Conservative Therapy. Treatment of acute pancreatitis is primarily focused on supportive care, including aggressive hydration, pain management, management of metabolic complications, and minimization of pancreatic stimulation. Treatment and control of pain are very important. IV morphine may be used. Pain medications may be combined with an antispasmodic agent. However, atropine and other anticholinergic drugs should be avoided when paralytic ileus is present because they can decrease GI mobility, thus further exacerbating the problem. Other medications that relax smooth muscles (spasmolytics), such as nitroglycerin or papaverine, may be used. Supplemental O_2 is used to maintain O_2 saturation greater than 95%. In patients with severe pancreatitis, serum glucose levels are closely monitored for hyperglycemia.

TABLE 43-18   Interprofessional Care

Acute Pancreatitis

Diagnostic Assessment
- History and physical examination
- Serum amylase and lipase
- Blood glucose
- Serum calcium
- Serum triglycerides
- Flat plate of the abdomen
- Abdominal ultrasound
- Endoscopic ultrasound (EUS)
- Magnetic resonance cholangiopancreatography (MRCP)
- Endoscopic retrograde cholangiopancreatography (ERCP)
- Contrast-enhanced CT of pancreas
- Chest x-ray

Management
- NPO with NG tube to suction
- Albumin (if shock present)
- IV calcium gluconate (10%) (if tetany present)
- Lactated Ringer's solution

Drug Therapy
- Pain medication (e.g., morphine)
- Proton pump inhibitor (e.g., omeprazole [Prilosec])
- Antibiotics (if necrotizing pancreatitis)

TABLE 43-19   Drug Therapy

Acute and Chronic Pancreatitis

Drug	Mechanism of Action
Acute Pancreatitis	
Morphine	Relief of pain
Antispasmodics (e.g., dicyclomine [Bentyl])	↓ Vagal stimulation, motility, pancreatic outflow (↓ volume and concentration of bicarbonate and enzyme secretion) Contraindicated in paralytic ileus
Carbonic anhydrase inhibitor (acetazolamide)	↓ Volume and bicarbonate concentration of pancreatic secretion
Antacids	Neutralization of gastric hydrochloric (HCl) acid secretion ↓ Production and secretion of pancreatic enzymes and bicarbonate
Proton pump inhibitors (e.g., omeprazole [Prilosec])	↓ HCl acid secretion (HCl acid stimulates pancreatic activity)
Chronic Pancreatitis	
Pancreatic enzyme products (pancrelipase [Pancrease, Zenpep, Creon, Viokace])	Replacement therapy for pancreatic enzymes
Insulin	Treatment for diabetes mellitus or hyperglycemia, if needed

If shock is present, blood volume replacements are used. Plasma or plasma volume expanders such as dextran or albumin may be given. Fluid and electrolyte imbalances are corrected with lactated Ringer's solution or other electrolyte solutions. Central venous pressure readings may be used to assist in determining fluid replacement requirements. Vasoactive drugs such as dopamine (Intropin) may be used to increase systemic vascular resistance in patients with ongoing hypotension.

CHECK YOUR PRACTICE

You are a nurse working in the emergency department. Your patient is a 45-yr-old woman who is admitted with acute abdominal pain in her left upper quadrant. She is diagnosed with acute pancreatitis. She tells you, "I've been waiting in this emergency room for 8 hours and I'm starving. Why can't I get something to eat? My pain is so bad; I think it's becoming worse because you won't give me food."
- How would you respond?
- What information and teaching would you provide her?

It is important to reduce or suppress pancreatic enzymes to decrease stimulation of the pancreas and allow it to rest. This is accomplished in several ways. First, the patient is NPO. Second, NG suction may be used to reduce vomiting and gastric distention and to prevent gastric acidic contents from entering the duodenum. In addition, certain drugs may be used to suppress gastric acid secretion (Table 43-19). With resolution of the pancreatitis, the patient resumes oral intake. For the patient with severe acute pancreatitis who does not resume oral intake, enteral nutrition support may be initiated.

The inflamed and necrotic pancreatic tissue is a good medium for bacterial growth. In patients with acute necrotizing pancreatitis, infection is the leading cause of morbidity and mortality. Therefore it is important to prevent infections. Because many of the organisms come from the intestine, enteral feeding reduces the risk of necrotizing pancreatitis. Monitor the patient closely so that antibiotic therapy can be instituted early if necrosis and infection occur. Endoscopic- or CT-guided percutaneous aspiration with Gram stain and culture may be performed.

Surgical Therapy. When the acute pancreatitis is related to gallstones, an urgent ERCP plus endoscopic *sphincterotomy* (severing of the muscle layers of the sphincter of Oddi) may be done. This may be followed by laparoscopic cholecystectomy to reduce the potential for recurrence. Surgical intervention may also be indicated when the diagnosis is uncertain and for patients who do not respond to conservative therapy.

Those with severe acute pancreatitis may require drainage of necrotic fluid collections. This is done surgically, under CT guidance, or endoscopically. Percutaneous drainage of a pseudocyst can be performed, and a drainage tube is left in place.

Drug Therapy. Several different drugs are used to prevent and treat problems associated with pancreatitis (Table 43-19). Currently there are no drugs that cure pancreatitis.

Nutritional Therapy. Initially the patient with acute pancreatitis is on NPO status to reduce pancreatic secretion. Depending on the severity of the pancreatitis, enteral feedings via nasojejunal tube are initiated. Because of infection risk, parenteral nutrition is reserved for patients who cannot tolerate enteral nutrition (see Chapter 39). If IV lipids are ordered, blood triglyceride levels must be monitored. In cases of moderate to severe pancreatitis, the patient may require enteral feeding via a jejunal feeding tube.

When food is allowed, small, frequent feedings are given. The diet is usually high in carbohydrate content because that is the least stimulating to the exocrine portion of the pancreas. Suspect intolerance to oral foods when the patient reports pain, has increasing abdominal girth, or has elevations in serum amylase and lipase levels. Supplemental fat-soluble vitamins may be given.

❖ NURSING MANAGEMENT: ACUTE PANCREATITIS

◆ Nursing Assessment

Subjective and objective data that should be obtained from a person with acute pancreatitis are presented in Table 43-20.

TABLE 43-20   Nursing Assessment

Acute Pancreatitis

Subjective Data

Important Health Information

Past health history: Biliary tract disease, alcohol use, abdominal trauma, duodenal ulcers, infection, metabolic disorders
Medications: Thiazides, nonsteroidal antiinflammatory drugs
Surgery or other treatments: Surgical procedures on the pancreas, stomach, duodenum, or biliary tract. Endoscopic retrograde cholangiopancreatography (ERCP)

Functional Health Patterns

Health perception–health management: Chronic alcohol use, fatigue
Nutritional-metabolic: Nausea and vomiting, anorexia
Activity-exercise: Dyspnea
Cognitive-perceptual: Severe midepigastric or left upper quadrant pain that may radiate to the back, aggravated by food and alcohol intake and unrelieved by vomiting

Objective Data

General

Restlessness, anxiety, low-grade fever

Integumentary

Flushing, diaphoresis, discoloration of abdomen and flanks, cyanosis, jaundice. Decreased skin turgor, dry mucous membranes

Respiratory

Tachypnea, basilar crackles

Cardiovascular

Tachycardia, hypotension

Gastrointestinal

Abdominal distention, tenderness, and muscle guarding. Diminished bowel sounds

Possible Diagnostic Findings

↑ Serum amylase and lipase, leukocytosis, hyperglycemia, hypocalcemia, abnormal ultrasound and CT scans of pancreas, abnormal ERCP or MRCP

Nursing Diagnoses

Nursing diagnoses for the patient with acute pancreatitis may include, but are not limited to, the following:

- Acute pain *related to* distention of pancreas, peritoneal irritation, obstruction of biliary tract, and ineffective pain and comfort measures
- Deficient fluid volume *related to* nausea, vomiting, restricted oral intake, and fluid shift into the retroperitoneal space
- Imbalanced nutrition: less than body requirements *related to* anorexia, dietary restrictions, nausea, loss of nutrients from vomiting, and impaired digestion
- Ineffective health management *related to* lack of knowledge of preventive measures, diet restrictions, alcohol intake restriction, and follow-up care

Additional information on nursing diagnoses for the patient with acute pancreatitis is presented in eNursing Care Plan 43-3 available on the website for this chapter.

Planning

The overall goals are that the patient with acute pancreatitis will have (1) relief of pain, (2) normal fluid and electrolyte balance, (3) minimal to no complications, and (4) no recurrent attacks.

Nursing Implementation

Health Promotion.
The major factors involved in health promotion are (1) assessment of the patient for predisposing and etiologic factors and (2) encouragement of early treatment of these factors to prevent acute pancreatitis. Encourage early diagnosis and treatment of biliary tract disease, such as cholelithiasis. Encourage the patient to eliminate alcohol intake, especially if he or she has had any previous episodes of pancreatitis. Recurrent attacks of pancreatitis may become milder or disappear with the discontinuance of alcohol use.

Acute Care.
During the acute phase, it is important to monitor vital signs. Hemodynamic stability may be compromised by hypotension, fever, and tachypnea. Monitor the response to IV fluids. Also closely monitor fluid and electrolyte balance. Frequent vomiting, along with gastric suction, may result in decreased chloride, sodium, and potassium levels.

Respiratory failure may develop in the patient with severe acute pancreatitis. Assess respiratory function (e.g., lung sounds, O_2 saturation levels). If ARDS develops, the patient may require intubation and mechanical ventilation support.

> ⚠ **SAFETY ALERT**   **Respiratory Distress in Acute Pancreatitis**
> - Assess for respiratory distress in the patient with severe acute pancreatitis.
> - Listen to lung sounds and monitor O_2 saturation on a regular basis.

Because hypocalcemia can also occur, observe for symptoms of tetany, such as jerking, irritability, and muscular twitching. Numbness or tingling around the lips and in the fingers is an early indicator of hypocalcemia. Assess the patient for a positive Chvostek's sign or Trousseau's sign (see Fig. 16-15). Calcium gluconate (as ordered) should be given to treat symptomatic hypocalcemia. Hypomagnesemia may also develop, necessitating the monitoring of serum magnesium levels.

Because abdominal pain is a prominent symptom of pancreatitis, a major focus of your care is the relief of pain. Pain and restlessness can increase the metabolic rate. In addition, acute pain can contribute to hemodynamic instability. Morphine may be used for pain relief. Assess and document the duration of pain relief. Measures such as comfortable positioning, frequent changes in position, and relief of nausea and vomiting assist in reducing the restlessness that usually accompanies the pain. Assuming positions that flex the trunk and draw the knees up to the abdomen may decrease pain. A side-lying position with the head elevated 45 degrees decreases tension on the abdomen and may help ease the pain.

For the patient who is on NPO status or has an NG tube, provide frequent oral and nasal care to relieve the dryness of the mouth and nose. Oral care is essential to prevent parotitis. Also if the patient is taking anticholinergics to decrease GI secretions, the mouth will be especially dry. If the patient is taking antacids to neutralize gastric acid secretion, they should be sipped slowly or inserted in the NG tube.

Observe for fever and other manifestations of infection in the patient with acute pancreatitis. Respiratory tract infections are common, which causes the patient to take shallow, guarded abdominal breaths. Measures to prevent respiratory tract infections include turning, coughing, deep breathing, and assuming a semi-Fowler's position.

Other important assessments are observation for signs of paralytic ileus, renal failure, and mental changes. Determine the blood glucose level to assess damage to the β cells of the islets of Langerhans in the pancreas.

If patients have surgery to drain necrotic fluid or treat a cyst, they may require special wound care for an anastomotic leak or a fistula. To prevent skin irritation, use skin barriers (e.g., Stomahesive, Karaya Paste, or Colly-Seel), pouching, and drains. In addition to protecting the skin, pouching also permits a more accurate determination of fluid and electrolyte losses and increases patient comfort. Sterile pouching systems are available. Consult with a clinical specialist or wound, ostomy, and continence nurse (WOCN).

◆ **Ambulatory Care.** After acute pancreatitis, the patient may require home care follow-up. Because of loss of physical and muscle strength, physical therapy may be needed. Continued care to prevent infection and detect any complications is important. Counseling regarding abstinence from alcohol is important to prevent the patient from experiencing future attacks of acute pancreatitis and development of chronic pancreatitis. Because cigarettes can stimulate the pancreas, smoking should be avoided.

Dietary teaching should include restriction of fats because they stimulate the secretion of cholecystokinin, which then stimulates the pancreas. Carbohydrates are less stimulating to the pancreas and are encouraged. Also instruct the patient to avoid crash dieting and bingeing because they can precipitate attacks.

Teach the patient and caregiver to recognize and report symptoms of infection, diabetes mellitus, or steatorrhea (foul-smelling, fatty stools). These changes indicate possible ongoing destruction of pancreatic tissue and pancreatic insufficiency and may require exogenous enzyme supplementation. Teach the patient and caregiver about the prescribed regimen, including the importance of taking the required medications and following the recommended diet.

◆ **Evaluation**

The expected outcomes are that the patient with acute pancreatitis will

- Have adequate pain control
- Maintain adequate fluid balance
- Be knowledgeable about treatment regimen to restore health
- Get help for alcohol dependence and smoking cessation (if appropriate)

Additional information on expected outcomes for the patient with acute pancreatitis is presented in eNursing Care Plan 43-3 available on the website for this chapter.

CHRONIC PANCREATITIS

Chronic pancreatitis is a continuous, prolonged, inflammatory, and fibrosing process of the pancreas. The pancreas is progressively destroyed as it is replaced by fibrotic tissue. Strictures and calcifications may also occur in the pancreas.

Etiology and Pathophysiology

Chronic pancreatitis can be due to chronic alcohol use; obstruction caused by cholelithiasis (gallstones), tumor, pseudocysts, or trauma; and systemic diseases (e.g., systemic lupus erythematosus), autoimmune pancreatitis, and cystic fibrosis. Some patients may not have an identifiable risk factor (idiopathic pancreatitis). Chronic pancreatitis may follow acute pancreatitis, but it may also occur in the absence of any history of an acute condition.

The most common cause of obstructive pancreatitis is inflammation of the sphincter of Oddi associated with cholelithiasis. Cancer of the ampulla of Vater, duodenum, or pancreas can also cause this type of chronic pancreatitis.

The most common cause of nonobstructive pancreatitis (the most common type of chronic pancreatitis) is chronic alcohol use. There is inflammation and sclerosis, mainly in the head of the pancreas and around the pancreatic duct. In some people who drink alcohol, a genetic factor may predispose them to the direct toxic effect of the alcohol on the pancreas.

Clinical Manifestations

As with acute pancreatitis, a major manifestation of chronic pancreatitis is abdominal pain. The patient may have episodes of acute pain, but it usually is chronic (recurrent attacks at intervals of months or years). The attacks may become more and more frequent until they are almost constant, or they may diminish as pancreatic fibrosis develops. The pain is located in the same areas as in acute pancreatitis but is usually described as a heavy, gnawing feeling or sometimes as burning and cramp-like. The pain is not relieved with food or antacids.

Other clinical manifestations include symptoms of pancreatic insufficiency, including malabsorption with weight loss, constipation, mild jaundice with dark urine, steatorrhea, and diabetes mellitus. The steatorrhea may become severe, with voluminous, foul-smelling, fatty stools. Some abdominal tenderness may be present.

Chronic pancreatitis is also associated with a variety of complications, including pseudocyst formation, bile duct or duodenal obstruction, pancreatic ascites or pleural effusion, splenic vein thrombosis, pseudoaneurysms, and pancreatic cancer.

Diagnostic Studies

Confirming the diagnosis of chronic pancreatitis can be challenging. The diagnosis is based on the patient's signs and symptoms, laboratory studies, and imaging. In chronic pancreatitis, the levels of serum amylase and lipase may be elevated slightly or not at all, depending on the degree of pancreatic fibrosis. Serum bilirubin and alkaline phosphatase levels may be increased. There is usually mild leukocytosis and an elevated sedimentation rate.

ERCP is used to visualize the pancreatic and common bile ducts. Imaging studies such as CT, MRI, MRCP, abdominal ultrasound, and EUS are useful in patients with chronic pancreatitis. These procedures show a variety of changes, including calcifications, ductal dilation, pseudocysts, and enlargement of the pancreas.

Stool samples are examined for fecal fat content. Deficiencies of fat-soluble vitamins and cobalamin, glucose intolerance, and possibly diabetes may also be found in those with chronic pancreatitis. A secretin stimulation test may be used to assess the degree of pancreatic dysfunction (see Chapter 38).

Interprofessional Care

When the patient with chronic pancreatitis experiences an acute attack, the therapy is identical to that for acute pancreatitis. At other times the focus is on prevention of further attacks, relief of pain, and control of pancreatic exocrine and endocrine insufficiency. It sometimes takes frequent doses of analgesics (morphine or fentanyl patch [Duragesic]) to relieve the pain if dietary measures and enzyme replacement are not effective.

Diet, pancreatic enzyme replacement, and control of diabetes are ways to control the pancreatic insufficiency. Small, bland, frequent meals that are low in fat content are recommended to decrease pancreatic stimulation. Smoking is associated with accelerated progression of chronic pancreatitis. Also teach the patient not to consume alcohol and caffeinated beverages.

Pancreatic enzyme products such as pancrelipase (Pancrease, Zenpep, Creon, Viokace) contain amylase, lipase, and trypsin and are used to replace the deficient pancreatic enzymes. They are usually enteric coated to prevent their breakdown or inactivation by gastric acid. Bile salts are sometimes given to facilitate the absorption of the fat-soluble vitamins (A, D, E, and K) and prevent further fat loss. If diabetes develops, it is controlled with insulin (more commonly) or oral hypoglycemic agents. Acid-neutralizing drugs (e.g., antacids) and acid-inhibiting drugs (e.g., H_2-receptor blockers, proton pump inhibitors) may be given to decrease hydrochloric (HCl) acid secretion but have little overall effect on patient outcomes. Antidepressants, such as nortriptyline (Aventyl), have been shown to reduce the neuropathic pain associated with chronic pancreatitis.

Treatment of chronic pancreatitis sometimes requires endoscopic therapy or surgery. When biliary disease is present or obstruction or pseudocyst develops, surgery may be indicated. Surgical procedures can divert bile flow or relieve ductal obstruction. A choledochojejunostomy diverts bile around the ampulla of Vater, where there may be spasm or hypertrophy of the sphincter. In this procedure, the common bile duct is anastomosed into the jejunum. Another type of surgical diverting procedure is the Roux-en-Y pancreatojejunostomy, in which the pancreatic duct is opened and an anastomosis is made with the jejunum. Pancreatic drainage procedures can relieve ductal obstruction and are often done with ERCP. Some patients may undergo ERCP with sphincterotomy and/or stent placement at the site of obstruction. These patients require follow-up procedures such as ERCP to either exchange or remove the stent.

❖ NURSING MANAGEMENT: CHRONIC PANCREATITIS

Except during an acute episode, nursing management focuses on chronic care and health promotion. Instruct the patient to take measures to prevent further attacks. Dietary control, along with consistency of other treatment measures, such as taking pancreatic enzymes, is essential. The enzymes are usually taken with meals or a snack. Observe the patient's stools for steatorrhea to help determine the effectiveness of the enzymes. Instruct the patient and caregiver to monitor stool quality.

If diabetes has developed, instruct the patient regarding testing of blood glucose levels and drug therapy (see Chapter 48). Ensure that the patient who is taking antisecretory agents or antacids takes them as ordered to control gastric acidity. Antacids should be taken after meals and at bedtime.

The patient must avoid alcohol and may need assistance with this problem. If the patient is dependent on alcohol, referral to other agencies or resources may be necessary (see Chapter 10).

PANCREATIC CANCER

Annually in the United States an estimated 48,960 people are diagnosed with pancreatic cancer, and 40,560 people die from pancreatic cancer.[33] It is the fourth leading cause of death from cancer in the United States. The risk increases with age, with the peak incidence occurring between 65 and 80 years of age.

Most pancreatic tumors are adenocarcinomas originating from the epithelium of the ductal system. More than half of the tumors occur in the head of the pancreas. As the tumor grows, the common bile duct becomes obstructed, and obstructive jaundice develops. Tumors starting in the body or the tail often remain silent until their growth is advanced. The majority of cancers have metastasized at the time of diagnosis. The signs and symptoms of pancreatic cancer are often similar to those of chronic pancreatitis. The prognosis of a patient with cancer of the pancreas is poor. The majority of patients die within 5 to 12 months of the initial diagnosis, and the 5-year survival rate is less than 5%.[33]

Etiology and Pathophysiology

The cause of pancreatic cancer remains unknown. Risk factors for pancreatic cancer include chronic pancreatitis, diabetes mellitus, age, cigarette smoking, family history of pancreatic cancer, high-fat diet, and exposure to chemicals such as benzidine. African Americans have a higher incidence of pancreatic cancer than whites. The most firmly established environmental risk factor is cigarette smoking. Smokers are two to three times more likely to develop pancreatic cancer than nonsmokers. The risk is related to both the duration and amount of cigarettes smoked.

Clinical Manifestations

Common manifestations of pancreatic cancer include abdominal pain (dull, aching), anorexia, rapid and progressive weight loss, nausea, and jaundice. The most common manifestations of cancer of the head of the pancreas are pain, jaundice, and weight loss. Pruritus may accompany obstructive jaundice. In general, pain is common and is related to the location of malignancy. Extreme, unrelenting pain is related to extension of the cancer into the retroperitoneal tissues and nerve plexuses. The pain is frequently located in the upper abdomen or left hypochondrium and often radiates to the back. It is commonly related to eating, and it also occurs at night. Weight loss is due to poor digestion and absorption caused by lack of digestive enzymes from the pancreas.

Diagnostic Studies

Abdominal ultrasound or endoscopic ultrasound (EUS), spiral CT scan, ERCP, MRI, and MRCP are the most commonly used diagnostic imaging techniques for pancreatic diseases, including cancer. EUS involves imaging the pancreas with the use of an endoscope positioned in the stomach and duodenum. EUS also allows for fine-needle aspiration of the tumor for pathologic examination. CT scan is often the initial study and provides information on metastasis and vascular involvement of the tumor. ERCP allows visualization of the pancreatic duct and biliary system. When ERCP is used, pancreatic secretions and tissue can be collected for analysis of different tumor markers. MRI and MRCP may also be used for diagnosing and staging pancreatic cancer. A positron emission tomography (PET) scan or PET/CT scan may also be obtained to confirm a pancreatic cancer diagnosis and determine the stage at time of diagnosis. It is also used to monitor progress and response to therapy.

Tumor markers are used both for establishing the diagnosis of pancreatic adenocarcinoma and for monitoring the response to treatment. Cancer-associated antigen 19-9 (CA 19-9) is elevated in pancreatic cancer and is the most commonly used tumor marker. However, CA 19-9 can also be elevated in gallbladder cancer or in benign conditions such as acute and chronic pancreatitis, hepatitis, and biliary obstruction.

Interprofessional Care

Surgery provides the most effective treatment for cancer of the pancreas, but only 15% to 20% of patients have resectable tumors at the time of diagnosis. With the use of neoadjuvant chemotherapy (treatment before surgery), more patients can eventually become surgical candidates. The type of surgery depends on the size and location of the tumor. Pancreatic head tumors require the classic Whipple procedure or pancreatico-duodenectomy (Fig. 43-13), whereas pancreatic body and/or tail tumors require a distal pancreatectomy procedure. In the Whipple surgery, the proximal pancreas (proximal pancreatectomy), along with duodenum (duodenectomy), distal segment of the common bile duct and distal portion of the stomach (partial gastrectomy) are removed together followed by a surgical anastomosis of the pancreatic duct, common bile duct, and stomach to the jejunum. Occasionally, a total pancreatectomy is performed, which would cause diabetes and the patient would be dependent on exogenous insulin and pancreatic enzyme supplementation for life. If the pancreatic tumor cannot be removed surgically, palliative measures such as a cholecystojejunostomy to relieve biliary obstruction and/or endoscopically placed biliary stents can be used.

Radiation therapy alone has little effect on survival but may be effective for pain relief. External radiation is typically used, but implantation of internal radiation seeds into the tumor has also been used. The current role of chemotherapy in pancreatic cancer is limited and can have significant side effect profile. Chemotherapy usually consists of fluorouracil (5-FU) and gemcitabine (Gemzar) either alone or in combination with agents such as capecitabine (Xeloda), paclitaxel (Abraxane), erlotinib (Tarceva), or irinotecan (Onivyde). Erlotinib is a targeted therapy drug (see Table 15-13).

❖ NURSING MANAGEMENT: PANCREATIC CANCER

Because the patient with pancreatic cancer has many of the same problems as the patient with pancreatitis, nursing care includes many of the same measures (see sections on acute and chronic pancreatitis on pp. 999-1001 and 1003-1004). Provide symptomatic and supportive nursing care. This includes administration of medications and comfort measures to relieve pain. Psychologic support is essential, especially during times of anxiety or depression.

Adequate nutrition is an important part of the nursing care plan. Frequent and supplemental feedings may be necessary. Include measures to stimulate the appetite as much as possible and to manage anorexia, nausea, and vomiting. If the patient is undergoing radiation therapy, observe for adverse reactions such as anorexia, nausea, vomiting, and skin irritation.

The prognosis for a patient with pancreatic cancer is poor. A significant component of the nursing care is helping the patient and caregiver cope with the diagnosis and prognosis. Chapter 9 provides information on palliative and end-of-life care.

DISORDERS OF THE BILIARY TRACT

CHOLELITHIASIS AND CHOLECYSTITIS

The most common disorder of the biliary system is **cholelithiasis** (stones in the gallbladder) (Fig. 43-14). The gallstones may get lodged in the neck of the gallbladder or in the cystic duct. **Cholecystitis** (inflammation of the gallbladder wall) is usually associated with cholelithiasis and usually occurs together, but a person can have cholelithiasis without cholecystitis. Cholecystitis may present acutely or chronically.

Gallbladder disease is a common health problem in the United States. It has been estimated that up to 10% of American adults have cholecystitis caused by gallstones. The actual number is not known because many persons with stones are asymptomatic. *Cholecystectomy* (removal of the gallbladder) ranks among the most common surgical procedures performed in the United States.

Cholelithiasis is more common in women, especially multiparous women and women over 40 years of age. Postmenopausal women on estrogen replacement therapy and younger women on oral contraceptives are at an increased risk for gallbladder disease. Oral contraceptives affect cholesterol production and increase the likelihood of gallbladder cholesterol saturation. Other factors that increase the occurrence of gallbladder disease are a sedentary lifestyle, a familial tendency, and obesity. Obesity causes increased secretion of cholesterol in bile. The incidence of gallbladder disease is especially high in the Native American population, particularly in the Navajo and Pima tribes.

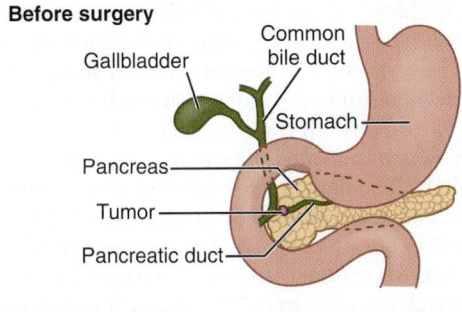

Before surgery

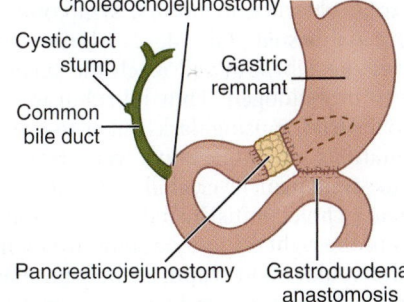

Whipple procedure

FIG. 43-13 Whipple procedure or radical pancreaticoduodenectomy. This surgical procedure involves resection of the proximal pancreas, adjoining duodenum, distal portion of the stomach, and distal portion of the common bile duct. An anastomosis of the pancreatic duct, common bile duct, and stomach to the jejunum is done. (From Butcher GP: *Gastroenterology: an illustrated colour text*, London, 2004, Churchill Livingstone.)

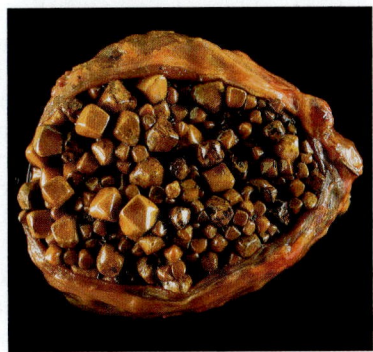

FIG. 43-14 Cholesterol gallstones in a gallbladder that was removed. (From Kumar V, Abbas AK, Aster JC, Fausto N: *Robbins and Cotran pathologic basis of disease*, ed 8, Philadelphia, 2010, Saunders.)

Etiology and Pathophysiology

Cholelithiasis. The cause of gallstones is unknown. Cholelithiasis develops when the balance that keeps cholesterol, bile salts, and calcium in solution is altered so that these substances precipitate. Conditions that upset this balance include infection and disturbances in the metabolism of cholesterol. In patients with cholelithiasis, the bile secreted by the liver is supersaturated with cholesterol (lithogenic bile). The bile in the gallbladder also becomes supersaturated with cholesterol. When bile is supersaturated with cholesterol, precipitation of cholesterol occurs in the gallbladder.

Other components of bile that precipitate into stones are bile salts, bilirubin, calcium, and protein. Mixed cholesterol stones, which are predominantly cholesterol, are the most common gallstones.

Changes in the composition of bile are significant in the formation of gallstones. Stasis of bile leads to progression of the supersaturation and changes in the chemical composition of the bile (biliary sludge). Immobility, pregnancy, and inflammatory or obstructive lesions of the biliary system decrease bile flow. Hormonal factors during pregnancy may cause delayed emptying of the gallbladder, resulting in stasis of bile.

The stones may remain in the gallbladder or migrate to the cystic duct or the common bile duct. They cause pain as they pass through the ducts, and they may lodge in the ducts and produce an obstruction. Small stones are more likely to move into a duct and cause obstruction. Table 43-21 depicts the changes and manifestations that occur when the stones obstruct the common bile duct. If the blockage occurs in the cystic duct, the bile can continue to flow into the duodenum directly from the liver. However, when the bile in the gallbladder cannot escape, this stasis of bile may lead to cholecystitis.

Cholecystitis. Cholecystitis is most commonly associated with obstruction caused by gallstones or biliary sludge. Cholecystitis in the absence of obstruction (*acalculous cholecystitis*) occurs most frequently in older adults and in patients who are critically ill. Acalculous cholecystitis is also associated with prolonged immobility and fasting, prolonged parenteral nutrition, and diabetes mellitus. The main cause of this illness is thought to be bile stasis. Critically ill patients are more predisposed because of increased bile viscosity due to fever and dehydration and because of prolonged absence of oral feeding resulting in a decrease or absence of cholecystokinin-induced gallbladder contraction. Other etiologic factors include adhesions, neoplasms, anesthesia, and opioids.

Once acalculous cholecystitis is established, secondary infection with enteric pathogens, including *Escherichia coli*, *Enterococcus faecalis*, *Klebsiella*, *Pseudomonas*, and *Proteus*, is common. Perforation occurs in severe cases.

Inflammation is the major pathophysiologic condition and may be confined to the mucous lining or involve the entire wall

TABLE 43-21 Manifestations of Obstructed Bile Flow

Manifestation	Etiology
Obstructive jaundice	No bile flow into duodenum, bilirubin accumulates in blood
Dark amber to brown urine, which foams when shaken	Increase in water soluble (conjugated) bilirubin elimination in urine
No urobilinogen in urine	No bilirubin reaching small intestine to be converted to urobilinogen
Clay-colored stools	Same as above
Pruritus	Deposition of bile salts in skin tissues
Intolerance for fatty foods (nausea, sensation of fullness, anorexia)	No bile in small intestine for fat digestion
Bleeding tendencies	Lack of or decreased absorption of vitamin K, resulting in decreased production of prothrombin
Steatorrhea	Undigested fatty components of food are eliminated in stool. Occurs because no bile in small intestine, thus preventing emulsion, digestion, and absorption of fat
Fever, chills, cholangitis	Bacterial reflux from biliary tract to systemic circulation

of the gallbladder. During an acute attack of cholecystitis, the gallbladder is edematous and hyperemic, and it may be distended with bile or pus. The cystic duct is also involved and may become occluded. The wall of the gallbladder becomes scarred after an acute attack. Decreased functioning will occur if large amounts of tissue become fibrotic.

Clinical Manifestations

Cholelithiasis may produce severe symptoms or none at all. Many patients have "silent cholelithiasis." The severity of symptoms depends on whether the stones are stationary or mobile and whether obstruction is present. When a stone is lodged in the ducts or when stones are moving through the ducts, spasms may result in response to the stone. This sometimes produces severe pain, which is termed *biliary colic,* even though the pain is rarely colicky. The pain is more often steady. The pain can be excruciating and accompanied by tachycardia, diaphoresis, and prostration. The severe pain may last up to an hour, and when it subsides, there is residual tenderness in the right upper quadrant. The attacks of pain frequently occur 3 to 6 hours after a high-fat meal or when the patient lies down.

When total obstruction occurs, symptoms related to bile blockage are manifested (Table 43-21). If the common bile duct is obstructed, no bilirubin will reach the small intestine to be converted to urobilinogen. Thus bilirubin will be excreted by the kidneys instead, causing dark amber to brown urine.

Manifestations of cholecystitis vary from indigestion to moderate to severe pain, fever, chills, and jaundice. Initial symptoms of acute cholecystitis include indigestion and pain and tenderness in the right upper quadrant, which may be referred to the right shoulder and scapula. The pain may be acute and be accompanied by nausea and vomiting, restlessness, and diaphoresis. Manifestations of inflammation include leukocytosis and fever. Physical findings include right upper quadrant or epigastrium tenderness and abdominal rigidity. Manifestations of chronic cholecystitis include a history of fat intolerance, dyspepsia, heartburn, and flatulence.

Complications

Complications of cholelithiasis and cholecystitis include gangrenous cholecystitis, subphrenic abscess, pancreatitis, *cholangitis* (inflammation of biliary ducts), biliary cirrhosis, fistulas, and rupture of the gallbladder, which can produce bile peritonitis. In older patients and those with diabetes, gangrenous cholecystitis and bile peritonitis are the most common complications of cholecystitis. *Choledocholithiasis* (stone in the common bile duct) may occur, producing symptoms of obstruction.

Diagnostic Studies

Ultrasound is commonly used to diagnose gallstones (see Table 38-11). It is especially useful for patients with jaundice (because it does not depend on renal function) and for patients who are allergic to contrast medium. ERCP allows for visualization of the gallbladder, cystic duct, common hepatic duct, and common bile duct. Bile taken during ERCP is sent for culture to identify possible infecting organisms.

Percutaneous transhepatic cholangiography is the insertion of a needle directly into the gallbladder duct followed by injection of contrast materials. It is generally done after ultrasound indicates a bile duct blockage.

Laboratory tests may reveal an increased WBC count as a result of inflammation. Both direct and indirect bilirubin levels may also be elevated, as is the urinary bilirubin level if an obstructive process is present (Table 43-3). Serum enzymes, such as alkaline phosphatase, ALT, and AST, may be elevated. Serum amylase is increased if there is pancreatic involvement.

Interprofessional Care

Once gallstones become symptomatic, definitive surgical intervention with cholecystectomy is usually indicated. However, in some cases, conservative therapy may be considered.

Conservative Therapy

Cholelithiasis. The treatment of gallstones depends on the stage of disease. Bile acids (cholesterol solvents) such as ursodeoxycholic acid (ursodiol) and chenodeoxycholic acid (chenodiol) are used to dissolve stones. However, the gallstones may recur. Gallstones are not usually treated with drugs because of the high use and success of laparoscopic cholecystectomy.

ERCP with endoscopic sphincterotomy (papillotomy) may be used for stone removal (Fig. 43-15). ERCP allows for visualization of the biliary system, dilation (balloon sphincteroplasty), and placement of stents and sphincterotomy. Special catheters with wire baskets or inflatable balloon tip may be used for stone removal.[34] When a stent is placed, it is generally removed or changed after a few months.

Extracorporeal shock-wave lithotripsy (ESWL) is an alternative treatment used when stones cannot be removed by endoscopic approaches. In ESWL a lithotriptor uses high-energy shock waves to disintegrate gallstones once they have been located by ultrasound. It usually takes 1 to 2 hours to disintegrate the stones. After they are broken up, the fragments pass through the common bile duct and into the small intestine. Usually ESWL and oral dissolution therapy are used together.

Cholecystitis. During an acute episode of cholecystitis, treatment focuses on pain control, control of possible infection with antibiotics, and maintenance of fluid and electrolyte balance (Table 43-22). Treatment is mainly supportive and focused on symptom management. If nausea and vomiting are severe, NG tube insertion and gastric decompression may be used to prevent further gallbladder stimulation. A cholecystostomy may be used to drain purulent material from the obstructed gallbladder. Opioids are given for pain management. Anticholinergics may be used to decrease GI secretions and counteract smooth muscle spasms.

Surgical Therapy. Laparoscopic cholecystectomy is the treatment of choice for symptomatic cholelithiasis. Approximately 90% of cholecystectomies are done laparoscopically. In this procedure, the gallbladder is removed through one to four small

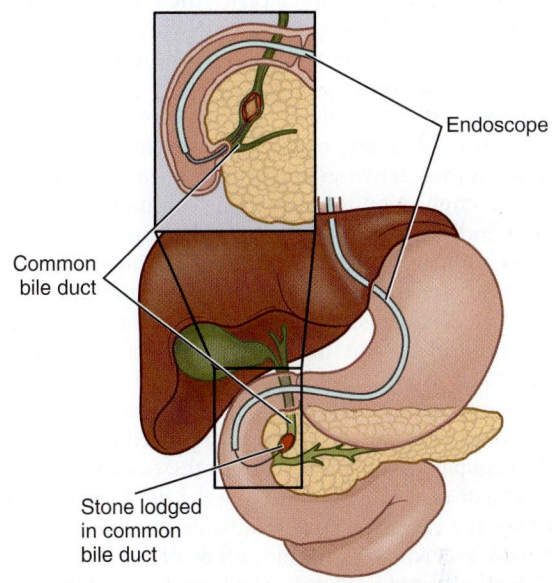

FIG. 43-15 During endoscopic sphincterotomy, an endoscope is advanced through the mouth and stomach until its tip sits in the duodenum opposite the common bile duct. *Inset,* After widening the duct mouth by incising the sphincter muscle, the physician advances a basket attachment into the duct and snags the stone.

TABLE 43-22 Interprofessional Care
Cholelithiasis and Acute Cholecystitis

Diagnostic Assessment
- History and physical examination
- Ultrasound
- Endoscopic retrograde cholangiopancreatography (ERCP)
- Percutaneous transhepatic cholangiography
- Liver function tests
- White blood cell count
- Serum bilirubin

Management
Conservative Therapy
- IV fluid
- NPO with NG tube, later progressing to low-fat diet
- Antiemetics
- Analgesics
- Fat-soluble vitamins (A, D, E, and K)
- Anticholinergics (antispasmodics)
- Antibiotics (for secondary infection)
- Transhepatic biliary catheter
- ERCP with sphincterotomy (papillotomy)
- Extracorporeal shock-wave lithotripsy

Dissolution Therapy
- ursodeoxycholic acid (ursodiol [Actigall])

Surgical Therapy
- Laparoscopic cholecystectomy
- Incisional (open) cholecystectomy

punctures in the abdomen. The surgeon makes a small cut below the umbilicus and inserts a needle into the area. CO_2 gas is passed into the abdomen to expand the area, which allows the surgeon to see the organs more clearly and provides more room to work. A laparoscope, which has a camera attached, and grasping forceps are inserted into the abdomen through the punctures. (The incision sites may vary.) Using closed-circuit monitors to view the abdominal cavity, the surgeon retracts and dissects the gallbladder and removes it with grasping forceps. This is a safe and routine procedure with minimal morbidity and quick recovery time.

Most patients have minimal postoperative pain and are discharged the day of surgery or the day after. They are usually able to resume normal activities and return to work within 1 week. The main complication is injury to the common bile duct. The few contraindications to laparoscopic cholecystectomy include peritonitis, cholangitis, gangrene or perforation of the gallbladder, portal hypertension, and serious bleeding disorders.

On selected patients an incisional (open) cholecystectomy may be performed. This involves removal of the gallbladder through a right subcostal incision. A T tube may be inserted into the common bile duct during surgery when a common bile duct exploration is part of the surgical procedure (Fig. 43-16). This ensures patency of the duct until the edema produced by the trauma of exploring and probing the duct has subsided. It also allows the excess bile to drain while the small intestine is adjusting to receiving a continuous flow of bile.

Transhepatic Biliary Catheter. The transhepatic catheter can be used preoperatively in biliary obstruction and in hepatic dysfunction secondary to obstructive jaundice. It can also be inserted for palliative care when inoperable liver, pancreatic, or bile duct carcinoma obstructs bile flow. The catheter is used when endoscopic drainage has been unsuccessful. The catheter is inserted percutaneously and allows for decompression of obstructed extrahepatic bile ducts so that bile can flow freely. After placement of the catheter into the obstructed duct internally, the external catheter is connected to a drainage bag. Patients should be encouraged to replace fluids lost in the drainage bag with electrolyte-rich drinks. The skin around the catheter insertion site should be cleansed daily with an antiseptic. Observe for bile leakage at the insertion site and any signs or symptoms of sudden abdominal pain, nausea, fever, or chills that may signal an occluded or malfunctioning drain.

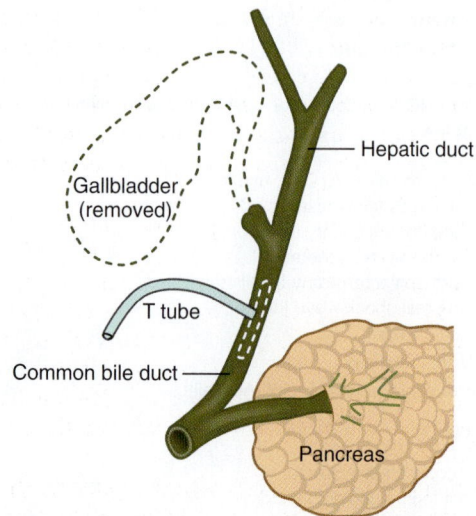

FIG. 43-16   Placement of T tube. *Dotted lines* indicate parts removed.

Drug Therapy. The most common drugs used in the treatment of gallbladder disease are analgesics, anticholinergics (antispasmodics), fat-soluble vitamins, and bile salts. Morphine may be used initially for pain management. Anticholinergics such as atropine and other antispasmodics may be used to relax the smooth muscle and decrease ductal tone.

If the patient has chronic gallbladder disease or any biliary tract obstruction, fat-soluble vitamins (A, D, E, and K) may be given. Bile salts may be administered to facilitate digestion and vitamin absorption.

Cholestyramine may provide relief from pruritus. Cholestyramine is a resin that binds bile salts in the intestine, increasing their excretion in the feces. It is administered in powder form, mixed with milk or juice. Side effects include nausea, vomiting, diarrhea or constipation, and skin reactions. Because cholestyramine may bind with other medications, check drug-to-drug interactions prior to administering.

Nutritional Therapy. People have fewer gallbladder problems if they eat smaller, more frequent meals with some fat at each meal to promote gallbladder emptying. If obesity is a problem, a reduced-calorie diet is indicated. The diet should be low in saturated fats (e.g., butter, shortening, lard) and high in fiber and calcium. Rapid weight loss should be avoided because it can promote gallstone formation.

After a laparoscopic cholecystectomy, instruct the patient to have liquids for the rest of the day and eat light meals for a few days. If an incisional cholecystectomy is done, the patient will progress from liquids to a regular diet once bowel sounds have returned. The amount of fat in the postoperative diet depends on the patient's tolerance of fat. A low-fat diet may be helpful if the flow of bile is reduced (usually only in the early postoperative period) or if the patient is overweight. Sometimes the patient is instructed to restrict fats for 4 to 6 weeks. Otherwise, no special dietary instructions are needed other than to eat nutritious meals and avoid excessive fat intake.

❖ NURSING MANAGEMENT: GALLBLADDER DISEASE

◆ Nursing Assessment

Subjective and objective data that should be obtained from a person with gallbladder disease are presented in Table 43-23.

◆ Nursing Diagnoses

Nursing diagnoses for the patient with gallbladder disease treated surgically include, but are not limited to, the following:
- Acute pain *related to* surgical procedure
- Ineffective health management *related to* lack of knowledge of diet and postoperative management

◆ Planning

The overall goals are that the patient with gallbladder disease will have (1) relief of pain and discomfort, (2) no complications postoperatively, and (3) no recurrent attacks of cholecystitis or cholelithiasis.

◆ Nursing Implementation

◆ **Health Promotion.** Be aware of predisposing factors for gallbladder disease in general health screening. Teach patients from ethnic groups in which the disease is more common, such as Native Americans, the initial manifestations and to see their HCP if these manifestations occur. Patients with chronic cholecystitis may not have acute symptoms and may not seek help until jaundice and biliary obstruction occur. Earlier detection

TABLE 43-23 Nursing Assessment
Cholecystitis or Cholelithiasis

Subjective Data

Important Health Information

Past health history: Obesity, multiparity, infection, cancer, extensive fasting, pregnancy

Medications: Estrogen or oral contraceptives

Surgery or other treatments: Previous abdominal surgery

Functional Health Patterns

Health perception–health management: Positive family history, sedentary lifestyle

Nutritional-metabolic: Weight loss, anorexia, indigestion, fat intolerance, nausea and vomiting, dyspepsia, chills

Elimination: Clay-colored stools, steatorrhea, flatulence. Dark urine

Cognitive-perceptual: Moderate to severe pain in right upper quadrant that may radiate to the back or scapula. Pruritus

Objective Data

General

Fever, restlessness

Integumentary

Jaundice, icteric sclera, diaphoresis

Respiratory

Tachypnea, splinting during respirations

Cardiovascular

Tachycardia

Gastrointestinal

Palpable gallbladder, abdominal guarding and distention

Possible Diagnostic Findings

↑ Serum liver enzymes, alkaline phosphatase, and bilirubin. Absence of urobilinogen in urine, ↑ urinary bilirubin, leukocytosis. Abnormal gallbladder ultrasound

---

in these patients is important so that they can be managed with a low-fat diet and monitored more closely.

◆ **Acute Care.** Nursing goals for the patient undergoing conservative therapy include treating pain, relieving nausea and vomiting, providing comfort and emotional support, maintaining fluid and electrolyte balance and nutrition, making accurate assessments to ensure effective treatment, and observing for complications.

The patient with acute cholecystitis or cholelithiasis frequently has severe pain. Give the drugs ordered to relieve the pain as required before it becomes more severe. Assess what drugs relieve the pain and how much medication is required. Observe for side effects of the drugs as part of the continued assessment. Nursing comfort measures, such as a clean bed, comfortable positioning, and oral care, are appropriate.

Some patients have more severe nausea and vomiting than others. For these patients, an NG tube and gastric decompression may be ordered. Eliminating intake of food and fluids also prevents further stimulation of the gallbladder. Oral hygiene, care of nares, accurate intake and output measurements, and maintenance of suction should be a part of the nursing care plan for this patient. For patients with less severe nausea and vomiting, antiemetics are usually adequate. When the patient is vomiting, provide comfort measures such as frequent mouth rinses. Remove any vomitus immediately from the patient's

view. If pruritus occurs with jaundice, measures to relieve itching are necessary and can include antihistamines or other treatments as previously discussed.

Assess for progression of the symptoms and development of complications. Observe for signs of obstruction of the ducts by stones. These include jaundice; clay-colored stools; dark, foamy urine; steatorrhea; fever; and increased WBC count.

When manifestations of obstruction are present (Table 43-21), bleeding may result from decreased prothrombin production by the liver. Common sites to observe for bleeding are the mucous membranes of the mouth, nose, gingivae, and injection sites. If injections are given, use a small-gauge needle and apply gentle pressure after the injection. Know the patient's prothrombin time and use it as a guide in the assessment process.

Assessment for infections includes monitoring vital signs. A temperature elevation with chills and jaundice may indicate choledocholithiasis.

Your care of the patient after ERCP with papillotomy includes assessment to detect complications such as pancreatitis, perforation, infection, and bleeding. Monitor the patient's vital signs. Abdominal pain, fever, and increasing amylase and lipase may indicate acute pancreatitis. The patient should be on bed rest for several hours and should be NPO until the gag reflex returns. Teach the patient the need for follow-up if the stent is to be removed or changed.

◆ *Postoperative Care.* Postoperative nursing care after a laparoscopic cholecystectomy includes monitoring for complications such as bleeding, making the patient comfortable, and preparing the patient for discharge. A common postoperative complaint is referred pain to the shoulder because of the CO_2 that is used to inflate the abdominal cavity during surgery. It may not be released or absorbed by the body. The CO_2 can irritate the phrenic nerve and diaphragm, causing some difficulty in breathing. Placing the patient in the Sims' position (on left side with right knee flexed) helps move the gas pocket away from the diaphragm. Encourage deep breathing along with movement and ambulation. The pain can usually be relieved by NSAIDs or codeine. The patient is allowed clear liquids and can walk to the bathroom to void. Most patients go home the same day.

Postoperative nursing care for incisional cholecystectomy focuses on adequate ventilation and prevention of respiratory complications. Other nursing care is the same as general postoperative nursing care (see Chapter 19).

If the patient has a T tube (Fig. 43-16), you must maintain bile drainage and monitor T-tube function and drainage. The T tube is usually connected to a closed gravity drainage system. If the Penrose or Jackson-Pratt drain or the T tube is draining large amounts of bile, it is helpful to use a sterile pouching system to protect the skin. Encourage the patient to replace fluids and electrolytes that are lost.

◆ **Ambulatory Care.** When the patient has conservative therapy, nursing management depends on the patient's symptoms and on whether surgical intervention is planned. Dietary teaching is usually necessary. The diet is usually low in fat, and sometimes a weight-reduction diet is also recommended. The patient may need to take fat-soluble vitamin supplements. Instruct the patient on observations that indicate obstruction (e.g., stool and urine changes, jaundice, pruritus). Explain the importance of continued health care follow-up.

The patient who undergoes a laparoscopic cholecystectomy is discharged soon after the surgery, so home care and teaching are important (Table 43-24).

TABLE 43-24   Patient & Caregiver Teaching
Postoperative Laparoscopic Cholecystectomy

The patient's postoperative teaching plan should include the following:

1. Remove the bandages on the puncture sites the day after surgery and you can shower.
2. Notify your surgeon if any of the following signs and symptoms occurs:
   - Redness, swelling, bile-colored drainage or pus from any incision
   - Severe abdominal pain, nausea, vomiting, fever, chills
3. You can gradually resume normal activities.
4. Return to work within 1 wk of surgery.
5. You can resume your usual diet, but a low-fat diet is usually better tolerated for several weeks after surgery.

After an incisional cholecystectomy, instruct the patient to avoid heavy lifting for 4 to 6 weeks. Usual sexual activities, including intercourse, can be resumed as soon as the patient feels ready, unless otherwise instructed by the HCP.

Sometimes the patient is required to remain on a low-fat diet for 4 to 6 weeks. If so, an individualized dietary teaching plan is necessary. A weight-reduction program may be helpful if the patient is overweight. Most patients tolerate a regular diet with no difficulties but should avoid excessive fats.

◆ **Evaluation**

The overall expected outcomes are that the patient with gallbladder disease will

- Appear comfortable and verbalize pain relief
- Verbalize knowledge of activity level and dietary restrictions

GALLBLADDER CANCER

Primary cancer of the gallbladder is uncommon. The majority of gallbladder carcinomas are adenocarcinomas. Annually an estimated 10,910 new cases of gallbladder cancer occur with an estimated 3700 deaths.[35] A relationship exists between cancer of the gallbladder and chronic cholecystitis and cholelithiasis.

The early symptoms of carcinoma of the gallbladder are insidious and are similar to those of chronic cholecystitis and cholelithiasis, which makes the diagnosis difficult. Later symptoms are usually those of biliary obstruction. Gallbladder cancer is twice as common in women as in men.[35]

Diagnosis and staging of gallbladder cancer are done using EUS, abdominal ultrasound, CT, MRI, and/or MRCP. Unfortunately, gallbladder cancer often is not detected until the disease is advanced. When it is found early, surgery can be curative. Several factors influence successful surgical outcomes, including the depth of cancer invasion, extent of liver involvement, venous or lymphatic invasion, and lymph node metastasis. Extended cholecystectomy with lymph node dissection has improved the outcomes for patients with gallbladder cancer.

When surgery is not an option, endoscopic stenting of the biliary tract can be done to reduce obstructive jaundice. Adjuvant therapies, including radiation therapy and chemotherapy, may be used depending on the disease state. Overall, cancer of the gallbladder has a poor prognosis.

Nursing management involves palliative care with special attention to nutrition, hydration, skin care, and pain relief. Nursing care measures used for patients with cholecystitis and cholelithiasis are frequently applied, as well as nursing care measures for the patient with cancer (see Chapter 15).

CASE STUDY
Cirrhosis of the Liver

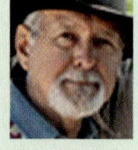

(©sbeagle/ iStock/ Thinkstock)

Patient Profile

M.B., a 58-yr-old male rancher who lives in rural Wyoming, is admitted with a diagnosis of cirrhosis of the liver. He has been vomiting for 2 days and noticed blood in the toilet when he vomits. He lives 40 miles from the nearest hospital. He had one of his ranch hands drive him to the hospital.

Subjective Data

- Has 2 children who live in New York. He has been estranged from them since his divorce 3 years ago
- Has had cirrhosis for 12 yr
- Acknowledges that he had been drinking heavily for 20 yr but has been sober for the past 2 yr
- Complains of anorexia, nausea, and abdominal discomfort

Objective Data

Physical Examination

- Has moderate ascites
- Has jaundice of sclera and skin
- Has 4+ pitting edema of the lower extremities
- Liver and spleen are palpable

Laboratory Values

- Total bilirubin: 15 mg/dL (257 mmol/L)
- AST: 190 U/L (3.2 μkat/L)
- ALT: 210 U/L (3.5 μkat/L)
- Platelets: 45,000/μL
- ECG is at right:

Discussion Questions

1. What are possible causes of cirrhosis? What type of cirrhosis does M.B. probably have?
2. Describe the pathophysiologic changes that occur in the liver as cirrhosis develops.
3. List M.B.'s clinical manifestations of liver failure. For each manifestation, explain the pathophysiologic basis.
4. Explain the significance of the results of his laboratory values and ECG findings.
5. If M.B. begins to manifest signs and symptoms of hepatic encephalopathy, what would you monitor? What measures should be instituted to control or decrease the encephalopathy?
6. What are possible causes of his gastrointestinal bleeding?
7. **Priority Decision:** Based on the assessment data, what are the priority nursing diagnoses? Are there any collaborative problems?
8. **Priority Decision:** What are the priority nursing interventions for a patient at this stage of his illness?
9. **Evidence-Based Practice:** M.B. discusses his prognosis with you. He says, "There is no hope. I might as well keep drinking." How would you respond to his statement?
10. **Safety:** Given the patient's bleeding history and current laboratory values, identify areas of injury risk and specify actions you will take to ensure patient safety.

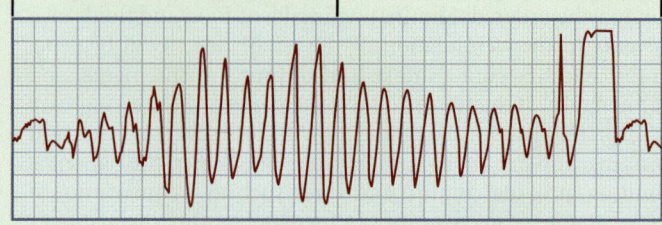

BRIDGE TO NCLEX EXAMINATION

The number of the question corresponds to the same-numbered outcome at the beginning of the chapter.

1. A patient with hepatitis A is in the acute phase. The nurse plans care for the patient based on the knowledge that
   a. pruritus is a common problem with jaundice in this phase.
   b. the patient is most likely to transmit the disease during this phase.
   c. gastrointestinal symptoms are not as severe in hepatitis A as they are in hepatitis B.
   d. extrahepatic manifestations of glomerulonephritis and polyarteritis are common in this phase.

2. A patient with acute hepatitis B is being discharged in 2 days. The discharge teaching plan should include instructions to
   a. avoid alcohol for the first 3 weeks.
   b. use a condom during sexual intercourse.
   c. have family members get an injection of immunoglobulin.
   d. follow a low-protein, moderate-carbohydrate, moderate-fat diet.

3. A patient has been told that she has elevated liver enzymes caused by nonalcoholic fatty liver disease (NAFLD). The nursing teaching plan should include
   a. having genetic testing done.
   b. recommending a heart-healthy diet.
   c. the necessity to reduce weight rapidly.
   d. avoiding alcohol until liver enzymes return to normal.

4. The patient with advanced cirrhosis asks why his abdomen is so swollen. The nurse's response is based on the knowledge that
   a. a lack of clotting factors promotes the collection of blood in the abdominal cavity.
   b. portal hypertension and hypoalbuminemia cause a fluid shift into the peritoneal space.
   c. decreased peristalsis in the GI tract contributes to gas formation and distention of the bowel.
   d. bile salts in the blood irritate the peritoneal membranes, causing edema and pocketing of fluid.

5. In planning care for a patient with metastatic liver cancer, the nurse should include interventions that
   a. focus primarily on symptomatic and comfort measures.
   b. reassure the patient that chemotherapy offers a good prognosis.
   c. promote the patient's confidence that surgical excision of the tumor will be successful.
   d. provide information necessary for the patient to make decisions regarding liver transplantation.

6. Nursing management of the patient with acute pancreatitis includes (select all that apply)
   a. checking for signs of hypocalcemia.
   b. providing a diet low in carbohydrates.
   c. giving insulin based on a sliding scale.
   d. observing stools for signs of steatorrhea.
   e. monitoring for infection, particularly respiratory tract infection.

7. A patient with pancreatic cancer is admitted to the hospital for evaluation of possible treatment options. The patient asks the nurse to explain the Whipple procedure that the surgeon has described. The explanation includes the information that a Whipple procedure involves
   a. creating a bypass around the obstruction caused by the tumor by joining the gallbladder to the jejunum.
   b. resection of the entire pancreas and the distal portion of the stomach, with anastomosis of the common bile duct and the stomach into the duodenum.
   c. removal of part of the pancreas, part of the stomach, the duodenum, and the gallbladder, with joining of the pancreatic duct, the common bile duct, and the stomach into the jejunum.
   d. radical removal of the pancreas, the duodenum, and the spleen, and attachment of the stomach to the jejunum, which requires oral supplementation of pancreatic digestive enzymes and insulin replacement therapy.

8. The nursing management of the patient with cholecystitis associated with cholelithiasis is based on the knowledge that
   a. shock-wave therapy should be tried initially.
   b. once gallstones are removed, they tend not to recur.
   c. the disorder can be successfully treated with oral bile salts that dissolve gallstones.
   d. laparoscopic cholecystectomy is the treatment of choice in most patients who are symptomatic.

9. Teaching in relation to home management after a laparoscopic cholecystectomy should include
   a. keeping the bandages on the puncture sites for 48 hours.
   b. reporting any bile-colored drainage or pus from any incision.
   c. using over-the-counter antiemetics if nausea and vomiting occur.
   d. emptying and measuring the contents of the bile bag from the T tube every day.

1. a, 2. b, 3. b, 4. b, 5. a, 6. a, e, 7. c, 8. d, 9. b

For rationales to these answers and even more NCLEX review questions, visit *evolve.elsevier.com/Lewis/medsurg*.

EVOLVE WEBSITE

evolve.elsevier.com/Lewis/medsurg
Review Questions (Online Only)
Key Points
Answer Keys for Questions
- Rationales for Bridge to NCLEX Examination Questions
- Answer Guidelines for Case Study on p. 1010
- Answer Guidelines for Managing Care of Multiple Patients Case Study (Section 8) on p. 1013
Student Case Studies
- Patient With Acute Pancreatitis and Septic Shock
- Patient With Cholelithiasis/Cholecystitis
- Patient With Cirrhosis
- Patient With Hepatitis

Nursing Care Plans
- eNursing Care Plan 43-1: Patient With Acute Viral Hepatitis
- eNursing Care Plan 43-2: Patient With Cirrhosis
- eNursing Care Plan 43-3: Patient With Acute Pancreatitis
Conceptual Care Map Creator
- Conceptual Care Map for Case Study on p. 1010
Audio Glossary
Content Updates

REFERENCES

1. Centers for Disease Control and Prevention: Viral hepatitis—Hepatitis A Information—United States. Retrieved from *www.cdc.gov/hepatitis/hav/havfaq.htm#general*.

2. Centers for Disease Control and Prevention: Viral hepatitis—Hepatitis B information—United States. Retrieved from *www.cdc.gov/hepatitis/hbv/hbvfaq.htm*.

3. Centers for Disease Control and Prevention: Viral hepatitis—CDC Recommendations for Specific Populations and Settings—United States. Retrieved from *www.cdc.gov/hepatitis/populations/api.htm*.

4. Centers for Disease Control and Prevention: Viral hepatitis—Hepatitis C information—United States. Retrieved from *www.cdc.gov/hepatitis/hcv/hcvfaq.htm#section3*.

5. American Cancer Society: Liver cancer. Retrieved from *www.cancer.org/cancer/livercancer/detailedguide/liver-cancer-risk-factors*.

6. Busch K, Thimme R: Natural history of chronic hepatitis B virus infection, *Med Microbiol Immunol* 204:5, 2015.

7. Castera L: Noninvasive assessment of liver fibrosis, *Dig Dis* 33:498, 2015.

*8. World Health Organization: Guidelines for the prevention, care and treatment for persons with chronic hepatitis B infection. Retrieved from *www.who.int/hiv/pub/hepatitis/hepatitis-b-guidelines/en/*.

9. Lucaciu LA, Dumitrascu DL: Depression and suicide ideation in chronic hepatitis C patients untreated and treated with interferon: prevalence, prevention, and treatment, *Ann Gastro* 28:1, 2015.

*10. American Association for the Study of Liver Diseases: Recommendations for testing, managing, and treating Hepatitis C—United States. Retrieved from *www.hcvguidelines.org/full-report/initial-treatment-hcv-infection*.

11. Centers for Disease Control and Prevention: Testing recommendations for hepatitis C virus infection. Retrieved from *www.cdc.gov/hepatitis/hcv/guidelinesc.htm*.

*12. Chalasani NP, Hayashi PH, Bonkovsky HL, et al: ACG Clinical Guideline: the diagnosis and management of idiosyncratic drug-induced liver injury, *Am J Gastroenterol* 109:950, 2014.

13. Trivedi PJ, Hirschfield GM: Treatment of autoimmune liver disease: current and future therapeutic options, *Ther Adv Chronic Dis* 4:119, 2013.

14. Hahn SH: Population screening for Wilson's disease, *Ann New York Acad Sci* 1:64, 2014.

15. Juran BD, Lazaridis KN: Environmental factors in primary biliary cirrhosis, *Semin Liver Dis* 34: 265, 2014.

16. Schwenger KP, Allard JP: Clinical approaches to non-alcoholic fatty liver disease, *World J Gastroenterol* 20:1712, 2014.

17. Centers for Disease Control and Prevention: Chronic liver disease and cirrhosis. Retrieved from *www.cdc.gov/nchs/fastats/liver-disease.htm*.

18. Iwakiri Y: Pathophysiology of portal hypertension, *Clin Liv Dis* 18:281, 2014.

19. Rajoriya N, Tripathi D: Historical overview and review of current day treatment in the management of acute variceal haemorrhage, *World J Gastroenterol* 20:6481, 2014.

20. Preveden T: Bacterial infections in patients with liver cirrhosis, *Med Pregl* 68:187, 2015.

21. Sharma P, Sharma BC: Management of overt hepatic encephalopathy, *J Clin Exp Hepatol* 5:S82, 2015.

22. Poorad FF: Presentation and complications associated with cirrhosis of the liver, *Curr Med Res Opin* 31:925, 2015.

23. Kodali S, McGuire BM: Diagnosis and management of hepatic encephalopathy in fulminant hepatic failure, *Clin Liver Dis* 19:565, 2015.

24. Toshikuni N, Arisawa T, Tsutsumi M: Nutrition and exercise in the management of liver cirrhosis, *World J Gastroenterol* 20:7286, 2014.

25. Raschi E, De Ponti F: Drug and herb-induced liver injury: progress, current challenges and emerging signals of post-marketing risk, *World J Hepatol* 7:1761, 2015.

26. Bernal W, Wendon J: Acute liver failure, *NEJM* 369:2525, 2013.

27. American Cancer Society: What are the key statistics about liver cancer? Retrieved from *www.cancer.org/cancer/livercancer/detailedguide/liver-cancer-what-is-key-statistics*.

28. You MW, Kim SY, Kim KW, et al: Recent advances in the imaging of hepatocellular carcinoma, *Clin Mol Hepatol* 21:95, 2015.

29. Tejeda-Maldonado J, Garcia-Juarez I, Aguirre-Valadez J, et al: Diagnosis and treatment of hepatocellular carcinoma: an update, *World J Hepatol* 7:362, 2015.

30. American Liver Foundation: More about organ donation. Retrieved from *dwww.liverfoundation.org/patients/organdonor/about*.

31. Kim IH: Aging and liver disease, *Curr Opin Gastroenterol* 31:184, 2015.

32. Talukdar R, Vege SS: Acute pancreatitis, *Curr Opin Gastroenterol* 31:374, 2015.

33. National Cancer Institute: Pancreatic cancer for health professionals. Retrieved from *www.cancer.gov/types/pancreatic/hp*.

34. Guda NM, Freeman ML: *Overview of ERCP complications: prevention and management in ERP and EUS*, New York, 2015, Springer.

*35. Aloia TA, Jarufe N, Javle M, et al: Gallbladder cancer: expert consensus statement, *HPB* 8:681, 2015.

*Evidence-based information for clinical practice.

CASE STUDY

Managing Care of Multiple Patients

You are working on the medical-surgical unit and have been assigned to care for the following five patients. You have one LPN and one UAP who are assigned to help you.

Patients

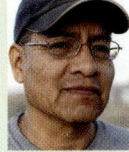

(©iStockphoto/ Thinkstock)

L.C. is a 58-yr-old Native American man admitted from the ED with acute abdominal pain. A CBC showed an Hgb of 6.8 g/dL and Hct of 20%. The WBC count is normal. A CT scan and colonoscopy indicated two medium-size tumors in the transverse colon. A hemicolectomy was performed. The adenocarcinoma had spread to the muscle of the colon wall, and there were two positive lymph nodes.

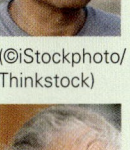

(©iStockphoto/ Thinkstock)

M.S. is a 70-yr-old white woman who was recently admitted to the unit with generalized weakness and malnutrition. She is 5 feet 4 inches tall and weighs 100 lb, with a 30-lb weight loss in past 2 months. Her PMH includes a recent thrombotic stroke with hemiparesis and dysphagia. She has had nothing by mouth for the past 24 hours and just started enteral nutrition via PEG tube.

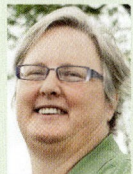

(©Christa Brunt/ iStock/ Thinkstock)

S.R. is a 48-yr-old white woman admitted with hip pain. She has a history of type 2 diabetes mellitus, hypertension, and osteoarthritis. She is 5 feet 4 inches tall and weighs 210 lb. Her most recent BP was 160/110 mm Hg. Her morning laboratory results reveal elevations in fasting blood glucose, total cholesterol, LDL cholesterol, and triglycerides. Her HDL cholesterol is low. Her cardiac enzymes and ECG are all within normal limits. She is scheduled to undergo a cardiac stress test at 10 AM.

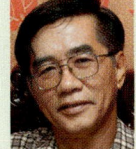

(©iStockphoto/ Thinkstock)

F.H., a 40-yr-old male immigrant from Vietnam, has a 1-yr history of epigastric distress. He underwent an upper endoscopy a few weeks ago, which revealed a duodenal ulcer and *H. pylori*. He was started on omeprazole, clarithromycin, and amoxicillin for 10 days. He came to the ED yesterday with complaints of severe epigastric pain and melena. His Hgb is 10.2 g/dL and Hct is 30%. He was admitted and put on a pantoprazole (Protonix) continuous infusion and is scheduled for a repeat EGD today.

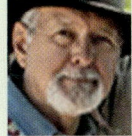

(©sbeagle/ iStock/ Thinkstock)

M.B. is a 58-yr-old man admitted with a diagnosis of upper GI bleeding. He has been vomiting for 2 days and noticed blood in the toilet when he vomits. He has had cirrhosis for 12 yr and admits to drinking heavily for 20 yr but has been sober for the past 2 yr. He currently complains of anorexia, nausea, and abdominal discomfort. He has moderate ascites, jaundice of sclera and skin, 4+ pitting edema of the lower extremities, and palpable liver and spleen. His bilirubin and liver enzymes are all elevated. His platelet and RBC counts are low.

Discussion Questions

1. **Priority Decision:** After receiving report, which patient should you see first? Provide a rationale for your decision.
2. **Teamwork and Collaboration:** Which tasks could you delegate to the LPN *(select all that apply)*?
   a. Assess L.C.'s dressing, pain level, and bowel sounds.
   b. Provide enteral tube feeding for M.S. if gastric residual <500 mL.
   c. Because she speaks Vietnamese, teach F.H.'s wife about his disease.
   d. Call M.B.'s health care provider regarding the morning laboratory results.
   e. Perform bedside glucometer reading and administer oral medications to S.R.
3. **Priority Decision:** As you are assessing M.B., the LPN informs you that F.H. just vomited a large amount of bright red blood. What initial action would be *most* appropriate?
   a. Have the LPN administer an antiemetic to F.H.
   b. Ask the LPN to notify F.H.'s health care provider.
   c. Leave M.B.'s room to perform a focused assessment on F.H.
   d. Ask the UAP to obtain a unit of packed RBCs from the blood bank.

Case Study Progression

When you enter F.H.'s room, he tells you that his pain actually feels somewhat relieved since he vomited. However, you note that his skin is cool and clammy, his BP is 90/54 mm Hg, and his heart rate is 116 bpm. You notify his HCP.

4. Which interventions would you expect the HCP to order for F.H. *(select all that apply)*?
   a. Stat hemoglobin and hematocrit
   b. Emergent endoscopy and endotherapy
   c. Discontinue the pantoprazole (Protonix) infusion
   d. Start a second IV site and administer 500 mL normal saline bolus
   e. Contact surgeon and notify operating room that patient is unstable and needs surgery
5. **Priority Decision:** After administering a bolus feeding of enteral nutrition to M.S., it would be *most* important to
   a. assess for gastric residual.
   b. obtain an abdominal x-ray.
   c. keep head of bed elevated 30 to 45 degrees.
   d. record the total amount of fluid administered.
6. Which intervention to treat ascites would you expect the HCP to order for M.B. *(select all that apply)*?
   a. Paracentesis
   b. 2 g sodium diet
   c. Diuretic therapy
   d. 1800 mL/day fluid restriction
   e. Shunt insertion from peritoneum to heart
7. **Management Decision:** As you enter the nurse's station, you overhear derogatory comments made by the UAP to the LPN about S.R.'s weight. Which response would be *most* appropriate?
   a. Report the incident to charge nurse for follow-up.
   b. Talk to the UAP to discuss possible HIPAA violation.
   c. Talk to S.R. to assess impact of UAP's bias on patient's self-image.
   d. Teach staff members to recognize obesity as a disease process.

SECTION 9

Problems of Urinary Function

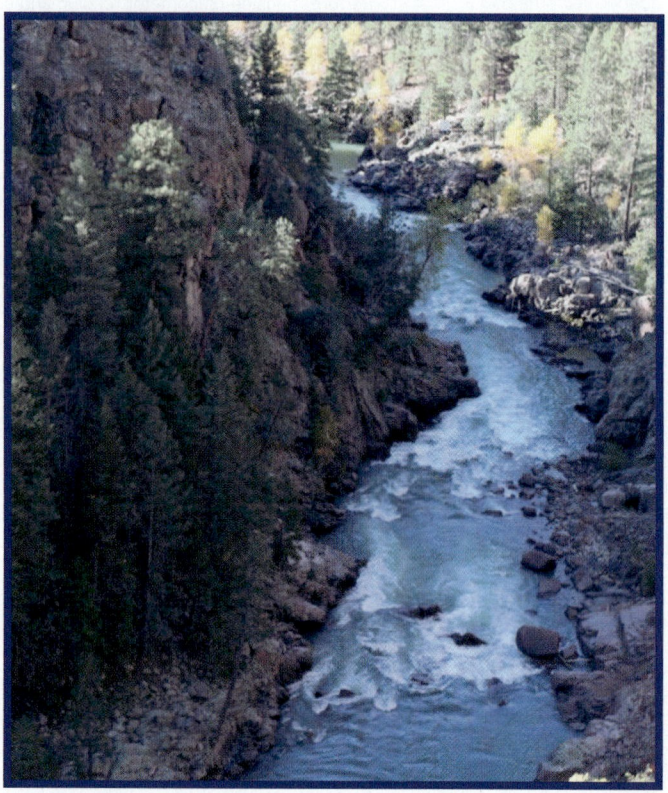

Peter Bonner

Sometimes ... if you lean over to watch the river slipping slowly away beneath you, you will suddenly know everything there is to be known.

Winnie the Pooh

44

Assessment of Urinary System

Suzanne Teresa Parsell

Life is really simple, but we insist on making it complicated.

Confucius

http://evolve.elsevier.com/Lewis/medsurg/

LEARNING OUTCOMES

1. Differentiate among the anatomic location and functions of the kidneys, ureters, bladder, and urethra.
2. Explain the physiologic events involved in the formation and passage of urine from glomerular filtration to voiding.
3. Obtain significant subjective and objective data related to the urinary system from a patient.
4. Link the age-related changes of the urinary system to the differences in assessment findings.
5. Perform a physical assessment of the urinary system using appropriate techniques.
6. Differentiate normal from abnormal findings of a physical assessment of the urinary system.
7. Describe the purpose, significance of results, and nursing responsibilities related to diagnostic studies of the urinary system.
8. Differentiate normal from abnormal findings of a urinalysis.

KEY TERMS

costovertebral angle (CVA), p. 1023
creatinine, Table 44-8, p. 1026
cystometrogram, Table 44-8, p. 1029

cystoscopy, Table 44-8, p. 1028
glomerular filtration rate (GFR), p. 1017
glomerulus, p. 1016

nephron, p. 1016
renal biopsy, Table 44-8, p. 1030

Adequate kidney function is essential to the maintenance of a healthy body. If a person has complete kidney failure and treatment is not provided, death is inevitable. This chapter discusses the structures and functions, assessment, and diagnostic studies of the urinary system.

STRUCTURES AND FUNCTIONS OF URINARY SYSTEM

The *upper urinary system* consists of two kidneys and two ureters. The *lower urinary system* consists of a urinary bladder and urethra (Fig. 44-1). Urine is formed in the kidneys, drains through the ureters to be stored in the bladder, and then passes out of the body through the urethra.

Kidneys

The kidneys are the principal organs of the urinary system. The primary functions of the kidneys are to (1) regulate the volume and composition of extracellular fluid (ECF) and (2) excrete waste products from the body. The kidneys also function to control BP, produce erythropoietin, activate vitamin D, and regulate acid-base balance.

Macrostructure. The paired kidneys are bean-shaped organs located retroperitoneally (behind the peritoneum) on either side of the vertebral column at about the level of the twelfth thoracic (T12) vertebra to the third lumbar (L3) vertebra. Each kidney weighs 4 to 6 oz (113 to 170 g) and is about 5 inches (12.5 cm) long. The right kidney, positioned at the level of the twelfth rib, is lower than the left. An adrenal gland lies on top of each kidney.

Each kidney is surrounded by a considerable amount of fat and connective tissue that cushions, supports, and maintains its position. A thin, smooth layer of fibrous membrane called the *capsule* covers the surface of each kidney. The capsule protects the kidney and serves as a shock absorber when this area is traumatized from a sudden force or strike. The *hilus* on the medial side of the kidney serves as the entry site for the renal artery and nerves and as the exit site for the renal vein and ureter.

The *parenchyma* (actual tissue) of the kidney can be visualized on a longitudinal section of the kidney (Fig. 44-2). The outer layer is the *cortex* and the inner layer is the *medulla*. The medulla consists of a number of pyramids. The apices (tops) of these pyramids are called *papillae*, through which urine passes to enter the calyces. The minor calyces widen and merge to form

Reviewed by Janie Corbitt, RN, MLS, Retired Instructor of Nursing, Milledgeville, Georgia; Deborah Erickson, RN, PhD, Associate Professor and Graduate Coordinator, Department of Nursing, Bradley University, Peoria, Illinois; Shari Gould, RN, MSN, Associate Professor of Nursing, Victoria College, Victoria, Texas; and Marci Langenkamp, RN, MS, Associate Professor of Nursing, Edison Community College, Piqua, Ohio.

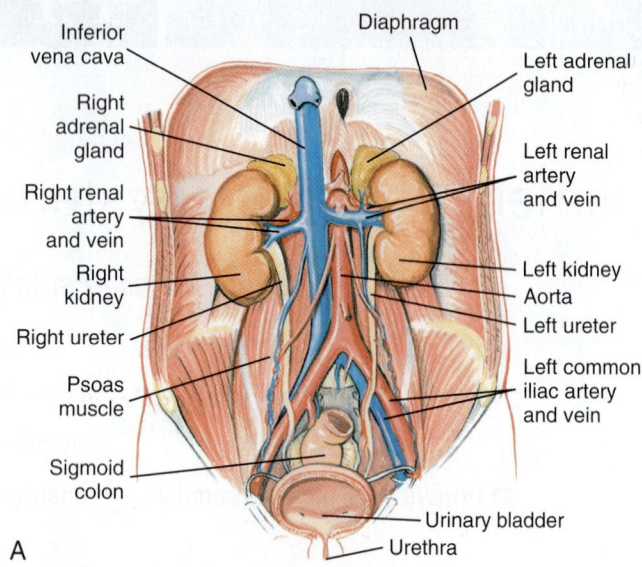

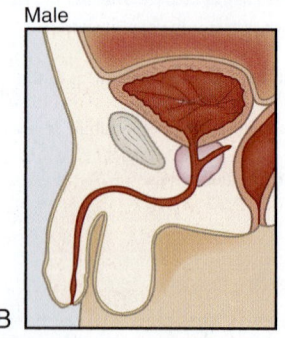

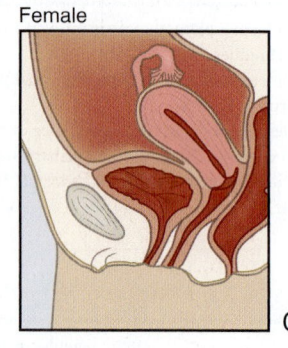

FIG. 44-1 Organs of the urinary system. **A,** Upper urinary tract in relation to other anatomic structures. **B,** Male urethra in relation to other pelvic structures. **C,** Female urethra.

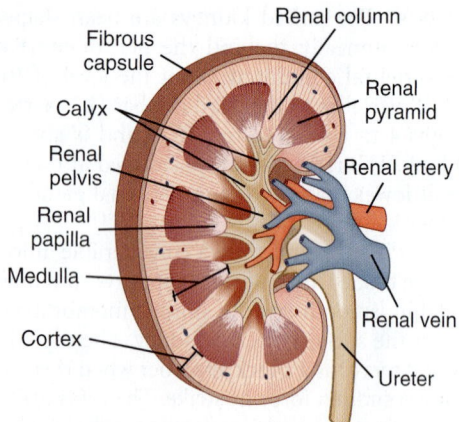

FIG. 44-2 Longitudinal section of the kidney.

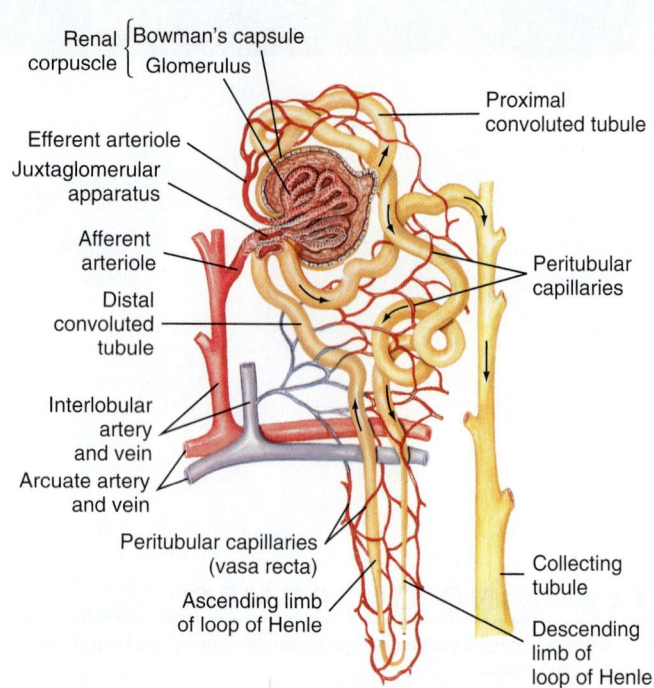

FIG. 44-3 The nephron is the basic functional unit of the kidney. This illustration of a single nephron unit also shows the surrounding blood vessels. (Modified from Thibodeau GA, Patton KT: *The human body in health and disease,* ed 4, St Louis, 2005, Mosby.)

major calyces, which form a funnel-shaped sac called the *renal pelvis.* The minor and major calyces transport urine to the renal pelvis, from which it drains through the ureter to the bladder. The renal pelvis can store a small volume of urine (3 to 5 mL).

Microstructure. The nephron is the functional unit of the kidney. Each kidney contains approximately 1 million nephrons. Each nephron is composed of the glomerulus, Bowman's capsule, and a tubular system. The tubular system consists of the proximal convoluted tubule, loop of Henle, distal

convoluted tubule, and collecting tubules (Fig. 44-3). The glomerulus, Bowman's capsule, proximal tubule, and distal tubule are located in the cortex of the kidney. The loop of Henle and collecting tubules are located in the medulla. Several collecting tubules join to form a single collecting duct. The collecting ducts eventually merge into a pyramid that empties via the papilla into a minor calyx.

Blood Supply. Blood flow to the kidneys, approximately 1200 mL/min, accounts for 20% to 25% of the cardiac output. Blood reaches the kidneys via the renal artery, which arises from the aorta and enters the kidney through the hilus. The renal artery divides into secondary branches and then into still smaller branches, each of which forms an afferent arteriole. The afferent arteriole divides into a capillary network, the glomerulus, which is a collection of up to 50 capillaries (Fig. 44-3). The capillaries of the glomerulus unite in the efferent arteriole. This efferent arteriole splits to form a capillary network, the peritubular capillaries, which surround the tubular system. All peritubular capillaries drain into the venous system; the renal vein empties into the inferior vena cava.

Physiology of Urine Formation. Urine formation is the outcome of a complex, multistep process of filtration, reabsorption, secretion, and excretion of water, electrolytes, and metabolic waste products. Although urine formation is the result of this process, the primary functions of the kidneys are to filter the blood and maintain the body's internal homeostasis.

Glomerular Function. Urine formation begins at the glomerulus, where blood is filtered. The glomerulus is a semipermeable membrane that allows filtration (Fig. 44-3). The hydrostatic pressure of the blood within the glomerular capillaries causes a portion of blood to be filtered across the semipermeable membrane into Bowman's capsule, where the filtered portion of the blood (glomerular filtrate) begins to pass down to the tubule. Filtration is more rapid in the glomerulus than in ordinary

TABLE 44-1   Functions of Nephron Segments

Segment	Function
Glomerulus	Selective filtration.
Proximal tubule	Reabsorption of 80% of electrolytes and water, glucose, amino acids, HCO_3^-. Secretion of H^+ and creatinine.
Loop of Henle	Reabsorption of Na^+ and Cl^- in ascending limb and water in descending loop. Concentration of filtrate.
Distal tubule	Secretion of K^+, H^+, ammonia. Reabsorption of water (regulated by ADH) and HCO_3^-. Regulation of Ca^{2+} and PO_4^{2-} by parathyroid hormone. Regulation of Na^+ and K^+ by aldosterone.
Collecting duct	Reabsorption of water (ADH required).

ADH, Antidiuretic hormone.

tissue capillaries because the glomerular membrane is porous. The ultrafiltrate is similar in composition to blood except that it lacks blood cells, platelets, and large plasma proteins. Under normal conditions, the capillary pores are too small to allow the loss of these large blood components. However, in many kidney diseases, capillary permeability is increased, which permits plasma proteins and blood cells to pass into the urine.

The amount of blood filtered each minute by the glomeruli is expressed as the glomerular filtration rate (GFR). The normal GFR is about 125 mL/min. The peritubular capillary network reabsorbs most of the glomerular filtrate before it reaches the end of the collecting duct. Therefore only 1 mL/min (on average) is excreted as urine.

Tubular Function. Since the glomerular membrane is a selective filtration membrane that filters primarily by size, provision is made for the reabsorption of essential materials and excretion of nonessential ones (Table 44-1). The tubules and collecting ducts carry out these functions by means of reabsorption and secretion. *Reabsorption* is the passage of a substance from the lumen of the tubules through the tubule cells and into the capillaries. This process involves both active and passive transport mechanisms. Tubular *secretion* is the passage of a substance from the capillaries through the tubular cells into the lumen of the tubule. Reabsorption and secretion cause numerous changes in the composition of the glomerular filtrate as it moves through the entire length of the tubule.

In the proximal convoluted tubule, about 80% of the electrolytes are reabsorbed. Normally, all the glucose, amino acids, and small proteins are reabsorbed. As reabsorption continues in the loop of Henle, water is conserved, which is important for concentrating the filtrate. The descending loop is permeable to water and moderately permeable to sodium, urea, and other solutes. In the ascending limb, chloride ions (Cl^-) are actively reabsorbed, followed by passive reabsorption of sodium ions (Na^+). About 25% of the filtered sodium is reabsorbed in the ascending limb.

Two important functions of the distal convoluted tubules are final regulation of water balance and acid-base balance. Antidiuretic hormone (ADH) is required for water reabsorption in the kidney and is important in water balance. ADH makes the distal convoluted tubules and collecting ducts permeable to water. This allows water to be reabsorbed into the peritubular capillaries and eventually returned to the circulation.

Decreases in plasma osmolality are detected in the anterior hypothalamus by osmoreceptors. These osmoreceptors send

neural input to *superoptic nuclei cells* in the hypothalamus. These superoptic nuclei cells have neuronal axons that terminate in the posterior pituitary gland and act to inhibit secretion of ADH. In the absence of ADH, the tubules are essentially impermeable to water. Thus any water in the tubules leaves the body as urine.

Aldosterone (released from the adrenal cortex) acts on the distal tubule to cause reabsorption of Na^+ and water. In exchange for Na^+, potassium ions (K^+) are excreted. The secretion of aldosterone is influenced by both circulating blood volume and plasma concentrations of Na^+ and K^+.

Acid-base regulation involves reabsorbing and conserving most of the bicarbonate (HCO_3^-) and secreting excess hydrogen ions (H^+). The distal tubule has different ways to maintain the pH of ECF within a range of 7.35 to 7.45 (see Chapter 16).

Myocyte cells in the right atrium secrete a hormone, atrial natriuretic peptide (ANP), in response to atrial distention, which is a result of an increase in plasma volume. ANP acts on the kidneys to increase sodium excretion. At the same time, ANP inhibits renin, ADH, and the action of angiotensin II on the adrenal glands, thereby suppressing aldosterone secretion. These combined effects of ANP result in the production of a large volume of dilute urine. Furthermore, secretion of ANP causes relaxation of the afferent arteriole, thus increasing the GFR.

The renal tubules are also involved in calcium balance. Parathyroid hormone (PTH) is released from the parathyroid gland in response to low serum calcium levels. PTH maintains serum calcium levels by causing increased tubular reabsorption of calcium ions (Ca^{2+}) and decreased tubular reabsorption of phosphate ions (PO_4^{2-}). In kidney disease, the effects of PTH may have a major effect on bone metabolism.

Vitamin D is a hormone that can be obtained in the diet or synthesized by the action of ultraviolet radiation on cholesterol in the skin. These forms of vitamin D are inactive and require two more steps to become metabolically active. The first step in activation occurs in the liver; the second step occurs in the kidneys. Active vitamin D is essential for the absorption of calcium from the gastrointestinal (GI) tract. The patient with kidney failure (also called *renal failure*) has a deficiency of the active metabolite of vitamin D and manifests problems of altered calcium and phosphate balance (see Chapter 47).

In summary, the basic function of nephrons is to cleanse blood plasma of unnecessary substances. After the glomerulus has filtered the blood, the tubules select the unwanted from the wanted portions of tubular fluid. Essential constituents are returned to the blood, and dispensable substances pass into urine.

Other Functions of Kidneys. The kidneys perform vital functions through participation in red blood cell (RBC) production and BP regulation. Erythropoietin is a hormone produced in the kidneys and secreted in response to hypoxia and decreased renal blood flow. Erythropoietin stimulates RBC production in the bone marrow. A deficiency of erythropoietin occurs in kidney failure, leading to anemia.

Renin is important in the regulation of BP. Renin is produced and secreted by the kidney's juxtaglomerular cells (Fig. 44-4). Renin is released into the bloodstream in response to decreased renal perfusion, decreased arterial BP, decreased ECF, decreased serum Na^+ concentration, and increased urinary Na^+ concentration. The plasma protein angiotensinogen (from the liver) is activated to angiotensin I by renin. Angiotensin I is

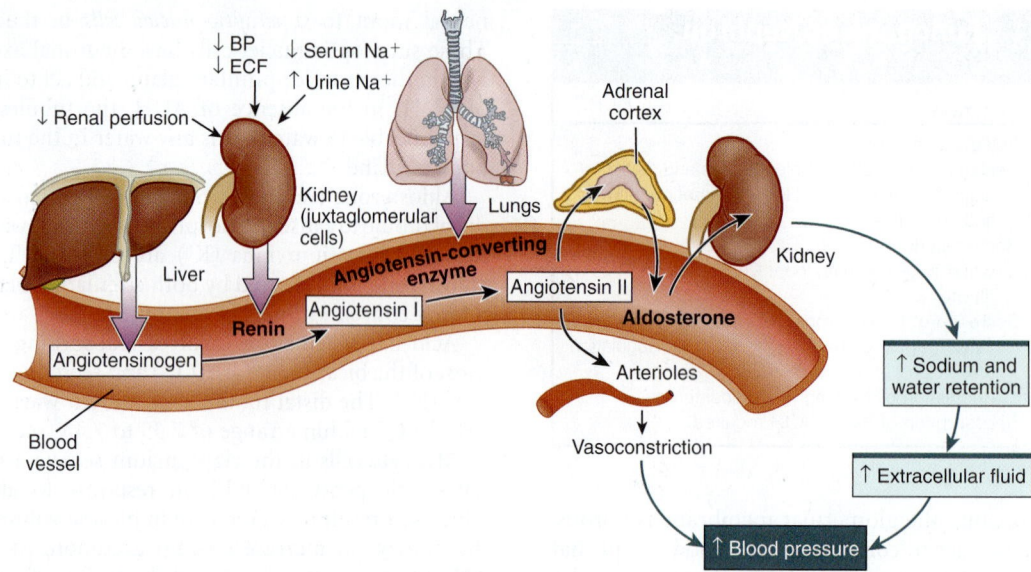

FIG. 44-4   Renin-angiotensin-aldosterone system. (Modified from Herlihy B, Maebius N: *The human body in health and disease*, ed 4, Philadelphia, 2011, Saunders.)

subsequently converted to angiotensin II by angiotensin-converting enzyme (ACE). ACE is located on the inner surface of all blood vessels, with particularly high levels in the vessels of the lungs. Angiotensin II stimulates the release of aldosterone from the adrenal cortex, which causes Na$^+$ and water retention, leading to increased ECF volume. Angiotensin II also causes increased peripheral vasoconstriction. Release of renin is inhibited by an elevation in BP. Excessive renin production caused by impaired renal perfusion may be a contributing factor in the etiology of hypertension (see Chapter 32).

Most body tissues synthesize prostaglandins (PGs) from the precursor arachidonic acid in response to appropriate stimuli. (See Chapter 11 and Fig. 11-2 for a more detailed discussion of PGs.) In the kidney, PG synthesis (primarily PGE$_2$ and PGI$_2$) occurs primarily in the medulla. These PGs have a vasodilating action, thus increasing renal blood flow, and promoting Na$^+$ excretion. They counteract the vasoconstrictive effect of substances such as angiotensin and norepinephrine. Renal PGs may have a systemic effect in lowering BP by decreasing systemic vascular resistance. The significance of renal PGs is related to the kidneys' role in causing hypertension. In renal failure with a loss of functioning tissue, these renal vasodilator factors are also lost, which may contribute to hypertension (see Chapter 46).

Ureters

The ureters are tubes that carry urine from the renal pelvis to the bladder (Fig. 44-1). Arranged in a meshlike outer layer, circular and longitudinal smooth muscle fibers contract to promote the peristaltic, one-way flow of urine through the ureters. Distention, neurologic and endocrine influences, and drugs can affect these muscle contractions. Each ureter is approximately 10 to 12 inches (25 to 30.5 cm) long and 0.08 to 0.3 inches (0.2 to 0.8 cm) in diameter.

The narrow area where each ureter joins the renal pelvis is termed the *ureteropelvic junction* (UPJ). Subsequently, the ureters insert into either side of the bladder base at the *uretero-vesical junctions* (UVJs). Because the ureteral lumens are narrowest at these junctions, the UPJ and UVJ are often sites of obstruction. The narrow ureteral lumens can be easily obstructed

internally (e.g., urinary calculi) or externally (e.g., tumors, adhesions, inflammation). Sympathetic and parasympathetic nerves, along with the vascular supply, surround the mucosal lining of the ureters. Stimulation of these nerves during passage of a stone may cause acute, severe pain, termed *renal colic*.

Because the renal pelvis holds only 3 to 5 mL of urine, kidney damage can result from a backflow of more than that amount of urine. The UVJ relies on the ureter's angle of bladder insertion and muscle fiber attachments with the bladder to prevent the backflow (*reflux*) of urine, which predisposes a person to an ascending infection. The distal ureter enters the bladder laterally at its base, courses along obliquely through the bladder wall for about 1.5 cm, and intermingles with muscle fibers of the bladder base. Circular and longitudinal bladder muscle fibers adjacent to the imbedded ureter help secure it. When bladder pressure rises (e.g., during voiding or coughing), muscle fibers that the ureter shares with the bladder base contract first, promoting ureteral lumen closure. Next, the bladder contracts against its base, ensuring UVJ closure and prevention of urine reflux through the junction.

Bladder

The urinary bladder is a stretchable (able to fill at relatively low pressures) organ positioned behind the symphysis pubis and anterior to the vagina and rectum (Fig. 44-5). Its primary functions are to serve as a reservoir for urine and to eliminate waste products from the body. Normal adult urine output is approximately 1500 mL/day, which varies with food and fluid intake. The volume of urine produced at night is less than half of that formed during the day because of hormonal influences (e.g., ADH). This diurnal pattern of urination is normal. Typically, an individual will urinate five or six times during the day and occasionally at night.

The *trigone* is the triangular area formed by the two ureteral openings and bladder neck at the base of the bladder. The trigone is attached to the pelvis by many ligaments and does not change its shape during bladder filling or emptying. The bladder muscle (*detrusor*) is composed of layers of intertwined smooth muscle fibers capable of considerable distention during bladder filling and contraction during emptying. It is attached

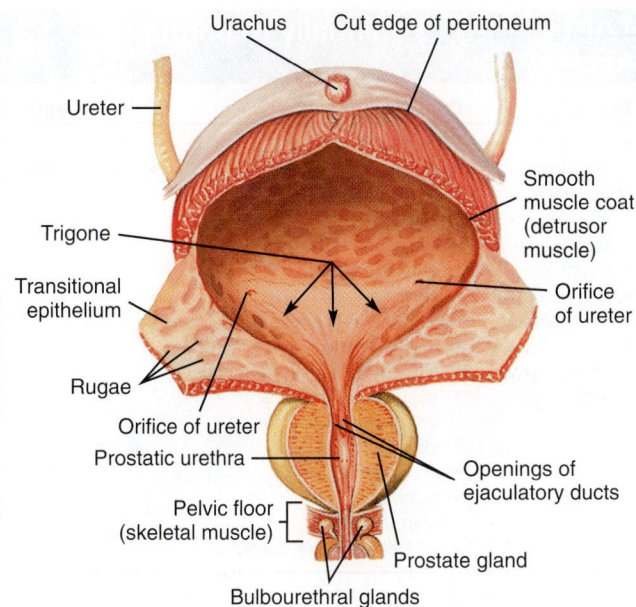

FIG. 44-5 Urinary bladder of a male. (Modified from Thibodeau GA, Patton KT: *Anatomy and physiology,* ed 6, St Louis, 2007, Mosby.)

to the abdominal wall by an umbilical ligament, the *urachus.* As a result of this attachment, as the bladder fills it rises toward the umbilicus. The dome and the anterior and lateral aspects of the bladder expand and contract.

On average, 200 to 250 mL of urine in the bladder cause moderate distention and the urge to urinate. When the quantity of urine reaches approximately 400 to 600 mL, the person feels uncomfortable. Bladder capacity varies with the individual but generally ranges from 600 to 1000 mL. Evacuation of urine is termed *urination, micturition,* or *voiding.*

The bladder has the same mucosal lining as that of the renal pelvises, ureters, and bladder neck. The bladder is lined by transitional cell epithelium and is referred to as the *urothelium.* Unique to the urinary tract, the urothelium is resistant to absorption of urine. This means that after waste products (produced by the kidneys) have left the kidneys, they cannot be reabsorbed in the urinary system. Microscopically, urothelium is only several cells deep. However, as urine enters the bladder, these cells can stretch to accommodate filling. As the bladder empties, the urothelium resumes its multicellular layer formation.

Transitional cell cancers occurring in one section of the urinary tract can easily metastasize to other urinary tract areas given that the mucosal lining throughout the urinary tract is the same. Malignant cells may move down from upper urinary tract cancers and embed in the bladder, or large bladder tumors can invade the ureter. Cancer recurrence within the bladder is common.

Urethra

The urethra is a small tube that incorporates the smooth muscle of the bladder neck and extends to the striated muscle of the external meatus. The urethra's primary functions are to (1) control voiding and (2) serve as a conduit for urine from the bladder to the outside of the body during voiding.

The female urethra is 1 to 2 inches (2.5 to 5 cm) long and lies behind the symphysis pubis but anterior to the vagina (Fig. 44-1, *C*). The male urethra, which is about 8 to 10 inches

(20 to 25 cm) long, originates at the bladder neck and extends the length of the penis (Fig. 44-1, *B*).

Urethrovesical Unit

Together, the bladder, urethra, and pelvic floor muscles form what is called the *urethrovesical unit.* Voluntary control of this unit is defined as *continence.* Stimulating and inhibiting impulses are sent from the brain through the thoracolumbar (T11 to L2) and sacral (S2 to S4) areas of the spinal cord to control voiding. Distention of the bladder stimulates stretch receptors within the bladder wall. Impulses are transmitted to the sacral spinal cord and then to the brain, causing a desire to urinate.

If it is not appropriate to void at a given time, inhibitor impulses in the brain are stimulated and transmitted back through the thoracolumbar and sacral nerves innervating the bladder. In a coordinated fashion, the detrusor muscle accommodates to the pressure (does not contract) while the sphincter and pelvic floor muscles tighten (contract) to resist bladder pressure.

If voiding is appropriate, cerebral inhibition is voluntarily suppressed, and impulses are transmitted via the spinal cord for the bladder neck, sphincter, and pelvic floor muscles to relax and for the bladder to contract. The sphincter closes and the detrusor muscle relaxes when the bladder is empty.

Any disease or trauma that affects the function of the brain, spinal cord, or nerves that directly innervate the bladder, bladder neck, external sphincter, or pelvic floor can affect bladder function. These conditions include diabetes mellitus, multiple sclerosis, paraplegia, and tetraplegia (quadriplegia). Drugs affecting nerve transmission also can affect bladder function.

Gerontologic Considerations: Effects of Aging on Urinary System

Anatomic changes in the aging kidney include a 20% to 30% decrease in size and weight between ages 30 and 90 years. By the seventh decade of life, 30% to 50% of glomeruli have lost their function.[1] Atherosclerosis accelerates the decrease of renal size with age. Despite these changes, older individuals maintain body fluid homeostasis unless they encounter diseases or other physiologic stressors.

Physiologic changes in the aging kidney include decreased renal blood flow, due in part to atherosclerosis, resulting in a decreased GFR. Alterations in hormone levels (including ADH, aldosterone, and ANP) result in decreased urinary concentrating ability and alterations in the excretion of water, sodium, potassium, and acid. Under normal conditions, the aging kidney is able to maintain homeostasis. However, after abrupt changes in blood volume, acid load, or other insults, the kidney may not be able to function effectively because much of its renal reserve has been lost.[2,3]

Physiologic changes also occur in the aging urethra and bladder. The female urethra, bladder, vagina, and pelvic floor undergo a loss of elasticity and muscle support. Consequently, older women are more prone to bladder infections and incontinence.

The prostate surrounds the proximal urethra. As men age, the prostate enlarges and may affect urinary patterns, causing hesitancy, retention, slow stream, and bladder infections.

Constipation, often experienced by older adults, can also affect urination. Partial urethral obstruction may occur because of the rectum's close proximity to the urethra.

TABLE 44-2   Gerontologic Assessment Differences

Urinary System

Gerontologic Changes	Differences in Assessment Findings
Kidney	
• ↓ Amount of renal tissue	• Less palpable
• ↓ Number of nephrons and renal blood vessels. Thickened basement membrane of Bowman's capsule and glomeruli	• ↓ Creatinine clearance, ↑ BUN level, ↑ serum creatinine
• ↓ Function of loop of Henle and tubules	• Alterations in drug excretion, nocturia, loss of normal diurnal excretory pattern because of ↓ ability to concentrate urine; less concentrated urine
Ureter, Bladder, and Urethra	
• ↓ Elasticity and muscle tone	• Palpable bladder after urination because of retention
• Weakening of urinary sphincter	• Stress incontinence (especially during Valsalva maneuver), dribbling of urine after urination
• ↓ Bladder capacity and sensory receptors	• Frequency, urgency, nocturia, overflow incontinence
• Estrogen deficiency leading to thin, dry vaginal tissue	• Stress or overactive bladder, dysuria
• ↑ Prevalence of unstable bladder contractions	• Overactive bladder
• Prostatic enlargement	• Hesitancy, frequency, urgency, nocturia, straining to urinate, retention, dribbling

TABLE 44-3   Potentially Nephrotoxic Agents

Antibiotics	Other Drugs	Other Agents
• amikacin	• captopril	• Gold
• amphotericin B	• cimetidine	• Heavy metals
• bacitracin	• cisplatin	
• cephalosporins	• cocaine	
• gentamicin	• cyclosporine	
• neomycin	• ethylene glycol	
• polymyxin B	• heroin	
• streptomycin	• lithium	
• sulfonamides	• methotrexate	
• tobramycin	• nitrosoureas (e.g., carmustine)	
• vancomycin	• nonsteroidal antiinflammatory drugs (e.g., ibuprofen, indomethacin)	
	• phenacetin	
	• quinine	
	• rifampin	
	• salicylates (large quantities)	

CASE STUDY

Patient Introduction

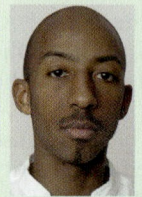

A.K. is a 28-yr-old African American man who comes to the emergency department (ED) in acute distress with complaints of severe abdominal pain. The pain began about 6 hr ago after he finished a 10-mile run as part of his training for a marathon. He says that the pain has steadily increased, he is nauseated, and his urine is a dark, smoky color.

(©iStockphoto/Thinkstock)

Discussion Questions

1. What are the possible causes of A.K.'s abdominal pain, nausea, and urine color?
2. What would be your priority assessment of A.K.?

You will learn more about A.K. and his condition as you read through this assessment chapter.

(See p. 1023 for more information on A.K.)

Answers available at *http://evolve.elsevier.com/Lewis/medsurg*.

Age-related changes in the urinary system and differences in assessment findings are presented in Table 44-2.

ASSESSMENT OF URINARY SYSTEM

Subjective Data

Important Health Information

Past Health History. Question the patient about the presence or history of diseases that are related to renal or other urologic problems. Some of these diseases are hypertension, diabetes mellitus, gout and other metabolic problems, connective tissue disorders (e.g., systemic lupus erythematosus, systemic sclerosis [scleroderma]), skin or upper respiratory tract infections of streptococcal origin, tuberculosis, viral hepatitis, congenital disorders, neurologic conditions (e.g., stroke, back injury), or trauma. Note specific urinary problems such as cancer, infections, benign prostatic hyperplasia, and calculi.

Medications. An assessment of the patient's current and past use of medications is important. This should include over-the-counter drugs, prescription medications, and herbs. Drugs affect the urinary tract in several ways. Many drugs are known to be nephrotoxic (Table 44-3). Certain drugs may alter the quantity and character of urine output (e.g., diuretics). A number of drugs change the color of urine such as phenazopyridine (Pyridium) (urine turns orange) and nitrofurantoin (Macrodantin) (urine turns dark yellow to brown). Anticoagulants may cause hematuria. Many antidepressants, calcium channel blockers, antihistamines, and drugs used for neurologic and musculoskeletal disorders affect the ability of the bladder or sphincter to contract or relax normally.

Surgery or Other Treatments. Ask the patient about previous hospitalizations related to renal or urologic diseases and all urinary problems during past pregnancies. Inquire about the duration, severity, and patient's perception of any problem and its treatment. Document past surgeries, particularly pelvic surgeries, or urinary tract instrumentation (e.g., catheterization). Ask the patient about any radiation or chemotherapy treatment for cancer.

Functional Health Patterns. Key questions to ask a patient with problems related to the renal system are listed in Table 44-4.

Health Perception–Health Management Pattern. Ask about the patient's general health, particularly when a disorder affecting the kidneys is suspected. Abnormal kidney function may be suspected if the patient reports changes in weight or appetite, excess thirst, fluid retention, headache, pruritus, blurred vision, or "feeling tired all the time." Similarly, an older patient may report malaise and nonlocalized abdominal discomfort as the only symptoms of a urinary tract infection (UTI). In older adults with a UTI, family members may report that the patient is disoriented or has increased confusion.

A patient's occupational history is an important consideration, because exposure to certain chemicals can affect the urinary system. Phenol and ethylene glycol are examples of

TABLE 44-4 Health History
Urinary System

Health Perception–Health Management
- How is your energy level compared with 1 yr ago?
- Do you notice any visual changes?*
- Have you ever smoked? If yes, how many packs per day?

Nutritional-Metabolic
- How is your appetite?
- Has your weight changed over the past yr?*
- Do you take vitamins, herbs, or any other supplements?*
- How much and what kinds of fluids do you drink daily?
- How many dairy products and how much meat do you eat?
- Do you drink coffee? Colas? Tea?
- Do you eat chocolate?
- Do you spice your food heavily?*

Elimination
- Are you able to sit through a 2-hr meeting or ride in a car for 2 hr without urinating?
- Do you awaken at night with the desire to urinate? If so, how many times does this occur during an average night?
- Do you ever notice blood in your urine?* If so, at what point in the urination does it occur?
- Do you ever pass urine when you do not intend to? When?
- Do you use special devices or supplies for urine elimination or control?*
- How often do you move your bowels?
- Do you ever experience constipation?
- Do you frequently experience diarrhea? Do you ever have problems controlling your bowels? If so, do you have problems controlling the passage of gas? Watery or liquid stool? Solid stool?

Activity-Exercise
- Have you noticed any changes in your ability to perform your usual daily activities?*
- Do certain activities aggravate your urinary problem?*
- Has your urinary problem caused you to alter or stop any activity or exercise?*
- Do you require assistance in moving or getting to the bathroom?*

Sleep-Rest
- Do you awaken at night from an urge to urinate?* How does this disturb your sleep?
- Do you awaken at night from pain or other problems and urinate as a matter of routine before returning to sleep?*
- Do you experience daytime sleepiness and fatigue as a result of nighttime urination?*

Cognitive-Perceptual
- Do you ever have pain when you urinate?* If so, where is the pain?

Self-Perception–Self-Concept
- How does your urinary problem make you feel about yourself?
- Do you perceive your body differently since you have developed a urinary problem?

Role-Relationship
- Does your urinary problem interfere with your relationships with family or friends?*
- Has your urinary problem caused a change in your job status or affected your ability to carry out job-related responsibilities?*

Sexuality-Reproductive
- Has your urinary problem caused any change in your sexual pleasure or performance?*
- Do hygiene concerns interfere with sexual activities?

Coping–Stress Tolerance
- Do you feel able to manage the problems associated with your urinary problem? If not, explain.
- What strategies are you using to cope with your urinary problem?

Values-Beliefs
- Has your present illness affected your belief system?*
- Are your treatment decisions related to your urinary problem in conflict with your value system?*

*If yes, describe.

nephrotoxic chemicals. Aromatic amines and some organic chemicals may increase the risk of bladder cancers. Textile workers, painters, hairdressers, and industrial workers have an increased incidence of bladder cancer.[4]

Obtain a smoking history. Cancer occurs more frequently in cigarette smokers than in nonsmokers. Cigarette smoking is a major risk factor for bladder and kidney cancer.

Information about places where a patient has lived is important. Persons living in certain parts of the United States (Great Lakes, Southwest, Southeast) have a higher than normal incidence of urinary calculi, possibly caused by the higher mineral content of the soil and water. A person living in Middle Eastern countries or Africa can acquire certain parasites that can cause cystitis or bladder cancer.

GENETIC RISK ALERT
- Polycystic kidney disease and congenital urinary tract abnormalities (e.g., Alport syndrome [congenital nephritis]) are genetic disorders.
- A family history of certain renal or urologic problems increases the likelihood of similar problems occurring in the patient.
- For any disease the patient has reported in the health history, ask if other family members also have/had the same or similar diseases.

Nutritional-Metabolic Pattern. The usual quantity and types of fluid a patient drinks are important in relation to urinary tract disease. Dehydration may contribute to UTIs, calculi formation, and kidney failure. Large intake of particular foods, such as dairy products or foods high in proteins, may also lead to calculi formation. Asparagus may cause the urine to smell musty, and red urine caused by beet ingestion may be mistaken for bloody urine. Caffeine, alcohol, carbonated beverages, some artificial sweeteners, or spicy foods often aggravate urinary inflammatory diseases. Green tea and some herbal teas also cause diuresis. An unexplained weight gain may be the result of fluid retention secondary to a renal problem. Anorexia, nausea, and vomiting can dramatically affect fluid status and require careful monitoring. Obtain information related to vitamin and mineral supplements and herbal therapies. The patient may not think of these supplements and therapies when listing over-the-counter drugs.

Elimination Pattern. Questions about urine elimination patterns are the cornerstone of the health history in the patient with a lower urinary tract disorder. This line of inquiry begins with a question of how the patient manages urine elimination. Most patients eliminate urine by spontaneous voiding. Therefore ask about daytime (diurnal) voiding frequency and

TABLE 44-5	**Manifestations of Urinary System Disorders**				
	SPECIFIC MANIFESTATIONS RELATED TO URINARY SYSTEM				
General Manifestations	**Edema**	**Pain**	**Patterns of Urination**	**Urine Output**	**Urine Composition**
• Fatigue • Headaches • Blurred vision • Elevated BP • Anorexia • Nausea and vomiting • Chills • Itching • Excessive thirst • Change in body weight • Cognitive changes	• Facial (periorbital) • Ankle • Ascites • Anasarca (generalized edema) • Sacral	• Dysuria • Flank or costovertebral angle • Groin • Suprapubic	• Frequency • Urgency • Hesitancy of stream • Change in stream • Retention • Dysuria • Nocturia • Incontinence • Stress incontinence • Dribbling	• Anuria • Oliguria • Polyuria	• Concentrated • Dilute • Hematuria • Pyuria • Color (red, brown, yellowish green)

the frequency of nocturia. Pelvic organ prolapse, particularly advanced anterior vaginal prolapse, may cause suprapubic pressure, frequency, urgency, and incontinence secondary to urinary retention. Query patients about additional bothersome lower urinary tract symptoms, including urgency, incontinence, or urinary retention. Table 44-5 lists some of the common manifestations of urinary tract disorders.

Changes in the color and appearance of urine are often significant and should be evaluated. If blood is visible in the urine, determine if it occurs at the beginning of, throughout, or at the end of urination. This is more difficult for the female patient.

Investigate bowel function. Problems with fecal incontinence may signal neurologic causes for bladder problems because of shared nerve pathways. Constipation and fecal impaction can partially obstruct the urethra, causing inadequate bladder emptying, overflow incontinence, and infection.

Determine the patient's method of managing a urinary problem. A patient may already be using a catheter or collection device. Sometimes a patient has to assume a particular position to urinate or perform maneuvers such as pressing on the lower abdomen (Credé's method) or straining (Valsalva maneuver) to empty the bladder.

Activity-Exercise Pattern. Assess the patient's level of activity. A sedentary person is more likely to have stasis of urine than an active individual and thus can be predisposed to infection and calculi. Demineralization of bones in an individual with limited physical activity can cause increased urine calcium precipitation.

An active person may find that increasing activity aggravates the urinary problem. The patient who has had prostate surgery or who has weakened pelvic floor muscles may leak urine when attempting particular activities such as running. Some men develop chronic inflammatory prostatitis or epididymitis after heavy lifting or long-distance driving.

Sleep-Rest Pattern. Nocturia is a common and a particularly bothersome lower urinary tract symptom that often leads to sleep deprivation, daytime sleepiness, and fatigue. It occurs in multiple disorders affecting the lower urinary tract, including urinary incontinence, urinary retention, and interstitial cystitis. Nocturia may also be related to polyuria secondary to kidney disease, poorly controlled diabetes mellitus, alcoholism, excessive fluid intake, liver disease, heart failure, or obstructive sleep apnea.

When assessing nocturia, determine whether the need to urinate causes the person to arise from sleep or whether pain or other symptoms interrupt sleep, and the person urinates as a matter of habit before returning to bed. Up to one episode of nocturia is considered normal in younger adults, and up to two episodes are acceptable in adults ages 65 years or older. If an older adult has more than two voidings during the night, assess the amount and timing of fluid intake. This information will help determine whether further investigation is needed.

Cognitive-Perceptual Pattern. Assess the level of mobility, visual acuity, and dexterity as these are important factors to evaluate in a patient with urologic problems, particularly when urine retention or incontinence is a problem. Determine if the patient is alert, is able to understand instructions, and can recall the instructions when necessary.

If urinary incontinence is present, elicit a thorough history of the problem to help determine the type of incontinence. Ask how the patient has managed the problem in the past. Recognize that incontinence is often distressing and embarrassing. Discuss the problem with the patient with sensitivity in a nonjudgmental manner.

A frequent symptom of renal and urologic problems is pain, including dysuria, groin pain, costovertebral pain, and suprapubic pain. Assess pain and document the location, character, and duration. The absence of pain when other urinary symptoms exist is also significant. Many urinary tract cancers are painless in the early stages.

Self-Perception–Self-Concept Pattern. Problems associated with the urinary system, such as incontinence, urinary diversion procedures, and chronic fatigue (may indicate anemia), can result in loss of self-esteem and a negative body image.

Role-Relationship Pattern. Urinary problems can affect many aspects of a person's life, including the ability to work and relationships with others. These factors have important implications for future treatment and management of the patient's condition.

Urinary system problems may be serious enough to cause problems in job-related and social situations. Chronic dialysis therapy often makes regular employment or management of home and family responsibilities difficult. Concurrent poor health and negative body image can seriously alter existing roles.

Sexuality-Reproductive Pattern. Assess the effect of renal problems on the patient's sexual satisfaction. Problems related to personal hygiene and fatigue can negatively affect sexual relationships. Although urinary incontinence is not directly associated with sexual dysfunction, it often has a devastating effect on self-esteem and social and intimate relationships. Counseling of both the patient and partner may be indicated.

CASE STUDY—cont'd

Subjective Data

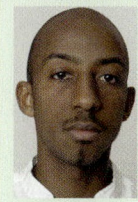

(©iStockphoto/ Thinkstock)

A focused subjective assessment of A.K. revealed the following information:

PMH: History of one isolated incidence of possible gout 6 yr ago. He stopped drinking alcohol with no further occurrence. Appendectomy 12 yr ago.

Medications: None.

Health Perception–Health Management: A.K. states that he is usually healthy. He does not smoke or drink alcohol. He has never experienced this type of pain before. Describes the pain as being sharp and colicky (coming in waves). Rates the pain as 9 on a scale of 0-10.

Nutritional-Metabolic: A.K. is currently on a high-protein diet as he trains for the marathon. He eats a lot of chicken, beef, and seafood. He drinks milk-based protein shakes and water after exercising but admits that he does not think he drinks enough to replace fluid loss from perspiration. He drinks coffee for energy but denies eating chocolate or other sweets. He also avoids sodas.

Elimination: Denies any history of difficulty with urination or constipation or diarrhea. This is the first time he has ever noticed a change of color in his urine.

Activity-Exercise: Prides himself on his ability to exercise and run without difficulty.

Sleep-Rest: Does not awaken at night to urinate.

Cognitive-Perceptual: Denies pain on urination.

Self-Perception–Self-Concept: Believes he is able to monitor self and maintain healthy lifestyle.

Coping–Stress Tolerance: Worried that this pain may interfere with his marathon training.

Discussion Questions

1. What type of assessment would be most appropriate for A.K.: comprehensive, focused, or emergency? On what basis did you make that decision?
2. What assessment questions will you ask him?
3. Which subjective assessment findings are of most concern to you? You will learn more about the physical examination of the urinary system in the next section.

(See p. 1024 for more information on A.K.)

Answers available at *http://evolve.elsevier.com/Lewis/medsurg.*

Objective Data

Physical Examination

Inspection. Assess for changes in the following:
- *Skin:* Pallor, yellow-gray cast, excoriations, changes in turgor, bruises, texture (e.g., rough, dry skin) (see Table 22-9 for assessment of dark-skinned individuals)
- *Mouth:* Stomatitis, ammonia breath odor
- *Face and extremities:* Generalized edema, peripheral edema
- *Abdomen:* Abdominal contour for midline mass in lower abdomen (may indicate bladder distention and urinary retention) or unilateral mass (occasionally seen in adults, indicating enlargement of one or both kidneys from large tumor or polycystic kidney)
- *Weight:* Weight gain secondary to edema. Weight loss and muscle wasting in kidney failure
- *General state of health:* Fatigue, lethargy, and diminished alertness

Palpation. The kidneys are posterior organs protected by the abdominal organs, ribs, and heavy back muscles. A landmark useful in locating the kidneys is the **costovertebral angle (CVA)** formed by the rib cage and the vertebral column. The normal-sized

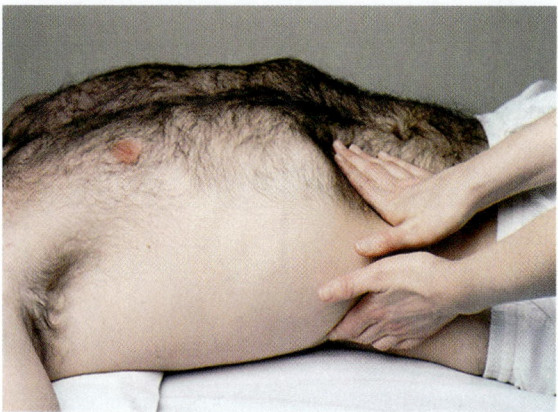

FIG. 44-6 Palpating the right kidney. (From Brundage DJ: *Renal disorders,* St Louis, 1992, Mosby.)

TABLE 44-6 Normal Physical Assessment of Urinary System
• No costovertebral angle tenderness
• Nonpalpable kidney and bladder
• No palpable masses

left kidney is rarely palpable because the spleen lies directly on top of it. Occasionally the lower pole of the right kidney is palpable.

To palpate the right kidney, place your left (anterior) hand behind and support the patient's right side between the rib cage and the iliac crest (Fig. 44-6). Elevate the right flank with the left hand. Use your right hand to palpate deeply for the right kidney. The lower pole of the right kidney may be felt as a smooth, rounded mass that descends on inspiration. If the kidney is palpable, note its size, contour, and tenderness. Kidney enlargement is suggestive of neoplasm or other serious renal pathologic conditions.

The urinary bladder is normally not palpable unless it is distended with urine. If the bladder is full, it may be felt as a smooth, round, firm organ and is sensitive to palpation.

Percussion. Tenderness in the flank area may be detected by fist percussion *(kidney punch).* This technique is performed by striking the fist of one hand against the dorsal surface of the other hand, which is placed flat along the posterior CVA margin (Fig. 44-7). Normally this type of percussion should not elicit pain. If CVA tenderness and pain are present, it may indicate a kidney infection or polycystic kidney disease.[5]

A bladder is not normally percussible until it contains at least 150 mL of urine. If the bladder is full, dullness is heard above the symphysis pubis. A distended bladder may be percussed as high as the umbilicus.

Auscultation. Use the diaphragm of the stethoscope to auscultate the bowels, since they may also affect the urinary system.

Table 44-6 shows how to record the normal physical assessment findings of the urinary system. Table 44-7 describes assessment abnormalities of the urinary system. Assessment findings may vary in the older adult. Table 44-2 presents the age-related changes in the urinary system and differences in assessment findings. Use a *focused assessment* to evaluate the status of previously identified urinary system problems and to monitor for signs of new problems (see Table 3-7). A focused assessment of the urinary system is presented in the box on p. 1024.

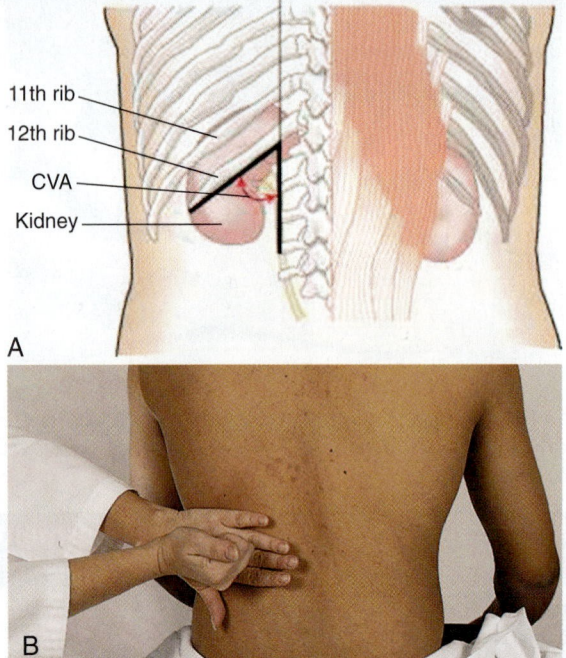

A

B

FIG. 44-7 A, Costovertebral angle. **B,** Indirect fist percussion of the costovertebral angle (CVA). To assess the kidney, place one hand over the twelfth rib at the CVA on the back. Thump that hand with the ulnar edge of the other fist. (*A,* From Jarvis C: *Physical examination and health assessment,* ed 7, St Louis, 2016, Saunders. *B,* From Jarvis C: *Physical examination and health assessment,* ed 6, St Louis, 2012, Saunders.)

11th rib
12th rib
CVA
Kidney

FOCUSED ASSESSMENT

Urinary System

Use this checklist to ensure that the key assessment steps have been done.

Subjective

Ask the patient about any of the following and note responses.

Painful urination	Y	N
Changes in color of urine (blood, cloudy)	Y	N
Change in characteristics of urination (diminished, excessive)	Y	N
Problems with frequent nighttime urination (nocturia)	Y	N

Objective: Diagnostic

Check the following laboratory results for critical values.

Blood urea nitrogen	✓
Serum creatinine	✓
Urinalysis	✓
Urine culture and sensitivity	✓

Objective: Physical Examination

Inspect

Abdomen	✓
Urinary meatus for inflammation or discharge	✓

Palpate

Abdomen for bladder distention, masses, or tenderness	✓

Percuss

Costovertebral angle for tenderness	✓

Objective Data: Physical Examination

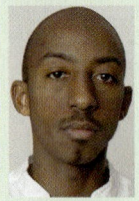

(©iStockphoto/ Thinkstock)

A focused assessment of A.K. reveals the following:
A.K. is lying on the ED stretcher with his knees bent and drawn to his abdominal area. He appears restless and keeps moving from back to side in an effort to reduce his discomfort. Vital signs as follows: BP 156/70, apical pulse 108, respiratory rate 24, temperature 37.4°C, O₂ saturation 96% on room air. Awake, alert, and oriented × 3. Lungs clear to auscultation. Apical pulse regular. Abdomen nondistended with + bowel sounds in all four quadrants. No rebound tenderness. Positive left costovertebral tenderness. Voiding small amounts of dark, smoky urine.

Discussion Questions

1. What should be included in the physical assessment? What would you be looking for?
2. Which physical assessment findings are of most concern to you?
3. Based on the results of the subjective and physical assessment findings, what diagnostic studies do you think may be ordered for A.K.?

You will learn more about diagnostic studies related to the urinary system in the next section.

(See p. 1031 for more information on A.K.)

DIAGNOSTIC STUDIES OF URINARY SYSTEM

Numerous diagnostic studies are used to assess problems of the urinary system. Tables 44-8 and 44-9 describe the most common studies, and select studies are described in more detail in the following text.

Many radiologic studies require the use of a bowel preparation the evening before the study to clear the lower GI tract of feces and flatus. Because the kidneys lie in a retroperitoneal location, the contents of the colon may obstruct visualization of the urinary tract. If the bowel preparation fails to adequately evacuate the lower GI tract, the study may be unsuccessful and may have to be rescheduled. Commonly used bowel preparations include enemas, magnesium citrate, and bisacodyl (Dulcolax) tablets or suppositories. In patients with kidney failure, some bowel preparations, such as magnesium citrate and Fleet enema, should not be used because magnesium cannot be excreted by the kidneys (see Chapter 46). Iodine-based contrast media used in some diagnostic studies may cause allergic reactions[6] (Table 44-8).

When a patient has undergone diagnostic studies on consecutive days, it is important to prevent dehydration. The patient is at risk for dehydration related to consecutive days of being NPO, extended time in the radiology department, and bowel preparations. Severe dehydration, especially in debilitated or older patients and patients with diabetes may lead to acute kidney injury. When a patient is scheduled for diagnostic studies, ensure that the patient is properly hydrated and given adequate nourishment between studies. Also check with the HCP regarding insulin dosage for diabetic patients who are placed on NPO status.

Urine Studies

Urinalysis. *Urinalysis* (Tables 44-8 and 44-9) is one of the first studies done to evaluate disorders of the urinary tract. Results

Text continued on p. 1031

TABLE 44-7 Assessment Abnormalities
Urinary System

Finding	Description	Possible Etiology and Significance
Anuria	Technically no urination (24-hr urine output <100 mL)	Acute kidney injury, end-stage renal disease, bilateral ureteral obstruction
Burning on urination	Stinging pain in urethral area	Urethral irritation, urinary tract infection, urethral calculus
Dysuria	Painful or difficult urination	Sign of urinary tract infection, interstitial cystitis, urethral calculus, and wide variety of pathologic conditions
Enuresis	Involuntary nocturnal urination	Symptomatic of lower urinary tract disorder
Frequency	Increased incidence of urination	Acutely inflamed bladder, retention with overflow, excess fluid intake, intake of bladder irritants, urethral calculus
Hematuria	Blood in the urine	Cancer of genitourinary tract, blood dyscrasias, kidney disease, urinary tract infection, stones in kidney or ureter, medications (anticoagulants)
Hesitancy	Delay or difficulty in initiating urination	Partial urethral obstruction, benign prostatic hyperplasia
Incontinence	Inability to voluntarily control discharge of urine	Neurogenic bladder, bladder infection, injury to external sphincter
Nocturia	Frequency of urination at night	Kidney disease with impaired concentrating ability, bladder obstruction, heart failure, diabetes mellitus, finding after renal transplant, excessive evening and nighttime fluid intake
Oliguria	Diminished amount of urine in a given time (24-hr urine output of 100-400 mL)	Severe dehydration, shock, transfusion reaction, kidney disease, end-stage renal disease
Pain	Suprapubic pain (related to bladder), urethral pain (irritation of bladder neck), flank (CVA) pain	Infection, urinary retention, foreign body in urinary tract, urethritis, pyelonephritis, renal colic or stones
Pneumaturia	Passage of urine containing gas	Fistula connections between bowel and bladder, gas-forming urinary tract infections
Polyuria	Large volume of urine in a given time	Diabetes mellitus, diabetes insipidus, chronic kidney disease, diuretics, excess fluid intake, obstructive sleep apnea
Retention	Inability to urinate even though bladder contains excessive amount of urine	Finding after pelvic surgery, childbirth, catheter removal, anesthesia; urethral stricture or obstruction; neurogenic bladder
Stress incontinence	Involuntary urination with increased pressure (sneezing or coughing)	Weakness of sphincter control, lack of estrogen, urinary retention

CVA, Costovertebral angle.

TABLE 44-8 Diagnostic Studies
Urinary System

Study	Description and Purpose	Nursing Responsibility
Urine Studies		
Urinalysis	General examination of urine to establish baseline information or provide data to establish a tentative diagnosis and determine whether further studies are needed (Table 44-9).	*Before:* Wash perineal area before collecting specimen. *During:* Try to obtain first urinated morning specimen. *After:* Ensure specimen is examined within 1 hr of urinating.
Creatinine clearance	Creatinine is a waste product of protein breakdown (primarily body muscle mass). Clearance of creatinine by kidney approximates the GFR. Creatinine clearance is calculated as follows: $$\text{Creatinine clearance} = \frac{\text{Urine creatinine (mg/dL)} \times \text{Urine volume (mL/min)}}{\text{Serum creatinine (mg/dL)}}$$ *Reference interval:* 70-135 mL/min/1.73 m² (corrected for body surface area).	*During:* Collect 24-hr urine specimen. Discard first urination when test is started. Save urine from all subsequent urinations for 24 hr. Instruct patient to urinate at end of 24 hr and add specimen to collection. Ensure that serum creatinine is determined during 24-hr period.
Composite urine collection	Measures specific components, such as electrolytes, glucose, protein, 17-ketosteroids, catecholamines, creatinine, and minerals. Composite urine specimens are collected over a period ranging from 2 to 24 hr.	*During:* Instruct the patient to urinate and discard this first urine specimen. Note this time as the start of the test. Save all urine from subsequent urinations in a container for designated period. At end of period, ask patient to urinate, and this urine is added to container. Remind patient to save all urine during study period. Specimens may have to be refrigerated or preservatives added to container used for collecting urine.
Urine culture ("clean catch," "midstream")	Confirms suspected urinary tract infection and identifies causative organisms. *Normally,* bladder is sterile, but urethra contains bacteria and a few WBCs. *Reference interval:* If properly collected, stored, and handled: <10³ organisms/mL usually indicates no infection. 10³-10⁵/mL is usually not diagnostic and test may have to be repeated. >10⁵/mL indicates infection.	*During:* Use sterile container for collection of urine. Touch only outside of container. *For women:* separate labia with one hand and clean meatus with other hand, using at least three sponges (saturated with cleansing solution) in a front-to-back motion. *For men:* retract foreskin (if present) and cleanse glans with at least three cleansing sponges. (Replace foreskin after cleaning.) After cleaning, instruct patient to start urinating and then continue voiding in sterile container. (The initial voided urine flushes out most contaminants in the urethra and perineal area.) Catheterization may be needed if patient is unable to cooperate with procedure.

Continued

TABLE 44-8 **Diagnostic Studies**

Urinary System—cont'd

Study	Description and Purpose	Nursing Responsibility
Urine Studies—cont'd		
Concentration test	Evaluates renal concentration ability. Measured by specific gravity readings. *Reference interval:* 1.003-1.030.	*Before:* Instruct patient to fast after given time in evening (in usual procedure). *During:* Collect three urine specimens at hourly intervals in morning.
Residual urine	Determines amount of urine left in bladder after urinating. Finding may be abnormal in problems with bladder innervation, sphincter impairment, BPH, or urethral strictures. *Reference interval:* ≤50 mL urine (increases with age).	*During:* Immediately after patient urinates, catheterize patient or use bladder ultrasound equipment. If a large amount of residual urine is obtained, HCP may want catheter left in bladder.
Protein determination		
• Dipstick (Albustix, Combistix)	Detects protein (primarily albumin) in urine. *Reference interval:* 0-trace.	*During:* Dip end of stick in urine and read result by comparison with color chart on label as directed. Grading is from 0 to 4+. Interpret with caution. Positive result may not indicate significant proteinuria. Some medications may give false-positive readings.
• Quantitative protein test	A 24-hr collection gives a more accurate indication of amount of protein in urine. Persistent proteinuria usually indicates glomerular kidney disease. *Reference interval:* <150 mg/24 hr (mainly albumin).	*During:* Perform 24-hr urine collection as above.
Urine cytologic study	Identifies abnormal cellular structures that occur with bladder cancer. Also used to follow the progress of bladder cancer after treatment.	*During:* Obtain specimens by voiding, catheterization, or bladder irrigation. Do not use morning's first voided specimen because epithelial cells may change in appearance in urine held in bladder overnight. *After:* Specimen should be fresh or brought to laboratory within the hour. An alcohol-based fixative is then added to preserve the cellular structure.
Blood Studies		
Blood urea nitrogen (BUN)	Used to detect renal problems. Concentration of urea in blood is regulated by rate at which kidney excretes urea. Nonrenal factors may cause an increased BUN (e.g., rapid cell destruction from infections, fever, GI bleeding, trauma, athletic activity and excessive muscle breakdown). *Reference interval:* 6-20 mg/dL (2.1-7.1 mmol/L).	*During:* Explain test and watch for postpuncture bleeding.
Creatinine	More reliable than BUN as a determinant of renal function. Creatinine is end product of muscle and protein metabolism and is released at a constant rate. *Reference interval:* 0.6-1.3 mg/dL (53-115 µmol/L).	*During:* Explain test and watch for postpuncture bleeding.
BUN/creatinine ratio	Increased ratio may be due to conditions that decrease blood flow to kidneys (e.g., heart failure, dehydration), GI bleeding, or increased dietary protein. A decreased ratio may occur with liver disease (due to decreased urea formation) and malnutrition. *Reference interval:* 12:1 to 20:1.	*During:* Explain test and watch for postpuncture bleeding
Uric acid	Used as screening test for disorders of purine metabolism but can also indicate kidney disease. Values depend on renal function, rate of purine metabolism, and dietary intake of food rich in purines. *Female:* 2.3-6.6 mg/dL (137-393 µmol/L). *Male:* 4.4-7.6 mg/dL (262-452 µmol/L).	*During:* Explain test and watch for postpuncture bleeding.
Sodium	Main extracellular electrolyte determining blood volume. Values usually stay within normal range until late stages of renal failure. *Reference interval:* 135-145 mEq/L (135-145 mmol/L).	*During:* Explain test and watch for postpuncture bleeding.
Potassium	Kidneys are responsible for excreting majority of body's potassium. In kidney disease, K^+ determinations are critical because K^+ is one of the first electrolytes to become abnormal. Elevated K^+ levels >6 mEq/L can lead to muscle weakness and cardiac dysrhythmias. *Reference interval:* 3.5-5.0 mEq/L (3.5-5.0 mmol/L).	*During:* Explain test and watch for postpuncture bleeding.
Calcium (total)	Main mineral in bone and aids in muscle contraction, neurotransmission, and clotting. In kidney disease, decreased reabsorption of Ca^{2+} leads to renal osteodystrophy. *Reference interval:* 8.6-10.2 mg/dL (2.15-2.55 mmol/L).	*During:* Explain test and watch for postpuncture bleeding.

TABLE 44-8 **Diagnostic Studies**

Urinary System—cont'd

Study	Description and Purpose	Nursing Responsibility
Phosphorus	Phosphorus balance is inversely related to Ca^{2+} balance. In kidney disease, phosphorus levels are elevated because the kidney is the primary excretory organ. *Reference interval:* 2.4-4.4 mg/dL (0.78-1.42 mmol/L).	*During:* Explain test and watch for postpuncture bleeding.
Bicarbonate	Most patients in renal failure have metabolic acidosis and low serum HCO_3^- levels. *Reference interval:* 22-26 mEq/L (22-26 mmol/L).	*During:* Explain test and watch for postpuncture bleeding.
Radiologic Procedures		
Kidneys, ureters, bladder (KUB)	X-ray examination of abdomen and pelvis delineates size, shape, and position of kidneys, ureter, and bladder. Radiopaque stones and foreign bodies can be seen.	*Before:* No special preparation needed.
Computed tomography (CT) scan (CT urogram)	Provides visualization of kidneys, ureters, and bladder. Can detect tumors, abscesses, suprarenal masses (e.g., adrenal tumors), and obstructions. Can be done with or without contrast media. Contrast is iodine based.*	*Before:* Explain procedure to patient. Ask patient about iodine sensitivity. Corticosteroids (prednisone) may be used to prevent an allergic reaction to contrast. *During:* Instruct the patient to lie still during the procedure while the machine takes precise transaxial images. Sedation may be required if patient is unable to cooperate.
Renal arteriogram (angiogram)	Visualizes renal blood vessels. Can assist in diagnosing renal artery stenosis (Fig. 44-8), additional or missing renal blood vessels, and renovascular hypertension. Can assist in differentiating between a renal cyst and renal tumor. Also included in workup of a potential renal transplant donor. A catheter is inserted into the femoral artery and passed up the aorta to level of renal arteries (Fig. 44-9). Contrast media is injected to outline renal blood supply.*	*Before:* Cathartic or enema may be used the night before. Before injection of contrast material, assess for iodine sensitivity. Tell patient a transient warm feeling may be felt along the course of blood vessel when contrast media is injected. *After:* Place a pressure dressing over femoral artery injection site. Observe site for bleeding and inflammation. Have patient maintain bed rest with affected leg straight. Take peripheral pulses in the involved leg every 30-60 min to detect occlusion of blood flow (from thrombus or emboli).
Renal ultrasound	Used to detect renal or perirenal masses (tumors, cysts) and obstructions. Small external ultrasound probe is placed on patient's skin. Conductive gel is applied to skin. Noninvasive procedure involves passing sound waves into body structures and recording images as they are reflected back. Computer interprets tissue density based on sound waves and displays it in picture form. It can be used safely in patients with renal failure.	*Before:* Explain procedure to patient. A bowel preparation is not required. *During:* Because radiation exposure is avoided, a number of images can be obtained and repeat studies can be done over a brief period. Images can be obtained from both prone and supine positions.
Intravenous pyelogram (IVP)	Visualizes urinary tract after IV injection of contrast media. Size and shape of kidneys, ureters, and bladder can be evaluated. Cysts, tumors, and ureteral obstructions (strictures) cause a distortion in normal appearance of these structures. Patient with decreased renal function should not have IVP because contrast media can be nephrotoxic. (Currently procedure is seldom performed.)	*Before:* Cathartic or enema given night before. Assess patient for iodine sensitivity to avoid anaphylactic reaction. *During:* Procedure involves lying on table and having serial x-rays taken. Advise patient that during injection of contrast material, warmth, flushed face, and a salty taste may be experienced. *After:* Force fluids (if permitted) to flush out contrast media.

*N-acetylcysteine, a renal vasodilator and antioxidant, is sometimes administered to reduce the incidence of contrast-induced nephropathy; it can be given by oral or IV route.

Continued

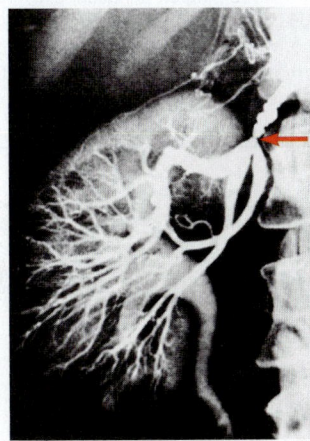

FIG. 44-8 Renal arteriogram showing stenosis of the right renal artery *(arrow)*. (From Brundage DJ: *Renal disorders,* St Louis, 1992, Mosby.)

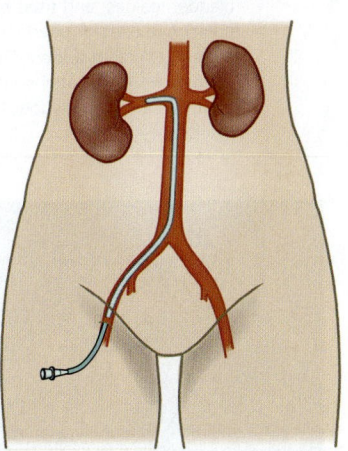

FIG. 44-9 Catheter insertion for a renal arteriogram.

TABLE 44-8   Diagnostic Studies

Urinary System—cont'd

Study	Description and Purpose	Nursing Responsibility
Radiologic Procedures—cont'd		
Antegrade pyelogram (nephrostogram)	Evaluates upper urinary tract when patient has allergy to contrast media, decreased renal function, or abnormalities that prevent passage of a ureteral catheter. Contrast media may be injected percutaneously into renal pelvis or via a nephrostomy tube that is already in place when determining tube function or ureteral integrity after trauma or surgery.*	*Before:* Explain procedure and prepare patient as for IVP. *During and after:* Watch for signs of complications (e.g., hematuria, infection, hematoma).
Retrograde pyelogram	X-ray of urinary tract taken after injection of contrast material into kidneys. It may be done if an IVP does not visualize the urinary tract or if patient is allergic to contrast media or has decreased renal function. A cystoscope is inserted and ureteral catheters are inserted through it into renal pelvis. Contrast media is injected through catheters.*	*Before:* Prepare patient as for IVP. Inform patient that pain may be experienced from distention of pelvis and discomfort from cystoscope. Inform patient that anesthesia may be given for procedure. *After:* Complications are similar to those for cystoscopy (see cystoscopy later in table).
Magnetic resonance imaging (MRI)	Useful for visualization of kidneys. Not proven useful for detecting urinary calculi or calcified tumors. Computer-generated films rely on radiofrequency waves and alteration in magnetic field.	*Before:* Explain procedure to patient. Have patient remove all metal objects. Patients with a history of claustrophobia may need to be sedated. Contraindications: presence of implanted magnetic clips or prosthesis and pacemakers
Magnetic resonance angiography	Allows visualization of renal vasculature. Gadolinium-enhanced studies allow visualization of renal artery.	Same as above. Does not require femoral artery puncture
Cystogram	Visualizes bladder and evaluates vesicoureteral reflux. Evaluates patients with neurogenic bladder and recurrent urinary tract infections. Can also delineate abnormalities of bladder (e.g., diverticula, calculi, tumors). Contrast media is instilled into bladder via cystoscope or catheter.	*Before:* Explain procedure to patient. *During:* If done via cystoscope, follow nursing care related to cystoscopy.
Urethrogram	Similar to a cystogram. Contrast media is injected retrograde into urethra to identify strictures, diverticula, or other urethral pathologic conditions. When urethral trauma is suspected, a urethrogram is done before catheterization.	*Before:* Explain procedure to patient.
Voiding cystourethrogram (VCUG)	Voiding study of bladder opening (bladder neck) and urethra. Bladder is filled with contrast media. Fluoroscopic films are taken to visualize bladder and urethra. After urination, another film is taken to assess for residual urine. Can detect abnormalities of lower urinary tract, urethral stenosis, bladder neck obstruction, vesicoureteral reflux, and prostatic enlargement.	*Before:* Explain procedure to patient.
Loopogram	Detects obstructions, anastomotic leaks, stones, reflux, and other uropathologic features when patient has a urinary pouch or ileal conduit. Because urinary diversions are created with bowel, there is risk of absorption of contrast media.	*Before:* Explain procedure to patient. *During:* Closely monitor patient for reactions to the contrast media.
Endoscopy		
Cystoscopy	Inspects interior of bladder with a tubular lighted scope (cystoscope) (Fig. 44-10). Can be used to insert ureteral catheters, remove calculi, obtain biopsy specimens of bladder lesions, and treat bleeding lesions. Lithotomy position is used. Procedure may be done using local or general anesthesia, depending on patient's needs and condition. Complications include urinary retention, urinary tract hemorrhage, bladder infection, and perforation of bladder.	*Before:* Force fluids or give IV fluids if general anesthesia is to be used. Ensure consent form is signed. Explain procedure to patient. Give preoperative medication. *After:* Explain that burning on urination, pink-tinged urine, and urinary frequency are expected effects. Observe for bright red bleeding, which is not normal. Assist with ambulation because orthostatic hypotension may occur. Offer warm sitz baths, heat, mild analgesics to relieve discomfort.

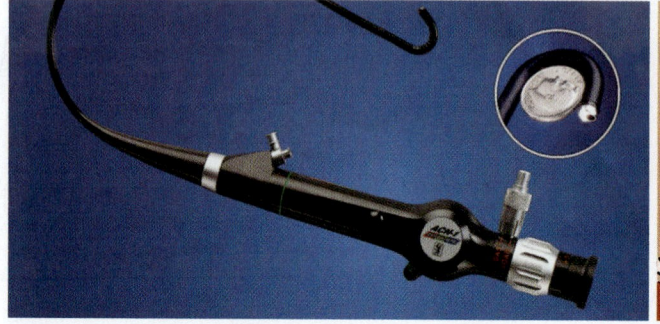
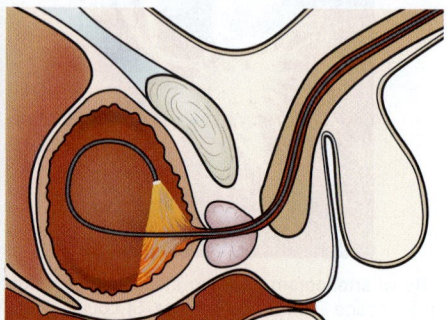

FIG. 44-10   Cystoscopic examination of the bladder in a man. **A,** Flexible cystonephroscope. **B,** Scope inserted into bladder. (*A,* Courtesy Circon Corporation, Santa Barbara, Calif.)

TABLE 44-8 Diagnostic Studies

Urinary System—cont'd

Study	Description and Purpose	Nursing Responsibility
Urodynamic Studies		
Urine flow study (uroflow)	Measures urine volume in a single voiding expelled in a period of time. Used to (1) assess the degree of outflow obstruction caused by such conditions as BPH or stricture, (2) assess bladder or sphincter dysfunction effects on voiding, and (3) evaluate effects of treatment for lower urinary tract problems. Graphic displays can illustrate straining and intermittent flow patterns or other abnormal voiding disorders. *Normal maximum flow rate:* Men: 20-25 mL/sec; women: 25-30 mL/sec. Volume voided and the patient's age can affect the flow rate.	*Before:* Explain procedure to patient. *During:* Ask the patient to start the test with a comfortably full bladder, urinate into a designated container, and try to empty completely. *After:* Measure residual urine volume immediately after a urinary flow study because this will help identify degree of chronic urinary retention that is often associated with abnormal flow patterns.
Cystometrogram	Evaluates bladder's capacity to contract and expel urine. Involves insertion of catheter and instillation of water or saline solution into bladder. Measurements of pressure exerted against bladder wall are recorded. If abdominal pressure is measured, a second tube is inserted into rectum or vagina. This tube is attached to a small fluid-filled balloon to allow pressure recording.	*Before:* Explain procedure to patient. *During:* Ask patient about sensations of bladder filling, usually including the first desire (urge) to urinate, a strong desire to urinate, and perception of bladder fullness. *After:* Observe patient for manifestations of urinary tract infection after procedure.
Sphincter electromyography (EMG)	Recording of electrical activity created when nervous system stimulates muscle tissue. By placing needles, percutaneous wires, or patches near the urethra, pelvic floor muscle activity can be assessed. During the cystometrogram, sphincter EMG is used to identify voluntary pelvic floor muscle contractions and response of these muscles to bladder filling, coughing, and other provocative maneuvers.	*Before:* Explain procedure to patient.
Voiding pressure flow study	Combines a urinary flow rate, cystometric pressures (intravesical, abdominal, and detrusor pressures), and sphincter EMG for detailed evaluation of micturition. It is completed by assisting the patient to a specialized toilet to urinate while the various pressure tubes and EMG apparatus remain in place.	*Before:* Explain procedure to patient.
Videourodynamics	Combination of cystometrogram, sphincter EMG, and/or urinary flow study with anatomic imaging of the lower urinary tract, typically via fluoroscopy. Used in selected cases to identify an obstructive lesion and characterize anatomic changes in bladder and lower urinary tract	*Before:* Explain procedure to patient.
Radionuclide cystography (RNC)	Detects and grades vesicoureteral reflux. Similar to VCUG with a small dose of radioisotope tracer instilled into the bladder via urethral catheter. More sensitive than VCUG, and radiation dose is 1/1000 that of the VCUG.	*Before:* Explain procedure to patient as in VCUG.
Whitaker study	Measures the pressure differential between renal pelvis and bladder. Ureteral obstruction can be assessed. Percutaneous access is gained to renal pelvis by placing a catheter in renal pelvis. A catheter is also placed in bladder. Fluid is perfused through the percutaneous tube or needle at a rate of 10 mL/min. Pressure data are then collected. Pressure measurements are combined with fluoroscopic imaging to identify the level of obstruction.	*Before:* Explain procedure to patient.
Renal Scan	Evaluates anatomic structures, perfusion, and function of kidneys. IV radioactive isotopes are injected. Radiation detector probes are placed over kidney and scintillation counter monitors radioactive material in kidney. Radioisotope distribution in kidney is scanned and mapped. Shows location, size, and shape of kidney and assesses blood flow, glomerular filtration, tubular function, and urinary excretion. Abscesses, cysts, and tumors may appear as cold spots because of nonfunctioning tissue. Also monitors function of a transplanted kidney	*Before:* Requires no dietary or activity restriction. Inform patient that no pain or discomfort should be experienced during test.

Continued

TABLE 44-8   Diagnostic Studies
Urinary System—cont'd

Study	Description and Purpose	Nursing Responsibility
Renal Biopsy	Obtains renal tissue for examination to determine type of kidney disease or to follow progress of kidney disease. Technique is usually done as a skin (percutaneous) biopsy through needle insertion into lower lobe of kidney. Can be performed with CT or ultrasound guidance. Absolute contraindications are bleeding disorders, single kidney, and uncontrolled hypertension. Relative contraindications include suspected renal infection, hydronephrosis, and possible vascular lesions.	*Before:* Type and crossmatch patient for blood. Ensure consent form is signed. Assess coagulation status through patient history, medication history, CBC, hematocrit, prothrombin time, and bleeding and clotting time. Patient should not be taking aspirin or warfarin (Coumadin). *After:* Apply pressure dressing and keep patient on affected side for 30-60 min. Bed rest for 24 hr. Vital signs every 5-10 min, first hour. Assess for flank pain, hypotension, decreasing hematocrit, ↑ temperature, chills, urinary frequency, dysuria, and gross or microscopic hematuria. Urine dipstick can be used to test for bleeding in urine. Inspect biopsy site for bleeding. Instruct patient to avoid lifting heavy objects for 5-7 days and to not take anticoagulant drugs until allowed by HCP.

BPH, Benign prostatic hyperplasia, *GFR,* glomerular filtration rate.

TABLE 44-9   Diagnostic Studies
Urinalysis

Test	Normal	Abnormal Finding	Possible Etiology and Significance
Color	Amber yellow	Dark, smoky color	Hematuria.
		Yellow-brown to olive green	Excessive bilirubin.
		Orange-red or orange-brown	phenazopyridine (Pyridium).
		Cloudiness of freshly voided urine	Urinary tract infection (UTI).
		Colorless urine	Excessive fluid intake, kidney disease, or diabetes insipidus.
Odor	Aromatic	Ammonia-like odor	Urine allowed to stand.
		Unpleasant odor	Urinary tract infection.
Protein	Random protein (dipstick): 0-trace	Persistent proteinuria	Characteristic of acute and chronic kidney disease, especially involving glomeruli. Heart failure.
	24-hr protein (quantitative): <150 mg/day		In absence of disease: high-protein diet, strenuous exercise, dehydration, fever, emotional stress, contamination by vaginal secretions.
Glucose	None	Glycosuria	Diabetes mellitus, low renal threshold for glucose reabsorption (if blood glucose level is normal). Pituitary disorders.
Ketones	None	Present	Altered carbohydrate and fat metabolism in diabetes mellitus and starvation; dehydration, vomiting, severe diarrhea.
Bilirubin	None	Present	Liver disorders. May appear before jaundice is visible (see Chapter 43).
Specific gravity	1.003-1.030	Low	Dilute urine, excessive diuresis, diabetes insipidus.
	Maximum concentrating ability of kidney in morning urine (1.025-1.030)	High	Dehydration, albuminuria, glycosuria.
		Fixed at about 1.010	Renal inability to concentrate urine; end-stage renal disease.
Osmolality	300-1300 mOsm/kg (300-1300 mmol/kg)	<300 mOsm/kg	Tubular dysfunction. Kidney lost ability to concentrate or dilute urine (not part of routine urinalysis).
		>1300 mOsm/kg	
pH	4.0-8.0 (average, 6.0)	>8.0	UTI. Urine allowed to stand at room temperature (bacteria decompose urea to ammonia).
		<4.0	Respiratory or metabolic acidosis.
RBCs	0-4/hpf	>4/hpf	Calculi, cystitis, neoplasm, glomerulonephritis, tuberculosis, kidney biopsy, UTI, trauma.
WBCs	0-5/hpf	>5/hpf	UTI or inflammation.
Casts	None	Present	Molds of the renal tubules that may contain protein, WBCs, RBCs, or bacteria. Noncellular casts (hyaline in appearance) occasionally found in normal urine.
	Occasional hyaline		
Culture for organisms	No organisms in bladder <10^4 organisms/mL result of normal urethral flora	Bacteria counts >10^5/mL	Urinary tract infection; most common organisms are *Escherichia coli,* enterococci, *Klebsiella, Proteus,* and streptococci.

hpf, High-powered field.

from the urinalysis may indicate possible abnormalities, suggest the need for further studies, or provide evidence of progression in a previously diagnosed disorder.

Although a specimen may be collected at any time of the day for a routine urinalysis, it is best to obtain the first specimen urinated in the morning. This concentrated specimen is more likely to contain abnormal constituents if they are present in the urine. The specimen should be examined within 1 hour of urinating. Otherwise, bacteria multiply rapidly, RBCs hemolyze, *casts* (molds of renal tubules) disintegrate, and the urine becomes alkaline as a result of urea-splitting bacteria. If it is not possible to send the specimen to the laboratory immediately, refrigerate it. However, to obtain the best results, coordinate specimen collection with routine laboratory hours.

Creatinine Clearance. A common test used to analyze urinary system disorders is creatinine clearance. **Creatinine** is a waste product produced by muscle breakdown. Urinary excretion of creatinine is a measure of the amount of active muscle tissue in the body, not of body weight. Therefore individuals with larger muscle mass have higher values. Because almost all creatinine in the blood is normally excreted by the kidneys, creatinine clearance is the most accurate indicator of renal function. The result of a creatinine clearance test closely approximates that of the GFR. A blood specimen for serum creatinine determination should be obtained during the period of urine collection.

Creatinine levels remain remarkably constant for each person because they are not significantly affected by protein ingestion, muscular exercise, water intake, or rate of urine production. Normal creatinine clearance values range from 70 to 135 mL/min (Table 44-8). After age 40, the creatinine clearance rate decreases at a rate of about 1 mL/min/yr.

Urodynamic Studies

Urodynamic studies measure urinary tract function. Urodynamic tests study the storage of urine within the bladder and the flow of urine through the urinary tract to the outside of the body.[7] A combination of techniques may be used for a detailed assessment of urinary function (Table 44-8).

CASE STUDY—cont'd

Objective Data: Diagnostic Studies

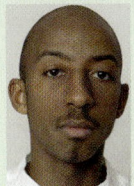

(©iStockphoto/Thinkstock)

The HCP orders the following initial diagnostic studies for A.K.:
- CBC, basic metabolic panel (electrolytes, BUN, creatinine)
- Urinalysis, culture if indicated
- Renal ultrasound

Although A.K.'s laboratory results are all within normal limits, his renal ultrasound identifies calculi in the left ureter. There is no hydronephrosis at present. The HCP prescribes IV opioids for pain management and admits A.K. to a medical unit for further observation.

Discussion Questions
1. Which diagnostic study results are abnormal?
2. Which diagnostic study results are of most concern to you?

Answers available at *http://evolve.elsevier.com/Lewis/medsurg.*

BRIDGE TO NCLEX EXAMINATION

The number of the question corresponds to the same-numbered outcome at the beginning of the chapter.

1. A renal stone in the pelvis of the kidney will alter the function of the kidney by interfering with the
   a. structural support of the kidney.
   b. regulation of the concentration of urine.
   c. entry and exit of blood vessels at the kidney.
   d. collection and drainage of urine from the kidney.

2. A patient with kidney disease has oliguria and a creatinine clearance of 40 mL/min. These findings most directly reflect abnormal function of
   a. tubular secretion.
   b. glomerular filtration.
   c. capillary permeability.
   d. concentration of filtrate.

3. The nurse identifies a risk for urinary calculi in a patient who relates a past health history that includes
   a. hyperaldosteronism.
   b. serotonin deficiency.
   c. adrenal insufficiency.
   d. hyperparathyroidism.

4. Diminished ability to concentrate urine, associated with aging of the urinary system, is attributed to
   a. a decrease in bladder sensory receptors.
   b. a decrease in the number of functioning nephrons.
   c. decreased function of the loop of Henle and tubules.
   d. thickening of the basement membrane of Bowman's capsule.

5. During physical assessment of the urinary system, the nurse
   a. cannot palpate the left kidney
   b. palpates an empty bladder as a small nodule.
   c. finds a dull percussion sound when 100 mL of urine is present in the bladder.
   d. palpates above the symphysis pubis to determine the level of urine in the bladder.

6. Normal findings expected by the nurse on physical assessment of the urinary system include *(select all that apply)*
   a. nonpalpable left kidney.
   b. auscultation of renal artery bruit.
   c. CVA tenderness elicited by a kidney punch.
   d. no CVA tenderness elicited by a kidney punch.
   e. palpable bladder to the level of the pubic symphysis.

7. A diagnostic study that indicates renal blood flow, glomerular filtration, tubular function, and excretion is a(n)
   a. IVP.
   b. VCUG.
   c. renal scan.
   d. loopogram.

8. On reading the urinalysis results of a dehydrated patient, the nurse would expect to find
   a. a pH of 8.4.
   b. RBCs of 4/hpf.
   c. color: yellow, cloudy.
   d. specific gravity of 1.035.

1. d, 2. b, 3. d, 4. c, 5. a, 6. a, d, 7. c, 8. d

For rationales to these answers and even more NCLEX review questions, visit *http://evolve.elsevier.com/Lewis/medsurg.*

EVOLVE WEBSITE

http://evolve.elsevier.com/Lewis/medsurg

Review Questions (Online Only)
Key Points
Answer Keys for Questions
• Rationales for Bridge to NCLEX Examination Questions
• Answer Guidelines for Case Study on pp. 1020, 1023, 1024 and 1031
Conceptual Care Map Creator
Audio Glossary
Content Updates

REFERENCES

1. Baldea AJ: Effect of aging on renal function plus monitoring and support, *Surg Clin North Am* 95(1):71, 2015.
2. Wang X, Bonventre JV, Parrish AR: The aging kidney: increased susceptibility to nephrotoxicity, *Int J Mol Sci* 15(9):15358, 2014.
3. Verma V, Kant R, Sunnoqrot N, et al: Proteinuria in the elderly: evaluation and management, *Int Urol Nephrol* 44(6):1745, 2012.
4. DeSouza K, Chowdhury S, Hughes S: Prompt diagnosis key in bladder cancer, *Practitioner* 258(1767):23, 2014.
5. Jarvis C: *Physical examination and health assessment*, ed 7, St Louis, 2016, Saunders.
6. Prasad V, Gandhi D, Stokum C, et al: Incidence of contrast material-induced nephropathy after neuroendovascular procedures, *Radiology* 273(3):853, 2014.
7. Danforth TL, Ginsberg DA: Neurogenic lower urinary tract dysfunction: how, when, and with which patients do we use urodynamics? *Urol Clin North Am* 41(3):445, 2014.

45

Renal and Urologic Problems

Suzanne Teresa Parsell

Happiness is never stopping to think if you are.

Palmer Sondreal

http://evolve.elsevier.com/Lewis/medsurg/

LEARNING OUTCOMES

1. Differentiate the pathophysiology, clinical manifestations, interprofessional care, and drug therapy of cystitis, urethritis, and pyelonephritis.
2. Explain the nursing management of urinary tract infections.
3. Describe the immunologic mechanisms involved in glomerulonephritis.
4. Differentiate the clinical manifestations and nursing and interprofessional management of acute poststreptococcal glomerulonephritis, Goodpasture syndrome, and chronic glomerulonephritis.
5. Describe the common causes, clinical manifestations, interprofessional care, and nursing management of nephrotic syndrome.
6. Compare and contrast the etiology, clinical manifestations, interprofessional care, and nursing management of various types of urinary calculi.

7. Differentiate the common causes and management of renal trauma, renal vascular problems, and hereditary kidney diseases.
8. Describe the clinical manifestations and nursing and interprofessional management of kidney cancer and bladder cancer.
9. Describe the common causes and management of urinary incontinence and urinary retention.
10. Differentiate among urethral, ureteral, suprapubic, and nephrostomy catheters with regard to indications for use and nursing responsibilities.
11. Explain the nursing management of the patient undergoing nephrectomy or urinary diversion surgery.

KEY TERMS

Renal and urologic disorders encompass a wide spectrum of problems. The diverse causes of these disorders may involve infectious, immunologic, obstructive, metabolic, collagen-vascular, traumatic, congenital, neoplastic, and neurologic mechanisms. This chapter discusses specific disorders of the upper urinary tract (kidneys and ureter) and lower urinary tract (bladder and urethra). Acute kidney injury and chronic kidney disease are discussed in Chapter 46.

INFECTIOUS AND INFLAMMATORY DISORDERS OF URINARY SYSTEM

URINARY TRACT INFECTION

Urinary tract infections (UTIs) are the most common bacterial infection in women.[1] Inflammation of the urinary tract may be caused by a variety of disorders, but bacterial infection is by far the most common. The bladder and its contents are free from bacteria in the majority of healthy people. Nevertheless, a minority of otherwise healthy individuals have some bacteria colonizing the bladder. This condition is called *asymptomatic bacteriuria* and does not justify screening or treatment except in pregnant women.

Escherichia coli (*E. coli*) is the most common pathogen causing a UTI (Table 45-1) and is seen primarily in women.[2] Bacterial counts of 10^5 colony-forming units per milliliter (CFU/mL) or higher typically indicate a clinically significant UTI. However, counts as low as 10^2 to 10^3 CFU/mL in a person with signs and symptoms are indicative of UTI.

Although fungal and parasitic infections may also cause UTIs, this is uncommon. UTIs from these causes are sometimes found in patients who are immunosuppressed, have diabetes mellitus, have kidney problems, or have undergone multiple courses of antibiotic therapy. These types of UTIs may also be

Reviewed by Janie Corbitt, RN, MLS, Retired Instructor of Nursing, Milledgeville, Georgia; Rowena W. Elliott, RN, PhD, CNN, CNE, AGNP-C, FAAN, Associate Professor, University of Southern Mississippi, College of Nursing, Hattiesburg, Mississippi; Deborah Erickson, RN, PhD, Associate Professor and Graduate Coordinator, Department of Nursing, Bradley University, Peoria, Illinois; Shari Gould, RN, MSN, Associate Professor of Nursing, Victoria College, Victoria, Texas; and Marci Langenkamp, RN, MS, Associate Professor of Nursing, Edison Community College, Piqua, Ohio.

found in persons who live in or have traveled to certain developing countries.

Classification of Urinary Tract Infection

A UTI can be broadly classified as an upper or lower UTI according to its location within the urinary system (Fig. 45-1). Infection of the upper urinary tract (involving the renal parenchyma, pelvis, and ureters) typically causes fever, chills, and flank pain, whereas a UTI confined to the lower urinary tract does not usually have systemic manifestations.

Specific terms are used to further delineate the location of a UTI. For example, pyelonephritis implies inflammation (usually caused by infection) of the renal parenchyma and collecting system, cystitis indicates inflammation of the bladder, and urethritis means inflammation of the urethra. Urosepsis

TABLE 45-1 Causes of Urinary Tract Infections

• Escherichia coli*	• Pseudomonas
• Enterococcus	• Staphylococcus
• Klebsiella	• Serratia
• Enterobacter	• Candida albicans†
• Proteus	

*Causative microorganism for urinary tract infection (UTI) in 80% of cases without urinary tract structural abnormalities or calculi.
†Typically identified as the causative microorganism for UTI associated with the use of broad-spectrum antibiotic therapy or in patients with an indwelling catheter.

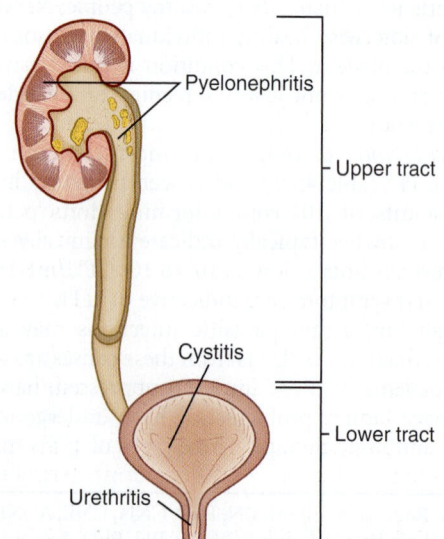

FIG. 45-1 Sites of infectious processes in the upper and lower urinary tracts.

is a UTI that has spread systemically and is a life-threatening condition requiring emergency treatment.

Classifying a UTI as complicated or uncomplicated is also useful. *Uncomplicated* UTIs occur in an otherwise normal urinary tract and usually only involve the bladder. *Complicated* UTIs include those infections in which the patient has coexisting obstruction, stones, or catheters; abnormal GU tract; or diabetes or neurologic diseases. They can also occur when a person has developed resistance to antibiotics, is immunocompromised, or has pregnancy-induced changes. The term *complicated UTI* also applies to a recurrent infection. The individual with a complicated infection is at risk for pyelonephritis, urosepsis, and renal damage.

Etiology and Pathophysiology

The urinary tract above the urethra is normally sterile. Several mechanical and physiologic defense mechanisms assist in maintaining sterility and preventing UTIs. These defenses include normal voiding with complete emptying of the bladder, ureterovesical junction competence, and ureteral peristaltic activity that propels urine toward the bladder. Antibacterial characteristics of urine are maintained by an acidic pH (less than 6.0), high urea concentration, and abundant glycoproteins that interfere with the growth of bacteria. An alteration in any of these defense mechanisms increases the risk for a UTI (Table 45-2).

The organisms that usually cause UTIs are introduced via the ascending route from the urethra and originate in the perineum. Most infections are caused by gram-negative bacilli normally found in the gastrointestinal (GI) tract. However, gram-positive organisms such as streptococci, enterococci, and *Staphylococcus saprophyticus* can also cause UTIs.

A common factor contributing to ascending infection is urologic instrumentation (e.g., catheterization, cystoscopic examinations). Instrumentation allows bacteria that are normally present at the opening of the urethra to enter into the urethra or bladder. Sexual intercourse promotes "milking" of bacteria from the vagina and perineum and may cause minor urethral trauma that predisposes women to UTIs.

Rarely do UTIs result from a hematogenous route, where blood-borne bacteria secondarily invade the kidneys, ureters, or bladder from elsewhere in the body. There must be prior injury to the urinary tract, such as obstruction of the ureter, damage caused by stones, or renal scars, for a kidney infection to occur from hematogenous transmission.

Catheter-associated urinary tract infections (CAUTIs) are the most common health care–associated infection (HAI). The cause of CAUTIs is often *E. coli* and, less frequently, *Pseudomonas* organisms. Most often these infections are underrecognized and undertreated, leading to extended hospital stays, increased health care costs, and patient morbidity and mortality.[3]

Clinical Manifestations

Clinical manifestations of UTIs range from painful urination in uncomplicated urethritis or cystitis to severe systemic illness associated with abdominal or back pain, fever, sepsis, and decreased kidney function in some cases of pyelonephritis.

Lower urinary tract symptoms are experienced in patients who have UTIs of the upper urinary tract, as well as those confined to the lower tract. Symptoms are related to either bladder storage or bladder emptying. These symptoms are presented in Table 45-3.

TABLE 45-2 Risk Factors for Urinary Tract Infections

Factors Increasing Urinary Stasis

- Intrinsic obstruction (stone, tumor of urinary tract, urethral stricture, BPH)
- Extrinsic obstruction (tumor, fibrosis compressing urinary tract)
- Urinary retention (e.g., neurogenic bladder)
- Renal impairment

Foreign Bodies

- Urinary tract calculi
- Catheters (indwelling, external condom catheter, ureteral stent, nephrostomy tube, intermittent catheterization)
- Urinary tract instrumentation (cystoscopy)

Anatomic Factors

- Congenital defects leading to obstruction or urinary stasis
- Fistula (abnormal opening) exposing urinary stream to skin, vagina, or fecal stream
- Shorter female urethra and colonization from normal vaginal flora
- Obesity

Factors Compromising Immune Response

- Aging
- Human immunodeficiency virus infection
- Diabetes mellitus

Functional Disorders

- Constipation
- Voiding dysfunction with detrusor sphincter dyssynergia

Other Factors

- Pregnancy
- Menopause
- Multiple sex partners (women)
- Use of spermicidal agents, contraceptive diaphragm (women), bubble baths, feminine sprays
- Poor personal hygiene
- Habitual delay of urination ("nurse's bladder," "teacher's bladder")

TABLE 45-3 Lower Urinary Tract Symptoms (LUTS)

Symptoms	Description
Emptying Symptoms	
Hesitancy	• Difficulty starting urine stream • Delay between initiation of urination (because of urethral sphincter relaxation) and beginning of flow of urine • Diminished urinary stream
Intermittency	• Interruption of urinary stream while voiding
Postvoid dribbling	• Urine loss after completion of voiding
Urinary retention or incomplete emptying	• Inability to empty urine from bladder • Caused by atonic bladder or obstruction of urethra • Can be acute or chronic
Dysuria	• Painful or difficult urination
Storage Symptoms	
Urinary frequency	• More than eight times in 24-hr period • Often <200 mL each voiding
Urgency	• Sudden, strong, or intense desire to void immediately • Commonly accompanied by frequency
Incontinence	• Involuntary or accidental urine loss or leakage
Nocturia	• Awakened by urge to void two or more times during sleep • May be diurnal or nocturnal depending on sleep schedule
Nocturnal enuresis	• Adults: loss of urine during sleep

Diagnostic Studies

In a patient suspected of having a UTI, initially obtain a dipstick urinalysis to identify the presence of nitrites (indicating bacteriuria), white blood cells (WBCs), and leukocyte esterase (an enzyme present in WBCs, indicating pyuria). These findings can be confirmed by microscopic urinalysis. After confirmation of bacteriuria and pyuria, a urine culture may be obtained. A urine culture is indicated in complicated or HAI UTIs, persistent bacteriuria, or frequently recurring UTIs (more than two or three episodes per year). Urine may also be cultured when the infection is unresponsive to empiric therapy or the diagnosis is questionable.

A voided midstream technique (*clean-catch urine sample*) is preferred for obtaining a urine culture in most circumstances. For women, teach them to spread the labia and wipe the periurethral area from front to back using a moistened, clean gauze sponge (no antiseptic is used because it could contaminate the specimen and cause false positives). Instruct them to keep the labia spread, start voiding, and collect the specimen 1 to 2 seconds after voiding starts. For men, instruct them to wipe the glans penis around the urethra and collect the specimen 1 to 2 seconds after voiding begins.

Refrigerate urine immediately on collection. The urine should be cultured within 24 hours of refrigeration. A specimen obtained by catheterization provides more accurate results than a clean-catch specimen. When an adequate clean-catch specimen cannot be readily obtained, a catheterization may be necessary.

A urine culture is accompanied by *sensitivity testing* to determine the bacteria's susceptibility to a variety of antibiotic drugs. The results of this test allow the HCP to select an antibiotic

These symptoms include dysuria, frequent urination (more than every 2 hours), urgency, and suprapubic discomfort or pressure. The urine may contain grossly visible blood (hematuria) or sediment, giving it a cloudy appearance. Flank pain, chills, and fever indicate an infection involving the upper urinary tract (pyelonephritis). People with significant bacteriuria may have no symptoms or may have nonspecific symptoms such as fatigue or anorexia.

Remember that these symptoms, considered characteristic of a UTI, are often absent in older adults. Older adults tend to experience nonlocalized abdominal discomfort rather than dysuria and suprapubic pain. In addition, they may have cognitive impairment or generalized clinical deterioration. Because older adults are less likely to experience a fever with a UTI, the value of body temperature as an indicator of a UTI is unreliable.[4]

Multiple factors may produce LUTS similar to the symptoms of a UTI. For example, patients with bladder tumors or those receiving intravesical chemotherapy or pelvic radiation usually experience urinary frequency, urgency, and dysuria. Interstitial cystitis/painful bladder syndrome (discussed on pp. 1040-1041) also produces urinary symptoms that are similar to and sometimes confused with a UTI.

known to be capable of destroying the bacteria causing a UTI in a specific patient.

Imaging studies of the urinary tract are indicated in selected cases. An ultrasound or CT scan (CT urogram) may be obtained when obstruction of the urinary system is suspected or UTIs recur.

Interprofessional Care

Once a UTI has been diagnosed, appropriate antimicrobial therapy is initiated. An antibiotic may be selected based on the HCP's best judgment (empiric therapy) or the results of sensitivity testing.

The interprofessional care and drug therapy of UTIs are summarized in Table 45-4. Uncomplicated cystitis can be treated using a short-term course of antibiotics, typically for 3 days. In contrast, complicated UTIs require treatment for a longer period of time, lasting 7 to 14 days or more.[7,8]

Many residents of long-term care facilities, especially women, have chronic asymptomatic bacteriuria. However, usually only symptomatic UTIs are treated.

First-choice drugs to empirically treat uncomplicated or initial UTIs are trimethoprim/sulfamethoxazole (Bactrim), nitrofurantoin (Macrodantin), and fosfomycin (Monurol).[5] Trimethoprim/sulfamethoxazole has the advantages of being relatively inexpensive and taken twice daily. A disadvantage is

---

TABLE 45-4 Interprofessional Care
Urinary Tract Infection

Diagnostic Assessment
- History and physical examination
- Urinalysis (obtain midstream, "clean-catch" voided specimen)
- Urine for culture and sensitivity (if indicated)
- Imaging studies of urinary tract (if indicated): CT scan (CT urogram), ultrasound, cystoscopy

Management
Uncomplicated UTI
- Patient teaching
- Adequate fluid intake (six 8-oz glasses/day)

Drug Therapy
- Phenazopyridine
- Antibiotics
  - trimethoprim/sulfamethoxazole (Bactrim)
  - trimethoprim alone (in patients with sulfa allergy)
  - nitrofurantoin (Macrodantin, Macrobid)
  - fosfomycin (Monurol)

Recurrent UTI
- Repeat urinalysis
- Urine culture and sensitivity testing
- Adequate fluid intake (six 8-oz glasses/day)
- Repeat patient teaching
- Imaging studies of urinary tract (if indicated): see above

Drug Therapy
- Antibiotic: trimethoprim/sulfamethoxazole, nitrofurantoin
- Sensitivity-guided antibiotic therapy: ampicillin, amoxicillin, first-generation cephalosporin, fluoroquinolones
- Consider 3- to 6-mo trial of suppressive or prophylactic antibiotic regimen
- Consider postcoital antibiotic prophylaxis: trimethoprim/sulfamethoxazole, nitrofurantoin, cephalexin

---

E. coli resistance to trimethoprim/sulfamethoxazole, which is an increasing problem in the United States. Nitrofurantoin is normally given three or four times daily, but a long-acting preparation (Macrobid) is available that is taken twice daily.

Other antibiotics that may be used to treat uncomplicated UTI include ampicillin, amoxicillin, and cephalosporins. The fluoroquinolones are used to treat complicated UTIs. These drugs include ciprofloxacin (Cipro), levofloxacin (Levaquin), ofloxacin, and gatifloxacin. In patients with UTIs secondary to fungi, amphotericin or fluconazole (Diflucan) is the preferred therapy.

> **DRUG ALERT** Nitrofurantoin (Furadantin, Macrodantin)
> - Avoid sunlight. Use sunscreen and wear protective clothing.
> - Notify HCP immediately if fever, chills, cough, chest pain, dyspnea, rash, or numbness or tingling of fingers or toes develops.

A urinary analgesic such as oral phenazopyridine may relieve discomfort caused by severe dysuria. Phenazopyridine is an azo dye excreted in urine, where it exerts a topical analgesic effect on the urinary tract mucosa. Teach patients that this drug causes the urine to turn orange or red.

Prophylactic or *suppressive antibiotics* are sometimes given to patients who have repeated UTIs. A low dose of TMP/SMX, nitrofurantoin, or another antibiotic may be taken daily to prevent recurring UTIs, or a single dose may be taken before an event likely to provoke a UTI, such as sexual intercourse. Although suppressive therapy is often effective on a short-term basis, this strategy is limited because of the risk of antibiotic resistance, which ultimately leads to breakthrough infections with increasingly virulent pathogens.

❖ NURSING MANAGEMENT: URINARY TRACT INFECTION

◆ Nursing Assessment

Subjective and objective data that should be obtained from a patient with a UTI are presented in Table 45-5.

◆ Nursing Diagnoses

Nursing diagnoses for the patient with a UTI may include, but are not limited to, the following:
- Impaired urinary elimination *related to* the effects of UTI
- Readiness for enhanced health management

Additional information on nursing diagnoses for the patient with a UTI is presented in eNursing Care Plan 45-1 (available on the website for this chapter).

◆ Planning

The overall goals are that the patient with a UTI will have (1) relief from bothersome, (2) no upper urinary tract involvement, and (3) no recurrence.

◆ Nursing Implementation

◆ **Health Promotion.** It is important to recognize individuals who are at risk for a UTI. These people include debilitated persons, older adults, patients who are immunocompromised (e.g., cancer, human immunodeficiency virus [HIV], diabetes mellitus), and patients treated with immunosuppressive drugs or corticosteroids. Health promotion activities, particularly for these individuals, can help decrease the frequency of infections and provide for early detection of infection. Health promotion activities include teaching preventive measures such as (1) emptying the bladder regularly and completely,

TABLE 45-5 Nursing Assessment
Urinary Tract Infection

Subjective Data
Important Health Information
Past health history: Previous urinary tract infection. Urinary calculi, reflux, strictures, or retention. Neurogenic bladder, pregnancy, benign prostatic hyperplasia, bladder cancer, sexually transmitted infection.
Medications: Antibiotics, anticholinergics, antispasmodics
Surgery or other treatments: Recent urologic instrumentation (catheterization, cystoscopy)

Functional Health Patterns
Health perception–health management: Urinary hygiene practices. Lassitude, malaise
Nutritional-metabolic: Nausea, vomiting, anorexia. Chills
Elimination: Urinary frequency, urgency, hesitancy. Dysuria, nocturia
Cognitive-perceptual: Suprapubic or low back pain, costovertebral tenderness, bladder spasms, dysuria, burning on urination
Sexuality-reproductive: Multiple sex partners (women), use of spermicidal agents or contraceptive diaphragm (women)

Objective Data
General
Fever, chills, dysuria
Atypical presentation in older adults: afebrile, absence of dysuria, loss of appetite, altered mental status

Urinary
Hematuria. Cloudy, foul-smelling urine. Tender, enlarged kidney

Possible Diagnostic Findings
Leukocytosis. UA positive for bacteria, pyuria, RBCs, WBCs, and nitrites. Positive urine culture. Ultrasound, CT scan (CT urogram), VCUG, and cystoscopy indicating urinary tract abnormalities

VCUG, Voiding cystourethrogram.

TABLE 45-6 Patient & Caregiver Teaching
Urinary Tract Infection

When teaching a patient and caregiver measures to prevent a recurrence of a urinary tract infection (UTI), include the following.
1. Take all antibiotics as prescribed. Symptoms may improve after 1-2 days of therapy, but organisms may still be present.
2. Practice appropriate hygiene, including the following:
   • Carefully clean the perineal region by separating the labia when cleansing.
   • Wipe from front to back after urinating.
   • Cleanse with warm soapy water after each bowel movement.
3. Empty the bladder before and after sexual intercourse.
4. Urinate regularly, approximately every 3-4 hr during the day.
5. Maintain adequate fluid intake.
6. Avoid vaginal douches and harsh soaps, bubble baths, powders, and sprays in the perineal area.
7. Report to the HCP symptoms or signs of recurrent UTI (e.g., fever, cloudy urine, pain on urination, urgency, frequency).
8. Consider drinking unsweetened cranberry juice (8 oz three times a day) or taking cranberry extract tablets 300-400 mg/day for UTI prevention. (This practice may not be effective with every patient.)

procedures. Wash your hands before and after contact with each patient. Wear gloves for care of urinary catheters. The American Nurses Association offers an evidenced-based clinical tool for decreasing CAUTI (*http://nursingworld.org/CAUTI-Tool*). Special measures for the care of urethral catheters are discussed in Table 45-21 later in this chapter on p. 1062.

◆ **Acute Care.** Acute care for a patient with a UTI includes ensuring adequate fluid intake if it is not contraindicated. Maintaining adequate fluid intake may be difficult because of the patient's perception that fluid intake will worsen the discomfort and urinary frequency associated with a UTI. Tell patients that fluids will increase frequency of urination at first but will also dilute the urine, making the bladder less irritable. Fluids will help flush out bacteria before they have a chance to colonize in the bladder. Caffeine, alcohol, citrus juices, chocolate, and highly spiced foods or beverages should be avoided because they are potential bladder irritants.

Application of local heat to the suprapubic area or lower back may relieve the discomfort associated with a UTI. Advise the patient to apply a heating pad (turned to its lowest setting) against the back or suprapubic area. A warm shower or sitting in a tub of warm water filled above the waist can also provide temporary relief.

Instruct the patient about the prescribed drug therapy, including side effects. Emphasize the importance of taking the full course of antibiotics. Often patients stop antibiotic therapy once symptoms disappear. This can lead to inadequate treatment and recurrence of infection or bacterial resistance to antibiotics.

Sometimes a second drug or a reduced dosage of drug is ordered after the initial course to suppress bacterial growth in patients susceptible to recurrent UTI. Instruct the patient to monitor for signs of improvement (e.g., cloudy urine becomes clear) and a decrease in or cessation of symptoms. Teach patients to promptly report any of the following to their HCP: (1) persistence of bothersome LUTS beyond the antibiotic treatment course, (2) onset of flank pain, or (3) fever.

◆ **Ambulatory Care.** Home care for the patient with a UTI should emphasize the importance of adhering to the drug regimen. Your responsibility is to teach the patient and caregiver about the need for ongoing care (Table 45-6). This includes taking

(2) evacuating the bowel regularly, (3) wiping the perineal area from front to back after urination and defecation, and (4) drinking an adequate amount of liquid each day.

To estimate the amount of fluid intake a person should have in 24 hours, take the person's weight in pounds and divide that number in half. The result is the number of ounces of fluid a person should have per day. Thus a 150-pound person would require 75 oz/day. The person will obtain about 20% of this fluid from food, which leaves 60 oz (1775 mL) obtained by drinking, or just over seven 8-oz glasses of fluid.

Daily intake of cranberry juice or cranberry tablets or capsules may reduce the number of UTIs. It is thought that enzymes found in cranberries inhibit attachment of urinary pathogens (especially *E. coli*) to the bladder wall.[6]

Routine and thorough perineal hygiene is important for all hospitalized patients, especially when a bedpan is used, after a bowel movement, or if fecal incontinence is present. Answer call lights quickly and offer the bedpan or urinal to bedridden patients at frequent intervals. These measures can prevent incontinence and decrease the number of incontinent episodes.

◆ **Prevention of CAUTI.** All patients undergoing instrumentation of the urinary tract are at risk for developing CAUTI. You have a major role in the prevention of these infections. Avoidance of unnecessary catheterization and early removal of indwelling catheters are the most effective means for reducing CAUTI. Always follow aseptic technique during these

antimicrobial drugs as ordered, maintaining adequate daily fluid intake, voiding regularly (approximately every 3 to 4 hours), urinating before and after intercourse, and temporarily discontinuing the use of a diaphragm.

If treatment is complete and the symptoms are still present, instruct the patient to get follow-up care. Recurrent symptoms because of bacterial persistence or inadequate treatment typically occur within 1 to 2 weeks after completion of therapy. If the patient has followed the treatment regimen, a relapse indicates the need for further evaluation.

◆ Evaluation

The expected outcomes are that the patient with a UTI will
- Experience normal urinary elimination patterns
- Report relief of bothersome urinary tract symptoms
- Verbalize knowledge of treatment regimen

Additional information on the expected outcomes for the patient with a UTI is presented in eNursing Care Plan 45-1 (available on the website for this chapter).

ACUTE PYELONEPHRITIS

Etiology and Pathophysiology

Pyelonephritis is an inflammation of the renal parenchyma (Fig. 45-2) and collecting system (including the renal pelvis). The most common cause is bacterial infection, but fungi, protozoa, or viruses can also infect the kidney.[7]

Urosepsis is a systemic infection arising from a urologic source. Its prompt diagnosis and effective treatment are critical because it can lead to septic shock and death unless promptly treated. (Septic shock is discussed in Chapter 65.)

Pyelonephritis usually begins with colonization and infection of the lower urinary tract via the ascending urethral route. Bacteria normally found in the intestinal tract, such as *E. coli* or *Proteus, Klebsiella,* or *Enterobacter* species, frequently cause pyelonephritis. A preexisting factor is often present such as *vesicoureteral reflux* (retrograde [backward] movement of urine from lower to upper urinary tract) or dysfunction of the lower urinary tract (e.g., obstruction from benign prostatic hyperplasia [BPH], stricture, urinary stone). For residents of long-term

care facilities, CAUTI is a common cause of pyelonephritis and urosepsis.

Acute pyelonephritis commonly starts in the renal medulla and spreads to the adjacent cortex. One of the most important risk factors for acute pyelonephritis is pregnancy-induced physiologic changes in the urinary system. Recurring episodes of pyelonephritis, especially in the presence of obstructive abnormalities, can lead to *chronic pyelonephritis* (discussed later).

Clinical Manifestations and Diagnostic Studies

The clinical manifestations of acute pyelonephritis vary from mild fatigue to the sudden onset of chills; fever; vomiting; malaise; flank pain; and the LUTS characteristic of cystitis, including dysuria, urgency, and frequency. *Costovertebral tenderness* to percussion (costovertebral angle [CVA] pain) is typically present on the affected side. Although the clinical manifestations may subside within a few days, even without specific therapy, bacteriuria and pyuria usually persist.

Urinalysis results indicate pyuria, bacteriuria, and varying degrees of hematuria. WBC casts may be found in the urine, indicating involvement of the renal parenchyma. A complete blood count shows leukocytosis and a shift to the left with an increase in bands (immature neutrophils). Urine cultures must be obtained when pyelonephritis is suspected. In patients with more severe illness who are hospitalized, blood cultures are usually done as well.

Ultrasounds of the urinary system may be performed to identify anatomic abnormalities, hydronephrosis, renal abscesses, or an obstructing stone. CT urograms are also used to assess for signs of infection in the kidney and complications of pyelonephritis, such as impaired renal function, scarring, chronic pyelonephritis, or abscesses.

Interprofessional Care

The diagnostic tests and interprofessional care of acute pyelonephritis are summarized in Table 45-7. Patients with severe infections or complicating factors such as nausea and vomiting with dehydration require hospitalization.

The patient with mild symptoms may be treated as an outpatient with antibiotics for 14 to 21 days (Table 45-7). Parenteral antibiotics are often given initially in the hospital to rapidly establish high serum and urinary drug levels.[7] When initial treatment resolves acute symptoms and the patient is able to tolerate oral fluids and drugs, the person may be discharged on a regimen of oral antibiotics for an additional 14 to 21 days. Symptoms and signs typically improve or resolve within 48 to 72 hours after starting therapy.

Relapses may be treated with a 6-week course of antibiotics. Antibiotic prophylaxis may also be used for recurrent infections. The effectiveness of therapy is evaluated based on the presence or absence of bacterial growth on urine culture.

Urosepsis is characterized by bacteriuria and bacteremia (bacteria in blood). Close observation and vital sign monitoring are essential. Prompt recognition and treatment of septic shock may prevent irreversible damage or death.

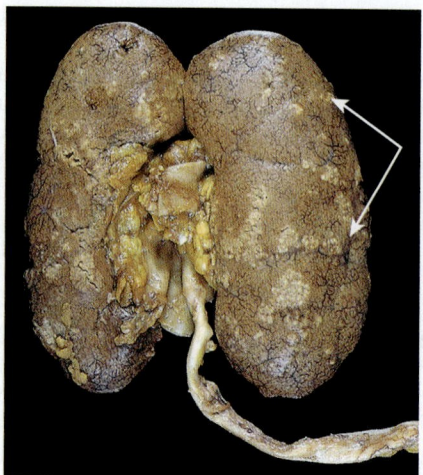

FIG. 45-2 Acute pyelonephritis. Cortical surface shows grayish white areas of inflammation and abscess formation *(arrows)*. (From Kumar V, Abbas AK, Aster JC, et al: *Robbins and Cotran pathologic basis of disease,* ed 8, Philadelphia, 2010, Saunders.)

❖ NURSING MANAGEMENT: ACUTE PYELONEPHRITIS

◆ Nursing Assessment

Subjective and objective data that should be obtained from a patient with pyelonephritis are similar to those for the patient with a UTI (Table 45-5).

TABLE 45-7 Interprofessional Care
Acute Pyelonephritis

Diagnostic Assessment
- History and physical examination
- Urinalysis
- Urine for culture and sensitivity
- Imaging studies: ultrasound (initially), CT scan (CT urogram), cystoscopy, VCUG
- CBC count with WBC differential
- Blood culture (if bacteremia is suspected)
- Percussion for flank (costovertebral angle [CVA]) pain

Management
Mild Symptoms
- Outpatient management or short hospitalization
  - Adequate fluid intake
  - Nonsteroidal antiinflammatory drugs (NSAIDs) or antipyretic drugs
  - Follow-up urine culture and imaging studies

Drug Therapy
- Empirically selected broad-spectrum antibiotics: ampicillin, vancomycin combined with an aminoglycoside (e.g., tobramycin, gentamicin)
- Switch to sensitivity-guided therapy: trimethoprim/sulfamethoxazole (Bactrim) when results of urine and blood culture are available
- Fluoroquinolones: ciprofloxacin (Cipro), ofloxacin, gatifloxacin

Severe Symptoms
- Hospitalization
- Adequate fluid intake (parenteral initially; switch to oral fluids as nausea, vomiting, and dehydration subside)
- NSAIDs or antipyretic drugs to reverse fever and relieve discomfort
- Follow-up urine culture and imaging studies

Drug Therapy
- Parenteral antibiotics
  - Empirically selected broad-spectrum antibiotics: ampicillin, vancomycin combined with an aminoglycoside (e.g., tobramycin, gentamicin)
  - Switch to sensitivity-guided antibiotic therapy when results of urine and blood culture are available
- Oral antibiotics when patient tolerates oral intake

VCUG, Voiding cystourethrogram.

◆ Nursing Diagnoses

Nursing diagnoses for the patient with pyelonephritis include, but are not limited to, those for the patient with a UTI (see p. 1036).

◆ Planning

The overall goals are that the patient with pyelonephritis will have (1) normal renal function, (2) normal body temperature, (3) no complications, (4) relief of pain, and (5) no recurrence of symptoms.

◆ Nursing Implementation

Health promotion and maintenance measures are similar to those for cystitis (see pp. 1036-1037). Early treatment for cystitis can prevent ascending infections. Because patients with structural abnormalities of the urinary tract are at high risk for infection, stress the need for regular medical care.

Nursing interventions vary depending on the severity of symptoms. These interventions include teaching the patient about the disease process with emphasis on (1) continuing medications as prescribed, (2) having a follow-up urine culture, and (3) recognizing manifestations of recurrence or relapse (Table 45-6). In addition to antibiotic therapy, encourage the patient to drink at least eight glasses of fluid every day, even after the infection has been treated. Rest will increase patient comfort.

The patient who has frequent relapses or reinfections may be treated with long-term, low-dose antibiotics. Making certain the patient understands the rationale for therapy is important to increase adherence.

◆ Evaluation

The expected outcomes for the patient with pyelonephritis are the same as for UTI (see p. 1038).

CHRONIC PYELONEPHRITIS

In *chronic pyelonephritis* the kidneys become small, atrophic, and shrunken and lose function due to fibrosis (scarring). Chronic pyelonephritis is usually the result of recurring infections involving the upper urinary tract. However, it may also occur in the absence of an existing infection, recent infection, or history of UTIs.

Radiologic imaging and a biopsy, rather than clinical features, are used to confirm the diagnosis of chronic pyelonephritis. Imaging studies reveal a small, fibrotic kidney. The collecting system may be small or hydronephrotic. Biopsy results indicate the loss of functioning nephrons, infiltration of the parenchyma with inflammatory cells, and fibrosis.

The level of renal function in chronic pyelonephritis depends on whether one or both kidneys are affected, the extent of scarring, and the presence of coexisting infection. Chronic pyelonephritis often progresses to end-stage renal disease (ESRD) even if the underlying infection is successfully treated. Nursing and interprofessional management of the patient with chronic kidney disease is discussed in Chapter 46.

URETHRITIS

Urethritis is an inflammation of the urethra. Causes of urethritis include a bacterial or viral infection, *Trichomonas* and monilial infection (especially in women), chlamydial infection, and gonorrhea (especially in men).

In men, the causes of urethritis are usually sexually transmitted. Purulent discharge usually indicates a gonococcal urethritis, whereas a clear discharge typically signifies a nongonococcal urethritis. (Sexually transmitted infections are discussed in Chapter 52.) Urethritis also produces bothersome LUTS, including dysuria, urgency, and frequent urination, similar to those seen with cystitis.

In women, urethritis is difficult to diagnose. It often produces bothersome LUTS, but urethral discharge may not be present.

Treatment of urethritis is based on identifying and treating the cause and providing symptomatic relief. Drugs used for bacterial infections include trimethoprim/sulfamethoxazole, doxycycline (Vibramycin), ceftriaxone (Rocephin), and nitrofurantoin. Metronidazole (Flagyl) and clotrimazole (Mycelex) may be used for treating *Trichomonas* infection. Drugs such as nystatin or fluconazole may be used for monilial infections. In chlamydial infections, doxycycline may be used. Women with negative urine cultures and no pyuria usually do not respond to antibiotics.

Warm sitz baths may temporarily relieve bothersome symptoms. Instruct the patient to avoid using vaginal deodorant sprays, properly cleanse the perineal area after bowel movements and urination, and avoid sexual intercourse until symptoms subside. Teach patients with sexually transmitted urethritis to refer their sex partners for evaluation and testing if they had sexual contact in the 60 days preceding the onset of the patient's symptoms or diagnosis.

URETHRAL DIVERTICULA

Urethral diverticula are localized outpouchings of the urethra. Most often they result from enlargement of obstructed periurethral glands. In women, who have a higher incidence than men, the diverticula protrude into the anterior vaginal wall. The rare cases reported in males generally have been associated with lower urinary tract congenital anomalies or surgical trauma.

The periurethral glands are found along the entire length of the urethra, with the majority draining into the distal third of the urethra. Skene's glands are the largest of these glands. Causes of urethral diverticuli include urethral trauma from childbearing, urethral instrumentation, urethral dilation, and infection with gonococcal organisms.

Symptoms of urethral diverticuli include dysuria, postvoid dribbling, frequent urination (more often than every 2 hours), urgency, suprapubic discomfort or pressure, dyspareunia, and a feeling of incomplete bladder emptying. Urinary incontinence is frequently present. However, many women have no symptoms.

The urine may contain gross blood (hematuria) or sediment, which gives it a cloudy appearance. An anterior vaginal wall mass may be felt on physical examination. When palpated, the mass is often quite tender and expresses purulent discharge through the urethra.

Radiographic studies such as voiding cystourethrography (VCUG) can be used to confirm the diagnosis. Additional studies include ultrasound and MRI to determine the size of the diverticulum in relation to the urethral lumen.

Surgical options include transurethral incision of the diverticular neck, marsupialization (creation of a permanent opening) of the diverticular sac into the vagina (often referred to as a *Spence procedure*), and surgical excision. Stress urinary incontinence, infection, bleeding, and urethral-vaginal fistula are potential complications of the surgery.

INTERSTITIAL CYSTITIS/PAINFUL BLADDER SYNDROME

Interstitial cystitis (IC) is a chronic, painful inflammatory disease of the bladder characterized by symptoms of urgency, frequency, and pain in the bladder and/or pelvis. *Painful bladder syndrome* (PBS) is suprapubic pain related to bladder filling. The term *IC/PBS* refers to cases of urinary pain that cannot be attributed to other causes such as infection or urinary calculi. IC/PBS is more common in women than men. It affects about 3.3 million women and 1.6 million men.[8]

The etiology of IC/PBS remains unknown and is likely multifactorial. Possible causes include neurogenic hypersensitivity of the lower urinary tract, alterations in mast cells in the muscle and/or mucosal layers of the bladder, infection with an unusual organism (e.g., slow-growing virus), or production of a toxic substance in the urine.

The bladder wall may be irritated and inflamed and can become scarred. *Glomerulations* (superficial ulcerations with pinpoint bleeding) and Hunner's ulcers may occur on the bladder wall.

Clinical Manifestations and Diagnostic Studies

The two primary clinical manifestations of IC/PBS are pain and bothersome LUTS (e.g., frequency, urgency). People with severe cases may urinate as often as 60 times in a day including nighttime urination. The pain is usually located in the suprapubic area but may involve the vagina, labia, or entire perineal region, including the rectum and anus. The pain varies from moderate to severe and is exacerbated by bladder filling, postponed urination, physical exertion, pressure against the suprapubic area, certain foods, or emotional distress. The pain is transiently relieved by urination. Bothersome LUTS are similar to a UTI, and the condition is often misdiagnosed as a recurring or chronic UTI or, in men, chronic prostatitis.

The patient experiences periods of remission and exacerbation of the pain and bothersome voiding symptoms. Women often report that pain occurs premenstrually and is aggravated by sexual intercourse or emotional stress. Some patients experience symptoms that disappear altogether after a period of weeks to months, whereas others have persistent symptoms over months to years.

IC/PBS is a diagnosis of exclusion. A careful history and physical examination are necessary to rule out other disorders that produce similar symptoms, such as UTI or endometriosis. Urine cultures do not find any bacteria or other organisms in the urine. Furthermore, people with IC/PBS do not respond to antibiotic therapy. Cystoscopic examination may reveal a small bladder capacity and glomerulations, but these findings are frequently not present in patients with IC/PBS.

Interprofessional Care

Because the etiology of IC/PBS is unknown, no single treatment consistently reverses or relieves symptoms. Various therapies have been effective, including nutritional and drug therapy. Surgical therapy is rarely indicated.

Elimination of foods and beverages that are likely to irritate the bladder may provide some relief from symptoms. Typical bladder irritants include caffeine; alcohol; citrus products; aged cheeses; nuts; foods containing vinegar, curries, or hot peppers; and foods or beverages likely to lower urinary pH (including fruits such as cranberries). Recipes and menus for a well-balanced diet that is specifically designed to avoid bladder-irritating foods and beverages are available at the website for the Interstitial Cystitis Association (*www.ichelp.org*).

An over-the-counter (OTC) dietary supplement called *calcium glycerophosphate* (Prelief) alkalinizes the urine and can provide relief from the irritating effects of certain foods. This agent may be particularly helpful when dining away from home, where the patient has less control over food preparation.

Because stress can exacerbate or cause flare-ups of IC/PBS symptoms, stress management techniques such as relaxation breathing and imagery (see Chapter 6) may be helpful. Using lubrication or altering positions may decrease pain associated with sexual intercourse.

Two tricyclic antidepressants, amitriptyline and nortriptyline, are used to reduce the burning pain and urinary frequency. Pentosan (Elmiron) is the only oral agent approved for the treatment of patients with symptoms of IC. It enhances the protective effects of the glycosaminoglycan layer of the bladder and relieves pain associated with IC/PBS by reducing the irritative effects of urine on the bladder wall. These drugs are used to provide relief over time (weeks to months) but do not provide the immediate relief that may be needed for an acute exacerbation of symptoms. A short course of opioid analgesics may be used for immediate relief.

Dimethyl sulfoxide (DMSO) can be directly instilled into the bladder through a small catheter. This drug desensitizes pain receptors in the bladder wall. Heparin and hyaluronic acid also may be instilled into the bladder to relieve IC/PBS symptoms. Like pentosan, they are thought to enhance the protective properties of the glycosaminoglycan layer of the bladder. Instillations are often administered with lidocaine, which rapidly desensitizes the bladder wall, helping the patient tolerate instillation of additional heparin or hyaluronic acid and providing transient relief from pain.

Several surgical procedures can be used to relieve severe, debilitating pain. Fulguration and resection of Hunner's ulcers are possible surgical treatments. Surgical urinary diversion, such as an ileal conduit, is used when other measures fail. Unfortunately, some patients have reported pain within the urinary diversion, possibly indicating that some factor in the urine may contribute to IC/PBS in certain cases.

❖ NURSING MANAGEMENT: INTERSTITIAL CYSTITIS/PAINFUL BLADDER SYNDROME

Assess the characteristics of the pain associated with IC/PBS. Ask the patient about specific dietary or lifestyle factors that exacerbate or alleviate pain, and assess the intensity of the pain. Instruct the patient to keep a bladder log or voiding diary over a period of at least 3 days to determine voiding frequency and patterns of nocturia. Keeping a pain record at the same time may be useful.

A UTI may occur during the course of IC/PBS management because of diagnostic instrumentation and frequent bladder instillations. A UTI is likely to produce an acute exacerbation of bothersome LUTS and urinary frequency, as well as dysuria (not typically associated with IC/PBS) and odorous urine, possibly with hematuria.

Instruct the patient to maintain good nutrition, particularly in light of the broad dietary restrictions often necessary to control IC-related pain. Advise the patient to take a multivitamin containing no more than the recommended dietary allowance for essential vitamins and to avoid high-potency vitamins, because they may irritate the bladder. Advise the patient to avoid clothing that creates suprapubic pressure, including pants with tight belts or restrictive waistlines. Educational materials about diet, ways to cope with the need for frequent urination, and strategies for coping with the emotional burden of IC/PBS are available from the Interstitial Cystitis Association (www.ichelp.com). Reassurance that IC/PBS is a real condition experienced by others and that it can be treated may relieve the anxiety, anger, guilt, and frustration related to experiences of chronic pain and voiding dysfunction in the absence of a clear-cut diagnosis and treatment strategy.

GENITOURINARY TUBERCULOSIS

Genitourinary tuberculosis (GUTB) is usually secondary to TB of the lung. In a small percentage of patients with pulmonary TB, the tubercle bacilli reach the kidneys via the bloodstream. Onset occurs 5 to 8 years after the primary lung infection.[9,10]

When the kidney is initially infected with bacilli, the patient is often asymptomatic. Sometimes the patient complains of fatigue and develops a low-grade fever. As the lesions ulcerate, infection descends to the bladder and other genitourinary organs. Then the patient experiences cystitis, frequent urination, burning on voiding, and epididymitis (in men).

Symptoms of a UTI are the first manifestations in the majority of patients with renal TB. However, the urinalysis and urine culture show sterile pyuria (WBCs but no organisms are present). Renal lesions may calcify as they heal. Infrequently, renal colic, lumbar and iliac pain, and hematuria may be present.

Tuberculin skin test results are positive in most patients, but this finding only indicates that the person has had previous inhalation of mycobacteria rather than active disease. A diagnosis of renal TB is based on finding tubercle bacilli in the urine.

Radiographic tests that may be done include CT urogram and voiding cystourethrogram (VCUG). These studies help determine the extent and severity of the disease.

Long-term complications of GUTB depend on the duration of the disease. Scarring of the renal parenchyma, hydronephrosis, and the development of ureteral strictures occur. The earlier treatment is initiated, the less likely renal failure will develop. The patient may require long-term urologic follow-up. Nursing and interprofessional management of the patient with TB is discussed in Chapter 27.

IMMUNOLOGIC DISORDERS OF KIDNEY

GLOMERULONEPHRITIS

Immunologic processes involving the urinary tract predominantly affect the renal glomerulus. The disease process results in glomerulonephritis (inflammation of the glomeruli), which affects both kidneys equally and is the third leading cause of ESRD in the United States. Although the glomerulus is the primary site of inflammation, tubular, interstitial, and vascular changes also occur.

A variety of conditions can cause glomerulonephritis, ranging from kidney infections to systemic diseases (Table 45-8). Glomerulonephritis can be acute or chronic. With *acute glomerulonephritis,* symptoms come on suddenly and may be temporary or reversible. An example of this is acute poststreptococcal glomerulonephritis (discussed in the next section). *Chronic glomerulonephritis* is slowly progressive glomerulonephritis generally leading to irreversible renal failure (discussed later in this chapter).

Acute Poststreptococcal Glomerulonephritis

Acute poststreptococcal glomerulonephritis (APSGN) is a common type of acute glomerulonephritis. It is most common in children and young adults, but all age groups can be affected. APSGN develops about 1 to 2 weeks after an infection of the tonsils, pharynx, or skin (e.g., streptococcal sore throat, impetigo) by nephrotoxic strains of group A β-hemolytic streptococci.[11] The person produces antibodies to the streptococcal antigen. Although the specific mechanism is not known, tissue injury occurs as the antigen-antibody complexes are deposited in the glomeruli, complement is activated (see Chapter 11), and inflammation results.

The clinical manifestations of APSGN include generalized body edema, hypertension, oliguria, hematuria with a smoky or rusty appearance, and proteinuria. Fluid retention occurs as a

TABLE 45-8   Causes or Risk Factors for Glomerulonephritis

Cause or Risk Factor	Description	Cause or Risk Factor	Description
Infections		**IgA nephropathy**	• Results from deposits of immunoglobulin A (IgA) in the glomeruli. • Characterized by recurrent episodes of hematuria.
Poststreptococcal glomerulonephritis	• GN may develop 1-2 wk after a streptococcal throat infection or, rarely, a skin infection (impetigo). • Antibodies (Ab) to strep antigen (Ag) develop and the Ag-Ab deposit in the glomeruli, causing inflammation.		
		Vasculitis	
		Polyarteritis	• Autoimmune disease that affects small and medium blood vessels. • Can affect any organ but common in heart, kidneys, and intestines.
Infective endocarditis	• Bacteria can cause an infection of one or more of the heart valves (see Chapter 36). • People at risk include those with a heart defect, such as a damaged or artificial heart valve. • Bacterial endocarditis is associated with GN, but the exact cause is not known.	Wegener's granulomatosis	• Form of vasculitis affecting small and medium blood vessels. • Most commonly affects kidneys, lungs, and upper respiratory tract.
		Conditions Causing Scarring of Glomeruli	
Viral infections	• Viral infections can trigger GN. • Common viruses include human immunodeficiency virus (HIV) and hepatitis B and hepatitis C viruses.	Diabetic nephropathy	• Primary cause of end-stage renal disease in the United States (see Chapter 46). • Microvascular changes of diffuse glomerulosclerosis involving thickening of the glomerular basement membrane.
Immune Diseases		Hypertension	• Nephrosclerosis is a complication of hypertension. • GN can also cause hypertension.
Systemic lupus erythematosus (SLE)	• Autoimmune disorder characterized by the involvement of several tissues and organs, particularly joints, skin, and kidneys (see Chapter 64). • GN frequently occurs in SLE and has a poor prognosis.	Focal segmental glomerulosclerosis	• Characterized by scattered scarring of glomeruli. • May result from another disease or occur for unknown reasons.
		Other Causes	
Scleroderma	• Disease of unknown etiology characterized by widespread alterations of connective tissue and vascular lesions in many organs (see Chapter 64). • In the kidney, vascular lesions are associated with fibrosis. Severity of renal involvement varies.	Amyloidosis	• Caused by infiltration of tissues with amyloid (hyaline substance). • Hyaline bodies consist largely of protein. • Kidney involvement is common, and proteinuria is often the first clinical manifestation.
Goodpasture syndrome	• Autoimmune disorder that causes lung and kidney disease. • Causes bleeding into lungs and GN.	Illegal drug use	• People who use these drugs are at increased risk for GN.

GN, Glomerulonephritis.

result of decreased glomerular filtration. Initially edema appears in low-pressure tissues, such as those around the eyes (*periorbital edema*), but later it progresses to involve the total body as ascites or peripheral edema in the legs. Smoky urine indicates bleeding in the upper urinary tract. The degree of proteinuria varies with the severity of the glomerulonephropathy. Hypertension primarily results from increased extracellular fluid volume. The patient with APSGN may have abdominal or flank pain. In other cases, the patient may be asymptomatic, and the problem is found on routine urinalysis.

More than 95% of patients with APSGN recover completely or improve rapidly with conservative management. Accurate recognition and assessment are critical, since chronic glomerulonephritis can develop if the patient is not treated appropriately.

The diagnosis of APSGN is based on a complete history and physical examination. An immune response to the streptococci is often demonstrated by assessment of antistreptolysin-O (ASO) titers. The finding of decreased complement components (especially C3 and CH50) indicates an immune-mediated response. A renal biopsy may be done to confirm the disease.

Dipstick urinalysis and urine sediment microscopy reveal erythrocytes in significant numbers. Erythrocyte casts are highly suggestive of APSGN. Proteinuria may range from mild to severe. Blood tests include blood urea nitrogen (BUN) and serum creatinine to assess the extent of renal impairment.

❖ NURSING AND INTERPROFESSIONAL MANAGEMENT: ACUTE POSTSTREPTOCOCCAL GLOMERULONEPHRITIS

The management of APSGN focuses on symptomatic relief. Rest is recommended until the signs of glomerular inflammation (proteinuria, hematuria) and hypertension subside. Edema is treated by restricting sodium and fluid intake and by administrating diuretics. Severe hypertension is treated with antihypertensive drugs. Dietary protein intake may be restricted if there is evidence of an increase in nitrogenous wastes (e.g., elevated BUN). The dietary protein restriction varies with the degree of proteinuria. Low-protein, low-sodium, fluid-restricted diets are discussed in Chapter 46.

Antibiotics should be given only if the streptococcal infection is still present. Corticosteroids and cytotoxic drugs have not been shown to be of value in the treatment of APSGN.

One of the most important ways to prevent APSGN is to encourage early diagnosis and treatment of sore throats and skin lesions. If streptococci are found in the culture, treatment with appropriate antibiotic therapy (usually penicillin) is essential. Encourage the patient to take the full course of antibiotics to ensure that the bacteria have been eradicated. Good personal hygiene is an important factor in preventing the spread of cutaneous streptococcal infections.

In most cases, recovery from the acute glomerulonephritis is complete. However, if progressive involvement occurs and chronic glomerulonephritis develops, ESRD results.

Goodpasture Syndrome

Goodpasture syndrome is an autoimmune disease characterized by antibodies that attack the glomerular and alveolar basement membrane. Damage to the kidneys and lungs results when binding of the antibody causes an inflammatory reaction mediated by complement activation (see Chapter 11).

Goodpasture syndrome is a rare disease that is found primarily in young male smokers. The clinical manifestations include flu-like symptoms with pulmonary symptoms such as cough, mild shortness of breath, hemoptysis, crackles, and pulmonary insufficiency. Renal involvement causes hematuria, weakness, pallor, anemia, and renal failure. Pulmonary hemorrhage usually occurs and may precede glomerular abnormalities by weeks or months.

Current management includes corticosteroids, immunosuppressive drugs (e.g., cyclophosphamide, azathioprine [Imuran]), plasmapheresis (see Chapter 13), and dialysis. Plasmapheresis removes the circulating anti–glomerular basement membrane (GBM) antibodies, and immunosuppressive therapy inhibits further antibody production. Renal transplantation can be attempted after the circulating anti-GBM antibody titer decreases. Although the disease may recur in the transplanted kidney, this is not a contraindication to transplantation.

Nursing management appropriate for a critically ill patient who is experiencing acute kidney injury (see Chapter 46) and respiratory distress (see Chapter 67) is instituted. Death is often secondary to hemorrhage in the lungs and respiratory failure.

Rapidly Progressive Glomerulonephritis

Rapidly progressive glomerulonephritis (RPGN) is a type of glomerular disease characterized by rapid, progressive loss of renal function over days to weeks. In contrast, chronic glomerulonephritis develops insidiously and progresses over many years. The manifestations of RPGN are hypertension, edema, proteinuria, hematuria, and red blood cell (RBC) casts.

RPGN can occur in a variety of situations: (1) as a complication of inflammatory or infectious disease (e.g., APSGN), (2) as a complication of a systemic disease (e.g., systemic lupus erythematosus), (3) as an idiopathic disease, or (4) with the use of certain drugs (e.g., penicillamine).

Treatment is directed toward correction of fluid overload, hypertension, uremia, and inflammatory injury to the kidney. Treatment includes corticosteroids, cytotoxic agents, and plasmapheresis. Dialysis therapy and transplantation are used as maintenance therapy for the patient with RPGN. After kidney transplantation, RPGN may recur.

Chronic Glomerulonephritis

Chronic glomerulonephritis is a syndrome that reflects the end stage of glomerular inflammatory disease. Most types of glomerulonephritis and nephrotic syndrome can eventually lead to chronic glomerulonephritis. Some people who develop chronic glomerulonephritis have no history of kidney disease.

Frequently the cause of chronic glomerulonephritis is not found. Infrequently, it is an inherited disorder (e.g., Alport syndrome [see p. 1052]).

With chronic glomerulonephritis, symptoms develop slowly over time. Patients are often unaware that progressive kidney impairment is occurring. They do not realize that they have severe kidney impairment until a diagnostic evaluation is done. Chronic glomerulonephritis is often discovered coincidentally with the finding of an abnormality on a urinalysis or elevated BP.

The syndrome is characterized by proteinuria, hematuria, and the slow development of uremia (see Chapter 46) as a result of decreasing renal function. Chronic glomerulonephritis progresses insidiously toward ESRD in 2 to 30 years.

Clinical manifestations of glomerulonephritis include varying degrees of hematuria (ranging from microscopic to gross) and urinary excretion of various formed elements, including RBCs, WBCs, and casts. Proteinuria and elevated BUN and serum creatinine levels are other findings. Sometimes fatigue may be a presenting symptom.

The patient's history provides important information related to glomerulonephritis. Assess exposure to drugs, immunizations, microbial infections, and viral infections such as hepatitis. Also evaluate the patient for more generalized conditions involving immune disorders, such as systemic lupus erythematosus and scleroderma. Commonly the patient has no recollection or history of any renal problems.

Ultrasound and CT scan are generally preferred as diagnostic measures. However, a renal biopsy may be performed to determine the exact cause of the glomerulonephritis.

Treatment is supportive and symptomatic. Management of chronic kidney disease is discussed in Chapter 46.

NEPHROTIC SYNDROME

Nephrotic syndrome results when the glomerulus is excessively permeable to plasma protein, causing proteinuria that leads to low plasma albumin and tissue edema.

Etiology and Clinical Manifestations

Some of the common causes of nephrotic syndrome are listed in Table 45-9. About one third of patients with nephrotic syndrome have a systemic disease such as diabetes or systemic lupus erythematosus.[12]

The characteristic manifestations of nephrotic syndrome include peripheral edema, massive proteinuria, hypertension, hyperlipidemia, hypoalbuminemia, and foamy urine. Characteristic laboratory findings include decreased serum albumin, decreased total serum protein, and elevated serum cholesterol. The increased glomerular membrane permeability found in nephrotic syndrome is responsible for the massive excretion of protein in the urine. This results in decreased serum protein and subsequent edema formation. Ascites and *anasarca* (massive generalized edema) develop if there is severe hypoalbuminemia.

The diminished plasma oncotic pressure from the decreased serum proteins stimulates hepatic lipoprotein synthesis, which results in hyperlipidemia. Initially, cholesterol and low-density lipoproteins are elevated. Later the triglyceride level is also increased. Fat bodies (fatty casts), which commonly appear in the urine, cause foamy urine.

Immune responses are altered in nephrotic syndrome. As a result, infection is a primary cause of morbidity and mortality.

TABLE 45-9	Causes of Nephrotic Syndrome
Primary Glomerular Disease	**Infections**
• Membranous proliferative glomerulonephritis	• Bacterial (streptococcal, syphilis)
• Primary nephrotic syndrome	• Viral (hepatitis, human immunodeficiency virus, mononucleosis)
• Focal glomerulonephritis	
• Inherited nephrotic disease	• Protozoal (malaria)
Extrarenal Causes	**Neoplasms**
Multisystem Disease	• Hodgkin's lymphoma
• Systemic lupus erythematosus	• Solid tumors of lungs, colon, stomach, breast
• Diabetes mellitus	
• Amyloidosis	• Leukemias
Allergens	**Drugs**
• Bee sting	• penicillamine
• Pollen	• Nonsteroidal antiinflammatory drugs (NSAIDs)
	• captopril heroin

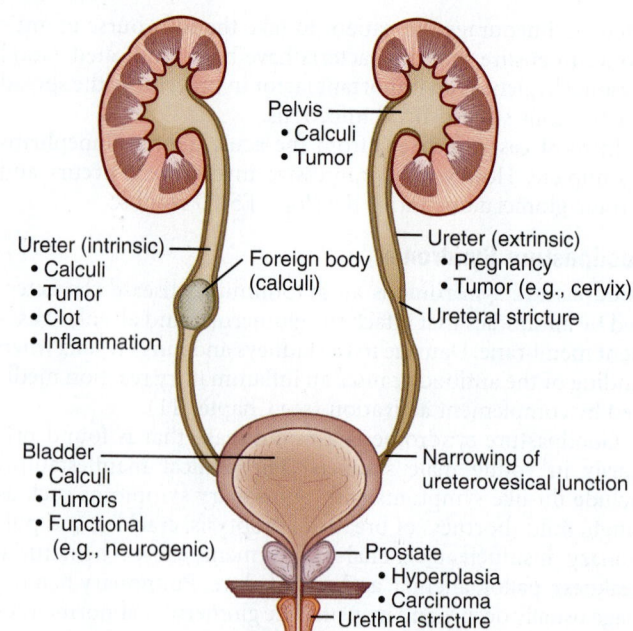

FIG. 45-3 Sites and causes of upper and lower urinary tract obstruction.

Calcium and skeletal abnormalities may occur, including hypocalcemia, blunted calcium response to parathyroid hormone, hyperparathyroidism, and osteomalacia.

With nephrotic proteinuria, hypercoagulability results from the urinary loss of anticoagulant proteins. Hypercoagulability with thromboembolism is a serious complication of nephrotic syndrome. The renal vein is the most common site for thrombus formation. Pulmonary emboli occur in about 40% of nephrotic patients with thrombosis.

❖ NURSING AND INTERPROFESSIONAL MANAGEMENT: NEPHROTIC SYNDROME

Specific treatment of nephrotic syndrome depends on the cause. The goals are to cure or control the primary disease and relieve the symptoms. Corticosteroids and cyclophosphamide may be used for the treatment of nephrotic syndrome. Prednisone has been effective to varying degrees for some causes of nephrotic syndrome (e.g., membranous glomerulonephritis, lupus nephritis). Management of diabetes and treatment of edema are measures used for nephrotic syndrome related to diabetes.

Management of the edema includes the cautious use of angiotensin-converting enzyme inhibitors; nonsteroidal antiinflammatory drugs (NSAIDs); and a low-sodium (2 to 3 g/day), moderate-protein (1 to 2 g/kg/day) diet. If urine protein losses are high (more than 10 g/day), additional protein may be recommended.

Dietary salt restrictions are a key to managing edema. Some individuals may need thiazide or loop diuretics.

The treatment of hyperlipidemia includes lipid-lowering agents, such as colestipol (Colestid) and lovastatin (see Table 33-5). If thrombosis is detected, anticoagulant therapy may be needed.

A major nursing intervention for a patient with nephrotic syndrome focuses on the management of edema. Assess the edema by weighing the patient daily, accurately recording intake and output, and measuring abdominal girth or extremity size. Compare this information on a daily basis to assess the effectiveness of treatment. Clean the edematous skin carefully. Avoid trauma to the skin. Monitor the effectiveness of diuretic therapy.

Patients with nephrotic syndrome are usually anorexic and have the potential to become malnourished from the excessive loss of protein in the urine. Serve small, frequent meals in a pleasant setting to encourage better dietary intake.

Because the patient with nephrotic syndrome is susceptible to infection, teach the patient to avoid exposure to persons with known infections. Support for the patient, especially helping them cope with an altered body image, is essential because of the embarrassment and shame often associated with the edematous appearance.

OBSTRUCTIVE UROPATHIES

Urinary obstruction refers to any anatomic or functional condition that blocks or impedes the flow of urine (Fig. 45-3). It may be congenital or acquired. Damaging effects from urinary tract obstruction affect the system above the level of the obstruction. The severity of these effects depends on the location, duration of obstruction, amount of pressure or dilation, and presence of urinary stasis or infection. Infection increases the risk of irreversible damage.[13]

When obstruction occurs at the level of the bladder neck or prostate, significant bladder changes can occur. Detrusor muscle fibers *hypertrophy* (increase in size) to contract harder to push urine out a narrower pathway. Over a long period, the detrusor loses its ability to compensate for this resistance, eventually leading to large residual urine volume in the bladder.

When *bladder outlet obstruction* is present, pressure increases during bladder filling or storage and can be transmitted to the ureter. This pressure leads to *reflux* (backflow of urine), **hydroureter** (ureteral dilation and distention), vesicoureteral reflux (backflow [backward movement] of urine from the lower to upper urinary tract), and **hydronephrosis** (dilation or enlargement of the renal pelvises and calyces) (Fig. 45-4). Chronic pyelonephritis and renal atrophy may develop. If only one kidney is obstructed, the other kidney may try to compensate by hypertrophy.

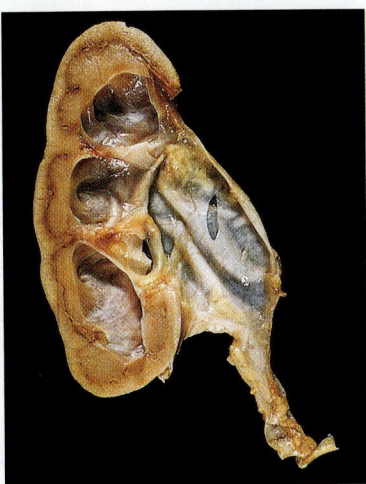

FIG. 45-4 Hydronephrosis of the kidney. Note the marked dilation of the pelvis and calyces and thinning of the renal parenchyma. (From Kumar V, Abbas AK, Aster JC, et al: *Robbins and Cotran pathologic basis of disease*, ed 8, Philadelphia, 2010, Saunders.)

Partial obstruction may occur in the ureter or at the ureteropelvic junction (UPJ) (where the renal pelvis narrows into the ureter). If the pressure remains low or moderate, the kidney may continue to dilate with no noticeable loss of function. The risk of pyelonephritis is increased because of urinary stasis and reflux. If only one kidney is involved and the other kidney is functioning, the patient may be asymptomatic.

If both kidneys or only one functioning kidney is involved (e.g., if the patient has only one kidney), alterations in renal function (e.g., increased BUN or serum creatinine levels) are found. Progressive obstruction can lead to renal failure. Treatment requires locating and relieving the blockage. This can include insertion of a tube (e.g., urethral or ureteral), surgical correction of the primary problem, or diversion of the urinary stream above the level of blockage.

URINARY TRACT CALCULI

Each year an estimated 1 million to 2 million people in the United States have **nephrolithiasis** (kidney stone disease). In the United States the incidence of urinary stone disease is highest in the Southeast and Southwest, followed by the Midwest. Except for struvite (magnesium ammonium phosphate) stones associated with UTI, stone disorders are more common in men than in women. The majority of patients are between 20 and 55 years of age.[13]

Stone formation is more frequent in whites than in African Americans. The incidence is also higher in persons with a family history of stone formation. Stones can recur in up to 50% of patients. Stone formation occurs more often in the summer months, thus supporting the role of dehydration in this process.

GENDER DIFFERENCES

Urinary Tract Calculi

Men	Women
• Urinary calculi disorders (except for struvite stones) are more common in men.	• Struvite stones associated with urinary tract infection are more common in women than in men.

TABLE 45-10 Risk Factors for Urinary Tract Calculi

Metabolic
- Abnormalities that result in increased urine levels of calcium, oxalate uric acid, or citric acid

Climate
- Warm climates that cause increased fluid loss, low urine volume, and increased solute concentration in urine

Diet
- Large intake of dietary proteins that increases uric acid excretion
- Excessive amounts of tea or fruit juices that elevate urinary oxalate level
- Large intake of calcium and oxalate
- Low fluid intake that increases urinary concentration

Genetic Factors
- Family history of stone formation, cystinuria, gout, or renal acidosis
- Lifestyle
- Sedentary occupation, immobility

Etiology and Pathophysiology

Many factors are involved in the incidence and type of stone formation, including metabolic, dietary, genetic, climatic, lifestyle, and occupational influences (Table 45-10). Although many theories have been proposed, no single theory can account for stone formation in all cases. Crystals, when in a supersaturated concentration, can precipitate and unite to form a stone. Keeping urine dilute and free flowing reduces the risk of recurrent stone formation in many individuals.

A mucoprotein is formed in the kidneys as a matrix for the stone. Urinary pH, solute load, and inhibitors in the urine affect the formation of stones. The higher the pH (alkaline), the less soluble are calcium and phosphate. The lower the pH (acidic), the less soluble are uric acid and cystine. When a substance is not very soluble in fluid, it is more likely to precipitate out of solution.

Other important factors in the development of stones include obstruction with associated urinary stasis and UTI with urea-splitting bacteria (e.g., *Proteus, Klebsiella, Pseudomonas,* and some species of staphylococci). These bacteria cause the urine to become alkaline and contribute to the formation of struvite stones. Infected stones, entrapped in the kidney (Fig. 45-5), may assume a staghorn configuration as the stone branches to occupy a large portion of the collecting system. These stones can lead to a renal infection, hydronephrosis, and loss of kidney function.

Genetic factors may also contribute to urine stone formation. Cystinuria, an autosomal recessive disorder, is characterized by a markedly increased excretion of cystine.

Types of Urinary Calculi

The term **calculus** refers to the stone, and *lithiasis* refers to stone formation. The five major categories of stones are (1) calcium phosphate, (2) calcium oxalate, (3) uric acid, (4) cystine, and (5) struvite (magnesium ammonium phosphate) (Table 45-11). Although calcium stones are the most common, stone composition may be mixed. Calculi can be found in various locations in the urinary tract (Figs. 45-3 and 45-5).

TABLE 45-11 Types of Urinary Tract Calculi

Characteristics	Predisposing Factors	Treatment
Calcium Oxalate*		
Small, often possible to get trapped in ureter. More frequent in men than in women. *Incidence:* 35%-40%	Idiopathic hypercalciuria, hyperoxaluria, independent of urinary pH, family history	Increase hydration. Reduce dietary oxalate.† Give thiazide diuretics. Give cellulose phosphate to chelate calcium and prevent GI absorption. Give potassium citrate to maintain alkaline urine. Give cholestyramine to bind oxalate. Give calcium lactate to precipitate oxalate in GI tract. Reduce daily sodium intake.
Calcium Phosphate		
Mixed stones (typically), with struvite or oxalate stones. *Incidence:* 8%-10%	Alkaline urine, primary hyperparathyroidism	Treat underlying causes and other stones.
Struvite (Magnesium Ammonium Phosphate)		
Three or four times as common in women as men. Always associated with urinary tract infections. Large staghorn type (usually) (Fig. 45-5). *Incidence:* 10%-15%	Urinary tract infections (usually *Proteus*)	Administer antimicrobial agents, acetohydroxamic acid. Use surgical intervention to remove stone. Take measures to acidify urine.
Uric Acid		
Predominant in men, high incidence in Jewish men. *Incidence:* 5%-8%	Gout, acidic urine, inherited condition	Reduce urinary concentration of uric acid. Alkalinize urine with potassium citrate. Administer allopurinol. Reduce dietary purines.†
Cystine		
Genetic autosomal recessive defect. Defective absorption of cystine in GI tract and kidney, excess concentrations causing stone formation. *Incidence:* 1%-2%	Acidic urine	Increase hydration. Give α-penicillamine and tiopronin to prevent cystine crystallization. Give potassium citrate to maintain alkaline urine.

*Calcium stones can exist as calcium oxalate, calcium phosphate, or a mixture of both. Calcium stones account for the majority of all stones.
†See Table 45-12: Nutritional Therapy: Urinary Tract Calculi.

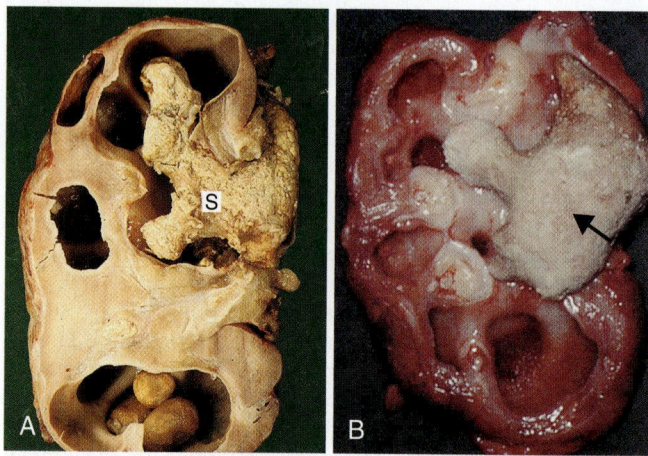

FIG. 45-5 A, Renal staghorn calculus. The renal pelvis is filled with a large calculus that is shaped to its contours, resembling the horns of a stag *(S)*. **B,** Imbedded staghorn calculus *(arrow)* in hydronephrotic, infected, nonfunctioning kidney. (**A,** From Stevens A, Lowe JS, Scott I: *Core pathology: illustrated review in color,* ed 3, London, 2009, Mosby Ltd. *B,* From Bullock N, Doble A, Turner W, et al: *Urology: an illustrated colour text,* London, 2008, Churchill Livingstone.)

Clinical Manifestations

The first symptom of a kidney stone is usually severe pain that begins suddenly. Typically, a person feels a sharp pain in the flank area, back, or lower abdomen. People describe the pain as the most excruciating that a person can endure. *Renal colic* is the term used for the sharp, severe pain, which results from the stretching, dilation, and spasm of the ureter in response to the obstructing stone. Nausea and vomiting may occur due to the severe pain.

Urinary stones cause clinical manifestations when they obstruct urinary flow. Common sites of obstruction are at the UPJ and ureterovesical junction (UVJ). The type of pain is determined by the location of the stone. If the stone is nonobstructing, pain may be absent. If the obstruction is in a calyx or at the UPJ, the patient may experience dull costovertebral flank pain or renal colic. Pain resulting from the passage of a calculus down the ureter is intense and colicky.

Patients with renal colic have a hard time being still. They go from walking to sitting to lying down, and then they repeat the process. Some people refer to this as the *kidney stone dance.*

The patient may be in mild shock with cool, moist skin. As a stone nears the UVJ, pain moves around toward the abdomen and down toward the lower quadrant. Men may experience testicular pain, whereas women may complain of labial pain. Both men and women may experience pain in the groin. The patient may also have manifestations of UTI with dysuria, fever, and chills.

Diagnostic Studies

Noncontrast helical (spiral) CT scan is commonly used in patients with renal colic. It is quick and noninvasive and requires no IV contrast. In some situations, ultrasound is used. A complete urinalysis helps confirm the diagnosis of a urinary stone by assessing for hematuria, crystalluria, and urinary pH.

Retrieval and analysis of the stones are important in the diagnosis of the underlying problem contributing to stone formation. The patient's serum calcium, phosphorus, sodium, potassium, bicarbonate, uric acid, BUN, and creatinine levels are also measured. A careful history should include any previous episodes of stone formation, prescribed and OTC medications, dietary supplements, and family history of urinary calculi. Measurement of urine pH is useful in the diagnosis of struvite stones and renal tubular acidosis (tendency to alkaline or high pH) and uric acid stones (tendency to acidic or low pH). Patients who experience recurrent stone formation should have a 24-hour urinary measurement of calcium, phosphorus, magnesium, sodium, oxalate, citrate, sulfate, potassium, uric acid, and total volume.

Interprofessional Care

Evaluation and management of a patient with renal calculi consist of two concurrent approaches. The first approach is directed toward management of the acute attack by treating the pain, infection, and/or obstruction. Administer opioids to relieve renal colic pain. Most stones are 4 mm or less in size and will probably pass spontaneously. However, it may take weeks for a stone to pass.

Tamsulosin (Flomax) or terazosin, α-adrenergic blockers that relax the smooth muscle in the ureter, can be used to facilitate stone passage. These drugs are also used to relax the muscle tissue in the prostate in men with BPH.

The second approach is directed toward evaluation of the cause of the stone formation and prevention of further stone development. Obtain information from the patient, including a family history of stone formation; geographic residence; nutritional assessment, including the intake of vitamins A and D; activity pattern (active or sedentary); history of prolonged illness with immobilization or dehydration; and any history of disease or surgery involving the GI or genitourinary tract.

Therapy for active stone formers requires a comprehensive management approach, with the primary emphasis on teaching. Adequate hydration, dietary sodium restrictions, dietary changes, and drugs are used to minimize urinary stone formation (Table 45-11). Depending on the specific problem underlying the stone formation, various drugs are prescribed. These drugs prevent stone formation in various ways, including altering urine pH, preventing excessive urinary excretion of a substance, or correcting a primary disease (e.g., hyperparathyroidism).

Treatment of struvite stones requires control of infection. This may be difficult if the stone remains in place. In addition to antibiotics, acetohydroxamic acid may be used to treat kidney infections that result in the continual formation of struvite stones. Acetohydroxamic acid inhibits the chemical action caused by the persistent bacteria and thus retards struvite stone formation. The stone may have to be removed surgically if the infection cannot be controlled.[14]

Endourology, lithotripsy, or open surgical stone removal may be used in the following situations: (1) stones too large for spontaneous passage (usually greater than 7 mm); (2) stones associated with bacteriuria or symptomatic infection; (3) stones causing impaired renal function; (4) stones causing persistent pain, nausea, or paralytic ileus; (5) inability of patient to be treated medically; and (6) patient with only one kidney.[15]

Endourologic Procedures. If the stone is located in the bladder, a cystoscopy is done to remove small stones. For large stones (Fig. 45-6), a *cystolitholapaxy* is done. In this procedure, large stones are broken up with an instrument called a *lithotrite* (stone crusher). The bladder is then irrigated and the crushed stones washed out. A *cystoscopic lithotripsy* uses an ultrasonic lithotrite to pulverize (break up) stones. Complications associated with these cystoscopic procedures include hemorrhage, retained stone fragments, and infection.

Flexible *ureteroscopes*, inserted via a cystoscope, can be used to remove stones from the renal pelvis and upper urinary tract. Ultrasonic, laser, or electrohydraulic lithotripsy may be used in conjunction with the ureteroscope to pulverize the stone.

In *percutaneous nephrolithotomy*, a nephroscope is inserted into the kidney pelvis through a track (using a sheath) in the skin. The track is created in the patient's back. The kidney stones can be fragmented using ultrasound, electrohydraulic, or laser lithotripsy. The stone fragments are removed, and the pelvis is irrigated. A percutaneous nephrostomy tube is usually left in place to make sure that the ureter is not obstructed. Complications include bleeding, injury to adjacent structures, and infection.

Lithotripsy. Lithotripsy is a procedure used to eliminate calculi from the urinary tract. Lithotripsy techniques include (1) laser lithotripsy, (2) extracorporeal shock-wave lithotripsy (ESWL), (3) percutaneous ultrasonic lithotripsy, and (4) electrohydraulic lithotripsy. *Laser lithotripsy* is used to fragment ureteral and large bladder stones (bladder stones are described earlier). To access ureteral stones, a ureteroscope is used to get close to the stone. A small fiber is inserted up the endoscope so that the tip (which emits the laser energy) can come in contact with the stone. A holmium laser in direct contact with the stone is commonly used. The intense energy breaks the stone into small pieces, which can be extracted or flushed out. Because of the type of laser energy, no other tissue is affected. This minimally invasive treatment usually requires general anesthesia.

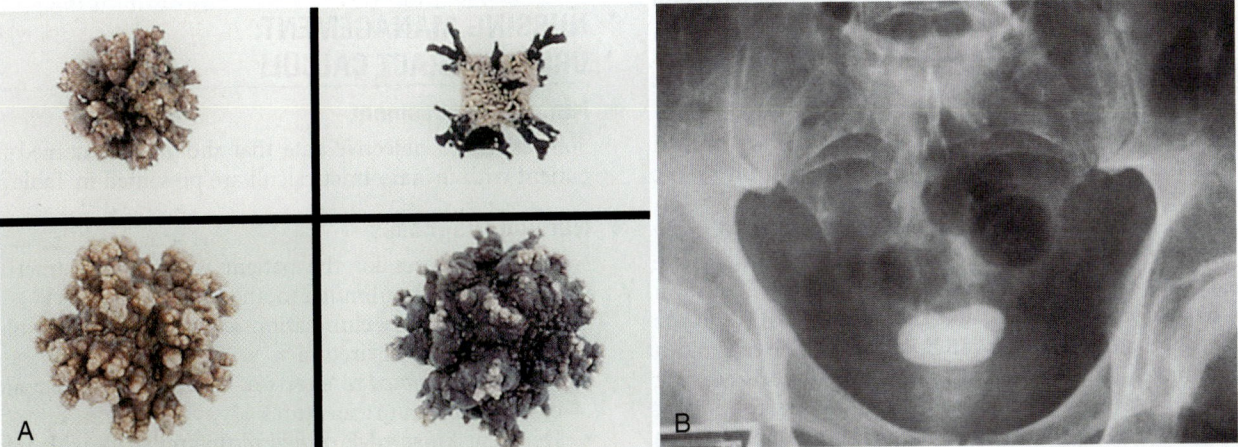

FIG. 45-6 **A,** Calcium oxalate stones. **B,** Plain abdominal x-ray showing large bladder calculus. (From Bullock N, Doble A, Turner W, et al: *Urology: an illustrated colour text*, London, 2008, Churchill Livingstone.)

In *extracorporeal shock-wave lithotripsy (ESWL),* a noninvasive procedure, the patient is anesthetized (spinal or general) to ensure that he or she maintains the same position during the procedure. Fluoroscopy or ultrasound is used to focus the lithotripter on the affected kidney, and a high-voltage spark generator produces high-energy acoustic shock waves that shatter the stone without damaging the surrounding tissues. The stone is broken into fine sand (*steinstrasse*) and excreted in the urine.

In *percutaneous ultrasonic lithotripsy* an ultrasonic probe is placed in the renal pelvis via a percutaneous nephroscope inserted through a small incision in the flank and is then positioned against the stone. The patient is given general or spinal anesthesia for this procedure. The probe produces ultrasonic waves, which break the stone into sandlike particles.

In *electrohydraulic lithotripsy* the probe is positioned directly on a stone, but it breaks the stone into small fragments that are removed by forceps or suction. A continuous saline irrigation flushes out the stone particles, and all of the outflow drainage is strained so that the particles can be analyzed. The calculi can also be removed by basket extraction. Complications are rare but they include hemorrhage, sepsis, and abscess formation. Postoperatively, the patient usually experiences moderate to severe colicky pain. The first few times that the patient urinates,

the urine is bright red. As the bleeding subsides, the urine becomes dark red or a smoky color. Antibiotics are usually administered after the procedure to reduce the risk of infection.

Hematuria is common after lithotripsy procedures. A self-retaining ureteral stent is often placed after the procedure to facilitate passage of sand (shattered stone) and prevent sand buildup within the ureter, which may lead to obstruction. The stent is typically removed within 2 weeks following lithotripsy. If a stone is large or positioned in the mid or distal ureter, additional treatment, such as surgery, may be necessary.

Surgical Therapy. A small group of patients require open surgical procedures. The primary indications for surgery include pain, infection, and obstruction. The type of open surgery performed depends on the location of the stone. A *nephrolithotomy* is an incision into the kidney to remove a stone. A *pyelolithotomy* is an incision into the renal pelvis for stone removal. If the stone is located within the ureter, a *ureterolithotomy* is performed. A *cystotomy* may be indicated for bladder calculi. For open surgery on the kidney or ureter, a flank incision directly below the diaphragm and across the side is usually preferred. The most common complications after surgical procedures for stone removal are related to hemorrhage.

Nutritional Therapy. To manage an obstructing stone, the patient should drink adequate fluids to avoid dehydration. Forcing excessive fluids is not advised, since this has not proved effective in facilitating spontaneous passage (excretion) of stones via the urine. Forcing fluids may also increase the pain or precipitate the development of renal colic.

After an episode of urolithiasis, encourage a high fluid intake (approximately 3 L/day) to produce a urine output of at least 2 L/day. High urine output prevents supersaturation of minerals (i.e., dilutes the concentration of urine) and promotes excretion of minerals within the urine, thus preventing stone formation. Increasing fluid intake is particularly important for patients at risk for dehydration, including those who (1) are active in sports, (2) live in a dry climate, (3) perform physical exercise, (4) have a family history of stone formation, or (5) work outside or in an occupation that requires a great deal of physical activity. Water is the preferred fluid. Limit consumption of colas, coffee, and tea because high intake of these beverages tends to increase the risk of recurring urinary calculi.

A low-sodium diet is recommended, since high-sodium intake increases calcium excretion in the urine. Foods high in calcium, oxalate, and purines are presented in Table 45-12.

❖ NURSING MANAGEMENT: URINARY TRACT CALCULI

◆ Nursing Assessment

Subjective and objective data that should be obtained from a patient with urinary tract calculi are presented in Table 45-13.

◆ Nursing Diagnoses

Nursing diagnoses for the patient with urinary tract calculi include, but are not limited to, the following:

- Impaired urinary elimination *related to* trauma or obstruction of ureters or urethra
- Acute pain *related to* effects of stones and inadequate pain control or comfort measures
- Deficient knowledge *related to* unfamiliarity with information resources and lack of experience with urinary stones

TABLE 45-12   Nutritional Therapy

Urinary Tract Calculi

Depending on the type of calculi, modify the diet to decrease foods that are high in the substance that is the cause of the calculi.

Purine*
High: Sardines, herring, mussels, liver, kidney, goose, venison, meat soups, sweetbreads
Moderate: Chicken, salmon, crab, veal, mutton, bacon, pork, beef, ham

Calcium
High: Milk, cheese, ice cream, yogurt, sauces containing milk; all beans (except green beans), lentils; fish with fine bones (e.g., sardines, kippers, herring, salmon); dried fruits, nuts; Ovaltine, chocolate, cocoa

Oxalate
High: Dark roughage, spinach, rhubarb, asparagus, cabbage, tomatoes, beets, nuts, celery, parsley, runner beans; chocolate, cocoa, instant coffee, Ovaltine, tea; Worcestershire sauce

*Uric acid is a waste product from purine in food.

Additional information on nursing diagnoses for the patient with urinary tract calculi is presented in eNursing Care Plan 45-2 (on the website for this chapter).

◆ Planning

The overall goals are that the patient with urinary tract calculi will have (1) relief of pain, (2) no urinary tract obstruction, and (3) knowledge of ways to prevent recurrence of stones.

◆ Nursing Implementation

Most people who have had urinary stones can lower their risk of recurrence by changing their lifestyle and dietary habits. Adequate fluid intake is important to produce a urine output of approximately 2 L/day. Consult with the HCP about specific recommendations for fluid intake in a given person. The moderately active, ambulatory person should drink about 3 L/day. Fluid intake must be higher in the active person who works outdoors or who regularly engages in athletic activities.

Preventive measures for a person who is on bed rest or is relatively immobile for a prolonged time include maintaining an adequate fluid intake, turning the patient every few hours, and helping the patient sit or stand, if possible, to maximize urinary flow.

Additional preventive measures focus on reducing metabolic or secondary risk factors. For example, dietary restriction of purines may be helpful for the patient at risk for developing uric acid stones. Teach the patient the dosage, scheduling, and potential side effects of drugs used to reduce the risk of stone formation (Table 45-11). Some patients may be taught to self-monitor urinary pH or urine output.

Pain management and patient comfort are primary nursing responsibilities when managing a patient who has an obstructing stone and renal colic (see eNursing Care Plan 45-2). To ensure that any spontaneously passed stones are retrieved, strain all urine voided by the patient using a gauze or a urine strainer. Encourage ambulation to promote movement of the stone from the upper to the lower urinary tract. To ensure safety, tell the patient who is experiencing acute renal colic to ask for assistance when ambulating, particularly if opioid analgesics are being given.

TABLE 45-13   Nursing Assessment

Urinary Tract Calculi

Subjective Data
Important Health Information
Past health history: Recent or chronic UTI. Immobilization. Previous urinary tract stones, obstruction, or kidney disease with urinary stasis. Gout, benign prostatic hyperplasia (BPH), hyperparathyroidism, chronic diarrhea
Medications: Prior use of medication for prevention of stones or treatment of UTI, allopurinol, analgesics, loop diuretics, thiazide diuretics
Surgery or other treatments: External urinary diversion, long-term indwelling urinary catheter

Functional Health Patterns
Health perception–health management: Family history of renal calculi, sedentary lifestyle
Nutritional-metabolic: Nausea, vomiting. Dietary intake of purines, excessive calcium ingestion, salt excess, oxalates, phosphates. Low fluid intake. Chills
Elimination: Decreased urine output, urinary urgency, frequency, feeling of bladder fullness
Cognitive-perceptual: Acute, severe, colicky pain in flank, back, abdomen, groin, or genitalia. Burning on urination, dysuria. Anxiety

Objective Data
General
Guarding, back pain, fever, dehydration

Integumentary
Warm, flushed skin or pallor with cool, moist skin (mild shock)

Gastrointestinal
Abdominal distention, absence of bowel sounds

Urinary
Oliguria, hematuria, tenderness on palpation of renal areas, passage of stone or stones

Possible Diagnostic Findings
↑ BUN and serum creatinine levels. Urinalysis indicating RBCs, WBCs, pyuria, crystals, casts, minerals, bacteria. ↑ Uric acid, calcium, phosphorus, oxalate, or cystine values on 24-hr urine sample. Calculi or anatomic changes on KUB x-ray. Direct visualization of obstruction on cystoureteroscopy

KUB, Kidneys, ureters, bladder; *UTI,* urinary tract infection.

◆ Evaluation

The expected outcomes are that the patient with urinary calculi will
- Maintain free flow of urine with minimal hematuria
- Report satisfactory pain relief
- Verbalize understanding of disease process and measures to prevent recurrence

Additional information on expected outcomes for the patient with urinary calculi is presented in eNursing Care Plan 45-2 (on the website for this chapter).

STRICTURES

A **stricture** is a narrowing of the lumen of the ureter or urethra.

Ureteral Strictures

Ureteral strictures can affect the entire length of the ureter, from the UPJ to UVJ. These strictures are usually secondary to adhesions or scar formation (following surgery or radiation) or they may be due to extrinsic factors such as large tumors in the peritoneal cavity. Depending on its severity, ureteral obstruction can threaten the function of the kidney.

Clinical manifestations of a ureteral stricture include mild to moderate colic. This pain may be moderate to severe in intensity if the patient consumes a large volume of fluids (such as alcohol) over a brief period. Infection is unusual unless a calculus or foreign object such as a stent or nephrostomy tube is present.

The discomfort and obstruction of a ureteral stricture may be temporarily bypassed by placing a stent using endoscopy or by diverting urinary flow via a nephrostomy tube inserted into the renal pelvis of the affected kidney. Definitive correction requires dilation with a balloon or catheter. If the stricture is severe or recurs after initial balloon or catheter dilation, it is surgically incised using an endoscopic procedure (*endoureterotomy*). In selected cases an open surgical approach may be required to excise the stenotic area and re-anastomose the ureter to the contralateral ureter (*ureteroureterostomy*) or to the renal pelvis. Alternatively, distal ureteral strictures may be treated by a *ureteroneocystostomy* (reimplantation of the ureter into the bladder wall).

Urethral Strictures

A *urethral stricture* is the result of fibrosis or inflammation of the urethral lumen. Causes of urethral strictures include trauma, urethritis (particularly after gonococcal infection), surgical intervention or repeated catheterizations (iatrogenic), or a congenital defect of the urethra. Once the process of inflammation and fibrosis begins, the lumen of the urethra narrows and its compliance (ability to close or open in response to bladder filling or micturition) is compromised. Meatal stenosis, a narrowing of the urethral opening, is also common.

Clinical manifestations associated with a urethral stricture include a diminished force of the urinary stream, straining to void, sprayed stream, postvoid dribbling, or a split urine stream. The patient may report feelings of incomplete bladder emptying with urinary frequency and nocturia. Moderate to severe obstruction of the bladder outlet may lead to acute urinary retention. The patient may report a history of urethritis, difficulty with insertion of a urinary catheter, or trauma involving the penis or the perineum. However, many patients are unable to recall any such events, thus leading to a diagnosis of an idiopathic stricture. A history of UTI is common, particularly if the stricture involves the distal urethra. Retrograde urethrography (RUG) and VCUG are used to identify stricture length, location, and caliber.

Initial management of a stricture is focused on dilation. A metal instrument (urethral sound) may be placed, or a series of progressively large stents (filiforms and followers) can be placed into the urethra to expand its lumen in a stepwise fashion. Although this process is initially successful, stenosis frequently recurs. Recurrences may be managed by teaching the patient to repeatedly dilate the urethra by self-catheterization using a soft (coudé-tip, red rubber) catheter every few days. Alternatively, an endoscopic or open surgical procedure (*urethroplasty*) may be a more definitive therapy for an obstructive urethral stricture. Shorter strictures may be treated by resection of the fibrotic area followed by re-anastomosis of the urethra. Longer strictures may require the use of a skin flap as a substitute urethral segment.

RENAL TRAUMA

Renal trauma can be blunt or penetrating. *Blunt trauma* is the most common cause. Injury to the kidney should be considered in sports injuries, motor vehicle collisions, and falls. Renal trauma is especially likely when the patient injures the abdomen, flank, or back. *Penetrating injuries* may result from violent encounters (e.g., gunshot or stabbing incidents). The majority of incidents occur in men younger than 30 years of age.

Clinical findings include a history of trauma to the area of the kidneys. Gross or microscopic hematuria may be present. Diagnostic studies include urinalysis, ultrasound, CT, or MRI evaluation. Renal arteriography may also be used. Both the injured kidney and the uninvolved kidney should be evaluated. The severity of renal trauma depends on the extent of the injury. Treatments range from bed rest, fluids, and analgesia to exploratory surgery and repair or nephrectomy.

Nursing interventions depend on the type of renal trauma and the extent of any associated injuries. Interventions related to renal trauma include the following: (1) assess the cardiovascular status and monitor for shock, especially in a penetrating injury; (2) ensure adequate fluid intake and monitor intake and output; (3) provide for pain relief and comfort measures; and (4) assess for hematuria and myoglobinuria.

RENAL VASCULAR PROBLEMS

Vascular problems involving the kidney include (1) nephrosclerosis, (2) renal artery stenosis, and (3) renal vein thrombosis.

NEPHROSCLEROSIS

Nephrosclerosis is sclerosis of the small arteries and arterioles of the kidney. The decreased blood flow results in ischemia and necrosis of parts of the kidney. *Benign nephrosclerosis*, which usually occurs in adults 30 to 50 years of age, is caused by vascular changes resulting from hypertension and from atherosclerosis. Atherosclerotic vascular changes account for most of the loss of renal function associated with aging. The degree of nephrosclerosis is directly related to the severity of hypertension. In the early stages, the patient with benign nephrosclerosis may have normal renal function, with the only detectable abnormality being hypertension.

Accelerated nephrosclerosis (malignant nephrosclerosis) is associated with malignant hypertension, which is characterized by a sharp increase in BP with a diastolic pressure greater than 130 mm Hg. The patient is usually a young adult, with a male-to-female predominance of 2:1. Renal insufficiency progresses rapidly.

Treatment for benign nephrosclerosis is the same as that for essential hypertension (see Chapter 32). Malignant nephrosclerosis is treated with aggressive antihypertensive therapy (see Chapter 32). The availability and use of antihypertensive drugs have improved the prognosis for patients with benign and malignant nephrosclerosis. Kidney disease, and subsequent renal failure, is a major complication of hypertension. The prognosis for a patient with untreated or refractory malignant hypertension is poor, with the major cause of death related to renal failure.

RENAL ARTERY STENOSIS

Renal artery stenosis is a partial occlusion of one or both renal arteries and their major branches. It can be due to atherosclerotic narrowing or fibromuscular hyperplasia. Renal artery stenosis, which accounts for 1% to 2% of all cases of hypertension, is a cause of secondary hypertension.

When hypertension develops rather abruptly, renal artery stenosis should be considered as a possible cause, especially in patients under 30 or over 50 years of age and in patients with no family history of hypertension. This contrasts with the age distribution for primary hypertension, which is 30 to 50 years of age.

Diagnostic tests used to assess for renal artery stenosis include a renal ultrasound, CT scan, MRI, and renal arteriogram (the best diagnostic tool).

The goals of therapy are to control BP and restore perfusion to the kidney. Percutaneous transluminal renal angioplasty is the procedure of choice, especially in older patients who are poor surgical risks.

Surgical revascularization of the kidney is indicated when decreased blood flow causes renal ischemia or when renovascular hypertension is present. Revascularization of the kidney may result in the patient becoming normotensive. The surgical procedure usually involves anastomosis between the kidney and another major artery, usually the splenic artery or aorta. In selected cases of unilateral renal involvement, unilateral nephrectomy may be indicated.

RENAL VEIN THROMBOSIS

Renal vein thrombosis may occur unilaterally or bilaterally. Causes include trauma, extrinsic compression (e.g., tumor, aortic aneurysm), renal cell cancer, pregnancy, contraceptive use, and nephrotic syndrome.

The patient has symptoms of flank pain, hematuria, or fever or has nephrotic syndrome. Anticoagulation (e.g., heparin, warfarin [Coumadin]) is important to treat the high incidence of pulmonary emboli. Corticosteroids may be used for the patient with nephrotic syndrome. Surgical thrombectomy may be performed instead of or along with anticoagulation.

HEREDITARY KIDNEY DISEASES

Hereditary kidney (or renal) diseases involve developmental abnormalities of the renal parenchyma. Most inherited structural abnormalities are cystic. However, cysts may also develop as a result of obstructive uropathies, metabolic problems, or neurologic diseases. Cysts may be evaluated to rule out tumors.

POLYCYSTIC KIDNEY DISEASE

Polycystic kidney disease (PKD) is the most common life-threatening genetic disease in the world, affecting 600,000 people in the United States. PKD accounts for 10% to 15% of chronic kidney disease.[16]

Genetic Link

PKD has two hereditary forms: manifestations in childhood or adulthood. The childhood form of PKD is a rare autosomal recessive disorder that is often rapidly progressive (see the Genetics in Clinical Practice box). The adult form of PKD is an autosomal dominant disorder (see Figs. 12-4 and 12-5). If one parent has the disease, there is a 50% chance that the disease will pass to the child.

Adult PKD is latent for many years and is usually manifested between 30 and 40 years of age.[17] It involves both kidneys and occurs in both men and women. The cortex and medulla are filled with large, thin-walled cysts that are several millimeters to several centimeters in diameter (Fig. 45-7). The cysts enlarge and destroy surrounding tissue by compression. The cysts are filled

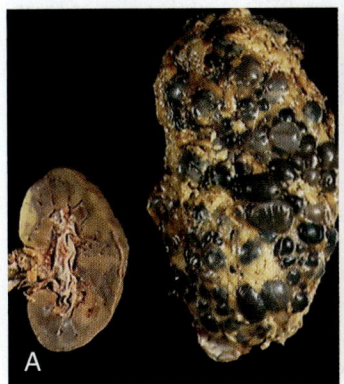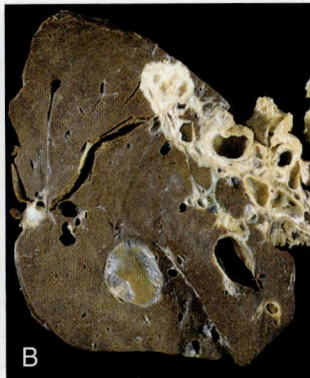

FIG. 45-7 A, Comparison of polycystic kidney with normal kidney. **B,** Cysts in the liver. (*A,* From Brundage DJ: *Renal disorders,* St Louis, 1992, Mosby. *B,* From Kumar V, Abbas AK, Fausto N: *Robbins and Cotran pathologic basis of disease,* ed 7, Philadelphia, 2005, Saunders.)

GENETICS IN CLINICAL PRACTICE

Polycystic Kidney Disease (PKD)

	Adult	Child
Genetic basis	Autosomal dominant	Autosomal recessive
Incidence	1 in 400-1000	1 in 10,000-20,000
Gene location	• *PKD1* gene on chromosome 16 and *PKD2* gene on chromosome 4 • Genes code for polycystins (proteins that promote normal kidney development and function) • Mutations in genes lead to formation of thousands of cysts that disrupt the normal function of kidneys and other organs	• Polycystic kidney and hepatic disease (*PKHD1*) gene on chromosome 6 • Gene codes for fibrocystin • Mutations in gene leads to cyst formation
Genetic testing	DNA testing available	DNA testing available*
Age of onset	Ages 30-40	Infancy or childhood
Clinical implications	• Multisystem involvement • Systemic hypertension occurs in 60%-80% of patients • Increased risk for cerebral aneurysms • Families at risk should be screened	• Up to 30%-50% of affected newborns die shortly after birth • If infant survives the newborn period, chances of survival are good, but about one third need dialysis or transplantation by age 10 yr

*Genetic testing is also available on fertilized embryos before implantation. This allows embryos free of the disorder to be placed into the uterus.

with fluid and may contain blood or pus. PKD kidneys examined during autopsy appear as if they are filled with golf balls.

Early in the disease, patients are generally asymptomatic. Symptoms appear when the cysts begin to enlarge. Often the first manifestations of PKD are headaches; hypertension; hematuria (from rupture of cysts); or a feeling of pain or heaviness in the back, side, or abdomen. However, the first manifestation can also be a UTI or urinary calculi.

Chronic pain is one of the most common problems experienced by individuals with PKD. The pain can be constant and severe. Bilateral, enlarged kidneys are often palpable on physical examination. Many people have no symptoms, and the disease is not diagnosed.

PKD can also affect the liver (liver cysts [Fig. 45-7]), heart (abnormal heart valves), blood vessels (aneurysms), and intestines (diverticulosis). The most serious complication is a cerebral aneurysm, which can rupture.

Diagnosis is based on clinical manifestations, family history, ultrasound (best screening measure), or CT scan (provides a more precise scan). The disease usually progresses from loss of kidney function to ESRD by age 60 in 50% of patients.[16]

❖ NURSING AND INTERPROFESSIONAL MANAGEMENT: POLYCYSTIC KIDNEY DISEASE

There is no specific treatment for PKD. A major aim of treatment is to prevent or treat infections of the urinary tract. Nephrectomy may be necessary if pain, bleeding, or infection becomes a chronic, serious problem. Dialysis and kidney transplant may be needed to treat ESRD (see Chapter 47).

When the patient begins to experience progressive renal failure, the interventions depend on the remaining renal function. Nursing measures are those used for management of ESRD. They include diet modification, fluid restriction, drugs (e.g., antihypertensives), and assistance for the patient and family in coping with the chronic disease process and financial concerns.

The patient who has adult PKD often has children by the time the disease is diagnosed. The patient needs appropriate counseling regarding plans for having more children. In addition, genetic counseling should be provided for the children.

> ### ❓ CHECK YOUR PRACTICE
>
> You are doing a rotation in the dialysis unit. You have been doing vital sign checks on a 45-yr-old man who receives dialysis three times/week. When you ask him why he is on dialysis, he tells you that he has polycystic kidney disease. After further discussion, he tells you that he only has one son who is now 23 years old, but they are estranged. He does not want to tell him about his medical problems or why he is on dialysis.
> • How would you respond to this patient?

MEDULLARY CYSTIC DISEASE

Medullary cystic disease is a hereditary disorder that occurs in two forms. The *autosomal recessive form* is associated with renal failure before age 20. The *autosomal dominant form* is associated with renal failure after age 20.

Most cysts are located in the medulla. The kidneys are asymmetric in shape and are significantly scarred. Defects in the kidneys' concentrating ability result in polyuria. Other clinical manifestations include hypertension, progressive renal failure, severe anemia, and metabolic acidosis. Genetic counseling may

be helpful in family planning. Treatment measures are those related to ESRD (see Chapter 46).

ALPORT SYNDROME

Alport syndrome, also known as *chronic hereditary nephritis*, is an inherited disease that primarily affects the glomeruli. The basic defect is a mutation in a gene for collagen that results in altered synthesis of the glomerular basement membrane.[18]

There are three genetic types of Alport syndrome: sex-linked, autosomal recessive type, and autosomal dominant type. In sex-linked (the most common type) the earliest manifestation is hematuria. These patients also have progressive hearing loss and deformities of the lens of the eye. The other types of Alport syndrome cause hematuria but not deafness or lens deformities.

Males are affected earlier and more severely than females. The disease is often diagnosed in the first decade of life. Alport syndrome causes progressive kidney damage, leading to kidney failure. Children with the autosomal recessive type of Alport syndrome develop kidney failure, usually by their teens or young adult years. People with autosomal dominant Alport syndrome usually live well into middle age before kidney failure develops.

Treatment is supportive. Corticosteroids and cytotoxic drugs are not effective. Kidney transplantation is usually very successful in people with Alport syndrome and is considered the best treatment. The disease does not recur after kidney transplantation.

█ URINARY TRACT TUMORS

KIDNEY CANCER

Kidney cancer arises from the cortex or pelvis (and calyces). Tumors from these areas may be benign or malignant. However, malignant tumors are more common. In the United States, about 61,560 new cases of kidney cancer are diagnosed each year, and about 14,080 people die from kidney cancer.[19]

Renal cell carcinoma (adenocarcinoma) is the most common type of kidney cancer (Fig. 45-8). This type of tumor occurs

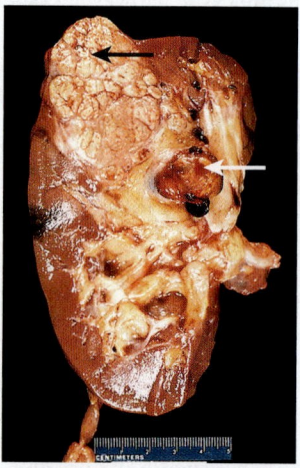

FIG. 45-8 Cross section of kidney with renal cell carcinoma. The carcinoma *(black arrow)* is on the pole of the kidney. Note that the renal vein is involved and thrombosed *(white arrow)*. (From Kumar V, Abbas AK, Fausto N: *Robbins and Cotran pathologic basis of disease,* ed 7, Philadelphia, 2005, Saunders.)

twice as often in men as in women and is typically discovered when the person is 50 to 70 years of age. Cigarette smoking is the most significant risk factor for the development of renal cell carcinoma. An increased incidence has also been found in first-degree relatives of people who have or had renal cell carcinoma. Other risk factors include obesity; hypertension; and exposure to asbestos, cadmium, and gasoline. Risk for kidney cancer is also increased in individuals who have acquired cystic disease of the kidney associated with ESRD (see Chapter 46).

Clinical Manifestations and Diagnostic Studies

Early stage kidney cancer usually has no symptoms, so many patients go undiagnosed until the disease has significantly progressed. Many kidney cancers are diagnosed as incidental findings on imaging studies used to evaluate symptoms for unrelated conditions.

Kidney tumors can cause symptoms by compressing, stretching, or invading structures near or within the kidney. The most common presenting manifestations are hematuria, flank pain, and a palpable mass in the flank or abdomen. Other clinical manifestations include weight loss, fever, hypertension, and anemia.

About 30% of patients have metastasis at the time of diagnosis. Local extension of kidney cancer into the renal vein and vena cava is common (Fig. 45-8). The most common sites of metastases include lungs, liver, and long bones.

CT scan is commonly used in the diagnosis and can detect small kidney tumors. Ultrasound examinations have improved the ability to differentiate between a solid mass tumor and a cyst. This is significant because the majority of masses detected on imaging are cysts. Angiography, biopsy, and MRI are also used in the diagnosis of renal tumors. Radionuclide isotope scanning is used to detect metastases.

❖ NURSING AND INTERPROFESSIONAL MANAGEMENT: KIDNEY CANCER

Preventive measures, such as quitting smoking, maintaining a healthy weight, controlling BP, and reducing or avoiding exposure to toxins, can help reduce the incidence of kidney cancer. Patients in high-risk groups should be aware of their increased risk for kidney cancer. Teach them about early manifestations (e.g., hematuria, hypertension). A cure for kidney cancer may be possible when it is detected early and treated.

Interprofessional care of the patient with kidney cancer is presented in Table 45-14. Staging of renal carcinoma provides a basis for determining treatment options. The following is a simple description of staging of kidney cancer:

Stage I: The tumor can be up to 7 cm in diameter but is confined to the kidney.

Stage II: The tumor is larger than a stage I tumor but is still confined to the kidney.

Stage III: The tumor extends beyond the kidney to the surrounding tissue and may also have spread to a nearby lymph node.

Stage IV: Cancer spreads outside the kidney to multiple lymph nodes or to distant parts of the body, such as bones, brain, liver, or lung.

The treatment of choice for some renal cancers is a partial nephrectomy (for smaller tumors), simple total nephrectomy, or a radical nephrectomy (for larger tumors). Radical nephrectomy involves removal of the kidney, adrenal gland,

TABLE 45-14 Interprofessional Care

Renal Cancer

Diagnostic Assessment	Management
• History and physical examination	• Surgical therapy
• Urinalysis	• Partial nephrectomy
• Ultrasound	• Radical nephrectomy
• CT scan (CT urogram)	• Ablation
• MRI	• Cryoablation
• Renal biopsy	• Radiofrequency ablation
• Renal scan	• Radiation therapy
• Angiography	• Chemotherapy
	• Immunotherapy
	• Targeted therapy

surrounding fascia, part of the ureter, and draining lymph nodes. Nephrectomy can be performed by a conventional (open) approach or laparoscopically (see discussion of nephrectomy on p. 1063). Other treatment options include cryoablation (freezing technique) and radiofrequency ablation (destroying tumor by using radiofrequency heat). These procedures can be used when surgery is not an option (e.g., patient has co-morbid conditions) and for small renal tumors.

Kidney cancer is relatively resistant to most chemotherapy drugs and radiation therapy. Chemotherapy is used as a treatment in metastatic disease.[20] These drugs include 5-fluorouracil (5-FU), floxuridine, and gemcitabine (Gemzar). Radiation therapy is used palliatively in inoperable cases and when there is metastasis to bone or lungs.

Immunotherapy, including α-interferon and interleukin-2 (IL-2), is another treatment in metastatic disease. (The use of α-interferon and IL-2 is discussed in Chapter 15.) Another type of drug used as immunotherapy is nivolumab (Opdivo). This drug targets PD-1, a protein on T cells that normally helps keep these cells from attacking other cells in the body. By blocking PD-1, this drug boosts the immune response against cancer cells. This can shrink some tumors or slow their growth.

Targeted therapy is the preferred treatment for metastatic kidney cancer. Kinase inhibitors, one class of targeted therapies, block certain proteins (kinases) that play a role in tumor growth and cancer progression. Kinase inhibitors include sunitinib (Sutent), sorafenib (Nexavar), cabozantinib (Cabometyx), and axitinib (Inlyta). Bevacizumab (Avastin) and pazopanib (Votrient) inhibit the formation of new blood vessel growth to the tumor. Temsirolimus (Torisel) and everolimus (Afinitor) inhibit a specific protein known as the *mechanistic target of rapamycin (mTOR)*. These drugs are presented in Table 15-13, and the mechanisms of action are shown in Fig. 15-16. The diagnosis of cancer is devastating. In kidney cancer the disease can already be metastasized by the time a person is diagnosed. (The nursing care of the patient with cancer is discussed in Chapter 15.)

BLADDER CANCER

About 74,000 new cases of bladder cancer are diagnosed annually, and about 16,000 deaths related to bladder cancer are reported every year. Cancer of the bladder is most common between ages 60 and 70 years and is four times more common in men than in women.[19]

The most frequent malignant tumor of the urinary tract is transitional cell carcinoma of the bladder. Most bladder tumors are papillomatous growths within the bladder (Fig. 45-9).

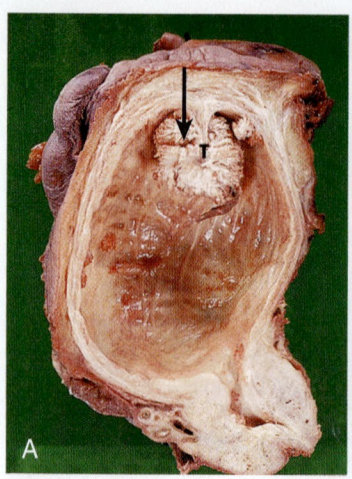 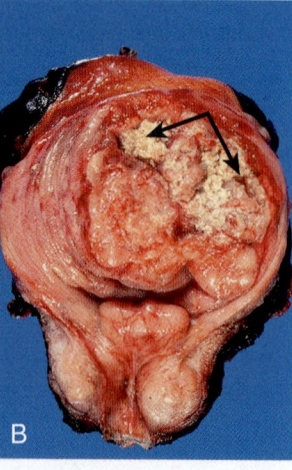

FIG. 45-9 **A,** Papillary transitional cell carcinoma *(T)* seen arising from the dome of the bladder as a cauliflower-like lesion *(arrow).* **B,** Opened bladder showing bladder cancer at an advanced stage. Yellow areas represent ulcerations and necrosis *(arrows).* (*A,* From Stevens A, Lowe J: *Pathology: illustrated review in colour,* ed 2, London, 2000, Mosby. *B,* From Kumar V, Abbas AK, Fausto N: *Robbins and Cotran pathologic basis of disease,* ed 7, Philadelphia, 2005, Saunders.)

About one half of bladder cancers are related to cigarette smoking. Other risk factors include exposure to dyes used in the rubber and other industries. Also at increased risk for bladder cancer are women treated with radiation for cervical cancer, patients who received cyclophosphamide, and patients who take the diabetes drug pioglitazone (Actos).

Individuals with chronic, recurrent renal calculi (often bladder) and chronic lower UTIs have an increased risk of squamous cell cancer of the bladder. Patients who have indwelling catheters for long periods are also at an increased risk to develop bladder cancer.

Clinical Manifestations and Diagnostic Studies

Microscopic or gross, painless hematuria (chronic or intermittent) is the most common clinical manifestation of bladder cancer. Bladder irritability with dysuria, frequency, and urgency may also occur.

When cancer is suspected, obtain urine specimens to identify any cancer or atypical cells. Exfoliated cells from the bladder's epithelial surface can be detected in voided specimens. Other urine tests assess for specific factors associated with bladder cancer, such as bladder tumor antigens.

Bladder cancers can be detected using CT, ultrasound, or MRI. The presence of cancer is confirmed by cystoscopy and biopsy. Cystoscopy with biopsy is the most reliable test for detecting bladder tumors.

❖ NURSING AND INTERPROFESSIONAL MANAGEMENT: BLADDER CANCER

The majority of bladder cancers are diagnosed at an early stage when the cancer is treatable. Before a treatment regimen is started, bladder cancers are graded based on the cell type and staged based on the extent and invasiveness of the cancer. A grading system is used to classify the malignant potential of tumor cells, using a scale from well differentiated (closely resembling the normal tissue) to undifferentiated (poorly differentiated) (see pp. 240-241 in Chapter 15).

The clinical staging of bladder cancer is determined by the depth of invasion of the bladder wall and surrounding tissue.

TABLE 45-15	Interprofessional Care

Bladder Cancer

Diagnostic Assessment	Management
• History and physical examination • Urinalysis • Urine cytology studies • Cystoscopy with biopsy • Ultrasound • CT scan	• Surgical therapy • Transurethral resection with fulguration • Laser photocoagulation • Open loop resection with fulguration • Cystectomy (segmental, partial, or radical) • Radiation therapy • Intravesical immunotherapy • Bacille Calmette-Guérin (BCG) • α-interferon (Intron A) • Intravesical chemotherapy • mitomycin • thiotepa • valrubicin (Valstar) • Systemic chemotherapy and immunotherapy

The following is a simple description of staging of bladder cancer:

Stage I: Cancer is in the inner lining of the bladder but has not invaded the bladder muscle wall.

Stage II: Cancer has invaded the bladder wall but is still confined to bladder.

Stage III: Cancer has spread through the bladder wall to surrounding tissue. It may also have spread to the prostate in men or the uterus or vagina in women.

Stage IV: Cancer has spread to the lymph nodes and other organs, such as lungs, bones, or liver.

Interprofessional care of bladder cancer includes surgery, radiation, chemotherapy, and intravesical therapy (Table 45-15).

◆ Surgical Therapy

Surgical therapies include a variety of procedures. *Transurethral resection of the bladder tumor* (TURBT) is used for superficial lesions of the bladder's inner lining. A wire loop inserted through the cystoscope is used to cauterize (with electric current or laser) and kill the cancer cells. This procedure is also used to control bleeding in the patient who is a poor operative risk or who has advanced tumors. The primary disadvantage of this approach is destruction of the tumor so that pathologic evaluation for grading and staging cannot be completed.

A *segmental cystectomy (partial cystectomy)* is used to treat larger tumors or those that involve only one area of the bladder. A portion of the bladder wall containing the tumor is removed along with a margin of normal tissue.

When the tumor is invasive or involves the trigone (the area where the ureters insert into the bladder) and the patient is free from metastasis beyond the pelvic area, a radical cystectomy is the treatment of choice. A *radical cystectomy* involves removal of the bladder, prostate, and seminal vesicles in men and the bladder, uterus, cervix, urethra, and ovaries in women. After a radical cystectomy, a new way must be created for urine to leave the body. This surgical technique is called a *urinary diversion* (discussed on pp. 1064-1065 later in this chapter).

Postoperative instructions for any of these surgical procedures include drinking a large volume of fluid for the first week after the procedure. Teach the patient to monitor the color and consistency of the urine. The urine is pink for the first several days after the procedure, but it should not be bright red or contain blood clots. Approximately 7 to 10 days after tumor resection, the patient may observe dark red or rust-colored flecks in the urine. These may be from the healing tumor resection site.

Administer opioid analgesics for a brief period after the procedure, along with stool softeners. Also help the patient and family cope with fears about cancer, surgery, and sexuality. Emphasize the importance of regular follow-up care. Follow-up cystoscopies are required on a regular basis after surgery for bladder cancer.

◆ Radiation Therapy, Chemotherapy, and Immunotherapy

Radiation therapy can be used in combination with cystectomy or as the primary therapy when the cancer is inoperable or the patient refuses surgery. Chemotherapy drugs used in treating invasive bladder cancer include cisplatin, vinblastine, doxorubicin, and methotrexate. Atezolizumab (Tecentriq) is a type of immunotherapy that enhances the immune response against the bladder cancer cells.

◆ Intravesical Therapy

Chemotherapy with local instillation of immunotherapy or chemotherapy can be delivered directly into the bladder by a urethral catheter.[21] *Intravesical therapy* is usually initiated at weekly intervals for 6 to 12 weeks. The drug is instilled directly into the patient's bladder and retained for about 2 hours. The patient's bladder must be empty before instillation. Change the patient's position every 15 minutes during the instillation for maximum contact in all areas of the bladder. Maintenance therapy after the initial induction regimen may be beneficial.

Bacille Calmette-Guérin (BCG), a weakened strain of *Mycobacterium bovis,* is the treatment of choice for carcinoma in situ. BCG stimulates the immune system rather than acting directly on cancer cells in the bladder. When BCG fails, α-interferon in addition to BCG may be used. Other treatments that can be used when BCG fails include mitomycin and valrubicin (chemotherapy antibiotics) and thiotepa (an alkylating agent).[22]

Most patients have irritative voiding symptoms and hemorrhagic cystitis after intravesical therapy. Thiotepa can significantly reduce WBC and platelet counts in some individuals when absorbed into the circulation from the bladder wall. BCG may cause flu-like symptoms, increased urinary frequency, hematuria, or systemic infection. Other side effects of chemotherapy (e.g., nausea, vomiting, hair loss) are not experienced with intravesical chemotherapy.

Encourage patients to increase their daily fluid intake and to quit smoking. Assess the patient for secondary UTI, and stress the need for routine urologic follow-up. The patient may have fears or concerns about sexual activity or bladder function that must be addressed. Because of the high rate of disease recurrence and progression in bladder cancer, follow-up studies are very important.

▌ BLADDER DYSFUNCTION

URINARY INCONTINENCE

Urinary incontinence (UI) is an involuntary leakage of urine. Although incontinence is more prevalent among older women and older men, it is not a natural consequence of aging. UI has traditionally been viewed as a social or hygienic problem, but it also has a major effect on quality of life and contributes to serious health problems, especially in older adults.

Etiology and Pathophysiology

UI occurs when bladder pressure exceeds urethral closure pressure. Anything that interferes with bladder or urethral sphincter

control can result in UI. Using the acronym *DRIP*, the causes can include *D:* delirium, dehydration, depression; *R:* restricted mobility, rectal impaction; *I:* infection, inflammation, impaction; and *P:* polyuria, polypharmacy. Patients may have more than one type of incontinence (Table 45-16).

Diagnostic Studies

The basic evaluation for UI includes a focused history, physical assessment, and bladder log or voiding record whenever possible. Obtain information related to the onset of UI, factors that provoke urinary leakage, and associated conditions. Pay special attention to factors known to produce transient UI, particularly when the onset of urine loss is relatively sudden. Begin the physical examination with an assessment of general health and functional issues associated with urination, including mobility, dexterity, and cognitive function.

A pelvic examination includes careful inspection of the perineal skin for signs of erosion or rashes related to UI and existence of pelvic organ prolapse. Also evaluate local innervation and pelvic floor muscle strength, including a digital examination of the pelvic floor muscle to determine weakness or tension. Whenever possible, ask the patient to keep a bladder log or voiding diary documenting the timing of urinations, episodes of urinary leakage, and frequency of nocturia for a period of 1 to 7 days. This record can be kept by nursing staff if the person is in an inpatient or long-term care facility.

A urinalysis is used to identify possible factors contributing to transient UI (e.g., UTI, diabetes mellitus). Measure postvoid residual (PVR) urine in the patient undergoing evaluation for UI. The PVR volume is obtained by asking the patient to urinate, followed by catheterization or use of a bladder ultrasound within a relatively brief period (preferably 10 to 20 minutes).

Urodynamic testing is indicated in selected cases of UI. Imaging studies of the upper urinary tract (e.g., ultrasound) are obtained when UI is associated with UTIs or evidence of upper urinary tract involvement.

Interprofessional Care

Many cases of incontinence can be cured or significantly improved. Transient, reversible factors are initially corrected, followed by management of the type of UI (Table 45-16). In general, less invasive treatments are attempted before more invasive methods (e.g., surgery). Nevertheless, the choice of the initial treatment is individualized, based on patient preference, the type and severity of UI, and associated anatomic defects.

Several behavioral therapies may be used to improve UI (Table 45-17). Pelvic floor muscle training (Kegel exercises) is used to manage stress, urge, or mixed UI[23] (Table 45-18). Biofeedback is used to help the patient identify, isolate, contract,

TABLE 45-16 Types of Urinary Incontinence

Description	Causes	Treatment
Stress Incontinence* • Sudden increase in intraabdominal pressure causes involuntary passage of urine. • Can occur during coughing, laughing, sneezing, or physical activities such as heavy lifting, exercising. • Leakage usually is in small amounts and may not be daily.	• Most common in women with relaxed pelvic floor musculature (from delivery, use of instrumentation during vaginal delivery, or multiple pregnancies). • Structures of female urethra atrophy when estrogen decreases. • Prostate surgery for BPH or prostate cancer.	• Pelvic floor muscle exercises (e.g., Kegel exercises), weight loss if obese, cessation of smoking, topical estrogen products, external condom catheters or penile clamp in men, surgery • Urethral inserts, patches, or bladder neck support devices (e.g., incontinence pessary) to correct underlying problem
Urge Incontinence* • Often referred to as overactive bladder. • Occurs randomly when involuntary urination is preceded by urinary urgency. • Leakage is periodic but frequent and usually in large amounts. • Nocturnal frequency and incontinence are common.	• Caused by uncontrolled contraction or overactive detrusor muscle. • Bladder escapes central inhibition and contracts reflexively. • Conditions include: • Nervous system disorders (e.g., stroke, Alzheimer's disease, brain tumor, Parkinson's disease) • Bladder disorders (e.g., carcinoma in situ, radiation effects, interstitial cystitis) • Interference with spinal inhibitory pathways (e.g., malignant growth in spinal cord, spondylosis) • Bladder outlet obstruction or conditions of unknown etiology	• Treatment of underlying cause • Biobehavioral interventions (bladder retraining with urge suppression, decrease in dietary irritants, bowel regularity, pelvic floor muscle exercises) • Anticholinergic drugs (Table 45-19) • Mirabegron (Myrbetriq) • Calcium channel blockers (Table 45-19) • Containment devices (e.g., external condom catheters) • Vaginal estrogen creams • Absorbent products
Overflow Incontinence • Occurs when pressure of urine in overfull bladder overcomes sphincter control. • Leakage of small amounts of urine is frequent throughout day and night. • Urination may also occur frequently in small amounts. • Bladder remains distended and is usually palpable.	• Disorder is caused by bladder or urethral outlet obstruction (bladder neck obstruction, urethral stricture, pelvic organ prolapse) or by underactive detrusor muscle caused by myogenic or neurogenic factors (e.g., herniated disc, diabetic neuropathy). • May also occur after anesthesia and surgery (e.g., hemorrhoidectomy, herniorrhaphy, cystoscopy). • Neurogenic bladder (flaccid type).	• Urinary catheterization to decompress bladder • Implementation of Credé or Valsalva maneuver • 5α-Reductase inhibitors (Table 45-19) to decrease outlet resistance • α-Adrenergic blockers (Table 45-19) • Bethanechol (Urecholine) to enhance bladder contractions • Intravaginal device such as a pessary to support prolapse • Intermittent catheterization • Surgery to correct underlying problem
Reflex Incontinence • Condition occurs when no warning or stress precedes periodic involuntary urination. • Urination is frequent, moderate in volume, and occurs equally during day and night.	• Spinal cord lesion above S2 interferes with central nervous system inhibition. • Disorder results in detrusor hyperreflexia and interferes with pathways coordinating detrusor contraction and sphincter relaxation.	• Treatment of underlying cause • Bladder decompression to prevent ureteral reflux and hydronephrosis • Intermittent self-catheterization • Diazepam (Valium) or baclofen (Lioresal) to relax external sphincter • Prophylactic antibiotics • Surgical sphincterotomy
Incontinence After Trauma or Surgery • In women, vesicovaginal or urethrovaginal fistula may occur. • In men, alteration in continence control involves proximal urethral sphincter (bladder neck and prostatic urethra) and distal urethral sphincter (external striated muscle).	• Fistulas may occur during pregnancy, after delivery of baby, as a result of hysterectomy or invasive cancer of cervix, or after radiation therapy. • Incontinence is a postoperative complication of transurethral, perineal, or retropubic prostatectomy.	• Surgery to correct fistula • Urinary diversion surgery to bypass urethra and bladder • External condom catheter • Penile clamp • Placement of artificial implantable sphincter
Functional Incontinence • Loss of urine resulting from cognitive, functional, or environmental factors.	• Older adults often have problems that affect balance and mobility (e.g., severe arthritis). • Cognitive problems (e.g., dementia).	• Modifications of environment or care plan that facilitates regular, easy access to toilet and promotes patient safety • Includes better lighting, removal of scatter rugs, ambulatory assistance equipment, clothing alterations, timed voiding, different toileting equipment

*Patients can have a combination of stress and urge incontinence, referred to as mixed incontinence.

TABLE 45-17   Interventions for Urinary Incontinence

Intervention	Description
Lifestyle Modifications	Self-management strategies to reduce or eliminate risk factors, including the following: • Smoking cessation • Weight reduction • Good bowel regimen • Reduction of bladder irritants (e.g., caffeine, aspartame artificial sweetener, citrus juices) • Fluid modifications for those with urge incontinence
Scheduled Voiding Regimens	
Timed voiding	Toileting on a fixed schedule (typically every 2-3 hr during waking hours).
Habit retraining	Scheduled toileting with adjustments of voiding intervals (longer or shorter) based on the individual's voiding pattern.
Prompted voiding	Scheduled toileting that requires prompts to void from a caregiver (typically every 3 hr). Used in conjunction with operant conditioning techniques to reward individuals for maintaining continence and appropriate toileting.
Bladder retraining and urge-suppression strategies	Scheduled toileting with progressive voiding intervals. Includes teaching of urge-control strategies using relaxation and distraction techniques, self-monitoring, reinforcement techniques, and other strategies such as conscious contraction of pelvic floor muscles.
Pelvic Floor Muscle Rehabilitation	
Pelvic floor muscle (Kegel) exercises or training	Table 45-18.
Vaginal weight training	Active retention of vaginal weights (devices designed and shaped to exercise and strengthen pelvic floor muscles) at least twice a day. Typically used in combination with pelvic floor muscle exercises.

Intervention	Description
Biofeedback	See Complementary & Alternative Therapies box on p. 1057.
Electrical stimulation	Application of low-voltage electric current to sacral and pudendal afferent fibers through vaginal, anal, or surface electrodes. Used to inhibit bladder overactivity and improve awareness, contractility, and efficiency of pelvic muscle contraction.
Anti-Incontinence Devices	
Intravaginal support devices (pessaries and bladder neck support prostheses)	Devices support bladder neck, relieve minor pelvic organ prolapse, and change pressure transmission to the urethra.
Intraurethral occlusive device (urethral plug)	Single-use device that is worn in the urethra to provide mechanical obstruction to prevent urine leakage. Removed for voiding.
Intraurethral valve pump	Replaceable urinary prosthesis for use in women who have impaired detrusor contractility (cannot contract muscles necessary to push urine out of the bladder). Draws urine out to empty bladder and blocks urine flow when continence is desired.
Incontinence clamps (penile compression devices)	Mechanical fixed compression applied to the penis to prevent any flow or leakage via the urethra. Must be released to void.
Containment Devices	
External collection devices	External catheter (condom) systems (e.g., penile sheaths) direct urine into a drainage bag. Most commonly used by men.
Absorbent products	Variety of reusable and disposable pads and undergarment systems.

COMPLEMENTARY & ALTERNATIVE THERAPIES

Biofeedback

Scientific Evidence

Biofeedback has been shown to be helpful in treating a variety of medical conditions: urinary incontinence, asthma, Raynaud's disease, irritable bowel syndrome, hot flashes, nausea and vomiting associated with chemotherapy, headaches, hypertension, and seizure disorders.

Nursing Implications

• Feedback from monitoring equipment can teach patients to control certain involuntary body responses, such as urinary incontinence.
• Although biofeedback is considered safe, patients should consult a qualified professional before using biofeedback.

and relax the pelvic muscles (see the Complementary & Alternative Therapies box on this page).

Drug Therapy. Drug therapy varies according to the UI type (Table 45-19). In stress UI, drugs have a limited role in the management. α-Adrenergic agonists can be used to increase bladder sphincter tone and urethral resistance, but they have limited benefit. In urge and reflex UI, drugs play a key management role.

Anticholinergic drugs (muscarinic receptor blockers) block the action of acetylcholine at muscarinic receptors. They relax the bladder muscle and inhibit overactive detrusor contractions (Table 45-19). Side effects of these drugs include dry mouth and eyes, constipation, blurred vision, and sleepiness.

Botox (onabotulinumtoxin A) can be used in the treatment of UI as a result of detrusor overactivity. Botox is injected into the bladder, resulting in relaxation of the bladder, an increase in its storage capacity, and a decrease in UI.

 DRUG ALERT   Tolterodine (Detrol)
• Overdosage can result in severe anticholinergic effects.
• These effects include GI cramping, diaphoresis, blurred vision, and urinary urgency.

Surgical Therapy. Surgical techniques also vary depending on the type of UI. Surgical correction of stress UI is aimed at making the urinary structures more receptive to intraabdominal pressure and augmenting the urethral resistance of the internal sphincter. It may involve repositioning the urethra and/or creating a backboard of support to stabilize the urethra and bladder neck and make them more receptive to changes in intraabdominal pressure. Another technique for stress UI

TABLE 45-18   Patient Teaching

Pelvic Floor Muscle (Kegel) Exercises

Include the following instructions when teaching the patient to perform Kegel exercises.

What Is the Pelvic Floor Muscle?

- Your pelvic floor muscle provides support for your bladder and rectum and, in women, the vagina and uterus.
- If it weakens or is damaged, it cannot support these organs and their position can change.
- This causes problems with the normal bladder and rectal function.
- If you have a weak pelvic floor muscle, you may want to do special exercises to make the muscle stronger, prevent unwanted urine leakage, and lessen urinary urgency.

Finding the Pelvic Floor Muscle

- Without tensing the muscles of your leg, buttocks, or abdomen, imagine that you are trying to control the passing of gas or pinching off a stool.
- Or imagine you are in an elevator full of people and you feel the urge to pass gas. What do you do?
- You tighten or pull in the ring of muscle around your rectum—your pelvic floor muscle.
- You should feel a lifting sensation in the area around the vagina or a pulling in of your rectum.

How to Do the Exercises

There are two different kinds of exercises—short squeezes and long squeezes.

1. To do the *short squeezes,* tighten your pelvic floor muscle quickly, squeeze hard for 2 sec, and then relax the muscle. Also, when you have strong urinary urges, try to tighten your pelvic floor muscle quickly and hard several times in a row until the urge passes.
2. To do the *long squeezes,* tighten the muscle for 5-10 sec before you relax.

Do both of these exercises 40-50 times each day.

When to Do These Exercises

- You can do these exercises anytime and anywhere.
- You can do these exercises in any position, but sitting or lying down may be the easiest.

How Long Does It Take Before I Notice a Change?

After 4-6 wk of doing these exercises, you should start to see less urine leakage and urinary urgency.

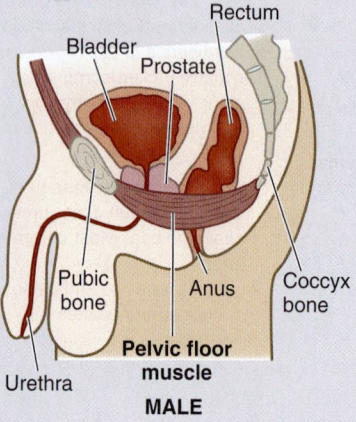

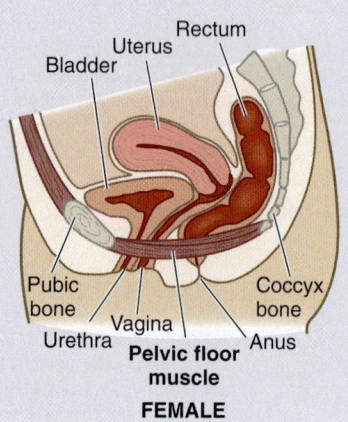

Courtesy Diane Newman.

augments the urethral resistance of the intrinsic sphincter with a sling or periurethral injectable.

Retropubic colposuspension and pubovaginal sling placement appear to be most effective. Typically, both procedures are performed through low transverse incisions. Complications specific to the retropubic suspensions include postoperative voiding dysfunction, urgency, and vaginal prolapse.

Placement of a suburethral sling, using the person's own fascia, cadaveric fascia, or a synthetic material, is also used to correct stress UI in women. Complications include vascular and bowel injury, urinary retention, mesh or sling erosion, infection, urgency, and bladder perforation. Suburethral slings have success rates comparable to those of colposuspensions or slings and are associated with shorter recovery periods. An artificial urethral sphincter can be used in men with intrinsic sphincter deficiency and severe stress UI.

Alternatively, one of several bulking agents can be injected underneath the mucosa of the urethra to correct stress UI in women or men. Bulking agents include glutaraldehyde cross-linked bovine collagen (GAX collagen), small silicone beads (Durasphere), or polytetrafluoroethylene (Teflon). Because of the risk of migration of Teflon particles, GAX collagen or Durasphere injections are most commonly used today. Although treatment with suburethral compounds avoids the risk associated with open surgery, reinjection is typically required after several years.

In artificial sphincter surgery, the bladder sphincter that no longer works is replaced with an artificial one. A silicone inflatable ring is placed around the urethra (internally), and the patient inflates it to stop the flow and deflates it when the need to empty occurs. The patient must be able to work the pump that is placed internally. This procedure is usually used only as a last resort and in a patient who is cognitively aware and able to participate in the use of the artificial sphincter.

❖ NURSING MANAGEMENT: URINARY INCONTINENCE

It is important to recognize both the physical and emotional problems associated with UI. Maintain and enhance the patient's dignity, privacy, and feelings of self-worth. This is a two-step approach: (1) containment devices to manage existing urinary leakage and (2) a definitive plan to reduce or resolve the factors leading to UI.

Management options are reviewed in Tables 45-17 and 45-18. They include lifestyle interventions such as teaching the patient about consumption of an adequate volume of fluids

TABLE 45-19 Drug Therapy

Voiding Dysfunction*

Class and Mechanism of Action	Drug
Anticholinergics (Muscarinic Receptor Blockers)	
Reduce overactive bladder contractions in urge urinary incontinence	oxybutynin (Ditropan XL, Oxytrol Transdermal System)
Relax bladder muscle during filling and improves the storage capacity of bladder	tolterodine (Detrol, Detrol LA)
	trospium chloride
	solifenacin (VESIcare)
	darifenacin (Enablex)
	flavoxate
α-Adrenergic Blockers	
Reduce urethral sphincter resistance to urinary outflow	doxazosin (Cardura)
	terazosin
	tamsulosin (Flomax)
	alfuzosin (Uroxatral)
5α-Reductase Inhibitors	
Suppress androgen resulting in epithelial atrophy and decrease in prostate size	finasteride (Proscar)
	dutasteride (Avodart)
α-Adrenergic Agonists	
Increase urethral resistance	phenylpropanolamine
	pseudoephedrine
β₃-Adrenergic Agonist	
Improves bladder's storage capacity by relaxing bladder muscle during filling	mirabegron (Myrbetriq)
Tricyclic Antidepressants	
Reduce sensory urgency and burning pain of interstitial cystitis	imipramine (Tofranil)
	amitriptyline
Reduce overactive bladder contractions	
Calcium Channel Blockers	
Reduce smooth muscle contraction strength	nifedipine
	diltiazem (Cardizem)
May reduce burning pain of interstitial cystitis	verapamil (Calan)
Hormone Therapy	
Local application reduces urethral irritation and increases host defenses against UTI	estrogen cream (Premarin, Estrace)
	estrogen vaginal ring (Estring)
	estrogen vaginal tablets (Vagifem)

*The type of drug therapy depends on the type of incontinence.

CHECK YOUR PRACTICE

You are doing BP and glucose screening at the community senior center. While you are checking the BP on a 78-year-old woman, she starts to sob quietly. You tell her that her BP is 134/84 and gently place your hand on her arm. You ask her what is wrong. She tells you, "I have to pee all the time. I soak the bed and my husband won't sleep with me anymore. I am washing sheets and my clothes all the time. Our whole house smells like urine."
• How would you respond to her?

and reduction or elimination of bladder irritants (particularly caffeine and alcohol) from the diet. Advise the patient to maintain a regular, flexible schedule of urination (usually every 2 to 3 hours while awake). Advise patients to quit smoking because this habit increases the risk of stress UI. Counsel patients about the relationship among constipation, UI, and urinary retention.

Aggressive management of constipation is recommended, beginning with ensuring adequate fluid intake, increasing dietary fiber, lightly exercising, and judiciously using stool softeners. (The management of constipation is discussed in Chapter 42.)

Behavioral treatments include scheduled voiding regimens (timed voiding, habit training, and prompted voiding), bladder retraining, and pelvic floor muscle training. Assess strategies that the patient uses to contain UI and offer alternative devices when indicated. When attempting to manage UI, many women use feminine hygiene pads, and many men and women use household products such as rags, paper towels, or folded toilet tissue. Unfortunately, none of these products is adequately designed to wick urine away from the skin, prevent soiling of clothing, and reduce or eliminate odor.

Instead, provide information on products specifically designed to contain urine. For example, patients with mild to moderate UI often benefit from incontinent pads containing superabsorbent material, designed to absorb many times its weight in water. Patients with higher-volume urine loss or those with both urinary and fecal incontinence may benefit from disposable or reusable incontinence protective underwear, briefs, or pad/pant systems.

In inpatient or long-term care facilities, nursing management of UI includes maximizing toilet access. This assistance may take the form of offering the urinal or bedpan or assisting the patient to the bathroom every 2 to 3 hours or at scheduled times. Ensure that toilets are accessible to patients and provide privacy to allow effective urine elimination.

TEAMWORK & COLLABORATION

Caring for the Incontinent Patient

All members of the interprofessional care team are responsible for decreasing the risk for incontinence and preventing complications such as skin breakdown in patients who are experiencing incontinence.

Role of Nursing Personnel
Registered Nurse (RN)
• Assess for risk factors for incontinence or urinary retention.
• Determine type of incontinence that patient is experiencing.
• Develop plan of care to decrease incontinence.
• Teach patient ways to decrease incontinence such as pelvic floor muscle (Kegel) exercises.
• Assist patient in choosing appropriate products to contain urine.

Licensed Practical/Vocational Nurse (LPN/LVN)
• Use bladder scanner to estimate the postvoid residual volume (PVR).
• Catheterize patient and measure PVR.
• Administer medications to decrease incontinence or urinary retention.

Unlicensed Assistive Personnel (UAP)
• Assist incontinent patient to commode or bedpan at regular intervals.
• Clean patient and provide skin care.
• Notify RN about new-onset incontinence in a previously continent patient.

URINARY RETENTION

Urinary retention is the inability to empty the bladder when a person voids (micturition) or the accumulation of urine in the bladder because of an inability to urinate. In certain cases, it is associated with urinary leakage or postvoid dribbling, called *overflow UI*. *Acute urinary retention* is the total inability to pass urine via micturition. It is a medical emergency. *Chronic urinary retention* is an incomplete bladder emptying despite urination. The postvoid residual (PVR) volumes in patients with chronic urinary retention vary widely. Normal PVR is between 50 and 75 mL. Findings over 100 mL indicate the need to repeat the measurement. An abnormal PVR in the older patient of more than 200 mL obtained on two separate occasions requires further evaluation. Even smaller volumes may justify further evaluation when the patient has recurring UTIs or lower urinary tract symptoms suggestive of UTI.

Etiology and Pathophysiology

Urinary retention is caused by two different dysfunctions of the urinary system: bladder outlet obstruction and deficient detrusor (bladder muscle) contraction strength. *Bladder outlet obstruction* leads to urinary retention when the blockage is so severe that the bladder can no longer evacuate its contents despite a detrusor contraction. A common cause of obstruction in men is an enlarged prostate.

Deficient detrusor contraction strength leads to urinary retention when the muscle is no longer able to contract with enough force or for a sufficient time to completely empty the bladder. Common causes of deficient detrusor contraction strength are neurologic diseases affecting sacral segments 2, 3, and 4; long-standing diabetes mellitus; overdistention; chronic alcoholism; and drugs (e.g., anticholinergic drugs).

Diagnostic Studies

The diagnostic studies for urinary retention are the same as the ones for UI (see p. 1055).

Interprofessional Care

Behavioral therapies that were described for UI may also be used in the management of urinary retention. Scheduled toileting and double voiding may be effective in chronic urinary retention with moderate PVR volumes. *Double voiding* is an attempt to maximize bladder evacuation. The patient is asked to urinate, sit on the toilet for 3 to 4 minutes, and urinate again before exiting the bathroom.

For acute or chronic urinary retention, catheterization may be required. Intermittent catheterization allows the patient to remain free of an indwelling catheter with its associated risk of UTI and urethral irritation. In some situations, an indwelling catheter is preferred (e.g., if the patient is unwilling or unable to perform intermittent catheterization). An indwelling catheter is also used when urethral obstruction makes intermittent catheterization uncomfortable or infeasible.

Drug Therapy. Several drugs may be administered to promote bladder evacuation. For the patient with obstruction at the level of the bladder neck, an α-adrenergic blocker may be prescribed. These drugs relax the smooth muscle of the bladder neck, the prostatic urethra, and possibly the rhabdosphincter, diminishing urethral resistance. Examples of α-adrenergic blockers are listed in Table 45-19. They are indicated in patients with BPH, bladder neck dyssynergia (muscle incoordination), or detrusor sphincter dyssynergia.

Surgical Therapy. Surgical interventions are used to manage urinary retention caused by obstruction. Transurethral or open surgical techniques are used to treat benign or malignant prostatic enlargement, bladder neck contracture, urethral strictures, or dyssynergia of the bladder neck. Pelvic reconstruction using an abdominal or transvaginal approach can correct bladder outlet obstruction in women with severe pelvic organ prolapse.

Unfortunately, surgery has a minimal role in the management of urinary retention caused by deficient detrusor contraction strength. Attempts to create a bladder stimulator (implanted device capable of stimulating micturition) have proved largely unsuccessful because of the difficulty in achieving a coordinated detrusor contraction associated with pelvic muscle and striated sphincter relaxation.

❖ **NURSING MANAGEMENT: URINARY RETENTION**

Acute urinary retention is a medical emergency that requires prompt recognition and bladder drainage. Insert a catheter (as ordered) unless otherwise directed. Use a catheter with a retention balloon in anticipation of the need for an indwelling catheter.

Teach the patient with acute urinary retention (and the patient predisposed to these episodes) strategies to minimize risk, including avoiding intake of large volumes of fluid over a brief period. Instead, advise the patient to drink small amounts throughout the day. In addition, instruct the patient (if chilled) to warm up before attempting to urinate and to avoid excessive alcohol intake because it leads to polyuria and a diminished awareness of the need to urinate until the bladder is distended.

Advise the patient who is unable to urinate to drink a cup of coffee or brewed caffeinated tea to create or maximize urinary urgency. Tell patients that sitting in a tub of warm water or taking a warm shower may also help them urinate. If these measures do not lead to successful urination, advise the patient to seek immediate care.

Patients with chronic urinary retention may be managed by behavioral methods, indwelling or intermittent catheterization, surgery, or drugs. Scheduled toileting and double voiding are the primary behavioral interventions used for chronic retention. Scheduled toileting is used to reduce rather than expand bladder capacity. In this case, ask the patient to void every 3 to 4 hours regardless of the desire to urinate. This intervention is particularly useful in the patient with chronic overdistention, diabetes mellitus, or chronic alcoholism characterized by a large bladder capacity and diminished or delayed sensations of bladder filling and urgency.

CATHETERIZATION

INDICATIONS FOR AND COMPLICATIONS OF CATHETERIZATION

Indications for short-term urinary catheterization are listed in Table 45-20. Unacceptable reasons for catheterization include (1) routine acquisition of a urine specimen for laboratory analysis and (2) convenience of the nursing staff or the patient's family. The risk of CAUTI is too high to allow catheterization of a patient for the convenience of hospital personnel or family members.

Complications that are seen more frequently with long-term use (more than 30 days) of indwelling catheters include CAUTI, bladder spasms, periurethral abscess, chronic pyelonephritis, urosepsis, urethral trauma or erosion, fistula or stricture formation, and calculi. Catheterization for sterile urine specimens may occasionally be necessary when patients have a history of

TABLE 45-20 Indications for Urinary Catheterization

Indwelling Catheter

* Relief of urinary retention caused by lower urinary tract obstruction, paralysis, or inability to void
* Bladder decompression preoperatively and operatively for lower abdominal or pelvic surgery
* Facilitation of surgical repair of urethra and surrounding structures
* Splinting of ureters or urethra to facilitate healing after surgery or other trauma in area
* Accurate measurement of urine output in critically ill patient
* Contamination of stage III or IV pressure ulcers with urine that has impeded healing, despite appropriate personal care for the incontinence
* Terminal illness or severe impairment, which makes positioning or clothing changes uncomfortable, or which is associated with intractable pain

Intermittent (Straight, in and Out) Catheter

* Relief of urinary retention caused by lower urinary tract obstruction, paralysis, or inability to void
* Study of anatomic structures of urinary system
* Urodynamic testing
* Collection of sterile urine sample in selected situations
* Instillation of medications into bladder
* Measurement of residual urine after urination (postvoid residual [PVR]) if portable ultrasound not available

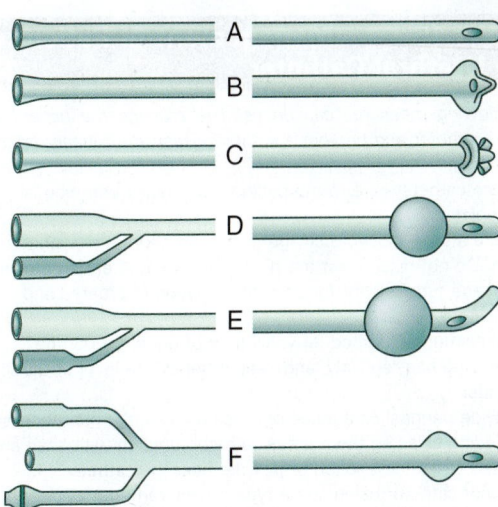

FIG. 45-10 Types of urinary catheters. **A,** Simple urethral catheter. **B,** Mushroom-tip de Pezzer catheter (can be for suprapubic catheterization). **C,** Wing-tip Malecot catheter (wings hold catheter in place for temporary drainage). **D,** Indwelling urethral catheter with inflated balloon. **E,** Indwelling Tiemann catheter with coudé-tip (slightly curved tip allows for passage past obstruction). **F,** Three-way indwelling catheter (third lumen can be used for irrigation).

large a catheter is tissue erosion secondary to excessive pressure on the meatus or urethra.

TYPES OF CATHETERS

Four routes are used for urinary tract catheterization: urethral, ureteral, suprapubic, and via a nephrostomy tube.

Urethral Catheterization

Urethral catheterization, the most common route of catheterization, involves the insertion of a catheter through the external meatus into the urethra, past the internal sphincter, and into the bladder. Table 45-21 summarizes important principles in the management of the patient with an indwelling urethral catheter.

complicated UTI. A catheter should be the final resort to provide the patient with a dry environment to prevent skin breakdown and protect dressings or skin lesions.

Urinary catheterization is commonly used in the management of the hospitalized patient. However, it is not without serious complications. As previously discussed on p. 1034, CAUTIs are the most common HAI. Scrupulous aseptic technique is mandatory when a urinary catheter is inserted. After insertion, maintenance and protection of the closed drainage system are major nursing responsibilities. Do not routinely irrigate the catheter; this should be done only if ordered.

While the patient has a catheter in place, maintain patency of the catheter, manage fluid intake, provide for the patient's comfort and safety, and prevent infection. Address the psychologic implications of urinary drainage. Patient concerns can include embarrassment related to exposure of the body, an altered body image, and fear that care of the catheter will result in increased dependency.

CATHETER CONSTRUCTION

Catheter materials include Teflon-coated latex, silicone elastomer, and hydrogel-coated silicone. Catheters coated with silver or antimicrobial agents may prevent UTIs.

Catheters vary in construction materials, tip shape (Fig. 45-10), and size of the lumen. A coudé-tip catheter is commonly used in men. Catheters are sized according to the French scale. Each French unit (F) equals 0.33 mm of diameter. The diameter listed is the internal diameter of the catheter. The size used varies with the patient's size and the purpose of catheterization. In women, urethral catheter sizes 14F to 16F are the most common. In men, sizes 14F to 18F are used. Balloon sizes are either 5 or 30 mL. The primary problem resulting from too

TEAMWORK & COLLABORATION
Urinary Catheters

Role of Nursing Personnel
Registered Nurse (RN)

* Determine need for catheterization, but HCP must order.
* Choose appropriate type and size of catheter.
* Insert catheter in patient with urethral trauma, pain, or obstruction.
* Develop plan of care to decrease risk for infection in patient with indwelling catheter.

Licensed Practical/Vocational Nurse (LPN/LVN)

* Insert intermittent or indwelling catheter for uncomplicated patients.
* Irrigate the catheter if obstruction is suspected in stable patients (e.g., in long-term care).

Unlicensed Assistive Personnel (UAP)

* Provide perineal care around the catheter with soap and water.
* Anchor the catheter in place (upper thigh in women and lower abdomen in men).
* Notify RN about changes in skin condition, especially around meatus.

TABLE 45-21   Management of Patient With Urethral Catheter

The following measures can be used to manage the patient with a urethral catheter and prevent a catheter-associated urinary tract infection (CAUTI).

1. Teach catheter care to the patient, particularly one who is ambulatory.
2. Use a sterile, closed drainage system in short-term catheterization. Do not disconnect the distal urinary catheter and proximal drainage tube except for catheter irrigation (if ordered and indicated).
3. Maintain unobstructed downhill flow of urine. Empty the collecting bag regularly, and keep it below the level of the bladder.
4. Provide perineal care (once or twice a day and when necessary), including cleaning the meatus-catheter junction with soap and water. Do not use lotion or powder near the catheter.
5. Anchor catheter using some type of securement device. Anchor catheter to upper thigh in women and lower abdomen in men to prevent catheter movement and urethral tension.
6. Use sterile technique whenever the collecting system is open. If frequent irrigations are necessary in short-term catheterization to maintain catheter patency, a triple-lumen catheter may be preferable, permitting continuous irrigations within a closed system.
7. If ordered, aspirate small volumes of urine for culture from the catheter sampling port by means of a sterile syringe and needle. First prepare the puncture site with an antiseptic solution.
8. When the patient is catheterized for less than 2 wk, routine catheter change is not necessary. For long-term use of an indwelling catheter, replace the catheter based on patient assessment and not on a routine changing schedule.
9. With long-term use of a catheter, a leg bag may be used. If the collection bag is reused, wash it in soap and water and rinse thoroughly. When it is not reused immediately, fill it with ½ cup of vinegar and drain. The vinegar is effective against *Pseudomonas* and other organisms and eliminates odors.
10. Remove the catheter as early as possible. Intermittent catheterization and external catheters are alternatives that may be associated with fewer cases of bacteriuria and UTI than chronic indwelling urethral catheters.

Ureteral Catheters

The *ureteral catheter* is placed through the ureters into the renal pelvis. The catheter is inserted either (1) by being threaded up the urethra and bladder to the ureters under cystoscopic observation or (2) by surgical insertion through the abdominal wall into the ureters. The ureteral catheter is used after surgery to splint the ureters and to prevent them from being obstructed by edema. Record the urine volume from the ureteral catheter separately from that of other urinary catheters.

The patient is often kept on bed rest while a ureteral catheter is in place until specific orders indicate that ambulation is permitted. The self-retaining ureteral catheter is often inserted after a lithotripsy procedure or when ureteral obstruction from adjacent tumors or fibrosis threatens renal function. The double-J ureteral catheter is frequently used and allows the patient to ambulate. One end coils up in the kidney pelvis, while the other coils in the bladder.

Check the placement of the ureteral catheter frequently and avoid tension on the catheter. The catheter drains urine from the renal pelvis, which has a capacity of 3 to 5 mL. If the volume of urine in the renal pelvis increases, tissue damage to the pelvis will result from pressure. Do not clamp the ureteral catheter. If the HCP orders irrigation of the ureteral catheter, use strict aseptic technique. If the output is decreased, notify the HCP immediately. Check the drainage often (at least every 1 or 2 hours). It is normal for some urine to drain around the ureteral catheter into the bladder. Accurately record the urine output from the ureteral and urethral catheters. Sometimes a ureteral catheter may be used as a stent and is not expected to drain. It is important to check with the HCP as to the type of catheter and what to expect.

Suprapubic Catheters

Suprapubic catheterization is the simplest and oldest method of urinary diversion. The two methods of insertion of a suprapubic catheter into the bladder are (1) through a small incision in the abdominal wall and (2) by the use of a trocar. A suprapubic catheter is placed while the patient is under general anesthesia for another surgical procedure or at the bedside with a local anesthetic. The catheter may be sutured into place. Tape the catheter to prevent dislodgment. The care of the tube and catheter is similar to that of the urethral catheter. A pectin-base skin barrier (e.g., Stomahesive) is effective in protecting the skin around the insertion site from breakdown.

The suprapubic catheter is used in temporary situations such as bladder, prostate, and urethral surgery. The suprapubic catheter is also used on a long-term basis in selected patients.

A suprapubic catheter is prone to poor drainage because of mechanical obstruction of the catheter tip by the bladder wall, sediment, and clots. To ensure patency of the tube (1) prevent tube kinking by coiling the excess tubing and maintaining gravity drainage, (2) have the patient turn from side to side, and (3) milk the tube. If these measures are not effective, obtain an order from the HCP to irrigate the catheter using sterile technique.

If the patient experiences bladder spasms that are difficult to control, urinary leakage may result. Oxybutynin or other oral antispasmodics or belladonna and opium (B&O) suppositories may be prescribed to decrease bladder spasms.

Nephrostomy Tubes

The *nephrostomy tube* (catheter) is inserted on a temporary basis to preserve renal function when a ureter is completely obstructed. The tube is inserted through a small flank incision directly into the pelvis of the kidney and attached to connecting tubing for closed drainage. The principle is the same as with the ureteral catheter—that is, the catheter should never be kinked, compressed, or clamped. If the patient complains of excessive pain in the area or if there is excessive drainage around the tube, check the catheter for patency. If irrigation is ordered, use strict aseptic technique. Gently instill no more than 5 mL of sterile saline solution at one time to prevent overdistention of the kidney pelvis and renal damage. Infection and secondary stone formation are complications associated with the insertion of a nephrostomy tube.

Intermittent Catheterization

An alternative approach to a long-term indwelling catheter is *intermittent catheterization,* often referred to as "straight" catheterization or "in-and-out" catheterization. The main goal of intermittent catheterization is to prevent urinary retention, stasis, and compromised blood supply to the bladder caused by prolonged pressure.[24]

It is being used with increasing frequency in conditions such as neurogenic bladder (e.g., spinal cord injuries, chronic neurologic diseases) or bladder outlet obstruction in men. This type of catheterization is used in the oliguric and anuric phases of acute kidney injury to reduce the possibility of infection from an indwelling catheter. Intermittent catheterization is also used postoperatively after a surgical procedure to treat UI.

The technique consists of inserting a urethral catheter into the bladder every 3 to 5 hours. Some patients perform intermittent catheterization only once or twice a day to measure residual urine and to ensure an empty bladder.

The techniques and protocols for intermittent catheterization vary. Catheters can be sterile (single use) or clean (multiple use). Catheters can be coated (prelubricated) or uncoated. Available data on intermittent catheterization do not provide convincing evidence that any specific technique (sterile or clean), catheter type (coated or uncoated), method (single-use or multiple-use), person (self or other), or strategy is better than any other for all clinical settings.[24]

The design of single-use, self-lubricating, silicone-coated (closed-sterile) systems is useful for patients who have recurrent UTIs or need to catheterize while at work or during travel. Instruct patients to wash and rinse the catheter and their hands with soap and water before and after catheterization. Lubricant is necessary for men and may make catheterization more comfortable for women. The catheter may be inserted by the patient, caregiver, or HCP.

Sterile technique is used for catheterization in the hospital or long-term care facility. For home care, a clean technique that includes good hand washing with soap and water is used. Teach the patient to observe for signs of UTI so that treatment can be started early. If indicated, some patients are placed on a regimen of prophylactic antibiotics. Urethral damage from intermittent catheterization in men is similar to problems seen with indwelling catheterization. Complications include urethritis, urethral sphincter damage (especially if there is a forceful catheterization against a closed sphincter), urethral stricture, and creation of a false passage.

SURGERY OF THE URINARY TRACT

RENAL AND URETERAL SURGERY

The most common indications for nephrectomy are a renal tumor, polycystic kidneys that are bleeding or severely infected, massive traumatic injury to the kidney, and the elective removal of a kidney from a donor to be transplanted. Surgery involving the ureters and kidneys is most commonly performed to remove calculi that become obstructive, correct congenital anomalies, and divert urine when necessary.

Surgical Procedure

Nephrectomy can be performed by a conventional (open) approach or laparoscopically. In the open approach, an incision of about 6 to 10 in is made through several layers of muscle. The incision can be made in the flank or abdominal area.

Laparoscopic Nephrectomy. *Laparoscopic nephrectomy* can be performed in selected situations to remove a diseased kidney. Laparoscopic nephrectomy can also be used to obtain a kidney from a living donor to be transplanted into a person with end-stage renal disease (ESRD). A laparoscopic nephrectomy is performed using five puncture sites. One incision is to view the kidney, and another is to dissect it. The laparoscope contains a miniature camera so that the surgeons can watch what they are doing on a video monitor. Once dissected, the kidney is maneuvered into a nylon impermeable sack and then safely removed from the patient. Compared with conventional nephrectomy, the laparoscopic approach is less painful, involves a shorter hospital stay, and has a much faster recovery.

Preoperative Management

The basic needs of the patient undergoing renal and ureteral surgery are similar to those of any patient who experiences surgery (see Chapters 17 through 19). In addition, it is important preoperatively to ensure adequate fluid intake and a normal electrolyte balance. Tell the patient that, if there is a flank incision, surgery will require a hyperextended, side-lying position. This position frequently causes the patient to experience muscle aches after surgery. If a nephrectomy is planned, it is important that the patient have one working kidney to maintain normal renal function.

Postoperative Management

Specific postoperative needs of a patient are related to urine output, respiratory status, and abdominal distention.

Urine Output. In the immediate postoperative period, measure and record the urine output at least every 1 or 2 hours. Measure drainage from the various catheters and record it separately. Do not clamp or irrigate the catheter or tube without a specific order. The total urine output should be at least 0.5 mL/kg/hr. It is important to assess for urine drainage on the dressing and to estimate this amount. Observe and monitor the color and consistency of urine. Urine with increased amounts of mucus, blood, or sediment may occlude the drainage tubing or catheter.

Weigh the patient daily using the same scale, and have the patient wear similar clothing and dressings each time. A significant change in daily weight can indicate retention of fluids, which places the patient at cardiovascular risk for developing heart failure. Retention of fluids can increase the work required of the remaining kidney to perform its functions.

Respiratory Status. A nephrectomy can be performed through a flank incision just below the diaphragm. Postoperatively, it is important to ensure adequate ventilation. The patient is often reluctant to turn, cough, and deep breathe because of the incisional pain. Give adequate pain medication to ensure the patient's comfort and ability to perform coughing and deep-breathing exercises. Frequently, additional respiratory devices such as an incentive spirometer are used every 2 hours while the patient is awake. In addition, early and frequent ambulation helps to maintain adequate respiratory function.

Abdominal Distention. Abdominal distention is present to some degree in most patients who have had surgery on their kidneys or ureters. It is most commonly due to paralytic ileus caused by manipulation and compression of the bowel during surgery. Oral intake is restricted until bowel sounds are present (usually 24 to 48 hours after surgery). IV fluids are given until the patient can take oral fluids. Progression to a regular diet follows.

URINARY DIVERSION

Urinary diversion may be performed with or without cystectomy. Urinary diversion procedures are performed to treat cancer of the bladder, neurogenic bladder, congenital anomalies, strictures, trauma to the bladder, and chronic infections

TABLE 45-22   Urinary Diversion Surgery

Description	Advantages	Disadvantages	Special Considerations
Ileal Conduit Ureters are implanted into part of ileum or colon that has been resected from intestinal tract. Abdominal stoma is created.	Relatively good urine flow with few physiologic alterations.	External appliance necessary to continually collect urine.	Surgical procedure is complex. Postoperative complications may be increased. Reabsorption of urea by ileum occurs. Meticulous attention is necessary to care for stoma and collecting device.
Cutaneous Ureterostomy Ureters are excised from bladder and brought through abdominal wall, and stoma is created. Ureteral stomas may be created from both ureters, or ureters may be brought together and one stoma created.	No need for major surgery as required with ileal conduit.	External appliance necessary because of continuous urine drainage. Possibility of stricture or stenosis of small stoma.	Periodic catheterizations may be required to dilate stomas to maintain patency.
Nephrostomy Catheter is inserted into pelvis of kidney. Procedure may be done to one or both kidneys and may be temporary or permanent. It is most frequently done in advanced disease as palliative procedure.	No need for major surgery.	High risk of renal infection. Predisposition to calculus formation from catheter.	Nephrostomy tube may have to be changed every month. Never clamp the catheter.

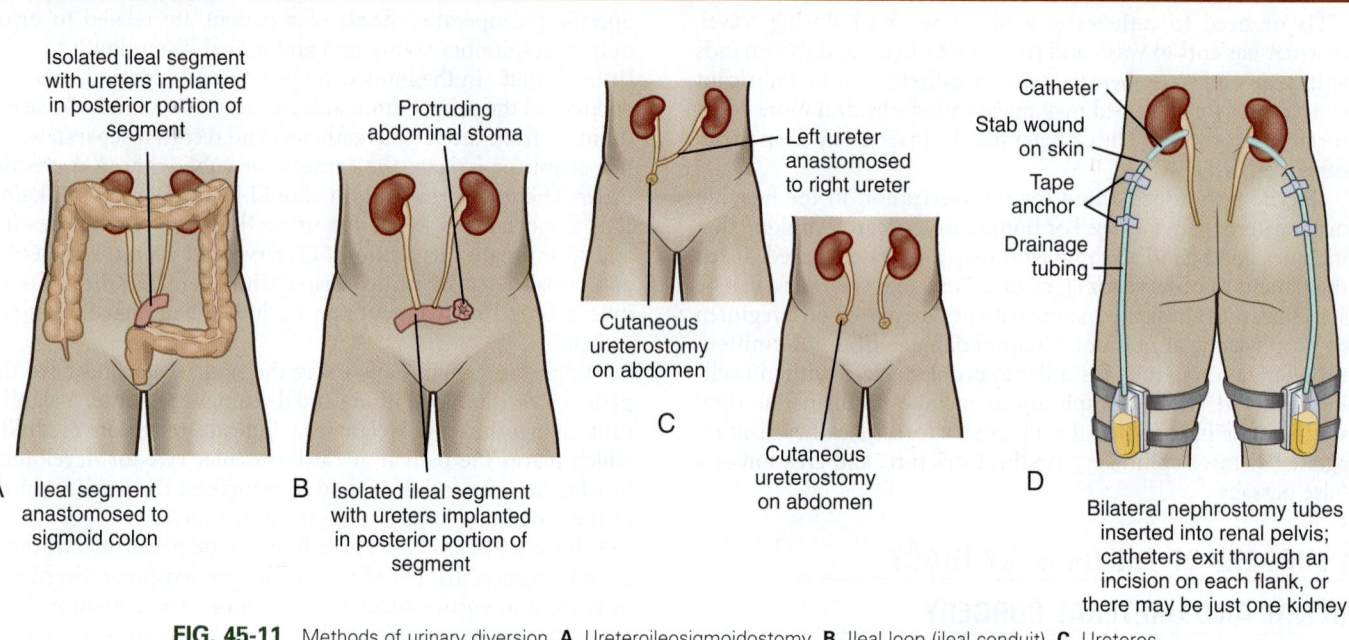

FIG. 45-11   Methods of urinary diversion. **A,** Ureteroileosigmoidostomy. **B,** Ileal loop (ileal conduit). **C,** Ureterostomy (transcutaneous ureterostomy and bilateral cutaneous ureterostomies). **D,** Nephrostomy.

with deterioration of renal function. Numerous urinary diversion techniques and bladder substitutes are possible, including an incontinent urinary diversion, a continent urinary diversion catheterized by the patient, or an orthotopic bladder so that the patient voids urethrally.[25] Types of surgical procedures for urinary diversion are presented in Table 45-22 and Fig. 45-11.

Incontinent Urinary Diversion

Incontinent urinary diversion is diversion to the skin, requiring an appliance. The simplest form is the cutaneous ureterostomy, but scarring and strictures of the ureter have led to the use of ileal or colonic conduits. The most commonly performed incontinent urinary diversion procedure is the **ileal conduit** (ileal loop). In this procedure a 6- to 8-in (15- to 20-cm) segment of the ileum is converted into a conduit for urinary drainage. The colon (colon conduit) can be used instead of the ileum. The ureters are anastomosed into one end of the conduit, and the other end of the bowel is brought out through the abdominal wall to form a stoma (Fig. 45-12). Although the

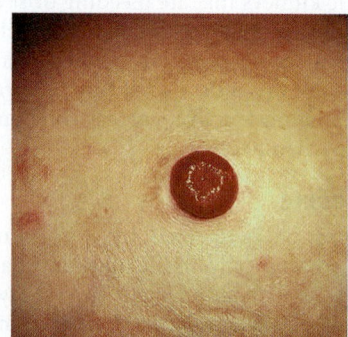

FIG. 45-12   Urinary stoma. Symmetric, no skin breakdown, protrudes about 1.5 cm. Mucosa is healthy red. This configuration is flat when the patient is upright or supine. (Courtesy Lynda Brubacher, Virginia Mason Hospital, Seattle, Wash.)

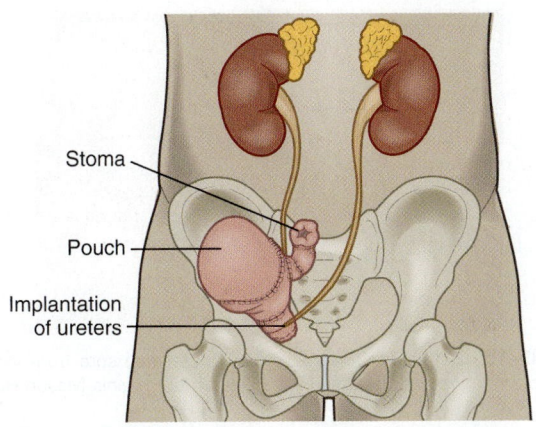

FIG. 45-13 Creation of a Kock pouch with implantation of ureters into one intussuscepted portion of the pouch and creation of a stoma with the other intussuscepted portion.

segment of bowel remains supported by the mesentery, it is completely isolated from the intestinal tract. The bowel is anastomosed and continues to function normally.

Because there is no valve and no voluntary control over the stoma, drops of urine flow from the stoma every few seconds, requiring a permanent external collecting device. The visible stoma and need for external collection devices are disadvantages of this procedure. The lifelong need to care for and deal with the stoma and collection devices may be psychologically difficult. These problems have led to the increasing use of continent diversions and orthotopic bladder substitutes.

Continent Urinary Diversions

A *continent urinary diversion* is an intraabdominal urinary reservoir that can be catheterized or that has an outlet controlled by the anal sphincter. Continent diversions are internal pouches created similarly to the ileal conduit. Reservoirs are constructed from the ileum, ileocecal segment, or colon. Large segments of bowel are altered to prevent peristaltic action. A continence mechanism is formed between this large, low-pressure reservoir and the stoma by intussuscepting a portion of bowel. In this way, a patient does not leak involuntarily. The patient with a continent reservoir needs to self-catheterize every 4 to 6 hours but does not need to wear external attachments. Patients may wear a small bandage on the stoma to collect any mucous drainage or excess drainage. Examples of continent diversions are the Kock (Fig. 45-13), Mainz, Indiana, and Florida pouches. The main difference among the various diversions is the segment of bowel used. For example, the Indiana pouch uses the right colon as a reservoir and has become a popular form of continent urinary diversion.

Orthotopic Bladder Reconstruction

Orthotopic bladder reconstruction, or orthotopic neobladder, is the construction of a new bladder in the bladder's normal anatomic position, with discharge of urine through the urethra. The reconstruction or neobladder can be derived from various segments of the intestines to create a low-pressure reservoir. An isolated segment of the distal ileum is often preferred. Various procedures include the hemi-Kock pouch, Studer pouch, and W-shaped ileoneobladder. In these procedures the bowel is surgically reshaped to become a neobladder. The ureters and urethra are sutured into the neobladder.

Orthotopic bladder reconstruction has become a more viable option for both men and women if cancer does not involve the bladder neck or urethra. Ideal candidates for this procedure have normal renal and liver function, longer than 1- to 2-year life expectancy, adequate motor skills, and no history of inflammatory bowel disease or colon cancer. Obese patients and those with inflammatory bowel disease are not good candidates for this procedure. The advantage of orthotopic bladder substitution is that it allows for natural micturition. Incontinence is a possible problem with this technique, and intermittent catheterization may be required.

❖ NURSING MANAGEMENT: URINARY DIVERSION

◆ Preoperative Management

Teaching is important for the patient awaiting cystectomy and urinary diversion surgery. Assess the patient's ability and readiness to learn before initiating a teaching program. If the patient is not ready to learn, modify the teaching plan. The patient's anxiety and fear may be decreased by providing more information. However, the anxiety and fear may also interfere with learning. Involve the patient's caregiver and family in the teaching process.

Discuss the psychosocial aspects of living with a stoma (including clothing, changes in body image and sexuality, exercise, and odor). This may allay some fears. Teach the patient with a continent diversion (e.g., Indiana pouch) to catheterize at least every 6 hours and irrigate the pouch daily. The patient with an orthotopic neobladder may have problems with incontinence. Discuss patient's' concerns about sexual activities and let them know that counseling is available. A wound, ostomy, and continence nurse (WOCN) should be involved in the preoperative phase of the patient's care. A visit from an ostomate can be helpful. Additional interventions are presented in eNursing Care Plan 45-3 for the patient with an ileal conduit (on the website for this chapter).

◆ Postoperative Management

Plan the nursing interventions during the postoperative period to prevent surgical complications such as postoperative atelectasis and shock (see Chapter 19). After pelvic surgery, there is an increased incidence of thrombophlebitis, small bowel obstruction, and UTI. With removal of part of the bowel, the incidence of paralytic ileus and small bowel obstruction is increased, the patient is kept on NPO status, and a nasogastric tube may be needed for a few days.

Prevent injury to the stoma and maintain urine output. Advise the patient that mucus in the urine is a normal occurrence. The mucus is secreted by the mucosa of the intestine (which is used to create the ileal conduit) in response to the irritating effect of urine. Encourage a high fluid intake to "flush" the ileal conduit or continent diversion.

When an ileal conduit is created, provide meticulous care for the skin around the stoma. Alkaline encrustations with dermatitis may occur when alkaline urine comes in contact with exposed skin (Fig. 45-14). The urine is kept acidic to prevent alkaline encrustations. Other common peristomal skin problems include yeast infections, product allergies, and shearing-effect excoriations. Changing appliances (pouches) is described in Table 45-23. A properly fitting appliance is essential to prevent skin problems. The appliance should be about 0.1 in (0.2 cm) larger than the stoma. It is normal for the stoma to shrink within the first few weeks after surgery.

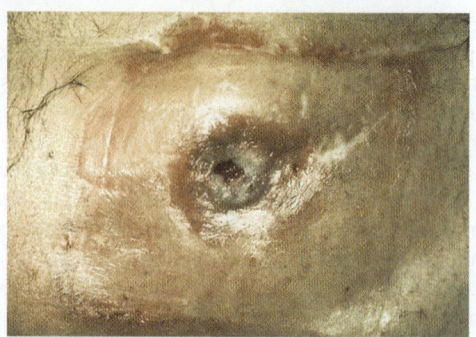

FIG. 45-14   Ammonia salt encrustation secondary to alkaline urine. (Courtesy Lynda Brubacher, Virginia Mason Hospital, Seattle, Wash.)

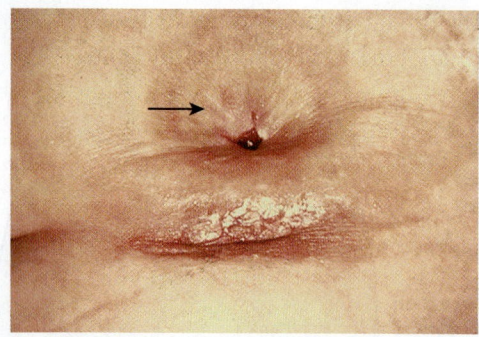

FIG. 45-15   Retracted urinary stoma with pressure sore from faceplate above stoma *(arrow)*. (Courtesy Lynda Brubacher, Virginia Mason Hospital, Seattle, Wash.)

TABLE 45-23   Patient & Caregiver Teaching
Ileal Conduit Appliances

Include the following instructions when teaching a patient or a caregiver how to change an ileal conduit appliance.

Temporary Appliance
1. Cut hole in pouch to fit over stoma (pouch 0.1 in [0.2 cm] larger than stoma).
2. Remove old pouch.
3. Clean area gently and remove old adhesive.
4. Wash area with warm water.
5. Place wick (rolled-up 4 × 4-in pad) over stoma to keep area dry during rest of procedure.
6. Dry skin around stoma.
7. Apply tincture of benzoin or other skin protectant around stoma to area where pouch will be placed.
8. Apply pouch by first smoothing its edges toward side and lower portion of body.
9. Remove wick and complete application of bag.
10. If patient is usually in bed, apply bag so that it lies toward side of body.
11. If patient is ambulatory, apply bag so that it lies vertically.
12. Connect drainage tubing to pouch.
13. Keep drainage pouch on same side of bed as stoma.

Permanent Appliance*
1. Keep appliance in place for 2-14 days.
2. Change appliance when fluid intake has been restricted for several hours.
3. Sit or stand in front of mirror.
4. Moisten edge of faceplate with adhesive solvent and gently remove.
5. Clean skin with adhesive solvent.
6. Wash skin with warm water (may be done while showering).
7. Dry skin and inspect.
8. Place wick (rolled-up 4 × 4-in pad) over stoma to keep skin free of urine.
9. Apply skin cement to faceplate and skin.
10. Place appliance over stoma.
11. Wash removed appliance with soap and lukewarm water; soak in distilled vinegar; rinse with lukewarm water and air dry.

*Many disposable appliances with self-adhesive backing are used as permanent appliances.

Patients with a neobladder may have postoperative urinary retention and require catheterization. It may take up to 6 months for them to regain bladder control. Patients empty their neobladders by relaxing their outlet sphincter muscles and bearing down with their abdominal muscles. Since there is no longer neurologic feedback between the reservoir and the brain, the patient should not expect a normal desire to void. To avoid bladder overdistention, patients should void at least every 2 to 4 hours, sit during voiding, and practice pelvic floor muscle relaxation to aid voiding. Follow-up x-ray studies include a "pouchogram" 3 to 4 weeks after surgery to assess for healing.

Acceptance of the surgery and of alterations in body image is needed to ensure the patient's best adjustment. Meeting and sharing feelings with similar patients can enhance a patient's adjustment to a urinary diversion. Patient concerns include fear that the stoma will be offensive to others and will interfere with sexual, personal, professional, and recreational activities. Advise the patient that few activities will be restricted as a result of the urinary diversion.

Discharge teaching after an ileal conduit includes instructing the patient about symptoms of obstruction or infection and care of the ostomy. The patient with an ileal conduit is fitted for a permanent appliance 7 to 10 days after surgery. It may have to be refitted at a later time, depending on the degree of stoma healing and shrinkage.

Appliances are made of a variety of products, including natural and synthetic rubbers, plastics, and metals. Most appliances have a faceplate that adheres to the skin, a collecting pouch, and an opening to drain the pouch. The faceplate may be secured to the skin with glues, adhesives, or adherent synthetic wafers. Some appliances do not require adhesives, but their design relies on pressure to keep the pouch in place. If improperly fitted or applied, the faceplate may cause skin problems (Fig. 45-15). Inform the patient and caregiver about where to purchase supplies, emergency telephone numbers, and location of ostomy clubs, and follow-up visits with a WOCN. Follow-up with an HCP is imperative to monitor the patient's recovery, detect any complications, and assess renal function.

CASE STUDY
Painful Bladder and Frequent Urination

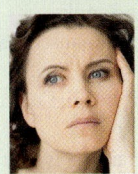

(©marilook/ iStock/ Thinkstock)

Patient Profile
L.T., a 38-yr-old white woman, is seen in the nurse practitioner's office for the eighth time in the past year for a history of pelvic pain with urinary frequency during the day, nocturia, and urgency to void. All urine cultures have been negative for bacteria. An evaluation by her gynecologist was negative for possible endometriosis.

Subjective Data
- Has a history of suprapubic and vaginal pain and urinary frequency and urgency. Bladder pain increases with bladder filling
- Reports this is her third attack of suprapubic pain and painful urination in 2 months
- Constant pain and discomfort has been physically and emotionally exhausting
- Is worried that she has cancer and no one cares
- Has had four pregnancies with uneventful vaginal deliveries
- Her menstrual cycles are normal. Her husband had a vasectomy, although they rarely have sexual intercourse because she experiences pain with intercourse
- She has a bowel movement every day. Denies constipation and/or diarrhea
- Recalls having many UTIs as a child

Objective Data
Physical Examination
- Lungs are clear. BP 132/86. Heart rate 86/min. Respiratory rate 18/min. Abdomen soft, tender in suprapubic region.

Diagnostic Studies
- Urinalysis: normal
- Urine cytology: ordered to rule out cancer
- Referral to urologist for cystoscopy

Interprofessional Care
- Cystoscopy results indicate glomerulations and Hunner's ulcers
- Diagnosis: interstitial cystitis
- Urologist prescribes pentosan (Elmiron)
- Follow-up in 4 weeks

Discussion Questions
1. After taking the patient's history, would you consider a UTI as a cause of her symptoms? Why or why not?
2. What additional testing and patient information would help to determine a definitive diagnosis?
3. What is the significance of the cystoscopy findings?
4. What is the rationale for the use of pentosan (Elmiron)?
5. *Patient-Centered Care:* How can you help L.T. deal with her diagnosis and treatment regimen?
6. *Priority Decision:* What are the priority nursing diagnoses for L.T.?
7. *Teamwork and Collaboration:* Why is it important to get a dietitian involved in the care of L.T.?
8. *Evidence-Based Practice:* L.T. asks you how she can control her interstitial cystitis. How would you respond?

Answers available at *http://evolve.elsevier.com/Lewis/medsurg.*

BRIDGE TO NCLEX EXAMINATION

The number of the question corresponds to the same-numbered outcome at the beginning of the chapter.

1. In teaching a patient with pyelonephritis about the disorder, the nurse informs the patient that the organisms that cause pyelonephritis *most* commonly reach the kidneys through
   a. the bloodstream.
   b. the lymphatic system.
   c. a descending infection.
   d. an ascending infection.
2. The nurse teaches the female patient who has frequent UTIs that she should
   a. take tub baths with bubble bath.
   b. urinate before and after sexual intercourse.
   c. take prophylactic sulfonamides for the rest of her life.
   d. restrict fluid intake to prevent the need for frequent voiding.
3. The immunologic mechanisms involved in acute poststreptococcal glomerulonephritis include
   a. tubular blocking by precipitates of bacteria and antibody reactions.
   b. deposition of immune complexes and complement along the GBM.
   c. thickening of the GBM from autoimmune microangiopathic changes.
   d. destruction of glomeruli by proteolytic enzymes contained in the GBM.

4. One of the nurse's *most* important roles in relation to acute post-streptococcal glomerulonephritis is to
   a. promote early diagnosis and treatment of sore throats and skin lesions.
   b. encourage patients to obtain antibiotic therapy for upper respiratory tract infections.
   c. teach patients with APSGN that long-term prophylactic antibiotic therapy is necessary to prevent recurrence.
   d. monitor patients for respiratory symptoms that indicate the disease is affecting the alveolar basement membrane.
5. The edema that occurs in nephrotic syndrome is due to
   a. increased hydrostatic pressure caused by sodium retention.
   b. decreased aldosterone secretion from adrenal insufficiency.
   c. increased fluid retention caused by decreased glomerular filtration.
   d. decreased colloidal osmotic pressure caused by loss of serum albumin.
6. A patient is admitted to the hospital with severe renal colic. The nurse's *first priority* in management of the patient is to
   a. administer opioids as prescribed.
   b. obtain supplies for straining all urine.
   c. encourage fluid intake of 3 to 4 L/day.
   d. keep the patient NPO in preparation for surgery.
7. The nurse recommends genetic counseling for the children of a patient with
   a. nephrotic syndrome.
   b. chronic pyelonephritis.
   c. malignant nephrosclerosis.
   d. adult-onset polycystic kidney disease.

8. The nurse identifies a risk factor for kidney and bladder cancer in a patient who relates a history of
   a. aspirin use.
   b. tobacco use.
   c. chronic alcohol abuse.
   d. use of artificial sweeteners.

9. In planning nursing interventions to increase bladder control in the patient with urinary incontinence, the nurse includes
   a. teaching the patient to use Kegel exercises.
   b. clamping and releasing a catheter to increase bladder tone.
   c. teaching the patient biofeedback mechanisms to suppress the urge to void.
   d. counseling the patient concerning choice of incontinence containment device.

10. A patient with a ureterolithotomy returns from surgery with a nephrostomy tube in place. Postoperative nursing care of the patient includes
    a. encouraging the patient to drink fruit juices and milk.
    b. encouraging fluids of at least 2 to 3 L/day after nausea has subsided.
    c. irrigating the nephrostomy tube with 10 mL of normal saline solution as needed.
    d. notifying the physician if nephrostomy tube drainage is more than 30 mL/hr.

11. A patient has had a cystectomy and ileal conduit diversion performed. Four days postoperatively, mucous shreds are seen in the drainage bag. The nurse should
    a. notify the physician.
    b. notify the charge nurse.
    c. irrigate the drainage tube.
    d. document it as a normal observation.

1. d, 2. b, 3. b, 4. a, 5. d, 6. a, 7. d, 8. b, 9. a, 10. b, 11. d

For rationales to these answers and even more NCLEX review questions, visit *http://evolve.elsevier.com/Lewis/medsurg*.

ⓔ EVOLVE WEBSITE

http://evolve.elsevier.com/Lewis/medsurg
Review Questions (Online Only)
Key Points
Answer Keys for Questions
- Rationales for Bridge to NCLEX Examination Questions
- Answer Guidelines for Case Study on p. 1067
Student Case Studies
- Patient With Bladder Cancer and Urinary Diversion
- Patient With Glomerulonephritis and Acute Kidney Injury
Nursing Care Plans
- eNursing Care Plan 45-1: Patient With a Urinary Tract Infection
- eNursing Care Plan 45-2: Patient With Urinary Tract Calculi
- eNursing Care Plan 45-3: Patient With an Ileal Conduit
Conceptual Care Map Creator
Audio Glossary
Content Updates

REFERENCES

1. National Kidney and Urologic Diseases Information Clearinghouse: Kidney and urologic diseases statistics for the United States. Retrieved from *www.niddk.nih.gov/health-information/health-topics/urologic -disease/urinary-tract-infections-in-adults/Pages/facts.aspx*.
2. Brusch JL, Bavaro MF, Cunha BA, et al: Cystitis in females. Retrieved from *http://emedicine.medscape.com/article/233101-overview*.
3. American Association of Nurses: ANA CAUTI Prevention Tool. Retrieved from *http://nursingworld.org/ANA-CAUTI-Prevention -Tool*.
4. Nazarko L: Recurrent urinary tract infection in older women: an evidence-based approach, *Br J Community Nurs* 18(8):407, 2013.
5. Wang A, Nizran P, Malone MA, et al: Urinary tract infections, *Prim Care* 40(3):687, 2013.
*6. Wang C, Fang C, Chen N, et al: Cranberry-containing products for prevention of urinary tract infections in susceptible populations: a systematic review and meta-analysis of randomized controlled trials, *Arch Intern Med* 172:988, 2012.
7. Neumann I, Moore P: Pyelonephritis (acute) in non-pregnant women, *BMJ Clin Evid* Nov 4, 2014. pii: 0807.
8. National Institute for Diabetes and Digestive and Kidney Diseases: Interstitial cystitis/painful bladder syndrome. Retrieved from *www.niddk.nih.gov/health-information/health-topics/urologic-disease/ interstitial-cystitis-painful-bladder-syndrome/Pages/facts.aspx*.

9. Lessnau K, Kim ED, Pais VM: Tuberculosis of the genitourinary system: overview of GUTB. Retrieved from *http://emedicine.medscape.com/ article/450651-overview*.
10. Soliman MS: Tuberculosis of the genitourinary system. Retrieved from *http://emedicine.medscape.com/article*.
11. Ralph AP, Carapetis JR: Group A streptococcal diseases and their global burden, *Curr Top Microbiol Immunol* 368:1, 2013.
12. Cohen EP, Batuman V: Nephrotic syndrome clinical presentation. Retrieved from *http://emedicine.medscape.com/article/244631-clinical*.
13. National Institute of Diabetes and Digestive and Kidney Diseases: Kidney stones in adults. Retrieved from *www.niddk.nih.gov/health-information/ health-topics/urologic-disease/kidney-stones-in-adults/Pages/facts.aspx*.
14. Flannigan R, Choy WH, Chew B, et al: Renal struvite stones— pathogenesis, microbiology, and management strategies, *Nat Rev Urol* 11(6):333, 2014.
15. Slater RC, Ost M: Percutaneous stone removal: new approaches to access and imaging, *Curr Urol Rep* 16(5):501, 2015.
16. Paul BM, Vanden Heuvel GB: Kidney: polycystic kidney disease, *Wiley Interdiscip Rev Dev Biol* 3(6):465, 2014.
17. Alam A: Risk factors for progression in ADPKD, *Curr Opin Nephrol Hypertens* 24(3): 290, 2015.
18. National Kidney Foundation: Alport syndrome. Retrieved from *www.kidney.org/atoz/content/Alport*.
19. American Cancer Society: Cancer facts and figures 2015. Retrieved from *www.cancer.org/research/cancerfactsstatistics/allcancerfactsfigures/index*.
20. Puente VA, Alonso G, Moreno J, et al: New challenges in kidney cancer management: integration of surgery and novel therapies, *Curr Treat Option Oncol* 16(3):337, 2015.
21. Kim JW, Tomita Y, Trepel J, et al: Emerging immunotherapies for bladder cancer, *Curr Opin Oncol* 27:191, 2015.
*22. Houghton BB, Chalasani V, Hayne D, et al: Intravesical chemotherapy plus bacille Calmette-Guérin in non-muscle invasive bladder cancer: a systematic review with meta-analysis, *BJU Int* 111:977, 2013.
*23. Shin DC, Shin SH, Lee MM, et al: Pelvic floor muscle training for urinary incontinence in female stroke patients: a randomized, controlled and blinded trial, *Clin Rehabil* 30(3):259, 2016.
24. Newman DK, Willson M: Review of intermittent catheterization and current best practices. Retrieved from *www.medscape.com/ viewarticle/745908_10*.
25. National Institute for Diabetes and Digestive and Kidney Diseases: Urinary diversion. Retrieved from *www.niddk.nih.gov/health-information/ health-topics/urologic-disease/urinary-diversion/Pages/facts.aspx*.

*Evidence-based information for clinical practice.

Acute Kidney Injury and Chronic Kidney Disease

Hazel A. Dennison

> *The greatest healing therapy is friendship and love.*
>
> *Hubert H. Humphrey*

ℯ http://evolve.elsevier.com/Lewis/medsurg/

LEARNING OUTCOMES

1. Differentiate between acute kidney injury and chronic kidney disease.
2. Identify criteria used in the classification of acute kidney injury using the acronym RIFLE (*Risk, Injury, Failure, Loss, End-*stage renal disease).
3. Describe the clinical course of acute kidney injury.
4. Explain the interprofessional care and nursing management of a patient with acute kidney injury.
5. Define chronic kidney disease and delineate its five stages based on the glomerular filtration rate.
6. Identify risk factors that contribute to the development of chronic kidney disease.
7. Summarize the significance of cardiovascular disease in individuals with chronic kidney disease.
8. Explain the conservative interprofessional care for and the related nursing management of the patient with chronic kidney disease.
9. Differentiate among renal replacement therapy options for individuals with end-stage renal disease.
10. Compare and contrast nursing interventions for individuals on peritoneal dialysis and hemodialysis.
11. Discuss the role of nurses in the management of individuals who receive a kidney transplant.

KEY TERMS

acute kidney injury (AKI), p. 1069
acute tubular necrosis (ATN), p. 1071
anuria, p. 1071
arteriovenous fistula (AVF), p. 1087
arteriovenous grafts (AVGs), p. 1088
automated peritoneal dialysis (APD), p. 1086
azotemia, p. 1069

chronic kidney disease (CKD), p. 1075
CKD mineral and bone disorder (CKD-MBD), p. 1078
continuous ambulatory peritoneal dialysis (CAPD), p. 1086
continuous renal replacement therapy (CRRT), p. 1091

dialysis, p. 1084
end-stage renal disease (ESRD), p. 1076
hemodialysis (HD), p. 1084
oliguria, p. 1071
peritoneal dialysis (PD), p. 1084
uremia, p. 1076

Kidney failure (also called *renal failure*) is the partial or complete impairment of kidney function. It results in an inability to excrete metabolic waste products and water, and it contributes to disturbances of all body systems. Kidney failure can be classified as acute or chronic (Table 46-1). Acute kidney injury (AKI) has a rapid onset. Chronic kidney disease (CKD) is linked with the development of cardiovascular (CV) disease.

ACUTE KIDNEY INJURY

Acute kidney injury (AKI) is the term used to encompass the entire scope of the syndrome, ranging from a slight deterioration in kidney function to severe impairment. AKI is characterized by a rapid loss of kidney function. This loss is accompanied by a rise in serum creatinine and/or a reduction in urine output.

The severity of dysfunction can range from a small increase in serum creatinine or reduction in urine output to the development of **azotemia** (an accumulation of nitrogenous waste products [urea nitrogen, creatinine] in the blood).

Although AKI is potentially reversible, it has a high mortality rate.[1] AKI usually affects people with other life-threatening conditions[2] (Table 46-2). Most commonly, AKI follows severe, prolonged hypotension or hypovolemia or exposure to a nephrotoxic agent.

AKI can develop over hours or days with progressive elevations of blood urea nitrogen (BUN), creatinine, and potassium with or without a reduction in urine output. Hospitalized patients develop AKI at a high rate (1 in 5) and have a high mortality rate. When AKI develops in patients in intensive care units (ICUs), the mortality rate can be as high as 70% to 80%.[3,4]

Reviewed by Rowena W. Elliott, RN, PhD, CNN, CNE, AGNP-C, FAAN, Associate Professor, University of Southern Mississippi, College of Nursing, Hattiesburg, Mississippi; Shari Gould, RN, MSN, Associate Professor of Nursing, Victoria College, Victoria, Texas; Sharon Haas, RN, MSN, CDN, Instructor, College of Nursing, Cardinal Stritch University, Milwaukee, Wisconsin; and Rebecca Personett, RN, PhD, NEA-BC, Professor of Nursing, North Central Texas College, Gainesville, Texas and Brookhaven College, Dallas, Texas.

Etiology and Pathophysiology

The causes of AKI, which are multiple and complex, are categorized as prerenal, intrarenal (or intrinsic), and postrenal causes (Table 46-2 and Fig. 46-1).

Prerenal. *Prerenal* causes of AKI are factors that reduce systemic circulation, causing a reduction in renal blood flow. The decrease in blood flow leads to decreased glomerular perfusion and filtration of the kidneys.

It is important to distinguish prerenal oliguria from the oliguria of intrarenal AKI. In prerenal oliguria there is no damage to the kidney tissue (parenchyma). The oliguria is caused by a decrease in circulating blood volume (e.g., severe dehydration, heart failure [HF], decreased cardiac output). Prerenal oliguria is readily reversible with appropriate treatment.[5] With a decrease in circulating blood volume, autoregulatory mechanisms that increase angiotensin II, aldosterone, norepinephrine, and antidiuretic hormone attempt to preserve blood flow to essential organs. Prerenal azotemia results in a reduction in the excretion of sodium (less than 20 mEq/L), increased sodium and water retention, and decreased urine output.

Prerenal conditions contribute to intrarenal AKI. If decreased perfusion persists for an extended time, the kidneys lose their ability to compensate and damage to kidney parenchyma occurs (intrarenal damage).

Intrarenal. *Intrarenal* causes of AKI (Table 46-2) include conditions that cause direct damage to the kidney tissue, resulting in impaired nephron function. The damage from intrarenal causes usually results from prolonged ischemia, nephrotoxins (e.g., aminoglycoside antibiotics, contrast media), hemoglobin released from hemolyzed red blood cells (RBCs), or myoglobin released from necrotic muscle cells.

Nephrotoxins can cause obstruction of intrarenal structures by crystallizing or by causing damage to the epithelial cells of

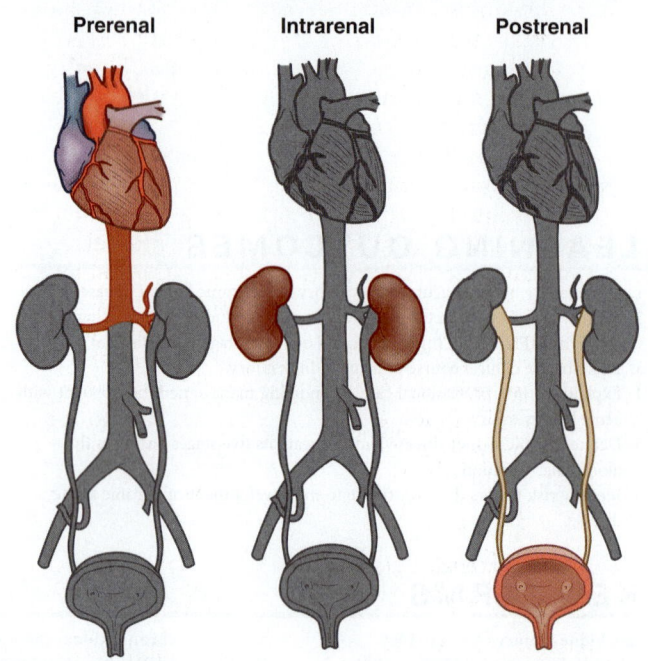

FIG. 46-1 Prerenal, intrarenal, and postrenal causes of acute kidney injury (AKI).

TABLE 46-1 Comparison of Acute Kidney Injury and Chronic Kidney Disease

	Acute Kidney Injury	Chronic Kidney Disease
Onset	Sudden	Gradual, often over many years
Most common cause	Acute tubular necrosis	Diabetic nephropathy
Diagnostic criteria	Acute reduction in urine output and/or	GFR <60 mL/min/1.73 m² for >3 mo and/or
	Elevation in serum creatinine	Kidney damage >3 mo
Reversibility	Potentially	Progressive and irreversible
Primary cause of death	Infection	Cardiovascular disease

GFR, Glomerular filtration rate.

TABLE 46-2 Common Causes of Acute Kidney Injury

Prerenal	Intrarenal	Postrenal
Hypovolemia • Dehydration • Hemorrhage • GI losses (diarrhea, vomiting) • Excessive diuresis • Hypoalbuminemia • Burns **Decreased Cardiac Output** • Cardiac dysrhythmias • Cardiogenic shock • Heart failure • Myocardial infarction **Decreased Peripheral Vascular Resistance** • Anaphylaxis • Neurologic injury • Septic shock **Decreased Renovascular Blood Flow** • Bilateral renal vein thrombosis • Embolism • Hepatorenal syndrome • Renal artery thrombosis	**Nephrotoxic Injury** • Drugs: aminoglycosides (gentamicin, amikacin), amphotericin B • Contrast media • Hemolytic blood transfusion reaction • Severe crush injury • Chemical exposure: ethylene glycol, lead, arsenic, carbon tetrachloride **Interstitial Nephritis** • Allergies: antibiotics (sulfonamides, rifampin), nonsteroidal antiinflammatory drugs, ACE inhibitors • Infections: bacterial (acute pyelonephritis), viral (CMV), fungal (candidiasis) **Other Causes** • Prolonged prerenal ischemia • Acute glomerulonephritis • Thrombotic disorders • Toxemia of pregnancy • Malignant hypertension • Systemic lupus erythematosus	• Benign prostatic hyperplasia • Bladder cancer • Calculi formation • Neuromuscular disorders • Prostate cancer • Spinal cord disease • Strictures • Trauma (back, pelvis, perineum)

ACE, Angiotensin-converting enzyme; *CMV,* cytomegalovirus.

the tubules. Hemoglobin and myoglobin can block the tubules and cause renal vasoconstriction. Diseases of the kidney such as acute glomerulonephritis and systemic lupus erythematosus may also cause AKI.

Acute tubular necrosis (ATN) is the most common intrarenal cause of AKI and is primarily the result of ischemia, nephrotoxins, or sepsis. Ischemic and nephrotoxic ATN is responsible for 90% of intrarenal AKI cases.[6,7] Severe kidney ischemia causes a disruption in the basement membrane and patchy destruction of the tubular epithelium. Nephrotoxic agents cause necrosis of tubular epithelial cells, which slough off and plug the tubules. ATN is potentially reversible if the basement membrane is not destroyed and the tubular epithelium regenerates.

ATN is the most common cause of AKI for hospitalized patients.[7] Risks associated with the development of ATN while in the hospital include major surgery, shock, sepsis, blood transfusion reaction, muscle injury from trauma, prolonged hypotension, and nephrotoxic agents (Table 46-2).

Postrenal. *Postrenal* causes of AKI involve mechanical obstruction in the outflow of urine. As the flow of urine is obstructed, urine refluxes into the renal pelvis, impairing kidney function. The most common postrenal causes are benign prostatic hyperplasia, prostate cancer, calculi, trauma, and extrarenal tumors. Bilateral ureteral obstruction leads to *hydronephrosis* (kidney dilation), increase in hydrostatic pressure, and tubular blockage, resulting in a progressive decline in kidney function. If bilateral obstruction is relieved within 48 hours of onset, complete recovery is likely. Prolonged obstruction can lead to tubular atrophy and irreversible kidney fibrosis. Postrenal causes of AKI account for less than 10% of AKI cases.[8]

Clinical Manifestations

Prerenal and postrenal AKI that has not caused intrarenal damage usually resolves quickly with treatment. When parenchymal damage occurs due to either prerenal or postrenal causes, or when parenchymal damage occurs directly as with intrarenal causes, AKI has a prolonged course. Clinically, AKI may progress through phases: oliguric, diuretic, and recovery. When a patient does not recover from AKI, then CKD may develop.

The RIFLE classification is used to describe the stages of AKI (Table 46-3). *Risk*, the first stage of AKI, is followed by *Injury*, which is the second stage. Then AKI increases in severity to the final, or third, stage, *Failure*. The two outcome variables are *Loss* and *End-stage renal disease*.[9,10]

Oliguric Phase. The most common manifestations of AKI are discussed in this section.

Urinary Changes. The most common initial manifestation of AKI is oliguria, a reduction in urine output to less than 400 mL/day. Nonoliguria AKI indicates a urine output greater than 400 mL/day. Oliguria usually occurs within 1 to 7 days of the injury to the kidneys. If the cause is ischemia, oliguria often occurs within 24 hours. In contrast, when nephrotoxic drugs are involved, the onset may be delayed for as long as 1 week. The oliguric phase lasts on average about 10 to 14 days but can last months in some cases. The longer the oliguric phase lasts, the poorer the prognosis for complete recovery of kidney function.[1]

About 50% of patients will not be oliguric, making the initial diagnosis more difficult.[7] Changes in urine output generally do not correspond to changes in glomerular filtration rate (GFR). However, changes in urine output are often helpful in differentiating the etiology of AKI. For example, anuria (no urine output) is usually seen with urinary tract obstruction, oliguria is commonly seen with prerenal causes, and nonoliguric AKI is seen with acute interstitial nephritis and ATN.[8]

A urinalysis may show casts, RBCs, and white blood cells (WBCs). The casts are formed from mucoprotein impressions of the necrotic renal tubular epithelial cells, which slough

TABLE 46-3	**RIFLE Classification for Staging Acute Kidney Injury**		
Stage	**GFR Criteria**	**Urine Output Criteria**	**Clinical Example**
Risk	Serum creatinine increased × 1.5 OR GFR decreased by 25%	Urine output <0.5 mL/kg/hr for 6 hr	• 68-yr-old African American woman with type 2 diabetes, hypertension, CAD, and CKD. • Scheduled to undergo emergency coronary artery bypass graft. • Serum creatinine is 1.8 mg/dL (increased) and she weighs 60 kg. • Calculated GFR is 35 mL/min/1.73 m². • She has Stage 3b CKD.
Injury	Serum creatinine increased × 2 OR GFR decreased by 50%	Urine output <0.5 mL/kg/hr for 12 hr	• During surgery, she experiences hypotension for a sustained period. • Acute tubular necrosis is diagnosed. • After surgery: Serum creatinine is 3.6 mg/dL and urine output is reduced to 28 mL/hr
Failure	Serum creatinine increased × 3 OR GFR decreased by 75% OR Serum creatinine >4 mg/dL with acute rise ≥0.5 mg/dL	Urine output <0.3 mL/kg/hr for 24 hr (oliguria) OR Anuria for 12 hr	• 72 hours after surgery and in ICU develops ventilator-associated pneumonia and sepsis. • Serum creatinine rises to 5.2 mg/dL and urine output drops to 10 mL/hr. • BP remains low despite dopamine therapy.
Loss	Persistent acute kidney failure. Complete loss of kidney function >4 wk	—	• Continuous venovenous hemodialysis is started. • After 3 wk of therapy she has a cardiopulmonary arrest and does not survive.
End-Stage Renal Disease	Complete loss of kidney function >3 mo	—	—

GFR, Glomerular filtration rate.

into the tubules. Urinary specific gravity (measure of the concentration of solutes in the urine) is normally 1.003 to 1.030. Urine osmolality is used to measure the number of dissolved particles in the urine. Urine osmolality range is 300 to 1300 mOsm/kg. As a measure of urine concentration, it is more accurate than specific gravity.

In kidney failure, a urinalysis may show a specific gravity fixed at around 1.010 and urine osmolality at about 300 mOsm/kg (300 mmol/kg). This is the same specific gravity and osmolality of plasma, thus reflecting tubular damage with a loss of concentrating ability by the kidney. Proteinuria may be present if kidney failure is related to glomerular membrane dysfunction.

Fluid Volume. Hypovolemia (volume depletion) has the potential to exacerbate all forms of AKI. Fluid replacement is often sufficient to treat many forms of AKI, especially prerenal causes. When urine output decreases, fluid retention occurs. The severity of the manifestations depends on the extent of the fluid overload. In the case of reduced urine output (anuria and oliguria), the neck veins may become distended with a bounding pulse. Edema and hypertension may develop. Fluid overload can eventually lead to heart failure, pulmonary edema, and pericardial and pleural effusions.

Metabolic Acidosis. In the normal kidney, excess hydrogen ions are excreted to maintain a physiologic balance of the blood pH. The impaired kidneys cannot excrete hydrogen ions or the acid products of metabolism. Serum bicarbonate production is decreased because of defective reabsorption and regeneration of bicarbonate ions. Serum bicarbonate is depleted through buffering of acidic hydrogen ions and metabolic end products. The patient with severe acidosis may develop Kussmaul respirations (rapid, deep respirations) in an effort to compensate by increasing the exhalation of CO_2.

Sodium Balance. Damaged tubules cannot conserve sodium. The urinary excretion of sodium may increase, resulting in normal or below-normal levels of serum sodium. Excessive intake of sodium should be avoided because it can lead to volume expansion, hypertension, and HF. Uncontrolled hyponatremia or water excess can lead to cerebral edema.

Potassium Excess. The kidneys normally excrete 80% to 90% of the body's potassium. In AKI the serum potassium level increases because the kidney's normal ability to excrete potassium is impaired. Hyperkalemia risk is increased if AKI is caused by massive tissue trauma because the damaged cells release additional potassium into the extracellular fluid. Bleeding and blood transfusions may cause cellular destruction, releasing more potassium into the extracellular fluid. Metabolic acidosis worsens hyperkalemia as hydrogen ions enter the cells, and potassium is driven out of the cells into the extracellular fluid.

While patients with hyperkalemia are often asymptomatic, some may complain of weakness with severe hyperkalemia. Because cardiac muscle is intolerant of acute increases in potassium, emergency treatment of hyperkalemia is needed.

Acute or rapid development of hyperkalemia may result in clinical signs that are apparent on electrocardiogram (ECG). These changes include peaked T waves, widening of the QRS complex, and ST segment depression. Progressive changes in the ECG that are related to increasing potassium levels are depicted in Fig. 16-14.

Hematologic Disorders. Several hematologic disorders are found in patients with AKI. Hospital-acquired AKI often occurs in patients who have multiorgan failure. Leukocytosis is often present with AKI. The most common cause of death in AKI is

infection. The most common sites of infection are the urinary and respiratory systems.

Waste Product Accumulation. The kidneys are the primary excretory organs for urea (an end product of protein metabolism) and creatinine (an end product of endogenous muscle metabolism). BUN and serum creatinine levels are elevated in kidney disease. An elevated BUN level can also be caused by dehydration; corticosteroids; or catabolism resulting from infections, fever, severe injury, or GI bleeding. The best serum indicator of AKI is creatinine because it is not significantly altered by other factors.

Neurologic Disorders. Neurologic changes can occur as the nitrogenous waste products accumulate in the brain and other nervous tissue. The manifestations can be as mild as fatigue and difficulty concentrating, and escalate to seizures, stupor, and coma.

Diuretic Phase. During the diuretic phase of AKI, daily urine output is usually around 1 to 3 L but may reach 5 L or more. The nephrons are still not fully functional even as urine output increases. The high urine volume is caused by osmotic diuresis from the high urea concentration in the glomerular filtrate and the inability of the tubules to concentrate the urine. In this phase, the kidneys have recovered their ability to excrete wastes but not to concentrate the urine. Hypovolemia and hypotension can occur from massive fluid losses.

Patients who develop an oliguric phase will have greater diuresis as kidney function returns. Large losses of fluid and electrolytes require the patient be monitored for hyponatremia, hypokalemia, and dehydration. The diuretic phase may last 1 to 3 weeks. Near the end of this phase, the patient's acid-base, electrolyte, and waste product (BUN, creatinine) values stabilize.

Recovery Phase. The recovery phase begins when the GFR increases, allowing the BUN and serum creatinine levels to decrease. Major improvements occur in the first 1 to 2 weeks of this phase, but kidney function may take up to 12 months to stabilize. The outcome of AKI is influenced by the patient's overall health, severity of kidney injury, and number and type of complications. Some individuals do not recover and progress to end-stage renal disease. The older adult is less likely to have a complete recovery of kidney function. Patients who recover may achieve clinically normal kidney function but remain in an early stage of CKD.

Diagnostic Studies

A thorough history is essential for diagnosing the etiology of AKI. Consider prerenal causes when there is a history of dehydration, hypotension, or blood loss. Suspect intrarenal causes if the patient has been exposed to potentially nephrotoxic drugs or contrast media used in a radiologic study. Postrenal causes are suggested by a history of changes in the urinary stream, stones, benign prostatic hyperplasia, or bladder or prostate cancer.

Although changes in urine output and serum creatinine occur relatively late in the course of AKI, they are known diagnostic indicators. An increase in serum creatinine may not be evident until there is a loss of more than 50% of kidney function. The rate of increase in serum creatinine is also important as a diagnostic indicator in determining the severity of injury.

Urinalysis is an important diagnostic test. Urine sediment containing abundant cells, casts, or proteins suggests intrarenal disorders. The urine osmolality, sodium content, and specific gravity help in differentiating the causes of AKI. Urine sediment may be normal in both prerenal and postrenal AKI. In

TABLE 46-4 Interprofessional Care
Acute Kidney Injury

Diagnostic Assessment
- History and physical examination
- Identification of precipitating cause
- Serum creatinine and BUN levels
- Serum electrolytes
- Urinalysis
- Renal ultrasound
- Renal scan
- CT scan

Management
- Treatment of precipitating cause
- Fluid restriction (600 mL plus previous 24-hr fluid loss)
- Nutritional therapy
- Adequate protein intake (0.6-2 g/kg/day) depending on degree of catabolism
- Enteral nutrition
- Parenteral nutrition
- Dietary restrictions (potassium, phosphate, sodium)
- Measures to lower potassium (if elevated) (Table 46-5)
- Calcium supplements or phosphate-binding agents
- Initiation of dialysis (if necessary)
- Continuous renal replacement therapy (if necessary)

TABLE 46-5 Therapies for Elevated Potassium Levels

Regular Insulin IV
- Potassium moves into cells when insulin is given.
- IV glucose is given concurrently to prevent hypoglycemia.
- When effects of insulin diminish, potassium shifts back out of cells.

Sodium Bicarbonate
- Therapy can correct acidosis and cause a shift of potassium into cells.

Calcium Gluconate IV
- Generally used in advanced cardiac toxicity (with evidence of hyperkalemic ECG changes).
- Calcium raises the threshold for excitation, resulting in dysrhythmias.

Hemodialysis
- Most effective therapy to remove potassium.
- Works within a short time.

Sodium Polystyrene Sulfonate (Kayexalate)
- Cation-exchange resin is administered by mouth or retention enema.
- When resin is in the bowel, potassium is exchanged for sodium.
- Therapy removes 1 mEq of potassium per gram of drug.
- It is mixed in water with sorbitol to produce osmotic diarrhea, allowing for evacuation of potassium-rich stool from body.

Dietary Restriction
- Potassium intake is limited to 40 mEq/day.
- Primarily used to prevent recurrent elevation. Not used for acute elevation.

Patiromer (Veltassa)
- Oral suspension that binds potassium in GI tract.
- It is used to treat chronic kidney disease.
- It should not be used as an emergency drug for life-threatening hyperkalemia.
- It has a delayed onset of action.

intrarenal problems, hematuria, pyuria, and crystals may be seen. To establish a diagnosis of AKI, other testing may be required (Table 46-4). A kidney ultrasound is often the first test done, since it provides imaging without exposure to potentially nephrotoxic contrast agents. It is useful for evaluating for possible kidney disease and obstruction of the urinary collection system. A renal scan can assess abnormalities in kidney blood flow, tubular function, and the collecting system. A CT scan can identify lesions, masses, obstructions, and vascular anomalies. A renal biopsy is considered the best method for confirming intrarenal causes of AKI.

Obtaining an MRI or magnetic resonance angiography (MRA) study with the contrast media gadolinium is not advised in patients with kidney failure. Administration of gadolinium can be potentially fatal.

In patients with normal kidney function, administration of contrast media poses minimal risk. In patients with kidney disease, *contrast-induced nephropathy* (CIN) can occur when contrast media for diagnostic studies causes nephrotoxic injury. In patients with diabetes receiving metformin, the drug should be held for 48 hours prior to and after the use of contrast media to decrease the risk of lactic acidosis. The best way to avoid CIN is to avoid exposure to contrast media by using other diagnostic tests such as ultrasound. If contrast media must be administered to a high-risk patient, the patient needs to have optimal hydration and the lowest possible dose of the contrast agent. Nursing interventions to ensure adequate fluid intake and hydration can decrease the risks associated with contrast media. Other treatment options to prevent CIN remain controversial such as administration of bicarbonate or sodium chloride solutions or prophylactic administration of *N*-acetylcysteine.

Interprofessional Care

Because AKI is potentially reversible, the primary goals of treatment are to eliminate the cause, manage the signs and symptoms, and prevent complications while the kidneys recover (Table 46-4). The first step is to determine if there is adequate intravascular volume and cardiac output to ensure adequate perfusion of the kidneys. Diuretic therapy may be administered and usually includes loop diuretics (e.g., furosemide [Lasix], bumetanide [Bumex]) or an osmotic diuretic (e.g., mannitol). If AKI is already established, forcing fluids and diuretics will not be effective and may be harmful. Closely monitor fluid intake during the oliguric phase of AKI.

The general rule for calculating the fluid restriction is to add all losses for the previous 24 hours (e.g., urine, diarrhea, emesis, blood) plus 600 mL for insensible losses (e.g., respiration, diaphoresis). For example, if a patient excreted 300 mL of urine on Tuesday with no other losses, the fluid allocation on Wednesday would be 900 mL.

Hyperkalemia is one of the most serious complications in AKI because it can cause life-threatening cardiac dysrhythmias. The various therapies used to treat elevated potassium levels are listed in Table 46-5. Both insulin and sodium bicarbonate serve as temporary measures for treatment of hyperkalemia by promoting a transient shift of potassium into the cells. Potassium will eventually diffuse back into the bloodstream. Calcium gluconate raises the threshold at which dysrhythmias occur, temporarily stabilizing the myocardium. Only sodium polystyrene sulfonate (Kayexalate) and dialysis actually remove potassium from the body. Never give sodium polystyrene sulfonate to a patient with a paralytic ileus as bowel necrosis can occur.

Conservative therapy may be all that is necessary until kidney function improves. If conservative therapy is not effective in treating AKI, then *renal replacement therapy* (RRT) is used. Controversy exists about the timing of RRT in AKI.[11] The most common indications for RRT in AKI are (1) volume overload, resulting in compromised cardiac and/or pulmonary status; (2) elevated serum potassium level; (3) metabolic acidosis (serum bicarbonate level less than 15 mEq/L [15 mmol/L]); (4) BUN level greater than 120 mg/dL (43 mmol/L); (5) significant change in mental status; and (6) pericarditis, pericardial effusion, or cardiac tamponade. Although laboratory values provide rough parameters, the best guideline is the clinical status of the patient.

Of the several RRT therapy options available, there is no consensus regarding the best approach.[10] Even though peritoneal dialysis (PD) is considered a viable option for RRT, it is not frequently used. Intermittent hemodialysis (HD) and continuous renal replacement therapy (CRRT) have both been used effectively.

CRRT is provided continuously over approximately 24 hours through cannulation of a vein or catheter placement. CRRT has much slower blood flow rates compared with intermittent HD. HD is the method of choice when changes are required emergently. It is technically more complicated because specialized staff and equipment and a vascular access are required. It also requires anticoagulation therapy to prevent the patient's blood from clotting when the blood makes contact with the extracorporeal dialysis circuit. Rapid fluid shifts during HD may cause hypotension. (RRT and CRRT are discussed later in this chapter on pp. 1091-1092.)

Nutritional Therapy. The goal of nutritional management in AKI is to provide adequate calories to prevent catabolism despite restrictions that prevent electrolyte and fluid disorders and azotemia. Nutritional intake must maintain adequate caloric intake (providing 30 to 35 kcal/kg and 0.8 to 1.0 g of protein per kilogram of desired body weight) to prevent the breakdown of body protein.

Adequate energy should primarily be from carbohydrate and fat sources to prevent ketosis from endogenous fat breakdown and gluconeogenesis from muscle protein breakdown. Essential amino acids may be supplemented. Potassium and sodium are regulated in accordance with plasma levels. Sodium is restricted as needed to prevent edema, hypertension, and HF. Dietary fat intake is increased so that the patient receives at least 30% to 40% of total calories from fat. Fat emulsion IV infusions given as a nutritional supplement provide a good source of nonprotein calories (see Chapter 39). If a patient cannot maintain adequate oral intake, enteral nutrition is the preferred route for nutritional support (see Chapter 39). When the gastrointestinal (GI) tract is not functional, parenteral nutrition is necessary to provide adequate nutrition. The patient treated with parenteral nutrition may need daily HD or CRRT to remove the excess fluid. Concentrated formulas of parenteral nutrition are available to minimize fluid volume.

❖ NURSING MANAGEMENT: ACUTE KIDNEY INJURY

◆ Nursing Assessment

Monitor vital signs, weight, and fluid intake and output. Daily monitoring of a patient's urine output has prognostic implications and is crucial for determining therapy and daily fluid volume replacement. Examine the urine for color, specific gravity, glucose, protein, blood, and sediment. Assess the patient's general appearance, including skin color, edema, neck vein distention, and bruises. If a patient is receiving dialysis, observe the access site for inflammation and exudate. Evaluate the patient's mental status and level of consciousness. Examine the oral mucosa for dryness and inflammation. Auscultate the lungs for crackles and wheezes or diminished breath sounds. Monitor the heart for an S_3 gallop, murmurs, or a pericardial friction rub. Assess ECG readings for dysrhythmias. Review laboratory values and diagnostic test results. All of the previous data are essential for developing an interprofessional plan of care.[12]

◆ Nursing Diagnoses

Nursing diagnoses and a potential complication for the patient with AKI include, but are not limited to, the following:

- Risk for infection *related to* invasive lines, uremic toxins, and altered immune responses secondary to kidney injury
- Excess fluid volume *related to* kidney injury and fluid retention
- Fatigue *related to* anemia, metabolic acidosis, and uremic toxins
- Anxiety *related to* disease processes, therapeutic interventions, and uncertainty of prognosis
- Potential complication: dysrhythmias *related to* electrolyte imbalances

◆ Planning

The overall goals are that the patient with AKI will (1) completely recover without any loss of kidney function, (2) maintain normal fluid and electrolyte balance, (3) have decreased anxiety, and (4) adhere to and understand the need for careful follow-up care.

◆ Nursing Implementation

◆ **Health Promotion.** Prevention and early recognition of AKI are the most important components of care. Prevention is directed primarily toward identifying and monitoring high-risk populations, controlling exposure to nephrotoxic drugs and industrial chemicals, and preventing prolonged episodes of hypotension and hypovolemia. In the hospital, the factors that increase the risk for developing AKI are preexisting CKD, older age, massive trauma, major surgical procedures, extensive burns, cardiac failure, sepsis, or obstetric complications.

Carefully monitor the patient's weight, intake and output, and fluid and electrolyte balance. Assess and record extrarenal losses of fluid from vomiting, diarrhea, hemorrhage, and increased insensible losses. Prompt replacement of significant fluid losses helps prevent ischemic tubular damage associated with trauma, burns, and extensive surgery. Intake and output records and the patient's weight provide valuable indicators of fluid volume status. Aggressive diuretic therapy for the patient with fluid overload from any cause can lead to a reduction in renal blood flow.

Monitor kidney function in individuals who are taking drugs that are potentially nephrotoxic (see Table 44-3). Nephrotoxic drugs should be used sparingly in the high-risk patient. When these drugs must be used, they should be given in the smallest effective doses for the shortest possible periods. Caution the patient about abuse of over-the-counter analgesics (especially nonsteroidal antiinflammatory drugs [NSAIDs]) as these may worsen kidney function in the patient with mild CKD.

Angiotensin-converting enzyme (ACE) inhibitors can also decrease perfusion pressure and cause hyperkalemia. If other measures such as diet modification, diuretics, and sodium bicarbonate cannot control the hyperkalemia, ACE inhibitors may have to be reduced or eliminated. However, ACE inhibitors are frequently used to prevent proteinuria and progression of kidney disease, especially in patients with diabetes.[13]

◆ **Acute Care.** The patient with AKI is critically ill and may have co-morbid diseases or conditions (e.g., diabetes, CV disease) in addition to kidney injury. Focus on the patient holistically, since he or she will have many physical and emotional needs. Usually the changes caused by AKI arise suddenly. The patient needs assistance in understanding that kidney disease may affect the entire body's functions.

You have an important role in managing fluid and electrolyte balance during the oliguric and diuretic phases. Observe and record accurate intake and output. Take daily weights with the same scale at the same time each day to detect excessive gains or losses of body fluid (1 kg is equivalent to 1000 mL of fluid). Assess for the common signs and symptoms of hypervolemia (in the oliguric phase) or hypovolemia (in the diuretic phase), potassium and sodium disturbances, and other electrolyte imbalances that may occur in AKI (see Chapter 16).

Because infection is the leading cause of death in AKI, meticulous aseptic technique is critical. Protect the patient from other individuals with infectious diseases. Be alert for local manifestations of infection (e.g., swelling, redness, pain) as well as systemic manifestations (e.g., fever, malaise, leukocytosis).

If a patient with renal failure has an infection, it is important to recognize that the temperature may not always be elevated. Patients with kidney failure have a blunted febrile response to an infection (e.g., pneumonia). If antibiotics are used to treat an infection, the type, frequency, and dosage must be carefully considered because the kidneys are the primary route of excretion for many antibiotics. Dosages may be altered depending on the patient's level of kidney function if the drug is primarily eliminated by the kidneys. Nephrotoxic drugs (see Table 44-3) should be used judiciously.

Perform skin care and take measures to prevent pressure ulcers as mobility may be impaired. Mouth care is important to prevent stomatitis, which develops when ammonia (produced by bacterial breakdown of urea) in saliva irritates the mucous membranes.

INFORMATICS IN PRACTICE

Computer Monitoring of Antibiotic Safety

- Many patients receiving antibiotic therapy are at risk for kidney failure.
- Set the computer to alert you about elevated creatinine levels and, if possible, send you a text message.
- With earlier notification of the HCP, medications can be stopped or doses adjusted and the patient's kidney function preserved.

◆ **Ambulatory Care.** Recovery from AKI is highly variable and depends on whether other body systems fail, the patient's general condition and age, the length of the oliguric phase, and the severity of nephron damage. Protein and potassium intake should be regulated in accordance with kidney function. Regular evaluation of kidney function through appropriate follow-up is necessary. Teach the patient the signs and symptoms of recurrent kidney disease. Emphasize measures to prevent the recurrence of AKI.

The long-term convalescence of 3 to 12 months may cause psychosocial and financial hardships for the patient, caregiver, and family. Make appropriate referrals for counseling. If the kidneys do not recover, the patient will need to transition to life on chronic dialysis or possible future transplantation.

◆ Evaluation

The expected outcomes are that the patient with AKI will
- Regain and maintain normal fluid and electrolyte balance
- Adhere to the treatment regimen
- Experience no complications
- Have a complete recovery

Gerontologic Considerations: Acute Kidney Injury

The glomerular filtration rate declines with age. In older adults, impaired function of other organ systems from CV disease or diabetes mellitus can increase the risk of developing AKI. The aging kidney is less able to compensate for changes in fluid volume, solute load, and cardiac output.

Although the causes of AKI in older adults are similar to younger adults, they are at an increased risk for AKI. Dehydration is a predisposing factor and tends to occur much more frequently in older adults. Dehydration can occur from polypharmacy (diuretics, laxatives, and drugs that suppress appetite or consciousness), acute febrile illnesses, and immobility from being bedridden.

Other common causes of AKI in the older adult include hypotension, diuretic therapy, aminoglycoside therapy, obstructive disorders (e.g., prostatic hyperplasia), surgery, infection, and contrast media. Mortality rates are similar for older and younger patients. Patients over 65 years of age are less likely to recover from AKI. Despite this, a patient's chronologic age is not a barrier to offering renal replacement therapy.[11]

CHRONIC KIDNEY DISEASE

Chronic kidney disease (CKD) involves progressive, irreversible loss of kidney function. More than 26 million American adults have CKD, and a million more are at increased risk. One of every nine Americans has CKD. Over half a million Americans are receiving treatment (dialysis, transplant) for ESRD. Despite all the technologic advances in life-sustaining treatment with dialysis, patients with ESRD have a high mortality rate. As the stage of kidney disease progresses, the mortality rate also increases. Mortality rates are as high as 19% to 24% for individuals with ESRD on dialysis.[14,15]

Although CKD has many different causes, the leading causes are diabetes (about 50%) and hypertension (about 25%). Less common etiologies include glomerulonephritis, cystic diseases, and urologic diseases.[16] (Kidney diseases are discussed in Chapter 45.)

CKD is much more common than AKI (Table 46-1). The increasing prevalence of CKD has been partially attributed to increased risk factors, including an aging population, increased rates of obesity, and increased incidence of diabetes and hypertension.

Because the kidneys are highly adaptive, kidney disease is often not recognized until there has been considerable loss of nephrons. Individuals with CKD are frequently asymptomatic, resulting in CKD being underdiagnosed and untreated. It has

TABLE 46-6   Stages of Chronic Kidney Disease

Description	GFR (mL/min/1.73 m^2)	Clinical Action Plan
Stage 1 Kidney damage with normal or ↑ GFR	≥90	Diagnosis and treatment CVD risk reduction Slow progression
Stage 2 Kidney damage with mild ↓ GFR	60-89	Estimation of progression
Stage 3a Moderate ↓ GFR	45-59	Evaluation and treatment of complications
Stage 3b Moderate ↓ GFR	30-44	More aggressive treatment of complications
Stage 4 Severe ↓ GFR	15-29	Preparation for renal replacement therapy (dialysis, kidney transplant)
Stage 5 Kidney failure	<15 (or dialysis)	Renal replacement therapy (if uremia present and patient desires treatment)

Source: Kidney Disease: Improving Global Outcomes (KDIGO) CKD Work Group. KDIGO 2012 Clinical Practice Guideline for the Evaluation and Management of Chronic Kidney Disease, *Kidney Inter Suppl* 3(1):1, 2013.

been estimated that about 70% of people with CKD are unaware that they have the disease.[14]

Kidney Disease Improving Global Outcomes (KDIGO) Clinical Practice Guidelines defines CKD as either the presence of kidney damage or a decreased GFR less than 60 mL/min/1.73 m^2 for longer than 3 months. The classification of CKD is presented in Table 46-6. The last stage of kidney disease, **end-stage renal disease (ESRD)**, occurs when the GFR is less than 15 mL/min. At this point, renal replacement therapy (dialysis or transplantation) is required to maintain life.

The prognosis and course of CKD are highly variable depending on the etiology, patient's condition and age, and adequacy of health care follow-up. Some individuals live normal, active lives with kidney disease, whereas others may rapidly progress to ESRD (stage 5).

Since 1972, the United States has covered the majority of the costs of providing dialysis through Medicare benefits. Under Title XVIII of the Social Security Act, ESRD was recognized as a disability. Medicare pays for 80% of eligible charges, with the remaining being paid for by state or private insurance or out of pocket.[15]

Clinical Manifestations

As kidney function deteriorates, all body systems become affected. The clinical manifestations are a result of retained urea, creatinine, phenols, hormones, electrolytes, and water. **Uremia** is a syndrome in which kidney function declines to the point that symptoms may develop in multiple body systems (Fig. 46-2). It often occurs when the GFR is 15 mL/min or less. The manifestations of uremia vary among patients according to the cause of the kidney disease, co-morbid conditions, age, and degree of adherence to the prescribed medical regimen. Many

patients are tolerant of the changes caused by declining kidney function because they occur gradually.

Urinary System. In the early stages of CKD, patients usually do not report any change in urine output. Since diabetes is the primary cause of CKD, polyuria may be present, but not necessarily as a consequence of kidney disease. As CKD progresses, patients have increasing difficulty with fluid retention and require diuretic therapy. After a period on dialysis, patients may develop anuria.

Metabolic Disturbances

Waste Product Accumulation. As the GFR decreases, the BUN and serum creatinine levels increase. The BUN is increased not only by kidney disease but also by protein intake, fever, corticosteroids, and catabolism. For this reason, serum creatinine clearance determinations (calculated GFR) are considered more accurate indicators of kidney function than BUN or creatinine (Table 46-8). Significant elevations in BUN contribute to development of nausea, vomiting, lethargy, fatigue, impaired thought processes, and headaches.

Altered Carbohydrate Metabolism. Defective carbohydrate metabolism is caused by impaired glucose metabolism, resulting from cellular insensitivity to the normal action of insulin. Mild to moderate hyperglycemia and hyperinsulinemia may occur.

❓ **CHECK YOUR PRACTICE**

You are working in a community-based dialysis unit. One of your patients is a 56-yr-old woman who has been on HD for 3 weeks. You are reviewing her medications with her and she is surprised that her dose of glargine insulin has been decreased. She tells you, "I have been a diabetic for 30 years, and this is the first time ever that my dose of insulin has been decreased."
- How would you respond?

Insulin and glucose metabolism may improve (but not to normal values) after the initiation of dialysis. Patients with diabetes who develop uremia may require less insulin than before the onset of CKD. Insulin, which depends on the kidneys for excretion, remains in the circulation longer. As a result, individuals who required insulin before starting dialysis may require

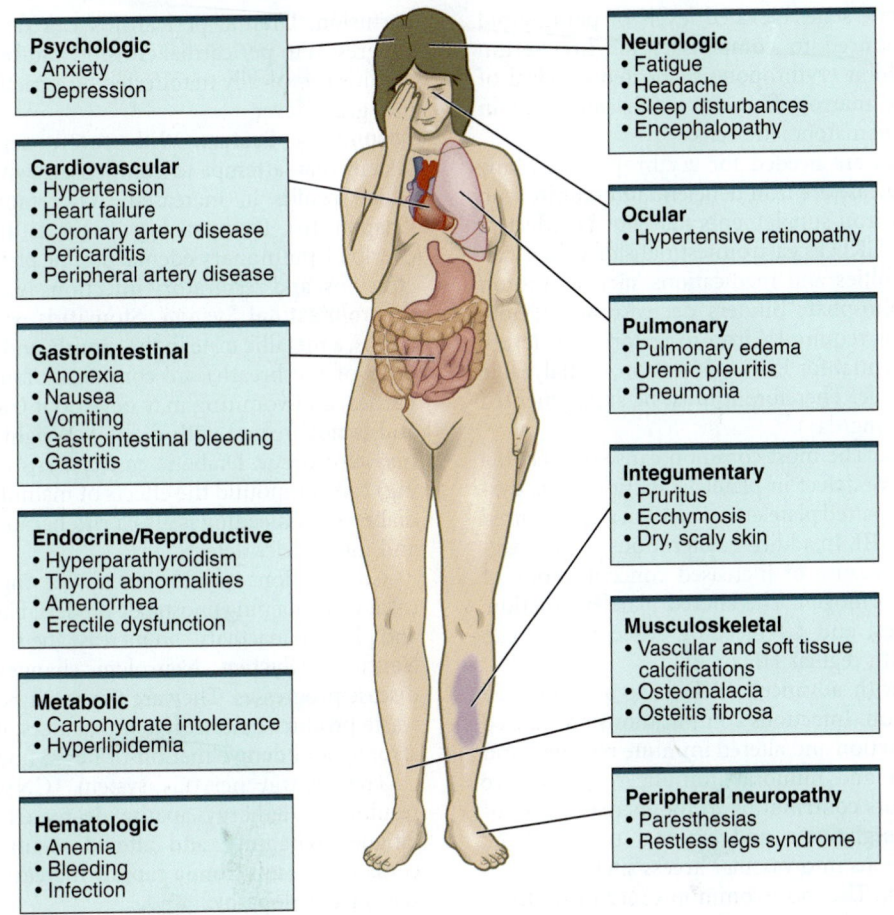

Psychologic
- Anxiety
- Depression

Cardiovascular
- Hypertension
- Heart failure
- Coronary artery disease
- Pericarditis
- Peripheral artery disease

Gastrointestinal
- Anorexia
- Nausea
- Vomiting
- Gastrointestinal bleeding
- Gastritis

Endocrine/Reproductive
- Hyperparathyroidism
- Thyroid abnormalities
- Amenorrhea
- Erectile dysfunction

Metabolic
- Carbohydrate intolerance
- Hyperlipidemia

Hematologic
- Anemia
- Bleeding
- Infection

Neurologic
- Fatigue
- Headache
- Sleep disturbances
- Encephalopathy

Ocular
- Hypertensive retinopathy

Pulmonary
- Pulmonary edema
- Uremic pleuritis
- Pneumonia

Integumentary
- Pruritus
- Ecchymosis
- Dry, scaly skin

Musculoskeletal
- Vascular and soft tissue calcifications
- Osteomalacia
- Osteitis fibrosa

Peripheral neuropathy
- Paresthesias
- Restless legs syndrome

FIG. 46-2   Possible clinical manifestations of chronic kidney disease.

less insulin therapy when they start dialysis and their kidney disease progresses. Insulin dosing must be individualized and glucose levels monitored carefully.

Elevated Triglycerides. Hyperinsulinemia stimulates hepatic production of triglycerides. Many patients with uremia develop dyslipidemia, with increased very-low-density lipoproteins (VLDLs), increased low-density lipoproteins (LDLs), and decreased high-density lipoproteins (HDLs). The altered lipid metabolism is related to decreased levels of the enzyme lipoprotein lipase, which is important in the breakdown of lipoproteins. Most patients with CKD die from CV disease.[17]

Electrolyte and Acid-Base Imbalances

Potassium. Hyperkalemia is a serious electrolyte disorder associated with kidney failure. Fatal dysrhythmias have been reported when the serum potassium level reaches 7 to 8 mEq/L (7 to 8 mmol/L). Hyperkalemia results from the decreased excretion of potassium by the kidneys, the breakdown of cellular protein, bleeding, and metabolic acidosis. Potassium may also come from foods, dietary supplements, drugs, and IV infusions.

Sodium. Sodium may be elevated, normal, or low in kidney disease. Because of impaired sodium excretion, sodium along with water is retained. If large quantities of water are retained, dilutional hyponatremia occurs. Sodium retention can contribute to edema, hypertension, and HF. Sodium intake must be individually determined but is generally restricted to 2 g/day.

Calcium and Phosphate. Calcium and phosphate alterations are discussed in the section on the musculoskeletal system on pp. 1078-1079.

Magnesium. Magnesium is primarily excreted by the kidneys. Hypermagnesemia is generally not a problem unless the patient is ingesting magnesium (e.g., milk of magnesia, magnesium citrate, antacids containing magnesium). Clinical manifestations of hypermagnesemia can include absence of reflexes, decreased mental status, cardiac dysrhythmias, hypotension, and respiratory failure.

Metabolic Acidosis. Metabolic acidosis results from the kidneys' impaired ability to excrete excess acid and from defective reabsorption and regeneration of bicarbonate. The average adult produces 80 to 90 mEq of acid per day. This acid is normally buffered by bicarbonate. In kidney disease, plasma bicarbonate, which is an indirect measure of acidosis, usually falls to a new steady state at around 16 to 20 mEq/L (16 to 20 mmol/L). The decreased plasma bicarbonate reflects its use in buffering metabolic acids. The bicarbonate level generally does not progress below this level because hydrogen ion production is usually balanced by buffering from demineralization of the bone (the phosphate buffering system).

Hematologic System

Anemia. A normocytic, normochromic anemia is associated with CKD. Anemia in CKD is due to decreased production of the hormone erythropoietin by the kidneys. Erythropoietin normally stimulates precursor cells in the bone marrow to produce RBCs (erythropoiesis). Other factors contributing to anemia are nutritional deficiencies, decreased RBC life span, increased hemolysis of RBCs, frequent blood samplings, and bleeding from the GI tract. For patients receiving maintenance hemodialysis (HD), blood loss in the dialyzer may also contribute to the anemic state. Elevated levels of parathyroid hormone (PTH) (produced to compensate for low serum calcium levels) can inhibit erythropoiesis, shorten survival of RBCs, and cause bone marrow fibrosis, which can result in decreased numbers of hematopoietic cells.

Sufficient iron stores are needed for erythropoiesis. Many patients with kidney disease are iron deficient and require iron supplementation. Oral iron supplements may not be effective for the individual with CKD as gastrointestinal side effects can cause adherence difficulties and medications such as proton pump inhibitors or phosphate binders decrease absorption. Patients on dialysis may require IV iron to restore iron levels. Folic acid, which is essential for RBC maturation, is dialyzable because it is water soluble. Therefore it must be supplemented in the diet (folic acid 1 mg/day).[18]

Bleeding Tendencies. The most common cause of bleeding in uremia is a qualitative defect in platelet function. This dysfunction is caused by impaired platelet aggregation and impaired release of platelet factor III. In addition, alterations in the coagulation system occur because of increased concentrations of both factor VIII and fibrinogen. The altered platelet function, hemorrhagic tendencies, and GI bleeding susceptibility can usually be corrected with regular HD or PD.

Infection. Patients with advanced CKD have an increased susceptibility to infection. Infectious complications are caused by changes in WBC function and altered immune response and function. Both cellular and humoral immune responses are suppressed. Other factors contributing to the increased risk of infection include hyperglycemia and external trauma (e.g., catheters, needle insertions into vascular access sites).

Cardiovascular System. The most common cause of death in patients with CKD is CV disease. Leading causes of death are myocardial infarction, ischemic heart disease, peripheral arterial disease, HF, cardiomyopathy, and stroke.[17] CV disease and CKD are so closely linked that if patients develop cardiac events (e.g., myocardial infarction, HF), kidney function is evaluated. Traditional CV risk factors such as hypertension and elevated lipids are common in CKD patients.

CV disease may also be related to nontraditional CV risk factors such as vascular calcification and arterial stiffness. The calcium deposits in the vascular medial layer are associated with stiffening of the blood vessels. The mechanisms involved are multifactorial. They include (1) vascular smooth muscle cells changing into chondrocytes or osteoblast-like cells, (2) high total body amount of calcium and phosphate resulting from abnormal bone metabolism, (3) impaired renal excretion, and (4) drug therapies to treat the bone disease (e.g., calcium phosphate binders).[19]

Hypertension, which is prevalent in patients with CKD, is both a cause and a consequence of CKD. Hypertension is aggravated by sodium retention and increased extracellular fluid volume.[20] In some individuals, increased renin production contributes to hypertension (see Fig. 44-4). Hypertension and diabetes mellitus are contributing risk factors for vascular complications.[21] Long-standing hypertension, extracellular fluid volume overload, and anemia contribute to development of left ventricular hypertrophy that may eventually lead to cardiomyopathy and HF. Hypertension can cause retinopathy, encephalopathy, and nephropathy. Because of the many effects of hypertension, BP control is one of the most important therapeutic goals in the management of CKD.

Patients with CKD are susceptible to cardiac dysrhythmias that result from hyperkalemia and decreased coronary artery perfusion. Uremic pericarditis can develop and occasionally progresses to pericardial effusion and cardiac tamponade. Pericarditis is typically manifested by a friction rub, chest pain, and low-grade fever.

Respiratory System. With severe acidosis, the respiratory system may attempt to compensate with Kussmaul breathing, which results in increased CO_2 removal by exhalation (see Chapter 16). Dyspnea may occur as a manifestation of fluid overload, pulmonary edema, uremic pleuritis (pleurisy), pleural effusions, and respiratory infections (e.g., pneumonia).

Gastrointestinal System. Stomatitis with exudates and ulcerations, a metallic taste in the mouth, and *uremic fetor* (a urinous odor of the breath) are commonly found in CKD. Anorexia, nausea, and vomiting may develop if CKD progresses to ESRD and is not treated with dialysis. Weight loss and malnutrition may also occur. Diabetic *gastroparesis* (delayed gastric emptying) can compound the effects of malnutrition for patients with diabetes. GI bleeding is also a risk because of mucosal irritation and the platelet defect.

Constipation may be due to the ingestion of iron salts or calcium-containing phosphate binders. Limitations on fluid intake and physical inactivity can increase the risk of constipation.

Neurologic System. Neurologic changes are expected as kidney disease progresses. They are the result of increased nitrogenous waste products, electrolyte imbalances, metabolic acidosis, and atrophy and demyelination of nerve fibers.

The central nervous system (CNS) becomes depressed, resulting in lethargy, apathy, decreased ability to concentrate, fatigue, irritability, and altered mental ability. Seizures and coma may result from a rapidly increasing BUN and hypertensive encephalopathy.

Peripheral neuropathy is initially manifested by a slowing of nerve conduction to the extremities. Individuals with advanced stage 5 CKD may complain of restless legs syndrome (see Chapter 58), described as "bugs crawling inside the leg." Paresthesias are most often experienced in the feet and legs and may be described by the patient as a burning sensation. Eventually, motor involvement may lead to bilateral footdrop, muscular weakness and atrophy, and loss of deep tendon reflexes. Muscle twitching, jerking, *asterixis* (hand-flapping tremor), and nocturnal leg cramps may occur. In patients with diabetic neuropathy, symptoms can be compounded by uremic neuropathy.[21]

Dialysis should improve general CNS manifestations and may slow or halt the progression of neuropathies. Motor neuropathy may not be reversible. The treatment for neurologic problems is dialysis or transplantation. Altered mental status, a late manifestation of CKD stage 5, rarely occurs unless the patient has chosen not to have renal replacement therapy.

Musculoskeletal System. CKD mineral and bone disorder (CKD-MBD) develops as a systemic disorder of mineral and bone metabolism caused by progressive deterioration in kidney function (Fig. 46-3). Activated vitamin D is necessary to optimize absorption of calcium from the GI tract. As kidney function deteriorates, less vitamin D is converted to its active form, resulting in decreased serum levels. Low levels of active vitamin D result in decreased serum calcium levels.[19]

Serum calcium levels are regulated primarily by parathyroid hormone (PTH). When hypocalcemia occurs, the parathyroid gland secretes PTH, which stimulates bone demineralization, releasing calcium from the bones. Phosphate is released as well, leading to elevated serum phosphate levels. Hyperphosphatemia also results from decreased phosphate excretion by the

PATHOPHYSIOLOGY MAP

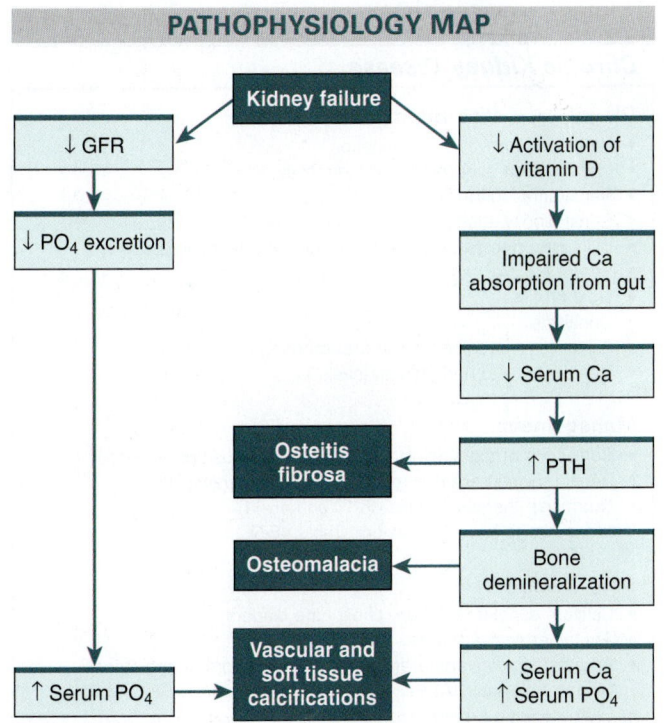

FIG. 46-3 Mechanisms of chronic kidney disease mineral and bone disorder (CKD-MBD). *GFR,* Glomerular filtration rate; *PTH,* parathyroid hormone.

kidneys. Hyperphosphatemia decreases serum calcium levels and further reduces the kidneys' ability to activate vitamin D.

Low serum calcium, elevated phosphate, and decreased vitamin D contribute to the stimulation of the parathyroid gland and excretion of PTH. PTH acts on the bone to increase remodeling and increase serum calcium levels. The accelerated rate of bone remodeling causes a weakened bone matrix and places the patient at a higher risk for fractures. Normally plasma calcium is found ionized or free (physiologically active form) or bound to protein.

A low ionized calcium level can lead to tetany (see Chapter 16). However, in kidney failure, it is unusual for hypocalcemia to be symptomatic. In the acidotic state associated with kidney failure, more calcium is in the ionized form than is bound to protein.

CKD-MBD is a common complication of CKD and results in skeletal complications, vascular and soft tissue (extraskeletal) complications. Skeletal complications include (1) *osteomalacia* (results from demineralization from slow bone turnover and defective mineralization of newly formed bone) and (2) *osteitis fibrosa* (decalcification of the bone and replacement of bone tissue with fibrous tissue).

Soft tissue complications result from vascular calcifications. Vascular calcifications are a significant contributing factor to CV disease. "Uremic red eye" is caused by the irritation from calcium deposits in the eye. Intracardiac calcifications can disrupt the conduction system and cause cardiac arrest.

Integumentary System. A small percentage of patients develop refractory pruritus that can have a devastating impact on their well-being and quality of life. Pruritus has multiple causes, including dry skin, calcium-phosphate deposition in the skin, and sensory neuropathy. Pruritus is more prevalent in patients receiving dialysis than in the earlier stages of CKD. The itching may be so intense that it can lead to bleeding or infection secondary to scratching. Uremic frost is an extremely rare condition in which urea crystallizes on the skin; this is usually seen only when BUN levels are extremely elevated (e.g., over 200 mg/dL).

Reproductive System. Both men and women can experience infertility and a decreased libido. Women usually have decreased levels of estrogen, progesterone, and luteinizing hormone, causing anovulation and menstrual changes (usually amenorrhea). Menses and ovulation may return after dialysis is started. Men experience loss of testicular consistency, decreased testosterone levels, and low sperm counts.

Sexual dysfunction may also be caused by anemia, which causes fatigue and decreased libido. In addition, peripheral neuropathy can cause impotence in men and anorgasmy in women. Additional factors that may cause changes in sexual function are psychologic problems (e.g., anxiety, depression), physical stress, and side effects of medications. Sexual function may improve with maintenance dialysis and may become normal with successful transplantation.

Patients who become pregnant while receiving dialysis have been able to carry a fetus to term, but there is significant risk to the mother and infant. Pregnancy in patients with a kidney transplant is more common, but there is still considerable risk to both the mother and fetus.

Psychologic Changes. Personality and behavioral changes, emotional lability, withdrawal, and depression are commonly observed in patients with CKD. Fatigue and lethargy contribute to the feeling of illness. The changes in body image caused by edema, integumentary disturbances, and access devices (e.g., fistulas, catheters) may lead to anxiety and depression. Decreased ability to concentrate and slowed mental activity can give the appearance of dullness and disinterest in the environment. The patient must also deal with significant changes in lifestyle, occupation, family responsibilities, and financial status. Long-term survival depends on medications, dietary restrictions, dialysis, and possibly transplantation. The patient also grieves the loss of kidney function and independence.

Diagnostic Studies

Because persistent proteinuria is usually the first indication of kidney damage, screening for CKD involves a dipstick evaluation of protein in the urine or evaluation for albuminuria, which is not detected with routine urinalysis. The urine of patients with diabetes must be examined for albuminuria if no protein is detected on routine urinalysis. A person with persistent proteinuria (1+ protein on standard dipstick testing two or more times over a 3-month period) should have further assessment of risk factors and a diagnostic workup with blood and urine tests to evaluate for CKD.

A urinalysis can detect RBCs, WBCs, protein, casts, and glucose. An ultrasound of the kidneys is usually done to detect any obstructions and determine the size of the kidneys. Other diagnostic studies (Table 46-7) help establish the diagnosis and cause of CKD. A kidney biopsy may be necessary to provide a definitive diagnosis.

Serum creatinine alone poorly reflects kidney function. GFR is the preferred measure to determine kidney function. Several GFR calculators are available. The two equations used most frequently to estimate GFR are the Cockcroft-Gault formula and Modification of Diet in Renal Disease (MDRD) Study equation (Table 46-8). MDRD is the preferred method.[22]

Interprofessional Care

The overall goals of CKD therapy are to preserve existing kidney function, reduce the risks of CV disease, prevent

EVIDENCE-BASED PRACTICE
Translating Research Into Practice

Do Nonpharmacologic Interventions Improve Sleep in Dialysis Patients?
Clinical Question
Among patients with end-stage renal disease on dialysis (P), what is the effect of cognitive behavioral therapy, physical exercise, and acupressure (I) versus control group (C) on sleep quality (O)?

Synthesis of Best Available Evidence
- Systematic review of randomized controlled trials (RCTs) and one prospective cohort study.
- 13 studies of patients (*n* = 1518) with end-stage renal disease dependent on dialysis. Interventions included cognitive behavioral therapy (CBT), physical exercise, and acupressure. Control groups included sleep hygiene and usual care. Outcome was sleep quality.
- Sleep latency and sleep disturbance improved with CBT. Sleep medication use declined with CBT.
- Aerobic exercise during dialysis may improve sleep quality for patients who also have restless leg syndrome.
- Trend was noted for CBT and improved daytime functioning and subjective sleep quality.
- Although acupressure appears promising to help with sleep, there are some concerns regarding the methodological quality of the studies.

Conclusion
- Nonpharmacologic interventions such as cognitive behavioral therapy (CBT), physical exercise, and acupressure can improve sleep quality in dialysis patients.

Implications for Nursing Practice
1. Why is it important to assess sleep quality in patients on dialysis who report poor quality of life?
2. How would you assist a patient who is on dialysis and experiencing sleep problems at night?
3. When sleep medications are minimally effective, what information would you share with a patient related to nonpharmacologic treatments?

Reference for Evidence
Yang B, Xy J, Xue Q, et al: Non-pharmacological interventions for improving sleep quality in patients on dialysis: systematic review and meta-analysis, *Sleep Med Rev* 23:68, 2015.

P, Patient population of interest; *I*, intervention or area of interest; *C*, comparison of interest or comparison group; *O*, outcomes of interest; *T*, timing (see p. 15).

TABLE 46-7 Interprofessional Care
Chronic Kidney Disease

Diagnostic Assessment
- History and physical examination
- Identification of reversible kidney disease
- Renal ultrasound, renal scan, CT scan
- Renal biopsy
- BUN, serum creatinine, and creatinine clearance levels
- Serum electrolytes
- Lipid profile
- Urinalysis
- Protein-to-creatinine ratio in first morning voided specimen
- Hematocrit and hemoglobin levels

Management
- Correction of extracellular fluid volume overload or deficit
- Renal replacement therapy (dialysis, kidney transplant)
- Nutritional therapy (Tables 46-10 and 46-11)
- Measures to lower potassium (Table 46-5)

Drug Therapy
- Calcium supplementation, phosphate binders, or both
- Antihypertensive therapy
- Angiotensin-converting enzyme (ACE) inhibitors or angiotensin receptor blockers (ARBs)
- Erythropoietin therapy
- Lipid-lowering drugs
- Adjustment of drug dosages to degree of renal function

TABLE 46-8 Indicators of Kidney Function

This example shows why serum creatinine alone is a poor indicator of kidney function. Calculation of GFR is considered the best index to estimate kidney function as indicated by the following example.

Estimation of GFR	TYPE OF PATIENT	
	76-Yr-Old African American Woman (Weight 56 kg)	28-Yr-Old African American Man (Weight 74 kg)
Serum creatinine	1.4 mg/dL	1.4 mg/dL
GFR, estimated by the Cockcroft-Gault formula*	30.2 mL/min	82.2 mL/min
GFR, estimated by MDRD equation†	47 mL/min/1.73 m²	64 mL/min/1.73 m²

Cr, Creatinine; *GFR*, glomerular filtration rate; *MDRD*, modification of diet in renal disease.
*Cockcroft-Gault GFR = $(140 - Age) \times (Weight\ in\ kilograms) \times (0.85\ if\ female)/(72 \times Cr)$.
†GFR as estimated by MDRD equation calculator can be accessed at *www.mdrd.com*.

Drug Therapy
Hyperkalemia. Multiple strategies are used to manage hyperkalemia (Table 46-5), including the restriction of high-potassium foods and drugs. Acute hyperkalemia may require treatment with IV glucose and insulin or IV 10% calcium gluconate.

Sodium polystyrene sulfonate, a cation-exchange resin, is commonly used to lower potassium levels in stage 4 CKD and can be administered on an outpatient basis. Sodium polystyrene sulfonate has an osmotic laxative action and ensures evacuation of the potassium from the bowel. Tell the patient to expect some diarrhea. Never give sodium polystyrene sulfonate to a patient with a hypoactive bowel (paralytic ileus) because fluid shifts could lead to bowel necrosis. As sodium polystyrene sulfonate exchanges sodium ions for potassium ions, observe the patient

---

complications, and provide for the patient's comfort (Table 46-9). Early recognition, diagnosis, and treatment can prevent the progression of kidney disease. It is important that patients with CKD receive appropriate referral to a nephrologist early in the course of the disease. Every effort is made to detect and treat potentially reversible causes of kidney failure (e.g., HF, dehydration, infections, nephrotoxins, urinary tract obstruction, glomerulonephritis, renal artery stenosis).

Patients with CKD have a high incidence of CV complications. A higher percentage of patients will die from CV disease than live to need dialysis. When a patient is diagnosed as having CKD, therapy is aimed at treating the CV disease in addition to slowing the progression of kidney disease (Table 46-7).

A focus on stages 1 through 4 (Table 46-6) before the need for dialysis (stage 5) includes the control of hypertension, hyperparathyroid disease, CKD-MBD, anemia, and dyslipidemia. The following section focuses primarily on the drug and nutritional aspects of care.

TABLE 46-9 Risk Factors for Chronic Kidney Disease

Risk Factors	Prevention and Management
Diabetes	Achieve optimal glycemic control.
Hypertension	Maintain BP in normal range with angiotensin-converting enzyme (ACE) inhibitors or angiotensin receptor blockers (ARBs).
Age >60 yr	Prevent insult or injury to kidneys.
Cardiovascular disease	Institute aggressive risk factor reduction.
Family history of CKD	Teach about increased risk and assist with appropriate screening (BP measurement, urinalysis).
Exposure to nephrotoxic drugs	Limit exposure and give sodium bicarbonate as treatment.
Ethnic minority (e.g., African American, Native American)	Teach about increased risk and assist with appropriate screening (BP measurement, urinalysis).

for sodium and water retention. If changes appear in the ECG such as peaked T waves and widened QRS complexes, dialysis may be required to remove excess potassium.

Patiromer (Veltassa) is an oral suspension that binds potassium in the GI tract and is used to treat hyperkalemia in individuals with CKD. It should not be used in emergency situations to treat hyperkalemia because of its delayed onset of action. Because this drug can also bind other oral medications, it needs to be given at least 6 hours before or 6 hours after other oral medications.

Hypertension. For some, the progression of CKD can be delayed by controlling hypertension. (Control and treatment of hypertension are discussed in Chapter 32.) Treatment of hypertension includes (1) weight loss (if indicated), (2) therapeutic lifestyle changes (e.g., exercise, avoidance of alcohol, smoking cessation), (3) diet recommendations (DASH Diet), and (4) administration of antihypertensive drugs. Most patients require two or more drugs to reach target BP.

Prescribed medications depend on whether the patient with CKD has diabetes. The ACE inhibitors and ARBs are used with patients with diabetes and those with nondiabetic proteinuria because they decrease proteinuria and possibly delay the progression of CKD. These medications must be used with caution as they can further decrease the GFR and increase serum potassium levels.

Measure the BP with the patient in the supine, sitting, and standing positions to monitor the effect of antihypertensive drugs. Teach the patient and caregiver how to monitor the BP at home and what readings require immediate intervention.

CKD-MBD. It is difficult to determine what type of bone disease a patient may have by just looking at the serum levels of calcium, phosphorus, PTH, and alkaline phosphatase. The gold standard for diagnosis is a bone biopsy.

Interventions for CKD-MBD include limiting dietary phosphorus, administering phosphate binders, supplementing vitamin D, and controlling hyperparathyroidism.[19] Phosphate intake is not usually restricted until the patient requires RRT. At that time, phosphate is usually limited to about 1 g/day, but dietary control alone is usually inadequate.

Phosphate binders include calcium-based binders: calcium acetate and calcium carbonate. They bind phosphate in the bowel and then are excreted in the stool. The administration of calcium may increase the calcium load and place the patient at increased risk for vascular calcifications. Therefore when calcium levels are increased or there is evidence of existing vascular or soft tissue calcifications, non–calcium-based phosphate binders may be used. These include lanthanum carbonate (Fosrenol), sevelamer carbonate (Renvela), and iron-based, calcium-free phosphate binders such as sucroferric oxyhydroxide (Velphoro) and ferric citrate (Auryxia).

To be most effective, administer phosphate binders with each meal. Constipation is a frequent side effect of phosphate binders, and stool softeners may be needed.

Because bone disease (osteomalacia) is associated with excess aluminum, aluminum preparations should be used with caution in patients with kidney disease. Do not use magnesium-containing antacids (e.g., Maalox, Mylanta) because magnesium depends on the kidneys for excretion.

Hypocalcemia is a problem in the later stages of CKD because of the inability of the GI tract to absorb calcium in the absence of active vitamin D. If hypocalcemia persists even if the serum phosphate levels are normal, then supplemental calcium and vitamin D should be given. Assess vitamin D levels to determine the need for supplementation. If the levels are low (serum values less than 30 ng/mL), vitamin D supplementation is recommended in the form of cholecalciferol.

Treatment of secondary hyperparathyroidism in ESRD patients requires the activated form of vitamin D because the kidneys no longer possess the ability to activate vitamin D. Active vitamin D is available as oral or IV calcitriol (Rocaltrol), IV paricalcitol (Zemplar), or oral or IV doxercalciferol (Hectorol), and can reduce the elevated levels of PTH. Cinacalcet (Sensipar), a calcimimetic agent, is used to control secondary hyperparathyroidism. Calcimimetics mimic calcium and increase the sensitivity of the calcium receptors in the parathyroid glands. As a result, the parathyroid glands detect calcium at lower serum levels and decrease PTH secretion.

If hyperparathyroid disease becomes severe despite medical management, a subtotal or total parathyroidectomy may be performed to decrease the synthesis and secretion of PTH. In most cases, a total parathyroidectomy is performed and parathyroid tissue is transplanted into the forearm. The transplanted cells produce PTH as needed. If production of PTH becomes excessive, some of the cells can be removed from the forearm.

Hypercalcemia may occur with calcium and vitamin D supplementation. If hypercalcemia occurs, vitamin D may be withheld and calcium-based phosphate binders replaced with noncalcium-based phosphate binders.

Anemia. Anemia in CKD is caused by a decreased production of erythropoietin by the kidneys. Exogenous erythropoietin (EPO) is used to treat anemia. It is available as epoetin alfa (Epogen, Procrit), which can be administered IV or subcutaneously, usually two or three times per week. Darbepoetin alfa (Aranesp) is longer acting and can be administered weekly or biweekly.

Hemoglobin and hematocrit levels may take 2 to 3 weeks to increase. Higher hemoglobin levels (more than 12 g/dL) and higher doses of EPO are associated with a higher rate of thromboembolic events and increased risk of death from serious CV events (heart attack, HF, stroke). The recommendation is to use the lowest possible dose of EPO to treat anemia.

Treatment of CKD-related anemia should be individualized with the goal being to reduce the need for blood transfusions.

There is no target hemoglobin or widely accepted EPO dosing strategy. Teach people who are prescribed EPO about the risks and benefits and allow them to make a decision regarding their treatment plan.

EPO can increase BP and is contraindicated in uncontrolled hypertension. The underlying mechanism is related to the hemodynamic changes (e.g., increased whole blood viscosity) that occurs as the anemia is corrected.

EPO therapy may lead to the development of iron deficiency from the increased demand for iron to support erythropoiesis. Iron supplementation is recommended if the plasma ferritin concentrations fall below 100 ng/mL. Most CKD patients receive iron supplementation.

Although iron can be administered by mouth or IV, the enteral route is limited due to GI side effects, which decrease patient adherence. Oral iron should not be taken at the same time as phosphate binders because calcium binds the iron, preventing its absorption. Tell the patient that iron may make the stool dark in color. Most patients receiving HD are prescribed IV iron sucrose injection (Venofer) or sodium ferric gluconate complex in sucrose injection (Ferrlecit). Supplemental folic acid (1 mg/day) is usually given because it is needed for RBC formation and is removed by dialysis.

Blood transfusions should be avoided in treating anemia unless the patient experiences an acute blood loss or has symptomatic anemia (i.e., dyspnea, excess fatigue, tachycardia, palpitations, chest pain). Transfusions increase the development of antibodies, thus making it more difficult to find a compatible donor for kidney transplantation. Multiple blood transfusions may lead to iron overload because each unit of blood contains about 250 mg of iron.

Dyslipidemia. Dyslipidemia, a risk factor for CV disease, is a common problem in CKD. Statins (HMG-CoA reductase inhibitors), such as atorvastatin (Lipitor), are used to lower LDL cholesterol levels (see Table 33-5). Statins should be used in patients with CKD (especially patients with diabetes) not yet on dialysis.

Fibrates (fibric acid derivatives), such as gemfibrozil (Lopid), are used to lower triglyceride levels (see Table 33-5) and can also increase HDLs. Specific drugs used in these classes depend on the individual patient response and HCP recommendation.

Complications of Drug Therapy. Many drugs are partially or totally excreted by the kidneys. CKD causes decreased elimination that leads to an accumulation of drugs and the potential for drug toxicity. Drug doses and frequency of administration are adjusted based on the severity of the kidney disease. Increased sensitivity may result as drug levels increase in the blood and tissues. Drugs of particular concern include digoxin, diabetic agents (metformin, glyburide), antibiotics (e.g., vancomycin, gentamicin), and opioid medications.

Nutritional Therapy

Protein Restriction. The current diet for the individual with CKD is designed to maintain good nutrition (Table 46-10). Calorie-protein malnutrition is a potential and serious problem that results from altered metabolism, anemia, proteinuria, anorexia, and nausea. Additional factors leading to malnutrition include depression and complex diets that restrict protein, phosphorus, potassium, and sodium. Frequent monitoring of laboratory parameters, especially serum albumin, prealbumin (may be a better indicator of recent or current nutritional status than albumin), and ferritin, and anthropometric measurements are necessary to evaluate nutritional status. All patients with CKD should be referred to a dietitian for nutritional teaching.

For the patient who is undergoing dialysis, protein is not routinely restricted (Table 46-10). For CKD stages 1 through 4, many HCPs encourage a diet with normal protein intake. Teach patients to avoid high-protein diets and supplements because they may overburden the diseased kidneys.[23]

Dietary protein guidelines for PD differ from those for HD because of protein loss through the peritoneal membrane. During PD, protein intake must be high enough to compensate for the losses so that the nitrogen balance is maintained. The recommended protein intake is at least 1.2 g/kg of ideal body weight (IBW) per day. This can be increased depending on the patient's individual needs.

For patients with malnutrition or inadequate caloric or protein intake, commercially prepared products that are high in protein but low in sodium and potassium are available (e.g., Nepro, Amin-Aid). As an alternative, liquid or powder breakfast drinks may be purchased at the grocery store.

Fluid Restriction. Water and any other fluids are not routinely restricted in patients with CKD stages 1 to 5 who are not receiving HD. In an effort to reduce fluid retention, diuretics are often used. Patients on HD have a more restricted fluid intake than patients receiving PD. For those receiving HD, as their urine output diminishes, fluids are restricted. Recommended fluid intake depends on the daily urine output. Generally, 600 mL (from insensible loss) plus an amount equal to the

---

TABLE 46-10   Nutritional Therapy

Chronic Kidney Disease*

	Pre-ESRD	Hemodialysis	Peritoneal Dialysis
Fluid allowance	As desired or depends on urine output	Urine output plus 600-1000 mL	Unrestricted if weight and BP controlled and residual renal function
Calories	30-35 kcal/kg/day	30-35 kcal/kg/day	25-35 kcal/kg/day (includes calories from dialysate glucose absorption)
Protein	Individualized or 0.6-1.0 g/kg/day (low protein)	1.2 g/kg/day	1.2-1.3 g/kg/day
Sodium	Individualized or 1-3 g/day	Individualized or 2-3 g/day	Individualized or 2-4 g/day
Potassium	Individualized based on laboratory values	Individualized or about 2-4 g/day	Usually not restricted
Phosphorus	Individualized or 1.0-1.8 g/day	Individualized or about 0.6-1.2 g/day	Individualized or about 0.6-1.2 g/day
Calcium	About 1000-1500 mg/day	Individualized	Individualized
Iron	Supplement recommended if receiving erythropoietin	Supplement recommended if receiving erythropoietin	Supplement recommended if receiving erythropoietin

*Diets must be individualized in accordance with needs.

TABLE 46-11 Nutritional Therapy

High-Potassium Foods*

Fruits	Vegetables	Other Foods
• Apricot, raw (medium)	• Baked beans	• Bran or bran products
• Avocado (¼ whole)	• Butternut squash	• Chocolate (1.5-2 oz)
• Banana (¼ whole)	• Refried beans	• Granola
• Cantaloupe	• Black beans	• Milk, all types (1 cup)
• Dried fruits	• Broccoli, cooked	• Nutritional supplements (use only under the direction of physician or dietitian)
• Grapefruit juice	• Carrots, raw	
• Honeydew	• Greens, except kale	
• Orange (medium)	• Mushrooms, canned	• Nuts and seeds (1 oz)
• Orange juice	• Potatoes, white and sweet	• Peanut butter (2 Tbsp)
• Prunes	• Spinach, cooked	• Salt substitutes, Lite Salt
• Raisins	• Tomatoes or tomato products	• Salt-free broth
	• Vegetable juices	• Yogurt

*Contain at least 200 mg/portion. Portion = ½ cup unless otherwise noted.
Source: National Kidney Foundation: Potassium and your CKD diet. www.kidney.org/atoz/content/potassium.cfm.

previous day's urine output is allowed for a patient receiving HD.

Foods that are liquid at room temperature (e.g., gelatin, ice) should be counted as fluid intake. The fluid allotment should be spaced throughout the day so that the patient does not become thirsty. Patients are advised to limit fluid intake so that weight gains are no more than 1 to 3 kg between dialyses (*interdialytic weight gain*).

Sodium and Potassium Restriction. Patients with CKD are advised to restrict sodium. Sodium-restricted diets may vary from 2 to 4 g/day. Instruct the patient to avoid high-sodium foods, such as cured meats, pickled foods, canned soups and stews, frankfurters, cold cuts, soy sauce, and salad dressings (see Chapter 34, Table 34-8). Potassium restriction depends on the kidneys' ability to excrete potassium. Salt substitutes should be avoided in potassium-restricted diets because they contain potassium chloride.

Dietary restrictions for potassium range from about 2 to 3 g (39 mg = 1 mEq). Teach patients receiving HD which foods are high in potassium and to avoid them (Table 46-11). Patients using PD do not usually need potassium restrictions and may even be prescribed oral potassium supplementation because of the loss of potassium with dialysis exchanges.

Phosphate Restriction. As kidney function deteriorates, phosphate elimination by the kidneys is diminished and the patient begins to develop hyperphosphatemia. By the time a patient reaches ESRD, phosphate is limited to approximately 1 g/day. Foods that are high in phosphate include meat, dairy products (e.g., milk, ice cream, cheese, yogurt), and foods containing dairy products (e.g., pudding). Many foods that are high in phosphate are also high in protein. Since patients on dialysis are encouraged to eat a diet containing protein, phosphate binders are essential to control the phosphate level.

❖ NURSING MANAGEMENT: CHRONIC KIDNEY DISEASE

◆ Nursing Assessment

Obtain a complete history of any existing kidney disease or family history of kidney disease. Some kidney disorders, including Alport syndrome and polycystic kidney disease,

have a genetic component. Other disorders that can lead to CKD are diabetes mellitus, hypertension, and systemic lupus erythematosus.

Because many drugs are potentially nephrotoxic, ask the patient about both current and past use of prescription and over-the-counter drugs and herbal preparations. Decongestants and antihistamines that contain pseudoephedrine and phenylephrine cause vasoconstriction and lead to an increase in BP. Magnesium and aluminum from antacids can accumulate in the body because they cannot be excreted. Some antacids contain high levels of salt, contributing to hypertension. In addition, antacids may interfere with the absorption of other medications.

NSAIDs (aspirin, ibuprofen, naproxen) can contribute to the development of AKI and progression of CKD, especially when taken in higher doses than recommended. If taken as prescribed, these analgesics are usually considered safe.

Assess the patient's dietary habits and discuss any problems regarding intake. Measure the patient's height and weight, and evaluate any recent weight changes.

The chronicity of kidney disease and the long-term treatment affect virtually every area of a person's life, including family relationships, social and work activities, self-image, and emotional state. Assess the patient's support systems. The choice of treatment modality may be related to support systems available.

◆ Nursing Diagnoses

Nursing diagnoses for CKD may include, but are not limited to, the following:

- Excess fluid volume *related to* impaired kidney function
- Risk for electrolyte imbalance *related to* impaired kidney function resulting in hyperkalemia, hypocalcemia, hyperphosphatemia, and altered vitamin D metabolism
- Imbalanced nutrition: less than body requirements *related to* restricted intake of nutrients (especially protein), nausea, vomiting, anorexia, and stomatitis

Additional information on nursing diagnoses for the patient with CKD is presented in eNursing Care Plan 46-1 (available on the website for this chapter).

◆ Planning

The overall goals are that a patient with CKD will (1) demonstrate knowledge of and ability to comply with the therapeutic regimen, (2) participate in decision making for the plan of care and future treatment modality, (3) demonstrate effective coping strategies, and (4) continue with activities of daily living within physiologic limitations.

◆ Nursing Implementation

◆ **Health Promotion.** Identify individuals at risk for CKD. At-risk individuals include those diagnosed with diabetes or hypertension and people with a history (or a family history) of kidney disease or repeated urinary tract infections. These individuals should have regular checkups that include a routine urinalysis and calculation of the estimated GFR.

People with diabetes need to have their urine checked for albuminuria if routine urinalysis is negative for protein. Advise patients with diabetes to report any changes in urine appearance (color, odor), frequency, or volume to the HCP. If a patient needs a potentially nephrotoxic drug, it is important to monitor kidney function with serum creatinine and BUN and GFR.

HEALTHY PEOPLE

Prevention and Detection of Chronic Kidney Disease

- Early detection and treatment are the primary methods for reducing chronic kidney disease.
- Monitor BP to detect elevations so that treatment can be started early.
- Treat hypertension appropriately and aggressively, since it is the second leading cause of chronic kidney disease.
- Ensure proper diagnosis and treatment of diabetes mellitus, since it is the leading cause of chronic kidney disease.

Individuals identified at risk must take measures to prevent or delay the progression of CKD. Most important are measures to reduce the risk or progression of CV disease. These include glycemic control for patients with diabetes (see Chapter 48); BP control (see Chapter 32); and lifestyle modifications, including smoking cessation.

◆ **Acute Care.** Most of the care of the patient with CKD occurs on an outpatient basis. In-hospital care is required for management of complications and for kidney transplantation (if applicable).

◆ **Ambulatory Care.** Encourage patients to participate in their care. Teach the patient and caregiver about the diet, drugs, and follow-up medical care (Table 46-12). The patient needs to understand the drugs and common side effects. Because patients with CKD take many medications, a pillbox organizer or a list of the drugs and the times of administration may be helpful. Instruct the patient to avoid over-the-counter medications such as NSAIDs and aluminum- and magnesium-based laxatives and antacids. Teach the patient to take daily BP readings and identify signs and symptoms of fluid overload, hyperkalemia, and other electrolyte imbalances.

TABLE 46-12   Patient & Caregiver Teaching

Chronic Kidney Disease

Include the following information in the teaching plan for the patient and caregiver.

1. Dietary (protein, sodium, potassium, phosphate) and fluid restrictions.
2. Difficulties in modifying diet and fluid intake.
3. Signs and symptoms of electrolyte imbalance, especially high potassium.
4. Alternative ways of reducing thirst, such as sucking on ice cubes, lemon, or hard candy.
5. Rationales for prescribed drugs and common side effects. *Examples:*
   - Phosphate binders (including calcium supplements used as phosphate barriers) should be taken with meals.
   - Calcium supplements prescribed to treat hypocalcemia should be taken on an empty stomach (but not at the same time as iron supplements).
   - Iron supplements should be taken between meals.
6. The importance of reporting any of the following:
   - Weight gain >4 lb (2 kg)
   - Increasing BP
   - Shortness of breath
   - Edema
   - Increasing fatigue or weakness
   - Confusion or lethargy
7. Need for support and encouragement. Share concerns about lifestyle changes, living with a chronic illness, and decisions about type of dialysis or transplantation.

The dietitian should meet with the patient and caregiver on a regular basis for diet planning. A diet history and consideration of cultural variations facilitate diet planning and adherence. The rate of progression of CKD is dependent on the type of kidney disease and presence of other co-morbid conditions. Specific nursing management of the patient with CKD is presented in eNursing Care Plan 46-1.

The patient can complete an evaluation for a kidney transplant prior to the need to initiate dialysis. Patients may receive a transplant before ever having to start dialysis. Even though transplantation offers the best therapeutic management for many ESRD patients, the critical shortage of donor organs limits this treatment option for many patients.

Most patients require either peritoneal dialysis (PD) or hemodialysis (HD). The majority of patients use HD as a modality. Explain to the patient and caregiver what is involved in PD or HD and home hemodialysis modalities, transplantation, and even the option for palliative care. Offer information about all treatment options so that the patient can be involved in the decision-making process, providing a sense of control over life-altering decisions. Inform the patient that even while on dialysis, transplant remains an option. Let the patient know that if a transplanted organ fails, the patient can return to dialysis.

It is important to respect the patient's choice to not receive treatment. Patients themselves often initiate the conversation about palliative care. Focus the discussion on moving from the curative approach to promotion of comfort care and consideration of hospice care. Listen to the patient and caregiver, allowing them to do most of the talking and pay special attention to their hopes and fears. (Palliative and end-of-life care is discussed in Chapter 9.)

◆ **Evaluation**

The expected outcomes are that the patient with CKD will maintain
- Fluid and electrolyte levels within normal ranges
- An acceptable weight with no more than a 10% weight loss
Additional information on expected outcomes is presented in eNursing Care Plan 46-1 (available on the website).

DIALYSIS

Dialysis is the movement of fluid and molecules across a semipermeable membrane from one compartment to another. Clinically, dialysis is a technique in which substances move from the blood through a semipermeable membrane and into a dialysis solution (*dialysate*). It is used to correct fluid and electrolyte imbalances and to remove waste products in kidney failure. It can also be used to treat drug overdoses.

The two methods of dialysis available are **peritoneal dialysis (PD)** and **hemodialysis (HD)** (Table 46-13). In PD the peritoneal membrane acts as the semipermeable membrane. In HD an artificial membrane (usually made of cellulose-based or synthetic materials) is used as the semipermeable membrane and is in contact with the patient's blood.

Dialysis is begun when the patient's uremia can no longer be adequately treated with conservative medical management. Generally dialysis is initiated when the GFR is less than 15 mL/min/1.73 m². This criterion can vary widely in different clinical situations, and the nephrologist determines when to start dialysis based on the patient's clinical status. Certain uremic

TABLE 46-13 Comparison of Peritoneal Dialysis and Hemodialysis

Advantages	Disadvantages
Peritoneal Dialysis (PD)	
• Immediate initiation in almost any hospital	• Bacterial or chemical peritonitis
• Less complicated than hemodialysis	• Protein loss into dialysate
• Portable system with CAPD	• Exit site and tunnel infections
• Fewer dietary restrictions	• Self-image problems with catheter placement
• Relatively short training time	• Hyperglycemia
• Usable in patient with vascular access problems	• Surgery for catheter placement
• Less cardiovascular stress	• Contraindicated in patient with multiple abdominal surgeries, trauma, unrepaired hernia
• Home dialysis possible	• Requires completion of education program
• Preferable for patient with diabetes	• Catheter can migrate
	• Best instituted with willing partner
Hemodialysis (HD)	
• Rapid fluid removal	• Vascular access problems
• Rapid removal of urea and creatinine	• Dietary and fluid restrictions
• Effective potassium removal	• Heparinization may be necessary
• Less protein loss	• Extensive equipment necessary
• Lowering of serum triglycerides	• Hypotension during dialysis
• Home dialysis possible	• Added blood loss that contributes to anemia
• Temporary access can be placed at bedside	• Specially trained personnel necessary
	• Surgery for permanent access placement
	• Self-image problems with permanent access

CAPD, Continuous ambulatory peritoneal dialysis.

complications, including encephalopathy, neuropathies, uncontrolled hyperkalemia, pericarditis, and accelerated hypertension, indicate a need for immediate dialysis.

Most patients with ESRD are treated with dialysis because (1) there is a lack of donated organs, (2) some patients are physically or mentally unsuitable for transplantation, or (3) some patients do not want transplants. An increasing number of individuals, including older adults and those with complex medical problems, are receiving maintenance dialysis. A patient's chronologic age is not a factor in determining candidacy for dialysis.

General Principles of Dialysis

Solutes and water move across the semipermeable membrane from the blood to the dialysate or from the dialysate to the blood in accordance with concentration gradients. The principles of diffusion, osmosis, and ultrafiltration are involved in dialysis (Fig. 46-4). *Diffusion* is the movement of solutes from an area of greater concentration to an area of lesser concentration. In kidney failure, urea, creatinine, uric acid, and electrolytes (potassium, phosphate) move from the blood to the dialysate with the net effect of lowering their concentration in the blood. RBCs, WBCs, and plasma proteins are too large to diffuse through the pores of the membrane. Small-molecular-weight substances can pass from the dialysate into a patient's blood, so the purity of the water used for dialysis is monitored and controlled.

Osmosis is the movement of fluid from an area of lesser concentration to an area of greater concentration of solutes.

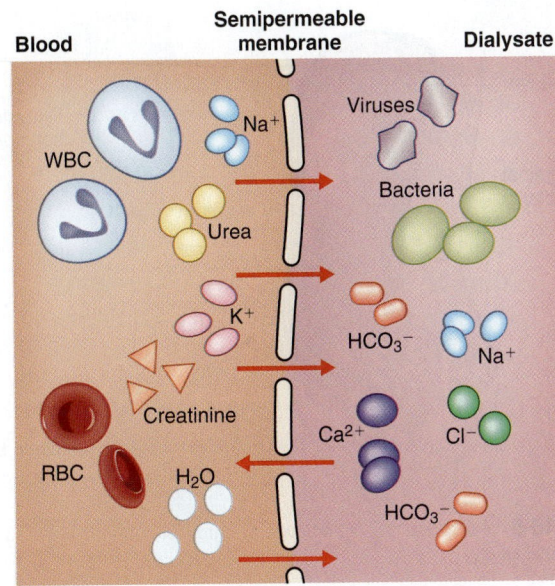

FIG. 46-4 Osmosis and diffusion across a semipermeable membrane.

Glucose is added to the dialysate and creates an osmotic gradient across the membrane, pulling excess fluid from the blood.

Ultrafiltration (water and fluid removal) results when there is an osmotic gradient or pressure gradient across the membrane. In PD, excess fluid is removed by increasing the osmolality of the dialysate (osmotic gradient) with the addition of glucose. In HD, the gradient is created by increasing pressure in the blood compartment (positive pressure) or decreasing pressure in the dialysate compartment (negative pressure). Extracellular fluid moves into the dialysate because of the pressure gradient. The excess fluid is removed by creating a pressure differential between the blood and the dialysate solution with a combination of positive pressure in the blood compartment or negative pressure in the dialysate compartment.

PERITONEAL DIALYSIS

Although PD was first used in 1923, it did not come into widespread use for chronic treatment until the 1970s with the development of soft, pliable peritoneal solution bags and the introduction of the concept of continuous PD. In the United States, approximately 12% of patients receiving dialysis treatments are on PD.

Catheter Placement

Peritoneal access is obtained by inserting a catheter through the anterior abdominal wall (Fig. 46-5). The catheter is about 24 inches (60 cm) long and has one or two Dacron cuffs. The cuffs act as anchors and prevent the migration of microorganisms into the peritoneum. Within a few weeks, fibrous tissue grows into the Dacron cuff, holding the catheter in place and preventing bacterial penetration into the peritoneal cavity. The tip of the catheter rests in the peritoneal cavity and has many perforations spaced along the distal end of the tubing, allowing fluid movement through the catheter.

The technique for catheter placement varies. It is usually placed surgically so that the catheter can be directly visualized, minimizing potential complications. Preparation of the patient for catheter insertion includes emptying the bladder and bowel, weighing the patient, and obtaining a signed consent form.

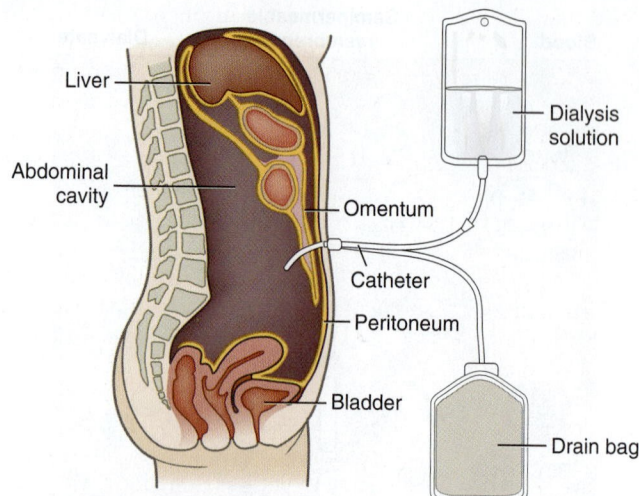

FIG. 46-5 Peritoneal dialysis showing peritoneal catheter inserted into peritoneal cavity.

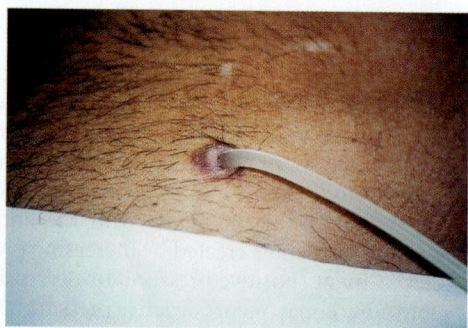

FIG. 46-6 Peritoneal catheter exit site. (Courtesy Mary Jo Holechek, Baltimore, Md.)

After placement, PD may be initiated immediately with low volume exchanges, or delayed for 2 weeks pending healing and sealing of the exit site. Once the catheter incision site is healed, the patient may shower and then pat the catheter and exit site dry.[24] Daily catheter care varies. Some patients just wash with soap and water and go without a dressing (Fig. 46-6), whereas others require daily dressing changes. Teach all patients to examine their catheter site for signs of infection. Showering is preferred to bathing.

Dialysis Solutions and Cycles

PD is accomplished by putting dialysis solution into the peritoneal space. The three phases of the PD cycle are inflow (fill), dwell (equilibration), and drain. The three phases are called an *exchange*. For manual PD, a period of about 30 to 50 minutes is required to complete an exchange. During *inflow,* a prescribed amount of solution, usually 2 L, is infused through an established catheter over about 10 minutes. The flow rate may be decreased if the patient has pain. After the solution has been infused, the inflow clamp is closed.

The next part of the cycle is the *dwell* phase, or equilibration, during which diffusion and osmosis occur between the patient's blood and peritoneal cavity. The duration of the dwell time can be brief lasting 20 or 30 minutes or up to 8 or more hours, depending on the method of PD.

Drain time takes 15 to 30 minutes and may be facilitated by gently massaging the abdomen or changing position. The cycle starts again with the infusion of another 2 L of solution.

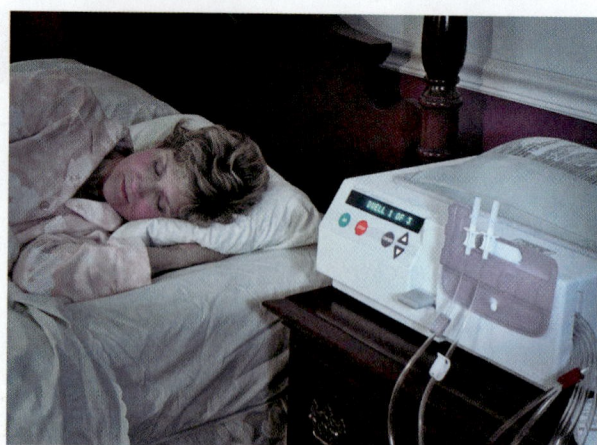

FIG. 46-7 Automated peritoneal dialysis that can be used while the patient is sleeping.

Dialysis solutions vary, and the choice of the exchange volume is primarily determined by the size of the peritoneal cavity. A larger person may require a 3-L exchange volume without any difficulty, whereas an average-size person typically uses a 2-L exchange. Smaller exchange volumes are used for patients with a smaller body, pulmonary compromise (the added pressure of the large volume may precipitate respiratory difficulty), or inguinal hernias.

Ultrafiltration (fluid removal) during PD depends on osmotic forces, with dextrose being the most commonly used osmotic agent in PD solutions. It is relatively safe and inexpensive but is associated with high rates of peritoneal glucose absorption leading to problems with hypertriglyceridemia, hyperglycemia, and long-term peritoneal membrane dysfunction.

Alternatives to dextrose PD solution include icodextrin and amino acid solutions. Icodextrin is a commercially available iso-osmolar preparation and induces ultrafiltration by its oncotic effect. Amino acid PD solutions are also available and used primarily for patients requiring nutritional supplementation.

Peritoneal Dialysis Systems

Automated Peritoneal Dialysis. Automated peritoneal dialysis (APD) is the most popular form of PD because it allows patients to do dialysis while they sleep. An automated device called a *cycler* is used to deliver the dialysate for APD (Fig. 46-7). The size of a cycler is similar to a DVD player. The automated cycler times and controls the fill, dwell, and drain phases. The machine cycles four or more exchanges per night with 1 to 2 hours per exchange. Alarms and monitors are built into the system to make it safe for the patient to sleep while dialyzing. The patient disconnects from the machine in the morning and usually leaves fluid in the abdomen during the day.

It is difficult to achieve the required solute and fluid clearance solely with nighttime APD. One or two daytime manual exchanges may be prescribed to ensure adequate dialysis.

Continuous Ambulatory Peritoneal Dialysis. Continuous ambulatory peritoneal dialysis (CAPD) is performed every few hours during the day. The patient may perform an exchange of 2 L of peritoneal dialysate four times daily, with dwell times averaging 4 hours. A common schedule includes exchanges at 7 AM, 12 noon, 5 PM, and 10 PM. In this procedure, the person instills 2 to 3 L of dialysate from a plastic bag into the peritoneal cavity through a disposable administration line.

In CAPD the bag and line can be disconnected after the instillation of the fluid. After the equilibration period, the line is reconnected to the catheter, the dialysate (effluent) is drained from the peritoneal cavity, and a new 2- to 3-L bag of dialysate solution is infused. In PD it is critical to maintain aseptic technique to avoid peritonitis. Several tubing connections and devices are commercially available to help in maintaining an aseptic system.

Complications of Peritoneal Dialysis

Exit Site Infection. Infection of the peritoneal catheter exit site is most commonly caused by *Staphylococcus aureus* or *Staphylococcus epidermidis* (from skin flora). Clinical manifestations of an exit site infection include redness at the site, tenderness, and drainage. Superficial exit site infections caused by these organisms are generally resolved with antibiotic therapy. If not treated immediately, subcutaneous tunnel infections may progress and may cause peritonitis, necessitating catheter removal.

Peritonitis. Peritonitis results from contact contamination or an exit site or tunnel infection. Most frequently peritonitis occurs because of improper technique when connections for exchanges are contaminated. Peritonitis is usually caused by *S. aureus* or *S. epidermidis*. Peritonitis infrequently results from bacteria in the intestine crossing into the peritoneal cavity.

The primary clinical manifestations of peritonitis are abdominal pain, rebound tenderness, and cloudy peritoneal effluent with a WBC count greater than 100 cells/μL (more than 50% neutrophils) or demonstration of bacteria in the peritoneal effluent by Gram stain or culture. GI manifestations of peritonitis may include diarrhea, vomiting, abdominal distention, and hyperactive bowel sounds. Fever may or may not be present. To determine if the peritoneal effluent is cloudy, drain the effluent and place the drained bag on reading material such as a newspaper. If you cannot read the print through the effluent, it is cloudy.

Cultures, Gram stain, and a WBC differential of the peritoneal effluent are used to confirm the diagnosis of peritonitis. Antibiotics can be given orally, IV, or intraperitoneally. In most cases, the patient is treated on an outpatient basis.

The formation of adhesions in the peritoneum can result from repeated infections and interferes with the peritoneal membrane's ability to act as a dialyzing surface. Repeated infections may require the removal of the peritoneal catheter and a temporary or permanent change of modality to HD.

Hernias. Because of increased intraabdominal pressure secondary to the dialysate volume, hernias can develop in predisposed individuals such as multiparous women and older men. After hernia repair, PD can often be resumed after several days using small dialysate volumes and keeping the patient supine.

Lower Back Problems. Increased intraabdominal pressure can cause or aggravate lower back pain. The lumbosacral curvature is increased by intraperitoneal infusion of dialysate. Orthopedic binders and a regular exercise program for strengthening the back muscles have been beneficial for some patients.

Bleeding. After peritoneal catheter placement, it is common for the PD effluent drained after the first few exchanges to be pink or slightly bloody secondary to the trauma associated with catheter insertion. Bloody effluent over several days or the new appearance of blood in the effluent can indicate active intraperitoneal bleeding. If this occurs, check the BP and hematocrit.

Blood may also be present in the effluent of women who are menstruating or ovulating, and this requires no intervention.

Pulmonary Complications. Atelectasis, pneumonia, and bronchitis may occur from repeated upward displacement of the diaphragm, resulting in decreased lung expansion. Longer dwell times increase the likelihood of pulmonary problems. Frequent repositioning and deep-breathing exercises can help. When the patient is lying in bed, elevate the head of the bed to prevent these problems.

Protein Loss. The peritoneal membrane is permeable to plasma proteins, amino acids, and polypeptides. These substances are lost in the dialysate fluid. The amount of loss is usually about 0.5 g/L of dialysate drainage, but it can be as high as 10 to 20 g/day. This loss may increase to as much as 40 g/day during episodes of peritonitis as the peritoneal membrane becomes more permeable. Unresolved peritonitis is associated with excessive protein loss that can result in malnutrition and may indicate the need to terminate PD temporarily or sometimes permanently.

Effectiveness of Chronic Peritoneal Dialysis

Learning the self-management skills required to do PD is usually accomplished in a 3- to 7-day training program. Mortality rates are similar between in-center HD patients and PD patients for the first few years. After about 2 years, mortality rates for patients receiving PD increase, especially for the older person with diabetes and patients with a prior history of CV disease.[24]

The primary advantage of PD is its simplicity and that it is a home-based program, increasing patient participation in their care. There is no need for special water systems, and equipment setup is relatively simple.

HEMODIALYSIS

Vascular Access Sites

Obtaining vascular access is one of the most difficult problems associated with HD. To perform HD, a very rapid blood flow is required, and access to a large blood vessel is essential. Enough time is needed for evaluation and consideration of the best arteriovenous access for HD. The types of vascular access include arteriovenous fistulas (AVFs), arteriovenous grafts (AVGs), and temporary vascular access.[25]

Arteriovenous Fistulas and Grafts. A subcutaneous arteriovenous fistula (AVF) is usually created in the forearm or upper arm with an anastomosis between an artery and a vein (usually cephalic or basilic) (Figs. 46-8, *A*, and 46-9). The fistula allows arterial blood to flow through the vein.

The vein becomes "arterialized," increasing in size and developing thicker walls. The arterial blood flow is essential to provide the rapid blood flow required for HD. As the fistula matures, it is more amenable to repeated venipunctures. Maturation may take 6 weeks to months. AVF should be placed at least 3 months before the need to initiate HD. The fistula is the preferred access for HD.[26]

Normally, a *thrill* (buzzing sensation) can be felt by palpating the fistula, and a *bruit* (rushing sound) can be heard with a stethoscope. The thrill and bruit are created by arterial blood moving at a high velocity through the vein.

AVFs are more difficult to create in patients with a history of severe peripheral vascular disease (e.g., people with diabetes), those with prolonged IV drug use, and obese women. For these individuals, a synthetic graft may be required.

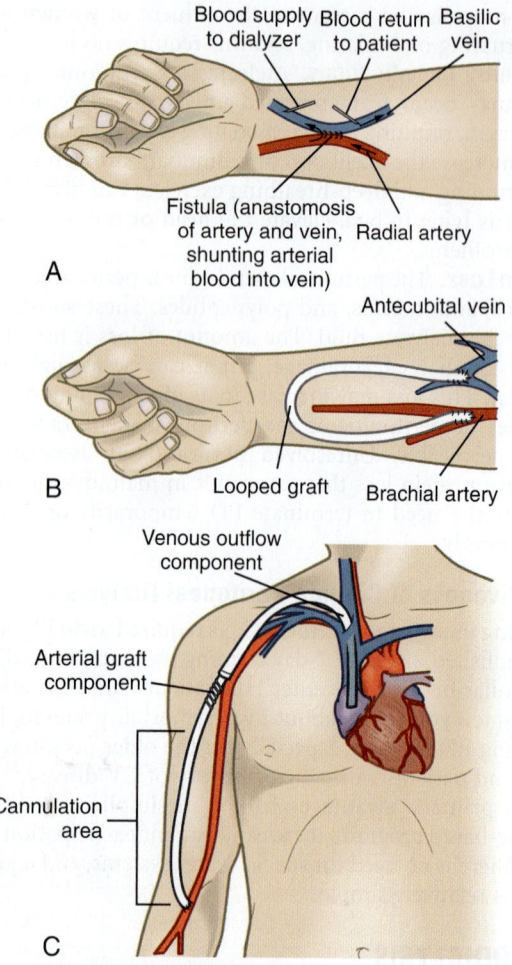

FIG. 46-8 Vascular access for hemodialysis. **A,** Arteriovenous fistula. **B,** Arteriovenous graft. **C,** HeRO graft.

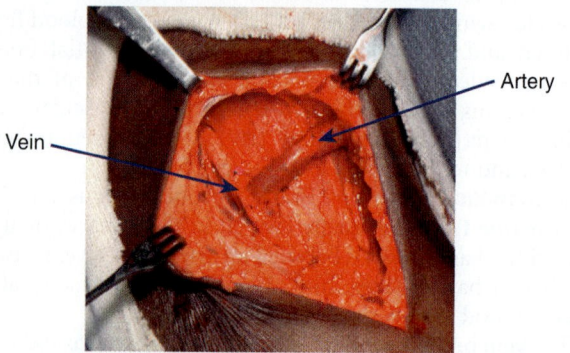

FIG. 46-9 Arteriovenous fistula created by anastomosing an artery and a vein. (Courtesy Dr. Stephen Van Voorst, MD.)

? CHECK YOUR PRACTICE

You are rotating to the inpatient dialysis unit today. It is your first experience working with HD patients. You are helping a hemodialysis tech "hook-up" a 56-yr-old man to HD. He has been on HD for 5 years secondary to polycystic kidney disease. You take his vital signs, palpate his AV fistula, and then use your stethoscope to auscultate the AV fistula. You are very concerned because you feel a super-strong pulse and hear a very loud "whoosh" sound. The patient turns to you and just smirks, "I bet you have never had a thrill like that."

• You are very flustered and not sure how to respond. What should you say to him?

Arteriovenous grafts (AVGs) are made of synthetic materials (polytetrafluoroethylene [PTFE, Teflon]) and form a "bridge" between the arterial and venous blood supplies. Grafts are placed under the skin and are surgically anastomosed between an artery (usually brachial) and a vein (usually antecubital) (Fig. 46-8, *B*). An interval of 2 to 4 weeks is usually necessary to allow the graft to heal but may be used earlier. Because grafts are made of artificial materials, they are more likely than AVFs to become infected, and they also have a tendency to be thrombogenic. When AVG infections occur, they may require surgical removal, since it is difficult to completely resolve the infection from the synthetic material.

A common problem in patients on HD is central venous stenosis (CVS) or occlusion. This is a serious issue and has a greater impact than peripheral venous stenosis because the central veins are the final pathway for blood flow to the heart. As CVS progresses, vascular access for HD is frequently lost.

HeRO graft (Hemodialysis Reliable Outflow) is a special bridge access used in patients when other access options are exhausted. It consists of two pieces: a reinforced tube to bypass blockages in veins and a dialysis graft anastomosed to an artery to be accessed for HD (Fig. 46-8, *C*). The *HeRO graft* is placed under the skin, like both a fistula and standard graft. The HeRO Graft bypasses the venous system to provide blood flow directly from a target artery to the heart. HeRO Graft is a graft but differs from a conventional AV graft since it has no venous anastomosis. It may be more difficult to auscultate the bruit or feel the thrill in this type of access because of the absence of a venous anastomosis.

Surgical creation of an arteriovenous access for HD has several risks, including development of distal ischemia *(steal syndrome)* and pain because too much of the arterial blood is being shunted or "stolen" from the distal extremity. Classic manifestations of steal syndrome are pain distal to the access site, numbness or tingling of fingers that may worsen during dialysis, and poor capillary refill. Aneurysms can also develop in the arteriovenous access and can rupture if left untreated.

> ⚠ **SAFETY ALERT   Arteriovenous Fistulas and Grafts**
> • Never perform BP measurements, insertion of IV lines, and venipuncture in the extremity with the vascular access.
> • These special precautions are taken to prevent infection and clotting of the vascular access.
> • When a patient is hospitalized, hang signs in patient's room or label the arm with a band that says "No BP, blood draws, or IV in this arm."

Temporary Vascular Access. When immediate vascular access is required, catheterization of the internal jugular or femoral vein is performed. A flexible catheter is inserted at the bedside into one of these large veins and provides access to the circulation without surgery (Fig. 46-10). The catheters usually have a double external lumen with an internal septum separating the two internal segments. One lumen is used for blood removal and the other for blood return (Fig. 46-11, *A* and *B*). Temporary catheters have high rates of infection, dislodgment, and malfunction. A patient should not be discharged from the hospital with a temporary catheter in place.

Long-term cuffed HD catheters are often used for temporary vascular access. These catheters provide temporary access while the patient is waiting for fistula placement or as long-term access when other forms of access have failed. This type of catheter exits on the upper chest wall and is tunneled subcutaneously to the internal or external jugular vein (Fig. 46-11, *C*).

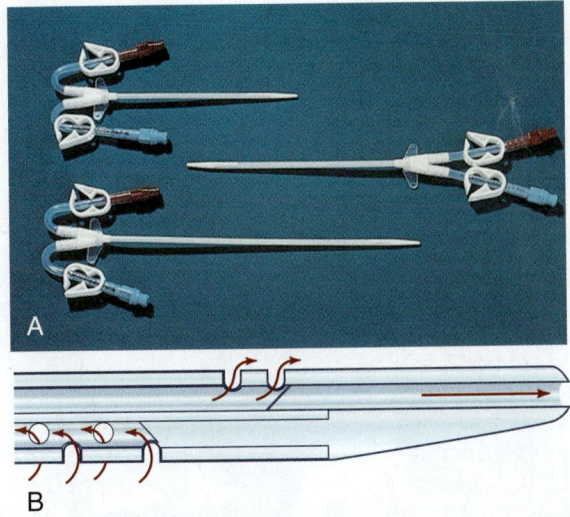

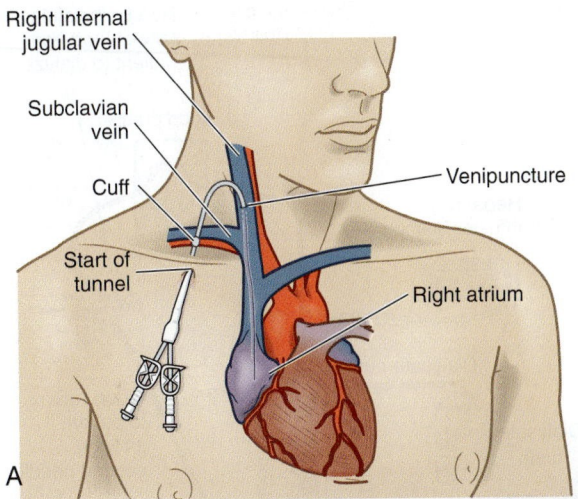

FIG. 46-10 Temporary double-lumen vascular access catheter for acute hemodialysis. **A,** Soft, flexible double-lumen tube is attached to a Y hub. **B,** The distance between the arterial intake lumen and the venous return lumen typically provides recirculation rates of 5% or less. (*A,* Courtesy Quinton Instrument Co., Seattle, Wash.)

The catheter tip rests in the right atrium. It has one or two subcutaneous Dacron cuffs that prevent infection from tracking along the catheter and anchor the catheter, thus eliminating the need for sutures.

Dialyzers

The HD dialyzer is a plastic cartridge that contains thousands of parallel hollow tubes or fibers. The fibers are semipermeable membranes made of cellulose-based or other synthetic materials. The blood is pumped into the top of the cartridge and is dispersed into all of the fibers. Dialysis fluid *(dialysate)* is pumped into the bottom of the cartridge and bathes the outside of the fibers. Ultrafiltration, diffusion, and osmosis occur across the pores of this semipermeable membrane. When the dialyzed blood reaches the end of the thousands of semipermeable fibers, it converges into a single tube that returns it to the patient. Dialyzers differ in surface area, membrane composition and thickness, clearance of waste products, and removal of fluid.

Procedure for Hemodialysis

The needles used for HD are large bore, usually 14 to 16 gauge, and are inserted into the fistula or graft to obtain vascular access. One needle is placed to pull blood from the circulation to the HD machine, and the other needle is used to return the dialyzed blood to the patient. The needles are attached via tubing to dialysis lines. If a patient has a catheter, the two blood lines are attached to the two catheter lumens. The needle closer to the fistula (red catheter lumen) is used to pull blood from the patient to the dialyzer using a blood pump. Blood is returned from the dialyzer to the patient through the second needle (blue catheter lumen).

When blood comes in contact with a foreign material (such as the dialyzer), it has a tendency to clot. Heparin is added to the blood to prevent clotting.

In addition to the dialyzer, a dialysate delivery and monitoring system is used (Fig. 46-12). This system pumps the dialysate through the dialyzer, countercurrent to the blood flow. To terminate the treatment, a saline solution is used to return the blood in the extracorporeal circuit back to the patient through

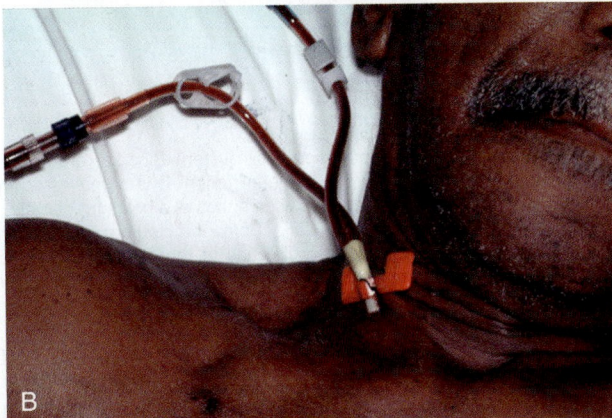

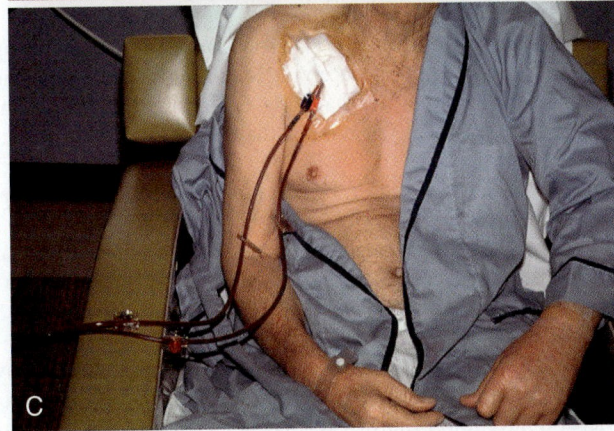

FIG. 46-11 **A,** Right internal jugular placement for a tunneled, cuffed semipermanent catheter. **B,** Temporary hemodialysis catheter in place. **C,** Long-term cuffed hemodialysis catheter. (*B* and *C,* Courtesy Dr. Stephen Van Voorst, MD.)

the vascular access. The needles are removed from the patient, and firm pressure is applied to the venipuncture sites until the bleeding stops.

Before beginning treatment, assess fluid status (weight, BP, peripheral edema, lung and heart sounds), condition of vascular access, and temperature. The difference between the last post-dialysis weight and the present predialysis weight determines the ultrafiltration or the amount of weight (from fluid) to be removed. While the patient is on dialysis, take vital signs at least every 30 to 60 minutes because rapid BP changes may occur.

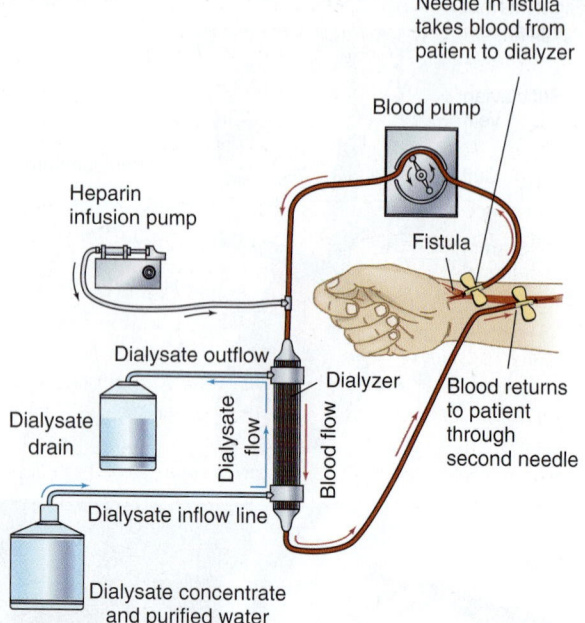

FIG. 46-12 Components of a hemodialysis system. Blood is removed via a needle inserted in a fistula or via catheter lumen. It is propelled to the dialyzer by a blood pump. Heparin is infused either as a bolus predialysis or through a heparin pump continuously to prevent clotting. Dialysate is pumped in and flows in the opposite direction of the blood. The dialyzed blood is returned to the patient through a second needle or catheter lumen. Old dialysate and ultrafiltrate are drained and discarded.

Settings and Schedules for Hemodialysis.

The majority of HD patients are treated in a community-based center and dialyze for 3 to 4 hours 3 days per week. Most people sleep, read, talk, or watch television during HD.

Other schedule options for HD are short daily HD and long nocturnal HD. The patient receiving long nocturnal HD has the advantage of sleeping while dialyzing. Each nocturnal treatment lasts 6 to 8 hours, and the patient dialyzes up to six times per week.

In addition to in-center HD, home HD is available (Fig. 46-13). The option for home HD often depends on a patient's family support. One of the main advantages of home HD is that it allows greater freedom in choosing dialysis times. In short daily HD, the patient dialyzes for $2\frac{1}{2}$ to 3 hours per session 5 to 6 days per week. Short daily HD is usually done at home.

Patients who choose daily dialysis or nocturnal dialysis may have fewer uremic symptoms, tend to require fewer medications, and have fewer dialysis-related side effects (e.g., hypotension, cramps). In addition, they have more autonomy. Although daily home HD offers the potential of significant health benefits, only about 2% of HD patients dialyze at home.

Complications of Hemodialysis

Hypotension. Hypotension that occurs during HD primarily results from rapid removal of vascular volume (hypovolemia), decreased cardiac output, and decreased systemic vascular resistance. The drop in BP during dialysis may precipitate light-headedness, nausea, vomiting, seizures, vision changes, and chest pain from cardiac ischemia. The usual treatment for hypotension includes decreasing the volume of fluid being removed and infusion of 0.9% saline solution.

Muscle Cramps. The cause of muscle cramps in HD is poorly understood. Factors associated with the development of muscle

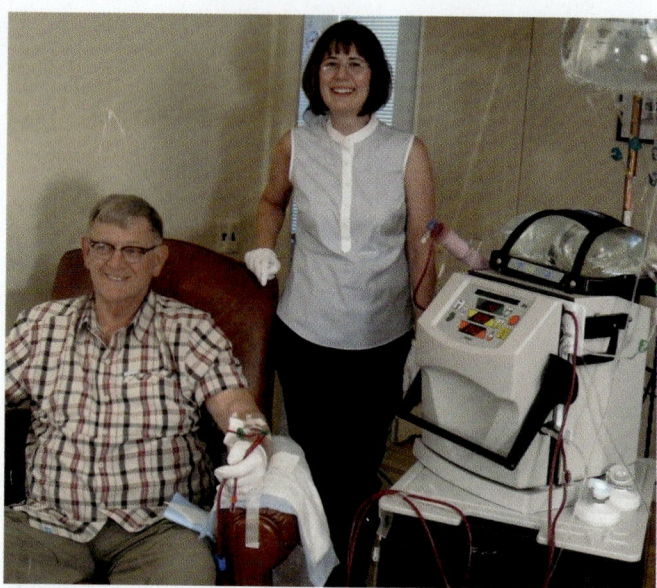

FIG. 46-13 Home hemodialysis is growing in popularity, and machines are more compact. (From NxStage Medical, Inc, Lawrence, Mass.)

✳ BECOMING A NURSE LEADER
Leadership vs. Management

Situation

Paula and Stacy, two nurses on a large dialysis unit, are discussing their dissatisfaction with their manager. Paula adamantly declares, "I never want to be a manager or a leader. I just want to be a nurse, take care of my patients, and go home at the end of my shift." Stacy responds, "All nurses need to be leaders." Paula fires back, "Not me!"

Points for Consideration

- Management and leadership are often lumped together. However, leadership roles are different from management responsibility.
- Both leadership and management are necessary for success in nursing today. You can be a leader without being a manager. Leadership has nothing to do with titles.
- *Leaders* create a vision of the future, communicate that vision effectively, and help team members commit to it. Leadership is an important skill for nurses at all levels.
- *Managers* are responsible for the functioning of their units, focusing on work and tasks. They must ensure there is sufficient staff that can provide safe, quality care. They maintain daily operations, stay within the unit budget, and meet strategic goals. However, the manager must also lead by exemplifying the mission, goals, and values of the organization to his or her staff, which will motivate them to strive for excellence.
- Nurse managers are expected to lead their team so that team members willingly participate, accept guidance, and carry out instruction.
- Education and training are required to be both a successful leader and manager. All too often in nursing, the best clinical nurses are promoted to managers without the benefit of formal training and mentoring.

Discussion Questions

1. Identify a situation in which you functioned as a leader.
2. What qualities could you develop personally and professionally to help you become a more effective nurse leader?

Reference

Baker J: Leadership from the trenches. Managing and leading in a competitive environment. Retrieved from *www.leadershipfrom thetrenches.com/2010/02/doing-the-right-thing.*

cramps include hypotension, hypovolemia, high ultrafiltration rate (large interdialytic weight gain), and low-sodium dialysis solution. Treatment includes reducing the ultrafiltration rate and administering fluids (saline, glucose, mannitol). Hypertonic saline is not recommended since the sodium load can be problematic. Hypertonic glucose administration is preferred.

Loss of Blood. Blood loss may result from blood not being completely rinsed from the dialyzer, accidental separation of blood tubing, dialysis membrane rupture, or bleeding after the removal of needles at the end of HD. If a patient has received too much heparin or has clotting problems, postdialysis bleeding can occur. It is essential to rinse back all blood, avoid excess anticoagulation, and hold firm but nonocclusive pressure on access sites until the risk of bleeding has passed.

Hepatitis. At one time, hepatitis B had an unusually high prevalence in dialysis patients, but the incidence today is low. Lower transfusion requirements, screening, and recommendations for vaccinations have lowered the incidence. Outbreaks of hepatitis B still occur, since transmission is attributed to breaks in infection control practices. To prevent transmission, all patients and personnel in dialysis units receive hepatitis B vaccine.

Currently, hepatitis C virus (HCV) is responsible for the majority of cases of hepatitis in dialysis patients. (Hepatitis is discussed in more detail in Chapter 43.) Approximately 8% to 10% of patients undergoing dialysis in the United States are positive for anti-HCV, which indicates a previous infection. Infection control precautions are mandated in care of the patient with hepatitis C to protect the patient and staff. (Infection control precautions are discussed in Chapter 14.) Currently no vaccine is available for hepatitis C.

Effectiveness of Hemodialysis

HD is still an imperfect therapy for management of ESRD. It cannot fully replace the normal functions of the kidneys. It can ease many of the symptoms of CKD and, if started early, can prevent certain complications. It does not alter the accelerated rate of CV disease and the related high mortality rate.

The yearly death rate of patients receiving maintenance dialysis remains high at an estimated 19% to 24%. The majority of deaths are caused by CV disease (stroke or myocardial infarction). Infectious complications are the second leading cause of death.[26]

Individual adaptation to maintenance HD varies considerably. Initially many patients feel positive about the dialysis because it makes them feel better and keeps them alive, but there is often great ambivalence about whether it is worthwhile. Dependence on a machine is a reality. In response to their illness, dialysis patients may be nonadherent or depressed and exhibit suicidal tendencies. The primary nursing goals are to (1) assist the patient to maintain a healthy self-image and (2) return the patient to the highest level of function possible, including returning to work.

CONTINUOUS RENAL REPLACEMENT THERAPY

Continuous renal replacement therapy (CRRT) is a method for treating AKI. It provides a means by which uremic toxins and fluids are removed while acid-base status and electrolytes are adjusted slowly and continuously in a hemodynamically unstable patient. The principle of CRRT is to dialyze patients in a more physiologic way (over 24 hours), just like the kidneys. CRRT is contraindicated if a patient has life-threatening manifestations

of uremia (hyperkalemia, pericarditis) that require rapid treatment. CRRT can be used in conjunction with HD.

Various types of CRRT are available (Table 46-14). CRRT most commonly uses the venovenous approaches of continuous venovenous hemofiltration (CVVH), continuous venovenous hemodialysis (CVVHD), and continuous venovenous hemodiafiltration (CVVHDF).

Vascular access for CRRT is achieved through the use of a double-lumen catheter (as used in HD [Fig. 46-10]) placed in the jugular or femoral vein. A blood pump propels the blood through the circuit. A highly permeable, hollow-fiber hemofilter removes plasma water and nonprotein solutes, which are collectively termed *ultrafiltrate*. The ultrafiltration rate (UFR) may range from 0 to 500 mL/hr. Under the influence of hydrostatic pressure and osmotic pressure, water and nonprotein solutes pass out of the filter into the extracapillary space and drain through the ultrafiltrate port into a collection device (drainage bag) (Fig. 46-14). The remaining fluid continues

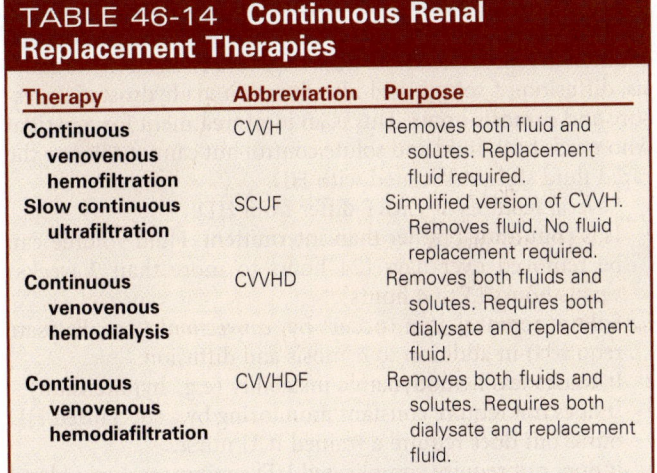

TABLE 46-14	**Continuous Renal Replacement Therapies**	
Therapy	**Abbreviation**	**Purpose**
Continuous venovenous hemofiltration	CVVH	Removes both fluid and solutes. Replacement fluid required.
Slow continuous ultrafiltration	SCUF	Simplified version of CVVH. Removes fluid. No fluid replacement required.
Continuous venovenous hemodialysis	CVVHD	Removes both fluids and solutes. Requires both dialysate and replacement fluid.
Continuous venovenous hemodiafiltration	CVVHDF	Removes both fluids and solutes. Requires both dialysate and replacement fluid.

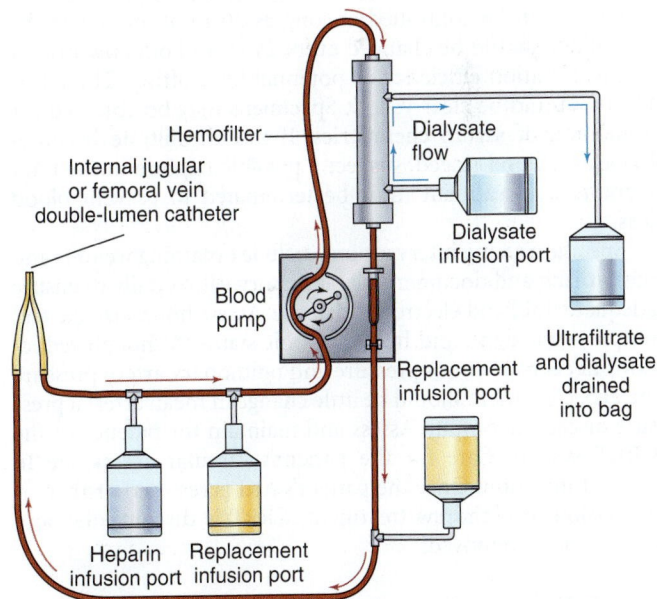

FIG. 46-14 Basic schematic of continuous venovenous therapies. Blood pump is required to pump blood through the circuit. Replacement ports are used for instilling replacement fluids and can be given prefilter or postfilter. Dialysate port is used for infusing dialysis solution. Regardless of modality, ultrafiltrate is drained via the ultrafiltration drain port.

through the filter and returns to the patient via the return port of the double-lumen catheter.

As ultrafiltrate drains out of the hemofilter, fluid and electrolyte replacements can be infused through a port located before or after the filter as the blood returns to the patient. Replacement fluid is designed to replace volume and solutes such as sodium, chloride, bicarbonate, and glucose. The infusion rate of replacement fluid is determined by the degree of fluid and electrolyte imbalance. Replacement fluid infused into the infusion port before the hemofilter allows for greater clearance of urea and can decrease filter clotting. The use of the infusion port located after the filter dilutes intravascular fluid, decreasing the concentration of unwanted solutes such as BUN, creatinine, and potassium. Anticoagulants are needed to prevent blood clotting and may be infused as a bolus at the initiation of CRRT or through an infusion port before the hemofilter.

The type of CRRT can be customized to the patient's needs. Some types involve the introduction of replacement fluids. CVVHD and CVVHDF use dialysate. Dialysis fluid is attached to the distal end of the hemofilter, and the fluid is pumped countercurrent to the blood flow (Fig. 46-14). As in hemodialysis, diffusion of solutes and ultrafiltration via hydrostatic pressure and osmosis occur. This is an ideal treatment for a patient who needs both fluid and solute control but cannot tolerate the rapid fluid shifts associated with HD.

Several features of CRRT differ from HD:

- It is continuous rather than intermittent. Fluid volume can be removed over days (24 hours to more than 2 weeks) versus hours (3 to 4 hours).
- Solute removal can occur by *convection* (no dialysate required) in addition to osmosis and diffusion.
- It causes less hemodynamic instability (e.g., hypotension).
- It does not require constant monitoring by a specialized HD nurse but does require a trained ICU nurse.
- It does not require complicated HD equipment, but a blood pump is needed for venovenous therapies.

CRRT can be continued as long as 30 to 40 days, but the hemofilter should be changed every 24 to 48 hours because of loss of filtration efficiency or potential for clotting. The ultrafiltrate should be clear yellow. Specimens may be obtained for evaluation of serum chemistries. If the ultrafiltrate becomes bloody or blood tinged, suspect a possible rupture in the filter membrane. Treatment must be terminated to prevent blood loss.

Specific nursing interventions include obtaining weights and monitoring and documenting laboratory values daily to ensure adequate fluid and electrolyte balance. Assess hourly intake and output, vital signs, and hemodynamic status. Although reductions in central venous pressure and pulmonary artery pressure are expected, there should be little change in mean arterial pressure or cardiac output. Assess and maintain the patency of the CRRT system. Care for the patient's vascular access site to prevent infection. Once the patient's AKI is resolved or there is a decision to withdraw treatment, CRRT is discontinued and the needle(s) removed.

WEARABLE ARTIFICIAL KIDNEY

While many improvements have been made for the care of ESRD patients, none has been able to replace a person's biologic kidneys. The wearable artificial kidney (WAK) has recently been developed and is approved for use to improve the quality of life of an ESRD patient.

The WAK is a miniaturized dialysis machine that can be worn on the body. The carrier resembles a tool belt. The device connects to a patient via a catheter. Like conventional dialysis machines, it is designed to filter the blood of ESRD patients. Unlike current portable or stationary dialysis machines, it can run continuously on batteries and is not plugged into an electrical outlet or attached to a water pipe. The present version weighs about 10 pounds, but future modifications could make it lighter and more streamlined.

KIDNEY TRANSPLANTATION

Major advances have been made in kidney transplantation since the first live donor kidney transplant was performed in 1954 between identical twins. These advances include organ procurement and preservation, surgical techniques, tissue typing and matching, immunosuppressant therapy, and prevention and treatment of graft rejection. (A general discussion of organ transplantation is in Chapter 13, pp. 207-210).

Even though kidney transplantation is the best treatment option available to patients with ESRD, fewer than 4% ever receive a transplant. This is because of the large disparity between the supply and demand for kidneys. Every year thousands are waiting for kidney transplants (more than 100,000 are currently on the list), yet only about 17,000 transplants take place every year. Most die while waiting. Transplantation from a deceased donor usually requires a prolonged waiting period with differences in waiting time depending on age, gender, and race. Average wait times in the United States for a cadaveric kidney usually range from 2 to 5 years.[27,28]

Kidney transplantation is very successful, with 1-year graft survival rates over 90% for deceased donor transplants and 95% for live donor transplants.[29] An advantage of kidney transplantation when compared with dialysis is that it reverses many of the pathophysiologic changes associated with renal disease. It also eliminates the dependence on dialysis and the accompanying dietary and lifestyle restrictions. Transplantation is also less expensive than dialysis after the first year.

Recipient Selection

Appropriate recipient selection is important for a successful outcome. Candidacy is determined by a variety of medical and psychosocial factors that vary among transplant centers. Some transplant programs exclude patients who are morbidly obese or who continue to smoke (despite smoking cessation interventions). A careful evaluation is completed in an attempt to identify and minimize potential complications after transplantation. Certain patients, particularly those with CV disease and diabetes mellitus, are considered high risk and must be carefully evaluated and then monitored closely after transplantation.

For a small number of patients who are approaching ESRD, a *preemptive transplant* (before dialysis is required) is possible if they have a living donor. This approach is most advantageous for patients with diabetes, who have a much higher mortality rate on dialysis than nondiabetics.

Contraindications to transplantation include disseminated malignancies, refractory or untreated cardiac disease, chronic respiratory failure, extensive vascular disease, chronic infection, and unresolved psychosocial disorders (e.g., nonadherence to medical regimens, alcoholism, drug addiction). Being HIV-positive or having hepatitis B or C is not a contraindication to transplantation.

Surgical procedures may be required before transplantation based on the results of the recipient evaluation. Coronary artery bypass or coronary angioplasty may be indicated for advanced coronary artery disease. Cholecystectomy may be necessary for patients with a history of gallstones, biliary obstruction, or cholecystitis. On rare occasions, bilateral nephrectomies are necessary for patients with refractory hypertension, recurrent urinary tract infections, or grossly enlarged kidneys from polycystic kidney disease. In general, the recipient's own kidneys do not have to be removed before he or she receives a kidney transplant.

Histocompatibility Studies

Histocompatibility studies, including human leukocyte antigen (HLA) testing and crossmatching, are discussed in Chapter 13 on pp. 206-207.

Donor Sources

Kidneys for transplantation may be obtained from compatible blood-type deceased donors, blood relatives, emotionally related (close and distant) living donors (e.g., spouses, distant cousins, etc.), and altruistic living donors who are known (friends) or unknown to the recipient.

Another option is *paired organ donation*, in which one donor/recipient pair who are incompatible or poorly matched with each other find another donor/recipient pair with whom they can exchange kidneys. Thus a spouse (person A) who wants to donate a kidney to his wife (person B) but is incompatible is paired with another donor/recipient pair involving a son with ESRD (person C) and his mother (person D). In this example, person A would donate his kidney to person C, and person D would donate her kidney to person B. Paired organ donation is the practice of matching biologically incompatible donor/recipient pairs to permit transplantation of both candidates with a well-matched organ.

Live Donors. Live donors undergo an extensive interprofessional evaluation to ensure that they are in good health and have no history of disease that would place them at risk for developing kidney disease or operative complications. Crossmatches are done at the time of the evaluation and about a week before the transplant to ensure that no antibodies to the donor are present or that the antibody titer is below the allowed level. Advantages of a live donor kidney include (1) better patient and graft survival rates regardless of histocompatibility match, (2) immediate organ availability, (3) immediate function because of minimal *cold time* (kidney out of body and not getting blood supply), and (4) the opportunity to have the recipient in the best possible medical condition because the surgery is elective.

The potential donor sees a nephrologist for a complete history and physical examination and laboratory and diagnostic studies. Laboratory studies include a 24-hour urine study for creatinine clearance and total protein, complete blood count, and chemistry and electrolyte profiles. Hepatitis B and C, HIV, and cytomegalovirus (CMV) testing is done to assess for transmitted diseases. An ECG and chest x-ray are also done. A renal ultrasound and renal arteriogram or three-dimensional CT scan is performed to ensure that the blood vessels supplying each kidney are adequate and that no anomalies exist and to determine selection of the kidney to be used in the transplant.

A transplant psychologist or social worker determines if the individual is emotionally stable and able to deal with the issues related to organ donation. All donors must be informed about the risks and benefits of donation, the potential short- and long-term complications, and what to expect during the hospitalization and recovery phases. Kidney donation is considered safe without any long-term health consequences. Although the costs of the evaluation and surgery are covered by the recipient's insurance, no compensation is available for lost wages during the posthospitalization recovery period. This period can last 6 weeks or longer.

When there is ABO incompatibility between a donor and recipient, paired donor exchange is a viable alternative. Another option for ABO incompatibility or a positive crossmatch between the donor and recipient is to use plasmapheresis to remove antibodies from the recipient. (Crossmatching is discussed in Chapter 13.) This allows transplant candidates to receive kidneys from live donors with blood types that have traditionally been considered incompatible. After the transplant, the patient undergoes additional plasmapheresis treatments.

Deceased Donors. Deceased (cadaver) kidney donors are relatively healthy individuals who have suffered an irreversible brain injury and are declared brain dead. The most common causes of injury are cerebral trauma from motor vehicle accidents or gunshot wounds, intracerebral or subarachnoid hemorrhage, and anoxic brain damage caused by cardiac arrest. The brain-dead donor must have effective CV function and be supported on a ventilator to preserve the organs.

Even if the donor carried a signed donor card, permission from the donor's legal next of kin is still requested after brain death is determined. That is why it is important for you to talk with your family about your wishes before losing the capacity to convey your desires.

In deceased kidney donation, the kidneys are removed and preserved. They can be preserved for up to 72 hours, but most transplant surgeons prefer to transplant kidneys before the cold time (time outside of the body when being transported from the deceased donor to the recipient) reaches 24 hours. Prolonged cold time increases the likelihood that the kidney will not function immediately, and acute tubular necrosis (ATN) may develop.

The United Network for Organ Sharing (UNOS) distributes deceased donor kidneys using an objective computerized point system. The ABO group, HLA typing, age, antibody level, and length of time waiting are entered into the national computer for each candidate. When a donor becomes available, the donor's key information is compared with the data of all patients awaiting transplantation locally and nationwide. Points are given for how close the HLA match is, how long the patient has been waiting, if the antibody level is unusually high, and if the recipient is younger than 19 years old. Extra points are given for high antibody levels because this can severely limit the number of donors with whom the patient will not have a positive crossmatch. The kidney is offered to the recipient with the most points in the local area. If no patients in the local area are suitable, the organ is then offered in the region and then in the nation. When a kidney arrives at the recipient's transplant center, a final crossmatch is done and must be negative for the deceased donor transplantation to proceed. (Crossmatching is discussed in Chapter 13.)

The only exception to the previous plan is if a patient needs an emergency transplant or if a donor and recipient match on all six HLA antigens (zero antigen mismatch). The patient meeting either one of these criteria goes to the top of the list. Emergency transplants are given priority because the patient is facing imminent death if not transplanted. If a zero antigen mismatch patient is identified nationally, since statistically these grafts have better survival rates, one of the donor kidneys must be sent to that recipient's transplant center regardless of location.

Surgical Procedure

Live Donor. Living donation accounts for nearly 27% of all kidney transplants in the United States, and most transplant centers regard them as the preferred donation modality.[27] The donor nephrectomy is performed by a transplant surgeon. The donor's surgery begins 1 to 2 hours before the recipient's surgery. The recipient is surgically prepared for the kidney transplant in a nearby operating room.

Laparoscopic donor nephrectomy is the most common technique for removing a kidney in a living donor. (Laparoscopic nephrectomy is discussed in Chapter 45.) After the kidney has been removed, it is flushed with a chilled, sterile electrolyte solution and prepared for immediate transplant into the recipient. The use of a laparoscopic donor nephrectomy procedure is

minimally invasive with fewer risks and shorter recovery time than an open procedure. The laparoscopic approach significantly decreases hospital stay, pain, operative blood loss, debilitation, and length of time off work. For these reasons, the number of people willing to donate a kidney has increased significantly.

For an *open (conventional) nephrectomy,* the donor is placed in the lateral decubitus position on the operating table so that the flank is exposed laterally. An incision is made at the level of the eleventh rib. The rib may have to be removed to provide adequate visualization of the kidney.

Kidney Transplant Recipient. The transplanted kidney is usually placed extraperitoneally in the iliac fossa. The right iliac fossa is preferred to facilitate anastomoses of the blood vessels and ureter and minimize the occurrence of paralytic ileus. A urinary catheter is placed into the bladder and an antibiotic solution is instilled to distend the bladder and decrease the risk of infection. A crescent-shaped incision is made extending from the iliac crest to the symphysis pubis (Fig. 46-15).

Rapid revascularization is critical to prevent ischemic injury to the kidney. The donor artery is anastomosed to the recipient's internal iliac (hypogastric) or external iliac artery. The donor vein is anastomosed to the recipient's external iliac vein. When the anastomoses are complete, the clamps are released, and blood flow to the kidney is reestablished. The kidney should become firm and pink. Urine may begin to flow from the ureter immediately. The donor ureter in most cases is then tunneled through the bladder submucosa before entering the bladder cavity and being sutured in place. This approach is called

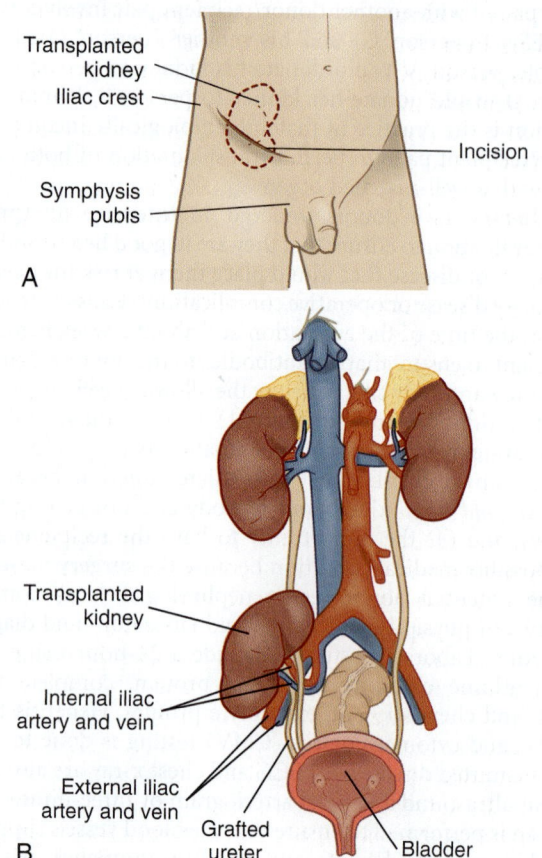

FIG. 46-15 A, Surgical incision for a renal transplant. **B,** Surgical placement of transplanted kidney.

ureteroneocystostomy. This allows the bladder wall to compress the ureter as it contracts for micturition, thereby preventing reflux of urine up the ureter into the transplanted kidney. The transplant surgery takes about 3 to 4 hours.

❖ NURSING MANAGEMENT: KIDNEY TRANSPLANT RECIPIENT

◆ Preoperative Care

Nursing care of the patient in the preoperative phase includes emotional and physical preparation for surgery. Because the patient and caregiver may have been waiting years for the kidney transplant, a review of the operative procedure and what can be expected in the immediate postoperative recovery period is necessary. Stress that there is a chance the kidney may not function immediately, and dialysis may be required for days to weeks. Review the need for immunosuppressive drugs and measures to prevent infection.

To ensure the patient is in optimal physical condition for surgery, an ECG, chest x-ray, and laboratory studies are ordered. Dialysis may be required before surgery for fluid overload or hyperkalemia. Because dialysis may be required after transplantation, the patency of the vascular access must be maintained. The vascular access extremity should be labeled "dialysis access, no procedures" to prevent use of the affected extremity for BP measurement, blood drawing, or IV infusions. A patient on PD must empty the peritoneal cavity of all dialysate solution before going to surgery and have the PD catheter capped.

◆ Postoperative Care

◆ **Live Donor.** Postoperative care for the donor is similar to that following open (conventional) or laparoscopic nephrectomy (see Chapter 45). Closely monitor renal function to assess for impairment and monitor the hematocrit to assess for bleeding. Donors usually experience more pain than the recipient. Donors who have had an open surgical approach may experience more pain than when a laparoscopic approach is used.

Donors who had an open approach are usually discharged from the hospital in 4 or 5 days and return to work in 6 to 8 weeks. With a laparoscopic approach, donors are discharged from the hospital in 2 to 4 days and return to work in 4 to 6 weeks. The donor is seen by the surgeon 1 to 2 weeks after discharge.

Nurses caring for the living donor must acknowledge the precious gift that this person has given. The donor has taken physical, emotional, and financial risks to assist the recipient. It is vital that the donor not be forgotten postoperatively. The donor will need support if the donated organ does not work immediately or for some reason fails.

◆ **Kidney Transplant Recipient.** The first priority during the postoperative period is maintenance of fluid and electrolyte balance. Because close monitoring is required, kidney transplant recipients spend the first 12 to 24 hours in the ICU. Large volumes of urine may be produced soon after the blood supply to the transplanted kidney is reestablished. This diuresis is due to the (1) new kidney's ability to filter BUN, which acts as an osmotic diuretic; (2) abundance of fluids administered during the operation; and (3) initial renal tubular dysfunction, which inhibits the kidney from concentrating urine normally. Urine output during this phase may be as high as 1 L/hr and gradually decreases as the BUN and serum creatinine levels return toward normal. Urine output is replaced with fluids milliliter for milliliter hourly for the first 12 to 24 hours.

Central venous pressure readings are essential for monitoring postoperative fluid status. Dehydration must be avoided to prevent subsequent renal hypoperfusion and renal tubular damage. Electrolyte monitoring to assess for the hyponatremia and hypokalemia often associated with rapid diuresis is critical. Treatment with potassium supplements or infusion of 0.9% normal saline may be indicated. IV sodium bicarbonate may also be required if the patient develops metabolic acidosis from a delay in the return of kidney function.

Acute tubular necrosis (ATN) in the transplanted kidney can occur because of prolonged cold times causing ischemic damage and the use of marginal cadaveric donors (those who are medically suboptimal). While the patient is in ATN, dialysis is required to maintain fluid and electrolyte balance. Some patients have high-output ATN with the ability to excrete fluid but not metabolic wastes or electrolytes. Other patients have oliguric or anuric ATN. These patients are at risk for fluid overload in the immediate postoperative period and must be assessed closely for the need for dialysis. The period of ATN can last anywhere from days to weeks, with gradually improving kidney function. Most patients with ATN are discharged from the hospital on dialysis. This is extremely discouraging for the patient, who needs reassurance that renal function usually improves. Dialysis is discontinued when urine output increases and serum creatinine and BUN begin to normalize.

A sudden decrease in urine output in the early postoperative period is a cause for concern. It may be due to dehydration, rejection, a urine leak, or obstruction. A common cause of early obstruction is a blood clot in the urinary catheter. Catheter patency must be maintained, since the catheter remains in the bladder for 3 to 5 days to allow the ureter-bladder anastomosis to heal. If blood clots are suspected, gentle catheter irrigation (if ordered) can reestablish patency.

With a hospital length of stay averaging 4 to 5 days, discharge planning and teaching needs must be identified and addressed early in the hospital course. Patient teaching ensures a smooth transition from the hospital to home and includes how to recognize signs of rejection, infection, and any complications of surgery. Frequent blood tests and clinic visits help detect rejection early.

Immunosuppressive Therapy

The goal of immunosuppression is to adequately suppress the immune response to prevent rejection of the transplanted kidney while maintaining sufficient immunity to prevent overwhelming infection. Immunosuppressive therapy is discussed in Chapter 13 and in Table 13-16.

Complications of Transplantation

Complications of PD, HD, and kidney transplantation are compared in Table 46-15.

Rejection. Rejection is one of the major problems following kidney transplantation. Rejection can be hyperacute, acute, or chronic. These types of rejection are discussed in Chapter 13 on pp. 208-209. Patients with chronic rejection may be placed on the transplant list to be retransplanted before dialysis is required.

Infection. Infection remains a significant cause of morbidity and mortality after transplantation.[29] The transplant recipient is at risk for infection because of suppression of the body's normal defense mechanisms by surgery, immunosuppressive drugs, and the effects of ESRD. Underlying systemic illness such as diabetes mellitus or systemic lupus erythematosus,

TABLE 46-15 Complications of Dialysis and Transplantation

Peritoneal Dialysis (PD)	Hemodialysis (HD)	Transplantation

• Exit site infection
• Peritonitis
• Abdominal pain
• Catheter outflow
• Hernias
• Lower back pain
• Cardiovascular disease
• Pulmonary problems
  • Atelectasis
  • Pneumonia
  • Bronchitis
• Protein loss
• Carbohydrate abnormalities
• Lipid abnormalities
• Encapsulating sclerosing peritonitis
	• Hypotension
	• Muscle cramps
	• Exsanguination
	• Hepatitis
	• Infection, including sepsis
	• Disequilibrium syndrome
	• Cardiovascular disease
		• Rejection of transplant
		  • Hyperacute
		  • Acute
		  • Chronic
		• Susceptibility to infection
		• Cardiovascular disease
		• Malignancies
		• Recurrence of kidney disease
		• Corticosteroid-related complications

malnutrition, and older age can further compound the negative effects on the immune response. The signs and symptoms of infection can be subtle. You must be astute in your observation and assessment of kidney transplant recipients because prompt diagnosis and treatment of infections improve patient outcomes.

The most common infections observed in the first month after transplantation are similar to those acquired by any postoperative patient, such as pneumonia, wound infections, IV line and drain infections, and urinary tract infections. Fungal and viral infections are common because of the patient's immunosuppressed state. Fungal infections include *Candida, Cryptococcus,* and *Aspergillus* organisms and *Pneumocystis jiroveci.* Fungal infections are difficult to treat, require prolonged treatment periods, and often involve the administration of nephrotoxic drugs. Transplant recipients usually receive prophylactic antifungal drugs to prevent these infections, such as clotrimazole, fluconazole (Diflucan), and trimethoprim/sulfamethoxazole (Bactrim).

Viral infections, including CMV, Epstein-Barr virus, herpes simplex virus (HSV), varicella-zoster virus, and polyomavirus (e.g., BK virus), can be primary infections or reactivations of existing disease. Primary infections occur as new infections after transplantation from an exogenous source such as the donated organ or a blood transfusion. Reactivation occurs when a virus exists in a patient and becomes reactivated after transplantation because of immunosuppression.

CMV is one of the most common viral infections. If a recipient has never had CMV and receives an organ from a donor with a history of CMV, antiviral prophylaxis will be administered (e.g., ganciclovir [Cytovene], valganciclovir [Valcyte]). To prevent HSV infections, oral acyclovir (Zovirax) is given for several months after the transplant.

Cardiovascular Disease. CV disease is the leading cause of death after renal transplantation.[29] Transplant recipients have an increased incidence of atherosclerotic vascular disease. Hypertension, dyslipidemia, diabetes mellitus, smoking, rejection, infections, and increased homocysteine levels (many of which existed prior to the transplant) can all contribute to CV disease. Immunosuppressants can worsen hypertension and dyslipidemia.

Teach the patient to control risk factors such as elevated cholesterol, triglycerides, and blood glucose and weight gain. Adherence to the prescribed antihypertensive regimen is essential not only to prevent CV events but also to prevent damage to the new kidney. (Hypertension is discussed in Chapter 32.)

Malignancies. The overall incidence of malignancies in kidney transplant recipients is greater than in the general population, primarily because of immunosuppressive therapy. Not only do immunosuppressants suppress the immune system to prevent rejection, but they also suppress the ability to fight infection and the production of abnormal cells such as cancer cells.

The most common types of cancer after transplant are (1) skin cancers: basal and squamous cell carcinoma and melanoma and (2) *posttransplant lymphoproliferative disorder (PTLD).* The majority of PTLDs are of B-cell origin, associated with Epstein-Barr virus (EBV), and cause aggressive lymphomas (Hodgkin's and non-Hodgkin's lymphoma). Most cases of PTLD occur within the first year of transplant.

Patients are also at risk for cancers of the colorectum, breast, cervix, liver, stomach, oropharynx, anus, vulva, and penis. Regular screening for cancer is an important part of the transplant recipient's preventive care. Advise the patient to avoid sun exposure by using protective clothing and sunscreens to minimize the incidence of skin cancers.

Recurrence of Original Kidney Disease. Recurrence of the original disease that destroyed the native kidneys occurs in some kidney transplant recipients. It is most common with certain types of glomerulonephritis, immunoglobulin A (IgA) nephropathy, diabetic nephropathy, and focal segmental sclerosis. Disease recurrence can result in the loss of a functioning kidney transplant. Patients must be advised before transplantation if they have a disease known to recur.

Corticosteroid-Related Complications. Aseptic necrosis of the hips, knees, and other joints can result from chronic corticosteroid therapy and renal osteodystrophy. Other significant problems related to corticosteroids include peptic ulcer disease, glucose intolerance and diabetes, cataracts, dyslipidemia, infections, and malignancies. The use of tacrolimus and other immunosuppressants has allowed corticosteroid doses to be much lower than they were in the past.

Many transplant programs have initiated corticosteroid-free drug regimens because of the problems of long-term corticosteroid use. Other centers withdraw patients from corticosteroids after transplantation. For patients who remain on corticosteroids, vigilant monitoring for side effects and early treatment are essential. (Corticosteroid therapy as immunosuppression is discussed in Chapter 13 on pp. 209-210.)

Gerontologic Considerations: Chronic Kidney Disease

The incidence of CKD in the United States is increasing most rapidly in older adults. The most common diseases leading to renal disease in older people are hypertension and diabetes.[30]

The care of older patients is particularly challenging, not only because of the normal physiologic changes of aging but also because of the disabilities, chronic diseases, and a number of co-morbid conditions that occur with aging. Physiologic changes include diminished cardiopulmonary function, bone loss, immunodeficiency, altered protein synthesis, impaired cognition, and altered drug metabolism. Malnutrition is common in these patients for a variety of reasons, including lack of mobility, lack of understanding of basic nutritional requirements, social isolation, physical disability, impaired cognitive function, and malabsorption problems.

When conservative therapy for CKD is no longer effective, the older patient needs to consider the best treatment modality based on his or her physical and emotional health, personal preferences, and availability of support. PD allows the patient to be more mobile and to enjoy an increased sense of control over the illness. PD causes less hemodynamic instability than HD but does require self-care or assistance from another person, which may not always be available.

Most individuals 65 years of age or older select treatment with in-center HD because of a lack of assistance in the home and reluctance to manage the technology of home HD or PD. Establishing vascular access for HD may be a concern in an older adult because of atherosclerotic changes. Although transplantation is an option, older adults must be carefully screened to ensure that the benefits of transplantation outweigh the risks.[31] Although a living donor is preferable, this may not be an option for many older patients.

The most common cause of death in older ESRD patients is CV disease (myocardial infarction, stroke), followed by withdrawal from dialysis. If a competent patient decides to withdraw from dialysis, it is essential to support the patient and family. Ethical issues (see the Ethical/Legal Dilemmas box) to consider in this situation include patient competency, benefit versus burden of treatment, and futility of treatment. Withdrawal from treatment is not a failure if the patient is well informed and comfortable with the decision.

Dialysis (especially PD) has been successfully used in older adults. Quality-of-life measures show no justification for excluding the older adult from dialysis programs. Rationing dialysis based on age alone is not a reasonable decision for health care professionals to make.

ETHICAL/LEGAL DILEMMAS
Withdrawing Treatment

Situation

L.R., a 70-yr-old patient with diabetes mellitus and end-stage renal disease, has been on dialysis for 10 yr. He tells you that he wants to discontinue his dialysis. His quality of life has diminished during the past 2 yr since his wife died. He is not a transplant candidate.

Ethical/Legal Points for Consideration

- Informed consent includes the legal right to refuse treatment. However, the right to refuse may be more difficult if (1) it is contrary to the wishes of family and friends, (2) the treatment still appears to have some effectiveness, and (3) the treatment has been in place for some time.
- Quality-of-life decisions often outweigh the benefit against the burden of treatment. When a treatment becomes too burdensome, the patient (if competent) may request to withdraw the treatment.
- It must be determined whether some other treatable problem, such as depression, may be clouding the patient's judgment.
- Although there is no ethical or legal difference between withdrawing treatment and withholding treatment, withdrawing treatment feels different because it requires an action.
- Some health care professionals become conflicted when they are asked to withdraw treatment, since they may think they are contributing to the patient's untimely death.
- If a decision is made to withdraw treatment, the interprofessional care team, patient, and family should develop an appropriate follow-up plan that includes palliative care and hospice support.

Discussion Questions

1. How should you respond to L.R.'s request?
2. What is the American Nurses Association's position on withdrawing or withholding treatment that no longer benefits the patient or causes suffering?

CASE STUDY
Chronic Kidney Disease

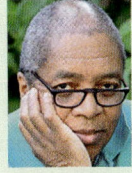
(©iStockphoto/ Thinkstock)

Patient Profile

M.B. is a 56-yr-old African American college professor. He is seen by his primary care provider for a routine physical examination. He has not been seen by a physician in a little over a year. He complains of generalized malaise, frequent urination, and "increasing thirst." His medical history is significant for borderline hypertension and dyslipidemia. He smokes one pack of cigarettes per day, and his efforts to quit have been unsuccessful.

Subjective Data

- Family history: father died of a heart attack at age 62, brother had coronary artery bypass graft (CABG) at age 50, mother died from complications of diabetes
- Becomes "winded" when walking from his car to his office at the university
- Wakes up at night to urinate and has more frequent urination
- Increasing thirst

Objective Data

Laboratory Data

- Calculated creatinine clearance using the MDRD equation: 42 mL/min/1.73 m²
- Serum creatinine 2.5 mg/dL
- BUN 35 mg/dL
- Serum glucose 264 mg/dL
- Hgb 13 g/dL
- Serum cholesterol 236 mg/dL

Physical Examination

- Weight 220 lb, height 5 ft 11 in
- BP 168/104 mm Hg

Discussion Questions

1. What do you think caused M.B.'s kidney disease?
2. What stage of chronic kidney disease does he have?
3. **Teamwork and Collaboration:** What are the most important treatment measures that the interprofessional team can provide for M.B.?
4. Identify the abnormal diagnostic study results and why each would occur.
5. **Patient-Centered Care:** What are the nursing interventions that would help promote M.B.'s self-management of his disease process?
6. **Priority Decision:** Based on the assessment data provided, what are the priority nursing diagnoses? Are there any collaborative problems?
7. **Teamwork and Collaboration:** How can the interprofessional team work together with M.B. to decide on the best form of renal replacement therapy?
8. **Evidence-Based Practice:** M.B. tells you that he has not been taking his BP medications regularly. When he asks you how important they are, what will you tell him?

BRIDGE TO NCLEX EXAMINATION

The number of the question corresponds to the same-numbered outcome at the beginning of the chapter.

1. Which descriptions characterize acute kidney injury (*select all that apply*)?
   a. Primary cause of death is infection.
   b. It almost always affects older people.
   c. Disease course is potentially reversible.
   d. Most common cause is diabetic nephropathy.
   e. Cardiovascular disease is most common cause of death.

2. RIFLE defines three stages of AKI based on changes in
   a. blood pressure and urine osmolality.
   b. fractional excretion of urinary sodium.
   c. estimation of GFR with the MDRD equation.
   d. serum creatinine or urine output from baseline.

3. During the oliguric phase of AKI, the nurse monitors the patient for (*select all that apply*)
   a. hypotension.
   b. ECG changes.
   c. hypernatremia.
   d. pulmonary edema.
   e. urine with high specific gravity.

4. If a patient is in the diuretic phase of AKI, the nurse must monitor for which serum electrolyte imbalances?
   a. Hyperkalemia and hyponatremia
   b. Hyperkalemia and hypernatremia
   c. Hypokalemia and hyponatremia
   d. Hypokalemia and hypernatremia

5. A patient is admitted to the hospital with chronic kidney disease. The nurse understands that this condition is characterized by
   a. progressive irreversible destruction of the kidneys.
   b. a rapid decrease in urine output with an elevated BUN.
   c. an increasing creatinine clearance with a decrease in urine output.
   d. prostration, somnolence, and confusion with coma and imminent death.

6. Nurses must teach patients at risk for developing chronic kidney disease. Individuals considered to be at increased risk include (*select all that apply*)
   a. older African Americans.
   b. patients more than 60 years old.
   c. those with a history of pancreatitis.
   d. those with a history of hypertension.
   e. those with a history of type 2 diabetes.

7. Patients with chronic kidney disease experience an increased incidence of cardiovascular disease related to (*select all that apply*)
   a. hypertension.
   b. vascular calcifications.
   c. a genetic predisposition.
   d. hyperinsulinemia causing dyslipidemia.
   e. increased high-density lipoprotein levels.

8. Nutritional support and management are essential across the entire continuum of chronic kidney disease. Which statements would be considered true related to nutritional therapy (*select all that apply*)?
   a. Fluid is not usually restricted for patients receiving peritoneal dialysis.
   b. Sodium and potassium may be restricted in someone with advanced CKD.
   c. Decreased fluid intake and a low-potassium diet are hallmarks of the diet for a patient receiving hemodialysis.
   d. Decreased fluid intake and a low-potassium diet are hallmarks of the diet for a patient receiving peritoneal dialysis.
   e. Decreased fluid intake and a diet with phosphate-rich foods are hallmarks of a diet for a patient receiving hemodialysis.

9. An ESRD patient receiving hemodialysis is considering asking a relative to donate a kidney for transplantation. In assisting the patient to make a decision about treatment, the nurse informs the patient that
   a. successful transplantation usually provides better quality of life than that offered by dialysis.
   b. if rejection of the transplanted kidney occurs, no further treatment for the renal failure is available.
   c. hemodialysis replaces the normal functions of the kidneys, and patients do not have to live with the continual fear of rejection.
   d. the immunosuppressive therapy following transplantation makes the person ineligible to receive other forms of treatment if the kidney fails.

10. To assess the patency of a newly placed arteriovenous graft for dialysis, the nurse should (*select all that apply*)
   a. monitor the BP in the affected arm.
   b. irrigate the graft daily with low-dose heparin.
   c. palpate the area of the graft to feel a normal thrill.
   d. listen with a stethoscope over the graft to detect a bruit.
   e. frequently monitor the pulses and neurovascular status distal to the graft.

11. A major advantage of peritoneal dialysis is
   a. the diet is less restricted and dialysis can be performed at home.
   b. the dialysate is biocompatible and causes no long-term consequences.
   c. high glucose concentrations of the dialysate cause a reduction in appetite, promoting weight loss.
   d. no medications are required because of the enhanced efficiency of the peritoneal membrane in removing toxins.

12. A kidney transplant recipient complains of having fever, chills, and dysuria over the past 2 days. What is the *first* action that the nurse should take?
   a. Assess temperature and initiate workup to rule out infection.
   b. Reassure the patient that this is common after transplantation.
   c. Provide warm cover for the patient and give 1 g acetaminophen orally.
   d. Notify the nephrologist that the patient has developed symptoms of acute rejection.

1. a, c, 2. d, 3. b, d, 4. c, 5. a, 6. a, b, d, e, 7. a, b, d, 8. a, b, c, 9. a, 10. c, d, e, 11. a, 12. a

For rationales to these answers and even more NCLEX review questions, visit *http://evolve.elsevier.com/Lewis/medsurg*.

REFERENCES

1. Workeneh BT, Agraharkar M, Gupta R: Acute kidney injury. 2014. Retrieved from *http://emedicine.medscape.com/article243492*.

2. Fournier M: Stemming the rising tide of acute kidney injury by obtaining a thorough history and conducting a careful assessment, you can help patients avoid this condition, *Am Nurse Today* 8(1):12, 2013.

3. Thakar CV, Christianson A, Almenoff P, et al: Degree of acute kidney injury before dialysis initiation and hospital mortality in critically ill patients, *Int J Nephrol* 2013:827459, 2013.

4. Zeng X, McMahon GM, Brunelli SM, et al: Incidence, outcomes, and comparisons across definitions of AKI in hospitalized individuals, *Clin J Am Soc Nephrol* 9(1):12, 2014.

5. Oh HJ, Shin DH, Lee MJ, et al: Urine output is associated with prognosis in patients with acute kidney injury requiring continuous renal replacement therapy, *J Crit Care* 28(4):379, 2013.

6. Libório AB, Leite TT, Neves FM, et al: AKI complications in critically ill patients: association with mortality rates and RRT, *Clin J Am Soc Nephrol* 10(1):21, 2015.

7. Bagshaw SM, Uchino S, Kellum JA, et al: Association between renal replacement therapy in critically ill patients with severe acute kidney injury and mortality, *J Crit Care* 28(6):1011, 2013.

8. Goldstein SL, Jaber BL, Faubel S, et al: AKI transition of care: a potential opportunity to detect and prevent CKD, *Clin J Am Soc Nephrol* 8(3):476, 2013.

9. Williams LM: Take aim at acute kidney injury with RIFLE criteria, *Nursing* 44:50, 2014.

10. Salgado G, Landa M, Masevicius D, et al: Acute renal failure according to the RIFLE and AKIN criteria: a multicenter study, *Med Intensiva* 38(5):271, 2014.

*11. Schneider AG, Bellomo R, Bagshaw SM, et al: Choice of renal replacement therapy modality and dialysis dependence after acute kidney injury: a systematic review and meta-analysis, *Intens Care Med* 39(6):987, 2013.

*12. Palevsky PM, Liu KD, Brophy PD, et al: KDOQI US commentary on the 2012 KDIGO clinical practice guideline for acute kidney injury, *Am J Kidney Dis* 61(5):649, 2013.

*13. James PA, Oparil S, Carter BL, et al: 2014 evidence-based guideline for the management of high blood pressure in adults: report from the panel members appointed to the Eighth Joint National Committee (JNC 8), *JAMA* 311(5):507, 2014.

*14. Inker LA, Astor BC, Fox CH, et al: KDOQI US commentary on the 2012 KDIGO clinical practice guideline for the evaluation and management of CKD, *Am J Kidney Dis* 63(5):713, 2014.

15. US Department of Health and Human Services: ESRD: general information, Centers for Medicare and Medicaid Services. Retrieved from *www.cms.gov/Medicare/End-Stage-Renal-Disease/ESRDGeneralInformation*.

16. United States Renal Data System: 2014 Annual data report: epidemiology of kidney disease in the United States. Bethesda, Md, 2014. National Institutes of Health, National Institute of Diabetes and Digestive and Kidney Diseases. Retrieved from *www.usrds.org/adr.aspx*.

17. Pilmore H, Dogra G, Roberts M, et al: Cardiovascular disease in patients with chronic kidney disease, *Nephrology* 19(1):3, 2014.

18. Drüeke TB: Anemia treatment in patients with chronic kidney disease, *N Engl J Med* 368:387, 2013.

19. Fang Y, Ginsberg C, Sugatani T, et al: Early chronic kidney disease–mineral bone disorder stimulates vascular calcification, *Kidney Int* 85(1):142, 2014.

20. Taler SJ, Agarwal R, Bakris GL, et al: KDOQI US commentary on the 2012 KDIGO clinical practice guideline for management of blood pressure in CKD, *Am J Kidney Dis* 62(2):201, 2013.

21. Afkarian M, Sachs MC, Kestenbaum B, et al: Kidney disease and increased mortality risk in type 2 diabetes, *J Am Soc Nephrol* 24(2):302, 2013.

22. National Kidney Foundation Kidney Disease Outcomes Quality Initiative (NKF KDOQI). Retrieved from *www.kidney.org/professionals/KDOQI/guidelines_commentaries*. 2015.

*23. Hernández Morante JJ, Sánchez-Villazala A, Cutillas RC, et al: Effectiveness of a nutrition education program for the prevention and treatment of malnutrition in end-stage renal disease, *J Ren Nutr* 24(1):42, 2014.

24. National Kidney and Urologic Diseases Information Clearinghouse: Treatment methods for kidney disease: peritoneal dialysis. Retrieved from *http://kidney.niddk.nih.gov/KUDiseases/pubs/peritoneal/index.aspx*.

25. Drew DA, Lok CE, Cohen JT, et al: Vascular access choice in incident hemodialysis patients: a decision analysis, *J Am Soc Nephrol* 26(1):183, 2015.

26. National Kidney and Urologic Diseases Information Clearinghouse: Treatment methods for kidney disease: hemodialysis. Retrieved from *http://kidney.niddk.nih.gov/KUDiseases/pubs/hemodialysis/index.aspx*.

27. United Network for Organ Sharing: 2012 annual report: the U.S. Scientific registry of transplant recipients and the organ procurement and transplantation network. Bethesda, Md, 2013, US Department of Health and Human Services.

28. Weir MR, Lerma EV: *Kidney transplantation: practical guide to management*, New York, 2014, Springer.

29. Reese PP, Bloom RD, Shults J, et al: Functional status and survival after kidney transplantation, *Transplantation* 97(2):189, 2014.

*30. Bolignano D, Mattace-Raso F, Sijbrands EJ, et al: The aging kidney revisited: a systematic review, *Ageing Res Rev* 14:65, 2014.

31. Haase M, Haase-Fielitz A: *Managing renal injury in the elderly patient*, New York, 2014, Springer.

*Evidence-based information for clinical practice.

CASE STUDY

Managing Care of Multiple Patients

You are working on the medical-surgical unit and have been assigned to care for the following four patients. You are also assigned to receive a new admission to the clinical unit. You have one UAP on your team to help you.

Patients

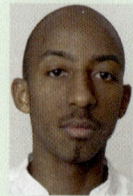

(©iStockphoto/ Thinkstock)

A.K., a 28-yr-old African American man, was admitted for observation after a renal ultrasound identified calculi in the left ureter. A.K. came to the ED with complaints of sharp, colicky left flank pain for which the HCP prescribed IV opioids. His last pain medication was given 2 hours ago. His current pain level is 4 on a scale of 1 to 10. He is voiding dark, smoky-colored urine. His vital signs are within normal limits. He has positive costovertebral tenderness.

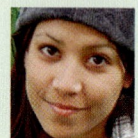

(©iStockphoto/ Thinkstock)

S.U., a 29-yr-old Hispanic woman with type 1 diabetes, was admitted with acute pyelonephritis following a recent UTI. She complains of bilateral flank pain and has abdominal tenderness to palpation. Her temperature is 101.5°F (38.6°C). Her urinalysis indicates pyuria and hematuria. Her WBC is elevated at 14,800/μL. Blood culture results are pending. IV antibiotics have been started. Most recent blood glucose is 195 mg/dL.

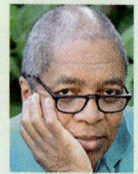

(©iStockphoto/ Thinkstock)

M.B., a 56-yr-old African American college professor, was admitted with uncontrolled hypertension. He was recently diagnosed with CKD. He smokes at least one pack of cigarettes per day and is experiencing some nicotine withdrawal symptoms. His BP on admission was 224/102 mm Hg. He is receiving IV metoprolol (Lopressor) 5 mg q4hr prn for SBP >180 mm Hg. His most recent BP 3 hr ago was 174/86 mm Hg. Most recent lab results indicate a BUN of 66 mg/dL and serum creatinine of 3.2 mg/dL.

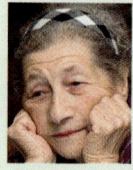

(©iStockphoto/ Thinkstock)

D.M., an 82-yr-old woman, was admitted to the ED with severe dehydration, heart failure, and acute kidney injury. Her daughter found her unconscious and lying on the floor. She is confused. Her serum potassium is 5.7 mEq/L. Her urine output for the past 8 hours was 90 mL.

Discussion Questions

1. *Priority Decision:* After receiving report, which patient should you see first? Second? Provide a rationale for your decision.
2. *Teamwork and Collaboration:* Which tasks could you delegate to the UAP *(select all that apply)?*
   a. Obtain vital signs on M.B.
   b. Strain A.K.'s voided urine.
   c. Report D.M.'s potassium level to the HCP.
   d. Measure D.M.'s urine output and report the results to the RN.
   e. Assess S.U. for manifestations of sepsis or diabetic ketoacidosis.

3. *Priority Decision and Teamwork and Collaboration:* As you are assessing D.M., the UAP informs you that M.B.'s blood pressure is 190/86. He is asymptomatic. Additionally, the charge nurse informs you that you will be receiving a patient with heart failure from the ED within the next 20 minutes. Which action would be *most* appropriate?
   a. Ask the charge nurse to assign the new admission to someone else.
   b. Have the UAP admit the new patient while you administer M.B.'s IV metoprolol.
   c. Call the ED and have them hold the new admission until after you have assessed all your patients.
   d. Ask the charge nurse to administer M.B.'s IV metoprolol while you complete your assessment of D.M. and then S.U.

Case Study Progression

As you complete your assessment of D.M., you notice her apical pulse is irregular. She has 1+ pitting edema in her lower extremities. Her BP is 160/90 mmHg, heart rate 108 bpm, and respiratory rate 28/min. Auscultation of D.M's lungs reveal crackles in the bases and O₂ saturation is 92% on room air. You notify her HCP.

4. Which interventions would you expect the HCP to order for D.M. *(select all that apply)?*
   a. Administer IV Kayexalate.
   b. Obtain arterial blood gas levels.
   c. Administer 40 mg of furosemide IV push.
   d. Prepare her for hemodialysis and notify her family.
   e. Obtain a 12-lead ECG and initiate continuous cardiac monitoring.
5. *Priority Decision:* Which nursing diagnosis would be of *highest* priority when planning care for A.K.?
   a. Risk for injury
   b. Impaired comfort
   c. Risk for infection
   d. Ineffective health management
6. Which statement would be *most* appropriate when teaching S.U. about her kidney infection?
   a. "The damage to your kidneys will likely require dialysis."
   b. "You will need to be in the hospital for a 2-week course of IV antibiotics."
   c. "It is very important that you maintain adequate hydration to flush your kidneys."
   d. "You will not need further antibiotics once you are discharged from the hospital."
7. *Management Decision:* As the UAP prepares the room for the patient being admitted from the ED, you overhear her telling a co-worker that she has to do all your work for you. What is your *best* initial action?
   a. Report the incident to the charge nurse for follow-up.
   b. Ask the UAP to discuss her concerns with you in private.
   c. Tell the UAP how much you appreciate and value her input on your team.
   d. Immediately clarify the situation by telling the UAP all the tasks you are completing.

Answers available at *http://evolve.elsevier.com/Lewis/medsurg.*

Problems Related to Regulatory and Reproductive Mechanisms

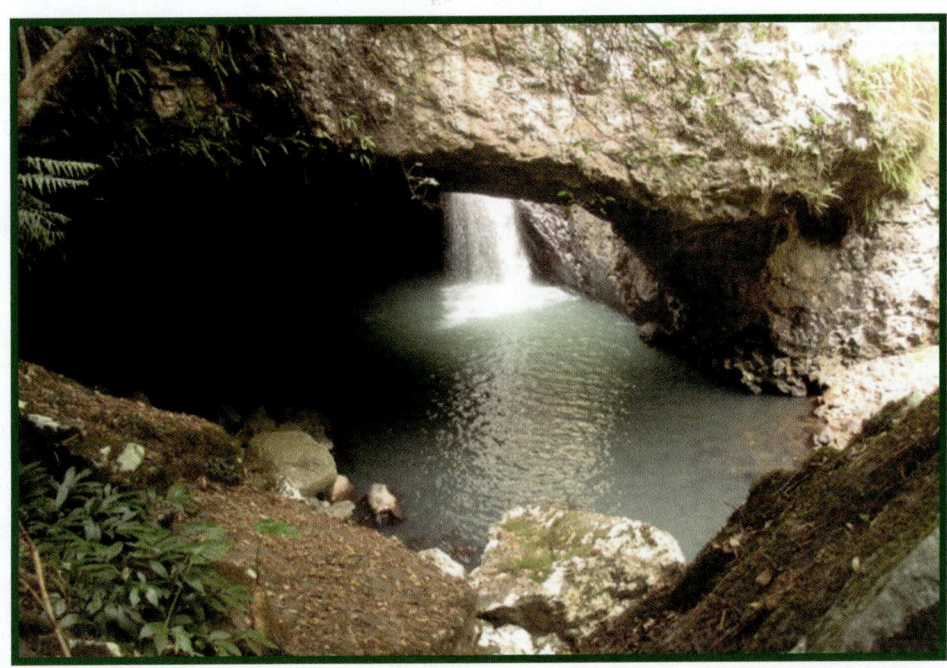

Peter Bonner

There's a river somewhere that flows through the lives of everyone.

Roberta Flack

47

Assessment of Endocrine System

Katherine A. Kelly

Success is walking from failure to failure with no loss of enthusiasm.

Winston Churchill

http://evolve.elsevier.com/Lewis/medsurg/

LEARNING OUTCOMES

1. Describe the common characteristics and functions of hormones.
2. Identify the locations of the endocrine glands.
3. Describe the functions of hormones secreted by the pituitary, thyroid, parathyroid, and adrenal glands and the pancreas.
4. Describe the locations and roles of hormone receptors.
5. Obtain significant subjective and objective assessment data related to the endocrine system from a patient.
6. Perform a physical assessment of the endocrine system using the appropriate techniques.
7. Link age-related changes in the endocrine system to differences in assessment findings.
8. Differentiate normal from common abnormal findings of a physical assessment of the endocrine system.
9. Describe the purpose, significance of results, and nursing responsibilities related to diagnostic studies of the endocrine system.

KEY TERMS

aldosterone, p. 1108
antidiuretic hormone (ADH), p. 1106
catecholamines, p. 1107
circadian rhythm, p. 1105
corticosteroid, p. 1107

cortisol, p. 1107
glucagon, p. 1108
growth hormone (GH), p. 1105
hormones, p. 1102
insulin, p. 1108

negative feedback, p. 1103
positive feedback, p. 1104
thyroxine (T_4), p. 1107
triiodothyronine (T_3), p. 1107
tropic hormones, p. 1105

STRUCTURES AND FUNCTIONS OF ENDOCRINE SYSTEM

Glands

Endocrine glands include the hypothalamus, pituitary, thyroid, parathyroids, adrenals, pancreas, ovaries, testes, and pineal gland (Fig. 47-1). These glands are able to make and release special chemical messengers called *hormones*. The endocrine system has five general functions. It has a role in reproductive and central nervous system development in the fetus, stimulating growth and development during childhood and adolescence, sexual reproduction, maintaining homeostasis, and responding to emergency demands.[1]

Hormones

Hormones are chemical substances produced by endocrine glands that control and regulate the activity of certain target cells or organs. Many are made in one part of the body and control and regulate the activity of certain cells or organs in another part of the body. The thyroid gland makes the hormone thyroxine, which affects many body tissues when released directly into the circulation. Other hormones act locally on cells where they are released and never enter the bloodstream. This local effect is called *paracrine action*. The action of sex steroids on the ovary is an example of paracrine action.

Most hormones have common characteristics, including (1) secretion in small amounts at variable but predictable rates; (2) regulation by feedback systems; and (3) ability to bind to specific target cell receptors. Table 47-1 summarizes the major hormones, the glands or tissues that synthesize the hormones, their target organs or tissues, and their functions.

There is a strong connection between the endocrine system and nervous system. *Catecholamines* (e.g., epinephrine), secreted by the adrenal gland, travel through the bloodstream and affect multiple organ systems. These same substances, when secreted by nerve cells in the brain and peripheral nervous system, act as neurotransmitters, sending important impulses across nerve synapses.[1]

Organs can act as endocrine glands by secreting hormones. For example, the kidneys secrete erythropoietin, a substance

Reviewed by Teresa J. Seright, RN, PhD, CCRN, Associate Teaching Professor, College of Nursing, Montana State University, Bozeman, Montana; and Crystal Sheaves, RN, MSN, APRN, FNP-BC, Senior Lecturer, West Virginia University School of Nursing, Charleston, West Virginia.

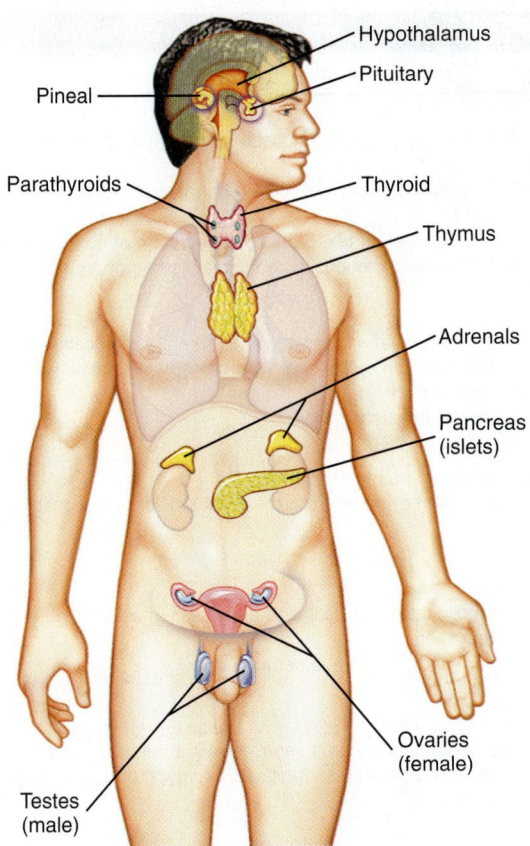

FIG. 47-1 Location of the major endocrine glands. The parathyroid glands lie on the posterior surface of the thyroid gland. (Modified from Patton KT, Thibodeau GA: *Anatomy and physiology,* ed 8, St Louis, 2013, Mosby.)

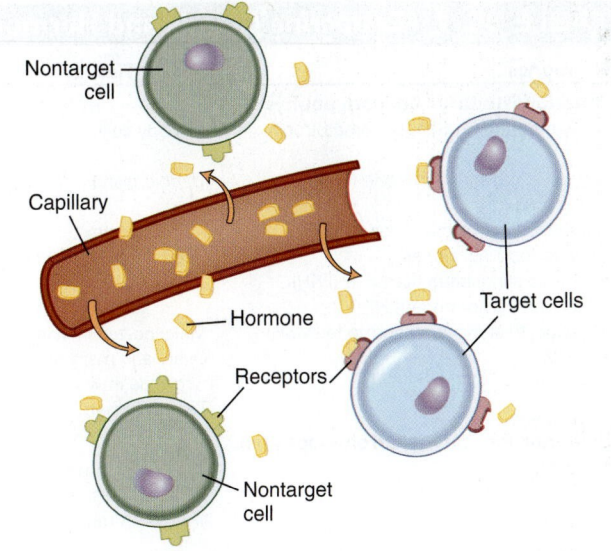

FIG. 47-2 The target cell concept. Hormones act only on cells that have receptors specific to that hormone, since the shape of the receptor determines which hormone can react with it. This is an example of the lock-and-key model of biochemical reactions.

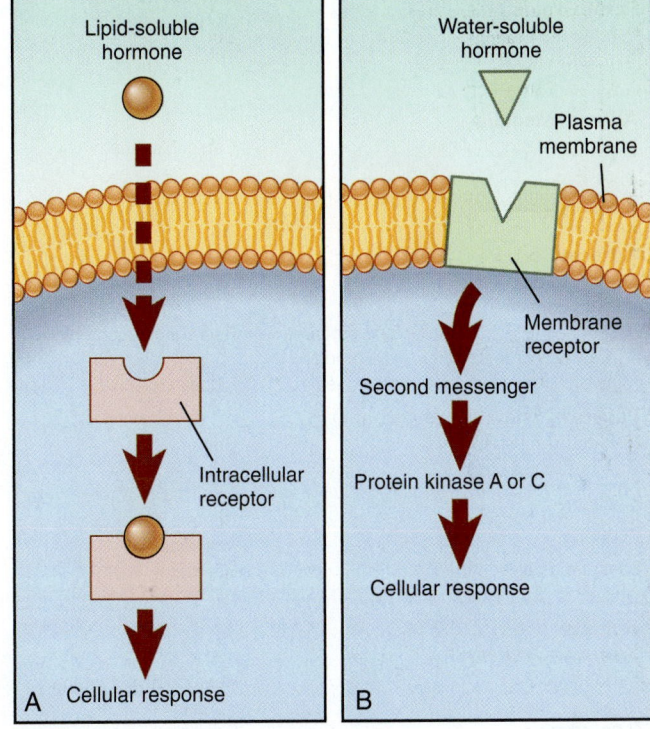

FIG. 47-3 **A,** Lipid-soluble hormones (e.g., steroid hormones) penetrate the cell membrane and interact with intracellular receptors. **B,** Water-soluble hormones (e.g., protein hormones) bind to receptors located in the cell membrane. The hormone-receptor interaction stimulates various cell responses. (Modified from McCance KL, Huether SE: *Pathophysiology: the biologic basis for disease in adults and children,* ed 6, St Louis, 2010, Mosby.)

that stimulates red blood cell production. The heart secretes atrial natriuretic peptide (ANP). The gastrointestinal (GI) tract secretes numerous peptide hormones (e.g., gastrin), which aid in digestion. These hormones are discussed in their respective assessment chapters.

Hormone Receptors. Hormones exert their effects by recognizing their target tissues and attaching to receptor sites in a "lock-and-key" type of mechanism. This means a hormone will act only on cells that have a receptor specific for that hormone (Fig. 47-2).

Lipid-Soluble and Water-Soluble Hormones. Hormones are classified by their chemical structure as either lipid soluble or water soluble. The differences in solubility become important in understanding how the hormone interacts with the target cell (Fig. 47-3). Lipid-soluble hormones (steroids, thyroid) are bound to plasma proteins as they travel to target cells. They cross the cell membrane by simple diffusion. Water-soluble hormones (insulin, growth hormone, prolactin) circulate freely in the blood and act directly on target tissues.

Regulation of Hormonal Secretion. Endocrine activity is controlled by specific mechanisms that either stimulate or inhibit hormone synthesis and secretion. These include positive and negative feedback, nervous system control, and physiologic rhythms.

Simple Feedback. Negative feedback relies on the blood level of a hormone or other chemical compound regulated by the hormone (e.g., glucose). It is the most common type of endocrine feedback system and results in the gland increasing or decreasing the release of a hormone. Negative feedback is

similar to the functioning of a thermostat. Cold air in a room activates the thermostat to release heat. Warm air signals the thermostat to turn off the heater. An example of negative feedback is calcium and parathyroid hormone (PTH) regulation. Low blood levels of calcium stimulate the parathyroid gland to release PTH. PTH acts on the bone, intestine, and kidneys to

TABLE 47-1   Endocrine Glands and Hormones

Hormones	Target Tissue	Functions
Anterior Pituitary (Adenohypophysis)		
Growth hormone (GH), or somatotropin	All body cells	Promotes protein anabolism (growth, tissue repair) and lipid mobilization and catabolism
Thyroid-stimulating hormone (TSH), or thyrotropin	Thyroid gland	Stimulates synthesis and release of thyroid hormones, growth and function of thyroid gland
Adrenocorticotropic hormone (ACTH)	Adrenal cortex	Fosters growth of adrenal cortex. Stimulates secretion of corticosteroids
Gonadotropic hormones	Reproductive organs	Stimulate sex hormone secretion, reproductive organ growth, reproductive processes
• Follicle-stimulating hormone (FSH)		
• Luteinizing hormone (LH)		
Melanocyte-stimulating hormone (MSH)	Melanocytes in skin	Increases melanin production in melanocytes to make skin darker
Prolactin	Ovary and mammary glands in women	Stimulates milk production in lactating women. Increases response of follicles to LH and FSH
	Testes in men	Stimulates testicular function in men
Posterior Pituitary (Neurohypophysis)		
Oxytocin	Uterus, mammary glands	Stimulates milk secretion, uterine contractility
Antidiuretic hormone (ADH), or vasopressin	Renal tubules, vascular smooth muscle	Promotes reabsorption of water from the renal tubules, vasoconstriction
Thyroid		
Thyroxine (T_4)	All body tissues	Precursor to T_3
Triiodothyronine (T_3)	All body tissues	Regulates metabolic rate of all cells and processes of cell growth and tissue differentiation
Calcitonin	Bone tissue	Regulates calcium and phosphorus serum levels
		Decreases serum Ca^{2+} levels
Parathyroids		
Parathyroid hormone (PTH), or parathormone	Bone, intestine, kidneys	Regulates calcium and phosphorus serum levels. Promotes bone demineralization and increases intestinal absorption of Ca^{2+}. Increases serum Ca^{2+} levels
Adrenal Medulla		
Epinephrine (adrenaline)	Catecholamine	Increases in response to stress. Enhances and prolongs effects of sympathetic nervous system
Norepinephrine (noradrenaline)	Catecholamine	Increases in response to stress. Enhances and prolongs effects of sympathetic nervous system
Adrenal Cortex		
Corticosteroids (e.g., cortisol, hydrocortisone)	All body tissues	Promote metabolism. Increased in response to stress. Antiinflammatory
Androgens (e.g., dehydroepiandrosterone [DGEA], androsterone) and estradiol	Reproductive organs	Promote growth spurt in adolescence, secondary sex characteristics, and libido in both sexes
Mineralocorticoids (e.g., aldosterone)	Kidney	Regulate sodium and potassium balance and thus water balance
Pancreas (Islets of Langerhans)		
Insulin (from β cells)	General	Promotes glucose transport from the blood into the cell
Amylin (from β cells)	Liver, stomach	Decreases gastric motility, glucagon secretion, and endogenous glucose release from liver. Increases satiety
Glucagon (from α cells)	General	Stimulates glycogenolysis and gluconeogenesis
Somatostatin	Pancreas	Inhibits insulin and glucagon secretion
Pancreatic polypeptide	General	Influences regulation of pancreatic exocrine function and metabolism of absorbed nutrients
Gonads		
Women: Ovaries		
Estrogen	Reproductive system, breasts	Stimulates development of secondary sex characteristics, preparation of uterus for fertilization and fetal development. Stimulates bone growth
Progesterone	Reproductive system	Maintains lining of uterus necessary for successful pregnancy
Men: Testes		
Testosterone	Reproductive system	Stimulates development of secondary sex characteristics, spermatogenesis

increase blood calcium levels. The increased blood calcium level then inhibits further PTH release (Fig. 47-4).

With **positive feedback**, increasing hormone levels cause another gland to release a hormone that then stimulates further release of the first hormone. A means to stop the release of the first hormone (e.g., follicle death) is required or its release will continue. The ovarian hormone estradiol operates by this type of feedback. Increased levels of estradiol produced by the follicle during the menstrual cycle result in the production and release of follicle-stimulating hormone (FSH) by the anterior pituitary. FSH causes further increases in estradiol until the death of the follicle. This results in a drop of FSH serum levels.

Nervous System Control. Nervous system activity directly affects some endocrine glands. Pain, fear, sexual excitement, and other stressors can stimulate the nervous system to modulate hormone secretion. For example, when stress is sensed or

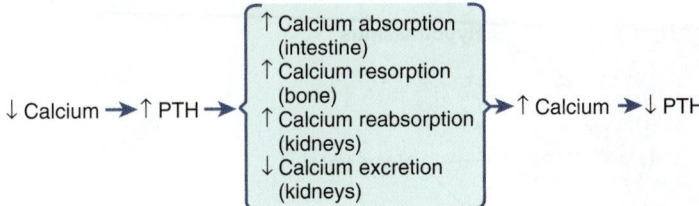

FIG. 47-4 Feedback mechanism between parathyroid hormone *(PTH)* and calcium.

perceived by the central nervous system (CNS), the sympathetic nervous system (SNS) secretes catecholamines (e.g., epinephrine), which maximize cardiac and lung function and vision to deal with the stress more effectively. Chronic exposure to some stressors can cause persistent elevation in heart rate and BP and changes in the endocrine system. This puts patients at risk for chronic disease such as hypertension and cardiac disease. Stress-related effects are discussed in Chapter 6.

Rhythms. A common physiologic rhythm is the circadian rhythm. It is a 24-hour rhythm that can be driven and altered by sleep-wake or dark-light 24-hour (diurnal) cycles. Hormone levels and the responsiveness of target tissues fluctuate predictably during these cycles.[2] Cortisol, produced by the adrenal cortex, rises early in the day, declines toward evening, and rises again toward the end of sleep to peak by morning (Fig. 47-5). Growth hormone (GH), thyroid-stimulating hormone (TSH), and prolactin levels peak during sleep. Reproductive cycles are often longer than 24 hours *(ultradian)*. An example is the menstrual cycle. These rhythms are an important factor when interpreting laboratory results for hormone levels.

Hypothalamus

Although many refer to the pituitary gland as the "master gland" of the endocrine system, most of its functions rely on its interrelationship with the hypothalamus, which lies adjacent to the pituitary gland. The hypothalamus releases substances that either stimulate or inhibit the formation and release of groups of hormones from the pituitary gland (Table 47-2). Examples of these hormones include corticotropin-releasing hormone and thyrotropin-releasing hormone. Somatostatin inhibits growth hormone release.

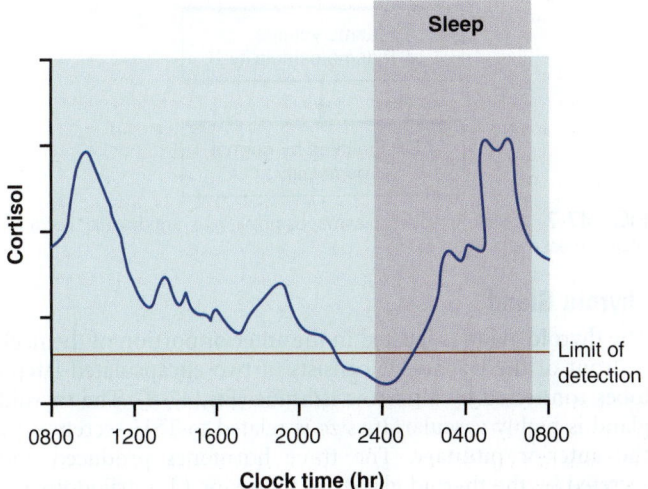

FIG. 47-5 Circadian rhythm of cortisol secretion.

TABLE 47-2 **Hormones of the Hypothalamus**
The following hormones from the hypothalamus target the anterior pituitary.
Releasing Hormones
• Corticotropin-releasing hormone (CRH)
• Thyrotropin-releasing hormone (TRH)
• Growth hormone–releasing hormone (GHRH), or somatotropin-releasing hormone
• Gonadotropin-releasing hormone (GnRH)
• Prolactin-releasing factor (PRF)
Inhibiting Hormones
• Somatostatin (inhibits growth hormone release)
• Prolactin-inhibiting factor (PIF)

The hypothalamus contains neurons that receive input from the CNS, including the brainstem, limbic system, and cerebral cortex. Neurons from the hypothalamus create a circuit to facilitate coordination of the endocrine system and autonomic nervous system (ANS). The hypothalamus also coordinates the expression of complex behavioral responses, such as anger, fear, and pleasure.

Pituitary

The pituitary gland *(hypophysis)* is located in the sella turcica under the hypothalamus at the base of the brain above the sphenoid bone (Fig. 47-1). The infundibular *(hypophyseal)* stalk connects the pituitary and hypothalamus. This stalk relays information between the hypothalamus and pituitary, creating a strong neuroendocrine connection. The pituitary consists of two major parts, the anterior lobe *(adenohypophysis)* and posterior lobe *(neurohypophysis)*. A smaller intermediate lobe produces melanocyte-stimulating hormone.

Anterior Pituitary. The anterior lobe of the pituitary accounts for 80% of the gland by weight. The hypothalamus regulates the anterior lobe through releasing and inhibiting hormones. These hypothalamic hormones reach the anterior pituitary through a network of capillaries known as the *hypothalamus-hypophyseal portal system*. The releasing and inhibiting hormones in turn affect the secretion of six hormones from the anterior pituitary (Fig. 47-6).

Several hormones secreted by the anterior pituitary are referred to as tropic hormones. Tropic hormones control the secretion of hormones by other glands. Thyroid-stimulating hormone (TSH) stimulates the thyroid gland to secrete thyroid hormones. Adrenocorticotropic hormone (ACTH) stimulates the adrenal cortex to secrete corticosteroids. Follicle-stimulating hormone (FSH) stimulates secretion of estrogen and the development of ova in women and sperm in men. Luteinizing hormone (LH) stimulates ovulation in women and secretion of sex hormones in both men and women. In men, LH is sometimes referred to as *interstitial cell–stimulating hormone (ICSH)*.

Growth hormone (GH) affects the growth and development of all body tissues. It has numerous biologic actions, including a role in protein, fat, and carbohydrate metabolism. *Prolactin*, or lactogenic hormone, stimulates breast development necessary for lactation after childbirth.

Posterior Pituitary. The posterior pituitary is composed of nerve tissue and is essentially an extension of the hypothalamus.

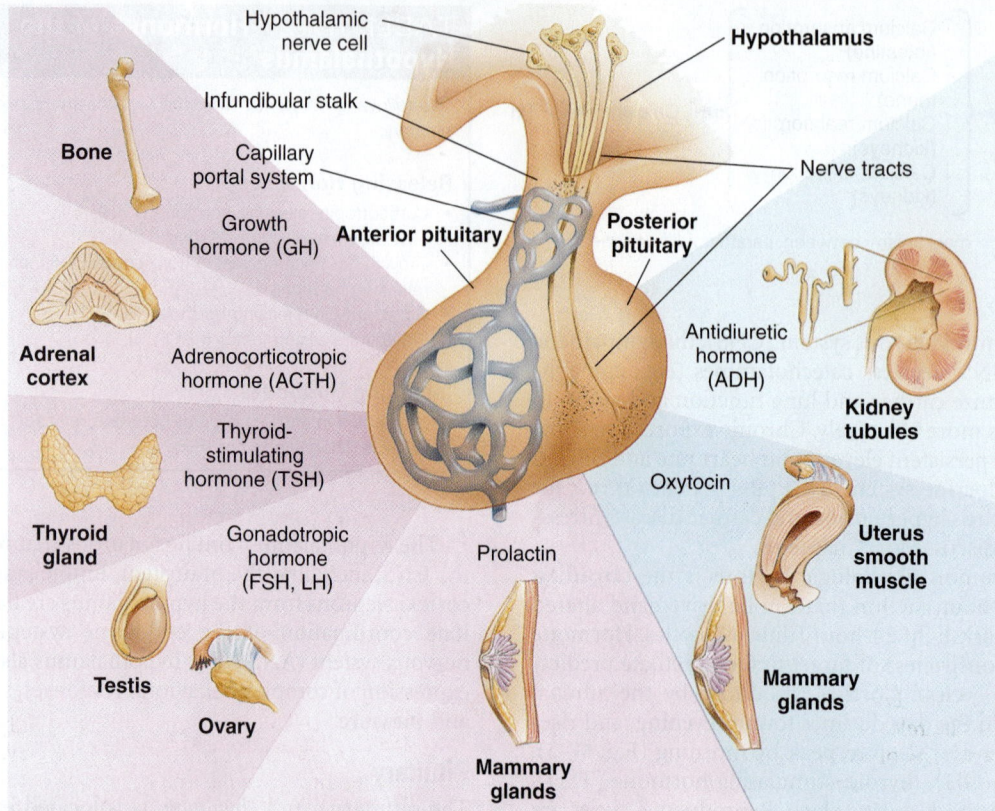

FIG. 47-6 Relationship between the hypothalamus, pituitary, and target organs. The hypothalamus communicates with the anterior pituitary via a capillary system and with the posterior pituitary via nerve tracts. The anterior and posterior pituitary hormones are shown with their target tissues. *FSH,* Follicle-stimulating hormone; *LH,* luteinizing hormone. (Modified from Patton KT, Thibodeau GA: *Anatomy and physiology,* ed 8, St Louis, 2013, Mosby.)

Communication between the hypothalamus and posterior pituitary occurs through nerve tracts known as the *median eminence.* The hormones secreted by the posterior pituitary, **antidiuretic hormone (ADH)** and oxytocin, are produced in the hypothalamus. These hormones travel down the nerve tracts from the hypothalamus to the posterior pituitary and are stored until the appropriate stimuli trigger their release (Fig. 47-6).

The major physiologic role of ADH (also called *arginine vasopressin*) is to regulate fluid volume. It causes the renal tubules to reabsorb water, making the urine more concentrated. A rise in *plasma osmolality* (a measure of solute concentration of circulating blood) and/or hypovolemia stimulates ADH secretion (Fig. 47-7). Increases in plasma osmolality cause specialized neurons in the hypothalamus, known as *osmoreceptors,* to stimulate ADH release from the posterior pituitary. Volume receptors in large veins, heart atria, and carotid arteries that sense pressure changes (from hypovolemia) also contribute to ADH control. When ADH release is inhibited, renal tubules do not reabsorb water, resulting in a more dilute urine. ADH is also a potent vasoconstrictor.

Pineal Gland

The pineal gland is located in the brain. It is composed of photoreceptive cells. Its primary function is the secretion of the hormone *melatonin.* Melatonin secretion increases in response to exposure to the dark and decreases in response to light exposure. The gland helps to regulate circadian rhythms and the reproductive system at the onset of puberty.

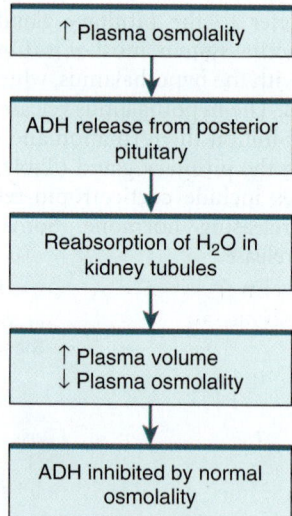

FIG. 47-7 Relationship of plasma osmolality to antidiuretic hormone *(ADH)* release and action.

Thyroid Gland

The thyroid gland is located in the anterior portion of the neck in front of the trachea. It consists of two encapsulated lateral lobes connected by a narrow isthmus (Fig. 47-8). The thyroid gland is highly vascular. Its size is related to TSH secretion by the anterior pituitary. The three hormones produced and secreted by the thyroid gland are thyroxine (T_4), triiodothyronine (T_3), and calcitonin.

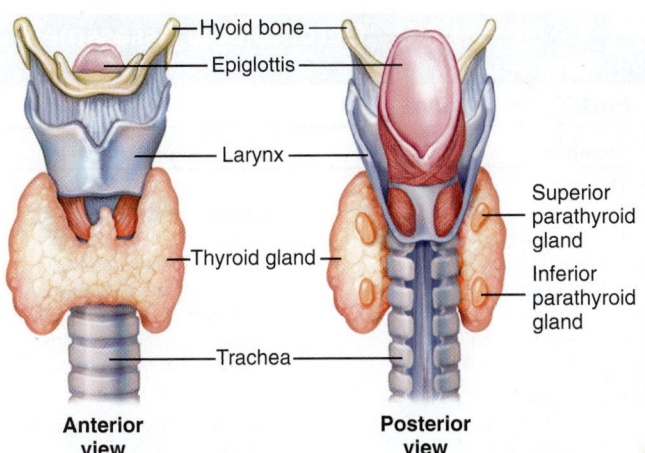

FIG. 47-8 Thyroid and parathyroid glands. Note the surrounding structures. (From Thibodeau GA, Patton KT: *The human body in health and disease*, ed 4, St Louis, 2005, Mosby.)

Thyroxine and Triiodothyronine. **Thyroxine (T_4)** accounts for 90% of thyroid hormone produced by the thyroid gland. However, **triiodothyronine (T_3)** is much more potent and has greater metabolic effects. The thyroid gland directly secretes about 20% of circulating T_3. The remainder comes from the conversion of T_4 after its release into the bloodstream. Iodine is necessary for the synthesis of both T_3 and T_4. Both hormones affect metabolic rate, caloric requirements, O_2 consumption, carbohydrate and lipid metabolism, growth and development, brain function, and other nervous system activities. More than 99% of thyroid hormones are bound to plasma proteins, especially thyroxine-binding globulin synthesized by the liver. Only the unbound "free" hormones are biologically active.

TSH from the anterior pituitary gland stimulates thyroid hormone production and release. When circulating levels of thyroid hormone are low, the hypothalamus releases thyrotropin-releasing hormone (TRH). TRH causes the anterior pituitary to release TSH. High circulating thyroid hormone levels inhibit the secretion of both TRH from the hypothalamus and TSH from the anterior pituitary gland.

Calcitonin. *Calcitonin* is made by C cells (parafollicular cells) of the thyroid gland in response to high circulating calcium levels. Calcitonin lowers serum calcium levels by (1) inhibiting the transfer of calcium from the bone to blood, (2) increasing calcium storage in bone, and (3) increasing renal excretion of calcium and phosphorus. Calcitonin and parathyroid hormone (PTH) regulate calcium balance.

Parathyroid Glands

Two pairs of parathyroid glands usually lie behind each thyroid lobe (Fig. 47-8). Although there are usually four glands, their number may range from two to six.

Parathyroid Hormone. The parathyroid glands secrete parathyroid hormone (PTH), also called *parathormone*. Its major role is to regulate serum calcium levels. PTH increases serum calcium levels by acting on bone, the kidneys, and indirectly on the GI tract. PTH stimulates the transfer of calcium from the bone into the blood. In the kidney, PTH promotes calcium reabsorption (moving calcium from the renal tubules back into the bloodstream) and phosphate excretion. In addition, PTH stimulates the renal conversion of vitamin D to its most active form (1,25-dihydroxyvitamin D_3). This form of vitamin D promotes absorption of calcium and phosphorus by the GI tract.

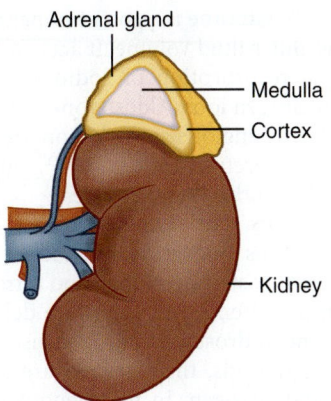

FIG. 47-9 The adrenal gland is composed of the adrenal cortex and the adrenal medulla.

PTH secretion is regulated by a negative feedback system. When the serum calcium level is low, PTH secretion increases. When the serum calcium level rises, PTH secretion falls. In addition, high levels of active vitamin D inhibit secretion of PTH, and low levels of magnesium stimulate PTH secretion.

Adrenal Glands

The adrenal glands are small, paired, highly vascular glands located on the upper portion of each kidney. Each gland consists of two parts: medulla and cortex (Fig. 47-9). Each part has distinct functions, and they act independently from one another.

Adrenal Medulla. The adrenal medulla is the inner part of the adrenal gland. It consists of sympathetic postganglionic neurons. The medulla secretes the **catecholamines** *epinephrine* (adrenaline), *norepinephrine* (noradrenaline), and *dopamine*. Catecholamines are considered neurotransmitters when secreted by neurons and hormones when secreted by the adrenal medulla. They are an essential part of the SNS's "fight or flight" response.

Adrenal Cortex. The adrenal cortex is the outer part of the adrenal gland. It secretes several steroid hormones, including *glucocorticoids, mineralocorticoids,* and *androgens.* Cholesterol is the precursor for steroid hormone synthesis. Glucocorticoids (e.g., cortisol) are named for their effects on glucose metabolism. They inhibit the inflammatory response and are considered antiinflammatory. Mineralocorticoids (e.g., aldosterone) are essential for maintaining fluid and electrolyte balance. The term **corticosteroid** refers to hormones synthesized by the adrenal cortex, excluding androgens.

Cortisol. **Cortisol**, the most abundant and potent glucocorticoid, is necessary to maintain life and protect the body from stress. It is secreted in a diurnal pattern (Fig. 47-5). A negative feedback mechanism controls cortisol secretion. The release of corticotropin-releasing hormone (CRH) from the hypothalamus stimulates the secretion of ACTH by the anterior pituitary.

One major function of cortisol is the regulation of blood glucose concentration by stimulating hepatic glucose formation *(gluconeogenesis).* Cortisol inhibits peripheral glucose use in the fasting state, inhibits protein synthesis, and stimulates the mobilization of glycerol and free fatty acids. It helps maintain vascular integrity and fluid volume through its action on mineralocorticoid receptors. Cortisol decreases the inflammatory response by stabilizing the membranes of cellular lysosomes and preventing increased capillary permeability. Stress, burns, infection, fever, acute anxiety, and hypoglycemia increase cortisol levels.

Aldosterone. Aldosterone is a potent mineralocorticoid that maintains extracellular fluid volume. It acts on the renal tubule to promote renal reabsorption of sodium and excretion of potassium and hydrogen ions. Aldosterone synthesis and secretion are stimulated by angiotensin II, hyponatremia, and hyperkalemia. Atrial natriuretic peptide (ANP) and hypokalemia inhibit aldosterone synthesis and release.

Adrenal Androgens. The adrenal cortex secretes small amounts of androgens that are converted to sex steroids in peripheral tissues: testosterone in men and estrogen in women. The most common adrenal androgens are dehydroepiandrosterone (DHEA) and androstenedione. Because they are precursors to other sex steroids, their actions are similar to those of testosterone and estrogen. In postmenopausal women, the major source of estrogen is from the peripheral conversion of adrenal androgen to estrogen.

Pancreas

The pancreas is a long, tapered, lobular, soft gland located behind the stomach and anterior to the first and second lumbar vertebrae. The pancreas has both exocrine and endocrine functions. The hormone-secreting portion of the pancreas is the *islets of Langerhans.* The islets account for less than 2% of the gland and consist of four types of hormone-secreting cells: α, β, delta, and F cells. α Cells make and secrete the hormone glucagon. β Cells make and secrete insulin and amylin. Delta cells make and secrete somatostatin. F (or PP) cells secrete pancreatic polypeptide.

Glucagon. Glucagon is released from pancreatic α cells and the gut in response to low blood glucose levels, protein ingestion, and exercise. Glucagon increases blood glucose, providing fuel for energy by stimulating glycogenolysis (breakdown of glycogen into glucose), gluconeogenesis (formation of glucose from non-carbohydrate molecules), and ketogenesis.[3] Glucagon and insulin function in a reciprocal manner to maintain normal blood glucose levels.

Insulin. Insulin is the principal regulator of metabolism and storage of ingested carbohydrates, fats, and proteins. Insulin facilitates glucose transport into cells, transport of amino acids across muscle membranes, and the synthesis of amino acids into protein in the peripheral tissues. However, the brain, nerves, lens of the eye, hepatocytes, erythrocytes, and cells in the intestinal mucosa and kidney tubules are not dependent on insulin for glucose uptake. After a meal, insulin is responsible for the utilization and storage of nutrients (*anabolism*). An increased blood glucose level is the major stimulus for insulin synthesis and secretion. Low blood glucose levels, glucagon, somatostatin, hypokalemia, and catecholamines usually inhibit insulin secretion.

 Gerontologic Considerations: Effects of Aging on Endocrine System

Normal aging has many effects on the endocrine system (Table 47-3). These include (1) decreased hormone production and secretion, (2) altered hormone metabolism and biologic activity, (3) decreased responsiveness of target tissues to hormones, and (4) alterations in circadian rhythms.

Assessing the effects of aging on the endocrine system may be difficult because the subtle changes of aging may mimic manifestations of endocrine disorders. Endocrine problems may manifest differently in an older adult than in a younger person. Older adults may have multiple co-morbidities and take

TABLE 47-3 Gerontologic Assessment Differences

Endocrine System

Changes	Clinical Significance
Thyroid	
Atrophy of thyroid gland	Increased incidence of hypothyroidism with aging
Decreased secretion of triiodothyronine (T_3), thyroxine (T_4), thyroid-stimulating hormone (TSH)	However, most older adults maintain adequate thyroid function.
Increased nodules	Thyroid hormone replacement dose lower in older adults
Parathyroid	
Increased secretion of PTH (parathyroid hormone)	Increased calcium resorption from bone
Increased basal level of PTH	Hypercalcemia, hypercalciuria (may reflect defective renal mechanism)
Adrenal Cortex	
Adrenal cortex becomes more fibrotic and slightly smaller	Decreased metabolic clearance rate for glucocorticoids
Decreased metabolism of cortisol	
Decreased plasma levels of adrenal androgens and aldosterone	
Adrenal Medulla	
Increased secretion and basal level of norepinephrine	Decreased responsiveness to β-adrenergic agonists and receptor blockers
Decreased β-adrenergic receptor response to norepinephrine	May partly explain increased incidence of hypertension with aging
Pancreas	
Increase in fibrosis and fatty deposits in pancreas	May partly contribute to increased incidence of diabetes mellitus with advanced aging
Increased glucose intolerance with decreased sensitivity to insulin	
Gonads	
Women: Decline in estrogen secretion	Experience symptoms associated with menopause Have increased risk for arteriosclerosis and osteoporosis
Men: Decline in testosterone secretion	Men may or may not experience symptoms

medications that alter the body's usual response to endocrine function. Symptoms of endocrine dysfunction such as fatigue, constipation, or mental impairment may be attributed to aging, resulting in delayed treatment.

ASSESSMENT OF ENDOCRINE SYSTEM

Endocrine dysfunction is generally the result of too much or too little of a specific hormone. The onset of symptoms is often gradual. The subtle or vague symptoms are often attributed to other physiologic or psychologic causes. Consequently, patients with endocrine dysfunction may present with fluid and electrolyte imbalances, altered tissue perfusion, inadequate coping mechanisms, alterations in cardiac rhythm, or changes in skin integrity that can be interpreted as many other conditions. Alternatively, patients may present with acute symptoms that are life threatening and demand immediate intervention.

CASE STUDY

Patient Introduction

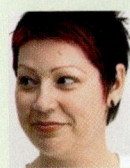

(©iStockphoto/ Thinkstock)

L.M. is a 35-yr-old Hispanic woman who comes to the clinic complaining of "just not feeling well." She is accompanied by H.H., her female partner. L.M. states that she has gained a lot of weight despite trying to watch her diet and just seems to be getting more and more tired. H.H. voices concerns about changes in her partner's energy level.

Discussion Questions

1. What are the possible causes of L.M.'s weight gain, fatigue, and irritability?
2. What would be your priority assessment of L.M.?
3. What questions would you ask L.M.?

You will learn more about L.M. and her condition as you read through this assessment chapter.

(See p. 1111 for more information on L.M.)

Answers available at *http://evolve.elsevier.com/Lewis/medsurg.*

GENETIC RISK ALERT

Pituitary
- Nephrogenic diabetes insipidus can be inherited as a sex-linked or autosomal disorder.

Thyroid
- Genetics has a role in many cases of hypothyroid and hyperthyroid disorders.
- Hashimoto's thyroiditis, the most common cause of hypothyroidism, and Graves' disease, a cause of hyperthyroidism, are autoimmune disorders. Both likely result from a combination of genetic and environmental factors.[4]

Multiple Endocrine Neoplasia
- Multiple endocrine neoplasia (MEN) involves tumors in two or more different endocrine glands.
- There are several types of MEN. Mutations of *MEN1, RET,* and *CDKN1B* genes determine the type.
- The features of MEN are relatively consistent within any one family.
- A common tumor associated with MEN type 2 is medullary thyroid carcinoma.[4]

Diabetes Mellitus
- Genetics has a strong role in the development of type 2 diabetes and to a lesser extent in type 1 diabetes.

Subjective Data

Information obtained from the patient can provide important clues as to the functioning of the endocrine system. You will need to obtain a thorough history from the patient and/or a caregiver if the patient's mental acuity is compromised.

Important Health Information

Past Health History. Patients with endocrine disorders often present with nonspecific complaints. The chief complaint may relate to not just one but a group of symptoms. The most common presenting problems include fatigue, weakness, menstrual irregularities, and weight changes. It is important to determine if the onset of symptoms has been gradual or sudden and what the patient has done about them.

Because some of the more general signs of dysfunction are the easiest to overlook, you must evaluate any reported or observed changes in weight, appetite, skin, libido, mental acuity, emotional stability, or energy levels.

Medications. Ask about the use of all medications (both prescription and over-the-counter drugs), herbs, and dietary supplements. Ask about the reason for taking the drug, the dosage, and the length of time the drug has been taken. In particular, ask about the use of hormone replacements. Knowing that the patient is currently taking hormone replacements such as insulin, thyroid hormone, or corticosteroids (e.g., prednisone) alerts the nurse to potential adverse drug events. For example, corticosteroids may increase blood glucose levels and cause bone loss with long-term use. Thyroid preparations may cause tachycardia or dysrhythmias. Drug-to-drug interactions and adverse effects of nonhormonal medications can contribute to endocrine problems.

Surgery or Other Treatments. Inquire about past medical, surgical, and obstetric history, including number of pregnancies and live births. Ask about traumatic events, birth weight, growth patterns, and stages of physical and emotional development. The depth of information required may vary depending on the presenting condition. For example, data regarding past radiation therapy to the head and neck are important when thyroid or pituitary dysfunction is suspected.

Functional Health Patterns. Key questions to ask the patient with an endocrine problem are summarized in Table 47-4.

Health Perception–Health Management Pattern. Heredity often plays an important role in the development of endocrine dysfunction. Ask about first-degree relatives with diabetes mellitus, thyroid disease, or endocrine gland cancers, since these conditions have a familial tendency. A genetic assessment of family members may be appropriate.

Nutritional-Metabolic Pattern. Changes in appetite and weight can indicate endocrine dysfunction. Weight loss with increased appetite may indicate hyperthyroidism or diabetes mellitus. Weight gain may indicate hypothyroidism or hypocortisolism. Obese persons are more likely to develop type 2 diabetes.

Ask if there have been problems with nausea, vomiting, or diarrhea. Difficulty swallowing or a change in neck size may indicate an enlarged thyroid gland. Increased SNS activity, including nervousness, palpitations, sweating, and tremors, may indicate thyroid dysfunction or a rare tumor of the adrenal medulla *(pheochromocytoma).* Heat or cold intolerance may indicate hyperthyroidism or hypothyroidism, respectively.

Ask about changes in the patient's skin, particularly on the face, neck, hands, or body creases. Changes in skin texture and skin that seems thicker or drier may indicate endocrine dysfunction. A patient with hypothyroidism or excess GH may have skin that feels coarse or leathery. Ask if the patient has noticed any change in the distribution of hair anywhere on the body.

Elimination Pattern. Because maintaining fluid balance is a major role of the endocrine system, questions related to fluid intake and elimination patterns may uncover endocrine dysfunction. For example, increased thirst and urination can indicate diabetes mellitus (pancreas disorder) or diabetes insipidus (pituitary disorder). Ask about the frequency and consistency of bowel movements. Frequent defecation may indicate hyperthyroidism or autonomic neuropathy of diabetes mellitus. Constipation occurs with hypothyroidism, hypoparathyroidism, and hypopituitarism.

Activity-Exercise Pattern. Determine if there are any acute or gradual changes in energy level or persistent fatigue. Changes in

---

TABLE 47-4   Health History

Endocrine System

Health Perception–Health Management
- What is your usual day like?
- Have you noticed any changes in your ability to perform your usual activities compared with last year? Five years ago?*

Nutritional-Metabolic
- What is your weight and height?
- How much do you want to weigh?
- Have there been any changes in your appetite or weight?*
- Have you noticed any changes in the distribution of the hair anywhere on your body?*
- Have you noticed any changes in the color of your skin, particularly on your face, neck, hands, or body creases?*
- Has the texture of your skin changed? For example, does it seem thicker and drier than it used to?*
- Have you noticed any difficulty swallowing, throat pain, or hoarseness? Is the top button on your shirt or blouse more difficult to button?*
- Do you feel more nervous than you used to? Do you notice your heart pounding or that you sweat when you do not think you should be sweating?*
- Do you have difficulty holding things because of shakiness of your hands?*
- Do you feel that most rooms are too hot or too cold? Do you frequently have to put on a sweater, or feel as though you need to open windows when others in the room seem comfortable?*
- Do you have or have you had any wounds that were slow to heal?*

Elimination
- Do you have to get up at night to urinate? If so, how many times? Do you keep water by your bed at night?
- Have you ever had a kidney stone?*
- Describe your usual bowel pattern. Have you noted any bowel changes?*
- Do you use anything, such as laxatives, to help you move your bowels?*

Activity-Exercise
- What is your usual activity pattern during a typical day?
- Do you have a planned exercise program? If yes, what is it and have you had to make any changes in this routine lately? If so, why and what kinds of changes?
- Do you experience fatigue with or without activity?*
- Have you had any trouble with breathing?*

Sleep-Rest
- How many hours do you sleep at night? Do you feel rested on awakening?
- Are you ever awakened by sweating during the night?*
- Do you have nightmares?*

Cognitive-Perceptual
- How is your memory? Have you noticed any changes?*
- Have you experienced any blurring or double vision?*
- When was your last eye examination?

Self-Perception–Self-Concept
- Have you noticed any changes in your physical appearance or size?*
- Are you concerned about your weight?*
- Do you feel you are able to do what you think you should be capable of doing? If not, why not?
- Does your health problem affect how you feel about yourself?*

Role-Relationship
- Do you have a support system or partner? Are you married? Do you have any children? Do you think you are able to take care of your family and home? If not, why not?
- Where do you work? What kind of work do you do? Are you able to do what is expected of you and what you expect of yourself?
- Are you retired? What type of work did you do before you retired? How do you spend your time now that you have retired?

Sexuality-Reproductive
Women
- When did you start to menstruate? Was this earlier or later than other women in your family?
- When was your last menstrual period? Do you have scant, heavy, or irregular menstrual flows?
- How many children have you had? How much did they weigh at birth? Were you told you had diabetes during any pregnancy?*
- Are you menopausal? If so, for how long?
- Are you attempting to get pregnant but cannot?*
- Are you postmenopausal? If so, do you have any bleeding from your uterus?

Men
- Have you noticed any changes in your ability to get and maintain an erection?*
- Are you trying to have children but cannot?*

Coping–Stress Tolerance
- What kind of stressors do you have?
- How do you deal with stress or problems?
- What is your support system? To whom do you turn when you have a problem?

Value-Belief
- Do you think medicine should still be taken even though you feel okay?
- Do any of your prescribed therapies cause any conflict in your value-belief system?*

*If yes, describe.

---

activity level can identify a patient with chronic fatigue secondary to hypothyroidism, hypocortisolism, or diabetes mellitus.

Sleep-Rest Pattern. Ask the patient how many hours he or she typically sleeps, and if he or she feels rested on awakening. Sleep disturbances can result from nocturia, nightmares, anxiety, depression, or insomnia that occurs with diabetes or thyroid dysfunction.

Cognitive-Perceptual Pattern. Memory deficits are apparent in hypothyroidism and occur with changes in sodium levels. Hyponatremia can occur because of inappropriate secretion of antidiuretic hormone (SIADH) or pituitary tumors. These issues can occur gradually, so it is sometimes difficult for

family members or care providers to identify changes in cognition. Gathering information from patient and family regarding memory, cognitive abilities, and balance can increase the chances of an earlier diagnosis.

Self-Perception–Self-Concept Pattern. Many endocrine disorders may affect a patient's self-esteem because of associated changes in physical appearance. For example, weight gain associated with hypothyroidism or exophthalmos and goiter associated with hyperthyroidism can cause problems related to body image.

Role-Relationship Pattern. Questions related to roles and relationships can highlight depression, chronic fatigue, and sleep disorders. With chronic fatigue, depression and anxiety, patients and their families will experience stressed relationships. Questions related to home life and the patient's ability to fulfill their role in the family will aid in the identification of these disorders.

Sexuality-Reproductive Pattern. Growth hormone, prolactin, LH, FSH, testosterone, and estrogen are regulated by the endocrine system. Therefore menstrual dysfunction, hirsutism, infertility, and growth disorders can be a result of endocrine disorders. Some women experience hypothyroidism during or after menopause. Other patients begin to develop type 2 diabetes during middle age when sex hormones are changing. Document the presence of abnormal secondary sex characteristics, such as facial hair *(hirsutism)* in women. Obtain a detailed history of menstruation and pregnancy. Menstrual dysfunction can occur with disorders of the ovaries and pituitary, thyroid, and adrenal glands. A history of large-birth-weight babies may indicate gestational diabetes, which may put the patient at a higher risk of developing type 2 diabetes later in life. Male sexual dysfunction may take the form of impotence, decreased libido, infertility, or the lack of development of secondary sexual characteristics. Retrograde ejaculation can occur in diabetes mellitus.

Coping–Stress Tolerance Pattern. Because stress exacerbates some endocrine conditions, ask patients about their stress level and usual coping patterns. Patients with adrenal insufficiency have difficulty dealing with stress. These patients are at risk for developing hypotension and fluid and electrolyte imbalance. Patients' perception of the impact of their condition and treatments on their lifestyle is significant.

Value-Belief Pattern. Determining a patient's ability to make lifestyle changes is an important nursing function. Identify the patient's value-belief patterns so that you can help to determine appropriate treatment regimens. This is particularly important in a condition such as diabetes mellitus, which may require major lifestyle changes. Other disorders, such as hypothyroidism or hypocortisolism, may be managed with medications but require lifelong monitoring with an HCP.

Objective Data

Most endocrine glands (with the exception of the thyroid and testes) are inaccessible to direct examination. Assessment can be accomplished using objective data, including physical examination and diagnostic tests. It is essential to understand the actions of hormones in order to assess the function of a gland by monitoring the target tissue.

Physical Examination. Specific clinical findings for the various endocrine problems are discussed in Chapters 48 and 49. Regardless of the type of endocrine dysfunction, use the following general examination.[5]

Take a full set of vital signs at the beginning of the examination. Variations in temperature, heart rate, and blood pressure can occur with a variety of endocrine-related problems.

Include a history of growth and development patterns, weight distribution and changes, and comparisons of these factors with normal findings. Calculate body mass index (BMI) to assess nutritional status.

Endocrine disorders may cause changes in mental and emotional status. Throughout the examination, assess the patient's orientation, alertness, memory, cognitive abilities, affect, personality, and anxiety and the appropriateness of his or her behavior.

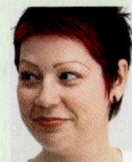
Integument. Assess the color and texture of the skin, hair, and nails. Note the overall skin color as well as pigmentation and possible ecchymosis (bruise). Decreased skin pigmentation can occur in hypopituitarism, hypothyroidism, and hypoparathyroidism. Hyperpigmentation, or "bronzing" of the skin

(particularly on knuckles, elbows, knees, genitalia, and palmar creases), is a classic finding in a form of adrenal insufficiency known as *Addison's disease.* Palpate the skin for texture and moisture. Examine hair distribution on the head, face, trunk, and extremities. Assess the hair's appearance and texture. Hair loss, excessive hair growth, or dull, brittle hair may indicate endocrine dysfunction. Assess for delayed wound healing.

Head. Inspect the size and contour of the head. Facial features should be symmetric. Hyperreflexia and facial muscle contraction upon percussion of the facial nerve *(Chvostek's sign)* may occur in hypoparathyroidism. Inspect the eyes for position, symmetry, and shape. Large and protruding eyes (exophthalmos) are associated with hyperthyroidism. Assess visual acuity using a Snellen eye chart. Visual field loss may indicate a pituitary tumor. In the mouth, inspect the buccal mucosa, condition of teeth, and tongue size. Note hair distribution on the scalp and face. Hearing loss is common in acromegaly from excess GH.[6]

Neck. The thyroid gland is not usually visible during inspection. A feature that distinguishes the thyroid from other masses in the neck is its upward movement on swallowing. Inspect the neck while the patient swallows a sip of water. The neck should appear symmetric without lumps or bulging.

Palpate the thyroid for its size, shape, symmetry, and tenderness and for any nodules. *Goiter,* an enlarged thyroid gland, can occur with hyper- or hypothyroidism. Be careful not to press too hard or massage an enlarged thyroid gland. This can cause a sudden release of thyroid hormone into an already overloaded system. An experienced clinician should perform palpation in patients with a known diagnosis of hyperthyroidism.

Perform palpation using a posterior or anterior approach. For *anterior palpation,* stand in front of the patient, with the patient's neck flexed. Place your thumb horizontally with the upper edge along the lower border of the cricoid cartilage. Then move your thumb over the isthmus as the patient swallows water. Place your fingers laterally to the anterior border of the sternocleidomastoid muscle, and palpate each lateral lobe before and while the patient swallows water.

For *posterior palpation,* stand behind the patient (Fig. 47-10). With the thumbs of both hands resting on the nape of the patient's neck, use your index and middle fingers of both hands to feel for the thyroid isthmus and for the anterior surfaces of the lateral lobes. To relax the neck muscles, ask the patient to flex the neck slightly forward and to the right. Displace the

thyroid cartilage to the right with your left hand and fingers. Palpate with your right hand after placing the thumb deep and behind the sternocleidomastoid muscle with the index and middle fingers in front of it. Ask the patient to swallow water, and feel for the thyroid to move up. In a normal person, the thyroid is often not palpable. If palpable, it usually feels smooth with a firm consistency. It is not tender with gentle pressure. If nodules, enlargement, asymmetry, or hardness (abnormal findings) are present, refer the patient for further evaluation. Auscultate the lateral lobes of an enlarged thyroid gland with the stethoscope bell to identify a *bruit,* a soft swishing sound that may indicate a goiter or hyperthyroidism.

Thorax. Inspect the thorax for shape and characteristics of the skin. Note the presence of breast gynecomastia in men. Auscultate lung sounds and heart sounds. Note any adventitious lung sounds (wheezing, diminished sounds) or extra heart sounds. Signs of fluid overload or heart failure may be present in patients with secretion of inappropriate antidiuretic hormone or hypothyroidism (SIADH).

Abdomen. Inspect the contour of the abdomen and note the symmetry and color. Cushing syndrome (hypercortisolism) causes the skin to be fragile, resulting in purple-blue striae across the abdomen. Note general obesity or truncal obesity. Auscultate bowel sounds.

Extremities. Assess the size, shape, symmetry, and general proportion of hands and feet. Patients with acromegaly from pituitary tumors may have large hands and feet. Inspect the skin for changes in pigmentation, lesions, and edema. Evaluate muscle strength and deep tendon reflexes. In the upper extremities, assess for tremors by placing a piece of paper on the outstretched fingers, palm down. Muscular spasms of the hand elicited on application of an occlusive BP cuff for 3 minutes *(Trousseau's sign)* may occur in hypoparathyroidism.

Genitalia. Inspect the genital hair distribution pattern, since it may be altered with hormone irregularities.

Assessment abnormalities related to the endocrine system are presented in Table 47-5. A focused assessment of the endocrine system is presented on p. 1114.

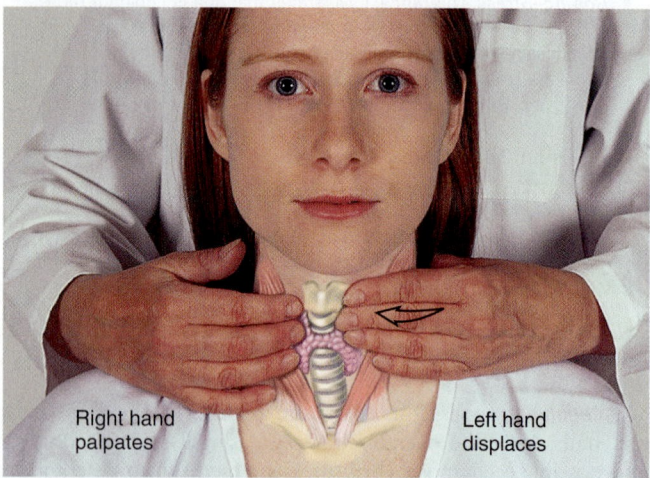

FIG. 47-10   Posterior palpation of the thyroid gland. (From Jarvis C: *Physical examination and health assessment,* ed 6, St Louis, 2012, Saunders.)

Right hand palpates

Left hand displaces

CASE STUDY—cont'd

Objective Data: Physical Examination

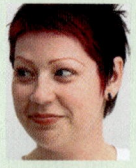

(©iStockphoto/ Thinkstock)

A focused assessment of L.M. reveals the following: L.M. is sitting on the edge of the examination table. She appears somewhat anxious. Her BP is 190/80, heart rate 84, respiratory rate 20, temp 98.6° F (37° C). Her weight is 160 lb, and she is 5 ft 4 inches tall. L.M.'s face is reddened and puffy, and she appears to have a lump on the back of her neck and shoulders. She has some acne on her face, along with some hair growth on her upper lip and chin area. Her abdomen is protruding, but her arms and legs are thin. She has +1 edema in her ankles bilaterally. There are several ecchymotic areas on her upper and lower extremities, as well as purple stretch marks on her abdomen.

Discussion Questions

1. Which physical assessment findings are of most concern to you?
2. Based upon the subjective and objective assessment data presented so far, what are three priority nursing diagnoses?
3. What diagnostic studies would you expect to be ordered?
   You will learn more about diagnostic studies related to the endocrine system in the next section.
   (See p. 1118 for more information on L.M.)

Answers available at *http://evolve.elsevier.com/Lewis/medsurg.*

TABLE 47-5 Assessment Abnormalities

Endocrine System

Finding	Description	Possible Etiology and Significance
Integument		
Hyperpigmentation	Darkening of the skin, particularly in creases and skinfolds	Addison's disease caused by increased secretion of melanocyte-stimulating hormone, acanthosis nigricans
Depigmentation (vitiligo)	Patchy areas of light skin	May be a marker of autoimmune endocrine disorders
Striae	Purplish red marks below the skin surface. Usually seen on abdomen, breasts, and buttocks	Cushing syndrome
Changes in skin texture	Thick, cold, dry skin	Hypothyroidism
	Thick, leathery, oily skin	Growth hormone excess (acromegaly)
	Warm, smooth, moist skin	Hyperthyroidism
Changes in hair distribution	Hair loss	Hypothyroidism, hyperthyroidism, decreased pituitary secretion
	Diminished axillary and pubic hair	Cortisol deficiency
	Hirsutism (excessive facial hair on women)	Cushing syndrome, prolactinoma (a pituitary tumor)
Skin ulceration	Areas of ulcerated skin, most commonly found on legs and feet	Peripheral neuropathy and peripheral vascular disease, which are contributory factors in the development of diabetic foot ulcers
Bruises easily	Multiple bruises over various parts of body	Cushing syndrome
Edema	Generalized edema	Mucopolysaccharide accumulation in tissue in hypothyroidism
Head and Neck		
Visual changes	Decreased visual acuity and/or decreased peripheral vision	Pituitary gland enlargement or tumor leading to pressure on optic nerve
Exophthalmos	Eyeball protrusion from orbits	Occurs in hyperthyroidism as a result of fluid accumulation in eye and retroorbital tissue
Moon face	Periorbital edema and facial fullness	Cushing syndrome as a result of increased cortisol secretion
Myxedema	Puffiness, periorbital edema, masklike affect	Hydrophilic mucopolysaccharides infiltrating dermis in patients with hypothyroidism
Goiter	Generalized enlargement of thyroid gland	Hyperthyroidism, hypothyroidism, iodine deficiency
Thyroid nodule(s)	Localized enlargement of thyroid gland	May be benign or malignant
Cardiovascular		
Chest pain	Angina caused by increased metabolic demands, effusions	Hyperthyroidism, hypothyroidism
Dysrhythmias	Tachycardia, atrial fibrillation	Hypothyroidism or hyperthyroidism, hypoparathyroidism or hyperparathyroidism, pheochromocytoma
Hypertension	Elevated BP caused by increased metabolic demands and catecholamines	Hyperthyroidism, pheochromocytoma, Cushing syndrome
Fluid overload or signs of heart failure	Crackles in the lungs, peripheral edema, shortness of breath	Syndrome of inappropriate antidiuretic hormone, hypothyroidism, myxedema
Musculoskeletal		
Changes in muscular strength or muscle mass	Generalized weakness and/or fatigue	Common symptoms associated with many endocrine problems, including pituitary, thyroid, parathyroid, and adrenal dysfunctions
		Diabetes mellitus, diabetes insipidus
	Decreased muscle mass	Specifically seen in those with growth hormone deficiency and in Cushing syndrome secondary to protein wasting
Enlargement of bones and cartilage	Coarsening of facial features. Increases in size of hands and feet over a period of several years	Gradual enlargement and thickening of bony tissue occurring with growth hormone excess in adults as seen in acromegaly secondary to pituitary dysfunction
Nutrition		
Changes in weight	Weight loss	Hyperthyroidism caused by increases in metabolism, type 1 diabetes mellitus, diabetic ketoacidosis
Altered glucose levels	Weight gain	Hypothyroidism, Cushing syndrome, type 2 diabetes mellitus
	Increased serum glucose	Diabetes mellitus, Cushing syndrome, growth hormone excess
Neurologic		
Lethargy	State of mental sluggishness or somnolence	Hypothyroidism
Tetany	Intermittent involuntary muscle spasms usually involving the extremities	Severe hypocalcemia that can occur with hypoparathyroidism
Seizure	Sudden involuntary contraction of muscles	Consequence of a pituitary tumor
		Hypervolemia and hyponatremia associated with syndrome of inappropriate antidiuretic hormone
		Complications of diabetes mellitus, severe hypothyroidism
Increased deep tendon reflexes	Hyperreflexia	Hyperthyroidism, hypoparathyroidism
Gastrointestinal		
Constipation	Passage of infrequent hard stools	Hypothyroidism, hyperparathyroidism

TABLE 47-5   Assessment Abnormalities

Endocrine System—cont'd

Finding	Description	Possible Etiology and Significance
Reproductive		
Changes in reproductive function	Menstrual irregularities, decreased libido, decreased fertility, impotence	Pituitary hypofunction, growth hormone excess, thyroid dysfunction, adrenocortical dysfunction
Other		
Polyuria	Excessive urine output	Diabetes mellitus (secondary to hyperglycemia) or diabetes insipidus (associated with decreased ADH)
Polydipsia	Excessive thirst	Extreme water losses in diabetes mellitus (with severe hyperglycemia), diabetes insipidus, dehydration
Decreased urine output	Decreased water reabsorption from kidney tubules	Syndrome of inappropriate antidiuretic hormone
Thermoregulation	Cold insensitivity Heat intolerance	Hypothyroidism caused by a slowing of metabolic processes Hyperthyroidism caused by excessive metabolism

FOCUSED ASSESSMENT

Endocrine System

Use this checklist to ensure the key assessment steps have been done.

Subjective

Ask the patient about any of the following and note responses.

Excessive or increased thirst	Y	N
Excessive or decreased urination	Y	N
Excessive hunger	Y	N
Intolerance to heat or cold	Y	N
Excessive sweating	Y	N
Recent weight gain or loss	Y	N

Objective: Diagnostic

Check the following laboratory results for critical values.

Potassium	✓
Glucose	✓
Sodium	✓
Glycosylated hemoglobin (A1C)	✓
Thyroid studies: TSH, T_3, T_4	✓
Serum osmolality	✓

Objective: Physical Examination

Inspect/Measure

Body temperature	✓
Height and weight	✓
Alertness and emotional state	✓
Skin for changes in color and texture	✓
Hair for changes in color, texture, and distribution	✓

Auscultate

Heart rate, BP	✓

Palpate

Extremities for edema	✓
Skin for texture and temperature	✓
Neck for thyroid size, shape	✓

T_3, Triiodothyronine; T_4, thyroxine; *TSH*, thyroid-stimulating hormone.

DIAGNOSTIC STUDIES OF ENDOCRINE SYSTEM

Diagnostic studies of the endocrine system are presented in Table 47-6. Pertinent findings from the history and physical examination guide the selection of diagnostic studies. Imaging studies can identify pituitary tumors, thyroid nodules, or adrenal tumors. Laboratory studies may include direct measurement of the hormone level or involve an indirect indication of gland function by evaluating blood or urine components affected by the hormone such as glucose or electrolytes. It is also possible to measure the releasing or stimulating hormone. For example, TSH can be measured to evaluate thyroid function.

Hormones with constant basal levels, such as T_4, can be assessed with a single measurement. Note the time of the sample collection on the laboratory slip. Information about night shift work is important for hormones with circadian or sleep-related secretion (e.g., cortisol). Evaluation of other hormones may require multiple blood samplings, such as in suppression tests (e.g., dexamethasone) and stimulation tests (e.g., glucose tolerance). In these situations, it is often necessary to obtain IV access to administer the testing medication and fluids and to draw multiple blood samples.

Disorders associated with the pituitary gland can manifest in a wide variety of ways because of the number of hormones produced. Many diagnostic studies evaluate these hormones either directly or indirectly.

A number of tests are available to evaluate thyroid function. The most sensitive and accurate laboratory test is the measurement of TSH. Thus it is often the first diagnostic test done to evaluate thyroid function.[7] Common additional tests ordered in the presence of an abnormal TSH level include total T_4, free T_4, and total T_3. Free T_4 is the unbound thyroxine and is a more accurate reflection of thyroid function than total T_4.

The only hormone secreted by the parathyroid glands is PTH. Because PTH regulates serum calcium and phosphate levels, abnormalities in PTH secretion are reflected by these levels. For this reason, diagnostic tests for the parathyroid gland typically include PTH, serum calcium, and serum phosphate levels.

Tests associated with the adrenal cortex function focus on measuring blood plasma and urine levels of the three types of hormones secreted: glucocorticoids, mineralocorticoids, and androgens. Urine studies often require a 24-hour urine collection to eliminate the impact of short-term fluctuations in plasma hormone levels.

The tests used to evaluate glucose metabolism are important in the diagnosis and management of diabetes mellitus. See Chapter 48 for information regarding diagnostic studies for diabetes mellitus.

TABLE 47-6 Diagnostic Studies

Endocrine System

Study	Purpose and Description	Nursing Responsibility
Pituitary Studies *Blood Studies*		
Growth hormone (GH) (somatotropin)	Evaluates GH secretion. Used to identify GH deficiency or GH excess. GH levels are affected by time of day, food intake, and stress. Difficult to interpret significance of isolated GH level. Further evaluation requires stimulation tests. *Reference interval:* Men: <4 ng/mL (<4.0 mcg/L), Women: <18 ng/mL (<18 mcg/L)	*Before:* Make sure that patient has been fasting. Emotional and physical stress may alter results. Indicate patient fasting status and recent activity level on the laboratory slip. *After:* Send blood sample to laboratory immediately.
Somatomedin C (insulin-like growth factor 1 [IGF-1])	Evaluates GH secretion. Provides a more accurate reflection of mean plasma concentration of GH because it is not subject to circadian rhythm and fluctuations. Low levels indicate GH deficiency. High levels indicate GH excess. *Reference interval:* 42-110 ng/mL	*Before:* Overnight fasting is preferred but not necessary.
Growth hormone (GH) stimulation	**Insulin tolerance test:** Regular insulin given IV and blood drawn at −30, 0, 30, 45, 60, and 90 min for measurement of glucose and GH. *Reference interval:* GH >5 mcg/L **Arginine-GHRH test:** GHRH bolus followed by 30-min infusion of arginine. *Reference interval:* GH >4.1 mcg/L	*Before:* Patient is NPO after midnight. Water is permitted on morning of test. Establish IV access for medication administration and blood sampling. *During:* Continually assess for hypoglycemia and hypotension. Keep 50% dextrose and 5% dextrose IV solution at the bedside in case severe hypoglycemia occurs.
Gonadotropins • Follicle-stimulating hormone (FSH) • Luteinizing hormone (LH)	Used to distinguish primary gonadal problems from pituitary insufficiency. In women, there are marked differences during menstrual cycle and in postmenopausal period. Levels are low in pituitary insufficiency and high in primary gonadal failure. **FSH Reference intervals** *Women:* Follicular phase: 1.37-9.9 mU/mL Ovulatory phase: 6.17-17.2 mU/mL Luteal phase: 1.09-9.2 mU/mL Postmenopause: 19.3-100.6 mU/mL *Men:* 1.42-15.4 mU/mL **LH Reference intervals** *Women:* Follicular phase: 1.68-15 IU/L Ovulatory phase: 21.9-56.6 IU/L Postmenopause: 14.2-52.3 IU/L *Men:* 1.24-7.8 IU/L	*Before:* Explain procedure to patient. *During:* Note on the laboratory slip time of menstrual cycle or whether woman is menopausal.
Water deprivation (restriction) (ADH stimulation)	Used to differentiate causes of diabetes insipidus (DI), including central DI, nephrogenic DI, and psychogenic polydipsia. ADH (vasopressin) is administered. In patients with central DI, urine osmolality increases after ADH. In patients with nephrogenic DI, no or minimal response to ADH.	*Before:* Obtain baseline weight and urine and plasma osmolality. Should be performed only if serum sodium is normal and urine osmolality is <300 mOsm/kg. *During:* Patient is NPO for test. Severe dehydration may occur with central or nephrogenic diabetes insipidus. Assess urine hourly for volume and specific gravity. Send hourly urine samples to laboratory for osmolality determination. Send blood samples for sodium and osmolality every 2 hr. Discontinue test and rehydrate if patient's weight drops >2 kg at any time. *After:* Rehydrate with oral fluids. Check orthostatic BP and pulse to ensure adequate fluid volume.
Radiologic Studies **Magnetic resonance imaging (MRI)**	Examination of choice for radiologic evaluation of the pituitary gland and hypothalamus. Used to identify tumors involving the hypothalamus or pituitary.	*Before:* Inform patient of the need to lie as still as possible during the test. Assess for contraindications, including pregnancy, presence of metal implants (e.g., pacemaker).
Computed tomography (CT) scan	Used to detect tumor and size of tumor. Oral and/or IV contrast medium may be used.	*Before:* Assess renal function before test. If IV contrast is used, check for iodine or shellfish allergy. Contrast medium may induce renal failure in at-risk patients.

Continued

TABLE 47-6   Diagnostic Studies

Endocrine System—cont'd

Study	Purpose and Description	Nursing Responsibility
Thyroid Studies *Blood Studies*		
Thyroid-stimulating hormone (TSH) (thyrotropin)	Measures TSH levels. Considered the most sensitive diagnostic test for evaluating thyroid dysfunction. *Reference interval:* 0.4-4.2 µU/mL (0.4-4.2 mU/L)	*Before:* Explain blood draw procedure to the patient. No specific preparations are necessary.
Triiodothyronine (T$_3$), total	Measures serum levels of T$_3$. Used to diagnose hyperthyroidism if T$_4$ levels are normal. *Reference interval: Ages 20-50:* 70-204 ng/dL (1.08-3.14 nmol/L) *Ages >50:* 40-181 ng/dL (0.62-2.79 nmol/L)	See above.
Thyroxine (T$_4$), total	Measures total serum level of T$_4$. Used to evaluate thyroid function and monitor thyroid therapy. *Reference interval:* 4.6-11.0 mcg/dL (59-142 nmol/L)	See above.
Free thyroxine (FT$_4$)	Measures active component of total T$_4$. Because level remains constant, considered better indicator of thyroid function than total T$_4$. *Reference interval:* 0.8-2.7 ng/dL (10-35 pmol/L)	*Before:* Tell patient that FT$_4$ levels may be measured until symptoms of hyperthyroidism have abated and levels have returned to normal.
Free triiodothyronine (FT$_3$)	Measures active component of total T$_3$. *Reference interval:* 260-480 pg/dL (4.0-7.4 pmol/L)	See above.
T$_3$ uptake (T$_3$ resin uptake)	Indirectly measures binding capacity of thyroid-binding globulin. *Reference interval:* 24%-34%	See above.
Thyroid antibodies (Ab) • Thyroid peroxidase (TPO) Ab • Thyroglobulin Ab • Thyroid-stimulating Ab	Measures levels of thyroid antibodies. Assists in the diagnosis of autoimmune thyroid disease and separates it from other forms of thyroiditis. One or more antibody tests may be ordered depending on symptoms.	See above.
Thyroglobulin	Identifies functioning thyroid tissue and thyroid cancer cells. Used primarily as a tumor marker for patients being treated for thyroid cancer. *Reference interval:* *Men:* 0.5-53 ng/mL *Women:* 0.5-43 ng/mL	See above.
Radiologic Studies **Ultrasound**	Evaluates thyroid nodule(s) to determine if it is a fluid-filled (cystic) or solid tumor and follows change over time.	*Before:* Explain that gel and a transducer will be used over the neck. The test lasts 15 min. No fasting or sedation required.
Thyroid scan and uptake	***Scan:*** Used to evaluate nodules of thyroid. Radioactive isotopes are given orally or IV. Scanner passes over thyroid and makes graphic record of radiation emitted. Normal thyroid scan reveals homogeneous pattern with symmetric lobes. Benign nodules appear as warm spots because they take up radionuclide. Malignant tumors appear as cold spots because they tend not to take up radionuclide. ***Radioactive iodine uptake (RAIU):*** Provides direct measure of thyroid activity. Evaluates function of thyroid nodules. Patient is given radioactive iodine either orally or IV. The uptake by the thyroid gland is measured with a scanner at several time intervals such as 2-4 hr and at 24 hr. The values of RAIU are expressed in percentage of uptake. *Reference interval:* For 2-4 hr: 3%-19% For 24 hr: 11%-30%	*Before:* Explain procedure to the patient. Reaction to iodine in allergic patients is rare because amount of iodine in preparation is minimal. *After:* Tell patient to drink increased amount of fluids for 24-48 hr unless contraindicated. Radionuclide will be eliminated in 6-24 hr.
Parathyroid Studies *Blood Studies*		
Parathyroid hormone (PTH)	Measures PTH level in serum. Must be interpreted in terms of concurrently drawn serum calcium level. *Reference interval:* 50-330 pg/mL (50-330 ng/L)	*Before:* Fasting specimen preferred. Inform patient that blood sample will be drawn. *After:* Keep sample on ice.
Calcium (total)	Used to detect bone and parathyroid disorders. Hypercalcemia can indicate primary hyperparathyroidism. Hypocalcemia can indicate hypoparathyroidism. *Reference interval:* 8.6-10.2 mg/dL (2.15-2.55 mmol/L)	See above.

TABLE 47-6 Diagnostic Studies

Endocrine System—cont'd

Study	Purpose and Description	Nursing Responsibility
Calcium (ionized)	Free form of calcium unaffected by variable serum albumin levels. *Reference interval:* 4.64-5.28 mg/dL (1.16-1.32 mmol/L)	See above.
Phosphate	Measures inorganic phosphorus. High levels indicate primary hypoparathyroidism or secondary causes (e.g., renal failure). Low levels indicate hyperparathyroidism. *Reference interval:* 2.4-4.4 mg/dL (0.78-1.42 mmol/L)	See above.
Radiologic Studies **Parathyroid scan**	Assists in identifying the number and location of parathyroid glands. Uses radioactive isotopes that are taken up by cells in parathyroid glands to obtain an image of the glands and any abnormally active areas.	*Before:* Explain procedure to the patient. No specific preparations are necessary.
Adrenal Studies ***Blood Studies*** **Cortisol (total)**	Measures amount of total cortisol in serum and evaluates status of adrenal cortex function. Cortisol has diurnal variation; levels are higher in morning than in evening. Stress and excessive physical activity produce elevated results. *Reference interval:* At 8 AM: 5-23 mcg/dL (138-635 nmol/L) At 4 PM: 3-16 mcg/dL (83-441 nmol/L)	*Before:* Sample should be drawn in morning. Note if patient does night shift work. Mark time of blood draw on laboratory slip.
Aldosterone	Used to assess for hyperaldosteronism. *Reference interval:* Upright posture: 7-30 ng/dL (0.19-0.83 nmol/L) Supine position: 3-16 ng/dL (0.08-0.44 nmol/L)	*Before:* Usually morning blood sample is preferred. Inform patient that the required position (supine or sitting/standing) must be maintained for 2 hr before specimen is drawn.
Adrenocorticotropic hormone (ACTH) (corticotropin)	Measures plasma level of ACTH. Since ACTH controls adrenal cortex secretion, levels help determine if underproduction or overproduction of cortisol is caused by adrenal gland or pituitary gland dysfunction. Diurnal levels correspond with variation of cortisol levels. Levels are higher in morning, lower in evening. *Reference interval:* Morning: <120 pg/mL (<26 pmol/L) Evening: <85 pg/mL (<19 pmol/L)	*Before:* Patient should be NPO after midnight. Do morning blood draw between 6-8 AM. *During:* Use prechilled blood tube and place on ice. *After:* Send to laboratory immediately.
ACTH stimulation with cosyntropin	Used to evaluate adrenal function. After baseline cortisol sample is drawn, give cosyntropin (synthetic ACTH) by IV bolus. Cortisol samples are drawn 30 and 60 min after bolus. Plasma cortisol at 60 min should increase by >7 mcg/dL from baseline.	*Before:* Obtain baseline cortisol level at beginning of cosyntropin infusion. *During:* Inject cosyntropin with a plastic syringe and collect blood samples in plastic heparinized tubes. Administer test with continuous-infusion method. Monitor site and rate of IV infusion. Ensure sample collection at appropriate times.
ACTH suppression (dexamethasone suppression)	Assesses adrenal function. Especially helpful if hyperactivity (Cushing syndrome) is suspected. *Overnight method:* Dexamethasone (Decadron) 1 mg (low dose) or 4 mg (high dose) is given at 11 PM to suppress secretion of corticotropin-releasing hormone. Plasma cortisol sample is drawn at 8 AM. *Reference interval:* Cortisol level <3 mcg/dL (<0.08 μmol/L) for low dose and <50% of baseline in high dose indicates normal adrenal response.	*Before:* Obtain a fasting specimen. Ensure accurate timing of medication and sample collection. Inform patient that blood sample will be taken. Do not test acutely ill patients or those under stress. Stress-stimulated ACTH may override suppression. Screen patient for drugs such as estrogen and corticosteroids that may give false-positive results.
Metanephrine	Screens for pheochromocytoma. A more accurate test than urinary vanillylmandelic acid (VMA) and catecholamine measurements.	*Before:* Ask about recent history of vigorous exercise, high levels of stress, or starvation (may artificially ↑ levels). Use of caffeine, alcohol, levodopa, lithium, nitroglycerin, acetaminophen, and medications containing epinephrine or norepinephrine can alter test results.
Urine Studies **17-Ketosteroids**	Measures androgen metabolites in urine and evaluates adrenocortical and gonadal function. *Reference interval:* Men: 6-20 mg/day (20-70 μmol/day) Women: 6-17 mg/day (20-60 μmol/day)	*Before:* Explain the 24-hr urine collection. Tell patient that specimen must be kept refrigerated or iced during entire collection period. Determine whether preservative is required.

Continued

TABLE 47-6 Diagnostic Studies

Endocrine System—cont'd

Study	Purpose and Description	Nursing Responsibility
Adrenal Studies—cont'd *Urine Studies—cont'd*		
Cortisol (free)	Measures free (unbound) cortisol. Preferred test to evaluate hypercortisolism. *Reference interval:* 20-90 mcg/24 hr (55-248 nmol/day)	*Before:* Explain the 24-hr urine collection and need to avoid stressful situations and excessive physical exercise. Assess for drug use (e.g., reserpine, diuretics, phenothiazines, insulin, amphetamines) that may alter results.
Vanillylmandelic acid (VMA)	Measures urinary excretion of catecholamine metabolite. Levels are increased in pheochromocytoma. *Reference interval:* 1.4-6.5 mg/24 hr (7-33 μmol/day)	*Before:* Keep 24-hr urine collection at pH <3.0 with HCl acid as preservative. Keep on ice. Consult with laboratory or HCP about patient discontinuing any drugs 3 days before urine collection.
Radiologic Studies **CT**	Abdominal CT is radiologic examination of choice for the adrenal gland. Used to detect tumor and size or metastatic spread. Oral and/or IV contrast medium may be used.	*Before:* Inform patient of procedure. Patient must lie still during the procedure. Assess renal function if IV contrast is used. Check for iodine or shellfish allergy.
MRI	Same as MRI above.	Same as MRI above.
Pancreatic Studies *Blood Studies*		
Fasting blood glucose (FBG)	Measures circulating glucose level. *Reference interval:* 70-99 mg/dL (3.9-5.5 mmol/L).	*Before:* Patient should fast 8–12 hr. Water intake is permitted. Many medications may influence results.
Oral glucose tolerance test (OGTT)	Used to evaluate abnormal FBG levels that do not clearly indicate diabetes. Patient drinks 75 g of glucose, samples for glucose are drawn at baseline and at 30, 60, and 120 min. Test takes 2 hr to complete. *Reference interval:* <100 mg/dL (5.5 mmol/L) at baseline, <200 mg/dL (11.1 mmol/L) at 30 and 60 min, and <140 mg/dL (7.8 mmol/L) at 120 min. Values >200 mg/dL (11.1 mmol/L) at 120 min are considered diagnostic for diabetes mellitus.	*Before:* Perform test on ambulatory patients after fasting 8-12 hr. Many drugs may influence results, including caffeine and smoking. Ensure that patient's diet 3 days before test includes 150-300 g of carbohydrate with intake of at least 1500 cal/day.
Glycosylated hemoglobin (A1C)	Indicates the amount of glucose linked to hemoglobin. Assesses long-term glycemic control during previous 3 mo. *Reference interval:* 4.0%-6.0% ADA treatment goal <7%	*Before:* Inform patient that fasting is not necessary and that blood sample will be drawn.
Urine Studies **Glucose**	Estimate amount of glucose in urine by using an enzymatic method. Dip dipstick into urine and read for color changes after 1 min. *Reference interval:* Negative	*Before:* Use freshly voided urine. Many drugs alter glucose readings. Follow directions exactly to avoid errors.
Ketones	Measures amount of acetone (a type of ketone) excreted in urine as result of incomplete fat metabolism. Tested with a dipstick as described above. Positive result can indicate lack of insulin and diabetic acidosis. *Reference interval:* Negative	*Before:* Use freshly voided urine specimen. Test is often done with glucose test. Follow directions exactly. Certain drugs can produce false-positive or false-negative results.
Radiologic Studies **CT**	Abdominal CT is the radiologic examination of choice for pancreas. Used to identify tumors or cysts. Oral and/or IV contrast medium may be ordered.	*Before:* Inform patient of procedure. Patient must lie still during the procedure. If IV contrast is used, check for iodine and shellfish allergy. Assess renal function if contrast is used.

ADA, American Diabetes Association; *ADH,* antidiuretic hormone; *GHRH,* growth hormone–releasing hormone.

CASE STUDY—cont'd

Objective Data: Diagnostic Studies

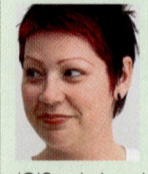
(©iStockphoto/ Thinkstock)

The health care provider orders the following initial diagnostic studies to be drawn in the morning after an 8-hr fast:
- CBC, basic metabolic panel (electrolytes, BUN, creatinine)
- Fasting blood glucose (FBG)
- TSH, free T₄
- Plasma cortisol levels
- Plasma ACTH levels

CBC results reveal a WBC of 12,200/μL and a decreased lymphocyte count at 800 cells/μL. The rest of the CBC is within normal limits (WNL). The FBG is 130 mg/dL. The plasma cortisol and ACTH levels are elevated. Thyroid studies are WNL.

Discussion Questions
1. Which diagnostic study results are of most concern to you?
2. Do you anticipate any additional diagnostic studies being ordered for L.M.?
3. What are the interprofessional team's priorities for L.M. at this time?

Answers available at *http://evolve.elsevier.com/Lewis/medsurg.*

BRIDGE TO NCLEX EXAMINATION

The number of the question corresponds to the same-numbered outcome at the beginning of the chapter.

1. A characteristic common to all hormones is that they
   a. circulate in the blood bound to plasma proteins.
   b. influence cellular activity of specific target tissues.
   c. accelerate the metabolic processes of all body cells.
   d. enter a cell to alter the cell's metabolism or gene expression.

2. A patient is receiving radiation therapy for cancer of the kidney. The nurse monitors the patient for signs and symptoms of damage to the
   a. pancreas.
   b. thyroid gland.
   c. adrenal glands.
   d. posterior pituitary gland.

3. A patient has a serum sodium level of 152 mEq/L (152 mmol/L). The normal hormonal response to this situation is
   a. release of ADH.
   b. release of ACTH.
   c. secretion of aldosterone.
   d. secretion of corticotropin-releasing hormone.

4. All cells in the body are believed to have intracellular receptors for
   a. insulin.
   b. glucagon.
   c. growth hormone.
   d. thyroid hormone.

5. When obtaining subjective data from a patient during assessment of the endocrine system, the nurse asks specifically about
   a. energy level.
   b. intake of vitamin C.
   c. employment history.
   d. frequency of sexual intercourse.

6. An appropriate technique to use during physical assessment of the thyroid gland is
   a. asking the patient to hyperextend the neck during palpation.
   b. percussing the neck for dullness to define the size of the thyroid.
   c. having the patient swallow water during inspection and palpation of the gland.
   d. using deep palpation to determine the extent of a visibly enlarged thyroid gland.

7. Endocrine disorders often go unrecognized in the older adult because
   a. symptoms are often attributed to aging.
   b. older adults rarely have identifiable symptoms.
   c. endocrine disorders are relatively rare in the older adult.
   d. older adults usually have subclinical endocrine disorders that minimize symptoms.

8. An abnormal finding by the nurse during an endocrine assessment would be (select all that apply)
   a. blood pressure of 100/70 mm Hg.
   b. excessive facial hair on a woman.
   c. soft, formed stool every other day.
   d. 3-lb weight gain over last 6 months.
   e. hyperpigmented coloration in lower legs.

9. A patient has a total serum calcium level of 3 mg/dL (1.5 mEq/L). If this finding reflects hypoparathyroidism, the nurse would expect further diagnostic testing to reveal
   a. decreased serum PTH.
   b. increased serum ACTH.
   c. increased serum glucose.
   d. decreased serum cortisol levels.

1. b, 2. c, 3. a, 4. d, 5. a, 6. c, 7. a, 8. b, e, 9. a

For rationales to these answers and even more NCLEX review questions, visit *http://evolve.elsevier.com/Lewis/medsurg*.

ⓔ EVOLVE WEBSITE

http://evolve.elsevier.com/Lewis/medsurg
NCLEX Review Questions (Online Only)
Key Points
Answer Keys for Questions
• Rationales for Bridge to NCLEX Examination Questions
• Answer Guidelines for the Case Study on pp. 1109, 1111, 1112, and 1118
Conceptual Care Map Creator
Audio Glossary
Supporting Media
• Animations
   • Overview of the Endocrine System
   • Thyroid and Parathyroid Glands
   • Thyroid Secretion
Supporting Media
Content Updates

REFERENCES

1. Huether SE, McCance KL: *Understanding pathophysiology*, ed 5, St Louis, 2014, Mosby.
*2. Gamble KL, Berry R, Frank SJ, et al: Circadian clock control of endocrine factors, *Nat Rev Endocrinol* 10:466, 2014.
3. McCance KL, Huether SE: *Pathophysiology: the biological basis for disease in adults & children*, ed 7, St Louis, 2014, Mosby.
4. Genetics Home Reference: Endocrine conditions. Retrieved from *http://ghr.nlm.nih.gov/conditionCategory/endocrine-system-hormones*.
5. Jarvis C: *Physical examination and health assessment*, ed 7, St Louis, 2015, Saunders.
*6. Aydin K, Ozturk B, Turkyilmaz MD, et al: Functional and structural evaluation of hearing loss in acromegaly, *Clin Endocrinol* 76:415, 2012.
7. Pagana K, Pagana T: *Mosby's manual of diagnostic and laboratory tests*, ed 5, St Louis, Mosby, 2014.

*Evidence-based information for clinical practice.

48

Diabetes Mellitus

Jane K. Dickinson

You don't have to let your life be destroyed by diabetes. You can reclaim your life.

Della Reese

http://evolve.elsevier.com/Lewis/medsurg/

LEARNING OUTCOMES

1. Describe the pathophysiology and clinical manifestations of diabetes mellitus.
2. Differentiate between type 1 and type 2 diabetes mellitus.
3. Describe the interprofessional care of a patient with diabetes mellitus.
4. Describe the role of nutrition and exercise in the management of diabetes mellitus.
5. Discuss the nursing management of a patient with newly diagnosed diabetes mellitus.
6. Describe the nursing management of a patient with diabetes mellitus in the ambulatory and home care settings.
7. Relate the pathophysiology of acute and chronic complications of diabetes mellitus to the clinical manifestations.
8. Explain the interprofessional care and nursing management of a patient with acute and chronic complications of diabetes mellitus.

KEY TERMS

dawn phenomenon, p. 1130
diabetes mellitus (DM), p. 1120
diabetic ketoacidosis (DKA), p. 1142
diabetic nephropathy, p. 1149
diabetic neuropathy, p. 1149

hyperosmolar hyperglycemic syndrome (HHS), p. 1145
impaired fasting glucose (IFG), p. 1123
impaired glucose tolerance (IGT), p. 1123
insulin resistance, p. 1123

intensive or physiologic insulin therapy, p. 1125
prediabetes, p. 1123
self-monitoring of blood glucose (SMBG), p. 1135
Somogyi effect, p. 1129

This chapter discusses the pathophysiology, clinical manifestations, complications, and interprofessional care of diabetes mellitus. To promote the patient's self-management of diabetes, you have a very important role in teaching both the patient and caregiver.

DIABETES MELLITUS

Diabetes mellitus (DM) is a chronic multisystem disease characterized by hyperglycemia related to abnormal insulin production, impaired insulin utilization, or both. Diabetes mellitus is a serious health problem throughout the world, and its prevalence is rapidly increasing. Currently in the United States an estimated 29.1 million people, or 9.3% of the population, have diabetes mellitus, and 86 million more people have prediabetes.[1] Approximately 8.1 million people with diabetes mellitus have not been diagnosed and are unaware that they have the disease. Diabetes mellitus is the seventh leading cause of death in the United States, but it is likely to be underreported.[2]

The long-term complications associated with diabetes can make it a devastating disease. Diabetes is the leading cause of adult blindness, end-stage renal disease, and nontraumatic lower limb amputations. It is also a major contributing factor to heart disease and stroke. Adults with diabetes have heart disease death rates two to four times higher than adults without diabetes. The risk for stroke is also two to four times higher among people with diabetes. In addition, more than half of adults with diabetes have hypertension and high cholesterol levels.[2]

Etiology and Pathophysiology

Current theories link the causes of diabetes, singly or in combination, to genetic, autoimmune, and environmental factors (e.g., virus, obesity). Regardless of its cause, diabetes is primarily a disorder of glucose metabolism related to absent or insufficient insulin supply and/or poor utilization of the insulin that is available.

The American Diabetes Association (ADA) recognizes four different classes of diabetes. The two most common are type 1 and type 2 diabetes mellitus (Table 48-1). The two other classes are gestational diabetes and other specific types of diabetes with various causes.

Normal Glucose and Insulin Metabolism. Insulin is a hormone produced by the β-cells in the islets of Langerhans of the pancreas. Under normal conditions, insulin is continuously released into the bloodstream in small increments, with increased release when food is ingested (Fig. 48-1). Insulin lowers blood glucose and facilitates a stable, normal glucose range of approximately 70 to 110 mg/dL (3.9 to 6.1 mmol/L). The average amount of

Reviewed by Cora Espina, RN, MN, ARNP, CWN, Nurse Practitioner, Inpatient Diabetes Consult Service and Diabetes Care Center, University of Washington Medical Center, Seattle, Washington; Carolyn Lyon, RN, MSN, Assistant Professor, Jefferson College of Health Science, Carilion Health System, Roanoke, Virginia; Lorraine Nowakowski-Grier, MSN, APRN, BC, CDE, Diabetes Nurse Practitioner, Christiana Care Health Services, Nursing Development and Education, Newark, Delaware; and Susan A. Sandstrom, RN, MSN, BC, CNE, Associate Professor in Nursing (retired), College of Saint Mary, Omaha, Nebraska.

TABLE 48-1	Comparison of Type 1 and Type 2 Diabetes Mellitus	
Factor	**Type 1 Diabetes Mellitus**	**Type 2 Diabetes Mellitus**
Age at onset	More common in young people but can occur at any age.	More common in adults but can occur at any age. Incidence is increasing in children.
Type of onset	Signs and symptoms usually abrupt, but disease process may be present for several years.	Insidious, may go undiagnosed for years.
Prevalence	Accounts for 5%-10% of all types of diabetes.	Accounts for 90%-95% of all types of diabetes.
Environmental factors	Virus, toxins.	Obesity, lack of exercise.
Primary defect	Absent or minimal insulin production.	Insulin resistance, decreased insulin production over time, and alterations in production of adipokines.
Islet cell antibodies	Often present at onset.	Absent.
Endogenous insulin	Absent.	Initially increased in response to insulin resistance. Secretion diminishes over time.
Nutritional status	Thin, normal, or obese.	Frequently overweight or obese. May be normal.
Symptoms	Polydipsia, polyuria, polyphagia, fatigue, weight loss without trying.	Frequently none. Fatigue, recurrent infections. May also experience polyuria, polydipsia, and polyphagia.
Ketosis	Prone at onset or during insulin deficiency.	Resistant except during infection or stress.
Nutrition therapy	Essential.	Essential.
Insulin	Required for all.	Required for some. Disease is progressive and insulin treatment may need to be added to treatment regimen.
Vascular and neurologic complications	Frequent.	Frequent.

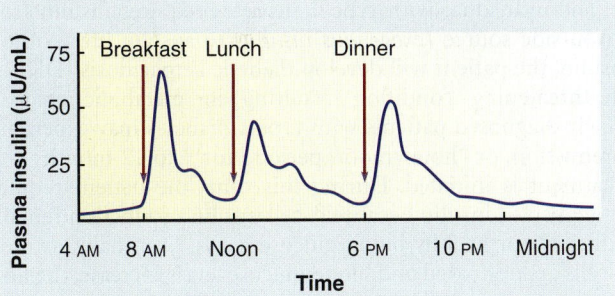

FIG. 48-1 Normal endogenous insulin secretion. In the first hour or two after meals, insulin concentrations rise rapidly in blood and peak at about 1 hour. After meals, insulin concentrations promptly decline toward preprandial values as carbohydrate absorption from the gastrointestinal tract declines. After carbohydrate absorption from the gastrointestinal tract is complete and during the night, insulin concentrations are low and fairly constant, with a slight increase at dawn.

insulin secreted daily by an adult is approximately 40 to 50 U, or 0.6 U/kg of body weight.

Insulin promotes glucose transport from the bloodstream across the cell membrane to the cytoplasm of the cell (Fig. 48-2). Cells break down glucose to make energy, and liver and muscle cells store excess glucose as glycogen. The rise in plasma insulin after a meal inhibits gluconeogenesis, enhances fat deposition of adipose tissue, and increases protein synthesis. For this reason, insulin is an *anabolic,* or storage, hormone. The fall in insulin level during normal overnight fasting facilitates the release of stored glucose from the liver, protein from muscle, and fat from adipose tissue.

Skeletal muscle and adipose tissue have specific receptors for insulin and are considered insulin-dependent tissues. Insulin is required to "unlock" these receptor sites, allowing the transport of glucose into the cells to be used for energy. Other tissues (e.g., brain, liver, blood cells) do not directly depend on insulin for glucose transport but require an adequate glucose supply for normal function. Although liver cells are not considered insulin-dependent tissue, insulin receptor sites on the liver facilitate hepatic uptake of glucose and its conversion to glycogen.

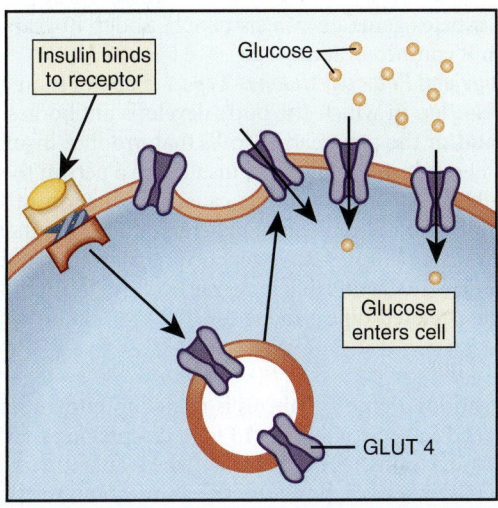

FIG. 48-2 Normal glucose metabolism. Insulin binds to receptors along the cell walls of muscle, adipose, and liver cells. Glucose transport proteins (GLUT 4) then attach to the cell wall and allow glucose to enter the cell, where it is either stored or used to make energy.

Other hormones (glucagon, epinephrine, growth hormone, and cortisol) work to oppose the effects of insulin and are referred to as *counterregulatory hormones.* These hormones increase blood glucose levels by (1) stimulating glucose production and release by the liver and (2) decreasing the movement of glucose into the cells. The counterregulatory hormones and insulin usually maintain blood glucose levels within the normal range by regulating the release of glucose for energy during food intake and periods of fasting.

Insulin is synthesized from a precursor, proinsulin. Enzymes split proinsulin to form insulin and C-peptide, and then the two substances are released in equal amounts. Therefore measuring C-peptide in serum and urine is a useful clinical indicator of pancreatic β-cell function.

Type 1 Diabetes Mellitus. *Type 1 diabetes mellitus,* formerly known as *juvenile-onset diabetes* or *insulin-dependent diabetes,* accounts for about 5% to 10% of all people with diabetes.

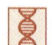

GENETICS IN CLINICAL PRACTICE

Types 1 and 2 Diabetes Mellitus and MODY

Type 1 Diabetes Mellitus	Type 2 Diabetes Mellitus	Maturity-Onset Diabetes of the Young (MODY)
Genetic Basis		
• Increased susceptibility (40%-50%) when one has specific human leukocyte antigens (HLA-DR3, HLA-DR4). • Polygenic (>40 genes influence susceptibility).	• Polygenic (>25 genes influence susceptibility).	• Autosomal dominant. • Monogenic (single gene). • Caused by mutations in any of six MODY genes (types 1-6). • Mutations in genes lead to β-cell dysfunction.
Risk to Offspring		
• Risk to offspring of mothers with diabetes is 1%-4%. • Risk to offspring of fathers with diabetes is 5%-6%. • When one identical twin has type 1 diabetes, the other gets the disease about 30%-40% of the time.	• Risk to offspring is 8%-14%. • When one identical twin has type 2 diabetes, the other gets it about 60%-75% of the time.	• If one parent has MODY, a child has a 50% chance of developing disease. • If one parent has MODY, a child has a 50% chance of being a carrier.
Clinical Implications		
• Disease is a result of complex interaction of genetic, autoimmune, and environmental factors.	• Disease is a result of complex genetic interactions, which are modified by environmental factors such as body weight and exercise.	• MODY accounts for 1% to 5% of people with diabetes. • Characterized by young age of onset (often before age 25). • Not associated with obesity or hypertension. • Treatment varies depending on the genetic mutation that caused MODY.

Type 1 diabetes generally affects people under 40 years of age, although it can occur at any age.[3]

Etiology and Pathophysiology. Type 1 diabetes is an autoimmune disorder, in which the body develops antibodies against insulin and/or the pancreatic β-cells that produce insulin. This eventually results in not enough insulin for a person to survive. Autoantibodies to the islet cells cause a reduction of 80% to 90% of normal function before hyperglycemia and other manifestations occur (Fig. 48-2). A genetic predisposition and exposure to a virus are factors that may contribute to the pathogenesis of immune-related type 1 diabetes.

Genetic Link

Predisposition to type 1 diabetes is related to human leukocyte antigens (HLAs). (See Chapter 13 for a discussion of HLAs and disease associations.) Theoretically, when an individual with certain HLA types is exposed to a viral infection, the β-cells of the pancreas are destroyed, either directly or through an autoimmune process. The HLA types associated with an increased risk for type 1 diabetes include HLA-DR3 and HLA-DR4 (Genetics in Clinical Practice box).

Idiopathic diabetes is a form of type 1 diabetes that is strongly inherited and not related to autoimmunity. It only occurs in a small number of people with type 1 diabetes, most often of Hispanic, African, or Asian ancestry.[3] *Latent autoimmune diabetes in adults* (LADA), a slowly progressing autoimmune form of type 1 diabetes, occurs in adults, and is often mistaken for type 2 diabetes.

Onset of Disease. In type 1 diabetes, the islet cell autoantibodies responsible for β-cell destruction are present for months to years before the onset of symptoms. Manifestations of type 1 diabetes develop when the person's pancreas can no longer produce sufficient amounts of insulin to maintain normal glucose. Once this occurs, the onset of symptoms is usually rapid, and patients often are initially seen with impending or actual ketoacidosis. The patient usually has a history of recent and sudden weight loss and the classic symptoms of *polydipsia* (excessive thirst), *polyuria* (frequent urination), and *polyphagia* (excessive hunger).

The individual with type 1 diabetes requires insulin from an outside source *(exogenous insulin)* to sustain life. Without insulin, the patient will develop diabetic ketoacidosis (DKA), a life-threatening condition resulting in metabolic acidosis. Newly diagnosed patients with type 1 diabetes may experience a remission, or "honeymoon period," for 3 to 12 months after treatment is initiated. During this time, the patient requires little injected insulin because β-cell insulin production remains sufficient for healthy blood glucose levels. Eventually, as more β-cells are destroyed and blood glucose levels increase, the honeymoon period ends and the patient will require insulin on a permanent basis.

Type 2 Diabetes Mellitus. *Type 2 diabetes mellitus was formerly known as adult-onset diabetes (AODM) or non–insulin-dependent diabetes (NIDDM).* Type 2 diabetes is, by far, the most prevalent type of diabetes, accounting for approximately 90% to 95% of patients with diabetes.[2] Many risk factors contribute to the development of type 2 diabetes, including being overweight or obese, being older, and having a family history of type 2 diabetes. Although the disease is seen less frequently in children, the incidence is increasing due to the increasing prevalence of childhood obesity. Type 2 diabetes is more prevalent in some ethnic populations. African Americans, Asian Americans, Hispanics, Native Hawaiians or other Pacific Islanders, and Native Americans have a higher rate of type 2 diabetes than whites.[4]

Etiology and Pathophysiology. Type 2 diabetes is characterized by a combination of inadequate insulin secretion and insulin resistance. The pancreas usually produces some *endogenous* (self-made) insulin. However, the body either does not produce enough insulin or does not use it effectively, or both. The presence of endogenous insulin is a major distinction between type 1 and type 2 diabetes. (In type 1 diabetes, there is an absence of endogenous insulin.)

Genetic Link

Although the genetics of type 2 diabetes is not yet fully understood, it is likely multiple genes are involved. Genetic mutations that lead to insulin resistance and a higher risk for obesity have been found in many people with type 2 diabetes. Individuals

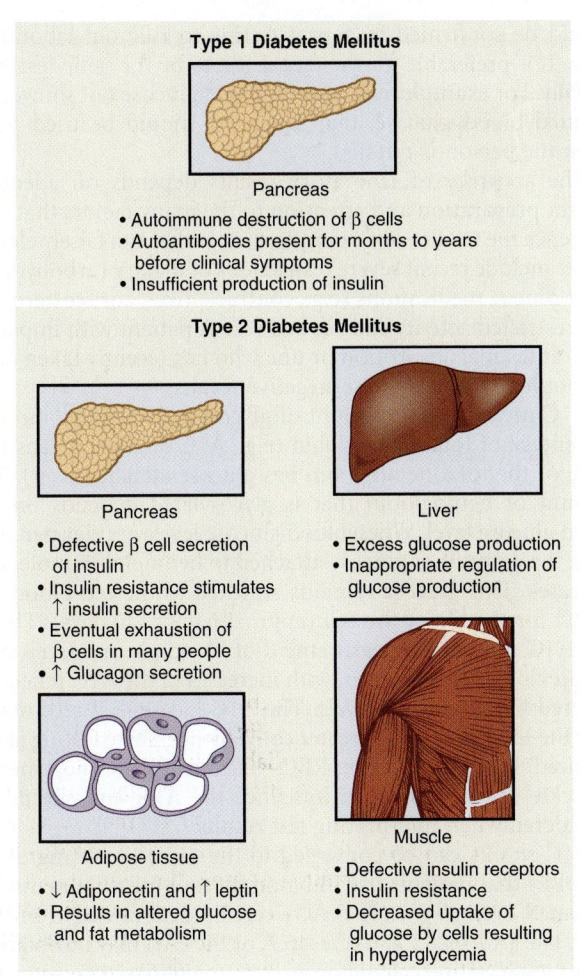

Type 1 Diabetes Mellitus

Pancreas

- Autoimmune destruction of β cells
- Autoantibodies present for months to years before clinical symptoms
- Insufficient production of insulin

Type 2 Diabetes Mellitus

Pancreas

- Defective β cell secretion of insulin
- Insulin resistance stimulates ↑ insulin secretion
- Eventual exhaustion of β cells in many people
- ↑ Glucagon secretion

Liver

- Excess glucose production
- Inappropriate regulation of glucose production

Adipose tissue

- ↓ Adiponectin and ↑ leptin
- Results in altered glucose and fat metabolism

Muscle

- Defective insulin receptors
- Insulin resistance
- Decreased uptake of glucose by cells resulting in hyperglycemia

FIG. 48-3   Altered mechanisms in type 1 and type 2 diabetes mellitus.

with a first-degree relative with the disease are 10 times more likely to develop type 2 diabetes.

Metabolic abnormalities have a role in the development of type 2 diabetes (Fig. 48-3). The first factor is **insulin resistance**, a condition in which body tissues do not respond to the action of insulin because insulin receptors are unresponsive, are insufficient in number, or both. Most insulin receptors are located on skeletal muscle, fat, and liver cells. When insulin is not properly used, the entry of glucose into the cell is impeded, resulting in hyperglycemia. In the early stages of insulin resistance, the pancreas responds to high blood glucose by producing greater amounts of insulin (if β-cell function is normal). This creates a temporary state of hyperinsulinemia that coexists with hyperglycemia.

A second factor in the development of type 2 diabetes is a marked decrease in the ability of the pancreas to produce insulin, as the β-cells become fatigued from the compensatory overproduction of insulin or when β-cell mass is lost. The underlying basis for the failure of β-cells to adapt is unknown. It may be linked to the adverse effects of chronic hyperglycemia or high circulating free fatty acids. In addition, the α-cells of the pancreas increase production of glucagon.

This leads to a third factor, which is inappropriate glucose production by the liver. Instead of properly regulating the release of glucose in response to blood levels, the liver does so in a haphazard way that does not correspond to the body's needs at the time.

A fourth factor is altered production of hormones and cytokines by adipose tissue *(adipokines)*. Adipokines secreted by adipose tissue appear to play a role in glucose and fat metabolism and are likely to contribute to the pathophysiology of type 2 diabetes.[5] Adipokines are thought to cause chronic inflammation, a factor involved in insulin resistance, type 2 diabetes, and cardiovascular disease (CVD). The two main adipokines believed to affect insulin sensitivity are adiponectin and leptin. Finally, the brain, kidneys, and gut also have roles in the development of type 2 diabetes, and scientists are continuously learning more about metabolic factors in the development of type 2 diabetes.[6]

Individuals with *metabolic syndrome* are at an increased risk for the development of type 2 diabetes. Metabolic syndrome has five components: elevated glucose levels, abdominal obesity, elevated BP, high levels of triglycerides, and decreased levels of high-density lipoproteins (HDLs) (see Table 41-10). An individual with three of the five components is considered to have metabolic syndrome.[7] Overweight individuals with metabolic syndrome can reduce their risk for diabetes through a program of weight loss and regular physical activity. (See Chapter 40 for a discussion of metabolic syndrome.)

Onset of Disease. The disease onset in type 2 diabetes is usually gradual. The person may go for many years with undetected hyperglycemia that may produce few, if any, symptoms. Many people are diagnosed on routine laboratory testing or when they undergo treatment for other conditions, and elevated glucose or glycosylated hemoglobin (A1C) levels are found. The signs and symptoms of hyperglycemia develop when about 50% to 80% of β-cells are no longer secreting insulin. At the time of diagnosis, the average person has had type 2 diabetes for 6½ years.

Prediabetes. Individuals diagnosed with prediabetes are at increased risk for the development of type 2 diabetes. **Prediabetes is defined as impaired glucose tolerance (IGT), impaired fasting glucose (IFG),** or both. It is an intermediate stage between normal glucose homeostasis and diabetes, in which the blood glucose levels are elevated but not high enough to meet the diagnostic criteria for diabetes. A diagnosis of IGT is made if the 2-hour oral glucose tolerance test (OGTT) values are 140 to 199 mg/dL (7.8 to 11.0 mmol/L).[3] IFG is diagnosed when fasting blood glucose levels are 100 to 125 mg/dL (5.56 to 6.9 mmol/L).

Persons with prediabetes usually do not have symptoms. However, long-term damage to the body, especially the heart and blood vessels, may already be occurring. It is important for patients to undergo screening and to understand risk factors for diabetes. Patients with prediabetes can take action to prevent or delay the development of type 2 diabetes. Encourage those with prediabetes to have their blood glucose and A1C checked regularly and monitor for symptoms of diabetes, such as fatigue, frequent infections, or slow healing wounds. Maintaining a healthy weight, exercising regularly, and making healthy food choices have all been found to reduce the risk of developing overt type 2 diabetes in people with prediabetes.

Gestational Diabetes. *Gestational diabetes* develops during pregnancy and occurs in about 4.6% to 9.2% of pregnancies in the United States.[8] Women with gestational diabetes have a higher risk for cesarean delivery, and their babies have increased risk for perinatal death, birth injury, and neonatal complications. Women who are at high risk for gestational diabetes are screened at the first prenatal visit.[9] Those at high risk include women who are obese, are of advanced maternal age, or have a family history of diabetes. Women with an average risk for gestational diabetes are screened using an OGTT at 24 to 28 weeks of gestation. Most women with gestational diabetes have normal glucose levels within 6 weeks postpartum. Be aware that women with a history of gestational diabetes have up to a 63% chance of developing type 2 diabetes within 16 years.[10] Gestational diabetes and management of the pregnant patient with diabetes are specialized areas not covered in detail in this chapter. Consult an obstetric text for more information.

Other Specific Types of Diabetes. Diabetes occurs in some people because of another medical condition or treatment of a medical condition that causes abnormal blood glucose levels. Conditions that may cause diabetes can result from injury to, interference with, or destruction of the β-cell function in the pancreas. These include Cushing syndrome, hyperthyroidism, recurrent pancreatitis, cystic fibrosis, hemochromatosis, and parenteral nutrition. Commonly used medications that can induce diabetes in some people include corticosteroids (prednisone), thiazides, phenytoin (Dilantin), and atypical antipsychotics (e.g., clozapine [Clozaril]). Diabetes caused by medical conditions or medications can resolve when the underlying condition is treated or the medication discontinued.

Clinical Manifestations

Type 1 Diabetes Mellitus. Because the onset of type 1 diabetes is rapid, the initial manifestations are usually acute. The classic symptoms are *polyuria, polydipsia,* and *polyphagia*. The osmotic effect of glucose produces the manifestations of polydipsia and polyuria. Polyphagia is a consequence of cellular malnourishment when insulin deficiency prevents utilization of glucose for energy. Weight loss may occur because the body cannot get glucose and turns to other energy sources, such as fat and protein. Weakness and fatigue may result because body cells lack needed energy from glucose. Ketoacidosis, a complication most common in those with untreated type 1 diabetes, is associated with additional clinical manifestations and is discussed later in this chapter.

Type 2 Diabetes Mellitus. The clinical manifestations of type 2 diabetes are often nonspecific, although it is possible that an individual with type 2 diabetes will experience some of the classic symptoms associated with type 1 diabetes, including polyuria, polydipsia, and polyphagia. Some of the more common manifestations associated with type 2 diabetes are fatigue, recurrent infections, recurrent vaginal yeast or candidal infections, prolonged wound healing, and visual changes.

Diagnostic Studies

The diagnosis of diabetes mellitus is made using one of the following four methods.
1. A1C of 6.5% or higher.
2. Fasting plasma glucose (FPG) level greater than or equal to 126 mg/dL (7.0 mmol/L). *Fasting* is defined as no caloric intake for at least 8 hours.
3. Two-hour plasma glucose level greater than or equal to 200 mg/dL (11.1 mmol/L) during an OGTT, using a glucose load of 75 g.
4. In a patient with classic symptoms of hyperglycemia (polyuria, polydipsia, unexplained weight loss) or hyperglycemic crisis, a random plasma glucose greater than or equal to 200 mg/dL (11.1 mmol/L).

If a patient is seen with a hyperglycemic crisis or clear symptoms of hyperglycemia (polyuria, polydipsia, polyphagia) with a random plasma glucose greater than or equal to 200 mg/dL, repeat testing is not warranted. Otherwise, criteria 1 through 3

should be confirmed by repeat testing to rule out laboratory error. It is preferable for the repeat test to be the same test used initially. For example, if a random blood glucose test showed an elevated blood glucose, that same test should be used again when the person is retested.

The accuracy of laboratory results depends on adequate patient preparation and attention to the many factors that may influence the results. For example, factors that can falsely elevate values include recent severe restrictions of dietary carbohydrate, acute illness, medications (e.g., contraceptives, corticosteroids), and restricted activity such as bed rest. A patient with impaired gastrointestinal absorption or one who has recently taken acetaminophen may have false-negative results.

A1C measures the amount of glycosylated hemoglobin as a percentage of total hemoglobin (e.g., A1C of 6.5% means that 6.5% of the total hemoglobin has glucose attached to it). The amount of hemoglobin that is glycosylated depends on the blood glucose level. When blood glucose levels are elevated over time, the amount of glucose attached to hemoglobin molecules increases. This glucose remains attached to the red blood cell (RBC) for the life of the cell (approximately 120 days). Therefore A1C provides a measurement of blood glucose levels over the previous 2 to 3 months, with increases in the A1C reflecting elevated blood glucose levels. The A1C has several advantages over the FPG, including greater convenience, since fasting is not required. Diseases affecting RBCs (e.g., iron deficiency anemia or sickle cell anemia) can influence the A1C and should be considered when interpreting test results.

A1C results can be converted to the same units (mg/dL or mmol/L) that patients use in blood glucose measurements. An *estimated average glucose* (eAG) can be determined from the A1C. The eAG = $28.7 \times A1C - 46.7$, or the eAG may be obtained by using an online calculator at *http://professional.diabetes.org/glucosecalculator.aspx*. For example, an A1C of 8.0% is equivalent to a glucose level of 183 mg/dL.

Teach patients with diabetes and prediabetes to have their A1C monitored regularly to determine the success of the current treatment plan and make changes in the plan if glycemic goals are not achieved. The ADA identifies an A1C goal for patients with diabetes of less than 7.0%. The American College of Endocrinology recommends an A1C of less than 6.5%. When the A1C is maintained at near-normal levels, the risk for the development of microvascular and macrovascular complications is greatly reduced. For individuals with prediabetes, monitoring the A1C can detect overt diabetes and provide feedback on efforts to prevent diabetes.

Fructosamine is another way to assess glucose levels. Fructosamine is formed by a chemical reaction of glucose with plasma protein. It reflects glycemia in the previous 1 to 3 weeks. Fructosamine levels may show a change in blood glucose levels before A1C does.

Islet cell autoantibody testing is primarily ordered to help distinguish between autoimmune type 1 diabetes and diabetes from other causes. Autoantibodies can develop to one or several of the autoantigens: GAD65, IA-2, or insulin.

Interprofessional Care

The goals of diabetes management are to reduce symptoms, promote well-being, prevent acute complications related to hyper- and hypoglycemia, and prevent or delay the onset and progression of long-term complications. These goals are most likely to be met when the patient is able to maintain blood glucose levels as near to normal as possible. Diabetes is a chronic disease that requires daily decisions about food intake, blood glucose monitoring, medication, and exercise. Patient teaching, which enables the patient to become the most active participant in his or her own care, is essential to achieve glycemic goals. Nutritional therapy, drug therapy, exercise, and self-monitoring of blood glucose are the tools used in the management of diabetes (Table 48-2).

The three major types of glucose-lowering agents (GLAs) used in the treatment of diabetes are insulin, oral agents (OAs), and noninsulin injectable agents. All individuals with type 1 diabetes require insulin. For some people with type 2 diabetes, a healthy eating plan, regular physical activity, and maintenance of healthy body weight are sufficient to attain optimal blood glucose levels. However, eventually most people with type 2 diabetes will require medication management because diabetes is a progressive disease.

Drug Therapy: Insulin

Exogenous (injected) insulin is needed when a patient has inadequate insulin to meet specific metabolic needs. People with type 1 diabetes require exogenous insulin to survive and often use multiple daily injections of insulin (often four or more) or continuous insulin infusion via an insulin pump to adequately manage blood glucose levels. People with type 2 diabetes may require exogenous insulin during periods of severe stress such as illness or surgery. In addition, since type 2 diabetes is a progressive disease, over time the combination of nutrition therapy, exercise, OAs, and noninsulin injectable agents may no longer adequately manage blood glucose levels. At that point, exogenous insulin would be added as part of the management plan. People with type 2 diabetes may also need up to four injections per day

to adequately maintain their blood glucose levels. Insulin pumps can also be used for patients with type 2 diabetes.

Types of Insulin. Today people use only genetically engineered human insulin made in laboratories. The insulin is derived from common bacteria (e.g., *Escherichia coli*) or yeast cells using recombinant deoxyribonucleic acid (DNA) technology. In the past, insulin was extracted from beef and pork pancreases, but these forms of insulin are no longer available.

Insulins differ by their onset, peak action, and duration (Fig. 48-4) and are categorized as rapid-acting, short-acting, intermediate-acting, and long-acting insulin (Table 48-3).

Insulin Regimens. Examples of insulin regimens are presented in Table 48-4. The insulin regimen that most closely mimics endogenous insulin production is the basal-bolus regimen, which uses rapid- or short-acting (bolus) insulin before meals and intermediate- or long-acting (basal) background insulin once or twice a day. The basal-bolus regimen is intensive or physiologic insulin therapy, consisting of multiple daily insulin injections together with frequent self-monitoring of blood glucose. The goal is to achieve a glucose level of 80 to 130 mg/dL before meals.

Other, less intense regimens can also promote healthy blood glucose levels for some people. Ideally, the patient and the HCP will work together to select a plan. The criteria for selection are based on the desired and feasible blood glucose levels and the patient's lifestyle, food choices, and activity patterns. If a less intense regimen is not giving the person optimal results, the HCP may encourage a more intense approach.

Mealtime Insulin (Bolus). To manage postprandial blood glucose levels, the timing of rapid- and short-acting insulin in relation to meals is crucial. Rapid-acting synthetic insulin analogs, which include lispro (Humalog), aspart (NovoLog), and glulisine (Apidra), have an onset of action of approximately 15 minutes and should be injected within 15 minutes of mealtime. The rapid-acting analogs most closely mimic natural insulin secretion in response to a meal.

TABLE 48-2 Interprofessional Care
Diabetes Mellitus

Diagnostic Assessment
- History and physical examination
- Blood tests, including fasting blood glucose, postprandial blood glucose, A1C, fructosamine, lipid profile, blood urea nitrogen and serum creatinine, electrolytes, islet cell autoantibodies
- Urine for complete urinalysis, albuminuria, and acetone (if indicated)
- Blood pressure
- ECG (if indicated)
- Funduscopic examination (dilated eye examination)
- Dental examination
- Neurologic examination, including monofilament test for sensation to lower extremities
- Ankle-brachial index (ABI) (if indicated) (see Table 37-3)
- Foot (podiatric) examination
- Monitoring of weight

Management
- Patient and caregiver teaching and follow-up programs
- Nutrition therapy (Table 48-8)
- Exercise therapy (Tables 48-9 and 48-10)
- Self-monitoring of blood glucose (SMBG) (Table 48-11)

Drug Therapy
- Insulin (Fig. 48-3 and Tables 48-3 and 48-4)
- Oral and noninsulin injectable agents (Table 48-7)
- Enteric-coated aspirin (81-162 mg/day)
- Angiotensin-converting enzyme (ACE) inhibitors (see Table 32-7)
- Angiotensin II receptor blockers (ARBs) (see Table 32-7)
- Antihyperlipidemic drugs (see Table 33-5)

TABLE 48-3 Drug Therapy
Types of Insulin

Classification	Examples*
Rapid-acting insulin	lispro (Humalog) aspart (NovoLog) glulisine (Apidra)
Short-acting insulin	regular (Humulin R, Novolin R)
Intermediate-acting insulin	NPH (Humulin N, Novolin N)
Long-acting insulin	glargine (Lantus) detemir (Levemir) degludec (Tresiba)
Combination therapy (premixed)	NPH/regular 70/30† (Humulin 70/30, Novolin 70/30) NPH/regular 50/50† (Humulin 50/50) lispro protamine/lispro 75/25† (Humalog Mix 75/25) lispro protamine/lispro 50/50† (Humalog Mix 50/50) aspart protamine/aspart 70/30† (NovoLog Mix 70/30) degludec/aspart 70/30 (Ryzodeg)
More concentrated insulin	Toujeo U-300 (insulin glargine) Humulin R U-500
Inhaled insulin	Afrezza

*Insulin preparations are clear solutions except for NPH and protamine-containing insulin, which are cloudy.
†These numbers refer to percentages of each type of insulin.

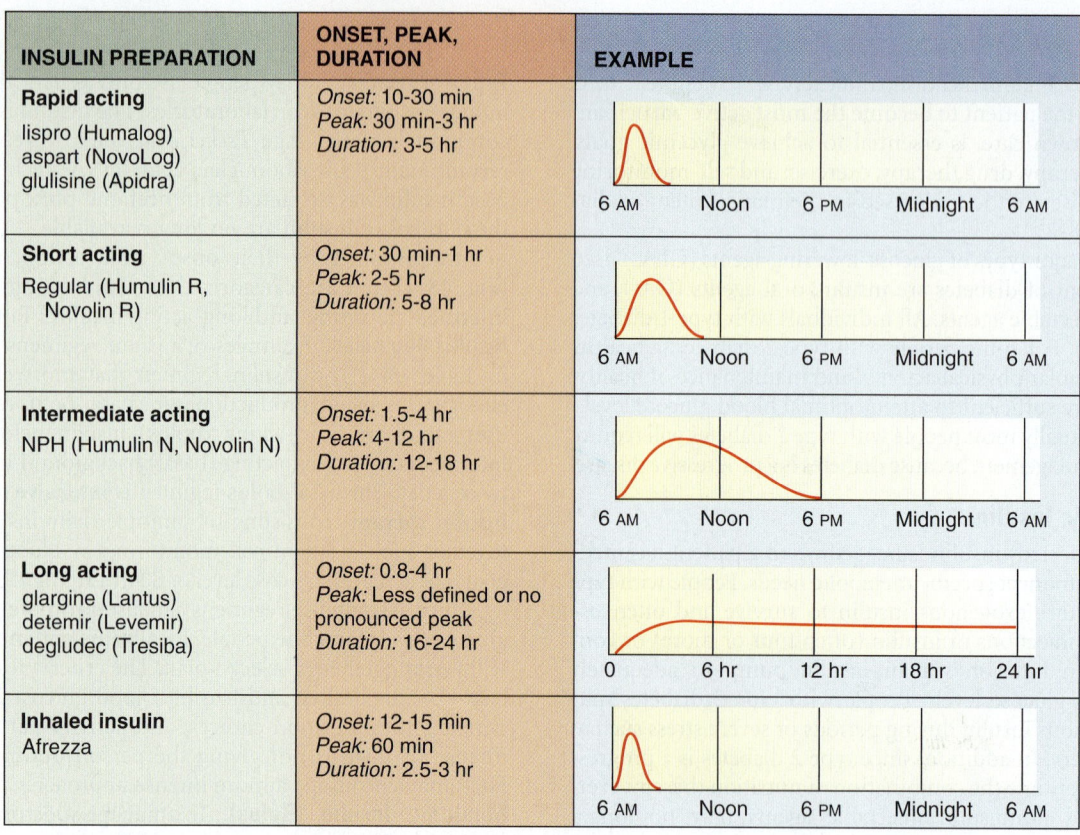

INSULIN PREPARATION	ONSET, PEAK, DURATION	EXAMPLE
Rapid acting lispro (Humalog) aspart (NovoLog) glulisine (Apidra)	*Onset:* 10-30 min *Peak:* 30 min-3 hr *Duration:* 3-5 hr	6 AM Noon 6 PM Midnight 6 AM
Short acting Regular (Humulin R, Novolin R)	*Onset:* 30 min-1 hr *Peak:* 2-5 hr *Duration:* 5-8 hr	6 AM Noon 6 PM Midnight 6 AM
Intermediate acting NPH (Humulin N, Novolin N)	*Onset:* 1.5-4 hr *Peak:* 4-12 hr *Duration:* 12-18 hr	6 AM Noon 6 PM Midnight 6 AM
Long acting glargine (Lantus) detemir (Levemir) degludec (Tresiba)	*Onset:* 0.8-4 hr *Peak:* Less defined or no pronounced peak *Duration:* 16-24 hr	0 6 hr 12 hr 18 hr 24 hr
Inhaled insulin Afrezza	*Onset:* 12-15 min *Peak:* 60 min *Duration:* 2.5-3 hr	6 AM Noon 6 PM Midnight 6 AM

FIG. 48-4 Commercially available insulin preparations showing onset, peak, and duration of action. Individual patient responses to each type of insulin are different and affected by many different factors.

Short-acting regular insulin has an onset of action of 30 to 60 minutes and is injected 30 to 45 minutes before a meal to ensure that the onset of action coincides with meal absorption. Because timing an injection 30 to 45 minutes before a meal is difficult for people to incorporate into their lifestyles, the flexibility that rapid-acting insulins offer is preferred by those taking insulin with their meals.[11] Short-acting insulin is also more likely to cause hypoglycemia because of a longer duration of action.

Long- or Intermediate-Acting (Basal) Background Insulin. In addition to mealtime insulin, people with type 1 diabetes use a long- or intermediate-acting basal (background) insulin to maintain blood glucose levels in between meals and overnight. Without 24-hour background insulin, people with type 1 diabetes are more prone to developing DKA. Many people with type 2 diabetes who use oral medications will also require insulin to adequately manage blood glucose levels.

The long-acting insulins include glargine (Lantus, Toujeo), detemir (Levemir), and degludec (Tresiba). This type of insulin is released steadily and continuously, and for many people does not have a peak of action. The action time for long-acting insulin varies (Fig. 48-4). Although they can be used for once-daily subcutaneous administration, detemir is often given twice daily. Because they lack peak action time, the risk for hypoglycemia from this type of insulin is greatly reduced. Glargine and detemir must not be diluted or mixed with any other insulin or solution in the same syringe. Ryzodeg 70/30 is a mixture of degludec and aspart (rapid-acting) insulin.

If oral agents and long-acting insulin are not adequate to achieve glycemic goals, mealtime insulin may also be added.

Intermediate-acting insulin (NPH) is also used as a basal insulin. It has a duration of 12 to 18 hours. The disadvantage of NPH is that it has a peak ranging from 4 to 12 hours, which can result in hypoglycemia. NPH can be mixed with short- and rapid-acting insulins. NPH insulin should never be given IV.

CHECK YOUR PRACTICE

You are preparing your patient's order for NPH insulin. When you look at the vial, you notice that it is cloudy. You are thinking that you should throw away the vial because it must be contaminated.
• Before you take this action, what should you do?

NPH, lispro protamine, and aspart protamine are cloudy insulins because they contain protamine. This substance decreases solubility, and as a result these insulins must be gently agitated before administration.

Combination Insulin Therapy. For those who want to use only one or two injections per day, a short- or rapid-acting insulin is mixed with intermediate-acting insulin in the same syringe. This allows the patient to have both mealtime and basal coverage without having to administer two separate injections. Although this may be more appealing to the patient, most patients achieve more optimal blood glucose levels with basal-bolus therapy. Patients may mix the two types of insulin themselves or may use a commercially premixed formula or pen (Table 48-3). Premixed formulas offer convenience to patients, who do not have to draw up and mix insulin from two different vials. This is especially helpful to those who lack the visual, manual, or cognitive skills to mix insulin themselves. However, the convenience of these formulas limits the potential for optimal blood glucose levels because there is less opportunity for flexible dosing based on need.

TABLE 48-4	Drug Therapy		
Insulin Regimens			

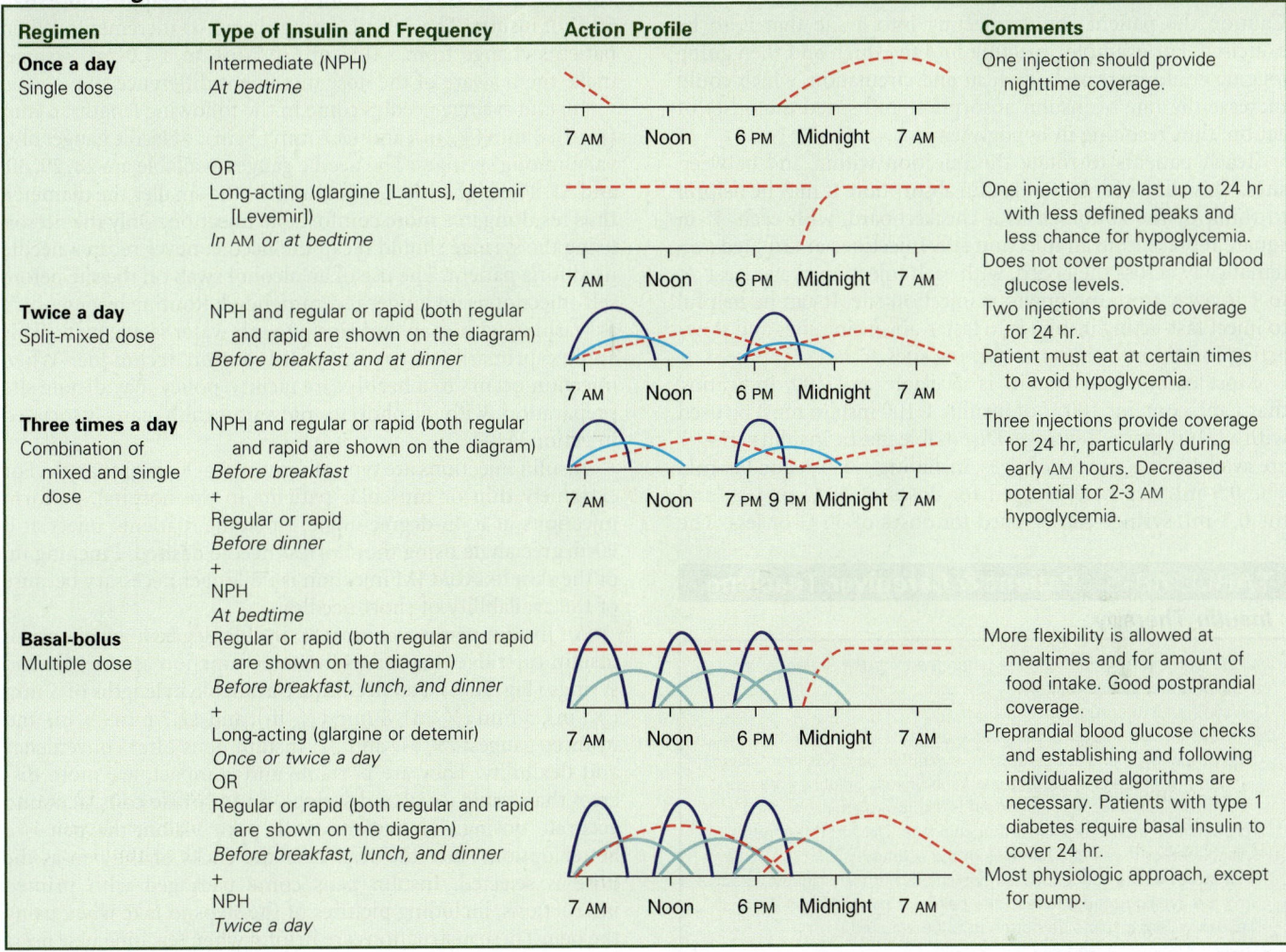

Regimen	Type of Insulin and Frequency	Action Profile	Comments
Once a day Single dose	Intermediate (NPH) *At bedtime* OR Long-acting (glargine [Lantus], detemir [Levemir]) *In AM or at bedtime*	7 AM · Noon · 6 PM · Midnight · 7 AM 7 AM · Noon · 6 PM · Midnight · 7 AM	One injection should provide nighttime coverage. One injection may last up to 24 hr with less defined peaks and less chance for hypoglycemia. Does not cover postprandial blood glucose levels.
Twice a day Split-mixed dose	NPH and regular or rapid (both regular and rapid are shown on the diagram) *Before breakfast and at dinner*	7 AM · Noon · 6 PM · Midnight · 7 AM	Two injections provide coverage for 24 hr. Patient must eat at certain times to avoid hypoglycemia.
Three times a day Combination of mixed and single dose	NPH and regular or rapid (both regular and rapid are shown on the diagram) *Before breakfast* + Regular or rapid *Before dinner* + NPH *At bedtime*	7 AM · Noon · 7 PM 9 PM Midnight 7 AM	Three injections provide coverage for 24 hr, particularly during early AM hours. Decreased potential for 2-3 AM hypoglycemia.
Basal-bolus Multiple dose	Regular or rapid (both regular and rapid are shown on the diagram) *Before breakfast, lunch, and dinner* + Long-acting (glargine or detemir) *Once or twice a day* OR Regular or rapid (both regular and rapid are shown on the diagram) *Before breakfast, lunch, and dinner* + NPH *Twice a day*	7 AM · Noon · 6 PM · Midnight · 7 AM 7 AM · Noon · 6 PM · Midnight · 7 AM	More flexibility is allowed at mealtimes and for amount of food intake. Good postprandial coverage. Preprandial blood glucose checks and establishing and following individualized algorithms are necessary. Patients with type 1 diabetes require basal insulin to cover 24 hr. Most physiologic approach, except for pump.

———— Rapid-acting (lispro, aspart, glulisine) insulin.
———— Short-acting (regular) insulin.
- - - - - - - Intermediate-acting (NPH) or long-acting (glargine, detemir) insulin.

Storage of Insulin. As a protein, insulin requires special storage considerations. Heat and freezing alter the insulin molecule and can make it less effective. Insulin vials and insulin pens currently in use may be left at room temperature for up to 4 weeks unless the room temperature is higher than 86° F (30° C) or below freezing (less than 32° F [0° C]). Prolonged exposure to direct sunlight should be avoided. A patient who is traveling in hot climates may store insulin in a thermos or cooler to keep it cool (not frozen). Store unopened insulin vials and insulin pens in the refrigerator.

Patients who are traveling or caregivers of patients who are sight impaired or who lack the manual dexterity to fill their own syringes may prefill insulin syringes. Prefilled syringes containing two different insulins are stable for up to 1 week when stored in the refrigerator, whereas syringes containing only one type of insulin are stable up to 30 days.[12]

Teach patients to store syringes in a vertical position with the needle pointed up to avoid clumping of suspended insulin in the needle. Before injection, gently roll prefilled syringes between the palms 10 to 20 times to warm the insulin and resuspend the particles. Some insulin combinations are not appropriate for prefilling and storage because the mixture can alter the onset, action, and/or peak times of either of the types.

Consult a pharmacy reference as needed when mixing and prefilling different types of insulin.

Administration of Insulin. Routine doses of insulin are administered by subcutaneous injection. Regular insulin can be given IV when immediate onset of action is desired. Insulin is not taken orally because it is inactivated by gastric fluids. Teach patients to avoid injecting insulin IM because rapid and unpredictable absorption could result in hypoglycemia.

Insulin Injection. The steps in administering a subcutaneous insulin injection are outlined in Table 48-5. Teach this technique to new insulin users and review it periodically with long-term users. Never assume that because the patient already uses insulin, he or she knows and practices the correct insulin injection technique. The patient may not have understood prior instructions, or changes in eyesight may result in inaccurate preparation. The patient may not see air bubbles in the syringe or may improperly read the scale on the syringe. The patient receiving mixed insulins in the same syringe needs to learn the proper technique for combining them if commercially prepared premixed insulins are not used.

The speed with which peak serum concentrations are reached varies with the anatomic site for injection. The fastest subcutaneous absorption is from the abdomen, followed by the arm, thigh, and buttock. Although the abdomen is often the preferred injection site, other sites also work well (Fig. 48-5). Caution the patient about injecting into a site that is to be exercised. For example, injecting into the thigh and then going jogging could increase body heat and circulation, which could increase the rate of insulin absorption and speed the onset of action, thus resulting in hypoglycemia.

Teach patients to rotate the injection within and between sites. This allows for better insulin absorption. It may be helpful to think of the abdomen as a checkerboard, with each ½-in square representing an injection site. Injections are rotated systematically across the board, with each injection site at least ½ to 1 in away from the previous injection site. It can be helpful to inject fast-acting insulin into faster-absorbing sites and slow-acting insulin into slower-absorbing sites.

Most commercial insulin is available as U100, indicating that 1 mL contains 100 U of insulin. U100 insulin must be used with a U100-marked syringe. Disposable plastic insulin syringes are available in a variety of sizes, including 1.0, 0.5, and 0.3 mL. The 0.5-mL size may be used for doses of 50 U or less, and the 0.3-mL syringe can be used for doses of 30 U or less. The

0.5- and 0.3-mL syringes are in 1-U increments. This provides more accurate delivery when the dose is an odd number. The 1.0-mL syringe is necessary for patients who require more than 50 U of insulin. The 1.0-mL syringe is in 2-U increments. When patients change from a 0.3- or a 0.5-mL to a 1.0-mL syringe, make them aware of the dose increment difference.

Insulin syringe needles come in the following lengths: 6 mm (¼ in), 8 mm (⁵⁄₁₆ in), and 12.7 mm (½ in).[13] Needle gauges also vary among syringes. The needle gauges available are 28, 29, 30, and 31. The higher the gauge number, the smaller the diameter, thus resulting in a more comfortable injection. Only the person using the syringe should recap the needle; never recap a needle used for a patient. The use of an alcohol swab on the site before self-injection is no longer recommended. Routine hygiene such as washing with soap and rinsing with water is adequate. This applies primarily to patient self-injection technique. When injection occurs in a health care facility, policy may dictate site preparation with alcohol to prevent health care–associated infection (HAI).

Insulin injections are typically given at a 90-degree angle. For extremely thin or muscular patients in the hospital, perform injections at a 45-degree angle. At home, patients inject at a 90-degree angle using the shortest needle desired. Pinching up of the skin to avoid IM injection is no longer necessary because of the availability of short needles.

An insulin pen is a compact portable device loaded with an insulin cartridge that serves the same function as a needle and syringe (Fig. 48-6). Pen needles are available in lengths of 4 mm (⁵⁄₃₂ in), 5 mm (³⁄₁₆ in), 8 mm (⁵⁄₁₆ in), and 12.7 mm (½ in) and in three gauges: 29, 31, and 32. Insulin pens offer convenience and flexibility. They are portable and compact, are more discreet than using a vial and syringe, and provide consistent and accurate dosing. For patients with poor vision, the pen is a better option, since they can hear the clicks of the pen as the dose is selected. Insulin pens come packaged with printed instructions, including pictures of the steps to take when using the pen. These instructions are helpful when teaching new users and reviewing technique with current users of a pen.

Insulin Pump. An *insulin pump* delivers a continuous subcutaneous insulin infusion through a small device worn on the belt, in a pocket, or under clothing. Insulin pumps use rapid-acting insulin, which is loaded into a reservoir or cartridge and connected via plastic tubing to a catheter inserted into the subcutaneous tissue. Insulet Corporation has an insulin pump that is a tubing-free system (Fig. 48-7). All insulin pumps are programmed to deliver a continuous infusion of rapid-acting insulin 24 hours a day, known as the *basal rate.* Basal insulin can be temporarily increased or decreased based on carbohy-

---

TABLE 48-5	**Patient & Caregiver Teaching**

Insulin Therapy

Include the following instructions when teaching the patient and caregiver about insulin therapy.

1. Wash hands thoroughly.
2. Always inspect insulin bottle before using it. Make sure that it is the proper type and concentration, expiration date has not passed, and top of bottle is in perfect condition. Insulin solutions (except for intermediate-acting insulins [NPH, lispro/protamine, aspart/protamine]) should look clear and colorless. Discard if it appears discolored or if you see particles in the solution.
3. For intermediate-acting insulins (which are normally cloudy), gently roll the insulin bottle between the palms of hands to mix the insulin. (Clear insulins do not need to be agitated.)
4. Select proper injection site (Fig. 48-5).
5. Ensure that the site is clean and dry.
6. Push the needle straight into the skin (90-degree angle). If you are very thin, muscular, or using an 8- or 12-mm needle, you may need to pinch the skin and/or use a 45-degree angle.
7. Push the plunger all the way down, leave needle in place for 5 sec to ensure that all insulin has been injected, and then remove needle.
8. Destroy and dispose of single-use syringe safely.

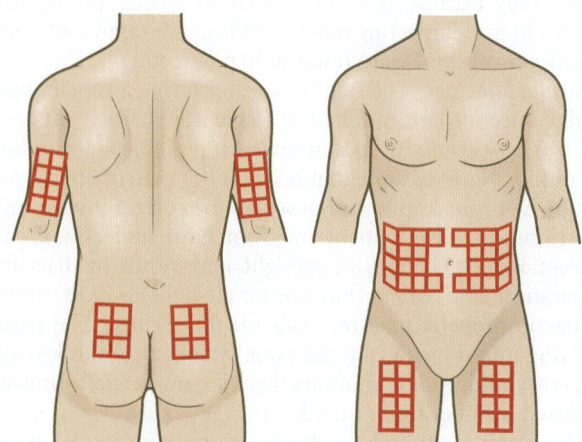

FIG. 48-5 Injection sites for insulin.

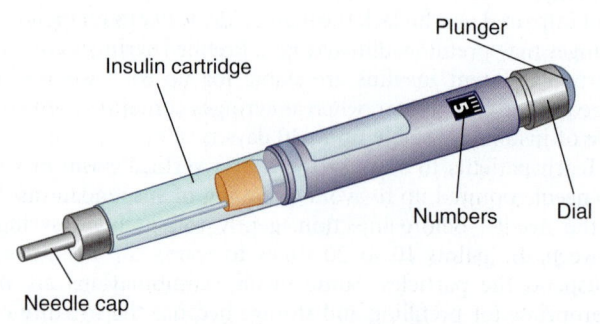

FIG. 48-6 Parts of insulin pen.

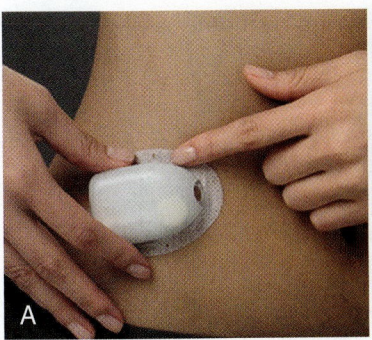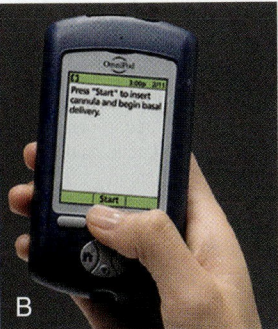

FIG. 48-7 **A,** OmniPod Insulin Management System. The Pod holds and delivers insulin. **B,** The Personal Diabetes Manager (PDM) wirelessly programs insulin delivery via the Pod. The PDM has a built-in glucose meter. (Courtesy of Insulet Corporation.)

drate intake, activity changes, or illness. Many individuals require different basal rates at different times of the day.

At mealtime, the user programs the pump to deliver a bolus infusion of insulin appropriate to the amount of carbohydrate ingested and an additional amount, if needed, to bring down or "correct" high preprandial blood glucose. The infusion set is changed every 2 to 3 days and placed in a new site to avoid infection and to promote good insulin absorption. Insulin pump users check their blood glucose level at least four times per day. Monitoring eight times or more per day is common.

A major advantage of the insulin pump is the potential for keeping blood glucose levels in a tighter range. This is possible because insulin delivery is similar to the normal physiologic pattern. Pumps offer users more flexibility with meal and activity patterns. Potential challenges of insulin pump therapy include infection at the insertion site, an increased risk for DKA if the insulin infusion is disrupted, the increased cost of the pump and supplies, and being attached to a device.[14]

Problems With Insulin Therapy. Problems associated with insulin therapy include hypoglycemia, allergic reactions, lipodystrophy, and the Somogyi effect. Hypoglycemia is discussed in detail later in this chapter. (Guidelines for assessing patients treated with insulin and other GLAs are presented in Table 48-6.)

Allergic Reactions. Local inflammatory reactions to insulin may occur, such as itching, erythema, and burning around the injection site. Local reactions may be self-limiting within 1 to 3 months or may improve with a low dose of antihistamine. A true insulin allergy, which is rare, is manifested by a systemic response with urticaria and possibly anaphylactic shock. Zinc or protamine used as a preservative in the insulin and the latex or rubber stoppers on the vials have been implicated in allergic reactions.

Lipodystrophy. Lipodystrophy (atrophy or hypertrophy of subcutaneous tissue) may occur if the same injection sites are used frequently. The use of human insulin has significantly reduced the risk for lipodystrophy. *Atrophy* is the wasting of subcutaneous tissue and presents as indentations in injection sites. *Hypertrophy,* a thickening of the subcutaneous tissue, eventually regresses if the patient does not use the site for at least 6 months. The use of hypertrophied sites may result in erratic insulin absorption.

Somogyi Effect and Dawn Phenomenon. Hyperglycemia in the morning may be due to the Somogyi effect. A high dose of insulin produces a decline in blood glucose levels during the

TABLE 48-6   Assessing the Patient Treated With Glucose-Lowering Agents

Category	Assessment
For Patient With Newly Diagnosed Diabetes or for Reevaluation of Drug Regimen	
Cognitive	• Is patient or caregiver able to understand why insulin or OAs are being used as part of diabetes management?
	• Is patient or caregiver able to understand concepts of asepsis, combining insulins, and side effects of medications?
	• Is patient able to remember to take >1 dose/day?
	• Does patient take medications at right times in relation to meals?
Psychomotor	• Is patient or caregiver physically able to prepare and administer accurate doses of the drugs?
Affective	• What emotions and attitudes are patient and caregiver displaying concerning diagnosis of diabetes and insulin or OA treatment?
For Follow-up of Patients Taking GLAs	
Effectiveness of therapy	• Is patient having symptoms of hyperglycemia?
	• Does blood glucose record show blood glucose levels in or out of the target range?
	• Is A1C in a healthy range and consistent with glucose records?
Side effects of therapy	• Is atrophy or hypertrophy present at injection sites?
	• Has patient had hypoglycemia? If so, how often? What time of day? What were the symptoms of hypoglycemia?
	• Are there complaints of nightmares, night sweats, or early morning headaches?
	• Has patient had a skin rash or GI upset since taking OAs?
	• Has patient gained or lost weight?
Self-management behaviors	• If patient is having hyperglycemia or hypoglycemia, how are those episodes managed?
	• Has patient determined reason for hyperglycemia or hypoglycemia?
	• How much insulin or OA is patient taking and at what time of day? Is patient adjusting insulin dose? Under what circumstances and by how much?
	• Has exercise pattern changed?
	• Is patient making healthy food choices? Are meals taken at times corresponding to peak insulin action?

A1C, Glycosylated hemoglobin; *GLA,* glucose-lowering agent; *OA,* oral agent.

night. As a result, counterregulatory hormones (e.g., glucagon, epinephrine, growth hormone, cortisol) are released, stimulating lipolysis, gluconeogenesis, and glycogenolysis, which in turn produce rebound hyperglycemia. The danger of this effect is that when blood glucose levels are measured in the morning, hyperglycemia is apparent and the patient (or the HCP) may increase the insulin dose.

If a patient is experiencing morning hyperglycemia, checking blood glucose levels between 2:00 and 4:00 AM for hypoglycemia will help determine if the cause is the Somogyi effect. The patient may report headaches on awakening and recall having night sweats or nightmares. A bedtime snack, a reduction in the dose of insulin, or both can help to prevent the Somogyi effect.

The dawn phenomenon is also characterized by hyperglycemia that is present on awakening. Two counterregulatory hormones (growth hormone and cortisol), which are excreted in increased amounts in the early morning hours, may be the cause of this phenomenon. The dawn phenomenon affects a majority of people with diabetes and tends to be most severe when growth hormone is at its peak in adolescence and young adulthood.

Careful assessment is required to document the Somogyi effect or dawn phenomenon because the treatment for each differs. The treatment for Somogyi effect is less insulin in the evening. The treatment for dawn phenomenon is an increase in insulin or an adjustment in administration time. Your assessment must include insulin dose, injection sites, and variability in the time of meals or insulin administration. Ask the patient to measure and document bedtime, nighttime (between 2:00 and 4:00 AM), and morning fasting blood glucose levels on several occasions. If the predawn levels are less than 60 mg/dL (3.3 mmol/L) and signs and symptoms of hypoglycemia are present, the insulin dosage should be reduced. If the 2:00 to 4:00 AM blood glucose is high, the insulin dosage should be increased. In addition, counsel the patient on appropriate bedtime snacks.

Inhaled Insulin. Afrezza, a rapid-acting inhaled insulin, is administered at the beginning of each meal or within 20 minutes after starting a meal. It is not a substitute for long-acting insulin. Afrezza must be used in combination with long-acting insulin in patients with type 1 diabetes. It is not recommended for the treatment of diabetic ketoacidosis or in patients who smoke. The most common adverse reactions are hypoglycemia, cough, and throat pain or irritation. Afrezza should not be used in patients with chronic lung disease, such as asthma or COPD, because bronchospasm can occur.

Drug Therapy: Oral and Noninsulin Injectable Agents

OAs and noninsulin injectable agents work to improve the mechanisms by which the body produces and uses insulin and glucose. These drugs work on three defects of type 2 diabetes: (1) insulin resistance, (2) decreased insulin production, and (3) increased hepatic glucose production. These drugs may be used in combination with agents from other classes or with insulin to achieve blood glucose goals. Oral and noninsulin injectable agents are listed in Table 48-7.

Biguanides. The most widely used oral diabetes agent is metformin, the only medication in the biguanide class available in the United States. Metformin is the most effective first-line treatment for type 2 diabetes.[15] Forms of metformin include Glucophage (immediate release), Glucophage XR (extended release), Fortamet (extended release), and Riomet (liquid form of metformin). The primary action of metformin is to reduce glucose production by the liver. It also enhances insulin sensitivity at the tissue level and improves glucose transport into the cells. Additionally, it has beneficial effects on plasma lipids.

Because it may cause moderate weight loss, metformin may be useful for people with type 2 diabetes and prediabetes who are overweight or obese. It is also used in the prevention of type 2 diabetes in those with prediabetes who are less than age 60 and have risk factors such as hypertension or a history of gestational diabetes.

Patients who are undergoing surgery or any radiologic procedures that involve the use of a contrast medium are instructed to temporarily discontinue metformin before surgery or the procedure. They should not resume the metformin until 48 hours afterward, once their serum creatinine has been checked and is normal.

DRUG ALERT Metformin

- Do not use in patients with kidney disease, liver disease, or heart failure. Lactic acidosis is a rare complication of metformin accumulation.
- IV contrast media that contain iodine pose a risk of acute kidney injury, which could exacerbate metformin-induced lactic acidosis.
- To reduce risk of kidney injury, discontinue metformin a day or two before the procedure.
- May be resumed 48 hours after the procedure, assuming kidney function is normal.
- Do not use in people who drink excessive amounts of alcohol.
- Take with food to minimize GI side effects.

Sulfonylureas. Sulfonylureas include glipizide (Glucotrol, Glucotrol XL), glyburide (DiaBeta, Glynase), and glimepiride (Amaryl). The primary action of the sulfonylureas is to increase insulin production by the pancreas. Therefore hypoglycemia is the major side effect with sulfonylureas.

Meglitinides. Like the sulfonylureas, repaglinide (Prandin) and nateglinide (Starlix) increase insulin production by the pancreas. However, because they are more rapidly absorbed and eliminated than sulfonylureas, they are less likely to cause hypoglycemia. When they are taken just before meals, pancreatic insulin production increases during and after the meal, mimicking the normal response to eating. Instruct patients to take meglitinides any time from 30 minutes before each meal right up to the time of the meal. These drugs should not be taken if a meal is skipped.

α-Glucosidase Inhibitors. Also known as "starch blockers," these drugs work by slowing down the absorption of carbohydrate in the small intestine. Acarbose (Precose) and miglitol (Glyset) are the available drugs in this class. Taken with the first bite of each main meal, they are most effective in lowering postprandial blood glucose. Their effectiveness is measured by checking 2-hour postprandial glucose levels.

Thiazolidinediones. Sometimes referred to as "insulin sensitizers," these agents include pioglitazone (Actos) and rosiglitazone (Avandia). They are most effective for people who have insulin resistance. These agents improve insulin sensitivity, transport, and utilization at target tissues. Because they do not increase insulin production, thiazolidinediones do not cause hypoglycemia when used alone. However, these drugs are rarely used today because of their adverse effects. Rosiglitazone is associated with adverse cardiovascular events (e.g., myocardial infarction) and can be obtained only through restricted access programs. Pioglitazone can worsen heart failure and is associated with an increased risk of bladder cancer.

Dipeptidyl Peptidase-4 (DPP-4) Inhibitors. Incretin hormones are released by the intestines throughout the day, but levels increase in response to a meal. When glucose levels are normal or elevated, incretins increase insulin synthesis and release from the pancreas, as well as decrease hepatic glucose production. The incretin hormones are normally inactivated by dipeptidyl peptidase-4 (DPP-4).

DPP-4 inhibitors (also known as *gliptins*) come in pill form and include sitagliptin (Januvia), saxagliptin (Onglyza), linagliptin (Tradjenta), and alogliptin (Nesina). DPP-4 inhibitors block the action of the DPP-4 enzyme, which is responsible for inactivating incretin hormones (gastric inhibitory peptide [GIP] and glucagon-like peptide-1 [GLP-1]). The result is an increase in insulin release, decrease in glucagon secretion,

TABLE 48-7 Drug Therapy
Oral Agents and Noninsulin Injectable Agents

Type	Mechanism of Action	Side Effects
Oral Agents		
Biguanides		
metformin (Glucophage, Glucophage XR, Riomet, Fortamet, Glumetza)	Decreases rate of hepatic glucose production. Augments glucose uptake by tissues, especially muscles.	Diarrhea, lactic acidosis. Must be held 1-2 days before IV contrast media given and for 48 hr after.
Sulfonylureas		
glipizide (Glucotrol, Glucotrol XL) glyburide (DiaBeta, Glynase) glimepiride (Amaryl)	Stimulate release of insulin from pancreatic islets. Decrease glycogenolysis and gluconeogenesis. Enhance cellular sensitivity to insulin.	Weight gain, hypoglycemia.
Meglitinides		
nateglinide (Starlix) repaglinide (Prandin)	Stimulate a rapid and short-lived release of insulin from the pancreas.	Weight gain, hypoglycemia.
α-Glucosidase Inhibitors		
acarbose (Precose) miglitol (Glyset)	Delay absorption of complex carbohydrates (starches) from GI tract.	Gas, abdominal pain, diarrhea.
Thiazolidinediones		
pioglitazone (Actos) rosiglitazone (Avandia)	Increase glucose uptake in muscle. Decrease endogenous glucose production.	Weight gain, edema. *pioglitazone:* may increase risk for bladder cancer and exacerbate heart failure. *rosiglitazone:* may increase risk for cardiovascular events (e.g., myocardial infarction, stroke).
Dipeptidyl Peptidase-4 (DPP-4) Inhibitors		
linagliptin (Tradjenta) saxagliptin (Onglyza) sitagliptin (Januvia) alogliptin (Nesina)	Enhance activity of incretins. Stimulate release of insulin from pancreatic β-cells. Decrease hepatic glucose production.	Pancreatitis, allergic reactions.
Dopamine Receptor Agonists		
bromocriptine (Cycloset)	Activates dopamine receptors in central nervous system. Unknown how it improves glycemic levels.	Orthostatic hypotension.
Sodium-Glucose Co-Transporter 2 (SGLT2) Inhibitors		
canagliflozin (Invokana) dapagliflozin (Farxiga) empagliflozin (Jardiance)	Decreases renal glucose reabsorption and increases urinary glucose excretion	Increased risk of genital and urinary tract infections. Hypoglycemia.
Combination Oral Therapy		
Glucovance	Same as for metformin and glyburide.	See side effects for individual drugs.
Duetact	Same as for pioglitazone and glimepiride.	Same as above.
Actoplus Met, Actoplus Met XR	Same as for metformin and pioglitazone.	Same as above.
Janumet, Janumet XR	Same as for metformin and sitagliptin.	Same as above.
Jentadueto	Same as for linagliptin and metformin.	Same as above.
PrandiMet	Same as for metformin and repaglinide.	Same as above.
Kombiglyze	Same as for saxagliptin and metformin.	Same as above.
Kazano	Same as for alogliptin and metformin.	Same as above.
Oseni	Same as for alogliptin and pioglitazone.	Same as above.
Glyxambi	Same as for empagliflozin and linagliptin.	Same as above.
Xigduo	Same as for dapagliflozin and metformin.	Same as above.
Synjardy	Same as metformin and empagliflozin.	Same as above.
Noninsulin Injectable Agents		
Glucagon-Like Peptide-1 (GLP-1) Receptor Agonists*		
exenatide (Byetta) exenatide extended-release (Bydureon) liraglutide (Victoza) albiglutide (Tanzeum) dulaglutide (Trulicity) lixisenatide (Adlyxin)	Stimulate release of insulin, decrease glucagon secretion, and slow gastric emptying. Increase satiety.	Nausea, vomiting, hypoglycemia, diarrhea, headache.
Amylin Analogs†		
pramlintide (Symlin)	Slows gastric emptying, decreases glucagon secretion and endogenous glucose output from liver. Increases satiety.	Hypoglycemia, nausea, vomiting, decreased appetite, headache.

*Administered subcutaneously.
†Administered subcutaneously only in abdomen or thigh.

and decrease in hepatic glucose production. Since the DPP-4 inhibitors are glucose dependent, they lower the potential for hypoglycemia. The main benefit of these drugs over other medications for diabetes with similar effects is the absence of weight gain as a side effect.

Sodium-Glucose Co-Transporter 2 (SGLT2) Inhibitors. Sodium-glucose co-transporter 2 (SGLT2) inhibitors work by blocking the reabsorption of glucose by the kidney, increasing glucose excretion, and lowering blood glucose levels. Drugs in this class include canagliflozin (Invokana), dapagliflozin (Farxiga), and empagliflozin (Jardiance).

Dopamine Receptor Agonist. Bromocriptine (Cycloset) is a dopamine receptor agonist that improves glycemic levels. The mechanism of action is unknown. Patients with type 2 diabetes are thought to have low levels of dopamine activity in the morning. These low levels of dopamine may interfere with the body's ability to control blood glucose. Bromocriptine increases dopamine receptor activity. It can be used alone or as an add-on to another type 2 diabetes treatment.

Combination Oral Therapy. Many combination drugs are currently available (Table 48-7). These drugs combine two different classes of medications to treat diabetes. One advantage of combination therapy is that the patient takes fewer pills, thus improving adherence to taking medications.

Glucagon-Like Peptide-1 Receptor Agonists. Exenatide (Byetta), exenatide extended-release (Bydureon), liraglutide (Victoza), albiglutide (Tanzeum), dulaglutide (Trulicity), and lixisenatide (Adlyxin) simulate GLP-1 (one of the incretin hormones), which is found to be decreased in people with type 2 diabetes. These drugs increase insulin synthesis and release from the pancreas, inhibit glucagon secretion, slow gastric emptying, and reduce food intake by increasing satiety.

These drugs may be used as monotherapy or adjunct therapy for patients with type 2 diabetes who have not achieved optimal glucose levels on OAs. These drugs are administered using a subcutaneous injection in a prefilled pen. In contrast to exenatide, which is given twice a day, and liraglutide, which is given once daily, dulaglutide, albiglutide, and Bydureon are given once every 7 days. The delayed gastric emptying that occurs with these medications may affect the absorption of oral medications. Advise patients to take fast-acting oral medications at least 1 hour before injecting a GLP-1 agonist drug.

 DRUG ALERT   Exenatide (Byetta)
• Acute pancreatitis and kidney problems have been associated with its use.

 DRUG ALERT   Liraglutide (Victoza) and Dulaglutide (Trulicity)
• Do not use in patients with a personal or family history of medullary thyroid cancer.
• Acute pancreatitis has been associated with its use.

Amylin Analogs. Pramlintide (Symlin) is the only available amylin analog. Amylin, a hormone secreted by the β-cells of the pancreas in response to food intake, slows gastric emptying, reduces glucagon secretion, and increases satiety.[12] Pramlintide is used in addition to mealtime insulin in patients with type 1 or type 2 diabetes who have elevated blood glucose levels on insulin therapy. It is only used concurrently with insulin and is not a replacement for insulin. Pramlintide is administered before major meals subcutaneously into the thigh or abdomen. It cannot be injected into the arm because absorption from this site is too variable. The drug cannot be mixed in the same syringe with insulin.

The concurrent use of pramlintide and insulin increases the risk of severe hypoglycemia during the 3 hours after injection, especially in patients with type 1 diabetes. Instruct patients to eat a meal with at least 250 calories and keep a form of fast-acting glucose on hand in the event that hypoglycemia develops. When pramlintide is used, the bolus dose of insulin should be reduced.

 DRUG ALERT   Pramlintide (Symlin)
• Can cause severe hypoglycemia when used with insulin.

Other Drugs Affecting Blood Glucose Levels. Both the patient and the HCP must be aware of drug interactions that can potentiate hypoglycemia and hyperglycemia effects. For example, β-adrenergic blockers can mask symptoms of hypoglycemia and prolong the hypoglycemic effects of insulin. Thiazide and loop diuretics can potentiate hyperglycemia by inducing potassium loss, although low-dose therapy with a thiazide is usually considered safe.

Nutritional Therapy

Individualized nutrition therapy, consisting of counseling, education, and ongoing monitoring, is a cornerstone of care for people with diabetes and prediabetes.[16] Changing eating habits can be challenging for many people. Achieving nutrition goals requires a coordinated team effort that takes into account the person's behavioral, cognitive, socioeconomic, cultural, and religious backgrounds and preferences. Because of these complexities, it is recommended that a dietitian with expertise in diabetes management work with the person who has diabetes. The dietitian starts with a nutrition assessment and develops an individualized food plan. Additional team members may include nurses, certified diabetes educators, clinical nurse specialists, HCPs, and social workers.

Guidelines from the ADA indicate that, within the context of an overall healthy eating plan, a person with diabetes can eat the same foods as a person who does not have diabetes. This means that the same principles of healthy nutrition that apply to the general population also apply to the person with diabetes. Table 48-8 describes nutrition guidelines for patients with diabetes. According to the ADA, the overall goal of nutrition therapy is to assist people with diabetes in making healthy nutritional choices that will lead to achieving and/or maintaining safe and healthy blood glucose levels. Additional specific goals include the following:

• Maintain blood glucose levels as close to normal as safely possible to prevent or reduce the risk for complications of diabetes.
• Achieve lipid profiles and BP levels that reduce the risk for CVD.
• Prevent or slow the rate of development of chronic complications of diabetes by modifying nutrient intake and lifestyle.
• Address individual nutrition needs while taking into account personal and cultural preferences and respecting the individual's willingness or ability to change eating and dietary habits.
• Maintain the pleasure of eating by encouraging a variety of healthy food choices.

Type 1 Diabetes Mellitus. People with type 1 diabetes base their meal planning on usual food intake and preferences balanced with insulin and exercise patterns. The patient coordinates insulin dosing with eating habits and activity pattern in mind. Day-to-day consistency in timing and amount of food eaten makes it much easier to manage blood glucose levels, especially for those individuals using conventional, fixed insulin

TABLE 48-8   Nutritional Therapy
Diabetes Mellitus

Component	Recommendations
Total carbohydrate	• Include carbohydrate from fruits, vegetables, grains, legumes, and low-fat milk. • Monitor by carbohydrate counting, exchange lists, or use of appropriate proportions. • Sucrose-containing food can be substituted for other carbohydrates in meal plan. • Fiber intake at 25-30 g/day. • Nonnutritive sweeteners are safe when consumed within FDA daily intake levels.
Protein	• Individualize goals. • High-protein diets are not recommended for weight loss.
Fat	• Individualize goals. • Minimize *trans* fat. • Dietary cholesterol <200 mg/day. • ≥2 servings of fish per week to provide polyunsaturated fatty acids.
Alcohol	• Limit to moderate amount (maximum 1 drink per day for women and 2 drinks per day for men). • Consume alcohol with food to reduce risk of nocturnal hypoglycemia in those using insulin or insulin secretagogues. • Moderate alcohol consumption has no acute effect on glucose and insulin concentrations, but carbohydrate taken with the alcohol (mixed drink) may raise blood glucose.

Source: Evert AB, Boucher JL, Cypress M: Nutrition therapy recommendations for the management of adults with diabetes, *Diabetes Care* 36(11): 3821, 2013.

regimens. Patients using rapid-acting insulin can adjust the dose before each meal based on the current blood glucose level and the carbohydrate content of the meal. Intensified insulin therapy, such as multiple daily injections or the use of an insulin pump, allows considerable flexibility in food selection and can be adjusted for alterations from usual eating and exercise habits.

Type 2 Diabetes Mellitus. Nutrition therapy in type 2 diabetes emphasizes achieving glucose, lipid, and BP goals. Modest weight loss has been associated with improved insulin resistance. Therefore weight loss is recommended for all individuals with diabetes who are overweight or obese.[16]

No one proven strategy or method can be uniformly recommended. A nutritionally adequate meal plan with appropriate serving sizes, a reduction of saturated and *trans* fats, and low carbohydrates can decrease calorie consumption. Spacing meals is another strategy that spreads nutrient intake throughout the day. A weight loss of 5% to 7% of body weight often improves blood glucose levels, even if desirable body weight is not achieved. Weight loss is best attempted by a moderate decrease in calories and an increase in caloric expenditure. Regularly exercising and adopting new behaviors and attitudes can facilitate long-term lifestyle changes. Monitoring of blood glucose levels, A1C, lipids, and BP provides feedback on how well the goals of nutrition therapy are being met.

Food Composition. A healthy balance of nutrients is essential to maintain blood glucose levels and overall health. Energy from food intake can be balanced with the patient's energy output. Patients plan their individual meal plan with their lifestyle and health goals in mind. The following are general recommendations for nutrient balance.

Carbohydrates. Carbohydrates include sugars, starches, and fiber. Carbohydrates provide important sources of energy, fiber, vitamins, and minerals and are therefore important to all people, including those with diabetes. Foods containing carbohydrates from whole grains, fruits, vegetables, and low-fat dairy are part of a healthy meal plan. The ADA recommends individualizing carbohydrate intake as there is no ideal number for all people with diabetes.

All individuals benefit from including dietary fiber as part of a healthy meal plan. The current recommendation for the general population is 25 to 30 g/day.[16]

Nutritive and nonnutritive sweeteners may be included in a healthy meal plan in moderation. Nonnutritive sweeteners include the sugar substitutes saccharine, aspartame, sucralose, neotame, and acesulfame-K.

Fats. Dietary fat provides energy, carries fat-soluble vitamins, and provides essential fatty acids. The ADA recommends individualizing saturated fat intake. Less than 200 mg/day of cholesterol and limited *trans* fats are also recommended as part of a healthy meal plan. Decreasing fat and cholesterol intake assists in reducing the risk for CVD. Healthy fats are those that come from plants, such as olives, nuts, and avocados.

Protein. The amount of daily protein in the diet for people with diabetes and normal renal function is the same as for the general population. The ADA recommends individualizing protein intake.

Alcohol. Alcohol inhibits gluconeogenesis (breakdown of glycogen to glucose) by the liver. This can cause severe hypoglycemia in patients on insulin or oral hypoglycemic medications that increase insulin secretion. Create a trusting environment where patients feel comfortable being honest about their use of alcohol because its use can make blood glucose more difficult to manage.

Moderate alcohol consumption can be safely incorporated into the meal plan if the person is monitoring blood glucose levels and if the patient is not at risk for other alcohol-related problems. Moderate consumption is defined as one drink per day for women and two drinks per day for men. A patient can reduce the risk for alcohol-induced hypoglycemia by eating carbohydrates when drinking alcohol. On the other hand, mixed drinks often contain sweetened mixers and can lead to elevated blood glucose levels. To decrease the carbohydrate content, recommend using sugar-free mixes and drinking dry, light wines.

Patient Teaching Related to Nutrition Therapy. Most often the dietitian initially teaches the principles of nutrition management. Whenever possible, work with dietitians as part of an interprofessional diabetes care team. Some patients who have limited insurance coverage or live in remote areas do not have access to a dietitian. In these cases, you may need to assume responsibility for teaching basic nutrition principles to patients with diabetes.

Carbohydrate counting is a meal planning technique used to keep track of the amount of carbohydrates eaten with each meal and per day. Advise patients to keep carbohydrates within a healthy range. The amount of total carbohydrates per day depends on blood glucose levels, age, weight, activity level, patient preference, and prescribed medications. A serving size of carbohydrates is 15 g. A typical adult usually starts with 45 to 60 g of carbohydrate per meal. For some patients, insulin doses are tailored to the number of carbohydrates that a patient will consume at the meal, with a set number of units of insulin given per gram of carbohydrate (e.g., 1 U/15 g carbohydrate, 2 U/25 g carbohydrate). Teach the patient about the foods that contain carbohydrates, how to read food labels, and appropriate serving sizes.

Diabetes exchange lists are another method for meal planning. Instead of counting carbohydrates, the individual is given a meal plan with specific numbers of helpings from a list of exchanges for each meal and snack. The exchanges are starches, fruits, milk, meat, vegetables, fats, and free foods. The patient chooses foods from the various exchanges based on the prescribed meal plan. This method may be easier for some patients than carbohydrate counting. It also encourages a well-balanced meal plan. Another advantage is that this approach helps the patient limit portion sizes and overall food intake, an important component of weight management.

MyPlate was developed by the U.S. Department of Agriculture (USDA) to represent national nutrition guidelines for people with or without diabetes. This simple method helps the patient visualize the amount of vegetables, starch, and meat that fills a 9-in plate. The recommendation is that each meal has one half of the plate filled with nonstarchy vegetables, one fourth filled with a starch, and one fourth filled with a protein (*www.diabetes.org/food-and-fitness/food/planning-meals/create-your-plate*). An 8-ounce glass of nonfat milk and a small piece of fresh fruit complete the meal.[17]

Whenever possible, include family members and caregivers in nutrition education and counseling, particularly the person who cooks for the household. However, the responsibility for maintaining a healthy eating plan still belongs to the person with diabetes. Reliance on another person to make health decisions interferes with the patient's ability to develop self-care skills, which are essential in the management of diabetes. Foster independence, even in patients with visual or cognitive impairment. It is also important to discuss traditional foods with the patient. Individualize food choices to take into account the patient's preferences and foods that are culturally appropriate.

Exercise

Regular, consistent exercise is an essential part of diabetes and prediabetes management.[18] The ADA recommends that people with diabetes engage in at least 150 min/wk (30 minutes, 5 days/week) of a moderate-intensity aerobic physical activity (Table 48-9). The ADA also encourages people with type 2 diabetes to perform resistance training three times a week in the absence of contraindications.[19]

Exercise decreases insulin resistance and can have a direct effect on lowering blood glucose levels. It also contributes to

weight loss, which further decreases insulin resistance. The therapeutic benefits of regular physical activity may result in a decreased need for diabetes medications to reach target blood glucose goals in people with type 2 diabetes. Regular exercise may also help reduce triglyceride and low-density lipoprotein (LDL) cholesterol levels, increase high-density lipoprotein (HDL), reduce BP, and improve circulation.[7]

Any new exercise program for patients with diabetes can be started after medical clearance. Patients start slowly with gradual progression toward the desired goal. Patients who use insulin, sulfonylureas, or meglitinides are at increased risk for hypoglycemia when they increase physical activity, especially if they exercise at the time of peak drug action or eat too little to maintain adequate blood glucose levels. This can also occur if a normally sedentary patient with diabetes has an unusually active day.

The glucose-lowering effects of exercise can last up to 48 hours after the activity, so it is possible for hypoglycemia to occur long after the activity. It is recommended that patients who use medications that can cause hypoglycemia schedule exercise about 1 hour after a meal or that they have a 10- to 15-g carbohydrate snack and check their blood glucose before exercising. They can eat small carbohydrate snacks every 30 minutes during exercise to prevent hypoglycemia. Patients using medications that place them at risk for hypoglycemia should always carry a fast-acting source of carbohydrate, such as glucose tablets or hard candies, when exercising. Table 48-10 describes exercise guidelines for patients with diabetes.

Although exercise is generally beneficial to blood glucose levels, strenuous activity can be perceived by the body as a stress, causing a release of counterregulatory hormones and a temporary elevation of blood glucose. In a person with type 1 diabetes

---

TABLE 48-9	**Activities That Affect Caloric Expenditure**	
Light Activity (100-200 kcal/hr)	**Moderate Activity (200-350 kcal/hr)**	**Vigorous Activity (400-900 kcal/hr)**
• Fishing • Light housework • Secretarial work • Teaching • Walking casually	• Active housework • Bicycling (light) • Bowling • Dancing • Gardening • Golf • Roller skating • Walking briskly	• Aerobic exercise • Bicycling (vigorous) • Hard labor • Ice skating • Outdoor sports • Running • Soccer • Tennis • Wood chopping

---

TABLE 48-10 Patient & Caregiver Teaching
Exercise for Patients With Diabetes Mellitus

Include the following information in the exercise teaching plan for the patient and caregiver.

1. Exercise does not have to be vigorous to be effective. The blood glucose–reducing effects of exercise can be attained with activity such as brisk walking.
2. The exercises selected should be enjoyable to foster regularity.
3. It is important to have properly fitting footwear.
4. The exercise session includes a warm-up period and a cool-down period. Start the exercise program gradually and increase slowly.
5. Exercise is best done after meals, when the blood glucose level is rising.
6. Exercise plans are individualized and monitored by the HCP.
7. It is important to self-monitor blood glucose levels before, during, and after exercise to determine the effect exercise has on blood glucose level at particular times of the day.
8. *Before exercise, if blood glucose ≤100 mg/dL,* eat a 15-g carbohydrate snack. After 15 to 30 min, recheck blood glucose levels. Delay exercise if <100 mg/dL.
9. *Before exercise, if blood glucose ≥250 mg/dL* in a person with type 1 diabetes and ketones are present, delay vigorous activity until ketones are gone. Drink fluids.
10. Exercise-induced hypoglycemia may occur several hours after the completion of exercise.
11. Taking a glucose-lowering medication does not mean that planned or spontaneous exercise cannot occur.
12. It is important to compensate for extensive planned and spontaneous activity by monitoring blood glucose levels to make adjustments in the insulin dose (if taken) and food intake.

who has hyperglycemia and ketones, exercise can worsen these conditions. Teach these patients to delay activity if the blood glucose level is over 250 mg/dL and ketones are present in the urine. If hyperglycemia is present without ketosis, it is not necessary to postpone exercise.[15]

EVIDENCE-BASED PRACTICE
Applying the Evidence

Education: Text Messaging and Diabetes

A.Y. is a 62-yr-old female recently diagnosed with type 2 diabetes. She understands the importance of maintaining blood glucose levels that are close to normal to reduce symptoms and prevent long-term complications. A.Y. tells you she wants to be an active participant in her care. You determine she is motivated and wants to learn the knowledge and skills necessary to manage her own care. You arrange for A.Y. to receive education text messages about diabetes as part of the teaching plan.

Making Clinical Decisions

Best Available Evidence. The delivery of education related to diabetes self-management may include remote electronic messages transmitted by mobile or cell phone. Electronic education text messaging can significantly improve glycemic levels in patients with type 2 diabetes, resulting in an almost 50% reduction in Hb A1C (A1C) levels.

Clinician Expertise. You know self-management diabetes education is effective in helping patients improve glycemic levels. You also know that education text messaging may be a useful method for delivering information to patients with chronic diseases who are managing their own care.

Patient Preferences and Values. A.Y. indicates strong interest in receiving text education messages 4 times/week from diabetes clinic that emphasize the importance of physical activity, blood glucose monitoring, and healthy food choices.

Implications for Nursing Practice

1. How can you use text messaging for communication with A.Y. related to her self-monitoring of blood glucose levels?
2. As you empower A.Y. to initially manage her care, why is it important for you to frequently assess A.Y.'s knowledge and skills?
3. What parameters will you use to assess if she is able to manage her own care?

Reference for Evidence

Saffari M, Ghanizadeh G, Koenig H: Health education via mobile text messaging for glycemic control in adults with type 2 diabetes: a systematic review and meta-analysis, *Prim Care Diabetes* 8:275, 2014.

Monitoring Blood Glucose

Self-monitoring of blood glucose (SMBG) is a critical part of diabetes management. By providing a current blood glucose reading, SMBG enables the patient to make decisions regarding food intake, activity patterns, and medication dosages. It also produces accurate records of daily glucose fluctuations and trends, and it alerts the patient to acute episodes of hyperglycemia and hypoglycemia. Furthermore, it provides patients with a tool for achieving and maintaining specific glycemic goals. SMBG is recommended for all patients who use insulin to manage their diabetes. Other patients with diabetes use SMBG to help achieve and maintain glycemic goals and monitor for acute fluctuations in blood glucose related to medications, food, and exercise.

The frequency of monitoring depends on several factors, including the patient's glycemic goals, type of diabetes,

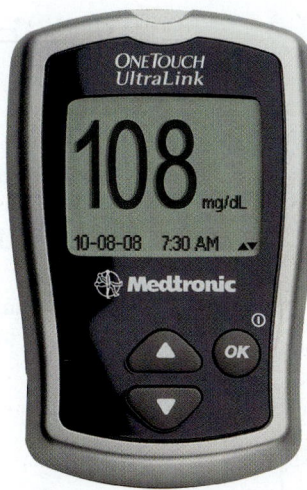

FIG. 48-8 Blood glucose monitors are used to measure blood glucose levels. Bayer Contour Link glucose meter. (Courtesy of Bayer Diabetes.)

medication regimen, patient's ability to check blood glucose independently, and patient's willingness and ability to do so. The recommendation for patients who use multiple insulin injections or insulin pumps is to monitor their blood glucose four or more times each day. Patients using less frequent insulin injections, noninsulin therapy, or nutrition management will monitor as often as needed to achieve their glycemic goals.[12]

Patients who perform SMBG use portable blood glucose monitors. A wide variety of blood glucose monitors are available (Fig. 48-8). Disposable lancets are used to obtain a small drop of capillary blood (usually from a finger stick) that is placed in a reagent strip. After a specified time, the monitor displays a digital reading of the capillary blood glucose value. The technology of SMBG is rapidly changing, with newer and more convenient systems being introduced on an ongoing basis.

Some systems allow the user to collect blood from alternative sites such as the forearm or palm. Alternate site use is not recommended with rapidly changing blood glucose readings, during pregnancy, or when symptoms of low blood glucose are present (Fig. 48-9). The data from some glucose monitors can be uploaded to a computer and reviewed by HCPs, allowing for more frequent and efficient adjustment of the plan of care if needed.

Continuous glucose monitoring (CGM) systems provide another route for monitoring glucose. Insulin pumps can also be matched with CGM (Fig. 48-10).

Using a sensor inserted subcutaneously, the systems display glucose values that are updated every 1 to 5 minutes. CGM assesses interstitial glucose, which lags behind blood glucose by up to 20 minutes.[20] The patient inserts the sensor using an automatic insertion device. Data are sent from the sensor to a transmitter, which displays the glucose value on either an insulin pump or a pager-like receiver. The continuous glucose monitor can be used with or without an insulin pump.

CGMs assist the patient and HCP to identify trends and patterns in glucose levels. In addition, they are useful for the management of insulin therapy or when continuous blood glucose readings are clinically important. The patient is alerted to episodes of hypoglycemia and hyperglycemia, thus allowing corrective action to be quickly taken. These systems still require finger-stick measurements using a blood glucose monitor to calibrate the sensor and to make treatment decisions.

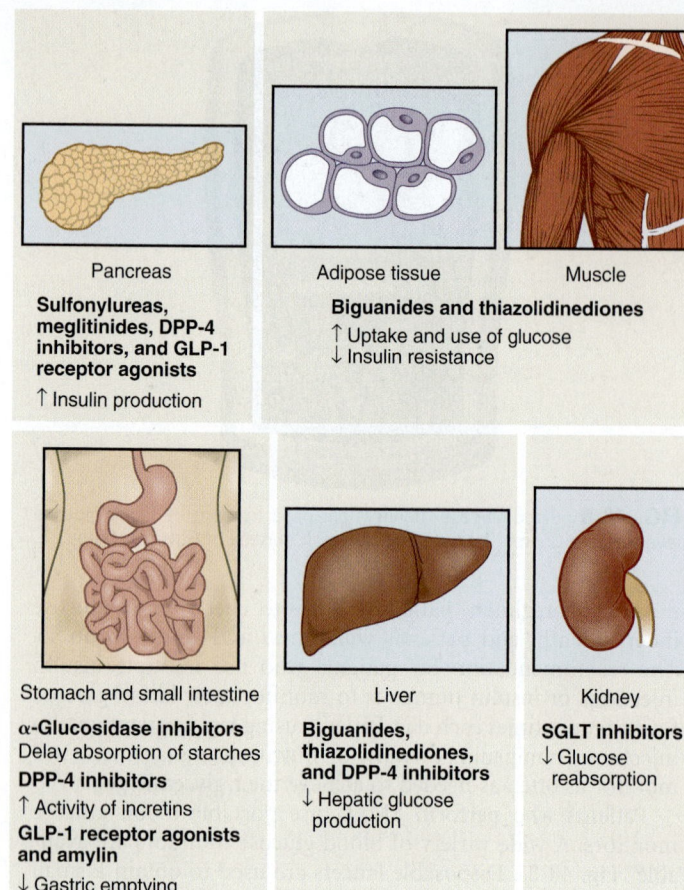

FIG. 48-9 Sites and mechanisms of action of type 2 diabetes drugs. *DDP-4*, Dipeptidyl peptidase; *GLP-1*, glucagon-like peptide-1; *SGLT*, sodium-glucose co-tranporter.

Pancreas

Sulfonylureas, meglitinides, DPP-4 inhibitors, and GLP-1 receptor agonists
↑ Insulin production

Adipose tissue — **Muscle**

Biguanides and thiazolidinediones
↑ Uptake and use of glucose
↓ Insulin resistance

Stomach and small intestine

α-Glucosidase inhibitors
Delay absorption of starches
DPP-4 inhibitors
↑ Activity of incretins
GLP-1 receptor agonists and amylin
↓ Gastric emptying

Liver

Biguanides, thiazolidinediones, and DPP-4 inhibitors
↓ Hepatic glucose production

Kidney

SGLT inhibitors
↓ Glucose reabsorption

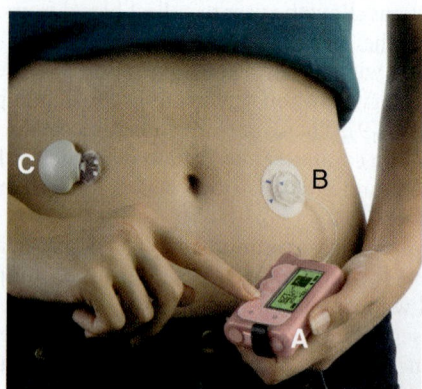

FIG. 48-10 The MiniMed® 530/730G with Enlite *(A)* delivers insulin through a thin plastic tubing to an infusion set, which has a cannula *(B)* that sits under the skin. Continuous glucose monitoring occurs through a tiny sensor *(C)* inserted under the skin. Sensor data are sent continuously to the insulin pump through wireless technology giving a more complete picture of glucose levels, which can lead to better treatment decisions and improved health. (MiniMed® 530G with Enlite® manufactured by the diabetes division of Medtronic, Inc.)

The blood glucose level reported by a laboratory is sometimes higher than the patient's home glucose monitor or the hospital's portable monitor. This is because some home monitors give capillary blood glucose values from whole blood (via finger stick), whereas tests performed in laboratories provide

---

TABLE 48-11   **Patient & Caregiver Teaching**
Self-Monitoring of Blood Glucose (SMBG)
Include the following instructions when teaching the patient and caregiver about SMBG. 1. Wash hands in warm water. It is not necessary to clean the site with alcohol, and it may interfere with test results. Finger should be dry before puncturing it. 2. If it is difficult to obtain an adequate drop of blood for testing, warm the hands in warm water or let the arms hang dependently for a few minutes before the finger puncture is made. 3. A lancing device is usually used. Place the lancet in the device, following the instructions that come with it. If the puncture is made on the finger, use the side of the finger pad rather than near the center. Fewer nerve endings are along the side of the finger pad. If an alternative site is used (e.g., forearm), special equipment may be needed. Refer to manufacturer's instructions for alternative site use, except during hypoglycemic episodes. 4. Set lancing device to make a puncture just deep enough to obtain a sufficiently large drop of blood. Unnecessarily deep punctures may cause pain and bruising. Current meters require very small amounts of blood. 5. Follow instructions on monitor for checking the blood. 6. Record results. Compare with personal target blood glucose goals.

plasma readings. Plasma samples, or venous samples, are approximately 10% to 12% higher. Most current monitors are automatically calibrated to give a "plasma" result (even though whole blood was used for the sample) so that the home readings can be more readily compared with laboratory values. It is important to read the literature accompanying a monitor to find out if it is displaying values as whole blood or plasma.

Because errors in monitoring technique can cause errors in management strategies, comprehensive patient teaching is essential. Initial instruction should be followed up with regular reassessment. Review the instructions that accompany each product. If a product has a control solution, teach patients to use and interpret control solutions. Control solution should be used when first using a blood glucose meter, when a new bottle of strips is used, or when there is a reason to believe that the readings are not correct. Table 48-11 lists the steps to include when teaching the patient how to perform SMBG.

People with type 1 diabetes often check their blood glucose before meals. This is because many patients use insulin pumps or multiple daily injections and base the insulin dose on the carbohydrates in a meal or make adjustments if the preprandial value is above or below target. Checking blood glucose 2 hours after the first bite of food helps a person determine if the bolus insulin dose was adequate for that meal.

Teach patients to monitor blood glucose whenever hypoglycemia is suspected so that immediate action can be taken. During times of illness, check blood glucose levels at 4-hour intervals to determine the effects of the illness on glucose levels. Teach the patient to monitor blood glucose before and after exercise to determine the effects of exercise on blood glucose levels. This is especially important in the patient with type 1 diabetes.

A patient who is visually impaired, cognitively impaired, or limited in manual dexterity needs careful evaluation of the degree to which SMBG can be performed independently. Nurses preparing patients for discharge from the hospital and nurses working in home health and outpatient settings may need to identify caregivers who can assume this responsibility. Adaptive devices are available to help patients with certain limitations. These include talking meters and other equipment for the visually impaired.

Bariatric Surgery

Bariatric surgery may be considered for patients with type 2 diabetes, especially if the diabetes or associated co-morbidities are difficult to manage with lifestyle and drug therapy. Patients with type 2 diabetes who have undergone bariatric surgery need lifelong lifestyle support and monitoring. (Bariatric surgery is discussed in Chapter 40.)

Pancreas Transplantation

Pancreas transplantation can be used as a treatment option for patients with type 1 diabetes. Usually it is done for patients who have end-stage renal disease and have had or plan to have a kidney transplant. Kidney and pancreas transplants are often performed together, or a pancreas may be transplanted after a kidney transplant. If renal failure is not present, the ADA recommends that pancreas transplantation be considered only for patients who exhibit the following three criteria: (1) a history of frequent, acute, and severe metabolic complications (e.g., hypoglycemia, hyperglycemia, ketoacidosis) requiring medical attention; (2) clinical and emotional problems with the use of exogenous insulin therapy that are so severe as to be incapacitating; and (3) consistent failure of insulin-based management to prevent acute complications.

Successful pancreas transplantation can improve quality of life for people with diabetes, primarily by eliminating the need for exogenous insulin, frequent blood glucose measurements, and the risks involved with hyper- and hypoglycemia. Transplantation can also eliminate the acute complications commonly experienced by patients with type 1 diabetes (e.g., hypoglycemia, hyperglycemia). However, pancreas transplantation is only partially successful in reversing the long-term renal and neurologic complications of diabetes. The patient will also require lifelong immunosuppression to prevent rejection of the organ. Complications can result from immunosuppressive therapy. (Immunosuppressive therapy is discussed in Chapter 13.)

Pancreatic islet cell transplantation is another potential treatment measure. During this procedure, the islets are harvested from the pancreas of a deceased organ donor. Most recipients require the use of two or more pancreases. The islets are infused via a catheter through the upper abdomen into the portal vein of the liver. With only the islets transplanted, pain and recovery time are diminished compared with whole pancreas transplants. Currently this procedure is experimental in the United States. Research is continuing to investigate the best ways to implant the islet cells and to prevent their rejection.

Culturally Competent Care: Diabetes Mellitus

Because culture can have a strong influence on dietary preferences and meal preparation practices, culturally competent care has special relevance for the patient with diabetes. For example, certain ethnic and cultural groups, such as Hispanics, Native Americans, African Americans, and Asians and Pacific Islanders have a high incidence of diabetes. The increased prevalence can be attributed to genetic predisposition, environmental factors, and dietary choices.

Explore the influences of culture on food choices and meal planning with the patient as part of the health history. When giving diet instructions, consider the patient's cultural

---

CULTURAL & ETHNIC HEALTH DISPARITIES
Diabetes Mellitus

- The highest incidence of diabetes is among Native Americans and Alaska Natives (16.5% are being treated for diabetes).
- Pima Indians in Arizona have the highest rate of diabetes in the world (50% of adults have diabetes).
- The rates of diabetes are: non-Hispanic whites 7.1%, Asian Americans 8.4%, Hispanics 11.8%, and non-Hispanic blacks 12.6%.
- Diabetes is 1.5 times more likely to cause death in Hispanics and 2.2 times more likely to cause death in African Americans than in non-Hispanic whites.
- Complications from diabetes are a major cause of death among Native Americans. Native Americans have a six times higher rate of end-stage renal disease and a four times higher rate of amputation than other ethnicities with diabetes.

---

food preferences. Nutrition resources specifically designed for members of different cultural groups are available from the ADA.

❖ NURSING MANAGEMENT: DIABETES MELLITUS

◆ Nursing Assessment

Table 48-12 provides initial subjective and objective data that you should obtain from a person with diabetes mellitus. After the initial assessment, perform periodic patient assessments on a regular basis.

◆ Nursing Diagnoses

Nursing diagnoses related to diabetes mellitus may include, but are not limited to, the following:
- Ineffective health management *related to* deficient knowledge of diabetes management and lack of understanding of diabetes management plan
- Risk for unstable blood glucose levels *related to* infrequent blood glucose monitoring and lack of following diabetes management plan
- Risk for injury *related to* decreased tactile sensation, episodes of hypoglycemia
- Risk for peripheral neurovascular dysfunction *related to* vascular effects of diabetes

Additional information on nursing diagnoses for the patient with diabetes is presented in eNursing Care Plan 48-1 available on the website.

◆ Planning

The overall goals are for the patient with diabetes mellitus to (1) engage in self-care behaviors to actively manage his or her diabetes, (2) experience few or no hyperglycemia or hypoglycemia emergencies, (3) maintain blood glucose levels at normal or near-normal levels, (4) prevent or minimize chronic complications related to diabetes, and (5) adjust lifestyle to accommodate the diabetes plan with a minimum of stress. The patient with diabetes needs to safely and effectively fit diabetes into life, rather than living life around diabetes.

◆ Nursing Implementation

◆ Health Promotion. Your role in health promotion is to identify, monitor, and teach the patient at risk for diabetes. Obesity is the primary risk factor for type 2 diabetes. The findings from the Diabetes Prevention Program indicated that a modest

TABLE 48-12 Nursing Assessment
Diabetes Mellitus

Subjective Data

Important Health Information

Past health history: Mumps, rubella, coxsackievirus, or other viral infections. Recent trauma, infection, or stress. Pregnancy, gave birth to infant >9 lb. Chronic pancreatitis, Cushing syndrome, acromegaly, family history of type 1 or type 2 diabetes mellitus

Medications: Use of and adherence to regimen with insulin or OAs, corticosteroids, diuretics, phenytoin (Dilantin)

Surgery or other treatments: Any recent surgery

Functional Health Patterns

Health perception–health management: Positive family history, malaise

Nutrition-metabolic: Obesity, weight loss (type 1), weight gain (type 2). Thirst, hunger, nausea and vomiting. Poor healing (especially involving the feet), eating habits in patients with previously diagnosed diabetes

Elimination: Constipation or diarrhea, frequent urination, frequent bladder infections, nocturia, urinary incontinence

Activity-exercise: Muscle weakness, fatigue

Cognitive-perceptual: Abdominal pain, headache, blurred vision, numbness or tingling of extremities, pruritus

Sexuality-reproductive: Erectile dysfunction, frequent vaginal infections, decreased libido

Coping–stress tolerance: Depression, irritability, apathy

Value-belief: Commitment to lifestyle changes involving diet, medication, and activity patterns

Objective Data

Eyes

Soft, sunken eyeballs.* History of vitreal hemorrhages, cataracts

Integumentary

Dry, warm, inelastic skin. Pigmented lesions (on legs), ulcers (especially on feet), loss of hair on toes, acanthosis nigricans

Respiratory

Rapid, deep respirations (Kussmaul respirations)*

Cardiovascular

Hypotension.* Weak, rapid pulse*

Gastrointestinal

Dry mouth, vomiting.* Fruity breath*

Neurologic

Altered reflexes, restlessness, confusion, stupor, coma

Musculoskeletal

Muscle wasting

Possible Findings

Serum electrolyte abnormalities. Fasting blood glucose level ≥126 mg/dL. Oral glucose tolerance test >200 mg/dL, random glucose ≥200 mg/dL. Leukocytosis. ↑ Blood urea nitrogen, creatinine, triglycerides, cholesterol, LDL, VLDL. ↓ HDL. A1C >6.0% (A1C >7.0% in those with diagnosed diabetes), glycosuria, ketonuria, albuminuria. Acidosis

A1C, Glycosylated hemoglobin; *HDL,* high-density lipoprotein; *LDL,* low-density lipoprotein; *OAs,* oral agents; *VLDL,* very-low-density lipoprotein.
*Indicates manifestations of diabetic ketoacidosis (DKA).

TABLE 48-13 Screening for Diabetes in Asymptomatic, Undiagnosed Individuals

Who to Screen

1. Consider screening all adults who are overweight (BMI >25 kg/m²) and have additional risk factors:
   - First-degree relative with diabetes
   - Physically inactive
   - Members of a high-risk ethnic population (e.g., African American, Hispanic, Native American, Asian American,* Pacific Islander)
   - Women who delivered a baby weighing >9 lb or were diagnosed with gestational diabetes mellitus
   - Hypertensive (≥140/90 mm Hg) or on therapy for hypertension
   - HDL cholesterol level ≤35 mg/dL (0.90 mmol/L) and/or a triglyceride level ≥250 mg/dL (2.82 mmol/L)
   - Women with polycystic ovary syndrome
   - A1C ≥5.7%, IGT, or IFG on previous screening
   - Other clinical conditions associated with insulin resistance (e.g., obesity, acanthosis nigricans)
2. In the absence of the above criteria, screening for diabetes should begin at age 45 yr regardless of weight.
3. If results are normal, screening should be repeated at least at 3-yr intervals, with consideration of more frequent screening depending on initial results and risk status.

What Measurements Are Used

To screen for diabetes or to assess risk of future diabetes, A1C, FPG, or 2-hour OGTT is appropriate.

Source: American Diabetes Association: Standards of Medical Care in Diabetes, *Diabetes Care* 39 (Suppl 1):S1, 2016.
A1C, Glycosylated hemoglobin; *BMI,* body mass index; *FPG,* fasting plasma glucose; *HDL,* high-density lipoprotein; *IFG,* impaired fasting glucose; *IGT,* impaired glucose tolerance; *OGTT,* oral glucose tolerance test.
*Consider screening in Asian Americans with a BMI of 23 kg/m² or higher.

weight loss of 5% to 7% of body weight and regular exercise of 30 minutes five times a week lowered the risk of developing type 2 diabetes up to 58%.[21]

The ADA recommends routine screening for type 2 diabetes for all adults who are overweight or obese (BMI greater than or equal to 25 kg/m²) or have one or more risk factors. For people who do not have risk factors for diabetes, screening should begin at age 45. Table 48-13 provides criteria to screen for prediabetes and diabetes. If results are normal, repeat screening at 3-year intervals.[3] Many factors put an individual at an increased risk for diabetes. These include age, ethnicity (being Native American, Hispanic, African American, Asian, Pacific Islander), obesity, having a baby that weighed more than 9 lb at birth, history of gestational diabetes, and a family history of diabetes. A diabetes risk test is available at *www.diabetes.org/risk-test.jsp.* The diabetes risk test determines if the person is at risk for prediabetes or diabetes based on the number of risk factors present.

♥ HEALTHY PEOPLE
Prevention and Early Detection of Diabetes Mellitus

- Increase level of exercise because physical activity reduces the risk of type 2 diabetes.
- Maintain a healthy weight because obesity increases the risk of type 2 diabetes.
- If overweight, lose weight and participate in a regular exercise program to reduce the risk of diabetes.
- Choose foods that are low in fat content, total calories, and processed foods and high in whole grains, fruits, and vegetables.
- If overweight and over age 45, get screened for diabetes.

◆ **Acute Care.** Acute situations involving the patient with diabetes include hypoglycemia, DKA, and hyperosmolar hyperglycemic syndrome (HHS). Nursing management for these situations is discussed in more detail later in this chapter. Other areas of acute care relate to management during acute illness and surgery.

◆ *Acute Illness and Surgery.* Both emotional and physical stress can increase the blood glucose level and result in hyperglycemia. Because stress is unavoidable, certain situations may require more intense treatment, such as extra insulin and more frequent blood glucose monitoring, to maintain glycemic goals and avoid hyperglycemia.

Acute illness, injury, and surgery are situations that may evoke a counterregulatory hormone response, resulting in hyperglycemia. Even common illnesses such as a viral upper respiratory tract infection or the flu can cause this response. Encourage patients with diabetes to check blood glucose at least every 4 hours during times of illness. Acutely ill patients with type 1 diabetes with a blood glucose greater than 240 mg/dL (13.3 mmol/L) should also check urine for ketones every 3 to 4 hours.

Teach patients to report to the HCP when glucose levels are over 300 mg/dL twice in a row or urine ketone levels are moderate to high. A patient with type 1 diabetes may need an increase in insulin to prevent DKA. Elevated blood glucose levels can lead to poor healing and infection. Insulin therapy may be required for a patient with type 2 diabetes to prevent or treat hyperglycemia symptoms and avoid an acute hyperglycemia emergency. In critically ill patients, insulin therapy may be started if the blood glucose is persistently greater than 180 mg/dL. These patients have a higher targeted blood glucose goal, which is usually 140 to 180 mg/dL. Food intake is important during times of stress and illness, when the body requires extra energy. If patients are able to eat normally, they can continue with their regular meal plan while increasing the intake of noncaloric fluids, such as water, sugar-free gelatin, and other decaffeinated beverages, and continue taking OAs, noninsulin injectable agents, and insulin as prescribed. When illness causes patients to eat less than normal, they can continue to take OAs, noninsulin injectable agents, and/or insulin as prescribed while supplementing food intake with carbohydrate-containing fluids. Examples include low-sodium soups, juices, and regular, sugar-sweetened decaffeinated soft drinks. It is important to tell the patient to contact an HCP if he or she is unable to keep down food or fluid.

During the intraoperative period, adjustments in the diabetes regimen can be planned to ensure safe and healthy blood glucose levels. The patient is given IV fluids and insulin (if needed) immediately before, during, and after surgery when there is no oral intake. Explain to the patient with type 2 diabetes who has been on OAs that this is a temporary measure, not a sign of worsening diabetes.

When caring for an unconscious surgical patient receiving insulin, be alert for signs of hypoglycemia such as sweating, tachycardia, and tremors. Frequent monitoring of blood glucose can prevent episodes of severe hypoglycemia.

◆ **Ambulatory Care.** Successful management of diabetes involves ongoing interaction among the patient, caregiver, and interprofessional team. It is important that a certified diabetes educator (CDE) be involved in the care of the patient and family. Because diabetes is a complex chronic condition, a great deal of patient contact takes place in outpatient and home settings. The major goal of patient care in these settings is to enable the patient (with the help of a caregiver as needed) to reach an optimal level of independence in self-care activities. Unfortunately, many patients with diabetes face challenges in reaching these goals. Diabetes increases the risk for other chronic conditions that can affect self-care activities. These include visual impairment, lower-extremity problems that affect mobility, and other functional limitations related to a stroke.

An important nursing function is to assess the ability of patients and caregivers in performing activities such as SMBG and insulin injection. Assistive devices for self-administration of insulin include syringe magnifiers, vial stabilizers, and dosing aids for the visually impaired. In some cases, referrals are made to help the patient achieve the self-care goal. These may include an occupational therapist, a social worker, a home care nurse, a home health aide, or a dietitian.

A diagnosis of diabetes affects the patient in many profound ways. Self-management of the disease is demanding. Patients with diabetes continually face lifestyle choices that affect the foods they eat, their activities, and demands on their time and energy. The requirements of scheduled meals, SMBG, medication, and insulin management may interfere with the patient's other responsibilities. Any change in the daily routine can be difficult. In addition, they face the challenge of preventing or dealing with the devastating complications of diabetes.

Careful assessment of what it means to the patient to have diabetes is a good starting point for teaching. The goals of teaching are mutually determined by the patient and you, based on individual needs and therapeutic requirements. Identify the patient's support system, and include them in planning, teaching, and counseling. When family members and other individuals close to the patient are included, they can support the patient's self-care behaviors. Additionally, they can provide care if self-care is not possible. Encourage the family and caregivers to provide emotional support and encouragement as the patient deals with the reality of living with a chronic disease.

Insulin Therapy. Nursing responsibilities for the patient receiving insulin include proper administration, assessment of the patient's response to insulin therapy, and teaching the patient about administration, storage, and side effects of insulin (Table 48-5). Table 48-6 lists guidelines for assessing a patient using glucose-lowering agents, including insulin and OAs.

Assessment of the patient who is a new user of insulin must include an evaluation of his or her ability to safely manage this therapy. This includes the ability to understand the interaction of insulin, food, and activity and to recognize and treat the symptoms of hypoglycemia appropriately. If the patient does not have the cognitive skills to do these things, identify and teach another responsible person. The patient or caregiver must have the cognitive and manual skills needed to prepare and inject insulin. Otherwise, additional resources will be needed to assist the patient. For patients with cognitive, physical, and other barriers, consider referral to a CDE because he or she has the specialized knowledge and skills to promote self-care behaviors for these patients.

Many patients are fearful when they first begin using insulin.[22] Some find it difficult to self-inject because they are afraid of needles or the pain associated with an injection. Others may think that the insulin is not necessary or that they will experience hypoglycemia after an injection. Explore the patient's underlying fears before beginning the teaching. Assessment of the patient's beliefs and concerns regarding starting insulin will guide the teaching, counseling, and plan of care. Having open discussion with patients, providing educational materials and programs, and working with a diabetes educator are all beneficial for patients starting insulin.

Follow-up assessment of the patient who has been using insulin therapy includes an inspection of injection sites for signs of lipodystrophy and other reactions, review of insulin preparation and injection technique, a history pertaining to the occurrence of hypoglycemia, and assessment of the patient's method for handling hypoglycemia. A review of the patient's recorded blood glucose readings is vital in assessing how the patient is doing and making any needed adjustments.

◆ *Oral and Noninsulin Injectable Agents.* Your responsibilities for the patient taking oral and noninsulin injectable agents are similar to those for the patient taking insulin. Proper administration of these drugs, assessment of the patient's use of and response to these drugs, and teaching the patient and family are all essential nursing actions.

Your assessment is valuable in determining the most appropriate drug for a patient. Factors such as the patient's mental status, eating habits, home environment, attitude toward diabetes, and medication history all play a significant role in determining the most appropriate drug. For example, frail older adults who live alone are at high risk for severe hypoglycemia because low blood glucose is frequently undetected or untreated in this population. This is especially true if the patient has cognitive impairment. In these cases, an OA that does not cause hypoglycemia, or a shorter-acting OA, would be most appropriate.

Patient teaching is essential. Some patients may assume that their diabetes is not a serious condition if they are only taking a pill to treat it. Instruct the patient that these agents will help manage blood glucose and help prevent serious long- and short-term complications of diabetes. Teach patients that OAs and noninsulin injectable agents are used in addition to food choices and activity as therapy for diabetes and the importance of following their meal and activity plans. Teach patients not to take extra pills if they have overeaten. If the patient uses sulfonylureas and metformin, instruct the patient about prevention, symptom recognition, and management of hypoglycemia.

◆ *Personal Hygiene.* The potential for infection requires diligent skin and dental hygiene practices. Because of the susceptibility to periodontal disease, encourage daily brushing and flossing in addition to regular visits to the dentist. When having dental work done, have the patient inform the dentist that he or she has diabetes.

Routine care includes regular bathing, with particular emphasis on foot care. Advise patients to inspect their feet daily, avoid going barefoot, and wear shoes that are supportive and comfortable. If cuts, scrapes, or burns occur, treat them promptly and monitor them carefully. Wash the area and apply a nonabrasive or nonirritating antiseptic ointment. Cover the area with a dry, sterile pad. Teach patients to notify the HCP immediately if the injury does not begin to heal within 24 hours or if signs of infection develop.

◆ *Medical Identification and Travel.* Instruct the patient to carry medical identification at all times indicating that he or she has diabetes. Police, paramedics, and many private citizens are aware of the need to look for this identification when working with sick or unconscious persons. Every person with diabetes is encouraged to wear a Medic Alert bracelet or necklace. An identification card (Fig. 48-11) can supply valuable information,

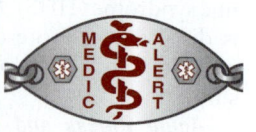

I have DIABETES

If unconscious or behaving abnormally, I may be having a reaction associated with diabetes or its treatment.

If I can swallow, give me a sweet drink, orange juice, LifeSavers, or low-fat milk.

If I do not recover promptly, call a physician or send me to the hospital.

If I am unconscious or cannot swallow, do not attempt to give me anything by mouth, but call 911 or send me to the hospital immediately.

FIG. 48-11 Medical alerts. A patient with diabetes should carry a card and wear a bracelet or necklace that indicates diabetes. If the patient with diabetes is unconscious, these measures will ensure prompt and appropriate attention.

such as the name of the HCP; the type of diabetes; and the type and dosage of insulin, noninsulin injectable agents, or OAs.

Travel for a patient with diabetes requires planning. Being sedentary for long periods may raise the person's glucose level. Encourage the patient to get up and walk at least every 2 hours to lower the risk for deep vein thrombosis and to prevent elevation of glucose levels. Teach the patient to have a full set of diabetes care supplies in the carry-on luggage when traveling by plane, train, or bus. This includes blood glucose monitoring equipment, insulin, noninsulin injectable agents, oral medications, and syringes or insulin pens.

When equipment such as syringes, lancing devices, insulin vials or pens, and insulin pumps are taken onto a commercial airliner, it is a good idea to have the professional printed pharmaceutical labels that accompany them. A letter from the prescribing HCP indicating medical necessity may prevent delays at security checkpoints. Notify screeners if an insulin pump is used so that they can inspect it while it is on the body, rather than removing it.

For patients who use insulin or OAs that can cause hypoglycemia, keep snack items and a quick-acting carbohydrate source for treating hypoglycemia in the carry-on luggage. Keep extra insulin available in case a bottle breaks or is lost. For longer trips, carry a full day's supply of food in the event of canceled flights, delayed meals, or closed restaurants. If the patient is planning a trip out of the country, it is wise to have a letter from the HCP explaining that the patient has diabetes and requires all the materials, particularly syringes, for ongoing health care.

When travel involves time changes, such as traveling coast to coast or across the International Date Line, the patient can contact the HCP to plan an appropriate insulin schedule. During travel, most patients find it helpful to keep watches set to the time of the city of origin until they reach their destination. The key to travel when taking insulin is to know the type of insulin being taken, its onset of action, the anticipated peak time, and mealtimes.

◆ *Patient and Caregiver Teaching.* The goals of diabetes self-management education are to match the level of self-management to the patient's individual ability so that he or she can become the most active participant possible. Patients who actively manage their diabetes care have better outcomes than those who do not. For this reason, an educational approach that facilitates informed decision making by the patient is advocated. Sometimes this is referred to as the *empowerment approach* to education.

Unfortunately, patients can encounter a variety of physical, psychologic, and emotional barriers when it comes to effectively managing their diabetes. These barriers may include feelings of

🌿 COMPLEMENTARY & ALTERNATIVE THERAPIES

Herbs and Supplements That May Affect Blood Glucose

Scientific Evidence*
- Herbs and supplements that may lower blood glucose include aloe, α-lipoic acid, cinnamon, chromium, garlic, and ginseng.
- However, many studies have been small and not well designed. Further research is needed.

Nursing Implications
- Teach patients to use herbs and supplements with caution, since they may affect blood glucose.
- Patients with diabetes mellitus should consult their health care provider before using herbs or nutritional supplements.
- Patients who use herbs should monitor their blood glucose levels carefully and regularly.

*Based on a systematic review of scientific literature. Retrieved from www.naturalstandard.com.

INFORMATICS IN PRACTICE

Patient Teaching Using Smart Phone Apps

- Teaching is a critical part of nursing care for patients with diabetes. Put some fun into patient teaching by using smart phone applications.
- Introduce patients to a variety of smart phone apps for healthy living and managing diabetes.
- Sample apps include Moves, Glucose Buddy, Diabetes Companion, Diabetes App, and Calorie King.

Based on list provided by American Diabetes Association. Retrieved from www.diabetesforecast.org/2014/Jan/app-happy.html.

inadequacy about one's own abilities, unwillingness to make the necessary behavioral changes, ineffective coping strategies, and cognitive deficits. If the patient is not able to manage the disease, a family member may be able to assume part of this role. If the patient or caregiver cannot make decisions related to diabetes management, consider a referral to a CDE, social worker, or other resources within the community. These resources can assist the patient and family in outlining a feasible treatment program that meets their capabilities.

An assessment of the patient's knowledge of diabetes and lifestyle preferences is useful in planning a teaching program. Tables 48-14 and 48-15 present guidelines to use for patient and caregiver teaching. Assess the patient's knowledge base frequently so that gaps in knowledge or incorrect or inaccurate ideas can be corrected.

The ADA offers resources for patients in the form of pamphlets, booklets, books, and a monthly magazine called *Diabetes Forecast*. Affiliates of the ADA are located in all states, and most can be reached by dialing 1-800-DIABETES (800-342-2383). The ADA publishes materials and sponsors conferences for health care professionals concerned with diabetes education, research, and management of patients. The ADA website (*www.diabetes.org*) has extensive information for the public and health care professionals. This organization also recognizes education programs that meet the national standards of diabetes education and can provide a list of these programs. Drug companies manufacturing diabetes-related products also have free educational materials for patients and HCPs. It is critical that

TABLE 48-14 Patient & Caregiver Teaching
Management of Diabetes Mellitus

Include the following instructions when teaching the patient and caregiver how to manage diabetes mellitus.

Component	What to Teach
Disease process	• Include an introduction about the pancreas and the islets of Langerhans. • Describe how insulin is made and what affects its production. • Discuss the relationship of insulin and glucose. • Explain the difference between type 1 and type 2 diabetes.
Physical activity	• Discuss the effect of regular exercise on the management of blood glucose, improvement of cardiovascular function, and general health.
Menu planning	• Stress the importance of a well-balanced diet as part of a diabetes management plan. • Explain the impact of carbohydrates on blood glucose levels.
Medication	• Ensure that the patient understands the proper use of prescribed medication (e.g., insulin [Table 48-5], OAs, and noninsulin injectables). • Account for a patient's physical limitations or inabilities for self-medication. If necessary, involve the family or caregiver in proper use of medication. • Discuss all side effects and safety issues regarding medication.
Monitoring blood glucose	• Teach correct blood glucose monitoring. • Include when to check blood glucose levels, how to record them, and how to adjust insulin levels if necessary.
Risk reduction	• Ensure that the patient understands and appropriately responds to the signs and symptoms of hypoglycemia and hyperglycemia (Table 48-16). • Stress the importance of proper foot care (Table 48-21), regular eye examinations, and consistent glucose monitoring. • Inform the patient about the effect that stress can have on blood glucose.
Psychosocial	• Help the patient identify resources that are available to facilitate the adjustment and answer questions about living with a chronic condition such as diabetes.

OAs, Oral agents.

you stay current in your diabetes knowledge so that you can effectively teach and support patients with diabetes.

◆ Evaluation

The expected outcomes are that the patient with diabetes mellitus will
- Verbalize key elements of the therapeutic regimen, including knowledge of disease and treatment plan
- Describe self-care measures that may prevent or slow progression of chronic complications
- Maintain a balance of nutrition, activity, and insulin availability that results in stable, safe, and healthy blood glucose levels
- Experience no injury resulting from decreased sensation in feet
- Implement measures to increase peripheral circulation

Additional information on expected outcomes for the patient with diabetes is presented in eNursing Care Plan 48-1 available on the website for this chapter.

TABLE 48-15 Patient & Caregiver Teaching

Instructions for Patients With Diabetes Mellitus

Include the following essential instructions for diabetes management for the patient and caregiver.

Blood Glucose

- Monitor your blood glucose at home and record results in a log.
- Take your insulin, OA, and/or noninsulin injectable agent as prescribed.
- Take insulin consistently, especially when you are sick.
- Keep an adequate supply of insulin on hand at all times.
- Obtain A1C blood test every 3-6 mo as an indicator of your long-term blood glucose levels.
- Be aware of symptoms of hypoglycemia and hyperglycemia.
- Carry some form of rapid-acting glucose at all times so that you can treat hypoglycemia quickly.
- Instruct family members how and when to use glucagon if patient becomes unresponsive because of hypoglycemia.

Exercise

- Learn how exercise and food affect your blood glucose levels.
- Remember that exercise will usually lower your blood glucose level.
- Begin an exercise program after approval from HCP.

Food

- Work with a dietitian to create an individualized meal plan.
- Make healthy food choices most of the time and eat regular meals at regular times.
- Choose foods low in saturated and *trans* fat. Know your cholesterol level.
- Limit the amount of alcohol you drink.
- Be aware that excessive amounts of alcohol may lead to unpredictable low blood glucose reactions.
- Avoid fad diets.
- Limit regular soda and fruit juice.

Other Guidelines

- Obtain an annual eye examination by an ophthalmologist.
- Obtain annual urine monitoring for protein.
- Examine your feet at home.
- Wear comfortable, well-fitting shoes to help prevent foot injury. Break in new shoes gradually.
- Always carry identification that says you have diabetes.
- Have other medical problems treated, especially high BP and high cholesterol.
- Have a yearly influenza vaccination.
- Quit or never start smoking cigarettes or using nicotine products.
- Avoid applying heat or cold directly to your feet.
- Avoid going barefoot.
- Keep skin moisturized by applying cream to surfaces of feet, but not between toes.

A1C, Glycosylated hemoglobin; *OA,* oral agent.

ACUTE COMPLICATIONS OF DIABETES MELLITUS

The acute complications of diabetes mellitus arise from events associated with hyperglycemia and hypoglycemia. Hyperglycemia occurs when there is not enough insulin working, and hypoglycemia occurs when there is too much insulin working. It is important for the HCP to distinguish between hyperglycemia and hypoglycemia because hypoglycemia worsens rapidly and is a serious threat if action is not immediately taken. Table 48-16 compares the manifestations, causes, management, and prevention of hyperglycemia and hypoglycemia.

EVIDENCE-BASED PRACTICE

Translating Research Into Practice

Can Exercise Improve Blood Pressure Levels in Patients With Diabetes?

Clinical Question

For adults with type 2 diabetes (P), what is the effect of structured exercise training (I) versus advice on physical activity (C) on blood pressure levels (O)?

Synthesis of Best Available Evidence

- Systematic review of randomized controlled trials (RCTs).
- 51 RCTs of patients (*n* = 9540) with type 2 diabetes receiving structured exercise training or physical activity advice only. Structured exercise was aerobic and/or resistance training. Activity advice was information provided on gradually increasing the frequency of moderate/vigorous activity up to 150 min/wk. Control groups received no exercise training or advice on activity. Outcome was BP level.

Conclusion

- All types of structured exercise training were associated with a reduction in both systolic and diastolic BP in patients with type 2 diabetes. Greatest decreases in BP occurred in structured exercise programs lasting >150 min/wk.
- Physical activity advice only is also associated with lowered BP levels.

Implications for Nursing Practice

1. Why is it important for patients with diabetes to seek non-pharmacological methods to decrease BP level?
2. What would you discuss with a patient who has an elevated BP and appears motivated to engage in a regular exercise program?
3. How will you facilitate the provision of physical activity information to patients with diabetes?

Reference for Evidence

Figueira F, Umpierre D, Cureau F, et al: Association between physical activity advice only or structured exercise training with blood pressure levels in patients with type 2 diabetes: a systematic review and meta-analysis, *Sports Med* 44:1557, 2014.

P, Patient population of interest; *I,* intervention or area of interest; *C,* comparison of interest or comparison group; *O,* outcomes of interest; *T,* timing (see p. 15).

DIABETIC KETOACIDOSIS

Etiology and Pathophysiology

Diabetic ketoacidosis (DKA) is caused by a profound deficiency of insulin and is characterized by hyperglycemia, ketosis, acidosis, and dehydration. It is most likely to occur in people with type 1 diabetes but may be seen in people with type 2 diabetes in conditions of severe illness or stress when the pancreas cannot meet the extra demand for insulin. Precipitating factors include illness and infection, inadequate insulin dosage, undiagnosed type 1 diabetes, poor self-management, and neglect.

When the circulating supply of insulin is insufficient, glucose cannot be properly used for energy. The body compensates by breaking down fat stores as a secondary source of fuel (Fig. 48-12). Ketones are acidic by-products of fat metabolism that can cause serious problems when they become excessive in the blood. Ketosis alters the pH balance, causing metabolic acidosis to develop. Ketonuria is a process that occurs when ketone bodies are excreted in the urine. During this process, electrolytes become depleted as cations are eliminated along with the anionic ketones in an attempt to maintain electrical neutrality.

TABLE 48-16   Comparison of Hyperglycemia and Hypoglycemia

Hyperglycemia	Hypoglycemia
Manifestations*	
• Elevated blood glucose†	• Blood glucose <70 mg/dL (3.9 mmol/L)
• Increase in urination	• Cold, clammy skin
• Increase in appetite followed by lack of appetite	• Numbness of fingers, toes, mouth
• Weakness, fatigue	• Rapid heartbeat
• Blurred vision	• Emotional changes
• Headache	• Headache
• Glycosuria	• Nervousness, tremors
• Nausea and vomiting	• Faintness, dizziness
• Abdominal cramps	• Unsteady gait, slurred speech
• Progression to DKA or HHS	• Hunger
	• Changes in vision
	• Seizures, coma
Causes	
• Illness, infection	• Alcohol intake without food
• Corticosteroids	• Too little food—delayed, omitted, inadequate intake
• Too much food	• Too much diabetes medication
• Too little or no diabetes medication	• Too much exercise without adequate food intake
• Inactivity	• Diabetes medication or food taken at wrong time
• Emotional, physical stress	• Loss of weight without change in medication
• Poor absorption of insulin	• Use of β-adrenergic blockers interfering with recognition of symptoms
Treatment	
• Get medical care	• Follow the Rule of 15 (see pp. 1146-1147).
• Continue diabetes medication as prescribed	• See Table 48-19 for treatment of hypoglycemia.
• Check blood glucose frequently and check urine for ketones; record results	
• Drink fluids at least on an hourly basis	
• Contact HCP regarding ketonuria	
Preventive Measures	
• Take prescribed dose of medication at proper time	• Take prescribed dose of medication at proper time
• Accurately administer insulin, noninsulin injectables, OA	• Accurately administer insulin, noninsulin injectables, OA
• Make healthy food choices	• Coordinate eating with medications
• Follow sick-day rules when ill	• Eat adequate food intake needed for calories for exercise
• Check blood glucose routinely	• Be able to recognize and know symptoms and treat them immediately
• Wear or carry diabetes identification	• Carry simple carbohydrates
	• Teach family and caregiver about symptoms and treatment
	• Check blood glucose routinely
	• Wear or carry diabetes identification

DKA, Diabetic ketoacidosis; *HHS,* hyperosmolar hyperglycemic syndrome; *OA,* oral agent.

*There is usually a gradual onset of symptoms in hyperglycemia and a more rapid onset in hypoglycemia. Many signs and symptoms of hyper- and hypoglycemia overlap. Signs and symptoms of hypoglycemia often change over time.

†Specific clinical manifestations related to elevated levels of blood glucose vary according to the patient.

PATHOPHYSIOLOGY MAP

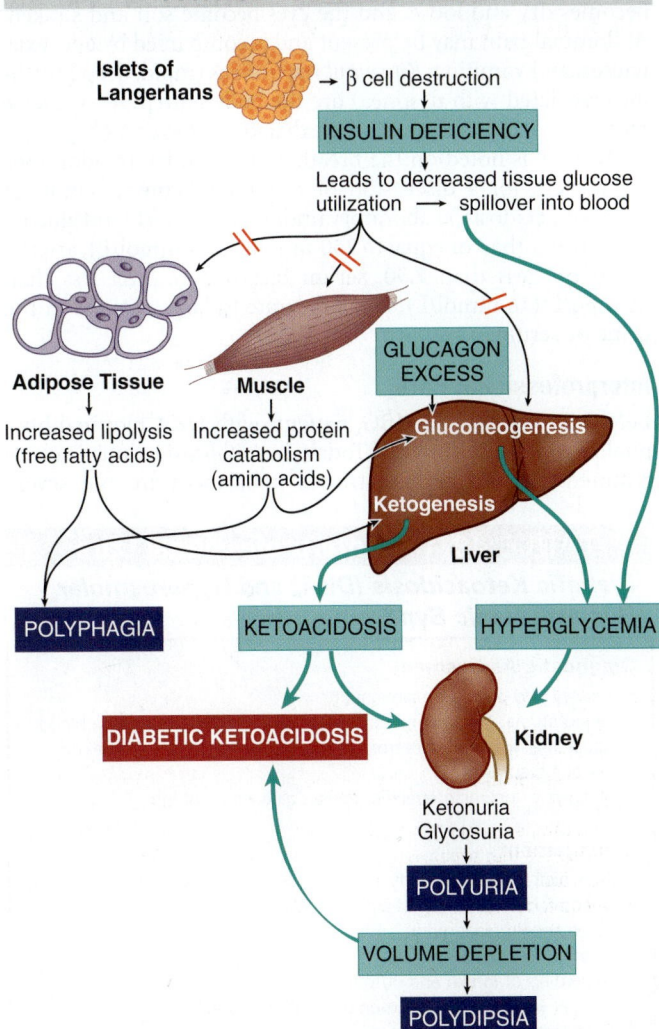

FIG. 48-12 Metabolic events leading to diabetic ketoacidosis. (From Kumar V, Abbas AK, Aster JC, Fausto N: *Robbins and Cotran pathologic basis of disease,* ed 8, Philadelphia, 2010, Saunders.)

Insulin deficiency impairs protein synthesis and causes excessive protein degradation. This results in nitrogen losses from the tissues. Insulin deficiency also stimulates the production of glucose from amino acids (from proteins) in the liver and leads to further hyperglycemia. Because of the deficiency of insulin, the additional glucose cannot be used and the blood glucose level rises further, adding to the osmotic diuresis.

If not treated, the patient will develop severe depletion of sodium, potassium, chloride, magnesium, and phosphate. Vomiting caused by the acidosis results in more fluid and electrolyte losses. Eventually, hypovolemia followed by shock will ensue. Renal failure, which may eventually occur from hypovolemic shock, causes the retention of ketones and glucose, and the acidosis progresses. Untreated, the patient becomes comatose as a result of dehydration, electrolyte imbalance, and acidosis. If the condition is not treated, death is inevitable.

Clinical Manifestations

Dehydration occurs in DKA with manifestations of poor skin turgor, dry mucous membranes, tachycardia, and orthostatic hypotension. Early symptoms may include lethargy and weakness. As the patient becomes severely dehydrated, the skin becomes dry and loose, and the eyes become soft and sunken. Abdominal pain may be present and accompanied by anorexia, nausea, and vomiting. *Kussmaul respirations* (rapid, deep breathing associated with dyspnea) are the body's attempt to reverse metabolic acidosis through the exhalation of excess CO_2.

Acetone is noted on the breath as a sweet, fruity odor. (See Chapter 16 for a discussion of respiratory compensation of metabolic acidosis.) Laboratory findings include a blood glucose level greater than or equal to 250 mg/dL (13.9 mmol/L), arterial blood pH less than 7.30, serum bicarbonate level less than 16 mEq/L (16 mmol/L), and moderate to large ketones in the urine or serum.

Interprofessional Care

Before the advent of SMBG, patients with DKA required hospitalization for treatment. Today, hospitalization may not be required. If fluid and electrolyte imbalances are not severe and blood glucose levels can be safely monitored at home, DKA may be managed on an outpatient basis (Table 48-17). Other factors to consider when deciding where the patient is managed include the presence of fever, nausea, vomiting, and diarrhea; altered mental status; the cause of the ketoacidosis; and availability of frequent communication with the HCP (every few hours). Patients with DKA who have an illness such as pneumonia or a urinary tract infection are usually admitted to the hospital.

DKA is a serious condition that proceeds rapidly and must be treated promptly. Refer to Table 48-18 for the emergency management of a patient with DKA. Because fluid imbalance is potentially life threatening, the initial goal of therapy is to establish IV access and begin fluid and electrolyte replacement. Typically, an infusion of 0.45% or 0.9% NaCl at a rate to restore urine output to 30 to 60 mL/hr and to raise BP constitutes the initial fluid therapy regimen. When blood glucose levels approach 250 mg/dL (13.9 mmol/L), add 5% to 10% dextrose to the fluid regimen to prevent hypoglycemia and a sudden drop in glucose that can be associated with cerebral edema. Overzealous rehydration, especially with hypotonic IV solutions, can result in cerebral edema.

The aim of fluid and electrolyte therapy is to replace extracellular and intracellular water and to correct deficits of sodium, chloride, bicarbonate, potassium, phosphate, magnesium, and nitrogen. Monitor patients with renal or cardiac compromise for fluid overload. Obtain a serum potassium level before starting insulin. If the patient is hypokalemic, insulin administration will further decrease the potassium levels, making early potassium replacement essential. Although initial serum potassium may be normal or high, levels can rapidly decrease once therapy starts as insulin drives potassium into the cells, leading to life-threatening hypokalemia.

IV insulin administration therapy is directed toward correcting hyperglycemia and hyperketonemia. Insulin is immediately started at 0.1 U/kg/hr by a continuous infusion. It is important to prevent rapid drops in serum glucose to avoid cerebral edema. A blood glucose reduction of 36 to 54 mg/dL/hr (2 to 3 mmol/L/hr) will avoid complications. Insulin allows water and potassium to enter the cell along with glucose and can lead

---

 TABLE 48-17   **Interprofessional Care**

Diabetic Ketoacidosis (DKA) and Hyperosmolar Hyperglycemic Syndrome (HHS)

Diagnostic Assessment

- History and physical examination
- Blood studies, including immediate blood glucose, complete blood count, pH, ketones, electrolytes, blood urea nitrogen, arterial or venous blood gases
- Urinalysis, including specific gravity, glucose, acetone

Management

- Administration of IV fluids
- IV administration of short-acting insulin
- Electrolyte replacement
- Assessment of mental status
- Recording of intake and output
- Central venous pressure monitoring (if indicated)
- Assessment of blood glucose levels
- Assessment of blood and urine for ketones
- ECG monitoring
- Assessment of cardiovascular and respiratory status

✚ **TABLE 48-18**   **Emergency Management**

Diabetic Ketoacidosis

Etiology	Assessment Findings	Interventions
• Undiagnosed diabetes mellitus • Inadequate treatment of existing diabetes mellitus • Insulin not taken as prescribed • Infection • Change in eating, insulin, or exercise plan • Malfunction of insulin pump/nondelivery of insulin	• Dry mouth • Thirst • Abdominal pain • Nausea and vomiting • Gradually increasing restlessness, confusion, lethargy • Flushed, dry skin • Eyes appearing sunken • Breath odor of ketones • Rapid, weak pulse • Labored breathing (Kussmaul respirations) • Fever • Urinary frequency • Serum glucose >250 mg/dL (13.9 mmol/L) • Glucosuria and ketonuria	**Initial** • Ensure patent airway. • Administer O_2 via nasal cannula or non-rebreather mask. • Establish IV access with large-bore catheter. • Begin fluid resuscitation with 0.9% NaCl solution 1 L/hr until BP stabilized and urine output 30-60 mL/hr. • Begin continuous regular insulin drip 0.1 U/kg/hr. • Identify history of diabetes, time of last food, and time and amount of last insulin injection. **Ongoing Monitoring** • Monitor vital signs, level of consciousness, cardiac rhythm, O_2 saturation, and urine output. • Assess breath sounds for fluid overload. • Monitor serum glucose and serum potassium. • Administer potassium to correct hypokalemia. • Administer sodium bicarbonate if severe acidosis (pH < 7.0). • Add dextrose to IV fluid for blood glucose <250 mg/dL.

CHECK YOUR PRACTICE

A 36-yr-old female patient was admitted to your unit with DKA. You are trying to regulate her IV rate. You know that too rapid administration of IV fluids and a rapid lowering of serum glucose can lead to cerebral edema. You also know that incorrect fluid replacement, especially with hypotonic fluids, can cause a sudden fall in serum sodium that can cause cerebral edema.
- What are the best clinical indicators of successful treatment of DKA?
- What is your role as a nurse in the care of this patient?

to a depletion of vascular volume and hypokalemia, so monitor the patient's fluid balance and potassium levels.

HYPEROSMOLAR HYPERGLYCEMIC SYNDROME

Hyperosmolar hyperglycemic syndrome (HHS) is a life-threatening syndrome that can occur in the patient with diabetes who is able to produce enough insulin to prevent DKA, but not enough to prevent severe hyperglycemia, osmotic diuresis, and extracellular fluid depletion (Fig. 48-13). HHS is less common than DKA (Table 48-17). It often occurs in patients over 60 years of age with type 2 diabetes.

Common causes of HHS are urinary tract infections, pneumonia, sepsis, any acute illness, and newly diagnosed type 2 diabetes. HHS is often related to impaired thirst sensation and/or a functional inability to replace fluids. There is usually a history of inadequate fluid intake, increasing mental depression, and polyuria.

The main difference between HHS and DKA is that the patient with HHS usually has enough circulating insulin so that ketoacidosis does not occur. Because HHS produces fewer symptoms in the earlier stages, blood glucose levels can climb quite high before the problem is recognized. The higher blood glucose levels increase serum osmolality and produce more severe neurologic manifestations, such as somnolence, coma, seizures, hemiparesis, and aphasia. Since these manifestations resemble a stroke, immediate determination of the glucose level is critical for correct diagnosis and treatment.

Laboratory values in HHS include a blood glucose level greater than 600 mg/dL (33.33 mmol/L) and a marked increase in serum osmolality. Ketone bodies are absent or minimal in both blood and urine.

Interprofessional Care

HHS is a medical emergency and has a high mortality rate. The management of DKA and HHS is similar and includes immediate IV administration of insulin and either 0.9% or 0.45% NaCl. HHS usually requires large volumes of fluid replacement. This should be accomplished slowly and carefully. Patients with HHS are commonly older and may have cardiac or renal compromise, requiring hemodynamic monitoring to avoid fluid overload during fluid replacement. When blood glucose levels fall to approximately 250 mg/dL (13.9 mmol/L), IV fluids containing dextrose are administered to prevent hypoglycemia.

Electrolytes are monitored and replaced as needed. Hypokalemia is not as significant in HHS as it is in DKA, although fluid losses may result in milder potassium deficits that require replacement. Assess vital signs, intake and output, tissue turgor, laboratory values, and cardiac monitoring to check the efficacy

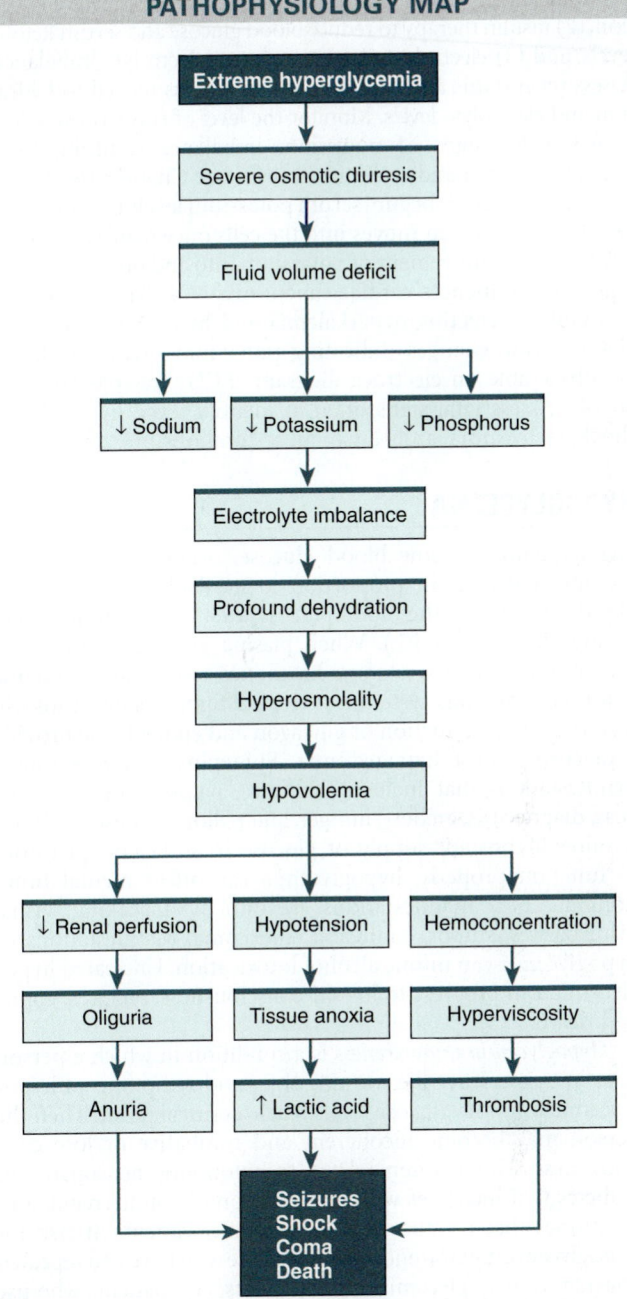

FIG. 48-13 Pathophysiology of hyperosmolar hyperglycemic syndrome. (Modified from Urden LD, Stacy KM, Lough ME: *Critical care nursing: diagnosis and management*, ed 6, St Louis, 2010, Mosby.)

of fluid and electrolyte replacement. This includes monitoring serum osmolality and frequently assessing cardiac, renal, and mental status. Once the patient is stabilized, initiate attempts to detect and correct the underlying cause.

❖ NURSING MANAGEMENT: DIABETIC KETOACIDOSIS AND HYPEROSMOLAR HYPERGLYCEMIC SYNDROME

Closely monitor the hospitalized patient with appropriate blood and urine tests. You are responsible for monitoring blood glucose and urine for output and ketones and using laboratory data to determine appropriate patient care.

Monitor the administration of (1) IV fluids to correct dehydration, (2) insulin therapy to reduce blood glucose and serum ketone levels, and (3) electrolytes given to correct electrolyte imbalance. Assess renal status and cardiopulmonary status related to hydration and electrolyte levels. Monitor the level of consciousness.

Assess for signs of potassium imbalance resulting from hypoinsulinemia and osmotic diuresis (see Chapter 16). When insulin treatment is begun, serum potassium levels may decrease rapidly as potassium moves into the cells once insulin becomes available. This movement of potassium into and out of extracellular fluid influences cardiac functioning. Cardiac monitoring is useful in detecting hyperkalemia and hypokalemia because characteristic changes indicating potassium excess or deficit are observable on electrocardiogram (ECG) tracings (see Fig. 16-14). Assess vital signs often to identify fever, hypovolemic shock, tachycardia, and Kussmaul respirations.

HYPOGLYCEMIA

Hypoglycemia, or low blood glucose, occurs when there is too much insulin in proportion to available glucose in the blood. This causes the blood glucose level to drop to less than 70 mg/dL (3.9 mmol/L). When plasma glucose drops below 70 mg/dL, counterregulatory hormones are released and the autonomic nervous system is activated. Suppression of insulin secretion and production of glucagon and epinephrine provide a defense against hypoglycemia. Epinephrine release causes manifestations that include shakiness, palpitations, nervousness, diaphoresis, anxiety, hunger, and pallor. Because the brain requires a constant supply of glucose in sufficient quantities to function properly, hypoglycemia can affect mental functioning. These manifestations are difficulty speaking, visual disturbances, stupor, confusion, and coma. Manifestations of hypoglycemia can mimic alcohol intoxication. Untreated hypoglycemia can progress to loss of consciousness, seizures, coma, and death.

Hypoglycemia unawareness is a condition in which a person does not experience the warning signs and symptoms of hypoglycemia until the glucose levels reach a critical point. Then the person may become incoherent and combative or lose consciousness. This is often related to autonomic neuropathy of diabetes that interferes with the secretion of counterregulatory hormones that produce these symptoms. Patients at risk for hypoglycemia unawareness include those who have had repeated episodes of hypoglycemia, older patients, and patients who use β-adrenergic blockers. Using intensive treatment to get tight blood glucose levels in patients who are at risk for hypoglycemia unawareness may not be an appropriate goal because a major drawback is hypoglycemia. These patients are usually managed with blood glucose goals that are somewhat higher than those of patients who are able to detect and manage the onset of hypoglycemia.

Causes of hypoglycemia are often related to a mismatch in the timing of food intake and the peak action of insulin or oral hypoglycemic agents that increase endogenous insulin secretion. The balance between blood glucose and insulin can be disrupted by administering too much insulin or medication, ingesting too little food, delaying the time of eating, and performing unusual amounts of exercise. Hypoglycemia can occur at any time, but most episodes occur when the OA or insulin is at its peak of action or when the patient's daily routine is disrupted without adequate adjustments in diet, medications, and

activity. Although hypoglycemia is more common with insulin therapy, it can occur with noninsulin injectable agents and OAs, and it may be severe and persist for an extended time because of the longer duration of action of these drugs.

Symptoms of hypoglycemia may occur when a very high blood glucose level falls too rapidly (e.g., a blood glucose level of 300 mg/dL [16.7 mmol/L] falling quickly to 180 mg/dL [10 mmol/L]). Although the blood glucose level is above normal by definition and measurement, the sudden metabolic shift can evoke hypoglycemia symptoms. Too vigorous management of hyperglycemia with insulin can cause this type of situation.

❖ NURSING AND INTERPROFESSIONAL MANAGEMENT: HYPOGLYCEMIA

Hypoglycemia can usually be quickly reversed with effective treatment. At the first sign of hypoglycemia, check the blood glucose if possible. If it is less than 70 mg/dL (3.9 mmol/L), immediately begin treatment for hypoglycemia. If the blood glucose is greater than 70 mg/dL, investigate other possible causes of the signs and symptoms. If the patient has manifestations of hypoglycemia and monitoring equipment is not available or the patient has a history of fluctuating blood glucose levels, hypoglycemia should be assumed and treatment initiated.

Follow the "Rule of 15" to treat hypoglycemia (Table 48-19). A blood glucose less than 70 mg/dL is treated by ingesting 15 g of a simple (fast-acting) carbohydrate, such as 4 to 6 oz of fruit juice or a regular soft drink. Commercial products such as gels or tablets containing specific amounts of glucose are convenient for carrying in a purse or pocket to be used in such situations. Recheck the blood glucose 15 minutes later. If the value is still

---

TABLE 48-19　Interprofessional Care

Hypoglycemia

Diagnostic Assessment
- History of hypoglycemia and symptoms.
- Blood glucose—immediately.

Management
- Determine cause of hypoglycemia (after correction of condition).

Conscious Patient
- Have patient eat or drink 15 g of quick-acting carbohydrate (4-6 oz of regular soda, 5-8 LifeSavers, 1 Tbsp syrup or honey, 4 tsp jelly, 4-6 oz orange juice, commercial dextrose products [per label instructions]).
- Wait 15 min. Then check blood glucose again.
- If blood glucose is still <70 mg/dL, have patient repeat treatment of 15 g of carbohydrate.
- Once the glucose level is stable and the next meal is more than 1 hr away, give patient additional food of carbohydrate plus protein or fat (e.g., crackers with peanut butter or cheese) after symptoms subside. Give additional food if patient is engaged in physical activity regardless of time until next meal.
- Immediately notify HCP or emergency service (if patient outside hospital) if symptoms do not subside after two or three administrations of quick-acting carbohydrate.

Worsening Symptoms or Unconscious Patient
- Subcutaneous or IM injection of 1 mg glucagon. IV administration of 20-50 mL of 50% glucose.

less than 70 mg/dL, ingest 15 g more of carbohydrate and recheck the blood glucose in 15 minutes. If no significant improvement occurs after two or three doses of 15 g of simple carbohydrate, contact the HCP. After an acute episode of hypoglycemia, have the patient ingest a complex carbohydrate after recovery to prevent repeat hypoglycemia.

Avoid treatment with carbohydrates that contain fat, such as candy bars, cookies, whole milk, and ice cream. The fat in those foods will slow the absorption of the glucose and delay the response to treatment. Avoid overtreatment with large quantities of quick-acting carbohydrates so that a rapid fluctuation to hyperglycemia does not occur.

In an acute care setting, patients with hypoglycemia may be treated with 20 to 50 mL of 50% dextrose IV push. If the patient is not alert enough to swallow and no IV access is available, another option is to administer 1 mg of glucagon by IM or subcutaneous injection. An IM injection in a site such as the deltoid muscle will result in a quicker response. Glucagon stimulates a strong hepatic response to convert glycogen to glucose and therefore makes glucose rapidly available. Nausea is a common reaction after glucagon injection. Therefore, to prevent aspiration if vomiting occurs, turn the patient on the side until he or she becomes alert. Patients with minimal glycogen stores will not respond to glucagon. This includes patients with alcohol-related hepatic disease, starvation, and adrenal insufficiency. Teach family members and others likely to be present when severe hypoglycemia occurs when and how to inject glucagon.

Once the acute hypoglycemia has been reversed, explore with the patient the reasons why the situation developed. This assessment may indicate the need for additional teaching of the patient and the family to avoid future episodes of hypoglycemia.

CHRONIC COMPLICATIONS OF DIABETES MELLITUS

ANGIOPATHY

Chronic complications associated with diabetes are primarily those of end-organ disease from damage to blood vessels (angiopathy) secondary to chronic hyperglycemia (Fig. 48-14). Angiopathy is one of the leading causes of diabetes-related deaths, with about 68% of deaths caused by CVD and 16% caused by strokes for those ages 65 or older.[23] These chronic blood vessel dysfunctions are divided into two categories: macrovascular complications and microvascular complications.

Several theories exist as to how and why chronic hyperglycemia damages cells and tissues. Possible causes include (1) the accumulation of damaging by-products of glucose metabolism, such as sorbitol, which is associated with damage to nerve cells; (2) the formation of abnormal glucose molecules in the basement membrane of small blood vessels such as those that circulate to the eyes and kidneys; and (3) a derangement in red blood cell function that leads to a decrease in oxygenation to the tissues.

The Diabetes Control and Complications Trial (DCCT), a landmark study in diabetes management, demonstrated that in patients with type 1 diabetes the risk for microvascular complications could be significantly reduced by keeping blood glucose levels as near to normal as possible for as much of the time as

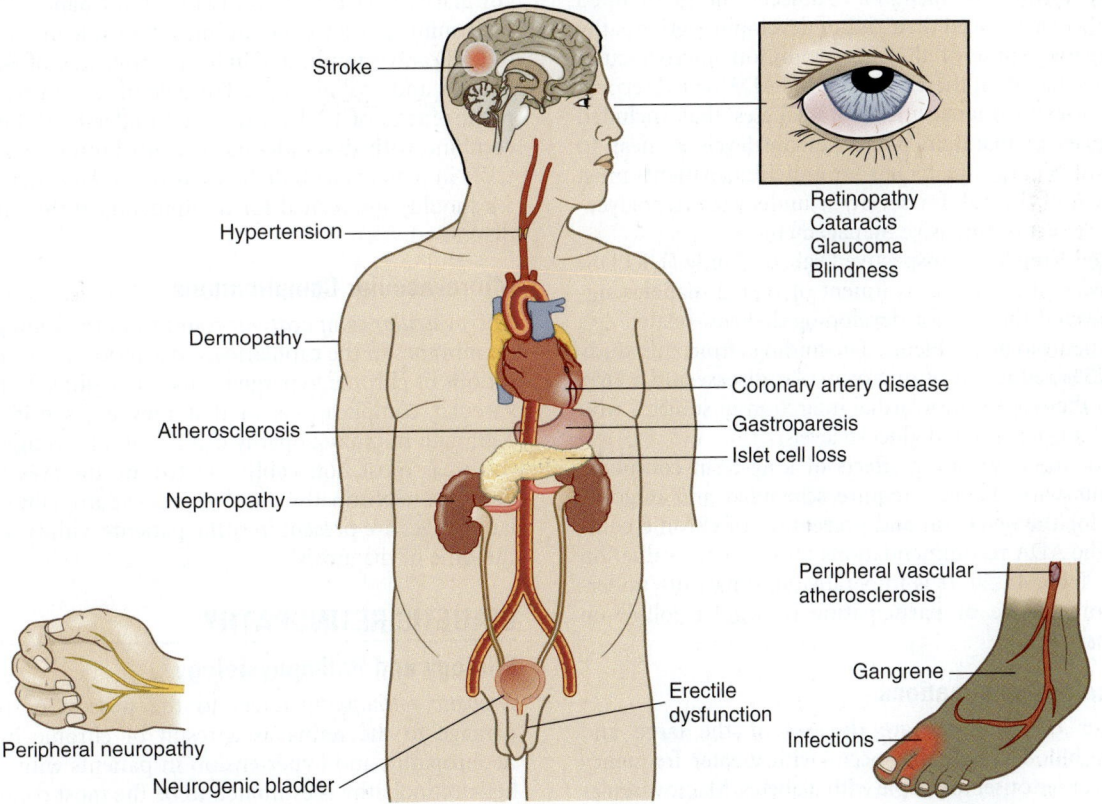

FIG. 48-14 Long-term complications of diabetes mellitus. (From Kumar V, Abbas AK, Aster JC, Fausto N: *Robbins and Cotran pathologic basis of disease*, ed 8, Philadelphia, 2010, Saunders.)

TABLE 48-20 Monitoring for Long-Term Complications of Diabetes Mellitus

Complication	Type of Examination	Frequency
Retinopathy	• Funduscopic: dilated eye examination • Fundus photography	• Annually
Nephropathy	• Urine for albuminuria • Serum creatinine	• Annually

Neuropathy (foot and lower extremities)	• Visual examination of foot
	
	• Comprehensive foot:
	  • Visual examination
	  • Sensory examination with monofilament and tuning fork
	  • Palpation (pulses, temperature, callus formation)
		• Daily by patient
		• Every visit to HCP
		• Annually*

Cardiovascular disease	• Risk factor assessment: hypertension, dyslipidemia, smoking, family history of premature coronary artery disease, and presence of albuminuria or • Exercise stress testing (may include stress ECG, stress echocardiogram, stress nuclear imaging)	• At least annually • As needed based on risk factors

Source: American Diabetes Association: Standards of medical care in diabetes, *Diabetes Care* 39 (Suppl 1):S1, 2016.
*If patients have a history of foot ulcers, loss of sensation in their feet, or other foot abnormalities, the recommendation is to have a foot exam at every visit.

possible (*tight or intensive therapy*).[24] Subjects who maintained tight glucose levels reduced their risk of developing retinopathy and nephropathy, some of the most common microvascular complications. Based on these findings, the ADA issued recommendations for the management of diabetes that included treatment goals to maintain blood glucose levels as near to normal as possible. Specific targets for individual patients must take into account the risk for severe or undetected hypoglycemia as a side effect of intensive management.

The United Kingdom Prospective Diabetes Study (UKPDS) demonstrated that intensive treatment of type 2 diabetes significantly lowered the risk for developing diabetes-related eye, kidney, and neurologic problems. The findings from this study included a 25% reduction of microvascular disease and a 16% reduction in the risk for myocardial infarction in subjects who maintained long-term blood glucose levels.[25]

Because of the devastating effects of long-term complications, patients with diabetes require scheduled and ongoing monitoring for the detection and prevention of chronic complications. The ADA recommendations for ongoing evaluation are listed in Table 48-20. It is imperative that patients understand the importance of participating in regular follow-up examinations.

Macrovascular Complications

Macrovascular complications are diseases of the large and medium-size blood vessels that occur with greater frequency and with an earlier onset in people with diabetes. Macrovascular diseases include cerebrovascular, cardiovascular, and peripheral vascular disease. Women with diabetes have a four to six times increased risk for CVD, and men with diabetes have a two to three times increased risk for CVD compared with those without diabetes.[4] Patients with diabetes can decrease several risk factors associated with macrovascular complications, such as obesity, smoking, hypertension, high fat intake, and sedentary lifestyle. Smoking, which is detrimental to health in general, is especially injurious to people with diabetes and significantly increases their risk for blood vessel and cardiovascular disease, stroke, and lower extremity amputation. The ADA recommends yearly screening for CVD risk factors in people with diabetes.[12]

Optimizing BP control in patients with diabetes is significant for the prevention of cardiovascular and renal disease. Treating hypertension in those with diabetes results in a decrease in macrovascular and microvascular complications. Hypertension in people with diabetes causes an increase in mortality greater than for those with hypertension without diabetes.[2] A target BP of less than 140/90 mm Hg is recommended for most patients with diabetes.[15]

Patients with diabetes have an increase in lipid abnormalities. This contributes to the increase in CVD seen in this population. The ADA recognizes that diabetes alone is a CVD risk factor. Therefore it recommends that all adults with diabetes take a statin. Dosing is based on the presence of age and additional atherosclerotic CVD risk factors. The ADA advocates lifestyle interventions, including nutritional therapy, exercise, weight loss, and smoking cessation to treat hyperlipidemia.

The ADA recommends BP screening at every routine visit for people with diabetes. They also recommend lifestyle advisement for BP greater than 130/80 and treatment for BP greater than 140/90. (Hypertension is discussed in Chapter 32, and coronary artery disease is discussed in Chapter 33.)

Insulin resistance has an important role in the development of CVD and is implicated in the pathogenesis of essential hypertension and dyslipidemia. The role of insulin resistance in the pathogenesis of CVD is not well understood, but it seems to combine with dyslipidemia in contributing to greater risk of CVD in patients with diabetes mellitus. All patients with diabetes should be screened for dyslipidemia at the time diabetes is diagnosed.

Microvascular Complications

Microvascular complications result from thickening of the vessel membranes in the capillaries and arterioles in response to conditions of chronic hyperglycemia. They differ from the macrovascular complications in that they are specific to diabetes. Although microangiopathy can be found throughout the body, the areas most noticeably affected are the eyes (retinopathy), kidneys (nephropathy), and nerves (neuropathy). Microvascular changes are present in some patients with type 2 diabetes at the time of diagnosis.

DIABETIC RETINOPATHY

Etiology and Pathophysiology

Diabetic retinopathy refers to the process of microvascular damage to the retina as a result of chronic hyperglycemia, nephropathy, and hypertension in patients with diabetes. Diabetic retinopathy is estimated to be the most common cause of new cases of adult blindness.[2]

Retinopathy can be classified as nonproliferative or proliferative. In *nonproliferative retinopathy,* the most common form, partial occlusion of the small blood vessels in the retina causes microaneurysms to develop in the capillary walls. The walls of these microaneurysms are so weak that capillary fluid leaks out, causing retinal edema and eventually hard exudates or intraretinal hemorrhages. This may cause mild to severe vision loss, depending on which parts of the retina are affected. If the center of the retina (macula) is affected, vision loss can be severe.

Proliferative retinopathy, the most severe form, involves the retina and vitreous. When retinal capillaries become occluded, the body compensates by forming new blood vessels to supply the retina with blood, a pathologic process known as *neovascularization.* These new vessels are extremely fragile and hemorrhage easily, producing vitreous contraction. Eventually light is prevented from reaching the retina as the vessels become torn and bleed into the vitreous cavity. The patient sees black or red spots or lines. If these new blood vessels pull the retina while the vitreous contracts, causing a tear, partial or complete retinal detachment will occur. If the macula is involved, vision is lost. Without treatment, more than half of patients with proliferative diabetic retinopathy will be blind.

Persons with diabetes are also prone to other visual problems. Glaucoma occurs as a result of the occlusion of the outflow channels secondary to neovascularization. This type of glaucoma is difficult to treat and often results in blindness. Cataracts develop at an earlier age and progress more rapidly in people with diabetes.

Interprofessional Care

The earliest and most treatable stages of diabetic retinopathy often produce no changes in the vision. Therefore patients with type 2 diabetes should have a dilated eye examination by an ophthalmologist or a specially trained optometrist at the time of diagnosis and annually thereafter for early detection and treatment. A person with type 1 diabetes should have a dilated eye examination within 5 years after the onset of diabetes and then repeated annually.

The best approach to the management of diabetes-related eye disease is to prevent it by maintaining healthy blood glucose levels and managing hypertension. Laser photocoagulation therapy is indicated to reduce the risk of vision loss in patients with proliferative retinopathy or macular edema and in some cases of nonproliferative retinopathy. Laser photocoagulation destroys the ischemic areas of the retina that produce growth factors that encourage neovascularization. A patient who develops vitreous hemorrhage and retinal detachment of the macula may need to undergo vitrectomy. *Vitrectomy* is the aspiration of blood, membrane, and fibers from the inside of the eye through a small incision just behind the cornea. (Photocoagulation and vitrectomy are discussed in Chapter 21.)

Iluvien (fluocinolone acetonide intravitreal implant) is used to treat retinopathy. It is an injectable micro-insert that provides sustained treatment through continuous delivery of corticosteroid fluocinolone acetonide for 36 months. Iluvien is injected in the back of the patient's eye with an applicator that uses a 25-gauge needle, which allows for a self-sealing wound.

Recent research has identified the importance of vascular endothelial growth factor (VEGF) in the development of diabetic retinopathy. Drugs injected into the eye that block the action of VEGF and reduce inflammation are currently being studied for their effectiveness in treating retinopathy.[26]

NEPHROPATHY

Diabetic nephropathy is a microvascular complication associated with damage to the small blood vessels that supply the glomeruli of the kidney. It is the leading cause of end-stage renal disease in the United States and is seen in 20% to 40% of people with diabetes. Risk factors for diabetes-related nephropathy include hypertension, genetic predisposition, smoking, and chronic hyperglycemia. Results of the DCCT and UKPDS research have demonstrated that kidney disease can be significantly reduced when near-normal blood glucose levels are maintained.[24,25]

Patients with diabetes are screened for nephropathy annually with a random spot urine collection to assess for albuminuria and measure the albumin-to-creatinine ratio. Serum creatinine is also measured to provide an estimation of the glomerular filtration rate and thus the degree of kidney function.

Patients with diabetes who have albuminuria receive either angiotensin-converting enzyme (ACE) inhibitor drugs (e.g., lisinopril [Prinivil, Zestril]) or angiotensin II receptor antagonists (e.g., losartan [Cozaar]). Both classifications of these drugs are used to treat hypertension and have been found to delay the progression of nephropathy in patients with diabetes.[12] Hypertension significantly accelerates the progression of nephropathy. Therefore aggressive BP management is indicated for all patients with diabetes. Keeping blood glucose levels in a healthy range is also critical in the prevention and delay of diabetes-related nephropathy. (See Chapter 32 for a discussion of hypertension and Chapter 46 for a discussion of renal failure.)

NEUROPATHY

Diabetic neuropathy is nerve damage that occurs because of the metabolic derangements associated with diabetes mellitus. About 60% to 70% of patients with diabetes have some degree of neuropathy.[2] The most common type of neuropathy affecting persons with diabetes is sensory neuropathy. This can lead to the loss of protective sensation in the lower extremities, and, coupled with other factors, significantly increases the risk for complications that result in a lower limb amputation. More than 60% of nontraumatic amputations in the United States occur in people with diabetes.[2] Screening for neuropathy begins at the time of diagnosis in patients with type 2 diabetes and 5 years after diagnosis in patients with type 1 diabetes.[12]

Etiology and Pathophysiology

The pathophysiologic processes of diabetes-related neuropathy are not well understood. Several theories exist, including metabolic, vascular, and autoimmune factors. The prevailing theory is that persistent hyperglycemia leads to an accumulation of sorbitol and fructose in the nerves that causes damage by an unknown mechanism. The result is reduced nerve conduction and demyelinization. Ischemic damage by chronic hyperglycemia in blood vessels that supply the peripheral nerves is also implicated in the development of diabetes-related neuropathy. Neuropathy can precede, accompany, or follow the diagnosis of diabetes.

Classification

The two major categories of diabetes-related neuropathy are *sensory neuropathy,* which affects the peripheral nervous system, and *autonomic neuropathy.* Each of these types can take on several forms.

Sensory Neuropathy. The most common form of sensory neuropathy is distal symmetric polyneuropathy, which affects the hands and/or feet bilaterally. This is sometimes referred to as *stocking-glove neuropathy.* Characteristics of distal symmetric polyneuropathy include loss of sensation, abnormal sensations, pain, and paresthesias. The pain, which is often described as burning, cramping, crushing, or tearing, is usually worse at night and may occur only at that time. The paresthesias may be associated with tingling, burning, and itching sensations. The patient may report a feeling of walking on pillows or numb feet. At times the skin becomes so sensitive (hyperesthesia) that even light pressure from bed sheets cannot be tolerated. Complete or partial loss of sensitivity to touch and temperature is common. Foot injury and ulcerations can occur without the patient ever having pain (Fig. 48-15). Neuropathy can also cause atrophy of the small muscles of the hands and feet, causing deformity and limiting fine movement.

Managing blood glucose is the only treatment for diabetes-related neuropathy. It is effective in many, but not all, cases. Drug therapy may be used to treat neuropathic symptoms, particularly pain. Medications commonly used include topical creams (e.g., capsaicin [Zostrix]), tricyclic antidepressants (e.g., amitriptyline), selective serotonin and norepinephrine reuptake inhibitors (e.g., duloxetine [Cymbalta]), and antiseizure medications (e.g., gabapentin [Neurontin], pregabalin [Lyrica]). Capsaicin is a moderately effective topical cream made from chili peppers. It depletes the accumulation of pain-mediating chemicals in the peripheral sensory neurons. The cream is applied three or four times a day.

At the start of therapy, symptoms usually increase, followed by relief of pain in 2 to 3 weeks. Tricyclic antidepressants are moderately effective in treating the symptoms of diabetic neuropathy. They work by inhibiting the reuptake of norepinephrine and serotonin, which are neurotransmitters believed to play a role in the transmission of pain through the spinal cord. Duloxetine is thought to relieve pain by increasing the levels of serotonin and norepinephrine, which improves the body's ability to regulate pain. Antiseizure medications decrease the release of neurotransmitters that transmit pain.[27]

Autonomic Neuropathy. Autonomic neuropathy can affect nearly all body systems and lead to hypoglycemia unawareness, bowel incontinence and diarrhea, and urinary retention. *Gastroparesis* (delayed gastric emptying) is a complication of autonomic neuropathy that can produce anorexia, nausea, vomiting, gastroesophageal reflux, and persistent feelings of fullness. Gastroparesis can trigger hypoglycemia by delaying food absorption. Cardiovascular abnormalities associated with autonomic neuropathy are postural hypotension, resting tachycardia, and painless myocardial infarction. Assess patients with diabetes for postural hypotension to determine if they are at risk for falls. Instruct the patient with postural hypotension to change from a lying or sitting position slowly.

Diabetes can affect sexual function in men and women. Erectile dysfunction (ED) in men with diabetes is well recognized and common, often being the first manifestation of autonomic neuropathy. ED in diabetes is also associated with other factors, including vascular disease, elevated blood glucose levels, endocrine disorders, psychogenic factors, and medications. Decreased libido is a problem for some women with diabetes. Candidal and nonspecific vaginitis is also common. ED or sexual dysfunction requires sensitive therapeutic counseling for both the patient and the patient's partner. (See Chapter 55 for a further discussion of ED.)

A neurogenic bladder may develop as the sensation in the inner bladder wall decreases, causing urinary retention. A patient with retention has infrequent voiding, difficulty voiding, and a weak stream of urine. Emptying the bladder every 3 hours in a sitting position helps prevent stasis and subsequent infection. Tightening the abdominal muscles during voiding and using the Credé maneuver (mild massage downward over the lower abdomen and bladder) may also help with complete bladder emptying. Cholinergic agonist drugs such as bethanechol (Urecholine) may be used. The patient may also need to learn self-catheterization (see Chapter 45).

COMPLICATIONS OF FEET AND LOWER EXTREMITIES

People with diabetes are at high risk for foot ulcerations and lower extremity amputations.[12] The development of diabetes-related foot complications can be the result of a combination of microvascular and macrovascular diseases that place the patient at risk for injury and serious infection (Fig. 48-16).

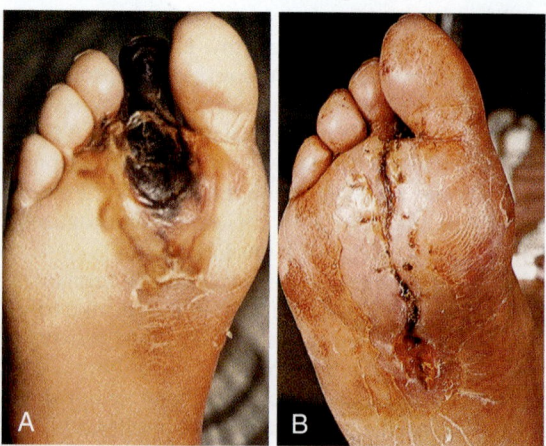

FIG. 48-16 The necrotic toe developed as a complication of diabetes. **A,** Before amputation. **B,** After amputation. (From Chew SL, Leslie D: *Clinical endocrinology and diabetes: an illustrated colour text,* Edinburgh, 2006, Churchill Livingstone.)

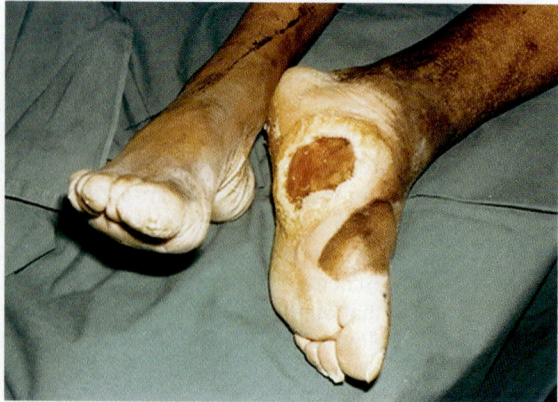

FIG. 48-15 Neuropathy: neurotrophic ulceration.

Sensory neuropathy and peripheral artery disease (PAD) are risk factors for foot complications. In addition, clotting abnormalities, impaired immune function, and autonomic neuropathy also have a role. Smoking is deleterious to the health of lower extremity blood vessels and increases the risk for amputation.

Sensory neuropathy is a major risk factor for lower extremity amputation in the person with diabetes. *Loss of protective sensation* (LOPS) often prevents the patient from being aware that a foot injury has occurred. Improper footwear and injury from stepping on foreign objects while barefoot are common causes of undetected foot injury in the person with LOPS.[12] Because the primary risk factor for lower extremity amputation is LOPS, annual screening using a *monofilament* is important. This is done by applying a thin, flexible filament to several spots on the plantar surface of the foot and asking the patient to report if it is felt. Insensitivity to a monofilament has been shown to greatly increase the risk for foot ulcers that can lead to amputation.

PAD increases the risk for amputation by causing a reduction in blood flow to the lower extremities. When blood flow is decreased, oxygen, white blood cells, and vital nutrients are not available to the tissues. Wounds take longer to heal, and the risk for infection increases. Signs of PAD include intermittent claudication, pain at rest, cold feet, loss of hair, delayed capillary filling, and dependent rubor (redness of the skin that occurs when the extremity is in a dependent position). The disease is diagnosed by history, ankle-brachial index (ABI) (see Table 37-3), and angiography. Management includes reduction of risk factors, particularly smoking, cholesterol intake, and hypertension. Bypass or graft surgery is indicated in some patients. (PAD is discussed in Chapter 37.)

If the patient has LOPS or PAD, aggressive measures must be taken to teach the patient how to prevent foot ulcers. These measures include the selection of proper footwear, including protective shoes. Teach the patient to carefully avoid injury to the foot, practice diligent skin and nail care, inspect the foot thoroughly each day, and treat small problems promptly. Guidelines for patient teaching are listed in Table 48-21.

Proper care of a foot ulcer is critical for wound healing. Several forms of treatment can be used. Casting can be done to redistribute the weight on the plantar surface of the foot. Wound care for the ulcer can include debridement, dressings, advanced wound healing products (becaplermin [Regranex]), vacuum-assisted closure, ultrasound, hyperbaric oxygen, and skin grafting.

Neuropathic arthropathy, or *Charcot's foot,* results in ankle and foot changes that ultimately lead to joint dysfunction and footdrop. These changes occur gradually and promote an abnormal distribution of weight over the foot, further increasing the chances of developing a foot ulcer as new pressure points emerge. Foot deformity should be recognized early and proper footwear fitted before ulceration occurs.

INTEGUMENTARY COMPLICATIONS

Up to two thirds of persons with diabetes develop skin problems.[12] Diabetes-related dermopathy, the most common diabetic skin lesion, is characterized by reddish brown, round or oval patches. They initially are scaly, then they flatten out and become indented. The lesions appear most frequently on the shins but can also be found on the front of the thighs, forearm, side of the foot, scalp, and trunk.

TABLE 48-21	**Patient & Caregiver Teaching***

Foot Care

Include the following instructions when teaching the patient and caregiver about foot care.

1. Wash feet daily with a mild soap and warm water. First test water temperature with elbow.
2. Pat feet dry gently, especially between toes.
3. Examine feet daily for cuts, blisters, swelling, and red, tender areas. Do not depend on feeling sores. If eyesight is poor, have others inspect feet.
4. Use lanolin on feet to prevent skin from drying and cracking. Do not apply between toes.
5. Use mild foot powder on sweaty feet.
6. Do not use commercial remedies to remove calluses or corns.
7. Cleanse cuts with warm water and mild soap, covering with clean dressing. Do not use iodine, rubbing alcohol, or strong adhesives.
8. Report skin infections or nonhealing sores to HCP immediately.
9. Cut toenails evenly with rounded contour of toes. Do not cut down corners. The best time to trim nails is after a shower or bath.
10. Separate overlapping toes with cotton or lamb's wool.
11. Avoid open-toe, open-heel, and high-heel shoes. Leather shoes are preferred to plastic ones. Wear slippers with soles. Do not go barefoot. Inspect socks and shoes for foreign objects before putting on.
12. Wear clean, absorbent (cotton or wool) socks or stockings that have not been mended. Colored socks must be colorfast.
13. Do not wear clothing that leaves impressions, hindering circulation.
14. Do not use hot water bottles or heating pads to warm feet. Wear socks for warmth.
15. Guard against frostbite.
16. Exercise feet daily either by walking or by flexing and extending feet in suspended position. Avoid prolonged sitting, standing, and crossing of legs.

*This teaching guide is also appropriate for patients with peripheral vascular problems.

Acanthosis nigricans is a manifestation of insulin resistance. It can appear as a velvety light brown to black skin thickening, predominantly seen on flexures, axillae, and the neck. *Necrobiosis lipoidica diabeticorum* usually appears as red-yellow lesions, with atrophic skin that becomes shiny and transparent revealing tiny blood vessels under the surface (Fig. 48-17). This condition is uncommon and occurs more frequently in young women. It may appear before other clinical signs or symptoms of diabetes. Because the thin skin is prone to injury, special care must be taken to protect affected areas from injury and ulceration.

INFECTION

A person with diabetes is more susceptible to infections because of a defect in the mobilization of white blood cells and an impaired phagocytosis by neutrophils and monocytes. Recurring or persistent infections such as *Candida albicans,* as well as boils and furuncles, in the undiagnosed patient often lead the HCP to suspect diabetes. Loss of sensation (neuropathy) may delay the detection of an infection.

Persistent glycosuria may predispose patients to bladder infections, especially patients with a neurogenic bladder. Decreased circulation resulting from angiopathy can prevent or delay the immune response. Antibiotic therapy has prevented infection from being a major cause of death in patients with diabetes. The

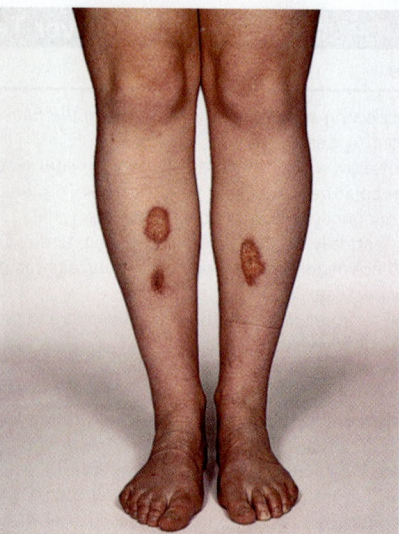

FIG. 48-17 Necrobiosis lipoidica diabeticorum. (From Chew SL, Leslie D: *Clinical endocrinology and diabetes: an illustrated colour text,* Edinburgh, 2006, Churchill Livingstone.)

treatment of infections must be prompt and vigorous. Teach patients to prevent infection by practicing good hand hygiene, avoiding exposure to individuals who have a communicable illness, and getting an annual influenza vaccine and pneumococcal vaccine. (Guidelines for pneumococcal vaccine are presented in Table 27-5.)

PSYCHOLOGIC CONSIDERATIONS

Patients with diabetes have high rates of depression, anxiety, and eating disorders. Depression contributes to diminished diabetes self-care, feelings of helplessness related to chronic illness, and poor outcomes.[12] Assess patients for manifestations of depression and/or diabetes distress.

Disordered eating behaviors (DEB) can occur in people with both type 1 and type 2 diabetes. DEBs include anorexia, bulimia, binge eating, excessive restriction of calories, and intense exercise. The greatest incidence of eating disorders is seen in females. Adolescent girls with diabetes are more than twice as likely to develop DEB than those who do not have diabetes.[28] Patients may intentionally decrease their dose of insulin or omit the dose. This is called "diabulimia" and leads to weight loss, hyperglycemia, and glycosuria because the food ingested cannot be used for energy without adequate insulin. Insulin omission and DEBs can have serious consequences, including retinopathy, neuropathy, lipid abnormalities, DKA, and death.[28]

Open communication is critical to identify these behaviors early. Patients with eating disorders need to be seen by a mental health professional with expertise in eating disorders and an understanding of diabetes management.

Gerontologic Considerations: Diabetes Mellitus

Diabetes is present in more than 25% of persons over 65 years of age, with this age group being the fastest-growing segment of the population developing diabetes.[2] Older people with diabetes have higher rates of premature death, functional disability, and coexisting illnesses such as hypertension and stroke than those without diabetes. The prevalence of diabetes increases with age. A major reason for this is that the process of aging is

Oral agents (OAs), noninsulin injectable agents, and insulin can be administered by licensed practical/vocational nurses (LPN/LVNs) (and in some states and settings by unlicensed assistive personnel [UAP]) to stable patients. In patients experiencing acute complications of diabetes mellitus (DM), actions such as insulin administration and infusion of IV fluids are done or directly supervised by a registered nurse (RN).

Role of Nursing Personnel
Registered Nurse (RN)
- Assess for risk factors for prediabetes and type 1 and type 2 DM.
- Teach the patient and caregiver about self-management of DM, including self-monitoring of blood glucose (SMBG), insulin, noninsulin injectables, OAs, nutrition, physical activity, and recognition and management of hypoglycemia.
- Develop a plan to avoid hypoglycemia or hyperglycemia in a patient with DM who is acutely ill or having surgery.
- Assess for acute complications and implement appropriate actions: hypoglycemia, diabetic ketoacidosis (DKA), and hyperosmolar hyperglycemic syndrome (HHS).
- Assess for chronic complications, including cardiovascular disease, retinopathy, nephropathy, neuropathy, and foot complications.
- Teach patient and caregiver about prevention and management of chronic complications related to diabetes.

Licensed Practical/Vocational Nurse (LPN/LVN)
- Administer OAs and routinely scheduled insulin regimens.
- Monitor the patient for symptoms of hypoglycemia, DKA, and HHS.
- In the ambulatory or home setting, monitor patient self-management of insulin, OAs, nutrition, and physical activity.
- Report concerns with patient self-management in the home setting to the RN.

Unlicensed Assistive Personnel (UAP)
- Check capillary blood glucose (CBG) levels (after being trained and evaluated in this procedure) and report values to the RN.
- Report changes in patient vital signs, urine output, behavior, or level of consciousness to the RN.
- In a community or home care setting, administer OAs and insulin to a stable patient (consider state nurse practice act and agency policy).

Role of Other Team Members
Dietitian
- Assess patient's knowledge of diabetes. Provide teaching about disease process as needed.
- Teach the patient and caregiver about nutrition and diet to self-manage DM and any complications (e.g., hypoglycemia).

associated with a reduction in β-cell function, decreased insulin sensitivity, and altered carbohydrate metabolism. Aging is also associated with a number of conditions that are more likely to be treated with medications that impair insulin action (e.g., corticosteroids, antihypertensives, phenothiazines). Undiagnosed and untreated diabetes is more common in older adults, partly because many of the normal physiologic changes of aging resemble those of diabetes, such as low energy levels, falls, dizziness, confusion, and chronic urinary tract infections.

Several factors are taken into account when determining glycemic goals for an older adult. One is that hypoglycemia unawareness is more common in older adults, making these patients more likely to suffer adverse consequences from blood glucose–lowering therapy. They may have delayed psychomotor function that could interfere with the ability to treat

ETHICAL/LEGAL DILEMMAS
Durable Power of Attorney for Health Care

Situation

G.V., a 64-yr-old woman, is admitted to the intensive care unit with heart failure. She has many complications from a long-term history of type 1 diabetes and hypertension, including a right leg above-the-knee amputation and blindness related to retinopathy. She severed ties with her family 30 yr ago. She has a life partner of 35 yr whom she designated as her proxy in her signed Durable Power of Attorney. She has stated many times that she would rather die than have renal dialysis. She has been sedated and intubated for 3 days. The physician plans to extubate her and resuscitate her so that dialysis can be initiated. Her brother shows up at the hospital and supports the physician's decision. Her partner disagrees with the decision. The physician refuses to recognize her partner as proxy because she is not a blood relative.

Ethical/Legal Points for Consideration

- The Patient Self-Determination Act (1990) requires all health care facilities receiving Medicare and Medicaid funding to make available advance directives allowing individuals to state their preferences or refusals of health care in the event that they are incapable of consenting for themselves.
- Durable Power of Attorney for health care is one type of advance directive in which people, when they are competent, identify someone else to make decisions for them, should they lose their decision-making ability in the future.
- The Living Will, another type of advance directive, permits individuals to state their own preferences and refusals.
- Many HCPs mistakenly think that proxies must be family members or blood relatives. Lesbian, gay, bisexual, and transgender (LGBT) individuals often have difficulty having their partnership recognized as valid, especially if the patient's family disputes their rights.
- Some families are deeply divided on decisions for their loved ones, and sometimes difficulties occur when money and property are also disputed. The passage of time may be an issue where the original documents were executed and then changes occurred (e.g., divorce, death or disability of the proxy, inability to contact the proxy, inability to find a valid original of the advance directive).
- Within your scope of nursing practice, you need to be informed as to decision-making laws and regulations in your own state and make advance directive documents available to patients. In addition, you need to (1) teach patients and their families about advance directives, (2) make sure that HCPs are aware of and follow advance directives, (3) assist the patient and family in communicating with the HCPs when a "No Code" order is requested, and (4) assist a conflicted family in obtaining appropriate counseling whenever necessary.*
- Counsel LGBT patients on the importance of having a health care proxy and a will to legally protect their end-of-life choices.

Discussion Questions

1. How would you handle a situation in which the family and surrogate decision maker disagree?
2. How can you assess the patient and family's understanding of durable power of attorney and assist them in understanding their role in decision making?
3. What should you do when a physician orders dialysis to be initiated when you know that this goes against the patient's advance directive?

*Advance directives are discussed in Table 9-6.

hypoglycemia. Other factors to consider in establishing glycemic goals for the older patient include the patient's own desire for treatment and coexisting medical problems such as cognitive impairment. Compounding the challenge, diabetes increases the rate of decline of cognitive function. Although it is generally agreed that treatment is indicated to prevent complications, intensive diabetes management may be difficult and dangerous to achieve, especially in older adults.

Meal planning and exercise are recommended as therapy for older adult patients with diabetes. This should take into account functional limitations that may interfere with physical activity and the ability to prepare meals. Because of the physiologic changes that occur with aging, the therapeutic outcome for the older adult with diabetes who receives OAs may be altered. Assess renal function and creatinine clearance in patients over 80 years of age taking metformin. Monitor those taking sulfonylurea drugs (e.g., glipizide) for hypoglycemia and renal and liver dysfunction. Insulin therapy may be instituted if OAs are not effective. However, it is important to recognize that older adults are more likely to have limitations in the manual dexterity and visual acuity necessary for accurate insulin administration. Insulin pens may be a safer alternative for older adults.

Patient education issues for the older patient include those related to altered vision, mobility, cognitive status, and functional ability. Plan patient teaching based on the individual's needs, using a slower pace with simple printed or audio materials in patients with cognitive and functional limitations. Include the family or caregivers in the teaching. Consider the patient's financial and social situation and the effect of multiple medications, eating habits, and quality-of-life issues.

CASE STUDY
Diabetic Ketoacidosis

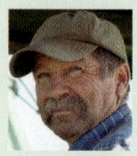

(©katrinaelena/
iStock/
Thinkstock)

Patient Profile
N.B., a 48-yr-old farmer, was admitted to the emergency department after he was found unconscious by his wife in their barn. They live 40 miles from the nearest health care facility.

Subjective Data (Provided by Wife)
- Was diagnosed with type 1 diabetes mellitus 15 years ago
- Was taking 50 U/day of insulin via insulin pump: 5 U of lispro insulin bolus with breakfast, 5 U bolus with lunch, and 10 U bolus with dinner plus 30 U of basal insulin
- Has history of gastroenteritis for 1 wk with vomiting and anorexia
- Stopped taking meal time boluses 2 days ago when he was unable to eat
- Has not changed his infusion set in 5 days

Objective Data
Physical Examination
- Breathing is deep and rapid
- Fruity acetone smell on breath
- Skin flushed and dry

Diagnostic Studies
- Blood glucose level 730 mg/dL (40.5 mmol/L)
- Blood pH 7.26

Discussion Questions
1. Briefly explain the pathophysiology of the development of diabetic ketoacidosis (DKA) in this patient.
2. What clinical manifestations of DKA does this patient exhibit?
3. What factors precipitated this patient's DKA?
4. **Priority Decision:** What is the priority nursing intervention for N.B.?
5. What distinguishes this case history from one of hyperosmolar hyperglycemic syndrome (HHS) or hypoglycemia?
6. **Priority Decision:** What is the priority teaching for this patient and his family?
7. What role should N.B.'s wife have in the management of his diabetes?
8. **Priority Decision:** Based on the assessment data presented, what are the priority nursing diagnoses? Are there any collaborative problems?
9. **Evidence-Based Practice:** N.B.'s wife asks you if she should have given her husband insulin when he got sick. How would you respond?
10. **Teamwork and Collaboration:** How can the interprofessional team be most effective in the care of N.B?
11. **Quality Improvement:** What outcomes would indicate that the interprofessional team was effective in the care of N.B.?

Answers and a corresponding concept map are available at http://evolve.elsevier.com/Lewis/medsurg.

BRIDGE TO NCLEX EXAMINATION

The number of the question corresponds to the same-numbered outcome at the beginning of the chapter.

1. Polydipsia and polyuria related to diabetes mellitus are primarily due to
   a. the release of ketones from cells during fat metabolism.
   b. fluid shifts resulting from the osmotic effect of hyperglycemia.
   c. damage to the kidneys from exposure to high levels of glucose.
   d. changes in RBCs resulting from attachment of excessive glucose to hemoglobin.

2. Which statement would be correct for a patient with type 2 diabetes who was admitted to the hospital with pneumonia?
   a. The patient must receive insulin therapy to prevent ketoacidosis.
   b. The patient has islet cell antibodies that have destroyed the pancreas's ability to produce insulin.
   c. The patient has minimal or absent endogenous insulin secretion and requires daily insulin injections.
   d. The patient may have sufficient endogenous insulin to prevent ketosis but is at risk for hyperosmolar hyperglycemic syndrome.

3. Analyze the following diagnostic findings for your patient with type 2 diabetes. Which result will need further assessment?
   a. A1C 9%
   b. BP 126/80 mm Hg
   c. FBG 130 mg/dL (7.2 mmol/L)
   d. LDL cholesterol 100 mg/dL (2.6 mmol/L)

4. Which statement by the patient with type 2 diabetes is accurate?
   a. "I will limit my alcohol intake to one drink."
   b. "I am not allowed to eat any sweets because of my diabetes."
   c. "I cannot exercise because I take a blood glucose-lowering medication."
   d. "The amount of fat in my diet is not important. Only carbohydrates raise my blood sugar."

5. You are caring for a patient with newly diagnosed type 1 diabetes. What information is *essential* to include in your patient teaching before discharge from the hospital *(select all that apply)*?
   a. Insulin administration
   b. Elimination of sugar from diet
   c. Need to reduce physical activity
   d. Use of a portable blood glucose monitor
   e. Hypoglycemia prevention, symptoms, and treatment

6. What is the *priority* action for the nurse to take if the patient with type 2 diabetes complains of blurred vision and irritability?
   a. Call the physician.
   b. Administer insulin as ordered.
   c. Check the patient's blood glucose level.
   d. Assess for other neurologic symptoms.

7. A patient with diabetes has a serum glucose level of 824 mg/dL (45.7 mmol/L) and is unresponsive. After assessing the patient, the nurse suspects diabetic ketoacidosis rather than hyperosmolar hyperglycemic syndrome based on the finding of
   a. polyuria.
   b. severe dehydration.
   c. rapid, deep respirations.
   d. decreased serum potassium.

8. Which are appropriate therapies for patients with diabetes mellitus *(select all that apply)*?
   a. Use of statins to reduce CVD risk
   b. Use of diuretics to treat nephropathy
   c. Use of ACE inhibitors to treat nephropathy
   d. Use of serotonin agonists to decrease appetite
   e. Use of laser photocoagulation to treat retinopathy

1. b, 2. d, 3. a, 4. a, 5. a, d, e, 6. c, 7. c, 8. a, c, e

For rationales to these answers and even more NCLEX review questions, visit *http://evolve.elsevier.com/Lewis/medsurg.*

EVOLVE WEBSITE

REFERENCES

1. American Diabetes Association: Statistics about diabetes. Retrieved from *www.diabetes.org/diabetes-basics/statistics*.
2. Centers for Disease Control and Prevention: 2014 National Diabetes Statistics Report. Retrieved from *www.cdc.gov/diabetes/data/statistics/2014StatisticsReport.html*.
3. American Diabetes Association: Diagnosis and classification of diabetes mellitus, *Diabetes Care* 39 (Suppl):S13, 2016.
4. Centers for Disease Control and Prevention: Diabetes public health resource: groups especially affected. Retrieved from *www.cdc.gov/diabetes*.
5. Dumore S, Brown J: The role of adipokines in β cell failure of type 2 diabetes, *J Endocrinol* 216:T37, 2013.
6. Bansal N: Prediabetes diagnosis and treatment: a review, *World J Diabetes* 6(2):296, 2015.
7. Ben-Shmuel S, Rostoker R, Scheinman EJ, et al: Metabolic syndrome, type 2 diabetes, and cancer: epidemiology and potential mechanisms, *Handb Exp Pharmacol* 233:355, 2016.
8. Centers for Disease Control and Prevention: Preventing chronic disease: prevalence estimates of gestational diabetes mellitus in the United States, pregnancy risk assessment monitoring system (PRAMS), 2014. Retrieved from *www.cdc.gov/pcd/issues/2014/13_0415.htm*.
*9. HAPO Study Cooperative Research Group: Hyperglycemia and adverse pregnancy outcomes, *N Engl J Med* 358:1991, 2008. (Classic)
*10. Schwartz N, Nachum Z, Green MS: The prevalence of gestational diabetes mellitus recurrence-effect of ethnicity and parity: a meta-analysis, *Am J Obstet Gynecol* 213:310, 2015.
11. Tran L, Zielinski A, Roach AH, et al: The pharmacologic treatment of type 2 diabetes: injectable medications, *Ann Pharmacother* 49:700, 2015.
12. American Association of Diabetes Educators: *The art and science of self-management education desk reference*, ed 3, Chicago, 2014, American Association of Diabetes Educators.
13. BD Diabetes: Syringe and needle sizes. Retrieved from *www.bd.com/us/products/category.asp*.
14. Joslin Diabetes Center: The advantages and disadvantages of an insulin pump, 2015. Retrieved from *www.joslin.org/info/the_advantages_and_disadvantages_of_an_insulin_pump.html*.
15. American Diabetes Association: Standards of medical care in diabetes, *Diabetes Care* 39 (Suppl 1):S1, 2016.
16. Evert AB, Boucher JL, Cypress M: Nutrition therapy recommendations for the management of adults with diabetes, *Diabetes Care* 36(11):3821, 2013.
17. American Diabetes Association: Food and fitness: create your plate. Retrieved from *www.diabetes.org/food-and-fitness/food*.
18. US Department of Health and Human Services: Physical activity guidelines advisory committee report. Retrieved from *www.cdc.gov/nccdphp/sgr/contents.htm*.
19. American Diabetes Association: Fitness, 2015. Retrieved from *www.diabetes.org/food-and-fitness/fitness*.
20. Cengiz E, Tamborlane W: A tale of two compartments: Interstitial versus blood glucose monitoring, *Diabetes Technol Ther* S-11, 2008. (Classic)
21. Ratner R: An update on the Diabetes Prevention Program, *Endocrine Pract* 12(Suppl 1):20, 2006. (Classic)
22. Kruger DF, LaRue S, Estepa P: Recognition of and steps to mitigate anxiety and fear of pain in injectable diabetes treatment, *Diabetes Metab Syndr Obes* 8:49, 2015.
23. Boucher J, Hurrell D: Cardiovascular disease and diabetes, *Diabetes Spectrum* 21:154, 2008. (Classic)
*24. Diabetes Control and Complications Trial Research Group: The effect of intensive treatment of diabetes on the development and progression of long-term complications in insulin-dependent diabetes mellitus, *N Engl J Med* 329:977, 1993. (Classic)
*25. UK Prospective Diabetes Study (UKPDS) Group: Intensive blood-glucose control with sulphonylureas or insulin compared with conventional treatment and risk of complications in patients with type 2 diabetes, *Lancet* 352:837, 1998. (Classic)
26. El-Shazly S, El-Bradey M, Tameesh M: Vascular endothelial growth factor gene polymorphism prevalence in patients with diabetic macular oedema and its correlation with anti-vascular endothelial growth factor treatment outcomes, *Clin Exp Opthalmol* 42:369, 2014.
*27. Javed S, Petropoulos N, Alam U, Malik, R: Treatment of painful diabetic neuropathy, *Ther Adv Chronic Dis* 6:15, 2015.
28. Pinhas-Hamiel O, Levy-Shraga Y: Eating disorders in adolescents with type 1 and type 2 diabetes, *Curr Diab Rep* 13:289, 2013.

*Evidence-based information for clinical practice.

49

Endocrine Problems

Katherine A. Kelly

The best way to cheer yourself up is to try to cheer somebody else up.

Mark Twain

ⓔ http://evolve.elsevier.com/Lewis/medsurg/

LEARNING OUTCOMES

1. Explain the pathophysiology, clinical manifestations, interprofessional care, and nursing management of the patient with an imbalance of hormones produced by the anterior pituitary gland.
2. Describe the pathophysiology, clinical manifestations, interprofessional care, and nursing management of the patient with an imbalance of hormones produced by the posterior pituitary gland.
3. Explain the pathophysiology, clinical manifestations, interprofessional care, and nursing management of the patient with thyroid dysfunction.
4. Describe the pathophysiology, clinical manifestations, interprofessional care, and nursing management of the patient with an imbalance of the hormone produced by the parathyroid glands.
5. Identify the pathophysiology, clinical manifestations, interprofessional care, and nursing management of the patient with an imbalance of hormones produced by the adrenal cortex.
6. Describe the pathophysiology, clinical manifestations, interprofessional care, and nursing management of the patient with an excess of hormones produced by the adrenal medulla.
7. List the side effects of corticosteroid therapy.
8. Describe common nursing assessments, interventions, rationales, and expected outcomes related to patient teaching for management of chronic endocrine problems.

KEY TERMS

acromegaly, p. 1156
Addison's disease, p. 1178
Cushing syndrome, p. 1174
diabetes insipidus (DI), p. 1161
exophthalmos, p. 1164
goiter, p. 1162
Graves' disease, p. 1163

hyperaldosteronism, p. 1180
hyperparathyroidism, p. 1171
hyperthyroidism, p. 1163
hypoparathyroidism, p. 1173
hypopituitarism, p. 1158
hypothyroidism, p. 1168
myxedema, p. 1169

pheochromocytoma, p. 1181
syndrome of inappropriate antidiuretic hormone (SIADH), p. 1159
thyroid cancer, p. 1171
thyroiditis, p. 1163
thyrotoxicosis, p. 1163

The endocrine system is made up of a number of organs and glands that are involved in the synthesis and secretion of hormones that affect every body system. Because these hormones have such a wide range of action, endocrine problems are associated with a variety of clinical manifestations. An endocrine problem often affects many aspects of a person's life.

DISORDERS OF ANTERIOR PITUITARY GLAND

The pituitary gland is considered the master gland of the endocrine system. The anterior pituitary gland secretes GH, prolactin, and the tropic hormones, ACTH, TSH, FSH, and LH. These hormones affect growth, sexual maturation, reproduction, metabolism, stress response, and fluid balance. As a result, pituitary gland disorders manifest in a variety of ways.

Tumors of the pituitary gland account for 5% to 20% of primary intracranial tumors.[1] The most common, the pituitary adenoma, is a slow-growing, benign tumor. It is generally found in adults between 40 and 60 years of age. Hypersecretory pituitary adenomas secrete an excess of a specific hormone causing manifestations related to the action of that hormone. The most common are prolactinomas and growth hormone and ACTH-secreting adenomas.[1]

ACROMEGALY

Acromegaly is a rare condition characterized by an overproduction of growth hormone (GH). Around four out of every 1 million adults in the United States are diagnosed annually.[2] It affects both genders equally. The mean age at the time of diagnosis is 40 to 45 years old.

Etiology and Pathophysiology

Acromegaly most often occurs because of a benign growth hormone–secreting pituitary adenoma. The excess GH results

Reviewed by Crystal Sheaves, RN, MSN, APRN, FNP-BC, Senior Lecturer, West Virginia University School of Nursing, Charleston, West Virginia; and Crystal R. Sherman, DNP, CNP, FNP-BC, APHN-BC, Assistant Professor of Nursing, Shawnee State University, Portsmouth, Ohio.

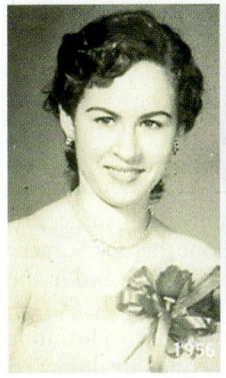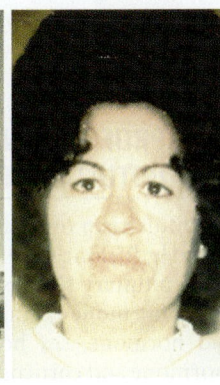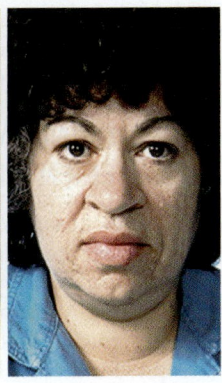

FIG. 49-1 Progressive development of facial changes associated with acromegaly. (Courtesy Linda Haas, Seattle, Wash.)

in an overgrowth of soft tissues and bones in the hands, feet, and face. Because the problem develops after epiphyseal closure, the bones of the arms and legs do not grow longer.

Clinical Manifestations

The changes resulting from excess GH in adults can occur slowly, over a number of years, and may go unnoticed by the person, family, and friends. Thickening and enlargement of the bony and soft tissues on the face, feet, and head occur (Fig. 49-1). Patients may experience proximal muscle weakness and joint pain that can range from mild to crippling. Carpal tunnel syndrome and peripheral neuropathy may be present.

Tongue enlargement results in dental problems and speech difficulties. The voice deepens because of hypertrophy of the vocal cords. Sleep apnea may occur because of upper airway narrowing and obstruction from increased amounts of pharyngeal soft tissues. The skin becomes thick, leathery, and oily with acne outbreaks.

Visual changes may occur due to pressure on the optic nerve from a pituitary adenoma. Headaches are common. Since GH antagonizes the action of insulin, glucose intolerance and manifestations of diabetes mellitus may occur, including *polydipsia* (increased thirst) and *polyuria* (increased urination).[3]

The life expectancy of those with acromegaly is reduced by 5 to 10 years. They are prone to cardiovascular disease, diabetes mellitus, and colorectal cancer.[4] Even if patients are cured or the disease is well controlled, manifestations such as joint pain and deformities often remain.

Diagnostic Studies

In addition to the history and physical examination, a diagnosis requires evaluating plasma insulin-like growth factor (IGF-1) levels and GH response to an oral glucose tolerance test (OGTT). IGF-1 mediates the peripheral actions of GH. As GH levels rise, so do IGF-1 levels. However, GH is released in a pulsatile fashion, requiring several samples to obtain an accurate assessment. Serum IGF-1 levels are more constant, giving a more reliable diagnostic measure of acromegaly. During an OGTT, GH concentration normally falls because glucose inhibits GH secretion. In acromegaly GH levels do not fall, and in some cases GH levels rise.

MRI or high-resolution CT scan with contrast media can detect pituitary adenomas. A complete eye examination, including visual fields, is done because a tumor may cause pressure on the optic chiasm or optic nerves.

❖ NURSING AND INTERPROFESSIONAL MANAGEMENT: ACROMEGALY

The patient's prognosis depends on the age at onset, age when treatment started, and tumor size. The overall goal is to return the patient's GH levels to normal. Treatment consists of surgery, radiation therapy, drug therapy, or a combination of these therapies. With treatment, bone growth can be stopped and tissue hypertrophy reversed. However, sleep apnea, diabetes, and cardiac complications may persist.

Surgery (hypophysectomy) is the treatment of choice. It offers the best chance for a cure and optimal symptom management, especially for smaller pituitary adenomas.[5] Surgery produces an immediate reduction in GH levels followed by a drop in IGF-1 levels within a few weeks. Patients with larger tumors or those with GH levels greater than 45 ng/mL may require adjuvant radiation or drug therapy. Surgery and radiation therapy for pituitary tumors are discussed later in this chapter on p. 1158.

Drug therapy is an option for patients whose surgery did not result in a cure and/or in combination with radiation therapy. The primary drug used is octreotide (Sandostatin), a somatostatin analog. It reduces GH levels to normal in many patients. Octreotide is given by subcutaneous injection three times a week. Long-acting somatostatin analogs, octreotide (Sandostatin LAR), pasireotide (Signifor, Signifor LAR), and lanreotide SR (Somatuline Depot), are available as IM injections given every 4 weeks. GH levels are measured every 2 weeks to guide drug dosing and then every 6 months until the desired response is obtained.

Dopamine agonists (e.g., bromocriptine, cabergoline) may be given alone or with somatostatin analogs if complete remission has not been achieved after surgery. These drugs reduce the secretion of GH from the tumor.

GH antagonists (e.g., pegvisomant [Somavert]) reduce the effect of GH in the body by blocking the hepatic production of IGF-1. Most patients taking this drug achieve normal IGF-1 levels with symptom improvement.[4]

Serial photographs showing improvement in appearance may be helpful to the patient's recovery. Psychosocial effects of acromegaly include body image disturbances, sexual dysfunction, and depression. Fatigue and sleep disturbances may persist after surgery. Patients will need strategies for dealing with these symptoms. Referral to a support group may be helpful.

EXCESSES OF OTHER TROPIC HORMONES

Excess secretion of prolactin or the tropic hormones (e.g., ACTH, TSH) by the anterior pituitary gland will cause other endocrine glands to overproduce certain hormones. An excess of these hormones (discussed later in the chapter) can cause significant disturbances in metabolism and general health.

A prolactin-secreting adenoma is known as a *prolactinoma*. Prolactinomas constitute about 40% of pituitary adenomas.[6] Women with prolactinomas frequently experience galactorrhea, anovulation, infertility, oligomenorrhea or amenorrhea, decreased libido, and hirsutism. In men, impotence, decreased sperm density, and libido may result. Compression of the optic chiasm can cause visual problems and signs of increased intracranial pressure, including headache, nausea, and vomiting.

Because prolactinomas do not typically progress in size, drug therapy is usually the first-line treatment. The dopamine agonists cabergoline and bromocriptine are used to treat prolactinomas. Surgery may be an option, depending on the extent and size of the tumor. Radiation therapy can reduce the risk of tumor recurrence for patients with large tumors.

HYPOFUNCTION OF PITUITARY GLAND

Hypopituitarism is a rare disorder that involves a decrease in one or more of the pituitary hormones. A deficiency of only one pituitary hormone is referred to as *selective hypopituitarism.* Total failure of the pituitary gland results in deficiency of all pituitary hormones—a condition referred to as *panhypopituitarism.* The most common hormone deficiencies associated with hypopituitarism involve GH and gonadotropins (i.e., LH, FSH).

Etiology and Pathophysiology

The usual cause of pituitary hypofunction is a pituitary tumor. Autoimmune disorders, infections, pituitary infarction (Sheehan syndrome), or destruction of the pituitary gland (from trauma, radiation, or surgical procedures) can also cause hypopituitarism. African Americans have a higher incidence of pituitary adenomas than other ethnic groups.[7]

Anterior pituitary hormone deficiencies can lead to end-organ failure. Deficiencies of TSH and ACTH are life threatening. ACTH deficiency can lead to acute adrenal insufficiency and hypovolemic shock from sodium and water depletion. (Acute adrenal insufficiency is discussed later in this chapter on pp. 1178-1179.)

Clinical Manifestations and Diagnostic Studies

The manifestations of hypopituitarism vary with the type and degree of dysfunction. Early manifestations associated with a space-occupying lesion include headaches, visual changes (decreased visual acuity or decreased peripheral vision), loss of smell, nausea and vomiting, and seizures. Manifestations associated with hyposecretion of the target glands vary widely (Table 49-1).

In addition to a history and physical examination, diagnostic studies such as MRI and CT can identify a pituitary tumor. Laboratory tests vary widely but generally involve the direct measurement of pituitary hormones (e.g., TSH) or an indirect determination of the target organ hormones (e.g., triiodothyronine [T_3], thyroxine [T_4]). (See Chapter 47 for more information regarding diagnostic studies.)

❖ NURSING AND INTERPROFESSIONAL MANAGEMENT: HYPOPITUITARISM

The treatment for hypopituitarism often consists of surgery or radiation therapy followed by lifelong hormone therapy. Surgery and radiation therapy for pituitary tumors are discussed in the next section. Appropriate hormone therapy is used (e.g., GH, corticosteroids, thyroid hormone, sex hormones). Hormone therapies for thyroid hormone and corticosteroids are discussed later in this chapter on p. 1169 and pp. 1179-1180.

Somatropin (Omnitrope, Genotropin, Humatrope), which is recombinant human GH, is used for long-term hormone therapy in adults with GH deficiency. These patients respond well to GH replacement and experience increased energy, increased lean body mass, a feeling of well-being, and improved body image. Mild to moderate side effects of GH include fluid retention with swelling in the feet and hands, myalgia, joint pain, and headache. GH is given daily as a subcutaneous injection (preferably in the evening). The dosing is variable because it is adjusted based on symptoms, IGF-1 levels, and the development of adverse effects.

Although gonadal deficiency is not life threatening, hormone therapy will improve sexual function and general well-being. It is contraindicated in those with certain medical conditions, such as phlebitis, pulmonary embolism, breast cancer in women, and prostate cancer in men. Estrogen and progesterone replacement therapy may be indicated for hypogonadal women to treat hot flashes, vaginal dryness, and decreased libido. (Hormone therapy for women is discussed in Chapter 53.) Testosterone is used to treat men with gonadotropin deficiency. The benefits achieved with testosterone therapy include a return of male secondary sex characteristics; improved libido; and increased muscle mass, bone mass, and bone density. (Hormone therapy for men is discussed in Chapter 54.)

PITUITARY SURGERY

A *hypophysectomy* is the surgical removal of the pituitary gland. It is the treatment of choice for tumors in the pituitary area, especially smaller pituitary adenomas. Most surgeries are done by an endoscopic *transsphenoidal* approach (Fig. 49-2). When the entire pituitary gland is removed, there is permanent loss of all pituitary hormones. The patient will require lifelong replacement therapy of thyroid hormone, sex hormones, and glucocorticoids.

Radiation therapy can reduce the size of a tumor before surgery. It is also used when surgery fails to produce a cure or when patients are poor candidates for surgery. Its full effects may not be noted for months to years. Radiation therapy may lead to hypopituitarism, which then requires lifelong hormone replacement therapy. Stereotactic radiosurgery (gamma knife surgery, proton beam, linear accelerator) is an option for small, surgically inaccessible pituitary tumors or in place of conventional radiation.

❖ NURSING MANAGEMENT: PITUITARY SURGERY

Postoperatively, assess the patient for the formation of a hematoma compressing the optic nerve or optic chiasma. Monitor

TABLE 49-1	Manifestations of Hypopituitarism
Hormone Deficiency	**Manifestations**
Growth hormone (GH)	Subtle, nonspecific findings: Truncal obesity, osteoporosis, decreased muscle mass and strength, weakness, fatigue, depression, or flat affect.
Follicle-stimulating hormone (FSH) and luteinizing hormone (LH)	*Women:* Menstrual irregularities, loss of libido, changes in secondary sex characteristics such as decreased breast size. *Men:* Testicular atrophy, diminished spermatogenesis, loss of libido, impotence, decreased facial hair and muscle mass.
Thyroid-stimulating hormone (TSH)	Mild form of primary hypothyroidism: Fatigue, cold intolerance, constipation, lethargy, weight gain.
Adrenocorticotropic hormone (ACTH)	Involves cortisol deficiency: Weakness, fatigue, headache, dry and pale skin, diminished axillary and pubic hair, lowered resistance to infection, fasting hypoglycemia.

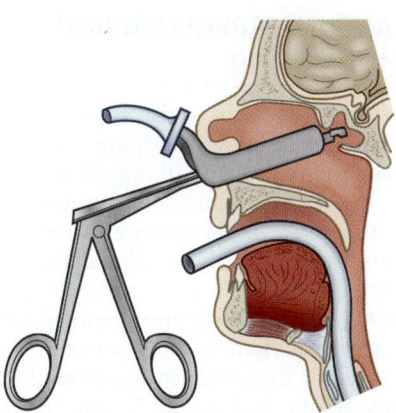

FIG. 49-2 Surgery on the pituitary gland is most commonly performed with the transsphenoidal approach. An incision is made in the inner aspect of the upper lip and gingiva. The sella turcica is entered through the floor of the nose and sphenoid sinuses.

 BECOMING A NURSE LEADER

Dealing With Conflict in the Workplace

Situation

It is your first 7 PM to 7 AM shift on a general medical unit. You quickly observe that Debbie and Carrie do not get along. In fact, they loudly bicker with each other the entire shift, and they refuse to watch each other's patients for breaks. Their relationship seems to negatively affect other team members. In addition, your patients want to know what is going on and why the nurses are so loud in the hallways. You are very uncomfortable and don't want to rock the boat, but you approach the charge nurse and are told, "Oh, everyone knows Debbie and Carrie don't get along. It's always like this."

Points for Consideration

- Some people will go to extreme lengths to avoid conflict. They may have so little confidence in their own communication skills that they fear losing control of their emotions and making the situation worse.
- People often avoid dealing with conflict in the workplace because they fear confronting others:
  - Afraid confronting them will make the situation worse
  - Afraid confrontation will hurt the relationship
  - Concerned that the other party will "attack"
  - Fear retribution in some way
- Help resolve conflict by choosing your words carefully and avoiding labeling people. Establish a win-win approach to help those in conflict view each other as partners.
- Model good conflict management behaviors by remaining neutral and being an active listener. Define the issue in neutral terms by taking personalities out of the problem. Invite the conflicting parties to suggest ways to reach an agreement, while adding objectivity to the situation.

Discussion Questions

1. As a new nurse on this shift, what actions can you take to resolve the conflict?
2. Why is decreased patient satisfaction likely to be an issue on this shift? What can be done about it by you and/or the nurse manager?

peripheral vision, visual acuity, extraocular movements, and pupillary response. Report changes immediately because timely intervention may prevent visual deterioration from becoming permanent.

CSF leaks and epistaxis are other common postoperative complications.[8] The surgeon may place a petroleum jelly–coated ribbon of gauze or a balloon-tipped catheter (like an indwelling urinary catheter) in the sphenoid sinus. It is usually removed after 24 hours. It can be left in for 2 to 3 days if there is concern for bleeding or CSF leak. It is important that the patient does not blow the nose for at least 48 hours after surgery and avoid vigorous coughing, sneezing, and straining at stool (Valsalva maneuver).

Monitor the "moustache" dressing regularly for any drainage. Check any clear drainage with a urine dipstick for glucose and protein. If present, notify the HCP of a possible CSF leak. A sample can be sent to the laboratory. A glucose level greater than 30 mg/dL (1.67 mmol/L) indicates CSF leakage from an open connection with the brain. If this happens, the patient is at increased risk for meningitis.

Complaints of persistent and severe generalized or supraorbital headache may indicate CSF leakage into the sinuses. A CSF leak usually resolves within 72 hours when treated with head elevation and bed rest. If the leak persists, daily spinal taps may be done to reduce pressure to below-normal levels.

Other postoperative measures include elevating the head of the patient's bed at all times to a 30-degree angle. This elevation avoids pressure on the sella turcica and decreases headaches. Monitor the pupillary response, speech patterns, and extremity strength to detect neurologic complications. Gentle mouth care every 4 hours is essential to keep the surgical area clean and free of debris. Advise the patient to avoid tooth brushing for at least 10 days to protect the suture line.

Fluid and electrolyte disturbances can occur from the development of diabetes insipidus (DI).[8] Transient DI may occur because of the loss of antidiuretic hormone (ADH), which is stored in the posterior lobe of the pituitary gland, or cerebral edema related to manipulation of the pituitary during surgery. To assess for DI, closely monitor urine output and measure specific gravity. Report a urine output of >200 mL/hour for more than 3 consecutive hours or a specific gravity level of <1.005. Patients with DI will have an elevated serum sodium and extreme thirst. DI is treated by giving desmopressin acetate (DDAVP). Fluid replacement may be necessary to avoid hypovolemia related to high urine output.

Syndrome of inappropriate ADH secretion (SIADH) can occur after any intracranial surgery. SIADH typically occurs later than DI, usually around the fourth postoperative day. It may occur due to manipulation of the pituitary and other structures causing release of ADH. The fluid retention caused by circulating ADH leads to dilutional hyponatremia. Sodium levels of less than 125 mEq/L will exhibit as headache, vomiting, and decreased level of consciousness. The manifestations and treatment of DI and SIADH are discussed in the next section.

ADH, cortisol, and thyroid hormone replacement are needed after a hypophysectomy. Teach the patient about the need for lifelong therapy. Surgery may result in permanent loss or deficiencies in follicle-stimulating hormone (FSH) and luteinizing hormone (LH). This can lead to decreased fertility. Assist the patient in working through the grieving process associated with these losses.

DISORDERS OF POSTERIOR PITUITARY GLAND

The hormones secreted by the posterior pituitary are antidiuretic hormone (ADH) and oxytocin. ADH, also referred to as *arginine vasopressin* (AVP) or vasopressin, plays a major role in the regulation of water balance and serum osmolarity (see Chapter 47). The two primary problems associated with ADH secretion are a result of either overproduction or underproduction of ADH. The overproduction of ADH results in a condition known as syndrome of inappropriate antidiuretic hormone

(SIADH). Underproduction of ADH results in a condition referred to as *diabetes insipidus* (DI).

SYNDROME OF INAPPROPRIATE ANTIDIURETIC HORMONE

Etiology and Pathophysiology

SIADH is the release of ADH despite normal or low plasma osmolarity (Fig. 49-3). ADH increases the permeability of the renal distal tubule and collecting duct, which leads to the reabsorption of water into the circulation. Extracellular fluid volume expands, plasma osmolality declines, glomerular filtration rate increases, and sodium levels decline (dilutional hyponatremia).[9] Thus the disorder is characterized by fluid retention, serum hypoosmolality, dilutional hyponatremia, hypochloremia, and concentrated urine in the presence of normal or increased intravascular volume.

This syndrome occurs more commonly in older adults. SIADH has various causes (Table 49-2). The most common cause is cancer, especially small cell lung cancer. Although SIADH tends to be self-limiting when caused by head trauma or drugs, it is chronic when associated with tumors or metabolic diseases.

Clinical Manifestations and Diagnostic Studies

The patient with SIADH experiences low urine output and increased body weight. Initially, the patient displays thirst, dyspnea on exertion, and fatigue. Mild hyponatremia causes muscle cramping, irritability, and headache. As the serum sodium level falls (usually below 120 mEq/L [120 mmol/L]), manifestations become more severe and include vomiting, abdominal cramps, and muscle twitching. As plasma osmolality and serum sodium levels continue to decline, cerebral edema may occur, leading to lethargy, confusion, seizures, and coma.

The diagnosis of SIADH is made by simultaneous measurements of urine and serum osmolality. Dilutional hyponatremia is indicated by a serum sodium less than 134 mEq/L, serum osmolality less than 280 mOsm/kg (280 mmol/kg), and urine specific gravity greater than 1.025. A serum osmolality much lower than the urine osmolality indicates the body is inappropriately excreting concentrated urine in the presence of dilute serum.

PATHOPHYSIOLOGY MAP

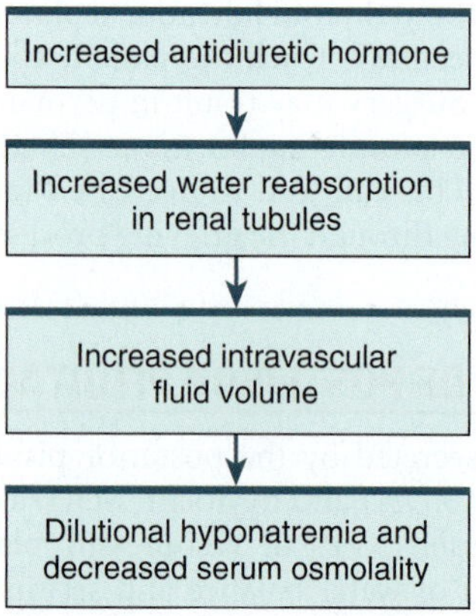

FIG. 49-3 Pathophysiology of syndrome of inappropriate antidiuretic hormone (SIADH). (Modified from Urden LD, Stacy KM, Lough ME: *Critical care nursing: diagnosis and management,* ed 6, St Louis, 2010, Mosby.)

❖ NURSING AND INTERPROFESSIONAL MANAGEMENT: SIADH

In your assessment of persons at risk and those who have confirmed SIADH, be alert for low urine output with a high specific gravity, a sudden weight gain without edema, or a decreased serum sodium level. Monitor intake and output, vital signs, and heart and lung sounds. Obtain daily weights. Observe for signs of hyponatremia, including seizures, headache, vomiting, and decreased neurologic function.

Once SIADH is diagnosed, treatment is directed at the underlying cause. Medications that stimulate ADH release should be avoided or discontinued (Table 49-2). If symptoms are mild and serum sodium is greater than 125 mEq/L (125 mmol/L), the only treatment may be a fluid restriction of 800 to 1000 mL/day. This restriction should result in weight reduction and a gradual rise in serum sodium concentration and osmolality. An improvement in symptoms should accompany normalization of serum sodium and osmolality. Provide the patient with frequent oral care and distractions to decrease discomfort related to thirst from the fluid restriction.

A loop diuretic such as furosemide (Lasix) may be used to promote diuresis. The serum sodium must be at least 125 mEq/L (125 mmol/L) because it may promote further sodium loss. Because furosemide increases potassium, calcium, and magnesium losses, supplements may be needed. Demeclocycline may also be given. This drug blocks the effect of ADH on the renal tubules, resulting in more dilute urine.

Initiate seizure and fall precautions if the patient has an altered sensorium or is having seizures. Position the head of the bed flat or elevated no more than 10 degrees to enhance venous return to the heart and increase left atrial filling pressure, thereby reducing the release of ADH. Frequent turning, positioning, and range-of-motion exercises are important to maintain skin integrity and joint mobility.

TABLE 49-2 Causes of SIADH

Malignant Tumors	Drug Therapy
• Small cell lung cancer	• carbamazepine (Tegretol)
• Pancreatic cancer	• chlorpropamide
• Lymphoid cancers (Hodgkin's lymphoma, non-Hodgkin's lymphoma, lymphocytic leukemia)	• General anesthesia agents
	• Opioids
	• oxytocin
• Thymus cancer	• Thiazide diuretics
• Prostate cancer	• Selective serotonin reuptake inhibitor (SSRI) antidepressants
• Colorectal cancer	• Tricyclic antidepressants
	• Chemotherapy drugs (vincristine, vinblastine, cyclophosphamide)
Central Nervous System Disorders	
• Head injury (skull fracture, subdural hematoma, subarachnoid hemorrhage)	**Miscellaneous Conditions**
• Stroke	• Hypothyroidism
• Brain tumors	• Lung infection (pneumonia, tuberculosis, lung abscess)
• Infection (encephalitis, meningitis)	• Chronic obstructive pulmonary disease
• Cerebral atrophy	• Positive pressure mechanical ventilation
• Guillain-Barré syndrome	• HIV
• Systemic lupus erythematosus	• Adrenal insufficiency

SIADH, Syndrome of inappropriate antidiuretic hormone.

In cases of severe hyponatremia (less than 120 mEq/L), especially in the presence of neurologic manifestations such as seizures, small amounts of IV hypertonic saline solution (3% sodium chloride) may be slowly given. It is important to correct hyponatremia slowly. The level should not increase by more than 8 to 12 mEq/L in the first 24 hours. Quickly increasing levels can cause osmotic demyelination syndrome with permanent damage to nerve cells in the brain.[9] A fluid restriction of 500 mL/day may be indicated for those with severe hyponatremia.

Vasopressor receptor antagonists (drugs that block the activity of ADH) are used to treat euvolemic hyponatremia in hospitalized patients. Two drugs are FDA-approved: conivaptan (Vapriosol) and tolvaptan (Samsca). Conivaptan is given IV; tolvaptan is given orally. Neither should be given to patients with liver disease because they worsen liver function.

Assist the patient with chronic SIADH in self-managing the treatment regimen. In chronic SIADH, a fluid restriction of 800 to 1000 mL/day is recommended. The use of ice chips or sugarless chewing gum helps to decrease thirst. Have the patient weigh daily to monitor changes in fluid balance. Have the patient supplement the diet with sodium and potassium, especially if loop diuretics are prescribed. Teach the patient the symptoms of fluid and electrolyte imbalances, especially those involving sodium and potassium (see Chapter 16).

DIABETES INSIPIDUS

Etiology and Pathophysiology

Diabetes insipidus (DI) is caused by a deficiency of production or secretion of ADH or a decreased renal response to ADH. The decrease in ADH results in fluid and electrolyte imbalances caused by increased urine output and increased plasma osmolality (Fig. 49-4). Depending on the cause, DI may be transient or a chronic, lifelong condition.

There are several types of DI (Table 49-3). Central DI is the most common form.

Clinical Manifestations

DI is characterized by polydipsia and polyuria. The primary characteristic of DI is the excretion of large quantities of urine (2 to 20 L/day) with a very low specific gravity (less than 1.005) and urine osmolality of less than 100 mOsm/kg (100 mmol/kg). Serum osmolality is elevated (usually greater than 295 mOsm/kg [295 mmol/kg]) because of hypernatremia (serum sodium greater than 145 mg/dL) caused by pure water loss in the kidneys. Most patients compensate for fluid loss by drinking large amounts of water so that serum osmolality remains normal or is moderately elevated. The patient may be tired from nocturia and experience generalized weakness. Uncorrected hypernatremia can cause brain shrinkage and intracranial bleeding.[9]

The onset of central DI is usually acute and accompanied by excessive fluid loss. After intracranial surgery, central DI has a triphasic pattern: the acute phase with an abrupt onset of polyuria, an interphase in which urine volume normalizes, and a third phase in which central DI may become permanent. The third phase occurs within 10 to 14 days postoperatively. Central DI that results from head trauma is often self-limiting and improves with treatment of the underlying problem. Although the clinical manifestations of nephrogenic DI are similar to those of central DI, the onset and amount of fluid loss are less dramatic.

Severe dehydration can result if oral fluid intake cannot keep up with urinary losses. The patient will have hypotension, tachycardia, and hypovolemic shock. Increasing serum osmolality and hypernatremia can cause central nervous system (CNS) manifestations, ranging from irritability and mental dullness to coma.

Diagnostic Studies

Patients with DI excrete dilute urine at a rate greater than 200 mL/hr with a specific gravity of less than 1.005. Identification of central DI requires a water deprivation test. Before the test, body weight, and urine osmolality, volume, and specific gravity are measured. The patient is deprived of water for 8 to 12 hours and then given desmopressin acetate (DDAVP) subcutaneously or nasally. Patients with central DI exhibit a dramatic increase in urine osmolality (from 100 to 600 mOsm/kg) and a significant decrease in urine volume. The patient with nephrogenic DI will not be able to increase urine osmolality to greater than 300 mOsm/kg.

Another test to differentiate central DI from nephrogenic DI is to measure the level of ADH after an analog of ADH (e.g., desmopressin) is given. If the cause is central DI, the kidneys will respond to the hormone by concentrating urine. If the kidneys do not respond in this way, then the cause is nephrogenic.

PATHOPHYSIOLOGY MAP

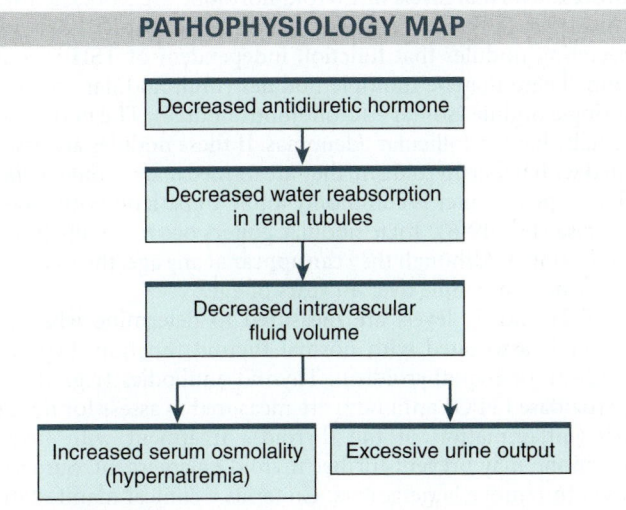

FIG. 49-4 Pathophysiology of diabetes insipidus (DI).

TABLE 49-3	Types of Diabetes Insipidus
Type	**Etiology**
Central (neurogenic) DI	Results from an interference with ADH synthesis, transport, or release *Examples:* Brain tumor, head injury, brain surgery, CNS infections
Nephrogenic DI	Results from inadequate renal response to ADH despite presence of adequate ADH *Examples:* Drug therapy (especially lithium), renal damage, hereditary renal disease
Primary DI	Results from excessive water intake *Examples:* Structural lesion in thirst center, psychologic disorder

❖ NURSING AND INTERPROFESSIONAL MANAGEMENT: DIABETES INSIPIDUS

Nursing management of the patient with DI includes early detection, maintaining adequate hydration, and patient teaching for long-term management. A therapeutic goal is maintaining fluid and electrolyte balance.

For central DI, fluid and hormone therapy is the cornerstone of treatment. Fluids are replaced orally or IV, depending on the patient's condition and ability to drink copious amounts of fluids. In acute DI, IV hypotonic saline or dextrose 5% in water (D_5W) is given and titrated to replace urine output. If IV glucose solutions are used, monitor serum glucose levels because hyperglycemia and glycosuria can lead to osmotic diuresis, which increases the fluid volume deficit. Monitoring BP, heart rate, urine output, level of consciousness, and specific gravity is essential and may be required hourly in the acutely ill patient. Assess for signs of acute dehydration. Maintain an accurate record of intake and output and daily weights to determine fluid volume status. Adjustments in fluid replacement should be made accordingly.

DDAVP, an analog of ADH, is the hormone replacement of choice for central DI. Another ADH replacement drug is aqueous vasopressin. DDAVP can be given orally, IV, subcutaneously, or as a nasal spray. Assess the response to DDAVP by monitoring pulse, BP, level of consciousness, intake and output, and specific gravity. Chlorpropamide and carbamazepine (Tegretol) are used to help decrease thirst associated with central DI.

Because the kidney is unable to respond to ADH in nephrogenic DI, hormone therapy has little effect. Instead, the treatment includes dietary measures (low-sodium diet) and thiazide diuretics (e.g., hydrochlorothiazide, chlorothiazide [Diuril]), which may reduce flow to the ADH-sensitive distal nephrons. Limiting sodium intake to no more than 3 g/day often helps decrease urine output. If a low-sodium diet and thiazide drugs are not effective, indomethacin (Indocin) may be prescribed. Indomethacin, a nonsteroidal antiinflammatory drug (NSAID), helps increase renal responsiveness to ADH.

DISORDERS OF THYROID GLAND

Alterations in thyroid function are among the most common endocrine disorders. The thyroid hormones, thyroxine (T_4) and triiodothyronine (T_3), regulate energy metabolism and growth and development. Disorders of the thyroid gland include goiter, benign and malignant nodules, inflammatory conditions leading to hyperthyroidism, and hypothyroidism (Fig. 49-5).

GOITER

A **goiter** is an enlarged thyroid gland. In a person with a goiter, the thyroid cells are stimulated to grow. This may result in an overactive thyroid (hyperthyroidism) or an underactive thyroid (hypothyroidism). The most common cause of goiter worldwide is a lack of iodine in the diet.[10] In the United States, where most people use iodized salt, goiter is more often due to the overproduction or underproduction of thyroid hormones or to nodules that develop in the gland itself. *Goitrogens* (foods or drugs that contain thyroid-inhibiting substances) can cause a goiter (Table 49-4).

A nontoxic goiter is a diffuse enlargement of the thyroid gland that does not result from a malignancy or inflammatory

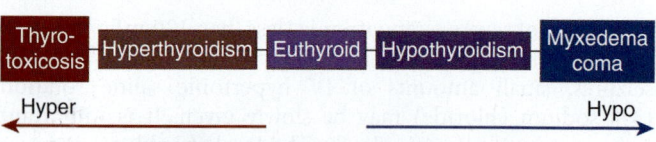

FIG. 49-5 Continuum of thyroid dysfunction.

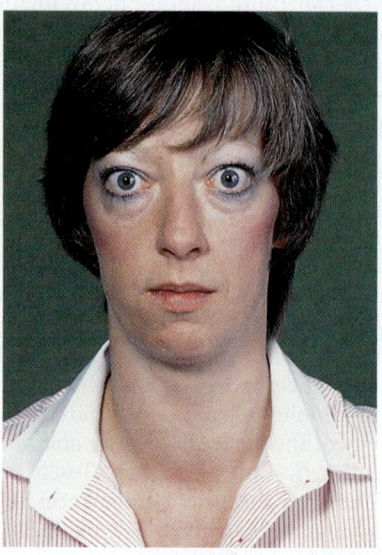

FIG. 49-6 Exophthalmos and goiter of Graves' disease. (From Forbes CD, Jackson WF: *Colour atlas and text of clinical medicine,* ed 3, London, 2003, Mosby.)

TABLE 49-4   Goitrogens

Thyroid Inhibitors	Select Foods
• propylthiouracil (PTU)	• Broccoli
• methimazole (Tapazole)	• Brussels sprouts
• Iodine in large doses	• Cabbage
	• Cauliflower
Other Drugs	• Kale
• Sulfonamides	• Mustard
• Salicylates	• Peanuts
• *p*-Aminosalicylic acid	• Strawberries
• lithium	• Turnips
• amiodarone (Cordarone)	

process. Normal levels of thyroid hormone are associated with this type of goiter. *Nodular goiters* are thyroid hormone–secreting nodules that function independent of TSH stimulation. There may be multiple nodules (multinodular goiter) or a single nodule (solitary autonomous nodule). The nodules are usually benign follicular adenomas. If these nodules are associated with hyperthyroidism, they are termed *toxic nodular goiters.* This type of goiter is commonly found in patients with Graves' disease (Fig. 49-6). Toxic nodular goiters occur equally in men and women. Although they can appear at any age, the frequency is greatest in people over 40 years of age.

TSH and T_4 levels are measured to determine whether a goiter is associated with normal thyroid function, hyperthyroidism, or hypothyroidism. Thyroid antibodies (e.g., thyroid peroxidase [TPO] antibody) are measured to assess for *thyroiditis* (inflammation of the thyroid). Treatment with thyroid hormone may prevent further thyroid enlargement. Surgery is used to remove large goiters. Goiter as a clinical manifestation of thyroid disorders is further discussed in the following sections.

THYROIDITIS

Thyroiditis, an inflammation of the thyroid gland, encompasses several clinical disorders.[11] It is a frequent cause of goiter. *Subacute granulomatous thyroiditis* is thought to be caused by a viral infection. *Acute thyroiditis* is due to bacterial or fungal infection. Subacute and acute forms of thyroiditis have an abrupt onset. The patient complains of pain localized in the thyroid or radiating to the throat, ears, or jaw. Other systemic manifestations include fever, chills, sweats, and fatigue.

Hashimoto's thyroiditis (chronic autoimmune thyroiditis) is caused by the destruction of thyroid tissue by antibodies.[11] It is the most common cause of hypothyroid goiters in the United States. Factors placing a person at higher risk include female gender, a positive family history, older age, and white ethnicity. The goiter, which is the hallmark of Hashimoto's thyroiditis, may develop gradually or rapidly. If it enlarges rapidly, it may compress structures in the neck (e.g., trachea, laryngeal nerves), changing the voice and affecting breathing. As thyroid tissue is destroyed by antibodies, there may be a transient phase of hyperthyroidism due to leaking thyroid hormone from the damaged tissues.

Silent, painless thyroiditis, which may be early Hashimoto's thyroiditis, can occur in postpartum women. This condition, which is usually seen in the first 6 months after delivery, may be due to an autoimmune reaction to fetal cells in the mother's thyroid gland.

T_4 and T_3 levels are initially elevated in subacute, acute, and silent thyroiditis but become depressed with time. Suppression of radioactive iodine uptake (RAIU) is seen in subacute and silent thyroiditis. In Hashimoto's thyroiditis, thyroid hormone levels are usually low and the TSH level is high. Antithyroid antibodies are present in Hashimoto's thyroiditis.

Recovery from acute or subacute thyroiditis may be complete in weeks or months without any treatment. If the thyroiditis is bacterial in origin, treatment may include specific antibiotics or surgical drainage. In the subacute and acute forms, NSAIDs (aspirin or naproxen [Aleve]) are used to relieve symptoms. With more severe pain, corticosteroids (e.g., prednisone up to 40 mg/day) can relieve discomfort. Propranolol (Inderal) or atenolol (Tenormin) may be used to treat the cardiovascular symptoms related to a hyperthyroid condition. Thyroid hormone therapy is indicated if the patient is hypothyroid.

Nursing care of the patient with thyroiditis includes patient teaching regarding the disease process and course of treatment. Teach the patient not to discontinue medications abruptly. Instruct the patient to remain under close health care supervision so that progress can be monitored. Tell the patient to report to the HCP any change in symptoms, such as difficulty breathing or swallowing, swelling to face and extremities, or rapid weight gain or loss. Teach those receiving thyroid hormone about the expected side effects of these drugs and measures to manage them (see p. 1170).

The patient with Hashimoto's thyroiditis is at risk for other autoimmune diseases such as Addison's disease, pernicious anemia, or Graves' disease. Teach the patient the signs and symptoms of these disorders, particularly Addison's disease.

HYPERTHYROIDISM

Hyperthyroidism is hyperactivity of the thyroid gland with sustained increase in synthesis and release of thyroid hormones.

Hyperthyroidism occurs in women more than men, with the highest frequency in persons 20 to 40 years old. The most common form of hyperthyroidism is Graves' disease. Other causes include toxic nodular goiter, thyroiditis, excess iodine intake, pituitary tumors, and thyroid cancer. Since hyperthyroidism may be precipitated by iodinated contrast media used in CT scans and other radiological studies, those who are at-risk for hyperthyroidism should be monitored closely after iodinated contrast media exposure.[12]

GENDER DIFFERENCES

Endocrine Problems

Men
- Ectopic ACTH production is more common in men.

Women
- Hyperthyroidism and hypothyroidism are more common in women than men.
- Graves' disease affects five times more women than men.
- Thyroid nodules and thyroid cancer affect up to four times as many women as men.
- Hyperparathyroidism affects twice as many women as men.
- Cushing disease and primary hyperaldosteronism are more common in women than men.

The term thyrotoxicosis refers to the physiologic effects or clinical syndrome of hypermetabolism resulting from excess circulating levels of T_4, T_3, or both.[13] Hyperthyroidism and thyrotoxicosis usually occur together. Subclinical hyperthyroidism occurs when the patient has a serum TSH level below 0.4 mU/L but normal T_4 and T_3 levels. Overt hyperthyroidism is defined by low or undetectable TSH and elevated T_4 and T_3 levels. The patient may or may not have symptoms of hyperthyroidism.

Etiology and Pathophysiology

Graves' Disease. Graves' disease is an autoimmune disease of unknown etiology characterized by diffuse thyroid enlargement and excess thyroid hormone secretion. Graves' disease accounts for 75% of the cases of hyperthyroidism. Women are five times more likely than men to develop Graves' disease. Precipitating factors such as insufficient iodine supply, cigarette smoking, infection, and stressful life events may interact with genetic factors to cause Graves' disease.

In Graves' disease the patient develops antibodies to the TSH receptor. These antibodies attach to the receptors and stimulate the thyroid gland to release T_3, T_4, or both. The excess release of thyroid hormones leads to the clinical manifestations associated with thyrotoxicosis. The disease is characterized by remissions and exacerbations, with or without treatment. It may progress to destruction of the thyroid tissue, ultimately causing hypothyroidism. Graves' disease is associated with the presence of other autoimmune disorders, including rheumatoid arthritis, pernicious anemia, systemic lupus erythematosus (SLE), Addison's disease, celiac disease, and vitiligo.

Clinical Manifestations

Clinical manifestations of hyperthyroidism are related to the effect of excess circulating thyroid hormone. It directly increases metabolism and tissue sensitivity to stimulation by the sympathetic nervous system.

Palpation of the thyroid gland may reveal a goiter. When the thyroid gland is excessively large, a goiter may be noted on inspection. Auscultating the thyroid gland may reveal bruits, a reflection of increased blood supply. Another common finding is *ophthalmopathy,* a term used to describe abnormal eye appearance or function. A classic finding in Graves' disease is **exophthalmos,** a protrusion of the eyeballs from the orbits that is usually bilateral (Fig. 49-6). Exophthalmos results from increased fat deposits and fluid (edema) in the orbital tissues and ocular muscles. The increased pressure forces the eyeballs outward. The upper lids are usually retracted and elevated, with the sclera visible above the iris. When the eyelids do not close completely, the exposed corneal surfaces become dry and irritated. Serious consequences, such as corneal ulcers and eventual loss of vision, can occur. The changes in the ocular muscles result in muscle weakness, causing diplopia.

Other manifestations of hyperthyroidism are summarized in Table 49-5. Abnormal laboratory findings are listed in Table 49-6. A patient in the early stages of hyperthyroidism may only exhibit weight loss and increased nervousness. *Acropachy* (clubbing of the digits) may occur with advanced disease (Fig. 49-7). Manifestations (e.g., palpitations, tremors, weight loss) in older adults with hyperthyroidism do not differ significantly from those of younger adults (Table 49-7). In older patients who are confused and agitated, dementia may be suspected and delay the diagnosis.

Complications

Acute thyrotoxicosis (also called *thyrotoxic crisis* or *thyroid storm*) is an acute, severe, and rare condition that occurs when excessive amounts of thyroid hormones are released into the

TABLE 49-6 Laboratory Results for Hyperthyroid and Hypothyroid Patients

| | | HYPOTHYROID | |
Test	Hyperthyroid	Primary	Secondary
Thyroid-stimulating hormone (TSH)	↓	↑	↓
T₄ (thyroxine)	↑	↓	↓
Total cholesterol	N	↑	↑
Low-density lipoproteins (LDLs)	↓	↑	↑
Triglycerides	N	↑	↑
Creatine kinase (CK)	N	↑	↑
Basal metabolic rate (BMR)	↑	↓	↓
Thyroid peroxidase (TPO) antibody	N	+ (in autoimmune hypothyroidism)	N

N, Normal; *+,* positive.

TABLE 49-5 Manifestations of Thyroid Dysfunction

Hyperfunction	Hypofunction
Cardiovascular System	
• Systolic hypertension	• Increased capillary fragility
• Increased rate and force of cardiac contractions	• Decreased rate and force of contractions
• Bounding, rapid pulse	• Varied changes in BP
• Increased cardiac output	• Cardiac hypertrophy
• Cardiac hypertrophy	• Distant heart sounds
• Systolic murmurs	• Anemia
• Dysrhythmias	• Heart failure
• Palpitations	• Angina
• Angina	
Respiratory System	
• Dyspnea on mild exertion	• Dyspnea
• Increased respiratory rate	• Decreased breathing capacity
Gastrointestinal System	
• Increased appetite, thirst	• Decreased appetite
• Weight loss	• Weight gain
• Increased peristalsis	• Nausea and vomiting
• Diarrhea, frequent defecation	• Constipation
• Increased bowel sounds	• Distended abdomen
• Splenomegaly	• Enlarged, scaly tongue
• Hepatomegaly	• Celiac disease
Integumentary System	
• Warm, smooth, moist skin	• Dry, thick, inelastic, cold skin
• Thin, brittle nails detached from nail bed (onycholysis)	• Thick, brittle nails
• Hair loss (may be patchy)	• Dry, sparse, coarse hair
• Clubbing of fingers (thyroid acropachy) (Fig. 49-7)	• Poor turgor of mucosa
• Palmar erythema	• Generalized interstitial edema
• Fine, silky hair	• Puffy face
• Premature graying (in men)	• Decreased sweating
• Diaphoresis	• Pallor
• Vitiligo	
• Pretibial myxedema (infiltrative dermopathy)	

Hyperfunction	Hypofunction
Musculoskeletal System	
• Fatigue	• Fatigue
• Weakness	• Weakness
• Proximal muscle wasting	• Muscular aches and pains
• Dependent edema	• Slow movements
• Osteoporosis	• Arthralgia
Nervous System	
• Difficulty focusing eyes	• Apathy
• Nervousness	• Lethargy
• Fine tremor of fingers and tongue	• Fatigue
• Insomnia	• Forgetfulness
• Lability of mood, delirium	• Slowed mental processes
• Restlessness	• Hoarseness
• Personality changes of irritability, agitation	• Slow, slurred speech
• Exhaustion	• Prolonged relaxation of deep tendon reflexes
• Hyperactive deep-tendon reflexes	• Stupor, coma
• Depression, fatigue	• Paresthesias
• Lack of ability to concentrate	• Anxiety, depression
• Stupor, coma	
Reproductive System	
• Menstrual irregularities	• Prolonged menstrual periods or amenorrhea
• Amenorrhea	
• Decreased libido	• Decreased libido
• Impotence in men	• Infertility
• Gynecomastia in men	
• Decreased fertility	
Other	
• Intolerance to heat	• Intolerance to cold
• Elevated basal temperature	• Increased susceptibility to infection
• Lid lag, stare	• Increased sensitivity to opioids, barbiturates, anesthesia
• Eyelid retraction	
• Exophthalmos	• Decreased hearing
• Goiter (Fig. 49-6)	• Goiter
• Rapid speech	• Sleepiness

circulation. Although considered a life-threatening emergency, death is rare when treatment is initiated early. Acute thyroiditis is thought to result from stressors (e.g., infection, trauma, surgery) in a patient with preexisting hyperthyroidism. Patients having a thyroidectomy are at risk because manipulation of the hyperactive thyroid gland results in an increase in hormones released.[14]

In acute thyrotoxicosis, all the symptoms of hyperthyroidism are prominent and severe. Manifestations include severe tachycardia, heart failure, shock, hyperthermia (up to 106°F [41.1°C]), agitation, delirium, seizures, abdominal pain, vomiting, diarrhea, and coma.

Diagnostic Studies

The two primary laboratory findings used to confirm the diagnosis of hyperthyroidism are low or undetectable TSH levels (<0.4 mU/L) and elevated free thyroxine (free T_4) levels. Total T_3 and T_4 levels may also be assessed, but they are not as definitive. Total T_3 and T_4 determine both free and bound (to protein) hormone levels. The free hormone is the only biologically active form of these hormones.

The RAIU test is used to differentiate Graves' disease from other forms of thyroiditis. The patient with Graves' disease shows a diffuse, homogeneous uptake of 35% to 95%, whereas the patient with thyroiditis shows an uptake of less than 2%.

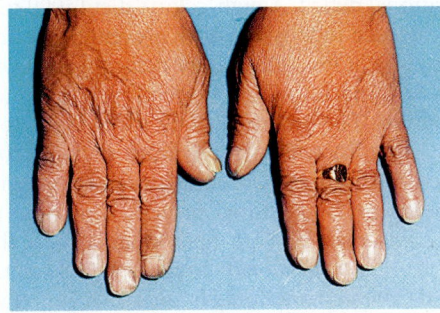

FIG. 49-7 Thyroid acropachy. Digital clubbing and swelling of fingers. (From Chew SL, Leslie D: *Clinical endocrinology and diabetes: an illustrated colour text*, Edinburgh, 2006, Churchill Livingstone.)

The person with a nodular goiter has an uptake in the high normal range.

Interprofessional Care

The goal of management of hyperthyroidism is to block the adverse effects of excessive thyroid hormone, suppress oversecretion of thyroid hormone, and prevent complications. There are several treatment options, including antithyroid medications, radioactive iodine therapy, and surgical intervention (Table 49-8). Supportive therapy is directed at managing respiratory distress, reducing fever, replacing fluid, and eliminating or managing the initiating stressor(s).

The choice of treatment is influenced by the patient's age and preferences, coexistence of other diseases, and pregnancy status. **Drug Therapy.** Drugs used in the treatment of hyperthyroidism include antithyroid drugs, iodine, and β-adrenergic blockers. These drugs are useful in treating thyrotoxic states, but they are not considered curative. Radiation therapy or surgery may ultimately be required.

Antithyroid Drugs. The first-line antithyroid drugs are propylthiouracil and methimazole (Tapazole).[13] These drugs inhibit the synthesis of thyroid hormones. Indications for use include Graves' disease in the young patient, hyperthyroidism during pregnancy, and the need to achieve a euthyroid state before surgery or radiation therapy. Propylthiouracil is generally used for patients who are in the first trimester of pregnancy, had an adverse reaction to methimazole, or require a rapid reduction in symptoms. Propylthiouracil is considered first-line therapy in thyrotoxicosis, since it also blocks the peripheral conversion of T_4 to T_3. An advantage of propylthiouracil is that it achieves the therapeutic goal of being euthyroid more quickly. However, it must be taken three times per day. Methimazole is given in a single daily dose.

Improvement usually begins 1 to 2 weeks after the start of drug therapy. Good results are usually seen within 4 to 8 weeks. Therapy is usually continued for 6 to 15 months to allow for spontaneous remission, which occurs in 20% to 40% of patients. Emphasize to the patient the importance of adhering to the

TABLE 49-7 Comparison of Hyperthyroidism in Younger and Older Adults

	Younger Adult	**Older Adult**
Common causes	Graves' disease in >90% of cases	Graves' disease or toxic nodular goiter
Common symptoms	Nervousness, irritability, weight loss, heat intolerance, warm moist skin	Anorexia, weight loss, apathy, lassitude, depression, confusion
Goiter	Present in >90% of cases	Present in about 50% of cases
Ophthalmopathy	Exophthalmos (Fig. 49-6) present in 20%-40% of cases	Exophthalmos less common
Cardiac features	Tachycardia and palpitations common, but without heart failure	Angina, dysrhythmia (especially atrial fibrillation with rapid ventricular response), heart failure may occur

TABLE 49-8 Interprofessional Care

Hyperthyroidism

Diagnostic Assessment
- History and physical examination
- Ophthalmologic examination
- ECG
- Laboratory tests
  - TSH levels, serum free T_4
  - Thyroid antibodies (e.g., thyroid peroxidase [TPO] antibody)
  - Total serum T_3 and T_4
- Radioactive iodine uptake (RAIU)

Management

Drug Therapy
- Antithyroid drugs
  - methimazole (Tapazole)
  - propylthiouracil
- Iodine (SSKI)
- β-Adrenergic receptor blockers
  - propranolol (Inderal)
  - atenolol (Tenormin) or metoprolol (Toprol)

Radiation Therapy
- Radioactive iodine

Surgical Therapy
- Subtotal thyroidectomy

Nutritional Therapy
- High-calorie, high-protein diet
- Frequent meals

drug regimen. Abruptly discontinuing drug therapy can result in a return of hyperthyroidism.

Iodine. Iodine is available as saturated solution of potassium iodine (SSKI) and Lugol's solution. Iodine is used with other antithyroid drugs to prepare the patient for thyroidectomy or for treatment of thyrotoxicosis. Rapidly giving large doses of iodine inhibits synthesis of T_3 and T_4 and blocks the release of these hormones into circulation. It also decreases the vascularity of the thyroid gland, making surgery safer and easier. The maximal effect is usually seen within 1 to 2 weeks. Because of a reduction in the therapeutic effect, long-term iodine therapy is not effective in controlling hyperthyroidism.

Iodine is mixed with water or juice, sipped through a straw, and given after meals. Assess the patient for signs of iodine toxicity, such as swelling of the buccal mucosa and other mucous membranes, excessive salivation, nausea and vomiting, and skin reactions. If toxicity occurs, discontinue iodine administration and notify the HCP.

β-Adrenergic Blockers. β-Adrenergic blockers are used for symptomatic relief of thyrotoxicosis. These drugs block the effects of sympathetic nervous stimulation, thereby decreasing tachycardia, nervousness, irritability, and tremors. Propranolol is usually given with antithyroid agents. Atenolol is the preferred β-adrenergic blocker for use in the hyperthyroid patient with asthma or heart disease.

Radioactive Iodine Therapy. Radioactive iodine (RAI) therapy is the treatment of choice for most nonpregnant adults. RAI damages or destroys thyroid tissue, thus limiting thyroid hormone secretion. RAI has a delayed response. The maximum effect may not be seen for up to 3 months. For this reason, the patient is usually treated with antithyroid drugs and propranolol before and for 3 months after starting RAI until the effects of radiation become apparent. Although RAI is usually effective, 80% of patients have posttreatment hypothyroidism, resulting in the need for lifelong thyroid hormone therapy. Teach the patient the symptoms of hypothyroidism and to seek medical help if these symptoms occur.

RAI therapy is usually given on an outpatient basis. A pregnancy test is done before starting therapy for all women who experience menstrual cycles. Tell the patient that radiation thyroiditis and parotiditis are possible and may cause dryness and irritation of the mouth and throat. Relief may be obtained with frequent sips of water, ice chips, or a salt and soda gargle three or four times per day. This gargle is made by dissolving 1 tsp of salt and 1 tsp of baking soda in 2 cups of warm water. The discomfort should subside in 3 to 4 days. A mixture of antacid (Mylanta or Maalox), diphenhydramine, and viscous lidocaine can be used to swish and spit, increasing patient comfort when eating.

To limit radiation exposure to others, teach the patient receiving RAI home precautions, including (1) using private toilet facilities if possible and flushing two or three times after each use; (2) separately laundering towels, bed linens, and clothes daily at home; (3) not preparing food for others that requires prolonged handling with bare hands; and (4) avoiding being close to pregnant women and children for 7 days after therapy.

Surgical Therapy. Thyroidectomy is indicated for those who have (1) a large goiter causing tracheal compression, (2) a lack of response to antithyroid therapy, or (3) thyroid cancer (Fig. 49-8). Additionally, surgery may be done when a person is not a candidate for RAI. One advantage that thyroidectomy has over RAI is a more rapid reduction in T_3 and T_4 levels. A *subtotal*

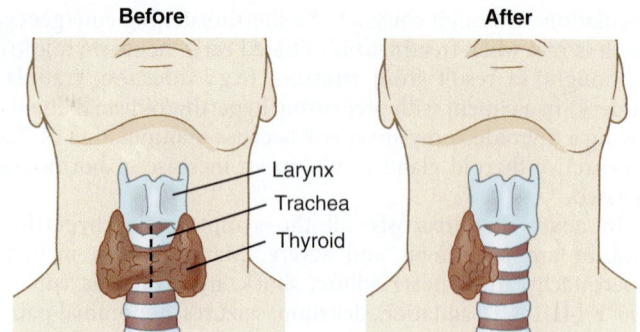

FIG. 49-8 Subtotal thyroidectomy. Part of the thyroid gland is removed.

thyroidectomy is the preferred surgical procedure, which involves removing a significant portion (90%) of the thyroid gland.

Some patients may undergo minimally invasive endoscopic or robotic thyroidectomy. Endoscopic thyroidectomy is an appropriate procedure for patients with small nodules (less than 3 cm) and no evidence of cancer. Robotic surgery is best for those who are not overweight and have small nodules on only one side of the gland. Advantages of endoscopic and robotic procedures over open thyroidectomy include less scarring, less pain, and a faster return to normal activity.

Nutritional Therapy. With the increased metabolic rate in hyperthyroid patients, there is a high potential for the patient to have a nutritional deficit. A high-calorie diet (4000 to 5000 cal/day) may be needed to satisfy hunger, prevent tissue breakdown, and decrease weight loss. This can be accomplished with six full meals a day and snacks high in protein, carbohydrates, minerals, and vitamins. The protein content should be 1 to 2 g/kg of ideal body weight. Increase carbohydrate intake to compensate for increased metabolism. Carbohydrates provide energy and decrease the use of body-stored protein. Teach the patient to avoid highly seasoned and high-fiber foods because these foods can further stimulate the already hyperactive GI tract. Have the patient avoid caffeine-containing liquids such as coffee, tea, and cola to decrease the restlessness and sleep disturbances associated with these fluids. Refer the patient to a dietitian for help in meeting individual nutritional needs.

❖ NURSING MANAGEMENT: HYPERTHYROIDISM

◆ Nursing Assessment

Subjective and objective data you should obtain from a person with hyperthyroidism are presented in Table 49-9.

◆ Nursing Diagnoses

Nursing diagnoses for the patient with hyperthyroidism include, but are not limited to, the following:
- Activity intolerance *related to* fatigue and heat intolerance
- Imbalanced nutrition: less than body requirements *related to* hypermetabolism and inadequate food intake

Additional information on nursing diagnoses is presented in eNursing Care Plan 49-1 for the patient with hyperthyroidism (available on the website for this chapter).

◆ Planning

The overall goals are that the patient with hyperthyroidism will (1) experience relief of symptoms, (2) have no serious complications related to the disease or treatment, (3) maintain nutritional balance, and (4) cooperate with the therapeutic plan.

◆ **Nursing Implementation**

◆ **Acute Care.** Patients with hyperthyroidism are usually treated in an outpatient setting. However, those who develop acute thyrotoxicosis or undergo thyroidectomy require hospitalization and acute care.

TABLE 49-9 Nursing Assessment

Hyperthyroidism

Subjective Data

Important Health Information

Past health history: Preexisting goiter. Recent infection or trauma, immigration from iodine-deficient area, autoimmune disease

Medications: Thyroid hormones, herbal therapies that may contain thyroid hormone

Functional Health Patterns

Health perception–health management: Positive family history of thyroid or autoimmune disorders

Nutritional-metabolic: Iodine intake, weight loss, increased appetite, thirst, nausea, vomiting

Elimination: Diarrhea, polyuria, sweating

Activity-exercise: Dyspnea on exertion, palpitations, muscle weakness, fatigue

Sleep-rest: Insomnia

Cognitive-perceptual: Chest pain, nervousness, heat intolerance, pruritus

Sexuality-reproductive: Decreased libido, impotence, gynecomastia (in men), amenorrhea (in women)

Coping–stress tolerance: Emotional lability, irritability, restlessness, personality changes, delirium

Objective Data

General Observation

Agitation, rapid speech and body movements, anxiety, restlessness, hyperthermia, enlarged or nodular thyroid gland

Eyes

Exophthalmos, eyelid retraction, infrequent blinking

Integumentary

Warm, diaphoretic, velvety skin. Thin, loose nails. Fine, silky hair and hair loss. Palmar erythema, clubbing, white pigmentation of skin (vitiligo), diffuse edema of legs and feet

Respiratory

Tachypnea, dyspnea on exertion

Cardiovascular

Tachycardia, bounding pulse, systolic murmurs, dysrhythmias, hypertension, bruit over the thyroid gland

Gastrointestinal

Increased bowel sounds. Increased appetite, diarrhea, weight loss, hepatosplenomegaly

Neurologic

Hyperreflexia; diplopia. Fine tremors of hands, tongue, eyelids

Musculoskeletal

Muscle wasting

Reproductive

Menstrual irregularities, infertility, impotence, gynecomastia in men

Possible Diagnostic Findings

↑ T_3, ↑ T_4, ↑ T_3 resin uptake, ↓ or undetectable TSH. Chest x-ray showing enlarged heart. ECG findings of tachycardia, atrial fibrillation.

Acute Thyrotoxicosis. Acute thyrotoxicosis is a systemic syndrome that requires aggressive treatment, often in an intensive care unit. Administer medications (previously discussed) that block thyroid hormone production and the sympathetic nervous system. Provide supportive therapy, including monitoring for cardiac dysrhythmias and decompensation, ensuring adequate oxygenation, and giving IV fluids to replace fluid and electrolyte losses. This is especially important in the patient who experiences fluid losses due to vomiting and diarrhea.

Ensuring adequate rest may be a challenge because of the patient's irritability and restlessness. Provide a calm, quiet room because increased metabolism and sensitivity of the sympathetic nervous system causes sleep disturbances. Other interventions may include (1) placing the patient in a cool room away from very ill patients and noisy, high-traffic areas; (2) using light bed coverings and changing the linen frequently if the patient is diaphoretic; and (3) encouraging and assisting with exercise involving large muscle groups (tremors can interfere with small-muscle coordination) to allow the release of nervous tension and restlessness. It is important to establish a supportive, trusting relationship to facilitate coping by a patient who is irritable, restless, and anxious.

If exophthalmos is present, there is a potential for corneal injury related to irritation and dryness. The patient may have orbital pain. To relieve eye discomfort and prevent corneal ulceration, apply artificial tears to soothe and moisten conjunctival membranes. Salt restriction may help reduce periorbital edema. Elevate the patient's head to promote fluid drainage from the periorbital area. The patient should sit upright as much as possible.

Dark glasses reduce glare and prevent irritation from smoke, air currents, dust, and dirt. If the eyelids cannot be closed, lightly tape them shut for sleep. To maintain flexibility, teach the patient to exercise the intraocular muscles several times a day by turning the eyes in the complete range of motion. Good grooming can help reduce the loss of self-esteem from an altered body image. If the exophthalmos is severe, treatment options include corticosteroids, radiation of retroorbital tissues, orbital decompression, or corrective lid or muscle surgery.

◆ **Thyroid Surgery.** When a subtotal thyroidectomy is the treatment of choice, the patient must be adequately prepared to avoid postoperative complications. Before surgery, antithyroid drugs, iodine, and β-adrenergic blockers may be given to achieve a euthyroid state. Iodine also reduces the vascularization of the thyroid gland, reducing the risk of hemorrhage.

Preoperatively, teach the patient about routine postoperative care and comfort and safety measures. Teach the patient the importance of performing leg exercises. Instruct the patient how to support the head manually while turning in bed, since this maneuver minimizes stress on the suture line after surgery. The patient should practice range-of-motion exercises of the neck. Tell the patient that talking is likely to be difficult for a short time after surgery.

◆ **Postoperative Care.** Postoperative complications include hypothyroidism, damage to or inadvertent removal of parathyroid glands, causing hypoparathyroidism and hypocalcemia, hemorrhage, injury to the recurrent or superior laryngeal nerve, thyrotoxicosis, and infection.[15] Recurrent laryngeal nerve damage leads to vocal cord paralysis. If both cords are paralyzed, spastic airway obstruction will occur, requiring an immediate tracheostomy.

!　**SAFETY ALERT** **Airway Obstruction**
- Although not common, airway obstruction after thyroid surgery is an emergency situation.
- O_2, suction equipment, and a tracheostomy tray should be readily available in the patient's room.

Respiration may become difficult because of excess swelling of the neck tissues, hemorrhage, and hematoma formation. *Laryngeal stridor* (harsh, vibratory sound) may occur during inspiration and expiration because of edema of the laryngeal nerve. Laryngeal stridor may also be related to tetany from hypocalcemia, which occurs if the parathyroid glands were removed or damaged during surgery. To treat tetany, IV calcium salts (e.g., calcium gluconate) should be available.

Important nursing interventions after a thyroidectomy include the following:

- Assess the patient every 2 hours for 24 hours for signs of hemorrhage or tracheal compression, such as irregular breathing, neck swelling, frequent swallowing, choking, blood on the dressings, and sensations of fullness at the incision site. Expect some hoarseness for 3 or 4 days after surgery because of edema.
- Place the patient in a semi-Fowler's position and support the patient's head with pillows. Avoid flexion of the neck and any tension on the suture lines.
- Monitor vital signs and calcium levels. Assess for signs of tetany secondary to hypoparathyroidism (e.g., tingling in toes, fingers, around the mouth; muscular twitching; apprehension) and any difficulty in speaking and hoarseness. Monitor Trousseau's sign and Chvostek's sign (see Fig. 16-15).
- Control postoperative pain by giving medication.

If postoperative recovery is uneventful, the patient ambulates within hours after surgery and is permitted fluids as soon as tolerated. A soft diet starts the day after surgery.

The appearance of the incision may be distressing to the patient. Reassure the patient that the scar will fade in color and eventually look like a normal neck wrinkle. A scarf, jewelry, a high collar, or other covering can effectively camouflage the scar.

◆ **Ambulatory Care.** The patient and caregiver must be aware that thyroid hormone balance should be monitored periodically. Most patients experience a period of relative hypothyroidism soon after surgery because of the substantial reduction in the size of the thyroid. However, the remaining tissue usually hypertrophies over time and recovers the capacity to produce hormones. The administration of thyroid hormone is avoided because the exogenous hormone inhibits pituitary production of TSH and delays or prevents the restoration of normal gland function and tissue regeneration.

To prevent weight gain, caloric intake must be substantially reduced below the amount that was required before surgery. Adequate iodine is necessary to promote thyroid function, but excesses can inhibit the thyroid gland. Seafood once or twice a week or normal use of iodized salt should provide sufficient iodine intake. Encourage regular exercise to stimulate the thyroid gland. Teach the patient to avoid high environmental temperatures because they inhibit thyroid regeneration.

Regular follow-up care is necessary. The patient should see the HCP biweekly for a month and then at least semiannually to assess thyroid function. Tell the patient who had a complete thyroidectomy about the need for lifelong thyroid hormone replacement. Teach the patient the signs and symptoms of thyroid failure and to seek medical care promptly if these develop.

◆ **Evaluation**

The expected outcomes are that the patient with hyperthyroidism will
- Experience relief of symptoms
- Have no serious complications related to the disease or treatment
- Cooperate with the therapeutic plan
- Maintain nutritional balance

Additional information on expected outcomes is presented in eNursing Care Plan 49-1 for the patient with hyperthyroidism (available on the website for this chapter).

HYPOTHYROIDISM

Hypothyroidism is a deficiency of thyroid hormone that causes a general slowing of the metabolic rate. About 4% of the U.S. population has mild hypothyroidism, with about 0.3% having more severe disease. Hypothyroidism is more common in women than men. Subclinical hypothyroidism occurs when the TSH is greater than 4.5 mU/L, but the thyroxine (T_4) levels are normal. Up to 10% of women older than 60 years have subclinical hypothyroidism.[16] Patients with overt hypothyroidism have elevated TSH and decreased thyroxine levels. Critically ill patients may present with nonthyroidal illness syndrome (NTIS).[17] Those with NTIS have low T_3, T_4, and TSH levels.

Etiology and Pathophysiology

Hypothyroidism can be classified as primary or secondary. *Primary hypothyroidism* is caused by destruction of thyroid tissue or defective hormone synthesis. *Secondary hypothyroidism* is caused by pituitary disease with decreased TSH secretion or hypothalamic dysfunction with decreased thyrotropin-releasing hormone (TRH) secretion. Hypothyroidism can be transient and related to thyroiditis or discontinuing thyroid hormone therapy.

Iodine deficiency is the most common cause of hypothyroidism worldwide. In the United States, the most common cause of primary hypothyroidism is atrophy of the thyroid gland. This atrophy is the end result of Hashimoto's thyroiditis or Graves' disease. These autoimmune diseases destroy the thyroid gland. Hypothyroidism may also develop after treatment for hyperthyroidism, specifically thyroidectomy or RAI therapy. Drugs such as amiodarone (Cordarone), which contains iodine, and lithium, which blocks hormone production, can cause hypothyroidism.

Hypothyroidism that develops in infancy (*cretinism*) is caused by thyroid hormone deficiencies during fetal or early neonatal life. All infants in the United States are screened for decreased thyroid function at birth.

Clinical Manifestations

Regardless of the cause, hypothyroidism has common features. It has systemic effects characterized by a slowing of body processes. Manifestations vary, depending on the severity and the duration of thyroid deficiency as well as the patient's age at the onset of the deficiency. Symptoms may develop over months to years, unless hypothyroidism occurs after a thyroidectomy, after thyroid ablation, or during treatment with antithyroid drugs.

The patient is often fatigued, lethargic, and experiences personality and mental changes, including impaired memory, slowed speech, decreased initiative, and somnolence. Many appear depressed. Weight gain is most likely a result of a decreased metabolic rate.

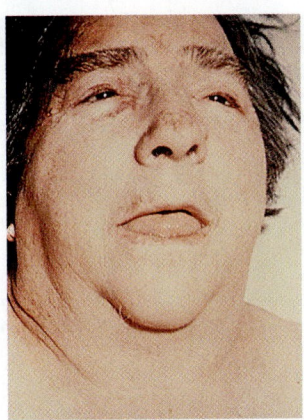

FIG. 49-9 Common features of myxedema. Dull, puffy skin; coarse, sparse hair; periorbital edema; and prominent tongue. (Courtesy Paul W. Ladenson, MD, The Johns Hopkins University and Hospital, Baltimore, Md. From Seidel HM, Ball JW, Dains JE, et al, editors: *Mosby's guide to physical examination*, ed 6, St Louis, 2006, Mosby.)

Hypothyroidism may cause significant cardiovascular problems, especially in a person with previous cardiovascular disorders. It is associated with decreased cardiac contractility and decreased cardiac output. Thus the patient may experience low exercise tolerance and shortness of breath on exertion. Increased serum cholesterol and triglyceride levels and the accumulation of mucopolysaccharides in the intima of small blood vessels can result in coronary atherosclerosis. Anemia is common.

Patients with severe, long-standing hypothyroidism may display myxedema, which alters the physical appearance of the skin and subcutaneous tissues with puffiness, facial and periorbital edema, and a masklike affect. Myxedema occurs due to the accumulation of hydrophilic mucopolysaccharides in the dermis and other tissues (Fig. 49-9). People with hypothyroidism may describe an altered self-image related to their disabilities and altered appearance. Other manifestations of hypothyroidism are summarized in Table 49-5.

In the older adult, the typical manifestations of hypothyroidism (fatigue, cold and dry skin, hoarseness, hair loss, constipation, and cold intolerance) may be attributed to normal aging. For this reason, the patient's symptoms may not raise suspicion of an underlying condition. Older adults who have confusion, lethargy, and depression should be evaluated for thyroid disease.

Complications

The mental sluggishness, drowsiness, and lethargy of hypothyroidism may progress gradually or suddenly to a notable impairment of consciousness or coma. This situation, termed *myxedema coma*, is a medical emergency. Myxedema coma can be precipitated by infection, drugs (especially opioids, tranquilizers, and barbiturates), exposure to cold, and trauma. It is characterized by subnormal temperature, hypotension, and hypoventilation. Cardiovascular collapse can result from hypoventilation, hyponatremia, hypoglycemia, and lactic acidosis. For the patient to survive myxedema coma, vital functions must be supported and IV thyroid hormone replacement administered.

Diagnostic Studies

The most reliable laboratory tests for thyroid function are TSH and free T$_4$. These values, correlated with symptoms obtained from the history and physical examination, confirm

TABLE 49-10   Interprofessional Care
Hypothyroidism

Diagnostic Assessment	Management
• History and physical examination • Serum TSH and free T$_4$ • Total serum T$_3$ and T$_4$ • Thyroid peroxidase (TPO) antibodies	• Thyroid hormone replacement (e.g., levothyroxine) • Monitor thyroid hormone levels and adjust dosage (if needed) • Nutritional therapy to promote weight loss • Patient and caregiver teaching (Table 49-11)

the diagnosis of hypothyroidism. Serum TSH levels help determine the cause of hypothyroidism. Serum TSH is high when the defect is in the thyroid and low when it is in the pituitary or the hypothalamus. The presence of thyroid antibodies suggests an autoimmune origin. Other abnormal laboratory findings are elevated cholesterol and triglycerides, anemia, and increased creatine kinase (Table 49-6).

Interprofessional Care

The treatment goal for a patient with hypothyroidism is restoration of a euthyroid state as safely and rapidly as possible with hormone therapy (Table 49-10). A low-calorie diet is indicated to promote weight loss or prevent weight gain.

Levothyroxine (Synthroid) is the drug of choice to treat hypothyroidism. In the young and otherwise healthy patient, the maintenance replacement dosage is adjusted according to the patient's response and laboratory findings. When initiating thyroid hormone therapy, the initial dosages are low to avoid increases in resting heart rate and BP. In the patient with compromised cardiac status, careful monitoring is needed when starting and adjusting the dosage because the usual dose may increase myocardial O$_2$ demand.[16] This may cause angina and cardiac dysrhythmias.

> **DRUG ALERT   Levothyroxine (Synthroid)**
> • Carefully monitor patients with cardiovascular disease who take this drug.
> • Monitor heart rate and report pulse greater than 100 beats/min or an irregular heartbeat.
> • Promptly report chest pain, weight loss, nervousness, tremors, and/or insomnia.

In a patient without side effects, the dose is increased at 4- to 6-week intervals as needed based on the TSH levels. It may take up to 8 weeks before the full effect of hormone therapy is seen. Levothyroxine has a peak of action of 1 to 3 weeks. It is important that the patient regularly take replacement medication. Lifelong thyroid therapy is usually required.

Liotrix is a synthetic mix of levothyroxine (T$_4$) and liothyronine (T$_3$) in a 4:1 combination. In contrast, liotrix has a faster onset of action with a peak of 2 to 3 days. Liotrix can be used in acutely ill patients with hypothyroidism.

❖ NURSING MANAGEMENT: HYPOTHYROIDISM

◆ Nursing Assessment

Careful assessment may reveal early and subtle changes in a patient suspected of having hypothyroidism. Note any previous history of hyperthyroidism and treatment with antithyroid medications, radioactive iodine, or surgery. Ask the patient about using iodine-containing medications (Table 49-4) and any changes in appetite, weight, activity level, speech, memory, and skin (e.g., increased dryness or thickening). Assess for cold intolerance, constipation, and signs of depression. Further assessment should focus on heart rate, tenderness over the thyroid gland, and edema in the extremities and face.

Nursing Diagnoses

Nursing diagnoses for the patient with hypothyroidism may include, but are not limited to, the following:

* Activity intolerance *related to* weakness and fatigue
* Constipation *related to* GI hypomotility
* Impaired memory *related to* hypometabolism

Additional information on nursing diagnoses is presented in the eNursing Care Plan 49-2 for the patient with hypothyroidism (available on the website for this chapter).

Planning

The overall goals are that the patient with hypothyroidism will (1) experience relief of symptoms, (2) maintain a euthyroid state, (3) maintain a positive self-image, and (4) comply with lifelong thyroid therapy.

Nursing Implementation

Health Promotion. Routine screening of thyroid function is not recommended in nonpregnant, asymptomatic adults. Risk factors for hypothyroidism include being female, white ethnicity, advancing age or having type 1 diabetes, Down syndrome, family history of thyroid disease, goiter, previous hyperthyroidism, and external beam radiation in the head and neck area.[18] High-risk populations should be screened for subclinical thyroid disease.

Acute Care. Most people with hypothyroidism are treated on an outpatient basis. The person who develops myxedema coma requires acute nursing care, often in an intensive care setting. Mechanical respiratory support and cardiac monitoring are frequently necessary.

Give thyroid hormone therapy and all other medications IV because severe gastric hypomotility may prevent the absorption of oral preparations. Monitor the core temperature for hypothermia that often occurs in myxedema and myxedema coma. Use gentle soap and moisturize frequently to prevent skin breakdown. Frequent position changes and a low-pressure mattress assist in maintaining skin integrity.

Monitor the patient's progress by assessing vital signs, body weight, fluid intake and output, and edema. Cardiac assessment is especially important because the cardiovascular response to hormone therapy determines the medication regimen. Note energy level and mental alertness, which should improve within 2 to 14 days and continue a steady progression to normal levels. Neurologic status and TSH levels are used to determine continuing treatment.

Ambulatory Care. Patient teaching regarding medication management and identification of complications is essential (Table 49-11). Initially the hypothyroid patient may have difficulty processing complex instructions. It is important to provide written instructions, repeat the information often, and assess the patient's comprehension level.

Stress the need for lifelong drug therapy and avoiding abrupt discontinuation of drugs. Caution patients against doubling up on doses for any reason. Some patients notice weight loss and are tempted to increase dosing to achieve a desired weight. Teach the patient the expected and unexpected side effects, including the signs and symptoms of hypothyroidism and hyperthyroidism

---

TABLE 49-11   Patient & Caregiver Teaching
Hypothyroidism

Include the following instructions when teaching the patient and caregiver about management of hypothyroidism.

1. Discuss the importance of thyroid hormone therapy.
   * Need for lifelong therapy
   * Taking thyroid hormone in the morning before food
   * Need for regular follow-up care
2. Caution the patient not to switch brands of the hormone unless prescribed, since the bioavailability of thyroid hormones may differ.
3. Emphasize the need for a comfortable, warm environment because of cold intolerance.
4. Teach measures to prevent skin breakdown. Soap should be used sparingly and lotion applied to skin.
5. Caution the patient, especially if an older adult, to avoid sedatives. If they must be used, suggest that the lowest dose be used. Caregiver should closely monitor mental status, level of consciousness, and respirations.
6. Discuss measures to minimize constipation, including
   * Gradual increase in activity and exercise
   * Increased fiber in diet
   * Use of stool softeners
   * Regular bowel elimination time
7. Tell patient to avoid using enemas because they produce vagal stimulation, which can be hazardous if cardiac disease is present.

(Table 49-5). The manifestations of overdose are the same as hyperthyroidism. Tell the patient to immediately contact an HCP if symptoms, such as orthopnea, dyspnea, rapid pulse, palpitations, chest pain, nervousness, or insomnia, are present.

The patient with diabetes mellitus should test his or her capillary blood glucose at least daily because the return to the euthyroid state frequently increases insulin requirements. Thyroid drugs potentiate the effects of anticoagulants and decrease the effect of digitalis compounds. Teach the patient the toxic signs and symptoms of these medications and the need to remain under close medical observation until stable. Medication interactions are an important reason for patients to consult their HCP before switching brands of thyroid replacement medication. Switching brands may alter bioavailability of the drug and physiologic response.

With treatment, striking transformations occur in both appearance and mental function. Most adults return to a normal state. Cardiovascular conditions and psychosis may persist despite corrections of the hormonal imbalance. Relapses occur if treatment is interrupted.

Evaluation

The expected outcomes are that the patient with hypothyroidism will

* Have relief from symptoms
* Maintain a euthyroid state as evidenced by normal thyroid hormone and TSH levels
* Avoid complications of therapy
* Adhere to lifelong therapy

Additional information on expected outcomes is presented in the eNursing Care Plan 49-2 for the patient with hypothyroidism (available on the website for this chapter).

THYROID NODULES AND CANCER

A *thyroid nodule* (growth in the thyroid gland) may be benign or malignant (thyroid cancer). More than 95% of all thyroid gland nodules are benign. Prevalence of thyroid nodule development increases with age. Benign nodules are usually not dangerous, but they can cause tracheal compression if they become too large.

Thyroid cancer is the most common type of cancer of the endocrine system. An estimated 62,450 new cases of thyroid cancer are diagnosed annually. The incidence of thyroid cancer has increased significantly in the past 25 years. It is the most rapidly increasing cancer in the United States. Thyroid cancer affects more women, and the incidence is higher in whites and Asian Americans.[19] Adults at risk include those who had head and neck radiation therapy during childhood, were exposed to radioactive fallout, or have a personal or family history of goiter.

Types of Thyroid Cancer

The four main types of thyroid cancer are papillary, follicular, medullary, and anaplastic. *Papillary* thyroid cancer is the most common type, accounting for about 70% to 80% of all thyroid cancers. Papillary cancer tends to grow slowly and spreads initially to lymph nodes in the neck.

Follicular thyroid cancer makes up about 15% of all thyroid cancers. It tends to occur in older patients. Follicular cancer first metastasizes into the cervical lymph nodes and then spreads to the neck, lungs, and bones.

Medullary thyroid cancer, which accounts for up to 10% of all thyroid cancers, is more likely to occur in families and be associated with other endocrine problems. It is diagnosed by genetic testing for a proto-oncogene called *RET*. Medullary thyroid cancer is a type of multiple endocrine neoplasia. It is often poorly differentiated and associated with early metastasis.

Anaplastic thyroid cancer, which is found in less than 2% of patients with thyroid cancer, is the most advanced and aggressive thyroid cancer. It is the least likely to respond to treatment and has a poor prognosis.

Clinical Manifestations and Diagnostic Studies

The primary manifestation of thyroid cancer is a painless, palpable nodule or nodules in an enlarged thyroid gland. Most nodules are found during routine palpation of the neck. The presence of firm, palpable, cervical masses suggests lymph node metastasis. Some patients may have difficulty swallowing or breathing because of tumor growth invading the trachea or esophagus. Hemoptysis and airway obstruction may occur if the trachea is involved. Patients with thyroid cancer generally are euthyroid.

Nodular enlargement of the thyroid gland or palpation of a mass requires further evaluation. Ultrasound is often the first test used. Follow-up testing may involve CT, MRI, positron emission tomography (PET), and ultrasound-guided fine-needle aspiration (FNA). FNA is indicated when a tissue sample for pathologic examination is necessary. A thyroid scan may be done. The scan shows whether nodules on the thyroid are "hot" or "cold." "Hot" tumors take up radioactive iodine and are nearly always benign. If the nodule does not take up the radioactive iodine, it appears as "cold" and has a higher risk of being malignant.

Elevations in serum calcitonin are associated with medullary thyroid cancer. In papillary and follicular cancers, serum thyroglobulin is elevated. In families with a history of medullary thyroid cancer, family members should be encouraged to get genetic testing done and have thyroid screening on a regular basis.

❖ NURSING AND INTERPROFESSIONAL MANAGEMENT: THYROID CANCER

Surgical removal of the tumor is the primary treatment for thyroid cancer.[19] Surgical procedures range from unilateral total lobectomy to near-total thyroidectomy with bilateral lobectomy. Lymph nodes in the neck may be removed to determine if the cancer has spread. RAI may be given to some patients to destroy any remaining cancer cells after surgery. RAI therapy has been shown to improve survival rates in patients with papillary and follicular thyroid cancer. External beam radiation may be given as palliative treatment for patients with metastatic thyroid cancer.

Many thyroid cancers are TSH dependent. Thyroid hormone therapy in high doses is often prescribed to inhibit pituitary secretion of TSH. Chemotherapy, including doxorubicin, may be used for advanced disease. Vandetanib (Caprelsa), lenvatinib (Lenvima), sorafenib tosylate (Nexavar), and cabozantinib (Cometriq) are targeted therapies used for metastatic thyroid cancer. These drugs inhibit tyrosine kinases, enzymes that are involved in growth of cancer cells.

Nursing care for the patient with thyroid cancer is similar to that of a patient undergoing thyroidectomy (see p. 1167). Because of the surgical site location and the potential for hypocalcemia, the patient requires frequent postoperative assessment. Assess the patient for airway obstruction, bleeding, and tetany, since the parathyroid gland may have been disturbed or removed during surgery.

MULTIPLE ENDOCRINE NEOPLASIA

Multiple endocrine neoplasia is an inherited condition characterized by hormone-secreting tumors.[20] It is caused by the mutation of one of two genes, *MEN1* or *RET*, that normally control cell growth. Tumors may develop in childhood or later in life.

The two major types of multiple endocrine neoplasia are type 1 and type 2. Both types are commonly inherited as autosomal dominant disorders. Persons with type 1 commonly have parathyroid gland hyperactivity (hyperparathyroidism). Other signs may include hyperactivity of the pituitary gland (prolactinoma) and pancreas (gastrinomas). In most cases the tumors are initially benign. Some tumors later become malignant. Persons with type 2 neoplasia often have medullary thyroid carcinoma. They may also develop pheochromocytoma (tumor of the adrenal glands). (Pheochromocytoma is discussed later in this chapter on p. 1181.)

Treatment of the tumor(s) may include conservative management (watchful waiting), medication to block the effects of excess hormone, and surgical removal of the gland and/or tumor. It is important for patients to have regular screening visits with their HCP so that new tumors may be detected early and existing tumors carefully monitored.

DISORDERS OF PARATHYROID GLANDS

HYPERPARATHYROIDISM

Etiology and Pathophysiology

Hyperparathyroidism is a condition involving an increased secretion of parathyroid hormone (PTH). PTH helps regulate

TABLE 49-12   Manifestations of Parathyroid Dysfunction

Hyperfunction	Hypofunction	Hyperfunction	Hypofunction
Cardiovascular System		**Visual System**	
• Hypertension	• Hypotension	• Impaired vision	• Eye changes, including
• Angina	• Edema	• Corneal calcification	lenticular opacities, cataracts,
• Dysrhythmias	• Dysrhythmias		papilledema
• Shortened ST segment	• Elongation of ST segment	**Gastrointestinal System**	
• Shortened QT interval	• Prolonged QT interval	• Vague abdominal pain	
• Increased digitalis effect	• Decreased cardiac output	• Anorexia	• Abdominal cramps
Neurologic System		• Nausea and vomiting	• Fecal incontinence (in older
• Lethargy, weakness, fatigue	• Weakness, fatigue	• Constipation	adult)
• Psychosis, depression	• Depression	• Pancreatitis	• Malabsorption
• Depressed reflexes	• Hyperreflexia, muscle	• Peptic ulcer disease	
• Personality changes	cramps	• Cholelithiasis	
• Irritability	• Personality changes	• Weight loss	
• Memory impairment	• Irritability	**Integumentary System**	
• Delirium, confusion, coma	• Memory impairment	• Skin necrosis	• Dry, scaly skin
• Headache	• Disorientation, confusion (in	• Moist skin	• Hair loss on scalp and body
• Poor coordination	older adult)		• Brittle nails, transverse
• Gait abnormalities	• Headache, increased		ridging
• Psychomotor retardation	intracranial pressure		• Lack of tooth enamel
• Paresthesias	• Tetany, seizures	**Musculoskeletal System**	
	• Positive Chvostek's and	• Weakness, fatigue	• Weakness, fatigue
	Trousseau's sign	• Skeletal pain	• Painful muscle cramps
	• Tremor	• Backache	• Skeletal x-ray changes,
	• Paresthesias of lips, hands,	• Pain on weight bearing	osteosclerosis
	feet	• Osteoporosis	• Soft tissue calcification
Renal/Urinary System		• Pathologic fractures of long bones	• Difficulty walking
• Hypercalciuria		• Compression fractures of spine	
• Kidney stones (nephrolithiasis)	• Urinary frequency	• Decreased muscle tone, muscle	
• Urinary tract infections	• Urinary incontinence	atrophy	
• Polyuria			

serum calcium and phosphate levels by stimulating bone resorption of calcium, renal tubular reabsorption of calcium, and activation of vitamin D. Thus oversecretion of PTH is associated with increased serum calcium levels. Primary hyperparathyroidism affects 25 of 100,000 persons per year.[21]

Hyperparathyroidism is classified as primary, secondary, or tertiary. *Primary hyperparathyroidism* is due to an increased secretion of PTH leading to disorders of calcium, phosphate, and bone metabolism. The most common cause is a benign tumor (adenoma) in the parathyroid gland. Patients who have previously undergone head and neck radiation have an increased risk of developing a parathyroid adenoma. Long-term lithium therapy is also associated with primary hyperparathyroidism. The peak incidence of primary hyperparathyroidism is in the 40s and 50s. Women are twice as likely to develop primary hyperparathyroidism as men.[21]

Secondary hyperparathyroidism is a compensatory response to conditions that induce or cause hypocalcemia, the main stimulus of PTH secretion. These conditions include vitamin D deficiencies, malabsorption, chronic kidney disease, and hyperphosphatemia.

Tertiary hyperparathyroidism occurs when there is hyperplasia of the parathyroid glands and a loss of negative feedback from circulating calcium levels. Thus there is autonomous secretion of PTH, even with normal calcium levels. This condition is seen in patients who have had a kidney transplant after a long period of dialysis treatment for chronic kidney disease (see Chapter 46).

Excess levels of circulating PTH usually lead to hypercalcemia and hypophosphatemia. Multiple body systems are affected

(Table 49-12). Decreased bone density can occur because of the effect of PTH on osteoclastic (bone resorption) and osteoblastic (bone formation) activity. In the kidneys the excess calcium cannot be reabsorbed, leading to increased urinary calcium levels (hypercalciuria). This urinary calcium, along with a large amount of urinary phosphate, can lead to calculi formation.

Clinical Manifestations and Complications

Clinical manifestations range from an asymptomatic person (diagnosed through testing for unrelated problems) to a patient with overt symptoms.[21] The manifestations are associated with hypercalcemia (Table 49-12). Loss of appetite, constipation, fatigue, emotional disorders, shortened attention span, and muscle weakness, particularly in the proximal muscles of the lower extremities, are often noted. Complications include osteoporosis, renal failure, kidney stones, pancreatitis, cardiac changes, and long bone, rib, and vertebral fractures.

Diagnostic Studies

PTH levels are elevated in patients with hyperparathyroidism. Serum calcium levels usually exceed 10 mg/dL (2.50 mmol/L). Because of its inverse relation with calcium, the serum phosphorus level is usually less than 3 mg/dL (0.1 mmol/L). Hypercalcemia in asymptomatic cases is often identified through a routine chemistry panel.

Elevations in other laboratory tests include urine calcium, serum chloride, uric acid, creatinine, amylase (if pancreatitis is present), and alkaline phosphatase (in the presence of bone disease). Bone density measurements may be used to detect bone loss. Conversely, those found to have bone loss on a screening dual-energy x-ray absorptiometry (DEXA) scan should be tested for hypercalcemia. MRI, CT, and/or ultrasound can detect an adenoma.

Interprofessional Care

The goal of treatment is to relieve symptoms and prevent complications caused by excess PTH. The choice of therapy depends on the urgency of the clinical situation, degree of hypercalcemia, and underlying cause of the disorder.

Surgical Therapy. The most effective treatment of primary and secondary hyperparathyroidism is surgical intervention. Surgery involves partial or complete removal of the parathyroid glands. The most commonly used procedure involves endoscopy and is done on an outpatient basis. Criteria for surgery include elevated serum calcium levels (more than 1 mg/dL above the upper limit of normal), hypercalciuria (greater than 400 mg/day), markedly reduced bone mineral density, overt symptoms (e.g., neuromuscular effects, nephrolithiasis), or those under age 50. Parathyroidectomy leads to a rapid reduction of high calcium levels.

Patients who have multiple parathyroid glands removed may undergo autotransplantation of normal parathyroid tissue in the forearm or near the sternocleidomastoid muscle. This allows PTH secretion to continue with normalization of calcium levels. If autotransplantation is not possible or if it fails, the patient will need to take calcium supplements for life.

Nonsurgical Therapy. A conservative approach is often used in patients who are asymptomatic or have mild symptoms of hyperparathyroidism. Ongoing care includes regular examination with measurements of serum PTH, calcium, phosphorus, alkaline phosphatase, creatinine and blood urea nitrogen (BUN) (to assess renal function), and urinary calcium excretion. Annual x-rays and DEXA scans are done to assess for metabolic bone loss. Continued ambulation and avoiding immobility are important. Dietary measures include high fluid and moderate calcium intake.

Severe hypercalcemia is managed with IV sodium chloride solution and loop diuretics such as furosemide to increase the urinary excretion of calcium. Several drugs help to lower calcium levels, but they do not treat the underlying problem. Bisphosphonates (e.g., alendronate [Fosamax]) inhibit osteoclastic bone resorption, normalizing serum calcium levels and improving bone mineral density. IV bisphosphonates (e.g., pamidronate [Aredia]) can rapidly lower serum calcium in patients with dangerously elevated levels. Phosphates are given if the patient has normal renal function and low serum phosphate levels.

Calcimimetic agents (e.g., cinacalcet [Sensipar]) increase the sensitivity of the calcium receptor on the parathyroid gland, resulting in decreased PTH secretion and calcium blood levels. They are useful in treating secondary hyperparathyroidism in those with chronic kidney disease on dialysis or in patients with parathyroid cancer.

❖ NURSING MANAGEMENT: HYPERPARATHYROIDISM

Nursing care for the patient after a parathyroidectomy is similar to that for a patient after thyroidectomy. The major postoperative complications are associated with hemorrhage and fluid and electrolyte disturbances. *Tetany,* a condition of neuromuscular hyperexcitability associated with sudden decrease in calcium levels, is another concern. It is usually apparent early in the postoperative period but may develop over several days. Mild tetany, characterized by unpleasant tingling of the hands and around the mouth, may be present but should decrease over time. If tetany becomes more severe (e.g., muscular spasms or laryngospasms), IV calcium may be given. IV calcium gluconate should be readily available for patients after parathyroidectomy in the event that acute tetany occurs.

Monitor intake and output to evaluate the patient's fluid status. Assess calcium, potassium, phosphate, and magnesium levels frequently, as well as Chvostek's and Trousseau's signs (see Fig. 16-15). Encourage mobility to promote bone calcification.

If surgery is not performed, treatment to relieve symptoms and prevent complications is initiated. Assist the patient with hyperparathyroidism to adapt the meal plan to his or her lifestyle. A referral to a dietitian may be useful. Because immobility can aggravate the bone loss, emphasize the importance of an exercise program. Encourage the patient to keep the regular follow-up appointments. Teach the patient the symptoms of hypocalcemia and hypercalcemia and to report them if they occur. Hypocalcemia and hypercalcemia are discussed in Chapter 16.

HYPOPARATHYROIDISM

Hypoparathyroidism is an uncommon condition associated with inadequate circulating PTH. It is characterized by hypocalcemia due to a lack of PTH to maintain serum calcium levels. PTH resistance at the cellular level may also occur *(pseudohypoparathyroidism).* This is caused by a genetic defect resulting in hypocalcemia despite normal or high PTH levels. It is often associated with hypothyroidism and hypogonadism.

The most common cause of hypoparathyroidism is iatrogenic. This may include accidental removal of the parathyroid glands or damage to the vascular supply of the glands during neck surgery (e.g., thyroidectomy). Idiopathic hypoparathyroidism resulting from the absence, fatty replacement, or atrophy of the glands is a rare disease. It usually occurs early in life and may be associated with other endocrine disorders. Affected patients may have antiparathyroid antibodies. Severe hypomagnesemia (e.g., malnutrition, chronic alcoholism, renal failure) also leads to a suppression of PTH secretion. Other causes of parathyroid deficiency include tumors and heavy metal poisoning.

The clinical features of acute hypoparathyroidism are due to hypocalcemia (Table 49-12). Sudden decreases in calcium concentration cause tetany, characterized by tingling of the lips and stiffness in the extremities. Painful tonic spasms of smooth and skeletal muscles can cause dysphagia and laryngospasms, which compromise breathing. Lethargy, anxiety, and personality changes may occur. Abnormal laboratory findings include decreased serum calcium and PTH levels and increased serum phosphate levels.

❖ NURSING AND INTERPROFESSIONAL MANAGEMENT: HYPOPARATHYROIDISM

Treatment goals for the patient with hypoparathyroidism are to treat acute complications such as tetany, maintain normal serum calcium levels, and prevent long-term complications. Emergency treatment of tetany after surgery requires the administration of IV calcium.

Give IV calcium slowly. Use ECG monitoring during calcium administration because high serum calcium levels can cause hypotension, serious cardiac dysrhythmias, or cardiac arrest. The patient who takes digoxin is particularly vulnerable. It is important to assess IV patency before administration. Calcium chloride can cause venous irritation and inflammation, and extravasation may cause cellulitis, necrosis, and tissue sloughing.

Rebreathing may partially relieve acute neuromuscular symptoms associated with hypocalcemia such as generalized muscle cramps or mild tetany. Instruct the patient (if cooperative) to breathe in and out of a paper bag or breathing mask. This reduces CO_2 excretion from the lungs, increases carbonic acid levels in the blood, and lowers the pH. A lower pH (acidic environment) enhances calcium ionization, which causes more total body calcium to be available in the active form.

> ### ❓ CHECK YOUR PRACTICE
>
> You are caring for a 56-yr-old man admitted 18 hours ago to your clinical unit. He had a total thyroidectomy for papillary thyroid cancer. As you are preparing to administer oral pain medication, he tells you he hopes he "doesn't have any trouble" taking the medication because his lips feel "a little numb."
> - What complication do you suspect could be occurring?
> - What assessments do you need to make at this time?
> - Describe the actions needed if this complication is occurring.

Teach the patient how to manage long-term drug and nutritional therapy. PTH replacement is not recommended because of the expense and need for parenteral administration. Most patients receive a regimen of oral calcium supplements (totaling 1.5 to 3 g/day in divided doses), magnesium supplements, and vitamin D.

Vitamin D is used to enhance intestinal calcium absorption. Vitamin D (e.g., dihydrotachysterol, 1,25-dihydroxycholecalciferol, or calcitriol [Rocaltrol]) increases calcium levels rapidly and is quickly metabolized. Rapid metabolism is desired because vitamin D is a fat-soluble vitamin and toxicity can cause irreversible renal impairment.

A high-calcium meal plan includes foods such as dark green vegetables, soybeans, and tofu. Tell the patient to avoid foods containing oxalic acid (e.g., spinach, rhubarb) because they inhibit the absorption of calcium. Teach the patient about the need for follow-up care, including monitoring of calcium levels three or four times a year.

DISORDERS OF ADRENAL CORTEX

Adrenal cortex steroid hormones have three main classifications: glucocorticoids, mineralocorticoids, and androgens. Glucocorticoids regulate metabolism, increase blood glucose levels, and are critical in the physiologic stress response. The primary glucocorticoid is cortisol. Mineralocorticoids regulate sodium and potassium balance. The primary mineralocorticoid is aldosterone. Androgens contribute to growth and development in both genders and to sexual development in women. The term *corticosteroid* refers to any one of these three types of hormones produced by the adrenal cortex.

CUSHING SYNDROME

Etiology and Pathophysiology

Cushing syndrome is a clinical condition that results from chronic exposure to excess corticosteroids, particularly glucocorticoids.[22] Several conditions can cause Cushing syndrome. The most common cause is iatrogenic administration of exogenous corticosteroids (e.g., prednisone). About 85% of the cases of endogenous Cushing syndrome are due to an ACTH-secreting pituitary adenoma (Cushing disease). Less common causes include adrenal tumors and ectopic ACTH production by tumors (usually of the lung or pancreas) outside of the hypothalamic-pituitary-adrenal axis. Cushing disease and primary adrenal tumors are more common in women in the 20- to 40-year-old age group. Ectopic ACTH production is more common in men.

Clinical Manifestations

Manifestations of Cushing syndrome occur in most body systems and are related to excess levels of corticosteroids (Table 49-13). Although signs of glucocorticoid excess usually predominate, symptoms of mineralocorticoid and androgen excess can occur.

Corticosteroid excess causes pronounced changes in physical appearance (Fig. 49-10). Weight gain, the most common feature, results from the accumulation of adipose tissue in the trunk (centripetal obesity), face ("moon face"), and cervical areas ("buffalo hump") (Fig. 49-11). Hyperglycemia occurs because of glucose intolerance (associated with cortisol-induced insulin resistance) and increased gluconeogenesis by the liver. Muscle wasting causes weakness, especially in the extremities. A loss of bone matrix leads to osteoporosis and back pain. The loss of collagen makes the skin weaker, thinner, and more easily bruised. Purplish red striae (usually depressed below the skin surface) appear on the abdomen, breast, or buttocks (Fig. 49-12). Catabolic processes lead to a delay in wound healing.

Mineralocorticoid excess may cause hypokalemia from potassium excretion and hypertension secondary to fluid retention. Adrenal androgen excess may cause severe acne, virilization in women, and feminization in men. Menstrual disorders and hirsutism in women and gynecomastia and impotence in men are seen more commonly in adrenal cancers.

Diagnostic Studies

Diagnosing Cushing syndrome begins with confirming elevated plasma cortisol levels. Three tests are used: (1) midnight or late-night salivary cortisol, (2) low-dose dexamethasone suppression test, and (3) 24-hour urine cortisol.[23] Urine cortisol levels higher than the normal range of 80 to 120 mcg/24 hr

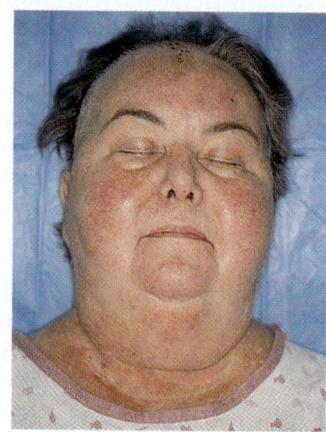

FIG. 49-10 Cushing syndrome. Facies include a rounded face ("moon face") with thin, reddened skin. Hirsutism may also be present. (From Seidel HM, Ball JW, Dains JE, et al: *Mosby's guide to physical examination*, ed 6, St Louis, 2006, Mosby.)

TABLE 49-13 Manifestations of Adrenocortical Dysfunction

System	Cushing Syndrome	Addison's Disease
Glucocorticoids		
General appearance	Truncal obesity, thin extremities, rounding of face (moon face), fat deposits on back of neck and shoulders (buffalo hump) (Fig. 49-11).	Weight loss, emaciation.
Integumentary	Thin, fragile skin, purplish red striae (Fig. 49-12). Petechial hemorrhages, bruises. Florid cheeks (plethora), acne, poor wound healing.	Bronzed or smoky hyperpigmentation of face, neck, hands (especially creases) (Fig. 49-13), buccal membranes, nipples, genitalia, and scars (if pituitary function normal). Vitiligo, alopecia.
Cardiovascular	Hypervolemia, hypertension, edema of lower extremities.	Hypotension, tendency to develop refractory shock, vasodilation.
Gastrointestinal	Increase in secretion of pepsin and HCl acid, risk of peptic ulcer disease, anorexia.	Anorexia, nausea and vomiting, cramping abdominal pain, diarrhea.
Renal/urinary	Glycosuria, hypercalciuria, risk for kidney stones.	
Musculoskeletal	Muscle wasting in extremities, fatigue, osteoporosis, awkward gait, back pain, weakness, compression fractures.	Fatigue.
Immune	Inhibition of immune response, suppression of allergic response.	Tendency for coexisting autoimmune diseases.
Metabolic	Hyperglycemia, negative nitrogen balance, dyslipidemia.	Hyponatremia, insulin sensitivity, fever.
Emotional	Euphoria, irritability, depression, insomnia, anxiety.	Depression, exhaustion or irritability, confusion, delusions.
Mineralocorticoids		
Fluid and electrolytes	Marked sodium and water retention, edema, marked hypokalemia, alkalosis.	Sodium loss, decreased volume of extracellular fluid, hyperkalemia, salt craving.
Cardiovascular	Hypertension, hypervolemia.	Hypovolemia, tendency toward shock, decreased cardiac output.
Androgens		
Integumentary	Hirsutism, acne, hyperpigmentation.	Decreased axillary and pubic hair (in women).
Reproductive	*Women:* Menstrual irregularities and enlargement of clitoris. *Men:* Gynecomastia and testicular atrophy.	*Women:* Decreased libido in women *Men:* No effect in men.
Musculoskeletal	Muscle wasting and weakness.	Decrease in muscle size and tone.

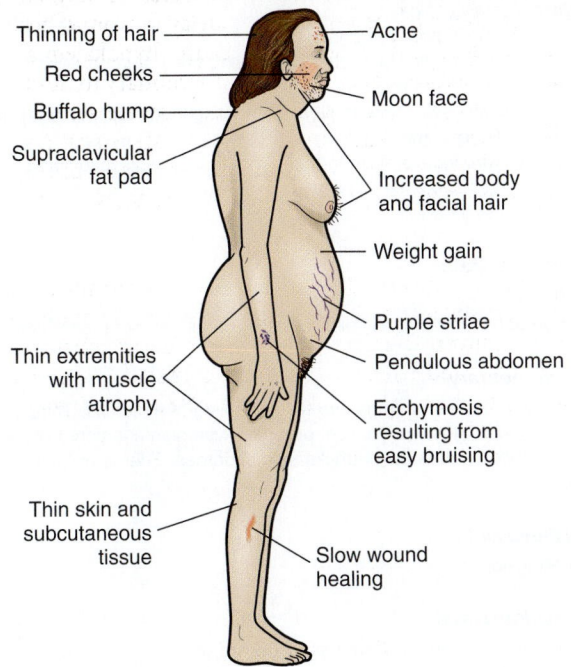

Thinning of hair
Red cheeks
Buffalo hump
Supraclavicular fat pad
Acne
Moon face
Increased body and facial hair
Weight gain
Purple striae
Pendulous abdomen
Ecchymosis resulting from easy bruising
Thin extremities with muscle atrophy
Thin skin and subcutaneous tissue
Slow wound healing

FIG. 49-11 Common characteristics of Cushing syndrome.

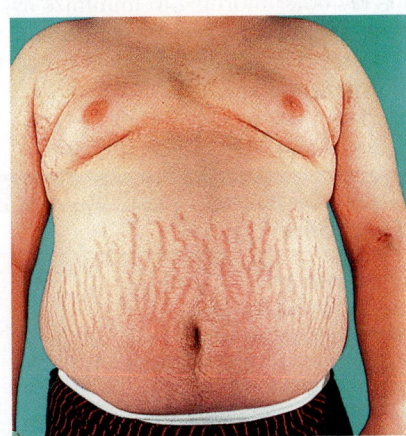

FIG. 49-12 Cushing syndrome. Truncal obesity; broad, purple striae; and easy bruising (left antecubital fossa). (From Chew SL, Leslie D: *Clinical endocrinology and diabetes: an illustrated colour text,* Edinburgh, 2006, Churchill Livingstone.)

indicate Cushing syndrome. Urine levels of 17-ketosteroids may be elevated. A CT scan or MRI of the pituitary and adrenal glands can detect a tumor.

Plasma ACTH levels may be low, normal, or elevated, depending on the underlying cause of Cushing syndrome. High or normal ACTH levels indicate Cushing disease, whereas low or undetectable levels indicate an adrenal or medication etiology. Other findings on diagnostic tests associated with, but not diagnostic of, Cushing syndrome include leukocytosis, lymphopenia, eosinopenia, hyperglycemia, glycosuria, hypercalciuria, and osteoporosis. Hypokalemia and alkalosis are seen in ectopic ACTH syndrome and adrenal carcinoma.

Interprofessional Care

The primary goal of treatment is to normalize hormone secretion. The specific treatment depends on the underlying cause (Table 49-14). If the underlying cause is a pituitary adenoma, the standard treatment is surgical removal of the pituitary tumor using the transsphenoidal approach.[23] (The transsphenoidal approach is discussed earlier in this chapter on p. 1158.) Radiation therapy is an option for patients who are not good surgical candidates.

Adrenalectomy is indicated for Cushing syndrome caused by adrenal tumors or hyperplasia. Occasionally, bilateral adrenalectomy is necessary. A laparoscopic approach is used unless a malignant adrenal tumor is suspected. An open surgical adrenalectomy is usually performed for adrenal cancer.

Patients with ectopic ACTH-secreting tumors are best managed by locating and removing the tumor (usually lung or pancreas). This is usually possible when the tumor is benign. When a tumor is malignant and it has already metastasized, surgical removal may not be possible or successful.

When the patient is a poor candidate for surgery or prior surgery has failed, then drug therapy may be attempted. The goal of drug therapy is to suppress the synthesis and secretion of cortisol from the adrenal gland (*medical adrenalectomy*). Drugs used include ketoconazole, aminoglutethimide, and mitotane. These are used cautiously because they are often toxic at the dosages needed to reduce cortisol secretion. Hydrocortisone or prednisone may be needed to avoid adrenal insufficiency. Mifepristone (Korlym) may be used to control hyperglycemia in patients with endogenous Cushing syndrome who have type 2 diabetes.

If Cushing syndrome has developed during the course of prolonged administration of corticosteroids (e.g., prednisone), the following alternatives may be tried: (1) gradually discontinuing corticosteroid therapy, (2) reducing the corticosteroid dose, and (3) converting to an alternate-day regimen. Gradual tapering of the corticosteroids is necessary to avoid potentially life-threatening adrenal insufficiency. In an alternate-day regimen, twice the daily dosage of a shorter-acting corticosteroid is given every other morning to minimize hypothalamic-pituitary-adrenal suppression, growth suppression, and altered appearance. This regimen is not used when the corticosteroids are given as hormone therapy.

TABLE 49-14   Interprofessional Care
Cushing Syndrome

Diagnostic Assessment
- History and physical examination
- Dexamethasone suppression test
- 24-hr urine for free cortisol and 17-ketosteroids
- Plasma and salivary cortisol levels
- Plasma ACTH levels
- Complete blood count (CBC) with WBC differential
- Blood chemistries for sodium, potassium, glucose
- CT scan, MRI

Management
Pituitary Adenoma
- Transsphenoidal resection
- Radiation therapy

Adrenocortical Adenoma, Carcinoma, or Hyperplasia
- Adrenalectomy (open or laparoscopic)
- Drug therapy (e.g., ketoconazole, aminoglutethimide, mitotane, mifepristone [Korlym])

Ectopic ACTH-Secreting Tumor
- Treatment of the tumor (surgical removal or radiation)

Exogenous Corticosteroid Therapy
- Discontinue or alter the dose of exogenous corticosteroids

❖ NURSING MANAGEMENT: CUSHING SYNDROME

◆ Nursing Assessment

Subjective and objective data that should be obtained from a patient with Cushing syndrome are presented in Table 49-15.

◆ Nursing Diagnoses

Nursing diagnoses for the patient with Cushing syndrome may include, but are not limited to, the following:
- Risk for infection *related to* lowered resistance to stress and suppression of immune system
- Risk for overweight *related to* increased appetite, high caloric content of foods, and inactivity

---

TABLE 49-15   Nursing Assessment
Cushing Syndrome

Subjective Data
Important Health Information
Past health history: Pituitary tumor (Cushing disease). Adrenal, pancreatic, or pulmonary neoplasms. GI bleeding, frequent infections
Medications: Corticosteroids

Functional Health Patterns
Health perception–health management: Malaise
Nutritional-metabolic: Weight gain, anorexia. Prolonged wound healing, easy bruising
Elimination: Polyuria
Activity-exercise: Weakness, fatigue
Sleep: Insomnia, poor sleep quality
Cognitive-perceptual: Headache. Back, joint, bone, and rib pain. Poor concentration and memory
Self-perception–self-concept: Negative feelings regarding changes in personal appearance
Sexuality-reproductive: Amenorrhea, impotence, decreased libido
Coping–stress tolerance: Anxiety, mood disturbances, emotional lability, psychosis

Objective Data
General
Truncal obesity, supraclavicular fat pads, buffalo hump, moon face

Integumentary
Plethora. Hirsutism of body and face, thinning of head hair. Thin, friable skin. Acne, petechiae, purpura, hyperpigmentation. Purplish red striae on breasts, buttocks, and abdomen. Edema of lower extremities

Cardiovascular
Hypertension

Musculoskeletal
Muscle wasting, thin extremities, awkward gait

Reproductive
Gynecomastia, testicular atrophy (in men), enlarged clitoris (in women)

Possible Diagnostic Findings
Hypokalemia, hyperglycemia, dyslipidemia, polycythemia, granulocytosis, lymphocytopenia, eosinopenia. ↑ plasma cortisol, ↑ salivary cortisol. High, low, or normal ACTH levels. Abnormal dexamethasone suppression test. ↑ Urine free cortisol, 17-ketosteroids. Glycosuria, hypercalciuria. Osteoporosis on x-ray

- Disturbed body image *related to* change in appearance from disease process
- Impaired skin integrity *related to* excess corticosteroids, immobility, and altered skin fragility

Additional information on nursing diagnoses is presented in eNursing Care Plan 49-3 for the patient with Cushing syndrome (available on the website for this chapter).

◆ Planning

The overall goals are that the patient with Cushing syndrome will (1) experience relief of symptoms, (2) avoid serious complications, (3) maintain a positive self-image, and (4) actively participate in the therapeutic plan.

◆ Nursing Implementation

◆ **Health Promotion.** Health promotion is focused on identifying patients at risk for Cushing syndrome. Patients receiving long-term, exogenous corticosteroids are at risk. Teaching related to using medications and monitoring side effects is an important preventive measure.

◆ **Acute Care.** The patient with Cushing syndrome is seriously ill. Because the therapy has many side effects, assessment focuses on signs and symptoms of hormone and drug toxicity and complicating conditions (e.g., cardiovascular disease, diabetes mellitus, infection). Monitor vital signs, daily weight, and glucose. Assess for possible infections. Because signs and symptoms of inflammation (e.g., fever, redness) may be minimal or absent, assess for pain, loss of function, and purulent drainage. Monitor for signs and symptoms of thromboembolic events such as pulmonary emboli (e.g., sudden chest pain, dyspnea, tachypnea).

Another important focus of nursing care is emotional support. Changes in appearance, such as truncal obesity, multiple bruises, hirsutism in women, and gynecomastia in men, can be distressing. The patient may feel unattractive, repulsive, or unwanted. You can help by remaining sensitive to the patient's feelings and offering respect and unconditional acceptance. Reassure the patient that the physical changes and much of the emotional lability will resolve when hormone levels return to normal.

If treatment involves surgical removal of a pituitary adenoma, an adrenal tumor, or one or both adrenal glands, nursing care will include preoperative and postoperative care.

◆ ***Preoperative Care.*** Before surgery the patient should be brought to optimal physical condition. Hypertension and hyperglycemia must be controlled. Hypokalemia must be corrected with diet and potassium supplements. A high-protein diet helps correct the protein depletion. Preoperative teaching depends on the type of surgical approach planned (hypophysectomy or adrenalectomy) and should include information regarding the anticipated postoperative care.

◆ ***Postoperative Care.*** Surgery on the adrenal glands poses great risks. Because the adrenal glands are vascular, the risk of hemorrhage is increased. In the postoperative period for both laparoscopic and open adrenalectomy, the patient may have a nasogastric tube, a urinary catheter, IV therapy, central venous pressure monitoring, and leg sequential compression devices to prevent emboli.

Manipulating glandular tissue during surgery may release large amounts of hormones into the circulation, producing marked fluctuations in the metabolic processes affected by these hormones. Postoperatively, BP, fluid balance, and electrolyte levels may be unstable due to these hormone fluctuations.

High doses of corticosteroids (e.g., hydrocortisone [Solu-Cortef]) are given IV during surgery and for several days afterward to ensure adequate responses to the stress of the procedure. If large amounts of endogenous hormone were released into the systemic circulation during surgery, the patient is likely to develop hypertension, increasing the risk of hemorrhage. High corticosteroid levels cause problems with glycemic control, increase susceptibility to infection, and delay wound healing.

The critical period for circulatory instability ranges from 24 to 48 hours after surgery. During this time you must constantly be alert for signs of corticosteroid imbalance. Report any rapid or significant changes in BP, respirations, or heart rate. Monitor fluid intake and output carefully and assess for potential imbalances. IV corticosteroids are given, and the dosage and flow rate are adjusted to the patient's clinical manifestations and fluid and electrolyte balance. Oral doses are given as tolerated. After IV corticosteroids are withdrawn, keep the IV line open for quick administration of corticosteroids or vasopressors. Obtain morning urine samples at the same time each morning for cortisol measurement to evaluate the surgery's effectiveness.

If corticosteroid dosage is tapered too rapidly after surgery, acute adrenal insufficiency may develop. Vomiting, increased weakness, dehydration, and hypotension are signs of hypocortisolism. In addition, the patient may complain of painful joints, pruritus, or peeling skin and may experience severe emotional disturbances. Report these signs and symptoms so that drug doses can be adjusted as necessary.

The patient is usually maintained on bed rest until the BP stabilizes. Be alert for subtle signs of postoperative infection because the usual inflammatory responses are suppressed. To prevent infection, provide meticulous care when changing the dressing and during any other procedures that involve access to body cavities, circulation, or areas under the skin.

◆ **Ambulatory Care.** Discharge instructions are based on the patient's lack of endogenous corticosteroids and resulting inability to react physiologically to stressors. Consider a home health nurse referral, especially for older adults, because of the need for ongoing evaluation and teaching. Instruct the patient to wear a Medic Alert bracelet at all times and carry medical identification and instructions in a wallet or purse. Teach the patient to avoid exposure to extreme temperatures, infections, and emotional disturbances. Stress may produce or precipitate acute adrenal insufficiency because the remaining adrenal tissue cannot meet an increased hormonal demand. Teach patients to adjust their corticosteroid replacement therapy in accordance with their stress levels. Consult with the patient's HCP to determine the parameters for dosage changes if this plan is feasible. If the patient cannot adjust his or her own medication or if weakness, fainting, fever, or nausea and vomiting occur, the patient should contact the HCP for a possible adjustment in corticosteroid dosage. Many patients require lifetime replacement therapy. However, patients should be prepared for it to take several months to adjust the hormone dose satisfactorily.

◆ Evaluation

The expected outcomes are that the patient with Cushing syndrome will

- Experience no signs or symptoms of infection
- Maintain weight appropriate for height
- Verbalize acceptance of appearance and treatment regimen
- Demonstrate healing of skin and maintenance of intact skin

Additional information on expected outcomes is presented in eNursing Care Plan 49-3 for the patient with Cushing syndrome (available on the website for this chapter).

ADRENOCORTICAL INSUFFICIENCY

Etiology and Pathophysiology

Adrenocortical insufficiency (hypofunction of the adrenal cortex) may be from a primary cause (Addison's disease) or a secondary cause (lack of pituitary ACTH secretion). In Addison's disease, all three classes of adrenal corticosteroids (glucocorticoids, mineralocorticoids, and androgens) are reduced. In secondary adrenocortical insufficiency, corticosteroids and androgens are deficient, but mineralocorticoids rarely are. ACTH deficiency may be caused by pituitary disease or suppression of the hypothalamic-pituitary axis because of the administration of exogenous corticosteroids.

Up to 80% of Addison's disease cases in the United States are caused by an autoimmune response.[24] Autoimmune adrenalitis causes the adrenal cortex to be destroyed by antibodies. This results in loss of glucocorticoid, mineralocorticoid, and adrenal androgen hormones. Addison's disease can be present along with other endocrine conditions. This is known as *autoimmune polyglandular syndrome*. It is most common in white females. Those with autoimmune adrenalitis often have other autoimmune disorders such as type 1 diabetes, autoimmune thyroid disease, pernicious anemia, and celiac disease.[25]

Although tuberculosis causes Addison's disease worldwide, it is now an uncommon cause in the United States. Other causes include amyloidosis, fungal infections (e.g., histoplasmosis), acquired immunodeficiency syndrome (AIDS), and metastatic cancer. Iatrogenic Addison's disease may be due to adrenal hemorrhage, often related to anticoagulant therapy, chemotherapy, ketoconazole therapy for AIDS, or bilateral adrenalectomy. Adrenal insufficiency most often occurs in adults younger than 60 years of age and affects both genders equally.

Clinical Manifestations

Because manifestations do not tend to become evident until 90% of the adrenal cortex is destroyed, the disease is often advanced before it is diagnosed. The manifestations have a slow (insidious) onset and include anorexia, nausea, progressive weakness, fatigue, and weight loss. Increased ACTH causes the striking feature of a bronze-colored skin hyperpigmentation. It is seen primarily in sun-exposed areas of the body; at pressure points; over joints; and in the creases, especially palmar creases (Fig. 49-13). The changes in the skin are most

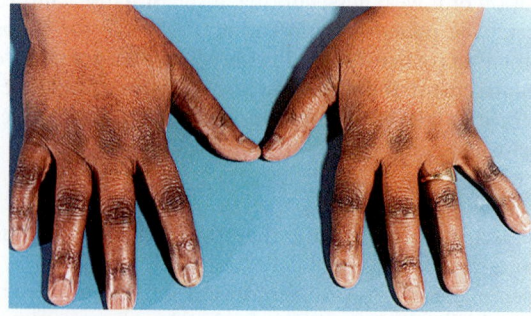

FIG. 49-13 Hyperpigmentation typically seen in Addison's disease. (From Chew SL, Leslie D: *Clinical endocrinology and diabetes: an illustrated colour text,* Edinburgh, 2006, Churchill Livingstone.)

likely due to increased secretion of β-lipotropin (which contains melanocyte-stimulating hormone [MSH]). This tropic hormone is increased because of decreased negative feedback and subsequent low corticosteroid levels. Other manifestations include abdominal pain, diarrhea, headache, orthostatic hypotension, salt craving, and joint pain. Irritability and depression may occur in primary adrenal hypofunction.

Patients with secondary adrenocortical hypofunction may have many signs and symptoms similar to those of patients with Addison's disease. However, they usually do not have hyperpigmented skin because ACTH levels are low.

Complications

Patients with adrenocortical insufficiency are at risk for acute adrenal insufficiency *(addisonian crisis),* a life-threatening emergency caused by insufficient adrenocortical hormones or a sudden sharp decrease in these hormones. Addisonian crisis is triggered by (1) stress (e.g., from infection, surgery, psychologic distress), (2) the sudden withdrawal of corticosteroid hormone therapy (which is often done by a patient who lacks knowledge of the importance of this therapy), (3) adrenal surgery, or (4) sudden pituitary gland destruction.

During acute adrenal insufficiency, the patient exhibits severe manifestations of glucocorticoid and mineralocorticoid deficiencies, including hypotension, tachycardia, dehydration, hyponatremia, hyperkalemia, hypoglycemia, fever, weakness, and confusion. Hypotension may lead to shock. Circulatory collapse associated with adrenal insufficiency is often unresponsive to the usual treatment (vasopressors and fluid replacement). GI manifestations include severe vomiting, diarrhea, and pain in the abdomen. Pain may occur in the lower back and legs.

Diagnostic Studies

The ACTH stimulation test is a common test to diagnose adrenal insufficiency. Baseline cortisol and ACTH levels are measured, and the patient is given an IV injection of synthetic ACTH (cosyntropin). Cortisol and ACTH levels are rechecked after 30 and 60 minutes. The normal response is a rise in blood cortisol levels. People with Addison's disease have little or no increase in cortisol levels. Those with primary adrenal insufficiency have a high ACTH level.[24]

When the response to the ACTH test is abnormal, a corticotropin-releasing hormone (CRH) stimulation test may be done. The patient is given an IV injection of synthetic CRH, and blood is taken after 30 and 60 minutes. Those with Addison's disease have high ACTH levels but no cortisol. People with secondary adrenal insufficiency due to pituitary or hypothalamus problems do not produce ACTH or have a delayed response.[25]

Other abnormal laboratory findings may include hyperkalemia, hypochloremia, hyponatremia, hypoglycemia, anemia, and increased BUN levels.[25] An ECG may show low voltage and peaked T waves caused by hyperkalemia. CT scans and MRI can identify causes other than autoimmune, including tumors, fungal infections, tuberculosis, or adrenal calcification.

Interprofessional Care

Treatment of adrenocortical insufficiency focuses on managing the underlying cause when possible. The mainstay is lifelong hormone therapy with glucocorticoids and mineralocorticoids (Table 49-16). Overall, patients who take their medications consistently can anticipate a normal life expectancy. Hydrocortisone,

TABLE 49-16	Interprofessional Care

Addison's Disease

Diagnostic Assessment
- History and physical examination
- ACTH stimulation test
- Serum cortisol and ACTH
- Urine cortisol and aldosterone
- CRH suppression test
- Serum electrolytes
- CT scan, MRI

Management
- Daily glucocorticoid (e.g., prednisone, hydrocortisone) replacement (two thirds on awakening in morning, one third in late afternoon)
- Daily mineralocorticoid (fludrocortisone) in morning
- Increased salt in the diet
- Androgen replacement with dehydroepiandrosterone (DHEA) for women
- Salt additives for excess heat or humidity
- Increased doses of glucocorticoid for stress situations (e.g., surgery, hospitalization)

TABLE 49-17	Patient & Caregiver Teaching

Addison's Disease

Include the following information in the teaching plan for patient with Addison's disease and the caregiver.
1. Names, dosages, and actions of drugs
2. Symptoms of overdosage and underdosage
3. Conditions requiring increased medication (e.g., trauma, infection, surgery, emotional crisis)
4. Course of action to take related to changes in medication
   - Increase in dose of corticosteroid
   - Administration of large dose of corticosteroid IM, including demonstration and return demonstration
   - Consultation with HCP
5. Prevention of infection and need for prompt and vigorous treatment of existing infections
6. Need for lifelong replacement therapy
7. Need for lifelong medical supervision
8. Need to carry medical identification
9. Prevention of falls
10. Adverse effects of corticosteroid therapy and prevention techniques
11. Special instruction for patients who are diabetics and management of blood glucose when taking corticosteroids

the most commonly used form of hormone therapy, has both glucocorticoid and mineralocorticoid properties. The dosage is increased in stressful situations to prevent addisonian crisis. Mineralocorticoids are replaced with fludrocortisone. Women need androgen replacement with dehydroepiandrosterone (DHEA) as their only source of androgen production is the adrenal glands.[25] Increased salt is added to the diet.

Addisonian crisis is a life-threatening emergency requiring aggressive management. Treatment is directed toward shock management and high-dose hydrocortisone replacement. Large volumes of 0.9% saline solution and 5% dextrose are given to reverse hypotension and electrolyte imbalances until BP returns to normal.

❖ NURSING MANAGEMENT: ADDISON'S DISEASE

◆ Nursing Implementation

◆ **Acute Care.** When the patient with Addison's disease is hospitalized, nursing management focuses on monitoring the patient while correcting fluid and electrolyte balance. Assess vital signs and neurologic status. Monitor for signs of fluid volume deficit and electrolyte imbalance. Obtain a daily weight and keep an accurate intake and output record. Take a complete medication history to determine drugs that can potentially interact with corticosteroids. These drugs include oral hypoglycemics, cardiac glycosides, oral contraceptives, anticoagulants, and NSAIDs.

Note changes in BP, weight gain, weakness, or other manifestations of Cushing syndrome. Guard the patient against exposure to infection and assist with daily hygiene. Protect the patient from noise, light, and environmental temperature extremes. The patient cannot cope with these stresses because of the inability to produce corticosteroids.

◆ **Ambulatory Care.** As a nurse, you have an important role in the long-term management of Addison's disease. The serious nature of the disease and the need for lifelong hormone therapy necessitate a comprehensive teaching plan. Table 49-17 outlines the major areas to include in a teaching plan.

Glucocorticoids are usually given in divided doses, two thirds in the morning and one third in the afternoon. Mineralocorticoids are given once daily, preferably in the morning. This schedule reflects normal circadian rhythm in endogenous hormone secretion and decreases the side effects associated with corticosteroid therapy. Teach patients using mineralocorticoid therapy (fludrocortisone) how to take their BP, increase salt intake, and report any significant changes to their HCP.

The patient with Addison's disease is unable to tolerate physical or emotional stress without additional exogenous corticosteroids. Long-term care revolves around recognizing the need for extra medication and techniques for stress management. Examples of situations requiring corticosteroid adjustment are fever, influenza, tooth extraction, and rigorous physical activity such as playing tennis on a hot day or distance running. Provide written and verbal instructions on when to change the dose. If vomiting or diarrhea occurs, as may happen with gastroenteritis, the patient should notify the HCP immediately, because electrolyte replacement and parenteral administration of cortisol may be necessary.

Teach patients the signs and symptoms of corticosteroid deficiency and excess (Cushing syndrome) and to report these signs to their HCP so that the drug dose can be adjusted. It is critical that the patient wear an identification bracelet (Medic Alert) and carry a wallet card stating the patient has Addison's disease so that appropriate therapy can be started in case of an emergency. The patient should carry an emergency kit at all times with 100 mg of IM hydrocortisone, syringes, and instructions for use. Teach the patient, caregiver, and significant others how to give an IM injection.

CORTICOSTEROID THERAPY

Corticosteroids are effective in treating many diseases and disorders (Table 49-18). However, the long-term administration of corticosteroids at therapeutic doses often leads to serious complications and side effects (Table 49-19). For this reason, corticosteroid therapy is not recommended for minor chronic conditions. Therapy should be reserved for diseases that have a risk of death or permanent loss of function and for conditions in which short-term therapy is likely to produce remission or

TABLE 49-18 Drug Therapy
Diseases/Disorders Treated With Corticosteroids

Hormone Therapy
- Adrenal insufficiency
- Congenital adrenal hyperplasia

Therapeutic Effect
Allergic Reactions
- Anaphylaxis
- Bee stings
- Contact dermatitis
- Drug reactions
- Serum sickness
- Urticaria

Connective Tissue Diseases
- Mixed connective tissue disorders
- Polymyositis
- Polyarteritis nodosa
- Rheumatoid arthritis
- Systemic lupus erythematosus

Neurologic Diseases
- Prevention of cerebral edema and increased intracranial pressure
- Head trauma

Gastrointestinal Diseases
- Inflammatory bowel disease
- Celiac disease

Endocrine Diseases
- Hypercalcemia
- Hashimoto's thyroiditis
- Thyrotoxicosis

Liver Diseases
- Alcoholic hepatitis
- Autoimmune hepatitis

Pulmonary Diseases
- Aspiration pneumonia
- Asthma
- Chronic obstructive pulmonary disease

Other Diseases or Disorders
- Skin diseases
- Cancer, leukemia, lymphoma
- Immunosuppression
- Inflammation
- Nephrotic syndrome

TABLE 49-19 Drug Therapy
Effects and Side Effects of Corticosteroids

- Hypokalemia may develop.
- Patient is predisposed to peptic ulcer disease.
- Skeletal muscle atrophy and weakness occur.
- Mood and behavior changes may be observed.
- Glucose intolerance predisposes patient to diabetes mellitus.
- Fat from extremities is redistributed to trunk and face.
- Hypocalcemia related to anti–vitamin D effect may occur.
- Healing is delayed, with increased risk for wound dehiscence.
- Susceptibility to infection is increased. Infection develops more rapidly and spreads more widely.
- Manifestations of inflammation, including redness, tenderness, heat, swelling, and local edema, are suppressed.
- Pituitary ACTH synthesis is suppressed. Corticosteroid deficiency is likely if hormones are withdrawn abruptly. Taper corticosteroid doses.
- BP increases because of excess blood volume and potentiation of vasoconstrictor effects. Hypertension predisposes patient to heart failure.
- Protein depletion decreases bone formation, density, and strength, leading to predisposition to pathologic fractures, especially compression fractures of the vertebrae (osteoporosis).

CHECK YOUR PRACTICE

You are working in the outpatient clinic. Your 39-yr-old female patient is experiencing Cushing syndrome secondary to high doses of prednisone use for her severe systemic lupus erythematosus. At her office visit today, she tells you, "I looked in the mirror this morning and did not recognize the fat, ugly woman looking back at me."
- How would you respond to her?

recovery. The potential benefits of treatment must always be weighed against the risks.

A beneficial effect of corticosteroids in one situation may be a harmful one in another. For example, decreasing inflammation in arthritis is an important therapeutic effect, but increasing the risk for infection is a harmful effect. Suppressing inflammation and the immune response may help save lives in persons with anaphylaxis and in those receiving an organ transplant, but it can reactivate latent tuberculosis and greatly reduce resistance to other infections and cancers. The vasopressive effect of corticosteroids is critical in enabling a person to function in stressful situations but can produce hypertension when used for drug therapy.

DRUG ALERT Corticosteroids
- Teach the patient not to abruptly discontinue these drugs.
- Monitor the patient for signs of infection.
- Have patients with diabetes closely monitor blood glucose.

Patients receive corticosteroid therapy for many reasons. Detailed instruction is necessary to ensure patient adherence. When corticosteroids are used as nonreplacement therapies, they are taken once daily or once every other day. They should be taken early in the morning with food to decrease gastric irritation. Because exogenous corticosteroid administration may suppress endogenous ACTH and therefore endogenous cortisol (suppression is time and dose dependent), emphasize the danger of abruptly stopping corticosteroid therapy to patients and caregivers. Corticosteroids taken for longer than 1 week will suppress adrenal production, and oral corticosteroids must be tapered. Ensure that increased doses of corticosteroids are prescribed in acute care or home care settings in situations of physical or emotional stress.

Corticosteroid-induced osteoporosis is an important concern for patients who receive corticosteroid treatment for prolonged periods (longer than 3 months).[26] Therapies to reduce bone resorption may include increased calcium intake, vitamin D supplementation, bisphosphonates (e.g., alendronate), and a low-impact exercise program. Further instruction and interventions to minimize the side effects and complications of corticosteroid therapy are outlined in Table 49-20.

HYPERALDOSTERONISM

Hyperaldosteronism (Conn's syndrome) is characterized by excessive aldosterone secretion. The main effects of aldosterone are (1) sodium retention and (2) potassium and hydrogen ion excretion. Thus the hallmark of this disease is hypertension with hypokalemic alkalosis. *Primary hyperaldosteronism* (PA) is most commonly caused by a small solitary adrenocortical adenoma. Occasionally multiple lesions are involved and are associated with bilateral adrenal hyperplasia.

PA affects women more than men and usually occurs between 30 and 50 years of age. A genetic link has been identified in some patients.[27] Up to 2% of all cases of hypertension are caused by PA. *Secondary hyperaldosteronism* occurs in response to a nonadrenal cause of elevated aldosterone levels such as renal artery stenosis, renin-secreting tumors, and chronic kidney disease.

Elevated aldosterone levels are associated with sodium retention and potassium excretion. Sodium retention leads to hypernatremia, hypertension, and headache. Edema does not usually occur because the rate of sodium excretion increases, which

TABLE 49-20 Patient & Caregiver Teaching

Corticosteroid Therapy

Include the following instructions when teaching the patient and caregiver to manage corticosteroid therapy.

1. Plan a diet high in protein, calcium (at least 1500 mg/day), and potassium and low in fat and concentrated simple carbohydrates, such as sugar, honey, syrups, and candy.
2. Identify measures to ensure adequate rest and sleep, such as daily naps and avoiding caffeine late in the day.
3. Develop and maintain an exercise program to help maintain bone integrity.
4. Recognize edema and ways to restrict sodium intake to <2000 mg/day if edema occurs.
5. Monitor glucose levels and recognize symptoms of hyperglycemia (e.g., polydipsia, polyuria, blurred vision). Report hyperglycemic symptoms or capillary glucose levels >120 mg/dL (10 mmol/L).
6. Notify HCP if experiencing heartburn after meals or epigastric pain that is not relieved by antacids.
7. See an eye specialist yearly to assess for cataracts.
8. Use safety measures such as getting up slowly from bed or a chair and use good lighting to avoid accidental injury.
9. Maintain good hygiene practices and avoid contact with persons with colds or other contagious illnesses to prevent infection.
10. Inform all HCPs about long-term corticosteroid use.
11. Recognize need for increased doses of corticosteroids in times of physical and emotional stress.
12. Never abruptly stop the corticosteroids because this could lead to addisonian crisis and possibly death.

prevents more severe sodium retention. Potassium wasting leads to hypokalemia, which causes generalized muscle weakness, fatigue, cardiac dysrhythmias, glucose intolerance, and metabolic alkalosis that may lead to tetany.

Hyperaldosteronism should be suspected in hypertensive patients with hypokalemia who are not being treated with diuretics. PA is associated with elevated plasma aldosterone levels, elevated sodium levels, decreased serum potassium levels, and decreased plasma renin activity. A CT scan or MRI can detect an adenoma.[27] If a tumor is not found, plasma 18-hydroxycorticosterone is measured after overnight bed rest. A level greater than 50 ng/dL indicates an adenoma.

❖ NURSING AND INTERPROFESSIONAL MANAGEMENT: PRIMARY HYPERALDOSTERONISM

The preferred treatment for PA is surgical removal of the adenoma (adrenalectomy). A laparoscopic approach is most often used. Before surgery, patients should be treated with potassium-sparing diuretics (spironolactone [Aldactone], eplerenone [Inspra]) and antihypertensive agents to normalize serum potassium levels and BP. Spironolactone and eplerenone block the binding of aldosterone to the mineralocorticoid receptor in the terminal distal tubules and collecting ducts of the kidney, thus increasing sodium and water excretion and potassium retention. Oral potassium supplements and sodium restrictions may be necessary. However, potassium supplementation and a potassium-sparing diuretic should not be started simultaneously because of the danger of hyperkalemia. Teach patients taking eplerenone to avoid grapefruit juice as it may increase potential for hyperkalemia.

Patients with bilateral adrenal hyperplasia are treated with a potassium-sparing diuretic (e.g., spironolactone) or aminoglutethimide, which blocks aldosterone synthesis. Calcium channel blockers may be used to control BP. Dexamethasone may be used to decrease adrenal hyperplasia.

Nursing care includes careful assessment of fluid and electrolyte balance (especially potassium) and cardiovascular status. Monitor BP frequently before and after surgery because unilateral adrenalectomy is successful in controlling hypertension in only 80% of patients with an adenoma. Tell patients receiving spironolactone about the possible side effects of gynecomastia, impotence, and menstrual disorders, as well as the signs and symptoms of hypokalemia and hyperkalemia. Teach patients how to monitor their own BP and the need for frequent monitoring. Stress the need for continued health supervision.

◼ DISORDERS OF ADRENAL MEDULLA

PHEOCHROMOCYTOMA

Pheochromocytoma is a rare condition caused by a tumor in the adrenal medulla. It affects the chromaffin cells, resulting in an excess production of catecholamines (epinephrine, norepinephrine). The most dangerous immediate effect of the disease is severe hypertension. If left untreated, it may lead to encephalopathy, diabetes mellitus, cardiomyopathy, multiple organ failure, and death. It is most commonly seen in young to middle-aged adults. Pheochromocytoma may be inherited in persons with multiple endocrine neoplasia.[28]

The most striking clinical features of pheochromocytoma are severe, episodic hypertension accompanied by severe, pounding headache; tachycardia with palpitations; profuse sweating; and unexplained abdominal or chest pain. Attacks can be induced by direct trauma, mechanical pressure to the tumor, stress (e.g., surgery, exercise, defecation, sexual intercourse, alcohol consumption, smoking), or many medications, including antihypertensives, opioids, radiologic contrast media, and tricyclic antidepressants. Attacks can last from a few minutes to several hours.

The simplest and most reliable diagnostic test for pheochromocytoma is measurement of urinary fractionated metanephrines (catecholamine metabolites) and fractionated catecholamines and creatinine, usually done as a 24-hour urine collection. Values are elevated in at least 95% of persons with pheochromocytoma. Serum catecholamines may be elevated during an "attack." CT scans and MRI can detect tumors. Avoid palpating the abdomen of a patient with suspected pheochromocytoma, since it may cause the sudden release of catecholamines and severe hypertension.

❖ NURSING AND INTERPROFESSIONAL MANAGEMENT: PHEOCHROMOCYTOMA

The primary treatment is surgical removal of the tumor. Treatment with α- and β-adrenergic receptor blockers is required preoperatively to control BP and prevent an intraoperative hypertensive crisis. Therapy begins with an α-adrenergic receptor blocker (e.g., doxazosin, prazosin, phenoxybenzamine) 10 to 14 days preoperatively to reduce BP.[28] After adequate α-adrenergic blockade, β-adrenergic receptor blockers (e.g., propranolol) are used to decrease tachycardia and dysrhythmias. If β-blockers are started too early, unopposed α-adrenergic stimulation can precipitate a hypertensive crisis. Therapy can cause orthostatic hypotension. Advise the patient to make postural changes cautiously.

Surgery is usually done using a laparoscopic approach. Removing the adrenal tumor usually cures the hypertension, but hypertension persists in about 10% to 30% of patients. If surgery is not an option, metyrosine (Demser) is used to decrease catecholamine production by the tumor.

Case finding is an important nursing role. Although pheochromocytoma is associated with a number of symptoms, the diagnosis is often missed. Any patient with hypertension accompanied by symptoms of sympathoadrenal stimulation should be referred to an HCP for definitive diagnosis. Assess the patient for the classic triad of symptoms of pheochromocytoma: severe pounding headache, tachycardia, and profuse sweating. Monitor the BP immediately if the patient is experiencing an "attack."

Make the patient as comfortable as possible. Monitor blood glucose levels to assess for diabetes mellitus. Patients need rest, nourishing food, and emotional support during this period. Preoperative and postoperative care is similar to that for any patient undergoing adrenalectomy. Note that BP fluctuations from catecholamine excesses tend to be severe and must be carefully monitored. Emphasize the importance of follow-up and routine BP monitoring because hypertension may persist even when the tumor is removed.

CASE STUDY

Graves' Disease

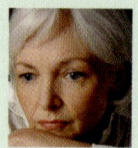

(©Hemera Technologies/ AbleStock.com/ Thinkstock)

Patient Profile

R.D., a 52-yr-old white woman, was admitted to the hospital with a high fever. Unable to find a source of infection, the HCP does an endocrine workup. R.D. is diagnosed with Graves' disease.

Subjective Data

- Reports recent job loss because she is no longer able to tolerate work-related stress
- Reports symptoms including fatigue, unintentional weight loss, insomnia, palpitations, and heat intolerance

Objective Data

Physical Examination

- Fever of 104°F (40°C)
- BP of 150/80 mm Hg, pulse of 116 beats/min, and respiratory rate of 26 breaths/min
- Hot, moist skin
- Fine tremors of the hands
- 4+ deep tendon reflexes and muscle strength of 1 to 2 out of 5

Interprofessional Care

- Subtotal thyroidectomy planned for 2 months later
- Started on methimazole and propranolol (Inderal LA)

Discussion Questions

1. What is the etiology of R.D.'s symptoms?
2. What diagnostic studies were probably ordered? What would the results have been to establish the diagnosis of Graves' disease?
3. Why was surgery delayed?
4. *Teamwork and Collaboration:* What is the interprofessional team's top priority at this time for R.D.?
5. *Quality Care:* What is the expected outcome associated with drug therapy?
6. *Priority Decision:* What are her priority teaching needs at this time?
7. *Patient-Centered Care:* What teaching will you provide after surgery so that R.D. can successfully self-manage her care?
8. *Priority Decision:* Based on the assessment data presented, what are the priority nursing diagnoses pertinent to this patient while hospitalized? Are there any collaborative problems?
9. *Evidence-Based Practice:* Why is R.D. counseled to give up her long-standing cigarette smoking habit?

Answers available at *http://evolve.elsevier.com/Lewis/medsurg*.

BRIDGE TO NCLEX EXAMINATION

The number of the question corresponds to the same-numbered outcome at the beginning of the chapter.

1. After a hypophysectomy for acromegaly, immediate postoperative nursing care should focus on
   a. frequent monitoring of serum and urine osmolarity.
   b. parenteral administration of a GH-receptor antagonist.
   c. keeping the patient in a recumbent position at all times.
   d. patient teaching regarding the need for lifelong hormone therapy.

2. A patient with a head injury develops SIADH. Manifestations the nurse would expect to find include
   a. hypernatremia and edema.
   b. muscle spasticity and hypertension.
   c. low urine output and hyponatremia.
   d. weight gain and decreased glomerular filtration rate.

3. The health care provider prescribes levothyroxine for a patient with hypothyroidism. After teaching regarding this drug, the nurse determines that further instruction is needed when the patient says
   a. "I can expect the medication dose may need to be adjusted."
   b. "I only need to take this drug until my symptoms are improved."
   c. "I can expect to return to normal function with the use of this drug."
   d. "I will report any chest pain or difficulty breathing to the doctor right away."

4. After thyroid surgery, the nurse suspects damage or removal of the parathyroid glands when the patient develops
   a. muscle weakness and weight loss.
   b. hyperthermia and severe tachycardia.
   c. hypertension and difficulty swallowing.
   d. laryngospasms and tingling in the hands and feet.

5. Important nursing intervention(s) when caring for a patient with Cushing syndrome include (*select all that apply*)
   a. restricting protein intake.
   b. monitoring blood glucose levels.
   c. observing for signs of hypotension.
   d. administering medication in equal doses.
   e. protecting patient from exposure to infection.

6. An important preoperative nursing intervention before an adrenalectomy for hyperaldosteronism is to
   a. monitor blood glucose levels.
   b. restrict fluid and sodium intake.
   c. administer potassium-sparing diuretics.
   d. advise the patient to make postural changes slowly.

7. To control the side effects of corticosteroid therapy, the nurse teaches the patient who is taking corticosteroids to
   a. increase calcium intake to 1500 mg/day.
   b. perform glucose monitoring for hypoglycemia.
   c. obtain immunizations due to high risk of infections.
   d. avoid abrupt position changes because of orthostatic hypotension.

8. The nurse teaches the patient that the *best* time to take corticosteroids for replacement purposes is
   a. once a day at bedtime.
   b. every other day on awakening.
   c. on arising and in the late afternoon.
   d. at consistent intervals every 6 to 8 hours.

1. a, 2. c, 3. b, 4. d, 5. b, e, 6. c, 7. a, 8. c

For rationales to these answers and even more NCLEX review questions, visit *http://evolve.elsevier.com/Lewis/medsurg*.

EVOLVE WEBSITE

REFERENCES

1. Kopczak A, Ulrich R, Günter KS: Advances in understanding pituitary tumors, *F1000Prime Reports* 6:2014.
2. Acromegaly. Retrieved from *www.niddk.nih.gov/health-information/health-topics/endocrine/acromegaly/Pages/fact-sheet.aspx*.
3. American Diabetes Association: Diagnosis and classification of diabetes mellitus, *Diabetes Care* 37:S81, 2014.
4. About acromegaly. Retrieved from *http://acromegaly.org/en/about/about-acromegaly*.
*5. Sarkar S, Rajaratnam S, Chacko G, et al: Endocrinological outcomes following endoscopic and microscopic transsphenoidal surgery in 113 patients with acromegaly, *Clin Neurol Neurosurg* 126:190, 2014.
*6. Brandon A, Miller A, Ioachimescu N, et al: Contemporary indications for transsphenoidal pituitary surgery, *World Neurosurg* 82:S147, 2014.
*7. Gittleman H, Ostrom Q, Farah P, et al: Descriptive epidemiology of pituitary tumors in the United States 2004-2009, *J Neurosurg* 121:527, 2014.
*8. Thomas J, Gadgil N, Samson S, et al: Prospective trial of a short hospital stay protocol after endoscopic endonasal pituitary adenoma surgery, *World Neurosurg* 81:576, 2014.
9. Braun M, Barstow C, Pyzocha N: Diagnosis and management of sodium disorders: hyponatremia and hypernatremia, *Am Fam Physician* 91:299, 2015.

*10. Zimmermann M, Boelaert K: Iodine deficiency and thyroid disorders, *Lancet Diabetes Endocrinol* 3:286, 2015.
11. Sweeney L, Stewart C, Gaitonde D: Thyroiditis: an integrated approach, *Am Fam Physician* 90:389, 2014.
*12. Lee S, Chang D, He X, et al: Urinary iodine excretion and serum thyroid function in adults after iodinated contrast administration, *Thyroid* 25:471, 2015.
13. Vaidya B, Pearce SH: Diagnosis and management of thyrotoxicosis, *BMJ* 349:5128, 2014.
*14. Chiha M: Thyroid storm: an updated review, *J Intens Care Med* 30:131, 2015.
*15. Orosco RK, Lin HW, Bhattacharyya N: Ambulatory thyroidectomy: a multistate study of revisits and complications, *Otolaryngol Head Neck Surg* 152:1017, 2015.
16. Nygaard B: Primary hypothyroidism, *Am Fam Physician* 91:359, 2015.
*17. Fliers E, Bianco A, Langouche L, et al: Endocrine and metabolic considerations in critically ill patients: thyroid function in critically ill patients, *Lancet*. Online June 11, 2015.
*18. Screening for thyroid disease: systematic evidence review. Retrieved from *www.ahrq.gov/clinic*.
19. Thyroid cancer. Retrieved from *www.cancer.org*.
20. Multiple endocrine neoplasia. Retrieved from *ghr.nlm.nih.gov/condition/multiple-endocrine-neoplasia*.
21. Michels T, Kelly K: Parathyroid disorders, *Am Fam Physician* 88:249, 2013.
*22. Lacroix A, Feelders R, Stratakis C, et al: Cushing's syndrome, *Lancet* 386:913, 2015.
*23. Raff H, Carroll T: Cushing's syndrome: from physiological principles to diagnosis and clinical care, *J Physiol* 593:493, 2015.
24. Michels A, Michels N: Addison disease: early detection and treatment principles, *Am Fam Physician* 89:563, 2014.
25. Addison's disease: adrenal insufficiency. Retrieved from *www.niddk.nih.gov/health-information/health-topics/endocrine/adrenal-insufficiency-addisons-disease/Pages/fact-sheet.aspx*.
26. Treating corticosteroid-induced bone loss. Retrieved from *www.arthritis.org/living-with-arthritis/treatments/medication/drug-types/corticosteroids/osteoporosis-bone-loss.php*.
27. Galati SJ: Primary aldosteronism: challenges in diagnosis and management, *Endocrinol Metab Clin North Am* 44:355, 2015.
28. Ahmed I, Jepegnanam C: Recognition and management of pheochromocytoma, *Anaesth Intens Care* 15:465, 2014.

*Evidence-based information for clinical practice.

50

Assessment of Reproductive System

Kim K. Choma

Happiness is not being pained in body or troubled in mind.

Thomas Jefferson

ⓔ http://evolve.elsevier.com/Lewis/medsurg/

LEARNING OUTCOMES

1. Describe the structures and functions of the male and female reproductive systems.
2. Summarize the functions of the major hormones essential for the functioning of the male and female reproductive systems.
3. Explain the physiologic changes during the stages of sexual response for both a man and a woman.
4. Link the age-related changes of the male and female reproductive systems to the differences in assessment findings.
5. Obtain significant subjective and objective data related to the male and female reproductive systems and information about sexual function from a patient.
6. Perform a physical assessment of the male and female reproductive systems using the appropriate techniques.
7. Differentiate normal from common abnormal findings of a physical assessment of the male and female reproductive systems.
8. Describe the purpose, significance of results, and nursing responsibilities related to diagnostic studies of the male and female reproductive systems.

KEY TERMS

amenorrhea, p. 1190
clitoris, p. 1187
ductus deferens, p. 1184
dyspareunia, p. 1194

epididymis, p. 1184
gonads, p. 1184
menarche, p. 1189
menopause, p. 1190

menstrual cycle, p. 1189
mons pubis, p. 1187
nulliparous, p. 1186
spermatogenesis, p. 1184

STRUCTURES AND FUNCTIONS OF MALE AND FEMALE REPRODUCTIVE SYSTEMS

The reproductive systems of males and females consist of primary (or essential) organs and secondary (or accessory) organs. The primary reproductive organs are referred to as gonads. The female gonads are the ovaries; the male gonads are the testes. The main purpose of the gonads is secretion of hormones and production of gametes (ova and sperm, sex cells that unite during fertilization to form a new cell called a *zygote*). Secondary (or accessory) organs begin their maturity at puberty under the influence of sex hormones and are responsible for (1) transporting and nourishing the ova (eggs) and sperm and (2) preserving and protecting the fertilized ova. Secondary (accessory) organs are discussed in the male and female reproductive portions of this chapter.

Male Reproductive System

The three primary roles of the male reproductive system are (1) production and transportation of sperm, (2) deposition of sperm in the female reproductive tract, and (3) secretion of hormones. The primary male reproductive organs are the testes. Secondary reproductive organs include ducts (epididymis, ductus deferens, ejaculatory duct, and urethra), sex glands

(prostate gland, Cowper's glands, and seminal vesicles), and the external genitalia (scrotum and penis)[1] (Fig. 50-1).

Testes. The paired testes are ovoid, smooth, firm organs measuring 1.4 to 2.2 in (3.5 to 5.6 cm) long and 0.8 to 1.2 in (2 to 3 cm) wide. They are within the scrotum, which is a loose protective sac composed of a thin outer layer of skin over a tough connective tissue layer. Within the testes, coiled structures known as seminiferous tubules form *spermatozoa* (immature sperm). The process of sperm production is called spermatogenesis. Interstitial cells of the testes lie between the seminiferous tubules and produce the male sex hormone testosterone.

Ducts. Sperm formed in the seminiferous tubules move through a series of ducts. These ducts transport sperm from the testes to the outside of the body. As sperm exit the testes, they enter and pass through the epididymis, ductus deferens, ejaculatory duct, and urethra.

The epididymis is a comma-shaped structure located on the posterosuperior aspect of each testis within the scrotum (see Figs. 50-1 and 50-2). It is a long, tightly coiled structure that measures about 20 ft in length.[1] The epididymis transports sperm as they mature. Sperm exit the epididymis through a long, thick tube known as the ductus deferens.

The ductus deferens (also known as the *vas deferens*) is continuous with the epididymis within the scrotal sac. It travels

Reviewed by Courtney Reinisch, RN, DNP, APN-BC, DCC, Clinical Associate Professor, Doctoral Candidate, School of Nursing, Rutgers University, Newark, New Jersey; and Crystal Sheaves, RN, MSN, APRN, FNP-BC, Senior Lecturer, West Virginia University School of Nursing, Charleston, West Virginia.

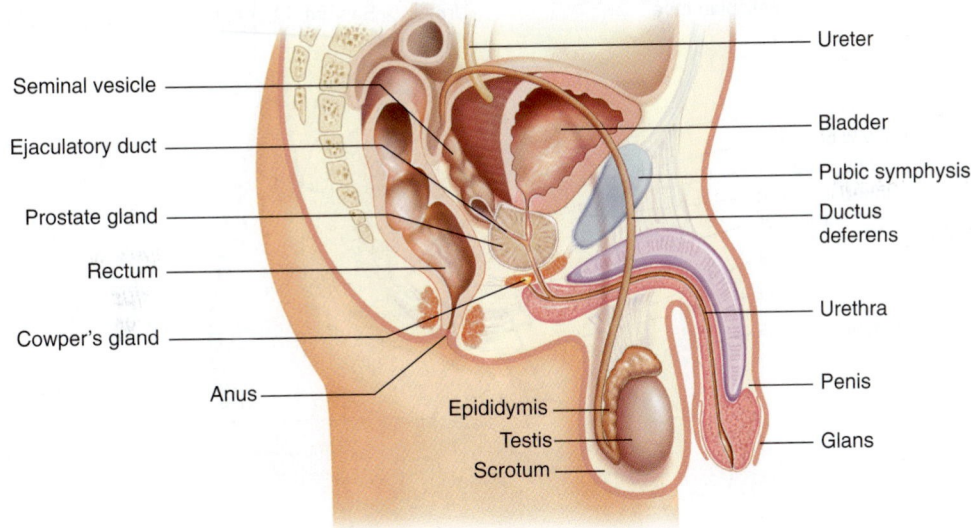

FIG. 50-1 Male reproductive tract. (Modified from Patton KT, Thibodeau GA: *Anatomy and physiology*, ed 8, St Louis, 2013, Mosby.)

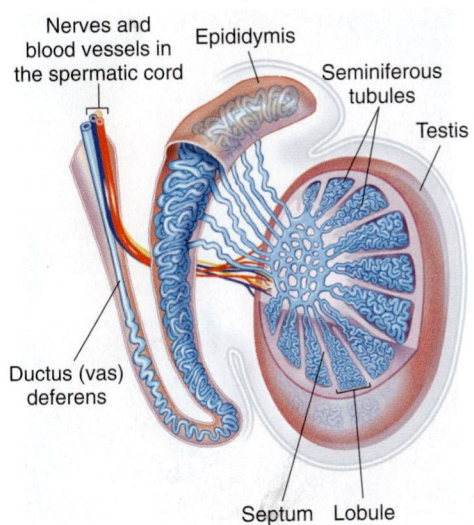

FIG. 50-2 Seminiferous tubules, testis, epididymis, and ductus (vas) deferens in the male. (Modified from Patton KT, Thibodeau GA: *Anatomy and physiology*, ed 8, St Louis, 2013, Mosby.)

upward through the scrotum and continues through the inguinal ring into the abdominal cavity. The spermatic cord is composed of a connective tissue sheath that encloses the ductus deferens, arteries, veins, nerves, and lymph vessels as it ascends up through the inguinal canal (Fig. 50-2). In the abdominal cavity, the ductus deferens travels up, over, and behind the bladder. Posterior to the bladder the ductus deferens joins the seminal vesicle to form the ejaculatory duct (Fig. 50-1).

The ejaculatory duct passes downward through the prostate gland, connecting with the urethra. The urethra extends from the bladder, through the prostate, and ends in a slit-like opening (the meatus) on the ventral side of the *glans*, the tip of the penis. During the process of ejaculation, sperm travel through the urethra and out of the penis.

Glands. The seminal vesicles, prostate gland, and Cowper's (bulbourethral) glands are the accessory glands of the male reproductive system. These glands produce and secrete seminal fluid *(semen)*, which surrounds the sperm and forms the *ejaculate.*

The seminal vesicles lie posterior to the bladder and between the rectum and bladder. The ducts of the seminal vesicles fuse with the ductus deferens to form the ejaculatory ducts that enter the prostate gland. The prostate gland lies beneath the bladder. Its posterior surface is in contact with the rectal wall. The prostate normally measures 0.8 in (2 cm) wide and 1.2 in (3 cm) long and is divided into the right and left lateral lobes and an anteroposterior median lobe. Cowper's glands lie on each side of the urethra and slightly posterior to it, just below the prostate. The ducts of these glands enter directly into the urethra.

Secretions from the seminal vesicles, prostate, and Cowper's glands make up most of the fluid in the ejaculate. These various secretions serve as a medium for the transport of sperm and create an alkaline, nutritious environment that promotes sperm motility and survival.

External Genitalia. The male external genitalia consist of the penis and scrotum. The penis consists of a shaft, and the tip is known as the *glans.* The glans is covered by a fold of skin, the prepuce (or foreskin), that forms at the junction of the glans and shaft of the penis. In circumcised males the prepuce has been removed. The shaft of the penis consists of erectile tissue composed of the corpus cavernosum, corpus spongiosum (fibrous sheath that encases the erectile tissue), and urethra. The skin covering the penis is thin, loose, and hairless.

Female Reproductive System

The three primary roles of the female reproductive system are (1) production of ova, (2) secretion of hormones, and (3) protection and facilitation of the development of the fetus in a pregnant female. Like the male, the female has primary and secondary reproductive organs. The primary reproductive organs in the female are the paired ovaries. Secondary reproductive organs include the ducts (fallopian tubes), uterus, vagina, sex glands (Bartholin's glands and breasts), and external genitalia (vulva).

Pelvic Organs

Ovaries. The ovaries are located on either side of the uterus, just behind and below the fallopian tubes (Fig. 50-3). The almond-shaped ovaries are firm and solid, approximately 0.6 in

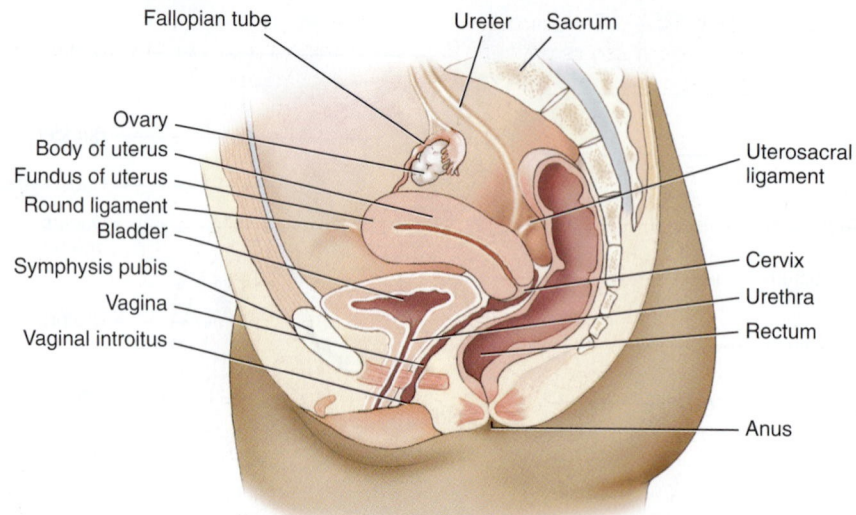

FIG. 50-3 Female reproductive tract. (Modified from McKenry L, Tessier E, Hogan M: *Mosby's pharmacology in nursing*, St Louis, 2006, Mosby.)

(1.5 cm) wide and 1.2 in (3 cm) long. Their functions include ovulation and secretion of the two major reproductive hormones: estrogen and progesterone.

The outer zone of the ovary contains follicles with germ cells, or *oocytes*. Each follicle contains a primordial (immature) oocyte surrounded by granulosa and theca cells. These two layers protect and nourish the oocyte until the follicle reaches maturity and ovulation occurs. However, not all follicles reach maturity. In a process termed *atresia*, most of the primordial follicles become smaller and are reabsorbed by the body. Thus the number of follicles declines from 1 million at birth to approximately 400,000 at *menarche* (first menstruation). This is the female's lifetime supply of sex cells. In contrast, males produce spermatocytes throughout their reproductive life cycle. As a woman ages, both the number and quality of the oocytes decline, with fewer than 500 oocytes actually released by ovulation during the reproductive years of the normal healthy woman.[2]

Fallopian Tubes. The fallopian tubes have two responsibilities: (1) transporting the ovum towards the uterus, allowing for fertilization, and (2) facilitating the passage of the ovum to the uterus for implantation. The tubes are uterine appendages that end by curling around the ovary. The distal ends of the fallopian tubes consist of fingerlike projections called *fimbriae*, which sweep the ovum from the ruptured ovarian follicle (ovulation) to the fallopian tube. The tubes, which average 4.8 in (12 cm) in length, extend from the fimbriae to the superior lateral borders of the uterus. Fertilization usually takes place within the outer one third of the fallopian tubes.[3]

Normally, each month during a woman's reproductive years, one ovarian follicle reaches maturity, and the ovum is ovulated, or expelled, from the ovary through the stimulus of the gonadotropic hormones: follicle-stimulating hormone (FSH) and luteinizing hormone (LH). The ovum then travels through a fallopian tube, where fertilization by sperm may occur (if sperm are present). An ovum can be fertilized up to 72 hours after its release.

Uterus. The uterus is a pear-shaped, hollow, muscular organ located between the bladder and rectum (Fig. 50-3). In the mature **nulliparous** (never pregnant) woman, the uterus is

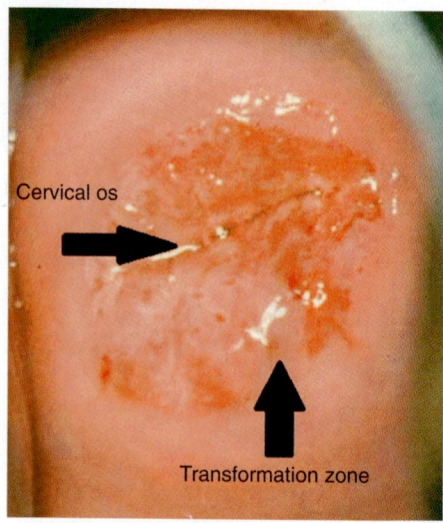

FIG. 50-4 Cervical os and squamocolumnar junction (transformation zone). (Courtesy Candy Tedschi, NP, Great Neck, NY.)

approximately 2.4 to 3.2 in (6 to 8 cm) long and 1.6 in (4 cm) wide. The uterine walls consist of an outer serosal layer, the *perimetrium;* a middle muscular layer, the *myometrium;* and an inner mucosal layer, the *endometrium.*

The uterus consists of the fundus, body (or corpus), and cervix (Fig. 50-3). The body makes up about 80% of the uterus and connects with the cervix at the isthmus, or neck. The cervix is the lower portion of the uterus that projects into the anterior wall of the vaginal canal. It makes up about 15% to 20% of the uterus in the nulliparous female. The cervix consists of the *ectocervix,* the outer portion that protrudes into the vagina, and the *endocervix,* the canal in the opening of the cervix. The opening of the cervix is referred to as the *cervical os* (Fig. 50-4).

The ectocervix is covered with squamous epithelial cells, which give it a smooth, pinkish appearance. The endocervix contains a lining of columnar epithelial cells, which give it a rough, reddened appearance. The junction at which the two types of epithelial cells meet is termed the *squamocolumnar junction* or the *transformation zone* (Fig. 50-4). Cells sampled from the squamocolumnar junction are examined as part of a Papanicolaou (Pap) test, which is a critical component of cervical cancer screening.

The cervical canal is 0.8 to 1.6 in (2 to 4 cm) long and is relatively tightly closed. However, the cervix allows sperm to enter the uterus through the cervical os and also allows menses to be expelled. The columnar epithelium, under hormonal influence, provides elasticity during labor. The cervix is able to stretch to allow passage of a fetus during the birth process. The entrance of sperm into the uterus is facilitated by mucus produced by the cervix under the influence of estrogen. Under normal conditions, the cervical mucus becomes watery, stretchy, and more abundant at ovulation. The postovulatory cervical mucus, under the influence of progesterone, is thick and inhibits sperm passage.

Vagina. The vagina is a tubular structure 3 to 4 in (7.6 to 10 cm) long that is lined with squamous epithelium. In reproductive-age women, the vagina has multiple transverse folds known as *rugae*. The secretions of the vagina consist of cervical mucus, desquamated epithelium, and, during sexual stimulation, a watery secretion. These fluids help protect against vaginal infection. The muscular and erectile tissue of the vaginal walls allows enough dilation and contraction to accommodate the passage of the fetus during labor, as well as penetration of the penis during intercourse. The anterior vaginal wall lies along the urethra and bladder. The posterior vaginal wall is adjacent to the rectum.

Pelvis. The female pelvis consists of four bones (two pelvic bones, sacrum, coccyx) held together by several strong ligaments. The pelvis in the female has a larger diameter and is circular, whereas a male pelvis is more heart shaped. The wider female pelvis plays an important role in *parturition* (childbirth), as the fetal head adapts its position to the pelvic dimensions during labor and delivery through rotation and flexion to pass through the pelvic inlet.[4]

External Genitalia. The external portion of the female reproductive system (Fig. 50-5), commonly called the *vulva*, consists of the mons pubis, labia majora, labia minora, clitoris, urethral meatus, Skene's glands, vaginal introitus (opening), and Bartholin's glands.

The **mons pubis** is a fatty layer lying over the pubic bone. It is covered with coarse hair that lies in a triangular pattern. The labia majora are folds of adipose tissue that form the outer borders of the vulva. The hairless labia minora form the borders of the vaginal orifice and extend anteriorly to enclose the clitoris.

The *vestibule* is the space between the labia minora that is observed when they are held apart. It extends from the clitoris to the *posterior forchette* (a mucous membrane band that connects the posterior ends of the labia minora to the vagina). The perineum is the area between the vagina and anus. The vaginal introitus (vaginal opening) is surrounded by thin membranous tissue called the *hymen*. It is usually perforated and has many variations in shape. In the adult woman the hymen usually appears as folds or hymenal tags *(carunculae myrtiformes)* and separates the external genitalia from the vagina. At the posterior aspect of the vagina, a tense band of mucous membrane connecting the posterior ends of the labia minora is referred to as the *posterior fourchette.*

The **clitoris** is erectile tissue that becomes engorged during sexual excitation. It lies anterior to the urethral meatus and the vaginal orifice and is usually covered by the prepuce. Clitoral stimulation is an important part of sexual activity for many women.

Ducts of the Skene's glands lie alongside the urinary meatus and are thought to help lubricate the urinary meatus.[5] The Bartholin's glands, located at the posterior and lateral aspects of the vaginal orifice, secrete a thin, mucoid material believed to contribute slightly to lubrication during sexual intercourse. These glands are not usually palpable unless sebaceous-like cysts form or they are swollen in the presence of an infection, such as a sexually transmitted infection (STI).

Breasts. The breasts are a secondary sex characteristic that develops during puberty in response to estrogen and progesterone. Cyclic hormonal changes lead to regular changes in breast tissue to prepare it for lactation when fertilization and pregnancy occur.

The breasts extend from the second to the sixth ribs. The extension of breast tissue into the upper-outer quadrant into the axilla is an area referred to as the *tail of Spence* (Fig. 50-6). The fully mature breast is dome shaped and contains a

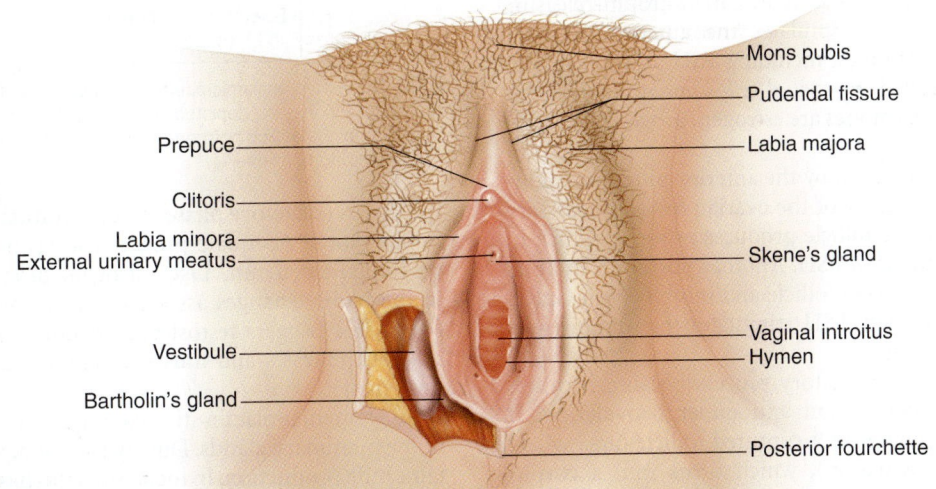

FIG. 50-5 External female genitalia. (Modified from Patton KT, Thibodeau GA: *Anatomy and physiology,* ed 8, St Louis, 2013, Mosby.)

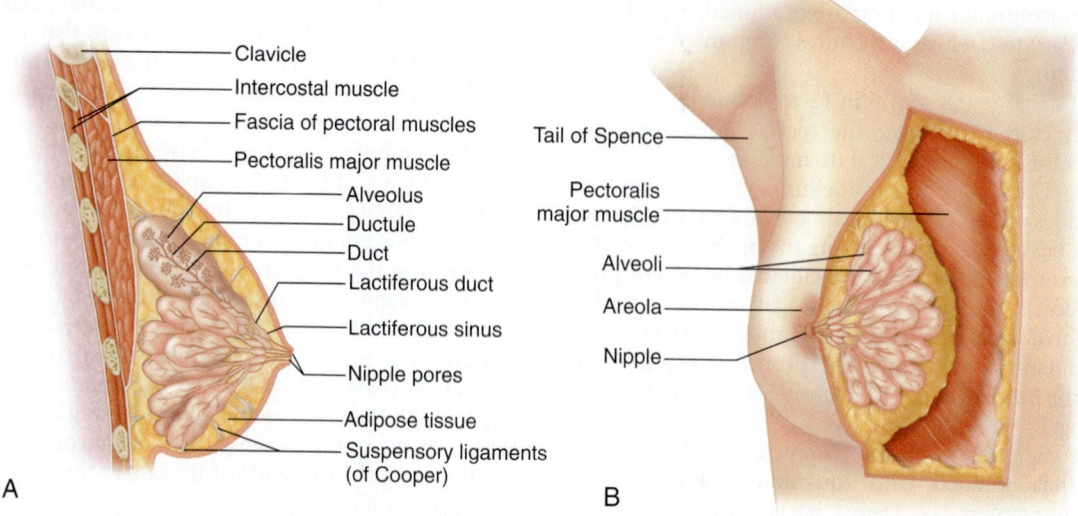

FIG. 50-6 The lactating female breast. **A,** Glandular structures are anchored to the overlying skin and the pectoralis muscle by suspensory ligaments of Cooper. Each lobule of glandular tissue is drained by a lactiferous duct that eventually opens through the nipple. **B,** Anterior view of a lactating breast. In nonlactating breasts, glandular tissue is less evident, with adipose tissue comprising most of the breast. (Modified from Patton KT, Thibodeau GA: *Anatomy and physiology,* ed 8, St Louis, 2013, Mosby.)

pigmented center termed the *areola.* The areolar region contains Montgomery's tubercles, which are similar to sebaceous glands and assist in lubricating the nipple. During lactation, the alveoli secrete milk. The milk then flows into a ductal system and is transported to the lactiferous sinuses. The nipple contains 15 to 20 tiny openings through which the milk flows during breastfeeding. The fibrous and fatty tissue that supports and separates the channels of the mammary duct system is primarily responsible for the varying sizes and shapes of the breasts in different individuals.

Neuroendocrine Regulation of Reproductive System

The hypothalamus, pituitary gland, and gonads secrete numerous hormones (Fig. 50-7). (Endocrine hormones are discussed in Chapter 47.) These hormones regulate the processes of ovulation, spermatogenesis (formation of sperm), and fertilization and the formation and function of the secondary sex characteristics. The hypothalamus secretes gonadotropin-releasing hormone (GnRH), which stimulates the anterior pituitary gland to secrete its hormones, including FSH and LH. LH in males is sometimes called *interstitial cell–stimulating hormone (ICSH).* The gonadal hormones are estrogen, progesterone, and testosterone.

In women, FSH production by the anterior pituitary stimulates the growth and maturity of the ovarian follicles necessary for ovulation. The mature follicle produces estrogen, which in turn suppresses the release of FSH. Another hormone, inhibin, is also secreted by the ovarian follicle and inhibits both GnRH and FSH secretion. In men, FSH stimulates the seminiferous tubules to produce sperm.

LH contributes to the ovulatory process because it causes follicles to complete maturation and undergo ovulation. It also affects the development of a ruptured follicle (area where ovum exited during ovulation), which turns into a corpus luteum from which progesterone is secreted. Progesterone plays a major role in the menstrual cycle, but most specifically in the secretory phase. It maintains the rich vascular state of

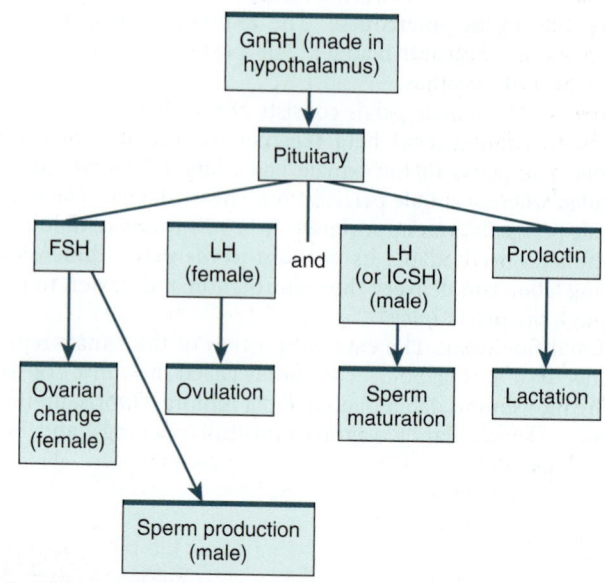

FIG. 50-7 Hypothalamic-pituitary-gonadal axis. Only the major pituitary hormone actions are depicted. *FSH,* Follicle-stimulating hormone; *GnRH,* gonadotropin-releasing hormone; *ICSH,* interstitial cell–stimulating hormone; *LH,* luteinizing hormone.

the uterus (secretory phase) in preparation for fertilization and implantation. Adequate progesterone is necessary to maintain an implanted ovum. Like estrogen, progesterone is involved in the bodily changes associated with pregnancy. In men, LH (or ICSH) triggers testosterone production by the interstitial cells of the testes and thus is essential for the full maturation of sperm.

In women, prolactin stimulates the development and growth of the mammary glands. During lactation, it initiates and maintains milk production. In men, prolactin has no known function.

In women, the gonadal hormones, estrogen and progesterone, are produced by the ovaries. Small amounts of an estrogen precursor are also produced in the adrenal cortices. Estrogen is

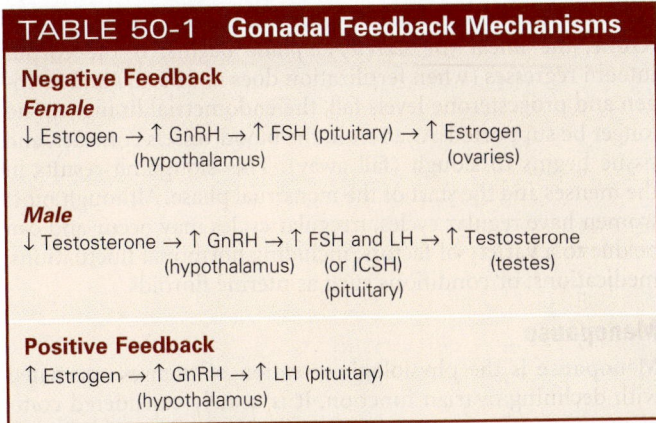

TABLE 50-1   Gonadal Feedback Mechanisms

Negative Feedback
Female
↓ Estrogen → ↑ GnRH → ↑ FSH (pituitary) → ↑ Estrogen
(hypothalamus)   (ovaries)

Male
↓ Testosterone → ↑ GnRH → ↑ FSH and LH → ↑ Testosterone
(hypothalamus)   (or ICSH)   (testes)
                  (pituitary)

Positive Feedback
↑ Estrogen → ↑ GnRH → ↑ LH (pituitary)
(hypothalamus)

FSH, Follicle-stimulating hormone; *GnRH,* gonadotropin-releasing hormone; *ICSH,* interstitial cell–stimulating hormone; *LH,* luteinizing hormone.

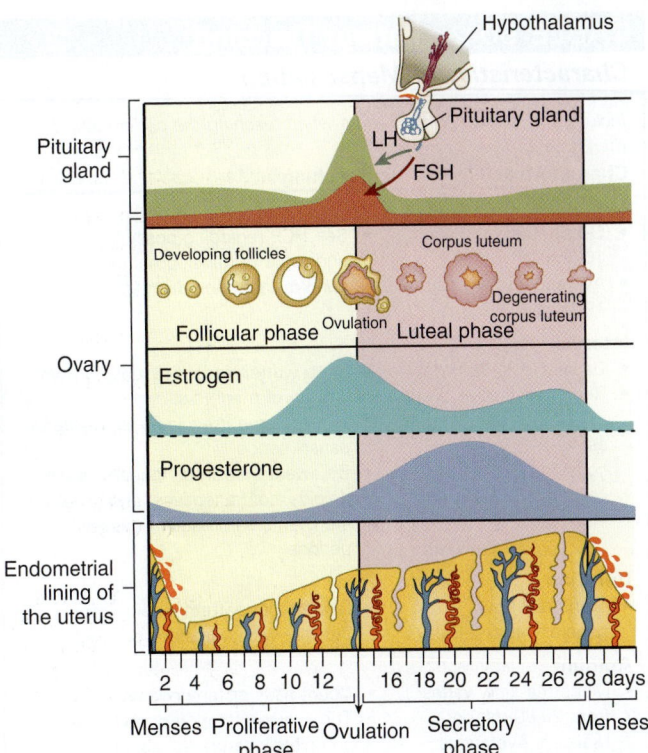

FIG. 50-8 Events of the menstrual cycle. The lines depict the changes in blood hormone levels, the development of the follicles, and the changes in the endometrium during the cycle. *FSH,* Follicle-stimulating hormone; *LH,* luteinizing hormone. (Modified from Patton KT, Thibodeau GA: *Anatomy and physiology,* ed 8, St Louis, 2013, Mosby.)

essential to the development and maintenance of the secondary sex characteristics, proliferative phase of the menstrual cycle immediately after menstruation, and uterine changes essential to pregnancy. In men, estrogen is produced predominantly in the adrenal cortices. The role and importance of estrogen in men are not well understood.

In men, the major gonadal hormone is testosterone, which is produced by the testes. Testosterone is responsible for the development and maintenance of secondary sex characteristics, as well as for adequate spermatogenesis. In women, androgens are produced in small amounts by the adrenal glands and ovaries.

The circulating levels of gonadal hormones are controlled primarily by a *negative feedback process.* Receptors within the hypothalamus and pituitary are sensitive to the circulating blood levels of the hormones (Table 50-1). Increased levels of hormones stimulate a hypothalamic response to decrease the high circulating levels. Likewise, low circulating levels provoke a hypothalamic response that increases the low circulating levels. For example, if the circulating level of testosterone in men is low, the hypothalamus is stimulated to secrete GnRH. This triggers the anterior pituitary to secrete greater amounts of FSH and LH, which in turn cause an increase in the production of testosterone. The high level of testosterone signals a decrease in the production of GnRH and thus of FSH and LH.

In women, however, there is a slight variation in the control of gonadal hormones. The circulating levels are controlled through a combination of both a negative and positive feedback system. A *negative feedback control* mechanism exists similar to that described above for men. When circulating estrogen levels are low, the hypothalamus is stimulated to increase its production of GnRH. GnRH stimulates the pituitary to secrete greater amounts of FSH and LH, resulting in higher levels of estrogen production by the ovaries. Reciprocally higher levels of circulating estrogen result in a decreasing secretion of GnRH and thus a decrease in the secretion of FSH by the pituitary.

Women also have a *positive feedback control* mechanism. Thus with increasing levels of circulating estrogen, a greater level of GnRH is produced, resulting in an increased level of LH from the pituitary. Likewise, lowered levels of estrogen result in a lowered level of LH.

Menarche

Menarche is the first episode of menstrual bleeding, indicating that a girl has reached puberty. Menarche usually occurs at

approximately 12 to 13 years of age but can occur as early as 10 years of age in some individuals. Menstrual cycles are often irregular for the first 1 to 2 years after menarche because of *anovulatory cycles* (cycles without ovulation).

Menstrual Cycle

The major functions of the ovaries are ovulation and the secretion of hormones. These functions are accomplished during the normal menstrual cycle, a monthly process mediated by the hormonal activity of the hypothalamus, pituitary gland, and ovaries. Menstruation occurs during each month in which an ovum is not fertilized (Fig. 50-8). The endometrial cycle is divided into three phases labeled in relation to uterine and ovarian changes: (1) the *proliferative,* or *follicular, phase;* (2) the *secretory,* or *luteal, phase;* and (3) the *menstrual,* or *ischemic, phase.* The length of the menstrual cycle ranges from 21 to 35 days, with an average of 28 days.

The menstrual cycle begins on the first day of menstruation, which usually lasts 4 to 6 days. The first day of the menstrual cycle is charted as the *LMP,* or last menstrual period. Table 50-2 includes characteristics of the menstrual cycle and related teaching. During menstruation, estrogen and progesterone levels are low, but FSH levels begin to increase. During the follicular phase, a single follicle matures fully under the stimulation of FSH. (The mechanism that ensures that usually only one follicle reaches maturity is not known.) The mature follicle stimulates estrogen production, causing a negative feedback with resulting decreased FSH secretion.

Although the initial stage of follicular maturation is stimulated by FSH, complete maturation and ovulation occur only in the presence of LH. When estrogen levels peak on about the

TABLE 50-2 Patient Teaching

Characteristics of Menstruation

Include the following information when teaching the patient about menstruation.

Characteristic	Teaching
Menarche • Occurs between ages 10 and 16 yr. • Average age at onset is 12-13 yr.	• See HCP regarding possible endocrine or developmental abnormality when delayed.
Interval • Usually is 21-35 days. • Regular cycles as short as 17 days or as long as 45 days are considered normal if pattern is consistent for individual.	• Keep written record to identify own pattern of menstrual cycle. • Expect some irregularity in perimenopausal period. • Be aware that drugs (phenothiazines, opioids, contraceptives) and stressful life events can result in missed periods.
Duration • Menstrual flow generally lasts 2-8 days.	• Realize that pattern is fairly constant but that wide variations do exist.
Amount • Menstrual flow varies from 20-80 mL per menses. Average is 30 mL. • Amount varies among women and in same woman at different times. • It is usually heaviest first 2 days.	• Count pads or tampons used per day. • The average tampon or pad (when completely saturated) absorbs 20-30 mL. • Very heavy flow is indicated by complete soaking of two pads in 1-2 hr. • Flow increases and then gradually decreases in perimenopausal period. • IUD or drugs such as anticoagulants and thiazides can produce heavy menses. • Women with uterine fibroids may also experience increased or heavy menses.
Composition • Menstrual discharge is mixture of endometrium, blood, mucus, and vaginal cells. • It is dark red and less viscous than blood and usually does not clot.	• Clots indicate heavy flow or vaginal pooling.

IUD, Intrauterine device.

twelfth day of the cycle, there is a surge of LH, which triggers ovulation a day or two later. After ovulation (maturation and release of an ovum), LH promotes the development of the corpus luteum, a temporary functional cyst that forms with the ruptured follicle.

The fully developed corpus luteum continues to secrete estrogen and initiates progesterone secretion. If fertilization occurs, high levels of estrogen and progesterone continue to be secreted because of the continued activity of the corpus luteum from stimulation by human chorionic gonadotropin (hCG). If fertilization does not take place, menstruation occurs because of a decrease in estrogen production and progesterone withdrawal.

During the *follicular phase,* the endometrial lining of the uterus also undergoes change. As more estrogen is produced, the endometrial lining undergoes proliferative changes, including an increase in the length of blood vessels and glandular tissue.

With ovulation and the resulting increased levels of progesterone, the *luteal* (or *secretory*) *phase* begins. If the corpus luteum regresses (when fertilization does not occur) and estrogen and progesterone levels fall, the endometrial lining can no longer be supported. As a result, the blood vessels contract, and tissue begins to slough (fall away). This sloughing results in the menses and the start of the menstrual phase. Although most women have regular cycles, irregular cycles may occur and can be due to a variety of factors, including hormonal fluctuations, medications, or conditions such as uterine fibroids.

Menopause

Menopause is the physiologic cessation of menses associated with declining ovarian function. It is usually considered complete after 1 year of amenorrhea (absence of menstruation). (Menopause is discussed in Chapter 53.)

Phases of Sexual Response

The sexual response is a complex interplay of psychologic and physiologic phenomena and is influenced by a number of variables (e.g., stress, illness). The changes that occur during sexual excitement are similar for men and women. Masters and Johnson described the sexual response in terms of the excitement, plateau, orgasmic, and resolution phases.[6]

Male Sexual Response. The penis and urethra are essential to the transport of sperm into the vagina and cervix during intercourse. This transport is facilitated by penile erection in response to sexual stimulation during the *excitement phase.* Erection results from the filling of the large venous sinuses within the erectile tissue of the penis. In the flaccid state the sinuses hold only a small amount of blood, but during the erection stage they are congested with blood. Because the penis is richly endowed with sympathetic, parasympathetic, and pudendal nerve endings, it is readily stimulated to erection. The loose skin of the penis becomes taut as a result of the venous congestion. This erectile tautness allows for easy insertion into the vagina.

As the man reaches the *plateau phase,* the erection is maintained, and the penis increases in diameter as a result of a slight increase in vasocongestion. Testicle size also increases. Sometimes the glans penis becomes more reddish purple.

The subsequent contraction of the penile and urethral musculature during the *orgasmic phase* propels the sperm outward through the meatus. In this process, termed *ejaculation,* sperm are released into the ductus deferens during contractions. Sperm advance through the urethra, where fluids from the prostate and seminal vesicles are added to the ejaculate. The sperm continue their path through the urethra, receiving a small amount of fluid from the Cowper's glands, and are finally ejaculated through the urinary meatus. *Orgasm* is characterized by the rapid release of the vasocongestion and muscular tension (myotonia) that have developed. The rapid release of muscular tension (through rhythmic contractions) occurs primarily in the penis, prostate gland, and seminal vesicles. After ejaculation, a man enters the *resolution phase.* The penis undergoes involution, gradually returning to its unstimulated, flaccid state.

Female Sexual Response. The changes that occur in a woman during sexual excitation are similar to those in a man. In response to stimulation, the clitoris becomes congested and vaginal lubrication increases from secretions from the cervix, Bartholin's glands, and vaginal walls. This initial response is the excitation phase.

As excitation is maintained in the plateau phase, the vagina expands and the uterus is elevated. In the orgasmic phase, contractions occur in the uterus from the fundus to the lower uterine segment. There is a slight relaxation of the cervical os, which helps the entrance of the sperm, and rhythmic contractions of the vagina. Muscular tension is rapidly released through rhythmic contractions in the clitoris, vagina, and uterus. This phase is followed by a resolution phase, in which these organs return to their preexcitation state. However, women do not have to go through the resolution (refractory) recovery state before they can be orgasmic again. They can be multi-orgasmic without resolution between orgasms.

Gerontologic Considerations: Effects of Aging on Reproductive Systems

With advancing age, changes occur in the male and female reproductive systems (Table 50-3). In women many of these changes are related to the altered estrogen production that is associated with menopause.[7] A reduction in circulating estrogen and other sex steroids in postmenopausal women is associated with breast and genital atrophy, reduction in bone mass, and increased rate of atherosclerosis. Vaginal dryness may occur, which can lead to urogenital atrophy and changes in the composition of vaginal *microbiome* (the aggregate of microorganisms and their genetic material in a particular environment).[8]

Testosterone levels decline in men as they age. Manifestations of hormonal decline are more gradual in men and can be physical, psychologic, or sexual. Some of the changes include an increase in prostate size and a decrease in testosterone level, sperm production, muscle tone of the scrotum, and size and firmness of the testicles. Erectile dysfunction and sexual dysfunction occur in some men as a result of these changes.

Gradual changes resulting from advancing age occur in the sexual responses of men and women. The cumulative effects of these changes, as well as the negative social attitude toward sexuality in older adults, can affect the sexual practices of older adults. Many factors affect sexuality in later life. Illness, disability, medicines, and surgeries can affect a person's ability to participate in sexual activities.

Nurses play an important role in providing accurate and unbiased information about sexuality and age. Emphasize the normalcy of sexual activity in older adults and refer them to resources that address such issues.

ASSESSMENT OF MALE AND FEMALE REPRODUCTIVE SYSTEMS

Subjective Data

Important Health Information. In addition to general health information, elicit information specifically relating to the reproductive system. Reproduction and sexual issues are often considered extremely personal and private. Develop trust with the patient to elicit such information. A professional demeanor is important when taking a reproductive or sexual history. Be sensitive, use gender-neutral terms when asking about partners, and maintain an awareness of a patient's culture and beliefs. Begin with the least sensitive information (e.g., menstrual history) before asking questions about more sensitive issues such as sexual practices or STIs.

TABLE 50-3 Gerontologic Assessment Differences

Reproductive Systems

Structure	Changes	Assessment Findings Abnormalities
Male		
Breasts	Enlargement	Gynecomastia (abnormal enlargement).
Penis	Decreased subcutaneous fat	Easily retractable foreskin (if uncircumcised). Decrease in size. Fewer sustained erections.
Prostate	Benign hyperplasia	Enlargement, urinary obstruction, incontinence.
Testes	Decreased testosterone production	Decrease in size, firmness.
Female		
Breasts	Decreased subcutaneous fat, increased fibrous tissue, decreased skin turgor	Less resilient, looser, more pendulous tissue. Decreased size. Duct around nipple may feel like stringy strand.
Ovaries	Decreased ovarian function	Nonpalpable ovaries normal postmenopause.
Urethra	Decreased muscle tone, mucosal thinning	Possible urinary tract infections, painful urination (dysuria), urgency, frequency, incontinence.
Uterus	Decreased thickness of myometrium	Uterine prolapse.
Vagina	Atrophy of tissue, decreased muscle tone, alkaline pH	Mucosa becomes pale, dry, smooth and thins. Vagina narrows and shortens.
Vulva	Decreased skin turgor	Atrophy. Decreased amount of pubic hair. Decreased size of clitoris and labia.

CASE STUDY

Patient Introduction

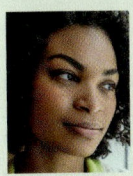

A.K. is a 30-yr-old African American, divorced, single mother who is being evaluated for irregular and heavy menses with clots for the past several months. She has frequent migraine headaches. She takes the following medications: topiramate (Topamax) 100 mg orally once daily, sumitriptan (Imitrex) 100 mg orally PRN migraine, oral contraceptive pills orally once daily, consistent with use and timing.

(©Benjamin A. Peterson/Mother Image/mother image/Fuse/Thinkstock)

Discussion Questions

1. What are the possible causes for A.K.'s irregular and heavy menstrual bleeding?
2. What type of assessment would you anticipate for A.K.: comprehensive? focused? emergency?

You will learn more about A.K. and her condition as you read through this assessment chapter.

(See p. 1195 for more information on A.K.)

Answers available at *http://evolve.elsevier.com/Lewis/medsurg*.

GENDER DIFFERENCES

Effects of Aging on Sexual Function

Men	Women
• Increased stimulation necessary for erection • Decreased force of ejaculation • Decreased ability to attain or sustain erection • Decreased size and rigidity of the penis at full erection • Decreased libido and interest in sex	• Decreased vaginal lubrication • Decreased sensitivity with labia shrinking and more clitoris exposed • Difficulty in maintaining arousal • Difficulty in achieving orgasm after stimulation • Decreased libido and interest in sex

Past Health History. The past health history should include information about major illnesses, hospitalizations, immunizations, and surgeries. Inquire about any infections involving the reproductive system, including STIs. Also take a complete obstetric and gynecologic history from the female patient.

Common pediatric illnesses that affect reproductive function are mumps and rubella. The occurrence of mumps in young men has been associated with an increase in sterility. Bilateral testicular atrophy may occur secondary to mumps-related orchitis. In the health history ask male patients if they have had mumps, have been immunized with the mumps vaccine, or have any indications of sterility.

Rubella is of primary concern to women of childbearing age. If rubella occurs during the first 3 months of pregnancy, the possibility of congenital anomalies is increased. For this reason, you should encourage immunization for all women of child-bearing age who have not been immunized for rubella or have not already had the disease. (Rubella immunity can be determined by antibody titers.) However, women should not be immunized if they are already pregnant.[9] Advise women to avoid becoming pregnant for 28 days after vaccination.

Question the patient regarding current health status and any acute or chronic health problems. Co-morbidities are often related to problems with the reproductive system. Chronic illnesses such as cardiovascular disease, respiratory disorders, anemia, cancer, and kidney and urinary tract disorders may affect the reproductive system and sexual functioning.

Ask questions relating to possible endocrine disorders, particularly diabetes mellitus (DM), hypothyroidism, and hyperthyroidism, because these disorders directly interfere with women's menstrual cycles and with sexual performance. Men who have DM may experience erectile dysfunction and retrograde ejaculation. In women with uncontrolled DM, pregnancy may pose significant health risks to both the woman and unborn fetus.

Determine if the patient has a history of a stroke. In men, strokes may cause physiologic or psychologic erectile dysfunction. Men who have suffered a myocardial infarction (MI) may experience erectile dysfunction because of fear that sexual activity could precipitate another MI. Post MI medication, such as β-blockers, may affect a man's ability to achieve an erection.[10] Although most patients have concerns about sexual activity after an MI, many are not comfortable expressing these fears to the nurse. Be sensitive to this concern.

Medications. Document all prescription and over-the-counter medications that the patient is taking, including the reason for the medication, dosage, and length of time that the medication has been taken. Ask the patient about the use of herbal products and dietary or nutritional supplements.

Particularly relevant in the assessment of the reproductive system is the use of diuretics (sometimes prescribed for premenstrual edema), psychotropic agents (which may interfere with sexual performance), and antihypertensives (some of which may cause erectile dysfunction). Patients who use drugs such as amlodipine (Norvasc), lisinopril (Prinivil), propranolol (Inderal), and clonidine (Catapres) must be closely assessed for these problems. Also note the use of drugs such as alcohol, marijuana, barbiturates, amphetamines, or phencyclidine hydrochloride (PCP [also called "angel dust"]), which can have serious behavioral or physiologic effects on the reproductive system.

In women, document the use of hormonal contraceptives or other hormone therapy (HT). The long-term use of combined hormone therapy (specifically a combination of oral conjugated equine estrogen and a progestin called *medroxyprogesterone acetate*) appears to increase the risk of stroke, breast cancer, deep vein thrombosis, gallbladder disease, and urinary incontinence in postmenopausal women.[11] The short-term use of HT appears to be appropriate for women experiencing moderate to severe menopausal symptoms. Women who use tobacco have a much higher risk of clotting disorders. (HT is discussed in Chapter 53.)

A history of cholecystitis and hepatitis is important because these conditions may be contraindications for the use of oral contraceptives. Cholecystitis is often aggravated by oral contraceptives, and chronic active inflammation of the liver generally precludes the use of estrogen products because they are metabolized by the liver. Chronic obstructive pulmonary disease may be a contraindication to oral contraceptive use because progesterone thickens respiratory secretions.

Surgery or Other Treatments. Note any surgical procedures in the health history. Examples of surgical procedures involving the female reproductive system are listed in Table 53-15. Also document any therapeutic or spontaneous abortions and type of intervention (e.g., medical versus surgical abortion).

Functional Health Patterns. The key questions to ask a patient with a reproductive problem are presented in Table 50-4.

Health Perception–Health Management Pattern. Two of the primary focuses of a health pattern are the patient's perception of his or her own health and measures that the patient takes to maintain health. Specifically, ask about self-examination practices and screenings. Mammography (based on current guidelines [see Chapter 51]), Pap tests, and clinical breast examinations are integral to a woman's health.

Men are at risk for testicular and prostate cancer. However, controversy exists regarding the benefits of routine screening for these cancers.[12] Patients should discuss the benefits and risks of screening with their primary care provider.

GENETIC RISK ALERT

- Breast, ovarian, uterine, and prostate cancer have known genetic risk factors.
- Having a first-degree relative with any of these cancers significantly increases the risk of cancer for the patient.
- The risk increases if several family members have been affected with these cancers over succeeding generations.
- Individuals with a known hereditary predisposition to breast or ovarian cancer can use this information to make informed decisions about how to minimize their risks.

Family history is also an important component of this health pattern. Inquire about a history of cancer, particularly cancer of the reproductive organs. Determine if the patient has a familial tendency for diabetes mellitus, hypothyroidism, hyperthyroidism, hypertension, stroke, angina, MI, endocrine disorders, or anemia.

Assessment of the reproductive system is incomplete without knowledge of the patient's lifestyle choices. Determine whether a patient has smoked or is currently smoking, the amount (if any) of alcohol consumption, or if the patient uses illicit drugs. Risks associated with smoking include ectopic pregnancy, spontaneous abortion, an increased risk of perinatal mortality and morbidity, placental abnormalities, preterm delivery, and congenital facial defects of the fetus.[13] In addition, smoking increases the risk of morbidity and mortality in women who

TABLE 50-4   Health History

Reproductive System

Health Perception–Health Management
- How would you describe your overall health?
- Describe the health of your family members. Any history of breast, uterine, ovarian, or prostate cancer?*

Women
- Do you perform self breast examination? Any concerns?
- What was the date of your last Pap test and the results?*
- Any prior abnormalities with your Pap tests?
- What was the date of your last mammogram and the results?*
- Any prior abnormalities with your mammograms?

Men
- Do you perform testicular self-examination? Any concerns?

Nutritional-Metabolic
- Describe what you usually eat and drink.
- Have you experienced any changes in weight?*
- How do you feel about your current weight?
- Do you take any nutritional supplements, such as calcium or vitamins?*
- Do you have any dietary restrictions?*

Elimination
- Do you experience problems with urination (e.g., pain, burning, dribbling, incontinence, frequency)?*
- Have you had bladder infections? If so, when? How often?
- Do you experience problems with bowel movements?*
- Do you experience any constipation, loose stools, or blood with stools?*
- Do you use laxatives?*

Activity-Exercise
- What activities do you typically do each day?
- Do you have enough energy for your desired activities?
- Can you dress yourself? Feed yourself? Walk without help?

Sleep-Rest
- How many hours do you typically sleep each night?
- Do you feel rested after sleep?
- Do you experience any problems associated with sleeping?*

Cognitive-Perceptual
- Are you able to read and write?
- Do you experience problems with dizziness?*
- Do you experience pain? If yes, where?
- Do you experience pain during sexual activity or intercourse?*

Self-Perception–Self-Concept
- How would you describe yourself?
- Have there been any recent changes that have made you feel differently about yourself?*
- Are you experiencing any problems that are affecting your sexuality?*

Role-Relationship
- Describe your living arrangements. With whom do you live?
- Do you have a significant other? If yes, is this relationship satisfying?
- Are you experiencing any role-related problems in your family?* At work?*
- What are the relationships among your family members?

Sexuality-Reproductive
- Are you sexually active? If so, how many partners do you have?
- What kind of sex do you engage in (e.g., oral, vaginal, anal)?
- How do you protect yourself against sexually transmitted infections and unwanted pregnancy?
- Are you satisfied with your present means of sexual expression? If not, explain.
- Have you experienced any recent changes in your sexual practices?*

Women
- How old were you when you had your first menstrual period? (Menarche)
- What was the first day of your last menstrual period?
- Describe your period. How many days does it last? How often does it come (for example, every 28 days)?
- Do you experience pain with your period? Do you pass clots?
- Do you feel your flow is heavy or excessive?
- How old were you when you went through menopause?
- Have you experienced any postmenopausal bleeding or spotting?*
- Pregnancy history: How many times have you been pregnant? How many living children do you have? Have you ever had any miscarriages or abortions? Did they require medical intervention?

Men
- Do you experience any difficulty with obtaining or sustaining an erection?

Coping–Stress Tolerance
- Have there been any major changes in your life within the past couple of years?*
- What is stressful in your life right now?
- How do you handle health problems when they occur?

Value-Belief
- What beliefs do you have about your health and illnesses?
- Do you use home remedies?*
- Is religion an important part of your life?*
- Do you think that any of your personal beliefs or values may be compromised because of your treatment?*

*If yes, describe.

use oral contraceptives. Smoking in women is also associated with early menopause.[8] Decreased sperm counts and erectile dysfunction are seen in male smokers. Finally, smoking is a known cofactor for persistence of *human papillomavirus* (HPV) infection and anogenital cancers among men and women.[14]

Document the patient's allergies, especially if the patient is allergic to sulfonamides, macrolides, cephalosporins, tetracyclines, penicillin, or latex. Sulfonamides, macrolides, cephalosporins, tetracyclines, and penicillin are used frequently in the treatment of reproductive and genitourinary problems such as STIs and urinary

tract infections (UTIs). Silicone and latex are commonly used in diaphragms and condoms. An allergy to these substances precludes their use as contraceptive methods.

Nutritional-Metabolic Pattern. Anemia is a common problem in women in their reproductive years, particularly during pregnancy and the postpartum period. Evaluate the adequacy of the diet with this condition in mind. Iron deficiency anemia is the most common cause of anemia in menstruating females.

Take a thorough nutritional and psychologic history to assess for the presence of an eating disorder. Anorexia nervosa can cause amenorrhea and subsequent problems, such as osteoporosis, that are related to menopause. Obesity can be related to polycystic ovarian syndrome and may be a precursor to type 2 DM.

From early adolescence, counsel women regarding adequate calcium and vitamin D intake to prevent osteoporosis. Estimate the patient's daily calcium intake to determine whether supplementation is needed. Evaluate folic acid intake for women in their reproductive years because a deficiency can result in spina bifida and other neural tube defects in the fetus.[15]

Elimination Pattern. Many gynecologic problems can result in genitourinary problems. Urinary incontinence is common in older women. Factors associated with female incontinence include relaxation of the pelvic musculature caused by multiple births, advancing age, fibroid tumors, DM, obesity, and weight gain. Use of condoms, diaphragms, and spermicides is associated with an increased risk of UTIs. In addition, vaginal infections such as bacterial vaginosis (BV) can facilitate the growth of *Escherichia coli,* which causes the majority of UTIs.[16] Men may suffer from urethritis, an inflammation of the urethra, which may be caused by an STI. Urethritis can cause painful urination. Benign prostatic hyperplasia (BPH) is a common problem of older men. It can alter normal urination by causing retention or difficulty in initiating the urinary stream.

Activity-Exercise Pattern. Record the amount, type, and intensity of activity and exercise. Lack of weight-bearing exercise is an important factor in the development of osteoporosis, especially in postmenopausal women. Adolescent females who engage in excessive leanness sports may experience *female athlete triad,* characterized by secondary amenorrhea, low energy availability, and osteoporosis.[17] Anemia can result in fatigue and activity intolerance and interfere with satisfactory performance of activities of daily living.

Sleep-Rest Pattern. Sleep patterns for women may be affected during the postpartum period and also while raising young children. Hot flashes and sweating that are often present during perimenopause can cause serious sleep interruption when the woman awakens in a drenching sweat. The need to change her nightgown and bedding further disrupts her sleep. Insomnia is also a common complaint of perimenopausal women. Daytime fatigue often results from such sleep disruptions. In men, sleep disturbances may be caused by frequent urination at night associated with prostate enlargement or hormone therapy for prostate cancer.

Cognitive-Perceptual Pattern. Pelvic pain is associated with various gynecologic disorders such as pelvic inflammatory disease, ovarian cysts, and endometriosis. Dyspareunia (painful intercourse) can be particularly problematic for women in the postmenopausal period. The pain associated with intercourse can create a reluctance to participate in sexual activity and strain relationships with sexual partners. Refer women with dyspareunia to their HCPs.

Self-Perception–Self-Concept Pattern. Changes that occur with aging, such as pendulous breasts and vaginal dryness in women and decreased size of the penis in men, may lead to emotional distress. The subtle changes associated with sexuality and advancing age may alter the self-concept of many persons.

Role-Relationship Pattern. Obtain information regarding the family structure and occupation. Question the patient regarding recent changes in work-related relationships or family conflict. Determine the patient's role in the family as a starting point to determine family dynamics.

Roles and relationships are affected by changes within the family. The addition of a new baby may change family dynamics. Role-relationship patterns change as children begin their careers and move away from home. Another change occurs when people lose their jobs at midlife or retire.

Sexuality-Reproductive Pattern. The extent and depth of the interview about a patient's sexuality depend primarily on the interviewer's expertise and on the patient's needs and willingness to discuss the topic. Before taking a sexual history, assess your comfort with your own sexuality, because any discomfort in questioning becomes obvious to the patient. Carry out interviews in an environment that provides reassurance, confidentiality, and a nonjudgmental attitude. Begin with the least sensitive areas of questioning and then move to more sensitive areas.

For women, obtain a menstrual and a chronologic obstetric history. The menstrual history includes the first day of the last menstrual period, description of menstrual flow, age of menarche, and, if applicable, age at menopause. Menstrual history data are used in the detection of pregnancy, infertility, and numerous other gynecologic problems. Have the patient explicitly describe changes in her usual menstrual pattern to determine whether the change is transient and unimportant or connected with a more serious gynecologic problem. Terminology that describes abnormal uterine bleeding patterns is discussed in Chapter 53.

Identify changes in menstrual patterns associated with the use of contraceptive pills, intrauterine devices (IUDs), birth control patches, vaginal rings, progestin-only implants, or medroxyprogesterone injections. Contraceptive pills usually decrease the amount and duration of flow, whereas some intrauterine devices can increase menstrual flow.[18] Some IUDs may be used for both contraception as well as a nonsurgical treatment for heavy menstrual bleeding.

The obstetric history includes the number of pregnancies, full-term births, preterm births, stillbirths, living children, and abortions (including spontaneous [miscarriage], ectopic, or induced). Document the course of each pregnancy, including the duration of each pregnancy, date of delivery, problems that may have occurred with each pregnancy, and any medical or surgical interventions that were needed.

A sexual history should include information regarding sexual activity, beliefs, and practices. Explore the (1) gender of the patient's partners (does the patient have sex with men? women? both?), (2) frequency and type of sexual activity (penile-vaginal, penile-rectal, receptive rectal, oral), (3) number of partners and protective measures against STI, and (4) contraceptive methods (if applicable). Determine the patient's knowledge of safe sexual practices. A history of multiple sex partners and unprotected sex increases the risk of contracting an STI. For a woman, this can increase the risk of pelvic inflammatory disease, which can compromise her ability to become pregnant.

Table 50-5 outlines *The 5 Ps of Sexual Health* approach for taking a sexual history that was developed by the Centers for Disease Control and Prevention. Never make an assumption about a patient's sexual orientation. Ask both men and women about their general satisfaction with their sexuality. Question the patient about sexual beliefs and practices and whether orgasm is achieved. Explore any unexplained change in sexual practices or performance. Problems of the reproductive system can cause physiologic or psychologic problems that can lead to painful intercourse, erectile dysfunction, sexual dysfunction, or infertility.

Coping–Stress Tolerance Pattern. The stress related to situations such as pregnancy or menopause increases dependence on support systems. Determine whom the support people are in

TABLE 50-5   Sexual History Format

The Five Ps of Taking a Sexual History*

The 5 Ps	Questions
1. Partners	Are you currently sexually active? (yes or no) • Do you have sex with men, women, or both? • In the past 2 months, with how many partners have you had sex? • In the past 12 months, with how many partners have you had sex?
2. Practices	To understand your risk for STIs, I need to understand the kind of sex you have had recently. • Genital (penis in the vagina) • Anal (penis in the anus) • Oral (mouth on penis, vagina, or anus)
3. Protection from STIs	Do you and your partner(s) use any protection against STIs? • What kind? • How often?
4. Past history of STIs	Have you ever been diagnosed with an STI? • What type? • When? • How were you treated?
5. Prevention of pregnancy	Are you or your partner trying to get pregnant? • If not, what are you doing to prevent pregnancy?

*This guide may need to be modified to be culturally appropriate for some patients based on culture or gender dynamics.
Adapted from www.cdc.gov/STI/treatment/sexualhistory.pdf.

the patient's life. The diagnosis of an STI can cause stress for the patient and partner. Explore ways to manage this stress with the patient by encouraging them to verbalize their fears and concerns.

Value-Belief Pattern. Sexual and reproductive functioning is closely related to cultural, religious, moral, and ethical values. Be aware of your own beliefs in these areas, and recognize and sensitively react to the patient's personal beliefs associated with reproductive and sexuality issues.

Objective Data

Physical Examination: Male. The examination of the male external genitalia by the nurse includes inspection and palpation of the pubis, penis, and scrotum. An examination may be performed with the patient lying or standing. The standing position is generally preferred. Sit in front of the standing patient. Use gloves during examination of the male genitalia.

If breast cancer is suspected or there is a strong family history of breast cancer in a male patient, a clinical breast examination is conducted in the same pattern for a male patient as a female breast examination (see Fig. 51-1).

Pubis. Assess for hair distribution and presence of body lice. Normally, the hair is in a diamond-shaped pattern and coarser than scalp hair. The absence of hair is not a normal finding unless the man is shaving or waxing the pubic hair. Carefully assess the skin for irritation and inflammation.

Penis and Scrotum. Inspect the penis for any lesions, bleeding, or swelling. Also note the location of the urethral meatus and the presence or absence of a foreskin. If present, the foreskin should be retracted to note any redness, discharge, irritation, lesions, or swelling from the meatus. Replace the foreskin over the glans after observation. Inspect the scrotum by lifting each testis to inspect all sides of the scrotal sac. Palpate the testes for tenderness or masses. The left testis usually hangs lower than the right. An

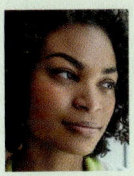
undescended testis (*cryptorchidism*) is a major risk factor for testicular cancer and a potential cause of male infertility.[19]

Anus. Note if the buttocks have any lesions, swelling, or inflammation. Spread the buttocks apart with both hands to expose the anus. Inspect the anal sphincter and perineal regions for fissures, lesions, masses, and hemorrhoids. The anus should be free from inflammation or skin changes.

Physical Examination: Female. With a chaperone present, physical examination of women often begins with inspection and palpation of the breasts and axillae and then proceeds to the abdomen and genitalia. Examination of the abdomen provides an opportunity to detect pain or any masses that may involve the genitourinary system. Abdominal examination is discussed in Chapter 38.

Breasts. First examine the breasts by visual inspection. With the patient seated, observe the breasts for symmetry, size, shape, skin color, vascular patterns, dimpling, and unusual lesions. Ask the patient to put her arms at her sides, arms overhead, lean forward, and press hands on hips. Observe for any abnormalities during these maneuvers. Palpate the axillae and clavicular areas for enlarged lymph nodes.

After the patient assumes a supine position, place a pillow under her back on the side to be examined. Ask the patient to put her arm above and behind her head. These maneuvers flatten breast tissue and make palpation easier. Then palpate the breast in a systematic fashion, preferably using a vertical line (see Fig. 51-1). Use the distal finger pads of the index, middle, and ring fingers for palpation. Include the axillary tail of Spence in the examination. This area of the breast lies adjacent to the upper outer quadrant, which is where most breast malignancies develop (see Fig. 51-1). Finally, palpate the area around the areolae for masses. Document the color, consistency, and odor of any discharge.

External Genitalia. The examination of a woman's genitalia by the nurse includes inspection and palpation of the mons pubis, vulva, and anus. Use gloves for the examination. Assess for hair distribution, presence of body lice, lesions, erythema, edema, or discharge. Many women remove hair from the genital region via shaving, waxing, or laser hair removal and may develop folliculitis (infection of the hair follicle). Separate the labia to fully inspect the clitoris, urethral meatus, and vaginal orifice. Spread the buttocks apart to inspect the anus for fissures, lesions, and hemorrhoids.

Internal Pelvic Examination. This part of the examination is usually performed by clinicians with advanced or specialized training. During the speculum examination, the examiner observes the walls of the vagina and cervix for inflammation, discharge, polyps, and suspicious growths. If indicated, a Pap test and specimens for culture and microscopic examination are obtained. After the speculum examination, a bimanual examination is performed to assess the size, shape, and consistency of the uterus and ovaries. The tubes are not normally palpable.

Table 50-6 provides an example of a recording format for the physical assessment findings for the male and female reproductive systems. Tables 50-7 through 50-9 summarize assessment abnormalities of the breasts, female reproductive system, and male reproductive system, respectively.

A *focused assessment* is used to evaluate the status of previously identified reproductive problems and to monitor for signs of new problems (see Table 3-7). A focused assessment of the reproductive system is presented in the box on this page.

CASE STUDY—cont'd

Objective Data: Physical Examination

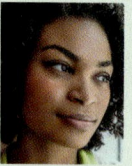

(©Benjamin A. Peterson/Mother Image/mother image/Fuse/Thinkstock)

Focused assessment of A.K. reveals the following: BP is 118/76 mmHg; her pulse is 70 beats per minute and regular. Skin warm and dry without lesions. No cyanosis of lips, mucous membranes, or nail beds. Thyroid is not enlarged. Cardiac examination is normal. Abdomen soft and nontender. External genitalia examination is normal. Bimanual examination performed by the physician is negative for cervical motion tenderness, adnexal masses, or pain. Uterus is enlarged, approximately 14 weeks in size, and boggy.

Discussion Questions

1. Based on the subjective and objective assessment findings, what diagnostic tests would you anticipate being ordered for A.K.?
   You will learn more about diagnostic studies related to the reproductive system in the next section.
   (See p. 1202 for more information on A.K.)

Answers available at *http://evolve.elsevier.com/Lewis/medsurg.*

DIAGNOSTIC STUDIES OF REPRODUCTIVE SYSTEMS

The most commonly used diagnostic studies in the assessment of the reproductive systems are summarized in Table 50-10. Diagnostic studies of the endocrine system may also be done in a person with a reproductive system problem (see Table 47-6).

Text continued on p. 1202

TABLE 50-6 Normal Physical Assessment of Reproductive System

Male	Female
Breasts	
Nipples soft. No lumps, nodules, swelling, or enlarged tissue noted.	Symmetric without dimpling. Nipples soft. No drainage, retraction, or lesions noted. No masses or tenderness. No lymphadenopathy.
External Genitalia	
Diamond-shaped hair distribution. No penile lesions or discharge noted. Scrotum symmetric, no masses, descended testes. No inguinal hernia.	Triangular hair distribution. Genitalia dark pink, no lesions, redness, swelling, or inflammation in perineal region. No vaginal discharge noted. No tenderness with palpation of Skene's ducts and Bartholin's glands.
Anus	
No hemorrhoids, fissures, or lesions noted.	No hemorrhoids, fissures, or lesions noted.

FOCUSED ASSESSMENT

Reproductive System

Use this checklist to ensure the key assessment steps have been done.

Subjective

Ask the patient about any of the following and note responses.

Vaginal or vulvar: discharge, lesions, itching, unusual bleeding, odor	Y	N
Penile pain, lesions, discharge	Y	N
Medications: oral contraceptives, antihypertensives, psychotropics, hormones	Y	N
Clinical examinations of reproductive systems (breast, pelvis, testicular, prostate) and results	Y	N
Pain: abdomen, pelvis, or genitalia	Y	N

Objective: Diagnostic

Check the following for results and critical values.

Serum hCG	✓
Serum PSA	✓
Culture and sensitivity	✓
Hormone studies (testosterone, progesterone, estrogen, FSH, LH)	✓
STI results (e.g., *Chlamydia*, gonorrhea)	✓
In office testing (e.g., wet mounts, pH assessment)	✓
Mammography and/or ultrasound of breasts	✓
Ultrasound: abdominal, pelvic, transvaginal, prostate	✓

Objective: Physical Examination

Inspect

External genitalia for erythema, swelling, discharge, lesions	✓
Breasts for swelling, dimpling, retraction, drainage, erythema, skin changes, masses,	✓

Palpate

Breast tissue for masses or tenderness	✓
External genitalia: tenderness, pain	✓

hCG, Human chorionic gonadotropin; *PSA,* prostate-specific antigen; *STIs,* sexually transmitted infections.

TABLE 50-7   Assessment Abnormalities

Breast

Finding	Description	Possible Etiology and Significance
Nipple inversion or retraction	Recent onset, erythematous, pain, unilateral.	Abscess, inflammation, cancer.
	Recent onset (usually within past year), unilateral presentation, lack of tenderness.	Neoplasm.
Nipple secretions		
• Galactorrhea (female)	Milky, no relationship to lactation, unilateral or bilateral, intermittent or consistent presentation.	Drug therapy, particularly phenothiazines, tricyclic antidepressants, methyldopa. Hypofunction or hyperfunction of thyroid or adrenal glands. Tumors of hypothalamus or pituitary gland. Excessive estrogen. Prolonged suckling or breast foreplay.
• Galactorrhea (male)	Milky, bilateral presentation.	Chorioepithelioma of testes, manifestation of pituitary tumor.
• Purulent	Gray-green or yellow color. Frequent unilateral presentation. Association with pain, erythema, induration, nipple inversion.	Puerperal (after birth) mastitis (inflammatory condition of breast) or abscess.
	Same as above but usually without nipple inversion.	Infected sebaceous cyst.
• Serous discharge	Clear appearance, unilateral or bilateral, intermittent or consistent presentation.	Intraductal papilloma.
• Dark green or multicolored discharge	Thick, sticky, and frequently bilateral.	Ductal ectasia (dilation of mammary ducts).
• Serosanguineous or bloody drainage	Unilateral presentation.	Papillomatosis (widespread development of nipple-like growths), intraductal papilloma, carcinoma (male and female).
Scaling or irritation of nipple	Unilateral or bilateral presentation, crusting, possible ulceration.	Paget's disease, eczema, infection.
Nodules, lumps, or masses	Multiple, bilateral, well-delineated, soft or firm, mobile cysts. Pain. Premenstrual occurrence.	Fibrocystic changes.
	Rubbery consistency, fluid-filled interior, pain.	Ductal ectasia.
	Soft, mobile, well-delineated cyst, absence of pain.	Lipoma, fibroadenoma.
	Erythema, tenderness, induration.	Infected sebaceous cysts, abscesses.
	Usually singular, hard, irregularly shaped, poorly delineated, nonmobile.	Neoplasm.
Dimpling of breast	Unilateral, recent onset, no pain.	Neoplasm.

TABLE 50-8   Assessment Abnormalities

Female Reproductive System

Finding and Description	Possible Etiology and Significance
Vulvar Discharge	
White, thick, curdy, frequent itching and inflammation, lack of odor or yeast-like smell	Candidiasis (*Candida* or yeast infection), vaginitis
Thin gray or white, copious flow, malodorous or fishy, vulvar irritation	Bacterial vaginosis infection
Frothy green or yellow color; malodorous	*Trichomonas vaginalis*
Bloody discharge	*Chlamydia trachomatis* or *Neisseria gonorrhoeae* infection, menstruation, trauma, cancer
Vulvar Erythema	
Bright or beefy red color, itching	*Candida albicans*, allergy, chemical vaginitis
Reddened base, painful vesicles or ulcerations	Genital herpes
Macules or papules, itching	Chancroid, contact dermatitis, scabies, pediculosis
Vulvar Growths	
Soft, fleshy growth, nontender	Condyloma acuminatum
Flat and warty appearance, nontender	Condyloma latum
Same as either of above, possible pain	Neoplasm
Reddened base, vesicles, and small erosions; pain	Lymphogranuloma venereum, genital herpes, chancroid
Indurated, firm ulcers, no pain	Chancre (syphilis), granuloma inguinale
Abdominal Pain or Tenderness	
Intermittent or consistent tenderness in right or left lower quadrant	Salpingitis (infection of fallopian tube), ectopic pregnancy, ruptured ovarian cyst, PID, tubal or ovarian abscess
Periumbilical location, consistent occurrence	Cystitis, endometritis (inflammation of endometrium), ectopic pregnancy

PID, Pelvic inflammatory disease.

TABLE 50-9   Assessment Abnormalities
Male Reproductive System

Finding and Description	Possible Etiology and Significance
Penile Growths or Masses	
Indurated, smooth, disklike appearance. Absence of pain. Singular presentation	Chancre
Papular to irregularly shaped ulceration with pus, lack of induration	Chancroid
Ulceration with induration and nodularity	Cancer
Flat, wartlike nodule	Condyloma latum
Elevated, fleshy, moist, elongated projections with single or multiple projections	Condyloma acuminatum
Localized swelling with retracted, tight foreskin	Paraphimosis (inability to replace foreskin to its normal position after retraction), trauma
Vesicles, Erosions, or Ulcers	
Painful, erythematous base. Vesicular or small erosions	Genital herpes, balanitis (inflammation of glans penis), chancroid
Painless, singular, small erosion with eventual lymphadenopathy	Lymphogranuloma venereum, cancer
Scrotal Masses	
Localized swelling with tenderness, unilateral or bilateral presentation	Epididymitis (inflammation of epididymis), testicular torsion, orchitis (mumps)
Swelling, tenderness	Incarcerated hernia
Swelling without pain. Unilateral or bilateral presentation. Translucent, cordlike or wormlike appearance	Hydrocele (accumulation of fluid in outer covering of testes), spermatocele (firm, sperm-containing cyst of epididymis), varicocele (dilation of veins that drain testes), hematocele (accumulation of blood within scrotum)
Firm, nodular testes or epididymis. Frequent unilateral presentation	Tuberculosis, cancer
Penile Discharge	
Clear to purulent color, minimal to copious flow	Urethritis or gonorrhea, *Chlamydia trachomatis* infection, trauma
Penile or Scrotal Erythema	
Macules and papules	Scabies, pediculosis
Inguinal Masses	
Bulging unilateral presentation during straining	Inguinal hernia
1- to 3-cm nodules	Lymphadenopathy

TABLE 50-10   Diagnostic Studies
Male and Female Reproductive Systems

Study	Description and Purpose	Nursing Responsibility
Urine and Blood Studies		
Anti-mullerian hormone (AMH)	Measures ovarian function. Level reflects size of the remaining egg supply ("ovarian reserve"). May be done when a woman has manifestations of polycystic ovarian syndrome (PCOS). Used to monitor AMH-producing ovarian tumor. Females with higher AMH have a better response to ovarian stimulation during fertility treatments. Females 13-45 years: 0.9-9.5 ng/mL Females >45 years: <1.0 ng/mL	*Before:* Inform patient that blood sample will be drawn. *After:* Observe venipuncture site for bleeding or hematoma formation.
Estradiol	Measures ovarian function. Useful in assessing estrogen-secreting tumors and states of precocious female puberty. May be used to confirm perimenopausal status. Increased serum estradiol levels in men may be indicative of testicular tumors. *Female:* Follicular phase: 20-150 pg/mL (73-1285 pmol/L) Luteal phase: 30-450 pg/mL (110-1652 pmol/L) Postmenopause: ≤20 pg/mL (≤73 pmol/L) *Male:* 10-50 pg/mL (37-184 pmol/L)	Same as above.
Fluorescent treponemal antibody absorption (FTA-Abs)	Detects antibodies to syphilis. *Reference interval:* Negative or nonreactive.	Same as above.

TABLE 50-10 Diagnostic Studies

Male and Female Reproductive Systems—cont'd

Study	Description and Purpose	Nursing Responsibility
Follicle-stimulating hormone (FSH)	Assesses gonadal function and abnormal levels may indicate pituitary tumors or dysfunction. Increased in menopause. May be used to validate menopausal status. In 24-hr urine samples: *Female:* Follicular phase: 2-15 U/24 hr Midcycle: 8-60 U/24 hr Luteal phase: 2-10 U/24 hr Postmenopause: 35-100 U/24 hr *Male:* 3-11 U/24 hr In blood: *Female:* Follicular phase: 1.37-9.9 mU/mL Ovulatory phase: 6.17-17.2 mU/mL Luteal phase: 1.09-9.2 mU/mL Postmenopause: 19.3-100.6 mU/mL *Male:* 1.42-15.4 mU/mL	Same as above.
Human chorionic gonadotropin (hCG)	Detects pregnancy. Also detects hydatidiform mole and chorioepithelioma (in men and women). Can be done in urine or blood. *Qualitative:* Negative *Quantitative:* <5 mIU/mL (<5 IU/L) *(males and nonpregnant females)*	*Before:* Obtain menstrual history from patient, including birth control methods. *During:* Urine tests can be purchased over the counter or used in HCP office.
Luteinizing hormone (LH)	Associated with ovulation in women and testosterone production in men. Particularly useful in women in the workup of infertility and menstrual irregularities. *Female: Premenopause:* 5-25 IU/L With higher peaks at ovulation *Female: Postmenopause:* 14-52.3 IU/L *Male:* 1.8-8.6 IU/L	*Before:* Inform patient that blood sample will be drawn. *After:* Observe venipuncture site for bleeding or hematoma formation.
Prolactin	Detects pituitary dysfunction that can cause amenorrhea, decreased libido, and impotence. *Female:* 3.8-23.2 ng/mL (3.8-23.2 mg/L) *Male:* 3.0-14.7 ng/mL (3.0-14.7 mg/L)	Same as above.
Progesterone	Used to assess infertility, monitors success of drugs for infertility or the effect of treatment with progesterone, determines whether ovulation is occurring, and diagnoses problems with adrenal glands and some types of cancer. *Female:* Follicular phase: 15-70 ng/dL (0.5-2.2 nmol/L) Luteal phase: 200-2500 ng/dL (6.4-79.5 nmol/L) Postmenopause: <40 ng/dL (1.28 nmol/L) *Male:* 13-97 ng/dL (0.4-3.1 nmol/L)	Same as above.
Prostate-specific antigen (PSA)	Detects prostate cancer. Also used to monitor response to therapy. *Reference interval:* <4 ng/mL (<4 mcg/L)	Same as above.
Rapid plasma reagin (RPR) (agglutination)	Screening test for syphilis. Test is most sensitive during secondary stage. *Reference interval:* Negative or nonreactive	Same as above.
Testosterone	Detects tumors and developmental anomalies of the testicles. Used to assess male infertility. In 24-hr urine samples: *Female:* 2-12 mcg/24 hr (6.9-41.6 nmol/24 hr) *Male:* 40-135 mcg/24 hr (139-469 nmol/24 hr) In blood: *Female:* 15-70 ng/dL (0.52-2.43 nmol/L) *Male:* 280-1100 ng/dL (10.4-38.17 nmol/L)	Same as above. *Before:* Obtain health history to eliminate potential sources of inaccuracy of results (e.g., use of corticosteroids or barbiturates, hypo- or hyperthyroidism). In males, can also be measured in saliva.
Cultures, Smears, and Nucleic Acid Amplification Tests		
Dark-field microscopy	Direct examination of specimen obtained from potential syphilitic lesion (chancre) is performed to detect *Treponema pallidum*.	*During:* Avoid direct skin contact with open lesion.
Wet mounts	Direct microscopic examination of specimen of vaginal discharge is performed immediately after collection. Determines presence or absence and number of *Trichomonas* organisms, bacteria, white and red blood cells, and candidal buds or hyphae.	*Before:* Explain procedure and purpose to patient. Instruct patient not to douche before examination. *During:* Prepare for collection of specimens (glass slide, cover slips, 10%-20% potassium hydroxide [KOH] solution, sodium chloride [NaCl] solution, and applicators).

Continued

TABLE 50-10   Diagnostic Studies
Male and Female Reproductive Systems—cont'd

Study	Description and Purpose	Nursing Responsibility
Cultures, Smears, and Nucleic Acid Amplification Tests—*cont'd*		
Cultures	Specimens from urine or vaginal, urethral, or cervical discharge are cultured to assess for gonorrhea or *Chlamydia* organisms. Rectal and throat cultures may also be taken, depending on data obtained from sexual history.	*Before:* Obtain specific contact and sexual history, including oral and rectal intercourse. *During:* Obtain urethral specimen from men before they void.
Nucleic acid amplification test (NAAT)	Nonculture test used to identify small amounts of DNA or RNA in test samples with sensitivity similar to culture tests. Uses ligase or polymerase chain reaction that amplifies the signal of the nucleic acids in the test sample so that they are easier to identify. Can be done on a wide variety of samples, including vaginal, endocervical, urethral, and urine specimens. Preferred method to test for gonorrhea, *Chlamydia,* and trichomoniasis.	*During:* Do not require special handling of specimens and are easier to perform than cell cultures.
Gram stain	Used for rapid detection of gonorrhea. Presence of gram-negative intracellular diplococci generally warrants treatment. Not highly accurate for women. Also a valid alternative for *Chlamydia* testing.	Same as culture.
Cytologic Studies		
Papanicolaou (Pap) test	Microscopic study of exfoliated cervical cells to detect abnormal cells. *Conventional cytology* entails fixing cells directly to a slide at the time of collection and sending the slide to the laboratory for interpretation. In *liquid-based cytology* the specimen is sent to the laboratory in a liquid solution that preserves it and is processed for microscopic evaluation at the laboratory. Testing for human papillomavirus (HPV) may be done on specimen obtained for liquid-based Pap test (see Chapter 53).	*Before:* Obtain data about menstrual history and current hormone therapy use. Instruct women that best time to schedule examination is 10-14 days after the first day of LMP and to avoid vaginal medications, lubricants, contraceptives, or douches 2 days prior to test.
Nipple discharge test	Cytologic study of nipple discharge.	*Before:* Find out if patient is taking hormonal preparations or other drugs, is breastfeeding, or has a history of amenorrhea. Document this information.
Radiologic Studies		
Mammography	X-ray image used to assess breast tissue. Detects benign and malignant masses. (Screening guidelines for mammography are discussed in Chapter 51.)	*Before:* Instruct patient to avoid use of deodorants, antiperspirants, powders, lotions, or creams under the arms or on breasts. Try to schedule test the week after menses when breasts are least likely to be tender.
Ultrasound (US) (breast, pelvic, testicular, transvaginal [TV], rectal [TRUS])	Measures and records high-frequency sound waves as they pass through tissues of variable density. Breast US useful in detecting fluid-filled masses and for follow-up screening after mammography in women with dense breast tissue. In women, pelvic and TV US useful to detect pelvic masses such as ectopic pregnancy, ovarian cysts, fibroids, and other pelvic masses. In men, US used to detect testicular masses and testicular torsion. Transrectal ultrasound (TRUS) is useful for diagnosing prostate tumors.	*Before:* Instruct patient that a full bladder is required for a pelvic ultrasound.
Ultrasound-guided biopsy	Use of ultrasound guidance while performing a biopsy. Ultrasound is used to direct the biopsy needle into the region of interest and obtain a sample of tissue. Removal of small tissue sample to diagnose infection, inflammation, or mass.	*Before:* Inform patient of purpose for this procedure. It is usually done as an outpatient procedure. *After:* Instruct patient to monitor for signs and symptoms of infection at biopsy site.
CT scan of pelvis	Detects tumors in the pelvis.	*Before:* Inform patient of procedure. *During:* Patient must lie still during the procedure. If IV contrast medium is used, check for iodine allergy.
MRI	Radio waves and magnetic field are used to assess soft tissue. Useful after an abnormal mammogram or in women with dense breast tissue. Breast MRI may be used in addition to mammography to detect breast cancer in women at high risk for breast cancer. Also used to diagnose abnormalities in female and male reproductive systems.	*Before:* Screen patient for metal parts and pacemaker. Inform patient the procedure is painless. Patient must lie still during the procedure.
Invasive Procedures		
Hysteroscopy	Allows visualization of uterine lining through insertion of scope through cervix. Used mainly to diagnose and treat abnormal bleeding such as polyps and fibroids. Biopsy may be taken during procedure. May be used as part of infertility assessment.	*Before:* Explain purpose and method of procedure and that it may be done in the physician's office or an outpatient setting. Inform patient that mild cramping and slight bloody discharge after procedure is normal.

TABLE 50-10 Diagnostic Studies

Male and Female Reproductive Systems—cont'd

Study	Description and Purpose	Nursing Responsibility
Hysterosalpingogram	Involves instillation of contrast media through cervix into uterine cavity and subsequently through fallopian tubes. X-ray images taken to detect abnormalities of uterus and its adnexa (ovaries and tubes) as contrast progresses through them. Most useful in diagnostic assessment of fertility (e.g., to detect adhesions near ovary, abnormal uterine shape, blockage of tubal pathways).	*Before:* Inform patient about procedure and that it may be fairly uncomfortable. Contrast medium is used. *After:* Inform patient she may experience slight vaginal bleeding and cramping. Monitor for foul-smelling vaginal discharge, severe pain, fever, or chills.
Colposcopy	Direct visualization of cervix with binocular microscope that allows magnification of cervix and study of cellular abnormalities. Used as follow-up for abnormal Pap test and for examination of women exposed to DES in utero. Biopsy(ies) of cervix may be taken during examination. Also used to assess for vaginal or vulvar dysplasia.	*Before:* Instruct patient about this procedure. Inform patient that this examination is similar to speculum examination.
Conization	Cone-shaped sample of squamocolumnar tissue of cervix is removed for direct study.	*Before:* Explain purpose and method of procedure and that it requires use of surgical facilities and anesthesia. *After:* Instruct patient to avoid sexual intercourse and tampons for about 3-4 wk. Also discuss necessity for 3-wk follow-up.
Loop electrosurgical excision procedure (LEEP)	Excision of cervical tissue via an electrosurgical instrument. Diagnoses and treats cervical dysplasia. Minimal amount of tissue removed and preserves childbearing ability.	*Before:* Explain purpose and method of procedure and that it may be done in the physician's office. Patient may feel slight tingling or abdominal cramping during procedure. *After:* Tell patient that discharge, bleeding, and cramping may occur for 1-3 days after procedure.
Culdotomy, culdoscopy, and culdocentesis	*Culdotomy* is an incision made through posterior fornix of cul-de-sac and allows visualization of peritoneal cavity (i.e., uterus, tubes, and ovaries). *Culdoscopy* can then be used to closely study these structures. This technique is valuable in fertility evaluations. Withdrawal of fluid *(culdocentesis)* allows examination of fluid.	*Before:* Explain purpose and method of procedure. Prepare patient for vaginal operation with preoperative instruction and sedation. *After:* Perform assessment of bleeding and discomfort after surgery.
Laparoscopy	Allows visualization of pelvic structures via fiberoptic scopes inserted through small abdominal incisions. Instillation of CO_2 into cavity improves visualization. Used in diagnostic assessment of uterus, tubes, and ovaries (Fig. 50-9, on following page). Often used for tubal sterilization or part of infertility assessment.	*Before:* Instruct patient about procedure, prepare abdomen, and reassure patient about sedation. Inform patient of probability of referred shoulder pain secondary to residual air in the abdomen.
Dilation and curettage (D&C)	Operative procedure that dilates cervix and allows curetting of endometrial lining. Used in assessment of abnormal bleeding and cytologic evaluation of lining.	*Before:* Instruct patient about procedure and sedation. *After:* Perform assessment of degree of bleeding (frequent pad check during first 24 hr).
Fertility Studies		
Semen analysis	Semen is assessed for volume (2-5 mL), viscosity, sperm count (>20 million/mL), sperm motility (60% motile), and percent of abnormal sperm (60% with normal structure).	*Before:* Instruct patient that no more than 1 hr should elapse between collection and examination of sample. Do not have any sexual activity that causes ejaculation 2-3 days before the test.
Basal body temperature assessment	Measurement indirectly indicates whether ovulation has occurred. (Temperature rises at ovulation and remains elevated during secretory phase of normal menstrual cycle.)	*Before:* Instruct woman to take temperature using special basal temperature thermometer (calibrated in tenths of degrees) every morning before getting out of bed. Instruct to record temperature on graph.
Hysterosalpingogram	Same as operative procedures.	Same as operative procedures.
Serum AMH, estradiol, FSH, progesterone	Same as blood studies.	Same as blood studies.
Urinary LH	Over-the-counter "ovulation predictor kits." Identifies midcycle LH surge that precedes ovulation by 1 to 2 days.	Inform patient to follow directions carefully of specific test used.

DES, Diethylstilbestrol; *IUD,* intrauterine device.

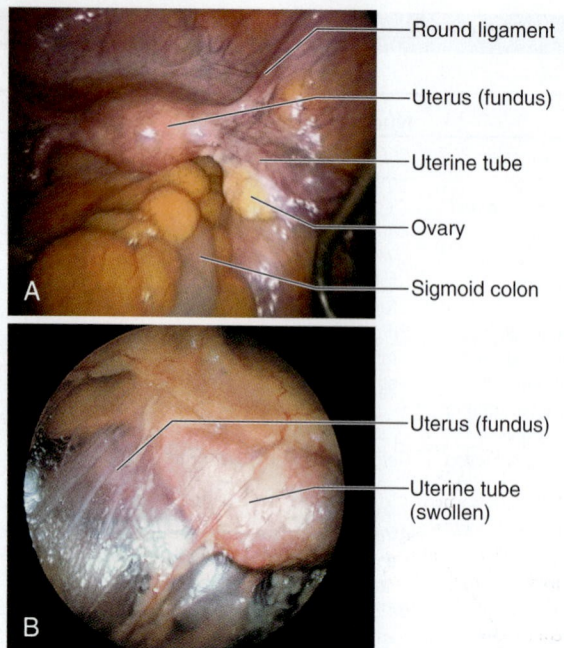

FIG. 50-9 Laparoscopic views of the female pelvis. **A,** Normal image. **B,** Pelvic inflammatory disease. (Note reddish inflammatory membrane covering and fixing the ovary and uterus to the surrounding structures.) (*A*, From Abrahams P, Marks S, Hutching R: *McMinn's color atlas of human anatomy,* ed 5, Philadelphia, 2003, Saunders. *B,* From Symonds EM, MacPherson MB: *Color atlas of obstetrics and gynecology,* London, 1994, Mosby Wolfe.)

CASE STUDY—cont'd

Objective Data: Diagnostic Studies

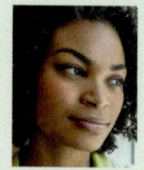

(©Benjamin A. Peterson/Mother Image/mother image/Fuse/Thinkstock)

The following laboratory and diagnostic tests are ordered for A.K.:
Urine pregnancy test, pelvic and transvaginal ultrasound, complete blood count (CBC), thyroid stimulating hormone (TSH), and iron studies.
Pregnancy test
CBC findings:
• Hemoglobin, 10.3 g/dL
• Hematocrit, 31%
Serum iron level, decreased
TSH, 2.3 IU/L
The pelvic and transvaginal ultrasound revealed a uterine fibroid. The patient is scheduled for a hysteroscopic myomectomy.

Discussion Questions

1. Which diagnostic and laboratory test results are of concern to you?
2. What additional patient teaching can you provide A.K. based on her diagnostic test results?

Answers available at *http://evolve.elsevier.com/Lewis/medsurg.*

BRIDGE TO NCLEX EXAMINATION

The number of the question corresponds to the same-numbered outcome at the beginning of the chapter.

1. A normal male reproductive function that may be altered in a patient who undergoes a orchiectomy (removal of testes) is
   a. production of GnRH
   b. production of testosterone.
   c. production of progesterone.
   d. production of seminal fluid.
2. Luteinizing hormone (LH) secretion by the anterior pituitary (*select all that apply*)
   a. results in ovulation.
   b. causes follicles to complete maturation.
   c. affects development of ruptured follicles.
   d. directly inhibits both GnRH and FSH secretion.
   e. stimulates testosterone production by interstitial cells of testes.
3. Male orgasm is characterized by
   a. resolution.
   b. increased testicular size.
   c. vasodilation and dystonia.
   d. vasocongestion and myotonia.
4. An age-related finding during the assessment of the older woman's reproductive system is
   a. dyspareunia.
   b. vaginal atrophy.
   c. nipple enlargement.
   d. increased vulvar skin turgor.
5. Significant information about a person's health history related to the reproductive system should include (*select all that apply*)
   a. tobacco use.
   b. intellectual status.
   c. current pain level.
   d. previous history of shingles.
   e. previous sexually transmitted infections.
6. Cultures used in the diagnosis of STIs can be obtained from (*select all that apply*)
   a. urine.
   b. vagina.
   c. urethra.
   d. rectum.
   e. endocervix.
7. An abnormal finding noted during physical assessment of the male reproductive system is
   a. descended testes.
   b. symmetric scrotum.
   c. slight clear urethral discharge.
   d. the glans covered with prepuce.

8. The nurse is caring for a patient scheduled for an endometrial biopsy who is having difficulty becoming pregnant. The nurse explains to the woman that
   a. the outpatient procedure is usually done preovulation.
   b. bleeding and discharge is common 2 to 4 days after the procedure.
   c. a small sample of tissue is obtained to diagnose and treat cervical dysplasia.
   d. common changes in endometrial cells in relation to progesterone levels will be assessed.

1. b, 2, a, b, c, e, 3, d, 4, b, 5, a, c, 6, a, b, c, d, e, 7, c, 8, d

For rationales to these answers and even more NCLEX review questions, visit *http://evolve.elsevier.com/Lewis/medsurg*.

EVOLVE WEBSITE

http://evolve.elsevier.com/Lewis/medsurg
Review Questions (Online Only)
Key Points
Answer Keys for Questions
• Rationales for Bridge to NCLEX Examination Questions
• Answer Guidelines for the Case Study on pp. 1191, 1195, 1196, and 1202
Conceptual Care Map Creator
Audio Glossary
Supporting Media
• Animations
   • Ovulation
   • Reproductive System Overview
   • Spermatogenesis
Content Updates

REFERENCES

1. Thibodeau GA, Patton KT: *Structure and function of the body*, ed 14, St Louis, 2012, Mosby.
2. Strauss J. Barbieri R, editors: *Yen and Jaffe's reproductive endocrinology: physiology, pathophysiology and clinical management*, ed 7, Philadelphia, 2014, Saunders.
3. Lentz GM, Lobo RA, Gerhenson DM, et al: *Comprehensive gynecology*, ed 6, Philadelphia, 2012, Saunders.
4. Singh V: *Textbook of anatomy abdomen and lower limb*, vol 2, ed 2, New Delhi, 2014, Elsevier.
5. Gynecologic cysts. Retrieved from *www.merckmanuals.com/home/womens_health_issues/noncancerous_gynecologic_abnormalities/gynecologic_cysts.html*.
6. Masters WH, Johnson E: *Human sexual response*, Boston, 1966, Little Brown. (Classic)
7. Menopause. Retrieved from *www.womenshealth.gov/menopause/index.html?from=AtoZ*.
*8. The North American Menopause Society (NAMS). *Menopause practice: a clinician's guide*, ed 5, Mayfield Heights, Ohio, 2014, NAMS.
*9. Centers for Disease Control and Prevention. Guidelines for vaccinating pregnant women. 2013. Retrieved from *www.cdc.gov/vaccines/pubs/downloads/b_preg_guide.pdf*.
10. Aging changes in the male reproductive system. Retrieved from *www.nlm.nih.gov/medlineplus/ency/article/004017.htm*.
11. The American College of Obstetricians and Gynecologists: Patient education fact sheet: hormone therapy. Retrieved from *www.acog.org/-/media/For-Patients/pfs003.pdf?dmc=1&ts=20141029T1921516354*.
12. American Cancer Society: Can prostate cancer be found early? 2014. Retrieved from *www.cancer.org/cancer/prostatecancer/detailedguide/prostate-cancer-detection*.
13. Centers for Disease Control and Prevention: 2014 Surgeon General's Report: The health consequences of smoking—50 years of progress. Retrieved from *www.surgeongeneral.gov/library/reports/50-years-of-progress/full-report.pdf*.
14. Moscicki AB, Schiffman M, Burchell A, et al: Updating the natural history of human papillomavirus and anogenital cancers, *Vaccine* 30:F24, 2012.
15. Centers for Disease Control and Prevention: Folic acid recommendations. Retrieved from *www.cdc.gov/ncbddd/folicacid/recommendations.html*.
16. Foxman B: Urinary tract infection syndromes: occurrence, recurrence, bacteriology, risk factors, and disease burden, *Infect Dis Clin North Am* 28:1, 2014.
17. Barrack MT, Ackerman KE, Gibbs JC: Update on the female athlete triad, *Curr Rev Musculoskelet Med* 6:195, 2013.
18. Hubacher D, Chen PL, Park S: Side effects from the copper IUD: Do they decrease over time? *Contraception* 79:356, 2010.
19. Viatori M: Testicular cancer, *Semin Oncol Nurs* 28:180, 2012.

*Evidence-based information for clinical practice.

51

Breast Disorders

Darcy Burbage

People grow through experience if they meet life honestly and courageously. This is how character is built.

Eleanor Roosevelt

ⓔ http://evolve.elsevier.com/Lewis/medsurg/

LEARNING OUTCOMES

1. Summarize screening guidelines for the early detection of breast cancer.
2. Describe accurate clinical breast examination techniques, including inspection and palpation.
3. Explain the types, causes, clinical manifestations, and nursing and interprofessional management of common benign breast disorders.
4. Assess the risk factors for breast cancer.
5. Describe the pathophysiology and clinical manifestations of breast cancer.

6. Describe the interprofessional care and nursing management of breast cancer.
7. Specify the physical and psychologic preoperative and postoperative aspects of nursing management for the patient undergoing breast cancer surgery.
8. Explain the indications for reconstructive breast surgery, types and complications of reconstructive breast surgery, and nursing management after reconstructive breast surgery.

KEY TERMS

ductal ectasia, p. 1208
fibroadenoma, p. 1207
fibrocystic changes, p. 1207
galactorrhea, p. 1208

gynecomastia, p. 1208
intraductal papilloma, p. 1208
lumpectomy, p. 1213
lymphedema, p. 1214

mammoplasty, p. 1222
mastalgia, p. 1206
mastitis, p. 1206
Paget's disease, p. 1211

Breast disorders are a significant health concern for women. Whether the actual diagnosis is a benign condition or a malignancy, the initial discovery of a lump or change in the breast often triggers intense feelings of anxiety, fear, and denial.

The most frequently encountered breast disorders in women are fibrocystic changes, fibroadenoma, intraductal papilloma, ductal ectasia, and breast cancer. In a woman's lifetime, there is a 1 in 8 (12%) chance that she will be diagnosed with breast cancer.[1] Although rare, breast cancer does occur in men.

ASSESSMENT OF BREAST DISORDERS

Breast Cancer Screening Guidelines

Screening guidelines for the early detection of breast cancer vary depending on a woman's age and risk. For women at average risk for breast cancer, the following is recommended by the American Cancer Society:[2]

- Women should undergo regular screening mammography starting at age 45 years.

- Women aged 45 to 54 years should be screened annually.
- Women 55 years and older should transition to biennial screening or have the opportunity to continue screening annually.
- Women should continue screening mammography as long as their overall health is good and they have a life expectancy of 10 years or longer.
- The ACS does not recommend clinical breast examination for breast cancer screening among average-risk women at any age.

Women at increased risk of breast cancer (family history, genetic link, prior breast cancer, past history of thoracic radiation therapy, or certain atypical findings on a prior breast biopsy) should talk with their HCP about the benefits and limitations of starting mammography screening earlier, using breast magnetic resonance imaging (MRI), and having more frequent clinical breast examinations.[3]

Consistent breast self-examination (BSE) may facilitate breast self-awareness.[3] In recent years there has been some

Reviewed by Jane E. Lacovara, RN, MSN, CMSRN, Clinical Nurse Specialist-BC, Nursing Administration, University of Arizona Medical Center–University Campus, Tucson, Arizona; Karen Meneses, RN, PhD, FAAN, Professor and Associate Dean for Research, School of Nursing, University of Alabama at Birmingham, Birmingham, Alabama; Mary Schied, RN, MSN, OCN, CBCN, Breast Health Nurse, North Colorado Medical Center, Greeley, Colorado; Kathryn J. Trotter, DNP, CNM, FNP-C, Assistant Clinical Professor, Duke University Medical Center, Durham, North Carolina; and Deborah Kirk Walker, DNP, FNP-BC, NP-C, AOCN, Assistant Professor/Nurse Practitioner, Coordinator of Dual Adult–Gerontology Primary Care and Oncology Nurse Practitioner Specialty Track, University of Alabama at Birmingham School of Nursing, Birmingham, Alabama.

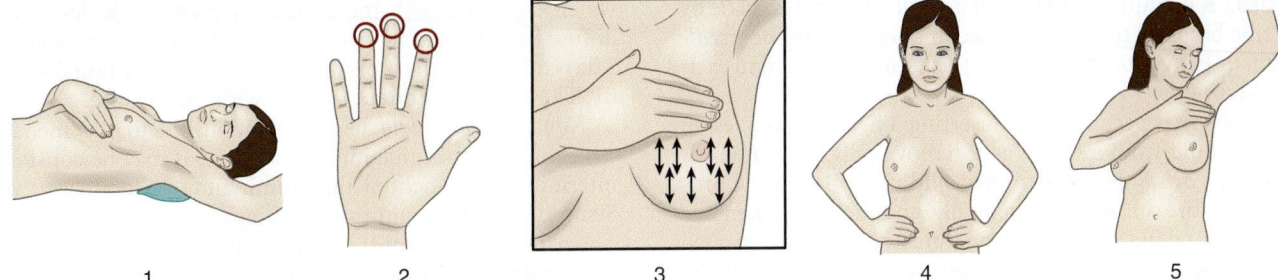

FIG. 51-1 Breast self-examination and patient instruction. *1,* Lie down and place your left arm behind your head. Lying down spreads breast tissue evenly and thinly over the chest wall, making it easier to feel the tissue. *2,* Use finger pads of three middle fingers on your right hand to feel for lumps in left breast. Use overlapping dime-sized circular motions to feel the breast tissue. Use three different levels of pressure to feel the breast tissue: light pressure to feel tissue closest to the skin; medium pressure to feel a little deeper; and firm pressure to feel tissue closest to the chest and ribs. A firm ridge in the lower curve of each breast is normal. *3,* The up-and-down (vertical) pattern is recommended for examining the entire breast. Move around the breast in an up-and-down pattern starting at an imaginary line straight down your side from the underarm (including the tail of Spence, which is the triangular breast tissue projecting into the axilla), and moving across the breast to the middle of the sternum. Examine the entire breast going down until you feel only ribs and up to the neck or clavicle. Repeat procedure while examining your right breast. *4,* Stand in front of a mirror. Place your hands firmly on your hips, which will tighten the pectoralis muscles. Look at your breasts for size, shape, redness, scaliness, or dimpling of the breast skin or nipple. *5,* Examine each underarm while standing or sitting with arm slightly raised. Check for any lump, hard knot, or thickening of tissue. (Source: American Cancer Society: How to examine your breasts. Retrieved from *www.cancer.org/cancer/breastcancer/moreinformation/breastcancerearlydetection/breast-cancer-early-detection-acs-recs-bse.*)

controversy regarding the value of BSE and its role in reducing mortality rates from breast cancer in women. While the benefit of BSE in reducing breast cancer deaths continues to be reviewed, BSE remains a useful technique in helping women develop awareness of how their breasts normally look and feel. Teach women beginning at age 20 the benefits and limitations of BSE and the importance of reporting breast changes (e.g., nipple discharge, a lump) to their HCP.[3]

When teaching the woman about BSE, include information related to potential benefits, limitations, and harm (chance of a false-positive test result). Allow time for questions about the procedure and a return demonstration. At every periodic health examination, ask the woman who is performing BSE to demonstrate her technique. For women who choose to perform BSE, the technique is described in Fig. 51-1.

Diagnostic Studies

Radiologic Studies. Several techniques can be used to screen for breast disorders or to help diagnose a suspicious physical finding. *Mammography* is a method used to visualize the breast's internal structure using x-rays (Fig. 51-2). This generally well-tolerated procedure can detect suspicious lumps that cannot be felt. Mammography has significantly improved the early and accurate detection of breast malignancies. Improved imaging technology has also reduced the radiation dose from mammography.

A comparison of current and prior mammograms may show early tissue changes. Because some tumors metastasize late, early detection by mammography allows for earlier treatment and the prevention of metastasis. In younger women, mammography is less sensitive because of the greater density of breast tissue, resulting in more false-negative results.

Digital mammography is a technique in which x-ray images are digitally coded and stored in a computer (Fig. 51-2). Digital mammograms are more accurate than traditional film mammography in younger women with dense breasts. The availability and associated costs of digital mammography are additional issues related to this technology.

Three-dimensional (3D) mammography, or tomosynthesis mammography, produces a 3D image of the breast. It provides a clearer view of overlapping breast tissue structures.

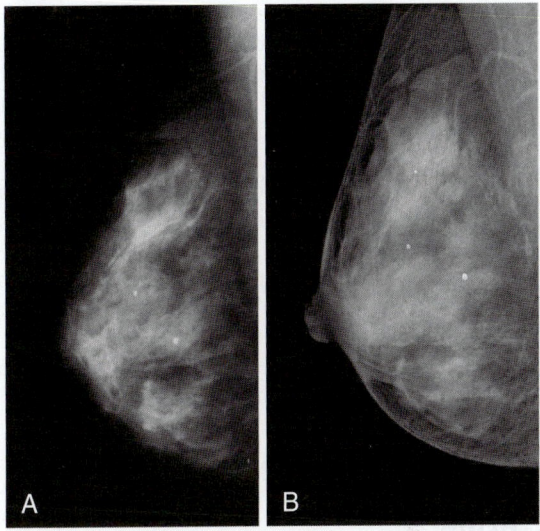

FIG. 51-2 Screening mammogram showing dense breast tissue and benign, scattered microcalcifications of a 57-year-old. **A,** Using conventional x-rays. **B,** Using digital x-rays. (From Adam A, Dixon AK, Grainger RG, et al: *Grainger and Allison's diagnostic radiology,* ed 5, St Louis, 2008, Churchill Livingstone.)

Calcifications are the most easily recognized mammogram abnormality (Fig. 51-2). These deposits of calcium crystals form in the breast for many reasons, such as inflammation, trauma, and/or aging. Although most calcifications are benign, they may also be associated with breast cancer.

About 10% to 15% of all breast cancers cannot be seen on mammography. They can be detected by palpation or additional breast imaging studies, such as ultrasound and MRI. If the clinical findings are suspicious and the mammogram is normal, an ultrasound or MRI may be used. Based on these additional findings, a biopsy may be done.

Ultrasound is used in conjunction with mammography to differentiate a solid mass from a cystic mass, to evaluate a mass in a pregnant or lactating woman, and to locate and biopsy a suspicious lesion. MRI is recommended as a screening tool in addition to mammography for women who are at risk for breast cancer (e.g., first-degree relative with a *BRCA* mutation).[3]

Biopsies. A definitive diagnosis of a suspicious area is made by analyzing biopsied tissue. Biopsy techniques include *fine-needle aspiration* (FNA), core (core needle), vacuum-assisted, and excisional biopsies.

FNA biopsy is performed by inserting a needle into a lesion to sample fluid from a breast cyst, remove cells from intercellular spaces, or sample cells from a solid mass. Before the procedure, the breast area is first locally anesthetized. Then the needle is placed into the breast, and fluid and cells are aspirated into a syringe. Three or four passes are usually made. If the results are negative with a suspicious lesion, an additional biopsy may be necessary.

A *core (core needle) biopsy* involves removing small samples of breast tissue using a hollow "core" needle. For palpable lesions, this is accomplished by fixing the lesion with one hand and performing a needle biopsy with the other. In the case of nonpalpable lesions, *stereotactic mammography, ultrasound, or MRI image guidance* is used. Stereotactic mammography uses computers to pinpoint the exact location of a breast mass based on mammograms. With ultrasound, the radiologist or surgeon watches the needle on the ultrasound monitor to help guide it to the area of concern. Because a core biopsy removes more tissue than an FNA, it is more accurate.

Vacuum-assisted biopsy is a version of core biopsy that uses a vacuum technique to help collect the tissue sample. In core biopsy, several separate needle insertions are used to acquire multiple samples. During vacuum-assisted biopsy, the needle is inserted only once into the breast, and the needle can be rotated, which allows for multiple samples through a single needle insertion.

Minimally invasive breast biopsies have become the standard of care for diagnosing abnormalities found either on imaging studies or through clinical examination. However, in some cases an *excisional biopsy* is recommended. An excisional biopsy is performed in an operating room.

BENIGN BREAST DISORDERS

MASTALGIA

Mastalgia (breast pain) is the most common breast-related complaint in women. The most common form is *cyclic mastalgia*, which coincides with the menstrual cycle.[4] It is described as diffuse breast tenderness or heaviness. Breast pain may last 2 or 3 days or most of the month and is related to hormonal sensitivity. The symptoms often decrease with menopause.

Noncyclic mastalgia has no relationship to the menstrual cycle and can continue into menopause. It may be constant or intermittent throughout the month and last for several years. Symptoms include a burning, aching, or soreness in the breast. The pain may be from trauma, fat necrosis, ductal ectasia, costochrondritis, or arthritic pain in the chest or neck radiating to the breast.

For patients with mastalgia, mammography and targeted ultrasound are frequently done to exclude cancer and provide information on the etiology of mastalgia. Although evidence supporting treatments for benign breast pain have yielded conflicting results, some relief for cyclic pain may occur by reducing intake of caffeine and dietary fat; taking vitamins E, A, B complex, gamma-linolenic acid (evening primrose oil); and continually wearing a supportive bra. Compresses, ice, analgesics, and antiinflammatory drugs may also help. Prescription medication such as oral contraceptives and danazol may also be used. However, the androgenic side effects of danazol (acne, edema, hirsutism) may make this therapy unacceptable for many women.

BREAST INFECTIONS

Mastitis

Mastitis is an inflammatory condition of the breast that occurs most frequently in lactating women (Table 51-1). *Lactational mastitis* manifests as a localized area that is erythematous, painful, and tender to palpation. Fever is often present. The infection develops when organisms (usually staphylococci) gain access to the breast through a cracked nipple. In its early stages, mastitis can be cured with antibiotics. Breastfeeding should continue unless an abscess is forming or purulent drainage is noted. The mother may wish to use a nipple shield or to hand-express milk from the involved breast until the pain subsides. The woman should see her HCP promptly to begin a course of antibiotic therapy. Any breast that remains red, tender, and not responsive to antibiotics requires follow-up care and evaluation for inflammatory breast cancer.[5]

TABLE 51-1	**Benign Breast Disorders***	
Disorder	**Risk Factors**	**Clinical Manifestations**
Lactational mastitis	Occurs in up to 10% of postpartum lactating mothers (both primipara and multipara), usually 2-4 wk after birth.	• Warm to touch, indurated, painful, often unilateral. • Most commonly caused by *Staphylococcus aureus*.
Fibrocystic changes	Most common between ages 35 and 50.	• Not usually discrete masses—nodularity instead. • Usually accompanied by cyclic pain and tenderness. • Mass(es) often cyclic in occurrence (movable, soft).
Cysts	Most common over age 35. Incidence decreases after menopause. Develop in 1 of every 14 women.	• Palpable fluid-filled mass (movable, soft). • Multiple cysts can occur and recur. • Rarely associated with breast cancer.
Fibroadenoma	Commonly occurs in 10% of all women ages 15-40.	• Palpable mass (firm, movable), usually 2-3 cm in size. • Rarely associated with breast cancer.
Fat necrosis	Many women report previous history of trauma to breast.	• Usually a hard, tender, mobile, indurated mass with irregular borders.
Ductal ectasia	Perimenopausal woman—most common in women in their 50s, previous lactation, inverted nipples.	• Fixation of nipple, usually accompanied by nipple discharge of thick gray material. • Often associated with breast pain.

*This list is not inclusive; other benign breast disorders are discussed in the text.

Lactational Breast Abscess

If lactational mastitis persists after several days of antibiotic therapy, a lactational breast abscess may have developed. In this condition, the skin may become red and edematous over the involved breast, often with a corresponding palpable mass, and the patient may have a fever. Antibiotics alone are insufficient treatment for a breast abscess. Ultrasound-guided drainage of the abscess or surgical incision and drainage are necessary. The drainage is cultured, sensitivities are obtained, and therapy with an appropriate antibiotic is begun. Breastfeeding can continue in most cases with ongoing treatment of the abscess.

FIBROCYSTIC CHANGES

Fibrocystic changes in the breast are a benign condition characterized by changes in breast tissue[5,6] (Fig. 51-3). Fibrocystic changes are the most common breast disorder.

The changes include the development of excess fibrous tissue, hyperplasia of the epithelial lining of the mammary ducts, proliferation of mammary ducts, and cyst formation. Fibrocystic changes are thought to be due to a heightened responsiveness of breast tissue to circulating estrogen and progesterone. These changes produce pain related to nerve irritation (from edema in the connective tissue) and fibrosis (from pinching of the nerve).

The use of the term *fibrocystic disease* is incorrect because the cluster of problems is actually an exaggerated response to hormonal influence. The terms *fibrocystic condition* or *fibrocystic complex* are more accurate.

Fibrocystic changes alone are not associated with increased breast cancer risk. Masses or nodularities can appear in both breasts. They are often found in the upper, outer quadrants and usually occur bilaterally.

Fibrocystic changes occur most frequently in women between 35 and 50 years of age but often begin as early as 20 years of age. Pain and nodularity often increase over time but tend to subside after menopause unless high doses of estrogen replacement are used. Fibrocystic changes most commonly occur in women with premenstrual abnormalities, nulliparous women, women with a history of spontaneous abortion, nonusers of oral contraceptives, and women with early menarche and late menopause. Symptoms related to fibrocystic changes often worsen in the premenstrual phase and subside after menstruation.

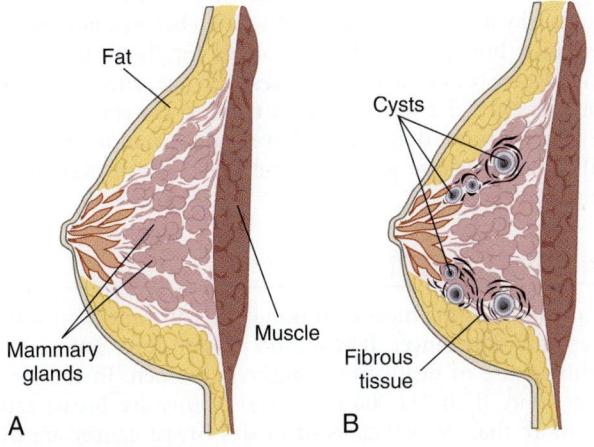

FIG. 51-3 A, Normal breast tissue. **B,** Fibrocystic breast tissue.

Manifestations of fibrocystic breast changes include one or more palpable lumps that are often round, well delineated, and freely movable within the breast (Table 51-1). Discomfort ranging from tenderness to pain may also occur. The lump is usually observed to increase in size and perhaps in tenderness before menstruation. Cysts may enlarge or shrink rapidly. Nipple discharge associated with fibrocystic breasts is often milky, watery-milky, yellow, or green.

Mammography may be helpful in distinguishing fibrocystic changes from breast cancer. However, in some women the breast tissue is so dense that it is difficult to obtain a mammogram. In these situations, ultrasound may be more useful in differentiating a fluid-filled cyst from a solid mass.

❖ NURSING AND INTERPROFESSIONAL MANAGEMENT: FIBROCYSTIC CHANGES

With the initial discovery of a discrete mass in the breast by a woman or her HCP, aspiration or biopsy may be indicated. If the nodularity is recurrent, a wait of 7 to 10 days may be planned in order to note any changes that may be related to the menstrual cycle. With large or frequent cysts, an excisional biopsy may be preferred over repeated aspiration. An excisional biopsy may be done if (1) no fluid is found on aspiration, (2) the fluid that is found is hemorrhagic, or (3) a residual mass remains after fluid aspiration. The biopsy is usually performed in an outpatient surgery unit.

Severe fibrocystic changes may make palpation of the breast more difficult. Teach the woman with cystic changes to maintain regular follow-up care with her HCP and encourage breast self-awareness and to report any changes found so that they can be evaluated.

Treatment for a fibrocystic condition is similar to that described earlier for mastalgia. Teach the woman with fibrocystic breasts that she may expect a recurrence of the cysts in one or both breasts until menopause and that the cysts may enlarge or become painful just before menstruation. Additionally, reassure her that the cysts do not "turn into" cancer. Advise her that any new lump that does not respond in a cyclic manner over 1 to 2 weeks should be examined by her HCP.

FIBROADENOMA

Fibroadenoma is a common cause of discrete benign breast lumps in young women. It generally occurs in women between 15 and 40 years of age. It is the most frequent cause of breast masses in women under 25 years of age.

The possible cause of fibroadenoma may be increased estrogen sensitivity in a localized area of the breast. Fibroadenomas are usually small (but can be large [2 to 3 cm]), painless, round, well delineated, and very mobile. They may be soft but are usually solid, firm, and rubbery in consistency. There is no accompanying retraction or nipple discharge. The fibroadenoma may appear as a single unilateral mass, although multiple bilateral fibroadenomas have been reported. Growth is slow and often ceases when the size reaches 2 to 3 cm. Size is not affected by menstruation. However, pregnancy can stimulate dramatic growth.

Fibroadenomas are easily detected by physical examination and may be visible on mammography and ultrasound. However, definitive diagnosis requires FNA, core, or excisional biopsy and tissue examination by a pathologist to exclude a malignancy.

Treatment of fibroadenomas can include observation with regular monitoring after a malignancy has been ruled out. In women over 35 years of age, all new lesions should be evaluated by breast ultrasound and possible biopsy.[3]

NIPPLE DISCHARGE

Nipple discharge may occur spontaneously or as a result of nipple manipulation. A milky secretion is due to inappropriate lactation (termed galactorrhea) and may be a result of certain medications or endocrine or neurologic disorders. Nipple discharge may also be idiopathic (no known cause).

Secretions can also be serous, bloody, or brown to green. A cytology slide may be made of the secretion to determine the specific cause and recommended treatment. Disorders associated with nipple discharge include benign breast conditions such as fibrocystic changes, intraductal papilloma, or ductal ectasia. In most cases, nipple discharge is not related to malignancy.

Intraductal Papilloma

An intraductal papilloma is a benign, soft, wartlike growth found in the mammary ducts. It is usually unilateral. Typically, the nipple has a bloody discharge that can be intermittent or spontaneous. Most intraductal papillomas are beneath the areola, and they may be difficult to palpate. They are usually found in women 40 to 60 years of age. A single duct or several ducts may be involved. Treatment includes excision of the papilloma and the involved duct or duct system. Papillomas are associated with a slightly increased risk (1.5 to 2 times) of developing breast cancer over the general population.[7]

Ductal Ectasia

Ductal ectasia (duct dilation) is a benign breast disease of perimenopausal and postmenopausal women involving the ducts in the subareolar area. It usually involves several bilateral ducts. Multicolored, sticky nipple discharge is the primary symptom. Ductal ectasia is initially painless but may progress to burning, itching, and pain around the nipple, as well as swelling in the areolar area. Inflammatory signs are often present, the nipple may retract, and the discharge may become bloody in more advanced disease. Ductal ectasia is not associated with malignancy. If an abscess develops, warm compresses and antibiotics are usually effective treatments. Therapy consists of close follow-up examinations or surgical excision of the involved ducts.

ATYPICAL HYPERPLASIA

Atypical hyperplasia is usually discovered after a biopsy is done to evaluate a suspicious area found on a mammogram or during a clinical breast examination. Atypical hyperplasia is found in either the ducts (atypical ductal hyperplasia) or in the lobules (atypical lobular hyperplasia). Both are associated with an increased risk of developing breast cancer. To follow up on a diagnosis of atypical hyperplasia an excisional biopsy or lumpectomy may be done to remove all of the affected tissue.[8]

GYNECOMASTIA IN MEN

Gynecomastia, a transient, noninflammatory enlargement of one or both breasts, is the most common breast problem in men. The condition is usually temporary and benign. Gynecomastia in itself is not a risk factor for breast cancer. The most common cause of gynecomastia is a disturbance of the normal ratio of active androgen to estrogen in plasma or within the breast itself.[9]

Gynecomastia can also occur in puberty. During puberty, there is often a transient relative imbalance between estrogen and testosterone, leading to gynecomastia. This condition usually resolves by age 18 years when adult androgen/estrogen ratios are achieved. The treatment of pubertal gynecomastia is reassurance of the parent and teenager regarding the benign nature of the condition.

Gynecomastia may also be a manifestation of other problems. It may accompany diseases such as testicular tumors, adrenal cancer, pituitary adenomas, hyperthyroidism, and liver disease. Gynecomastia may occur as a side effect of drug therapy, particularly with estrogen and androgen, digitalis, isoniazid, ranitidine (Zantac), and spironolactone (Aldactone). The use of heroin and marijuana can also cause gynecomastia.

Senescent Gynecomastia

Senescent gynecomastia occurs in many older men. A probable cause is the elevation in plasma estrogen in older adult men as the result of increased conversion of androgens to estrogens in peripheral circulation. Although initially unilateral, the tender, firm, centrally located enlargement may become bilateral. When gynecomastia is characterized by a discrete, circumscribed mass, it must be biopsied to differentiate it from the rarer breast cancer in males. Senescent hyperplasia requires no treatment and generally regresses within 6 to 12 months.

Gerontologic Considerations: Age-Related Breast Changes

The loss of subcutaneous fat and structural support and the atrophy of mammary glands often result in pendulous breasts in the postmenopausal woman. Encourage older women to wear a well-fitting bra. Adequate support can improve physical appearance and reduce pain in the back, shoulders, and neck. It can also prevent intertrigo (dermatitis caused by friction between opposing surfaces of skin). Sagging breasts can be surgically lifted (mastopexy).

The decrease in glandular tissue in older women makes a breast mass easier to palpate. This decreased density is likely a result of age-related decreases in estrogen. Rib margins may be palpable in a thin woman and can be confused with a mass. That is why it is so important that women become familiar with their own breasts and what is normal for them. Because the incidence of breast cancer increases with age, encourage breast awareness in older women. Teach them to (1) continue BSE if they are routinely doing it, (2) have annual mammograms and CBEs, and (3) have any breast-related concern evaluated by their HCP.

BREAST CANCER

Breast cancer is the most common cancer in American women except for skin cancer. It is second only to lung cancer as the leading cause of death from cancer in women. In the United States more than 231,000 new cases of invasive breast cancer and more than 60,000 cases of in situ breast cancer are diagnosed annually. An additional 2200 cases of breast cancer are diagnosed in men. Approximately 40,300 deaths occur each year related to breast cancer.[1]

The incidence of breast cancer is slowly decreasing, with a slight drop in the number of deaths related to breast cancer. This decline may be the result of the decreased use of hormone therapy after menopause. Breast cancer survivors are the largest group of any cancer survivors.[1] (Survivorship is discussed later in this chapter.)

Etiology and Risk Factors

Although the etiology is not completely understood, a number of risk factors are related to breast cancer (Table 51-2). Risk factors appear to be cumulative and interacting. Therefore the presence of multiple risk factors may greatly increase the overall risk, especially for people with a positive family history.

Risk Factors for Women. The risk factors most associated with breast cancer include female gender and advancing age. Women are at far greater risk than men, with 99% of breast cancers occurring in women. Increasing age also increases the risk of developing breast cancer. The incidence of breast cancer in women under 25 years of age is very low and increases gradually until age 60. After age 60, the incidence increases dramatically.

Hormonal regulation of the breast is related to the development of breast cancer, but the mechanisms are poorly understood. The hormones estrogen and progesterone may act as tumor promoters to stimulate breast cancer growth if malignant changes in the cells have already occurred. The Women's Health Initiative study showed that the use of combined hormone therapy (estrogen plus progesterone) increases the risk of breast cancer. It also showed that there was a risk of having a larger, more advanced breast cancer at diagnosis. The use of estrogen therapy alone for longer than 10 years (for women with a prior hysterectomy) increases a woman's long-term risk for breast cancer.[10] A link may exist between oral contraceptive use and increased risk of breast cancer for younger women.[11]

Modifiable risk factors include excess weight gain during adulthood, sedentary lifestyle, smoking, dietary fat intake, obesity, and alcohol intake. Environmental factors such as radiation exposure may also play a role.

Genetic Link

Family history of breast cancer is an important risk factor, especially if the involved family member also had ovarian cancer, was premenopausal, had bilateral breast cancer, or is a first-degree relative (i.e., mother, father, sister, brother, daughter). Having any first-degree relative with breast cancer increases a woman's risk of breast cancer 1.5 to 3 times, depending on age.[12,13] A breast cancer risk assessment tool for HCPs is available (www.cancer.gov/bcrisktool). Genetic counseling must be considered for an individual at high risk for breast cancer and appropriate referrals made.

About 5% to 10% of all breast cancers are hereditary. This means that specific genetic abnormalities that contribute to the development of breast cancer have been inherited (passed from parent to child). Most inherited cases of breast cancer are associated with mutations in two genes: *BRCA1* and *BRCA2* (*BRCA* stands for *BR*east *CA*ncer). Everyone has *BRCA* genes. The *BRCA1* gene, located on chromosome 17, is a tumor suppressor gene that inhibits tumor development when functioning normally. Women who have *BRCA1* mutations have a 40% to 80% lifetime chance of developing breast cancer. The *BRCA2* gene, located on chromosome 11, is another tumor suppressor gene. Women with a mutation of this gene have a similar risk of breast cancer.[12,13]

Mutations in *BRCA* genes may cause as many as 10% to 40% of all inherited breast cancers. As many as 1 in 200 to 400 women in the United States may be carriers for these genetic abnormalities. Women with *BRCA* mutations are also at higher risk for developing ovarian, colon, pancreatic, and uterine cancers.[12]

In addition to *BRCA* gene mutations, many other abnormal genes have been identified that increase a person's risk of developing breast cancer. These include the tumor suppressor genes *p53* and *PTEN* (which inhibit tumor development when functioning normally), *ATM* (which helps to repair damaged deoxyribonucleic acid [DNA]), *CHEK2* (which stops tumor growth), and *PALB2* (which partners with *BRCA* to suppress tumor growth).[14]

Most people who develop breast cancer do not have an abnormal breast cancer gene, nor do they have a family history of breast cancer. Ongoing research continues to investigate the role of genes in the development of breast cancer. (Genomics and genetics are discussed in Chapter 12.)

Risk Factors for Men. Predisposing risk factors for breast cancer in men include hyperestrogenism, a family history of breast cancer, and radiation exposure. A thorough examination of the

TABLE 51-2 Risk Factors for Breast Cancer

Risk Factor	Comments
Female	Women account for 99% of breast cancer cases.
Age ≥50 yr	Majority of breast cancers are found in postmenopausal women. After age 60, increase in incidence.
Hormone use	Use of estrogen and/or progesterone as hormone therapy, especially in postmenopausal women.
Family history	Breast cancer in a first-degree relative, particularly when premenopausal or bilateral, increases risk.
Genetic factors	Gene mutations (BRCA1, BRCA2, P53, PTEN, PALB2) play a role in 5%-10% of breast cancer cases.
Personal history of breast cancer, colon cancer, endometrial cancer, ovarian cancer	Personal history significantly increases risk of breast cancer, risk of cancer in other breast, and recurrence.
Early menarche (before age 12), late menopause (after age 55)	A long menstrual history increases the risk of breast cancer.
First full-term pregnancy after age 30, nulliparity	Prolonged exposure to unopposed estrogen increases risk for breast cancer.
Benign breast disease with atypical epithelial hyperplasia, lobular carcinoma in situ	Atypical changes in breast biopsy increase the risk of breast cancer.
Weight gain and obesity after menopause	Fat cells store estrogen, which increases the likelihood of developing breast cancer.
Exposure to ionizing radiation	Radiation damages DNA (e.g., prior treatment for Hodgkin's lymphoma).
Alcohol consumption	Women who drink ≥1 alcoholic beverage per day may have an increased risk of breast cancer.

Breast Cancer

Genetic Basis
- Mutations occur in *BRCA1* and/or *BRCA2* genes.
- Normally these genes are tumor suppressor genes involved in DNA repair.
- Transmission is autosomal dominant.
- Additional genes (e.g., *ATM, CHEK-2, p53, PTEN, PALB2*) may increase the risk of breast cancer.

Incidence
- Approximately 5% to 10% of breast cancers are related to *BRCA1* and *BRCA2* gene mutations.
- Women with *BRCA1* and *BRCA2* gene mutations have a 40% to 80% lifetime risk of developing breast cancer.
- *BRCA1* and *BRCA2* gene mutations are associated with early-onset breast cancer that is more likely to involve both breasts.
- Men with mutations in *BRCA1* and *BRCA2* have an increased risk of breast cancer and prostate cancer.
- Family history of both breast and ovarian cancer increases the risk of having a *BRCA* mutation.

Genetic Testing
- DNA testing is available for *BRCA1* and *BRCA2* gene mutations.
- Newer genetic tests are available to analyze an entire panel of genes in specific breast cancer patient populations.

Clinical Implications
- Most breast cancers (about 90%-95%) are not inherited. They are associated with genetic changes that occur after a person is born (somatic mutations). There is no risk of passing on the mutated gene to children.
- Bilateral oophorectomy and/or bilateral mastectomy reduces the risk of breast cancer and ovarian cancer in women with *BRCA1* and *BRCA2* mutations.
- Mutations in the *BRCA1* and *BRCA2* genes increase the risk of ovarian cancer.
- Genetic counseling and testing for *BRCA* mutations should be considered for patients whose personal or family history puts them at high risk for a genetic predisposition to breast cancer.

BRCA, BReast CAncer.

male breast should be a routine part of a physical examination. Men in *BRCA*-positive families should consider genetic testing. Men who test positive for a *BRCA* gene mutation should receive BSE training starting at the age of 35, a CBE every 6 months starting at the age of 35, and a baseline mammogram beginning at the age of forty. These men should also begin prostate screening at the age of 40 as they also have an increased risk of developing prostate cancer.[13]

Prophylactic Oophorectomy and Mastectomy. In women with *BRCA1* or *BRCA2* mutations, prophylactic bilateral oophorectomy can decrease the risk of breast cancer as well as ovarian cancer. Removing the ovaries lowers the risk of breast cancer because the ovaries are the main source of estrogen in a premenopausal woman. Removing the ovaries does not reduce the risk of breast cancer in postmenopausal women because the ovaries are not the main producers of estrogen in these women. A woman who has a high risk of developing breast cancer (i.e., related to factors such as family history and prior tissue biopsies) may choose (in consultation with her physician and genetic counselor) to undergo prophylactic bilateral mastectomy.

Younger women with hereditary (non-*BRCA*) early-stage, estrogen receptor–negative breast cancer may have a higher risk of developing a secondary primary breast cancer in the unaffected (contralateral) breast.[14] These women may also choose to have the unaffected breast removed prophylactically at the time of initial surgery for breast cancer or at a later time.

Pathophysiology

The main components of the breast are lobules (milk-producing glands) and ducts (milk passages that connect the lobules and the nipple). In general, breast cancer arises from the epithelial lining of the ducts *(ductal carcinoma)* or from the epithelium of the lobules *(lobular carcinoma)*. Breast cancers may be *in situ* (within the duct) or invasive (invading through the wall of the duct).

Metastatic breast cancer is breast cancer that has spread to other organs, with the most common sites being bone, liver, lung, and brain. Cancer growth rates can range from slow to rapid. Factors that affect cancer prognosis are tumor size, axillary node involvement (the more nodes involved, the worse the prognosis), tumor differentiation, estrogen and progesterone receptor status, and *human epidermal growth factor receptor 2* (HER-2) status. HER-2 is a protein that helps regulate cell growth.[15]

Types of Breast Cancer

Breast cancer is not just one disease, but a group of diseases characterized by different pathologic findings and clinical behaviors. Breast cancer can be classified as (1) ductal or lobular or other or (2) noninvasive or invasive (Table 51-3). It can also be classified based on hormonal status and genetic subtypes.

Noninvasive Breast Cancer. An estimated 20% of breast cancers are noninvasive. These intraductal cancers include *ductal carcinoma in situ* (DCIS) and *lobular carcinoma in situ* (LCIS). DCIS tends to be unilateral and may progress to invasive breast cancer if left untreated.

To determine treatment options for DCIS, the Oncotype DX Assay (a genomic test) can be used to (1) predict the risk of local recurrence or invasive carcinoma and (2) guide personalized treatment based on tumor biology.[16] Treatment options include breast-conserving treatment (lumpectomy), total mastectomy with or without sentinel lymph node biopsy, radiation therapy, and/or hormone therapy (e.g., tamoxifen).

The term *lobular carcinoma in situ* is somewhat misleading. Although women with LCIS are more likely to develop invasive breast cancer than women without LCIS, it is not considered to be a premalignant lesion. No surgical or radiation treatment is indicated for LCIS. Hormone therapy may be used as a preventive measure to reduce breast cancer risk for some patients.

Invasive Ductal Carcinoma. *Invasive (infiltrating) ductal carcinoma* is the most common type of breast cancer accounting for approximately 80% of all invasive breast cancers. It starts in the milk ducts and then breaks through the walls of the duct, invading the surrounding tissue. From there it may metastasize to

TABLE 51-3 Classification of Breast Cancer

Based on Tissue Type
- Ductal carcinoma (affects milk ducts)
  - Medullary
  - Tubular
  - Colloid (mucinous)
- Lobular carcinoma (affects milk-producing glands)
- Other
  - Inflammatory
  - Paget's disease
  - Phyllodes tumor

Based on Invasiveness

Noninvasive (In situ)
- Ductal carcinoma in situ (DCIS)
- Lobular carcinoma in situ (LCIS)

Invasive (Spreading to Other Locations)
- Invasive ductal carcinoma
- Invasive lobular carcinoma

Based on Hormone Receptor and Genetic Status

Estrogen and Progesterone Receptor Status
- Estrogen receptor positive
- Estrogen receptor negative
- Progesterone receptor positive
- Progesterone receptor negative

HER-2 Genetic Status
- HER-2 positive
- HER-2 negative

HER-2, Human epidermal growth factor receptor 2.

other parts of the body. Subtypes of invasive ductal carcinoma include medullary carcinoma, tubular carcinoma, colloid (mucinous) carcinoma, papillary carcinoma, and metaplastic carcinoma.

Invasive Lobular Carcinoma. *Invasive (infiltrating) lobular carcinoma* begins in the lobules (milk-producing glands) of the breast and accounts for approximately 10% to 15% of invasive breast cancers. The cancer cells can break out of the lobule and have the potential to metastasize to other areas of the body. Invasive lobular carcinoma usually presents as a subtle thickening in the upper outer quadrant of the breast. It is a type of breast cancer that is generally not detected by mammography.

Other Types of Breast Cancer

Inflammatory Breast Cancer. *Inflammatory breast cancer* is an aggressive and fast-growing breast cancer with a high risk for metastasis accounting for approximately 1% to 3% of all breast cancers. In the early stages, it is often mistaken for mastitis. However, the inflammatory changes do not improve with antibiotics, as the lymph channels in the skin of the breast are blocked by cancer cells. Because of skin involvement, the breast looks red, feels warm, and has a thickened appearance that is often described as resembling an orange peel *(peau d'orange)*. Sometimes the breast develops ridges and small bumps that look like hives. A breast mass may not be present and changes may not show up on mammograms, thus making diagnosis difficult. Inflammatory breast cancer is associated with a worse prognosis as compared to invasive ductal and lobular breast cancer.[17]

Paget's Disease. Paget's disease is a rare breast malignancy that starts in the breast ducts and spreads to the nipple and areola. It is rare, causing approximately 1% of all breast cancers (This is different from Paget's disease of the bone, which is discussed in Chapter 63.) Most women with Paget's disease have underlying ductal carcinoma. Only in rare cases is the cancer confined to the nipple.

Itching, burning, bloody nipple discharge with superficial skin erosion and ulceration may be present. Diagnosis of Paget's disease is confirmed by pathologic examination of the lesion. Nipple changes are often diagnosed as an infection or dermatitis, which can lead to treatment delays.

The treatment of Paget's disease is surgical removal of the involved tissue (central lumpectomy or mastectomy). Radiation therapy may also be used after surgery. The prognosis is good when the cancer is confined to the nipple.

Phyllodes Tumor. A phyllodes tumor is a rare tumor that develops in the connective tissue (stroma) of the breast as compared with invasive ductal or lobular carcinomas. Treatment for this tumor is usually mastectomy and if needed, chemotherapy.

Triple-Negative Breast Cancer. A patient whose breast cancer tests negative for all three receptors (estrogen, progesterone, and HER-2) has *triple-negative breast cancer.* (Receptor testing is discussed on pp. 1212-1213.) The incidence of triple-negative breast cancer is higher in African Americans, Hispanics, premenopausal women, and those with a *BRCA1* mutation. These patients tend to have more aggressive tumors with a poorer prognosis because these tumors do not respond to treatment.

These cancers do not usually respond to hormone therapy or therapy for the human epidermal growth factor receptor 2 (HER-2). Chemotherapy appears to be the most successful method for treating triple-negative breast cancer.

Clinical Manifestations

Breast cancer is usually detected as a lump or thickening in the breast or mammography abnormality. It occurs most often in the upper, outer quadrant of the breast, which is the location of most of the glandular tissue (Fig. 51-4). Breast cancers vary in their growth rate. If palpable, breast cancer is characteristically hard and may be irregularly shaped, poorly delineated, nonmobile, and nontender.

A small percentage of breast cancers cause nipple discharge. The discharge is usually unilateral and may be clear or bloody. Nipple retraction may occur. Peau d'orange may occur due to plugging of the dermal lymphatics. In large cancers, infiltration, induration, and dimpling (pulling in) of the overlying skin may also occur.

Complications

The main complication of breast cancer is recurrence (Table 51-4). Recurrence may be *local* or *regional* (skin or soft tissue near the mastectomy site, axillary or internal mammary lymph nodes) or distant (most commonly involving bone, lung, brain, and liver). However, metastatic disease can be found in any site in the body.

Widely disseminated or metastatic disease involves the growth of cancerous breast cells in parts of the body distant from the breast. Metastases primarily occur through the lymphatics, usually those of the axilla (Fig. 51-5). However, the cancer can spread to other parts of the body.

Diagnostic Studies

In addition to radiologic and biopsy studies used to diagnose breast cancer (see earlier discussion in this chapter on

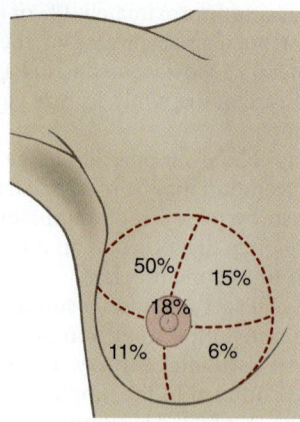

FIG. 51-4 Distribution of where breast cancer occurs.

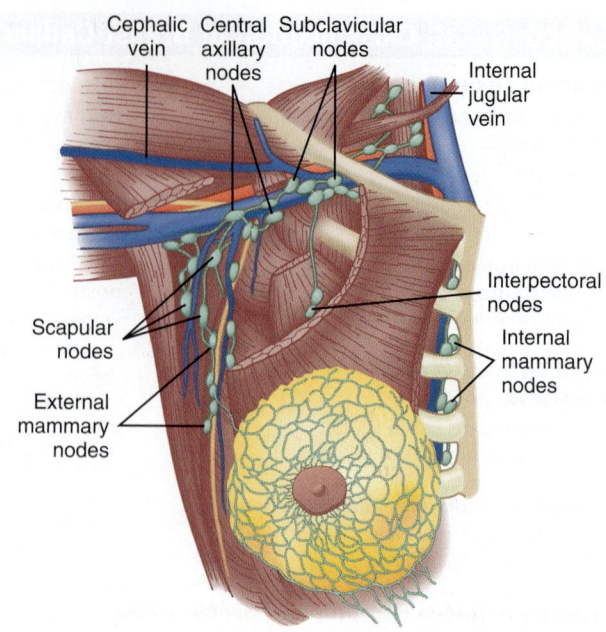

FIG. 51-5 Lymph nodes and drainage in the axilla. The sentinel lymph node is usually found in the external mammary nodes. A complete axillary dissection would remove all nodes. (From Donegan WL, Spratt JS: *Cancer of the breast*, ed 3, Philadelphia, 1988, Saunders.)

TABLE 51-4   Sites of Breast Cancer Recurrence and Metastasis

Site	Manifestations
Local Recurrence	
Skin, chest wall	Firm, discrete nodules. Occasionally pruritic, usually painless, commonly in or near a scar.
Regional Recurrence	
Lymph nodes	Enlarged nodes in axilla or supraclavicular area, usually nontender.
Distant Metastasis	
Skeletal	Localized pain of gradually increasing intensity, percussion tenderness at involved sites, pathologic fracture caused by involvement of bone cortex.
Spinal cord	Progressive back pain, localized and radiating. Change in bladder or bowel function. Loss of sensation in lower extremities.
Brain	Headache described as "different," unilateral sensory loss, focal muscular weakness, hemiparesis, incoordination (ataxia), nausea and vomiting unrelated to medication, cognitive changes.
Pulmonary (including lung nodules and pleural effusions)	Shortness of breath, tachypnea, nonproductive cough (not present in all patients).
Liver	Abdominal distention. Right lower quadrant abdominal pain sometimes radiating to scapular area. Nausea and vomiting, anorexia, weight loss. Weakness and fatigue. Hepatomegaly, ascites, jaundice. Peripheral edema. Elevated liver enzymes.
Bone marrow	Anemia, infection, increased bleeding, bruising, petechiae. Weakness, fatigue, mild confusion, light-headedness. Dyspnea.

pp. 1205-1206), other tests are used to predict the risk of local or systemic recurrence. These tests include axillary lymph node analysis, tumor size, estrogen and progesterone receptor status, cell-proliferative indices, and genomic assays.

Axillary Lymph Node Analysis. Axillary lymph node involvement is one of the most important prognostic factors in breast cancer. *Axillary lymph nodes* are often examined to determine if cancer has spread to the axilla on the side of the breast cancer

(Fig. 51-5). The more nodes involved, the greater the risk of recurrence.

A *sentinel lymph node biopsy* (SLNB) helps to identify the lymph node(s) that drain first from the tumor site (*sentinel node*). In SLNB a radioisotope and/or blue dye, which will travel the same route as the cancer, is injected into the affected breast. Then intraoperatively it is determined in which sentinel lymph nodes (SLNs) the radioisotope (using radioactive detector) or dye (visually see blue nodes) is located. A local incision is made in the axilla, and the surgeon dissects the blue-stained and/or radioactive SLNs. Generally, with a SLNB, one to four axillary lymph nodes are removed. The nodes are sent for pathologic analysis. If the SLNs are negative, no further axillary surgery is required.

If the SLNs are positive, a complete *axillary lymph node dissection* (ALND) may be done. In an ALND, the surgeon will typically remove 12 to 20 lymph nodes. SLNB is less invasive than ALND and is associated with lower morbidity rates and greater accuracy compared with ALND.

Tumor Size. *Tumor size* is a prognostic variable: the larger the tumor, the poorer the prognosis. The wide variety of biologic types of breast cancer explains the variability of disease behavior. In general, the more well differentiated (like the original cell type) the tumor, the less aggressive it is. The cells of poorly differentiated (unlike the original cell type) tumors appear morphologically disorganized, and they are more aggressive.

Estrogen and Progesterone Receptor Status. *Estrogen and progesterone receptor status* is another diagnostic test useful for decisions about both treatment and prognosis. Receptor-positive tumors (1) commonly show histologic evidence of being well differentiated, (2) frequently have a *diploid* (more normal) DNA content and low proliferative indices, (3) have a lower chance for recurrence, and (4) are frequently hormone dependent and responsive to hormone therapy. Receptor-negative tumors (1) are often poorly differentiated histologically, (2) have a high incidence of *aneuploidy* (abnormally high or low DNA content) and higher proliferative indices, (3) frequently recur, and (4) are usually unresponsive to hormone therapy. Ploidy status correlates with tumor aggressiveness. Diploid tumors have been shown to have a significantly lower risk of recurrence than aneuploid tumors.

Cell-Proliferative Indices. *Cell-proliferative indices* indirectly measure the rate of tumor cell proliferation. The percentage of tumor cells in the synthesis (S) phase of the cell cycle (see Chapter 15, Fig. 15-1) is another important prognostic indicator. Although cell-proliferative indices are not routinely performed as part of the breast cancer pathology evaluation, patients with cells that have high S-phase fractions have a higher risk for recurrence and earlier cancer death.

Genomic Assay. An important *genomic assay* is to determine HER-2, which is a prognostic indicator. Overexpression of this receptor has been associated with unusually aggressive tumor growth, a greater risk for recurrence, and a poorer prognosis in breast cancer.[15] HER-2 is overexpressed in about 10% to 20% of patients with breast cancer. The presence or absence of this marker assists in the selection and sequence of drug therapy and predicts the patient's response to treatment.

A *genomic* test uses a sample of the breast cancer tissue to analyze the activity of a group of genes that can affect how a cancer is likely to behave and respond to treatment. Knowing whether certain genes are present or absent, or overly active or not active enough, can provide information about the risk of recurrence and the likely benefit of chemotherapy or hormone therapy. The Oncotype DX test is the most commonly used genomic test. Other genomic tests are MammaPrint, Mammostrat, and Prosigna.

Interprofessional Care

A wide range of treatment options is available to the patient and HCPs making critical decisions about how to treat breast cancer (Table 51-5). Prognostic factors are considered when treatment decisions are made. The therapeutic regimen is often determined by the clinical stage and biology of the cancer.

Staging of Breast Cancer. The most widely accepted staging method for breast cancer is the TNM system.[18] This system uses tumor size (T), nodal involvement (N), and presence of metastasis (M) to determine the stage of disease. The stage of a breast cancer describes its size and the extent to which it has spread (Table 51-6).

The stages range from 0 to IV, with stage 0 being in situ cancer with no lymph node involvement and no metastasis. Further classification within these stages depends on the tumor size and number of lymph nodes involved. Stage IV indicates metastatic spread, regardless of tumor size or lymph node involvement. The presence or absence of malignant cells in lymph nodes remains a powerful prognostic factor related to local recurrence or metastasis after primary therapy.

Surgical Therapy. Surgery is considered the primary treatment for breast cancer. Table 51-7 describes the most common surgical procedures used to treat breast cancer. The most common surgical options for operable breast cancer are (1) breast conservation surgery (lumpectomy [segmental mastectomy]) and (2) mastectomy with or without reconstruction. Most women diagnosed with early stage breast cancer (tumors smaller than 5 cm) are candidates for either treatment choice as the overall survival rate with lumpectomy and radiation is the same as that with mastectomy.[19]

TABLE 51-5 Interprofessional Care

Breast Cancer

Diagnostic Assessment

Prediagnosis

- Health history, including risk factors
- Physical examination, including breast and lymph nodes
- Mammography
- Ultrasound (if indicated)
- Breast MRI (if indicated)
- Biopsy

Postdiagnosis

- Lymph node analysis
- Estrogen and progesterone receptor status
- Cell-proliferative indices
- HER-2 marker
- Genetic assays (e.g., MammaPrint or Oncotype DX)

Staging

- Complete blood count, platelet count
- Alkaline phosphatase
- Liver function tests
- Chest x-ray (if indicated)
- Bone scan (if indicated)
- CT scan of chest, abdomen, pelvis (if indicated)
- MRI (if indicated)
- PET/CT scan (if indicated)

Management

Surgical Therapy

- Breast-conserving surgery (lumpectomy) with SLNB and/or axillary lymph node dissection
- Simple (total) mastectomy with SLNB and/or axillary lymph node dissection
- Modified radical mastectomy
- Reconstructive surgery

Radiation Therapy

- External radiation
- Brachytherapy
- Palliative radiation therapy

Drug Therapy (Table 51-8)

- Chemotherapy
- Hormone therapy
- Immunotherapy
- Targeted therapy

SLNB, Sentinel lymph node biopsy.

It is important to note that breast reconstruction is an option for any woman undergoing surgical treatment for breast cancer. For women undergoing mastectomy, breast reconstruction can be performed at the time of the mastectomy or delayed for months or even years. Women may opt to not have reconstruction and choose to use a breast prosthesis instead.

Breast-Conserving Surgery. Breast-conserving surgery (also called lumpectomy) involves removal of the entire tumor along with a margin of normal surrounding tissue (Fig. 51-6, *A*). In some cases, it may take two to three additional surgeries to remove all the cancer from the margins. After surgery, radiation therapy is delivered to the entire breast, ending with a boost to the tumor bed. If the risk for recurrence is high, chemotherapy may be administered before radiation therapy.

Not everyone is a candidate for breast conservation surgery. Contraindications include breast size too small in relation to the tumor size to yield an acceptable cosmetic result, multifocal masses and calcifications, multicentric masses (in more than one quadrant), diffuse calcifications in more than one quadrant, or prior radiation therapy. In addition to these issues, the choice between mastectomy and breast conservation surgery depends on additional factors. Because of the time commitment (i.e., 6 to 7 weeks of daily radiation therapy treatments) and travel distances to access radiation therapy treatment facility, some patients may chose mastectomy over breast conservation surgery.

Axillary Lymph Node Analysis. Sentinel lymph node biopsy (SLNB) is the preferred standard for axillary lymph node analysis and staging. It was described on p. 1212. However, if the sentinel lymph node cannot be identified, or if the node is positive for cancer, ALND may have to be performed.

TABLE 51-6 Staging of Breast Cancer

Stage	Tumor Size	Lymph Node Involvement	Metastasis
0	TIS*	No	No
I	<2 cm	No	No
II			
A	No evidence of tumor ranging to 5 cm	No, or 1-3 axillary nodes and/or internal mammary nodes	No
B	Ranging from 2 to >5 cm	No, or 1-3 axillary nodes and/or internal mammary nodes	No
III			
A	No evidence of tumor ranging to >5 cm	Yes, 4-9 axillary nodes and/or internal mammary nodes	No
B	Any size with extension to chest wall or skin	Yes, 4-9 axillary nodes and/or internal mammary nodes	No
C	Any size	Yes, ≥10 axillary nodes, internal mammary nodes, or infraclavicular nodes	No
IV	Any size	Any type of nodal involvement	Yes

Modified from American Joint Committee on Cancer: AJCC cancer staging manual, ed 7. Retrieved from *www.cancerstaging.org/staging/changes2010.*
*TIS, Tumor in situ.

Lymphedema. **Lymphedema** (accumulation of lymph in soft tissue) can occur as a result of the lymph node sampling procedure or radiation therapy (Fig. 51-7). When the axillary nodes cannot return lymph fluid to the central circulation, the fluid accumulates in the arm, hand, or breast, causing obstructive pressure on the veins and venous return. The patient may experience heaviness, impaired motor function in the arm, and numbness and paresthesia of the fingers. Cellulitis and progressive fibrosis of the skin can result from untreated lymphedema. (See further discussion on lymphedema later in this chapter on p. 1220.)

Mastectomy. A *total* or *simple mastectomy* removes the entire breast. A *modified radical mastectomy* includes removal of the breast and axillary lymph nodes, but it preserves the pectoralis major muscle (Fig. 51-6, *B*). In a *nipple-sparing mastectomy*, the nipple and/or areola are left in place while the breast tissue under them is removed. Women who have a small cancer near the outer part of the breast, with no signs of cancer in the skin or near the nipple, may be able to have nipple-sparing surgery.[16]

For women who have a mastectomy, breast reconstruction can be performed immediately or it can be delayed. If the woman chooses, it may not be done at all. There are two main types of breast reconstruction procedures: implant reconstruction or tissue flap procedures (Table 51-7). Breast reconstructive surgery is discussed on pp. 1222-1224.

> ### ? CHECK YOUR PRACTICE
>
> You are working in the breast clinic and doing a postoperative assessment on a 56-yr-old woman who had a right radical mastectomy 6 weeks ago. She is complaining of sharp, prickly feelings in her right arm. She tells you, "I also feel pain in the breast that was removed. Am I going crazy? That breast is not even attached to my body anymore!"
> • How would you respond and what follow-up would you provide?

Post–Breast Therapy Pain Syndrome. *Post–breast therapy pain syndrome* (PBTPS) occurs in some people who have undergone procedures for breast cancer. Most commonly it is caused by injury to nerves during surgery. However, it can also be due to chemotherapy and radiation therapy. The most common theory for the onset of this syndrome is injury to intercostobrachial nerves, which are sensory nerves that exit the chest wall muscles and provide sensation to the shoulder and upper arm.

Because of its multiple causes, PBTPS symptoms can range from mild to debilitating.[20] Common symptoms include chest

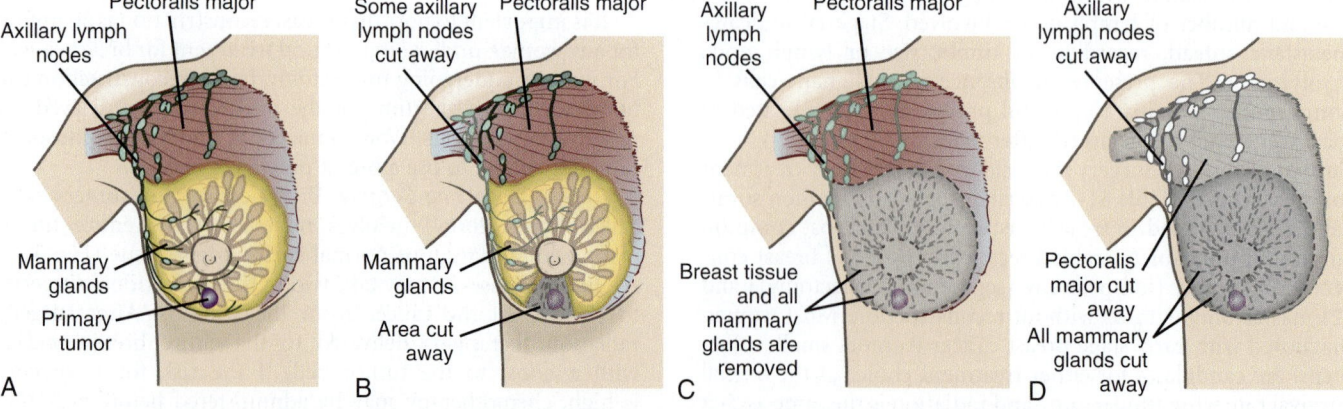

FIG. 51-6 Breast cancer surgery. **A,** Preoperative. **B,** Lumpectomy. **C,** Simple mastectomy. **D,** Modified radical mastectomy.

TABLE 51-7 Surgical Procedures for Breast Cancer

Procedure	Side Effects	Complications	Patient Issues
Breast-Conserving Surgery (Lumpectomy) With Radiation Therapy			
Wide excision of tumor, sentinel lymph node biopsy (SLNB) and/or axillary lymph node dissection (ALND) Radiation therapy	• Breast soreness • Breast edema • Skin reactions • Arm swelling • Sensory changes in breast and arm	*Short-term:* Moist desquamation,* hematoma, seroma, infection *Long-term:* Fibrosis, lymphedema,† myositis, pneumonitis,* rib fractures*	• Prolonged treatment* • Impaired arm mobility† • Change in texture and sensitivity of breast
Mastectomy			
Simple Mastectomy Removal of breast, preservation of pectoralis muscle with SLNB **Modified Radical Mastectomy** Removal of breast and pectoralis muscle with ALND	• Chest wall tightness, scar • Phantom breast sensations • Lymphedema • Sensory changes • Impaired range of motion	*Short-term:* Skin flap necrosis, seroma, hematoma, infection *Long-term:* Sensory loss, muscle weakness, lymphedema	• Loss of breast • Incision • Body image • Need for prosthesis • Impaired arm mobility
Breast Implants and Tissue Expansion			
Expander used to slowly stretch tissue. Saline gradually injected into reservoir over weeks to months Insertion of implant under musculofascial layer of chest wall	• Discomfort • Chest wall tightness	*Short-term:* Skin flap necrosis, wound separation, seroma, hematoma, infection *Long-term:* Capsular contractions, displacement of implant	• Altered body image • Prolonged physician visits to expand implants • Potential additional surgeries for nipple construction, symmetry
Breast Reconstruction Tissue Flap Procedures‡ ***Transverse Rectus Abdominis Musculocutaneous (TRAM) Flap***			
Musculocutaneous flap (muscle, skin, fat, blood supply) is transposed from abdomen to the mastectomy site May be done concurrently with mastectomy	• Pain related to two surgical sites and extensive surgery	*Short-term:* Delayed wound healing, infection, skin flap necrosis, abdominal hernia, hematoma	• Prolonged postoperative recovery
Deep Inferior Epigastric Artery Perforator (DIEP) Flap			
Free flap that transfers skin and fat from the abdomen to the chest. Differs from TRAM flap because no muscle is moved	• Requires more time in surgery than TRAM flap • Pain related to two surgical sites	If procedure fails, tissue flap may die and have to be completely removed If tissue dies, new reconstruction may not be done for 6-12 mo	• Patients may experience less pain and restriction of movement than with a TRAM flap.

*Specific to radiation therapy.
†If ALND (less likely with SLNB).
‡This list is not inclusive as additional breast reconstruction options are available to patients.

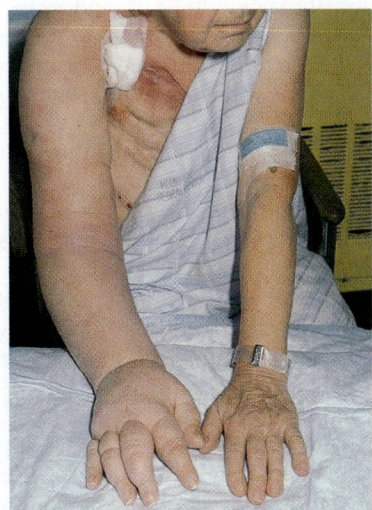

FIG. 51-7 Lymphedema. Accumulation of fluid in the tissue after excision of lymph nodes. (From Swartz MH: *Textbook of physical diagnosis: history and examination,* ed 6, Philadelphia, 2010, Saunders.)

and upper arm pain, tingling down the arm, continuous aching and burning, numbness, edema, shooting or pricking pain, and unbearable itching that persists beyond the normal 3-month healing time.

Treatment includes nonsteroidal antiinflammatory drugs (NSAIDs), low-dose antidepressants, EMLA (local anesthetics: lidocaine and prilocaine), and antiseizure drugs (e.g., gabapentin [Neurontin]). Other possible treatment modalities include biofeedback, physical therapy to prevent "frozen shoulder" syndrome as a result of inadequate movement, guided imagery, and psychologic counseling with a therapist trained in the management of chronic pain syndromes.

Phantom Breast Pain. *Phantom breast pain* is feeling pain in the breast after a mastectomy. Phantom breast pain can happen after the breast has been removed for the same reasons phantom limb sensation occurs after limb amputations. The brain continues to send signals to nerves in the breast area that were cut during surgery, even though the breast is no longer physically there.

Radiation Therapy. Radiation therapy is one form of *adjuvant (additional)* therapy that can be used after surgery. Radiation therapy may be used for breast cancer to (1) prevent local breast cancer recurrences after breast-conserving surgery; (2) prevent local and lymph node recurrences after mastectomy; or (3) relieve pain caused by local, regional, or distant spread of cancer.

External Radiation Therapy. When radiation therapy is a primary treatment, it is usually performed after surgery for the breast cancer. The decision to use radiation therapy after mastectomy is based on the probability that local residual cancer cells are present. Radiation of the axilla and/or supraclavicular nodes may be indicated when lymph nodes are involved to decrease the risk of axillary recurrence. Radiating a localized area will not prevent distant metastasis.

In traditional whole breast (and regional lymph nodes in some cases) radiation treatment, the area is radiated 5 days per week over the course of about 5 to 7 weeks. An external beam of radiation is used to deliver 1.8 Gy to 2 Gy daily fractions to an approximate total dose of 45 to 50 Gy (4500 to 5000 cGy). In patients who have had breast-conserving surgery, a "boost" is a dose of radiation delivered to the area in which the original tumor was located. It is given by external beam and adds five to eight more treatments to the total number given.

For some breast cancer patients, accelerated external beam radiation may be used. With this type of radiation, a shortened schedule of radiation therapy is given daily for 3 to 4 weeks for a total dose of 42.5 Gy.[17]

Fatigue, skin changes, and breast edema may be temporary side effects of external radiation therapy. (Nursing management of the patient receiving radiation therapy is discussed in Chapter 15.)

Brachytherapy. Brachytherapy (internal radiation) is used for partial-breast radiation as an alternative to traditional external radiation treatment for some patients with early stage breast cancer.[17] Radiation is delivered directly into the cavity left after a tumor is surgically removed by a lumpectomy. This approach is a minimally invasive way to deliver radiation. Because the radiation is concentrated and focused on the area with the highest risk for tumor recurrence, internal radiation only requires 5 days. Traditional external radiation treatments can take 5 to 7 weeks. Internal radiation therapy is primarily delivered using a multicatheter method or balloon-catheter system.

In the *multicatheter method* (e.g., SAVI) many very small catheters are placed in the breast at the site of the tumor. The SAVI is inserted through a small incision, and the catheter bundle expands uniformly. The ends of the catheters stick out through little holes in the skin. Small radioactive seeds are placed in the catheters. The seeds are left in place just long enough to deliver the radiation dose (e.g., 5 to 10 minutes). The tiny radioactive seeds are inserted only during treatment and then removed. The radiation does not remain in the body between treatments or after the final treatment is over.

In the *balloon-catheter system,* the balloon is placed where the tumor is located. The balloon is filled with fluid to keep it in place. Radioactive seeds are inserted (Fig. 51-8). Radiation is emitted by a tiny radioactive seed attached by a wire on the way to an afterloader, a computer-controlled machine. The seed travels through the MammoSite applicator into the inflated balloon. As with the multicatheter system, the radiation does not remain in the body between treatments or after the final treatment is over. Once the final session is completed, the balloon is deflated and the system is removed.

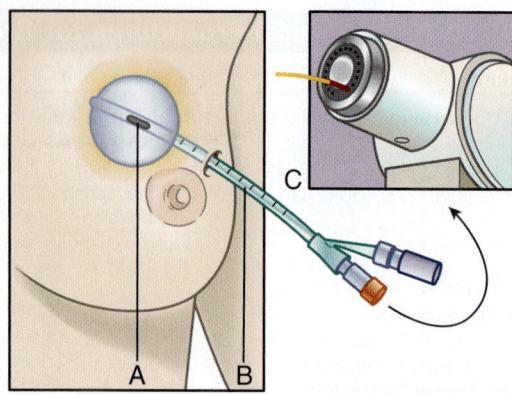

FIG. 51-8 High-dose brachytherapy for breast cancer. The MammoSite system involves the insertion of a single small balloon catheter *(B)* at the time of the lumpectomy or shortly thereafter into the tumor resection cavity (the space that is left after the surgeon removes the tumor). A tiny radioactive seed *(A)* is inserted into the balloon, connected to a machine called an *afterloader (C),* and delivers the radiation therapy.

Palliative Radiation Therapy. In addition to reducing the primary tumor mass with a resultant decrease in pain, radiation therapy is also used to treat symptomatic metastatic lesions in such sites as bone, soft tissue organs, brain, and chest. Radiation therapy often relieves pain and is successful in controlling recurrent or metastatic disease.

Drug Therapy. Drug therapy (systemic therapy) is treatment that travels through the bloodstream to all parts of the body, not just the cancer. Drug therapy includes chemotherapy, hormone therapy, immunotherapy, and targeted therapy.

When drug therapy is given before surgery, it is called *neoadjuvant therapy.* Neoadjuvant therapy is often used to shrink the size of the tumor enough to make surgical removal possible, or to allow for breast-conserving surgery in women who would have been recommended to have a mastectomy. Drug therapy after surgery is called *adjuvant therapy.* Drug therapy can decrease the rate of recurrence and increase the length of survival. Because of the risk for recurrent disease, nearly all patients with evidence of node involvement, particularly those who are hormone receptor negative, will have some type of drug therapy. Some patients, particularly those with a larger or more aggressive tumor, are known to be at higher risk for recurrent or metastatic disease. Drug therapy may be used for these patients even when there is no evidence of node involvement. Weighing the risks and benefits of drug therapy is a complex process.[17]

Chemotherapy. Chemotherapy is the use of cytotoxic drugs to destroy cancer cells. A combination of drugs is usually superior to the use of a single drug. Combination treatment is beneficial because the drugs have different mechanisms of action and work at different parts of the cell cycle.

When used in the neoadjuvant and adjuvant setting, chemotherapy is usually given for 3 to 6 months. However, when a patient has metastasis, chemotherapy may be given for the rest of the patient's life.

Common combination-therapy protocols in the adjuvant and neoadjuvant setting are (1) CMF: cyclophosphamide, methotrexate, and 5-fluorouracil (5-FU); (2) AC: doxorubicin and cyclophosphamide, with or without the addition of a taxane such as paclitaxel (Taxol) or docetaxel (Taxotere); or (3) CEF or CAF: cyclophosphamide, epirubicin (Ellence) or doxorubicin, and 5-FU.

DRUG ALERT Doxorubicin
- Monitor for signs of cardiotoxicity and heart failure (e.g., new onset of shortness of breath, pedal edema, decreased activity tolerance, dysrhythmias, ECG changes).
- Instruct patient not to have immunizations without HCP's approval.
- Instruct patient to avoid contact with those who recently received live virus vaccine.

Because healthy cells are also affected by chemotherapy, a variety of side effects accompany this treatment modality. The incidence and severity of common side effects are related to specific drug combination, drug schedule, and dosage. The most common side effects involve rapidly dividing cells in the gastrointestinal tract (nausea, anorexia, weight loss), bone marrow (anemia), and hair follicles (alopecia [hair loss]).

Cognitive changes during and after treatment, especially with chemotherapy, can occur in patients with cancer. This phenomenon is called *"chemobrain."* These changes include difficulties in concentration, memory, focus, and attention. (Cognitive changes in cancer are discussed in Chapter 15 on p. 256.)

Hormone Therapy. Estrogen can promote the growth of breast cancer cells if the cells are estrogen receptor positive. Hormone therapy can block the effect and source of estrogen, thus promoting tumor regression.

Both estrogen and progesterone receptor status assays have been developed to identify women whose breast cancers are likely to respond to hormone therapy. These assays predict whether hormone therapy is a treatment option. Chances of tumor regression are significantly greater in women whose tumors have estrogen and progesterone receptors.

Hormone therapy can (1) block estrogen receptors or (2) suppress estrogen synthesis by inhibiting aromatase, an enzyme needed for estrogen synthesis (Table 51-8). Premenopausal women with estrogen receptor (ER)–positive breast cancers may also benefit from the removal or suppression of their ovaries. Ovarian ablation can be accomplished surgically or by using luteinizing hormone releasing hormone (LHRH) analogs such as goserelin (Zoladex) or leuprolide (Lupron).

Estrogen receptor blockers. Estrogen receptor blockers include tamoxifen, toremifene (Fareston), and fulvestrant (Faslodex).

Tamoxifen has been the hormone therapy of choice in ER-positive women with all stages of breast cancer over the past 30 years. Tamoxifen may also be used in high-risk premenopausal and postmenopausal women to prevent breast cancer. The most common side effects of tamoxifen include hot flashes, mood swings, vaginal discharge and dryness, and other effects commonly associated with decreased estrogen. It also increases the risk of blood clots, cataracts, stroke, and endometrial cancer in postmenopausal women.

DRUG ALERT Tamoxifen
- Irregular vaginal bleeding or spotting may occur.
- Decreased visual acuity, corneal opacity, and retinopathy can occur in women receiving high doses (240-320 mg/day for >17 mo). These problems may be irreversible.
- Instruct patient to immediately report decreased visual acuity.
- Monitor for signs of deep vein thrombosis, pulmonary embolism, and stroke, including shortness of breath, leg cramps, and weakness.

Aromatase inhibitors. Aromatase inhibitor drugs interfere with the anastrozole enzyme aromatase, which is needed for

TABLE 51-8 Drug Therapy
Breast Cancer

Drug Class	Mechanism of Action	Indications
Hormone Therapy		
Estrogen Receptor Blockers		
tamoxifen	Blocks estrogen receptors (ERs)	ER-positive breast cancer in premenopausal and postmenopausal women Used as a preventive measure in high-risk premenopausal and postmenopausal women
toremifene (Fareston)	Blocks ERs	ER-positive breast cancer in postmenopausal women only
fulvestrant (Faslodex)	Blocks ERs	ER-positive breast cancer in postmenopausal women only
Aromatase Inhibitors		
anastrozole (Arimidex)	Prevents production of estrogen by inhibiting aromatase	ER-positive breast cancer in postmenopausal women only
letrozole (Femara)		
exemestane (Aromasin)		
Estrogen Receptor Modulator		
raloxifene (Evista)	In breast blocks the effect of estrogen In bone promotes effect of estrogen and prevents bone loss	Postmenopausal women
Immunotherapy and Targeted Therapy		
trastuzumab (Herceptin)	Blocks HER-2 receptor	HER-2-positive breast cancer
pertuzumab (Perjeta)		
lapatinib (Tykerb)	Inhibits HER-2 tyrosine kinase and EGFR tyrosine kinase	HER-2-positive breast cancer
ado-trastuzumab emtansine (Kadcyla)	trastuzumab connected to a chemotherapy drug called DM1	HER-2-positive breast cancer
everolimus (Afinitor)	Binds to mammalian target of rapamycin (mTOR), thereby suppressing T cell activation and proliferation	ER-positive, HER-2-negative breast cancer in postmenopausal women
palbociclib (Ibrance)	Kinase inhibitor	ER-positive, HER-2-negative breast cancer in postmenopausal women

EGFR, Epidermal growth factor receptor; *HER-2,* human epidermal growth factor receptor 2.

the synthesis of estrogen. These drugs include anastrozole, letrozole (Femara), and exemestane (Aromasin). They are used in the treatment of breast cancer in postmenopausal women. Aromatase inhibitors do not block the production of estrogen by the ovaries. Thus they are of little benefit and may be harmful in premenopausal women.

Aromatase inhibitors have different side effects than tamoxifen. They rarely cause blood clots, and they do not cause endometrial cancer. Because they block the production of estrogen in postmenopausal women, osteoporosis and bone fractures may occur. These drugs have been associated with night sweats, nausea, arthralgias, and myalgias.

Estrogen receptor modulator and others. Raloxifene (Evista) is a selective estrogen receptor modulator that produces both estrogen-agonistic effects on bone and estrogen-antagonistic effects on breast tissue. (Raloxifene is discussed in the section on osteoporosis in Chapter 63.)

Additional drugs that may be used to suppress hormone-dependent breast tumors include megestrol acetate (Megace), diethylstilbestrol (DES), and fluoxymesterone (Halotestin).

Immunotherapy and Targeted Therapy. As more is known about the genetic changes in breast cancer, drugs have been developed to specifically target cells that have altered gene expression. One of these genetic changes is the overexpression of HER-2. Tumors that overexpress the HER-2 protein tend to be more aggressive and are more likely to recur.

Trastuzumab (Herceptin) is a monoclonal antibody to HER-2. After the antibody attaches to the antigen, it is taken into the cells and eventually kills them. It can be used alone or in combination with chemotherapy agents. The most common side effects are flu-like symptoms (fever, chills, myalgia). Another possible, but more serious side effect, is damage to the heart.

DRUG ALERT   Trastuzumab (Herceptin)
- Use with caution in women with preexisting heart disease.
- Monitor for signs of ventricular dysfunction and heart failure.

Other drugs that target HER-2 include pertuzumab (Perjeta), ado-trastuzumab emtansine (Kadcyla), which is trastuzumab connected to a chemotherapy drug called DM1, and lapatinib (Tykerb), which works inside the cell by blocking the function of the HER-2 protein.

Drugs in other classes that are used to treat breast cancer include everolimus (Afinitor) and palbociclib (Ibrance). Everolimus works by blocking mTOR, a protein that normally promotes cell growth and division. Palbociclib is a kinase inhibitor that prevents cells from dividing, thus slowing cancer growth. (The use of immunotherapy and targeted therapy is discussed in Chapter 15.)

Culturally Competent Care: Breast Cancer

Differences exist in the incidence, mortality rates, and care issues among diverse racial and ethnic groups related to breast cancer (see Cultural & Ethnic Health Disparities box on this page). In addition, cultural differences may involve gender roles, health beliefs, religion, family structure, socioeconomic factors (e.g., poverty) and lack of health insurance. In addition, the lack of education may influence disparities related to access to health care and the use of recommended surveillance examinations.[21]

Cultural values strongly influence how individuals respond to and cope with breast cancer and treatment. Health beliefs and behaviors are influenced by diverse cultural norms. Breast cancer screening, diagnosis, and treatment are affected by the cultural values and meanings (body image, sexuality, modesty, motherhood) associated with the breasts. Women may delay screening or treatment for varying reasons, including an acceptance of disease as inevitable fate or "God's will," a mistrust of Western medicine, lack of health care benefits, fear, or the stigma of a cancer diagnosis.

🌐 CULTURAL & ETHNIC HEALTH DISPARITIES
Breast Cancer

- White women have a higher incidence of breast cancer than other ethnic groups.
- African American women have lower survival rates from breast cancer than white women, even when diagnosed at an early stage.
- Triple-negative breast cancer (negative for estrogen, progesterone, and HER-2 receptors) has a higher incidence in African American and Hispanic women.
- Breast cancer incidence and mortality rates are lower among Hispanic and Asian/Pacific Islander women than among white and African American women.
- Breast cancer is the most commonly diagnosed cancer among Hispanic women.
- Hispanic women, especially Mexican Americans, have the lowest rate of breast cancer screening of any ethnic group.
- Hispanic and African American women are more likely to be diagnosed at a later stage of breast cancer than white women.

HER-2, Human epidermal growth factor receptor 2.

❖ NURSING MANAGEMENT: BREAST CANCER

◆ Nursing Assessment

Many factors must be considered when assessing a patient with a breast problem. The history of the breast disorder assists in establishing a diagnosis. Investigate the presence of nipple discharge, pain, rate of growth of the lump, breast asymmetry, and correlation with the menstrual cycle.

Carefully document the size and location of the lump or lumps. Assess the physical characteristics of the lesion, such as consistency, mobility, and shape. If nipple discharge is present, note the color and consistency and whether it occurs from one or both breasts.

Subjective and objective data that should be obtained from an individual suspected of having or diagnosed with breast cancer are presented in Table 51-9.

◆ Nursing Diagnoses

Nursing diagnoses related to the care of a patient diagnosed with breast cancer vary. After diagnosis and before a treatment plan has been selected, the following nursing diagnoses would apply:
- Decisional conflict *related to* lack of knowledge about treatment options and their effects
- Fear and/or anxiety *related to* diagnosis of breast cancer
- Disturbed body image *related to* physical and emotional effects of treatment modalities

If surgery is planned, the nursing diagnoses may include, but are not limited to, those presented in eNursing Care Plan 51-1 (available on the website for this chapter).

◆ Planning

The overall goals are that the patient with breast cancer will (1) actively participate in the decision-making process related to treatment, (2) adhere to the therapeutic plan, (3) communicate about and manage the side effects of adjuvant therapy, (4) access and benefit from the support provided by significant others and HCPs, and (5) comply with recommended follow-up and surveillance after treatment.

◆ Nursing Implementation

Health Promotion. Review the risk factors in Table 51-2. People can reduce their risk factors by maintaining a healthy weight,

TABLE 51-9 Nursing Assessment

Breast Cancer

Subjective Data

Important Health Information

Past health history: Benign breast disease with atypical changes. Previous unilateral breast cancer. Menstrual history (early menarche with late menopause), pregnancy history (nulliparity or first full-term pregnancy after age 30). Previous endometrial, ovarian, or colon cancer. Hyperestrogenism and testicular atrophy (in men)

Medications: Hormones, especially as postmenopausal hormone therapy and in oral contraceptives. Infertility treatments

Surgery or other treatments: Exposure to therapeutic radiation (e.g., Hodgkin's lymphoma or thyroid radiation)

Functional Health Patterns

Health perception–health management: Family history of breast cancer (young age at diagnosis). History of abnormal mammogram or atypical prior biopsy. Palpable change found on BSE. Known BRCA mutation carrier, first-degree relative of *BRCA* carrier (but untested)

Nutritional-metabolic: Obesity; unexplained severe weight loss (possible indicator of metastasis)

Activity-exercise: Level of usual activity

Cognitive-perceptual: Changes in cognition, headache, bone pain (possible indicators of metastasis)

Sexuality-reproductive: Unilateral nipple discharge (clear, milky, or bloody). Change in breast contour, size, or symmetry

Coping–stress tolerance: Psychologic stress

Self-perception–self-concept: Anxiety regarding threat to self-esteem

Objective Data

General

Axillary and supraclavicular lymphadenopathy

Integumentary

Hard, irregular, nonmobile breast lump most often in upper, outer sector, possibly fixated to fascia or chest wall. Thickening of breast. Nipple inversion or retraction, erosion. Edema ("peau d'orange"), erythema, induration, infiltration, or dimpling (in later stages). Firm, discrete nodules at mastectomy site (possible indicator of local recurrence). Peripheral edema (possible indicator of metastasis)

Respiratory

Pleural effusions (possible indicator of metastasis)

Gastrointestinal

Hepatomegaly, jaundice, ascites (possible indicators of liver metastasis)

Possible Diagnostic Findings

Finding of mass or change in tissue on breast examination. Abnormal mammogram, ultrasound, or breast MRI. Positive results of FNA or surgical biopsy or similar results with a needle biopsy

BSE, Breast self-examination; *FNA,* fine-needle aspiration.

exercising regularly, limiting alcohol, eating nutritious food, and never smoking (or quitting if currently smoking).

Encourage people to adhere to the breast cancer screening guidelines presented on pp. 1204-1205. If a person is at high risk, he or she needs to develop an individualized plan with the HCP. Early detection can decrease the morbidity and mortality associated with breast cancer.

Along with these lifestyle choices, there are other risk-reduction options for individuals at high risk. Genetic testing for *BRCA* gene mutations is available. People with a strong family history of breast cancer should talk with their HCP about the possibility of genetic testing. Routine screening for genetic abnormalities in women without evidence of a strong family history of breast cancer is not warranted.

In women with an abnormal *BRCA1* or *BRCA2* gene, prophylactic oophorectomy may reduce their risk of developing breast cancer and ovarian cancer. In deciding whether and when to undergo this surgical procedure, women should receive counseling about the risks and benefits of prophylactic oophorectomy, including fertility issues.

Prophylactic surgery decisions require a great deal of thought, patience, and discussion with the HCP, genetic counselor, and family. Patients need to consider these options and make decisions with which they feel comfortable. Removing both breasts and ovaries at a young age does not eliminate the risk of breast cancer. A small risk exists that cancer can develop in the areas where the breasts used to be. Close follow-up is necessary, even after prophylactic surgery.

◆ **Acute Care.** The times of waiting for the initial biopsy results and waiting for the HCP to make treatment recommendations are difficult for patients and their families. Even after the HCP has discussed treatment options, the patient often relies on you to clarify and expand on these options. During this stressful time, the patient may not be coping effectively. Appropriate nursing interventions are to explore the patient's usual decision-making processes, help to evaluate the advantages and disadvantages of the options, provide information relevant to the decision, clarify unresolved issues with the HCP, and support the patient and family once the decision is made.

Regardless of the surgery planned, provide the patient with sufficient information to ensure informed consent. Some patients seek extensive, detailed information to maintain a sense of control, whereas others avoid information to decrease anxiety and fear. Be sensitive to the individual's need for and preferred type of information. These include (1) preoperative instructions on pain control and what to expect after surgery (e.g., reporting of complications, dressing and drain care, turning, coughing, deep breathing); (2) a review of mobility restrictions and postoperative exercises; and (3) explanation of the recovery period from the time of surgery until the first postoperative visit.

The woman who has breast-conserving surgery usually has an uncomplicated postoperative course with variable pain intensity. Pain depends primarily on the extent of the lymph node sampling procedure performed. If an ALND has been done or if the patient had a mastectomy, drains are generally left in place, and patients are discharged home with them. Teach the patient and family, with a return demonstration, how to manage the drains at home.

Most patients are discharged from the hospital within 24 to 48 hours after a mastectomy, depending on if reconstructive surgery was performed. Restoring arm function on the affected side after breast cancer surgery is a key nursing goal. Postoperative arm and shoulder exercises, which are started gradually, may begin prior to discharge (Fig. 51-9). These exercises are designed to prevent contractures and muscle shortening, maintain muscle tone, and improve lymph and blood circulation. The difficulty and pain encountered in performing what used to be simple tasks may cause frustration and depression. The goal of all exercise is a gradual return to full range of motion.

Treatment for Breast Cancer

C.P. is a 56-yr-old woman who was diagnosed with stage IIIA breast cancer. Her treatment plan is to receive neoadjuvant chemotherapy and then have surgery and radiation. C.P. tells you that she is anxious and will have surgery and radiation but does not want chemotherapy because she is afraid of the side effects.

Making Clinical Decisions

Best Available Evidence. The use of chemotherapy before surgery reduces the size and extent of the tumor, thus making the surgery more likely to succeed. It also reduces the consequences of a more extensive treatment that would be required if the tumor were not reduced.

Clinician Expertise. Neoadjuvant chemotherapy is usually recommended for stage IIIA breast cancer. The common side effects (e.g., nausea, vomiting, fatigue) can be managed with appropriate treatment.

Patient Preferences and Values. C.P. does not want chemotherapy and prefers to take her chances. If the cancer comes back, she will have chemotherapy.

Implications for Nursing Practice

1. Why is it important to discuss with C.P. why chemotherapy is recommended?
2. What information would you share with her regarding possible treatment side effects and how they can be managed?
3. You note her spouse appears attentive and supportive. How will you involve him in C.P.'s care?

Reference for Evidence

National Comprehensive Cancer Network: NCCN guidelines for patients. Stage III breast cancer. Retrieved from *www.nccn.org/patients/guidelines/stage_iii_breast/index.html*.

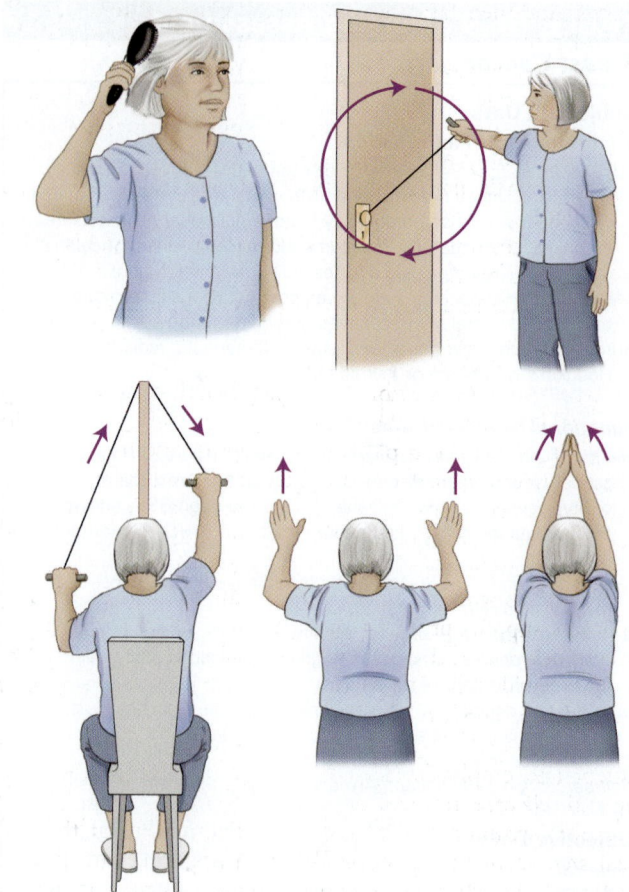

FIG. 51-9 Postoperative exercises for the patient with a mastectomy or lumpectomy with axillary lymph node sampling and/or dissection.

Postoperative discomfort can be minimized by administering analgesics regularly when the patient is in pain and about 30 minutes before initiating exercises. When the patient is able to shower, the warm water on the involved shoulder often relaxes the muscle and reduces joint stiffness.

Upper extremity lymphedema can occur at any point after treatment for breast cancer. Teach the patient measures to prevent and reduce lymphedema, including no BP readings, venipunctures, or injections on the affected arm. The affected arm should not be dependent for long periods. Caution should be used to prevent infection, burns, or compromised circulation on the affected side.

If trauma to the arm occurs, the area should be washed thoroughly with soap and water and observed. A topical antibiotic ointment and a bandage or other sterile dressing may be applied.

When the patient's lymphedema is acute (Fig. 51-7), complete decongestive therapy will be recommended. This therapy is performed by specially trained professionals and consists of a massage-like technique to mobilize the subcutaneous accumulation of fluid. This may be followed by use of compression bandaging and an intermittent pneumatic compression sleeve. The sleeve applies mechanical massage to the arm and facilitates lymph drainage up toward the heart. Elevation of the arm so that it is level with the heart and isometric exercises may be used to reduce the fluid in the arm. To maintain maximum volume reduction, the patient may need to wear a fitted compression sleeve during waking hours and preventively during air travel.

◆   ***Psychosocial Support.*** Throughout history, the female breast has been regarded as a symbol of beauty, femininity, sexuality, and motherhood. The potential loss of a breast, or part of a breast, may be devastating for many women because of the significant psychologic, social, sexual, and body image implications associated with it. For men diagnosed with breast cancer, isolation and embarrassment related to the diagnosis can occur. You must be aware of resources for men (*www.malebreastcancer.org*).

As difficult as it is to predict which patients will develop physical effects of treatment, it can be even more difficult to foresee the psychosocial effects of treatment. In some cases, psychosocial concerns may increase the physical effects of cancer, such as pain, fatigue, sleep disturbances, fear of recurrence, and cognitive changes.

Screening all cancer patients for psychosocial distress has been added to the Commission on Cancer accreditation requirements.[22] From the time of diagnosis through treatment, survivorship, or metastatic disease, the patient may exhibit signs of distress or tension (e.g., tachycardia, increased muscle tension, sleep disturbances, restlessness, changes in appetite or mood). Assess the patient's body language and affect during periods of high stress and indecision so that appropriate interventions, including referral to a mental health provider, can be initiated.

Remain sensitive to the complex psychologic impact that a diagnosis of cancer and subsequent breast surgery can have on patients and their families. With an accepting attitude and the offer of resources, you can help the patient cope with feelings of fear, anger, anxiety, and depression. You can help to:

- Provide a safe environment for the expression of feelings.
- Identify sources of support and strength, such as his or her partner, family, and spiritual or religious practices.
- Encourage the patient to identify and learn individual coping strengths.
- Promote communication between the patient and his or her family and friends.
- Provide accurate and complete answers to questions about the disease; treatment options; and reproductive, fertility, or lactation issues (if appropriate).
- Make resources available for mental health counseling.
- Offer information about local and national community resources. Referring patients to support resources, such as the Cancer Support Community, Breastcancer.org, or local breast cancer organizations, is invaluable. The American Cancer Society and National Cancer Institute can provide excellent materials to assist you in meeting the special needs of patients with breast cancer. In addition to in-person and online support programs, multiple free smart phone applications are available through national cancer organizations that provide reliable and current information for the patient and his or her family.

◆ **Ambulatory Care.** Explain the specific follow-up plan to the patient and emphasize the importance of ongoing monitoring and self-care. Immediately after surgery, advise the patient to report symptoms such as fever, inflammation at the surgical site, erythema, postoperative constipation, and unusual swelling. Other changes to report are new back pain, weakness, shortness of breath, and change in mental status, including confusion.

For women who have had a mastectomy without breast reconstruction, a variety of products are available. These include garments such as camisoles with soft breast prosthetic inserts or a fitted prosthesis with bra. Should the woman choose a breast prosthesis, a certified fitter can help her select a comfortable, more permanent weighted prosthesis and bra, generally at 4 to 8 weeks postoperatively. Your role is to present the choices and resources without judgment.

How the loss of part or all of the breast and cancer affect the patient's sexual identity, body image, and relationships can vary. If you are comfortable, initiate a discussion of sexuality by inviting questions about relationships or intimacy concerns. Often

the patient's partner and/or family members need help dealing with their emotional reactions to the diagnosis and surgery before they can provide effective support for the patient. There are no physical reasons why a mastectomy would prevent sexual satisfaction. A woman taking hormone therapy may have a decreased sexual drive or vaginal dryness. She may need to use lubrication to prevent discomfort during intercourse. Concerns about sexuality are not well addressed by many HCPs. If difficulty in adjustment or other problems develop, individual or couples counseling may be necessary to deal with the emotional component of a diagnosis of cancer.

COMPLEMENTARY & ALTERNATIVE THERAPIES

Imagery

Imagery is the use of one's mind to generate images that have a calming effect on the body.

Scientific Evidence*

- Good evidence for decreasing cancer pain and postoperative pain.
- Good evidence for treatment of migraine or tension headache in conjunction with standard medical care.

Nursing Implications

- Used by nurses to help patients promote relaxation, decrease stress, and manage pain.
- Should be used as a supplemental technique, not a replacement for medical care.

*Source: www.naturalstandard.com.

EVIDENCE-BASED PRACTICE
Translating Research Into Practice

Are Integrative Therapies Helpful During Breast Cancer Treatment?

Clinical Question

For women receiving breast cancer treatment (P), what is the effect of integrative therapy (I) versus usual care (C) on anxiety, depression, fatigue, and quality of life (O)?

Synthesis of Best Available Evidence

- Systematic review of randomized controlled trials (RCTs).
- 203 RCTs of patients receiving breast cancer treatments of surgery, chemotherapy, radiation therapy, and/or hormonal therapy. Intervention was the use of integrative therapies (complementary and alternative therapies) during treatment. Many therapies were examined including meditation, acupuncture, hypnosis, yoga, natural products (e.g., botanicals, minerals), relaxation with imagery, stress management, yoga, massage, music therapy, Tai Chi/qigong, and energy conservation. Outcomes included anxiety, stress reduction, pain, hot flashes, depression, fatigue, sleep, skin changes, and quality of life.
- *Strongest evidence:* Meditation, relaxation with imagery, and yoga decreased anxiety, depression, and fatigue and improved quality of life.
- *Moderate evidence:* Stress management, yoga, massage, music therapy, energy conservation, and meditation decreased stress, fatigue, anxiety, and depression and improved quality of life.

Conclusions

- Women use a variety of integrative therapies during breast cancer treatment.
- Meditation, yoga, relaxation with imagery, stress management, massage, music therapy, and energy conservation may be particularly helpful in managing symptoms and improving quality of life during treatment.

Implications for Nursing Practice

1. Why is it important for you to determine patient use of complementary and alternative therapies and document your findings?
2. How will you stay informed on evidence that supports or discourages the use of specific complementary and alternative therapies during breast cancer treatment?
3. How can you best help a patient who is exploring various complementary and alternative therapies to reduce treatment-related fatigue?
4. Why are patient preferences for complementary and alternative therapies an integral part of evidence-based practice?

Reference for Evidence

Greenlee H, Balneaves L, Carlson L, et al: Clinical practice guidelines on the use of integrative therapies as supportive care in patients treated for breast cancer, *J Natl Cancer Inst Monogr* 50: 346, 2014.

P, Patient population of interest; *I*, intervention or area of interest; *C*, comparison of interest or comparison group; *O*, outcomes of interest; *T*, timing (see p. 15).

Depression and anxiety may occur with the continued stress and uncertainty of a cancer diagnosis. A patient's self-esteem and identity may also be threatened. The support of family and friends and participation in a cancer support group and/or individual counseling are important aspects of care that may improve the patient's quality of life.

Almost 3 million breast cancer survivors are alive in the United States, making this population the largest group of cancer survivors. This number is expected to grow due to an aging population and improved methods for early detection and treatment. After treatment for breast cancer, the patient will have ongoing survivorship care.[22,23]

A history and physical examination is recommended one to four times per year as clinically appropriate for 5 years, then annually thereafter. In addition, advise breast cancer survivors to perform monthly BSE and chest wall self-examination, and report any changes to their HCP. Local recurrence of breast cancer is usually at the surgical site. Breast cancer survivors should have an annual mammogram. Other breast imaging studies such as a breast ultrasound or breast MRI should only be performed as an adjunct to mammography and not for annual routine surveillance. (Cancer survivorship is discussed in Chapter 15 on p. 266.)

◆ Evaluation

Expected outcomes are that the patient after breast cancer surgery will

- Identify activities that can reduce postoperative edema and improve mobility
- Use pain control measures appropriately
- Demonstrate effective use of coping strategies that provide reduction of anxiety
- Discuss feelings about and the meaning of changes in physical appearance
- Identify community and online resources, individual counseling resources, and support groups

Additional information on expected outcomes for the patient after breast cancer surgery is presented in eNursing Care Plan 51-1 (available on the website for this chapter).

 Gerontologic Considerations: Breast Cancer

A major risk for breast cancer is increasing age, and more than half of all breast cancers are diagnosed in women who are age 65 or older.[1] Older women are less likely to have mammograms. Screening and treatment decisions for breast cancer should be based on a woman's general health status rather than biologic age, since health status has a greater influence on tolerance to treatment and long-term prognosis. In addition to medical co-morbidities and life expectancy, treatment decisions for the older woman with breast cancer should be based on an assessment of nutritional and functional status; vision, gait, and balance; and the presence of delirium, dementia, or depression.

Breast cancer treatment is similar for older and younger patients, including the use of surgery, radiation therapy, and drug therapy. For healthy older women, breast cancer survival rates are similar to those of younger women when matched by cancer stage.

MAMMOPLASTY

Mammoplasty is the surgical change in the size or shape of the breast. It may be done electively for cosmetic purposes to either

---

✦ BECOMING A NURSE LEADER
Protecting Patient Privacy

Situation

During your clinical rotation on the oncology unit, Felicia, a fellow nursing student, asks you to take a photo of her with her patient, who is a famous TV newscaster. Felicia assures you that this photo will only be for her private collection. Later, you see the photo posted on Felicia's Facebook page with the caption: "Look who I took care of in the hospital today! Hope her treatments for breast cancer are successful."

Points for Consideration

- Privacy and confidentiality are basic rights in our society. As nurses, it is our ethical and legal obligation to safeguard those rights.
- *Privacy* is the right of individuals to keep information about themselves from being disclosed. *Confidentiality* is the principle that the information that a patient reveals to an HCP is private and has limits on how and when it can be disclosed to a third party.
- The Health Insurance Portability and Accountability Act (HIPAA) of 1996 privacy rule protects an individual's health information. This information includes the individual's past, present, or future physical or mental health or condition. If you violate HIPAA confidentiality laws by posting patient information online, you may be fired or lose your license.[1]
- The American Nurses Association Code of Ethics details that nurses promote, advocate for, and strive to protect the health, safety, and rights of patients.[2] This includes their right to privacy and confidentiality. The nurse has a duty to maintain confidentiality of all patient information. The patient's well-being could be jeopardized and the fundamental trust between patient and nurse destroyed.
- Our patients trust us with intimate details of their lives, and we should never post patient-related issues on any social media site.

Discussion Questions

1. What should you have done when asked to take a photo of the nursing student and her patient?
2. What consequences could happen to Felicia as a result of posting this photo and comment on Facebook?
3. What consequences could you face?

References

1. Tortorice J: What is right and wrong when it comes to posting medical pictures online? Retrieved from *www.ceufast.com/blog/julia-tortorice/what-is-right-and-wrong-when-it-comes-to-posting-medical-pictures-online*.
2. American Nurses Association: Code of ethics. Retrieved from *www.nursingworld.org/MainMenuCategories/EthicsStandards/CodeofEthicsforNurses/Code-of-Ethics.pdf*.

---

enlarge or reduce the size of the breasts. It may also be done to reconstruct the breast after a mastectomy.

A professional, nonjudgmental attitude and clear information about surgical breast options are most useful for women engaged in decision making about mammoplasty. The desire to change the appearance of the breasts has special significance for each woman as she attempts to alter or recreate her body image. Be aware of the cultural value that the woman places on the breast. Help the patient set realistic expectations about what mammoplasty can accomplish and about possible complications (e.g., hematoma formation, hemorrhage, infection). If an implant is involved, capsular contracture and loss of the implant are possible.

Breast Reconstruction

Breast reconstructive surgery is a type of surgery for women who have had all or part of a breast removed. It is done to

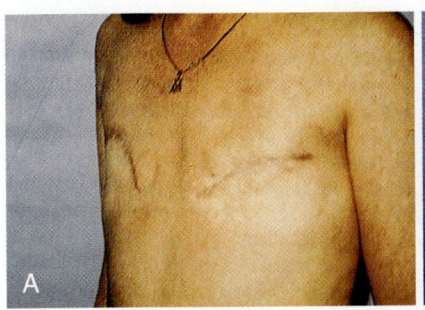 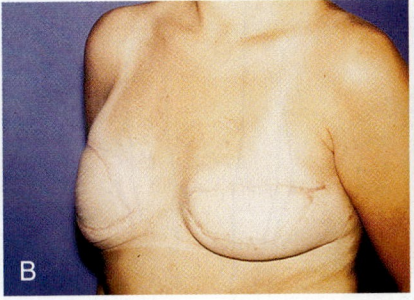 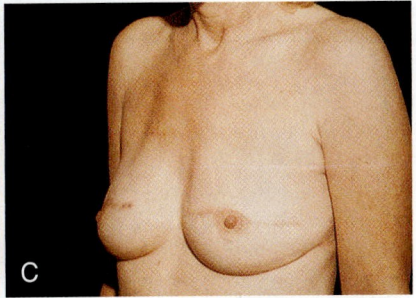

FIG. 51-10 A, Appearance of chest after bilateral mastectomy. **B,** Postoperative breast reconstruction before nipple-areolar reconstruction. **C,** Postoperative breast reconstruction after nipple-areolar reconstruction. (Courtesy Brian Davies, MD. From Fortunato N, McCullough S: *Plastic and reconstructive surgery,* St Louis, 1998, Mosby.)

achieve symmetry and to restore or preserve body image. It may be done simultaneously with a mastectomy or some time afterward. The timing of reconstructive surgery is individualized based on the patient's physical and psychologic needs.[24]

Indications. The main indication for breast reconstruction is to improve a woman's self-image, regain a sense of normalcy, and assist in coping with the loss of the breast. The contour of the breast is restored without the use of an external prosthesis. Reconstruction techniques cannot restore lactation, nipple sensation, or erectility. Although the breast will not fully resemble its premastectomy appearance, the reconstructed appearance usually represents an improvement over the mastectomy scar (Fig. 51-10).

Types of Reconstruction

Breast Implants and Tissue Expansion. Implants have a silicone shell filled with either silicone gel or saline.[25] Some newer types use a cohesive gel, which is a thicker silicone gel. Implant surgery can be done during one stage or two stages.

In the *one-stage procedure,* the implant is placed at the same time as the mastectomy. The implant is usually placed under the pectoralis muscle.

In the *two-stage procedure,* a tissue expander is inserted after the mastectomy. It is used to stretch the skin and muscle at the mastectomy site before inserting permanent implants (Fig. 51-11). The tissue expander is placed in a pocket under the pectoralis muscle, which protects the implant and provides soft tissue coverage. The tissue expander is minimally inflated and then gradually filled by weekly injections of sterile saline solution. This procedure stretches the skin and muscle and can be painful. A small magnet is embedded in most expanders to help locate the port where the fluid is injected. Therefore a woman should not have an MRI with a magnet in place.

The expander can be (1) surgically removed and a permanent implant is inserted or (2) remain in place to become the implant, thus eliminating the need for a second surgical procedure. Tissue expansion does not work well in individuals with extensive scar tissue from surgery or radiation therapy.

The body's natural response to the presence of a foreign substance is the formation of a fibrous capsule around the implant. If excessive capsular formation occurs as a result of infection, hematoma, trauma, or reaction to a foreign body, a contracture can develop, resulting in deformity. Although surgeons differ in their approaches to the prevention of contracture formation, gentle manual massage around the implant is

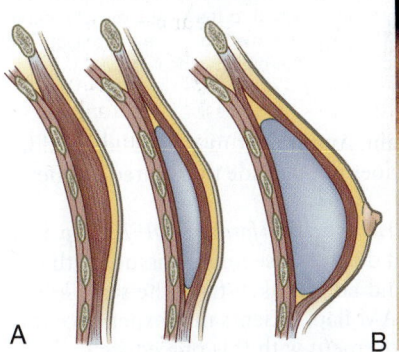 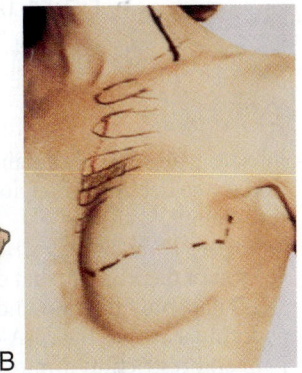

FIG. 51-11 A, Tissue expander with gradual expansion. **B,** Tissue expander in place after mastectomy. (*A,* Modified from Cameron J: *Current surgical therapy,* ed 5, St Louis, 1995, Mosby. *B,* Courtesy Brian Davies, MD. From Fortunato N, McCullough S: *Plastic and reconstructive surgery,* St Louis, 1998, Mosby.)

routine. Other adverse outcomes include wrinkling, scarring, asymmetry, pain, and infection at the incision site.[22]

Tissue Flap Procedures. Another type of breast reconstruction uses autologous (person's own) tissue to recreate a breast mound. In autologous breast reconstruction, tissue from the abdomen, back, thighs, or buttocks is used to create a reconstructed breast. The most common types of tissue flap procedures are *transverse rectus abdominis musculocutaneous (TRAM) flap, deep inferior epigastric artery perforator (DIEP) flap,* and *latissimus dorsi flap.*

The *transverse rectus abdominis musculocutaneous (TRAM) flap* is a frequently used flap operation. The rectus abdominis muscles are paired flat muscles running from the rib cage down to the pubic bone. Arteries running inside the muscles provide branches at many levels, and these branches supply the fat and skin across a large expanse of the abdomen.

There are two different types of TRAM: pedicle flap and free flap. In a pedicle flap, the tissue remains attached to the rectus muscle and is tunneled under the skin to the patient's chest (Fig. 51-12). In a free flap, the tissue is completely separated from the muscle and its blood supply and moved to the new place on the patient's chest.

The tissue is molded and fashioned to form a breast. The abdominal incision is closed, giving the patient a result that is similar to having an abdominoplasty ("tummy tuck"). This surgical procedure can last 6 to 8 hours with recovery taking 6 to 8 weeks. Some patients have reported pain and fatigue for up to 3 months. Complications include bleeding, seroma, hernia,

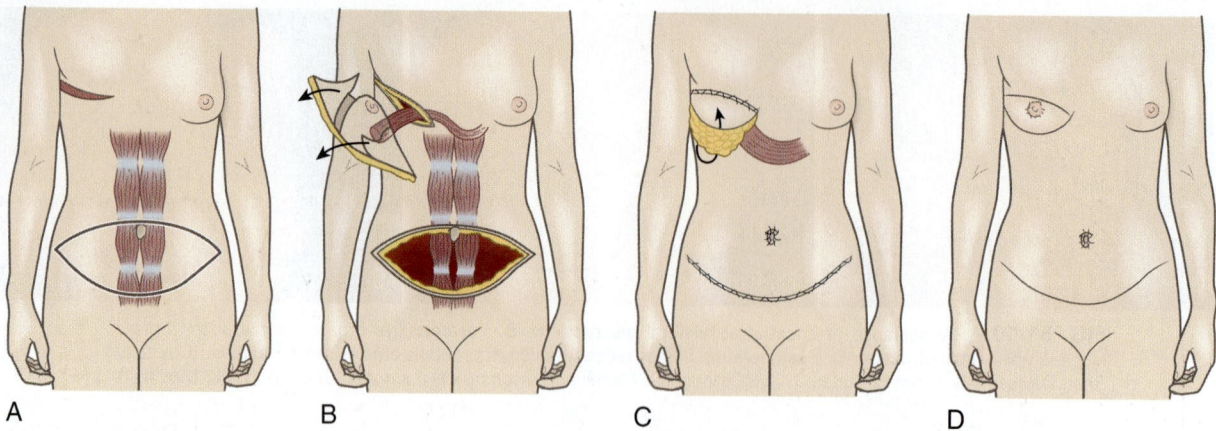

FIG. 51-12 Transverse rectus abdominis musculocutaneous (TRAM) flap. **A,** TRAM flap is planned. **B,** The abdominal tissue, while attached to the rectus muscle, nerve, and blood supply, is tunneled through the abdomen to the chest. **C,** The flap is trimmed to shape the breast. The lower abdominal incision is closed. **D,** Nipple and areola are reconstructed after the breast is healed.

infection, and low back pain. An implant may be used in addition to the flap if the flap does not provide the desired cosmetic result alone.

A *deep inferior epigastric artery perforator (DIEP) flap* is a version of the free flap that does not use muscle tissue. With the DIEP flap, only the skin and fat are taken from the same lower abdominal area as the TRAM flap. Patients may experience less pain and restriction of movement with this procedure.

In a *latissimus dorsi flap*, a block of skin and muscle from the patient's back is used to replace tissue removed during mastectomy. A small implant may be needed beneath the flap to gain reasonable breast shape and size. A disadvantage of this technique is an additional scar on the back.

Other types of breast reconstruction include gluteal free flap (tissue is used from buttocks, including the gluteal muscle) and transverse upper gracilis flap or inner thigh flap (tissue is taken from the bottom fold of the buttock extending into the inner thigh.)

Nipple-Areolar Reconstruction. Many patients undergoing breast reconstruction also have nipple-areolar reconstruction. Nipple reconstruction gives the reconstructed breast a much more natural appearance (Fig. 51-10, *C*). Nipple-areolar reconstruction is usually done a few months after breast reconstruction. Tissue to construct a nipple may be taken from the opposite breast or from a small flap of tissue on the reconstructed breast mound. The areola may be grafted from the labia, skin in the area of the groin, or lower abdominal skin. Tattooing may be done with a permanent pigmented dye. In some patients, a small implant may be placed under the completed nipple-areolar reconstruction to provide additional projection.

Breast Augmentation

In *augmentation mammoplasty* (procedure to enlarge the breasts), an implant is placed in a surgically created pocket between the capsule of the breast and pectoral fascia, or ideally under the pectoralis muscle. (Implants are discussed on p. 1223.)

Breast Reduction

For some women, large breasts can be a source of physical and psychologic discomfort. They can interfere with normal daily activities, such as walking, using a computer, and driving a car. The weight of large breasts can lead to back, shoulder, and neck problems, including degenerative nerve changes. Overly large breasts can interfere with self-esteem, self-image, and comfort in wearing some clothing. Reduction in the size of the breasts can have positive effects on the patient's psychologic and physical health.

Reduction mammoplasty is performed by resecting wedges of tissue from the upper and lower quadrants of the breast. The excess skin is removed, and the areola and nipple are relocated on the breast. Lactation can usually be accomplished if massive amounts of tissue are not removed and the nipples are left connected during surgery.

❖ NURSING MANAGEMENT: BREAST AUGMENTATION AND REDUCTION

Breast augmentation and breast reduction may be done in the outpatient surgical area or they may involve overnight hospitalization. General anesthesia is used. Drains are generally placed in the surgical site to prevent hematoma formation and then removed when drainage is under 20 to 30 mL/day. The drainage must be examined for color and odor to detect postoperative infection or hemorrhage. Also monitor the woman's temperature. Dressings should be changed as necessary using sterile technique.

After surgery, assure the woman that the breast's appearance will improve when healing is complete. Depending on physician preference, the patient may be instructed to wear a bra that provides good support continuously for 2 or 3 days after breast reduction or augmentation. Depending on the extent of the operation, most women resume normal activities within 2 to 3 weeks. Strenuous exercise may not be appropriate until several weeks later.

CASE STUDY
Breast Cancer

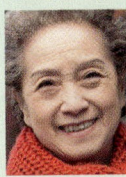

(©XiXinXing/ iStock/ Thinkstock)

Patient Profile

A.K., a 68-yr-old married Asian American woman, has been diagnosed with breast cancer. She is scheduled for surgery in the morning for a lumpectomy and sentinel lymph node biopsy with possible axillary node dissection.

Interprofessional Care
Preoperative

- When she is seen in the preoperative clinic 1 week before surgery, she is crying uncontrollably and says, "My husband does not want to look at me anymore. He is afraid of what I am going to look like with a flat chest."
- She says, "I cannot sleep and I just pace the floor at night."
- "My mother died of breast cancer when she was 60, and my sister got it when she was 40."
- Expresses concern that her two daughters (34 and 32) and their daughters are going to get "this horrible disease."

Operative Procedure

- A lumpectomy and sentinel lymph node biopsy are performed.
- A.K. has cancer cells in her sentinel lymph node.
- Axillary node dissection is then done, involving the removal of 12 nodes.

Postoperative

- Does not want to leave hospital. She wants to stay in bed.
- Swelling and restricted range of motion in right arm.
- Pain not controlled well with pain medication.

Follow-Up Findings and Treatment

- Two positive lymph nodes are found.
- Scheduled for outpatient chemotherapy followed by external radiation.

Discussion Questions

1. What in A.K.'s breast cancer experience with her family members may influence her coping response?
2. *Patient-Centered Care:* What information would you provide to A.K. about her surgery?
3. What complication did she develop after her surgery?
4. Which common postoperative exercises will A.K. need to practice after her surgery?
5. *Teamwork and Collaboration:* Which of the following personnel should provide this instruction to A.K.: registered nurse, licensed practical/vocational nurse, unlicensed assistive personnel?
6. What community resources are available to help A.K. and her family adjust to the change in her body and to cope with the diagnosis of cancer? How can you access these resources?
7. What information is important for you to provide to A.K. about her radiation treatment and chemotherapy?
8. *Priority Decision:* Based on the assessment data, what are the priority nursing diagnoses? Are there any collaborative problems?
9. What information is important for you to provide to A.K. and her daughters? What early detection measures are important for them to know?
10. *Evidence-Based Practice:* A.K. wants to know what the psychologic benefit may be for her daughters if they decide on a breast cancer genetic risk assessment.
11. *Patient-Centered Care:* How will you include cultural preferences in A.K.'s plan of care?
12. *Teamwork and Collaboration:* What types of referrals may be indicated for A.K.?
13. *Safety:* Describe specific nursing interventions aimed at minimizing risk of harm for A.K.
14. *Quality Improvement:* What outcomes would indicate nursing interventions were successful for A.K.?

Answers and a corresponding conceptual care map available at *http://evolve.elsevier.com/Lewis/medsurg.*

BRIDGE TO NCLEX EXAMINATION

The number of the question corresponds to the same-numbered outcome at the beginning of the chapter.

1. You are a community health nurse planning a program on breast cancer screening guidelines for women in the neighborhood. To best promote the participants' learning and adherence, you would include *(select all that apply)*
   a. a short audiotape on the BSE procedure.
   b. a packet of articles from the medical literature.
   c. written guidelines for mammography and CBE.
   d. a discussion of the value of early breast cancer detection.
   e. community resources where they can obtain an ultrasound and MRI.

2. In teaching a patient who wants to perform BSE, you inform her that the technique involves both the palpation of the breast tissue and
   a. palpation of cervical lymph nodes.
   b. hard squeezing of the breast tissue.
   c. a mammogram to evaluate breast tissue.
   d. inspection of the breasts for any changes.

3. You are caring for a young woman who has painful fibrocystic breast changes. Management of this patient would include
   a. scheduling a biopsy to rule out malignant changes.
   b. teaching that symptoms will probably subside if she stops using oral contraceptives.
   c. preparing her for surgical removal of the lumps, since they will become larger and more painful.
   d. explaining that restrictions of coffee and chocolate and supplements of vitamin E may relieve some discomfort.

4. When discussing risk factors for breast cancer with a group of women, you emphasize that the greatest known risk factor for breast cancer is
   a. being a woman over age 60.
   b. experiencing menstruation for 30 years or more.
   c. using hormone therapy for 5 years for menopausal symptoms.
   d. having a paternal grandmother with postmenopausal breast cancer.

5. A patient with breast cancer has a lumpectomy with sentinel lymph node biopsy that is positive for cancer. You explain that, of the other tests done to determine the risk for cancer recurrence or spread, the results that support the more favorable prognosis are *(select all that apply)*
   a. well-differentiated tumor.
   b. estrogen receptor–positive tumor.
   c. overexpression of HER-2 cell marker.
   d. involvement of two to four axillary nodes.
   e. aneuploidy status from cell proliferation studies.

6. A simple mastectomy has been scheduled for your patient with breast cancer. Postoperatively, to restore arm function on the affected side, you would
   a. apply heating pads or blankets to increase circulation.
   b. place daily ice packs to minimize the risk of lymphedema.
   c. teach passive exercises with the affected arm in a dependent position.
   d. emphasize regular exercises for the affected shoulder to increase range of motion.

7. Preoperatively, to meet the psychologic needs of a woman scheduled for a simple mastectomy, you would
   a. discuss the limitations of breast reconstruction.
   b. include her significant other in all conversations.
   c. promote an environment for expression of feelings.
   d. explain the importance of regular follow-up screening.

8. To prevent capsular formation after breast reconstruction with implants, teach the patient to
   a. gently massage the area around the implant.
   b. bind the breasts tightly with elastic bandages.
   c. exercise the arm on the affected side to promote drainage.
   d. avoid strenuous exercise until the implant has healed.

1, c, d, 2, d, 3, d, 4, a, 5, a, b, 6, d, 7, c, 8, a

For rationales to these answers and even more NCLEX review questions, visit *http://evolve.elsevier.com/Lewis/medsurg*.

ⓔ EVOLVE WEBSITE

http://evolve.elsevier.com/Lewis/medsurg
Review Questions (Online Only)
Key Points
Answer Keys for Questions
• Rationales for Bridge to NCLEX Examination Questions
• Answer Guidelines for Case Study(ies) on p. 1225
Student Case Study
• Patient With Breast Cancer
Nursing Care Plan
• eNursing Care Plan 51-1: Patient After Breast Surgery
Conceptual Care Map Creator
• Conceptual Care Map for Case Study on p. 1225
Audio Glossary
Content Updates

REFERENCES

1. American Cancer Society: Breast cancer facts and figures. Retrieved from *www.cancer.org/research/cancerfactsstatistics/breast-cancer-facts-figures*.
2. Oeffinger KC, Fontham ETH, Etzioni R, et al: Breast cancer screening for women at average risk : 2015 guideline update from the American Cancer Society, *JAMA* 314(15):1599, 2015.
*3. National Comprehensive Cancer Network (NCCN): NCCN Guidelines Version1.2014. Breast Cancer Screening and Diagnosis. Retrieved from *www.nccn.org/professionals/physician_gls/pdf/breast-screening.pdf*.
4. Mansel R: Management of breast pain. In Harris JR, Morrow M, Osborne CK, et al, editors: *Diseases of the breast*, ed 5, Philadelphia, 2014, Wolters Kluwer Health.
5. Twoon M, Ng NY, Thomson SE: Breast lumps, *BMJ* 349:g5275, 2014.
6. Collins LC, Schnitt S: Pathology of benign breast disorders. In Harris JR, Morrow M, Osborne CK, et al, editors: *Diseases of the breast*, ed 5, Philadelphia, 2014, Wolters Kluwer Health.
7. Fatemi Y, Hurley R, Grant C, et al: Challenges in the management of giant intraductal breast papilloma, *Clin Case Rep* 3(1):7, 2015.
8. Mayo Clinic: Atypical hyperplasia. Retrieved from *www.mayoclinic.org/diseases-conditions/atypical-hyperplasia/basics/definition/con-20032601*.
9. Braunstein G: Management of gynecomastia. In Harris JR, Morrow M, Osborne CK, et al, editors: *Diseases of the breast*, ed 5, Philadelphia, 2014, Wolters Kluwer Health.
*10. National Institutes of Health: Women's Health Initiative study. Retrieved from *www.nhlbi.nih.gov/whi*.
11. National Cancer Institute: Oral contraceptives and cancer risk. Retrieved from *www.cancer.gov/about-cancer/causes-prevention/risk/hormones/oral-contraceptives-fact-sheet*.
12. National Cancer Institute: BRCA1 and BRCA2: cancer risk and genetic testing. Retrieved from *www.cancer.gov/about-cancer/causes-prevention/genetics/brca-fact-sheet*.
*13. National Comprehensive Cancer Network (NCCN): NCCN Guidelines Version 2.2014. Genetic/Familial High-Risk Assessment: Breast and Ovarian. Retrieved from *www.nccn.org/professionals/physician_gls.pdf/genetics_screening.pdf*.
14. Breastcancer.org: Other abnormal gene testing. Retrieved from *www.breastcancer.org/symptoms/diagnosis/other-gene-testing*.
15. Zelnak AB, Wisinski KB: Management of patients with HER2-positive metastatic breast cancer: is there an optimal sequence of HER2-directed approaches? *Cancer* 121(1):17, 2015.
16. Oncotype testing for DCIS. Retrieved from *http://breast-cancer.oncotypedx.com/en-US/Patient-DCIS/WhatIsTheOncotypeDXCancerTest.aspx*.
*17. National Comprehensive Cancer Network (NCCN). NCCN Guidelines Version1.2015. Breast Cancer. Retrieved from *www.nccn.org/professionals/_gls.pdf/.pdf*.
18. Joint Committee on Cancer: AJCC cancer staging manual, ed 7. Retrieved from *www.cancerstaging.org*.
19. National Cancer Institute. Breast cancer treatment: Stage I, II, IIIA, and Operable Stage IIIC Breast Cancer. Retrieved from *www.cancer.gov/cancertopics/pdq/treatment/breast/healthprofessional*.
20. Post-breast therapy pain syndrome. Retrieved from *http://cancersupportivecare.com/neuropathicpain.php.org*.
21. Reeder-Hayes KE, Wheeler SB, Mayer DK: Health disparities across the breast cancer continuum, *Semin Oncol Nurs* 31(2):170, 2015.
22. American College of Surgeons Commission on Cancer (2012). Cancer Program Standards 2012, Version 1.1: Ensuring Survivor-Centered Care Manual, retrieved from *www.facs.org/cancer/coc/programstandards2012.html*.
23. Hulett JM, Armer JM, Stewart BR, et al: Perspectives of the breast cancer survivorship continuum: diagnosis through 30 months post-treatment, *J Pers Med* 5(2):174, 2015.
24. American Cancer Society: Types of reconstruction. Retrieved from *www.cancer.org/cancer/breastcancer/moreinformation/breastreconstructionaftermastectomy/breast-reconstruction-after-mastectomy-types-of-br-recon*.
25. Food and Drug Administration: Breast implants. Retrieved from *www.fda.gov/MedicalDevices/ProductsandMedicalProcedures/ImplantsandProsthetics/BreastImplants/default.htm*.

*Evidence-based information for clinical practice.

52

Sexually Transmitted Infections

Adena Bargad

They may forget your name, but they will never forget how you made them feel.

Maya Angelou

e http://evolve.elsevier.com/Lewis/medsurg/

LEARNING OUTCOMES

1. Identify factors contributing to the high rates of sexually transmitted infections (STIs) in the United States.
2. Describe the etiology, clinical manifestations, complications, and diagnostic studies for chlamydia, gonorrhea, trichomoniasis, genital herpes, genital warts, and syphilis.
3. Compare and contrast primary genital herpes with recurrent genital herpes.
4. Explain the interprofessional care and drug therapy of chlamydia, gonorrhea, trichomoniasis, genital herpes, genital warts, and syphilis.
5. Integrate the nursing assessment and nursing diagnoses for patients who have an STI.
6. Describe the nursing management of patients with STIs, including the teaching and counseling appropriate for each STI.
7. Summarize the nursing role in the prevention and control of STIs.

KEY TERMS

chlamydial infections, p. 1228
genital herpes, p. 1232
genital warts, p. 1234

gonorrhea, p. 1230
sexually transmitted infections (STIs), p. 1227

syphilis, p. 1235
trichomoniasis, p. 1231

Sexually transmitted infections (STIs) are infectious diseases that are spread through sexual contact with the penis, vagina, anus, mouth, or sexual fluids of an infected person. Mucosal tissues in the genitals (urethra in men, vagina in women), rectum, and mouth are especially susceptible to the bacteria and viruses that cause STIs. A list of common STIs is presented in Table 52-1.

Some STIs, such as genital human papillomavirus (HPV), may also be spread from direct skin-to-skin contact with an infected person. Other STIs, such as human immunodeficiency virus (HIV), may also be contracted via blood or blood products or be transmitted from mother to baby during pregnancy or labor and delivery. Some STIs may also be spread through *autoinoculation* (spread of infection by touching or scratching an infected area and transferring it to another part of the body). STIs cannot typically be transmitted from inanimate objects.

STIs are very common. It is estimated that nearly 20 million new infections occur in the United States each year. An estimated 110 million Americans are currently infected with one or more STIs.[1] Having one STI increases the risk of getting another. A person can have more than one STI at the same time.

All STIs have an incubation period, which refers to the time from initial infection to the time when symptoms first appear or screening tests for the infection are positive. This can lead to the transmission of disease from an asymptomatic (but infected) person to another person, even before any symptoms or signs begin.

In the United States, all cases of gonorrhea and syphilis, and, in most states, chlamydial infection must be reported to public health authorities for purposes of surveillance and partner notification. Surveillance and partner notification are a major part of the effort to prevent and control the spread of STIs. Nurses play an important role in STI reporting and are mandated to report these STIs to public health authorities. In spite of this requirement, many cases of these infections go unreported. Every year, only a small percentage of the estimated 20 million new STIs are reported.

FACTORS AFFECTING INCIDENCE OF STIs

Many factors contribute to the high rate of STIs. Earlier reproductive maturity and increased longevity make for a longer sexual life span. Other factors include (1) greater sexual freedom, (2) inconsistent or incorrect use of barrier methods (e.g., condoms) during sexual activity, and (3) the media's increasing emphasis on sexuality without mentioning safer sex. Substance

Reviewed by Suzanne Jed, MSN, FNP-BC, Senior Clinical Technical Advisor, International Training and Education Center for Health (I-TECH) South Africa, University of Washington, Pretoria, South Africa; Crystal Sheaves, RN, MSN, APRN, FNP-BC, Senior Lecturer, West Virginia University School of Nursing, Charleston, West Virginia; and Whitney Starr, MSN, FNP-BC, Assistant Professor, Division of Infectious Diseases, University of Colorado, Denver, Colorado.

TABLE 52-1 Causes of Sexually Transmitted Infections (STIs)

Sexually Transmitted Infection	Cause
Bacterial Infections	
Chlamydial	*Chlamydia trachomatis*
Gonorrhea	*Neisseria gonorrhoeae*
Syphilis	*Treponema pallidum*
Viral Infections	
Genital herpes	Herpes simplex virus (HSV 1 or 2)
Genital warts (*condylomata acuminata*)	Human papillomavirus (HPV)
Human immunodeficiency virus infection (HIV)	Human immunodeficiency virus (HIV) (see Chapter 14)
Acquired immunodeficiency syndrome (AIDS)	
Hepatitis B and C	Hepatitis B and C viruses (see Chapter 43)
Molluscum	*Molluscum contagiosum*
Parasitic/Protozoan Infection	
Trichomoniasis	*Trichomonas vaginalis*

TABLE 52-2 Risk Factors for STIs

High-Risk Populations
- Women
- Men who have sex with men
- Adolescents and young adults (age <25)
- Men and women in correctional facilities
- Victims of sexual assault

High-Risk Behaviors
- Having new or multiple sexual partners
- Having more than one sexual partner
- Having sexual partners who have had multiple partners
- Sharing needles used to inject drugs
- Alcohol or drug dependence or abuse (inhibits judgment)
- Inconsistent or incorrect use of condoms or other barrier methods

High-Risk Medical History
- Not being vaccinated for STIs that have vaccines
- Having one STI is a risk factor for getting another

use and abuse can further contribute to unsafe sexual practices by impairing judgment. Risk factors for STIs are presented in Table 52-2.

Urbanization and easier national and international travel are some of the more global changes that may contribute to increased opportunities for exposure to all infectious diseases, including STIs. Finally, certain groups of people are disproportionately affected by STIs, including youth under age 25 and those who are socially and economically disadvantaged.[1]

The rate of STIs is also reflected in trends in methods of contraceptive use. For example, the male condom is considered to be the best form of protection (other than abstinence) against STIs. Although condom use has increased in the United States, condoms are not frequently used in the general population for contraception. Only a small percentage of women use condoms as their method of contraception. It is important to note that hormone contraceptives (oral contraceptive pills, patch, injectables) and long-acting reversible contraceptives (e.g., intrauterine devices or implantable devices) provide no barrier protection against STIs.[2]

🌐 CULTURAL & ETHNIC HEALTH DISPARITIES
Sexually Transmitted Infections

Incidence of STIs
- *Chlamydial infection:* African Americans represent 52% of cases.
- *Syphilis:* African Americans represent 47% of cases, a rate 60 times higher than that of whites.
- *Herpes simplex virus-2:* More common in African Americans (39%) than whites (12%).
- *Gonococcal infection:* African Americans represent 69% of reported cases.

Factors Influencing Disparities
- Social and economic disadvantages can make it difficult for individuals to care for their overall health, including their sexual health.
- People who cannot afford basic necessities may have trouble accessing and affording quality sexual health services.
- Fear and distrust of HCPs and institutions can negatively affect racial and ethnic minorities from seeking health care.
- In ethnic communities where there is a high prevalence of STIs, it may be difficult to reduce the risk of infection because with any sexual encounter, a person faces a higher chance of encountering an infected partner than in those communities with a lower prevalence.

STIs CHARACTERIZED BY DISCHARGE, CERVICITIS, OR URETHRITIS

CHLAMYDIAL INFECTIONS

Chlamydial infection is the most common STI in the United States, with an estimated nearly 3 million new cases per year.[1]

Etiology and Pathophysiology

Chlamydial infections are caused by *Chlamydia trachomatis*, a gram-negative bacterium and intracellular pathogen. *Chlamydia* is transmitted through exposure to sexual fluids during vaginal, anal, or oral sex. Ejaculation does not have to occur for this infection to be transmitted. The incubation period for chlamydial infection is 1 to 3 weeks. Infection with *Chlamydia* does not confer immunity to future infection. This means that people who have been treated for chlamydial infection can be reinfected.

The most common site for infection in men is the urethra. Infections in the male urethra are called *urethritis*. The most common site for infection for women is the cervix. Infections in the female cervix are called *cervicitis*. Both men and women can get chlamydial infections of the rectum from anal sex. Because the vagina acts as a natural reservoir for infectious secretions, transmission of STIs is often more efficient from men to women than it is from women to men.

There are many strains of the *C. trachomatis* bacteria. Some of these strains can cause other sexually acquired infections, such as *nongonococcal urethritis* (NGU) or lymphogranuloma venereum (LGV).

Clinical Manifestations

Persons with chlamydial infection may have no symptoms. However, if symptoms develop in men, they may experience pain with urination or a urethral discharge. Rarely, men can have pain or swelling of the testicles caused by infection of the epididymis (Fig. 52-1). Symptoms of cervicitis in women include

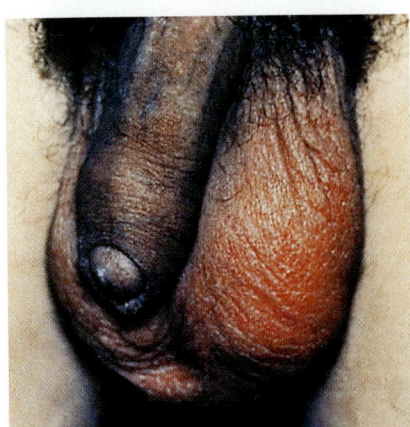

FIG. 52-1 Chlamydial epididymitis. Red, swollen scrotum. (From Morse S, Moreland A, Holmes K, editors: *Atlas of sexually transmitted diseases and AIDS*, London, 1996, Mosby-Wolfe.)

 TABLE 52-3 Interprofessional Care

Chlamydial Infections

Diagnostic Assessment
- History and physical examination
- Nucleic acid amplification test (NAAT)
- Testing for other STIs (gonorrhea, HIV, syphilis)

Management
- azithromycin (Zithromax) or doxycycline (Vibramycin)
- Alternative regimen: erythromycin, ofloxacin, or levofloxacin (Levaquin)
- Instruction on abstinence from sexual intercourse for 7 days after completing treatment
- Treatment of all sexual partners

mucopurulent discharge (mucus with pus), bleeding, dysuria, and pain with intercourse. Symptoms of rectal chlamydial infection can include rectal pain, discharge, and bleeding.

Complications

Complications often develop from poorly managed, inaccurately diagnosed, or undiagnosed chlamydial infections. Chlamydial infection is often not diagnosed until complications occur. While men rarely have long-term complications from chlamydial infection, epididymitis can result in male infertility. More commonly, chlamydial infections can affect a woman's reproductive tract, resulting in *pelvic inflammatory disease* (PID). PID can damage fallopian tubes and increases a woman's risk for an ectopic pregnancy (pregnancy outside of uterus), infertility, and chronic pelvic pain. The risk of developing PID increases with repeated chlamydial infection. The more episodes of PID, the more likely a woman will experience infertility.[3] Both men and women can develop a rare reactive arthritis, an autoimmune response to infection with *C. trachomatis*.

Diagnostic Studies

The preferred method for diagnosing chlamydial infection is through nucleic acid amplification testing (NAAT) (Table 52-3). NAAT is used to identify small amounts of DNA or RNA in test samples.

NAAT can be performed on endocervical or vaginal swabs from women, urethral swabs from men, and urine from both men and women. NAATs are also the recommended test for

EVIDENCE-BASED PRACTICE

Translating Research Into Practice

Is Home-Based STI Testing Effective?
Clinical Question
In females screened for sexually transmitted infections (P) what is the effectiveness of home-based self-sampling (I) versus clinic-based testing (C) on acceptability and specimen quality (O)?

Synthesis of Best Available Evidence
- Systematic review of randomized controlled trials (RCTs).
- 7 RCTs of females (*n* = 4042) 14 to 50 years old. Intervention was sampling method used to screen for sexually transmitted infections (STIs) of *Chlamydia*, gonorrhea, and trichomoniasis. Outcome was uptake or nonuptake of screening, which is the number of females screened as a proportion of all those that should have been screened. Also measured were acceptability of sampling method and quality of specimen obtained.
- Home-based STI testing had greater uptake compared to clinic-based testing and was the preferred screening method.
- Specimen quality did not differ according to sampling method used.

Conclusions
- Home-based testing increased screening uptake for STIs with no compromise in specimen quality.
- Greater ease (acceptability) occurred when specimens are obtained at home.

Implications for Nursing Practice
1. Why is home-based sampling important for younger females who do not want to attend a screening clinic?
2. How will you provide teaching to older women with STI symptoms who refuse clinic testing because "only young people get STIs"?
3. Why is it important for HCPs to learn new strategies to improve STI screening rates?

Reference for Evidence
Odesanmi TY, Wasti SP, Odesanmi OS, et al: Comparative effectiveness and acceptability of home-based and clinic-based sampling methods for sexually transmissible infections screening in females aged 14-50 years: a systematic review and meta-analysis, *Sexual Health* 10:559, 2013.

P, Patient population of interest; *I*, intervention or area of interest; *C*, comparison of interest or comparison group; *O*, outcomes of interest; *T*, timing (see p. 15).

rectal and oropharyngeal screening and diagnosis in these extragenital sites.[4]

Interprofessional Care

Because of the high prevalence of asymptomatic infections, regular screening for chlamydial infection in high-risk populations is recommended (Table 52-2). Anyone diagnosed and treated for chlamydial infection should be retested 3 months posttreatment to detect repeat infections.

Drug Therapy. The preferred treatment for chlamydial infection is a single dose of azithromycin or doxycycline for 7 days (Table 52-3). Instruct patients to abstain from sexual intercourse for 7 days after treatment and until all sexual partners have completed a full course of treatment. Advise patients to return if symptoms persist or recur.

 DRUG ALERT Doxycycline (Vibramycin)
- Patients on this drug should avoid unnecessary exposure to sunlight.
- Do not take with antacids, iron products, or dairy products.
- Pregnant women should not take doxycycline.

Any sexual partner within the preceding 60 days of diagnosis or onset of symptoms needs to be treated. Teach patients to return for testing 3 months after treatment to be sure that they have not been reinfected. Encourage patients to use condoms or barrier methods consistently and correctly every time they have sex.

? CHECK YOUR PRACTICE

You are working in a public health STI clinic. You are seeing a 28-yr-old woman for the second time in 2 months for recurrent vaginal discharge. The patient states she has not been with anyone else except her regular partner and she says, "I don't know why I have this again. The doctor gave me the pills and I took them."
- How would you respond?
- What do you think is causing her symptoms?

Unfortunately, there is a high rate of recurrence for chlamydial infections. This may be due to the fact that sexual partners of infected people may not be treated. This "ping-pong" effect (treatment, reexposure, and reinfection) can end only when infected partners are also treated. Because of this issue, the CDC recommends *Expedited Partner Therapy* (EPT). EPT means HCPs can provide medications or prescriptions to their patients with STIs to give to partners without actually examining the partner. The legality of EPT varies from state to state, but few states actually prohibit EPT. EPT is not routinely recommended for men who have sex with men (MSM) because of a higher risk for coexisting infections in partners of MSM, especially undiagnosed syphilis or HIV.[5]

GONOCOCCAL INFECTIONS

In the United States, approximately 800,000 gonococcal infections occur per year, making it the second most common STI.[1]

Etiology and Pathophysiology

Gonorrhea is caused by *Neisseria gonorrhoeae*, a gram-negative, diplococcus bacterium. Gonorrhea can be transmitted by exposure to sexual fluids during vaginal, anal, or oral sex, but ejaculation does not have to occur for gonorrhea to be transmitted. The incubation period is from a few days to 1 week. The infection confers no immunity to subsequent reinfection. The most common site for infection for men is the urethra and for women, the cervix. Both men and women can get gonorrheal infections of the rectum from anal sex or of the oropharynx from oral sex.

Clinical Manifestations

The initial site of infection in men is usually the urethra. Many men with gonorrhea are asymptomatic, while many others do report symptoms. The most common symptoms of gonococcal urethritis among men are dysuria, purulent urethral discharge (Fig. 52-2), or epididymitis. Most women who contract gonorrhea are asymptomatic or have minor symptoms that are often overlooked. For women, common symptoms are increased vaginal discharge, dysuria, frequency of urination, or bleeding after sex. Often, redness and swelling can occur at the cervix or urethra along with a purulent exudate (Fig. 52-3).

Both men and women can contract rectal gonorrhea during anal intercourse and oropharyngeal gonorrhea during oral sex. Symptoms of rectal gonorrhea may include mucopurulent rectal discharge, bleeding, pain, pruritus, and painful bowel movements.

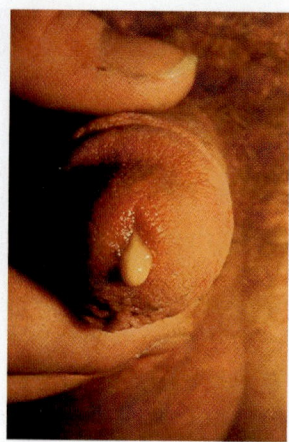

FIG. 52-2 Profuse, purulent drainage in a patient with gonorrhea. (From Marx J, Walls R, Hockberger R: *Rosen's emergency medicine: concepts and clinical practice,* ed 7, St Louis, 2010, Mosby.)

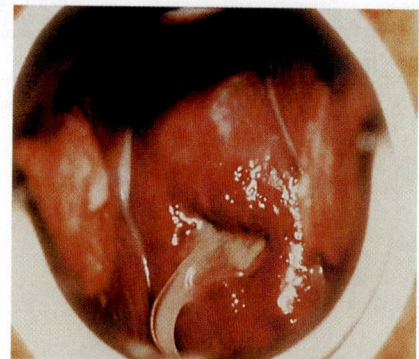

FIG. 52-3 Endocervical gonorrhea. Cervical redness and edema with discharge. (From Morse S, Moreland A, Holmes K, editors: *Atlas of sexually transmitted diseases and AIDS,* London, 1996, Mosby-Wolfe.)

Most patients with gonorrheal infections in the throat have few if any symptoms. Some may complain of a sore throat.

Complications

Because men are often symptomatic and seek treatment early in the course of gonorrhea infection, they are less likely to develop serious complications than women. The complication that can occur in men is epididymitis, which can result in infertility.

Because women who are asymptomatic seldom seek treatment, serious complications are more common for women and are usually the reason for seeking medical attention. Untreated gonorrhea can cause an infection in the Bartholin's glands (located internally on either side of the vaginal opening) and can also result in PID. PID increases risk for ectopic pregnancy, infertility, and chronic pelvic pain.

Although rare, both men and women can develop a disseminated gonococcal infection (DGI). DGI is associated with skin lesions, fever, arthralgia, arthritis, and/or endocarditis (Fig. 52-4).

Neonates can develop gonococcal conjunctivitis (*ophthalmia neonatorum*) from exposure to an infected mother during delivery that can result in permanent blindness. Almost all states have a law or a health department regulation requiring the use of a prophylactic treatment in the eyes of all newborns to prevent such infections. Because of both improved prenatal screening for gonorrhea and prophylactic treatment regimens, *ophthalmia neonatorum* caused by gonorrhea is relatively rare.

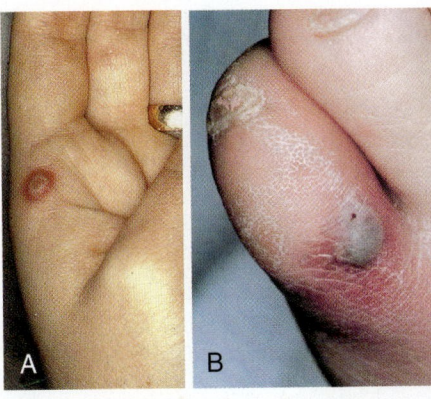

FIG. 52-4 Skin lesions with disseminated gonococcal infection. **A,** On the hand. **B,** On the fifth toe. (*A,* From Cohen J, Powderly WG: *Infectious diseases,* ed 2, St Louis, 2004, Mosby. *B,* From Mandell GL, Bennett JE, Dolin R: *Mandell, Douglas, and Bennett's principles and practice of infectious diseases,* ed 7, Philadelphia, 2010, Churchill Livingstone.)

GENDER DIFFERENCES
Sexually Transmitted Infections

Men	Women
• Syphilis more common, especially in men who have sex with men	• Anatomy increases risk for STI
• More likely to have symptoms	• Chlamydial infection three times more common
• Chlamydial infection results in few complications	• Gonorrhea, trichomoniasis, and HSV-2 more common
• Easier to diagnose because of less complex anatomy	• HPV is most common STI in women
• Less likely to seek medical care	• Have more frequent and serious complications related to STIs (e.g., PID, infertility, ectopic pregnancy, untreated syphilis in pregnant women can result in infant death)

Adapted from Centers for Disease Control and Prevention: 10 Ways STDs impact women differently than men. Retrieved from *www.cdc.gov/nchhstp/newsroom/docs/STDs-Women-042011.pdf.*
HSV-2, Herpes simplex type 2; *PID,* pelvic inflammatory disease; *STIs,* sexually transmitted infections.

Diagnostic Studies

Diagnosis of any STI requires an accurate sexual history, a physical exam, and appropriate laboratory tests specific to each infection. For men, a presumptive diagnosis of gonorrhea is made if there is a history of sexual contact with a new or infected partner followed within a few days by urethral discharge. For women, making a diagnosis of gonorrhea on the basis of symptoms is difficult. Most women are asymptomatic or have complaints that may be confused with other conditions, such as chlamydial or urinary tract infection.

As with chlamydial infection, NAATs are used for detecting gonorrhea. Culture may also be used to diagnose infection. Gram stains of urethral secretions may also be used, but the sensitivity of gram stain is not as good as other methods.

Interprofessional Care

Drug Therapy. Because of a short incubation period and high rates of infectivity, treatment for gonorrhea is often given without waiting for positive test results. The first-line treatment for gonorrhea is dual therapy with ceftriaxone (Rocephin) given IM with oral azithromycin (Table 52-4). Over the years, *N. gonorrhoeae* has developed resistance to many classes of antibiotics, including fluoroquinolones (ciprofloxacin [Cipro],

TABLE 52-4 Interprofessional Care
Gonococcal Infections

Diagnostic Assessment
- History and physical examination
- Gram-stained smears of urethral or endocervical exudate
- Culture for *Neisseria gonorrhoeae*
- Nucleic acid amplification test (NAAT) to detect *N. gonorrhoeae*
- Testing for other STIs (syphilis, HIV, chlamydial infection)

Management
- Uncomplicated gonorrhea: ceftriaxone (Rocephin) IM with azithromycin (Zithromax)
- Treatment of sexual contacts
- Instruction on abstinence from sexual intercourse and alcohol during treatment
- Reexamination if symptoms persist or recur after completion of treatment

ofloxacin, levofloxacin [Levaquin]) and tetracyclines (doxycycline [Vibramycin]). Given the increasing rate of drug resistance, all patients with gonococcal infection must receive treatment with at least two antibiotics as a way of reducing or minimizing the chance of incomplete treatment to combat the potential for drug resistance. Patients treated with a preferred regimen but who have a persistently positive test 7 days after treatment need antibiotic sensitivity testing.

As with *C. trichomatis,* all sexual contacts of patients with gonorrhea should be evaluated and treated to prevent reinfection and further transmission. All sexual partners within 60 days of diagnosis should also be treated. Counsel patients to abstain from sexual intercourse during and one week after treatment. Review the ways to reduce risk of acquiring a repeat or new STI in the future.

TRICHOMONIASIS

Trichomoniasis, a type of STI caused by a protozoan, *Trichomonas vaginalis,* is one of the most common STIs in the world. Also known as "trich," this infection was often overlooked compared to other STIs. However, better testing methods have improved detection of trichomoniasis. Trichomoniasis is much more common among women than men, particularly among women with HIV.[6]

Etiology and Pathophysiology

Trichomonas vaginalis is a flagellate protozoan parasite. *Trichomonas* can be transmitted by exposure to sexual fluids during vaginal, anal, or oral sex, even if ejaculation does not occur. The incubation period for trichomoniasis is approximately 1 week to 1 month but can be much longer. The infection confers no immunity to future reinfection.

The most common site for infection in men is the urethra, and in women, the cervix. It is uncommon for *Trichomonas* to infect the rectum, and it is not known to infect the oropharynx. Routine screening for *T. vaginalis* should be considered for women in high-risk populations, including HIV-positive women and women seeking care for vaginal discharge.

Clinical Manifestations

The majority of people with trichomoniasis do not have symptoms. Men may report burning with urination or ejaculation or urethral discharge. Women with trichomoniasis may report painful urination, vaginal itching, painful intercourse, bleeding after sex, or a yellow-green discharge with a foul odor. On speculum exam, the cervix can have a "strawberry" appearance.

Complications

The main complications of untreated trichomoniasis are related to the inflammation and irritation that the infection causes in the genital tract. This irritation makes an infected person more likely to acquire or transmit another STI, particularly HIV. While gonorrhea and chlamydial infection are responsible for the vast majority of PID, trichomoniasis infection is associated with PID in women with HIV.

Diagnostic Studies

Diagnosis of trichomoniasis can be achieved by several methods. The preferred method is nucleic acid amplification testing (NAAT) of vaginal or endocervical secretions, or urine. Other methods include culture, point of care testing, or direct visualization of trichomonads under the microscope. Identification of motile trichomonads in the vaginal secretions confirms infection. Tests can be done on liquid-based cervical Pap samples. In men, NAAT testing is recommended.[7]

Interprofessional Care

Drug Therapy. Patients and their partners should be treated with either metronidazole (Flagyl) or tinidazole (Tindamax). Instruct patients to abstain from sexual intercourse for 7 days after treatment and until all sexual partners have completed a full course of treatment. Advise patients to return if symptoms persist or recur. Any sexual partner within the preceding 60 days should be treated. Teach patients to use condoms or other barrier methods with every sexual contact. Because of a high rate of recurrence of trichomoniasis, repeat testing 3 months after treatment is recommended.

STIs CHARACTERIZED BY GENITAL LESIONS OR ULCERS

GENITAL HERPES INFECTIONS

Genital herpes infection is a lifelong, incurable infection that is very common. There are two strains of herpes that cause genital infections, herpes simplex virus type 1 (HSV-1) and herpes simplex virus type 2 (HSV-2). Although both forms of HSV may cause genital infection, HSV-1 is more commonly associated with oral lesions, and HSV-2 is more common in the genitals. However, an increasing proportion of genital herpes infections is caused by HSV-1.[8]

More than 24 million people in the United States have HSV-2. Nearly 800,000 new infections occur annually. Rates of new infections are high, partly due to the fact that an estimated 80% of those infected with genital HSV-2 have never received a clinical diagnosis and are unaware that they are capable of transmitting the virus.[1] The prevalence of new genital HSV-2 infections is twice as high among women compared to men.

Etiology and Pathophysiology

HSV-1 and HSV-2 are strains of herpesvirus that cause genital herpes. Having one type does not confer immunity against getting the other type. The virus enters through the mucous membranes or breaks in the skin during contact with an infected

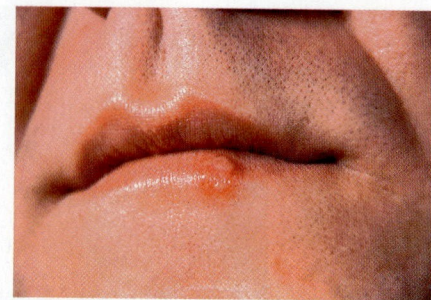

FIG. 52-5 Herpes simplex virus (HSV) to the lips. (From Centers for Disease Control and Prevention. Courtesy Dr. Hermann.)

person. The virus reproduces inside the cell and spreads to the surrounding cells. Then the virus enters the peripheral or autonomic nerve endings and ascends to the sensory or autonomic nerve ganglion near the infection site, where it often becomes dormant. Viral reactivation (recurrence) may occur when the virus descends to that initial site of infection, either the mucous membranes or skin.

When a person is infected with HSV-1 or HSV-2, the virus persists within the individual for life. Transmission of either strain of HSV occurs through direct contact with skin or mucous membranes when an infected individual is symptomatic. HSV-1 and HSV-2 can also be transmitted without any symptoms being apparent, called *asymptomatic shedding*. It is impossible to predict when asymptomatic shedding will occur.

HSV type 1 (HSV-1) was primarily associated with orolabial disease, commonly known as "cold sores" or "fever blisters" (Fig. 52-5) and HSV-2 with genital disease. However, there has been a shift in understanding that either HSV-1 or HSV-2 can cause genital or orolabial infections. In most cases, HSV-1 infections are more common "above the waist," involving the gingivae, dermis, upper respiratory tract, and, rarely the CNS. HSV-2 almost always infects sites "below the waist," the genital tract or perineum. It is important to understand that there is no absolute, single site for either virus. Among young women, HSV-1 is more commonly associated with genital infection than HSV-2.[9]

Clinical Manifestations

Primary Episode. A *primary (initial) episode* of genital herpes has an incubation of 2 days to 2 weeks. The vast majority of people do not have any recognizable symptoms of primary HSV genital infection. If symptoms do occur, they follow a series of stages. During the *prodromal stage*, the period before lesions appear, the patient may have burning, itching, or tingling at the site of inoculation. In the *vesicular stage*, few to multiple small, often painful vesicles (blisters) may appear on the buttock, inner thigh, penis, scrotum, vulva, perineum, perianal region, vagina, or cervix. The vesicles contain large quantities of infectious viral particles.

Next in the *ulcerative stage*, the lesions rupture and form shallow, moist ulcerations. In the *final stage*, spontaneous crusting and epithelialization of the erosions occur (Fig. 52-6). Primary infections also tend to be associated with local inflammation and pain, regional (inguinal node) lymphadenopathy and systemic flu-like symptoms, including fever, headache, malaise, and myalgia. Urination may be painful from the urine touching active lesions. The whole process from prodrome to healing varies and can take approximately 3 weeks.

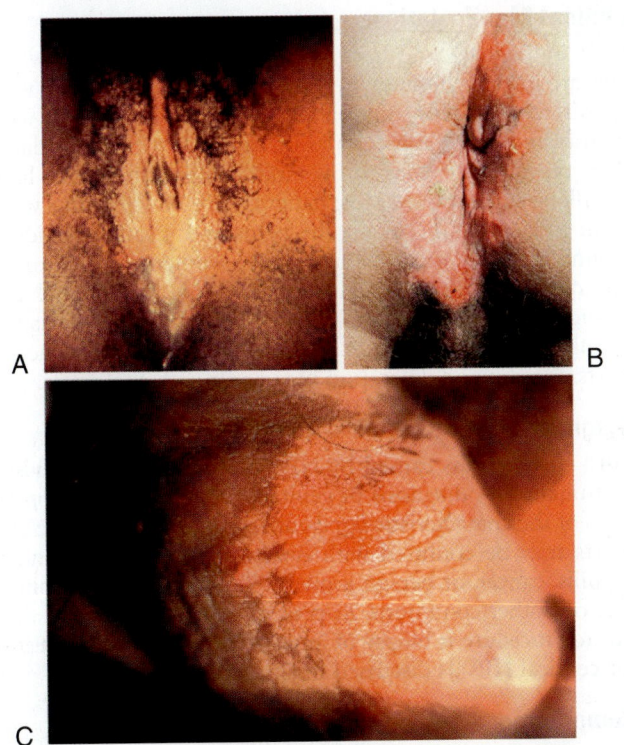

FIG. 52-6 Unruptured vesicles of herpes simplex virus type 2 (HSV-2). **A,** Vulvar area. **B,** Perianal area. **C,** Penile herpes simplex, ulcerative stage. (*A* and *C,* From Centers for Disease Control and Prevention. Courtesy Susan Lindsley. *B,* From Morse S, Moreland A, Holmes K, editors: *Atlas of sexually transmitted diseases and AIDS,* London, 1996, Mosby-Wolfe.)

Autoinoculation can occur if active lesions are touched or scratched, causing additional and potentially recurrent infection at extragenital sites.

Recurrent Episodes. *Recurrent genital herpes* occurs in many individuals during the year following the primary episode. The symptoms of recurrent episodes are less severe, and the lesions usually heal more quickly. HSV-1 genital infections recur less frequently than HSV-2 genital infections, and over time, both decrease in frequency.

Common triggers of recurrence include stress, fatigue, sunburn, general illness, immunosuppression, and menses. Many patients can predict a recurrence by noticing the prodromal symptoms of tingling, burning, and itching at the site where the lesions will recur. The greatest risk for transmitting infection exists when active lesions are present. However, it is possible to transmit the virus when no visible lesions or symptoms are present. The majority of HSV transmission occurs during these asymptomatic periods.[8]

Complications

Both HSV-1 and HSV-2 can cause rare but serious complications, such as blindness, encephalitis (inflammation of the brain), and aseptic meningitis (inflammation of the linings of the brain). Autoinoculation can result in the development of extragenital lesions in the buttocks, groin, thighs, fingers, and eyes. Genital ulcers increase the risk of acquiring HIV, and HSV lesions can be more severe and more persistent in HIV-infected patients.

Pregnant women with HSV can transmit the virus to the baby, most commonly if the virus is shed while the infant passes though the birth canal. Women with a primary episode of HSV near the time of delivery have the highest risk of transmitting genital herpes to the neonate. The virus can infect the neonate's skin, eyes, mouth, or the CNS or become disseminated and cause significant morbidity and mortality. An active genital lesion at the time of delivery is usually an indication for cesarean delivery.[10]

In addition to the physiologic complications associated with HSV infection, one of the most serious consequences for people diagnosed with genital herpes is the overall impact it can have on their psychologic well-being, their relationships, and their sexual lives. You can help teach patients to understand how to talk to sexual partners about HSV. Refer patients who need counseling. Teach patients with herpes that it is a manageable condition and help them to understand their treatment options.

Diagnostic Studies

Diagnosis of genital herpes is often based on the patient's reported symptoms and then confirmation by visual exam. Culture from direct lesion samples can be used to diagnose HSV and differentiate between HSV-1 and HSV-2. Highly accurate blood tests for antibodies are available for HSV-1 and HSV-2. These antibodies usually appear by 12 weeks after exposure.

Interprofessional Care

Drug Therapy. Although not a cure, antiviral medications can shorten the duration of HSV viral shedding, shorten the healing time of genital lesions, and reduce the frequency of outbreaks by 75%.[9] Treatment of HSV infection should be started before diagnostic results are available because early treatment reduces the duration of the ulcers and risk of transmission (Table 52-5).

Three antiviral agents are available for the treatment of HSV: acyclovir, valacyclovir, and famciclovir. These drugs inhibit herpetic viral replication and are prescribed for both primary and recurrent infections. These antiviral medications can also be used on a daily basis as suppressive therapy to decrease

TABLE 52-5 Interprofessional Care
Genital Herpes
Diagnostic Assessment
• History and physical examination
• Antibody assay for HSV type
• Viral isolation by tissue culture
Management
Primary (Initial) Infection
• acyclovir (Zovirax), famciclovir (Famvir), or valacyclovir (Valtrex)
Recurrent Episodic Infection
• acyclovir, famciclovir, or valacyclovir
• Identify triggering factors
• Abstinence from sexual contact while lesions are present
• Symptomatic care
• Confidential counseling and testing for HIV
Suppressive Therapy
• acyclovir, famciclovir, or valacyclovir
Severe Infection
• acyclovir IV until clinical improvement, followed by oral antiviral therapy

frequent recurrences. Teach patients with active outbreaks to maintain good genital hygiene and wear loose-fitting cotton undergarments.

The primary goal is to keep lesions clean and dry. Techniques to reduce pain on urination include pouring water onto the perineal area while voiding to dilute the urine or voiding in the shower. Pain may require a local anesthetic such as lidocaine gel or analgesics such as ibuprofen, acetaminophen, acetaminophen with codeine, or aspirin. Ice packs to the affected area can provide some relief.

IV acyclovir is reserved for severe or life-threatening infections in which hospitalization is required for the treatment of disseminated infections, central nervous system infections (meningitis), or pneumonitis.

GENITAL WARTS

Genital warts *(condylomata acuminata)* are caused by the human papillomavirus (HPV). There are approximately 150 papillomavirus types. More than 40 types can be sexually transmitted. Some of these can cause warts on the skin, while others can cause cancers of the genital tract or oropharynx. Ninety percent of genital warts are caused by HPV types 6 and 11. About 360,000 people get genital warts each year. Most sexually active men and women will get some type of HPV at some point in their lives.[1] In most states, genital warts are not a reportable infection. (HPV infection of the cervix is discussed in Chapter 53.)

Etiology and Pathophysiology

HPV is transmitted by skin-to-skin contact, most commonly during vaginal, anal, or oral sex, but it can be transmitted during nonpenetrative sexual activity. The basal epithelial cells infected with HPV undergo transformation and proliferation to form a warty growth (Fig. 52-7). The incubation period of the virus can range from weeks to months to years. Infection with one type of HPV does not prevent infection with another type.

In general, genital HPV infection is considered transient (virus is "cleared" or resolves spontaneously usually after 1 to 2 years). However, HPV infection can also persist even when the warts themselves are not visible after treatment. It is unclear whether removing visible genital warts helps a person to clear the virus, cure the virus, or reduces a person's ability to transmit the virus.[11]

Clinical Manifestations

Most individuals who have HPV infection do not know that they are infected because they are asymptomatic. Genital warts are discrete single or multiple papillary growths that are white to gray and pink-flesh colored or can be brownish on darker skin types. They may grow and coalesce to form large, cauliflower-like masses. Most patients have 1 to 10 genital warts.

In men, warts occur on the penis and scrotum, inside or around the anus, or in the urethra. In women, warts occur on the inner thighs, vulva, vagina, or cervix, in the perianal area, including in the internal anal canal (Fig. 52-7). There are usually no other signs or symptoms. Itching may occur with anogenital warts. Bleeding on defecation may occur with anal warts.

Diagnostic Studies

Most early lesions caused by HPV are undetectable by visual examination. A diagnosis of genital warts can be made on the basis of the characteristic appearance of the lesions (Fig. 52-7). Warts may be confused with *condylomata lata* of secondary syphilis, cancer, or benign growths. Testing should be done to rule out other conditions. At present, the only definitive diagnostic procedure is biopsy of any questionable growth. Testing for cervical HPV is discussed in Chapter 53.

Complications

Genital warts have few long-term complications. Approximately 90% of warts are caused by noncancerous strains of HPV. However, certain strains of HPV (types 16 and 18) can lead to cancer of the cervix, vagina, vulva, penis, rectum, and throat or pharynx. For some individuals, HPV lesions can cause psychosocial burden due to the cosmetic appearance of lesions on the genitals or the need for long courses of HPV-related treatment. During pregnancy, genital warts tend to grow rapidly and increase in size.

Interprofessional Care

HPV Vaccines. It may be possible to eradicate some of the oncogenic HPV types over the next few decades, particularly if both girls and boys are vaccinated.[11,12] Currently three vaccines are available to protect against HPV. A quadrivalent vaccine (Gardasil) protects against types 6, 11, 16, and 18; a bivalent vaccine (Cervarix) offers protection against HPV types 16 and 18; and a 9-valent vaccine (Gardasil 9) protects against HPV types 6, 11, 16, 18 and five other HPV types. These vaccines are

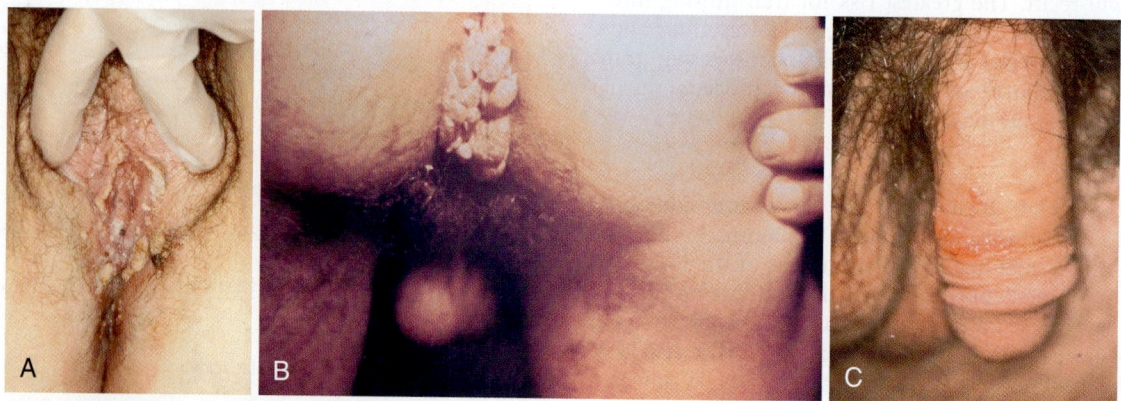

FIG. 52-7 Genital warts. **A,** Severe vulvar warts. **B,** Perineal wart. **C,** Multiple genital warts of the glans penis. (*A,* From Centers for Disease Control and Prevention. Courtesy Joe Millar. *B,* From Centers for Disease Control and Prevention. Courtesy Dr. Wiesner. *C,* From Centers for Disease Control and Prevention. Courtesy Susan Lindsley.)

given in three IM doses over a 6-month period and have few side effects. The CDC recommends that all children, males and females, be vaccinated at age 11 to 12, but vaccination can be started as early as age 9. The bivalent and quadrivalent vaccines are approved for persons up to age 26. The 9-valent vaccine is approved for girls 9 to 26 and boys 9 to 15.

These vaccines do not treat active HPV infection. Ideally, individuals should receive the vaccine before the start of sexual activity, but even those who are infected with HPV can still get protection against HPV types not already acquired. The HPV vaccine reduces the risk of anal cancer and may also protect against oropharynx cancer.[11]

EVIDENCE-BASED PRACTICE
Applying the Evidence

HPV Vaccine and Young Men

T.N. is a 19-yr-old man who is being seen in the health care center for signs and symptoms of a urinary tract infection. After reviewing his health history, you learn he has not received the human papillomavirus (HPV) vaccine. When asked, he shares with you that he is sexually active and that he does not need to get the vaccine because his girlfriend already has.

Making Clinical Decisions

Best Available Evidence. Males ages 9 to 26 can get vaccinated with Gardasil to reduce the incidence of anogenital HPV infections, which are caused by HPV types 6, 11, 16, or 18. Gardasil protects against the two HPV types (6 and 11) that cause 90% of genital warts.

Clinician Expertise. You know younger men may be unaware of expanded recommendations for Gardasil, which was originally approved to prevent cervical, vulvar, and vaginal cancer in females ages 9 through 26.

Patient Preferences and Values. T.N. states he never has unprotected sex and does not like injections.

Implications for Nursing Practice

1. Why is it important to discuss the risks and benefits of the vaccine with T.N.?
2. How would you respond to T.N., who has heard that if you are already sexually active the vaccine will not be effective?

Reference for Evidence

Centers for Disease Control: HPV vaccination. Retrieved from *www.cdc.gov/vaccines/vpd-vac/hpv* and Centers for Disease Control: HPV-associated cancers statistics. Retrieved from *www.cdc.gov/cancer/hpv/statistics/index.htm.*

Drug Therapy. Treatment of genital warts is hampered by the high proportion of asymptomatic infections and lack of curative treatment. The primary goal when treating visible genital warts is the removal of symptomatic warts.

Treatment consists of chemical or ablative (removal with laser or electrocautery) methods. One common treatment is the use of trichloroacetic acid (TCA) or bichloroacetic acid (BCA) applied directly to the wart surface. Petroleum jelly is applied to the surrounding normal skin to minimize irritation before a small amount of TCA or BCA is applied to the wart with a cotton swab. A sharp, stinging pain is often felt with initial acid contact, but this quickly subsides.

Patient-managed treatment is also an option. Podofilox liquid and gel are available by prescription (Condylox, Condylox Gel). The patient applies the solution or gel for 3 successive days. Treatment can be repeated for up to 4 weeks or until resolution

of the lesions. Imiquimod (Aldara) cream is an immune response modifier that is applied at bedtime, three times a week for up to 16 weeks. Sinecatechin (Veregen) ointment (made from extract of green tea leaves) is applied three times weekly.

The removal of warts may or may not decrease infectivity. Genital warts are difficult to treat and often require multiple office visits. The therapy should be modified if a patient has not improved after three treatments or if the warts have not completely disappeared after six treatments.

If the warts do not regress with any of these therapies, treatments such as cryotherapy with liquid nitrogen, electrocautery, laser therapy, intralesional use of α-interferon, and surgical excision may be indicated. Because treatment does not destroy the virus, merely the infected tissue, recurrence and reinfection are possible, and careful long-term follow-up is advised.

SYPHILIS

Syphilis is a sexually transmitted bacterial infection that can cause serious long-term complications if not treated effectively. Over 55,000 cases of syphilis are reported annually in the United States. There has been a shift in the population most affected by syphilis, with rates highest among young men 20 to 29 years old, with 75% of cases reported among MSM.[1]

Etiology and Pathophysiology

Syphilis is caused by *Treponema pallidum*, a bacterial spirochete. It is transmitted via direct contact with a syphilitic lesion called a *chancre* that can occur externally on the genitals, anus, or lips, or internally in the vagina, rectum, or mouth or tongue (Fig. 52-8). The transmission of this bacterium occurs during vaginal, anal, or oral sex. The incubation period for syphilis can range from 10 to 90 days (average 21 days). Having the infection does not confer immunity to future infection, even after successful treatment. An infected pregnant woman can transmit syphilis to her fetus during her pregnancy and is at high risk for stillbirth or having babies who develop complications after birth, including seizures and death.

Clinical Manifestations

Syphilis is called "*The Great Pretender*" because it can infect many organs in the body and present with a variety of signs and symptoms that can mimic a number of other diseases. Consequently, compared with other STIs, syphilis is more difficult to recognize. If it is not diagnosed and treated, specific clinical stages are characteristic of the progression of the disease (Table 52-6). It can take weeks to years to progress through all of the stages. At each stage, if no treatment is initiated, the disease will progress to the next stage.

Complications

Complications of the disease occur mostly in late syphilis. The gummas of late syphilis may produce irreparable damage to skin, bone, or liver. In cardiovascular syphilis, the resulting aneurysm may press on structures such as the intercostal nerves, causing pain. The possibility of a rupture exists as the aneurysm increases in size. Scarring of the aortic valve results in aortic valve insufficiency and eventually heart failure. Neurosyphilis occurs when *T. pallidum* invades the central nervous system. It can occur at any of the stages of syphilis. Visual impairment, *tabes dorsalis* (progressive locomotor ataxia), and dementia are extreme manifestations and are rare.

TABLE 52-6   Stages of Syphilis

Primary

- *Infectivity:* Highly infectious
- Single or multiple chancres (painless indurated lesions) of penis, vulva, lips, mouth, vagina, and rectum) (Fig. 52-8). Occurs 10-90 days after inoculation
- Regional lymphadenopathy (draining of the microorganisms into the lymph nodes)
- Exudate and blood from chancre are highly infectious
- *Duration of stage:* 3-6 wk

Secondary

- *Infectivity:* Highly infectious
- Occurs a few weeks after primary chancre heals
- Flu-like symptoms: malaise, fever, sore throat, headaches, fatigue, arthralgia, generalized adenopathy
- Mucous patches in mouth (Fig. 52-9), tongue, or cervix
- Symmetric, nonpruritic rash bilaterally that appears on trunk, palms, and/or soles (Fig. 52-10)
- *Condylomata lata* (moist, weeping papules) in the anogenital area
- Weight loss, alopecia
- *Duration of stage:* 1-2 yr

Latent

- *Infectivity:* Early (<1 yr)–Infectious; Late (≥1 yr)–Noninfectious
- Absence of signs or symptoms
- Diagnosis based on positive specific treponemal antibody test together with normal CSF and absence of clinical manifestations
- *Duration of stage:* Throughout life or progression to late stage

Late

- *Infectivity:* Noninfectious
- Occurs 1-20 years after initial infection
- Gummas (chronic, destructive lesions affecting any organ of body, especially skin, bone, liver, mucous membranes) (Fig. 52-11)
- *Cardiovascular:* Aneurysms, heart valve insufficiency, heart failure, aortitis
- *Neurosyphilis:* Can occur at any stage of syphilis
- *General paresis:* Personality changes from minor to psychotic, tremors, physical and mental deterioration
- *Tabes dorsalis* (ataxia, areflexia, paresthesias, lightning pains, damaged joints)
- *Duration of stage:* Chronic (without treatment), possibly fatal

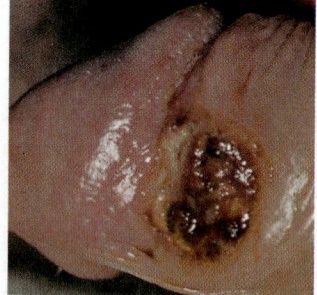

FIG. 52-8 Primary syphilis chancre. (From Forbes CD, Jackson WF. *Color atlas and text of clinical medicine*, ed 3, London, 2003, Mosby.)

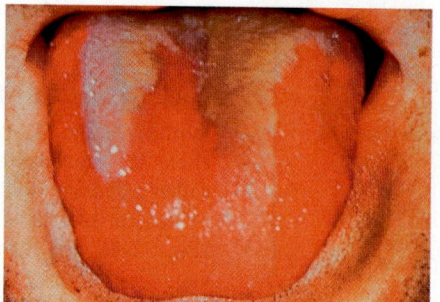

FIG. 52-9 Secondary syphilis. Mucous patch in the mouth. (From Mandell GL, Bennett JE, Dolin R: *Mandell, Douglas, and Bennett's principles and practice of infectious diseases*, ed 7, Philadelphia, 2010, Churchill Livingstone.)

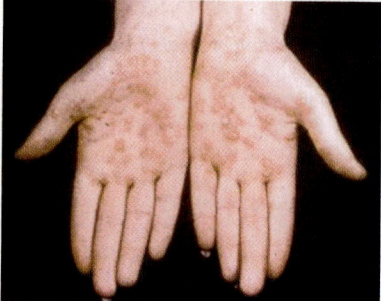

FIG. 52-10 Secondary syphilis. Palmar rash. (From Centers for Disease Control and Prevention Public Health Image Library. Courtesy Robert Sumpter.)

Chancres on the genitalia enhance HIV transmission. Patients with HIV and syphilis appear to be at greatest risk for clinically significant CNS involvement and may require more intensive treatment than do other patients with syphilis.

Diagnostic Studies

Syphilis is most commonly diagnosed by a blood test. Tests for syphilis are classified as those performed for screening and those performed for confirmation of a positive screening test. Nontreponemal tests used for screening detect antibodies that are not specific for syphilis. Nontreponemal tests include the Venereal Disease Research Laboratory (VDRL) test and the rapid plasma reagin (RPR) test. These screening tests usually become positive 10 to 14 days after the appearance of a chancre. The fluorescent treponemal antibody absorption (FTA-Abs) test and the *T. pallidum* particle agglutination (TP-PA) test are called *treponemal tests* because they specifically detect treponemal antibodies. These treponemal tests are used for confirming the diagnosis.[13]

False-negative and false-positive test results do occur with the nontreponemal tests (VDRL, RPR). A false-negative result may be obtained during primary syphilis if the test is done before the individual has had time to produce antibodies. A false-positive finding may occur if patients have various other diseases or conditions. Positive nontreponemal test results

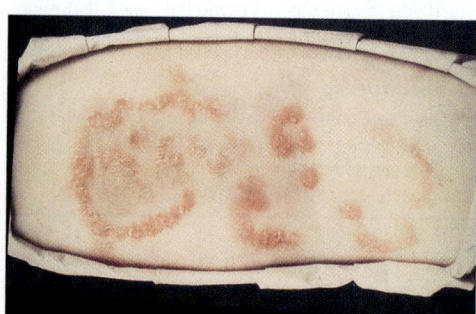

FIG. 52-11 Destructive skin gummas associated with tertiary syphilis. (From Cohen J, Powderly WG: *Infectious diseases*, ed 2, St Louis, 2004, Mosby.)

are always confirmed by more specific treponemal tests to rule out other causes. In the cerebrospinal fluid (CSF), changes such as an increased WBC count, increased total protein, and a positive treponemal antibody test are diagnostic of neurosyphilis.[13]

If treatment with antibiotics is initiated early in the course of the disease on the basis of the history and the symptoms, the serologic testing may not indicate syphilis. Once a person has tested positive for syphilis, these findings may remain positive for an indefinite period in spite of successful treatment.

TABLE 52-7   Interprofessional Care
Syphilis

Diagnostic Assessment
- History and physical examination
- Dark-field microscopy
- Nontreponemal and/or treponemal serologic testing
- Testing for other STIs (HIV, gonorrhea, chlamydial infection)

Management
- Antibiotic therapy
  - penicillin G benzathine (Bicillin LA)
  - doxycycline (Vibramycin) or tetracycline (when penicillin is contraindicated)
- Confidential counseling and testing for HIV infection
- Surveillance
- Repeat of nontreponemal tests at 6 and 12 months
- Examination of cerebrospinal fluid at 1 yr*

*If treatment involves alternative antibiotics or treatment failure has occurred.

Interprofessional Care

Because of the serious complications associated with untreated syphilis, screening programs for high-risk groups are important for reducing morbidity and mortality. The evaluation of all patients with syphilis should also include HIV testing, and the CDC recommends annual syphilis testing for HIV patients[13] (Table 52-7).

Drug Therapy. Management of syphilis is aimed at initiating treatment early and eradicating the syphilitic organisms. Penicillin G benzathine (Bicillin LA) is the recommended treatment for all stages (Table 52-7). When penicillin is contraindicated, doxycycline or tetracycline may be used. Aqueous procaine penicillin G is the treatment of choice for neurosyphilis. Treatment cannot reverse damage that is already present in the later stages of the disease. All sexual contacts from the preceding 90 days should be treated presumptively. Reexamination and follow-up testing are recommended every 6 months for up to 2 years.[13]

❖ NURSING MANAGEMENT: STIs

◆ Nursing Assessment

Subjective and objective data that should be obtained from a person with an STI are presented in Table 52-8. Assess the patient's risk for contracting an STI. Questions to ask include number of partners, types of partners ("Do you have sex with men, women, or both?"), type of birth control used (if applicable), use of condoms or other barrier methods, history of an STI, use of drugs and alcohol, exchange of sex for drugs or money, and risk for violence and personal safety. Plan teaching based on the responses to these questions.

Interpersonal skills necessary for this interview include respect, compassion, and a nonjudgmental attitude. Tailor your counseling to the individual. Do not assume that older people are not at risk: sex and sexuality are dynamic across the life cycle, and sexually active older individuals can be at risk for STIs.[14]

❓ CHECK YOUR PRACTICE

You are working on the medicine unit caring for a 68-yr-old man admitted for IV penicillin for neurosyphilis. The nurse that you are working with says, "I can't believe a man that old could get a sexually transmitted infection."
- How would you respond?
- What should you discuss with your colleague?

TABLE 52-8   Nursing Assessment
Sexually Transmitted Infections

Subjective Data
Important Health Information
Sexual health history: Sexual activity with individuals with STIs, past history of STIs, multiple sexual partners, unsafe sexual practices
Medications: Allergy to any antibiotics

Functional Health Patterns
Health perception–health management: Unsafe sexual practices, drug and/or alcohol use
Nutritional-metabolic: Nausea, vomiting, anorexia. Pharyngitis, oral lesions, chills. Alopecia
Elimination: Dysuria, urinary frequency, urethral discharge, pain with bowel movements
Cognitive-perceptual: Arthralgia, headache, painful, burning lesions, itching or irritation at infected site
Sexuality-reproductive: Dyspareunia, vaginal or penile discharge, bleeding with sex, genital or perianal lesions

Objective Data
General
Fever, lymphadenopathy (generalized or inguinal)

Integumentary
Syphilis: Primary: Painless, indurated genital, oral, or perianal lesions
Secondary: Bilateral, symmetric rash on palms, soles, or entire body. Mucous patches on mouth or tongue; alopecia
Genital herpes: Painful genital or anal vesicular lesions
Genital warts: Single or multiple gray or white genital or anal warts

Gastrointestinal
Rectal discharge, rectal lesions

Urinary
Urethral discharge, erythema

Reproductive
Cervical mucopurulent discharge, cervical erythema, cervical bleeding; penile purulent discharge, epididymitis, proctitis, genital lesions

Possible Diagnostic Findings
Chlamydia: Positive culture or NAAT cervical, urethral, anal, oropharyngeal, or urine samples
Gonorrhea: Positive cultures or NAAT from cervical, urethral, anal, oropharyngeal, or urine samples
Genital herpes: Positive HSV-1 or HSV-2 serum antibody test. Positive culture from active lesion indicating HSV-1 or HSV-2
Syphilis: Positive findings on VDRL and RPR, spirochetes on dark-field microscopy
Trichomoniasis: Positive increased pH and positive motile protozoa on wet prep of discharge. Positive FDA-approved rapid test or liquid-based Pap positive for trichomoniasis.

HSV-1, Herpes simplex virus type 1; *HSV-2,* herpes simplex virus type 2; *NAAT,* nucleic acid amplification test; *RPR,* rapid plasma reagin; *STIs,* sexually transmitted infections; *VDRL,* Venereal Disease Research Laboratory.

◆ Nursing Diagnoses

Nursing diagnoses for the patient with an STI include, but are not limited to, the following:
- Risk for infection *related to* lack of knowledge about modes of STI transmission, failure to practice safer sex, and engaging in other high-risk behaviors
- Anxiety *related to* impact of the condition on relationships, long-term effects of infection, and lack of knowledge regarding the infection

- Ineffective health maintenance *related to* lack of knowledge about disease process and transmission, inadequate follow-up measures, and possibility of reinfection

◆ Planning

The overall goals are that the patient with an STI will (1) demonstrate understanding of the mode of transmission of STIs and the risks associated with STIs, (2) complete treatment and return for appropriate follow-up, (3) notify or assist in notification of sexual contacts about their need for testing and treatment, (4) abstain from intercourse until infection is resolved, and (5) demonstrate knowledge of safer sex practices.

◆ Nursing Implementation

◆ **Health Promotion.** Many approaches to stopping the spread of STIs have been met with varying degrees of success. Be prepared to discuss "safer" sex practices with all patients, not only those who are perceived to be at risk. These practices include abstinence, monogamy, avoidance of high-risk sexual behaviors, and the correct use of condoms and other barriers with every sexual act. Sexual abstinence is the only certain method of avoiding all STIs, but few people consider this a feasible alternative to sexual expression. Limiting sexual contacts to a well-established, monogamous relationship in which both partners are tested regularly for STIs can reduce the risk of contracting an STI. Addressing issues related to drug and alcohol dependence or abuse is important for the promotion of healthy sexual behavior.

Be prepared to teach special populations, such as MSM, women who have sex with women (WSW), and transgender persons, about their particular risks (Table 52-9). A teaching guide for the patient with an STI is presented in Table 52-10.

◆ *Measures to Prevent Infection.* Encourage patients to take notice of a sexual partner's genitalia before sex, paying attention to any discharge, sores, blisters, or rashes. Help patients to be aware of specific signs and symptoms of infection. This can assist them to make good decisions about whether to continue a sexual interaction with safer-sex modifications or to elect not to have sexual relations at all. Remind patients that most STIs may have no symptoms but can still be transmitted. Also emphasize with patients that when they have sex, they are exposed to the infections of everyone with whom their partner has ever had sex.

Proper use of a condom provides a highly effective mechanical barrier to infection. Partners should openly discuss any objections to condom usage, such as interference with spontaneity and the presence of a barrier. Information about the mechanics of sexual arousal and incorporating a condom into sex can help in overcoming the individual's or partner's resistance to its use. Refusing sexual activity with any partner who will not use a condom is a safe and legitimate option.

The *female condom,* a lubricated polyurethane sheath designed for vaginal use, is another option for some individuals. Remind patients to avoid the spermicide nonoxynol 9 (N-9), which can be used alone to prevent pregnancy or as a condom lubricant. Nonoyxnol 9 is one of the least effective methods of birth control when used alone and can act as an irritant to the vagina and rectum, increasing the risk for acquiring an STI.

◆ *Screening Programs.* Screening programs are an effective means of identifying, treating, preventing, and controlling the spread of STIs. At present, there are CDC-recommended screening programs for certain populations, including young people, MSM, pregnant women, and anyone at increased risk for

---

TABLE 52-9   Understanding Risk for STIs in Special Populations

When dealing with the following populations at risk for STIs, it is important to consider cultural, behavioral, and other risk factors that may place them at increased risk for STIs or not receiving appropriate screening.

Women Who Have Sex with Women (WSW)

- WSW should not be presumed to be at low or no risk for STIs based on sexual orientation.
- Self-identified WSW report having had sex with men and indicate that they may continue this practice in the future.
- WSW are at risk for acquiring bacterial, viral, and protozoal infections from current and prior partners, both male and female.
- Practices involving digital-vaginal or digital-anal contact, particularly with shared penetrative sex items, present a possible means for transmission of infected cervicovaginal secretions.
- Female-to-female transmission of *Chlamydia,* trichomoniasis, HIV, HPV, HSV, and syphilis have all been reported.
- Report of same-sex behavior in women should not deter HCPs from screening for all STIs.

Men Who Have Sex with Men (MSM)

- MSM are at higher risk for HIV, syphilis, hepatitis C, and other viral and bacterial STIs compared to the general population.
- Rates of rectal gonorrhea infection are increasing in MSM, particularly in HIV-infected MSM.
- HCPs should assess risk for STIs among MSM patients and be comfortable asking questions about sexual practices, including anal sex.

Transgender Individuals

- Transgender man is a term used to describe a person born anatomically female but who identifies as male. Transgender woman is a term used to describe a person born anatomically male but who identifies as female.
- Rates of certain STIs, including HIV, are higher among transgender women, compared to the general population.
- Not all transgender persons have had genital reassignment surgery and may still have the genitals they were assigned at birth. Therefore these individuals should be screened for STIs based on both risk history and current anatomy. For example, a transgender man may still have a vagina and cervix.
- HCPs must remain aware of their patients' gender identity, current anatomy, and screen patients based on risk history and sexual behaviors.

Source: Centers for Disease Control, Sexually Transmitted Disease Treatment Guidelines, 2015, *www.cdc.gov/std/tg2015/specialpops.htm.*

---

exposure to an STI (new partners, nonmonogamous relationships, not using condoms/barriers).[7]

◆ *Case Finding.* Interviewing and case finding are other methods used to control the spread of STIs. These activities are directed toward locating and examining all sexual contacts of patients with reportable STIs so that effective treatment can be initiated. Public health professionals, often nurses, are aware of the social implications of these diseases and the need for discretion in locating partners. Sexual contacts are not informed about the origin of the information naming them as a contact so that patient privacy mandates are ensured.

Partner notification and treatment impose a heavy burden on public health departments and, as a result, the notification often becomes the responsibility of the infected partner. The infected partner may choose not to inform sexual partners, and the partners may choose not to seek treatment.

◆ *Educational and Research Programs.* Actively encourage your community to provide better education about STIs for its citizens. High-risk populations (e.g., young people under age 25,

TABLE 52-10 Patient Teaching
Sexually Transmitted Infections

When teaching the patient with sexually transmitted infections:
1. Explain precautions to take such as
   - Using condoms and other barrier methods with every sexual encounter
   - Being monogamous
   - Asking potential partners about sexual history
   - Asking potential partners if they have been tested for STIs
   - Avoiding sex with partners who use IV drugs or who have visible oral, inguinal, genital, perineal, or anal lesions
   - Voiding and washing genitalia and surrounding area after sex to flush out some organisms and potentially reduce exposure infection
2. Explain the importance of taking all antibiotics and/or antiviral agents as prescribed. Symptoms will improve after 1-2 days of therapy, but organisms may still be present.
3. Teach patients about the need for treatment of sexual partners to prevent transmission and reinfection.
4. Instruct patients to abstain from sexual intercourse during treatment and to use condoms or other barrier methods when sexual activity is resumed to prevent spread of infection and reinfection.
5. Explain the importance of follow-up examination and retesting at least once after treatment if appropriate to confirm complete cure and prevent relapse.
6. Allow patients and partners to verbalize concerns to clarify areas that need explanation.
7. Instruct patient about symptoms of complications and need to report problems to ensure proper follow-up and early treatment of reinfection.
8. Inform patient regarding state of infectivity to prevent a false sense of security, which may result in careless sexual practices and poor personal hygiene.
9. Inform patients about health department requirements for reporting certain STIs.

MSM) should be a prime target for such educational programs. STI rates are also rising in older adults.[14] Older adults are less likely to use condoms and often have a hard time initiating discussion of sexual health issues.

Knowledge and understanding can decrease the incidence of STIs. The HPV vaccine that protects against genital warts and cervical cancer should be encouraged for boys and girls before the start of sexual activity. Accurate and current information may help reduce parental fears related to the vaccine. Consider stressing the prevention of cancer as a reason for the vaccine, which may be more productive and less controversial, thus making the parent and adolescent more receptive.

◆ **Acute Care**

◆ *Psychologic Support.* The diagnosis of an STI may be met with a variety of emotions, such as shame, guilt, anger, and a desire for vengeance. Encourage the patient to verbalize feelings. Couples in marital or committed relationships are confronted with an added problem when an STI is diagnosed if they must face the implication of possible sexual activity outside the relationship. The STI raises other concerns about their relationship and may serve as an incentive for further problem solving. A referral for professional counseling to explore the ramifications of an STI in their relationship may be indicated.

A patient who has genital herpes is faced with the fact that repeated infections can occur and that no cure is available. This can be frustrating and disruptive to the patient's physical, emotional, social, and sexual life. Help the patient identify and avoid any factors that may precipitate the condition. Inform the patient that the frequency and severity of recurrences will decrease over time.

ETHICAL/LEGAL DILEMMAS
Confidentiality and HIPAA

Situation

P.H., a 22-yr-old woman, is informed of the positive results of a test for chlamydial infection. You advise her to tell her sexual partners that she has this disease. She refuses to tell her boyfriend because he will know that she has had sex with another partner. You later learn that the nursing student who was in the clinic for the day, who is a friend of the boyfriend, hinted to him that he should have STI testing.

Ethical/Legal Points for Consideration

- Each state has requirements for reporting communicable diseases and other health-related data. Inform the patient of the reporting requirements for communicable diseases.
- Nurses and other HCPs have both a legal and an ethical obligation to maintain confidentiality of patient information. The Health Insurance Portability and Accountability Act (HIPAA) ensures the privacy of personal health information.
- The duty to maintain confidentiality is not absolute and may be limited, as necessary, to protect the patient or other parties, or by law or regulation such as mandated reporting for safety or public health reasons.[1]
- Your primary obligation is to the patient seeking care. Patient teaching is one way to establish a partnership with this woman. Share information about the effects of the disease if it is not treated, the consequences of reinfection, and the effect of the disease on others who may not know that they are infected. Then encourage the patient to inform her partners of the diagnosis for the good of everyone, and discuss the option of expedited partner therapy (EPT) where applicable.*

Discussion Questions

1. What are your state's requirements for reportable conditions?
2. In your opinion, what is the best way to balance the needs of an individual patient with those of the general public?
3. What are the risks to the institution for the breach of confidentiality and HIPAA?

Reference

1. Code of Ethics for Nurses. *www.nursingworld.org/ MainMenuCategories/EthicsStandards/Ethics-Position-Statements.*

*EPT is discussed on p. 1230.

Genital warts involve a prolonged course of treatment. The patient can become frustrated and distressed because of frequent office visits, associated costs, potential for unpleasant side effects as a result of treatment, and effects of the infection on future health and sexual relationships. Support and a willingness to listen to the patient's concerns are needed. Local or online support groups are available for almost all STIs. Help patients to connect with support groups.

◆ *Follow-Up.* If you work in public health facilities, clinics, or other outpatient settings, you are more likely to care for a patient with an STI than if you work in a hospital setting. Whatever the setting, as a nurse you are in a position to explain and interpret treatment measures such as the purpose and possible side effects of prescribed drugs and the need for follow-up care (Table 52-10).

Frequently, single-dose treatment for gonorrhea, chlamydial infection, and syphilis helps prevent the problems associated with nonadherence with drug therapy. Give special instructions to the patient requiring multiple-dose therapy to complete the prescribed regimen. Also inform the patient about problems resulting from nonadherence. All patients should return to the treatment center for a repeat culture from the infected sites or for serologic testing at designated times to determine the effectiveness of the treatment. Explaining to the patient that cures are not always obtained on the first treatment can reinforce the need for a follow-up visit. Also advise the patient to inform sexual partners of the need for testing and treatment, regardless of whether they are free of symptoms or experiencing symptoms.

Hygiene Measures. Emphasize to the patient with an STI the importance of certain hygiene measures, such as frequent hand washing. Tell the patient not to itch or scratch infection sites in order to avoid autoinoculation of STIs that can be spread to other parts of the body that way. Washing with soap and water as well as voiding after sex may theoretically provide some benefit in decreasing the exposure to STIs but certainly does not provide adequate protection against transmission. Teach patients that douching after sex is never recommended, as it can push bacteria higher into the reproductive tract or undermine local immune responses.

Sexual Activity. Sexual abstinence is indicated during the communicable phase of any STI, and long-term precautions must be taken with those STIs that are chronic or recurrent. Emphasize that even single-dose treatments can take up to 1 week to be effective and thus the patient is infectious during this period. Emphasize to the patient the importance of using condoms or other barrier methods to help prevent the spread of infection and reinfection. Also encourage condom or other barrier methods use after treatment to prevent future exposure to infection. Remind patients that complications can follow if unprotected sexual activity occurs before treatment completion. Patients need to discuss re-treatment or continued treatment with an HCP. During treatment, the patient can also choose to relate to a partner in an intimate way that avoids penetrative, oral-genital contact, or skin-to-skin contact.

◆ **Ambulatory Care.** Because many STIs are cured with a single dose or short course of antibiotic therapy, many patients are casual about the outcome of these infections. The consequences of this attitude can include delays in treatment, non-adherence with instructions, and subsequent development of complications. The complications are serious and costly and can include future infertility.

Surgery and prolonged therapy are indicated for many patients with infection-related complications. Major surgical procedures such as resection of an aneurysm or aortic valve replacement may be necessary to treat cardiovascular problems caused by syphilis. Pelvic surgery and procedures to correct fertility problems secondary to an STI may be necessary and, if not successful, patients may require assisted reproductive technologies to achieve future pregnancy. Because young people ages 15 to 24 represent about 50% of new STIs annually, it is important to know that almost every state and the District of Columbia have laws that allow minors to consent to STI services without parental involvement (the minimum age varies by state).[1]

◆ **Evaluation**

Expected outcomes for the patient with an STI are that the patient will

- Understand the course, modes of transmission, and treatment options for the STI
- Understand the potential long-term complications of the infection
- Demonstrate compliance with medication regimens and the follow-up protocol
- Understand the importance of partner notification and treatment
- Experience no reinfection and understand STI risk-reducing behaviors and practices

CASE STUDY

Gonococcal and Chlamydial Infection

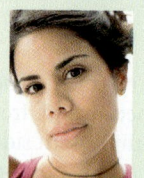

(©Eyecandy Images/ Thinkstock)

Patient Profile

C.R. is a 24-yr-old Hispanic woman who is seen at the outpatient clinic with complaints of increased yellow vaginal discharge and bleeding after sex for the past 2 weeks. She is sexually active with a new partner. She was treated in the past for chlamydial infection at age 20.

Subjective Data

- She and her partner use condoms "sometimes"
- Last menstrual period was 3 weeks ago and she does not use a birth control method
- Noticed her partner had some unusual discharge before they had sex
- Appears anxious and teary

Objective Data

- Cervix: erythematous
- Mucopurulent cervical discharge
- Urine pregnancy test is negative
- Nucleic acid amplification testing (NAAT) of the cervix is positive for both *Neisseria gonorrhoeae* and *Chlamydia trachomatis*

Interprofessional Care

- ceftriaxone 250 mg IM × 1 dose
- azithromycin 1 g PO × 1 dose

Discussion Questions

1. What were C.R.'s risk factors for acquiring gonorrhea and chlamydial infection?
2. What complications could occur if C.R.'s infections are not treated?
3. **Priority Decision:** What is the priority of care for C.R.?
4. **Patient-Centered Care:** What instructions should C.R. receive to ensure successful treatment? To prevent reinfection? To prevent further transmission of the infection?
5. **Teamwork and Collaboration:** Which nursing personnel should be responsible for teaching C.R. what she needs to know about other sexually transmitted infections (STIs): RN, LPN/LVN, UAP?
6. **Patient-Centered Care:** What impact is her diagnosis likely to have on C.R.'s self-image? On her relationship with her sexual partner?
7. **Safety:** C.R. tells you she is worried about how her partner will react when she discloses this information. What safety precautions should be considered?
8. **Priority Decision:** Based on the assessment data presented, what are the priority nursing diagnoses?
9. **Evidence-Based Practice:** C.R. mentions she is using the spermicide nonoxynol-9 (N-9) to protect herself against STIs. Would you advise her to continue to use it?

BRIDGE TO NCLEX EXAMINATION

The number of the question corresponds to the same-numbered outcome at the beginning of the chapter.

1. The individual with the lowest risk for sexually transmitted pelvic inflammatory disease is a woman who uses
   a. oral contraceptives.
   b. barrier methods of contraception.
   c. an intrauterine device for contraception.
   d. Norplant implant or injectable Depo-Provera for contraception.

2. The nurse is obtaining a subjective data assessment from a woman reported as a sexual contact of a man with chlamydial infection. The nurse understands that symptoms of chlamydial infection in women
   a. are frequently absent.
   b. are similar to those of genital herpes.
   c. include a macular palmar rash in the later stages.
   d. may involve chancres inside the vagina that are not visible.

3. A primary HSV infection differs from recurrent HSV episodes in that *(select all that apply)*
   a. only primary infections are sexually transmitted.
   b. symptoms are less severe during recurrent episodes.
   c. transmission of the virus to a fetus is less likely during primary infection.
   d. systemic manifestations such as fever and myalgia are more common in primary infection.
   e. lesions from recurrent HSV are more likely to transmit the virus than lesions from primary HSV.

4. Explain to the patient with gonorrhea that treatment will include both ceftriaxone and azithromycin because
   a. azithromycin helps prevent recurrent infections.
   b. some patients do not respond to oral drugs alone.
   c. coverage with more than one antibiotic will prevent reinfection.
   d. the increasing rates of drug resistance requires the use of at least two drugs.

5. In assessing patients for STIs, the nurse needs to know that many STIs can be asymptomatic. Which STIs can be asymptomatic *(select all that apply)*?
   a. Syphilis
   b. Gonorrhea
   c. Genital warts
   d. Genital herpes
   e. Chlamydial infection

6. To prevent the infection and transmission of STIs, the nurse's teaching plan would include an explanation of
   a. the appropriate use of oral contraceptives.
   b. sexual positions that can be used to avoid infection.
   c. the necessity of annual Pap tests for patients with HPV.
   d. sexual practices that are considered high-risk behaviors.

7. Provide emotional support to a patient with an STI by
   a. offering information on how safer sexual practices can prevent STIs.
   b. showing concern when listening to the patient who expresses negative feelings.
   c. reassuring the patient that the disease is highly curable with appropriate treatment.
   d. helping the patient who received an STI from his or her sexual partner in forgiving the partner.

1. b, 2. a, 3. b, d, 4. d, 5. a, b, c, d, e, 6. d, 7. b

For rationales to these answers and even more NCLEX review questions, visit *http://evolve.elsevier.com/Lewis/medsurg.*

REFERENCES

1. Centers for Disease Control and Prevention: Sexually transmitted disease surveillance, 2013. Retrieved from *www.cdc.gov/std/stats13/default.htm.*
2. Daniels K, Daugherty J, Jones J: Current contraceptive status among women aged 15–44: United States, 2011–2013. *NCHS Data Brief,* No. 173, 2014. Retrieved from *www.cdc.gov/nchs/data/databriefs/db173.pdf.*
3. Centers for Disease Control and Prevention: STDs and infertility. Retrieved from *www.cdc.gov/std/infertility.*
4. Centers for Disease Control and Prevention: Recommendations for the laboratory-based detection of *Chlamydia trachomatis* and *Neisseria gonorrhoeae*—2014, *MMWR* 63(No. RR-2), 2014.
5. Centers for Disease Control and Prevention: Sexually transmitted diseases: expedited partner therapy 2015. Retrieved from *www.cdc.gov/std/ept/legal/default.htm.*
6. Lewis D: Trichomoniasis, *Medicine* 42:369, 2014.
*7. Centers for Disease Control and Prevention: Sexually transmitted diseases treatment guidelines 2015, *MMWR* 64(3):1, 2015.
8. Hofstetter AM: Current thinking on genital herpes, *Curr Opin Infect Dis* 27:75, 2014.
9. Garland S: Vulvovaginal disease: genital herpes, *Best Pract Res Clin Obstet Gynaecol* 26:1098, 2014.
10. James SH, Kimberlin DW: Neonatal herpes simplex virus infection: epidemiology and treatment, *Clin Perinatol* 42:47, 2015.
11. Centers for Disease Control and Prevention: HPV. Retrieved from *www.cdc.gov/std/hpv/default.htm*
12. Crossignani P, De Stefani A, Fara GM, et al: Towards eradication of HPV infection through universal specific vaccination, *BMC Public Health* 13:642, 2013.
13. Centers for Disease Control and Prevention: Syphilis. Retrieved from *www.cdc.gov/std/syphilis/stdfact-syphilis-detailed.htm.*
14. Poynten IM, Grulich AE, Templeton DJ: Sexually transmitted infections in older populations, *Curr Opin Infect Dis* 26:80, 2013.

*Evidence-based information for clinical practice.

53

Female Reproductive and Genital Problems

Amy McKeever, Kim K. Choma

A woman is the full circle. Within her is the power to create, nurture, and transform.

Diane Mariechild

🄴 http://evolve.elsevier.com/Lewis/medsurg/

LEARNING OUTCOMES

1. Summarize the etiologies of infertility and the strategies for diagnosis and treatment of the infertile woman.
2. Describe the etiology, clinical manifestations, interprofessional care, and nursing management of menstrual problems and abnormal uterine bleeding.
3. Identify the risk factors, clinical manifestations, and nursing and interprofessional management of ectopic pregnancy.
4. Describe the changes related to menopause and the interprofessional care and nursing management of the patient with menopausal symptoms.
5. Describe the assessment, interprofessional care, and nursing management of women with pelvic inflammatory disease and endometriosis.
6. Explain the clinical manifestations, diagnostic studies, interprofessional care, including surgical therapy for cervical, endometrial, ovarian, and vulvar cancers.
7. Summarize the preoperative and postoperative nursing management of the patient requiring surgery of the female reproductive system.
8. Differentiate among the common problems that occur with cystoceles, rectoceles, and fistulas and the related interprofessional care and nursing management.
9. Summarize the clinical manifestations of sexual assault and the appropriate nursing and interprofessional management of the patient who has been sexually assaulted.

KEY TERMS

abnormal uterine bleeding (AUB), p. 1246
abortion, p. 1243
amenorrhea, p. 1246
cystocele, p. 1262
dysmenorrhea, p. 1245
ectopic pregnancy, p. 1247

endometriosis, p. 1253
hysterectomy, p. 1254
infertility, p. 1242
leiomyomas, p. 1254
menopause, p. 1248
pelvic inflammatory disease (PID), p. 1251

perimenopause, p. 1248
premenstrual syndrome (PMS), p. 1244
sexual assault, p. 1263
uterine prolapse, p. 1261

INFERTILITY

Infertility is the inability to conceive after at least 1 year of regular unprotected intercourse. Approximately 15% of couples in North America are infertile.[1]

Etiology and Pathophysiology

Infertility may be caused by either female or male or combined factors. (Conditions that cause male infertility are discussed in Chapter 54.) In some cases, the cause of infertility may not be identified.

Female infertility may be due to problems with ovulation, the fallopian tubes, or conditions that affect the uterus or cervix. In women, the risk for infertility begins around age 30. By the time a woman reaches the age of 40, the chances of conceiving are 10% or less. For both genders, chronic diseases, genital infections, and exposure to environmental toxins can affect fertility.

Diagnostic Studies

Couples who are being evaluated for infertility usually have a detailed history and physical examination. Based on the findings from the history and physical examination, additional diagnostic testing may be ordered (Table 53-1). Formal evaluation of the infertile couple is usually conducted after 1 year of regular unprotected intercourse. Earlier evaluation may occur in women over age 35 or based on medical or physical findings, such as a history of irregular menstrual cycles or if the partner has a known fertility problem.

A comprehensive evaluation of the female reproductive system includes cervical, uterine, endometrial, tubal, peritoneal, and ovarian factors that may be the source of infertility. A

Reviewed by Adena Bargad, PhD, CNM, Assistant Professor, Columbia University Medical Center, Director, Sub-Specialty Program in Women's Health, Columbia University School of Nursing, New York, New York; Courtney Reinisch, RN, DNP, APN-BC, DCC, Clinical Associate Professor, School of Nursing, Rutgers University, Newark, New Jersey; and Crystal Sheaves, RN, MSN, APRN, FNP-BC, Senior Lecturer, West Virginia University School of Nursing, Charleston, West Virginia.

TABLE 53-1 Interprofessional Care

Infertility

Diagnostic Assessment
- History and physical examination of both partners, including psychosocial functioning
- Review of menstrual and gynecologic history
- Assessment of possible sexually transmitted infections
- Hormone levels
  - Serum hormone levels (e.g., FSH, LH, prolactin)
  - Urinary LH
- Pap test
- Ovulatory study
- Tubal patency study
  - Hysterosalpingogram
- Postcoital test
  - Cervical mucus
  - Sperm penetration assay
  - Semen analysis
- Pelvic ultrasound
- Genetic screening

Management
- Hormone therapy
- Drug therapy (Table 53-2)
- Intrauterine insemination
- Assisted reproductive technologies (ARTs)

FSH, Follicle-stimulating hormone; *LH,* luteinizing hormone.

TABLE 53-2 Drug Therapy

Infertility

Drug	Mechanism of Action
Selective Estrogen Receptor Modulator	
clomiphene (Clomid)	Stimulates hypothalamus to ↑ production of GnRH, which ↑ release of LH and FSH. End result is stimulation of ovulation.
Menotropins (Human Menopausal Gonadotropin)	
Pergonal	Product made of FSH and LH to
Repronex	promote the development and
Humegon	maturation of follicles in ovaries.
Follicle-Stimulating Hormone Agonists	
urofollitropin (Bravelle)	Stimulate follicle growth and
follitropin (Gonal-f)	maturation by mimicking the body's natural FSH.
GnRH Antagonists	
cetrorelix (Cetrotide)	Prevent premature LH surges and
ganirelix	premature ovulation in women undergoing ovarian stimulation.
GnRH Agonists	
leuprolide (Lupron)	Suppress release of LH and FSH with
nafarelin (Synarel)	continuous use. May also be used in the treatment of endometriosis.
Human Chorionic Gonadotropin (hCG)	
Pregnyl	Induces ovulation by stimulating
Profasi	release of eggs from follicles.
Novarel	

FSH, Follicle-stimulating hormone; *GnRH,* gonadotropin-releasing hormone; *LH,* luteinizing hormone.

TABLE 53-3 Types of Spontaneous Abortion

Type	Description
Complete abortion	All products of conception (POC) are expelled
Incomplete abortion	Parts of POC are retained
Inevitable abortion	Cervix is open and pregnancy loss cannot be prevented
Infected (septic) abortion	Endometrium (uterine lining) and POC become infected
Missed abortion	Fetus has died but has not been expelled
Threatened abortion	Unexplained bleeding with or without pain. Suggests pregnancy loss may occur

semen sample is required to determine if the cause is related to the male partner.

❖ NURSING AND INTERPROFESSIONAL MANAGEMENT: INFERTILITY

Infertility management depends on the cause. If the cause is due to ovarian function, supplemental hormone therapy may be required. Table 53-2 provides a review of drugs commonly used for women experiencing infertility.

Assisted reproductive technology (ART) can be used to help women who are experiencing difficulty becoming pregnant. ART includes fertility medications, artificial insemination, and surrogacy. Different types of ART include (1) in vitro fertilization (IVF); (2) gamete intrafallopian transfer (GIFT); (3) zygote intrafallopian transfer (ZIFT); (4) donor gametes; and (5) freezing of ova. Some types of ART, such as IVF, are expensive and can be emotionally stressful. Assisting couples experiencing infertility is critical. You can provide teaching about the physiology of reproduction and an overview of infertility evaluation and treatments.

EARLY PREGNANCY LOSS

Early pregnancy loss is a term used to describe the loss of a pregnancy before 20 weeks gestation.[2] Abortion is another term that is used to describe the loss of pregnancy. Abortions are classified as *spontaneous* (those occurring naturally [e.g., miscarriage]) or *induced* (those occurring as a result of medical intervention). *Miscarriage* is the common term for the unintended loss of a pregnancy.

Spontaneous Abortion

Spontaneous abortion is the natural loss of pregnancy before 20 weeks of gestation (Table 53-3). Nearly 20% of pregnancies can result in miscarriage, a loss that can be devastating for both the mother and her partner. Fetal chromosomal abnormalities account for many miscarriages before 8 weeks of gestation. Other causes of spontaneous abortions include endocrine abnormalities, maternal infection, uterine abnormalities (e.g., uterine fibroids, endometriosis), immunologic factors, and environmental factors.

Treatment to prevent spontaneous abortion is limited. Although bed rest and avoidance of vaginal intercourse are often recommended, there is no evidence that these measures improve the outcome. Women are advised to report any bleeding to their HCP.

If the pregnancy is not viable, two types of management are considered: expectant management or medical management. *Expectant management* refers to monitoring the patient to see if the *products of conception* (POC) are expelled naturally without complications. *Medical management* may be indicated if the POCs do not pass completely or bleeding becomes

TABLE 53-4   Methods for Inducing Abortions

Method	Length of Pregnancy	Description
Medical vacuum aspiration	Usually up to 2 wk after first missed period	Catheter is inserted through cervix into uterus, and suction is applied. Contents of uterus are aspirated.
Suction aspiration (curettage)	Up to 12 wk	Cervix is dilated, uterine aspirator is introduced, and suction is applied, removing contents of uterus.
Dilation and evacuation (D&E)	10-16 wk (approximate)	Cervix is dilated and contents of uterus are removed by vacuum cannula and use of other instruments as needed.
Mifepristone (Mifeprex) with misoprostol (Cytotec)	Up to 49-63 days*	Mifepristone is administered orally, followed by misoprostol orally 48 hr later.

*FDA recommends 49 days. The American Congress of Obstetricians and Gynecologists guidelines indicate it is safe to use up to 63 days.

excessive. This may involve a *dilation and curettage (D&C)* or the use of medications to expel the remaining contents from the uterus. The D&C involves surgically dilating the cervix and scraping the endometrium of the uterus to empty the contents of the uterus.

Women who experience moderate-to-heavy bleeding and the passage of clots during pregnancy may require emergency care at a hospital. Vital signs and blood loss are monitored along with an assessment of her psychologic well-being. Any heavy bleeding, severe pain, or fever that occurs after medical management should be reported to the HCP. Ovulation can occur as soon as 2 weeks after early pregnancy loss, and normal menses should return within 4 to 6 weeks.

Provide grief support as the couple deals with the psychologic distress of their loss. Encourage them to verbalize their feelings and refer them to a pregnancy loss support group.

Induced Abortion

Induced abortion is an elective termination of a pregnancy.[3] Several methods can be used for induced abortions (Table 53-4). Deciding which method to use depends on the length of the pregnancy and the woman's condition.

Once the decision is made to have an abortion, the woman and her partner need support and acceptance. Prepare the patient for what to expect both emotionally and physically. Grief and sadness are normal emotions after an abortion. Nursing care for a women who terminates her pregnancy includes assessment of a woman's need for counseling and support, providing for privacy, maintaining her physical comfort, and monitoring her vital signs.

After the abortion, teach the patient the signs and symptoms of possible complications, such as abnormal vaginal bleeding, severe abdominal cramping, fever, and foul-smelling drainage. Also stress to the patient that as soon as 1 week after having an abortion she is able to become pregnant again. Normal menstruation returns in 4 to 6 weeks.

Instruct patients to refrain from intercourse and putting anything into the vagina for 1 week after the abortion. (The one exception is for women who use NuvaRing birth control.) Oral contraception can be started the day of the abortion or 1 to 2 weeks after the procedure, depending on the patient's needs and desires.

PROBLEMS RELATED TO MENSTRUATION

The normal menstrual cycle is discussed in Chapter 50. After *menarche* (onset of menses), the menstrual cycle may be irregular during the first few years as well as the years preceding menopause. Although most women have a predictable menstrual cycle, considerable normal variation exists among women

in cycle length and in duration, amount, and character of the menstrual flow (see Table 50-2). During the perimenopausal period as ovarian function begins to diminish, women may note a change in their menstrual patterns.

PREMENSTRUAL SYNDROME

Premenstrual syndrome (PMS) refers to a group of symptoms that occur during a woman's menstrual cycle. Many women experience symptoms of PMS. The syndrome includes a variety of physical, psychologic, and somatic symptoms that may be severe enough to affect interpersonal relationships, professional responsibilities, academic performance, and social activities.

As many as 150 symptoms have been associated with PMS. *Premenstrual dysphoric disorder* (PMDD) is the term used to describe PMS associated with a severe mood disorder.

Etiology and Pathophysiology

The cause of PMS is not well understood. PMS is probably due to a combination of biologic and psychosocial factors. Genetics, imbalances in hormones and neurotransmitters (e.g., serotonin), and nutritional deficiencies have all been thought to be causes of PMS.

Clinical Manifestations

PMS is extremely variable in its clinical manifestations, frequency, and severity among women. Symptoms may also vary from one cycle to another. Common symptoms include breast discomfort, peripheral edema, abdominal bloating, sensation of weight gain, episodes of binge eating, headaches, anxiety, depression, irritability and moodiness, back pain, insomnia, menstrual cramps, fatigue, and generalized muscle pain.

Diagnostic Studies and Interprofessional Care

A focused health history and physical examination are performed to identify any underlying conditions such as thyroid dysfunction, uterine fibroids, anemia, nutritional and vitamin deficiencies, autoimmune disorders, endometriosis, and/or depression that may account for the symptoms.

To accurately diagnose PMS or PMDD, four factors are critical: (1) consistency of the syndrome complex, (2) occurrence of the symptoms in the luteal phase and resolution after the beginning of menses, (3) documented ovulatory cycles, and (4) symptoms that disrupt the woman's life.

A holistic approach to managing PMS symptoms for women includes stress management, dietary changes, exercise, teaching, and cognitive behavioral therapy.

Drug Therapy. Selective serotonin reuptake inhibitors (SSRIs), such as sertraline (Zoloft) and fluoxetine (Prozac, Sarafem), have provided relief to women who suffer from symptoms of anxiety, irritability, and mood changes associated with PMS. Many women choose to take oral contraceptives and/or NSAIDs to reduce cramping and back pain. Vitamin B₆, calcium, and magnesium have been recommended for mood changes associated with PMS.

> ### ? CHECK YOUR PRACTICE
>
> You are working in the GYN outpatient clinic. Your patient is a 28-yr-old woman who is being seen for symptoms of PMS. She tells you, "My PMS has gotten so bad lately that I spend the entire day in bed due to pain. I am very anxious and overwhelmed. I can't function like this anymore."
> - How would you respond?
> - What are things she can do to relieve symptoms?

❖ NURSING MANAGEMENT: PREMENSTRUAL SYNDROME

Nursing care for the patient with PMS includes teaching her about the symptoms associated with PMS and how to manage them (Table 53-5). Acknowledging that she has PMS can be therapeutic and empowering. Teaching the woman's partner about the nature of PMS helps the partner better understand PMS and its effects. Provide the patient with support and reassure her that PMS is not an emotional disorder, but one that has a physiologic basis and one that can be managed.

DYSMENORRHEA

Dysmenorrhea is painful menses with abdominal cramping. The two types of dysmenorrhea are *primary* (no pathologic condition exists) and *secondary* (pelvic disease is the underlying cause). Dysmenorrhea is one of the most common gynecologic problems.

Etiology and Pathophysiology

Primary dysmenorrhea begins in the first few years after menarche, typically with the onset of regular menstrual cycles. It is usually related to elevated levels of prostaglandin, a hormone that is found in the endometrium. Stimulation of the endometrium by estrogen and progesterone results in a dramatic increase in prostaglandin production. Prostaglandin stimulates the uterus to contract. Uterine contractions and constriction of small endometrial blood vessels result in tissue ischemia and increased sensitization of the pain receptors. This results in painful menstrual cramps. As menstruation continues, prostaglandin levels decrease each day, and menstrual cramping lessens.

Secondary dysmenorrhea usually occurs after adolescence, most commonly at 30 to 40 years of age and worsens as a woman ages. Common pelvic conditions that cause secondary dysmenorrhea include endometriosis, chronic pelvic inflammatory disease, and uterine fibroids. Because secondary dysmenorrhea can be caused by many conditions, the clinical manifestations and severity vary. However, painful menses is the primary manifestation.

Clinical Manifestations

Clinical manifestations of dysmenorrhea include menstrual pain that is most severe during the first few days of menses. Painful menstruation rarely lasts more than 2 days. Typical symptoms reported by women include lower, colicky abdominal pain, frequently radiating to the lower back and upper thighs. Nausea, diarrhea, fatigue, and headache may also occur.

Secondary dysmenorrhea usually occurs after the woman has little to no pain during the menstrual cycle. The pain, which may be unilateral, is generally more constant and continues longer than in primary dysmenorrhea. Depending on the cause, symptoms such as *dyspareunia* (painful intercourse), painful defecation, or irregular bleeding may occur at times other than menstruation.

Diagnostic Studies

Evaluating a patient for dysmenorrhea begins with a complete health history and pelvic examination. A probable diagnosis of primary dysmenorrhea is given if the history reveals an onset shortly after menarche with symptoms that are associated only with menses. The pelvic examination is otherwise normal. If the HCP finds an underlying cause of dysmenorrhea, the diagnosis is secondary dysmenorrhea.

❖ NURSING AND INTERPROFESSIONAL MANAGEMENT: DYSMENORRHEA

Treatment for primary dysmenorrhea includes pharmacologic and nonpharmacologic therapy. Nonsteroidal antiinflammatory drugs (NSAIDs) (e.g., naproxen [Naprosyn]) inhibit prostaglandins. Oral contraceptives (OCPs) may also be used to decrease estrogen and progesterone. This results in lower prostaglandin levels, decreased monthly endometrial lining proliferation, and decreased menstrual flow.

Nonpharmacologic interventions include applying heat to the lower abdomen or back and physical exercise. Regular exercise helps to reduce prostaglandin production. Acupuncture and transcutaneous nerve stimulation may be used for women who have inadequate relief from drugs or who prefer not to take drugs.

Treatment of secondary dysmenorrhea depends on the etiology. Some individuals with secondary dysmenorrhea are helped by the approaches used for primary dysmenorrhea. However, if a gynecologic abnormality is the main cause of secondary dysmenorrhea, then treating the underlying gynecologic abnormality is the priority. For example, women with endometriosis who have secondary dysmenorrhea may benefit from taking OCPs. Nursing interventions include teaching women with dysmenorrhea about the cause, symptoms, and treatment. This will

---

TABLE 53-5 Interprofessional Care

Premenstrual Syndrome (PMS)

Diagnostic Assessment
- History and physical examination
- Symptom diary

Management
- Stress management
- Nutritional therapy
- Aerobic exercise

Drug Therapy
- Diuretics
- Prostaglandin inhibitors (e.g., ibuprofen)
- Selective serotonin reuptake inhibitors (e.g., sertraline [Zoloft])
- Combined oral contraceptives

provide women with a basis for coping with this common problem and increase feelings of self-control. Advise women that during acute pain, relief may be obtained by applying heat to the abdomen or back and taking NSAIDs. Also suggest noninvasive pain-relieving practices such as relaxation breathing and guided imagery, yoga, and meditation. Other measures to reduce the discomfort of dysmenorrhea include regular exercise and good nutrition.

ABNORMAL UTERINE BLEEDING

Abnormal uterine bleeding (AUB) is any change in a woman's menstrual flow, including volume, duration, or cycle pattern. AUB can be classified based on the cause of bleeding (Fig. 53-1). *Heavy menstrual bleeding* (HMB) (instead of the term *menorrhagia*) describes excessive bleeding. *Intermenstrual bleeding* (instead of the term *metrorrhagia*) refers to bleeding between regular menstrual cycles.

Chronic AUB is classified as uterine bleeding that is abnormal in volume, timing, or regularity and has been present for most of the past 6 months. *Acute AUB* is an episode of heavy bleeding that requires immediate treatment.

In reproductive-age women, the causes of AUB may include uterine fibroids, polyps, ovulatory dysfunction, endometrial problems, or cancer. Other causes of AUB may include bleeding disorders (e.g., thrombocytopenia), leukemia, medications, eating disorders, or liver failure.[4] For postmenopausal women, endometrial cancer must be considered whenever bleeding or spotting is experienced after her menstrual bleeding has ceased for 1 year or longer.

Anovulation is the most common reason for missing menses. Ovulation is often erratic for several years after menarche and before menopause. Bleeding in between periods (spotting) is also common for women who start taking oral contraceptives. If spotting continues beyond the first few months on oral contraceptives, a different pill formulation may be prescribed. Spotting with long-acting progestin therapies (e.g., intrauterine devices [IUDs], Nexplanon implant, progestin-only pills [levonorgestrel, norethindrone], progesterone injections [medroxyprogesterone-Depo-Provera] is also common and not usually associated with any serious complications.

Amenorrhea is the absence or abnormal interruption of menstruation (Table 53-6). *Primary amenorrhea* refers to the failure of menstrual cycles to begin by 16 years of age. *Secondary amenorrhea* occurs when menstrual cycles stop for 3 to 6 months in menstruating women. Primary amenorrhea is often associated with chromosomal or congenital abnormalities. Many causes of secondary amenorrhea can be attributed to primary ovarian insufficiency, polycystic ovary syndrome (PCOS), hypothalamic disorders, and hyperprolactinemia.

Diagnostic Studies and Interprofessional Care

Once it is determined that a patient has AUB, the HCP will determine if the AUB is related to a structural cause or nonstructural cause. A comprehensive history and physical examination are done to determine the cause of AUB (Table 53-7). Laboratory evaluation and diagnostic procedures are based on findings from the history and physical examination. Treatment depends on the cause of the problem, degree of threat to the patient's health, her quality of life, and whether children are desired in the future.

TABLE 53-6   Causes of Amenorrhea

Natural Amenorrhea
- Pregnancy
- Breastfeeding
- Menopause

Lifestyle
- Stress
- Excessive exercise
- Low body weight
- Acute and chronic illness

Hormonal Imbalance
- Polycystic ovary syndrome (PCOS)
- Pituitary tumors
- Thyroid dysfunction

Medications
- Antipsychotics
- Antihypertensives
- Chemotherapy
- Antidepressants
- Hormone therapy (oral or injectable contraceptives, intrauterine devices)

Structural Problems
- Damage or scarring to reproductive organs from infection, trauma, radiation

Genetic
- Congenital absence of reproductive organ(s)
- Turner's syndrome

TABLE 53-7   Interprofessional Care

Abnormal Uterine Bleeding

Diagnostic Assessment
- History, including surgical history and medication history
- Pelvic examination
- Age of menarche/menopause
- Bleeding patterns and perceived severity of bleeding (clots, soaking through clothing)
- Evaluation for manifestations of obesity/hirsutism (suggestive of polycystic ovary syndrome)
- Pregnancy test
- Complete blood count (CBC)
- Thyroid-stimulating hormone (TSH)
- STI screening
- Screening for bleeding disorders (if indicated)
- Imaging studies and tissue sampling
  - Transvaginal/pelvic ultrasound
  - Saline infusion sonohysterography
  - MRI
  - Hysteroscopy
  - Endometrial biopsy

Management
Based on etiology of problem, may include:
- Oral contraceptives
- Hormonal therapy
- Nonsteroidal antiinflammatory drugs
- Mirena IUD

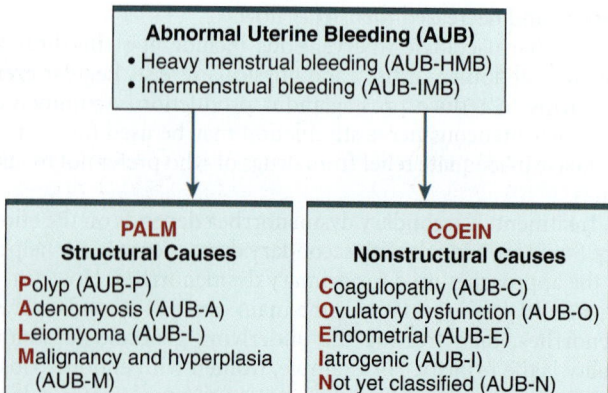

FIG. 53-1   PALM-COEIN classification system for abnormal uterine bleeding. (Used with permission. The American College of Obstetricians and Gynecologists: *Practice Bulletin* 128:1, 2012.)

Combined oral contraceptives may be prescribed for a woman with amenorrhea to ensure regular shedding of the endometrium. Tranexamic acid (Lysteda) may be used to treat heavy menstrual bleeding. This drug stabilizes a protein that helps blood to clot. The use of tranexamic acid is contraindicated in women who use combined oral contraceptives.

Estradiol valerate/dienogest (Natazia) is the only combined oral contraceptive approved for treatment of heavy menstrual bleeding. It may be given to women who desire an oral contraceptive to prevent pregnancy. Other options for treatment of heavy menstrual bleeding include nonsteroidal antiinflammatory drugs (NSAIDs) and the Mirena IUD (progestin IUD).

❖ NURSING MANAGEMENT: ABNORMAL UTERINE BLEEDING

Teach women about the characteristics of the menstrual cycle to help them identify variations (see Table 50-2). This knowledge can decrease apprehension and dispel misconceptions about the menstrual cycle. Encourage the patient to report excessive bleeding, passing of clots, and unusually long duration of menstrual cycles.

Teach women to avoid the prolonged use of superabsorbent tampons that can increase the risk of toxic shock syndrome (TSS). TSS is an acute life-threatening condition caused by a toxin from *Staphylococcus aureus*. TSS causes high fever, vomiting, diarrhea, weakness, myalgia, and a sunburn-like rash.

ECTOPIC PREGNANCY

An ectopic pregnancy is the implantation of the fertilized ovum anywhere outside the uterus. Almost all ectopic pregnancies occur within the fallopian tube. Approximately 3% of all pregnancies are ectopic (Fig. 53-2). Ectopic pregnancy is a life-threatening condition. Early detection can lead to successful management as well as reduced morbidity and mortality.

Etiology and Pathophysiology

Ectopic pregnancy can be caused by blockage of the fallopian tube(s) or reduction of tubal peristalsis that impedes or delays the fertilized ovum from passing to the uterus. After the fertilized egg implants itself in the fallopian tube, the growth of the gestational sac expands the tubal wall and eventually the fallopian tube ruptures. This leads to manifestations of acute peritonitis 6 to 8 weeks after the last normal menstrual period. Often the woman presents to the HCP or the emergency department (ED) due to bleeding and/or pelvic pain or pressure.

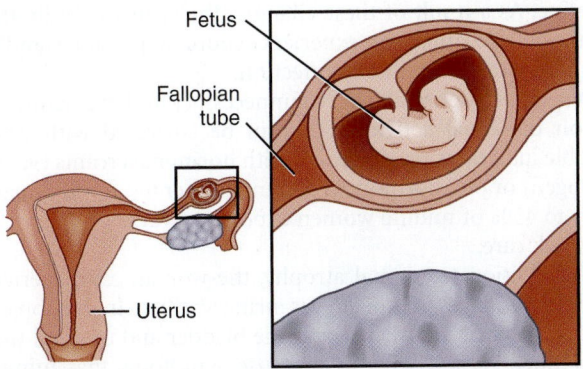

FIG. 53-2 Ectopic pregnancy occurring in the fallopian tube.

Risk factors or causes for ectopic pregnancy include a history of pelvic inflammatory disease, prior ectopic pregnancy, current progestin-releasing IUD, and prior pelvic or tubal surgery. Additional risk factors include procedures used in infertility treatment (e.g., IVF, embryo transfer, ovulation induction).

Clinical Manifestations

The classic manifestations of ectopic pregnancy are abdominal or pelvic pain, missed menses, and/or irregular vaginal bleeding. Other manifestations include morning sickness, breast tenderness, gastrointestinal disturbance, malaise, and syncope.

Pelvic and/or abdominal pain is almost always present and is caused by distention of the fallopian tube. The character of the pain varies among women and can be colicky or vague, unilateral or bilateral.

Symptom severity does not necessarily correlate with the extent of vaginal bleeding. The vaginal bleeding that may accompany ectopic pregnancy is usually described as spotting. However, bleeding may be heavier and can be confused with menses. If tubal rupture occurs, there is risk of hemorrhage and hypovolemic shock. This situation is an emergency.

Diagnostic Studies

Diagnosing an ectopic pregnancy can be challenging because of the clinical manifestations. If an HCP suspects an ectopic pregnancy, a pelvic examination should be performed along with a serum pregnancy test (quantitative human chorionic gonadotropin β-hCG). If the patient is in stable condition, a combination of serial measurements of serum β-hCG and vaginal ultrasound is indicated to monitor the ectopic pregnancy.

❓ CHECK YOUR PRACTICE

You are working in the ED. Your patient is a 29-yr-old woman who presented with acute abdominal pain. She has had in vitro fertilization. Her pain is 7 (on 0 to 10 pain scale). The HCP suspects an ectopic pregnancy. She is crying, "I am going to lose this baby, and we have been trying so hard to have one."
- As her nurse, what are your priorities?
- How would you respond to her?

❖ NURSING AND INTERPROFESSIONAL MANAGEMENT: ECTOPIC PREGNANCY

There are two ways to treat ectopic pregnancies: drug therapy or surgery.[5] Drug therapy is used (1) when an ectopic pregnancy is confirmed on ultrasound, (2) the woman is hemodynamically stable, (3) the woman is compliant with the required follow-up, and (4) the pregnancy is small and the fallopian tube has not ruptured.

Methotrexate therapy is the drug therapy of choice. Methotrexate stops the growth of rapidly dividing cells, such as embryonic, fetal, and early placenta cells. Methotrexate can be given as a single shot or as several injections. The most common side effect of methotrexate is cramping abdominal pain. It usually occurs during the first 2 to 3 days of treatment. Other side effects may include vaginal bleeding, nausea, vomiting, indigestion, or dizziness.

Serum β-hCG levels are determined on posttreatment days 4 and 7. A 15% reduction in β-hCG is expected. Weekly β-hCG are performed until negative. If at any time serum β-hCG levels plateau or increase, methotrexate may be repeated. If an ectopic

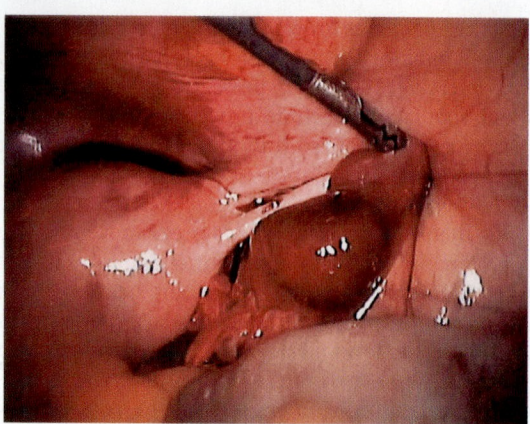

FIG. 53-3 Laparoscopic treatment of ectopic pregnancy in the right fallopian tube. (From Katz V: *Comprehensive gynecology*, ed 5, St Louis, 2007, Mosby.)

TABLE 53-8	**Manifestations of Perimenopause and Postmenopause**
Perimenopause	**Postmenopause**
• Irregular menstrual cycles	• Cessation of menses
• Occasional vasomotor symptoms (e.g., hot flashes)	• Vasomotor instability (e.g., hot flashes and night sweats)
• Mood changes	• Atrophy of genitourinary tissue (e.g., vaginal epithelium)
• Sleep disturbances	• Stress and urge incontinence
• Vaginal dryness	• Breast tenderness
	• Atrophy of genitourinary tissue with decreased support
	• Osteoporosis

TABLE 53-9	**Manifestations of Estrogen Deficiency**	
Vasomotor	**Musculoskeletal**	
• Hot flashes	• Increased fracture rate, especially vertebral bodies but also humerus, distal radius, and upper femur	
• Night sweats		
Genitourinary		
• Atrophic vaginitis	**Cardiovascular**	
• Dyspareunia secondary to poor lubrication	• Decreased high-density lipoproteins (HDLs)	
• Incontinence	• Increased low-density lipoproteins (LDLs)	
Psychologic		
• Emotional lability	**Other**	
• Change in sleep pattern	• Diminished collagen content of skin	
• Decreased REM sleep	• Breast tissue changes	

REM, Rapid eye movement.

pregnancy continues after 2 or 3 doses of methotrexate, surgical treatment is needed to remove the ectopic pregnancy.

If surgery is needed, a conservative approach that limits damage to the reproductive system is the goal. If the pregnancy is small, the pregnancy is removed laparoscopically (Fig. 53-3). If the tube ruptures, emergent surgery is required to stabilize the patient.

Nursing care includes closely monitoring vital signs and observing for signs of shock. Provide patient teaching to prepare her for the diagnostic procedures and drug therapy. Explain the side effects of methotrexate and tell her to avoid NSAIDs. Follow-up with weekly β-hCG measurements is required. If the patient requires laparoscopic surgery, provide patient teaching and emotional support.

PERIMENOPAUSE AND POSTMENOPAUSE

Perimenopause is a normal life transition for women that begins with the first signs of change in menstrual cycles and ends after cessation of menses. Menstrual changes can include shorter cycles, less frequent cycles, lighter cycles, or heavier cycles.

Menopause is a normal physiologic cessation of menses associated with declining ovarian function that ends in cessation of the menstrual cycle and ovulation. *Natural menopause* is diagnosed retrospectively after 12 months of no periods. The average age for a woman is 52 years, but the age can vary from 40 to 58 years.

Induced menopause occurs as a result of surgical intervention to remove the ovaries or from side effects of chemotherapy, radiation therapy, or other drugs. *Postmenopause* is a term that refers to the time in a woman's life after menopause.

Clinical Manifestations

Clinical manifestations of perimenopause and menopause are presented in Table 53-8. Perimenopause is a time of erratic hormonal fluctuation and irregular menstrual cycles. With the decrease in function of the ovaries, estrogen levels drop and hot flashes and other symptoms begin. The signs and symptoms of diminished estrogen are listed in Table 53-9.

The loss of estrogen plays a significant role in the cause of age-related alterations. Changes most critical to a woman's well-being are the increased risks for coronary artery disease

(CAD) and osteoporosis (secondary to bone density loss). Other changes include a redistribution of fat, a tendency to gain weight more easily, muscle and joint pain, loss of skin elasticity, changes in hair amount and distribution, and atrophy of external genitalia and breast tissue.

Vasomotor instability (hot flashes) and irregular menses are the two main clinical manifestations associated with menopause. A hot flash is a sudden sensation of intense heat along with perspiration and flushing. Other manifestations of menopause include atrophy of the vagina. Vaginal atrophy is due to decreased estrogen levels related to the loss of ovarian function. Decreased estrogen causes thinning of the vaginal mucosa and disappearance of rugae, which results in a decrease in vaginal secretions and causes the vaginal secretions to become more alkaline. As a result of these changes, the vagina is easily traumatized, the woman can experience more dyspareunia, and she can be more susceptible to infection.

Vaginal atrophy can lead to unnecessary and premature cessation of sexual activity. This can be corrected with water-soluble lubricants or, if needed, with hormonal creams (vaginal estrogen) or oral hormone replacement therapy. Approximately 20% to 45% of midlife women experience vaginal atrophy, but few seek care.

In addition to vaginal atrophy, the woman can experience atrophic changes in the lower urinary tract. In menopause, bladder capacity decreases, and the bladder and urethral tissue lose tone. These changes can cause symptoms that mimic a bladder infection (e.g., dysuria, urgency, frequency) when no infection is present. Decreasing blood serum estrogen levels can cause an array of physical and cognitive changes during menopause that include depression, irritability, insomnia, and memory loss.

EVIDENCE-BASED PRACTICE
Translating Research Into Practice

Is Sleep Disturbance Associated With Menopausal Stage?

Clinical Question

For women who are premenopausal, perimenopausal, or postmenopausal (P), what is the association between menopausal stage (I) and sleep disturbance (O)?

Synthesis of Best Available Evidence

- Systematic review and meta-analysis of cross-sectional, cohort, and experimental studies.
- Included 24 studies of community-dwelling midlife women ($n = 63{,}542$) in various stages of natural menopause, including premenopausal, perimenopausal, and postmenopausal stages. Also included women with surgical menopause. Women from ethnically diverse backgrounds included white, Asian (Chinese and Japanese), Iranian, and Hispanic.
- Significant association was found between perimenopausal and postmenopausal stages and higher rates of sleep disturbance.
- Surgical menopause had stronger link to sleep disturbance than natural menopause.
- Asian and white women had more increased sleep disturbance compared than other ethnic groups when comparing perimenopausal to premenopausal and postmenopausal to premenopausal stages.

Conclusions

- Sleep disturbance is associated with menopausal stage.
- Association between menopausal stage and sleep disturbance may be influenced by a women's ethnicity.

Implications for Nursing Practice

1. What would you advise a woman who is in the perimenopausal stage and asks if her sleep problems are "normal"?
2. Why is it important for health care professionals to be knowledgeable of menopausal attitudes and beliefs when caring for ethnically diverse women with sleep problems?

Reference for Evidence

Xu Q, Lang C: Examining the relationship between subjective sleep disturbance and menopause: a systematic review and meta-analysis, *Menopause* 21:1301, 2014.

P, Patient population of interest; *I*, intervention or area of interest; *C*, comparison of interest or comparison group; *O*, outcomes of interest; *T*, timing (see p. 15).

Interprofessional Care

The diagnosis of menopause should be made only after careful consideration of other possible causes for a woman's symptoms. Follicle-stimulating hormone (FSH) levels may be done to confirm a diagnosis of menopause. (The FSH levels are increased in menopause.) Because of the hormonal fluctuations that occur before menopause, routine testing of the serum FSH level to establish a diagnosis is not indicated until the woman has stopped menstruating for 12 months.

Drug Therapy. Hormone replacement therapy (HRT) using estrogen, with or without progesterone, is prescribed for some women. Women may choose to use HRT for short-term symptom management and treatment for several years (4 to 5 years) of menopausal symptoms. The risks (e.g., increased risk

of breast and endometrial cancer, risk for blood clots) and benefits (e.g., minimizes bone loss, hot flashes, vaginal atrophic changes) must be carefully considered for an individual woman.[6]

Nonhormonal Therapy. Because of the risks associated with HRT some women choose to use nonhormonal and nonpharmacologic interventions to manage their symptoms. If a woman does not want to use HRT but has significant menopausal symptoms, other nonhormonal pharmacologic agents may be used. For example, the SSRI antidepressants, paroxetine (Paxil, Brisdelle), fluoxetine, and venlafaxine (Effexor XR), are an effective alternative to HRT to reduce hot flashes.

Clonidine (Catapres), an antihypertensive drug, and gabapentin (Neurontin), an antiseizure drug, have also been shown to manage vasomotor symptoms during menopause. Selective estrogen receptor modulators (SERMs), such as raloxifene (Evista), are also used to manage menopausal symptoms. SERMs have positive benefits of estrogen, such as preventing bone loss, without the negative effects that include risk for endometrial hyperplasia.

Nutritional Therapy. Good nutrition can decrease the risk of cardiovascular disease and osteoporosis in addition to assisting with vasomotor symptoms. A decrease in metabolic rate and careless eating habits can cause the weight gain and fatigue often attributed to menopause. An adequate intake of calcium and vitamin D helps maintain healthy bones and counteracts loss of bone density.

Postmenopausal women not taking supplemental HRT should have a daily calcium intake of at least 1500 mg. Women taking estrogen replacement need at least 1000 mg/day. Calcium supplements are best absorbed when taken with meals. Either dietary calcium or calcium supplements may be used (see Table 63-14).

COMPLEMENTARY & ALTERNATIVE THERAPIES
Herbs and Supplements for Menopause

Herb	Scientific Evidence	Nursing Implications
Black cohosh	Mixed evidence for use in the treatment of menopausal symptoms*	• Generally well tolerated in recommended doses for up to 6 mo. • Should not be used in people with a liver disorder.
Soy	Mixed evidence for treatment of menopausal symptoms*	• Women with a history of breast, ovarian, or uterine cancer or endometriosis should consult with their HCP before using soy or soy products. • Soy may interact with warfarin. Patients taking warfarin should consult with their HCP before using soy or soy products.

Source: *www.nlm.nih.gov/medlineplus/herbalmedicine.html#summary*.
*In general, the evidence for use of these herbs as treatments for menopause symptoms is limited by a lack of well-designed, controlled trials.

❖ NURSING MANAGEMENT: PERIMENOPAUSE AND POSTMENOPAUSE

Menopause is a time of great transition for a woman both physically and psychologically. Many women experience symptoms for years during the perimenopausal period while others transition without any difficulty. In addition, menopause may be occurring simultaneously with role changes in the woman's personal and professional life. The combination of menopause and these changes can cause great emotional distress or a renewed sense of self and well-being.

Women in their perimenopausal and menopausal years need a lot of emotional support. Provide reassurance that symptoms can be treated and managed with either hormonal or non-hormonal therapies. It is also important to teach them about strategies to prevent or reduce the risk of cardiovascular disease and osteoporosis.

INFECTIONS OF LOWER GENITAL TRACT

Etiology and Pathophysiology

The female genital tract is susceptible to different types of infections, especially if the pH of the genital tract is altered. In most women, the vaginal pH is typically below 4.5, which helps prevent certain bacterial infections from occurring. The pH level of the vagina is maintained through a combination of sufficient levels of estrogen and *Lactobacillus,* a naturally occurring bacteria that colonizes the vagina.

Infection and inflammation of the vagina, cervix, and vulva commonly occur when estrogen levels decrease and/or the presence of *Lactobacillus* is disrupted. Aging, poor nutrition, and drugs (e.g., antibiotics, oral contraceptives, corticosteroids) can affect the bacterial flora or mucosa, leading to alterations in the pH balance of the genital tract. For example, *Candida albicans* may be present in small numbers in the vagina. However, some women who take an antibiotic for another type of infection may experience an overgrowth of *Candida albicans,* leading to a condition called *vulvovaginal candidiasis* (more commonly referred to as "yeast infection").

Organisms gain entrance to the lower genital tract through contaminated hands, clothing, douching, and intercourse. Most lower genital tract infections are related to sexual intercourse. Intercourse can transmit organisms, injure tissue, and alter the acid-base balance of the vagina.

Table 53-10 presents the causes, manifestations, and interprofessional care of common infections of the female lower genital tract.

Clinical Manifestations

The clinical manifestations of lower genital tract infections depend on the type of infection. Abnormal vaginal discharge and reddened vulvar lesions are common clinical manifestations. Women with vulvovaginal candidiasis have a curd-like discharge accompanied with intense itching and pain with urination. Women who have bacterial vaginosis often produce vaginal discharge that has a fishy odor. Women with cervicitis may notice spotting (bleeding) after intercourse.

Common vulvar lesions include herpes infection and genital warts. Initial or primary herpes infections may be extremely painful. Herpes infections begin as a small vesicle followed by a superficial red, painful, ulcer. Genital warts, caused by the human papillomavirus (HPV), vary in appearance. Irregularly shaped "cauliflower" lesions are common. Genital warts are painless unless traumatized. (Herpes infection and genital warts are discussed in Chapter 52.)

Postmenopausal women may develop vulvar changes such as *lichen sclerosis.* This chronic inflammatory skin condition is associated with intense itching in the genital skin area (e.g., labia minora, clitoris). Although the lesions are white with a "tissue paper" appearance initially, scratching produces changes in the appearance. The cause is unknown.

Interprofessional Care

Evaluation of genital problems includes a history, physical examination, and appropriate laboratory and diagnostic studies. Because many problems relate to sexual activity, a sexual history is essential. The nature of the problem determines the extent of the evaluation. When ulcerative lesions are present, an HCP will usually obtain a culture for herpes and a blood test for syphilis.

TABLE 53-10	**Infections of the Lower Genital Tract**	
Infection and Etiology	**Manifestations**	**Drug Therapy**
Vulvovaginal Candidiasis		
Candida albicans (fungus)	Pruritus, thick white curd-like discharge.	Antifungal agents (e.g., miconazole [Monistat], clotrimazole [Gyne-Lotrimin, Mycelex] [available over the counter, in cream or suppository]). Fluconazole (Diflucan). Terconazole (Terazol) vaginal creams and suppositories.
Trichomonas Vaginitis		
Trichomonas vaginalis (protozoa)	Sexually transmitted. Pruritus, frothy greenish or gray discharge. Hemorrhagic spots on cervix or vaginal walls.	Metronidazole (Flagyl) or tinidazole (Tindamax) for patient and partner.
Bacterial Vaginosis		
Gardnerella vaginalis *Corynebacterium vaginale*	Watery discharge with fish-like odor. May or may not have other symptoms.	Oral or vaginal metronidazole (Flagyl), vaginal clindamycin (Clindesse), or oral tinidazole (Tindamax). *Lactobacillus acidophilus* taken orally by diet (e.g., yogurt, fermented soy products) or supplements can decrease unwanted vaginal bacteria.
Cervicitis		
Chlamydia trachomatis or *Neisseria gonorrhoeae* (most often)	Sexually transmitted. Mucopurulent discharge with postcoital spotting from cervical inflammation.	Based on cause. Common treatment includes azithromycin (Zithromax) and ceftriaxone (Rocephin). Treat patient and partner.
Severe Recurrent Vaginitis (more than four episodes per year)		
C. albicans (most often) or non-*albicans* strains	May be indication of HIV infection. All women who are unresponsive to first-line treatment should be offered HIV testing.	Drug appropriate to opportunistic organism.

KOH, Potassium hydroxide.

Genital warts are usually identified by their clinical appearance. Vulvar skin conditions may be examined by colposcopy and biopsy of the skin lesion.

Problems involving vaginal discharge are evaluated by examining the discharge under a microscope and obtaining cultures. To assess for cervicitis, specimens are obtained for chlamydial infection and gonorrhea. (Sexually transmitted infections [STIs] are discussed in Chapter 52.)

Drug therapy is based on the diagnosis (Table 53-10). Antibiotics taken as directed will cure bacterial infections. Teach patients how to properly take their medications and get follow-up care. Partners should be treated so that reinfection does not occur.

Women with vaginal conditions or cervical infection should abstain from intercourse for at least 1 week. Douching should be avoided. Sexual partners must be evaluated and treated if the patient is diagnosed with trichomoniasis, chlamydial infection, gonorrhea, syphilis, or HIV.

Treatment of vulvar skin conditions is symptomatic because no cures are available. Treatment involves controlling the itching and hence the scratching. High-potency topical corticosteroid ointment such as clobetasol (Temovate) helps relieve itching. Interrupting the "itch-scratch cycle" prevents further secondary damage to the skin.

❖ NURSING MANAGEMENT: INFECTIONS OF LOWER GENITAL TRACT

Teach women about common infections of the genital tract and how to reduce their risks for infection. Recognize symptoms that indicate a problem, and help women seek care in a timely manner. Discussing problems that concern the patient's genitalia or sexual intercourse is frequently difficult. Use a nonjudgmental attitude to make women feel more comfortable while empowering them to ask questions.

When a woman is diagnosed with a genital infection, ensure that she fully understands the treatment. Taking the full course of medication is especially important to decrease the chance of relapse. Because genitalia are such a private area, the use of graphs and models is especially helpful for patient teaching. When a woman is using a vaginal medication for the first time, show her the applicator and how to fill it. Also teach where and how the applicator should be inserted using visual aids or models. Vaginal creams should be inserted before going to bed so that the medication will remain in the vagina for a long period. Women using vaginal creams or suppositories may wish to use panty liners during the day when the residual medication may drain out.

PELVIC INFLAMMATORY DISEASE (PID)

Pelvic inflammatory disease (PID) is an infectious condition of the pelvic cavity that may involve the fallopian tubes (salpingitis), ovaries (oophoritis), and pelvic peritoneum (peritonitis). A tubo-ovarian abscess may also form (Fig. 53-4).

Etiology and Pathophysiology

PID is often the result of untreated cervical infection. The organism infecting the cervix can spread into the uterus, fallopian tubes, ovaries, and peritoneal cavity. *Chlamydia trachomatis* and *Neisseria gonorrhoeae* are the most common causative organisms of PID.[7] These organisms, as well as anaerobes,

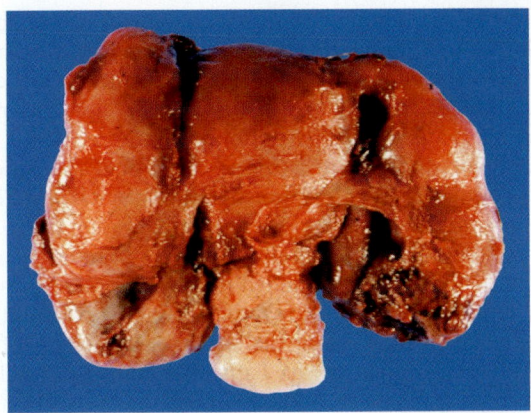

FIG. 53-4 Pelvic inflammatory disease. Acute infection of the fallopian tubes and the ovaries. The tubes and the ovaries have become an inflamed mass attached to the uterus. A tubo-ovarian abscess is also present. (From Kumar V, Abbas AK, Aster JC, Fausto N: *Robbins and Cotran pathologic basis of disease,* ed 8, Philadelphia, 2010, Saunders.)

mycoplasma, streptococci, and enteric gram-negative rods, gain entrance during sexual intercourse or after pregnancy termination, pelvic surgery, or childbirth. It is important to remember that not all cases of PID are the result of an STI.

Women at increased risk for chlamydial infections (e.g., younger than 24 years of age, have multiple sex partners, have a new sex partner) should be routinely tested for *Chlamydia*. Chlamydial infections can be asymptomatic and unknowingly transmitted during intercourse.

Clinical Manifestations

Lower abdominal pain is a common manifestation of PID. The pain typically starts gradually and then becomes constant. The intensity may vary from mild to severe. Movement such as walking can increase the pain. The pain is also frequently associated with intercourse. Spotting after intercourse and purulent cervical or vaginal discharge may also be noted. Fever and chills may be present.

Women with less acute symptoms often notice increased cramping pain with menses, irregular bleeding, and some pain with intercourse. Women who have mild symptoms may go untreated either because they did not seek care or the HCP misdiagnosed their complaints.

Complications

Complications of PID may include septic shock, perihepatitis, tubo-ovarian abscess, peritonitis, and embolism. PID can cause adhesions and strictures in the fallopian tubes, which may lead to ectopic pregnancy. After one episode of PID, the risk of having an ectopic pregnancy increases nearly 10 times. Further damage can obstruct the fallopian tubes and cause infertility.

Interprofessional Care

A pelvic examination assists in the diagnosis of PID. Women with PID have lower abdominal tenderness, adnexal tenderness, and positive cervical motion tenderness.

Diagnostic testing includes examination for *N. gonorrhoeae* and *C. trachomatis* and a pregnancy test to rule out an ectopic pregnancy. When the patient's pain or obesity compromises the pelvic examination, a vaginal ultrasound may be ordered.

PID is usually treated on an outpatient basis. The patient is given a combination of antibiotics to provide broad coverage against the causative organisms. With effective antibiotic therapy, the pain should subside. The patient should abstain from intercourse for 3 weeks. Her partner(s) must be examined and treated. An important part of care is physical rest and oral fluids. Reevaluation in 48 to 72 hours, even if symptoms are improving, is an essential part of outpatient care.

If outpatient treatment is unsuccessful or if the patient is acutely ill or in severe pain, admission to a hospital is indicated. If a tubo-ovarian abscess is present, hospitalization is also indicated. Maximum doses of IV antibiotics are given in the hospital. Corticosteroids may be added to the antibiotic regimen to reduce inflammation, allowing for faster recovery and optimizing the chances for subsequent fertility. Application of heat to the lower abdomen or sitz baths may improve circulation and decrease pain. Bed rest in a semi-Fowler's position promotes drainage of the pelvic cavity by gravity and may prevent the development of abscesses high in the abdomen. Analgesics to relieve pain and IV fluids to prevent dehydration are also used.

Surgery is indicated for abscesses that fail to resolve with IV antibiotics. The abscess may be drained by laparoscopy or laparotomy. In extreme cases of infection or severe chronic pelvic pain, a hysterectomy may be performed. When surgery is necessary, the capacity for childbearing is preserved whenever possible.

❖ NURSING MANAGEMENT: PELVIC INFLAMMATORY DISEASE

Subjective and objective data that should be obtained from the woman with PID are presented in Table 53-11. Prevention, early recognition, and prompt treatment of vaginal and cervical

TABLE 53-11   Nursing Assessment
Pelvic Inflammatory Disease
Subjective Data
Important Health Information
Past health history: Use of IUD. Previous PID, gonorrhea, or chlamydial infection. Multiple sexual partners. Exposure to partner with urethritis. Infertility
Medications: Use of and allergy to any antibiotics
Surgery or other treatments: Recent abortion or pelvic surgery
Functional Health Patterns
Health perception–health management: Malaise
Nutritional-metabolic: Nausea, vomiting; chills, fever
Elimination: Urinary frequency, urgency
Cognitive-perceptual: Lower abdominal and pelvic pain, low back pain, onset of pain just after a menstrual cycle. Dysmenorrhea, dyspareunia, dysuria, vulvar pruritus
Sexuality-reproductive: Abnormal vaginal bleeding and menstrual irregularity. Vaginal discharge
Objective Data
Reproductive
Mucopurulent cervicitis, vulvar maceration, vaginal discharge (heavy and purulent to thin and mucoid), tenderness on motion of cervix and uterus. Presence of inflammatory masses on palpation
Possible Diagnostic Findings
Leukocytosis, ↑ erythrocyte sedimentation rate, positive culture of secretions or endocervical fluid, pelvic inflammation and positive endometrial biopsy on laparoscopic examination, abscess or inflammation on ultrasonography

IUD, Intrauterine device; *PID,* pelvic inflammatory disease.

infections can help prevent PID and its serious complications. Provide accurate information about factors that place a woman at increased risk for PID. Urge women to seek medical attention for any unusual vaginal discharge or possible infection of their reproductive organs. Inform patients that not all vaginal discharge indicates infection, but early diagnosis and treatment of an infection, if present, can prevent serious complications. Teach patients methods to decrease the risk of getting STIs and to recognize the signs of infection in their partner(s).

The patient may feel guilty about having PID, especially if it is associated with an STI. She may also be concerned about the complications associated with PID, such as infertility, and the increased incidence of ectopic pregnancy. Discuss with the patient her feelings and concerns to help her cope with them more effectively.

For patients requiring hospitalization, you have an important role in implementing drug therapy, monitoring the patient's health status, and providing symptom relief and patient teaching. Record vital signs and the character, amount, color, and odor of the vaginal discharge. Explain the need for limiting activity, being in a semi-Fowler's position, and increasing fluid intake. Assess the degree of abdominal pain to determine the effectiveness of drug therapy.

CHRONIC PELVIC PAIN

Chronic pelvic pain refers to pain in the pelvic region (below the umbilicus and between the hips) that lasts 6 months or longer. The cause of chronic pelvic pain is often hard to find. Many different conditions can cause pelvic pain. Gynecologic etiologies include PID, endometriosis, ovarian cysts, uterine fibroids, pelvic adhesions, and ectopic pregnancies. Abdominal etiologies include irritable bowel syndrome, interstitial cystitis, appendicitis, and colitis. Psychologic factors (e.g., depression, chronic stress, history of sexual or physical abuse) may increase the risk of developing chronic pelvic pain. Emotional distress makes pain worse, and living with chronic pain contributes to emotional distress.

Chronic pelvic pain has many different clinical manifestations, including severe and steady pain, intermittent pain, dull and achy pain, pelvic pressure or heaviness, and sharp pain or cramping. In addition, pain may occur during intercourse or while having a bowel movement.

Determining the cause of chronic pelvic pain often involves a process of elimination. In addition to a detailed history and physical examination (including a pelvic examination), the patient may be asked to keep a journal of the onset of symptoms and any precipitating factors.

Diagnostic tests may include cultures from the cervix or vagina (used to detect STIs), ultrasound, CT scan, or MRI to detect abnormal structures or growths. Laparoscopy may be used to visualize the pelvic organs. This procedure is especially useful in detecting endometriosis and chronic PID.

If the cause of chronic pelvic pain is found, treatment focuses on that cause. If no cause can be found, treatment involves managing the pain. Over-the-counter pain medications (e.g., aspirin, ibuprofen, acetaminophen) may provide some relief. Sometimes stronger pain drugs may be needed. Birth control pills or other hormonal medications may help relieve cyclic pelvic pain related to menstrual cycles. If an infection is the source of the problem, antibiotics are used.

Tricyclic antidepressants (e.g., amitriptyline, nortriptyline [Pamelor]) have pain-relieving and antidepressant effects.

These drugs may help improve chronic pelvic pain even in women who do not have depression. The patient may be encouraged to get counseling for any emotional issues.

Laparoscopic surgery may be used to remove pelvic adhesions or endometrial tissue. As a last resort, a hysterectomy may be done.

ENDOMETRIOSIS

Endometriosis is a benign gynecologic condition in which endometrial tissue accumulates outside the endometrium. Endometriosis is a common gynecologic problem.

In endometriosis, the most frequent sites for endometrial tissue growth is in or near the ovaries, uterosacral ligaments, and uterovesical peritoneum (Fig. 53-5). The tissue responds to the hormones of the ovarian cycle and undergoes a "mini-menstrual cycle" similar to the uterine endometrium. Although it is not a life-threatening condition, endometriosis can cause considerable pain. Endometriosis can significantly affect a woman's quality of life and ability to conceive. It also increases the risk of ovarian cancer.

Etiology and Pathophysiology

Although the etiology of endometriosis is poorly understood, many theories have been proposed. Some of the theories include the possibility that the disorder may be due to retrograde (backward) flow of endometrial tissue. Instead of flowing out the cervix, the endometrial tissue flows through the fallopian tubes, depositing endometrial tissue into the pelvis.

Other theories have suggested that endometrial tissue is spread to the pelvic area through the lymph system or bloodstream. Another theory suggests that there is an increased sensitivity and production of prostaglandins, which are released prior to onset of menses. Other proposed causes include a genetic predisposition and altered immune function.

Clinical Manifestations

Patients with endometriosis have a wide range of clinical manifestations. The severity of symptoms does not always correlate with the degree of disease found. The most common manifestations are secondary dysmenorrhea, infertility, pelvic pain, painful intercourse, and irregular bleeding. Less common manifestations include backache, painful bowel movements, and pain with urination. With menopause, estrogen is no longer produced in the ovaries, and the symptoms may disappear.

Interprofessional Care

Endometriosis may be suspected based on a woman's history of the characteristic symptoms and the HCP's palpation of firm nodular lumps in the adnexa on bimanual examination. However, laparoscopy with a biopsy is necessary for a definitive diagnosis. MRI is now being used more frequently prior to surgery as a way to determine if the gynecologic symptoms the woman is experiencing are a result of endometriosis.

The treatment of endometriosis is influenced by the patient's age, desire for pregnancy, symptom severity, and extent and location of the disease. When symptoms are not disruptive, a "watch and wait" approach is used (Table 53-12). When endometriosis is identified as a probable cause of infertility, therapy proceeds more rapidly.

Drug Therapy. Drug therapy is used to reduce symptoms. Pain may be relieved with the use of NSAIDs such as ibuprofen, naproxen (Naprosyn), and diclofenac (Voltaren). The most common agent used to control symptoms and cause regression of endometrial tissue is combined oral contraceptives (OCPs). The continuous use of combined OCPs causes regression of endometrial tissue.

Another class of drugs used is GnRH agonists (e.g., leuprolide [Lupron], nafarelin [Synarel]). These drugs result in amenorrhea. Side effects are usually the same as those of menopause (hot flashes, vaginal dryness, emotional lability). Loss of bone density has also been reported in women who remain on the therapy longer than 6 months.

Endometriosis is controlled but not cured by drug therapy. Persistent lesions give rise to subsequent recurrences once the menstrual cycle is reestablished.

> **DRUG ALERT Leuprolide (Lupron)**
> - Assess patient for pregnancy before initiating therapy.
> - Monitor patient for dysrhythmias, palpitations.
> - Instruct patient to use nonhormonal contraceptive measures during therapy.

Surgical Therapy. The only cure for endometriosis is surgical removal of all endometrial tissue.[8] It involves removal or

TABLE 53-12 Interprofessional Care
Endometriosis

Diagnostic Assessment
- History and physical examination
- Pelvic examination
- Laparoscopy
- Pelvic ultrasound
- MRI

Management
Conservative Therapy
- Watch and wait

Drug Therapy
- Nonsteroidal antiinflammatory drugs (NSAIDs)
- Oral contraceptives
- danazol
- GnRH agonists (e.g., leuprolide [Lupron])

Surgical Therapy
- Laparotomy to remove implanted tissue and adhesions
- Total abdominal hysterectomy and bilateral salpingo-oophorectomy (TAH-BSO)

GnRH, Gonadotropin-releasing hormone.

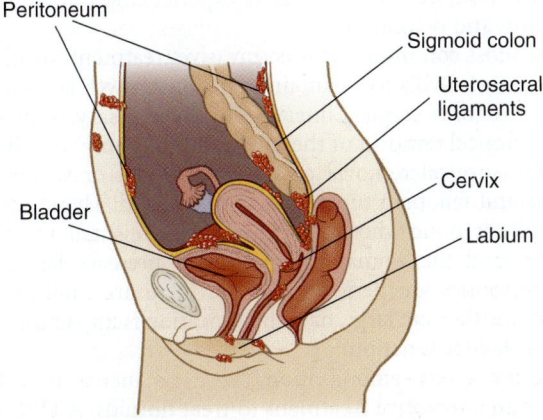
FIG. 53-5 Common sites of endometriosis.

Peritoneum

Sigmoid colon

Uterosacral ligaments

Cervix

Labium

Bladder

destruction of endometrial tissue and excision of adhesions by means of laparoscopic laser surgery or laparotomy. Definitive surgery involves removal of the uterus, fallopian tubes, ovaries, and as many endometrial implants as possible. GnRH agonist therapy can be given for 4 to 6 months to reduce the size of the lesions before surgery.

For women wishing to get pregnant, conservative surgical therapy is used to remove implants blocking the fallopian tube. Adhesions are removed from the tubes, ovaries, and pelvic structures. Efforts are made to conserve all tissues necessary to maintain fertility.

Patients should be actively involved in making the decision about preserving part or all of their ovaries, if surgically possible. Explore the patient's feelings about maintaining her ovarian function. The HCP should assess the woman's risk for ovarian cancer and provide this information for her consideration.

❖ NURSING MANAGEMENT: ENDOMETRIOSIS

Nursing care for the woman with endometriosis includes reassurance that endometriosis is not life threatening and treatment options exist. When the symptoms are less severe, teach the patient about comfort measures that may be helpful. If pharmacologic therapy is required, then teach her about the action and side effects of the prescribed medication. Psychologic support may be needed for women experiencing severe disabling pain, sexual difficulties secondary to dyspareunia, and infertility.

BENIGN TUMORS OF THE FEMALE REPRODUCTIVE SYSTEM

LEIOMYOMAS

Etiology and Pathophysiology

Leiomyomas (uterine fibroids) are benign smooth-muscle tumors (noncancerous) that occur during the childbearing years. Leiomyomas do not increase a woman's risk of endometrial cancer. They may be present inside the uterus within the endometrium, within the muscle of the uterus (myometrium), or outside on the surface of the uterus (subserosal). The size, shape, location, and number of leiomyomas vary among women. Some fibroids grow in spurts, while others slowly grow during the reproductive years (Fig. 53-6). Leiomyomas can

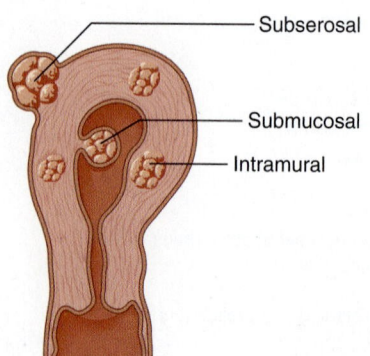

- Subserosal
- Submucosal
- Intramural

FIG. 53-6   Leiomyomas. Uterine section showing whorl-like appearance and locations of leiomyomas. (From McCance KL, Huether SE: *Pathophysiology: the biologic basis for disease in adults and children*, ed 6, St Louis, 2010, Mosby.)

occur at any age but are commonly found in women ages 30 to 40 years.

The etiology of leiomyomas is unknown. Their growth appears to depend on estrogen and progesterone because they grow during the reproductive years and undergo atrophy after menopause. In addition, leiomyomas contain more estrogen and progesterone receptors than normal uterine tissue. Thus they are more sensitive and grow in response to the release of these hormones.

In addition, genetics may play a role. Identical twins and women with mothers and sisters with leiomyomas have an increased risk. African American women seem to have increased incidence of leiomyomas and present with larger uterine fibroids and ones at an early age compared to other women. Other risk factors for fibroids include early age of menarche, alcohol use, and a diet high in red meat and low in green vegetables.

Clinical Manifestations

The majority of women who have uterine fibroids do not report any symptoms. Those who report clinical manifestations may have abnormal uterine bleeding (AUB), abdominal and pelvic pain (i.e., dull, heaving and or achy pain and with pelvic pressure), painful sexual intercourse, pressure or pain during urination, or frequent urination. If leiomyomas are large, some women will report constipation and difficulty passing stool. AUB can manifest as increased duration, more frequent, or increased menstrual bleeding. The pain associated with a leiomyoma seems to be caused from uterine blood vessel compression as the fibroid grows or from the fibroid pressing on surrounding organs.

❖ NURSING AND INTERPROFESSIONAL MANAGEMENT: LEIOMYOMAS

Clinical diagnosis is based on the characteristic pelvic examination findings of an enlarged uterus distorted by nodular masses. Ultrasound can confirm the diagnosis. In some cases, small leiomyomas are found during a hysteroscopy, laparoscopy, or hysterosalpingogram when a woman is having a comprehensive workup for other gynecologic conditions, especially infertility.

The treatment of uterine fibroids depends on the patient's clinical manifestations, patient's age, a woman's desire to conceive, and the location and size of the fibroid.[9] If the symptoms are minimal, the HCP may elect to follow the patient closely for a period of time. Treatment may be required if a woman is seeking conception, is experiencing AUB, has pelvic pain and pressure, has anemia, or if she is experiencing difficulty with urination and defecation.

The most common and least invasive treatment for fibroids is the use of OCPs to maintain and slow growth as well as to manage AUB. If surgical intervention is necessary, a myomectomy (surgical removal of the uterine fibroid only) or a hysterectomy (surgical removal of the uterus with or without the ovaries and fallopian tubes) may be indicated. Myomectomies are typically done when the leiomyomas are small and few in number and the woman would like to preserve her uterus. Hysterectomies are performed when there are multiple leiomyomas, if they are large, or if their location is impacting bowel and or bladder function.

Uterine artery embolization (UAE) is increasingly being used as an alternative treatment to treat fibroids. A UAE is the process by which embolic material (small plastic or gelatin beads) is injected into the uterine artery. This process blocks blood flow to the uterus and shrinks the fibroid.

OVARIAN CYSTS

Ovarian cysts are usually soft and surrounded by a thin capsule. Follicle and corpus luteum cysts are common ovarian cysts (Fig. 53-7). Multiple small ovarian follicles may occur in a condition called *polycystic ovary syndrome* (PCOS).

Ovarian cysts are often asymptomatic until they are large enough to cause pressure in the pelvis. Depending on the tumor's size and location, constipation, menstrual irregularities, urinary frequency, a full feeling in the abdomen, anorexia, an increase in abdominal girth, and peripheral edema may occur.

Pelvic pain may be present if the tumor is growing rapidly. Severe pain results when the cyst twists on its pedicle (ovarian torsion). In some cases, an ovarian cyst can rupture. A ruptured ovarian cyst is not only extremely painful, but it can lead to serious complications such as hemorrhage and infection.

Pelvic examination reveals a mass or an enlarged ovary. A pelvic ultrasound may be done to determine a diagnosis. In premenopausal women, ovarian cysts often resolve on their own. If the mass is cystic (does not appear cancerous) and smaller than 5 cm, the patient is asked to return for reexamination in 4 to 6 weeks. This is called "watchful waiting."

In postmenopausal women, watchful waiting may be an option depending on the results of the ultrasound. If the mass is cystic and greater than 5 cm or is solid, laparoscopic surgery or laparotomy is performed. Immediate surgery is necessary if ovarian torsion occurs, causing the ovary to rotate and cutting off circulation. Surgical techniques are used to save as much of the ovary as possible (if indicated).

Polycystic Ovary Syndrome

Polycystic ovary syndrome (PCOS) is a disorder that includes ovulatory dysfunction, polycystic ovaries, and hyperandrogenism.[10] It most commonly occurs in women under 30 years old and is a cause of infertility.

The etiology of this disorder is unknown and the treatment is based on symptoms. PCOS is thought to be due to the ovaries producing estrogen and excess testosterone but not progesterone. As a result of this hormonal imbalance, ovulation fails and multiple fluid-filled cysts develop from mature ovarian follicles (Fig. 53-8). Classic manifestations of PCOS include irregular menstrual periods, amenorrhea, hirsutism, and obesity (80% of women). Of these manifestations, obesity in particular has been associated with severe symptoms such as excess androgens, oligomenorrhea, amenorrhea, and infertility. Many women start with normal menstrual periods, which become irregular after 1 to 2 years, and then the periods become infrequent. If PCOS is left untreated, cardiovascular disease and abnormal insulin resistance with type 2 diabetes mellitus may develop.

Pelvic ultrasound reveals enlarged ovaries with multiple small cysts. Successful management includes early diagnosis and treatment to improve quality of life and decrease the risk of complications. OCPs are useful in regulating menstrual cycles. Hirsutism may be treated with spironolactone. Hyperandrogenism can be treated with flutamide and a GnRH agonist such as leuprolide. Metformin (Glucophage) reduces hyperinsulinemia, improves hyperandrogenism, and restores ovulation. For women wishing to become pregnant, fertility drugs (e.g., clomiphene [Clomid]) may be used to induce ovulation. If all other treatments are unsuccessful, a hysterectomy with bilateral salpingectomy and oophorectomy may be performed.

Nursing management of a woman with PCOS includes teaching about the importance of weight management and exercise to decrease insulin resistance. Obesity exacerbates the problems related to PCOS. Monitor lipid profile and fasting glucose levels. Hirsutism is cosmetically distressing for many women. Support the patient as she explores measures to remove unwanted hair (e.g., depilating agents, electrolysis). Stress the importance of regular follow-up care to monitor the effectiveness of therapy and to detect any complications.

CERVICAL POLYPS

Cervical polyps are benign pedunculated lesions that generally arise from the endocervical mucosa and are seen protruding through the cervical os during a speculum examination. Polyps are a characteristic bright cherry red and are soft and fragile. They are generally small, measuring less than 3 cm in length, and may be single or multiple. Their cause is unknown. Symptoms are usually not present, but intermenstrual bleeding after straining for a bowel movement and coitus can occur. Polyps are prone to infection.

When the polyp is small, it can be excised in an outpatient procedure. If the point of attachment of the polyp cannot be identified and is not accessible to cautery, a polypectomy is

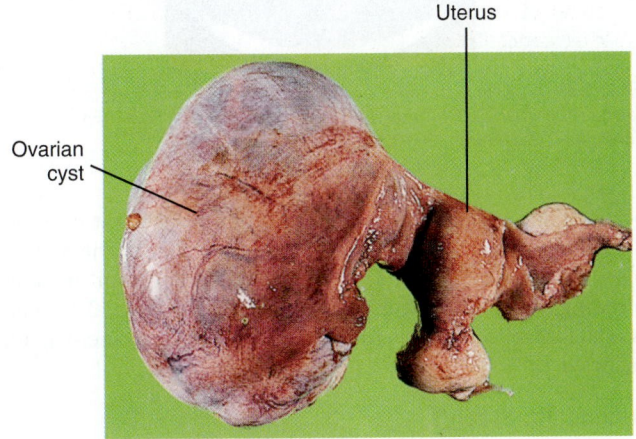

FIG. 53-7   Large ovarian cyst. (From Symonds EM, McPherson MBA: *Colour atlas of obstetrics and gynecology,* London, 1994, Mosby.)

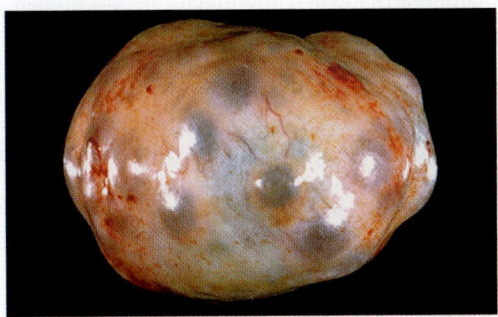

FIG. 53-8   Polycystic ovary syndrome. Multiple fluid-filled cysts in the ovary. (From Kumar V, Abbas A, Fausto N: *Robbins and Cotran pathologic basis of disease,* ed 7, Philadelphia, 2005, Saunders.)

performed in an operating room. All tissue removed is sent for pathologic review because polyps occasionally undergo malignant changes.

CANCERS OF THE FEMALE REPRODUCTIVE SYSTEM

CERVICAL CANCER

Approximately 12,900 women in the United States are diagnosed with cervical cancer and approximately 4100 women will die from cervical cancer each year. While Hispanic women are the most likely to be diagnosed with cervical cancer, African American women have the highest mortality rate from cervical cancer.[11]

Cervical cancer was once the most frequent cause of cancer death in women. However, with early detection (using Pap test), the mortality rate from cervical cancer has significantly declined.

🌐 CULTURAL & ETHNIC HEALTH DISPARITIES

Cancers of the Female Reproductive System

Ovarian Cancer
- Japanese women have a low incidence of ovarian cancer.
- However, second- and third-generation Japanese women in the United States have much higher rates, similar to those of white women born in the United States.

Endometrial Cancer
- Incidence is higher for white women and African American women than other ethnic groups.
- Mortality rate for African American women is nearly twice that of white women.

Cervical Cancer
- Incidence is higher among Hispanic, African American, and Native American women than among white women.
- Mortality rates are more than twice as high among African American women as among white women.

Etiology and Pathophysiology

Risk factors for cervical cancer include (1) infection with high-risk strains of human papillomavirus (HPV) 16 and 18, (2) immunosuppression, (3) low socioeconomic status, (4) chlamydia infection, and (5) smoking.[12]

The cervix is the lower third of the uterus that projects into the vagina and comprises glandular cells that line the uterine cavity and endocervical canal. Squamous epithelium lines the vagina and outer portion of the cervix. These two cell types meet and undergo a normal physiologic process known as *squamous metaplasia*, the transformation of columnar epithelium into squamous epithelium, resulting in an area called the *transformation zone*. This process begins at puberty and continues throughout a women's reproductive life cycle, with the transformation zone moving in and out the endocervical canal, depending upon her hormonal status and other factors. While the entire anogenital tract can be infected by HPV, the transformation zone is an area that is particularly susceptible to HPV-associated carcinogenesis.

Clinical Manifestations

Early cervical cancer generally has no symptoms. However, an unusual discharge, AUB, or postcoital bleeding eventually

---

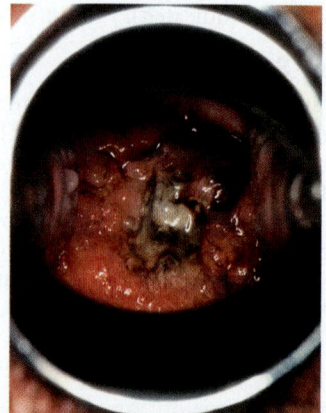

FIG. 53-9 Cervical cancer. View through a speculum inserted into the vagina. (From Drake RL, Vogl W, Mitchell AWM: *Gray's anatomy for students,* ed 2, Edinburgh, 2010, Churchill Livingstone.)

occurs. The discharge is usually thin and watery but becomes dark and foul smelling as the disease advances. The vaginal bleeding initially presents as spotting. As the tumor enlarges, bleeding becomes heavier and more frequent (Fig. 53-9). Pain is a late symptom and is followed by weight loss, anemia, and cachexia.

Diagnostic Studies

The two tests used for cervical cancer screening are the Papanicolaou (Pap) test and the HPV test. The Pap test identifies changes in cervical cells that may indicate precancerous changes. Cells are obtained from the cervix during a pelvic examination.

HPV testing can be used to identify the high-risk HPV types 16 and 18, which are associated with cervical cancer. To do the test, cervical scrapings are obtained and tested for viral DNA or RNA.

The use of these two tests to screen for cervical cancer may be referred to as cotesting. While the Pap test helps find cervical cell changes, the HPV test checks for the HPV virus that can cause these cell changes.

All women should begin cervical cancer screening at age 21. Women ages 21 to 29 years should get a Pap test every 3 years. Women between the ages of 30 and 65 should have a Pap test and HPV test every 5 years. This is the preferred approach, but the woman may choose to get a Pap test without an HPV test every 3 years.[13]

If both tests are negative, the risk for cervical cancer is very low and women can wait 5 years before another screening. HPV tests may also be used to provide more information when a Pap test has unclear results.

Women found to have an abnormal Pap test typically need a *colposcopy* (an examination of the cervical tissue under magnification). Typically a cervical biopsy is taken and sent for further analysis.

Interprofessional Care

Vaccination against HPV provides for primary prevention of cervical cancer. Inform both parents and patients about the need to complete the HPV vaccination series prior to first sexual contact.

Currently three vaccines are available to protect against HPV: (1) Gardasil protects against types 6, 11, 16, and 18; (2) Cervarix offers protection against HPV types 16 and 18; and (3) Gardasil 9 protects against HPV types 6, 11, 16, 18 and five other HPV types. These vaccines are given in three IM doses over a 6-month period and have few side effects. The CDC recommends that all children, males and females, be vaccinated at age 11 to 12, but vaccination can be started as early as age 9. (More specific information about HPV vaccines is discussed on p. 1234 in Chapter 52.)

Women diagnosed with cervical cancer are typically referred to an oncologist for treatment recommendations. Treatment options can include surgery or a combination of chemotherapy and radiation (Table 53-13). For patients with advanced disease, bevacizumab (Avastin), a targeted therapy drug, may be used in addition to cisplatin-based chemotherapy. Bevacizumab is an angiogenesis inhibitor and works by interfering with the blood vessels that supply nutrients to cancer cells. (Chemotherapy, radiation therapy, and targeted therapy are discussed in Chapter 15.)

ENDOMETRIAL CANCER

Endometrial cancer is the most common gynecologic malignancy. About 55,000 women are diagnosed each year with endometrial cancer, and 10,200 will die. If endometrial cancer is diagnosed in the early stage, it has a relatively low mortality rate, with survival rates over 95%.[11]

Etiology and Pathophysiology

The major risk factor for the development of endometrial cancer is exposure to estrogen, especially unopposed estrogen. Obesity is a risk factor because adipose cells store estrogen, thus

TABLE 53-13	**Staging and Treatment of Cervical Cancer**	
Stage	**Extent**	**Treatment**
0	In situ	Cervical conization, hysterectomy, cryosurgery, laser surgery
I	Confinement to cervix	Radiation, radical hysterectomy
II	Spread beyond cervix to upper two thirds of vagina but not to tissues around uterus	Radiation, cisplatin-based chemotherapy, radical hysterectomy
III	Spread to pelvic wall, involvement of lower third of vagina, and/or has caused kidney problems	Radiation, cisplatin-based chemotherapy
IV	Spread to other parts of the body such as bladder, rectum, liver, lungs, and bones	Radiation, surgery (e.g., pelvic exenteration), cisplatin-based chemotherapy

Modified from National Cancer Institute: Cancer cervical treatment: stages of cervical cancer. Retrieved from *www.cancer.gov/cancertopics/pdq/treatment/cervical/Patient/page2.*

increasing the amount of circulating estrogen. Additional risk factors include increasing age, never being pregnant, early menarche, late menopause, smoking, diabetes mellitus, and a personal or family history of hereditary nonpolyposis colorectal cancer (HNPCC) (see the Genetics in Clinical Practice box for HNPCC in Chapter 42 on p. 954). Pregnancy, use of oral contraceptives and IUDs, and physical exercise are associated with reduced risk.

Endometrial cancer arises from the lining of the endometrium within the uterus and most tumors are adenocarcinomas. If endometrial cancer is not diagnosed in early stages, it can invade the myometrium (muscle of the uterus) and the regional lymph nodes.

If metastasis occurs, the common sites include the lung, liver, bone, and brain. Prognosis depends on tumor size, cell type, degree of invasion into the myometrium, and any metastasis.[14]

Clinical Manifestations

Early clinical manifestations of endometrial cancer include abnormal uterine bleeding, especially in postmenopausal women. Later symptoms can include pain during urination or intercourse or in the pelvic area.

Interprofessional Care

No routine screening test is available for endometrial cancer. Most cases are diagnosed at an early stage because of postmenopausal bleeding.

An endometrial biopsy is the primary diagnostic test for identifying endometrial cancer. This procedure is typically performed in the office. For women who have or are at risk of developing HNPCC, the American Cancer Society recommends annual screening with an endometrial biopsy beginning at 35 years of age.[11]

Treatment of endometrial cancer in the early stage is a total hysterectomy and bilateral salpingo-oophorectomy with lymph node biopsies. (Various types of hysterectomies are shown in Fig. 53-10.) Surgery may be followed by external radiation either to the pelvis or abdomen or internal radiation (brachytherapy) intravaginally if there is local or distant metastasis.

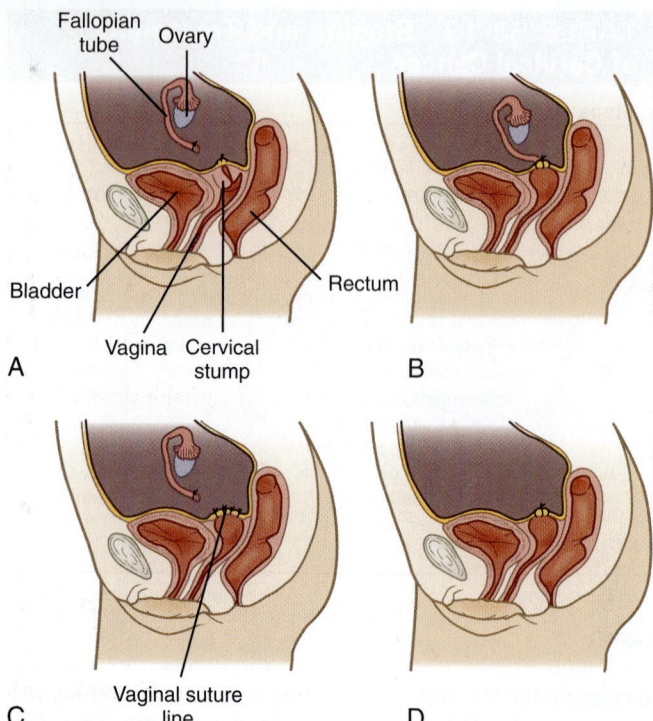

Fallopian tube   Ovary

Bladder

Rectum

Vagina   Cervical stump

A

B

Vaginal suture line

C

D

FIG. 53-10   Hysterectomies. **A,** Cross section of subtotal hysterectomy. Note that cervical stump, fallopian tubes, and ovaries remain. **B,** Cross section of total hysterectomy. Note that fallopian tubes and ovaries remain. **C,** Cross section of vaginal hysterectomy. Note that fallopian tubes and ovaries remain. **D,** Total hysterectomy, salpingectomy, and oophorectomy. Note that uterus, fallopian tubes, and ovaries are completely removed.

GENETICS IN CLINICAL PRACTICE

Ovarian Cancer

Genetic Basis
- Mutations in *BRCA1* and/or *BRCA2* genes.
- Normally these genes are tumor suppressor genes involved in DNA repair.
- Autosomal dominant transmission.
- Mutations passed down from either mother or father.

Incidence
- About 10% of cases of ovarian cancer are related to hereditary factors.
- Women with *BRCA1* mutations have a 25%-40% lifetime risk of developing ovarian cancer.
- Women with *BRCA2* mutations have a 10%-20% lifetime risk of developing ovarian cancer.
- Family history of both breast and ovarian cancer increases the risk of having a BRCA mutation.
- *BRCA* mutations occur in 10%-20% of patients with ovarian cancer who have no family history of breast or ovarian cancer.

Genetic Testing
- DNA testing is available for *BRCA1* and *BRCA2* genetic mutations.

Clinical Implications
- Bilateral oophorectomy reduces the risk of ovarian cancer in women with *BRCA1* and *BRCA2* mutations.
- Genetic counseling and testing for *BRCA* mutations should be considered for women whose personal or family history puts them at high risk for a genetic predisposition to ovarian cancer.

If the woman has advanced or recurrent disease, chemotherapy and hormonal therapy may be indicated. The 5- and 10-year survival rates are 82% and 79%, respectively.[11]

OVARIAN CANCER

Ovarian cancer is the most deadly gynecologic malignancy. Approximately 21,290 new cases of ovarian cancer are diagnosed each year, and about 14,200 women die. It is the fifth leading cause of cancer deaths in women in the United States. In most women, ovarian cancer is diagnosed when the disease is in the advanced stages.[11] It is most common in women between 55 and 65 years of age.

Etiology and Pathophysiology

The cause of ovarian cancer is not known. The major risk factor for ovarian cancer is family history (one or more first-degree relatives). A family history of breast or colon cancer is also a risk factor. Other risk factors include a personal history of breast or colon cancer and HNPCC (see the Genetics in Clinical Practice box on HNPCC in Chapter 42 on p. 954). **Genetic Link.** Women who have mutations of the *BRCA* genes have an increased susceptibility to ovarian cancer. The *BRCA* genes are tumor suppressor genes that inhibit tumor growth when functioning normally. When they mutate, they lose their tumor suppressor ability. This results in an increased risk for women to develop ovarian or breast cancer (see the Genetics in Clinical Practice box).

Women who have never been pregnant (nulliparity) are also at higher risk. Other risk factors include increasing age, high-fat diet, increased number of ovulatory cycles (usually associated with early menarche and late menopause), HRT, and possibly the use of infertility drugs.

Breastfeeding, multiple pregnancies, oral contraceptive use (more than 5 years), and early age at first birth seem to reduce the risk of ovarian cancer. These factors may have a protective effect because they reduce the number of ovulatory cycles and thus reduce the exposure to estrogen.

About 90% of ovarian cancers are epithelial carcinomas that arise from malignant transformation of the surface epithelial cells. Germ cell tumors account for another 10%. Histologic grading is important to determine the prognosis of the disease. Tumor cells are graded according to the level of differentiation, ranging from well differentiated (grade I) to poorly differentiated (grade III) to undifferentiated (grade IV). Grade IV cells have a poorer prognosis than the other grades.

Intraperitoneal dissemination is a common characteristic of ovarian cancer. It metastasizes to the uterus, bladder, bowel, and omentum. In advanced disease, it can spread to the stomach, colon, liver, and other parts of the body.

Clinical Manifestations

Early ovarian cancer usually has no obvious symptoms. Most clinical manifestations are vague and nonspecific. These include pelvic or abdominal pain, bloating, urinary urgency or frequency, and difficulty eating or feeling full quickly. Late stage disease typically presents with abdominal enlargement with ascites (fluid in the abdominal cavity), unexplained weight loss or gain, and menstrual changes.

Diagnostic Studies

No accurate screening test exists for early detection of ovarian cancer. Since early ovarian cancer has vague symptoms, yearly

TABLE 53-14	**Interprofessional Care**

Ovarian Cancer

Diagnostic Assessment
- History and physical examination
- Pelvic examination
- Abdominal and transvaginal ultrasound
- CA-125 level
- Laparotomy for diagnostic staging

Management
- Surgery
  - Abdominal hysterectomy and bilateral salpingo-oophorectomy with pelvic lymph node biopsies
  - Debulking for advanced disease
- Chemotherapy
  - Adjuvant and palliative
- Radiation therapy
  - Adjuvant and palliative

bimanual pelvic examinations should be performed to identify an ovarian mass (Table 53-14). Postmenopausal women should not have palpable ovaries, so a mass of any size should be considered suspicious. An abdominal or a transvaginal ultrasound can be done to detect ovarian masses. An exploratory laparotomy may be used to establish the diagnosis and stage the disease.

For women at high risk for ovarian cancer, screening using a combination of the tumor marker CA-125 and ultrasound is often recommended in addition to a yearly pelvic examination. The CA-125 test is positive in 80% of women with epithelial ovarian cancer. CA-125 is also used to monitor the course of the disease and response to treatment. Of concern is that levels of CA-125 may be elevated with other malignancies (e.g., pancreatic cancer) or with benign gynecologic conditions such as fibroids or endometriosis.

Interprofessional Care

Options for women identified as being at high risk based on family and health history include prophylactic removal of the ovaries and fallopian tubes and the use of OCPs.[15] Although oophorectomy significantly reduces the risk of ovarian cancer, it does not completely eliminate the possibility of the disease in the peritoneum.

The initial treatment for all stages of ovarian cancer is a total abdominal hysterectomy and bilateral salpingo-oophorectomy with omentectomy and removal of as much of the tumor as possible (i.e., tumor debulking). Depending on the differentiation of the cells and the stage of cancer, treatment options include intraperitoneal and systemic chemotherapy, intraperitoneal instillation of radioisotopes, and external abdominal and pelvic radiation therapy. The chemotherapy agents most commonly used are taxanes (paclitaxel or docetaxel) and platinum agents (carboplatin or cisplatin). (See Table 15-7 for a discussion of these drugs.)

Targeted therapy that is used to treat advanced ovarian cancer includes Bevacizumab (Avastin) (discussed on p. 1257) and olaparib (Lynparza). Olaparib is a poly ADP-ribose polymerase (PARP) inhibitor that blocks enzymes involved in repairing damaged DNA. It used for women with ovarian cancer that is associated with defective *BRCA* genes.

Overall the 5- and 10-year survival rates are 45% and 35%, respectively. The majority of patients with ovarian cancer are

diagnosed when the disease is advanced, for which the 5-year survival rate is 27%.[11]

VAGINAL CANCER

Vaginal cancers are rare, with about 4000 new cases reported annually.[11] They are usually found in women between ages 50 and 70. Vaginal tumors can be secondary sites or metastases of other gynecologic cancers, such as cervical or endometrial cancer. The most common type of vaginal cancer is squamous cell carcinoma. Intrauterine exposure to diethylstilbestrol (DES) places a woman at risk for clear cell adenocarcinoma of the vagina.

Treatment of vaginal cancer depends on the type of cells involved, stage of the disease, and the size and location of the tumor. Squamous cell carcinomas can be treated with both surgery and radiation.

VULVAR CANCER

Vulvar cancer is relatively rare, with about 5150 new cases reported annually.[11] Preinvasive lesions referred to as *vulvar intraepithelial neoplasia (VIN)* precede invasive vulvar cancer. The invasive form occurs mainly in women over 60 years of age, with the highest incidence being in women in their 70s.

Patients with vulvar cancer may have symptoms of vulvar itching or burning, pain, bleeding, or discharge. Women who are immunosuppressed and/or have diabetes mellitus, hypertension, or chronic vulvar dystrophies are at a higher risk for developing vulvar cancers. HPV DNA have been identified in some but not all vulvar cancers.

Diagnosis of vulvar cancer is based on physical examination, colposcopy, and biopsy results of the suspicious lesion. VIN can be treated topically with imiquimod cream (Aldara) or laser surgery. Surgery is the most common treatment for vulvar cancer with the goal to remove all the cancer without any loss of the woman's sexual function. In some cases, surgery to remove the lesion is performed.

If a woman has extensive lesions, a vulvectomy is recommended. Various types of vulvectomies are presented in Table 53-15. As adjuvant measures, the patient may have chemotherapy or radiation therapy after surgery.

❖ NURSING AND INTERPROFESSIONAL MANAGEMENT: CANCERS OF FEMALE REPRODUCTIVE SYSTEM

◆ Nursing Assessment

Malignant tumors of the female reproductive system can be found in the cervix, endometrium, ovaries, vagina, and vulva. A patient with any of these malignant tumors may experience a variety of clinical manifestations, including leukorrhea, irregular vaginal bleeding, vaginal discharge, abdominal pain and pressure, bowel and bladder dysfunction, and vulvar itching and burning. Assessment for these signs and symptoms is an important nursing responsibility.

◆ Nursing Diagnoses

Nursing diagnoses for the female patient with cancer of the reproductive system include, but are not limited to, the following:
- Anxiety *related to* threat of a malignancy and lack of knowledge about the disease process and prognosis

TABLE 53-15 Surgical Procedures Involving the Female Reproductive System

Type of Surgery	Description
Hysterectomy	
Total abdominal hysterectomy (TAH)	Uterus and cervix removed using abdominal incision (bikini cut).
Total abdominal hysterectomy and bilateral salpingo-oophorectomy (TAH-BSO)	Uterus, cervix, fallopian tubes, and ovaries removed using abdominal incision.
Radical hysterectomy	Panhysterectomy, partial vaginectomy, and dissection of lymph nodes in pelvis.
Vaginal hysterectomy	Uterus and cervix removed through a cut in the top of vagina.
Laparoscopic hysterectomy	Laparoscope (video camera and small surgical instruments).
• Laparoscopic-assisted vaginal hysterectomy (LAVH)	Incision made at top of vagina. Uterus and cervix removed through the vagina. Laparoscope inserted into abdomen to assist in the procedure.
• Laparoscopic supracervical hysterectomy	Uterus removed using only laparoscopic instruments. Cervix is left intact.
Myomectomy	Surgical removal of fibroid from the uterus, leaving the uterus in place.
Vulvectomy	Surgical procedure to remove part or all of the vulva.
• Skinning vulvectomy	Removal of top layer of vulvar skin where the cancer is found. Skin grafts from other parts of the body may be needed to cover the area.
• Simple vulvectomy	Entire vulva is removed.
• Radical vulvectomy	Entire vulva, including clitoris, labia majora and minora, and nearby tissue, is removed. Nearby lymph nodes may also be removed.
Vaginectomy	Removal of vagina.
Pelvic exenteration	Radical hysterectomy, total vaginectomy, removal of bladder with diversion of urinary system and resection of colon and rectum with colostomy.
Dilation and curettage	Dilation of cervix and scraping of endometrium.

- Acute pain *related to* pressure secondary to an enlarging tumor
- Disturbed body image *related to* loss of body part and loss of good health
- Ineffective sexuality pattern *related to* physiologic limitations and fatigue
- Grieving *related to* poor prognosis of advanced disease

◆ Planning

The overall goals are that the patient with cancer of the female reproductive system will (1) actively participate in treatment decisions, (2) achieve satisfactory pain and symptom management, (3) recognize and report problems promptly, (4) maintain preferred lifestyle as long as possible, and (5) continue to practice cancer detection strategies.

◆ Nursing Implementation

◆ Health Promotion. Through your contact with women in a variety of settings, teach women the importance of routine screening for cancers of the reproductive system. Cancer can be prevented when screening reveals precancerous conditions of the vulva, cervix, endometrium, and, rarely, the ovaries. Also routine screening increases the chance that a cancer will be found in an early stage.

Teaching women about risk factors for cancers of the reproductive system is also important. Limiting sexual activity during adolescence, using condoms, having fewer sexual partners, and not smoking reduce the risk of cervical cancer. When high-risk behaviors are identified, assist women in modifying their lifestyles to decrease risk.

⍰ CHECK YOUR PRACTICE

You are working in the preoperative surgery holding unit. Your patient is a 42-yr-old woman who is scheduled for a total abdominal hysterectomy for endometrial cancer. When you ask her how she is doing, she tells you that she's worried because "life will never be the same."

- How would you approach this situation? What do you think are her major concerns?

◆ Acute Intervention Related to Surgery. Various types of surgery of the female reproductive tract are presented in Table 53-15 and Fig. 53-10. All patients experience a degree of anxiety when contemplating surgery, but the prospect of major gynecologic surgery increases these concerns. Some women are relieved by the thought of no longer having menstrual periods or becoming pregnant.

Some women may focus on the effect the surgery will have on their reproductive and sexual functions. The ability to bear children may be associated with her perception of womanhood. Grief from this loss is normal.

Elicit the woman's feelings and concerns about her surgery. Assess each patient individually. Be willing to listen, since this can provide considerable psychologic support.

Preoperatively, prepare the patient physically for surgery with the standard perineal or abdominal preparation. A vaginal douche and enema may be given (based on the surgeon's preference). The bladder should be emptied before the patient is sent to the operating room. An indwelling catheter is commonly inserted preoperatively.

◆ Hysterectomy. Following a hysterectomy, abdominal distention may develop from the sudden release of pressure on the intestines when a large tumor is removed or from paralytic ileus secondary to anesthesia and pressure on the bowel. Food and fluids may be restricted if the patient is nauseated. Ambulation will help relieve flatus.

Take special care to prevent the development of deep vein thrombosis (DVT). Frequent changes of position, avoidance of the high Fowler's position, and avoidance of pressure under the knees minimize stasis and pooling of blood. Pay special attention to patients with varicosities. Encourage leg exercises to promote circulation.

Teach the patient what to expect after surgery (e.g., she will not menstruate). Instructions should include specific activity restrictions. Intercourse should be avoided until the wound is healed (about 4 to 6 weeks). However, intercourse is not contraindicated once healing is complete.

If a vaginal hysterectomy is performed, inform the patient that she may have a temporary loss of vaginal sensation. Reassure her that the sensation will return in several months.

Physical restrictions are limited for a short time. Heavy lifting should be avoided for 2 months. Teach her to avoid activities that may increase pelvic congestion, such as dancing and walking swiftly, for several months. However, activities such as swimming may be both physically and mentally helpful. Assure her that once healing is complete, all previous activity can be resumed.

◆ *Salpingectomy and Oophorectomy.* Postoperative care of the woman who has undergone removal of a fallopian tube (salpingectomy) or an ovary (oophorectomy) is similar to that for any patient having abdominal surgery. However, if a large ovarian cyst is removed, she may have abdominal distention caused by the sudden release of pressure in the intestines. An abdominal binder may provide relief until the distention subsides.

When both ovaries are removed (bilateral oophorectomy), surgical menopause results. The symptoms are similar to those of regular menopause but may be more severe because of the sudden withdrawal of hormones.

◆ *Vulvectomy.* It is important to recognize the extent of the vulvectomy and the significant effect it is likely to have on the patient's life. Because the surgery causes mutilation of the perineal area and the healing process is slow, the patient is likely to become discouraged. Provide opportunities for the patient to express her feelings and concerns about the operation.

Special attention to bowel and bladder care is needed. A low-residue diet and stool softeners prevent straining and wound contamination. An indwelling catheter is used to provide urinary drainage. Be careful not to dislodge the catheter because extensive edema makes its reinsertion difficult. Heavy, taut sutures are often used to close the wounds, resulting in severe discomfort. In other instances, the wound may be allowed to heal by granulation. Analgesics may be required to control pain. Carefully position the patient using strategically placed pillows to provide comfort. Anticoagulant therapy to prevent DVTs is commonly used.

Teach the patient specific instructions in self-care before discharge. Instruct her to report any unusual odor, fresh bleeding, breakdown of incision, or perineal pain. Home care nursing can benefit the patient during her adjustment period.

Sexual function is often retained. Whether clitoral sensation is retained may be critical to some women, particularly if it was a primary source of orgasmic satisfaction. Discussing alternative methods of achieving sexual satisfaction may be indicated.

◆ *Pelvic Exenteration.* When other forms of therapy fail to control the spread of cancer and no metastases have been found outside of the pelvis, pelvic exenteration may be performed. This radical surgery usually involves removal of the uterus, ovaries, fallopian tubes, vagina, bladder, urethra, and pelvic lymph nodes (Fig. 53-11). In some situations, the descending colon, rectum, and anal canal may also be removed. Candidates for this procedure are selected on the basis of their likelihood

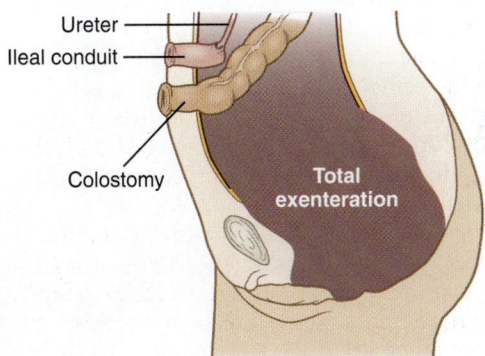

FIG. 53-11 Total exenteration is removal of all pelvic organs with creation of an ileal conduit and a colostomy.

of surviving the surgery and their ability to adjust to and accept the resulting limitations.

Postoperative care is similar to that of a patient who has had a radical hysterectomy, an abdominal perineal resection, and an ileostomy or a colostomy. The physical, emotional, and social adjustments to life required by the woman and her family are great. There are urinary or fecal diversions in the abdominal wall, a reconstructed vagina, and the onset of menopausal symptoms.

Assess the patient's physical and emotional adjustment to the changes in body image produced by the surgery and her ability to carry out any treatment measures. The patient's rehabilitative process should keep pace with her acceptance of the situation. You need to provide understanding and support during a long recovery period. Gently encourage the patient to regain her independence. She needs to verbalize her feelings about her altered body structure. Include her caregiver and family in the plan of care. Careful follow-up monitoring is needed so that early recurrence of the cancer can be identified and treated.

◆ **Acute Intervention With Radiation Therapy.** Instruct the patient who is to receive external radiation to urinate immediately before the treatment to minimize radiation exposure to the bladder. Advise her about radiation side effects, including enteritis and cystitis. These are natural reactions to radiation therapy and do not indicate an overdose. Fully inform the patient of the possible side effects and measures that can be used to reduce their impact.

Nursing management of the patient receiving internal radiation therapy requires special considerations. Do not stay in the immediate area any longer than is necessary to give proper care and attention. (Radiation therapy is discussed in Chapter 15.)

◆ **Evaluation**

The expected outcomes are that the patient with cancer of the female reproductive system will

- Actively participate in treatment decisions
- Achieve satisfactory pain and symptom management
- Recognize and report problems promptly
- Maintain preferred lifestyle as long as possible
- Continue to practice cancer detection strategies

PELVIC ORGAN PROLAPSE

The most common problems with pelvic support are uterine prolapse, cystocele, and rectocele. Although vaginal birth increases the risk for these problems, these conditions can occur in women who have never experienced childbirth. Obesity, chronic coughing, and straining during bowel movements can increase the likelihood of these problems. The decreased estrogen that normally accompanies perimenopause also decreases connective tissue support.

UTERINE PROLAPSE

Uterine prolapse is the downward displacement of the uterus into the vaginal canal (Fig. 53-12). Prolapse is rated by degrees. In first-degree prolapse the cervix rests in the lower part of the vagina. Second-degree prolapse means the cervix is at the vaginal opening. Third-degree prolapse means the uterus protrudes through the introitus.

Symptoms vary with the degree of prolapse. The patient may describe a feeling of "something coming down." She may have

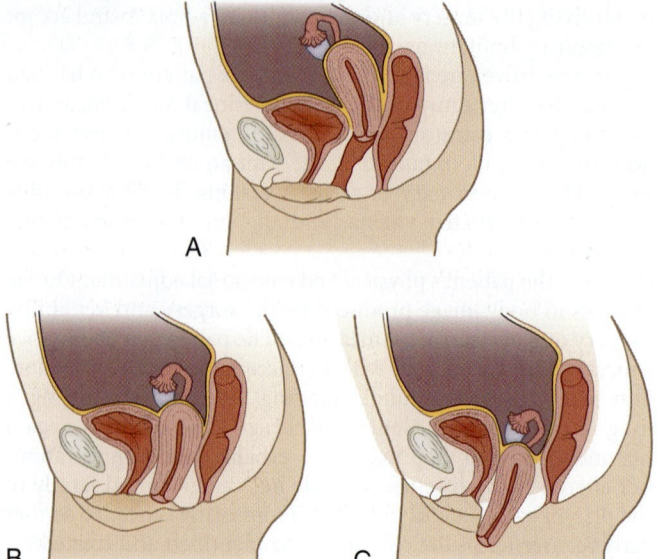

FIG. 53-12   Uterine prolapse. **A,** First-degree prolapse. **B,** Second-degree prolapse. **C,** Third-degree prolapse.

dyspareunia, a dragging or heavy feeling in the pelvis, backache, and bowel or bladder problems if a cystocele or rectocele is also present. Stress incontinence is a common and troubling problem. When third-degree uterine prolapse occurs, the protruding cervix and vaginal walls are subjected to constant irritation, and tissue changes may occur.

Therapy depends on the degree of prolapse and how much the woman's daily activities have been affected.[16] Pelvic muscle strengthening exercises (Kegel exercises) may be effective for some women (see Table 45-18). If not, a pessary may be used. A *pessary* is a device that is placed in the vagina to help support the uterus.[17] A wide variety of shapes exist, including rings, arches, and balls. Most are made of plastic or wire coated with plastic. When a woman first receives a pessary, she needs instructions on how to clean it. Pessaries that are left in place for long periods are associated with erosion, fistulas, and vaginal carcinoma.

If more conservative measures are not successful, surgery is indicated. Surgery generally involves a vaginal hysterectomy with anterior and posterior repair of the vagina and the underlying fascia.

CYSTOCELE AND RECTOCELE

Cystocele occurs when support between the vagina and bladder is weakened (Fig. 53-13). Similarly, a *rectocele* results from weakening between the vagina and rectum (Fig. 53-14). Cystocele and rectocele are common problems, and in many women they are asymptomatic.[18] With large cystoceles, complete emptying of the bladder can be difficult, predisposing women to bladder infections. A woman with a large rectocele may not be able to completely empty her rectum when defecating unless she helps push the stool out by putting her fingers in her vagina.

As with uterine prolapse, Kegel exercises (see Table 45-18) may be used to strengthen the weakened perineal muscles if the cystocele or rectocele is not too problematic. A pessary may be helpful for cystoceles.

Surgery designed to tighten the vaginal wall (colporrhaphy) is generally the method of treatment. A cystocele is corrected with a procedure called an *anterior colporrhaphy,* whereas a posterior colporrhaphy is done for a rectocele. If further surgery

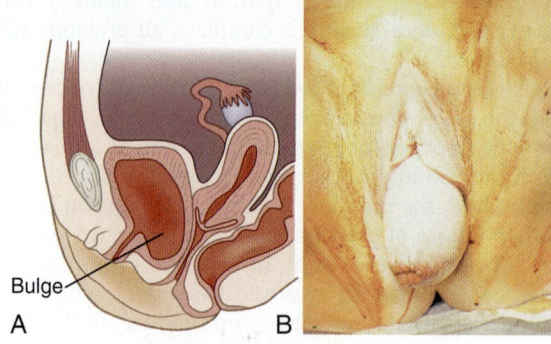

FIG. 53-13   **A,** Cystocele. **B,** Bladder has prolapsed into the vagina, causing a uterine prolapse.

is needed to relieve stress incontinence, procedures to support the urethra and restore the proper angle between the urethra and the posterior bladder wall are used.

❖ NURSING AND INTERPROFESSIONAL MANAGEMENT: PELVIC ORGAN PROLAPSE

Assist women to avoid or decrease problems with pelvic support by teaching them how to do Kegel exercises.[19] Women of all ages may benefit from these exercises. Instruct the patient to pull in or contract her muscles as if she were trying to stop the flow of urine, control the passing of gas, or pinch off a stool (see Table 45-18).

If vaginal surgery is necessary, the preoperative preparation usually includes a cleansing douche the morning of surgery. A cleansing enema is usually given when a rectocele repair is scheduled. A perineal shave may be done.

In the postoperative period, the goals of care are to prevent wound infection and pressure on the vaginal suture line. Perineal care must be done at least twice a day and after each urination or defecation. Apply an ice pack locally to help relieve the initial perineal discomfort and swelling. A disposable glove filled with ice and covered with a cloth works well to create an ice pack. Later, sitz baths may be used.

After an anterior colporrhaphy, an indwelling catheter is usually left in the bladder for 4 days to allow the local edema to subside. The catheter keeps the bladder empty, preventing strain on the sutures. Twice-daily catheter care with an antiseptic is generally done. To prevent constipation after a posterior colporrhaphy, a high-fiber diet and stool softener may be used.

Review discharge instructions before the patient leaves the hospital. These include the (1) use of douches or a mild laxative

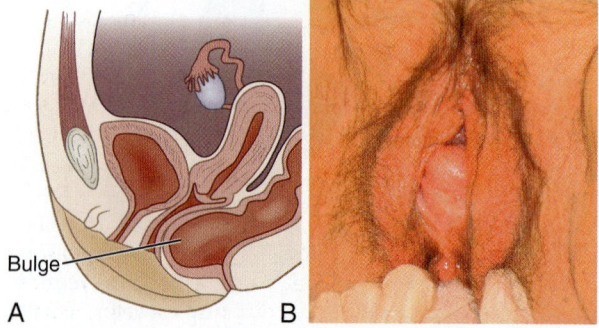

FIG. 53-14   **A,** Rectocele. **B,** Rectum has prolapsed into the vagina. (*B,* From Townsend CM: *Sabiston textbook of surgery,* ed 18, St Louis, 2009, Mosby.)

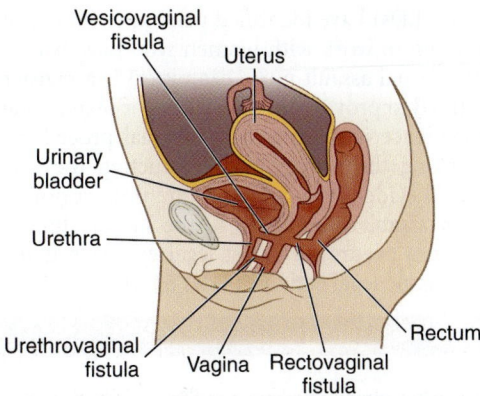

FIG. 53-15 Common fistulas involving the vagina.

as needed; (2) restrictions on heavy lifting and prolonged standing, walking, or sitting; and (3) avoidance of intercourse until the HCP gives permission. There may be a temporary loss of vaginal sensation, which can last for several months.

FISTULA

A *fistula* is an abnormal opening between internal organs or between an organ and the exterior of the body (Fig. 53-15). Gynecologic procedures cause most urinary tract fistulas. Other causes include injury during childbirth and disease processes, such as cancer. Fistulas may develop between the vagina and bladder, urethra, ureter, or rectum. When *vesicovaginal* fistulas (between the bladder and vagina) develop, some urine leaks into the vagina, whereas with *rectovaginal* fistulas (between the rectum and vagina), flatus and feces escape into the vagina. In both instances, excoriation and irritation of the vaginal and vulvar tissues occur and may lead to severe infections. In addition to wetness, offensive odors may develop, causing embarrassment and severely limiting socialization.

❖ NURSING AND INTERPROFESSIONAL MANAGEMENT: FISTULAS

Because small fistulas may heal spontaneously within a matter of months, treatment may not be needed. If the fistula does not heal, surgical repair is required. Inflammation and tissue edema must be eliminated before surgery is attempted, which may involve a wait of many months. The fistulectomy may result in the patient's having an ileal conduit or temporary colostomy. (See Chapter 45 for care of a patient with an ileal conduit and Chapter 42 for care of a patient with a colostomy.)

Surgical repair of fistulas is not always effective, even in the best conditions. Therefore supportive nursing care for the patient and her significant others is especially important.[20]

Perineal hygiene is of great importance both preoperatively and postoperatively. Cleanse the perineum every 4 hours. Warm sitz baths should be taken three times daily if possible. Change perineal pads frequently. Encourage the patient to maintain an adequate fluid intake.

Encouragement and reassurance are needed to help the patient cope with her problems. Postoperatively emphasize the avoidance of stress on the repaired areas and prevention of infection. Take care so that the indwelling catheter, usually in place for 7 to 10 days, is draining at all times. Urge oral fluids to provide for internal catheter irrigation. Use minimal pressure and strict asepsis if catheter irrigation becomes necessary.

The first stool after bowel surgery may be purposely delayed to prevent contamination of the wound. Later, give stool softeners or mild laxatives (as ordered).

SEXUAL ASSAULT

Sexual assault is the forcible perpetration of a sexual act on a person without his or her consent. It is a crime of violence and aggression. It can include any of the following actions: sodomy (anal or oral copulation with a person of the same or opposite sex), forced vaginal intercourse, assault with a foreign object, unwanted kissing, touching, or fondling as well as serial battery and rape. The Federal Bureau of Investigation's (FBI) definition of *rape* includes female or male victims who have experienced sexual assault that includes oral or anal penetration.

Sexual assault may be committed by a stranger or by an intimate partner. *Intimate partner violence (IPV)* is a major health problem in the United States.[21] Sexual assault that is perpetrated by a family member is termed *incest*. *Statutory rape* is consensual sexual intercourse with someone younger than a specific age. This age usually varies state to state, but most states use the criteria of a person younger than 16 years of age. Most states consider that an adolescent who is 16 years of age or older can consent to consensual sexual intercourse.

The involvement of children 14 years of age or younger in sexual activity either consensual or forced is termed *child sexual abuse*. Child sexual abuse is defined as the employment, persuasion, inducement, or enticement or even coercion of a person younger than 14 years of age in any sexually explicit conduct or simulation of sexual conduct. It also includes behaviors that are forced onto the child for the purpose of production of video material as well as rape, molestation, prostitution, or other forms of exploitation of children involving any sexual behavior.

Approximately 1.3 million rape or rape-related assaults occur to women annually. Approximately 18% of women reported that they had been victims of an attempted or completed rape during their lifetime. Most (80%) reported that they were victimized before the age of 25. Survivors suffer an array of physical and psychologic health consequences.[21]

Clinical Manifestations

Physical. Some female victims of assault experience more injuries than others. Factors that influence the severity of injury include the woman's age, if the perpetrator used a weapon, and if the victim knew the perpetrator. Physical injuries may include fractures, subdural hematomas, cerebral concussions, and intraabdominal injuries. In addition, sexual injuries may include bruising and lacerations of the perineum, hymen, vulva, vagina, cervix, and anus. Sexual assault also places women at risk for STIs and pregnancy.

Psychologic. Immediately after the assault, women may demonstrate signs of shock, numbness, denial, or withdrawal. Some women may seem unnaturally calm, while others may cry or express anger. Feelings of humiliation, degradation, embarrassment, anger, self-blame, and fear of another assault are commonly expressed.

These symptoms usually decrease after 2 weeks, and victims may appear to have adjusted. Yet any time from 2 to 3 weeks to months or years after the assault, symptoms may return and become more severe.

Rape trauma syndrome is a classification of posttraumatic stress disorder. Flashbacks, intrusive recall, sleep disturbances, gastrointestinal symptoms, and numbing of feelings are common initial symptoms. Women feel embarrassment, self-blame, and powerlessness. Later symptoms include mood swings, irritability, and anger. Feelings of despair, shame, and hopelessness may be internalized and lead to depression, and the risk of suicide may increase.[22]

Interprofessional Care

The highest priority for the victim of assault is her emotional and physical safety. Table 53-16 outlines the emergency management of the patient who has been sexually assaulted. Most emergency departments (EDs) have identified personnel who have received special training to work with women who have been assaulted. The SANE (sexual assault nurse examiner) is a registered nurse who is certified to provide care to victims of sexual assault, while ensuring evidence is safeguarded.[23] Special procedures are followed in taking the history and conducting the examination to preserve all evidence in case of future prosecution. When the victim of an assault is admitted to the ED or clinic, a specific chain of events occurs to collect legal evidence if the woman chooses to pursue legal action (Tables 53-16 and 53-17).

✚ TABLE 53-16   Emergency Management

Sexual Assault

Etiology	Assessment Findings	Interventions
• Sexual molestation • Sodomy • Assault involving genitalia (male or female) without consent	• Emotional or physical manifestations of shock • Hysteria • Crying • Anger • Silence • Decreased level of consciousness • Hyperventilation • Oral, vaginal, and rectal injuries • Extragenital injuries • Pain in genital or extragenital area	**Initial** • Treat shock and other urgent medical problems (e.g., head injury, hemorrhage, wounds, fractures). • Assess emotional state. • Contact support person (i.e., social worker, rape advocate, sexual assault nurse examiner). • Do *not* clean the patient until all evidence is collected. Make sure the patient does not wash, douche, urinate, brush teeth, or gargle. • Place sheet on floor. Then have patient stand on sheet to remove clothing. Place sheet with clothing in paper bag. • Obtain forensic evidence per local protocol (e.g., body hair, nail scrapings, tissue, dried semen, vaginal washing, blood samples). • Maintain chain of evidence for all legal specimens. Clearly label evidence and keep in locked cabinet until given to law enforcement agency. • Obtain baseline HIV, syphilis, and other STI screening. • Determine method of contraception, date of last menstrual period, and date of last tetanus immunization. • Consider tetanus prophylaxis if lacerations contain soil or dirt. • Vaccinate against hepatitis B if not already done. **Ongoing Monitoring** • Monitor vital signs and emotional status. • Provide clothing as needed. • Counsel patient regarding confidential HIV and STI testing.

HIV, Human immunodeficiency virus; *STI,* sexually transmitted infection.

TABLE 53-17   Evaluation of Alleged Sexual Assault

1. Medicolegal
• Valid written consent for examination, photographs, laboratory tests, release of information, and laboratory samples
• Appropriate "chain of evidence" documentation

2. History
• History of assault (who, what, when, where)
• Penetration, ejaculation, extragenital acts
• Activities since assault (e.g., changed clothes, bathed, douched)
• Inquire about safety
• Menstrual and contraceptive history
• Medical history
• Emotional status
• Current symptoms

3. General Physical Examination
• Vital signs and general appearance
• Extragenital trauma: mouth, breasts, neck
• Cuts, bruises, scratches (photographs taken)

4. Pelvic Examination
• Vulvar trauma, erythema. Hymen, anal, and rectal status
• Matted hairs or free hairs
• Vaginal examination with unlubricated speculum for discharge, blood, lacerations
• Uterine size
• Adnexa, especially hematomas

5. Laboratory Samples
• Vaginal vault content sampling
• Vaginal smears: microscope evaluation for trichomonads and semen
• Oral or rectal swabs and smears (if indicated)
• Blood samples: pregnancy test; serologic testing for syphilis, HIV, and hepatitis B infection
• Freeze serum sample for later testing
• Cultures: cervix and other areas (if indicated) for gonorrhea and chlamydial infection
• Fingernail scrapings
• Pubic hair scrapings
• Clipping of matted pubic hairs

6. Treatment
• Care of injuries and emotional trauma
• Prophylaxis for STIs, tetanus, and hepatitis B (see appropriate chapters)
• If appropriate, consider levonorgestrel (Plan-B One-Step) emergency contraceptive pill up to 72 hr after assault; follow-up for pregnancy test in 2-3 wk
• Testing for HIV, syphilis, and hepatitis B may be done at 6-8 wk
• Protection of legal rights
• Recommendation of continued follow-up and services of rape crisis center

The SANE nurse takes a comprehensive gynecologic and sexual history and an account of the assault (who, what, when, and where), as well as a general physical and pelvic examination. Laboratory tests are performed to identify sperm in the vagina and to screen for STIs or pregnancy. The patient is provided preventive treatment for pregnancy and STIs as well as treatment for injuries sustained in the assault.

Follow-up physical and psychologic care is recommended. Women should return weekly for the first month after the assault. This includes the time period when a woman's psychologic reactions may be the most severe.

❖ NURSING MANAGEMENT: SEXUAL ASSAULT

Nursing care for a sexual assault victim is complex. Provide emotional and nonjudgmental support. Obtain referrals as needed for follow-up care. Part of the role of the SANE nurse is to discuss the possibility of pregnancy and STIs, and offer the patient an emergency contraception pill as well as antibiotics (Table 53-18). A social worker or nurse case manager referral should be made by the primary nurse in the ED to assist the patient in follow-up with financial compensation to assist them in paying for emergency services as a result of the assault as well as for emotional injuries sustained from the assault and any missed work.

TABLE 53-18 Patient Teaching
Sexual Assault Prevention

Include the following instructions when teaching measures to prevent sexual assault.
1. Be proactive and take a self-defense class.
2. Be aware of date-rape drugs (e.g., GHB, Rohypnol, ketamine). Never leave your beverage unattended when socializing.
3. Place and maintain lights at all entrances to your home.
4. Keep your doors locked and do not open them to a stranger. Ask for identification if a service person comes to the door.
5. Do not advertise that you live alone. List only your initials with your last name in the telephone directory or on the mailbox. Never reveal to a caller that you are home alone.
6. Avoid walking alone in deserted areas. Walk to the parking lot with a friend. Be sure you see each other leave.
7. Have your keys ready as you approach your car or home.
8. Keep all doors locked and the windows up when driving.
9. Never get on an elevator with a suspicious person. Pretend you have forgotten something and get off.
10. Say what you mean in social situations. Be sure your voice and body language reflect your response.
11. Proceed with caution in online correspondence.
12. Carry a loud whistle and use it when you think you are in danger.
13. Yell "Fire!" if you are attacked and run toward a lighted area.

CASE STUDY

Uterine Fibroids and Endometrial Cancer

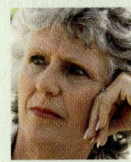

(©Wavebreakmedia/iStock/Thinkstock)

Patient Profile

T.J. is a 56-yr-old white woman who has lower pelvic discomfort and stress incontinence. She also has hypertension and type 2 diabetes. T.J. is the mother of four adult children. She has had abnormal uterine bleeding for 5 months. Large multiple uterine fibroids were diagnosed on ultrasound. She comes to the hospital for an abdominal hysterectomy.

Subjective Data
- Was initially reluctant about surgery
- Concerned about her dyspareunia and her husband's reaction to the surgery
- States she has pelvic discomfort and stress incontinence

Objective Data (Preoperative)
- BP 148/90 mm Hg, pulse 82 beats/min, respirations 14 breaths/min
- Height 5'6" Weight 175 lb.

Operative
- During surgery, abnormal-looking endometrial tissue was sent for pathologic analysis. The results were positive for endometrial cancer.
- Had total hysterectomy and bilateral salpingo-oophorectomy with lymph node biopsies. Five large fibroids were found in the uterus.

Postoperative Status
- Returned to room with indwelling urinary catheter in place
- Abdominal incision
- Sequential compression devices on lower extremities
- Patient-controlled analgesia (PCA) pump for pain management

Discussion Questions
1. Can the manifestations of uterine fibroids be differentiated from endometrial cancer?
2. *Patient-Centered Care:* Preoperatively T.J. asks you about the effect of the surgery on her sexuality. How would you respond, and what type of patient teaching would you do?
3. *Patient-Centered Care:* When she is told about the diagnosis of endometrial cancer, she is shocked. She cannot believe that was not discovered before surgery. How would you respond to her?
4. *Priority Decision:* What are priorities of care for T.J.?
5. *Safety:* When assessing T.J. after you got her out of bed, you note that her abdominal dressing is saturated with blood and she is complaining that she feels weak and dizzy. What would you do?
6. What other possible complications (including reasons for their development) can occur after an abdominal hysterectomy?
7. *Teamwork and Collaboration:* Which nursing personnel should be responsible for teaching T.J. related to her hypertension and diabetes: registered nurse, licensed practical/vocational nurse, unlicensed assistive personnel? What should she be taught?
8. *Priority Decision:* Based on the assessment data presented, what are the priority nursing diagnoses? Are there any collaborative problems?
9. *Evidence-Based Practice:* Her 37-yr-old daughter asks you if she is at risk for endometrial cancer. How would you respond?

Answers available at http://evolve.elsevier.com/Lewis/medsurg.

BRIDGE TO NCLEX EXAMINATION

The number of the question corresponds to the same-numbered outcome at the beginning of the chapter.

1. In telling a patient with infertility what she and her partner can expect, the nurse explains that
   a. ovulatory studies can help determine tube patency.
   b. a hysterosalpingogram is a common diagnostic study.
   c. the cause will remain unexplained for 40% of couples.
   d. if postcoital studies are normal, infection tests will be done.

2. An appropriate question to ask the patient with painful menstruation to differentiate primary from secondary dysmenorrhea is
   a. "Does your pain become worse with activity or overexertion?"
   b. "Have you had a recent personal crisis or change in your lifestyle?"
   c. "Is your pain relieved by nonsteroidal antiinflammatory medications?"
   d. "When in your menstrual history did the pain with your period begin?"

3. The nurse should advise the woman recovering from surgical treatment of an ectopic pregnancy that
   a. she has an increased risk for salpingitis.
   b. bed rest must be maintained for 12 hours to assist in healing.
   c. having one ectopic pregnancy increases her risk for another one.
   d. intrauterine devices and infertility treatments should be avoided.

4. To prevent or decrease age-related changes that occur after menopause in a patient who chooses not to take hormone therapy, the *most* important self-care measure to teach is
   a. maintaining usual sexual activity.
   b. increasing the intake of dairy products.
   c. performing regular aerobic, weight-bearing exercise.
   d. taking vitamin E and B-complex vitamin supplements.

5. In caring for a patient with endometriosis, the nurse teaches the patient that interventions used to treat or cure this condition may include (*select all that apply*)
   a. radiation.
   b. antibiotic therapy.
   c. oral contraceptives.
   d. surgical removal of tissue.
   e. total abdominal hysterectomy and salpingo-oophorectomy.

6. Nursing responsibilities related to the patient with endometrial cancer who has a total abdominal hysterectomy and salpingectomy and oophorectomy include
   a. maintaining absolute bed rest.
   b. keeping the patient in high Fowler's position.
   c. need for supplemental estrogen after removal of ovaries.
   d. encouraging movement and walking as much as tolerated.

7. Postoperative goals in caring for the patient who has undergone an abdominal hysterectomy include (*select all that apply*)
   a. monitoring urine output.
   b. changing position frequently.
   c. restricting all food for 24 hours.
   d. observing perineal pad for bleeding.
   e. encouraging leg exercises to promote circulation.

8. Postoperative nursing care for the woman with a gynecologic fistula includes (*select all that apply*)
   a. bed rest.
   b. bladder training.
   c. warm sitz baths.
   d. perineal hygiene.
   e. use of stool softeners.

9. The *first* nursing intervention for the patient who has been sexually assaulted is to
   a. treat urgent medical problems.
   b. contact support person for the patient.
   c. provide supplies for the patient to cleanse self.
   d. document bruises and lacerations of the perineum and the cervix.

1. b, 2. d, 3. c, 4. c, 5. c, d, e, 6. d, 7. a, b, d, e, 8. b, c, d, e, 9. a

For rationales to these answers and even more NCLEX review questions, visit *http://evolve.elsevier.com/Lewis/medsurg*.

ⓔ EVOLVE WEBSITE

http://evolve.elsevier.com/Lewis/medsurg
Review Questions (Online Only)
Key Points
Answer Keys for Questions
• Rationales for Bridge to NCLEX Examination Questions
• Answer Guidelines for Case Study on p. 1265
Student Case Study
• Patient With Endometrial Cancer
Nursing Care Plan(s)
• eNursing Care Plan 53-1: Patient Having Abdominal Hysterectomy
Conceptual Care Map Creator
Audio Glossary
Content Updates

REFERENCES

1. American Society for Reproductive Medicine: Defining infertility. Retrieved from *www.asrm.org/FACTSHEET_Defining_Infertility*.
2. American Congress of Obstetricians & Gynecologists: Early pregnancy loss. Retrieved from *www.acog.org/~/media/For%20Patients/faq090.pdf*.
3. American Congress of Obstetricians & Gynecologists: Retrieved from *www.acog.org/-/media/For-Patients/faq043.pdf?dmc=1&ts=201502 08T1033249676*.
4. Contraceptive technology update: classify the causes of abnormal uterine bleeding, 2014. Retrieved from *www.ctcfp.org/wp-content/uploads/Contraceptive-Technology-Update-1-2014.pdf*.
5. Tulundi T: Ectopic pregnancy: choosing a treatment and methotrexate therapy. Retrieved from *www.uptodate.com/contents/ectopic-pregnancy-choosing-a-treatment-and-methotrexate-therapy?source=search_result&search=ectopic+pregnancy&selectedTitle=2~150*.
*6. Shifren J, Gass L: The North American Menopause Society Recommendations for clinical care of midlife women, *Menopause* 21:1038, 2014.
7. CDC: Pelvic inflammatory disease (PID). Retrieved from *www.cdc.gov/std/pid/treatment.htm*.
8. Schenken R: Overview of the treatment of endometriosis. Retrieved from *www.uptodate.com/contents/overview-of-the-treatment-of-endometriosis?source=search_result&search=endometriosis&selectedTitle=1~150*.
9. Owen C, Armstrong A: Clinical management of leiomyoma, *Obstet Gynecol Clin North Am* 42:67, 2015.

*10. The Endocrine Society: Diagnosis and treatment of polycystic ovary syndrome: an endocrine society clinical practice guideline. Retrieved from *www.endocrine.org/~/media/endosociety/Files/Publications/Clinical%20Practice%20Guidelines/120513_PCOS_FinalA_2013.pdf.*

11. American Cancer Society: American Cancer Society: Cancer facts and figures 2015. Retrieved from *www.cancer.org/research/cancerfactsstatistics/allcancerfactsfigures/index.*

12. National Cancer Institute: A snapshot of cervical cancer: incidence and mortality. Retrieved from *www.cancer.gov/researchandfunding/snapshots/cervical.*

13. The American College of Obstetricians and Gynecologists: Cervical cancer screening. Retrieved from *www.acog.org/Patients/FAQs/Cervical-Cancer-Screening.*

14. American Cancer Society: Endometrial (uterine) cancer overview. Retrieved from *www.cancer.org/acs/groups/cid/documents/webcontent/003048-pdf.pdf.*

15. National Cancer Institute: Ovarian epithelial, fallopian tube, and primary peritoneal cancer treatment (PDQ). Retrieved from *www.cancer.gov/types/ovarian/patient/ovarian-epithelial-treatment-pdq.*

16. Anderson K, Davis K, Flynn B: Urinary incontinence and pelvic organ prolapse, *Med Clin North Am* 99:405, 2015.

17. Ding J, Chen C, Song X, et al: Successful use of ring pessary with support for advanced pelvic prolapse, *Int Urogynecol J* 26:1517, 2015.

18. Guzman Rojas R, Quintero C, Shek K, et al: Does childbirth play a role in the etiology of rectocele? *Int Urogynecol J* 26:737, 2015.

19. Alas A, Anger J: Management of apical pelvic organ prolapse, *Curr Urol Rep* 16:33-2015.

20. The Bowel and Bladder Foundation: Vaginal fistulas. Retrieved from *www.bladderandbowelfoundation.org/bladder/bladder-conditions-and-symptoms/vaginal-and-recto-vaginal-fistulas.*

21. Centers for Disease Control and Prevention: Intimate partner violence. Retrieved from *www.cdc.gov/violenceprevention/intimatepartnerviolence.*

22. American Congress of Obstetrics and Gynecologists: Sexual assault. Retrieved from *www.acog.org/Resources-And-Publications/Committee-Opinions/Committee-on-Health-Care-for-Underserved-Women/Sexual-Assault.*

23. Georgia Network to End Sexual Assault: Basic SANE training. Retrieved from *www.gnesa.org.*

*Evidence-based information for clinical practice.

54

Male Reproductive and Genital Problems

Susanne A. Quallich

Only those who risk going too far can possibly find out how far they can go.

T.S. Eliot

Ⓔ http://evolve.elsevier.com/Lewis/medsurg/

LEARNING OUTCOMES

1. Describe the pathophysiology, clinical manifestations, and interprofessional care of benign prostatic hyperplasia.
2. Describe the nursing management of benign prostatic hyperplasia.
3. Describe the pathophysiology, clinical manifestations, and interprofessional care of prostate cancer.
4. Explain the nursing management of prostate cancer.
5. Specify the pathophysiology, clinical manifestations, and nursing and interprofessional management of prostatitis and problems of the penis and scrotum.

6. Explain the clinical manifestations and interprofessional care of testicular cancer.
7. Describe the pathophysiology, clinical manifestations, and nursing and interprofessional management of problems related to male sexual function.
8. Summarize the psychologic and emotional implications related to male reproductive problems.

KEY TERMS

benign prostatic hyperplasia (BPH), p. 1268
epididymitis, p. 1284
erectile dysfunction (ED), p. 1286
orchitis, p. 1284
paraphimosis, p. 1283

phimosis, p. 1283
prostate cancer, p. 1275
prostatitis, p. 1282
radical prostatectomy, p. 1278
testicular cancer, p. 1285

testicular torsion, p. 1285
transurethral resection of the prostate
    (TURP), p. 1272
vasectomy, p. 1286

This chapter discusses problems of the male reproductive system. These involve a variety of structures, including the prostate, penis, urethra, ejaculatory duct, scrotum, testes, epididymis, ductus (vas) deferens, and rectum (Fig. 54-1).

PROBLEMS OF THE PROSTATE GLAND

BENIGN PROSTATIC HYPERPLASIA

Benign prostatic hyperplasia (BPH) is a condition in which the prostate gland increases in size, leading to disruption of the outflow of urine from the bladder through the urethra. Almost half of the men with BPH will have bothersome lower urinary tract symptoms (LUTS), such as difficulty starting a urine stream, a decreased flow of urine, or urinary frequency.[1] Research is not clear about whether having BPH leads to an increased risk of developing prostate cancer.[2,3]

Etiology and Pathophysiology

The etiology of BPH is not completely understood. However, hormonal changes associated with aging are believed to be contributing factors.[1] Dihydroxytestosterone (DHT), one of several sex hormones, stimulates prostate cell growth. Excess amounts of DHT can cause overgrowth of prostate tissue. As men age, they have a decrease in testosterone but continue to produce and accumulate high levels of DHT, resulting in prostate enlargement.

Another possible cause of BPH is an increased proportion of estrogen (as compared to testosterone). Throughout their lives, men produce both testosterone and small amounts of estrogen. As men age, the amount of active testosterone in the blood decreases, leaving a higher proportion of estrogen. A higher amount of estrogen within the prostate gland increases the activity of substances (including DHT) that promote prostate cell growth.

BPH usually develops in the inner part of the prostate. (Prostate cancer is most likely to develop in the outer part.) As the prostate enlarges, it gradually compresses the urethra, leading to partial or complete obstruction (Fig. 54-2). This compression of the urethra leads to the development of clinical manifestations. There is no direct relationship between prostate size and the severity of manifestations or degree of obstruction. The location of the enlargement is most significant in the development of obstructive symptoms (Fig. 54-3). For example, it is

---

Reviewed by Shari Gould, RN, MSN, Associate Professor of Nursing, Victoria College, Victoria, Texas; and Anthony R. Lutz, RN, MSN, A-GNP-C, Urology Nurse Practitioner, Carolinas Health Care System, Charlotte, North Carolina.

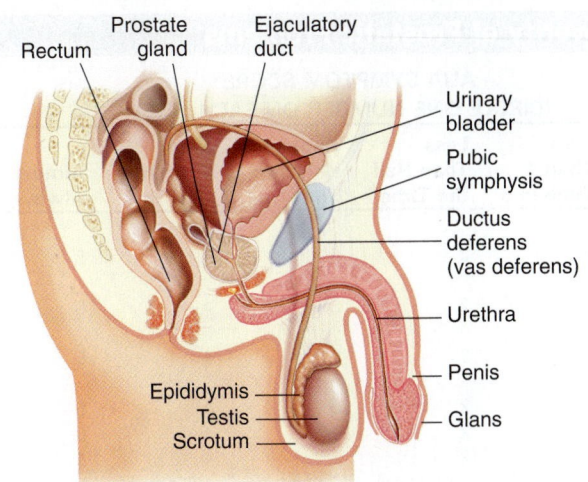

FIG. 54-1 Areas of the male reproductive system in which problems are likely to develop.

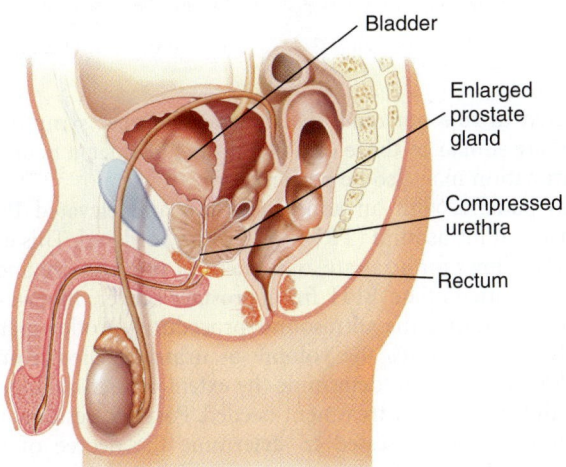

FIG. 54-2 Benign prostatic hyperplasia. The enlarged prostate compresses the urethra.

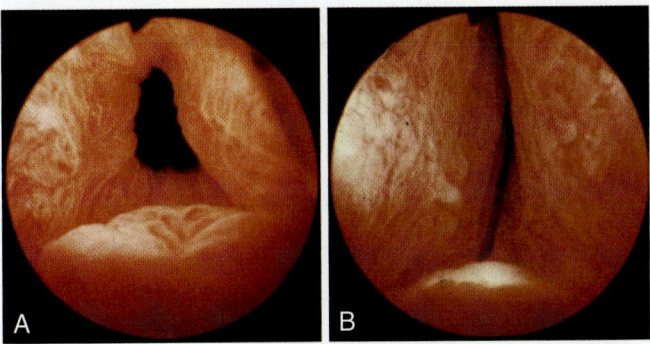

FIG. 54-3 Views of the prostate by cystoscopy. **A,** Normal appearance. **B,** Moderate benign prostatic hyperplasia with urethral obstruction. (From Townsend CM, Beauchamp RD, Evers BM, et al: *Sabiston textbook of surgery*, ed 19, Philadelphia, 2012, Saunders.)

possible for mild prostate enlargement to cause severe obstruction, or for extreme prostate enlargement to cause few obstructive symptoms.

Risk factors for BPH include aging, obesity (in particular increased waist circumference), lack of physical activity, alcohol consumption, erectile dysfunction, smoking, and diabetes.[4] A family history of BPH in a first-degree relative may also be a risk factor.

Clinical Manifestations

Manifestations of BPH occur gradually and may not be noticed until prostate enlargement has been present for some time. Early symptoms may not cause significant problems because the bladder can compensate for a small amount of resistance to urine flow. As the severity of urethral obstruction increases, the symptoms gradually worsen.

Symptoms can be divided into two groups: irritative and obstructive. *Irritative symptoms* include nocturia, urinary frequency, urgency, dysuria, bladder pain, and incontinence. These symptoms are associated with inflammation or infection. Nocturia is often the first symptom that the patient notices. *Obstructive symptoms,* caused by prostate enlargement, include a decrease in the caliber and force of the urinary stream, difficulty

in initiating a stream, intermittency (stopping and starting stream several times while voiding), and dribbling at the end of urination. These symptoms are due to the increased effort of the bladder as it tries to empty through the decreased diameter of the urethra. As a group, both irritative and obstructive symptoms are considered lower urinary tract symptoms (LUTS).

The American Urological Association (AUA) symptom index for BPH (Table 54-1) is a widely used tool to assess voiding symptoms associated with obstruction.[5] Although this tool is not diagnostic, it helps determine the extent of symptoms and provides guidelines for treatment.[6] Higher scores on this tool indicate greater symptom severity.

Complications

Complications of BPH are relatively rare. However, some men may experience acute urinary retention. This complication is manifested by the sudden and painful inability to urinate. Treatment involves the insertion of a catheter to drain the bladder. Surgery may be indicated in severe situations.

Urinary tract infection (UTI) can also be a complication of BPH. Since the bladder is unable to empty completely, bacteria can grow and cause infection within the urinary tract. In more severe cases, sepsis may also develop. Bladder calculi (stones) may develop in the bladder because of the alkalinization of the residual urine. Although bladder stones are more common in men with BPH, the risk of kidney stones is not significantly increased.

Additional complications include renal failure caused by *hydronephrosis* (distention of pelvis and calyces of the kidney by urine that cannot flow through the ureter to the bladder), pyelonephritis, and bladder damage if treatment for acute urinary retention is delayed.

Diagnostic Studies

A history and physical examination are important for diagnosis. (Diagnostic studies are outlined in Table 54-2.) A digital rectal examination (DRE) is done to estimate the prostate size, symmetry, and consistency. In BPH, the prostate is symmetrically enlarged, firm, and smooth.

Other diagnostic testing may include a urinalysis with culture to look for bacteria, white blood cells (WBCs), or microscopic hematuria, which indicate infection or inflammation.

A prostate-specific antigen (PSA) blood test may be done to screen for prostate cancer. However, PSA levels may be slightly elevated in patients with BPH. Serum creatinine levels may be

TABLE 54-1 **AUA Symptom Index to Determine Severity of Prostatic Problems**

	AUA SYMPTOM SCORE* (CIRCLE ONE NUMBER ON EACH LINE)					
Questions	Not At All	Less Than 1 Time in 5	Less Than Half the Time	About Half the Time	More Than Half the Time	Almost Always
Over the past month						
1. How often do you have the sensation that your bladder is not completely empty after you finish urinating?	0	1	2	3	4	5
2. How often do you have to urinate again, less than 2 hr after you finish urinating?	0	1	2	3	4	5
3. How often do you stop and start again several times when you urinate?	0	1	2	3	4	5
4. How often do you find it difficult to postpone urination?	0	1	2	3	4	5
5. How often do you have a weak urinary stream?	0	1	2	3	4	5
6. How often do you have to push or strain to begin urination?	0	1	2	3	4	5
7. How many times do you usually get up to urinate from the time you go to bed at night until the time you get up in the morning?	0 (None)	1 (1 time)	2 (2 times)	3 (3 times)	4 (4 times)	5 (5 times or more)
Sum of circled numbers (AUA Symptom Score): _____ *						

Source: Barry MJ, Fowler FJ, O'Leary MP, et al: The American Urological Association symptom index for benign prostatic hyperplasia, *J Urol* 148:1549, 1992. Used with permission.
AUA, American Urological Association.
*Score is interpreted as follows: 0-7, mild; 8-19, moderate; 20-35, severe.

TABLE 54-2 **Interprofessional Care**

Benign Prostatic Hyperplasia

Diagnostic Assessment
- History and physical examination
- Digital rectal examination (DRE)
- Urinalysis with culture
- Prostate-specific antigen (PSA)
- Serum creatinine
- Postvoid residual
- Transrectal ultrasound (TRUS)
- Uroflowmetry
- Cystoscopy

Management
Active Surveillance
- Annual PSA and DRE

Drug Therapy
- 5α-Reductase inhibitors (e.g., finasteride [Proscar], dutasteride [Avodart], dutasteride plus tamsulosin [Jalyn])
- α-Adrenergic receptor blockers (e.g., silodosin [Rapaflo], alfuzosin [Uroxatral], doxazosin [Cardura], prazosin [Minipress], terazosin, tamsulosin [Flomax])
- Erectogenic drugs (e.g., tadalafil [Cialis])

Minimally Invasive Therapy*
- Transurethral microwave thermotherapy (TUMT)
- Transurethral needle ablation (TUNA)
- Laser prostatectomy
- Transurethral electrovaporization of the prostate (TUVP)

Invasive (Surgery) Therapy*
- Transurethral resection of the prostate (TURP)
- Transurethral incision of the prostate (TUIP)
- Open prostatectomy

*See Table 54-3.

ordered to rule out renal insufficiency. Because symptoms of BPH are similar to those of a neurogenic bladder, a neurologic examination may also be performed.

In patients with an abnormal DRE and elevated PSA, a transrectal ultrasound (TRUS) is typically ordered. This examination allows for accurate assessment of prostate size and can help to differentiate BPH from prostate cancer. Biopsies can be taken during the ultrasound procedure. Uroflowmetry, a study that measures the volume of urine expelled from the bladder, is helpful to determine the extent of urethral blockage and thus the type of treatment needed. Postvoid residual urine volume is often assessed to determine the degree of urine flow obstruction. Cystoscopy, a procedure allowing internal visualization of the urethra and bladder, is performed if the diagnosis is unclear or to visualize the degree of prostatic enlargement.

Interprofessional Care

The goals of interprofessional care are to (1) restore bladder drainage, (2) relieve the patient's symptoms, and (3) prevent or treat the complications of BPH. Treatment is generally based on the degree to which the symptoms bother the patient or the presence of complications, rather than the size of the prostate. Alternatives to surgical intervention for some patients include drug therapy and minimally invasive procedures.

The most conservative treatment that may be recommended for some patients with BPH is referred to as *active surveillance*, or watchful waiting. When the patient has mild symptoms (AUA symptom scores of 0 to 7), a wait-and-see approach is taken. Teaching patients to make lifestyle changes can help relieve early or mild symptoms. Making dietary changes (decreasing intake of caffeine, artificial sweeteners, and spicy or acidic foods), avoiding drugs such as decongestants and anticholinergics, and restricting evening fluid intake may improve symptoms.

In addition, a timed voiding schedule may reduce or eliminate symptoms, thus eliminating the need for further intervention. If the patient begins to have signs or symptoms that indicate an increase in obstruction, further treatment is indicated.

Drug Therapy. Two classes of drugs that are used to treat BPH include 5α-reductase inhibitors and α-adrenergic receptor blockers. Combination therapy using both types of drugs may be more effective in reducing symptoms than using one drug alone.

5α-Reductase Inhibitors. 5α-Reductase inhibitors work by reducing the size of the prostate gland. Finasteride (Proscar) blocks the enzyme 5α-reductase, which is necessary for the conversion of testosterone to DHT (principal intraprostatic androgen). Prostate size is directly related to the amount of DHT. By blocking DHT, overly enlarged prostates can decrease in size. This class of medication is more effective for men with larger prostates who experience bothersome symptoms.

Finasteride is an appropriate treatment option for men who have a moderate to severe symptom score on the AUA symptom index (Table 54-1). Although most men who are treated with the drug have symptom improvement, it can take up to 6 months to be effective. These drugs must be taken on a regular basis to have an effect.

Serum PSA levels may be decreased by almost 50% when taking finasteride. Therefore to "correct" for the decrease caused by the finasteride, the HCP should double the PSA result. This allows for an accurate comparison to premedication levels to more accurately track trends in the PSA over time.

Dutasteride (Avodart) has the same effect on prostatic tissue as finasteride and is a dual inhibitor of 5α-reductase type 1 and 2 isoenzymes. (Finasteride inhibits only the type 2 isoenzyme.) The combination of a 5α-reductase inhibitor (dutasteride) and an α-adrenergic receptor blocker (tamsulosin) is available in a single oral medication (Jalyn).

In addition to decreasing the symptoms of BPH, finasteride, dutasteride, and Jalyn (finasteride plus tamsulosin) may also lower the risk of prostate cancer.[7] However, the use of these drugs in the prevention of prostate cancer has not been recommended. Patients with an increased PSA level while taking these medications should be referred to their HCP. Also encourage the patient to discuss the need for prostate cancer screening with the HCP.

> **DRUG ALERT** **Finasteride (Proscar)**
> * Women who may be or are pregnant should not handle tablets due to potential risk to male fetus (anomaly).

α-Adrenergic Receptor Blockers. α-Adrenergic receptor blockers are another drug treatment option for BPH. These medications selectively block α₁-adrenergic receptors, which are abundant in the prostate, and are increased in hyperplastic prostate tissue. Although nonspecific α-adrenergic blockers are more commonly used for the treatment of hypertension, these drugs promote smooth muscle relaxation in the prostate, thus facilitating urinary flow through the urethra.

Several α-adrenergic blockers are used, including silodosin (Rapaflo), alfuzosin (Uroxatral), doxazosin (Cardura), prazosin (Minipress), terazosin, and tamsulosin (Flomax). Although these drugs offer symptom relief of BPH by relaxing the smooth muscle of the prostate that surrounds the urethra, these medications do not decrease the overall size of the prostate.

Erectogenic Drugs. Tadalafil (Cialis) has been used in men who have symptoms of BPH alone or in combination with erectile dysfunction (ED). The drug has shown to be effective in reducing symptoms for both of these conditions.[8]

Herbal Therapy. Some patients take plant extracts such as saw palmetto (*Serenoa repens*). However, research indicates that saw palmetto has no benefit over a placebo.[9,10] Advise patients to discuss herbal therapies with their HCP.

Minimally Invasive Therapy. Minimally invasive therapies are becoming more common as an alternative to watchful waiting and invasive treatment (Table 54-3). They generally do not require hospitalization or catheterization and are associated with few adverse events. Many minimally invasive therapies have outcomes comparable to those of invasive techniques.[11]

Transurethral Microwave Thermotherapy. Transurethral microwave thermotherapy (TUMT) is an outpatient procedure that involves the delivery of microwaves directly to the prostate through a transurethral probe (probe inserted into the meatus and through the urethra). The microwaves increase the temperature of the prostate tissue to about 113° F (45° C). The heat causes death of tissue, thus relieving the obstruction. A rectal temperature probe is used during the procedure to ensure that the temperature in the rectum is kept below 110° F (43.5° C) to prevent rectal tissue damage. The procedure takes about 90 minutes.

Postoperative urinary retention is a common complication. Patients who have a TUMT are generally sent home with an indwelling catheter for 2 to 7 days to maintain urinary flow and to facilitate the passing of small clots or necrotic tissue. Antibiotics, pain medication, and bladder antispasmodic medications are used to treat and prevent postprocedure problems. The procedure is not appropriate for men with rectal problems. Anticoagulant therapy should be stopped 10 days before treatment. Mild side effects include occasional problems of bladder spasm, hematuria, dysuria, and retention.

Transurethral Needle Ablation. Transurethral needle ablation (TUNA) is another procedure that increases the temperature of prostate tissue, thus causing localized necrosis. TUNA differs from TUMT in that low-wave radiofrequency is used to heat the prostate. Only prostate tissue in direct contact with the needle is affected, which allows for more precise removal of the target tissue. The majority of the patients undergoing TUNA have an improvement in symptoms.

> **?** **CHECK YOUR PRACTICE**
>
> You are working in the preoperative unit and caring for a patient who is scheduled for a transurethral needle ablation for BPH. He appears anxious. He tells you, "I'm afraid of the pain after the procedure. They told me I might have to have a tube in my bladder. I don't know how I'll manage at home."
> * What type of information and teaching would you provide him?

This procedure is performed in an outpatient unit or physician's office using local anesthesia and IV or oral sedation. The TUNA procedure lasts approximately 30 minutes. The patient typically experiences little pain with an early return to regular activities. Complications include urinary retention, UTI, and irritative voiding symptoms (e.g., frequency, urgency, dysuria). Some patients require a urinary catheter for a short time. Patients often have hematuria for up to a week, and irritative voiding symptoms may persist for several weeks.

Laser Prostatectomy. The use of laser therapy through visual or ultrasound guidance is an effective alternative to transurethral resection of the prostate (TURP) in treating BPH. The laser beam is delivered transurethrally through a fiber instrument and is used for cutting, coagulation, and vaporization of prostatic tissue. There are a variety of laser procedures using different sources, wavelengths, and delivery systems. Retreatment rates are comparable to those of a TURP.[12]

TABLE 54-3 Treatment for Benign Prostatic Hyperplasia

Description	Advantages	Disadvantages
Minimally Invasive		
Transurethral Microwave Thermotherapy (TUMT)		
Use of microwave radiating heat to produce coagulative necrosis of the prostate.	• Outpatient procedure • Erectile dysfunction, urinary incontinence, and retrograde ejaculation are rare	• Potential for damage to surrounding tissue • Urinary catheter needed after procedure
Transurethral Needle Ablation (TUNA)		
Low-wave radiofrequency used to heat the prostate, causing necrosis.	• Outpatient procedure • Erectile dysfunction, urinary incontinence, and retrograde ejaculation are rare • Precise delivery of heat to desired area • Very little pain experienced	• Urinary retention common • Irritative voiding symptoms • Hematuria
Laser Prostatectomy		
Procedure uses a laser beam to cut or destroy part of the prostate. Different techniques are available: • Visual laser ablation of prostate (VLAP) • Contact laser • Photovaporization of prostate (PVP) • Interstitial laser coagulation (ILC)	• Short procedure • Comparable results to TURP • Minimal bleeding • Fast recovery time • Rapid symptom improvement • Very effective	• Catheter (up to 7 days) needed after procedure due to edema and urinary retention • Delayed sloughing of tissue • Takes several weeks to reach optimal effect • Retrograde ejaculation
Transurethral Electrovaporization of Prostate (TUVP)		
Electrosurgical vaporization and desiccation are used together to destroy prostatic tissue.	• Minimal risks • Minimal bleeding and sloughing	• Retrograde ejaculation • Intermittent hematuria
Invasive (Surgery)		
Transurethral Resection of Prostate (TURP)		
Use of excision and cauterization to remove prostate tissue via cystoscope. Remains the standard for treatment of BPH.	• Erectile dysfunction unlikely	• Bleeding • Retrograde ejaculation
Transurethral Incision of Prostate (TUIP)		
Involves transurethral incisions into prostatic tissue to relieve obstruction. Effective for men with small to moderate prostates.	• Outpatient procedure • Minimal complications • Low occurrence of erectile dysfunction or retrograde ejaculation	• Urinary catheter needed after procedure
Open Prostatectomy		
Surgery of choice for men with large prostates, bladder damage, or other complicating factors. Involves external incision with two possible approaches (see Fig. 54-6).	• Complete visualization of prostate and surrounding tissue	• Erectile dysfunction • Bleeding • Postoperative pain • Risk of infection

One common procedure is *visual laser ablation of the prostate* (VLAP), which uses the laser beam to produce deep coagulation necrosis. The affected prostate tissue gradually sloughs in the urinary stream. It takes several weeks before the patient reaches optimal results after this type of laser therapy. At the completion of VLAP, a urinary catheter is inserted to allow for drainage.

Contact laser techniques involve the direct contact of the laser with the prostate tissue, producing an immediate vaporization of the tissue. Blood vessels near the laser tip are immediately cauterized. Thus bleeding during the procedure is rare. A three-way catheter with slow-drip irrigation is placed immediately after the procedure for a short time. Typically the catheter is removed within 6 to 8 hours after the procedure. Advantages of this procedure over TURP include minimal bleeding both during and after the procedure, faster recovery time, and ability to perform the surgery on patients taking anticoagulants.

Photovaporization of the prostate (PVP) uses a high-power green laser light to vaporize prostate tissue. Improvements in urine flow and symptoms are almost immediate after the procedure. Bleeding is minimal, and a catheter is usually inserted for 24 to 48 hours afterward. PVP works well for larger prostate glands, but irritative voiding symptoms may persist for several weeks.

Another approach to laser prostatectomy is *interstitial laser coagulation* (ILC). The prostate is viewed through a cystoscope. A laser is used to quickly treat precise areas of the enlarged prostate by placement of interstitial light guides directly into the prostate tissue.

Invasive (Surgery) Therapy. Invasive treatment of symptomatic BPH involves surgery. The choice of the treatment approach depends on the size and location of the prostatic enlargement and patient factors such as age and surgical risk. Invasive treatments are summarized in Table 54-3.

Invasive therapy is indicated when a decrease in urine flow causes discomfort, persistent residual urine, acute urinary retention because of obstruction with no reversible precipitating cause, or hydronephrosis. Intermittent catheterization or insertion of an indwelling catheter can temporarily reduce symptoms and bypass the obstruction. However, avoid long-term catheter use because of the increased risk of infection.

Transurethral Resection of the Prostate. Transurethral resection of the prostate (TURP) is a surgical procedure involving the removal of prostate tissue using a resectoscope inserted through the urethra. TURP has long been considered the gold standard for surgical treatments of obstructing BPH. Results of a TURP are superior but at the cost of a longer hospital stay. The number of TURP procedures done in recent years has declined due to the development of less invasive technologies.[6]

In TURP no external surgical incision is made. A resectoscope is inserted through the urethra to excise and cauterize obstructing prostatic tissue (Fig. 54-4). A large three-way

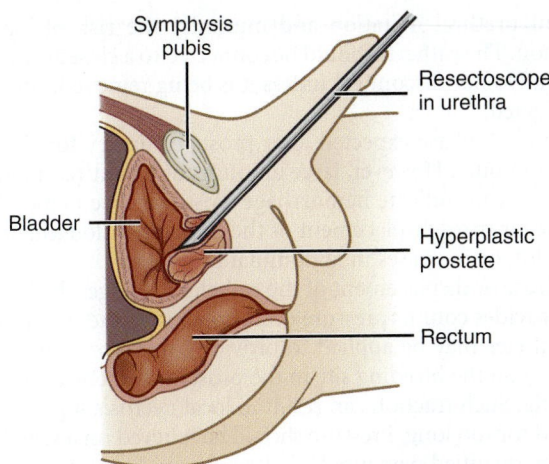

FIG. 54-4 Transurethral resection of the prostate.

indwelling catheter with a 30-mL balloon is inserted into the bladder after the procedure to provide hemostasis and to facilitate urinary drainage. The bladder is irrigated, either continuously or intermittently, usually for the first 24 hours to prevent obstruction from mucus and blood clots.

The outcome for the majority of patients is excellent, with marked improvements in symptoms and urinary flow rates. TURP is a surgical procedure with a relatively low risk, but caregivers must be vigilant for signs or symptoms of transurethral resection syndrome (TUR or TURP syndrome). This condition is manifested by nausea, vomiting, confusion, bradycardia, and hypertension. TUR syndrome is the result of hyponatremia due to longer operative times and prolonged intraoperative bladder irrigation.

Other postoperative complications include bleeding and clot retention. Because bleeding is a common complication, patients taking aspirin, warfarin (Coumadin), or other anticoagulants must discontinue these medications several days before surgery. BPH medications are also stopped after this procedure.

Transurethral Incision of the Prostate. Transurethral incision of the prostate (TUIP) is a surgical procedure done under local anesthesia for men with moderate to severe symptoms. Several small incisions are made into the prostate gland to expand the urethra, which relieves pressure on the urethra and improves urine flow. TUIP is an option for patients with a small or moderately enlarged prostate gland. TUIP has similar patient outcomes to TURP in relieving symptoms.

❖ NURSING MANAGEMENT: BENIGN PROSTATIC HYPERPLASIA

Because you will be most directly involved in care of patients with BPH having invasive therapies, the focus of nursing management in this section is on preoperative and postoperative care.

◆ Nursing Assessment

Subjective and objective data that should be obtained from a patient with BPH are presented in Table 54-4.

◆ Nursing Diagnoses

Nursing diagnoses for the patient with BPH preoperatively may include, but are not limited to, the following:
- Acute pain *related to* bladder distention secondary to enlarged prostate

TABLE 54-4 Nursing Assessment
Benign Prostatic Hyperplasia
Subjective Data
Important Health Information
Medications: Testosterone supplementation
Surgery or other treatments: Previous treatment for BPH
Functional Health Patterns
Health perception–health management: Knowledge of the condition
Nutritional-metabolic: Voluntary fluid restriction
Elimination: Urinary urgency, diminution in caliber and force of urinary stream. Hesitancy in initiating voiding. Postvoid dribbling, urinary retention, urinary incontinence
Sleep-rest: Nocturia
Cognitive-perceptual: Dysuria, sensation of incomplete voiding, bladder discomfort
Sexuality-reproductive: Anxiety about sexual dysfunction
Objective Data
General
Older adult male
Urinary
Distended bladder on palpation. Smooth, firm, elastic enlargement of prostate on rectal examination
Possible Diagnostic Findings
Enlarged prostate on ultrasonography, vesicle neck obstruction on cystoscopy, residual urine with postvoiding catheterization. White blood cells, bacteria, or microscopic hematuria with bladder infection. ↑ serum creatinine levels with renal involvement

- Risk for infection *related to* an indwelling catheter, urinary stasis, or environmental pathogens

Nursing diagnoses for the patient with BPH who has invasive therapy (surgery) are presented in eNursing Care Plan 54-1 (available on the website for this chapter).

◆ Planning

The overall preoperative goals for the patient having invasive procedures are to have (1) restoration of urinary drainage; (2) treatment of any UTI; and (3) understanding of the upcoming procedure, implications for sexual function and urinary control. The overall postoperative goals are to have (1) no complications, (2) restoration of urinary control, (3) complete bladder emptying, and (4) satisfying sexual expression.

◆ Nursing Implementation

◆ **Health Promotion.** The cause of BPH is largely attributed to the aging process.[13] Health promotion focuses on early detection and treatment. The American Urological Association (AUA) currently recommends that men age 55 to 69 have the greatest potential benefit from PSA screening. The recommended screening interval is every 2 years.[14] When symptoms of prostatic hyperplasia are present, further diagnostic screening may be necessary (Table 54-2).

Some men find that consuming alcohol, caffeine, or other bladder irritants tends to increase prostatic symptoms because the diuretic effect increases bladder distention. Compounds found in common cough and cold remedies such as pseudoephedrine (in Sudafed) and phenylephrine (in Allerest PE and Coricidin D) often worsen the symptoms of BPH. These drugs are α-adrenergic agonists that cause smooth muscle contraction. If this occurs, the patient should avoid these drugs.

Teach patients with obstructive symptoms to urinate every 2 to 3 hours and when they first feel the urge. This will minimize urinary stasis and acute urinary retention. Instruct patients to maintain a normal level of fluid so that they do not become dehydrated. The patient may believe that if he restricts his fluid intake, symptoms will be less severe, but this only increases the chances of an infection while concentrating his urine.

◆ **Acute Care.** The following discussion focuses on preoperative and postoperative care for the patient undergoing a TURP.

◆   *Preoperative Care.* Antibiotics are usually administered before any invasive GU procedure. Any infection of the urinary tract must be treated before surgery. Restoring urinary drainage and encouraging a high fluid intake (2 to 3 L/day unless contraindicated) are helpful in managing the infection. Prostatic obstruction may result in acute retention or inability to void. Urinary drainage must be restored before surgery.

A urethral catheter such as a coudé (curved-tip) catheter may be needed to restore bladder drainage. In many health care settings, 10 mL of sterile 2% lidocaine gel is injected into the urethra before insertion of the catheter. The lidocaine gel not only acts as a lubricant but also provides local anesthesia and helps open the urethral lumen. If a sizable obstruction of the urethra exists, the urologist may insert a filiform catheter with sufficient rigidity to pass the obstruction. Aseptic technique is important at all times to avoid introducing bacteria into the bladder. (Urinary catheters are discussed in Chapter 45.)

Patients may be concerned about the impact of the impending surgery on sexual function. Provide an opportunity for the patient and his partner to express their concerns. Inform the patient that his ejaculate volume may be decreased or absent after the procedure. Most types of prostatic surgery results in some degree of *retrograde ejaculation*, a condition in which some semen travels back into the bladder during orgasm instead of traveling out of the penis. This may decrease orgasmic sensations felt during ejaculation. Retrograde ejaculation is not harmful, and the semen is voided during the next urination.

◆   *Postoperative Care.* The main complications after surgery are hemorrhage, bladder spasms, urinary incontinence, and infection. Adjust the plan of care to the type of surgery, reasons for surgery, and patient's response to surgery.

After surgery the patient will have a standard catheter or a triple-lumen catheter. Bladder irrigation is typically done to remove clotted blood from the bladder and ensure drainage of urine. The bladder is irrigated either manually on an intermittent basis or more commonly as continuous bladder irrigation (CBI) with sterile normal saline solution or another prescribed solution. If the bladder is manually irrigated (if ordered), instill 50 mL of irrigating solution and then withdraw with a syringe to remove clots that may be in the bladder and catheter. Painful bladder spasms often occur as a result of manual irrigation.

With CBI, irrigating solution is continuously infused and drained from the bladder. The rate of infusion is based on the color of drainage. Ideally the urine drainage should be light pink without clots. Continuously monitor the inflow and outflow of the irrigant. If outflow is less than inflow, assess the catheter patency for kinks or clots. If the outflow is blocked and patency cannot be reestablished by manual irrigation, stop the CBI and notify the physician.

Use careful aseptic technique when irrigating the bladder because bacteria can easily be introduced into the urinary tract. Secure the catheter to the leg with tape or a catheter strap to

prevent urethral irritation and minimize the risk of bladder infection. The catheter should be connected to a closed-drainage system. Do not disconnect unless it is being removed, changed, or irrigated.

Blood clots are expected after prostate surgery for the first 24 to 36 hours. However, large amounts of bright red blood in the urine can indicate hemorrhage. Postoperative hemorrhage may occur from displacement of the catheter, dislodgment of a large clot, or increases in abdominal pressure.

Release or displacement of the catheter dislodges the balloon that provides counterpressure on the operative site. Traction on the catheter may be applied to provide counterpressure (tamponade) on the bleeding site in the prostate, thereby decreasing bleeding. Such traction can result in local necrosis if pressure is applied for too long. Pressure should be relieved on a scheduled basis by qualified personnel.

Activities that increase abdominal pressure should be avoided in the postoperative recovery period. These include sitting or walking for prolonged periods and straining to have a bowel movement (Valsalva maneuver).

Bladder spasms are a distressing complication for the patient after transurethral procedures. They occur as a result of irritation of the bladder mucosa from the insertion of the resectoscope, presence of a catheter, or clots leading to obstruction of the catheter. If bladder spasms develop, check the catheter for clots. If present, remove the clots by irrigation so that urine can

---

🔲 TEAMWORK & COLLABORATION
Patient Receiving Bladder Irrigation

Intermittent or continuous bladder irrigation (CBI) is usually required after invasive prostate surgery to prevent bladder obstruction by clots or mucus.

Role of Nursing Personnel
Registered Nurse (RN)

- Assess for bleeding and clots.
- Assess catheter patency by measuring intake and output and presence of bladder spasms.
- Manually irrigate catheter if bladder spasms or decreased outflow occurs.
- Discontinue CBI and notify physician if obstruction occurs.
- Teach patient Kegel exercises after catheter removal.
- Provide care instructions for patient discharged with indwelling catheter.

Licensed Practical/Vocational Nurse (LPN/LVN)

- Monitor catheter drainage for increased blood or clots.
- Increase flow of irrigating solution to maintain light pink color in outflow.
- Administer antispasmodics and analgesics as needed.

Unlicensed Assistive Personnel (UAP)

- Clean around catheter daily.
- Record intake and output.
- Notify RN if large amount of bright red blood is in urine.
- Report complaints of pain or bladder spasms to RN.

Role of Other Team Members
Physician or Advanced Practice Clinician (Nurse Practitioner or Physician Assistant)

- Assess for bleeding and clots.
- Assess and manage catheter if obstruction occurs.
- Order antispasmodics and analgesics as needed.

flow freely. Instruct the patient not to urinate around the catheter because this increases the likelihood of spasm. Belladonna and opium suppositories or other antispasmodics (e.g., oxybutynin [Ditropan XL]), along with relaxation techniques, are used to relieve the pain and decrease spasm.

The catheter is often removed 2 to 4 days after surgery. The patient should have a voiding trial after catheter removal. If he cannot urinate, he will have a catheter reinserted for a day or two or be taught to perform clean intermittent self-catheterization (see Chapter 45).

Sphincter tone may be poor immediately after catheter removal, resulting in urinary incontinence or dribbling. This is a common but distressing situation for the patient. Sphincter tone can be strengthened by having the patient practice Kegel exercises (pelvic floor muscle technique) 10 to 20 times per hour while awake. (Kegel exercises are discussed in Table 45-18.) Encourage the patient to practice starting and stopping the stream several times during urination. This helps the patient to target the correct pelvic floor muscles when performing Kegel exercises.

It can take several weeks to achieve urinary continence. In some instances, control of urine may never be fully regained. Continence can improve for up to 12 months. If continence has not been achieved by that time, the patient may be referred to a continence clinic. A variety of methods, including biofeedback, have been used to achieve positive results.

Teach the patient how to use a penile clamp, a condom catheter, or incontinence pads or briefs to avoid embarrassment from dribbling. In severe cases, an occlusive cuff that serves as an artificial sphincter can be surgically implanted to restore continence. Assist the patient in finding ways to manage the problem that allow him to continue socializing and interacting with others. (Urinary incontinence is discussed in Chapter 45.)

Observe the patient for signs of postoperative infection. If an external wound is present (from an open prostatectomy), assess the area for redness, heat, swelling, and purulent drainage. Special care must be taken if a perineal incision is present because of the proximity of the anus. Avoid rectal procedures, such as taking rectal temperatures and administering enemas. The insertion of well-lubricated belladonna and opium suppositories is acceptable.

Dietary intervention and stool softeners are important in the postoperative period to prevent the patient from straining while having bowel movements. Straining increases the intraabdominal pressure, which can lead to bleeding at the operative site. A diet high in fiber facilitates the passage of stool.

◆ **Ambulatory Care.** Discharge planning and home care issues are important aspects of care after prostate surgery. Patient teaching includes (1) caring for an indwelling catheter (if one is left in place); (2) managing urinary incontinence; (3) maintaining adequate oral fluid intake; (4) observing for signs and symptoms of urinary tract and wound infection; (5) preventing constipation; (6) avoiding heavy lifting (more than 10 lb [4.5 kg]); and (7) refraining from driving or intercourse after surgery as directed by the provider.

The patient may experience a change in sexual function after surgery. Many men experience retrograde ejaculation because of trauma to the internal urethral sphincter. Erectile dysfunction (ED) may occur if the nerves are cut or damaged during surgery. The patient may experience anxiety over the change because of a perceived loss of his sex role, self-esteem, or quality of sexual interaction with his partner. Discuss these changes with the patient and his partner and allow them to ask questions and express their concerns. Sexual counseling and treatment options may be necessary if ED becomes a chronic issue. (ED is discussed later in this chapter on pp. 1286-1288.)

Some patients experience concerns regarding change in sexual function, but this is not a universal concern. Recovery depends on the type of surgery performed and the interval of time between when symptoms first appeared and the date of surgery. It may take up to 1 year for complete sexual function to return.

The bladder may take up to 2 months to return to its normal capacity. Instruct the patient to drink at least 2 to 3 L of fluid per day and urinate every 2 to 3 hours to flush the urinary tract. Teach the patient to avoid or limit the amounts of bladder irritants such as caffeine products, citrus juices, and alcohol. Because the patient may experience incontinence or dribbling, he may incorrectly believe that decreasing fluid intake will relieve this problem.

Urethral strictures may result from instrumentation or catheterization. Treatment may include teaching the patient intermittent clean self-catheterization or having a urethral dilation.

Advise the patient to discuss the need for a yearly DRE with his HCP if he has had any procedure other than complete removal of the prostate. Hyperplasia or cancer can occur in the remaining prostatic tissue.

◆ **Evaluation**

The expected outcomes are that the patient with BPH who has surgery will
• Report satisfactory pain control
• Report improved urinary function with no pain or incontinence

Additional information on expected outcomes for the patient with BPH is presented in eNursing Care Plan 54-1.

PROSTATE CANCER

Prostate cancer is a malignant tumor of the prostate gland. Prostate cancer is the most common cancer among men, excluding skin cancer, and is the second leading cause of cancer death in men (exceeded only by lung cancer). Annually 220,800 men are diagnosed and 27,580 die. Men have a 1 in 7 risk of developing prostate cancer. Almost 2.9 million men in the United States are survivors of prostate cancer.[15]

Etiology and Pathophysiology

Prostate cancer is slow-growing, androgen-dependent cancer. It can spread by three routes: by direct extension, through the lymph system, or through the bloodstream. Spread by direct extension involves the seminal vesicles, urethral mucosa, bladder wall, and external sphincter. The cancer later spreads through the lymphatic system to the regional lymph nodes. The bloodstream seems to be the mode of spread to the axial skeleton: pelvic bones, head of the femur, lower lumbar spine, and finally liver and lungs.

Age, ethnicity, and family history are known risk factors for prostate cancer. (See the Cultural & Ethnic Health Disparities box.) The incidence of prostate cancer rises markedly after age 50 with a median age at diagnosis of 67 years old.[15] However, many cases occur in younger men who sometimes have a more aggressive type of cancer.

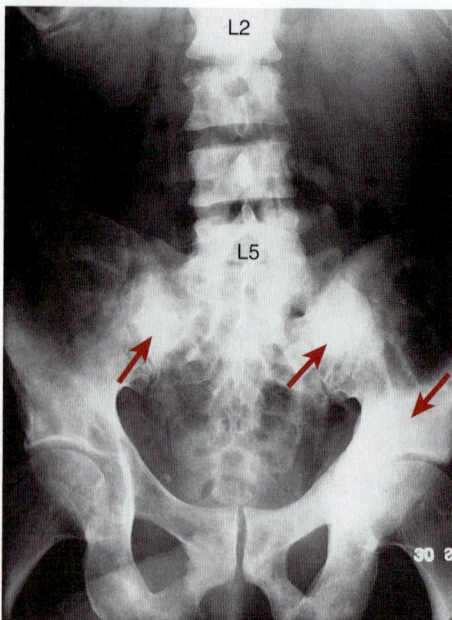

FIG. 54-5 Metastasis of prostate cancer to the pelvis and lumbar spine indicated by *arrows*. (From Mettler F: *Essentials of radiology,* ed 2, Philadelphia, 2004, Saunders.)

The incidence of prostate cancer is higher in African Americans than in any other ethnic group (except Jamaican men of African descent).[15] The reasons for the higher rate are unknown. African American men are likely to have more aggressive tumors at diagnosis and have higher mortality rates from prostate cancer. Differences in survival may be due to body composition, dietary factors, and endogenous hormones. It is not clear if smoking is a risk factor for prostate cancer. Neither is it clear if having BPH increases the risk of developing prostate cancer.[3]

Dietary factors and obesity may be associated with prostate cancer. A diet high in red and processed meat and high-fat dairy products along with a low intake of vegetables and fruits may increase the risk of prostate cancer.[15] Environment may also play a role, as there is an increased prevalence of prostate cancer in farmers and commercial pesticide applicators, possibly due to chemicals found in pesticides.[16]

 ### Genetic Link

Currently no known single gene causes prostate cancer. Some genes or gene mutations are more common in men with prostate cancer. From a genetics viewpoint, prostate cancer can be classified into three categories.

Most prostate cancers (about 75%) are considered *sporadic,* which means that damage to the genes occurs by chance after a person is born. Prostate cancer that runs in a family, called *familial prostate cancer,* is less common (about 20%). It occurs because of a combination of shared genes and shared environment or lifestyle factors. Familial prostate cancer is when two or more first-degree relatives (father, brother, son) are diagnosed with prostate cancer.

Hereditary (inherited) prostate cancer is rare (5% to 10%) and occurs when gene mutations are passed down in a family from one generation to the next. In hereditary prostate cancer, a family has any of the following characteristics: (1) three or more first-degree relatives with prostate cancer, (2) prostate cancer in three generations on the same side of the family, and (3) two or more close relatives (father, brother, son, grandfather, uncle, nephew) on the same side of the family diagnosed with prostate cancer before age 55.

Only genetic testing can determine whether a man has a genetic mutation. However, no genetic tests are available to determine if a man is predisposed to developing prostate cancer.

Having a family history does not mean that a man will develop prostate cancer; it indicates that he has an increased risk. Men with a family history of prostate cancer should talk with their HCP about their concerns. It is important for the HCP to obtain a detailed family history, including a family pedigree (see Figs. 12-4 and 12-5). Depending on the findings of the family history, a referral to a genetic counselor may be appropriate.

Hereditary breast and ovarian cancer (HBOC) syndrome is associated with mutations in the *BRCA1* and/or *BRCA2* genes (BRCA stands for *BR*east *CA*ncer). HBOC is most commonly associated with an increased risk of breast and ovarian cancer in women. However, men with HBOC also have an increased risk of breast cancer and prostate cancer. Mutations in *BRCA1* and *BRCA2* cause only a small percentage of familial prostate cancers. Genetic testing may be appropriate for families with prostate cancer that also have HBOC.

Clinical Manifestations and Complications

Prostate cancer may have no symptoms in the early stages. Eventually the patient may have LUTS similar to those of BPH. Pain in the lumbosacral area that radiates down to the hips or the legs, when combined with urinary symptoms, may indicate metastasis.

The tumor can spread to pelvic lymph nodes, bones, bladder, lungs, and liver. Once the tumor has spread to distant sites, the major problem becomes the management of pain. As the cancer spreads to the bones (common site of metastasis), pain can become severe, especially in the back and legs because of compression of the spinal cord and destruction of bone (Fig. 54-5).

Diagnostic Studies

Most men in the United States with prostate cancer are diagnosed by PSA screening. As prostate cancer screening has become more widespread, smaller cancers are being found in older men. In most cases, slow-growing cancers probably do not need to be treated. Many men live and die *with* prostate cancer, but most will not die *from* it.

Men have a chance to make an informed decision with their HCP about whether to be screened for prostate cancer. Men should be informed about the potential risks (e.g., subsequent evaluation and treatment that may be unnecessary) and benefits (early detection of prostate cancer) of PSA screening before being tested. After this discussion with their HCP, men who want to be screened may have an annual PSA test and DRE. On DRE, an abnormal prostate may feel hard, nodular, and asymmetric.

The AUA believes that men age 55 to 69 have the greatest potential benefit from PSA screening and recommend screening every 2 years.[14] Men at higher risk (African American men, men with a first-degree relative with prostate cancer) will have an individualized schedule for screening.

The American Cancer Society recommends that men should have a discussion with their HCP about screening for prostate cancer (as mentioned earlier). Men should not be screened unless they have received this information. The discussion about screening should take place at:

- Age 50 for men who are at average risk of prostate cancer and are expected to live at least 10 more years.
- Age 45 for men at high risk of developing prostate cancer. This includes African Americans and men who have a first-degree relative (father, brother, or son) diagnosed with prostate cancer at an early age (younger than age 65).
- Age 40 for men at even higher risk (those with more than one first-degree relative who had prostate cancer at an early age).

Elevated levels of PSA (normal level, 0 to 4 ng/mL [0 to 4 mcg/L]), a glycoprotein produced by the prostate, do not necessarily indicate prostate cancer. Mild elevations in PSA may occur with aging, BPH, recent ejaculation, constipation, acute or chronic prostatitis, or after long bike rides. In addition, cystoscopy, indwelling urethral catheters, and prostate biopsies may also produce transient elevations in PSA levels.

Neither PSA nor DRE is a definitive diagnostic test for prostate cancer. If PSA levels are continually elevated or if the DRE is abnormal, a biopsy of the prostate tissue is usually indicated. Biopsy of prostate tissue is necessary to confirm the diagnosis of prostate cancer. The biopsy is typically done using a transrectal approach. In a transrectal ultrasound (TRUS) procedure, an ultrasound probe enables the urologist to visualize abnormalities where the biopsy needles are going to be placed into the prostate. When a suspicious area is located, biopsy needles are inserted through the wall of the rectum into the prostate to obtain tissue samples. A pathologic examination of the specimen is done to assess for malignant changes.

Another approach for biopsies is to use an MRI/ultrasound fusion biopsy. In this approach, MRIs are fused with real-time, three-dimensional ultrasound. This new technique is more accurate than the traditional approach. Men who are candidates for this procedure are those who have a history of a previous negative ultrasound-guided biopsy and increasing PSA. This approach may also be used for men who are on active surveillance.

PSA is used not only to detect prostate cancer but also to monitor the success of treatment. When treatment has been successful, PSA levels should fall to undetectable levels. The regular measurement of PSA levels after treatment is important to evaluate the effectiveness of treatment and possible recurrence of prostate cancer.[17]

An elevated level of prostatic isoenzyme of serum acid phosphatase (prostatic acid phosphatase [PAP]) is another indicator of prostate cancer, especially if the cancer has spread outside of the prostate. With advanced prostate cancer, serum alkaline phosphatase is increased as a result of bone metastasis.

Other tests used to determine the location and extent of the spread of the cancer may include bone scan, CT scan, and MRI using an endorectal probe.

Interprofessional Care

Chemoprevention of prostate cancer is an active area of research. As discussed earlier in this chapter, finasteride and dutasteride used to treat BPH may reduce the chance of getting prostate cancer. Men who are concerned about prostate cancer should discuss with their HCP the potential risks and benefits of taking finasteride or dutasteride.

Early recognition and treatment are important to control tumor growth, prevent metastasis, and preserve quality of life. Most patients (93%) with prostate cancer are initially diagnosed when the cancer is at a local or regional stage.[15,18] The 5-year survival rate with an initial diagnosis at this stage is almost 100%.

The most common classification system for determining the extent of the prostate cancer is the tumor, node, and metastasis (TNM) system (Table 54-5). The tumor is graded on the basis of tumor histology using the Gleason scale.[19] The Gleason scale grades the tumor from 1 to 5 based on the degree of glandular differentiation. Grade 1 represents the most well-differentiated or lowest grade (most like the original cells), and grade 5 represents the most poorly differentiated (unlike the original cells) or highest grade. The two most commonly occurring patterns of cells are graded, and then the two scores are added together to create a Gleason score, which ranges from 2 to 10. The PSA level at diagnosis and the patient's Gleason score are used with the TNM system to determine the stage of the tumor, which is vital to determine treatment options.

The interprofessional care of the patient with prostate cancer depends on the stage of the cancer and the patient's overall health. None of these diagnostic options can predict the progression of prostate cancer, but at all stages, there is more than

		Lymph Node		PSA	Gleason
Stage	Tumor Size	Involvement	Metastasis	Level	Score
I	Not felt on DRE. Not seen by visual imaging.	No	No	<10	≤6
II	Felt on DRE. Seen by imaging. Tumor confined to prostate.	No	No	10-20	6-7
III	Cancer outside prostate. Possible spread to seminal vesicles.	No	No	Any level	Any score
IV	Any size.	Any nodal involvement.	Yes	Any level	Any score

TABLE 54-5 Staging of Prostate Cancer

DRE, Digital rectal examination.
Adapted from American Cancer Society: How is prostate cancer staged? Retrieved from *www.cancer.org/Cancer/ProstateCancer/DetailedGuide/prostate-cancer-staging.*

TABLE 54-6 Interprofessional Care

Prostate Cancer

Diagnostic Assessment
- History and physical examination
- Digital rectal examination (DRE)
- Prostate-specific antigen (PSA)
- Prostatic acid phosphatase (PAP)
- Transrectal ultrasound (TRUS)
- Biopsy of prostate and lymph nodes
- CT scan, MRI
- Bone scan (to evaluate for metastatic disease)

Management

Active Surveillance
- Annual PSA and DRE

Surgery
- Radical prostatectomy
- Cryotherapy
- Orchiectomy (for metastatic disease)

Radiation Therapy
- External beam for primary, adjuvant, and recurrent disease
- Brachytherapy

Drug Therapy
- Androgen deprivation therapy (Table 54-7)
- Chemotherapy for metastatic disease

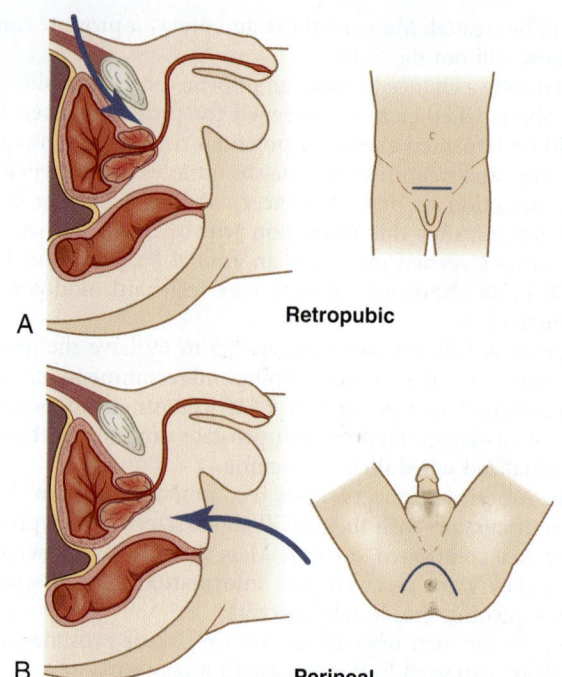

FIG. 54-6 Common approaches used to perform a prostatectomy. **A,** Retropubic approach involves a midline abdominal incision. **B,** Perineal approach involves an incision between the scrotum and the anus.

one possible treatment option (Table 54-6), depending on the stage, Gleason score, and PSA. The decision of which treatment course to pursue should be made jointly by patients, their partners, and the interprofessional care team.[17,18]

Active Surveillance. Prostate cancer is relatively slow growing. Therefore a conservative approach to management of prostate cancer is active surveillance, or "watchful waiting." This strategy is appropriate when the patient has (1) a life expectancy of less than 10 years (low risk of dying of the disease); (2) a low-grade, low-stage tumor; and (3) serious coexisting medical conditions. With active surveillance, patients are typically followed with frequent PSA measurements and DRE to monitor the progress of the disease. Significant changes in the PSA level or the DRE, or the development of symptoms, warrant a reevaluation of treatment options.

Surgical Therapy

Radical Prostatectomy. With **radical prostatectomy**, the entire prostate gland, seminal vesicles, and part of the bladder neck (ampulla) are removed. The entire prostate is removed because the cancer tends to be in many different locations within the gland. Retroperitoneal lymph node dissection is performed only on men with a high risk for metastatic disease. Surgery is usually not considered an option for advanced stage disease (except to relieve symptoms associated with obstruction) because metastasis has already occurred.

Traditional surgical approaches for a radical prostatectomy include retropubic and perineal resection (Fig. 54-6). With the *retropubic* approach, a low midline abdominal incision is made to access the prostate gland, and the pelvic lymph nodes can be dissected. With the *perineal* resection, an incision is made between the scrotum and anus.

A *robotic-assisted* (e.g., da Vinci system) prostatectomy is a type of surgery in which the surgeon sits at a computer console while controlling high-resolution cameras and microsurgical instruments. Robotics is being used more frequently since it allows for increased precision, visualization, and dexterity by the surgeon when removing the prostate gland. It results in less bleeding, less pain, and a faster recovery compared with other approaches.[20,21]

After surgery, the patient has a large indwelling catheter with a 30-mL balloon placed in the bladder via the urethra. A drain is left in the surgical site to aid in the removal of drainage from the area. This drain is typically removed after a couple of days. Because the perineal approach has a higher risk of postoperative infection (because of the location of the incision related to the anus), careful dressing changes and perineal care after each bowel movement are important for comfort and to prevent infection. Depending on the type of surgery, the length of hospital stay postoperatively ranges from 1 to 3 days.

Two major adverse outcomes after a radical prostatectomy are erectile dysfunction (ED) and urinary incontinence.[22] The incidence of ED depends on the patient's age, preoperative sexual function, whether nerve-sparing surgery was performed, and the surgeon's expertise. Sexual function after surgery tends to return gradually over at least 24 months or more, but phosphodiesterase type 5 (PDE5) medications may help improve sexual function.

Problems with urinary control may occur for the first few months after surgery because the bladder must be reattached to the urethra after the prostate is removed. Over time, the bladder adjusts and most men regain control.[22] Kegel exercises strengthen the urinary sphincter and may help improve continence. (Kegel exercises are presented in Table 45-18.) Other complications associated with surgery include hemorrhage, urinary retention, infection, wound dehiscence, deep vein thrombosis, and pulmonary emboli.

Nerve-Sparing Procedure. Near the prostate gland are neurovascular bundles that maintain erectile functioning. The preservation of these bundles during a prostatectomy is possible while still removing all of the cancer. Nerve-sparing prostatectomy is not indicated for patients with cancer outside of the prostate gland. Although the risk of ED is reduced with this procedure, there is no guarantee that potency will be maintained.

Cryotherapy. *Cryotherapy* (cryoablation) is a surgical technique for prostate cancer that destroys cancer cells by freezing the tissue. It has been used both as an initial treatment and as a second-line treatment after radiation therapy has failed. A TRUS probe is inserted to visualize the prostate gland. Probes containing liquid nitrogen are then inserted into the prostate. Liquid nitrogen delivers freezing temperatures, thus destroying the tissue. The treatment takes about 2 hours under general or spinal anesthesia and does not involve an abdominal incision.

Possible complications include damage to the urethra and, in rare cases, an urethrorectal fistula (an opening between the urethra and rectum) or a urethrocutaneous fistula (an opening between the urethra and skin). Tissue sloughing, ED, urinary incontinence, prostatitis, and hemorrhage can also occur.

Radiation Therapy. Radiation therapy is another common treatment option for prostate cancer. Radiation therapy may be the only treatment, or it may be used in combination with surgery or with hormone therapy. Salvage radiation therapy given for prostate cancer recurrence after a radical prostatectomy may improve survival in some men.

External Beam Radiation. External beam radiation is the most widely used method of delivering radiation treatments for men with prostate cancer. This therapy can be used to treat patients with prostate cancer confined to the prostate and/or surrounding tissue. Patients are usually treated on an outpatient basis 5 days a week for 4 to 8 weeks; each treatment lasts only a few minutes.

Side effects from radiation can be acute (occurring during treatment or within 90 days that follow) or delayed (occurring months or years after treatment). The most common side effects involve changes to the skin (dryness, redness, irritation, pain), gastrointestinal tract (diarrhea, abdominal cramping, bleeding, radiation proctitis), urinary tract (dysuria, frequency, hesitancy, urgency, nocturia), and sexual function.[23,24] Fatigue may also occur. In patients with localized prostate cancer, cure rates with external beam radiation are comparable to those with radical prostatectomy.[15]

Brachytherapy. *Brachytherapy* involves placing radioactive seed implants into the prostate gland, allowing higher radiation doses directly in the tissue while sparing the surrounding tissue (rectum and bladder). The radioactive seeds are placed in the prostate gland with a needle through a grid template guided by TRUS (Fig. 54-7) to ensure accurate placement of the seeds.

Because brachytherapy is a one-time outpatient procedure, many patients find this more convenient than external beam radiation treatment. Brachytherapy is best suited for patients with early stage disease. The most common side effect is the development of urinary irritative or obstructive problems. Some men may also experience ED. The AUA Symptom Index (Table 54-1) can be used to measure urinary function for patients undergoing brachytherapy and can be incorporated into postoperative nursing management. For those with more advanced tumors, brachytherapy may be offered in combination with external beam radiation treatment.[24] (Brachytherapy is further discussed in Chapter 15.)

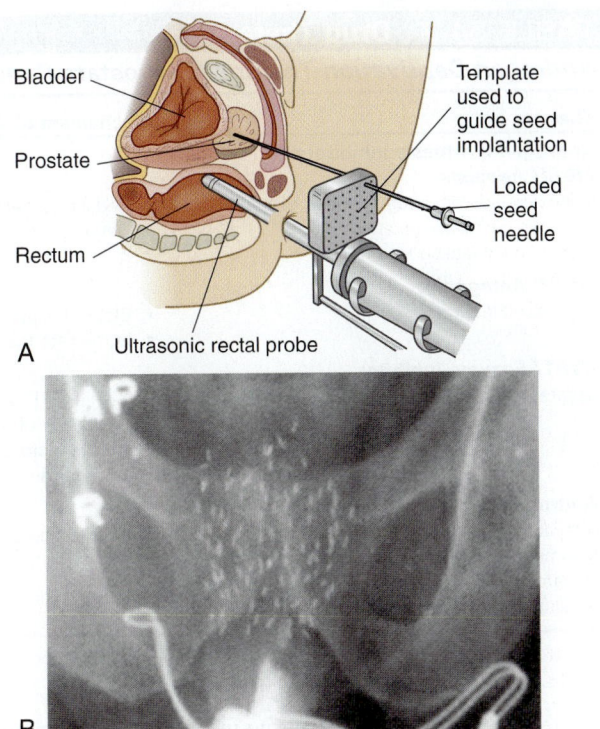

FIG. 54-7   A, Prostate brachytherapy. Implantation of radioactive seeds with a needle guided by ultrasound and a template grid. **B,** Radioactive seeds. (*B,* From Abeloff MD, Armitage JO, Niederhuber JE, et al, editors: *Abeloff's clinical oncology,* ed 4, 2008, Churchill Livingstone.)

Drug Therapy. The forms of drug therapy available for the treatment of advanced or metastatic prostate cancer are androgen deprivation (hormone) therapy, chemotherapy, or a combination of both.

Androgen Deprivation Therapy. Prostate cancer growth is largely dependent on the presence of androgens. *Androgen deprivation therapy* (ADT) reduces the levels of circulating androgens to reduce the tumor growth. Androgen deprivation can be produced by inhibiting androgen production or blocking androgen receptors (Table 54-7).

One of the biggest challenges with ADT is that almost all tumors treated become resistant to this therapy (*hormone refractory*) within a few years. An elevated PSA level is often the first sign that this therapy is no longer effective. Patients taking ADT have an increased risk of cardiovascular side effects, including elevated serum cholesterol and triglyceride levels and coronary artery disease.[25]

Osteoporosis and fractures may occur in prostate cancer patients receiving ADT. Drugs recommended to reduce bone mineral loss in these patients include zoledronic acid (Reclast) and raloxifene (Evista).[26] Denosumab (Prolia), a drug that slows the breakdown of bone, may also be used to increase bone mass in men with nonmetastatic prostate cancer.

Androgen synthesis inhibitors. The hypothalamus produces luteinizing hormone–releasing hormone (LH-RH), which stimulates the anterior pituitary to produce luteinizing hormone (LH) and follicle-stimulating hormone (FSH). LH stimulates the testicular Leydig cells to produce testosterone. *LH-RH agonists* super stimulate the pituitary, downregulating the LH-RH receptors, and leading to a refractory condition in which the anterior pituitary is unresponsive to LH-RH. These drugs cause an initial transient increase in LH and FSH;

TABLE 54-7 Drug Therapy
Androgen Deprivation Therapy for Prostate Cancer

Therapy	Mechanism of Action	Side Effects
Androgen Synthesis Inhibitors **LH-RH Agonists** leuprolide (Lupron, Lupron Depot, Eligard) goserelin (Zoladex) triptorelin (Trelstar)	• Reduce secretion of LH and FSH • Decrease testosterone production	• Hot flashes, gynecomastia, decreased libido, erectile dysfunction • Depression and mood changes
LH-RH Antagonist degarelix (Firmagon)	• Blocks LH receptors • Immediate testosterone suppression	• Pain, redness, and swelling at injection site • Elevated liver enzymes
CYP17 Enzyme Inhibitor abiraterone (Zytiga)	• Inhibits CYP17, an enzyme needed for production of testosterone • Inhibits testosterone synthesis from testes, adrenal glands, and prostate cancer cells	• Joint swelling, fluid retention • Muscle discomfort • Hot flashes • Diarrhea
Androgen Receptor Blockers bicalutamide (Casodex) flutamide nilutamide (Nilandron) enzalutamide (Xtandi)	• Block action of testosterone by competing with receptor sites	• Loss of libido, erectile dysfunction, and hot flashes • Breast pain and gynecomastia may also occur

FSH, Follicle-stimulating hormone; *LH,* luteinizing hormone; *LH–RH,* luteinizing hormone–releasing hormone.

testosterone abruptly rises resulting in a *flare.* Symptoms may worsen during this time. However, with continued administration, LH and testosterone levels are decreased.

LH-RH agonists include leuprolide (Lupron, Lupron Depot, Eligard), goserelin (Zoladex), and triptorelin (Trelstar) (Table 54-7). These drugs essentially produce a chemical castration similar to the effects of an orchiectomy. These drugs are given by subcutaneous or IM injections on a regular basis. Viadur is an implant that is placed subcutaneously and delivers leuprolide continuously for 1 year.

Degarelix is an *LH-RH antagonist* that lowers testosterone levels to castration levels. Unlike the LH-RH agonists, degarelix does not cause a testosterone flare because it acts directly to block LH and FSH receptors. It is given as a subcutaneous injection, and results are seen in 3 days.

Abiraterone (Zytiga) works by inhibiting an enzyme, CYP17, which is needed for the production of testosterone. This drug is given orally to men with castration-resistant prostate cancer, and improves overall survival by 4 to 5 months.

Androgen receptor blockers. Androgen receptor blockers are another classification of antiandrogen drugs that compete with circulating androgens at the receptor sites. Flutamide, nilutamide (Nilandron), bicalutamide (Casodex), and enzalutamide (Xtandi) are androgen receptor blockers. They are taken daily as an oral medication and can be used in combination with an LH-RH agonist (e.g., goserelin, leuprolide). Combining an androgen receptor blocker with an LH-RH agonist results in combined androgen blockade.

Chemotherapy. The use of chemotherapy has primarily been limited to treatment for those with hormone-refractory prostate cancer (HRPC) in late-stage disease. In HRPC the cancer is progressing despite treatment. This occurs in patients who have taken an antiandrogen for a certain period. The goal of chemotherapy is mainly palliative.

Some commonly used chemotherapy drugs for prostate cancer include docetaxel (Taxotere), cabazitaxel (Jevtana), paclitaxel (Abraxane), mitoxantrone, vinblastine, cyclophosphamide, and estramustine (Emcyt).

Men with advanced prostate cancer who have HRPC may receive a vaccine (sipuleucel-T [Provenge]). The vaccine stimulates the patient's system against the cancer and may prolong survival, although its exact mechanism is unknown. It prolongs survival by about 4 months but does not reduce tumor burden. It is individually prepared for each man by a process that combines his own white blood cells with granulocyte macrophage colony-stimulating factor (GMCSF), which then attacks the prostate tumor cells.

Radiotherapy. Radium-223 dichloride (Xofigo) can be used in the treatment of patients with castration-resistant prostate cancer, symptomatic bone metastases, and no known visceral metastatic disease. It is an alpha particle–emitting radiotherapy drug that mimics calcium and forms complexes with hydroxyapatite at areas of increased bone turnover, such as bone metastases.

Orchiectomy. A bilateral orchiectomy is the surgical removal of the testes that may be done alone or after prostatectomy. It is the gold standard for androgen deprivation, as there are no side effects to be managed, and it is very low cost when compared with other options. For advanced stages of prostate cancer, an orchiectomy is one treatment option for cancer control, with rapid relief of bone pain associated with advanced tumors.

Orchiectomy may also shrink the prostate, thus relieving urinary obstruction in the later stages of disease when surgery is not an option. After an orchiectomy, weight gain and loss of muscle mass can alter a man's physical appearance. These physical changes can affect self-esteem, leading to grief and depression. Because this procedure is permanent, many men prefer drug therapy over an orchiectomy. Currently orchiectomy is rarely performed.

Culturally Competent Care: Prostate Cancer

Nurses need to be aware of ethnic and cultural considerations when providing information about the risk for prostate cancer and screening recommendations. Consider not only the ethnic differences in the incidence of prostate cancer but also differences in health promotion practices.

African American men have the highest mortality rates from prostate cancer, in part because their prostate cancer often is more advanced at the time of diagnosis. Despite the availability of screening measures (PSA and DRE), African American men and those in lower socioeconomic groups may not access these services. This is only partially related to knowledge levels about prostate cancer. In comparison to white men, African American men with prostate cancer report more problems with financial access to transportation and health care costs, and they indicate using more religious coping strategies. White men are also perceived as receiving more favorable treatment from their HCPs than African Americans.[27]

Although exposure to electronic and print media is successful in informing some men about prostate cancer, the effectiveness differs significantly based on demographic variables such as ethnicity, age, education level, and socioeconomic level. Ideally, all men should be aware of the risks associated with prostate cancer and the screening methods available. Consider the best method to communicate this information to men of all cultures and ethnicities, while being aware of the changing guidelines, to promote understanding and participation in prostate cancer screening for men in at risk groups.

❖ NURSING MANAGEMENT: PROSTATE CANCER

◆ Nursing Assessment

Subjective and objective data that should be obtained from a patient with prostate cancer are presented in Table 54-8.

◆ Nursing Diagnoses

Nursing diagnoses for the patient with prostate cancer depend on the stage of the cancer. General nursing diagnoses may include, but are not limited to, the following.

- Decisional conflict *related to* numerous alternative treatment options
- Acute pain *related to* surgery, prostatic enlargement, bone metastasis, and bladder spasms
- Urinary retention and impaired urinary elimination *related to* obstruction of the urethra by the prostate and loss of bladder tone
- Sexual dysfunction *related to* effects of treatment
- Anxiety *related to* uncertain outcome of disease process on life and lifestyle and effect of treatment on sexual function

◆ Planning

The overall goals are that the patient with prostate cancer will (1) be an active participant in the treatment plan, (2) have satisfactory pain control, (3) follow the therapeutic plan, (4) understand the effect of the therapeutic plan on sexual function, and (5) find a satisfactory way to manage the impact on bladder and bowel function.

◆ Nursing Implementation

◆ **Health Promotion.** One of the most important roles in relation to prostate cancer is to encourage patients, in consultation with their HCPs, to have annual prostate screening (PSA and DRE). (The age at which to begin screening is discussed on pp. 1276-1277.) Because of their increased risk of prostate cancer, African American men and other men at high risk, such as those with a family history of prostate cancer, should discuss the need for annual PSA and DRE beginning at age 45.[15]

TABLE 54-8   Nursing Assessment

Prostate Cancer

Subjective Data

Important Health Information

Medications: Testosterone supplements. Use of any medications affecting urinary tract such as morphine, anticholinergics, monoamine oxidase inhibitors, and tricyclic antidepressants

Functional Health Patterns

Health perception–health management: Positive family history. Increasing fatigue and malaise

Nutritional-metabolic: High-fat diet. Anorexia, weight loss (possible indicators of metastasis)

Elimination: Hesitancy or straining to start stream, urinary urgency, frequency, retention with dribbling, weak stream, hematuria

Sleep-rest: Nocturia

Cognitive-perceptual: Dysuria. Low back pain radiating to legs or pelvis, bone pain (possible indicators of metastasis). Pain level

Self-perception–self-concept: Anxiety regarding self-concept

Objective Data

General

Older adult male. Pelvic lymphadenopathy (late sign)

Urinary

Distended bladder on palpation. Unilaterally hard, enlarged, fixed prostate on rectal examination

Musculoskeletal

Pathologic fractures (metastasis)

Possible Diagnostic Findings

Serum PSA. ↑ serum PAP (metastasis). Nodular and irregular prostate on ultrasonography, positive biopsy results. Anemia

PAP, Prostatic acid phosphatase; *PSA,* prostate-specific antigen.

◆ **Acute Care.** Preoperative and postoperative phases of radical prostatectomy are similar to surgical procedures for BPH (see pp. 1273-1275). Nursing interventions for the patient who undergoes radiation therapy and chemotherapy are discussed in Chapter 15. An additional consideration is the patient's psychologic response to a diagnosis of cancer. Provide sensitive, caring support for the patient and his family to help them cope with the diagnosis. Prostate cancer support groups are available for men and their families to encourage them to be active, informed participants in their own care.

◆ **Ambulatory Care.** Teach appropriate catheter care if the patient is discharged with an indwelling catheter in place. Instruct the patient to clean the urethral meatus with soap and water once a day; maintain a high fluid intake; keep the collecting bag lower than the bladder at all times; keep the catheter securely anchored to the inner thigh or abdomen; and report any signs of bladder infection, such as bladder spasms, fever, or hematuria.

If urinary incontinence is a problem, encourage the patient to practice pelvic floor muscle exercises (Kegel exercises) at every urination and throughout the day. Continuous practice during the 4- to 6-week healing process improves the success rate. Products used for incontinence specifically designed for men are available through home care product catalogs and retail stores. (Urinary incontinence is discussed in Chapter 45.)

Palliative and end-of-life care are often appropriate and beneficial to the patient with advanced disease and his family (see

Chapter 9). Common problems experienced by the patient with advanced prostate cancer include fatigue, bladder outlet obstruction and ureteral obstruction (caused by compression of the urethra and/or ureters from tumor mass or lymph node metastasis), severe bone pain and fractures (caused by bone metastasis), spinal cord compression (from spinal metastasis), and leg edema (caused by lymphedema, deep vein thrombosis, and other medical conditions). Nursing interventions must focus on all of these problems.

Pain management is one of the most important aspects of your care for these patients. Pain control involves ongoing pain assessment, administration of prescribed medications (both opioid and nonopioid agents), and nonpharmacologic methods of pain relief (e.g., relaxation breathing). (Pain management is further discussed in Chapter 8.)

◆ Evaluation

The outcomes are that the patient with prostate cancer will
- Be an active participant in the treatment plan
- Have satisfactory pain control
- Follow the therapeutic plan
- Understand the effect of the treatment on sexual function
- Find a satisfactory way to manage the impact on bladder or bowel function

PROSTATITIS

Etiology and Pathophysiology

Prostatitis is a broad term that describes a group of inflammatory and noninflammatory conditions affecting the prostate gland. Prostatitis is one of the most common urologic disorders. It is estimated that 12% of all men experience prostatitis in their lifetime.[28] Almost 2 million men are treated for prostatitis every year, and the most common type is nonbacterial.

The four categories of prostatitis syndromes are: (1) acute bacterial prostatitis, (2) chronic bacterial prostatitis, (3) chronic prostatitis/chronic pelvic pain syndrome, and (4) asymptomatic inflammatory prostatitis.

Both acute and chronic bacterial prostatitis generally result from organisms reaching the prostate gland by one of the following routes: ascending from the urethra, descending from the bladder, and invading via the bloodstream or the lymphatic channels. Common causative organisms are *Escherichia coli* (most common), *Klebsiella, Pseudomonas, Enterobacter, Proteus, Chlamydia trachomatis, Neisseria gonorrhoeae,* and group D streptococci.

Chronic bacterial prostatitis differs from acute prostatitis in that it involves recurrent episodes of infection. It is the most common reason for recurrent UTIs in adult men.

Chronic prostatitis/chronic pelvic pain syndrome describes a syndrome of prostate and urinary pain in the absence of an obvious infectious process. The etiology of this syndrome is not known. It may occur after a viral illness, or it may be associated with sexually transmitted infections (STIs), particularly in younger adults. A culture reveals no causative organisms, but leukocytes may be found in prostatic secretions.

Asymptomatic inflammatory prostatitis is usually diagnosed in individuals who have no symptoms but are found to have an inflammatory process in the prostate. These patients are usually diagnosed during the evaluation of other genitourinary tract problems. Leukocytes are present in the seminal fluid from the prostate, but the cause of this process is unclear.

Clinical Manifestations and Complications

Common manifestations of acute prostatitis include fever, chills, back pain, and perineal pain. In addition, acute urinary symptoms such as dysuria, urinary frequency, urgency, and cloudy urine may occur. The patient may progress to acute urinary retention caused by prostatic swelling if he remains untreated. With DRE, the prostate is extremely swollen, extremely tender, and boggy.

The complications of prostatitis are epididymitis and cystitis. Sexual function may be affected as manifested by postejaculation pain, libido problems, and ED. Prostatic abscess is also a potential, but uncommon, complication.

In chronic bacterial prostatitis and chronic prostatitis/chronic pelvic pain syndrome, manifestations are similar but generally milder than those of acute bacterial prostatitis. These include irritative voiding symptoms (frequency, urgency, dysuria), backache, perineal and pelvic pain, and ejaculatory pain. Obstructive symptoms are uncommon unless there is coexisting BPH.[29] With DRE, the prostate feels enlarged and soft or boggy and can be slightly tender with palpation. Chronic prostatitis can predispose the patient to recurrent UTIs.

The clinical features of prostatitis can mimic those of a UTI. However, it is important to remember that acute cystitis is not common in men.

Diagnostic Studies

Because patients with prostatitis have urinary symptoms, a urinalysis (UA) and urine culture are indicated. Often WBCs and bacteria are present. If the patient has a fever, WBC count and blood cultures are also indicated. The PSA test may be done to rule out prostate cancer. However, PSA levels are often elevated with prostatic inflammation. Thus it is not in itself considered diagnostic.

Microscopic evaluation and culture of expressed prostate secretion can be useful in the diagnosis of prostatitis. Expressed prostate secretion is obtained using a premassage and postmassage test.[29] The patient is asked to void into a specimen cup just before and just after a vigorous prostate massage. Prostatic massage (for expressed prostate secretion) should be avoided if acute bacterial prostatitis is suspected, since compression is extremely painful and can increase the risk of bacterial spread. TRUS has not been useful in the diagnosis of prostatitis. However, TRUS or MRI may be done to rule out an abscess in the prostate.

❖ NURSING AND INTERPROFESSIONAL MANAGEMENT: PROSTATITIS

Antibiotics commonly used for acute and chronic bacterial prostatitis include trimethoprim/sulfamethoxazole (Bactrim), ciprofloxacin (Cipro), ofloxacin, carbachol (Miostat), carbenicillin, cephalexin (Keflex), and doxycycline (Vibramycin) or tetracycline. Antibiotics are usually given orally for up to 4 weeks for acute bacterial prostatitis. However, if the patient has high fever or other signs of impending sepsis, he will be hospitalized and IV antibiotics given.

Men with chronic bacterial prostatitis may be given oral antibiotic therapy for 8 to 12 weeks. Antibiotics may be given for a lifetime if the patient is immunocompromised. A short course of oral antibiotics is usually prescribed for those with chronic prostatitis/chronic pelvic pain syndrome in case of bacterial infection. However, antibiotic therapy is often ineffective for patients whose prostatitis is not due to bacteria.

Although patients with acute and chronic bacterial prostatitis tend to experience a great amount of discomfort, the pain resolves as the infection is treated. However, they may have residual discomfort for several weeks after a course of antibiotics, as it takes time for the prostate to return to normal. Pain management for patients with chronic prostatitis/chronic pelvic pain syndrome is more difficult because the pain persists for weeks to months. No single approach has been shown to provide relief for everyone with this condition. Antiinflammatory agents (e.g., ibuprofen, indomethacin) may be used for pain control in prostatitis, but these drugs provide only moderate pain relief.

Warm sitz baths may help to relieve pain. Relaxation of muscle tissue in the prostate using α-adrenergic blockers (e.g., tamsulosin, alfuzosin) has been shown to be effective in reducing discomfort for some men.

Acute urinary retention can develop in acute prostatitis, requiring insertion of a urinary catheter. However, passage of a catheter through an inflamed urethra is contraindicated in acute prostatitis. The placement of a suprapubic catheter may then be indicated. Repetitive prostatic massage may be recommended as adjunct therapy for prostatitis for men. This potentially relieves congestion within the prostate by squeezing out excess prostatic secretions, providing pain relief. Similar to massage, measures to stimulate ejaculation (masturbation and intercourse) may help to drain the prostate and provide some relief.

Because the prostate can serve as a source of bacteria, fluid intake should be kept at a high level for all patients experiencing prostatitis. Encourage the patient to drink plenty of fluids, especially men with acute bacterial prostatitis because of the increased fluid needs associated with fever and infection. Management of fever is also an important nursing intervention.

PROBLEMS OF THE PENIS

Health problems of the penis are rare if STIs are excluded (see Chapter 52). Problems of the penis may be classified as congenital, problems of the prepuce, problems with the erectile mechanism, and cancer.

CONGENITAL PROBLEMS

Hypospadias is a urologic abnormality in which the urethral meatus is located on the ventral surface of the penis anywhere from the corona to the perineum. Possible causes are hormonal influences in utero, environmental factors, and genetic factors. Surgical repair of hypospadias, especially those that are closest to the scrotum or perineum, is usually done while the boy is young. Surgery may be necessary if it is associated with *chordee* (a painful downward curvature of the penis during erection) or if it prevents intercourse or normal urination. Surgery may be considered for cosmetic reasons or emotional well-being in older boys and adult men.

PROBLEMS OF PREPUCE

Problems of the prepuce (foreskin) in the United States are not common because circumcision (surgical removal of the foreskin of the penis) has been a routine procedure for many male infants.

Phimosis is a tightness or constriction of the foreskin around the head of the penis, making retraction difficult (Fig. 54-8, *A*). It is caused by chronic inflammation of the foreskin, usually

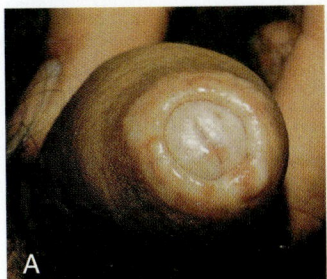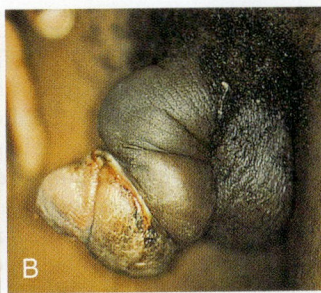

FIG. 54-8 A, Phimosis: inability to retract the foreskin due to secondary lesions on the prepuce. **B,** Paraphimosis: ulcer with edema from foreskin remaining contracted over the prepuce (foreskin).

associated with poor hygiene techniques that allow bacterial and yeast organisms to become trapped under the foreskin. Topical corticosteroid cream, with or without an antifungal, applied two or three times daily to the exterior and interior of the tip of the foreskin may be effective in the initial treatment of any inflammation. Definitive treatment is either circumcision or a dorsal slit surgical procedure.

Paraphimosis is tightness of the foreskin resulting in the inability to pull it forward from a retracted position and preventing normal return over the glans. It is a urologic emergency, as a sufficiently tight retracted phimotic ring will compromise arterial flow to the glans. An ulcer can develop if the foreskin remains contracted (Fig. 54-8, *B*). Paraphimosis can occur when the foreskin is pulled back during bathing, use of urinary catheters, or intercourse and is not placed back in the forward position. Replacement of the foreskin after careful cleaning helps to prevent this condition. The goal of treatment is to return the foreskin to its natural position over the glans penis through manual reduction. One strategy involves pushing the glans back through the prepuce by applying constant thumb pressure while the index fingers pull the prepuce over the glans. Ice and/or hand compression on the foreskin, glans, and penis may be done before this technique to reduce edema. Treatment may include antibiotics or warm soaks. Definitive treatment is either circumcision or a dorsal slit.

PROBLEMS OF ERECTILE MECHANISM

Priapism is a painful erection lasting longer than 6 hours that may constitute a medical emergency. Priapism is caused by complex vascular and neurologic factors that result in an obstruction of venous outflow in the penis. Conditions that may be associated with priapism include sickle cell disease, diabetes mellitus, trauma to the spinal cord, degenerative lesions of the spine, and drugs (e.g., cocaine, trazodone). Vasoactive drugs (e.g., alprostadil) injected into the corpora cavernosa for ED can also cause priapism. Complications include penile tissue necrosis caused by lack of blood flow or hydronephrosis from bladder distention. With immediate medical treatment, the risk of permanent ED is low.

Treatment varies depending on the cause. In patients with sickle cell disease, a blood exchange transfusion may be done, whereas other patients may be treated with sedatives, an injection of a smooth muscle relaxant directly into the penis, or aspiration and irrigation of the corpora cavernosa with a large-bore needle.

Peyronie's disease is caused by plaque formation in one of the corpora cavernosa of the penis that results in inelasticity during erection. The palpable, nontender, hard plaque formation may occur spontaneously or result from trauma to the penile shaft. The plaque prevents adequate blood flow into the spongy tissue, which results in a curvature during erection. The condition is not dangerous but can result in painful erections, ED, or embarrassment. Patients may improve slightly over time, stabilize, or need surgery. Collagenase clostridium histolyticum (Xiaflex) is a series of injections into the plaque that can reduce the curvature over the course of the injections and allows men to avoid surgery.

CANCER OF PENIS

Cancer of the penis is rare in the United States. More than 95% are squamous cell carcinoma. It occurs more commonly in men who have human papillomavirus (HPV) infection and phimosis or uncircumcised men.[30] The tumor may appear as a superficial ulceration or a pimple-like nodule. Pain is not a usual complaint, and this contributes to a delay in seeking treatment. The nontender warty lesion may be mistaken for a genital wart. Treatment in the early stages is laser removal of the growth. A radical resection of the penis may be done if the cancer has spread. Surgery, radiation, or chemotherapy may be attempted, depending on the extent of the disease, lymph node involvement, or metastasis.

PROBLEMS OF SCROTUM AND TESTES

It is important for the patient to see his HCP if he feels any scrotal lumps or painful areas in his scrotum or testes. He would be unable to distinguish normal variations from cancer when performing self-examination, and an incidental finding of a "scrotal lump" results in high anxiety for the patient.

INFLAMMATORY AND INFECTIOUS PROBLEMS

Skin Problems

The skin of the scrotum is susceptible to a number of common skin diseases. The most common are fungal infections, dermatitis (neurodermatitis, contact dermatitis, seborrheic dermatitis), and parasitic infections (scabies, lice). These conditions involve discomfort for the patient but are associated with few severe complications (see Chapter 23).

Epididymitis

Epididymitis is an acute, painful inflammatory process of the epididymis (Fig. 54-9), which is often due to an infectious process, trauma, or urinary reflux down the ductus (vas) deferens. It is usually unilateral. Swelling may progress to the point that the epididymis and testis are indistinguishable. In men younger than 35 years of age, the most common cause is gonorrhea or chlamydial infection; in men greater than 35 the most common cause is *E. coli*. BPH and prostatitis are common contributors in older men.

The use of antibiotics is important for both partners if the transmission is through sexual contact. Encourage patients to refrain from sexual intercourse until treatment is complete. If they do engage in intercourse, a condom should be used. Conservative treatment consists of elevation of the scrotum, ice packs, and analgesics. Ambulation places the scrotum in a dependent position and increases pain. Acute tenderness subsides within 1 week, although some discomfort and swelling may last for weeks or months.

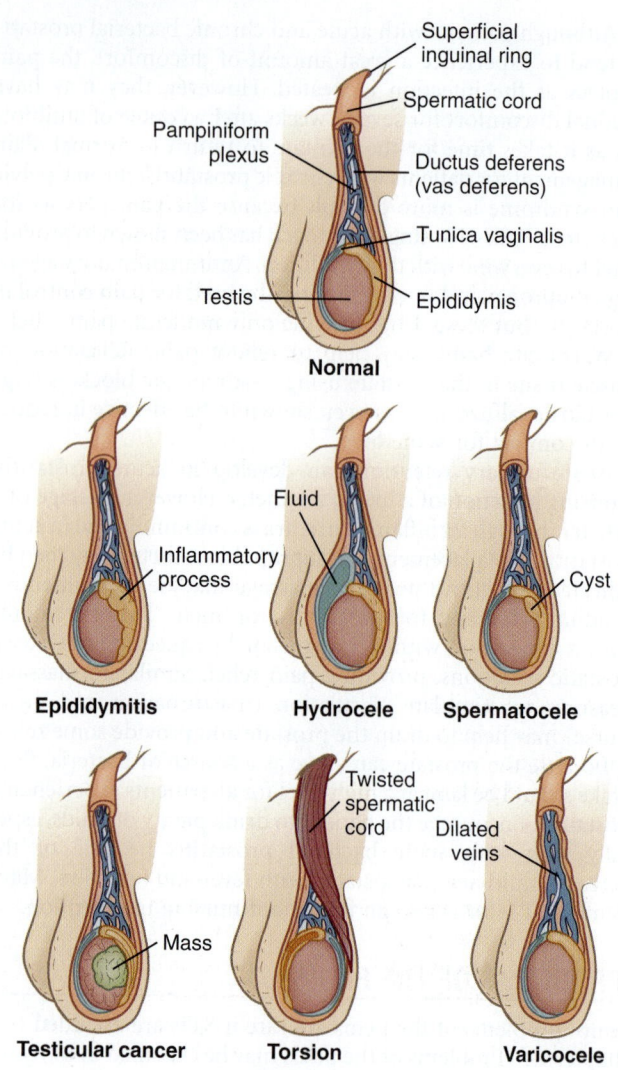

FIG. 54-9   Scrotal masses.

Orchitis

Orchitis refers to an acute inflammation of the testis. In orchitis, the testis is painful, tender, and swollen. It generally occurs after an episode of bacterial or viral infection such as mumps, pneumonia, tuberculosis, or syphilis. It can also be a side effect of epididymitis, trauma, infectious mononucleosis, influenza, catheterization, or complicated UTI. Mumps orchitis is a condition contributing to infertility that could be avoided by childhood vaccination against mumps. Treatment is similar to that for epididymitis.

CONGENITAL PROBLEMS

Cryptorchidism (undescended testes) is failure of the testes to descend into the scrotal sac before birth. It is the most common congenital testicular condition and is more common on the right. It may occur bilaterally or unilaterally and may be a contributing factor to male infertility if corrective surgery is not done by 2 years of age. The incidence of testicular cancer is also higher if the condition is not corrected before puberty. Surgery is performed to locate and suture the testis or testes to the scrotum.

ACQUIRED PROBLEMS

Hydrocele

A *hydrocele* is a nontender, fluid-filled mass that results from interference with lymphatic drainage of the scrotum and swelling of the tunica vaginalis that surrounds the testis (Fig. 54-10; also Fig. 54-9). Diagnosis is aided by shining a flashlight through the scrotum (transillumination). No treatment is indicated unless the swelling becomes large and uncomfortable, in which case surgical repair of the hydrocele is performed. Hydrocele repair is avoided in men who have not started their family or seek to add to their family as repair can contribute to subfertility or infertility.

Spermatocele

A *spermatocele* is a firm, sperm-containing cyst of the epididymis that may be visible with transillumination (Fig. 54-9). The cause is unknown, and these structures can become large, tense and painful, and their size can wax and wane with time. Spermatocele repair is also avoided in men who have not started their family or seek to add to their family as repair can contribute to subfertility or infertility.

Varicocele

A *varicocele* is a dilation of the veins that drain the testes (Fig. 54-9). The scrotum can feel wormlike when palpated if the venous dilation is significant. However, this is dependent on the examiner's experience and skill. The cause of the problem is unknown.

A varicocele is usually located on the left side of the scrotum as a consequence of retrograde blood flow from the left renal vein. Surgery can be considered if the patient is infertile, as varicoceles are associated with 40% to 50% of cases of infertility. Sperm is thought to be damaged by varicoceles via an undetermined mechanism. Repair of the varicocele may be through injection of a sclerosing agent or by surgical ligation of the spermatic vein. Untreated varicoceles are not associated with any long-term health risk.

Testicular Torsion

Testicular torsion involves a twisting of the spermatic cord that supplies blood to the testes and epididymis (Fig. 54-9). It is considered a surgical emergency. It is most commonly seen in males younger than age 20. It can occur spontaneously, as a result of trauma, or as a result of an anatomic abnormality. The patient experiences severe, sudden onset of scrotal pain, tenderness, swelling, nausea, and vomiting. Urinary symptoms, fever, and WBCs or bacteria in the urine are absent. The pain does not usually subside with rest or elevation of the scrotum.

In testicular torsion, the cremasteric reflex is absent on the side of the swelling. Normal anatomic landmarks are lost due to tissue edema.

A nuclear scan of the testes or Doppler ultrasound is typically performed to assess blood flow within the testicle. Decreased or absent blood flow confirms the diagnosis. Torsion is an emergency if the blood supply to the affected testicle is not restored within 4 to 6 hours. Ischemia to the testis will occur, leading to necrosis. Unless the torsion resolves spontaneously, surgery to untwist the cord and restore the blood supply must be performed emergently.

TESTICULAR CANCER

Etiology and Pathophysiology

Testicular cancer is rare, accounting for less than 1% of all cancers found in males. It is the most common type of cancer in young men between 15 and 44 years of age. In the United States about 8430 new cases occur annually with a median age at diagnosis of 33 years old.[15,31]

Testicular tumors are more common in males who have had undescended testes (cryptorchidism) or a family history of testicular cancer or anomalies. Other predisposing factors include orchitis, human immunodeficiency virus (HIV) infection, maternal exposure to exogenous estrogen, and testicular cancer in the contralateral (other) testis.

Most testicular cancers develop from two types of embryonic germ cells: seminomas and nonseminomas. Although seminoma germ cell cancers are the most common, they are the least aggressive. Nonseminoma testicular germ cell tumors are rare but very aggressive. Non–germ cell tumors arise from other testicular tissue and include Leydig cell and Sertoli cell tumors. These account for less than 10% of testicular cancers.

Clinical Manifestations and Complications

Testicular cancer may have a slow or rapid onset depending on the type of tumor (Fig. 54-9). The patient may notice a painless lump in his scrotum, scrotal swelling, and a feeling of heaviness. The scrotal mass usually is nontender and firm. Some patients complain of a dull ache or heavy sensation in the lower abdomen, perianal area, or scrotum. Acute pain is the initial symptom in about 10% of patients. Manifestations associated with advanced disease are varied and include lower back or chest pain, cough, and dyspnea.

Diagnostic Studies

Palpation of the scrotal contents is the first step in diagnosing testicular cancer. A cancerous mass is firm and does not transilluminate. Ultrasound of the testes is indicated whenever testicular cancer is suspected (e.g., palpable mass) or when persistent or painful testicular swelling is present. If a testicular neoplasm is suspected, blood is obtained to determine the serum levels of α-fetoprotein (AFP), lactate dehydrogenase (LDH), and human chorionic gonadotropin (hCG).[32] (The tumor markers AFP and hCG are discussed in Chapter 15.)

A chest x-ray and CT scan of the abdomen and pelvis are done to detect metastasis. Anemia may be present, and liver function levels may be elevated in metastatic disease.

❖ NURSING AND INTERPROFESSIONAL MANAGEMENT: TESTICULAR CANCER

Testicular cancer is one of the most curable types of cancer. Interprofessional care generally involves a radical orchiectomy

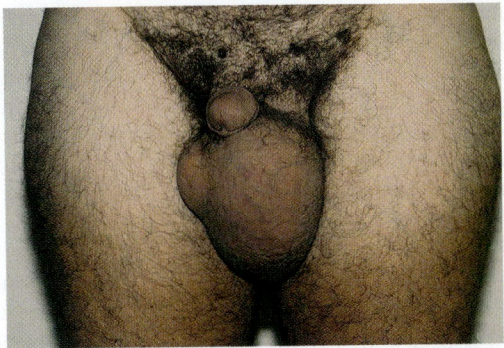

FIG. 54-10 Hydrocele. (From Swartz MH: *Textbook of physical diagnosis*, ed 6, Philadelphia, 2010, Saunders.)

(surgical removal of the affected testis, spermatic cord, and regional lymph nodes). Some patients with early stage disease do not need further treatment after an orchiectomy. Retroperitoneal lymph node dissection and removal may also be done in early stage disease. These nodes are the primary route for metastasis.

Postorchiectomy treatment may also involve surveillance, radiation therapy, or chemotherapy, depending on the stage of the cancer. Radiation therapy is mainly used for patients with a seminoma, which is very sensitive to radiation. Radiation does not work well for nonseminomas.

Testicular germ cell tumors are more sensitive to systemic chemotherapy than any other adult solid tumor. Chemotherapy protocols use a combination of agents, including bleomycin, etoposide, ifosfamide (Ifex), and cisplatin. Retroperitoneal lymph node dissection may be done after chemotherapy as adjunct therapy in patients with advanced testicular cancer.[33]

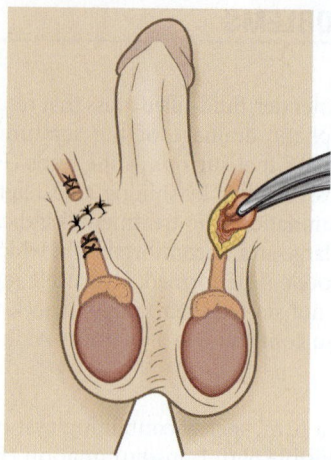

FIG. 54-11 Vasectomy procedure. The ductus deferens is ligated or resected for the purpose of sterilization.

CHECK YOUR PRACTICE

You are working on the urologic oncology unit caring for a 24-yr-old man who recently underwent orchiectomy for testicular cancer. He appears quiet and nonengaged when you assess him. He says, "I'm never going to have a normal sex life."
- How would you respond? What kind of support or information would you provide?

The prognosis for patients with testicular cancer in recent years has greatly improved, and 95% of the patients obtain complete remission if the disease is detected in the early stages. As a result of treatment successes, a majority of men with testicular cancer are long-term survivors.

However, some of the drugs used to treat testicular cancer can cause serious long-term side effects. These include pulmonary toxicity, kidney damage, nerve damage (which can cause numbness and tingling), and hearing loss (from nerve damage). Secondary malignancies can occur as a result of chemotherapy (see Chapter 15).

All patients with testicular cancer, regardless of pathology or stage, require surveillance and regular physical examinations, chest x-rays, CT scans, and assessment of hCG and AFP. The goal is to detect relapse when the tumor burden is minimal.

Pretreatment subfertility or impaired fertility is identified at diagnosis. In treatment of testicular cancer, chemotherapy with cisplatin and/or pelvic radiation often damages the testicular germ cells.[33] However, spermatogenesis can return in some patients. Because of the high risk for infertility, the cryopreservation of sperm in a sperm bank before treatment begins should be sensitively discussed and recommended for the man with testicular cancer. Ejaculatory dysfunction may result from retroperitoneal lymph node dissection. These issues may be hard to discuss with the newly diagnosed patient. Men may think that the disease is a threat to their masculinity and self-worth.

SEXUAL FUNCTION

VASECTOMY

Vasectomy is the bilateral surgical ligation or resection of the ductus deferens performed for the purpose of sterilization (Fig. 54-11). The procedure requires only 15 to 30 minutes and is usually performed with the patient under local anesthesia on an outpatient basis. Although vasectomy is considered a permanent form of sterilization, successful vasectomy reversals *(vaso-vasotomy, vasoepididymostomy)* are common.

After vasectomy, the patient should not notice any difference in the look or feel of the ejaculate because its major components are seminal and prostatic fluid. The patient must use an alternative form of contraception until semen examination reveals no sperm. Sperm cells continue to be produced by the testes but are stored in the epididymis and reabsorbed by the body rather than being passed through the ductus deferens. Vasectomy does not affect the production of hormones, ability to ejaculate, or physiologic mechanisms related to erection or orgasm. Psychologic adjustment may be a problem after surgery. It may be difficult for the patient to separate vasectomy from castration at a subconscious level. Some men may develop psychogenic ED or may feel the need to become more sexually active than they were in the past to prove their masculinity.

ERECTILE DYSFUNCTION

Erectile dysfunction (ED) is the inability to attain or maintain an erection that allows satisfactory sexual activity. Although sexual function is a topic that many individuals are uncomfortable discussing, health care professionals must be able and willing to address ED.

ED is a condition that is significant because of its prevalence, with more than 10 million men in the United States estimated to have ED. It can occur at any age, although the incidence increases with age. In fact, it is estimated that about 50% of all men between ages 40 and 70 have at least some degree of ED. Regardless of age, ED is increasing in all sexually active males. In younger men, the increase is attributed to substance abuse (e.g., recreational drugs, alcohol) or stress and anxiety. Middle-aged men are more likely to experience ED due to chronic medical conditions (e.g., diabetes, hypertension) or treatment for these conditions (e.g., antihypertensive drugs) that may cause ED.

Etiology and Pathophysiology

ED can be due to many factors (Table 54-9). Common causes include diabetes, vascular disease, side effects from medications, result of surgery (e.g., prostatectomy), trauma, chronic illness, stress, difficulty in a relationship, or depression. Since ED results

TABLE 54-9 Risk Factors for Erectile Dysfunction*

Vascular
- Atherosclerosis
- Hypertension
- Peripheral vascular disease

Drug Induced
- Alcohol
- Antiandrogens
- Antihypertensives
- Antilipidemic agents
- Major tranquilizers (diazepam [Valium], alprazolam [Xanax])
- Marijuana, cocaine
- Nicotine
- Tricyclic antidepressants (e.g., amitriptyline [Elavil])

Endocrine
- Diabetes mellitus
- Hypogonadism
- Obesity

Genitourinary
- Radical prostatectomy
- Renal failure

Neurologic
- Cerebrovascular disease
- Diabetes mellitus
- Parkinson's disease
- Trauma to the spinal cord
- Tumors or transection of spinal cord

Psychologic
- Anxiety
- Depression
- Stress

Other
- Aging

*Table is not all-inclusive.

TABLE 54-10 Interprofessional Care
Erectile Dysfunction

Diagnostic Assessment
- History and physical examination
- Sexual history
- Serum glucose and lipid profile
- Testosterone, prolactin, and thyroid hormone levels
- Nocturnal penile tumescence and rigidity testing
- Vascular studies

Management
- Modify reversible causes
- Sexual counseling

Drug Therapy
- sildenafil (Viagra)
- vardenafil (Levitra, Staxyn)
- tadalafil (Cialis)
- avanafil (Stendra)

Devices and Implants
- Vacuum erection device (VED)
- Intraurethral medication pellet
- Intracavernosal self-injection
- Penile implants

from reduced blood flow to the penis, there is a potential association with cardiovascular disease (CVD) because the risk factors for both of these disorders are the same.

Normal physiologic age-related changes are associated with changes in erectile function and may be an underlying cause of ED for some men. Table 50-3 lists age-related changes in sexual function. Explain these age-related changes (if necessary) to reassure an anxious older man regarding normal changes in his sexual abilities. (The male sexual response is discussed in Chapter 50.)

Clinical Manifestations and Complications

The typical symptom of ED is a patient's self-report of problems associated with erectile activity, describing an inability to attain or maintain an erection. The symptoms may occur only occasionally, may be continual with a gradual onset, or may occur with a sudden onset. A gradual onset of symptoms is usually associated with physiologic factors, whereas a sudden or rapid onset of symptoms may be associated with psychologic issues. It is not uncommon for younger men who seek care for ED to be diagnosed with diabetes, hypertension, depression, or cholesterol abnormalities during their evaluation for ED.

A man's inability to perform sexually can cause great distress in his interpersonal relationships and may interfere with his concept of himself as a man. It can also affect the relationship between the man and his partner. Problems with ED can lead to a number of personal issues, including anger, anxiety, and depression.

Diagnostic Studies

The first step in diagnosis and management of ED begins with a thorough sexual, health, and psychosocial history. Self-administered assessment and treatment-related questionnaires have been developed and may prove useful as primary screening tools. For example, the International Index of Erectile Function (IIEF) identifies a man's response to five key areas of male sexual function: erectile function, orgasmic function, sexual desire, intercourse satisfaction, and overall satisfaction.[34]

Second, a physical examination should focus on secondary sexual characteristics, noting if secondary sexual characteristics reflect the individual's chronologic age (Tanner stage). A DRE should be done to assess prostate size, consistency, and presence of nodules. Assessment of BP with palpation and auscultation of the femoral arteries and peripheral pulses should also be included.

Further examination or diagnostic testing is typically based on findings from the history and physical examination. A serum glucose and lipid profile is recommended to rule out diabetes mellitus. Hormonal levels for testosterone, prolactin, LH, and thyroid hormones may help identify endocrine-related problems. PSA level and a complete blood count may help to identify other diseases.

Other diagnostic tests may be done to diagnose ED. Nocturnal penile tumescence and rigidity testing is a noninvasive method that involves the continuous measurement of penile circumference and axial rigidity during sleep. Such measurements are used to differentiate between physiologic or psychogenic causes of ED. Vascular studies, including penile arteriography, penile blood flow study, and duplex Doppler ultrasound studies, are used to assess penile blood inflow and outflow. These tests help to identify vascular problems interfering with erection.

Interprofessional Care

The goal of ED therapy is for the patient and his partner to achieve a satisfactory sexual relationship. The treatment for ED can be based on the underlying cause, but generally men are moved directly into treatment without a costly workup. A variety of treatment options are available (Table 54-10). Advise patients that none of the options will restore ejaculation or tactile sensations if they were absent before treatment.

It is important to determine if ED is reversible before treatment is started. For example, if ED appears to be a side effect of prescribed drugs, alternative treatments can be explored. With an established diagnosis of testicular failure (hypogonadism), androgen replacement therapy may be part of the prescribed treatment.

For individuals who have ED that is psychologic in nature, counseling for the patient (with or without his partner) is recommended. This counseling should be carried out by a qualified sex therapist.

Erectogenic Drugs. Sildenafil (Viagra), tadalafil (Cialis), vardenafil (Levitra, Staxyn), and avanafil (Stendra) are erectogenic drugs.[35,36] These drugs are phosphodiesterase type 5 (PDE5) inhibitors that cause smooth muscle relaxation and increased blood flow into the corpus cavernosum, thus promoting penile erection. They are taken orally before sexual activity. These drugs have been found to be generally safe and effective for the treatment of most types of ED but are ineffective in the absence of arousal.

Side effects of these drugs include headaches, dyspepsia, flushing, and nasal congestion. Additional rare side effects are blurred or blue-green visual disturbances, sudden hearing loss, and an erection lasting more than 4 hours (priapism). Instruct the patient to seek immediate medical attention if any of these reactions occur. Because these drugs may potentiate the hypotensive effect of nitrates, they are contraindicated for individuals taking nitrates (e.g., nitroglycerin).

 DRUG ALERT   Phosphodiesterase Type 5 (PDE5) Inhibitors
- Should not be used with nitrates (nitroglycerin) in any form.
- Can potentiate hypotensive effects of nitrates.

Vacuum Erection Devices. Vacuum erection devices (VEDs) are suction devices that can be applied to the flaccid penis to produce an erection by pulling blood up into the corporeal bodies. A penile ring or constrictive band is placed around the base of the penis to retain venous blood, thereby preventing the erection from subsiding.

Intraurethral Devices and Intracavernosal Injections. Intraurethral devices include the use of vasoactive drugs administered as a topical gel or a medication pellet inserted into the urethra using a medicated urethral system for erection (MUSE) device. Intracavernosal self-injections may also be performed, which should be injected directly into the corpus cavernosum while taking care to avoid the corpus spongiosum.

Alprostadil (Caverject, Edex) is a vasoactive drug that enhances blood flow into the penile arteries. It can be given either by injection or as a transurethral pellet (suppository). When given as a suppository, the drug is placed into the opening at the tip of the penis. When injected, a needle and syringe is used to inject the drug directly into the penis. Trimix (a combination product) includes alprostadil, papaverine, and phentolamine.

Penile Implants. Implantation requires surgery but can sometimes be accomplished in an outpatient setting. The devices are implanted into the corporeal bodies to provide an erection firm enough for penetration. The inflatable implant consists of cylinders in the penis, a small pump in the scrotum, and a reservoir in the lower abdomen. The main complications associated with penile prostheses are infection, erosions, and rarely, mechanical failure.

Sexual Counseling. Sexual counseling can be recommended at any point during treatment for ED and may be most valuable in cases with a component of psychogenic ED. Counseling should address psychologic or interpersonal factors that may enhance sexual expression, as well as other factors that are of concern. Counseling can be effective for an individual patient, but it can include his partner, particularly if he is involved in a long-term relationship.[37]

❖ NURSING MANAGEMENT: ERECTILE DYSFUNCTION

The man experiencing ED requires a great deal of emotional support for both himself and his partner. Men often do not feel comfortable discussing their problems with others because of their perceptions of society's expectations of a man's sexual abilities. Reassure the patient that confidentiality will be maintained. The majority of men delay seeking medical assistance and may expect immediate solutions to their problems. The interprofessional care team should provide a support system and accurate information.

Conducting routine health assessments on men seeking any form of medical treatment places you in a unique position. It provides an opportunity to ask the patient questions pertaining to general health, as well as sexual health and function. Given the opportunity, men will be less hesitant to answer these questions when they know that someone cares and can address their concerns.

Be aware that increasing numbers of men are seeking alternate methods for obtaining medications to treat their ED. This can include compounding pharmacies and online pharmacies. Seeking alternate methods can be due to both the cost of these medications and lack of insurance coverage for ED.

HYPOGONADISM

Hypogonadism is a gradual decline in androgen secretion that occurs in most men as they age. The primary male androgen that is reduced is testosterone (Fig. 54-12). This has also been called *late onset hypogonadism* or *hypogonadism of old age*, but it can begin as early as age 40. It is unclear what causes a decline in testosterone, but obesity has been identified as one contributing factor.

Manifestations associated with low testosterone include decreased libido, fatigue, ED, depression and mood swings, and sleep disturbances. Since many of these manifestations can be associated with aging, some patients may not mention this to their HCP, or the HCP may not recognize these manifestations as signs of low testosterone. Long-term effects of low testosterone include loss of muscle mass and strength, which may contribute to an increased risk of falls and fractures.

Hypogonadism is diagnosed with a blood test and a physical examination. Normal serum testosterone levels can range from 280 to 1100 ng/dL. Replacement testosterone therapy is considered once levels drop below 200 ng/dL.[38] Therapy may be started earlier depending on severity of symptoms. Testosterone replacement therapy (TRT) should not be started until the patient, in consultation with his HCP, considers the risks and benefits of therapy. Potential risks of TRT include lowered levels of high-density lipoprotein (HDL) cholesterol, increased hematocrit, and worsening sleep apnea, although these are uncommon. Since TRT may cause increased growth of prostate tissue, TRT is contraindicated in patients with unmanaged BPH

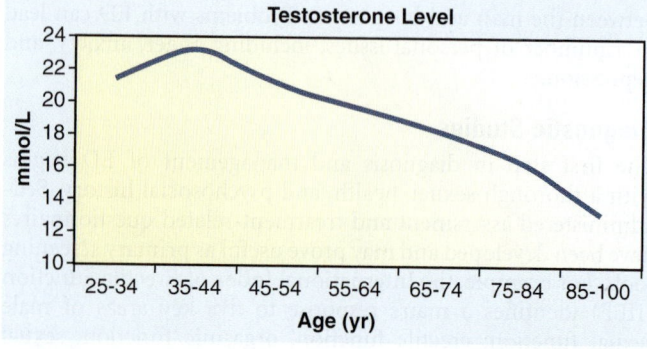

FIG. 54-12   Changes in testosterone plasma level in men as they age.

or prostate cancer. Before treatment is initiated, a DRE and PSA test should be performed. Once TRT begins, patients should be closely monitored by their HCP.

Replacement therapy is available in different forms, including injection, transdermal, topical, buccal, or intranasal preparations. Oral TRT is not approved for use in the United States.[39] IM injections such as testosterone cypionate (Depo-Testosterone) and testosterone enanthate (Delatestryl) are available in varying doses. These drugs create a cyclic rise and fall in serum testosterone levels with the highest levels 2 or 3 days after the injection. Testosterone levels slowly decrease until the next injection. One of the side effects of this form of TRT is that men may complain of mood swings with these fluctuations.

Transdermal preparations, including patches and gels (e.g., Androderm, Testim), are more commonly prescribed. They are generally applied to the skin daily at product-specific sites, including the back, arm, and abdomen. Skin irritation is a common side effect. Testosterone may also be given as a buccal tablet (Striant) or intranasally (Natesto).

Emphasize to the patient the importance of hand washing with soap and water after applying testosterone preparations to the skin. Covering the area with clothing until the preparation has dried is recommended.

Women of childbearing age and children should avoid direct contact with testosterone products. Testosterone may cause early signs of puberty in young children and changes (virilization) in the external genitalia of a female fetus.

INFERTILITY

Infertility in a couple is defined as the inability to conceive after 1 year of frequent unprotected intercourse. Infertility is a disorder of a couple, not of one individual. For this reason, both partners must be involved in determining the cause of infertility. In 20% to 30% of cases, infertility is caused primarily by factors involving the man.[40]

Male infertility can be caused by disorders of the hypothalamic-pituitary system, disorders of the testes, and abnormalities of the ejaculatory system. The physical causes of infertility can be divided into three categories: pretesticular, testicular, and posttesticular. The *pretesticular* or endocrine causes occur only in

about 3% of the cases and can generally be treated with medication or surgery.

Testicular problems make up 50% of the cases. The most common cause of male infertility is a varicocele. Other factors that influence the testes include infection (e.g., mumps virus, STIs, bacterial infections), congenital anomalies, drugs, radiation, substance abuse (alcohol, nicotine, drugs), and environmental hazards.

Posttesticular causes account for approximately 5% to 7% of the cases, with obstruction, infection, and the result of a surgical procedure being the primary causes. The remaining 40% are classified as *idiopathic,* or of unknown causes.

A careful health history and examination may reveal the cause of a patient's infertility. Thus the history is a starting point for determining cause and treatment. The history should include age; occupation; past injury, surgery, or infections to the genital tract; lifestyle issues such as hot tubs, weight training, or wearing tight undergarments; sexual practices; frequency of intercourse; and emotional factors such as stress levels and the desire for children. Document the use of drugs, such as chemotherapeutic agents, anabolic steroids or testosterone, sulfasalazine (Azulfidine), cimetidine (Tagamet HB), and recreational drugs, since these drugs can reduce the sperm count. A physical examination may identify a varicocele, Peyronie's disease, or other physical findings.

The first test in the male infertility evaluation is a semen analysis to determine sperm concentration, motility, and morphology. Hormone studies are also helpful in determining the etiology, including plasma testosterone and serum LH and FSH measurements. Be tactful in dealing with the male patient undergoing infertility studies. Many cultures equate fertility and masculinity. Both male and female partners should undergo evaluation simultaneously to avoid potential treatment delays for the couple.

Treatment options for the man include drugs, conservative lifestyle changes (e.g., avoidance of scrotal heat, substance abuse, high stress), in vitro fertilization techniques, and corrective surgery. Infertility can seriously strain a relationship, and the couple may require counseling and discussion of alternatives if conception is not achieved. (Female infertility is discussed in Chapter 53.)

CASE STUDY
Benign Prostatic Hyperplasia With Acute Urinary Retention

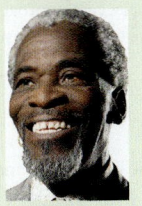
(©IPGGutenberg-UKLtd/iStock/Thinkstock)

Patient Profile
B.G., a 60-yr-old married African American man, comes to the ED because of an inability to void for the past 13 hours and pain in the lower abdomen.

Subjective Data
- Complains of the urge to void
- Is restless, anxious, and agitated

Objective Data
- Has prostate enlargement on digital rectal examination
- Has hematuria, bacteria, and WBCs in urine
- Has a tender and palpable bladder above the umbilicus
- PSA test: 5 ng/mL

Interprofessional Care
- Indwelling catheter inserted by a urology resident
- Admitted to the hospital for observation

Discussion Questions
1. What risk factors for prostate problems are present in B.G.?
2. Explain the etiology of the manifestations that B.G. exhibited.
3. What are possible reasons for B.G.'s elevated PSA level?
4. Discuss the drug and surgical options available to B.G.
5. *Patient-Centered Care:* B.G. asks you about the effect of the various surgical options on his ability to have sex. How would you respond and what type of teaching would you provide?
6. *Priority Decision:* Based on the assessment data, what are the priority nursing diagnoses? Are there any collaborative problems?
7. *Priority Decision:* What is the priority nursing intervention for B.G.?
8. *Patient-Centered Care:* On further assessment, you note that B.G. has a nursing diagnosis of decisional conflict. How would you help him resolve this conflict related to treatment options, and how would you teach him about these options?
9. *Evidence-Based Practice:* What information would you offer to B.G. when he asks if he should start taking saw palmetto to prevent future UTIs?

BRIDGE TO NCLEX EXAMINATION

The number of the question corresponds to the same-numbered outcome at the beginning of the chapter.

1. Symptoms of BPH are *primarily* caused by
   a. obstruction of the urethra.
   b. untreated chronic prostatitis.
   c. decreased bladder compliance.
   d. excessive secretion of testosterone.

2. Postoperatively, a patient who has had a laser prostatectomy has continuous bladder irrigation with a three-way urinary catheter with a 30-mL balloon. When he complains of bladder spasms with the catheter in place, the nurse should
   a. deflate the balloon to 10 mL to decrease bulk in the bladder.
   b. deflate the balloon and then reinflate to ensure that it is patent.
   c. encourage the patient to try to have a bowel movement to relieve colon pressure.
   d. explain that this feeling is normal and that he should not try to urinate around the catheter.

3. Which factors would place a patient at a higher risk for prostate cancer *(select all that apply)*?
   a. Older than 65 years
   b. Asian or Native American
   c. Long-term use of an indwelling urethral catheter
   d. Father diagnosed and treated for early stage prostate cancer
   e. Previous history of undescended testicle and testicular cancer

4. A patient scheduled for a prostatectomy for prostate cancer expresses the fear that he will have erectile dysfunction. In responding to this patient, the nurse should keep in mind that
   a. erectile dysfunction can occur even with a nerve-sparing procedure.
   b. the most common complication of this surgery is postoperative bowel incontinence.
   c. retrograde ejaculation affects sexual function more frequently than erectile dysfunction.
   d. preoperative sexual function is the most important factor in determining postoperative erectile dysfunction.

5. The nurse explains to the patient with chronic bacterial prostatitis who is undergoing antibiotic therapy that *(select all that apply)*
   a. all patients require hospitalization.
   b. pain will lessen once treatment has ended.
   c. course of treatment is generally 2 to 4 weeks.
   d. long-term therapy may be indicated in immunocompromised patient.
   e. if the condition is unresolved and untreated, he is at risk for prostate cancer.

6. In assessing a patient for testicular cancer, the nurse understands that the manifestations of this disease often include
   a. acute back spasms and testicular pain.
   b. rapid onset of scrotal swelling and fever.
   c. fertility problems and bilateral scrotal tenderness.
   d. painless mass and heaviness sensation in the scrotal area.

7. The nurse should explain to the patient who has erectile dysfunction (ED) that *(select all that apply)*
   a. the most common cause is benign prostatic hypertrophy.
   b. ED may be due to medications or conditions such as diabetes.
   c. only men who are over 65 years or older benefit from PDE5 inhibitors.
   d. there are medications and devices that can be used to help with erections.
   e. this condition is primarily due to anxiety and best treated with psychotherapy.

8. To decrease the patient's discomfort related to discussing his reproductive organs, the nurse should
   a. relate his sexual concerns to his sexual partner.
   b. arrange to have male nurses care for the patient.
   c. maintain a nonjudgmental attitude toward his sexual practices.
   d. use technical terminology when discussing reproductive function.

1. a, 2. d, 3. a, d, 4. a, 5. b, d, 6. d, 7. b, d, 8. c

For rationales to these answers and even more NCLEX review questions, visit *http://evolve.elsevier.com/Lewis/medsurg*.

EVOLVE WEBSITE

http://evolve.elsevier.com/Lewis/medsurg
Review Questions (Online Only)
Key Points
Answer Keys for Questions
- Rationales for Bridge to NCLEX Examination Questions
- Answer Guidelines for Case Study on p. 1289
- Answer Guidelines for Managing Care of Multiple Patients Case Study (Section 10) on p. 1292

Student Case Study
- Patient With Benign Prostatic Hyperplasia

Nursing Care Plan
- eNursing Care Plan 54-1: Patient Having Prostate Surgery

Conceptual Care Map Creator
Audio Glossary
Supporting Media
- Animations
  - Prostatectomy
  - Vasectomy

Content Updates

REFERENCES

1. Rosenberg M, Witt E, Miner M, et al: A practical primary care approach to lower urinary tract symptoms caused by benign prostatic hyperplasia (BPH-LUTS), *Can J Urol* 21 (Suppl 2):12, 2014.
2. Weight C, Kim S, Jacobson D, et al: The effect of benign lower urinary tract symptoms on subsequent prostate cancer testing and diagnosis, *Eur Urol* 63:1021, 2013.
3. Ørsted D, Bojesen S: The link between benign prostatic hyperplasia and prostate cancer, *Nat Review Urol* 10:49, 2013.
4. American Urological Association Foundation: What is benign prostatic hyperplasia (BPH)? Retrieved from *www.urologyhealth.org/urologic-conditions/benign-prostatic-hyperplasia-(bph)*.
5. Barry M, Fowler F, O'Leary M, et al: The American Urologic Association symptom index for benign prostatic hyperplasia, *J Urol* 148:1549, 1992. (Classic)
*6. American Urological Association: American Urological Association Guideline: Management of benign prostatic hyperplasia (BPH). Retrieved from *www.auanet.org/education/guidelines/benign-prostatic-hyperplasia.cfm*.
7. National Cancer Institute: Prostate cancer prevention trial, National Institutes of Health. Retrieved from *www.cancer.gov*.

8. Brock G, McVary K, Roehrborn C, et al: Direct effects of tadalafil on lower urinary tract symptoms versus indirect effects mediated through erectile dysfunction symptom improvement: integrated data analyses from 4 placebo controlled clinical studies, *J Urol* 191:405, 2014.

9. Barry M, Cantor A, Roehrborn C, et al: Relationships among participant international prostate symptom score, benign prostatic hyperplasia impact index changes and global ratings of change in a trial of phytotherapy in men with lower urinary tract symptoms, *J Urol* 189:987, 2013.

10. Andriole G, McCullum-Hill C, Sandhu G, et al: The effect of increasing doses of saw palmetto fruit extract on serum prostate specific antigen: analysis of the CAMUS randomized trial, *J Urol* 189:486, 2013.

*11. Cornu J, Ahyai S, Bachmann A, et al: A systematic review and meta-analysis of functional outcomes and complications following transurethral procedures for lower urinary tract symptoms resulting from benign prostatic obstruction: an update, *Eur Urol* 67:1066, 2015.

12. Chughtai B, Simma-Chiang V, Lee R, et al: Trends and utilization of laser prostatectomy in ambulatory surgical procedures for the treatment of benign prostatic hyperplasia in New York State (2000-2011), *J Endourol* 29:700, 2015.

13. National Kidney and Urologic Diseases Information Clearinghouse: Prostate enlargement: benign prostatic hyperplasia, US Department of Health and Human Services. Retrieved from *www.niddk.nih.gov/health-information/health-topics/urologic-disease/benign-prostatic-hyperplasia-bph/pages/facts/aspx.*

*14. American Urological Association (2013). PSA Testing for the Pretreatment Staging and Posttreatment Management of Prostate Cancer: 2013 Revision of 2009 Best Practice Statement. Retrieved from *www.auanet.org/education/guidelines/prostate-specific-antigen.cfm.*

15. American Cancer Society: What are the key statistics about prostate cancer? Retrieved from *www.cancer.org/cancer/prostatecancer/detailedguide/prostate-cancer-key-statistics.*

16. Alavanja M, Ross M, Bonner M: Increased cancer burden among pesticide applicators and others due to pesticide exposure, *CA Cancer J Clin* 63:120, 2013.

*17. Skolarus T, Wolf A, Erb N, et al: American Cancer Society prostate cancer survivorship care guidelines, *CA Cancer J Clin* 64:225, 2014.

18. National Institutes of Health, National Cancer Institute: Treatment choices for men with early-stage prostate cancer. Retrieved from *www.cancer.gov/types/prostate/patient/prostate-treatment-pdq.*

19. Brimo F, Montironi R, Egevad L, et al: Contemporary grading for prostate cancer: implications for patient care, *Eur Urol* 63:892, 2013.

*20. Gandaglia G, Sammon J, Chang S, et al: Comparative effectiveness of robot-assisted and open radical prostatectomy in the postdissemination era, *J Clin Oncol* 32:1419, 2014.

*21. Sukumar S, Rogers C, Trinh Q, et al: Oncological outcomes after robot-assisted radical prostatectomy: long-term follow-up in 4803 patients, *BJU Int* 114:824, 2014.

22. Steineck G, Bjartell A, Hugosson J, et al: Degree of preservation of the neurovascular bundles during radical prostatectomy and urinary continence 1 year after surgery, *Eur Urol* 67:559, 2015.

23. Chen R, Chang P, Vetter R, et al: Recommended patient-reported core set of symptoms to measure in prostate cancer treatment trials, *J Natl Cancer Inst* 106:7, 2014.

*24. Smolska-Ciszewska B, Miszczyk L, Bialas B, et al: The effectiveness and side effects of conformal external beam radiotherapy combined with high-dose-rate brachytherapy boost compared to conformal external beam radiotherapy alone in patients with prostate cancer, *Radiat Oncol* 10:60, 2015.

*25. Gandaglia G, Sun M, Popa I, et al: The impact of androgen-deprivation therapy (ADT) on the risk of cardiovascular (CV) events in patients with non-metastatic prostate cancer: a population-based study, *BJU Int* 114:E82, 2014.

*26. Limburg C, Maxwell C, Mautner B: Prevention and treatment of bone loss in patients with nonmetastatic breast or prostate cancer who receive hormonal ablation therapy, *Clin J Oncol Nurs* 18:223, 2014.

*27. Dilori C, Steenland K, Goodman M, et al: Differences in treatment-based beliefs and coping between African American and white men with prostate cancer, *J Commun Health* 36:505, 2011.

28. National Institute of Diabetes and Digestive and Kidney Disorders Information Clearinghouse: Prostatitis: inflammation of the prostate. Retrieved from *www.niddk.nih.gov/healht-information/health-topics/urologic-disease/prostatitis-disorders-of-the-prostate/pages/facts.aspx.*

*29. Wagenlehner F, van Till J, Magri V, et al: National Institutes of Health chronic prostatitis symptoms index (NIH-CPSI) symptom evaluation in multinational cohorts of patients with chronic prostatitis/chronic pelvic pain syndrome, *Eur Urol* 63:953, 2013.

30. Inman B, Stewart S, Kattan M: Staging and risk stratification in penile cancer. In Spiess PE, editor: *Penile cancer*, New York, 2013, Humana Press.

31. Znaor A, Lortet-Tieulent J, Jemal A, et al: International variations and trends in testicular cancer incidence and mortality, *Eur Urol* 65:1095, 2014.

32. Hanna N, Einhorn L: Testicular cancer-discoveries and updates, *N Eng J Med* 371: 2005-16, 2014.

*33. Bujan L, Walschaerts M, Moinard N, et al: Impact of chemotherapy and radiotherapy for testicular germ cell tumors on spermatogenesis and sperm DNA: a multicenter prospective study from the CECOS network, *Fertil Steril* 100:673, 2013.

34. Rosen R, Riley A, Wagner G, et al. The International Index of Erectile Function (IIEF): a multidimensional scale for assessment of erectile dysfunction, *Urology* 49:822, 1997. (Classic)

35. Porst H, Burnett A, Brock G, et al: SOP conservative (medical and mechanical) treatment of erectile dysfunction, *J Sex Med* 10:130, 2013.

36. Smith W, McCaslin I, Gokce A, et al: PDE5 inhibitors: considerations for preference and long-term adherence, *Int J Clin Pract* 67:768, 2013.

*37. Schmidt H, Munder T, Gerger H, et al: Combination of psychological intervention and phosphodiesterase-5 inhibitors for erectile dysfunction: a narrative review and meta-analysis, *J Sex Med* 11:1376, 2014.

*38. Buvat J, Maggi M, Guay A, et al: Testosterone deficiency in men: systematic review and standard operating procedures for diagnosis and treatment, *J Sex Med* 10:245, 2013.

39. Basaria S: Male hypogonadism, *Lancet* 383:1250, 2014.

*40. American Urological Association (2011). The optimal evaluation of the infertile male: Best practice statement reviewed and validity confirmed 2011. Retrieved from *www.auanet.org/education/guidelines/male-infertility-d.cfm.*

*Evidence-based information for clinical practice.

CASE STUDY

Managing Care of Multiple Patients

You are working on the medical-surgical unit and have been assigned to care for the following six patients. You have one LPN and one UAP on your team to help you.

Patients

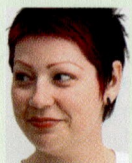

L.M. is a 35-yr-old Hispanic woman who went to the clinic 3 days ago complaining of "just not feeling well." She was admitted to the hospital for treatment of hypertension caused by newly diagnosed Cushing syndrome. She has been depressed and crying because of her physical appearance. Her most recent BP was 164/94 mm Hg.

(©iStockphoto/ Thinkstock)

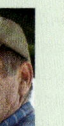

N.B. is a 48-yr-old farmer admitted to the ICU 2 days ago with a diagnosis of diabetic ketoacidosis. He was transferred to the clinical unit yesterday evening. His fasting blood glucose level this morning is 296 mg/dL.

(©iStockphoto/ Thinkstock)

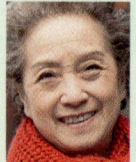

A.K. is a 68-yr-old Asian American woman recently diagnosed with adenocarcinoma of her right breast. She had a lumpectomy and axillary node dissection yesterday. She has a Jackson-Pratt drain in her right chest. Her last pain medication was administered 1 hour ago, at which time she rated her pain as a 7 on a scale of 0-10.

(©XiXinXing/ iStock/ Thinkstock)

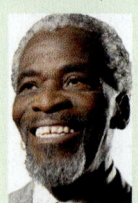

B.G. is a 60-yr-old African American man who was admitted to the hospital because of an inability to void for 13 hours and pain in the lower abdomen. He has a urinary tract infection and prostatic enlargement. An indwelling catheter was inserted by a urology resident. B.G. is scheduled to undergo a transurethral resection of his prostate (TURP) this morning.

(©IPGGutenberg-UKLtd/iStock/ Thinkstock)

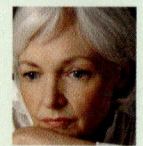

R.D. is a 52-yr-old white woman who was diagnosed with Graves' disease 2 months ago. She was treated with antithyroid medication for 2 months and underwent a subtotal thyroidectomy yesterday. In report it is noted that her voice has become slightly "hoarse" in the last hour.

(©Jupiterimages/ Photos.com/ Thinkstock)

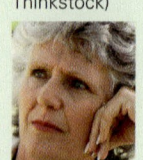

T.J. is a 56-yr-old white woman who underwent a total abdominal hysterectomy and bilateral salpingo-oophorectomy 1 day ago. She has a urinary catheter in place. Her vital signs are stable and she is not complaining of pain.

(©Wavebreak-media/iStock/ Thinkstock)

Discussion Questions

1. ***Priority Decision:*** After receiving report, which patient should you see first? Second? Provide a rationale.
2. ***Teamwork and Collaboration:*** Which tasks could you delegate to UAP *(select all that apply)?*
   a. Assist T.J. to ambulate in the hallway.
   b. Teach B.G. what to expect postoperatively.
   c. Take R.D.'s vital signs and report the results to you.
   d. Assess A.K.'s mastectomy incision for manifestations of infection.
   e. Listen to L.M. talk about her feelings while helping her with AM care.
3. ***Priority Decision and Teamwork and Collaboration:*** While you are assessing R.D., the LPN informs you that A.K.'s chest dressing is totally saturated with bloody drainage. Which *initial* action would be most appropriate?
   a. Ask the LPN to call the laboratory for a stat Hgb and Hct on A.K.
   b. Have the LPN reinforce the dressing with sterile 4 × 4 gauze pads.
   c. Have the LPN stay with R.D. while you assess the patency of A.K.'s Jackson-Pratt drain.
   d. Ask the LPN to stay with A.K. and the UAP to monitor R.D. while you call A.K.'s surgeon.

Case Study Progression

A.K.'s Jackson-Pratt drain was not functioning properly. You get it working and change the chest dressing. The incision is well approximated without signs of infection. When you leave the room, the Jackson-Pratt has a small amount of serosanguineous drainage in it. As you enter R.D.'s room you notice that the patient is having a carpal spasm on the same arm that the LPN is taking her BP on. You recognize this as a manifestation of hypocalcemia and notify the health care provider.

4. Which assessment findings would be *most* important to include in a discussion with the health care provider regarding R.D. *(select all that apply)?*
   a. Patient is anxious
   b. Hoarseness of voice
   c. Most recent Hgb and Hct
   d. Carpal spasm upon inflation of BP cuff
   e. Blood pressure of 138/76 and heart rate of 78
5. ***Priority Decision:*** Which intervention would be of *highest* priority in caring for L.M.?
   a. Assess her for fall risk.
   b. Assess her for signs and symptoms of hypoglycemia.
   c. Teach her the need for a high-carbohydrate, low-protein diet.
   d. Reassure her that her physical appearance will improve with treatment.
6. B.G. asks you what to expect when he returns from surgery. You explain that he will have a(n)
   a. dressing in his groin as well as a urinary catheter.
   b. 3-way urinary catheter connected to an irrigation system.
   c. patient-controlled analgesia (PCA) pump for pain control.
   d. abdominal and a perineal drain that will be recharged q4h.
7. ***Priority Decision and Management Decision:*** The LPN is assigned to administer medications to N.B., including his sliding scale Novolog insulin with breakfast. The UAP, who is also a senior nursing student, tells you that the LPN administered N.B.'s insulin at least 30 min after the patient ate his breakfast. What is your *best* initial action?
   a. Report the incident to the charge nurse for follow-up.
   b. Talk to the LPN about the importance of timely medication administration.
   c. Ask the LPN what time the insulin was given and when the patient ate breakfast.
   d. Ask the UAP to first discuss the concern with the LPN so as to follow proper channels of communication.

Problems Related to Movement and Coordination

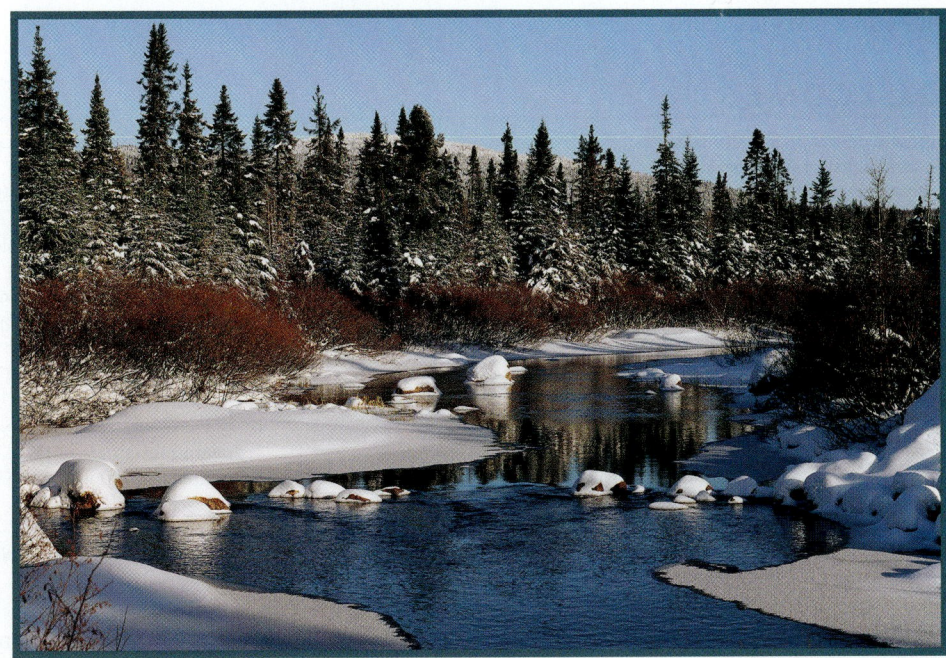

(©Stockbyte/Stockbyte/Thinkstock)

The river has taught me to listen; you will learn from it, too.
The river knows everything; one can learn everything from it.

Hermann Hesse

55

Assessment of Nervous System

Linda Littlejohns

It always seems impossible until it is done.

Nelson Mandela

℮ http://evolve.elsevier.com/Lewis/medsurg/

LEARNING OUTCOMES

1. Differentiate between the functions of neurons and glial cells.
2. Explain the anatomic location and functions of the cerebrum, brainstem, cerebellum, spinal cord, peripheral nerves, and cerebrospinal fluid.
3. Identify the major arteries supplying the brain.
4. Describe the functions of the 12 cranial nerves.
5. Compare the functions of the two divisions of the autonomic nervous system.
6. Link the age-related changes in the neurologic system to the differences in assessment findings.

7. Obtain significant subjective and objective data related to the nervous system from a patient.
8. Perform a physical assessment of the nervous system using the appropriate techniques.
9. Differentiate normal from abnormal findings of a physical assessment of the nervous system.
10. Describe the purpose, significance of results, and nursing responsibilities related to diagnostic studies of the nervous system.

KEY TERMS

autonomic nervous system (ANS), p. 1299
blood-brain barrier, p. 1299
central nervous system (CNS), p. 1294
cerebrospinal fluid (CSF), p. 1298
cranial nerves (CNs), p. 1299

dermatome, p. 1298
glial cells, p. 1294
lower motor neurons (LMNs), p. 1296
meninges, p. 1300
neurons, p. 1294

neurotransmitters, p. 1295
peripheral nervous system (PNS), p. 1294
reflex, p. 1296
synapse, p. 1295
upper motor neurons (UMNs), p. 1296

STRUCTURES AND FUNCTIONS OF NERVOUS SYSTEM

The nervous system is responsible for the control and integration of the body's many activities. It can be divided into the central nervous system and peripheral nervous system. The **central nervous system (CNS)** consists of the brain, spinal cord, and cranial nerves I and II. The **peripheral nervous system (PNS)** consists of cranial nerves III to XII, spinal nerves, and peripheral components of the **autonomic nervous system (ANS)**.

Cells of Nervous System

The nervous system is made up of two types of cells: neurons and supportive glial cells.

Neurons. **Neurons** are the primary functional unit of the nervous system. Although neurons come in many shapes and sizes, they share three characteristics: (1) *excitability,* or the ability to generate a nerve impulse; (2) *conductivity,* or the ability to transmit an impulse; and (3) *influence,* or the ability to influence other neurons, muscle cells, or glandular cells.

A typical neuron consists of a cell body, multiple dendrites, and an axon (Fig. 55-1). The *cell body* containing the nucleus and cytoplasm is the metabolic center of the neuron. *Dendrites* are short processes extending from the cell body that receive impulses or signals from other neurons and conduct them toward the cell body. The *axon* projects varying distances from the cell body. The axon carries nerve impulses to other neurons or to end organs, such as smooth and striated muscles and glands.

Many axons in the CNS and PNS are covered by a *myelin sheath,* a white, lipid protein substance that acts as an insulator for the conduction of impulses. Axons may be myelinated or unmyelinated, as in the case of smaller fibers.

Glial Cells. **Glial cells** (glia or neuroglia) provide support, nourishment, and protection to neurons. Glial cells constitute almost half of the brain and spinal cord mass. Glial cells are divided into microglia and macroglia. *Microglia,* specialized macrophages capable of phagocytosis, protect the neurons. These cells are mobile within the brain and multiply when the brain is damaged.

Types of *macroglial cells* include the astrocytes, oligodendrocytes, and ependymal cells. *Astrocytes* are found primarily in

Reviewed by Tara Back, RN, MSN, Instructor, Goldfarb School of Nursing at Barnes Jewish College, St. Louis, Missouri; Julia R. Popp, RN, MSN, Professor of Nursing, Owens Community College, Toledo, Ohio; and Crystal R. Sherman, DNP, CNP, FNP-BC, APHN-BC, Assistant Professor of Nursing, Shawnee State University, Portsmouth, Ohio.

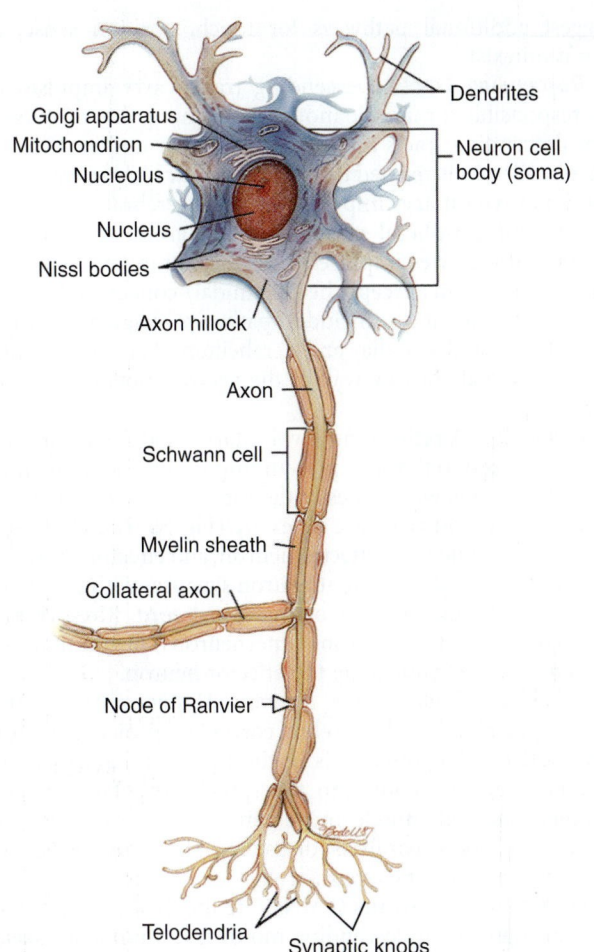

Golgi apparatus
Mitochondrion
Nucleolus
Nucleus
Nissl bodies
Dendrites
Neuron cell body (soma)
Axon hillock
Axon
Schwann cell
Myelin sheath
Collateral axon
Node of Ranvier
Telodendria
Synaptic knobs

FIG. 55-1 Structural features of neurons: dendrites, cell body, and axons. (Modified from Thibodeau GA, Patton KT: *Anatomy and physiology*, ed 8, St Louis, 2013, Mosby.)

gray matter and provide structural support to neurons. Their delicate processes form the *blood-brain barrier* with the endothelium of the blood vessels. They also play a role in *synaptic transmission* (conduction of impulses between neurons). When the brain is injured, astrocytes act as phagocytes for cleaning up neuronal debris. They help restore the neurochemical milieu and provide support for repair. Proliferation of astrocytes contributes to the formation of scar tissue *(gliosis)* in the CNS.

Oligodendrocytes are specialized cells that produce the myelin sheath of nerve fibers in the CNS and are found primarily in the white matter of the CNS. (*Schwann cells* myelinate the nerve fibers in the periphery.) *Ependymal cells* line the brain ventricles and aid in the secretion of cerebrospinal fluid (CSF).

Neuroglia are mitotic and can replicate. In general, when neurons are destroyed, the tissue is replaced by the proliferation of neuroglial cells. Most primary CNS tumors involve glial cells. Primary malignancies involving neurons are rare.

Nerve Regeneration

If the axon of the nerve cell is damaged, the cell attempts to repair itself. Damaged nerve cells attempt to grow back to their original destinations by sprouting many branches from the damaged ends of their axons. Axons in the CNS are generally less successful than peripheral axons in regeneration.[1]

Injured nerve fibers in the PNS can regenerate by growing within the protective myelin sheath of the supporting Schwann

cells if the cell body is intact and the environment is optimal.[1] The final result of nerve regeneration depends on the number of axon sprouts that join with the appropriate Schwann cell columns and reinnervate appropriate end organs.

Neurons have long been thought to be nonmitotic. That is, after being damaged, neurons could not be replaced. Although cell proliferation historically was not believed to be possible, recent evidence indicates a subset of glial cells (astrocytes) proliferate after certain injuries in the CNS, and neurogenesis may occur from stem cells.[2] These findings support the expectation that the patient will experience a certain amount of recovery after injury involving the neurons.

Nerve Impulse

The purpose of a neuron is to initiate, receive, and process messages about events both within and outside the body. The initiation of a neuronal message *(nerve impulse)* involves the generation of an action potential. A series of action potentials travel along the axon. When the impulse reaches the end of the nerve fiber, it is transmitted across the junction *(synapse)* between nerve cells by a chemical interaction involving neurotransmitters. This chemical interaction generates another set of action potentials in the next neuron. These events are repeated until the nerve impulse reaches its destination.

Because of its insulating capacity, myelination of nerve axons facilitates the conduction of an action potential. Many peripheral nerve axons have *nodes of Ranvier* (gaps in the myelin sheath) that allow an action potential to travel much faster by jumping from node to node. This is called *saltatory* (hopping) conduction. In an unmyelinated fiber, the wave of depolarization travels the entire length of the axon, with each portion of the membrane becoming depolarized in turn.

Synapse. A synapse is the structural and functional junction between two neurons. It is the point at which the nerve impulse is transmitted from one neuron to another. The nerve impulse also can be transmitted from neurons to glands or muscles. The essential structures of synaptic transmission are a presynaptic terminal, synaptic cleft, and receptor site on the postsynaptic cell (Fig. 55-2).

Neurotransmitters. Neurotransmitters are chemicals that affect the transmission of impulses across the synaptic cleft. *Excitatory neurotransmitters* (e.g., epinephrine, norepinephrine, glutamate) activate postsynaptic receptors that increase the likelihood that an action potential will be generated. *Inhibitory neurotransmitters* (e.g., serotonin, GABA, dopamine) activate postsynaptic receptors to decrease the likelihood that an action potential will be generated. Endorphins block pain transmission while substance P makes nerves more sensitive to pain.

In general, the net effect (excitatory or inhibitory) depends on the number of presynaptic neurons releasing neurotransmitters on the postsynaptic cell. A presynaptic cell that releases an excitatory neurotransmitter does not always cause the postsynaptic cell to depolarize enough to generate an action potential.

Neurotransmitters can be affected by drugs and toxins, which can modify their function or block their attachment to receptor sites on the postsynaptic membrane. When many presynaptic cells release excitatory neurotransmitters on a single neuron, the sum of their input is enough to generate an action potential. Neurotransmitters continue to combine with the receptor sites at the postsynaptic membrane until they are

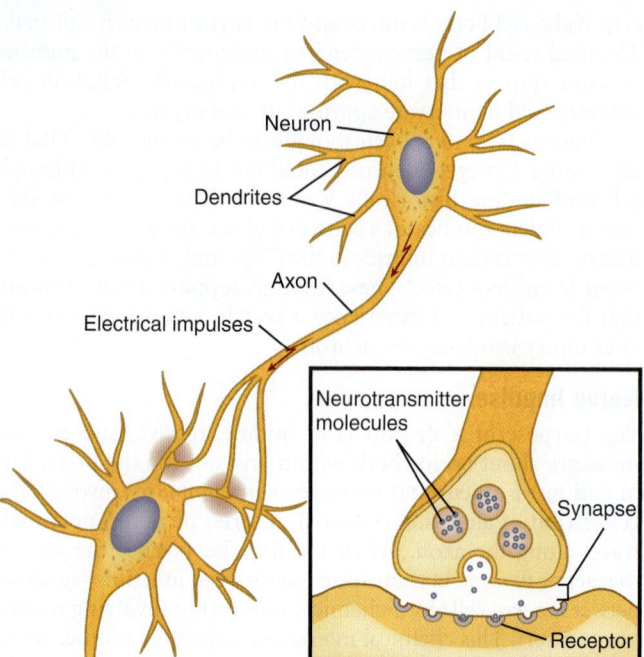

FIG. 55-2 Impulse generation between neurons. Synapse shown with neurotransmitters and receptors.

inactivated by enzymes, are taken up by the presynaptic endings, or diffuse away from the synaptic region. (See Chapter 56 for information regarding the use of cerebral microdialysis for measuring neurotransmitter levels in the cerebral cortex.)

Central Nervous System

The components of the CNS include the cerebrum (cerebral hemispheres), brainstem, cerebellum, and spinal cord.

Spinal Cord. The *spinal cord* is continuous with the brainstem and exits from the cranial cavity through the foramen magnum. A cross section of the spinal cord reveals gray matter that is centrally located in an H shape and surrounded by white matter. The gray matter contains the cell bodies of voluntary motor neurons, preganglionic autonomic motor neurons, and association neurons (interneurons). The white matter contains the axons of the ascending sensory and descending motor fibers. The myelin surrounding these fibers gives them their white appearance. The spinal pathways or tracts are named for the point of origin and the point of destination (e.g., spinocerebellar tract [ascending], corticospinal tract [descending]).

Ascending Tracts. In general, the ascending tracts carry specific sensory information to higher levels of the CNS. This information comes from special sensory receptors in the skin, muscles and joints, viscera, and blood vessels and enters the spinal cord by way of the dorsal roots of the spinal nerves. The fasciculus gracilis and the fasciculus cuneatus (commonly called the *dorsal* or *posterior columns*) carry information concerned with touch, deep pressure, vibration, position sense, and kinesthesia (appreciation of movement, weight, and body parts). The *spinocerebellar tracts* carry information about muscle tension and body position to the cerebellum for coordination of movement. The *spinothalamic tracts* carry pain and temperature sensations. Thus the ascending tracts are organized by sensory modality, as well as by anatomy.

Although the functions of these pathways are generally accepted, other ascending tracts may also carry sensory modalities. The signs and symptoms of various neurologic diseases suggest additional pathways for touch, position sense, and vibration exist.

Descending Tracts. Descending tracts carry impulses that are responsible for muscle movement. Among the most important descending tracts are the corticobulbar and corticospinal tracts, collectively termed the *pyramidal tract.* These tracts carry volitional (voluntary) impulses from the cerebral cortex to the cranial and peripheral nerves. Another group of descending motor tracts carries impulses from the extrapyramidal system (all motor systems except the pyramidal) concerned with voluntary movement. It includes pathways originating in the brainstem, basal ganglia, and cerebellum. The motor output exits the spinal cord by way of the ventral roots of the spinal nerves.

Reflex Arc. A **reflex** is an involuntary response to stimuli. In the spinal cord, reflex arcs play an important role in maintaining muscle tone, which is essential for body posture. The components of a monosynaptic reflex arc (Fig. 55-3) are a receptor organ, afferent neuron, effector neuron, and effector organ (e.g., skeletal muscle). The afferent neuron synapses with the efferent neuron in the gray matter of the spinal cord. More complex reflex arcs have other neurons (interneurons) in addition to the afferent neuron influencing the effector neuron.

Lower and Upper Motor Neurons. **Upper motor neurons (UMNs)** originate in the cerebral cortex and project downward. The corticobulbar tract ends in the brainstem, and the corticospinal tract descends into the spinal cord. These neurons influence skeletal muscle movement. UMN lesions generally cause weakness or paralysis, disuse atrophy, hyperreflexia, and increased muscle tone (spasticity).

Lower motor neurons (LMNs) are the final common pathway through which descending motor tracts influence skeletal muscle. The cell bodies of LMNs, which send axons to innervate the skeletal muscles of the arms, trunk, and legs, are located in the anterior horn of the corresponding segments of the spinal cord (e.g., cervical segments contain LMNs for the arms). LMNs for skeletal muscles of the eyes, face, mouth, and throat are located in the corresponding segments of the brainstem. These cell bodies and their axons make up the somatic motor components of the cranial nerves. LMN lesions generally cause weakness or paralysis, denervation atrophy, hyporeflexia or areflexia, and decreased muscle tone (flaccidity).

Brain. The *brain* has three major intracranial components: cerebrum, brainstem, and cerebellum.

Cerebrum. The *cerebrum* is composed of the right and left cerebral hemispheres and divided into four lobes: frontal, temporal, parietal, and occipital (Fig. 55-4). The functions of the cerebrum are multiple and complex (Table 55-1). The *frontal lobe* controls higher cognitive function, memory retention, voluntary eye movements, voluntary motor movement, and motor functions involved in speech production *(Broca's area).* The *temporal lobe* integrates somatic, visual, and auditory data and contains *Wernicke's receptive speech area.* (Language and potential functional deficits are described further in the discussion of stroke in Chapter 57 [Table 57-4]).

The *parietal lobe* interprets spatial information and contains the sensory cortex. Processing of sight takes place in the *occipital lobe.*

The division of the cerebrum into lobes is useful to delineate portions of the neocortex (gray matter), which makes up the outer layer of the cerebral hemispheres. Neurons in specific parts of the neocortex are essential for various highly complex

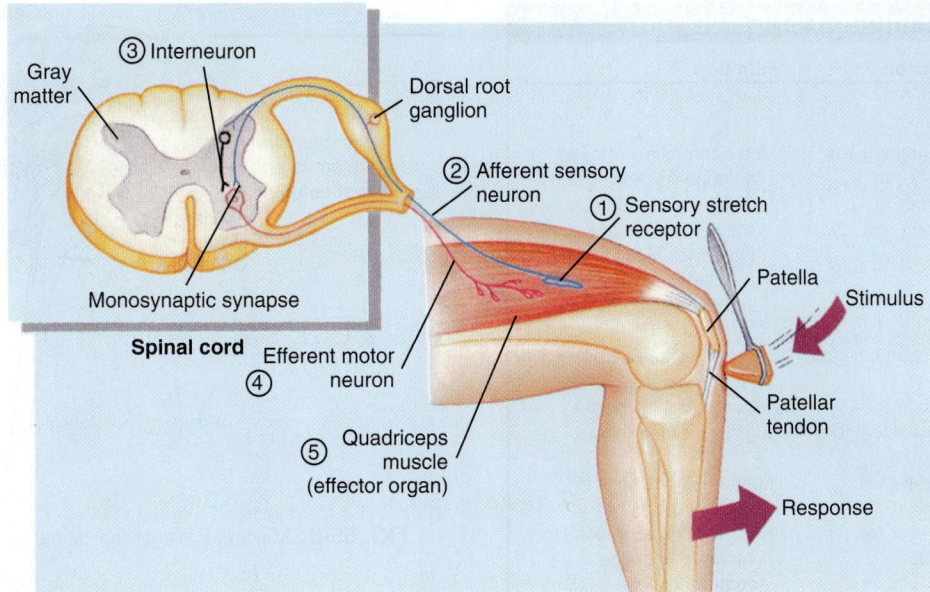

FIG. 55-3 Basic diagram of the patellar "knee jerk" reflex arc, including the *(1)* sensory stretch receptor, *(2)* afferent sensory neuron, *(3)* interneuron, *(4)* efferent motor neuron, and *(5)* quadriceps muscle (effector organ). (Modified from Thibodeau GA, Patton KT: *Anatomy and physiology*, ed 6, St Louis, 2007, Mosby.)

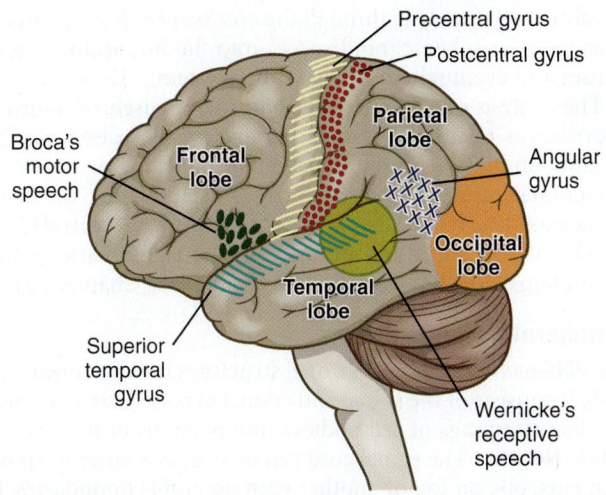

FIG. 55-4 Left hemisphere of cerebrum, lateral surface, showing major lobes and areas of the brain.

and sophisticated functions, such as language, memory, and appreciation of visual-spatial relationships.

The basal ganglia, thalamus, hypothalamus, and limbic system are also located in the cerebrum. The *basal ganglia* are a group of structures located centrally in the cerebrum and midbrain. Most of them are on both sides of the thalamus. The function of the basal ganglia includes the initiation, execution, and completion of voluntary movements, learning, emotional response, and automatic movements associated with skeletal muscle activity (e.g., swallowing saliva, blinking, and swinging the arms while walking).

The *thalamus* lies directly above the brainstem (Fig. 55-5) and is the major relay center for sensory input from the body, face, retina, and cochlear and taste receptors. Motor relay nuclei in the thalamus connect the cerebellum and basal ganglia to the frontal cortex.

The *hypothalamus* is located just inferior to the thalamus and slightly in front of the midbrain. It exerts a direct influence on

release of hormones from the anterior pituitary gland and has a rich capillary connection to this gland to assist in the transport of hormones. These hormones include thyroid-stimulating hormone, growth hormone, luteinizing hormone, and prolactin-releasing hormone, which play a role in regulating reproductive function. In contrast, the supraoptic and paraventricular neurons travel directly through the pituitary stalk to the posterior pituitary, where they release vasopressin and oxytocin. The hypothalamus contains the satiety center that regulates appetite. Subject to input from the limbic system, it also regulates body temperature, water balance (through influence on vasopressin secretion), circadian rhythm, and expression of emotion. The *limbic system* is located near the inner surfaces of the cerebral hemispheres and is concerned with emotion, aggression, feeding behavior, and sexual response.

Brainstem. The *brainstem* includes the midbrain, pons, and medulla (Fig. 55-5). Ascending and descending fibers to and from the cerebrum and cerebellum pass through the brainstem. The nuclei of cranial nerves III through XII are in the brainstem. The vital centers concerned with respiratory, vasomotor, and cardiac function are located in the medulla.

Also located in the brainstem is the *reticular formation,* a diffusely arranged group of neurons and their axons that extends from the medulla to the thalamus and hypothalamus. The functions of the reticular formation include relaying sensory information, influencing excitatory and inhibitory control of spinal motor neurons, and controlling vasomotor and respiratory activity. The *reticular activating system* (RAS) is a complex system that requires communication among the brainstem, reticular formation, and cerebral cortex. The RAS is responsible for regulating arousal and sleep-wake transitions. The brainstem also contains the centers for sneezing, coughing, hiccuping, vomiting, sucking, and swallowing.

Cerebellum. The *cerebellum* is located in the posterior cranial fossa inferior to the occipital lobe. The cerebellum coordinates voluntary movement and maintains trunk stability and equilibrium. The cerebellum receives information from the cerebral cortex, muscles, joints, and inner ear. It influences motor

TABLE 55-1	Function of Cerebrum	
Part	**Location**	**Function**
Cortical Areas		
Motor		
Primary	Precentral gyrus	Motor control and movement on opposite side of body
Supplemental	Anterior to precentral gyrus	Facilitates proximal muscle activity, including activity for stance and gait, and spontaneous movement and coordination
Sensory		
Somatic	Postcentral gyrus	Sensory response from opposite side of body
Visual	Occipital lobe	Registers visual images
Auditory	Superior temporal gyrus	Registers auditory input
Association areas	Parietal lobe	Integrates somatic and sensory input
	Posterior temporal lobe	Integrates visual and auditory input for language comprehension
	Anterior temporal lobe	Integrates past experiences
	Anterior frontal lobe	Controls higher-order processes (e.g., judgment, reasoning)
Language		
Comprehension	Wernicke's area in dominant posterior temporal lobe	Integrates auditory language (understanding of spoken words)
Expression	Broca's area in dominant frontal lobe	Regulates motor speech
Basal Ganglia	Near lateral ventricles of both cerebral hemispheres	Controls and refines learned and automatic movements
Thalamus	Below and slightly posterior to basal ganglia	Relays sensory and motor input to and from cerebrum
Hypothalamus	Below and anterior to thalamus	Regulates endocrine and autonomic functions
Limbic System	Lateral to hypothalamus	Influences emotional behavior and basic drives such as feeding and sexual behavior

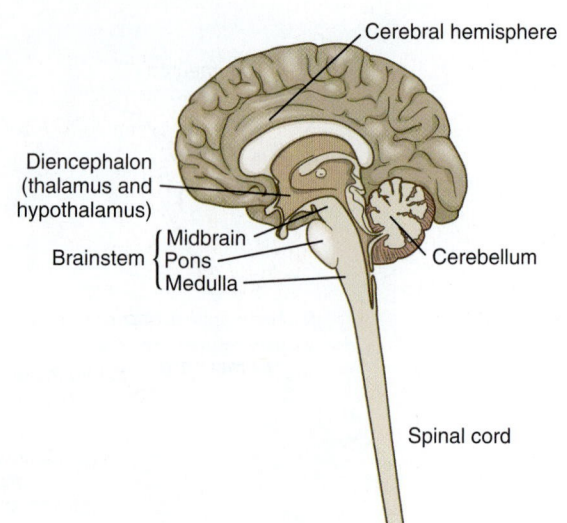

FIG. 55-5 Major divisions of the central nervous system (CNS).

the ventricles and central canal. Excessive buildup of CSF results in a condition known as *hydrocephalus*.

The CSF circulates throughout the ventricles and seeps into the subarachnoid space surrounding the brain and spinal cord. It is absorbed primarily through the *arachnoid villi* (tiny projections into the subarachnoid space) into the intradural venous sinuses and eventually into the venous system.

The analysis of CSF composition provides useful diagnostic information related to certain nervous system diseases. CSF pressure often is measured in patients with actual or suspected intracranial injury. Increased intracranial pressure, indicated by increased CSF pressure, can force downward (central) herniation of the brain and brainstem. The signs marking this event are part of the herniation syndrome (see Chapter 56).

Peripheral Nervous System

The PNS includes all the neuronal structures that lie outside the CNS. It consists of the spinal and cranial nerves, their associated ganglia (groupings of cell bodies), and portions of the ANS.

Spinal Nerves.   The spinal cord can be seen as a series of spinal segments, one on top of another with no visible boundaries. In addition to the cell bodies, each segment contains a pair of dorsal (afferent) sensory nerve fibers or roots and ventral (efferent) motor fibers or roots, which innervate a specific region of the body. This combined motor-sensory nerve is called a *spinal nerve* (Fig. 55-6). The cell bodies of the voluntary motor system are located in the anterior horn of the spinal cord gray matter. The cell bodies of the autonomic (involuntary) motor system are located in the anterolateral portion of the spinal cord gray matter. The cell bodies of sensory fibers are located in the dorsal root ganglia just outside the spinal cord. On exiting the spinal column, each spinal nerve divides into ventral and dorsal rami, a collection of motor and sensory fibers that eventually goes to peripheral structures (e.g., skin, muscles, viscera).

A **dermatome** is the area of skin innervated by the sensory fibers of a single dorsal root of a spinal nerve (Fig. 55-7). The dermatomes give a general picture of somatic sensory innervation by spinal segments. A *myotome* is a muscle group innervated by the primary motor neurons of a single ventral root. The dermatomes and myotomes of a given spinal segment overlap with those of adjacent segments because of the development of ascending and descending collateral branches of nerve fibers.

activity through axonal connections to the thalamus, motor cortex, and brainstem nuclei and their descending pathways.

Ventricles and Cerebrospinal Fluid. The ventricles are four interconnected fluid-filled cavities. The lower portion of the fourth ventricle becomes the central canal in the lower part of the brainstem. The spinal canal extends centrally through the full length of the spinal cord.

Cerebrospinal fluid (CSF) is produced largely in the choroid plexuses of the brain within the ventricles. It circulates within the subarachnoid space that surrounds the brain, brainstem, and spinal cord, cushioning the brain and spinal cord. CSF flows from the cranial cavity to the spinal cavity, carrying nutrients through both passive diffusion and active transport. CSF is produced at an average rate of about 500 mL/day. The ventricles and central canal are filled with an average of 150 mL at any given time. Changes in the rate of CSF production or absorption can occur, leading to a change in the volume within

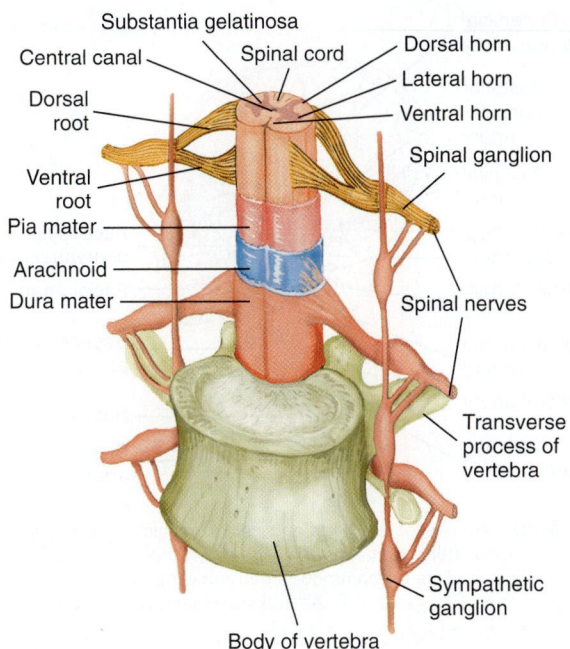

FIG. 55-6 Cross section of spinal cord showing attachments of spinal nerves and coverings of the spinal cord.

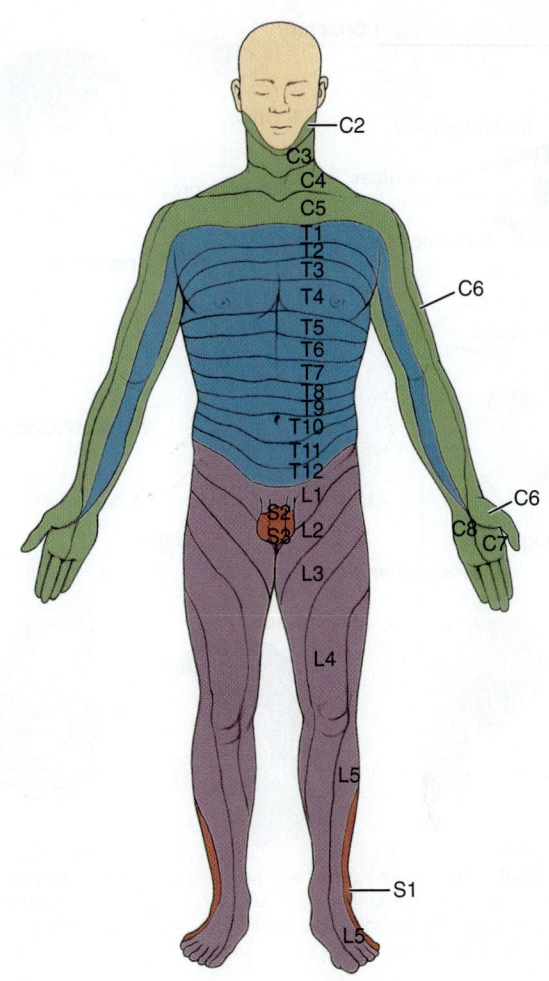

FIG. 55-7 Dermatomes of the body. (From Herlihy B: *The human body in health and illness*, ed 4, St Louis, 2011, Saunders.)

Cranial Nerves. The **cranial nerves (CNs)** are the 12 paired nerves composed of cell bodies with fibers that exit from the cranial cavity. Unlike the spinal nerves, which always have both afferent sensory and efferent motor fibers, some CNs are only sensory, some only motor, and some both.

Table 55-4 (later in this chapter) summarizes the motor and sensory components of the CNs. Fig. 55-8 shows the position of the CNs in relation to the brain and spinal cord. Just as the cell bodies of the spinal nerves are located in specific segments of the spinal cord, so are the cell bodies (nuclei) of the CNs located in specific segments of the brainstem. Exceptions are the nuclei of the olfactory and optic nerves. The primary cell bodies of the olfactory nerve are located in the nasal epithelium, and those of the optic nerve are in the retina.

Autonomic Nervous System. The **autonomic nervous system (ANS)** is divided into the sympathetic and parasympathetic systems. The ANS governs involuntary functions of cardiac muscle, smooth muscle, and glands through both efferent and afferent pathways. The two systems function together to maintain a relatively balanced internal environment. The preganglionic cell bodies of the *sympathetic nervous system* (SNS) are located in spinal segments T1 through L2. The major neurotransmitter released by the postganglionic fibers of the SNS is norepinephrine, and the neurotransmitter released by the preganglionic fibers is acetylcholine.

The preganglionic cell bodies of the *parasympathetic nervous system* (PSNS) are located in the brainstem and sacral spinal segments (S2 through S4). Acetylcholine is the neurotransmitter released at both preganglionic and postganglionic nerve endings.

SNS stimulation activates the mechanisms required for the "fight-or-flight" response that occurs throughout the body. In contrast, the PSNS is geared to act in localized and discrete regions. It conserves and restores the body's energy stores. The ANS provides dual and often reciprocal innervation to many structures. For example, the SNS increases the rate and force of heart contraction, and the PSNS decreases the rate and force.

Cerebral Circulation

Knowledge of the distribution of the brain's major arteries is essential for understanding and evaluating the signs and symptoms of cerebrovascular disease and trauma. The brain's blood supply arises from the internal carotid arteries (anterior circulation) and the vertebral arteries (posterior circulation), which are shown in Fig. 55-9.

The internal carotid arteries provide blood flow to the anterior and middle portions of the cerebrum. The vertebral arteries join to form the basilar artery and provide blood flow to the brainstem, cerebellum, and posterior cerebrum. The *Circle of Willis* is formed by communicating arteries that join the basilar and internal carotid arteries (Fig. 55-10). Although the Circle of Willis is considered a safety valve for blood flow, variations exist in 31% to 44% of patients.[3]

Superior to the Circle of Willis, three pairs of arteries supply blood to the left and right hemispheres. The anterior cerebral artery feeds the medial and anterior portions of the frontal lobes. The middle cerebral artery feeds the outer portions of the frontal, parietal, and superior temporal lobes. The posterior cerebral artery feeds the medial portions of the occipital and inferior temporal lobes. Venous blood drains from the brain through the dural sinuses, which form channels that drain into the two jugular veins.

Blood-Brain Barrier. The **blood-brain barrier** is a physiologic barrier between blood capillaries and brain tissue. This barrier

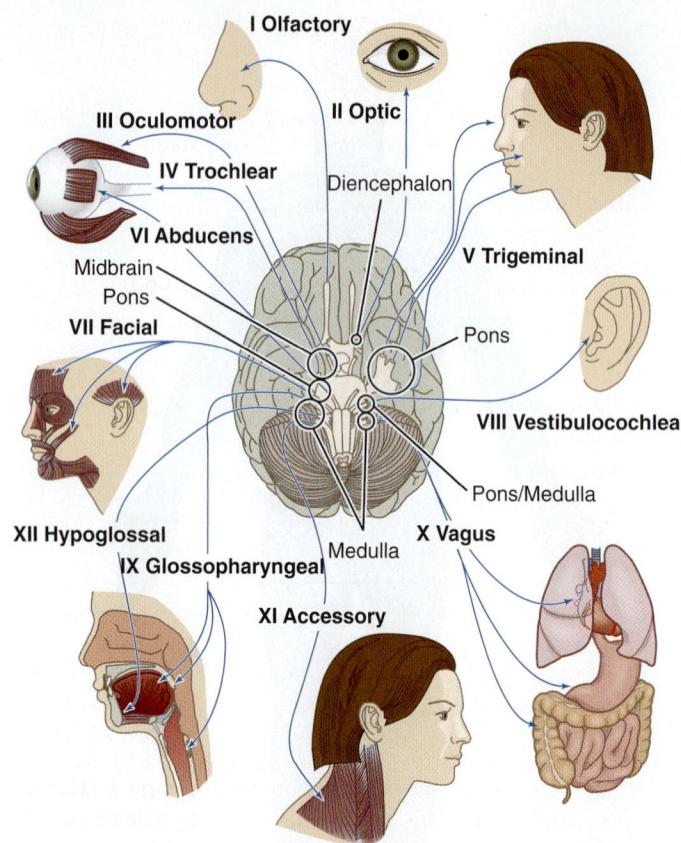

FIG. 55-8 The cranial nerves are numbered according to the order in which they leave the brain. (Redrawn from McCance KL, Huether SE: *Pathophysiology: the biologic basis for disease in adults and children,* ed 6, St Louis, 2010, Mosby.)

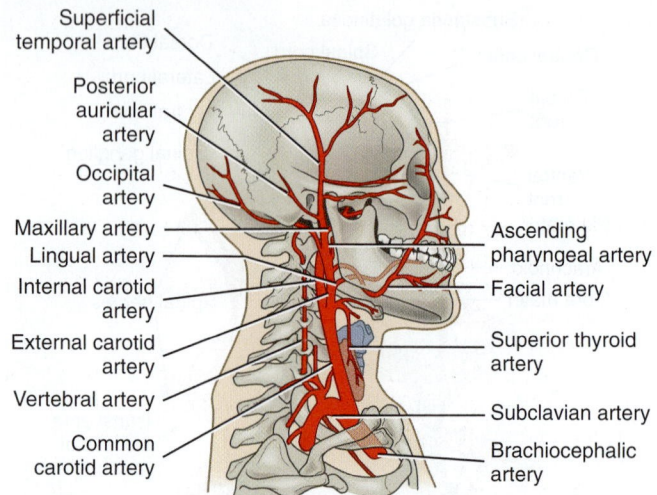

FIG. 55-9 Arteries of the head and neck. Brachiocephalic artery, right common carotid artery, right subclavian artery, and their branches. The major arteries to the head are the common carotid and vertebral arteries. (Modified from Thibodeau GA, Patton KT: *Anatomy and physiology,* ed 8, St Louis, 2013, Mosby.)

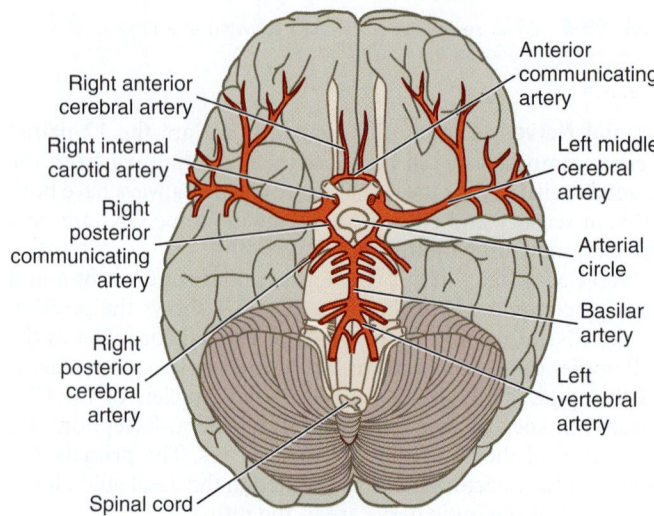

FIG. 55-10 Arteries at the base of the brain. The arteries that compose the Circle of Willis are the two anterior cerebral arteries joined to each other by the anterior communicating cerebral artery and to the posterior cerebral arteries by the posterior communicating arteries. (Modified from Thibodeau GA, Patton KT: *Anatomy and physiology,* ed 8, St Louis, 2013, Mosby.)

protects the brain from harmful agents, while allowing nutrients and gases to enter. The structure of brain capillaries differs from that of other capillaries, so substances that normally pass into most tissues are prevented from entering brain tissue. Lipid-soluble compounds enter the brain easily, whereas water-soluble and ionized drugs enter the brain and the spinal cord slowly. Thus the blood-brain barrier affects the penetration of drugs. Only certain drugs can enter the CNS from the bloodstream.

Protective Structures

Meninges. The **meninges** consist of three protective membranes that surround the brain and spinal cord: dura mater, arachnoid, and pia mater (Fig. 55-11). The thick *dura mater* forms the outermost layer. The *falx cerebri* is a fold of the dura that separates the two cerebral hemispheres and slows expansion of brain tissue in conditions such as a rapidly growing tumor or acute hemorrhage. The *tentorium cerebelli* is a fold of dura that separates the cerebral hemispheres from the posterior fossa (which contains the brainstem and cerebellum).

The *arachnoid* layer is a fragile, web-like membrane that lies between the dura mater and *pia mater* (the vascular innermost layer of the meninges). The area between the arachnoid layer and pia mater *(subarachnoid space)* is filled with CSF. Structures such as arteries, veins, and cranial nerves passing to and from the brain and skull must pass through the subarachnoid space. A larger subarachnoid space in the region of the third and fourth lumbar vertebrae is the area used to obtain CSF during a lumbar puncture.

Skull. The *skull* protects the brain from external trauma. It is composed of eight cranial bones and 14 facial bones. Although the top and sides of the inside of the skull are relatively smooth, the bottom surface is uneven. It has many ridges, prominences, and foramina (holes through which blood vessels and nerves enter the intracranial vault). The largest hole is the *foramen magnum,* through which the brainstem extends to the spinal cord. This foramen offers the only major space for the expansion of brain contents when increased intracranial pressure occurs.

Vertebral Column. The *vertebral column* protects the spinal cord, supports the head, and provides flexibility. The vertebral column is made up of 33 individual vertebrae: 7 cervical, 12 thoracic, 5 lumbar, 5 sacral (fused into one), and 4 coccygeal (fused into one). Each vertebra has a central opening through which the spinal cord passes. The vertebrae are held together by a series of ligaments. Intervertebral discs occupy the spaces between vertebrae, allowing movement of the column. Fig.

55-12 shows the natural curvature of the spinal column and its relation to the trunk.

Gerontologic Considerations: Effects of Aging on Nervous System

Several parts of the nervous system are affected by aging. In the CNS the gradual loss of neurons in certain areas of the brainstem, cerebellum, and cerebral cortex begins in early adulthood. With loss of neurons, the ventricles widen or enlarge, brain weight decreases, cerebral blood flow decreases, and CSF production declines.[4,5]

In the PNS, degenerative changes in myelin cause a decrease in nerve conduction. Coordinated neuromuscular activity, such as the maintenance of BP in response to changing from a lying to a standing position, is altered with aging. As a result, older adults are more likely to experience orthostatic hypotension. Similarly, coordination of neuromuscular activity to maintain body temperature also becomes less efficient with aging. Older adults are less able to adapt to extremes in environmental temperature and are more vulnerable to both hypothermia and hyperthermia.

Additional relevant changes associated with aging include decreases in memory, vision, hearing, taste, smell, vibration, position sense, muscle strength, and reaction time. Sensory changes, including decreases in taste and smell perception, may result in decreased dietary intake in the older adult.[6] Reduced hearing and vision can result in perceptual confusion. Problems with balance and coordination can put the older adult at risk for falls and subsequent fractures.[7] Changes in assessment findings result from age-related alterations in the various components of the nervous system (Table 55-2). Changes should not be attributed to aging without considering other underlying causes.

ASSESSMENT OF NERVOUS SYSTEM

Subjective Data

Important Health Information

Past Health History. When performing a neurologic examination, first determine if an emergency exists. For example, does the patient demonstrate decreasing level of consciousness? The neurologic assessment is performed when an abnormality is identified during screening or can be expected based on patient history. Is the patient a reliable historian and able to provide detailed information? If not, interview someone with firsthand knowledge of the patient's history and current complaint. Avoid suggesting symptoms or asking leading questions.

Second, the mode of onset and course of the illness are especially important aspects of the history. Often the nature of a neurologic disease process can be described by these facts alone. Obtain all pertinent data in the history of the present illness, especially data related to the characteristics and progression of the symptoms. In some cases, the history may include

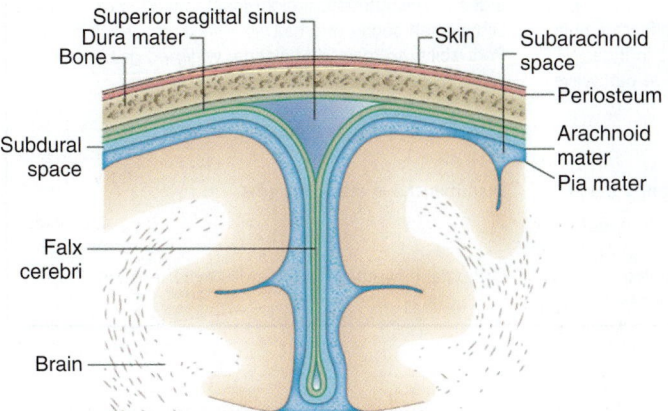

FIG. 55-11 Meninges.

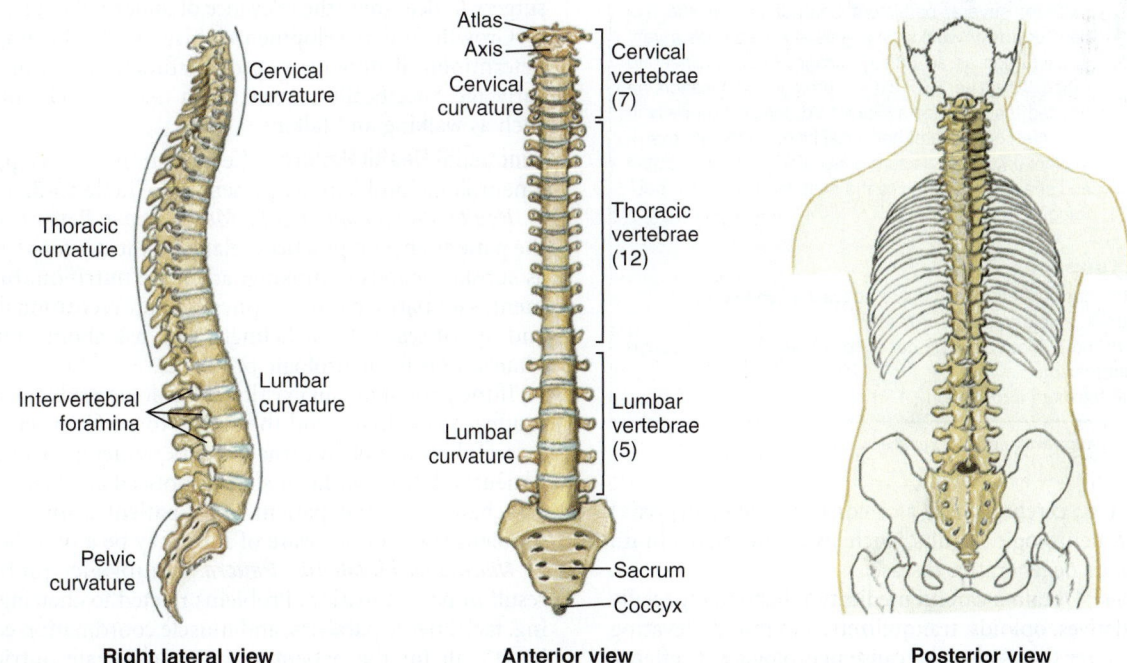

Right lateral view   **Anterior view**   **Posterior view**

FIG. 55-12 The vertebral column (three views). (Modified from Thibodeau GA, Patton KT: *Anatomy and physiology,* ed 8, St Louis, 2013, Mosby.)

TABLE 55-2 Gerontologic Assessment Differences

Nervous System

Component	Changes	Differences in Assessment Findings
Central Nervous System		
Brain	↓ Cerebral blood flow and metabolism	Alterations in mental functioning.
	↓ Efficiency of temperature-regulating mechanism	Impaired ability to adapt to environmental temperature.
	↓ Neurotransmitters, loss of neurons	Slowed conduction of nerve impulses, with slowed response time.
	↓ O₂ supply	Changes in gait and ambulation. Diminished kinesthetic sense.
	Cerebral tissue atrophy and ↑ size of ventricles	Altered balance, vertigo, syncope. ↑ Postural hypotension. Proprioception diminished. ↓ Sensory input.
Peripheral Nervous System		
Cranial and spinal nerves	Loss of myelin and ↓ conduction time	↓ Reaction time in specific nerves.
	Cellular degeneration, death of neurons	↓ Speed and intensity of neuronal reflexes.
Functional Divisions		
Motor	↓ Muscle bulk	Diminished strength and agility.
Sensory*	↓ Sensory receptors	Diminished sense of touch, pain, and temperature.
	↓ Electrical activity	Slowing of or alteration in sensory reception.
	Atrophy of taste buds	Signs of malnutrition, weight loss.
	Degeneration and loss of fibers in olfactory bulb	Diminished sense of smell.
	Degenerative changes in nerve cells in inner ear, cerebellum, and proprioceptive pathways	Poor ability to maintain balance, widened gait.
Reflexes	↓ Deep tendon reflexes	Below-average reflex score.
	↓ Sensory conduction velocity	Sluggish reflexes, slowed reaction time.
Reticular Formation		
Reticular activating system	Modification of hypothalamic function, ↓ stage IV sleep	Disturbances in sleep patterns.
Autonomic Nervous System		
Sympathetic nervous system and parasympathetic nervous system	Morphologic features of ganglia, slowed autonomic nervous system responses	Orthostatic hypotension, systolic hypertension.

*Specific changes related to the eye are listed in Table 20-1, and specific changes related to the ear are listed in Table 20-7.

CASE STUDY

Patient Introduction

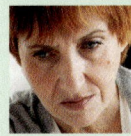

(©TatyanaGl/ iStock/ Thinkstock)

J.K. is a 57-yr-old white woman who went to see her HCP for severe, persistent headaches that she has had for a few weeks. She lives alone and has a very stressful job as an office manager in an engineering office. When her HCP did a neurologic examination, he noticed that she had a visual field deficit, especially in upper left quadrant of her visual field. During the examination, J.K. had a seizure in his office. 911 was called and she was admitted to the hospital. The on-call neurologist was notified.

Discussion Questions

1. What are the possible causes of J.K.'s headaches and seizure?
2. Is her condition stable or an emergency?
   You will learn more about J.K. and her condition as you read through this assessment chapter.
   (See p. 1304 for more information on J.K.)

Answers available at http://evolve.elsevier.com/Lewis/medsurg.

birth injury (e.g., cerebral palsy as a consequence of hypoxia) and/or other neurologic insults, such as a traumatic brain injury, stroke, or degenerative disease.

Medications. Obtain a careful medication history, especially the use of sedatives, opioids, tranquilizers, and mood-elevating drugs. Many other drugs also can cause neurologic side effects. Additionally, ask the patient to describe the medication regimen to determine adherence to prescribed therapies.

Surgery or Other Treatments. Inquire about any surgery involving any part of the nervous system, such as head, spine, or sensory organs. If a patient had surgery, determine the date, cause, procedure, recovery, and current status. Also note any history of eye surgery to determine the relevance of abnormal pupil assessment.

Growth and developmental history can be important in determining if nervous system dysfunction was present at an early age. Specifically inquire about major developmental tasks such as walking and talking.

Functional Health Patterns. Key questions to ask a patient with a neurologic problem are presented in Table 55-3.

Health Perception–Health Management Pattern. Ask about the patient's health practices related to the nervous system, such as substance abuse, smoking, adequate nutrition, BP management, safe participation in physical and recreational activities, and use of seat belts or helmets. Also ask about previous hospitalizations for neurologic problems.

If the patient has an existing neurologic problem, assess how it affects daily living and the ability to perform self-care. After a careful review of information, ask someone who knows the patient well whether he or she has noticed any mental or physical changes in the patient. The patient with a neurologic problem may not be aware of it or may be a poor historian.

Nutritional-Metabolic Pattern. Neurologic problems can result in poor nutrition. Problems related to chewing, swallowing, facial nerve paralysis, and muscle coordination could make it difficult for the patient to ingest adequate nutrients. Also, certain vitamins such as thiamine (B₁), niacin, and pyridoxine (B₆) are essential for the maintenance and health of the CNS.

TABLE 55-3 Health History

Nervous System

Health Perception–Health Management
- What are your usual daily activities?
- Do you use alcohol, tobacco, or recreational drugs?*
- What safety practices do you perform in a car? On a motorcycle? On a bicycle?
- Do you have hypertension? If so, how is it managed?
- Have you ever been hospitalized for a neurologic problem?*

Nutritional-Metabolic
- Are you able to feed yourself?
- Do you have any problems getting adequate nutrition because of chewing or swallowing difficulties, facial nerve paralysis, or poor muscle coordination?*
- Give a 24-hr dietary recall.

Elimination
- Do you have incontinence of your bowels or bladder?*
- Do you ever experience problems with urinary hesitancy, urgency, retention?*
- Do you postpone your bowel movements?*
- Do you take any medication to manage neurologic problems? If so, what?

Activity-Exercise
- Describe any problems you experience with usual activities and exercise as a result of a neurologic problem.
- Do you have weakness or lack of coordination?*
- Are you able to perform your personal hygiene needs independently?*

Sleep-Rest
- Describe your sleep pattern.
- When you have trouble sleeping, what do you do?

Cognitive-Perceptual
- Have you noticed any changes in your memory?*
- Do you experience dizziness, heat or cold sensitivity, numbness, or tingling?*
- Do you have chronic pain?*
- Do you have any difficulty with verbal or written communication?*
- Have you noticed any changes in vision or hearing?*

Self-Perception–Self-Concept
- How do you feel about yourself, about who you are?
- Describe your general emotional pattern.

Role-Relationship
- Have you experienced changes in roles such as spouse, parent, or breadwinner?*

Sexuality-Reproductive
- Are you dissatisfied with your sexual function?*
- Are problems related to your sexual function causing tension in an important relationship?*
- Do you feel the need for professional counseling related to your sexual function?*

Coping–Stress Tolerance
- Describe your usual coping pattern.
- Do you think your present coping pattern is adequate to meet the stressors of your life?*
- What needs are unmet by your current support system?

Value-Belief
- Describe any culturally specific beliefs and attitudes that may influence your care.

*If yes, describe.

GENETIC RISK ALERT

- Huntington's disease is a genetically transmitted, autosomal dominant disorder.
- Major neurologic disorders that may have a genetic basis are multiple sclerosis, headaches, Parkinson's disease, and Alzheimer's disease. The presence of these problems in a family history increases the likelihood of similar problems occurring in the patient.
- A careful family history may determine if a neurologic problem has a genetic basis.

Deficiencies in one or more of these vitamins could result in such nonspecific complaints as depression, apathy, neuritis, weakness, mental confusion, and irritability. Cobalamin (vitamin B_{12}) deficiency can occur in older adults, who may have problems with vitamin absorption from supplements as well as natural food sources such as meat, fish, and poultry. Untreated, cobalamin deficiency can cause mental function decline. In the patient with brain injury, early nutritional support can markedly improve outcomes.[8]

Elimination Pattern. Bowel and bladder problems often are associated with neurologic problems such as stroke, head injury, spinal cord injury, multiple sclerosis, and dementia. To plan appropriate interventions, determine if the bowel or bladder problem was present before or after the current neurologic event. Urinary retention and incontinence of urine and feces are the most common elimination problems associated with a neurologic problem or its treatment. For example, nerve root compression (as occurs in cauda equina conditions) leads to a sudden onset of incontinence. Document key details, such as number of episodes, accompanying sensations or lack of sensations, and measures to control the problem.

Activity-Exercise Pattern. Many neurologic disorders can cause problems in the patient's mobility, strength, and coordination. Neurologic problems can result in changes in the patient's usual activity and exercise patterns. These problems can also result in falls.[7] Assess the person's activities of daily living because neurologic diseases can affect the ability to perform motor tasks, which increases the possibility of injury.

Sleep-Rest Pattern. Sleep pattern alteration can be both a cause and a response to neurologic problems. Pain and reduced ability to change position because of muscle weakness and paralysis could interfere with sleep quality. Hallucinations resulting from dementia or drugs can also interrupt sleep. Carefully assess and document the patient's sleep pattern and bedtime routines.

Cognitive-Perceptual Pattern. Because the nervous system controls cognition and sensory integration, many neurologic disorders affect these functions.[9] Consider culture, age, and education when assessing communication because they play a role in the interaction among people. Assess memory, language, calculation ability, problem-solving ability, insight, and judgment. Ask the patient hypothetical questions such as, "What is a reasonable price for a cup of coffee?" or "What would you do if you saw a car crash outside your house?" Often a structured mental status questionnaire is used to evaluate these functions and provide baseline data.

Delirium is an acute and transient disorder of cognition that can be seen at any time during a patient's illness. As discussed in Chapter 59, delirium is often an early indicator of various illnesses (see Table 59-17). The Confusion Assessment Method tool is used to assess for delirium (see Table 59-18).

Assess a person's ability to use and understand language. Appropriateness of responses is a useful indicator of cognitive and perceptual ability. Determine the patient's understanding and ability to carry out necessary treatments. Neurologic-related cognitive changes can interfere with the patient's understanding of the disease and adherence to related treatment.

Pain is commonly associated with many neurologic problems, and is often the reason a patient seeks care. Carefully assess the patient's pain. (Pain and pain assessment are discussed in Chapter 8.)

Self-Perception–Self-Concept Pattern. Neurologic diseases can drastically alter a patient's control over life and create dependency on others for meeting daily needs. Also, the patient's physical appearance and emotional control can be affected. Sensitively inquire about the patient's evaluation of self-worth, perception of abilities, body image, and general emotional pattern.

Role-Relationship Pattern. Physical impairments such as weakness and paralysis can alter or limit participation in usual roles and activities. Cognitive changes can permanently alter a person's ability to maintain previous roles. These changes can dramatically affect the patient, caregiver, and family. Ask the patient if a role change has occurred (e.g., spouse or breadwinner) as a result of neurologic problems and determine how long it has lasted. Family members or caregivers should participate in decision making when neurologic deficits preclude the patient from decisions that will affect the role.

Sexuality-Reproductive Pattern. Assess the person's ability to participate in sexual activity because many neurologic disorders can affect sexual response. Cerebral lesions may inhibit the desire phase or the reflex responses of the excitement phase. The hypothalamus stimulates the pituitary gland to release hormones that influence sexual desire. Brainstem and spinal cord lesions may partially or completely interrupt the desire or ability to have intercourse. Neuropathies and spinal cord lesions may prevent reflex activities of the sexual response or affect sensation and decrease desire. Despite neurologically related changes in sexual function, many persons can achieve satisfying expression of intimacy and affection.

Coping–Stress Tolerance Pattern. The physical sequelae of a neurologic problem can strain a patient's coping ability. Often the problem is chronic and requires the patient to learn new coping skills. Assess if the patient's coping skills are adequate to deal with the stress of this problem. Also assess the patient's support system.

Value-Belief Pattern. Many neurologic problems have serious, long-term, life-changing effects. Determine what these effects are because they can strain the patient's belief system. Also determine if any religious or cultural beliefs could affect the planned treatment regimen.

Objective Data

Physical Examination. The standard neurologic examination helps determine the presence, location, and nature of nervous system disease. The examination assesses six categories of function: mental status, cranial nerve function, motor function, sensory function, cerebellar function, and reflexes.[10] Develop a consistent pattern of completing the neurologic examination to remember to include each element for every patient examination.

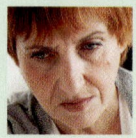
Mental Status. Assessment of mental status (cerebral function) gives a general impression of how the patient is functioning. It involves determining complex and high-level cerebral functions governed by many areas of the cerebral cortex. Complete most of the mental status examination during your interaction with the patient. For example, assess language and memory when asking the patient for details of the illness and significant past events. Consider the patient's age, cultural background, and level of education when evaluating mental status.

The components of the mental status examination include:

- *General appearance and behavior:* This component includes level of consciousness (awake, asleep, comatose), motor activity, body posture, dress and hygiene, facial expression, and speech pattern. A patient who has deficits in self-care as evidenced by poor grooming is more likely to have other cognitive deficits.
- *Cognition:* Note orientation to time, place, person, and situation, as well as memory, general knowledge, insight, judgment, problem solving, and calculation. Common questions are "Who were the last three presidents?" "Does a rock float on water?" "How much money is a quarter, two dimes, and a nickel?" Consider if the patient's plans and goals match the physical and mental capabilities. Note the presence of factors affecting intellectual capacity, such as cognitive impairment, hallucinations, delusions, and dementia.
- *Mood and affect:* Note any agitation, anger, depression, or euphoria, and the appropriateness of these states. Use suitable questions to reveal the patient's feelings.

Cranial Nerves. Testing each CN is an essential part of the neurologic examination (Table 55-4).

TABLE 55-4 Cranial Nerves: Function and Assessment

Nerve	Function	Assessment
I Olfactory	*Sensory:* from olfactory (smell)	Ask patient to close one nostril at a time and identify easily recognized odors (e.g., coffee). Any asymmetry in sense of smell is important.
II Optic	*Sensory:* from retina of eyes (vision)	Examine each eye independently. *Visual fields:* Position yourself opposite the patient. Ask him or her to look directly at the bridge of your nose and indicate when an object (finger, pencil tip) presented from the periphery of each of the visual fields is seen (Fig. 55-13). *Visual acuity:* Ask patient to read a Snellen chart. Record the number on the lowest line the patient can read with 50% accuracy. The patient who wears glasses should wear them during testing unless they are used only for close reading. If a Snellen chart is not available, ask the patient to read newsprint for gross assessment of acuity. Record the distance from patient to newsprint required for accurate reading.
III Oculomotor	*Motor:* to four eye movement muscles and levator palpebrae muscle *Parasympathetic:* smooth muscle in eyeball	Ask the person to hold the head steady and to follow the movement of your finger, pen, or penlight only with the eyes. Hold the target back about 12 inches so that the person can focus on it comfortably. Move the target to each of the six positions (right and up, right, right and down, left and up, left, left and down), hold it momentarily, and then move back to center. Progress clockwise. A normal response is parallel tracking of the object with both eyes. Check for pupillary constriction and *accommodation* (pupils constricting with near vision). To test pupillary constriction, shine a light into the pupil of one eye; look for ipsilateral constriction of the same pupil and contralateral (consensual) constriction of the opposite eye. Note the size and shape of the pupils. (The optic nerve must be intact for this reflex to occur.)
IV Trochlear	*Motor:* to one eye movement muscle, the superior oblique muscle	See testing for CN III. (Because the oculomotor [CN III], trochlear [CN IV], and abducens [CN VI] nerves help move the eye, they are tested together.)
V Trigeminal • Ophthalmic branch • Maxillary branch • Mandibular branch	 *Sensory:* from forehead, eye, superior nasal cavity *Sensory:* from inferior nasal cavity, face, upper teeth, mucosa of superior mouth *Sensory:* from surfaces of jaw, lower teeth, mucosa of lower mouth, and anterior tongue *Motor:* to muscles of mastication	*Sensory:* Have patient close eyes and identify light touch (cotton wisp) and pinprick in each of the three divisions (ophthalmic, maxillary, and mandibular) of nerve on both sides of face. *Motor:* Ask patient to clench teeth and then palpate masseter muscles just above the mandibular angle. Muscles should feel equally strong on both sides. *Corneal (blink) reflex:* Evaluates CN V and CN VII simultaneously. (Sensory component of this reflex [corneal sensation] is innervated by the ophthalmic division of CN V. The motor component [eye blink] is innervated by the facial nerve [CN VII]). Have patient look up and away. Then from the other side, lightly touch the cornea with cotton wisp. Look for normal blink reaction of both eyes. Repeat on other side.
VI Abducens	*Motor:* to the lateral rectus muscle of the eye (one eye movement)	See testing for CN III. (Because the oculomotor [CN III], trochlear [CN IV], and abducens [CN VI] nerves help move the eye, they are tested together.)
VII Facial	*Motor:* to facial muscles of expression and cheek muscle *Sensory:* taste from anterior two thirds of tongue	Ask patient to raise eyebrows, close eyes tightly, purse lips, draw back the corners of mouth in an exaggerated smile, and frown. Note any asymmetry in the facial movements because this can indicate damage to nerve.
VIII Vestibulocochlear • Vestibular branch • Cochlear branch	 *Sensory:* from equilibrium sensory organ (vestibular apparatus) *Sensory:* from auditory sensory organ (cochlea), hearing	 Not routinely tested unless the patient complains of dizziness, vertigo, or unsteadiness, or has auditory dysfunction. Have patient close eyes and indicate when he or she hears the rustling of your fingertips. For more precise assessment of hearing, perform the Weber and Rinne tests or use an audiometer (see Table 20-11).
IX Glossopharyngeal	*Sensory:* from pharynx and posterior tongue, including taste *Motor:* to superior pharyngeal muscles	The glossopharyngeal and vagus nerves (CN IX and X) are tested together because both innervate the pharynx. To test the gag reflex, touch the sides of the posterior pharynx or soft palate with a tongue blade. If the reflex is weak or absent, the patient is in danger of aspirating food or secretions. Another test for the awake, cooperative patient is to ask the patient to say "ah," and note the bilateral symmetry of elevation of the soft palate. If a patient has an endotracheal tube, the cough reflex (elicited when the suction catheter contacts the *carina* of the respiratory tree) is a method of assessing the vagus nerve.
X Vagus	*Sensory:* from much of viscera of thorax and abdomen *Motor:* to larynx and middle and inferior pharyngeal muscles *Parasympathetic:* to heart, lungs, most of digestive system	See testing for CN IX. (The glossopharyngeal and vagus nerves [CN IX and X] are tested together because both innervate the pharynx.)
XI Accessory	*Motor:* to sternocleidomastoid and trapezius muscles	Ask patient to shrug the shoulders and to turn head to either side against resistance. Sternocleidomastoid and trapezius muscles should contract smoothly. Note symmetry, atrophy, or fasciculation of muscle.
XII Hypoglossal	*Motor:* to muscles of tongue	Ask to protrude tongue, which should protrude in midline. Next ask the patient to move the tongue up and down and side to side. Finally, the patient should also be able to push the tongue to either side against the resistance of a tongue blade. Note any asymmetry, atrophy, or fasciculation.

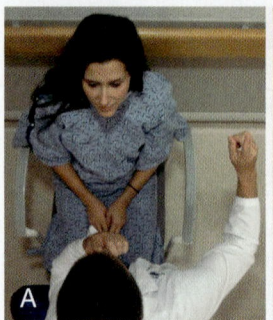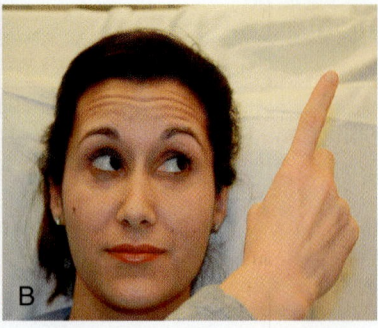

FIG. 55-13 **A,** Nurse checking visual fields. **B,** Nurse checking extraocular movement (EOM). (Courtesy DaiWai Olson, RN, PhD, CCRN, Dallas, Tex.)

Olfactory nerve. Chronic rhinitis, sinusitis, and heavy smoking may decrease the sense of smell. Disturbance in ability to smell may be associated with a tumor involving the olfactory bulb or may be the result of a basilar skull fracture that has damaged the olfactory fibers as they pass through the delicate cribriform plate of the skull. *Anosmia* (loss of sense of smell) also has been identified as an early sign in Parkinson's disease and Lewy body dementia.[11]

Optic nerve. Visual field defects may arise from lesions of the optic nerve, optic chiasm, or tracts that extend through the temporal, parietal, or occipital lobes. Visual field changes resulting from brain lesions include *hemianopsia* (one half of the visual field is affected), *quadrantanopsia* (one fourth of the visual field is affected), *bitemporal hemianopsia* (bilateral peripheral vision is affected), or monocular vision. It may be difficult to test acuity if the patient does not read English or is aphasic.

Oculomotor, trochlear, and abducens nerves. Because the oculomotor (CN III), trochlear (CN IV), and abducens (CN VI) nerves help move the eye, they are tested together (Table 55-4). With weakness or paralysis of one of the eye muscles, the eyes do not move together, and the patient has a *disconjugate gaze.* The presence and direction of *nystagmus* (fine, rapid jerking movements of the eyes) are observed at this time, even though this condition most often indicates vestibulocerebellar problems.

Because the oculomotor nerve exits at the top of the brainstem at the tentorial notch, it can be compressed easily by expanding mass lesions. When this occurs, sympathetic input to the pupil is unopposed; the pupil changes shape and becomes dilated. The lack of pupillary constriction is an early sign of central herniation (see Chapter 56).

Two abbreviations commonly used to record the reaction of the pupils are *PERRL* (Pupils are Equal [in size], Round, and Reactive to Light) and *PERRLA* (Pupils are Equal, Round, and Reactive to Light and Accommodation). The *PERRL* abbreviation is appropriate when accommodation cannot be assessed, as in an unconscious patient. Convergence and accommodation are tested by having the patient focus on the examiner's finger as it moves toward the patient's nose.

Another function of the oculomotor nerve is to keep the eyelid open. Damage to the nerve can cause *ptosis* (drooping eyelid), pupillary abnormalities, and eye muscle weakness.

Motor System. The motor system examination includes assessment of strength, tone, coordination, and symmetry of the major muscle groups. Test muscle strength by asking the patient to push and pull against the resistance of your arm as it opposes flexion and extension of the patient's muscle. Ask patient to offer resistance at the shoulders, elbows, wrists, hips, knees, and ankles. Mild weakness of the arm is demonstrated by downward drifting of the arm or pronation of the palm (*pronator drift*). The pronator drift test is particularly sensitive when the patient has a potential for vasospasm or increasing edema in one hemisphere of the cerebrum. Ask the patient to close the eyes and hold the arms out with palms facing up (as though he or she is holding a large pizza). The patient should hold this position for 30 seconds. Downward drift with palm pronation indicates a problem in the opposite motor cortex. Note any weakness or asymmetry of strength between the same muscle groups of the right and left sides.

Test muscle tone by passively moving the limbs through their range of motion. You should identify a slight resistance to these movements. Abnormal tone is described as *hypotonia* (flaccidity) or *hypertonia* (spasticity). Note any involuntary movements, such as tics, tremor, *myoclonus* (spasm of muscles), *athetosis* (slow, writhing, involuntary movements of extremities), *chorea* (involuntary, purposeless, rapid motions), and *dystonia* (impairment of muscle tone).

Test cerebellar function by assessing balance and coordination. A good screening test for both balance and muscle strength is to observe the patient's stature (posture while standing) and gait. Note the pace and rhythm of the gait, and observe for normal symmetric and oppositional arm swing. The patient's ability to ambulate helps to determine the level of nursing care required and the risk of falling.

The finger-to-nose test (having the patient alternately touch the nose, then touch the examiner's finger) and the heel-to-shin test (having the patient stroke the heel of one foot up and down the shin of the opposite leg) assess coordination and cerebellar function. Reposition your finger while the patient is touching the nose so that the patient must adjust to a new distance each time your finger is touched. These movements should be performed smoothly and accurately. Other tests include asking the patient to pronate and supinate both hands rapidly and to do a shallow knee bend, first on one leg and then on the other. Note dysarthria or slurred speech because it is a sign of incoordination of the speech muscles.

Sensory System. In the somatic sensory examination, several modalities are tested. Each modality is carried by a specific ascending pathway in the spinal cord before it reaches the sensory cortex. As a rule, perform the examination with the patient's eyes closed and avoid providing the patient with clues. Ask "How does this feel?" rather than "Is this sharp?" In the routine neurologic examination, sensory testing of the anterior torso, posterior torso, and the four extremities is sufficient. However, if a disturbance is identified in sensory function of the skin, the boundaries of that dysfunction should be carefully delineated along the dermatome.

Touch, pain, and temperature. Light touch is usually tested first using a cotton wisp or light pinprick. Gently touch each of the four extremities and ask the patient to indicate when he or she feels the stimulus. Test pain by alternately touching the skin with the sharp and dull end of a pin. Tell the patient to respond "sharp" or "dull." Evaluate each limb separately.

Extinction is assessed by simultaneously touching both sides of the body symmetrically. Normally, the simultaneous stimuli are both perceived (sensed). An abnormal response occurs when the patient perceives the stimulus on only one side. The other stimulus is *extinguished.*

The sensation of temperature (only to be assessed when the response to deep pain is abnormal) can be tested by applying tubes of warm and cold water to the skin and asking the patient to identify the stimuli with the eyes closed. If pain sensation is intact, assessment of temperature sensation may be omitted because both sensations are carried by the same ascending pathways.

Vibration sense. Assess vibration sense by applying a vibrating tuning fork to the fingernails and bony prominences of the hands, legs, and feet. Ask the patient if the vibration or "buzz" is felt. Then ask the patient to indicate when the vibration ceases.

Position sense. Assess position sense (*proprioception*) by placing your thumb and forefinger on either side of the patient's forefinger or great toe and gently moving his or her digit up or down. Ask the patient to close the eyes and indicate the direction in which the digit is moved.

Another test of proprioception is the Romberg test. Ask the patient to stand with feet together and then close his or her eyes. If the patient is able to maintain balance with the eyes open but sways or falls with the eyes closed (i.e., a positive Romberg test), vestibulocochlear dysfunction or disease in the posterior columns of the spinal cord may be indicated. Be aware of patient safety during this test.

Cortical sensory functions. Several tests evaluate cortical integration of sensory perceptions (which occurs in the parietal lobes). Explain these tests to the patient before performing them, while his or her eyes are still open. Assess *two-point discrimination* by placing the two points of a calibrated compass on the tips of the fingers and toes. The minimum recognizable separation is 4 to 5 mm in the fingertips and a greater degree of separation elsewhere. This test is important in diagnosing diseases of the sensory cortex and PNS.

Graphesthesia (ability to feel writing on skin) is tested by having the patient identify numbers traced on the palm of the hands. *Stereognosis* (ability to perceive the form and nature of objects) is tested by having the patient close the eyes and identify the size and shape of easily recognized objects (e.g., coins, keys, safety pin) placed in the hands.

Reflexes. Tendons have receptors that are sensitive to stretch. A reflex contraction of the skeletal muscle occurs when the tendon is stretched. In general, the biceps, triceps, brachioradialis, patellar, and Achilles tendon reflexes are tested. Initiate a simple muscle stretch reflex by briskly tapping the tendon of a stretched muscle, usually with a reflex hammer (Fig. 55-14). The response (muscle contraction of the corresponding muscle) is measured on a 0 to 5 scale as follows: 0 = absent reflex, 1 = weak response, seen only with reinforcement, 2 = normal response, 3 = brisk response, 4 = hyperreflexia with nonsustained clonus, and 5 = hyperreflexia with sustained clonus. *Clonus,* an abnormal response, is a continued rhythmic contraction of the muscle with continuous application of the stimulus.

Elicit the *biceps reflex,* with the patient's arm partially flexed and palm up, by placing your thumb over the biceps tendon in the antecubital space and striking the thumb with a hammer. The normal response is flexion of the arm at the elbow or contraction of the biceps muscle that can be felt by your thumb.

Elicit the *triceps reflex* by striking the triceps tendon above the elbow while the patient's arm is flexed. The normal response is extension of the arm or visible contraction of the triceps.

Elicit the *brachioradialis reflex* by striking the radius 3 to 5 cm above the wrist while the patient's arm is relaxed. The normal response is flexion and supination at the elbow or visible contraction of the brachioradialis muscle.

Elicit the *patellar reflex* by striking the patellar tendon just below the patella. The patient can be sitting or lying as long as the leg being tested hangs freely. The normal response is extension of the leg with contraction of the quadriceps.

Gently dorsiflex the patient's foot at the ankle. Elicit the *Achilles tendon reflex* by striking the Achilles tendon while the

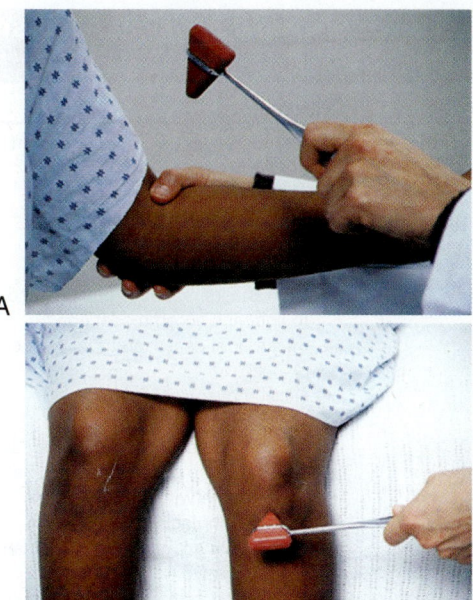

FIG. 55-14 The examiner strikes a swift blow over a stretched tendon to elicit a stretch reflex. **A,** Biceps reflex. **B,** Patellar reflex.

CASE STUDY—cont'd

Objective Data: Physical Examination

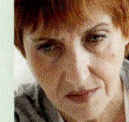

(©TatyanaGl/ iStock/ Thinkstock)

A physical assessment of J.K. reveals the following:
- BP 145/80, HR 78, RR 20, T 37°C
- Alert, oriented, and appropriate but anxious
- Strength 5/5 on all extremities
- Visual field deficits in upper left quadrant of visual field

Discussion Question

1. What should be included in the physical assessment? For what would you be looking?
2. Which physical assessment findings are of most concern to you?
3. Based on the results of the subjective and physical assessment, what diagnostic studies do you think may be ordered for J.K.?

You will learn more about diagnostic studies related to the neurologic system in the next section.

(See p. 1312 for more information on J.K.)

Answers available at *http://evolve.elsevier.com/Lewis/medsurg.*

---

patient's leg is flexed at the knee. The normal response is plantar flexion at the ankle.

A *focused assessment* is used to evaluate the status of previously identified neurologic problems and to monitor for signs of new problems (see Table 3-7). A focused assessment of the neurologic system is presented in the box.

Table 55-5 is an example of a normal neurologic physical assessment. Abnormal assessment findings of the neurologic system are presented in Table 55-6.

DIAGNOSTIC STUDIES OF NERVOUS SYSTEM

Numerous diagnostic studies are available to assess the nervous system (Table 55-7). CSF analysis provides information about a variety of CNS diseases. Normal CSF is clear, colorless, odorless, and free of red blood cells. It contains little protein. Normal CSF values are listed in Table 55-8. CSF may be obtained through lumbar puncture (most common) or ventriculostomy.

TABLE 55-5 Normal Physical Assessment of Nervous System*

Parameter	Findings
Mental status	• Alert and oriented, orderly thought processes. • Appropriate mood and affect.
Cranial nerves†	• Smell intact to soap or coffee. • Visual fields full to confrontation. • Intact extraocular movements. • No nystagmus. Pupils equal, round, reactive to light and accommodation. • Intact facial sensation to light touch and pinprick. • Facial movements full. • Hearing intact bilaterally. • Intact gag and swallow reflexes. Symmetric smile. Midline protrusion of tongue. • Full strength with head turning and shoulder shrugging.
Motor system	• Normal gait and station. Normal tandem walk. Negative Romberg test. • Normal and symmetric muscle bulk, tone, and strength. • Smooth performance of finger-nose, heel-shin movements.
Sensory system	• Intact sensation to light touch, position sense, pinprick, heat, and cold.
Reflexes‡	• Biceps, triceps, brachioradialis, patellar, and Achilles tendon reflexes 2/5 bilaterally. • Toes pointed down with plantar stimulation.

*If some portion of the neurologic examination was not done, this should be indicated (e.g., "Smell not tested").
†May also be recorded as "CN I to XII intact."
‡May also be recorded as drawing of stick figure indicating reflex strength at appropriate sites.

FOCUSED ASSESSMENT
Nervous System

Use this checklist to make sure the key assessment steps have been done.

Subjective
Ask the patient about any of the following and note responses.

Blackouts/loss of memory	Y	N
Weakness, numbness, tingling in arms or legs	Y	N
Headaches, especially new onset	Y	N
Loss of balance/coordination	Y	N
Orientation to person, place, time, and situation	Y	N

Objective: Diagnostic
Check the following diagnostic results for critical values.

Lumbar puncture	✓
CT or MRI of brain	✓
EEG	✓

Objective: Physical Examination
Inspect/Observe

General level of consciousness/orientation	✓
Oropharynx for gag reflex and soft palate movement	✓
Peripheral sensation of light touch and pinprick (face, hands, feet)	✓
Smell with coffee or soap	✓
Eyes for extraocular movements, PERRLA, peripheral vision, nystagmus	✓
Gait for smoothness and coordination	✓

Palpate

Strength of neck, shoulders, arms, and legs for fullness and symmetry	✓

Percuss

Reflexes	✓

CT, Computed tomography; *EEG,* electroencephalogram; *MRI,* magnetic resonance imaging; *PERRLA,* pupils equal, round, and reactive to light and accommodation.

TABLE 55-6 Assessment Abnormalities
Nervous System

Finding	Description	Possible Etiology and Significance
Mental Status		
Altered consciousness	Stuporous, mute, diminished response to verbal cues or pain	Intracranial lesions, metabolic disorder, psychiatric disorders
Anosognosia	Inability to recognize bodily defect or disease	Lesions in right parietal cortex
Speech		
Aphasia, dysphasia	Loss of or impaired language faculty (comprehension, expression, or both)	Left cerebral cortex lesion
Dysarthria	Lack of coordination in articulating speech	Cerebellar or cranial nerve lesion Antiseizure drugs, sedatives, hypnotic drug toxicity (including alcohol)
Eyes		
Anisocoria	Inequality of pupil size	Oculomotor nerve injury Sympathetic pathway injury
Diplopia	Double vision	Lesions affecting nerves of extraocular muscles, cerebellar damage
Homonymous hemianopsia	Loss of vision in one side of visual field	Lesions in the contralateral occipital lobe
Cranial Nerves		
Dysphagia	Difficulty in swallowing	Lesions involving motor pathways of CNs IX, X (including lower brainstem)
Ophthalmoplegia	Paralysis of eye muscles	Lesions in brainstem
Papilledema	"Choked disc," swelling of optic nerve head	Increased intracranial pressure

TABLE 55-6 Assessment Abnormalities

Nervous System—cont'd

Finding	Description	Possible Etiology and Significance
Motor System		
Apraxia	Inability to perform learned movements despite having desire and physical ability to perform them	Cerebral cortex lesion
Ataxia	Lack of coordination of movement	Lesions of sensory or motor pathways, cerebellum Antiseizure drugs, sedatives, hypnotic drug toxicity (including alcohol)
Dyskinesia	Impairment of voluntary movement, resulting in fragmentary or incomplete movements	Disorders of basal ganglia, idiosyncratic reaction to psychotropic drugs
Hemiplegia	Paralysis on one side	Stroke and other lesions involving contralateral motor cortex
Nystagmus	Jerking or bobbing of eyes as they track moving object	Lesions in cerebellum, brainstem, vestibular system Antiseizure drugs, sedatives, hypnotic toxicity (including alcohol)
Sensory System		
Analgesia	Loss of pain sensation	Lesion in spinothalamic tract or thalamus. Analgesic drugs
Anesthesia	Absence of sensation	Lesions in spinal cord, thalamus, sensory cortex, or peripheral sensory nerve. Anesthesia drugs
Paresthesia	Alteration in sensation	Lesions in the posterior column or sensory cortex
Astereognosis	Inability to recognize form of object by touch	Lesions in parietal cortex
Reflexes		
Extensor plantar response	Toes pointing up with plantar stimulation	Suprasegmental or upper motor neuron lesion
Deep tendon reflexes	Diminished or absent motor response	Lower motor neuron lesions
Spinal Cord		
Bladder dysfunction		
• Atonic (autonomous)	Absence of muscle tone and contractility, enlargement of capacity, no sensation of discomfort, overflow with large residual, inability to voluntarily empty	Early stage of spinal cord injury
• Hypotonic	More ability than atonic bladder but less than normal	Interruption of afferent pathways from bladder
• Hypertonic	Increased muscle tone, diminished capacity, reflex emptying, dribbling, incontinence	Lesions in pyramidal tracts (efferent pathways)
Paraplegia	Paralysis of lower extremities	Spinal cord transection or mass lesion (thoracolumbar region)
Tetraplegia (quadriplegia)	Paralysis of all extremities	Spinal cord transection or mass lesion (cervical region)

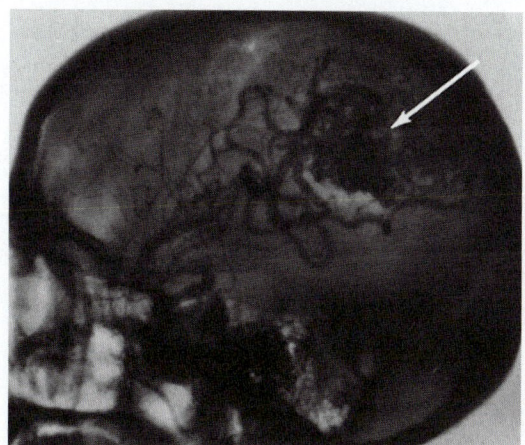

FIG. 55-15 Cerebral angiogram illustrating an arteriovenous malformation *(arrow)*. (From Chipps E, Clanin N, Campbell V: *Neurologic disorders,* St Louis, 1992, Mosby.)

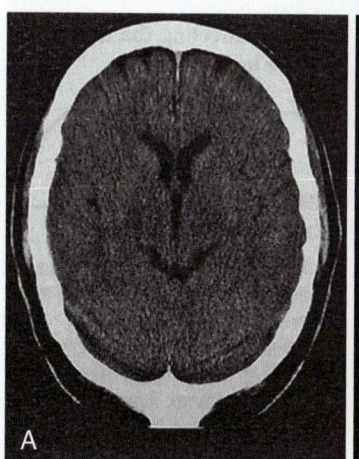 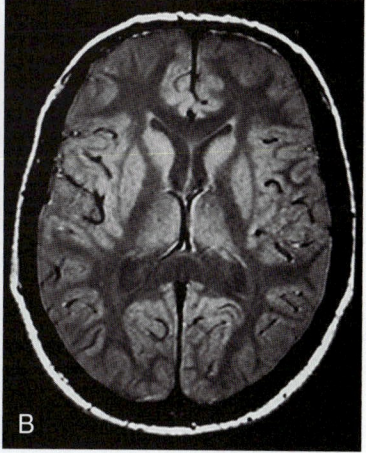

FIG. 55-16 Normal images of the brain. **A,** Computed tomography scan. **B,** Magnetic resonance imaging. (From Fuller G, Manford M: *Neurology: an illustrated colour text,* ed 3, New York, 2010, Churchill Livingstone.)

TABLE 55-7   Diagnostic Studies

Nervous System

Study	Description and Purpose	Nursing Responsibility
Cerebrospinal Fluid Analysis		
Lumbar puncture	CSF is aspirated by needle insertion in L3-4 or L4-5 interspace. Manometer is attached to needle to obtain CSF pressure. CSF is withdrawn in a series of tubes and sent for analysis (Table 55-8). Contraindicated in the presence of increased intracranial pressure (risk of downward herniation from CSF removal) or infection at site of puncture.	*Before:* Have patient void. Inform the patient that he or she may feel temporary, sharp pain or tingling radiating down the leg as a sterile needle is passed between 2 lumbar vertebrae. *During:* Most commonly, the patient is side lying. Seated position may also be used. Ensure labeling of CSF specimens in proper sequence. *After:* Encourage fluids. Monitor neurologic signs and VS. Monitor for headache intensity, meningeal irritation *(nuchal rigidity),* or signs and symptoms of local trauma (e.g., hematoma, pain). Administer analgesia as needed.
Radiology		
Skull and spine x-rays	Simple x-ray of skull and spinal column is done to detect fractures, bone erosion, calcifications, abnormal vascularity.	*Before:* Explain that procedure is noninvasive.
Cerebral angiography	Serial x-ray visualization of intracranial and extracranial blood vessels performed to detect vascular lesions (aneurysms, hematomas, arteriovenous malformations) and tumors of brain (Fig. 55-15 on p. 1309). Catheter is inserted into the femoral (sometimes brachial) artery and passed through the aortic arch into the base of a carotid or a vertebral artery for injection of contrast medium. Timed-sequence radiographic images are obtained as contrast flows through arteries, smaller vessels, and veins.	*Before:* Assess patient for stroke risk before procedure because thrombi may be dislodged during procedure. Withhold preceding meal. Explain that patient will have hot flush of head and neck when contrast medium is injected. Explain need to be absolutely still during procedure. *During:* Allergic (anaphylactic) reaction may occur from contrast medium. May require emergency resuscitation measures. *After:* Monitor neurologic signs and VS every 15-30 min for first 2 hr, every hour for next 6 hr, then every 2 hr for 24 hr. Maintain bed rest for 6 hr (1 hr if a closure device is used) and monitor for bleeding. Report any neurologic status changes.
CT scan	Provides a rapid means of obtaining radiographic images of the brain (Fig. 55-16, *A,* on p. 1309). Computer-assisted x-ray of multiple cross sections of body parts to detect problems such as hemorrhage, tumor, cyst, edema, infarction, brain atrophy, and other abnormalities. Contrast medium may be used to enhance visualization of brain structures.	*Before:* Assess for contraindications to contrast media, including allergy to shellfish, iodine, or dye. Explain appearance of scanner. Instruct patient to remain still during procedure.
• CT angiography (CTA)	Noninvasive imaging of vascular system (e.g., aneurysms). Evaluates blood volume, flow, and mean transit time as a measure of perfusion. Has fewer complications than cerebral angiography and is less expensive.	Similar to CT (see above).
MRI	Imaging of brain, spinal cord, and spinal canal by means of magnetic energy (Fig. 55-16, *B,* on p. 1309). Used to detect strokes, multiple sclerosis, tumors, trauma, herniation, and seizures. Provides greater detail than CT and improved resolution (detail) of intracranial structures. Takes a longer time to complete and may not be appropriate in life-threatening emergencies. Contrast medium may be used to enhance visualization. Advantage of MRI is that the contrast agent *gadolinium* has a lower incidence of allergy than iodine used in CT.	*Before:* Screen patient for metal parts and pacemaker in body. Instruct patient on need to lie very still for up to 1 hr. Sedation may be necessary if patient is claustrophobic.
• Magnetic resonance angiography (MRA)	Uses differential signal characteristics of flowing blood to evaluate extracranial and intracranial blood vessels. Provides both anatomic and hemodynamic information. Can be used in conjunction with contrast medium.	Similar to MRI (see above).
• Functional MRI (fMRI)	MRI technique that provides time-related (temporal) images that can be used to evaluate how the brain responds to various stimuli. Makes it possible to detect the brain areas that are involved in a task, process, or an emotion.	Similar to MRI (see above).
• MR spectroscopy (MRS)	Noninvasive test for measuring biochemical changes in the brain, especially the presence of tumors. Compares the chemical composition of normal brain tissue with abnormal tumor tissue. Can also be used to detect tissue changes in stroke and epilepsy.	Similar to MRI (see above).

TABLE 55-7 Diagnostic Studies

Nervous System—cont'd

Study	Description and Purpose	Nursing Responsibility
Positron emission tomography (PET)	Measures metabolic activity of brain to assess cell death or damage. Uses radioactive material that shows up as a bright spot on the image (see Fig. 15-7). Used for patients with stroke, Alzheimer's disease, seizure disorders, Parkinson's disease, and tumors.	*Before:* Explain procedure to patient. Explain that 2 IV lines will be inserted. Instruct patient not to take sedatives or tranquilizers. Have patient empty bladder before procedure. *During:* Patient may be asked to perform different activities during test.
Single-photon emission computed tomography (SPECT)	Method of scanning similar to PET, but using more stable substances and different detectors. Radiolabeled compounds are injected, and their photon emissions can be detected. Resulting images are accumulation of labeled compound. Used to visualize blood flow or O_2 or glucose metabolism in the brain. Useful in diagnosing strokes, brain tumors, and seizure disorders.	Similar to PET (see above).
Myelogram	X-ray of spinal cord and vertebral column after injection of contrast medium into subarachnoid space. Used to detect spinal lesions (e.g., herniated or ruptured disc, spinal tumor).	*Before:* Administer sedative as ordered. Instruct patient to empty bladder. Inform patient that test is performed with patient on tilting table that is moved during test. *After:* Patient should lie flat for a few hours. Encourage fluids. Monitor neurologic signs and VS. Headache, nausea, and vomiting may occur after procedure.
Electrographic Studies		
Electroencephalography (EEG)	Electrical activity of brain is recorded using scalp electrodes to evaluate seizure disorders, cerebral disease, CNS effects of systemic diseases, brain injury, brain death. Specific tests may be done to evaluate brain's electrical response to lights and loud noises.	*Before:* Inform patient procedure is noninvasive and without danger of electric shock. Determine if any medications (e.g., tranquilizers, antiseizure drugs) should be withheld. *After:* Resume medications and instruct patient to wash electrode paste out of hair after test.
Magnetoencephalography (MEG)	Uses a biomagnetometer to detect magnetic fields generated by neural activity. Can accurately pinpoint the part of the brain involved in a stroke, seizure, or other disorder or injury. Measures extracranial magnetic fields and scalp electric field (EEG).	*Before:* Explain procedure to patient. MEG, a passive sensor, does not make physical contact with patient.
Electromyography (EMG)	Recording of electrical activity associated with innervation of skeletal muscle. Needle electrodes are inserted into the muscle to record specific motor units. Normal muscle at rest shows no electrical activity. Electrical activity occurs only when the muscle contracts. Activity may be altered in diseases of muscle itself (e.g., myopathic conditions) or in disorders of muscle innervation (e.g., segmental or LMN lesions, peripheral neuropathic conditions).	*Before:* Explain procedure and inform patient that pain and discomfort are associated with insertion of needles.
Electroneurography (nerve conduction studies)	Measures conduction velocity of peripheral nerves. Involves applying a brief electrical stimulus to a distal portion of a sensory nerve and recording the resulting wave of depolarization at a point proximal to the stimulation. The time between the stimulus onset and the initial wave of depolarization at the recording electrode is measured. This is termed *nerve conduction velocity.* Damaged nerves have slower conduction velocities.	*Before:* Explain procedure to patient. For example, a stimulus can be applied to the forefinger and a recording electrode placed over the median nerve at the wrist will detect the speed of the conduction.
Evoked potentials	Electrical activity associated with nerve conduction along sensory pathways is recorded by electrodes placed on skin and scalp. A stimulus generates the impulse. Increases in the normal time from stimulus onset to a given peak (latency) indicate slowed nerve conduction or nerve damage. Used to diagnose disease (e.g., multiple sclerosis), locate nerve damage, and monitor function intraoperatively. Useful in diagnosing abnormalities of the visual or auditory systems because it indicates if a sensory impulse is reaching the appropriate part of brain.	*Before:* Explain procedure to patient and instruct to shampoo hair before test.

TABLE 55-7   Diagnostic Studies
Nervous System—cont'd

Study	Description and Purpose	Nursing Responsibility
Ultrasound		
Carotid artery duplex scan	Noninvasive study that evaluates the degree of stenosis of carotid and vertebral arteries. Combines ultrasound and Doppler technology. Probe is placed over the carotid artery and slowly moved along the course of common carotid artery. Frequency of reflected ultrasound signal corresponds to blood velocity. Increased blood flow velocity can indicate stenosis of a vessel.	*Before:* Explain procedure to patient.
Transcranial Doppler	Same technology as carotid duplex but evaluates blood flow velocities of intracranial blood vessels. Probe is placed on skin at various "windows" in the skull (areas in the skull that have only a thin bony covering) to record velocities of the blood vessels.	*Before:* Explain procedure to patient.
Biopsies (neurologic pathology tests)	Biopsy of brain, nerve, muscle, and artery with a needle or through a small incision. Brain biopsy is done primarily using stereotactic procedure. Local anesthesia is used at the site for all types of biopsy. Indications include tumors, infectious disease, degenerative diseases, weakness, and temporal artery for arteritis.	*Before:* Explain procedure to patient. *After:* Follow up with results of the biopsy and plans for surgery if needed.

CNS, Central nervous system; *CSF*, cerebrospinal fluid; *ICP*, intracranial pressure; *LMN*, lower motor neuron.

TABLE 55-8   Normal Cerebrospinal Fluid Values

Parameter	Normal Value
Specific gravity	1.007
pH	7.35
Appearance	Clear, colorless
Red blood cells (RBCs)	None
White blood cells (WBCs)	0-5 cells/µL (0-5 × 10⁶ cells/L)
Protein	
• Lumbar	15-45 mg/dL (0.15-0.45 g/L)
• Cisternal	15-25 mg/dL (0.15-0.25 g/L)
• Ventricular	5-15 mg/dL (0.05-0.15 g/L)
Glucose	40-70 mg/dL (2.2-3.9 mmol/L)
Microorganisms	None
Pressure	60-150 mm H₂O

White blood cells (WBCs): 0-5 cells/µL ($0\text{-}5 \times 10^6$ cells/L)

CASE STUDY—cont'd
Objective Data: Diagnostic Studies

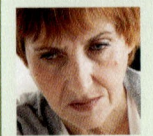

MRI/MRA results indicate a temporal-parietal glioblastoma that has extended into margins of the occipital lobes.

(©TatyanaGl/ iStock/ Thinkstock)

Discussion Questions
1. Are these the diagnostic studies that you expected to be ordered?
2. Why are these diagnostic study results of concern to you?

This case study is continued in Chapter 57 on p. 1366.

Answers available at *http://evolve.elsevier.com/Lewis/medsurg.*

BRIDGE TO NCLEX EXAMINATION

The number of the question corresponds to the same-numbered outcome at the beginning of the chapter.

1. In a patient with a disease that affects the myelin sheath of nerves, such as multiple sclerosis, the glial cells affected are the
   a. microglia.
   b. astrocytes.
   c. ependymal cells.
   d. oligodendrocytes.

2. Drugs or diseases that impair the function of the extrapyramidal system may cause loss of
   a. sensations of pain and temperature.
   b. regulation of the autonomic nervous system.
   c. integration of somatic and special sensory inputs.
   d. automatic movements associated with skeletal muscle activity.

3. During the admitting neurologic examination, the nurse determines the patient has speech difficulties as well as weakness of the right arm and lower face. The nurse would expect a CT scan to show pathology in the distribution of the
   a. basilar artery.
   b. left middle cerebral artery.
   c. right anterior cerebral artery.
   d. left posterior communicating artery.

4. A patient is seen in the emergency department after diving into the pool and hitting the bottom with a blow to the face that hyperextended the neck and scraped the skin off the nose. The patient also described "having double vision" when looking down. During the neurologic exam, the nurse finds the patient is unable to abduct either eye. The nurse recognizes this finding is related to
   a. a basal skull fracture.
   b. a stretch injury to bilateral CN VI.
   c. a stiff neck from the hyperextension injury.
   d. facial swelling from the scrape on the bottom of the pool.

5. Stimulation of the parasympathetic nervous system results in *(select all that apply)*
   a. constriction of the bronchi.
   b. dilation of skin blood vessels.
   c. increased secretion of insulin.
   d. increased blood glucose levels.
   e. relaxation of the urinary sphincters.

6. The nurse is assessing the muscle strength of an older adult patient. The nurse knows the findings cannot be compared with those of a younger adult because
   a. nutritional status is better in young adults.
   b. muscle bulk and strength decrease in older adults.
   c. muscle strength should be the same for all adults.
   d. most young adults exercise more than older adults.

7. A patient is admitted with a headache, fever, and general malaise. The HCP has asked that the patient be prepared for a lumbar puncture. What is a *priority* nursing action to avoid complications?
   a. Ensure that CT scan is performed prior to lumbar puncture.
   b. Assess laboratory results for changes in the white cell count.
   c. Provide acetaminophen for the headache and fever before the procedure.
   d. Administer antibiotics before the procedure to treat the potential meningitis.

8. During neurologic testing, the patient is able to perceive pain elicited by pinprick. Based on this finding, the nurse may omit testing for
   a. position sense.
   b. patellar reflexes.
   c. temperature perception.
   d. heel-to-shin movements.

9. A patient's eyes jerk while the patient looks to the left. The nurse will record this finding as
   a. nystagmus.
   b. CN VI palsy.
   c. ophthalmic dyskinesia.
   d. oculocephalic response.

10. The nurse is caring for a patient with peripheral neuropathy who is scheduled for EMG studies tomorrow morning. The nurse should
    a. ensure the patient has an empty bladder.
    b. instruct the patient about the risk of electric shock.
    c. ensure the patient has no metallic jewelry or metal fragments.
    d. instruct the patient that pain may be experienced during the study.

1. d, 2. d, 3. b, 4. b, 5. a, 6. b, 7. e, 8. c, 9. a, 10. d

For rationales to these answers and even more NCLEX review questions, visit *http://evolve.elsevier.com/Lewis/medsurg.*

EVOLVE WEBSITE

http://evolve.elsevier.com/Lewis/medsurg
Review Questions (Online Only)
Key Points
Answer Keys for Questions
- Rationales for Bridge to NCLEX Examination Questions
- Answer Guidelines for Case Study on pp. 1302, 1304, 1307, and 1312

Conceptual Care Map Creator
Audio Glossary
Supporting Media
- Animations
  - Cervical Nerves
  - Overview of Nervous System
  - Parts of the Brain
  - Synaptic Transmission
  - The Synapse
  - Vertebral Column and Spinal Nerves

Content Updates

REFERENCES

1. Arslantunali D, Dursun T, Yucel D, et al: Peripheral nerve conduits: technology update, *Med Devices (Auckl)* 2014:405, 2014.
2. Banerjee S, Bentley P, Hamady M, et al: Intra-arterial immunoselected CD34+ stem cells for acute ischemic stroke, *Stem Cells Trans Med* 3:1322, 2014.
3. Raghavendra R, Shirol VS, Daksha D, et al: Circle of Willis and its variations: morphometric study in adult human cadavers, *Int J Med Res Health Sci* 3:394, 2014.
4. Hafkemeijer A, Altmann-Schneider I, de Craen A, et al: Associations between age and gray matter volume in anatomical brain networks in middle-age to older adults, *Aging Cell* 13:1068, 2014.
5. Pedersen NL, Gerritsen L: Genetics of brain and cognitive aging: introduction to the special issue of neuropsychology review, *Neuropsychol Rev* 25(1):1, 2015.
6. NIH MedlinePlus: Aging changes in the senses. Retrieved from *www.nlm.nih.gov/medlineplus/ency/article/004013.htm.*
7. Quigley P, White S: Hospital-based fall program measurement and improvement in high reliability organizations, *Online J Issues Nurs* 18:2, 2013.
8. Gerber L, Chiu Y, Carney N, et al: Marked reduction in mortality of patients with severe traumatic brain injury, *J Neurosurg* 119:1583, 2013.
9. Saracoglu K: Patient safety and preoperative assessment of neurological status in neurosurgical patients, *Surg Curr Res* 4:e114, 2014.
10. Rank W: Performing a focused neurologic assessment, *Nursing* 43(12):37, 2013.
11. Donaghy P, McKeith I: The clinical characteristics of dementia with Lewy bodies and a consideration of prodromal diagnosis, *Alzheimers Res Ther* 6:46, 2014.

56

Acute Intracranial Problems

Linda Littlejohns

You can observe a lot by just watching.

Yogi Berra

ⓔ http://evolve.elsevier.com/Lewis/medsurg/

LEARNING OUTCOMES

1. Explain the physiologic mechanisms that maintain normal intracranial pressure.
2. Describe the common etiologies, clinical manifestations, and interprofessional care of the patient with increased intracranial pressure.
3. Describe the interprofessional and nursing management of the patient with increased intracranial pressure.
4. Differentiate types of head injury by mechanism of injury and clinical manifestations.
5. Describe the interprofessional care and nursing management of the patient with a brain injury.
6. Compare the types, clinical manifestations, and interprofessional care of patients with brain tumors.
7. Discuss the nursing management of the patient with a brain tumor.
8. Describe the nursing management of the patient undergoing cranial surgery.
9. Differentiate among the primary causes, interprofessional care, and nursing management of brain abscess, meningitis, and encephalitis.

KEY TERMS

brain abscess, p. 1338
cerebral edema, p. 1316
coma, p. 1317
concussion, p. 1327
contusion, p. 1328
diffuse axonal injury (DAI), p. 1327

encephalitis, p. 1341
epidural hematoma, p. 1328
Glasgow Coma Scale (GCS), p. 1323
head injury, p. 1326
intracerebral hematoma, p. 1329
intracranial pressure (ICP), p. 1314

meningitis, p. 1339
nuchal rigidity, p. 1339
subdural hematoma, p. 1329
unconsciousness, p. 1318

Acute intracranial problems include diseases and disorders that can increase intracranial pressure (ICP). This chapter discusses the mechanisms that maintain normal ICP and increase ICP. In addition, head injury, brain tumors, and cerebral inflammatory disorders are discussed.

INTRACRANIAL PRESSURE

Understanding the dynamics associated with ICP is important in caring for patients with many different neurologic problems. The skull is an enclosed space with three essential volume components: brain tissue, blood, and cerebrospinal fluid (CSF) (Fig. 56-1). The intracellular and extracellular fluids of brain tissue make up approximately 78% of this volume. Blood in the arterial, venous, and capillary network makes up 12% of the volume, and the remaining 10% is the volume of the CSF.

Primary versus secondary injury is another important concept in understanding ICP. *Primary injury* occurs at the initial time of an injury (e.g., impact of car accident, blunt-force

trauma) that results in displacement, bruising, or damage to any of the three components.

Secondary injury is the resulting hypoxia, ischemia, hypotension, edema, or increased ICP that follows the primary injury. Secondary injury, which could occur several hours to days after the initial injury, is a primary concern when managing brain injury. Nursing management of the patient with an acute intracranial problem must include management of secondary injury and thus increased ICP.

Regulation and Maintenance of Intracranial Pressure

Normal Intracranial Pressure. Intracranial pressure (ICP) is the hydrostatic force measured in the brain CSF compartment. Under normal conditions in which intracranial volume remains relatively constant, the balance among the three components (brain tissue, blood, CSF) maintains the ICP. Factors that influence ICP under normal circumstances are changes in (1) arterial pressure; (2) venous pressure; (3) intraabdominal and intrathoracic pressure; (4) posture; (5) temperature; and

Acknowledgment: We would like to acknowledge the contributions of Meg Zomorodi, RN, PhD, CNL, University of North Carolina at Chapel Hill School of Nursing, Chapel Hill, North Carolina to this chapter over the past three editions of the book.
Reviewed by Molly McNett, RN, PhD, CNRN, Director, Nursing Research, The MetroHealth System, Cleveland, Ohio and Meg Zomorodi, RN, PhD, CNL, Clinical Associate Professor, University of North Carolina at Chapel Hill School of Nursing, Chapel Hill, North Carolina.

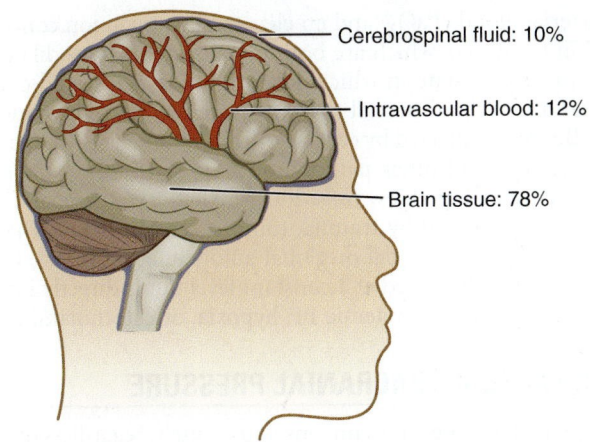

- Cerebrospinal fluid: 10%
- Intravascular blood: 12%
- Brain tissue: 78%

FIG. 56-1 Components of the brain.

TABLE 56-1	**Calculation of Cerebral Perfusion Pressure**

CPP = MAP − ICP

MAP = DBP + 1/3 (SBP − DBP)

OR

$$MAP = \frac{SBP + 2(DBP)}{3}$$

Example: Systemic BP = 122/84 mm Hg
MAP = 97 mm Hg
ICP = 12 mm Hg
CPP = 85 mm Hg

CPP, Cerebral perfusion pressure; *DBP,* diastolic blood pressure; *ICP,* intracranial pressure; *MAP,* mean arterial pressure; *SBP,* systolic blood pressure.

(6) blood gases, particularly CO_2 levels. The degree to which these factors increase or decrease the ICP depends on the brain's ability to adapt to changes.

The Monro-Kellie doctrine states that the three components must remain at a relatively constant volume within the closed skull structure. If the volume of any one of the three components increases within the cranial vault and the volume from another component is displaced, the total intracranial volume will not change.[1] This hypothesis is only applicable in situations in which the skull is closed. The hypothesis is not valid in persons with displaced skull fractures or hemicraniectomy.

ICP can be measured in the ventricles, subarachnoid space, subdural space, epidural space, or brain tissue using a pressure transducer.[2] Normal ICP ranges from 5 to 15 mm Hg. A sustained pressure greater than 20 mm Hg is considered abnormal and must be treated.

Normal Compensatory Adaptations. In applying the Monro-Kellie doctrine, the body can adapt to volume changes within the skull in three different ways to maintain a normal ICP. First, compensatory mechanisms can include changes in the CSF volume. The CSF volume can be changed by altering CSF absorption or production and by displacing CSF into the spinal subarachnoid space. Second, changes in intracranial blood volume can occur through the collapse of cerebral veins and dural sinuses, regional cerebral vasoconstriction or dilation, and changes in venous outflow. Third, brain tissue volume compensates through distention of the dura or compression of brain tissue.

Initially an increase in volume produces no increase in ICP as a result of these compensatory mechanisms. However, the ability to compensate for changes in volume is limited. As the volume increase continues, the ICP rises and decompensation ultimately occurs, resulting in compression and ischemia.

Cerebral Blood Flow

Cerebral blood flow (CBF) is the amount of blood in milliliters passing through 100 g of brain tissue in 1 minute. The global CBF is approximately 50 mL/min/100 g of brain tissue. The maintenance of blood flow to the brain is critical because the brain requires a constant supply of O_2 and glucose. The brain uses 20% of the body's O_2 and 25% of its glucose.[3]

Autoregulation of Cerebral Blood Flow. The brain regulates its own blood flow in response to its metabolic needs despite wide fluctuations in systemic arterial pressure. *Autoregulation* is the automatic adjustment in the diameter of the cerebral blood vessels by the brain to maintain a constant blood flow during changes in arterial blood pressure (BP). The purpose of autoregulation is to ensure a consistent CBF to provide for the metabolic needs of brain tissue and to maintain cerebral perfusion pressure within normal limits.

The lower limit of systemic arterial pressure at which autoregulation is effective in a normotensive person is a mean arterial pressure (MAP) of 70 mm Hg. Below this, CBF decreases, and symptoms of cerebral ischemia, such as syncope and blurred vision, occur. The upper limit of systemic arterial pressure at which autoregulation is effective is a MAP of 150 mm Hg. When this pressure is exceeded, the vessels are maximally constricted, and further vasoconstrictor response is lost.

The *cerebral perfusion pressure* (CPP) is the pressure needed to ensure blood flow to the brain. CPP is equal to the MAP minus the ICP (CPP = MAP − ICP) (see the example in Table 56-1). This formula is clinically useful, although it does not consider the effect of cerebrovascular resistance. Cerebrovascular resistance, generated by the arterioles within the cranium, links CPP and blood flow as follows:

$$CPP = Flow \times Resistance$$

When cerebrovascular resistance is high, blood flow to brain tissue is impaired. Transcranial Doppler is a noninvasive technique used in intensive care units (ICUs) to monitor changes in cerebrovascular resistance.

As the CPP decreases, autoregulation fails and CBF decreases. Normal CPP is 60 to 100 mm Hg. A CPP of less than 50 mm Hg is associated with ischemia and neuronal death. A CPP of less than 30 mm Hg results in ischemia and is incompatible with life.

Normally, autoregulation maintains an adequate CBF and perfusion pressure primarily by adjusting the diameter of cerebral blood vessels and metabolic factors that affect ICP. It is critical to maintain MAP when ICP is elevated.

Remember that CPP may not reflect perfusion pressure in all parts of the brain. There may be local areas of swelling and compression limiting regional perfusion pressure. Thus a higher CPP may be needed for these patients to prevent localized tissue damage. For example, a patient with an acute stroke may require a higher BP, increasing MAP and CPP, in order to increase perfusion to the brain and prevent further tissue damage.

Pressure Changes. The relationship of pressure to volume is depicted in the pressure-volume curve (Fig. 56-2). The curve is affected by the brain's compliance. *Compliance* is the expandability of the brain. It is represented as the volume increase for

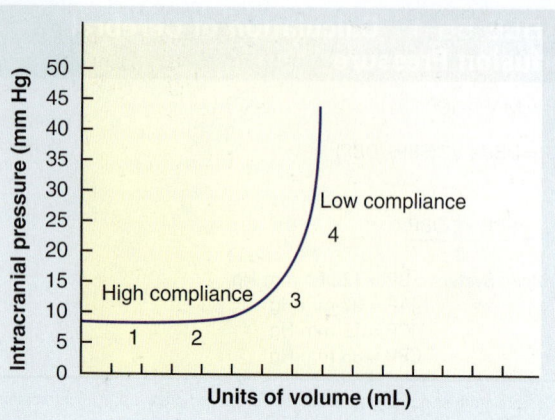

FIG. 56-2 Intracranial pressure-volume curve. (See text for descriptions of *1, 2, 3,* and *4*.)

each unit increase in pressure. With low compliance, small changes in volume result in greater increases in pressure.

$$Compliance = Volume/Pressure$$

The concept of the pressure-volume curve can be used to represent the stages of increased ICP. At stage 1 on the curve, there is high compliance. The brain is in total compensation, with accommodation and autoregulation intact. An increase in volume (brain tissue, blood, or CSF) does not increase the ICP.

At stage 2, the compliance is beginning to decrease, and an increase in volume places the patient at risk of increased ICP and secondary injury. At stage 3, there is significant reduction in compliance. Any small addition of volume causes a great increase in ICP. Compensatory mechanisms fail, there is a loss of autoregulation, and the patient exhibits manifestations of increased ICP (e.g., headache, changes in level of consciousness or pupil responsiveness).

With a loss of autoregulation, the body attempts to maintain cerebral perfusion by increasing systolic BP. However, decompensation is imminent. The patient's response is characterized by systolic hypertension with a widening pulse pressure, bradycardia with a full and bounding pulse, and altered respirations. This is known as *Cushing's triad* and is a neurologic emergency.

As the patient enters stage 4, the ICP rises to lethal levels with little increase in volume. *Herniation* occurs as the brain tissue is forcibly shifted from the compartment of greater pressure to a compartment of lesser pressure. In this situation, intense pressure is placed on the brainstem, and if herniation continues, brainstem death is imminent.

Factors Affecting Cerebral Blood Flow. CO_2, O_2, and hydrogen ion concentration affect cerebral blood vessel tone. An increase in the partial pressure of CO_2 in arterial blood ($PaCO_2$) relaxes smooth muscle, dilates cerebral vessels, decreases cerebrovascular resistance, and increases CBF. A decrease in $PaCO_2$ constricts cerebral vessels, increases cerebrovascular resistance, and decreases CBF.

Cerebral O_2 tension of less than 50 mm Hg results in cerebrovascular dilation. This dilation decreases cerebrovascular resistance, increases CBF, and increases O_2 tension. However, if O_2 tension is not increased, anaerobic metabolism begins, resulting in an accumulation of lactic acid. As lactic acid increases and hydrogen ions accumulate, the environment becomes more acidic. Within this acidic environment, further vasodilation occurs in a continued attempt to increase blood flow. The combination of a severely low partial pressure of O_2

in arterial blood (PaO_2) and an elevated hydrogen ion concentration (acidosis), which are both potent cerebral vasodilators, may produce a state in which autoregulation is lost and compensatory mechanisms fail to meet tissue metabolic demands.

CBF can be affected by cardiac or respiratory arrest, systemic hemorrhage, and other pathophysiologic states (e.g., diabetic coma, encephalopathies, infections, toxicities). Regional CBF can also be affected by trauma, tumors, cerebral hemorrhage, or stroke. When regional or global autoregulation is lost, CBF is no longer maintained at a constant level but is directly influenced by changes in systemic BP, hypoxia, or catecholamines.

INCREASED INTRACRANIAL PRESSURE

Any patient who becomes unconscious acutely, regardless of the cause, should be suspected of having increased ICP.

Mechanisms of Increased Intracranial Pressure

Increased ICP is a potentially life-threatening situation that results from an increase in any or all of the three components (brain tissue, blood, CSF) within the skull. Elevated ICP is clinically significant because it diminishes CPP, increases risks of brain ischemia and infarction, and is associated with a poor prognosis.[4] Common causes of increased ICP include a mass (e.g., hematoma, contusion, abscess, tumor) and cerebral edema (associated with brain tumors, hydrocephalus, head injury, or brain inflammation).

These cerebral insults, which may result in hypercapnia, cerebral acidosis, impaired autoregulation, and systemic hypertension, increase the formation and spread of cerebral edema. This edema distorts brain tissue, further increasing the ICP, and leads to even more tissue hypoxia and acidosis. Fig. 56-3 illustrates the progression of increased ICP.

It is critical to maintain CBF to preserve tissue and thus minimize secondary injury. Sustained increases in ICP result in brainstem compression and herniation of the brain from one compartment to another.

Displacement and herniation of brain tissue can cause a potentially reversible process to become irreversible. Ischemia and edema are further increased, compounding the preexisting problem. Compression of the brainstem and cranial nerves may be fatal. (Fig. 56-4 illustrates types of herniation.) Herniation forces the cerebellum and brainstem downward through the foramen magnum. If compression of the brainstem is unrelieved, respiratory arrest will occur due to compression of the respiratory control center in the medulla.

Cerebral Edema

As shown in Table 56-2, there are a variety of causes of cerebral edema (increased accumulation of fluid in the extravascular spaces of brain tissue). Regardless of the cause, cerebral edema results in an increase in tissue volume that can increase ICP. The extent and severity of the original insult are factors that determine the degree of cerebral edema.

There are three types of cerebral edema: vasogenic, cytotoxic, and interstitial. The same patient may have more than one type.

Vasogenic Cerebral Edema. *Vasogenic cerebral edema*, the most common type of cerebral edema, occurs mainly in the white matter and is characterized by leakage of large molecules from the capillaries into the surrounding extracellular space. This results in an osmotic gradient that favors the flow of fluid from the intravascular to extravascular space. A variety of insults,

PATHOPHYSIOLOGY MAP

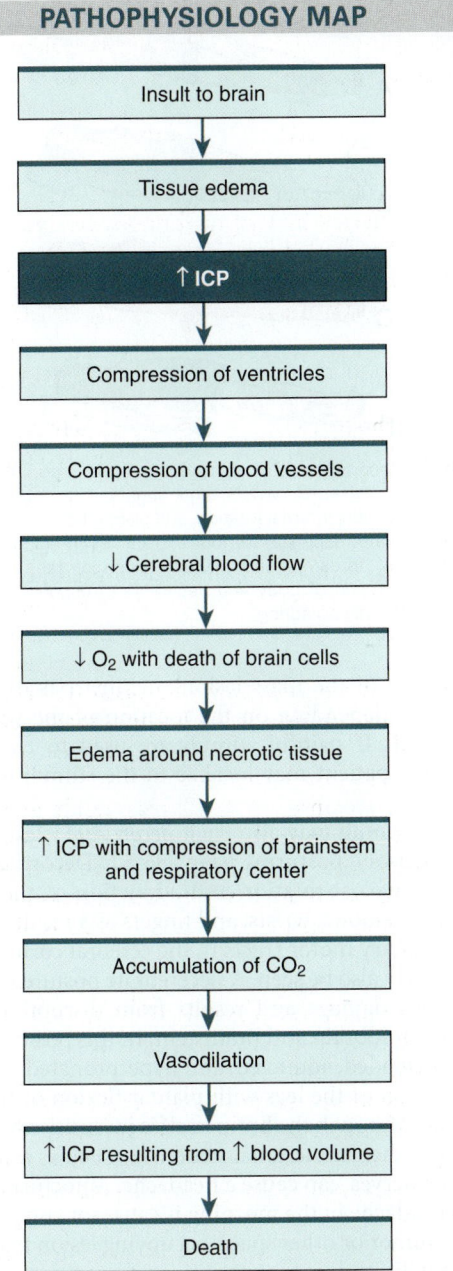

FIG. 56-3   Progression of increased intracranial pressure (ICP).

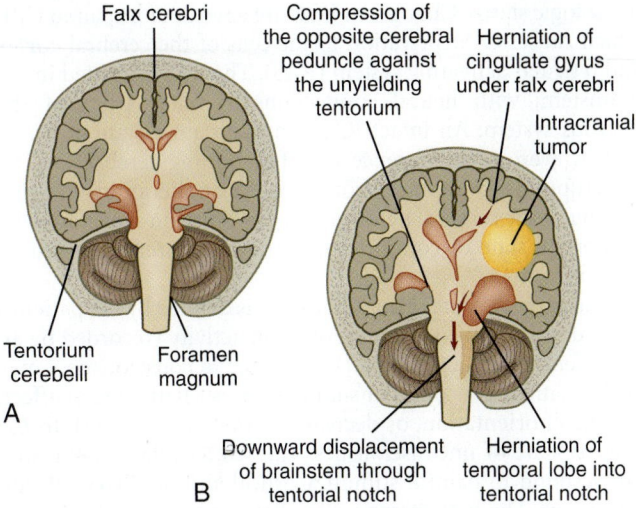

FIG. 56-4   Herniation. **A,** Normal relationship of intracranial structures. **B,** Shift of intracranial structures. (Modified from McCance KL, Huether SE: *Pathophysiology: the biologic basis for disease in adults and children,* ed 6, St Louis, 2010, Mosby.)

TABLE 56-2   Causes of Cerebral Edema

Mass Lesions	Cerebral Infections
• Brain abscess	• Encephalitis
• Brain tumor (primary or metastatic)	• Meningitis
• Hematoma (intracerebral, subdural, epidural)	**Vascular Insult**
• Hemorrhage (intracerebral, cerebellar, brainstem)	• Anoxic and ischemic episodes
	• Cerebral infarction (thrombotic or embolic)
Head Injuries and Brain Surgery	• Venous sinus thrombosis
• Contusion	**Toxic or Metabolic Encephalopathic Conditions**
• Hemorrhage	
• Posttraumatic brain swelling	• Hepatic encephalopathy
	• Lead or arsenic intoxication
	• Uremia

such as brain tumors, abscesses, and ingested toxins, may cause an increase in the permeability of the blood-brain barrier and produce an increase in the extracellular fluid volume. The speed and extent of the spread of the edema fluid are influenced by the systemic BP, site of the brain injury, and extent of the blood-brain barrier defect.

This edema may produce a continuum of symptoms ranging from headache to disturbances in consciousness, including coma (profound state of unconsciousness) and focal neurologic deficits.

It is important to recognize that although a headache may seem to be a benign symptom, in cases of cerebral edema it can quickly progress to coma and death. Therefore you must be vigilant in your assessment.

Cytotoxic Cerebral Edema. *Cytotoxic cerebral edema* results from disruption of the integrity of the cell membranes. It develops from destructive lesions or trauma to brain tissue, resulting in cerebral hypoxia or anoxia and syndrome of inappropriate antidiuretic hormone (SIADH) secretion. In this type of edema, the blood-brain barrier remains intact. Cerebral edema occurs as a result of a fluid and protein shift from the extracellular space directly into the cells, with subsequent swelling and loss of cellular function.

Interstitial Cerebral Edema. *Interstitial cerebral edema* is usually a result of hydrocephalus. *Hydrocephalus* is a buildup of fluid in the brain and is manifested by ventricular enlargement. It can be due to excess CSF production, obstruction of flow, or an inability to reabsorb the CSF. Hydrocephalus treatment usually consists of a ventriculostomy or ventriculoperitoneal shunt. (Management of hydrocephalus is discussed later in this chapter.)

Clinical Manifestations

The clinical manifestations of increased ICP can take many forms, depending on the cause, location, and rate of increases in ICP.

Change in Level of Consciousness. The *level of consciousness* (LOC) is the most sensitive and reliable indicator of the patient's neurologic status. Changes in LOC are a result of impaired CBF, which causes O_2 deprivation to the cells of the cerebral cortex and reticular activating system (RAS). The RAS is located in the brainstem, with neural connections to many parts of the nervous system. An intact RAS can maintain a state of wakefulness even in the absence of a functioning cerebral cortex. Interruptions of impulses from the RAS or alterations in functioning of the cerebral hemispheres can cause **unconsciousness** (abnormal state of complete or partial unawareness of self or environment).

The patient's state of consciousness is defined by the patient's clinical responses and pattern of brain activity (recorded by an electroencephalogram [EEG]). A change in consciousness may be dramatic (as in coma) or subtle (such as a flattening of affect, change in orientation, or decrease in level of attention). In the deepest state of unconsciousness (i.e., coma), the patient does not respond to painful stimuli. Corneal and pupillary reflexes are absent. The patient cannot swallow or cough and is incontinent of urine and feces. The EEG pattern demonstrates suppressed or absent neuronal activity.

Changes in Vital Signs. Changes in vital signs are caused by increasing pressure on the thalamus, hypothalamus, pons, and medulla.

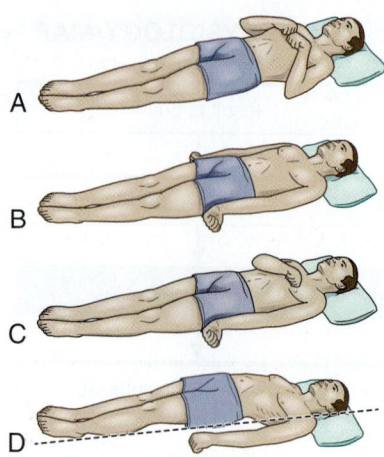

FIG. 56-5 Decorticate and decerebrate posturing. **A,** Decorticate response. Flexion of arms, wrists, and fingers with adduction in upper extremities. Extension, internal rotation, and plantar flexion in lower extremities. **B,** Decerebrate response. All four extremities in rigid extension, with hyperpronation of forearms and plantar flexion of feet. **C,** Decorticate response on right side of body and decerebrate response on left side of body. **D,** Opisthotonic posturing.

CHECK YOUR PRACTICE

You are monitoring the vital signs of an 82-yr-old female who was admitted for a head injury after she fell while walking on the sidewalk. She hit her head on a fire hydrant. She was confused on admission, but vital signs were stable at BP 150/86, pulse 84, respirations 14/minute. Two hours after admission, her vital signs are now BP 166/74, pulse 54, respirations 10-16/minute.
• What is your interpretation of her vital signs?

Manifestations such as *Cushing's triad* (systolic hypertension with a widening pulse pressure, bradycardia with a full and bounding pulse, and irregular respirations) may be present but often do not appear until ICP has been increased for some time or is suddenly and markedly increased (e.g., head trauma). Always recognize Cushing's triad as a medical emergency, since this is a sign of brainstem compression and impending death. A change in body temperature may also occur because increased ICP affects the hypothalamus.

Ocular Signs. Compression of cranial nerve (CN) III, the oculomotor nerve, results in dilation of the pupil on the same side *(ipsilateral)* as the mass lesion, sluggish or no response to light, inability to move the eye upward and adduct, and ptosis of the eyelid. These signs can be the result of the brain shifting from midline, compressing the trunk of CN III, and paralyzing the muscles controlling pupillary size and shape. In this situation, a fixed, unilateral, dilated pupil is considered a neurologic emergency that indicates herniation of the brain.

Other cranial nerves may also be affected, such as the optic (CN II), trochlear (CN IV), and abducens (CN VI) nerves. Signs of dysfunction of these cranial nerves include blurred vision, diplopia, and changes in extraocular eye movements. *Central herniation* may initially manifest as sluggish but equal pupil response. *Uncal herniation* may cause a dilated unilateral pupil. *Papilledema* (an edematous optic disc seen on retinal examination) is also noted and is a nonspecific sign associated with persistent increases in ICP.

Decrease in Motor Function. As the ICP continues to rise, the patient manifests changes in motor ability. A *contralateral*

(opposite side of the mass lesion) hemiparesis or hemiplegia may develop, depending on the location of the source of the increased ICP. If painful stimuli are used to elicit a motor response, the patient may localize to the stimuli or withdraw from it.

Noxious stimuli may also elicit *decorticate* (flexor) or *decerebrate* (extensor) posturing (Fig. 56-5). Decorticate posture consists of internal rotation and adduction of the arms with flexion of the elbows, wrists, and fingers as a result of interruption of voluntary motor tracts in the cerebral cortex. Extension of the legs may also be seen. A decerebrate posture may indicate more serious damage and results from disruption of motor fibers in the midbrain and brainstem. In this position, the arms are stiffly extended, adducted, and hyperpronated. There is also hyperextension of the legs with plantar flexion of the feet.

Headache. Although the brain itself is insensitive to pain, compression of other intracranial structures, such as arteries, veins, and cranial nerves, can cause a headache. A nocturnal headache and/or a headache in the morning is cause for concern and may indicate a tumor or other space-occupying lesion that is causing increased ICP. Straining, agitation, or movement may accentuate the pain.

Vomiting. Vomiting, usually not preceded by nausea, is often a nonspecific sign of increased ICP. This is called *unexpected vomiting* and is related to pressure changes in the cranium. Projectile vomiting may also occur and is related to increased ICP.

Complications

The major complications of uncontrolled increased ICP are inadequate cerebral perfusion and cerebral herniation (Fig. 56-4). To better understand cerebral herniation, two important structures in the brain must be described. The *falx cerebri* is a thin wall of dura that folds down between the cortex, separating the two cerebral hemispheres. The *tentorium cerebelli* is a rigid fold of dura that separates the cerebral hemispheres from the cerebellum (Fig. 56-4). It is called the *tentorium* (meaning tent) because it forms a tentlike cover over the cerebellum.

Tentorial herniation (central herniation) occurs when a mass lesion in the cerebrum forces the brain to herniate downward through the opening created by the brainstem. *Uncal herniation* occurs when there is lateral and downward herniation. *Cingulate herniation* occurs when there is lateral displacement of brain tissue beneath the falx cerebri.

Diagnostic Studies

Diagnostic studies can be used to identify the cause of increased ICP (Table 56-3). CT and MRI are used to differentiate the many conditions that can cause increased ICP and to assess the effect of treatment.

Additional tests include EEG, cerebral angiography, ICP measurement, brain tissue oxygenation measurement via the LICOX catheter (described later), transcranial Doppler studies, and evoked potential studies. Positron emission tomography (PET) is also used to diagnose the cause of increased ICP. In general, a lumbar puncture is not performed when increased ICP is suspected. The reason for this is that cerebral herniation could occur from the sudden release of the pressure in the skull from the area above the lumbar puncture.

In some institutions, a hand-held near-infrared scanner (Infrascanner) is used to detect life-threatening intracranial bleeding. The scanner directs a wavelength of light that can penetrate tissue and bone. Blood from intracranial hematomas absorbs the light differently than other areas of the brain.

Monitoring ICP and Cerebral Oxygenation

Indications for Intracranial Pressure Monitoring. ICP monitoring is used to guide clinical care when the patient is at risk for or has elevations in ICP.[4] It may be used in patients with a variety of neurologic insults, including hemorrhage, stroke, tumor, infection, or traumatic brain injury. ICP should be monitored in patients admitted with a Glasgow Coma Scale (GCS) score of 8 or less and an abnormal CT scan or MRI. These results indicate that the patient may have bleeding, contusion, edema, or other problems. (The GCS is presented later in Table 56-5.)

Methods of Measuring ICP. Patients with conditions known to elevate ICP, except those with irreversible problems or advanced neurologic disease, usually undergo ICP monitoring in an ICU. Multiple methods and devices are available to monitor ICP in various sites (Fig. 56-6).

The gold standard for monitoring ICP is the *ventriculostomy,* in which a specialized catheter is inserted into the lateral ventricle and coupled to an external transducer (Figs. 56-7 and 56-8). This technique directly measures the pressure within the ventricles, facilitates removal and/or sampling of CSF, and allows for intraventricular drug administration. In this system the transducer is external, and it is important to ensure that the transducer of the ventriculostomy is level with the foramen of Monro (interventricular foramen). The ventriculostomy system must also be at the ideal height (Fig. 56-9, *A*). A reference point for this foramen is the tragus of the ear. Every time the patient is repositioned, the system must be assessed to ensure it is level.

The *fiberoptic catheter,* an alternative technology, uses a sensor transducer located within the catheter tip. The sensor tip is placed within the ventricle or the brain tissue and provides a direct measurement of brain pressure.

The *air pouch/pneumatic technology,* another system for monitoring ICP, has an air-filled pouch at the tip of the catheter that maintains a constant volume. The pressure changes within the cranium are transmitted through the changes exerted on this pouch to the monitor.

ICP is represented on the monitor as a mean pressure in mm Hg. If a CSF drainage device is in place, the drain must be closed for at least 6 minutes to ensure an accurate reading. Record the waveform strip along with other pressure monitoring waveforms. The normal ICP waveform has three phases (Fig. 56-7

TABLE 56-3 Interprofessional Care

Increased Intracranial Pressure

Diagnostic Assessment

- History and physical examination
- Vital signs, neurologic assessments, ICP measurements
- Skull, chest, and spinal x-ray studies
- CT scan, MRI, cerebral angiography, EEG, PET
- Transcranial Doppler studies
- Infrascanner
- ECG
- Evoked potential studies
- Laboratory studies, including CBC, coagulation profile, electrolytes, serum creatinine, ABGs, ammonia level, drug and toxicology screen, CSF analysis (for protein, WBC, and glucose)*

Management

- Elevation of head of bed to 30 degrees with head in a neutral position
- Intubation and mechanical ventilation
- ICP monitoring
- Cerebral oxygenation monitoring (PbtO₂, SjvO₂)
- Maintenance of PaO₂ ≥100 mm Hg
- Maintenance of fluid balance and assessment of osmolality
- Maintenance of systolic arterial pressure between 100 and 160 mm Hg
- Maintenance of CPP >60 mm Hg
- Reduction of cerebral metabolism (e.g., high-dose barbiturates)

Drug Therapy

- Osmotic diuretic (mannitol)
- Hypertonic saline
- Antiseizure drugs (e.g., phenytoin [Dilantin])
- Corticosteroids (dexamethasone) for brain tumors, bacterial meningitis
- Histamine (H₂)-receptor antagonist (e.g., cimetidine) or proton pump inhibitor (e.g., pantoprazole [Protonix]) to prevent GI ulcers and bleeding

CPP, Cerebral perfusion pressure; *ICP,* intracranial pressure; *PaO₂,* partial pressure of O₂ in arterial blood; *PbtO₂,* pressure of O₂ in brain tissue; *SjvO₂,* jugular venous O₂ saturation.
*A lumbar puncture to obtain CSF for analysis should not be done if there is a possibility of herniation.

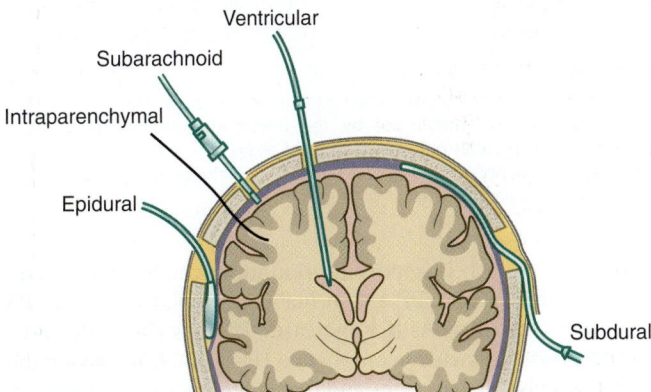

FIG. 56-6 Coronal section of brain showing potential sites for placement of intracranial pressure monitoring devices.

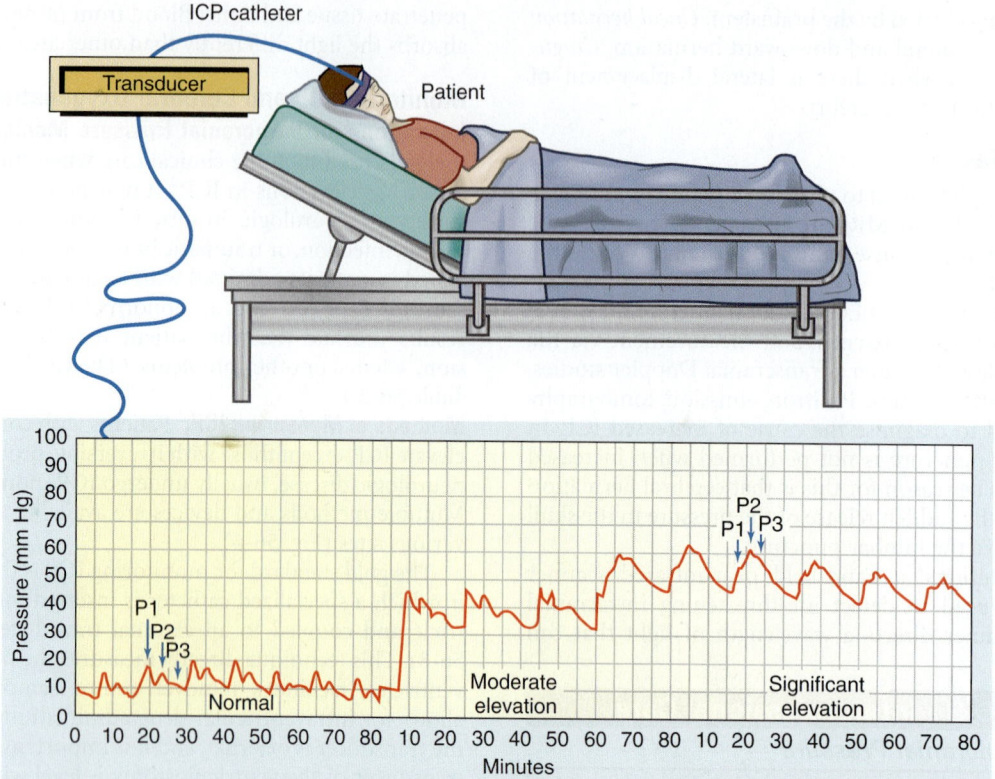

FIG. 56-7 Intracranial pressure (ICP) monitoring can be used to continuously measure ICP. The ICP tracing shows normal, elevated, and plateau waves. At high ICP, the P2 peak is higher than the P1 peak, and the peaks become less distinct and plateau. (Modified from Copstead-Kirkhorn LC, Banasik JL: *Pathophysiology*, ed 5, St Louis, 2013, Mosby.)

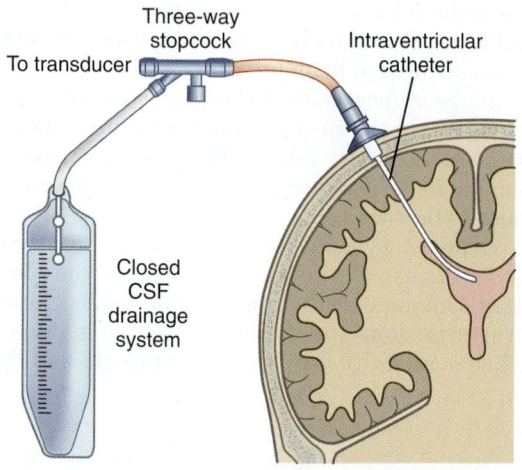

FIG. 56-8 Ventriculostomy in place. Cerebrospinal fluid (CSF) can be drained via a ventriculostomy when intracranial pressure (ICP) exceeds the upper pressure parameter set by the physician. Intermittent drainage involves opening the three-way stopcock to allow CSF to flow into the drainage bag for brief periods (30 to 120 seconds) until the pressure is below the upper pressure parameters.

TABLE 56-4	**Normal Intracranial Pressure Waveforms***
Waveform	**Meaning**
P1 Percussion wave	Represents arterial pulsations. Normally the highest of the three waveforms.
P2 Rebound wave or tidal wave	Reflects intracranial compliance or relative brain volume. When P2 is higher than P1, intracranial compliance is compromised.
P3 Dicrotic wave	Follows dicrotic notch. Represents venous pulsations. Normally the lowest waveform.

*See Fig. 56-7.

ICP elevation, either as a mean increase in pressure or as an abnormal waveform configuration.

Inaccurate ICP readings can be caused by CSF leaks around the monitoring device, obstruction of the intraventricular catheter (from tissue or blood clot), a difference between the height of the catheter and the transducer, kinks in the tubing, and incorrect height of the drainage system relative to the patient's reference point. Bubbles or air in the tubing can also dampen the waveform.

Infection is a serious complication with ICP monitoring. Factors that contribute to the development of infection include ICP monitoring more than 5 days, use of a ventriculostomy, a CSF leak, and a concurrent systemic infection. Routinely assess the insertion site, use aseptic technique, and monitor the CSF for a change in drainage color or clarity.

Cerebrospinal Fluid Drainage. With the ventricular catheter, it is possible to control ICP by removing CSF (Fig. 56-8). The

and Table 56-4). It is important to monitor the ICP waveform, as well as the mean CPP. When ICP is normal, P1, P2, and P3 resemble a staircase. As ICP increases, P2 rises above P1, indicating poor ventricular compliance (Fig. 56-7). Consider the rate at which changes occur and the patient's clinical condition. Neurologic deterioration may not occur until ICP elevation is pronounced and sustained. Immediately report to the HCP any

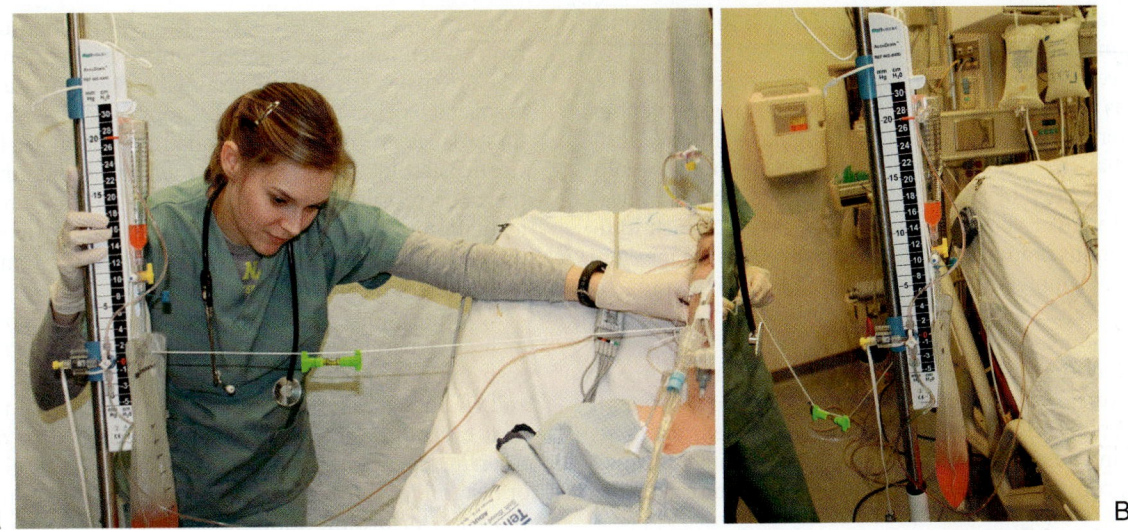

FIG. 56-9   A, Leveling a ventriculostomy. **B,** Cerebrospinal fluid is drained into a drainage system. (Courtesy Meg Zomorodi, RN, PhD, CNL, Raleigh, N.C.)

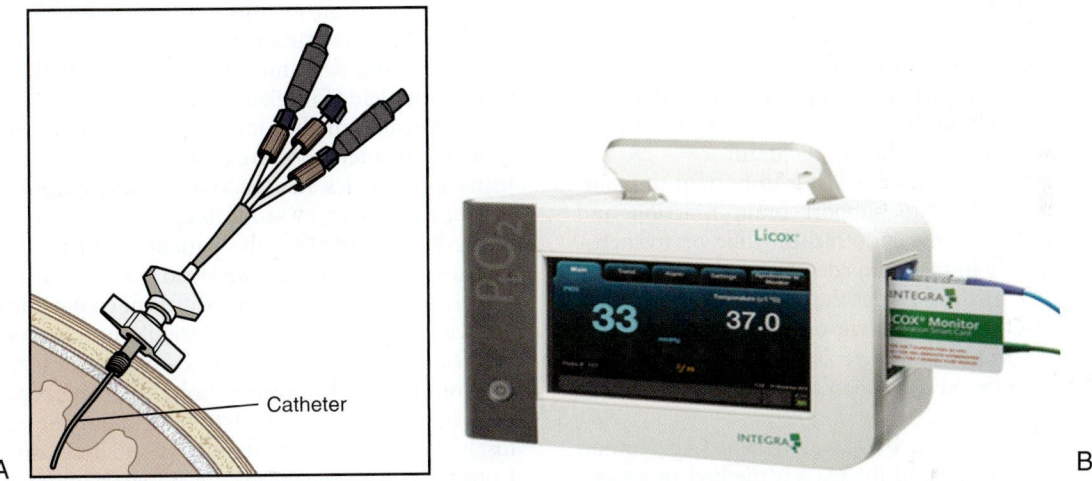

FIG. 56-10   A, The LICOX brain tissue O_2 system involves insertion of a catheter. **B,** The system measures O_2 in the brain ($PbtO_2$), brain tissue temperature, and intracranial pressure. (*B,* Permission granted by Integra Life-Sciences Corporation, Plainsboro, N.J.)

HCP typically orders a specific level at which to initiate drainage (e.g., if ICP is greater than 20 mm Hg) and the frequency of drainage (intermittent or continuous). When the ICP is above the indicated level, the ventriculostomy system is opened by turning a stopcock and allowing the drainage of CSF, thus relieving pressure inside the cranial vault (Fig. 56-9, *B*).

The two options for CSF drainage are intermittent or continuous. If intermittent drainage is ordered, open the ventriculostomy system at the indicated ICP and allow CSF to drain for 2 to 3 minutes. Then close the stopcock to return the ventriculostomy to a closed system. If continuous ICP drainage is ordered, carefully monitor the volume of CSF drained. Keep in mind that normal CSF production is about 20 to 30 mL/hr, with a total CSF volume of about 150 mL within the ventricles and subarachnoid space. It is also recommended that a sign be posted above the patient's bed to notify anyone before turning, moving, or suctioning the patient to prevent the removal of too much CSF, which can result in other complications.

Strict aseptic technique during dressing changes or sampling of CSF is imperative to prevent infection. The system must remain intact to ensure that the ICP readings are accurate because treatment is initiated based on the pressures.

Complications of this type of drainage system include ventricular collapse, infection, and herniation or subdural hematoma formation from rapid decompression. Although it is generally recognized that CSF removal decreases ICP and improves CPP, guidelines for CSF removal are not universally accepted but are typically based on institution or HCP preference.[5]

Cerebral Oxygenation Monitoring. Technology is available to measure cerebral oxygenation and assess perfusion. Three intracranial devices used in ICU settings are the LICOX catheter, Neurovent catheter, and jugular venous bulb catheter.

The LICOX and Neurovent catheters are placed in viable (healthy) white matter of the brain (Fig. 56-10). These catheters can measure brain oxygenation and temperature. These systems provide continuous monitoring of the pressure of O_2 in brain tissue ($PbtO_2$). The normal range for $PbtO_2$ is 20 to 40 mm Hg. A lower-than-normal $PbtO_2$ level is indicative of ischemia.[6] These catheters can also measure brain temperature.

A cooler brain temperature (96.8° F [36° C]) may produce better outcomes.

Jugular venous bulb oximetry, which measures global O_2 extraction, is also used in some institutions. The jugular venous bulb catheter is placed in the internal jugular vein and positioned so that the catheter tip is located in the jugular bulb. Placement is verified by an x-ray. This catheter provides a measurement of jugular venous O_2 saturation ($SjvO_2$), which indicates total venous brain tissue extraction of O_2. This is a measure of cerebral O_2 supply and demand. The normal $SjvO_2$ range is 55% to 75%. Values less than 50% demonstrate impaired cerebral oxygenation.[7]

In addition to measuring ICP and brain oxygenation, many clinicians are now looking at multimodality monitoring in traumatic brain injury and intracranial hypertension. This technology includes brain microdialysis (measurement of small molecules), continuous EEG, and blood flow monitoring.

Interprofessional Care

The goals of interprofessional care (Table 56-3) are to (1) identify and treat the underlying cause of increased ICP and (2) support brain function. The earlier the condition is recognized and treated, the better the patient outcome. A careful history is an important diagnostic aid in the search for the underlying cause. The underlying cause of increased ICP is usually an increase in blood (hemorrhage), brain tissue (tumor or edema), or CSF (hydrocephalus) in the brain.

For any patient with increased ICP, it is important to maintain adequate oxygenation to support brain function and prevent secondary injury. An endotracheal tube or tracheostomy may be necessary to maintain adequate ventilation. Arterial blood gas (ABG) analysis guides the O_2 therapy. The goal is to maintain the PaO_2 at greater than or equal to 100 mm Hg and to keep $PaCO_2$ in normal range at 35 to 45 mm Hg. The patient may need to be on a mechanical ventilator to ensure adequate oxygenation.

If increased ICP is caused by a mass lesion (e.g., tumor, hematoma), surgical removal of the mass is the best treatment (see the sections on brain tumors and cranial surgery later in this chapter). In aggressive situations, a craniectomy (removal of part of skull) may be performed to reduce ICP and prevent herniation (see head injury section for further details).

Drug Therapy. Drug therapy plays an important part in the management of increased ICP. Mannitol (Osmitrol) (25%) is an osmotic diuretic given IV. Mannitol decreases the ICP in two ways: plasma expansion and osmotic effect. The immediate plasma-expanding effect reduces the hematocrit and blood viscosity, thereby increasing CBF and cerebral O_2 delivery. A vascular osmotic gradient is created by mannitol. Thus fluid moves from the tissues into the blood vessels, reducing the ICP because of the decrease in the total brain fluid content. Monitor fluid and electrolyte status when osmotic diuretics are used. Mannitol may be contraindicated if renal disease is present and if serum osmolality is elevated.

Hypertonic saline solution is another drug treatment used to manage increased ICP. It produces massive movement of water out of edematous swollen brain cells and into blood vessels. This movement of water out of the brain can reduce swelling and improve cerebral blood flow. Hypertonic solution infusion requires frequent monitoring of BP and serum sodium levels because intravascular fluid volume excess can occur. Hypertonic saline infusion has been shown to be just as effective as mannitol

when treating increased ICP, and both are often used concurrently when caring for a patient with a severe brain injury.[8]

Corticosteroids (e.g., dexamethasone) are used to treat vasogenic edema surrounding tumors and abscesses. However, these drugs are not recommended for traumatic brain injury. Corticosteroids stabilize the cell membrane and inhibit the synthesis of prostaglandins (see Fig. 11-2), thus preventing the formation of proinflammatory mediators. Corticosteroids also improve neuronal function by improving CBF and restoring autoregulation.

Complications associated with the use of corticosteroids include hyperglycemia, increased incidence of infections, and gastrointestinal (GI) bleeding. Regularly monitor fluid intake and sodium levels, and perform blood glucose monitoring at least every 6 hours until hyperglycemia is ruled out. Patients receiving corticosteroids should concurrently be given antacids or histamine (H_2)-receptor blockers (e.g., cimetidine, ranitidine [Zantac]) or proton pump inhibitors (e.g., omeprazole [Prilosec], pantoprazole [Protonix, Protonix IV]) to prevent GI ulcers and bleeding.

Metabolic demands such as fever (greater than 100.4° F [38° C]), agitation or shivering, pain, and seizures can also increase ICP. The interprofessional team should plan to reduce these metabolic demands to lower the ICP in the at-risk patient. Monitor patients for seizure activity. They may need prophylactic antiseizure medication. Fever should be well controlled to maintain a temperature of 96.8° to 98.6° F (36° to 37° C) by using antipyretics (e.g., acetaminophen), cool baths, cooling blankets, ice packs, or intravascular cooling devices as necessary. However, avoid letting the patient shiver or shake, since this increases the metabolic workload on the brain. If this occurs, sedatives may be needed or a different cooling method selected.

Manage pain while being careful not to oversedate or overmedicate. Finally, the patient should remain in a quiet, calm environment with minimal noise and interruptions. Observe the patient for signs of agitation, irritation, or frustration. Also teach the caregiver and family about decreasing stimulation. Coordinate with the interprofessional team to minimize procedures that may produce agitation.

Drug therapy for reducing cerebral metabolism may be an effective strategy to control ICP. Reducing the metabolic rate decreases the CBF and therefore the ICP. High doses of barbiturates (e.g., pentobarbital, thiopental) are used in patients with increased ICP refractory to other treatments. Barbiturates decrease cerebral metabolism, causing a decrease in ICP and a reduction in cerebral edema. When this treatment is used, monitor the patient's ICP, blood flow, and EEG. Barbiturate dosing is typically based on analysis of the bedside EEG tracing and the ICP. The HCP orders the barbiturate infusion at a rate that achieves a desired level of brain wave suppression as a means to control ICP. Total *burst suppression,* recognized by the absence of spikes showing brain activity on the EEG monitor, indicates that maximal therapeutic effect has been achieved.

Nutritional Therapy. Regardless of their state of consciousness, patients must have their nutritional needs met. Because malnutrition promotes continued cerebral edema, maintenance of optimal nutrition is imperative. The patient with increased ICP is in a hypermetabolic and hypercatabolic state that increases the need for glucose as fuel for metabolism of the injured brain. If the patient cannot maintain an adequate oral intake, other means of meeting the nutritional requirements, such as enteral feedings or parenteral nutrition, should be initiated.

Early feeding after brain injury may improve patient outcome.[9] Nutritional replacement should begin within 3 days after injury to reach full nutritional replacement within 7 days after the injury is sustained. (Nutritional therapy is discussed in Chapter 39.) Feedings or supplements should be guided by the patient's fluid and electrolyte status and metabolic needs. The patient should remain in a normovolemic fluid state. Continuously evaluate the patient based on clinical factors such as urine output, insensible fluid loss, serum and urine osmolality, and serum electrolytes.

IV 0.9% sodium chloride is the preferred solution for administration of piggyback medications. If 5% dextrose in water or 0.45% sodium chloride is used, serum osmolarity decreases and an increase in cerebral edema may occur.

❖ NURSING MANAGEMENT: INCREASED INTRACRANIAL PRESSURE

◆ Nursing Assessment

Subjective data about the patient with increased ICP can be obtained from the patient, caregiver, or family member who is familiar with the patient. Learn appropriate neurologic assessment techniques. Describe the LOC by noting the specific behaviors observed. Assess the LOC using the Glasgow Coma Scale (Table 56-5). Also assess body functions, especially circulation and respiration.

◆ **Glasgow Coma Scale.** The Glasgow Coma Scale (GCS) is a quick, practical, and standardized system for assessing the LOC. The three areas assessed in the GCS are the patient's ability to (1) open the eyes when a verbal or painful stimulus is applied, (2) speak, and (3) obey commands. Specific assessments evaluate the patient's response to varying degrees of stimulus. Three indicators of response are evaluated: (1) opening of the eyes, (2) best verbal response, and (3) best motor response (Table 56-5).

Specific behaviors observed as responses to the testing stimulus are given a numeric value. Your responsibility is to elicit the best response on each of the scales: the higher the scores, the higher the level of brain functioning. The subscale scores are particularly important if a patient is untestable in one area. For example, severe periorbital edema may make eye opening impossible.

The total GCS score is the sum of the numeric values assigned to each of the three areas evaluated. The highest GCS score is 15 for a fully alert person, and the lowest possible score is 3. A GCS score of 8 or less generally indicates coma, and mechanical ventilation should be considered. Plot the results of the GCS scores on a graph, which can be used to determine whether the patient is stable, improving, or deteriorating.

The GCS offers several advantages in the assessment of the unconscious patient. It allows different health care professionals to arrive at the same conclusion regarding the patient's status and can be used to discriminate between different or changing states.

Although the GCS is the gold standard assessment tool for LOC, other scales such as the *Full Outline of Unresponsiveness (FOUR) scale* are also used in the clinical setting.[10] In cases of stroke or hemorrhage associated with increased ICP, use the NIH Stroke Scale (Table 57-10). Other components of the neurologic assessment include cranial nerve assessment and motor and sensory testing.

◆ **Neurologic Assessment.** Compare the pupils with one another for size, shape, movement, and reactivity (Fig. 56-11). If the

TABLE 56-5 Glasgow Coma Scale

Appropriate Stimulus	Response	Score
Eyes Open		
• Approach to bedside	Spontaneous response.	4
• Verbal command	Opening of eyes to name or command.	3
• Pain	Lack of opening of eyes to previous stimuli but opening to pain.	2
	Lack of opening of eyes to any stimulus.	1
	Untestable.*	U
Best Verbal Response		
• Verbal questioning with maximum arousal	Appropriate orientation, conversant. Correct identification of self, place, yr, and mo.	5
	Confusion. Conversant, but disorientation in one or more spheres.	4
	Inappropriate or disorganized use of words (e.g., cursing), lack of sustained conversation.	3
	Incomprehensible words, sounds (e.g., moaning).	2
	Lack of sound, even with painful stimuli.	1
	Untestable.*	U
Best Motor Response		
• Verbal command (e.g., "raise your arm, hold up two fingers")	Obedience of command.	6
• Pain (pressure on proximal nail bed)	Localization of pain, lack of obedience but presence of attempts to remove offending stimulus.	5
	Flexion withdrawal,* flexion of arm in response to pain without abnormal flexion posture.	4
	Abnormal flexion, flexing of arm at elbow and pronation, making a fist.	3
	Abnormal extension, extension of arm at elbow usually with adduction and internal rotation of arm at shoulder.	2
	Lack of response.	1
	Untestable.*	U

oculomotor nerve (CN III) is compressed, the pupil on the affected side *(ipsilateral)* becomes larger until it fully dilates. If ICP continues to increase, both pupils dilate.

Test pupillary reaction with a penlight. The normal reaction is brisk constriction when the light is shone directly into the eye. Also note a consensual response (slight constriction in the opposite pupil) at the same time. A sluggish reaction can indicate early pressure on CN III. A fixed pupil unresponsive to light stimulus usually indicates increased ICP. However, note that there are other causes of a fixed pupil, including direct injury to CN III, previous eye surgery, administration of atropine, and use of mydriatic eye drops.

In some hospitals, clinicians are using a handheld device *(pupillometer)* to measure the pupil reactivity and size. The device removes any subjectivity from the pupil evaluation.

Evaluation of other cranial nerves can be included in the neurologic assessment. (Cranial nerve assessment is presented in Table 55-4.)

Eye movements controlled by CN III, IV, and VI can be examined in the patient who is awake and able to follow

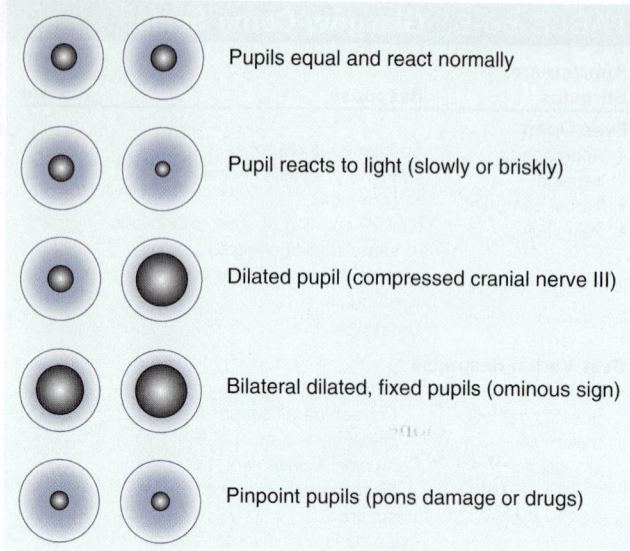

FIG. 56-11 Pupillary check for size and response.

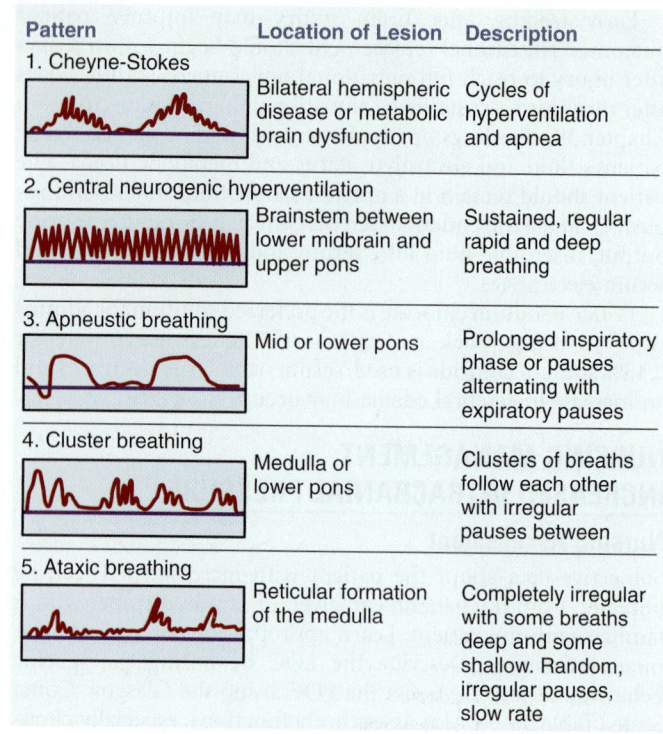

FIG. 56-12 Common abnormal respiratory patterns associated with coma.

commands and can be used to assess the function of the brainstem. Testing the corneal reflex gives information about the functioning of CN V and VII. If this reflex is absent, initiate routine eye care to prevent corneal abrasion (see Chapter 21).

Eye movements of the uncooperative or unconscious patient can be elicited by reflex with the use of head movements (oculocephalic) and caloric stimulation (oculovestibular). To test the oculocephalic reflex (doll's eye reflex), turn the patient's head briskly to the left or right while holding the eyelids open. A normal response is movement of the eyes across the midline in the direction opposite that of the turning. Next, quickly flex and then extend the neck. Eye movement should be opposite to the direction of head movement—up when the neck is flexed and down when it is extended. Abnormal responses can help locate the intracranial lesion. This test should not be attempted if a cervical spine problem is suspected.

Test motor strength by asking the awake and cooperative patient to squeeze your hands to compare strength in the hands. The pronator drift test is an excellent measure of strength in the upper extremities. The patient raises the arms in front of the body with the palms facing upward and eyes closed. If there is any weakness in the upper extremity, the palmar surface turns downward and the arm drifts down. This would indicate a problem in the opposite motor cortex. Asking the patient to raise the foot from the bed or to bend the knees up in bed is a good assessment of lower extremity strength. Test all four extremities for strength and for any asymmetry in strength or movement.

Assess the motor response of the unconscious or uncooperative patient by observation of spontaneous movement. If no spontaneous movement is possible, apply a pain stimulus to the patient, and note the response. Resistance to movement during passive range-of-motion exercises is another measure of strength. Do not include hand squeezing as part of the assessment of motor movement in the unconscious or uncooperative patient, since this is a reflex action and can misrepresent the patient's status.

Also record the vital signs, including BP, pulse, respiratory rate, and temperature. Be aware of Cushing's triad, which indicates severely increased ICP. Besides recording respiratory rate, also note the respiratory pattern. Specific respiratory patterns are associated with severely increased ICP (Fig. 56-12).

◆ Nursing Diagnoses

Nursing diagnoses for the patient with increased ICP include, but are not limited to, the following:

- Decreased intracranial adaptive capacity *related to* decreased cerebral perfusion or increased ICP
- Risk for ineffective cerebral tissue perfusion *related to* reduction of venous and/or arterial blood flow and cerebral edema
- Risk for disuse syndrome *related to* altered LOC, immobility, and altered nutritional intake

Additional information on nursing diagnoses for patients with increased ICP is presented in eNursing Care Plan 56-1 (available on the website for this chapter).

◆ Planning

The overall goals for the patient with increased ICP are to (1) maintain a patent airway; (2) have ICP within normal limits; (3) have normal fluid, electrolyte, and nutritional balance; and (4) prevent complications secondary to immobility and decreased LOC.

◆ Nursing Implementation

◆ Acute Care

◆   ***Respiratory Function.*** Maintaining a patent airway is critical in the patient with increased ICP and is a primary nursing responsibility. As the LOC decreases, the patient is at an increased risk of airway obstruction from the tongue dropping back and occluding the airway or from accumulation of secretions.

> **! SAFETY ALERT**   **Altered Breathing**
> - Be alert to altered breathing patterns in a patient with increased ICP.
> - Snoring sounds indicate obstruction and require immediate intervention.

Remove accumulated secretions by suctioning as needed. An oral airway facilitates breathing and provides an easier suctioning route in the comatose patient. In general, any patient with a GCS of 8 or less or an altered LOC who is unable to maintain a patent airway or effective ventilation needs intubation and mechanical ventilation.

Prevent hypoxia and hypercapnia to minimize secondary injury. Proper positioning of the head is important. Elevation of the head of the bed to 30 degrees enhances respiratory exchange and aids in decreasing cerebral edema. Suctioning and coughing cause transient decreases in the PaO_2 and increases in the ICP. Keep suctioning to a minimum and less than 10 seconds in duration, with administration of 100% O_2 before and after to prevent decreases in the PaO_2. To avoid cumulative increases in the ICP with suctioning, limit suctioning to two passes per suction procedure, if possible. Patients with elevated ICP are at risk for lower CPP during suctioning.

Try to prevent abdominal distention, since it can interfere with respiratory function. Insertion of a nasogastric tube to aspirate the stomach contents can prevent distention, vomiting, and possible aspiration. However, in patients with facial and skull fractures, a nasogastric tube is contraindicated unless a basilar skull fracture (at base of skull) has been ruled out, and oral insertion of a gastric tube is preferred.

Pain, anxiety, and fear related to the primary injury, therapeutic procedures, or noxious stimuli can increase ICP and BP, thus complicating the management and recovery of the brain-injured patient. The appropriate choice or combination of sedatives, paralytics, and analgesics for symptom management presents a challenge to the ICU team. Administration of these agents may alter the neurologic state, thus masking true neurologic changes. It may be necessary to temporarily suspend drug therapy to appropriately assess neurologic status. The choice, dose, and combination of agents may vary depending on the patient's history, neurologic state, and overall clinical presentation.

Opioids, such as morphine sulfate and fentanyl (Sublimaze), are rapid-onset analgesics with minimal effect on CBF or O_2 metabolism. The IV anesthetic sedative propofol (Diprivan) is used in the management of anxiety and agitation in the ICU because of its rapid onset and short half-life. An accurate neurologic assessment can be performed soon after turning off the infusion of propofol. Dexmedetomidine (Precedex), an α_2-adrenergic agonist, is used for continuous IV sedation of intubated and mechanically ventilated patients in the ICU setting for up to 24 hours. When using continuous IV sedatives, be aware of the side effects of these drugs, especially hypotension, since this can result in a lower CPP value.

Nondepolarizing neuromuscular blocking agents (e.g., vecuronium, cisatracurium besylate [Nimbex]) are useful for achieving complete ventilatory control in the treatment of refractory intracranial hypertension. Because these agents paralyze muscles without blocking pain or noxious stimuli, they are used in combination with sedatives, analgesics, or benzodiazepines.

Benzodiazepines, although useful for sedation, are usually avoided in the management of the patient with increased ICP because of the hypotensive effect and long half-life, unless they are used as an adjunct to neuromuscular blocking agents.

Frequently monitor and evaluate the ABG values, and take measures to maintain the levels within prescribed or acceptable parameters (see Chapter 25). The appropriate ventilatory support can be ordered on the basis of the PaO_2 and $PaCO_2$ values.

◆ *Fluid and Electrolyte Balance.* Fluid and electrolyte disturbances can have an adverse effect on ICP. Closely monitor IV fluids with the use of an accurate IV infusion control device or pump. Intake and output, with insensible losses and daily weights taken into account, are important parameters in the assessment of fluid balance.

Make electrolyte determinations daily, and discuss any abnormal values with the HCP. It is especially important to monitor serum glucose, sodium, potassium, magnesium, and osmolality.

Monitor urine output to detect problems related to diabetes insipidus and SIADH. Diabetes insipidus is caused by a decrease in antidiuretic hormone (ADH). It results in increased urine output and hypernatremia. The usual treatment of diabetes insipidus is fluid replacement, vasopressin, or desmopressin acetate (DDAVP) (see Chapter 49). If it is not treated, severe dehydration will occur.

SIADH is caused by an excess secretion of ADH. SIADH results in decreased urine output and dilutional hyponatremia. It may result in cerebral edema, changes in LOC, seizures, and coma. (Treatment of SIADH is described in Chapter 49.)

◆ *Monitoring ICP.* ICP monitoring is used in combination with other physiologic parameters to guide the care of the patient and assess the patient's response to treatment. Valsalva maneuver, coughing, sneezing, suctioning, hypoxemia, and arousal from sleep are factors that can increase ICP. Be alert to these factors and attempt to minimize them.

◆ *Body Position.* Maintain the patient with increased ICP in the head-up position. The head should be maintained in a midline position, avoiding extreme neck flexion. This position can cause venous obstruction and contribute to elevated ICP. Adjust the body position to decrease the ICP and improve the CPP. Elevation of the head of the bed promotes drainage from the head and decreases the vascular congestion that can produce cerebral edema. However, raising the head of the bed above 30 degrees may decrease the CPP by lowering systemic BP. Carefully evaluate the effects of elevation of the head of the bed on both the ICP and CPP. Position the bed so that it lowers the ICP while optimizing the CPP and other indices of cerebral oxygenation.

Take care to turn the patient with slow, gentle movements because rapid changes in position may increase the ICP. Prevent discomfort in turning and positioning the patient because pain or agitation also increases pressure. Increased intrathoracic pressure contributes to increased ICP by impeding the venous return. Thus coughing, straining, and the Valsalva maneuver should be avoided. Avoid extreme hip flexion to decrease the risk of raising the intraabdominal pressure, which increases ICP. Turn the patient at least every 2 hours.

Decorticate or decerebrate posturing is a reflex response in some patients with increased ICP. Turning, skin care, and even passive range of motion can elicit the posturing reflexes. Provide the physical care to minimize complications of immobility, such as atelectasis and contractures.

◆ *Protection From Injury.* The patient with increased ICP and decreased LOC needs protection from self-injury. Confusion, agitation, and the possibility of seizures increase the risk for injury. Use restraints judiciously in the agitated patient. If restraints are absolutely necessary to keep the patient from removing tubes or falling out of bed, they should be secure enough to be effective, and observe the skin area under the restraints regularly for irritation. Agitation may increase with the use of restraints, which indicates the need for other measures to protect the patient from injury. Light sedation with agents such as midazolam or lorazepam (Ativan) may be needed. Having a family member stay with the patient may have a calming effect.

For the patient with seizures or the patient at risk for such activity, institute seizure precautions. These include padded side rails, an airway at the bedside, suction readily available, accurate and timely administration of antiseizure drugs, and close observation. The use of prophylactic antiseizure drugs has been controversial as their use may not decrease seizures.[11]

The patient can benefit from a quiet, nonstimulating environment. Always use a calm, reassuring approach. Touch and talk to the patient, even one who is in a coma.

◆ *Psychologic Considerations.* In addition to carefully planned physical care, also be aware of the psychologic well-being of patients and their families. Anxiety over the diagnosis and the prognosis can be distressing to the patient, caregiver and family, and nursing staff. Your competent and assured manner in performing care is reassuring to everyone involved. Short, simple explanations are appropriate and allow the patient and caregiver to acquire the amount of information they desire. There is a need for support, information, and teaching of both patients and families. Assess the family members' desires to assist in providing care for the patient and allow for their participation as appropriate. Encourage interprofessional management (social work, chaplain, etc.) of the patient and family in decision making as much as possible.

◆ **Evaluation**

The expected outcomes are that the patient with increased ICP will
- Maintain ICP and cerebral perfusion within normal parameters
- Experience no serious increases in ICP during or after care activities
- Experience no complications of immobility

Additional expected outcomes for the patient with increased ICP are addressed in eNursing Care Plan 56-1 (available on the website for this chapter).

HEAD INJURY

Head injury includes any injury or trauma to the scalp, skull, or brain. A serious form of head injury is *traumatic brain injury* (TBI). Statistics regarding the occurrence of head injuries are incomplete because many victims die at the injury scene or because the condition is considered minor and health care services are not sought. In U.S. hospital emergency departments, an estimated 1.7 million persons are treated and released with TBI. Fifty thousand people die and 275,000 persons are hospitalized with TBI. Of individuals hospitalized, 20% of the patients die.[12] At least 5.3 million Americans (2% of the U.S. population) currently live with disabilities resulting from TBI (*www.braintrauma.org*).

The most common causes of head injury are falls and motor vehicle accidents. Other causes of head injury include firearms, assaults, sports-related trauma, recreational injuries, and war-related injuries.[13] Males are twice as likely to sustain a TBI as females.

Head trauma has a high potential for a poor outcome. Deaths from head trauma occur at three points after injury: immediately after the injury, within 2 hours after injury, and approximately 3 weeks after injury.[13] The majority of deaths after a head injury occur immediately after the injury, either from the direct head trauma or from massive hemorrhage and shock. Deaths occurring within a few hours of the trauma are caused by progressive worsening of the brain injury or internal bleeding.[14]

Deaths occurring 3 weeks or more after the injury result from multisystem failure. Expert nursing care in the weeks after the injury is crucial in decreasing the mortality risk and in optimizing patient outcomes.[15]

Types of Head Injuries

Scalp Lacerations. *Scalp lacerations* are an easily recognized type of external head trauma. Because the scalp contains many blood vessels with poor constrictive abilities, most scalp lacerations are associated with profuse bleeding. Even relatively small wounds can bleed significantly. The major complications associated with scalp laceration are blood loss and infection.

Skull Fractures. *Skull fractures* frequently occur with head trauma. Skull fractures can be described in several ways: (1) linear or depressed; (2) simple, comminuted, or compound; and (3) closed or open (Table 56-6). Fractures may be closed or open, depending on the presence of a scalp laceration or extension of the fracture into the air sinuses or dura. The type and severity of a skull fracture depend on the velocity, momentum, direction and shape (blunt or sharp) of the injuring agent, and site of impact.

The location of the fracture determines the clinical manifestations (Table 56-7). For example, a basilar skull fracture is a specialized type of linear fracture involving the base of the skull. Manifestations can evolve over the course of several hours; vary with the location and severity of fracture; and may include cranial nerve deficits, Battle's sign (postauricular ecchymosis), and periorbital ecchymosis (raccoon eyes) (Fig. 56-13). This fracture generally is associated with a tear in the dura and subsequent leakage of CSF.

Rhinorrhea (CSF leakage from the nose) or *otorrhea* (CSF leakage from the ear) generally confirms that the fracture has traversed the dura (Fig. 56-13). Rhinorrhea may also manifest as postnasal sinus drainage. The significance of rhinorrhea may be overlooked unless the patient is specifically assessed for this finding. The risk of meningitis is high with a CSF leak, and antibiotics should be administered as a preventive measure.

Two methods of testing can be used to determine whether the fluid leaking from the nose or ear is CSF. The first method

TABLE 56-6	Types of Skull Fractures	
Type	**Description**	**Cause**
Linear	Break in continuity of bone without alteration of relationship of parts	Low-velocity injuries
Depressed	Inward indentation of skull	Powerful blow
Simple	Linear or depressed skull fracture without fragmentation or communicating lacerations	Low to moderate impact
Comminuted	Multiple linear fractures with fragmentation of bone into many pieces	Direct, high-momentum impact
Compound	Depressed skull fracture and scalp laceration with communicating pathway to intracranial cavity	Severe head injury

TABLE 56-7   Manifestations of Skull Fractures

Location	Manifestations
Frontal fracture	Exposure of brain to contaminants through frontal air sinus, possible association with air in forehead tissue, CSF rhinorrhea, or pneumocranium (air between cranium and dura mater)
Orbital fracture	Periorbital ecchymosis (raccoon eyes), optic nerve injury
Temporal fracture	Boggy temporal muscle because of extravasation of blood, oval-shaped bruise behind ear in mastoid region (Battle's sign), CSF otorrhea, middle meningeal artery disruption, epidural hematoma
Parietal fracture	Deafness, CSF or brain otorrhea, bulging of tympanic membrane caused by blood or CSF, facial paralysis, loss of taste, Battle's sign
Posterior fossa fracture	Occipital bruising resulting in cortical blindness, visual field defects, rare appearance of ataxia or other cerebellar signs
Basilar skull fracture	CSF or brain otorrhea, bulging of tympanic membrane caused by blood or CSF, Battle's sign, tinnitus or hearing difficulty, rhinorrhea, facial paralysis, conjugate deviation of gaze, vertigo

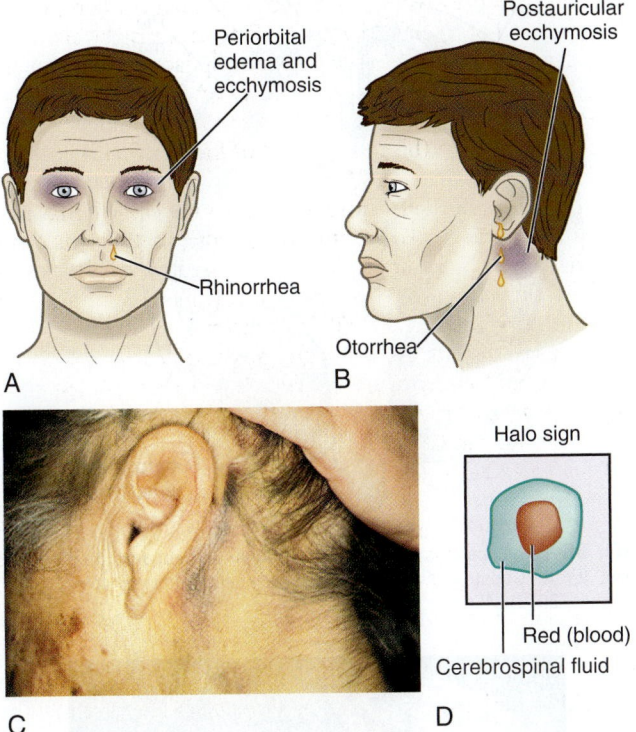

FIG. 56-13 **A,** Raccoon eyes and rhinorrhea. **B,** Battle's sign (postauricular ecchymosis) with otorrhea. **C,** Battle's sign. **D,** Halo or ring sign (see text). (*C,* From Bingham BJG, Hawke M, Kwok P: *Clinical atlas of otolaryngology,* St Louis, 1992, Mosby.)

is to test the leaking fluid with a Dextrostix or Tes-Tape strip to determine whether glucose is present. CSF gives a positive reading for glucose. If blood is present in the fluid, testing for glucose is unreliable because blood also contains glucose. In this event, look for the *halo* or *ring* sign (Fig. 56-13, *D*). Allow the leaking fluid to drip onto a white gauze pad (4 × 4) or towel, and then observe the drainage. Within a few minutes, the blood coalesces into the center, and a yellowish ring encircles the blood if CSF is present. Note the color, appearance, and amount of leaking fluid because both tests can give false-positive results.

The major potential complications of skull fractures are intracranial infections, hematoma, and meningeal and brain tissue damage. Note that in cases where a basilar skull fracture is suspected, an orogastric tube should be inserted rather than a nasogastric tube.

Head Trauma. Brain injuries are categorized as diffuse (generalized) or focal (localized). In a *diffuse* injury (e.g., concussion, diffuse axonal injury), damage to the brain cannot be localized to one particular area. In a *focal injury* (e.g., contusion, hematoma), damage can be localized to a specific area of the brain. Brain injury can be classified as *minor* (GCS 13 to 15), *moderate* (GCS 9 to 12), and *severe* (GCS 3 to 8).

Diffuse Injury. Concussion (a sudden transient mechanical head injury with disruption of neural activity and a change in the LOC) is considered a minor diffuse head injury. The patient may or may not lose total consciousness with this injury.

Typical signs of concussion include a brief disruption in LOC, amnesia regarding the event (retrograde amnesia), and headache. The manifestations are generally of short duration. If the patient has not lost consciousness, or if the loss of consciousness lasts less than 5 minutes, the patient is usually discharged from the care facility with instructions to notify the HCP if symptoms persist or if behavioral changes are noted.

Postconcussion syndrome may develop in some patients, usually anywhere from 2 weeks to 2 months after the injury. Manifestations include persistent headache, lethargy, personality and behavioral changes, shortened attention span, decreased short-term memory, and changes in intellectual ability. This syndrome can significantly affect the patient's abilities to perform activities of daily living.

Although concussion is generally considered benign and usually resolves spontaneously, the signs and symptoms may be the beginning of a more serious, progressive problem, especially in a patient with a history of prior concussion or head injury. At the time of discharge, it is important to give the patient and caregiver instructions for observation and accurate reporting of symptoms or changes in neurologic status.

Diffuse axonal injury. Diffuse axonal injury (DAI) is widespread axonal damage occurring after a mild, moderate, or severe TBI. The damage occurs primarily around axons in the subcortical white matter of the cerebral hemispheres, basal ganglia, thalamus, and brainstem.[16] Initially, DAI was believed to occur from the tensile forces of trauma that sheared axons, resulting in axonal disconnection. There is increasing evidence that axonal damage is not preceded by an immediate tearing of the axon from the traumatic impact, but rather the trauma changes the function of the axon, resulting in axon swelling and disconnection. This process takes approximately 12 to 24 hours to develop and may persist longer.

The clinical signs of DAI are varied but may include a decreased LOC, increased ICP, decortication or decerebration, and global cerebral edema. Approximately 90% of patients with DAI remain in a persistent vegetative state.[16] Patients with DAI who survive the initial event are rapidly triaged to an ICU, where they will be vigilantly watched for signs of increased ICP and treated accordingly (as previously discussed).

Focal Injury. Focal injury can be minor to severe and can be localized to an area of injury. Focal injury consists of lacerations, contusions, hematomas, and cranial nerve injuries.

Lacerations involve actual tearing of the brain tissue and often occur in association with depressed and open fractures and penetrating injuries. Tissue damage is severe, and surgical repair of the laceration is impossible because of the nature of brain tissue. Medical management consists of antibiotics (until meningitis is ruled out) and prevention of secondary injury related to increased ICP. If bleeding is deep into the brain tissue, focal and generalized signs develop.

When major head trauma occurs, many delayed responses are seen, including hemorrhage, hematoma formation, seizures, and cerebral edema. Intracerebral hemorrhage is generally associated with cerebral laceration. This hemorrhage manifests as a space-occupying lesion accompanied by unconsciousness, hemiplegia on the contralateral side, and a dilated pupil on the ipsilateral side. As the hematoma expands, signs of increased ICP become more severe. Subarachnoid hemorrhage and intraventricular hemorrhage can also occur secondary to head trauma.

A contusion is bruising of the brain tissue within a focal area. It is usually associated with a closed head injury. A contusion may contain areas of hemorrhage, infarction, necrosis, and edema, and it frequently occurs at a fracture site.

With contusion, the phenomenon of *coup-contrecoup injury* is often noted (Fig. 56-14), and injuries can range from minor to severe. Damage from coup-contrecoup injury occurs when the brain moves inside the skull due to high-energy or high-impact injury mechanisms. Contusions or lacerations occur both at the site of the direct impact of the brain on the skull *(coup)* and at a second area of damage on the opposite side away from injury *(contrecoup)*, leading to multiple contused areas. *Contrecoup* injuries tend to be more severe, and overall patient prognosis depends on the amount of bleeding around the contusion site.

Contusions may continue to bleed or rebleed and appear to "blossom" on subsequent CT scans of the brain. Bleeding worsens the neurologic outcome. Neurologic assessment may demonstrate focal and generalized manifestation, depending on the contusion's size and location. Seizures can occur as a result of a brain contusion, particularly when the injury involves the frontal or temporal lobes. Anticoagulant use and coagulopathy are associated with increased hemorrhage, more severe head injury, and an increased mortality rate.[17] This is especially important when considering older individuals who are taking anticoagulants. If they fall, their contusion is likely to be more severe due to the use of anticoagulants. Risk for falls should be assessed in all patients taking anticoagulants (see Table 62-1).

Complications

Epidural Hematoma.

An epidural hematoma results from bleeding between the dura and inner surface of the skull (Figs. 56-15 and 56-16). An epidural hematoma is a neurologic emergency and is usually associated with a linear fracture crossing a major artery in the dura, causing a tear. It can have a venous or an arterial origin. Venous epidural hematomas are associated with a tear of the dural venous sinus and develop slowly. With arterial hematomas, the middle meningeal artery lying under the temporal bone is often torn. Hemorrhage occurs into the epidural space, which lies between the dura and inner surface of the skull (Fig. 56-15). Because this is an arterial hemorrhage, the hematoma develops rapidly.

Classic signs of an epidural hematoma include an initial period of unconsciousness at the scene, with a brief lucid interval followed by a decrease in LOC. Other manifestations may be a headache, nausea and vomiting, or focal findings. Rapid surgical intervention to evacuate the hematoma and prevent

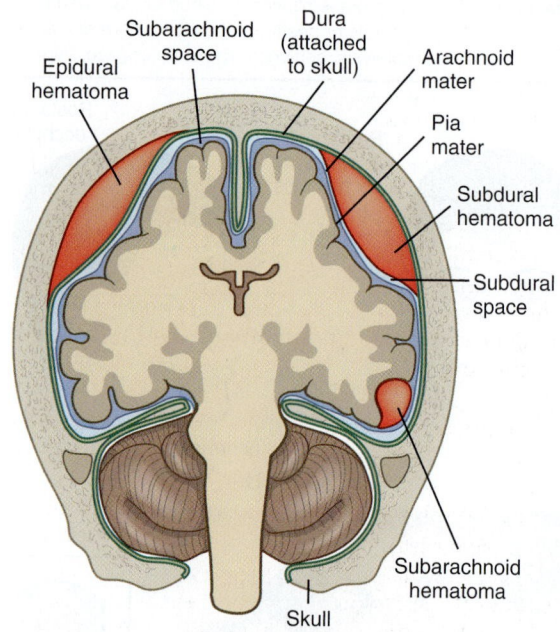

FIG. 56-15 Locations of epidural, subdural, and subarachnoid hematomas. (From Copstead-Kirkhorn LC, Banasik JL: *Pathophysiology*, ed 4, St Louis, 2010, Mosby.)

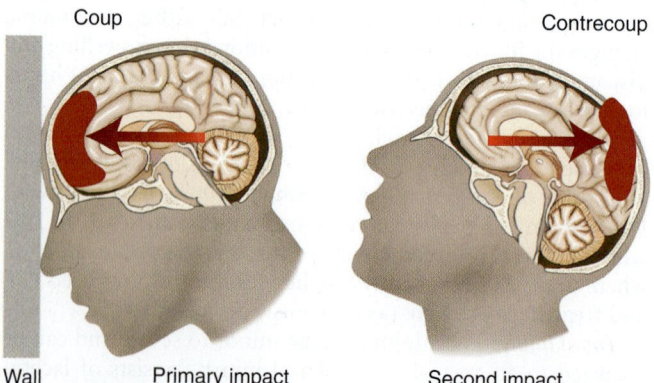

FIG. 56-14 Coup-contrecoup injury. After the head strikes the wall, a coup injury occurs as the brain strikes the skull (primary impact). The contrecoup injury (the second impact) occurs when the brain strikes the skull surface opposite the site of the original impact.

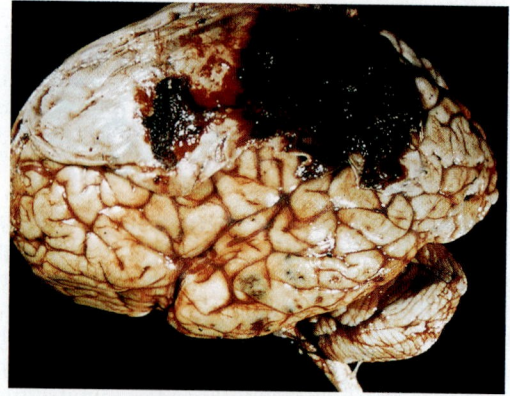

FIG. 56-16 Epidural hematoma covering a portion of the dura. Multiple small contusions are seen in the temporal lobe. (From Kumar V, Abbas AK, Aster JC, Fausto N: *Robbins and Cotran pathologic basis of disease*, ed 8, Philadelphia, 2010, Saunders.)

TABLE 56-8	Types of Subdural Hematomas	
Occurrence After Injury	**Progression of Symptoms**	**Treatment**
Acute 24-48 hr after severe trauma.	Immediate deterioration.	Craniotomy, evacuation, and decompression.
Subacute 48 hr to 2 wk after severe trauma.	Alteration in mental status as hematoma develops. Progression dependent on size and location of hematoma.	Evacuation and decompression.
Chronic Weeks or months, usually >20 days after injury. Often injury seemed trivial or was forgotten by patient.	Nonspecific, nonlocalizing progression. Progressive alteration in LOC.	Evacuation and decompression, membranectomy.

LOC, Level of consciousness.

cerebral herniation, along with medical management for increasing ICP, can dramatically improve outcomes.

Subdural Hematoma. A subdural hematoma occurs from bleeding between the dura mater and arachnoid layer of the meninges (Fig. 56-15). A subdural hematoma usually results from injury to the brain tissue and its blood vessels. The veins that drain from the surface of the brain into the sagittal sinus are the source of most subdural hematomas. Because it is usually venous in origin, the subdural hematoma may be slower to develop. However, a subdural hematoma may be caused by an arterial hemorrhage, in which case it develops more rapidly. Subdural hematomas may be acute, subacute, or chronic (Table 56-8).

An *acute subdural hematoma* manifests within 24 to 48 hours of the injury.[18] The signs and symptoms are similar to those associated with brain tissue compression in increased ICP and include decreasing LOC and headache. The size of the hematoma determines the patient's clinical presentation and prognosis. The patient's appearance may range from drowsy and confused to unconscious. The ipsilateral pupil dilates and becomes fixed if ICP is significantly elevated. Blunt force injuries that produce acute subdural hematomas may also cause significant underlying brain injury, resulting in cerebral edema. The resulting increase in ICP from the cerebral edema can cause an increased morbidity and mortality risk despite surgical intervention to evacuate the hematoma.

A *subacute subdural hematoma* usually occurs within 2 to 14 days of the injury. After the initial bleeding, a subdural hematoma may appear to enlarge over time as the breakdown products of the blood draw fluid into the subdural space.

A *chronic subdural hematoma* develops over weeks or months after a seemingly minor head injury.[19] Chronic subdural hematomas are more common in older adults because of a potentially larger subdural space as a result of brain atrophy. With atrophy, the brain remains attached to the supportive structures, but tension is increased, and it is subject to tearing. Because the subdural space is larger, the presenting complaint is focal symptoms (specific to a certain area of the brain), rather than signs of increased ICP.[20] Chronic alcoholics are also prone to cerebral atrophy and subsequent development of subdural hematoma because of an increased incidence of falls.

Diagnosis of a subdural hematoma in the older adult may be delayed because symptoms mimic other health problems in this age group, such as somnolence, confusion, lethargy, and memory loss. The manifestations of a subdural hematoma are often misinterpreted as vascular disease (stroke, transient ischemic attack [TIA]) or dementia.

Intracerebral Hematoma. Intracerebral hematoma occurs from bleeding within the brain tissue in approximately 16% of head injuries. It usually occurs within the frontal and temporal lobes, possibly from rupture of intracerebral vessels at the time of injury. The size and location of the hematoma are key determinants of the patient's outcome.

Diagnostic Studies and Interprofessional Care

CT scan is the best diagnostic test to evaluate for head trauma because it allows for rapid diagnosis and intervention in the acute care setting. MRI, PET, and evoked potential studies may also be used in the diagnosis and differentiation of head injuries. An MRI scan is more sensitive than the CT scan in detecting small lesions. Transcranial Doppler studies allow for the measurement of cerebral blood flow (CBF) velocity. A cervical spine x-ray series, CT scan, or MRI of the spine may also be indicated, since cervical spine trauma often occurs at the same time as a head injury. In general, the diagnostic studies are similar to those used for a patient with increased ICP (Table 56-3).

Emergency management of the patient with a head injury is presented in Table 56-9. In addition to measures to prevent secondary injury by treating cerebral edema and managing increased ICP, the principal treatment of head injuries is timely diagnosis and surgery (if necessary). For the patient with concussion and contusion, observation and management of increased ICP are the primary management strategies.

The treatment of skull fractures is usually conservative. For depressed fractures and fractures with loose fragments, a craniotomy is necessary to elevate the depressed bone and remove the free fragments. If large amounts of bone are destroyed, the bone may be removed (craniectomy), and a cranioplasty will be needed later (see the section on cranial surgery later in this chapter).

In cases of large acute subdural and epidural hematomas or those associated with significant neurologic impairment, the blood must be removed through surgical evacuation. A craniotomy is generally performed to visualize and allow control of the bleeding vessels. Burr-hole openings may be used in an

✚ **TABLE 56-9   Emergency Management**

Head Injury

Etiology	Assessment Findings	Interventions
Blunt • Motor vehicle collision • Fall • Assault • Sports injury **Penetrating** • Gunshot wound • Arrow	**Surface Findings** • Scalp lacerations • Fracture or depressions in skull • Bruises or contusions on face, Battle's sign (bruising behind ears) • Raccoon eyes (dependent bruising around eyes) **Respiratory** • Central neurogenic hyperventilation • Cheyne-Stokes respirations • Decreased O$_2$ saturation • Pulmonary edema **Central Nervous System** • Unequal or dilated pupils, photophobia • Asymmetric facial movements • Garbled speech, abusive speech • Confusion • Decreased level of consciousness • Combativeness • Involuntary movements • Seizures • Bowel and bladder incontinence • Flaccidity • Depressed or hyperactive reflexes • Decerebrate or decorticate posturing • GCS score <12 • CSF leaking from ears or nose	**Initial** • If unresponsive, assess circulation, airway, and breathing. • If responsive, monitor airway, breathing, and circulation. • Assume neck injury with head injury. • Stabilize cervical spine. • Administer O$_2$ via non-rebreather mask. • Establish IV access with two large-bore catheters to infuse normal saline or lactated Ringer's solution. • Intubate if GCS score <8. • Control external bleeding with sterile pressure dressing. • Remove patient's clothing. **Ongoing Monitoring** • Maintain normothermia using blankets, warm IV fluids, as necessary. • Monitor vital signs, level of consciousness, O$_2$ saturation, cardiac rhythm, GCS score, pupil size and reactivity. • Anticipate need for intubation if gag reflex is impaired or absent. • Assess for rhinorrhea, otorrhea, scalp wounds. • Administer fluids cautiously to prevent fluid overload and increasing ICP.

GCS, Glasgow Coma Scale, *ICP,* intracranial pressure.

extreme emergency for a more rapid decompression, followed by a craniotomy. A drain may be placed postoperatively for several days to prevent reaccumulation of blood. In cases in which extreme swelling is expected (e.g., DAI, hemorrhage), a craniectomy may be performed, which involves removing a piece of skull to reduce the pressure inside the cranial vault, thus reducing the risk of herniation.

❖ NURSING MANAGEMENT: HEAD INJURY

◆ Nursing Assessment

A patient with a head injury always has the potential to develop increased ICP, which is associated with higher mortality rates and poorer functional outcomes. Objective data are obtained by applying the GCS (Table 56-5), assessing and monitoring the neurologic status, and determining whether a CSF leak has occurred. (Nursing assessment related to increased ICP is discussed on pp. 1323-1324.) Nursing assessment of the patient with a head injury is presented in Table 56-10.

◆ Nursing Diagnoses

Nursing diagnoses and a potential complication for the patient who has sustained a head injury may include, but are not limited to, the following:

• Risk for ineffective cerebral tissue perfusion *related to* interruption of CBF associated with cerebral hemorrhage, hematoma, and edema
• Hyperthermia *related to* increased metabolism, infection, and hypothalamic injury
• Impaired physical mobility *related to* decreased LOC
• Anxiety *related to* abrupt change in health status, hospital environment, and uncertain future

• Potential complication: increased ICP *related to* cerebral edema and hemorrhage

◆ Planning

The overall goals are that the patient with an acute head injury will (1) maintain adequate cerebral oxygenation and perfusion; (2) remain normothermic; (3) achieve control of pain and discomfort; (4) be free from infection; (5) have adequate nutrition; and (6) attain maximal cognitive, motor, and sensory function.

◆ Nursing Implementation

◆ **Health Promotion.** One of the best ways to prevent head injuries is to prevent car and motorcycle accidents. The use of helmets by cyclists has led to fewer TBIs. The use of car seat belts and child car seats is also associated with reduced TBI mortality rates.

Be active in campaigns that promote driving safety, and speak to driver education classes regarding the dangers of unsafe driving and of driving after drinking alcohol and using drugs. Wearing seat belts in cars and helmets for riding on motorcycles is the most effective measure for increasing survival after crashes. Protective helmets should also be worn by lumberjacks, construction workers, athletes who play contact sports, miners, horseback riders, bicycle riders, snowboarders, skiers, and skydivers. Additionally, individuals who are at risk for falls (e.g., older adults) should be evaluated for safety in the home, since falls are the second leading cause of head injuries.

◆ **Acute Care.** Management at the injury scene can have a significant impact on the outcome of the head injury. Emergency management of head injury is presented in Table 56-9. The general goal of nursing management of the head-injured patient

TABLE 56-10 Nursing Assessment
Head Injury

Subjective Data
Important Health Information
Past health history: Mechanism of injury: motor vehicle collision, sports injury, industrial incident, assault, falls
Medications: Anticoagulant medications

Functional Health Patterns
Health perception–health management: Alcohol or recreational drugs. Risk-taking behaviors
Cognitive-perceptual: Headache, mood or behavioral change, mentation changes, aphasia, dysphasia, impaired judgment
Coping–stress tolerance: Fear, denial, anger, aggression, depression

Objective Data
General
Altered mental status

Integumentary
Lacerations, contusions, abrasions, hematoma, Battle's sign, periorbital edema and ecchymosis, otorrhea, exposed brain matter

Respiratory
Rhinorrhea, impaired gag reflex, inability to maintain a patent airway. Impending herniation: altered/irregular respiratory rate and pattern

Cardiovascular
Impending herniation: Cushing's triad (systolic hypertension with widening pulse pressure, bradycardia with full and bounding pulse, irregular respirations)

Gastrointestinal
Vomiting, projectile vomiting, bowel incontinence

Urinary
Bladder incontinence

Reproductive
Uninhibited sexual expression

Neurologic
Altered level of consciousness, seizure activity, pupil dysfunction, cranial nerve deficit(s)

Musculoskeletal
Motor deficit/impairment, weakness, palmar drift, paralysis, spasticity, decorticate or decerebrate posturing, muscular rigidity or increased tone, flaccidity, ataxia

Possible Diagnostic Findings
Location and type of hematoma, edema, skull fracture, and/or foreign body on CT scan and/or MRI; abnormal EEG; positive toxicology screen or alcohol level, ↓ or ↑ blood glucose level; ↑ ICP

ICP, Intracranial pressure.

ETHICAL/LEGAL DILEMMAS
Brain Death

Situation
The emergency nurse receives a radio call from emergency response system (ERS) personnel about R.G., a young man involved in a motorcycle crash. He was not wearing a helmet and has a large open skull fracture. Transport from the accident scene was delayed by 45 min as a result of a severe thunderstorm and traffic congestion. On the way to the hospital, R.G. exhibits fixed, dilated pupils and experiences cardiac arrest. Estimated arrival at the hospital is still an additional 45 min as a result of the severe weather. EMS personnel request permission to stop resuscitation efforts.

Ethical/Legal Points for Consideration
- Criteria for brain death include coma or unresponsiveness, absence of brainstem reflexes, and apnea (see Chapter 9).
- The definition of death has changed with the advent of new technology, monitoring devices, and interventions.
- A circumstance that influences the manner in which a state of death is determined is the customary practice or best practice for the specific situation.
- In a situation in which the professional responsible for determining a state of death is in remote contact with the patient, but the monitoring devices available provide virtual contact with the patient, a remote diagnosis of death may be legally acceptable.
- Brain death criteria do not address patients in a permanent vegetative state, since the brainstem activity in these patients is adequate to maintain heart and lung function.
- CPR is inappropriate when survival is not expected or if the patient is expected to survive without the ability to communicate. Quantitative futility implies that survival is not expected after CPR under given circumstances. In the absence of mitigating factors, prolonged resuscitative efforts are unlikely to be successful and can be discontinued if there is no return of spontaneous circulation at any time during 30 minutes of cumulative advanced life support.
- It is ethical for ED personnel to discontinue treatment initiated by ERS personnel in the prehospital setting, provided that there is valid, after-the-fact evidence that these interventions are now inappropriate.

Discussion Questions
1. What are your feelings about cessation of brain function vs. cessation of heart and lung function as the criteria for death of a patient?
2. What are your state's laws or practices about stopping cardiopulmonary resuscitation (CPR) efforts by ERS personnel in the field?
3. When brain death has occurred, what is your obligation for teaching the family or significant other regarding organ donation?

is to maintain cerebral oxygenation and perfusion and prevent secondary cerebral ischemia.

Surveillance or monitoring for changes in neurologic status is critically important because the patient's condition may deteriorate rapidly, necessitating emergency surgery. Appropriate preoperative and postoperative nursing interventions are initiated if surgery is anticipated. Because of the close association between hemodynamic status and cerebral perfusion, be aware of any coexisting injuries or conditions.

Explain the need for frequent neurologic assessments to both the patient and caregiver. Behavioral manifestations associated with head injury can result in a frightened, disoriented patient who is combative and resists help. Your approach should be calm and gentle. A family member may be available to stay with the patient and thus decrease anxiety and fear. One of the most important needs of the caregiver and family members in the acute injury phase is information about the patient's diagnosis, treatment plan, and rationale for the interventions. Other teaching points are presented in Table 56-11.

Perform neurologic assessments at intervals based on the patient's condition. The GCS is useful in assessing the LOC (Table 56-5). Report any indications of a deteriorating neurologic state, no matter how subtle, such as a decreasing LOC or

TABLE 56-11   Patient & Caregiver Teaching
Head Injury

Include the following instructions when teaching the patient and caregiver about care during the first 2 or 3 days after a head injury.

1. Notify your HCP immediately if experiencing signs and symptoms that may indicate complications. These include the following:
   - Increased drowsiness (e.g., difficulty arousing, confusion)
   - Nausea or vomiting
   - Worsening headache or stiff neck
   - Seizures
   - Vision difficulties (e.g., blurring) or sensitivity to light (photophobia)
   - Behavioral changes (e.g., irritability, anger)
   - Motor problems (e.g., clumsiness, difficulty walking, slurred speech, weakness in arms or legs)
   - Sensory disturbances (e.g., numbness)
   - A heart rate <60 beats/min
2. Have someone stay with you.
3. Abstain from alcohol.
4. Check with your HCP before taking drugs that may increase drowsiness, including muscle relaxants, tranquilizers, and opioid pain medications.
5. Avoid driving, using heavy machinery, playing contact sports, and taking hot baths.

decreasing motor strength, to the HCP. Monitor the patient's condition closely.

The major focus of nursing care for the brain-injured patient relates to increased ICP (see eNursing Care Plan 56-1). However, some problems may require specific nursing intervention.

Eye problems may include loss of the corneal reflex, periorbital ecchymosis and edema, and diplopia. Loss of the corneal reflex may necessitate administering lubricating eye drops or taping the eyes shut to prevent abrasion. Periorbital ecchymosis and edema decrease with time, but cold and, later, warm compresses provide comfort and hasten the process. Diplopia can be relieved by use of an eye patch. Consider a consult with an ophthalmologist.

Hyperthermia may occur from injury to or inflammation of the hypothalamus. Elevations in body temperature can result in increased CBF, cerebral blood volume, and ICP. Increased metabolism secondary to hyperthermia increases metabolic waste, which in turn produces further cerebral vasodilation. Avoid hyperthermia with a goal of a temperature of 96.8° to 98.6° F (36° to 37° C) as the standard of care. Use interventions to reduce temperature as previously discussed (see p. 1322) in conjunction with sedation as necessary to prevent shivering.

If CSF rhinorrhea or otorrhea occurs, inform the HCP immediately. The head of the bed may be raised to decrease the CSF pressure so that a tear can seal. A loose collection pad may be placed under the nose or over the ear. Do not place a dressing in the nasal or ear cavities and document the amount of drainage each shift. Instruct the patient not to sneeze or blow the nose. Do not use nasogastric tubes. Do not perform nasotracheal suctioning on these patients because of the high risk of meningitis.

Nursing measures specific to the care of the immobilized patient, such as those related to bladder and bowel function, skin care, and infection, are also indicated. Nausea and vomiting may be a problem and can be alleviated by antiemetic drugs. Headache can usually be controlled with acetaminophen or small doses of codeine.

If the patient's condition deteriorates, intracranial surgery may be necessary (see the section on cranial surgery later in this chapter). A burr-hole opening or craniotomy may be indicated,

depending on the underlying injury that is causing the problems. The emergency nature of the surgery may hasten the usual preoperative preparation. Consult with the neurosurgeon to determine specific preoperative nursing measures.

The patient is often unconscious before surgery, making it necessary for a family member to sign the consent form for surgery. This is a difficult and frightening time for the patient's caregiver and family and requires sensitive nursing management. The suddenness of the situation makes it especially difficult for the family to cope. Use the interprofessional team, including social workers, to assist the patient and family throughout the hospitalization and recovery time.

◆ **Ambulatory Care.** Once the condition has stabilized, the patient is usually transferred for acute rehabilitation management. There may be chronic problems related to motor and sensory deficits, communication, memory, and intellectual functioning. Many of the principles of nursing management of the patient with a stroke are appropriate for these patients (see Chapter 57).

Conditions that may require nursing and interprofessional management include poor nutritional status, bowel and bladder management, spasticity, dysphagia, deep vein thrombosis, and hydrocephalus. The patient's outward appearance is not a good indicator of how well he or she will ultimately function in the home or work environment. The outward physical appearance does not necessarily reflect what has happened in the brain.

Seizure disorders may occur in patients with nonpenetrating head injury. Seizures may develop during the first week after the head injury, but some patients may not develop a seizure disorder until years later. Antiseizure drugs may be used prophylactically to manage posttraumatic seizure activity, but this practice is controversial as previously discussed on p. 1326.

The mental and emotional sequelae of brain trauma are often the most incapacitating problems. One of the consequences of TBI is that the person may not realize that a brain injury has occurred. Many of the patients with head injuries who have been comatose for more than 6 hours undergo some personality change. They may suffer loss of concentration and memory and defective memory processing. Personal drive may decrease. Apathy may increase. Euphoria and mood swings, along with a seeming lack of awareness of the seriousness of the injury, may occur. The patient's behavior may indicate a loss of social restraint, judgment, tact, and emotional control.

Progressive recovery may continue for years. Specific nursing management in the posttraumatic phase depends on specific residual deficits. Being able to return to work and maintaining employment is one of the challenges during the recovery period.[21]

In all cases, the family must be given special consideration. They need to understand what is happening and be taught appropriate interaction patterns. Provide guidance and referrals for financial aid, child care, and other personal needs. Assist the family in involving the patient in family activities whenever possible. Help the patient and family remain hopeful. The family often has unrealistic expectations of the patient as the coma begins to recede. The family expects full return to pretrauma status. In reality, the patient usually experiences a reduced awareness and ability to interpret environmental stimuli. Prepare the family for the patient's emergence from coma and explain that the process of awakening often takes several weeks. In addition, arrange for social work and chaplain consultations for the family.

When it is the time for discharge planning, the patient, caregiver, and family may benefit from specific posthospitalization instructions to avoid family-patient friction. Special "no" policies that may be appropriately suggested by the neurosurgeon, neuropsychologist, and nurse include no drinking of alcoholic beverages, no driving, no use of firearms, no working with hazardous implements and machinery, and no unsupervised smoking. Family members, particularly spouses, go through role transition as the role changes from that of spouse to that of caregiver. (The stresses and needs of family caregivers are discussed in Chapter 4.)

◆ **Evaluation**

The expected outcomes are that the patient with a head injury will
- Maintain normal CPP
- Achieve maximal cognitive, motor, and sensory function
- Experience no infection or hyperthermia

BRAIN TUMORS

Annually there are an estimated 23,400 newly diagnosed people with brain tumors in the United States. The brain is also a frequent site for metastasis from other sites.[22] Males have a slightly higher incidence of brain tumors than females. Brain tumors are more commonly seen in middle-aged persons, but they may occur at any age.

CULTURAL & ETHNIC HEALTH DISPARITIES

Brain Tumors

- Whites have a higher incidence of malignant brain tumors than African Americans.
- White males have the highest incidence of malignant brain tumors.
- African Americans have a higher incidence of benign brain tumors (e.g., meningiomas) than whites.

Types

Brain tumors can occur in any part of the brain or spinal cord. Tumors of the brain may be *primary,* arising from tissues within the brain, or *secondary,* resulting from a metastasis from a malignant neoplasm elsewhere in the body.[23] Metastatic brain tumors are the most common brain tumor. The cancers that most commonly metastasize to the brain are lung and breast.

Primary brain tumors are generally classified according to the tissue from which they arise (Table 56-12). Meningiomas are the most common primary brain tumor. Other common brain tumors are gliomas (e.g., astrocytoma, glioblastoma [most common form of glioma]).

More than half of brain tumors are malignant. They infiltrate the brain tissue and are not amenable to complete surgical removal. Other tumors may be histologically benign but are located such that complete removal is not possible.

Brain tumors rarely metastasize outside the central nervous system (CNS) because they are contained by structural (meninges) and physiologic (blood-brain) barriers. Table 56-12 compares the most common brain tumors. A glioblastoma and meningioma are shown in Fig. 56-17.

Clinical Manifestations and Complications

The clinical manifestations of brain tumors depend mainly on their location and size (Table 56-13). The rate of growth and appearance of manifestations depend on the location, size, and mitotic rate of the cells of the tissue of origin. Fig. 56-18 illustrates the functional areas of the cerebral cortex and can be used as a guide to correlate the clinical manifestations with the location of the tumor, as indicated by an alteration in the function controlled by the affected area.

Wide ranges of possible clinical manifestations are associated with brain tumors. Headache is a common problem. Tumor-related headaches tend to be worse at night and may awaken the patient. The headaches are usually dull and constant but occasionally throbbing. Seizures are common in gliomas and brain metastases. Brain tumors can cause nausea and vomiting from increased ICP. Cognitive dysfunction, including memory problems and mood or personality changes, is another common manifestation, especially in patients with brain metastases. Muscle weakness, sensory losses, aphasia, and visual-spatial dysfunction are also manifestations of brain tumors.

If the tumor mass obstructs the ventricles or occludes the outlet, ventricular enlargement (hydrocephalus) can occur. As the brain tumor expands, it may also produce manifestations of increased ICP, cerebral edema, or obstruction of the CSF pathways. Unless treated, all brain tumors eventually cause death from increasing tumor volume leading to increased ICP.

TABLE 56-12	**Types of Brain Tumors**	
Type	**Tissue of Origin**	**Characteristics**
Gliomas		
• Astrocytoma	Supportive tissue, glial cells, and astrocytes	Can range from low-grade to moderate-grade malignancy.
• Glioblastoma	Primitive stem cell (glioblast)	Highly malignant and invasive. Among the most devastating of primary brain tumors.
• Oligodendroglioma	Oligodendrocytes	Benign (encapsulation and calcification).
• Ependymoma	Ependymal epithelium	Range from benign to highly malignant. Most are benign and encapsulated.
• Medulloblastoma	Primitive neuroectodermal cell	Highly malignant and invasive. Metastatic to spinal cord and remote areas of brain.
Meningioma	Meninges	Can be benign or malignant. Most are benign.
Acoustic neuroma (Schwannoma)	Cells that form myelin sheath around nerves. Commonly affects cranial nerve VIII	Many grow on both sides of the brain. Usually benign or low-grade malignancy.
Pituitary adenoma	Pituitary gland	Usually benign.
Hemangioblastoma	Blood vessels of brain	Rare and benign. Surgery is curative.
Primary central nervous system lymphoma	Lymphocytes	Increased incidence in transplant recipients and acquired immunodeficiency syndrome (AIDS) patients.
Metastatic tumors	Lungs and breast (most common)	Malignant.

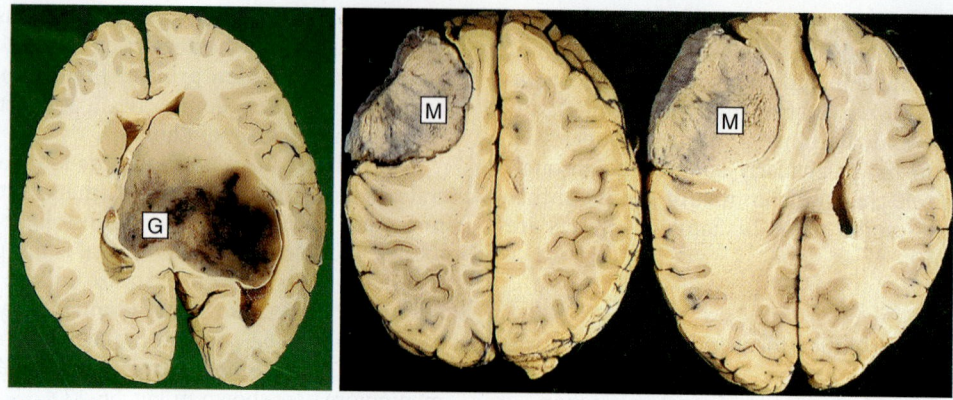

FIG. 56-17   **A,** A large glioblastoma *(G)* arises from one cerebral hemisphere and has grown to fill the ventricular system. **B,** Meningioma. These two different sections from different levels in the same brain show a meningioma *(M)* compressing the frontal lobe and distorting underlying brain. (From Stevens A, Lowe J: *Pathology: illustrated review in colour,* ed 2, London, 2000, Mosby.)

TABLE 56-13   **Manifestations of Brain Tumors**

Tumor Location	Manifestations
Cerebral hemisphere	
• Frontal lobe (unilateral)	Unilateral hemiplegia, seizures, memory deficit, personality and judgment changes, visual disturbances.
• Frontal lobe (bilateral)	Symptoms associated with unilateral frontal lobe tumors. Ataxic gait.
• Parietal lobe	Speech disturbance (if tumor is in the dominant hemisphere), inability to write, spatial disorders, unilateral neglect.
• Occipital lobe	Vision disturbances and seizures.
• Temporal lobe	Few symptoms. Seizures, dysphagia, hallucinations, auras.
Subcortical	Hemiplegia. Other symptoms may depend on area of infiltration.
Meningeal tumors	Symptoms associated with compression of the brain and depend on tumor location.
Metastatic tumors	Headache, nausea, or vomiting (occur from ↑ ICP). Other symptoms depend on tumor location.
Thalamus and sellar tumors	Headache, nausea, vision disturbances, papilledema, and nystagmus (occur from ↑ ICP). Diabetes insipidus may occur.
Fourth ventricle and cerebellar tumors	Headache, nausea, and papilledema (occur from ↑ ICP). Ataxic gait and changes in coordination.
Cerebellopontine tumors	Tinnitus and vertigo, deafness.
Brainstem tumors	Headache on awakening, drowsiness, vomiting, ataxic gait, facial muscle weakness, hearing loss, dysphagia, dysarthria, "crossed eyes" or other visual changes, hemiparesis.

ICP, Intracranial pressure.

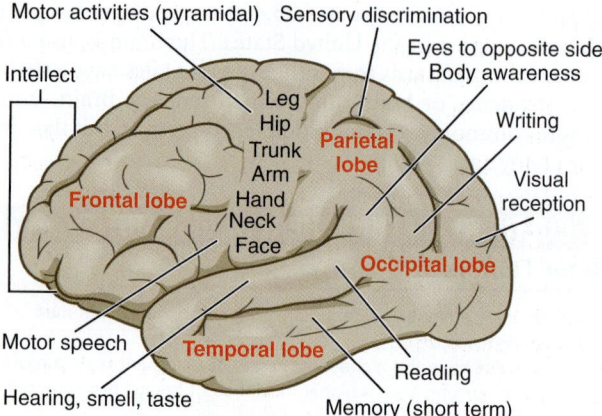

FIG. 56-18   Each area of the brain controls a particular activity.

The sensitivity of techniques such as MRI and PET scans allows for detection of small tumors and may provide more reliable diagnostic information than a CT scan. CT with contrast and MRI are used to identify the lesion's location. Other tests include magnetic resonance spectroscopy, functional MRI, and single-photon emission computed tomography (SPECT). The EEG is useful for ruling out seizures but is of less importance. A lumbar puncture is seldom diagnostic and carries with it the risk of cerebral herniation. Cerebral angiography can be used to determine blood flow to the tumor and further localize the tumor. Other studies are done to rule out a primary lesion elsewhere in the body. Endocrine studies are helpful when a pituitary adenoma is suspected (see Chapter 49).

The correct diagnosis of a brain tumor can be made by obtaining tissue for histologic study. In most patients, tissue is obtained at the time of surgery. Computer-guided stereotactic biopsy is also an option. A smear or frozen section can be performed in the operating room for a preliminary interpretation of the histologic type. With this information, the neurosurgeon can make a better decision about the extent of surgery.

Interprofessional Care

Treatment goals are aimed at (1) identifying the tumor type and location, (2) removing or decreasing tumor mass, and (3) preventing or managing increased ICP.

Surgical Therapy. Surgical removal is the preferred treatment for brain tumors (see the section on cranial surgery later in this

Diagnostic Studies

An extensive history and a comprehensive neurologic examination must be done in the workup of a patient with a suspected brain tumor. A careful history and physical examination may provide data with respect to location. New onset of seizures or adult-onset migraines may be indicative of a brain tumor and should be investigated. Diagnostic studies are similar to those used for a patient with increased ICP (Table 56-3).

chapter). Stereotactic surgical techniques are used with greater frequency to perform a biopsy and remove small brain tumors. The outcome of surgical therapy depends on the tumor's type, size, and location. Meningiomas and oligodendrogliomas can usually be completely removed, whereas the more invasive gliomas and medulloblastomas may only be partially removed. Computer-guided stereotactic biopsy, ultrasound, functional MRI, and cortical mapping can be used to localize brain tumors intraoperatively.

Complete surgical removal of brain tumors is not always possible because the tumor is not always accessible or may involve vital parts of the brain. Surgery can reduce tumor mass, which decreases ICP, provides relief of symptoms, and extends survival time.

Ventricular Shunts. Hydrocephalus due to a tumor obstructing the CSF flow can be treated with the placement of a ventricular shunt. A catheter with one-way valves is placed in the lateral ventricle and then tunneled under the skin to drain CSF into the peritoneal cavity. Rapid decompression of ICP can cause total body collapse and weakness, including a headache that may be prevented by gradually introducing the patient to the upright position.

Manifestations of shunt malfunction, which are related to increased ICP, include decreasing LOC, restlessness, headache, blurred vision, or vomiting. This may necessitate shunt revision or replacement. Infection may also occur, as exhibited by high fever, persistent headache, and stiff neck. Antibiotics are used to treat the infection. In some situations, the shunt must be replaced and CSF drainage managed with an extraventricular drainage system while the infection is treated.

Radiation Therapy and Stereotactic Radiosurgery. Radiation therapy may be used as a follow-up measure after surgery. Radiation seeds can also be implanted into the brain. Cerebral edema and rapidly increasing ICP may be a complication of radiation therapy, but these problems can be managed with high doses of corticosteroids (dexamethasone, prednisone, or methylprednisolone [Solu-Medrol]). (Radiation therapy is discussed in Chapter 15.)

Stereotactic radiosurgery is a method of delivering a highly concentrated dose of radiation to a precise location within the brain. Stereotactic radiosurgery may be used when conventional surgery has failed or is not an option because of the tumor location. (Radiosurgery is discussed on p. 1337.)

Chemotherapy and Targeted Therapy. The effectiveness of chemotherapy has been limited by the difficulty with getting drugs across the blood-brain barrier, tumor cell heterogeneity, and tumor cell drug resistance. Chemotherapy drugs called *nitrosoureas* (e.g., carmustine, lomustine) are used to treat brain tumors. Normally the blood-brain barrier prohibits the entry of most drugs into the brain. The most malignant tumors cause a breakdown of the blood-brain barrier in the area of the tumor, thus allowing chemotherapy agents to be used to treat the malignancy. Chemotherapy-laden biodegradable wafers (e.g., Gliadel wafer [polifeprosan with carmustine implant]) implanted at the time of surgery can deliver chemotherapy directly to the tumor site. Other drugs being used include methotrexate and procarbazine (Matulane). One method used to deliver chemotherapy drugs directly to the CNS is intrathecal administration via an Ommaya reservoir.

Temozolomide (Temodar) is an oral chemotherapy agent that can cross the blood-brain barrier. In contrast with many traditional chemotherapy drugs, which require metabolic activation to exert their effects, temozolomide can convert spontaneously to a reactive agent that directly interferes with tumor growth. It does not interact with other drugs commonly taken by patients with brain tumors, such as antiseizure medications, corticosteroids, and antiemetics.

 DRUG ALERT Temozolomide (Temodar)
- Causes myelosuppression. Before using, it is recommended that absolute neutrophil count be ≥1500/μL and platelet count be ≥100,000/μL.
- To reduce nausea and vomiting, take on empty stomach.

Bevacizumab (Avastin) is used to treat patients with glioblastoma that continues to progress after standard therapy. Bevacizumab is a targeted therapy that inhibits the action of vascular endothelial growth factor, which helps form new blood vessels. These vessels can feed a tumor, helping it to grow, and can also provide a pathway for cancer cells to circulate in the body. (Targeted therapy is discussed in Chapter 15 and Table 15-13.)

Other Therapies. A medical device system, OpTune System, is used to treat glioblastoma that recurs or progresses after receiving chemotherapy and radiation therapy. With this system, electrodes are placed on the surface of the patient's scalp to deliver low-intensity, changing electrical fields called *tumor treatment fields* (TTFs) to the tumor site.

❖ NURSING MANAGEMENT: BRAIN TUMORS

◆ Nursing Assessment

Structure the initial assessment to provide baseline data of the patient's neurologic status. Use this information to design a realistic, individualized care plan. Assess the patient's LOC, motor abilities, sensory perception, integrated function (including bowel and bladder function), and balance and proprioception. In addition, assess the coping abilities of the patient, caregiver, and family. Watching a patient perform activities of daily living and listening to the patient's conversation can be part of the neurologic assessment. Having the patient or caregiver explain the problem can be helpful to determine the patient's limitations and obtain information about the patient's insight into the problems. Record all initial data to provide a baseline for comparison to determine whether the patient's condition is improving or deteriorating.

Interview data are as important as the actual physical assessment. Ask questions about the medical history, intellectual abilities and educational level, and history of nervous system infections and trauma. Determine the presence of seizures, syncope, nausea and vomiting, and headaches or other pain to help better plan care for the patient.

◆ Nursing Diagnoses

Nursing diagnoses and collaborative problems for the patient with a brain tumor may include, but are not limited to, the following:

- Risk for ineffective cerebral tissue perfusion *related to* cerebral edema
- Acute pain (headache) *related to* cerebral edema and increased ICP
- Anxiety *related to* diagnosis and treatment
- Potential complications: seizures *related to* abnormal electrical activity of the brain and increased ICP *related to* tumor and failure of normal compensatory mechanisms

◆ Planning

The overall goals are that the patient with a brain tumor will (1) maintain normal ICP, (2) maximize neurologic functioning, (3) achieve control of pain and discomfort, and (4) be aware of the long-term implications with respect to prognosis and cognitive and physical functioning.

◆ Nursing Implementation

A primary or metastatic tumor of the frontal lobe can cause behavioral and personality changes. Loss of emotional control, confusion, disorientation, memory loss, impulsivity, and depression may be signs of a frontal lobe lesion. These behavioral changes are often not perceived by the patient but can be disturbing and even frightening to the caregiver and family. These changes can also cause a distancing to occur between the family and patient. Assist the caregiver and family in understanding what is happening to the patient, and support the family.

The confused patient with behavioral instability can be a challenge. Protecting the patient from self-harm is an important part of nursing care. Essential techniques in the care of these patients include close supervision of activity, use of side rails, judicious use of restraints, appropriate sedative medications, padding of the rails and the area around the bed, and a calm, reassuring approach.

Perceptual problems associated with frontal and parietal lobe tumors contribute to a patient's disorientation and confusion. Minimize environmental stimuli, create a routine, and use reality orientation for the confused patient. Tumors in the temporal lobe can cause hallucinations, which may be confused with dementia or delirium in the hospitalized patient.

Seizures, which often occur with brain tumors, are managed with antiseizure drugs. Also use seizure precautions for the patient's protection. Some behavioral changes seen in the patient with a brain tumor are a result of seizure disorders and can improve with adequate seizure control. Patients at risk for seizures may be unable to drive, so be aware of the extra resources needed and collaborate with the social worker and family. (Seizure disorders are discussed in Chapter 58.)

Motor and sensory dysfunctions interfere with activities of daily living. Alterations in mobility must be managed. Encourage the patient to provide as much self-care as physically possible. Self-image often depends on the patient's ability to participate in care within the limitations of the physical deficits.

Language deficits can also occur in patients with brain tumors. Motor (expressive) or sensory (receptive) dysphasia may occur. The disturbance in communication can be frustrating for the patient and may interfere with your ability to meet the patient's needs. Make attempts to establish a communication system that can be used by both the patient and staff.

Nutritional intake may be decreased because of the patient's inability to eat, loss of appetite, or loss of desire to eat. Assess the patient's nutritional status, and ensure adequate nutritional intake. Encourage the patient to eat. Some patients may need enteral or parenteral nutrition (see Chapter 39). The patient with a brain tumor who undergoes cranial surgery requires complex nursing care (discussed in the next section).

Provide help and support during the adjustment phase and in long-range planning. Social work and home health nurses may be needed to assist the caregiver with discharge planning and to help the family adjust to role changes and psychosocial and socioeconomic factors. Issues related to palliative and end-of-life care must be discussed with both the patient and family (see Chapter 9).

◆ Evaluation

The expected outcomes are that the patient with a brain tumor will

- Achieve control of pain, vomiting, and other discomforts
- Maintain ICP within normal limits
- Demonstrate maximal neurologic function (cognitive, motor, sensory) given the location and extent of the tumor
- Maintain optimal nutritional status
- Accept the long-term consequences of the tumor and its treatment

CRANIAL SURGERY

Indications for cranial surgery are related to brain tumors, CNS infection (e.g., abscess), vascular abnormalities, craniocerebral trauma, seizure disorder, or intractable pain (Table 56-14).

Types

Various types of cranial surgical procedures are presented in Table 56-15.

Craniotomy. Depending on the location of the pathologic condition, a *craniotomy* may be frontal, parietal, occipital, temporal, suboccipital, or a combination of any of these. The surgeon drills a set of burr holes and uses a saw to connect the holes to remove the bone flap. Sometimes operating microscopes are used to magnify the site. After surgery, the bone flap is secured with small plates or wired shut. Sometimes drains are placed to remove fluid and blood. Patients are usually cared for in an ICU until stable.

TABLE 56-14	**Indications for Cranial Surgery**	
Indication	**Cause**	**Surgical Procedure**
Brain abscess	Bacteria that caused intracranial infection	Excision or drainage of abscess
Hydrocephalus	Overproduction of CSF, obstruction to flow, defective reabsorption	Placement of ventriculoperitoneal or (rarely) ventriculoatrial shunt
Brain tumors	Benign or malignant cell growth	Excision or partial resection of tumor
Intracranial bleeding	Rupture of cerebral vessels because of trauma or stroke	Surgical evacuation through burr holes or craniotomy
Skull fractures	Trauma to skull	Debridement of fragments and necrotic tissue, elevation and realignment of bone fragments
Arteriovenous (AV) malformation	Congenital tangle of arteries and veins (frequently in middle cerebral artery)	Excision of malformation
Aneurysm repair	Dilation of weak area in arterial wall (usually near anterior portion of circle of Willis)	Dissection and clipping or coiling of aneurysm

CSF, Cerebrospinal fluid.

TABLE 56-15	Types of Cranial Surgery
Type	**Description**
Burr hole	Opening into the cranium with a drill. Used to remove localized fluid and blood beneath the dura.
Craniotomy	Opening into cranium with removal of bone flap and opening the dura to remove a lesion, repair a damaged area, drain blood, or relieve ↑ ICP.
Craniectomy	Excision into the cranium to cut away bone flap.
Cranioplasty	Repair of cranial defect resulting from trauma, malformation, or previous surgical procedure. Artificial material used to replace damaged or lost bone.
Stereotactic procedure	Precise localization of a specific area of the brain using a frame or frameless system based on three-dimensional coordinates. Procedure is used for biopsy, radiosurgery, or dissection.
Shunt procedures	Alternate pathway to redirect cerebrospinal fluid from one area to another using a tube or implanted device. Examples include ventricular shunt and Ommaya reservoir.

ICP, Intracranial pressure.

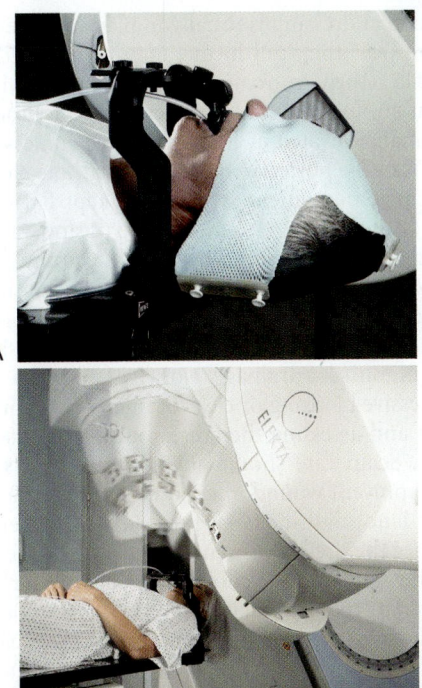

FIG. 56-19   A, Patient in a stereotactic frame. **B,** Elekta's Fraxion head frame helps ensure accuracy and precision in stereotactic radiation therapy (SRT) of cancer targets in the brain and cranium. (Courtesy Elekta.)

Stereotactic Radiosurgery. Stereotactic procedures use precision apparatus (often computer guided) to help the physician precisely target an area of the brain. Stereotactic biopsy can be performed to obtain tissue samples for histologic examination. CT scanning and MRI are used to image the targeted tissue. With the patient under general or local anesthesia, the surgeon drills a burr hole or creates a bone flap for an entry site and then introduces a probe and biopsy needle. Stereotactic procedures are used for removal of small brain tumors and abscesses, drainage of hematomas, ablative procedures for extrapyramidal diseases (e.g., Parkinson's disease), and repair of arteriovenous malformations. A major advantage of the stereotactic approach is a reduction in damage to surrounding tissue.

Stereotactic radiosurgery is not a form of surgery in the traditional sense. Instead, radiosurgery uses precisely focused radiation to destroy tumor cells and other abnormal growths in the brain. Computers create three-dimensional images of the brain, and these images are used to guide the focused radiation while the patient's head is held still in a stereotactic frame (Fig. 56-19). Radiosurgical techniques can use ionizing radiation generated by a linear accelerator, gamma knife, or CyberKnife. In these procedures, a high dose of cobalt radiation is delivered to precisely targeted tumor tissue. The dose of radiation is delivered in a single treatment lasting a few hours or in multiple sessions. Side effects of stereotactic radiosurgery may include fatigue, headache, and nausea.

In combination with stereotactic procedures to identify and localize tumor sites, surgical lasers can be used to destroy tumors. Three surgical lasers currently used are the carbon dioxide, argon, and neodymium:yttrium-aluminum-garnet (Nd:YAG) lasers. All three work by creating thermal energy, which destroys the tissue on which it is focused. Laser therapy also provides the benefit of reducing damage to surrounding tissue.

❖ NURSING MANAGEMENT: CRANIAL SURGERY

◆ Nursing Implementation

◆ **Acute Care.** The general preoperative and postoperative nursing care for the patient undergoing cranial surgery is similar regardless of the cause. Nursing management is similar to that for the patient with increased ICP (presented in eNursing Care Plan 56-1). The patient (if conscious and coherent), caregiver, and family will be concerned about the potential physical and emotional problems that can result from surgery. The uncertainty regarding prognosis and outcome requires compassionate nursing care in the preoperative period.

Preoperative teaching is important in allaying the fears of the patient, caregiver, and family, and also in preparing them for the postoperative period. Provide general information concerning the type of operation that will be performed and what can be expected immediately after the operation. Explain that some hair may be shaved to allow for better exposure and to prevent contamination. The hair is usually removed in the operating room after induction of anesthesia. Also inform the family that the patient will be taken to an ICU or to a special care unit after surgery.

The primary goal of care after cranial surgery is prevention of increased ICP. (Nursing management of the patient with increased ICP is presented on pp. 1323-1326.) Frequent assessment of the patient's neurologic status is essential during the first 48 hours. In addition to the neurologic functions, closely monitor fluid and electrolyte levels and serum osmolality to detect changes in sodium regulation, the onset of diabetes insipidus, or severe hypovolemia. Turning and positioning the patient may depend on the site of the operation.

Monitor the patient for pain and nausea. Although the brain itself does not possess pain receptors, patients often report headache caused by edema or pain at the incision site. Control pain with short-acting opioids and monitor neurologic status. Nausea and vomiting are common after surgery and are usually treated with antiemetics. The use of promethazine is discouraged because it can increase somnolence, thus altering the accuracy of a neurologic assessment.

The surgical dressing is usually in place for a few days. With an incision over the skull in the anterior or middle fossa, the patient will return from the operating room with the head elevated at an angle of 30 to 45 degrees. The head of the bed should remain elevated at least 30 degrees unless the surgical approach is in the posterior fossa or a burr hole has been made. In these cases, the patient is generally kept flat or at a slight elevation (10 to 15 degrees) during the postoperative phase.

If a bone flap has been removed (craniectomy), do not position the patient on the operative side. A sign should be placed at the head of the bed, alerting everyone of the craniectomy site and position of the surgical site. Observe the dressing for color, odor, and amount of drainage. Notify the surgeon immediately of any excessive bleeding or clear drainage. Checking drains for placement and assessing the area around the dressing are also important. Scalp care should include meticulous care of the incision to prevent wound infection. Cleanse the area and treat it in accordance with hospital protocol or the neurosurgeon's orders. Once the dressing is removed, use an antiseptic soap for washing the scalp. The psychologic impact of hair removal can be alleviated by the use of a wig, turban, scarves, or cap. For the patient who is receiving radiation, instruct the patient to use a sunblock and head covering if any exposure to the sun is anticipated.

◆ **Ambulatory Care.** The rehabilitative potential for a patient after cranial surgery depends on the reason for the surgery, postoperative course, and patient's general state of health. Base your nursing interventions on a realistic appraisal of these factors. An overall goal is to foster independence for as long as possible and to the highest degree possible.

Specific rehabilitation potential cannot be determined until cerebral edema and increased ICP subside postoperatively. Take care to maintain as much function as possible through measures such as careful positioning, meticulous skin and mouth care, regular range-of-motion exercises, bowel and bladder care, and adequate nutrition.

Referrals may be made to other specialists on the interprofessional team. For example, the speech therapist may be helpful to the patient who has a speech problem, or the physical therapist may provide an exercise plan to regain functional deficits. Address the needs and problems of each patient individually because many variables affect the plan. The patient's mental and physical deterioration, including seizures, personality disorganization, apathy, and wasting, is difficult for both family and health care professionals to watch. Cognitive and emotional residual deficits are often harder to accept than are motor and sensory losses.

INFLAMMATORY CONDITIONS OF THE BRAIN

Brain abscesses, meningitis, and encephalitis are the most common inflammatory conditions of the brain and spinal cord (Table 56-16). Inflammation can be caused by bacteria, viruses, fungi, and chemicals (e.g., contrast media used in diagnostic tests, blood in the subarachnoid space). CNS infections may occur via the bloodstream, by extension from a primary site, or along cranial and spinal nerves.

The mortality rate for inflammatory conditions of the brain is approximately 10% to 30% in the general population, with higher rates in older patients. Up to 19% of those who recover can have long-term neurologic deficits, including hearing loss.[24]

ETHICAL/LEGAL DILEMMAS
Withholding Treatment

Situation

C.J., a 26-yr-old patient in a permanent vegetative state, is diagnosed with her fifteenth bladder infection. As her home care nurse, you must determine whether to seek antibiotics for this infection. The family members have expressed a concern that no heroic measures be used to extend the biologic life of their daughter and sister. However, they have been unwilling to withdraw the existing treatment, which is enteral nutrition through a gastrostomy tube. Should antibiotics be withheld?

Ethical/Legal Points for Consideration

- Patients in a persistent vegetative state do not recover.
- The primary legal issue here is who has the legal right to refuse or consent to treatment for this incapacitated patient. You need to know if a guardian has been appointed by the court or if her parents retain a form of guardianship to make health care decisions for her.
- You also need to know when the vegetative state began; that is, did the patient ever have the right to consent having reached the age of majority as a competent adult, or did the vegetative state begin while she was a minor? If the patient did become a competent adult before the vegetative state, did she ever express any preference for quality-of-life and end-of-life decision making?
- The courts have widespread legal precedents for accepting the decision of the patient's guardian or parents or the patient's clearly expressed preferences for quality-of-life decision making.
- Life-sustaining treatment is any treatment that serves to prolong life without reversing the underlying medical condition. Life-sustaining treatment may include, but is not limited to, mechanical ventilation, renal dialysis, chemotherapy, antibiotics, and artificial nutrition and hydration.
- There is no ethical distinction between withdrawing and withholding life-sustaining treatment. If there is not adequate evidence of the incompetent patient's preferences and values, the decision should be based on the best interests of the patient (i.e., what outcome would most likely promote the patient's well-being).

Discussion Questions

1. How would you approach C.J.'s family?
2. What are your feelings about providing nutrition, hydration, and treatments that will prolong life in a patient for whom there is no hope of recovery?
3. What options are available to the family for the care of their daughter once a decision is made about withholding antibiotics?

BRAIN ABSCESS

Brain abscess is an accumulation of pus within the brain tissue that can result from a local or systemic infection. Direct extension from an ear, tooth, mastoid, or sinus infection is the primary cause. Other causes for brain abscess formation include spread from a distant site (e.g., pulmonary infection, bacterial endocarditis), skull fracture, and prior brain trauma or surgery. Streptococci and *Staphylococcus aureus* are the primary infective organisms.

Manifestations of brain abscess, which are similar to those of meningitis and encephalitis, include headache, fever, and nausea and vomiting. Signs of increased ICP may include drowsiness, confusion, and seizures. Focal symptoms may reflect the local area of the abscess. For example, visual field defects or psychomotor seizures are common with a temporal lobe abscess, whereas an occipital abscess may be accompanied by visual impairment and hallucinations. CT and MRI are used to diagnose a brain abscess.

TABLE 56-16	Comparison of Cerebral Inflammatory Conditions		
	Meningitis	**Encephalitis**	**Brain Abscess**
Cause	Bacteria (*Streptococcus pneumoniae*, *Neisseria meningitidis*, group B streptococci, viruses, fungi)	Bacteria, fungi, parasites, herpes simplex virus (HSV), other viruses (e.g., West Nile virus)	Streptococci, staphylococci through bloodstream
CSF (Reference Interval)			
• Pressure (70-150 mm H$_2$O)	Increased *Bacterial:* 200-500 *Viral:* ≤250	Normal to slight increase	Increased
• WBC count (0-5 cells/µL)	*Bacterial:* >1000/µL (mainly neutrophils) *Viral:* 25-500/µL (mainly lymphocytes)	500/µL, neutrophils (early), lymphocytes (later)	25-300/µL (neutrophils)
• Protein (15-45 mg/dL [0.15-0.45 g/L])	*Bacterial:* >500 mg/dL *Viral:* 50-500 mg/dL	Slight increase	Normal
• Glucose (40-70 mg/dL [2.2-3.9 mmol/L])	*Bacterial:* Decreased 5-40 *Viral:* Normal or low >40	Normal	Low or absent
• Appearance	*Bacterial:* Turbid, cloudy *Viral:* Clear or cloudy	Clear	Clear
Diagnostic Studies	CT scan, Gram stain, smear, culture, PCR*	CT scan, EEG, MRI, PET, PCR, IgM antibodies to virus in serum or CSF	CT scan
Treatment	Antibiotics, dexamethasone, supportive care, prevention of ↑ ICP	Supportive care, prevention of ↑ ICP, acyclovir (Zovirax) for HSV	Antibiotics, incision and drainage Supportive care

CSF, Cerebrospinal fluid; *ICP*, intracranial pressure; *PCR*, polymerase chain reaction.
*PCR is used to detect viral RNA or DNA.

Antimicrobial therapy is the primary treatment for brain abscess. Other manifestations are treated symptomatically. If drug therapy is not effective, the abscess may have to be drained or removed if it is encapsulated.

Nursing measures are similar to those for management of meningitis or increased ICP. If surgical drainage or removal is the treatment of choice, nursing care is similar to that described under cranial surgery.

BACTERIAL MENINGITIS

Meningitis is an acute inflammation of the meningeal tissues surrounding the brain and spinal cord. Meningitis usually occurs in fall, winter, or early spring and is often secondary to viral respiratory disease. Older adults and persons who are debilitated are affected more frequently than the general population. College students living in dormitories and individuals living in institutions (e.g., prisoners) have a high risk for contracting meningitis. Untreated bacterial meningitis has a mortality rate near 100%.[25]

Etiology and Pathophysiology

Streptococcus pneumoniae and *Neisseria meningitidis* are the leading causes of bacterial meningitis. *Neisseria meningitides* has at least 13 different subtypes (serogroups) with five of them (A, B, C, Y, W) causing most cases. *Haemophilus influenzae* was once the most common cause of bacterial meningitis. However, the use of *H. influenzae* vaccine has resulted in a significant decrease in meningitis related to this organism.

The organisms usually gain entry to the CNS through the upper respiratory tract or bloodstream. However, they may enter by direct extension from penetrating wounds of the skull or through fractured sinuses in basilar skull fractures.

The inflammatory response to the infection tends to increase CSF production with a moderate increase in ICP. In bacterial meningitis the purulent secretions produced quickly spread to other areas of the brain through the CSF and cover the cranial nerves and other intracranial structures. If this process extends into the brain parenchyma or if concurrent encephalitis is present, cerebral edema and increased ICP become more of a problem. Closely observe all patients with meningitis for manifestations of increased ICP, which is thought to be a result of swelling around the dura and increased CSF volume.

Clinical Manifestations

Fever, severe headache, nausea, vomiting, and **nuchal rigidity** (neck stiffness) are key signs of meningitis. Photophobia, a decreased LOC, and signs of increased ICP may also be present. Coma is associated with a poor prognosis and occurs in 5% to 10% of patients with bacterial meningitis. Seizures occur in one third of all cases. The headache becomes progressively worse and may be accompanied by vomiting and irritability.

If the infecting organism is a meningococcus, a skin rash is common, and petechiae may be seen on the trunk, lower extremities, and mucous membranes. A *Tumbler test* can be done by pressing the base of a drinking glass against the rash. The rash does not blanch or fade under pressure.

Complications

The most common acute complication of bacterial meningitis is increased ICP. Most patients have increased ICP, and it is the major cause of an altered mental status. Another complication of bacterial meningitis is residual neurologic dysfunction.

Dysfunction often occurs involving many cranial nerves. Cranial nerve irritation can have serious sequelae. The optic nerve (CN II) is compressed by increased ICP. Papilledema is often present, and blindness may occur. When the oculomotor (CN III), trochlear (CN IV), and abducens (CN VI) nerves are irritated, ocular movements are affected. Ptosis, unequal pupils, and diplopia are common. Irritation of the trigeminal nerve (CN V) results in sensory losses and loss of the corneal reflex. Irritation of the facial nerve (CN VII) results in facial paresis. Irritation of the vestibulocochlear nerve (CN VIII) causes tinnitus, vertigo, and deafness. The dysfunction usually disappears within a few weeks. However, hearing loss may be permanent after bacterial meningitis.

Hemiparesis, dysphasia, and hemianopsia may also occur. These signs usually resolve over time. If they do not, a cerebral abscess, subdural empyema, subdural effusion, or persistent meningitis is suspected. Acute cerebral edema may cause seizures, CN III palsy, bradycardia, hypertensive coma, and death.

Headaches may occur for months after the diagnosis of meningitis until the irritation and inflammation have completely resolved. It is important to implement pain management for chronic headaches.

A noncommunicating hydrocephalus may occur if the exudate causes adhesions that prevent the normal flow of CSF from the ventricles. CSF reabsorption by the arachnoid villi may also be obstructed by the exudate. In this situation, surgical implantation of a shunt is the only treatment.

Waterhouse-Friderichsen syndrome is a complication of meningococcal meningitis. The syndrome is manifested by petechiae, disseminated intravascular coagulation (DIC), adrenal hemorrhage, and circulatory collapse. DIC and shock, which are some of the most serious complications of meningitis, are associated with meningococcemia. (DIC is discussed in detail in Chapter 30.)

Diagnostic Studies

When a patient has manifestations suggestive of bacterial meningitis, a blood culture and CT scan should be done. Diagnosis is usually verified by doing a lumbar puncture with analysis of the CSF. A lumbar puncture should be completed only after the CT scan has ruled out an obstruction in the foramen magnum in order to prevent a fluid shift resulting in herniation.

Specimens of the CSF, sputum, and nasopharyngeal secretions are taken for culture before the start of antibiotic therapy to identify the causative organism. A Gram stain is done to detect bacteria. The predominant white blood cell type in the CSF during bacterial meningitis is neutrophils (Table 56-16).

X-rays of the skull may demonstrate infected sinuses. CT scans and MRI may be normal in uncomplicated meningitis. In other cases, CT scans may reveal evidence of increased ICP or hydrocephalus.

Interprofessional Care

Bacterial meningitis is a medical emergency. Rapid diagnosis based on history and physical examination is crucial because the patient is usually in a critical state when health care is sought. When meningitis is suspected, antibiotic therapy is begun after the collection of specimens for cultures, even before the diagnosis is confirmed (Table 56-17).

Ampicillin, penicillin, vancomycin, cefuroxime (Ceftin), cefotaxime (Claforan), ceftriaxone (Rocephin), ceftizoxime, and ceftazidime are some commonly prescribed drugs for treating bacterial meningitis. Dexamethasone (a corticosteroid) may also be prescribed before or with the first dose of antibiotics. Collaborate with the HCP to manage the headache, fever, and nuchal rigidity often associated with meningitis.

❖ NURSING MANAGEMENT: BACTERIAL MENINGITIS

◆ Nursing Assessment

Initial assessment should include vital signs, neurologic assessment, fluid intake and output, and evaluation of the lungs and skin.

TABLE 56-17 Interprofessional Care

Bacterial Meningitis

Diagnostic Assessment	Management

• History and physical examination
• Analysis of CSF (for protein, WBC, and glucose), Gram stain, and culture
• CBC, coagulation profile, electrolyte levels, glucose, platelet count
• Blood culture
• CT scan, MRI, PET scan
• Skull x-ray studies
	• Rest
	• IV fluids
	• Hypothermia
	
	Drug Therapy
	• IV antibiotics
	  • ampicillin, penicillin
	  • cephalosporin (e.g., cefotaxime [Claforan], ceftriaxone [Rocephin])
	• codeine for headache
	• dexamethasone
	• acetaminophen or aspirin for temperature >100.4° F (38° C)
	• phenytoin IV
	• mannitol (Osmitrol) IV for diuresis

CSF, Cerebrospinal fluid; *PET,* positron emission tomography.

◆ Nursing Diagnoses

Nursing diagnoses for the patient with bacterial meningitis may include, but are not limited to, the following:

• Decreased intracranial adaptive capacity *related to* decreased cerebral perfusion or increased ICP
• Risk for ineffective cerebral tissue perfusion *related to* reduction of blood flow and cerebral edema
• Hyperthermia *related to* infection
• Acute pain *related to* headache and muscle aches

Additional information on nursing diagnoses for the patient with bacterial meningitis is presented in eNursing Care Plan 56-2 (available on the website for this chapter).

Planning

The overall goals for the patient with bacterial meningitis are to (1) return to maximal neurologic functioning, (2) resolve the infection, and (3) control pain and discomfort.

◆ Nursing Implementation

◆ **Health Promotion.** Prevention of respiratory tract infections through vaccination programs for pneumococcal pneumonia and influenza is important. Meningococcal vaccines are available that protect against all serogroups of meningococcal disease that are most commonly seen in the United States, but they will not prevent all cases. Three kinds of meningococcal vaccines available in the United States include:

• Meningococcal conjugate vaccines (MCV4) (Menactra, MenHibrix, Menveo)
• Meningococcal polysaccharide vaccine (MPSV4) (Menomune)
• Serogroup B meningococcal vaccines (Bexsero and Trumenba)

Early and vigorous treatment of respiratory tract and ear infections is important. Persons who have close contact with anyone who has bacterial meningitis should be given prophylactic antibiotics.

◆ **Acute Care.** The patient with bacterial meningitis is usually acutely ill. The fever is high, and head pain is severe. Irritation of the cerebral cortex may result in seizures. The changes in mental status and LOC depend on the degree of increased ICP.

Assess and record vital signs, neurologic status, fluid intake and output, skin, and lung fields at regular intervals based on the patient's condition.

Head and neck pain secondary to movement requires attention. Codeine provides some pain relief without undue sedation for most patients. Assist the patient to a position of comfort, often curled up with the head slightly extended. The head of the bed should be slightly elevated. A darkened room and a cool cloth over the eyes relieve the discomfort of photophobia.

For the patient with delirium, additional low lighting may be necessary to decrease hallucinations. All patients suffer some degree of mental distortion and hypersensitivity, and they may be frightened and misinterpret the environment. Make every attempt to minimize environmental stimuli and prevent injury. A familiar person at the bedside may have a calming effect. Be efficient with care but also convey an attitude of caring and of unhurried gentleness. The use of touch and a soothing voice to give simple explanations of activities is helpful. If seizures occur, make appropriate observations and take protective measures. Administer antiseizure drugs such as phenytoin (Dilantin) or levetiracetam (Keppra) as ordered. Problems associated with increased ICP must be managed (see the section on increased ICP earlier in this chapter).

Fever must be vigorously treated because it increases cerebral edema and the frequency of seizures. In addition, neurologic damage may result from an extremely high temperature over a prolonged time. Acetaminophen or aspirin may be used to reduce fever. However, if the fever is resistant to aspirin or acetaminophen, more vigorous means are necessary, such as a cooling blanket. Take care not to reduce the temperature too rapidly because shivering may result, causing a rebound effect and increasing the temperature. Wrap the extremities in soft towels or a blanket covered with a sheet to reduce shivering (which can raise ICP). If a cooling blanket is not available or desirable, tepid sponge baths with water may be effective in lowering the temperature. Protect the skin from excessive drying and injury and prevent breaks in the skin.

Because high fever greatly increases the metabolic rate and thus insensible fluid loss, assess the patient for dehydration and adequacy of fluid intake. Diaphoresis further increases fluid losses, which should be noted on the output record. Calculate replacement fluids as 800 mL/day for respiratory losses and 100 mL for each degree of temperature above 100.4° F (38° C). Supplemental feeding (e.g., enteral nutrition) to maintain adequate nutritional intake may be necessary. Follow the designated antibiotic schedule to maintain therapeutic blood levels.

Meningitis generally requires respiratory isolation until the cultures are negative. Meningococcal meningitis is highly contagious, whereas other causes of meningitis may pose minimal to no infection risk with patient contact. However, standard precautions are essential to protect the patient and nurse.

◆ **Ambulatory Care.** After the acute period has passed, the patient requires several weeks of convalescence before resuming normal activities. In this period, stress the importance of adequate nutrition, with an emphasis on a high-protein, high-calorie diet in small, frequent feedings.

Muscle rigidity may persist in the neck and backs of the legs. Progressive range-of-motion exercises and warm baths are useful. Have the patient gradually increase activity as tolerated, but encourage adequate rest and sleep.

Residual effects can result in sequelae such as dementia, seizures, deafness, hemiplegia, and hydrocephalus. Assess vision, hearing, cognitive skills, and motor and sensory abilities after recovery, with appropriate referrals as indicated. Throughout the acute and convalescent periods, be aware of the anxiety and stress experienced by the caregiver and other family members.

◆ **Evaluation**

The expected outcomes are that the patient with bacterial meningitis will
- Demonstrate appropriate cognitive function
- Be oriented to person, place, and time
- Maintain body temperature within normal range
- Report satisfaction with pain control

Additional information on expected outcomes for the patient with bacterial meningitis is provided in eNursing Care Plan 56-2.

VIRAL MENINGITIS

The most common causes of viral meningitis are enteroviruses, arboviruses, human immunodeficiency virus, and herpes simplex virus (HSV). Enteroviruses are most often spread through direct contact with respiratory secretions. Viral meningitis usually manifests as a headache, fever, photophobia, and stiff neck.[24] The fever may be moderate or high.

The Xpert EV test is used to rapidly diagnose viral meningitis. A sample of CSF is used to determine if enterovirus is present, and results are available within hours of symptom onset.[26]

The CSF can be clear or cloudy, and the typical finding is lymphocytosis (Table 56-16). Organisms are not seen on Gram stain or acid-fast smears. Polymerase chain reaction (PCR) used to detect viral-specific deoxyribonucleic acid (DNA) or ribonucleic acid (RNA) is a highly sensitive method for diagnosing CNS viral infections.

Antibiotics should be administered after the lumbar puncture while awaiting the results of the CSF analysis. Antibiotics are the best defense for bacterial meningitis and can be easily discontinued if the meningitis is found to be viral.

Viral meningitis is managed symptomatically because the disease is self-limiting. Full recovery from viral meningitis is expected. Rare sequelae include persistent headaches, mild mental impairment, and incoordination.

ENCEPHALITIS

Encephalitis, an acute inflammation of the brain, is a serious, and sometimes fatal, disease. In the United States, encephalitis is responsible for about 20,000 cases and 1400 deaths annually.[27]

Encephalitis is usually caused by a virus. Many different viruses have been implicated in encephalitis. Some of the viruses are associated with certain seasons of the year and endemic to certain geographic areas.

Ticks and mosquitoes transmit epidemic encephalitis. Examples include eastern equine encephalitis, La Crosse encephalitis, St. Louis encephalitis, West Nile encephalitis, and western equine encephalitis.[27] Nonepidemic encephalitis may occur as a complication of measles, chickenpox, or mumps. HSV encephalitis is the most common cause of acute nonepidemic viral encephalitis. Cytomegalovirus encephalitis is a common complication in patients with acquired immunodeficiency syndrome (AIDS).

Clinical Manifestations and Diagnostic Studies

The onset of infection is typically nonspecific, with fever, headache, nausea, and vomiting. Encephalitis can be acute or subacute. Signs of encephalitis appear on day 2 or 3 and may vary from minimal alterations in mental status to coma. Virtually any CNS abnormality can occur, including hemiparesis, tremors, seizures, cranial nerve palsies, personality changes, memory impairment, amnesia, and dysphasia.

Early diagnosis and treatment of viral encephalitis are essential for favorable outcomes. Diagnostic findings related to viral encephalitis are shown in Table 56-16. Brain imaging techniques include CT, MRI, and PET. PCR tests allow for early detection of HSV and West Nile encephalitis. West Nile virus should be strongly considered in adults over 50 years old who develop encephalitis or meningitis in summer or early fall. The best diagnostic test for West Nile virus is a blood test that detects viral RNA. This test is also used in screening blood, organs, cells, and tissues that have been donated.

❖ NURSING AND INTERPROFESSIONAL MANAGEMENT: ENCEPHALITIS

Prevention of encephalitis requires mosquito control, including cleaning rain gutters, removing old tires, draining bird baths, and removing water where mosquitoes can breed. In addition, insect repellent should be used during mosquito season.

Interprofessional and nursing management of encephalitis, including West Nile virus infection, is symptomatic and supportive. In the initial stages of encephalitis, many patients require intensive care.

Acyclovir (Zovirax) and vidarabine (Vira-A) are used to treat encephalitis caused by HSV infection. Acyclovir has fewer side effects than vidarabine and is often the preferred treatment. Use of these antiviral agents has been shown to reduce mortality rates, although neurologic complications may not be reduced. For maximal benefit, antiviral agents should be started before the onset of coma. Treat seizure disorders with antiseizure drugs. Prophylactic treatment with antiseizure drugs may be used in severe cases of encephalitis. Treatment of cytomegalovirus encephalitis in AIDS patients is discussed in Chapter 14.

CASE STUDY

Traumatic Brain Injury

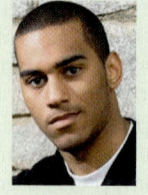
(©Comstock/ Thinkstock)

Patient Profile

C.G. is a 24-yr-old African American man who has just returned from a 15-month Army deployment to Afghanistan. He comes to the outpatient clinic with a report of chronic headaches (pain rating of 8 [0-10 point scale]) and difficulty sleeping. His wife has noticed some personality changes since his return from deployment and is concerned that he has posttraumatic stress disorder (PTSD).

Subjective Data

* Reports that he has been depressed lately but attributes it to headache and difficulty returning home.
* Headache is worse in the morning or when he lies down.
* Uses tobacco and drinks coffee throughout the day.
* Has difficulty sleeping.
* Reports "incidents" of heavy combat and blasts with a loss of consciousness. Cannot remember how many times. Unable to obtain a more through history as he becomes quite agitated.

Objective Data

* During your assessment, you note that C.G. is looking around the room and jumps when the phone rings next door.
* Loss of short-term memory (remembers one of three items).
* Heart rate ranges from 100 to 130 beats/min.
* ECG strip is shown below:

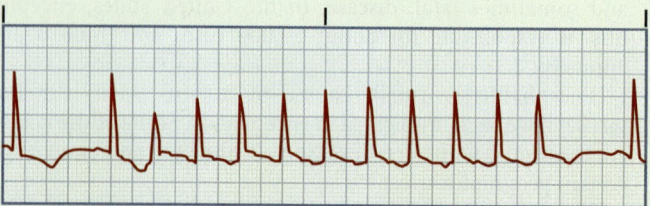

* Systolic BP ranges from 120 to 160 mm Hg.
* Right pupil, 3 mm sluggishly reactive; left pupil, 3 mm briskly reactive.

Diagnostic Studies

* CT of the head: negative for skull fracture, hematoma, or hemorrhage. Cerebral edema is noted with cingulate herniation on the right side.
* MRI performed following CT. Results indicate mild diffuse axonal injury.

Discussion Questions

1. What could be the cause of C.G.'s hypertension, tachycardia, and ECG rhythm?
2. In addition to PTSD, what do his clinical manifestations suggest?
3. *Priority Decision:* What are the priority nursing interventions that should be implemented?
4. *Teamwork and Collaboration:* How can the interprofessional team work together to meet his needs?
5. *Safety:* Are there any safety concerns for this patient or his wife?
6. *Priority Decision:* Based on the assessment data presented, what are the priority nursing diagnoses? Are there any collaborative problems?
7. *Evidence-Based Practice:* What interventions and support can help his wife?

Answers available at *http://evolve.elsevier.com/Lewis/medsurg.*

BRIDGE TO NCLEX EXAMINATION

The number of the question corresponds to the same-numbered outcome at the beginning of the chapter.

1. Vasogenic cerebral edema increases intracranial pressure by
   a. shifting fluid in the gray matter.
   b. altering the endothelial lining of cerebral capillaries.
   c. leaking molecules from the intracellular fluid to the capillaries.
   d. altering the osmotic gradient flow into the intravascular component.

2. A patient with intracranial pressure monitoring has a pressure of 12 mm Hg. The nurse understands that this pressure reflects
   a. a severe decrease in cerebral perfusion pressure.
   b. an alteration in the production of cerebrospinal fluid.
   c. the loss of autoregulatory control of intracranial pressure.
   d. a normal balance between brain tissue, blood, and cerebrospinal fluid.

3. A nurse plans care for the patient with increased intracranial pressure with the knowledge that the *best* way to position the patient is to
   a. keep the head of the bed flat.
   b. elevate the head of the bed to 30 degrees.
   c. maintain patient on the left side with the head supported on a pillow.
   d. use a continuous-rotation bed to continuously change patient position.

4. The nurse is alerted to a possible acute subdural hematoma in the patient who
   a. has a linear skull fracture crossing a major artery.
   b. has focal symptoms of brain damage with no recollection of a head injury.
   c. develops decreased level of consciousness and a headache within 48 hours of a head injury.
   d. has an immediate loss of consciousness with a brief lucid interval followed by decreasing level of consciousness.

5. During admission of a patient with a severe head injury to the emergency department, the nurse places the *highest* priority on assessment for
   a. patency of airway.
   b. presence of a neck injury.
   c. neurologic status with the Glasgow Coma Scale.
   d. cerebrospinal fluid leakage from the ears or nose.

6. A patient is suspected of having a brain tumor. The signs and symptoms include memory deficits, visual disturbances, weakness of right upper and lower extremities, and personality changes. The nurse recognizes that the tumor is *most* likely located in the
   a. frontal lobe.
   b. parietal lobe.
   c. occipital lobe.
   d. temporal lobe.

7. Nursing management of a patient with a brain tumor includes *(select all that apply)*
   a. discussing with the patient methods to control inappropriate behavior.
   b. using diversion techniques to keep the patient stimulated and motivated.
   c. assisting and supporting the family in understanding any changes in behavior.
   d. limiting self-care activities until the patient has regained maximum physical functioning.
   e. planning for seizure precautions and teaching the patient and the caregiver about antiseizure drugs.

8. The nurse on the clinical unit is assigned to four patients. Which patient should she assess *first*?
   a. Patient with a skull fracture whose nose is bleeding
   b. Older patient with a stroke who is confused and whose daughter is present
   c. Patient with meningitis who is suddenly agitated and reporting a headache of 10 on a 0-to-10 scale
   d. Patient who had a craniotomy for a brain tumor and who is now 3 days postoperative and has had continued vomiting

9. A nursing measure that is indicated to reduce the potential for seizures and increased intracranial pressure in the patient with bacterial meningitis is
   a. administering codeine for relief of head and neck pain.
   b. controlling fever with prescribed drugs and cooling techniques.
   c. keeping the room dark and quiet to minimize environmental stimulation.
   d. maintaining the patient on strict bed rest with the head of the bed slightly elevated.

1. b, 2. d, 3. b, 4. c, 5. a, 6. a, 7. c, e, 8. c, 9. b

For rationales to these answers and even more NCLEX review questions, visit *http://evolve.elsevier.com/Lewis/medsurg.*

ⓔ EVOLVE WEBSITE

http://evolve.elsevier.com/Lewis/medsurg
Review Questions (Online Only)
Key Points
Answer Keys for Questions
- Rationales for Bridge to NCLEX Examination Questions
- Answer Guidelines for Case Study on p. 1342

Student Case Studies
- Patient With Head Injury
- Patient With Meningitis

Nursing Care Plans
- eNursing Care Plan 56-1: Patient With Increased Intracranial Pressure
- eNursing Care Plan 56-2: Patient With Meningitis

Conceptual Care Map Creator
Audio Glossary
Supporting Media
- Animation
  - Parts of the Brain Controlling Body Function

Content Updates

REFERENCES

1. Cushing H: *Studies in intracranial physiology and surgery,* London, 1925, Oxford University Press. (Classic)
2. Miller C, Torbey M: *Neurocritical care monitoring,* New York, 2015, Demos Medical Publishing.
3. Seidman R: Cerebrovascular disease, Stonybrook University Medical Center. Retrieved from *www.stonybrookmedicalcenter.org/pathology/ neuropathology/chapter2.*
4. Perez-Barcena J, Llompart-Pou JA, O'Phelan KH: Intracranial pressure monitoring and management of intracranial hypertension, *Crit Care Clin* 30(4):735, 2014.
*5. Olson D, Zomorodi M, Britz G, et al: Continuous cerebral spinal fluid drainage associated with complications in patients admitted with subarachnoid hemorrhage, *J Neurosurg* 119(4):974, 2013.
6. Oddo M, Le Roux P: Brain oxygen. In Le Roux P, Levine J, Kofke W, editors: *Monitoring in neurocritical care,* Philadelphia, 2013, Saunders.
7. Stochetti N, Magnoni S, Zanier E: My paper 20 years later: cerebral venous oxygen saturation studied with bilateral samples in the internal

jugular veins, Intensive Care Medicine. Retrieved from *www.ncbi.nlm.nih.gov/pubmed/25614058*.

*8. Surani S, Lockwood G, Macias M, et al: Hypertonic saline in elevated intracranial pressure: past, present, and future, *J Intens Care Med* 30:1, 2015.

9. Wang X, Dong Y, Han X, et al: Nutritional support for patients sustaining traumatic brain injury: A systematic review and meta-analysis of prospective studies, *PLoS One* 8(3): ee58838, 2013. Retrieved from *www.ncbi.nlm.nih.gov/pmc/articles/PMC3602547*.

*10. Jalali R, Rezaei M: A comparison of the Glasgow Coma Scale Score with Full Outline of Unresponsiveness Scale to predict patients' traumatic brain injury outcomes in intensive care units, *Crit Care Res Prac* 2014 Article ID 289803. Retrieved from *www.hindawi.com/journals/ccrp/2014/289803*.

*11. Bhullar I, Johnson D, Paul J, et al: More harm than good: Antiseizure prophylaxis after traumatic brain injury does not decrease seizure rates but may inhibit functional recovery, *J Trauma Acute Care Surgery* 76(1):54, 2014.

12. Faul M, Xu L, Wald M, et al: Traumatic brain injury in the United States: emergency department visits, hospitalizations, and deaths 2002-2006, Atlanta. Centers for Disease Control and Prevention, National Center for Injury Prevention and Control. Retrieved from *www.cdc.gov/traumaticbraininjury/pdf/blue_book.pdf*.

13. Centers for Disease Control and Prevention: Traumatic brain injury in the United States fact sheet. Retrieved from *www.cdc.gov/traumaticbraininjury/get_the_facts.html*.

14. American Association of Neurological Surgeons: Traumatic brain injury: fact sheets. Retrieved from *www.aans.org/patientinformation/conditionsandtreatments/traumaticbraininjury.aspx*.

15. Lump D: Managing patients with severe traumatic brain injury, *Nursing* 44(3):30, 2014.

16. Wasserman J, Koenigsberg RA: Diffuse axonal injury. Retrieved from *http://emedicine.medscape.com/article/339912-overview*.

17. Hyatt KS: Mild traumatic brain injury, *AJN* 114:36, 2014.

18. Phan N, Hemphill J: Management of acute severe traumatic brain injury. Retrieved from *www.uptodate.com/contents/management_of_acute_traumatic_brain_injury*.

19. Bauman M, McCourt TR: Assessing and managing patients with chronic subdural hematoma, *Am Nurse Today* 9:38, 2014.

20. Chronic subdural hematoma. Retrieved from *www.nlm.nih.gov/medlineplus/ency/article/000781.html*.

*21. Waljas M, Iverson G, Lange R, et al: Return to work following mild traumatic brain injury, *J Head Trauma Rehab* 29(5):443, 2014.

22. National Cancer Institute: Brain tumor, approved by the US National Institutes of Health. Retrieved from *www.cancer.gov/cancertopics/types/brain*.

23. University of Pittsburgh: Types of brain tumors. Retrieved from *www.neurosurgery.pitt.edu/neuro_oncology/brain/types.html*.

24. Centers for Disease Control and Prevention: Meningitis questions and answers. Retrieved from *www.cdc.gov/meningitis/about/fac/html*.

25. Miller A: Fire up to beat the threat of bacterial meningitis, *Nursing* 43(12):52, 2013.

26. Nordqvist C: Rapid test approved by FDA. Retrieved from *www.medicalnewstoday.com/articles/65448.php*.

27. Venkatesan A, Tunkel A, Bloch K, et al: Case definitions, diagnostic algorithms, and priorities in encephalitis: consensus statement of the international encephalitis consortium, *Clin Infect Dis* 57(8):1114, 2013.

*Evidence-based information for clinical practice.

57

Stroke

Meg Zomorodi

If I have the belief that I can do it, I shall surely acquire the capacity to do it even if I may not have it at the beginning.

Gandhi

http://evolve.elsevier.com/Lewis/medsurg/

LEARNING OUTCOMES

1. Describe the incidence of and risk factors for stroke.
2. Explain mechanisms that affect cerebral blood flow.
3. Compare and contrast the etiology and pathophysiology of ischemic and hemorrhagic strokes.
4. Correlate the clinical manifestations of stroke with the underlying pathophysiology.
5. Identify diagnostic studies performed for patients with strokes.
6. Differentiate among the interprofessional care, drug therapy, and surgical therapy for patients with ischemic strokes and hemorrhagic strokes.
7. Describe the acute nursing management of a patient with a stroke.
8. Describe the rehabilitative nursing management of a patient with a stroke.
9. Explain the psychosocial impact of a stroke on the patient, caregiver, and family.

KEY TERMS

aneurysm, p. 1349
aphasia, p. 1351
brain attack, p. 1345
cerebrovascular accident (CVA), p. 1345
dysarthria, p. 1351

dysphasia, p. 1351
embolic stroke, p. 1349
hemorrhagic strokes, p. 1349
intracerebral hemorrhage, p. 1349
ischemic stroke, p. 1348

stroke, p. 1345
subarachnoid hemorrhage (SAH), p. 1349
thrombotic stroke, p. 1348
transient ischemic attack (TIA), p. 1347

Stroke occurs when there is (1) *ischemia* (inadequate blood flow) to a part of the brain or (2) *hemorrhage* (bleeding) into the brain that results in death of brain cells. In a stroke, functions such as movement, sensation, thinking, talking, or emotions that were controlled by the affected area of the brain are lost or impaired. The severity of the loss of function varies according to the location and extent of the brain damage.

The terms brain attack and cerebrovascular accident (CVA) are also used to describe stroke. The term *brain attack* communicates the urgency of recognizing the warning signs of a stroke and treating it as a medical emergency, as would be done with a heart attack (Table 57-1). After the onset of a stroke, immediate medical attention is crucial to decrease disability and the risk of death.

Stroke is a major public health concern. An estimated 7 million people over the age of 20 in the United States have had a stroke.[1] With an aging population, a further increase in the incidence of stroke can be expected. However, stroke can occur at any age. About 34% of strokes occur in people younger than 65 years old.[2]

Stroke is currently the fifth most common cause of death in the United States. More than 137,000 deaths occur annually from stroke.[3] While death due to stroke has been reduced, stroke is the leading cause of serious long-term disability. About 800,000 people have a stroke each year, with 15% to 30% with permanent disability.[4]

Common long-term disabilities include *hemiparesis* (partial paralysis on one side), inability to walk, complete or partial dependence for activities of daily living (ADLs), *aphasia* (dysfunction in communication), and depression. In addition to the physical, cognitive, and emotional impact of the stroke on the stroke survivor, the stroke affects the lives of the stroke victim's caregiver and family.[5] A stroke is a lifelong change for both the stroke survivor and family. Be mindful of this impact when caring for patients who survive stroke.

Reviewed by Carol Annesser, RN, MSN, BC, CNE, Assistant Professor of Nursing, Mercy College of Ohio, Toledo, Ohio; Regina Gonzalez-Lama, RN, MS, Lecturer, College of Staten Island–CUNY, Staten Island, New York; Linda Littlejohns, RN, MSN, CNRN, FAAN, Neuroscience Clinical Nurse Consultant, San Juan Capistrano, California; Molly McClelland, RN, PhD, ACNS-BC, CMSRN, Associate Professor of Nursing, College of Health Professions, University of Detroit Mercy, Detroit, Michigan; and Kathy Morrison, RN, MSN, CNRN, SCRN, Stroke Program Manager, Neuroscience Institute, Penn State Hershey Medical Center, Hershey, Pennsylvania.

TABLE 57-1 Patient & Caregiver Teaching

FAST for Warning Signs of Stroke

FAST is an easy way to remember the signs of stroke. Include the following information in the teaching plan for a patient at risk for stroke and the patient's caregiver.

F	Face drooping	Does one side of the face droop or is it numb? Ask the person to smile. Is the smile uneven?
A	Arm weakness	Is one arm weak or numb? Ask the person to raise both arms. Does one arm drift downward?
S	Speech difficulties	Is speech slurred? Is the person unable to speak or hard to understand? Ask the person to repeat a simple sentence like "The sky is blue." Is the sentence repeatedly correctly?
T	Time	Time is CRITICAL! If someone shows any of these signs (even if they go away), call 911 and get the person to the hospital. Note the time when the signs first appeared.

In addition, the following should be reported:
- Sudden trouble seeing in one or both eyes
- Sudden trouble walking, dizziness, loss of balance or coordination
- Sudden, severe headache with no known cause

Source: American Stroke Association: FAST. Retrieved from *www.strokeassociation.org/STROKEORG/WarningSigns/Stroke-Warning-Signs-and-Symptoms_UCM_308528_SubHomePage.jsp.*

PATHOPHYSIOLOGY OF STROKE

Anatomy of Cerebral Circulation

Blood is supplied to the brain by two major pairs of arteries: internal carotid arteries (anterior circulation) and vertebral arteries (posterior circulation). The carotid arteries branch to supply most of the (1) frontal, parietal, and temporal lobes; (2) basal ganglia; and (3) part of the diencephalon (thalamus and hypothalamus). The major branches of the carotid arteries are the middle cerebral and anterior cerebral arteries. The vertebral arteries join to form the basilar artery, which branches to supply the middle and lower parts of the temporal lobes, occipital lobes, cerebellum, brainstem, and part of the diencephalon. The main branch of the basilar artery is the posterior cerebral artery. The anterior and posterior cerebral circulation is connected at the *Circle of Willis* by the anterior and posterior communicating arteries (Fig. 57-1). (Fig. 55-10 illustrates the arteries at the base of the brain.) Genetic variations in this area are common, and all connecting vessels may not be present.

Regulation of Cerebral Blood Flow

The brain requires a continuous supply of blood to provide the O_2 and glucose that neurons need to function. Blood flow must be maintained at 750 to 1000 mL/min (55 mL/100 g of brain tissue), or 20% of the cardiac output, for optimal brain functioning. If blood flow to the brain is totally interrupted (e.g., cardiac arrest), neurologic metabolism is altered in 30 seconds, metabolism stops in 2 minutes, and cellular death occurs in 5 minutes.

The brain is normally well protected from changes in mean systemic arterial BP over a range from 50 to 150 mm Hg by a mechanism known as *cerebral autoregulation.* This involves changes in the diameter of cerebral blood vessels in response to changes in pressure so that the blood flow to the brain stays constant. When cerebral ischemia occurs, cerebral autoregulation may be impaired, making the brain dependent on systemic BP. CO_2 is a potent cerebral vasodilator. Changes in arterial CO_2 levels have a dramatic effect on cerebral blood flow (increased

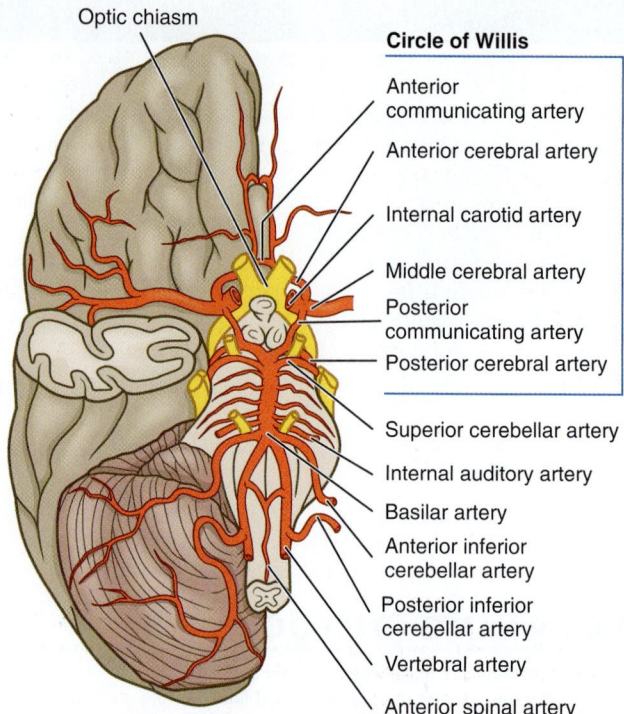

FIG. 57-1 Cerebral arteries and the circle of Willis. The top of the temporal lobe has been removed to show the course of the middle cerebral artery.

CO_2 levels increase cerebral blood flow, and decreased CO_2 levels decrease cerebral blood flow). Very low arterial O_2 levels (partial pressure of arterial O_2 less than 50 mm Hg) or increases in hydrogen ion concentration also increase cerebral blood flow.

Factors that affect blood flow to the brain include systemic BP, cardiac output, and blood viscosity. During normal activity, O_2 requirements vary considerably, but changes in cardiac output, vasomotor tone, and distribution of blood flow normally maintain adequate blood flow to the brain. Cardiac output has to be reduced by one third before cerebral blood flow is reduced. Changes in blood viscosity affect cerebral blood flow, with decreased viscosity increasing blood flow.

Collateral circulation may develop over time to compensate for a decrease in cerebral blood flow. An area of the brain can potentially receive blood supply from another blood vessel even if blood supply from the original vessel has been cut off (e.g., because of thrombosis). In other words, the vessels in the brain make an "alternate route" for blood flow to reach damaged areas, thus preventing a stroke.

Intracranial pressure (ICP) also influences cerebral blood flow. Increased ICP causes brain compression and reduced cerebral blood flow. One of your major goals when caring for a stroke patient is to reduce secondary injury related to increased ICP (see Chapter 56).

RISK FACTORS FOR STROKE

The most effective way to decrease the burden of stroke is prevention and teaching, especially about risk factors. Risk factors can be divided into nonmodifiable and modifiable. Stroke risk increases with multiple risk factors. Thus primary prevention of stroke, and reduction of these risk factors, can dramatically reduce the morbidity and mortality of stroke.[6]

Nonmodifiable Risk Factors

Nonmodifiable risk factors include age, gender, ethnicity or race, and family history or heredity. Stroke risk increases with age, doubling each decade after 55 years of age. Two thirds of all strokes occur in individuals older than 65 years, but stroke can occur at any age. Strokes are more common in men, but more women die from stroke than men. Because women tend to live longer than men, they have more opportunity to suffer a stroke.[2]

African Americans have twice the incidence of stroke and a higher death rate from stroke compared to any other ethnic group. This may be related in part to a higher incidence of hypertension, obesity, and diabetes mellitus in African Americans.[2]

⊕ CULTURAL & ETHNIC HEALTH DISPARITIES

Stroke

African Americans

- Have a higher incidence of strokes than whites.
- Have a rate of first strokes that is almost twice that of any other ethnic group.
- Are three times more likely than whites to have an ischemic stroke and four times more likely to have a hemorrhagic stroke.
- Experience increased rates of hypertension, diabetes mellitus, and sickle cell anemia, which may be related to their high incidence of strokes.
- Have a higher incidence of smoking and obesity than whites, which are two risk factors for stroke.
- Are twice as likely to die from a stroke as whites.

Other Ethnicities

- Hispanics, Native Americans, and Asian Americans have a higher incidence of strokes than whites.
- Diabetes (an important risk factor for strokes) has a high incidence among Hispanics.
- Native Americans are more likely than whites to have at least two risk factors for stroke.

Genetic risk factors are important in the development of all vascular diseases, including stroke. A person with a family history of stroke has an increased risk of having a stroke. Genes encoding products involved in lipid metabolism, thrombosis, and inflammation are believed to be potential genetic factors for stroke. Individuals who have at least two first-degree relatives with a history of subarachnoid hemorrhage or aneurysm should be screened to rule out anomalies in their cerebral vasculature.[7]

Modifiable Risk Factors

Modifiable risk factors are those that can potentially be altered through lifestyle changes and medical treatment, thus reducing the risk of stroke. Ninety percent of strokes are a result of modifiable risk factors.[7] Modifiable risk factors include hypertension, heart disease, diabetes mellitus, smoking, obesity, sleep apnea, metabolic syndrome, lack of physical exercise, poor diet, and drug and alcohol abuse.

Hypertension is the single most important modifiable risk factor, but it is still often undetected and inadequately treated. Increases in systolic and diastolic BP independently increase the risk of stroke. Stroke risk can be reduced by up to 50% with appropriate treatment of hypertension. New recommendations by the American Heart Association include home BP monitoring with a goal of SBP less than 140 mm Hg.[4,7]

Heart disease, including atrial fibrillation, myocardial infarction, cardiomyopathy, cardiac valve abnormalities, and cardiac congenital defects, is also a risk factor for stroke. Atrial fibrillation is responsible for about 25% of all strokes.[8] The incidence of atrial fibrillation increases with age. Oral anticoagulants (e.g., warfarin, dabigatran [Pradaxa]) and adherence to these medications play an important role in the prevention of stroke.[4,7]

Diabetes mellitus is a significant risk factor for stroke. The risk for stroke in people with diabetes mellitus is five times higher than in the general population.[8]

Increased serum cholesterol and smoking are risk factors for stroke. Smoking nearly doubles the risk of ischemic stroke, and smokers are four times as likely to have a hemorrhagic stroke than nonsmokers.[6] The risk associated with smoking decreases substantially over time after the smoker quits. After 5 to 10 years of no tobacco use, former smokers have the same risk of stroke as nonsmokers.

The effect of alcohol on stroke risk appears to depend on the amount consumed. Women who drink more than one alcoholic drink per day and men who drink more than two alcoholic drinks per day are at higher risk for hypertension, which increases their chance of stroke. Illicit drug use, especially cocaine use, has been associated with stroke risk.[7]

A waist circumference to hip circumference ratio equal to or above the mid-value for the population increases the risk of ischemic stroke threefold. In addition, obesity is also associated with hypertension, high blood glucose, and elevated blood lipid levels, all of which increase the risk of stroke.[6] An association of physical inactivity and increased stroke risk is present in both men and women, regardless of ethnicity. Benefits of physical activity can occur with even light to moderate regular activity. The American Stroke Association recommends 40 minutes of exercise 3 to 4 days per week in order to reduce risk of stroke.[7] Nutrition teaching is important for the individual at risk for stroke, since a diet high in fat and low in fruits and vegetables may increase stroke risk.

The early forms of birth control pills that contained high levels of progestin and estrogen increased a woman's chance of experiencing a stroke, especially if the woman also smoked heavily. Newer, low-dose oral contraceptives have lower risks for stroke except in those individuals who have hypertension and smoke.

Women who experience migraine with aura are at an increased risk for stroke. The American Heart Association recommends smoking cessation and alternatives to estrogen oral contraceptives for these women to reduce the incidence of stroke.[4,7]

Other conditions that may increase the risk for strokes include inflammatory conditions (rheumatoid arthritis), sickle cell disease, lack of exercise, and obesity.[6]

Transient Ischemic Attack

Another risk factor associated with stroke is a history of a **transient ischemic attack (TIA)**. A TIA is a transient episode of neurologic dysfunction caused by focal brain, spinal cord, or retinal ischemia, but without acute infarction of the brain. Clinical symptoms typically last less than 1 hour. In the past, TIAs were operationally defined as any focal cerebral ischemic event with symptoms lasting less than 24 hours.

However, it is important to teach the patient to seek treatment for any stroke symptoms, since there is no way to predict if a TIA will resolve or if it is in fact the development of a stroke. In general, one third of individuals who experience a TIA do not experience another event, one third have additional TIAs, and one third progress to stroke.[9]

TIAs may be due to microemboli that temporarily block the blood flow. TIAs are a warning sign of progressive cerebrovascular disease. The signs and symptoms of a TIA depend on the blood vessel that is involved and the area of the brain that is ischemic. If the carotid system is involved, patients may have a temporary loss of vision in one eye (*amaurosis fugax*), transient hemiparesis, numbness or loss of sensation, or a sudden inability to speak. Signs of a TIA involving the vertebrobasilar system may include tinnitus, vertigo, darkened or blurred vision, diplopia, ptosis, dysarthria, dysphagia, ataxia, and unilateral or bilateral numbness or weakness.

? CHECK YOUR PRACTICE

You are talking with your uncle at your family reunion. He knows that you are a nurse and seems very eager to talk with you. He tells you that earlier this morning he was having problems talking, got dizzy, and then "blanked" out for a while. He found himself just lying on the floor in his room.
- He says, "I think it is just all the excitement of the reunion, but what do you think?"

A TIA should be treated as a medical emergency as it is usually a precursor to ischemic stroke.

Teach people at risk for TIAs to seek medical attention immediately with any stroke-like symptom and to identify the time of onset of symptoms.

TYPES OF STROKE

Unlike a TIA, in which ischemia occurs without infarction, a stroke results in infarction (cell death). Strokes are classified as ischemic or hemorrhagic based on the cause and underlying pathophysiologic findings (Fig. 57-2 and Table 57-2).

Ischemic Stroke

An ischemic stroke results from inadequate blood flow to the brain from partial or complete occlusion of an artery.[10] Ischemic strokes are further divided into thrombotic and embolic strokes.

Thrombotic Stroke. A thrombotic stroke occurs from injury to a blood vessel wall and formation of a blood clot (Fig. 57-2, *A*).

The lumen of the blood vessel becomes narrowed and, if it becomes occluded, infarction occurs. Thrombosis develops readily where atherosclerotic plaques have already narrowed blood vessels. Thrombotic stroke, which is the result of thrombosis or narrowing of the blood vessel, is the most common cause of stroke, accounting for about 60% of strokes.[2] Thrombotic strokes are more common in older individuals, especially those with high cholesterol, atherosclerosis, or diabetes. A

TABLE 57-2	**Types of Stroke**	
Gender and Age	**Warning and Onset**	**Prognosis**
Ischemic		
Incidence: Accounts for 87% of strokes		
Thrombotic		
Men more than women Oldest median age	*Warning:* TIA (30%-50% of cases) *Onset:* Often during or after sleep	Stepwise progression, signs and symptoms develop slowly, usually some improvement, recurrence in 20%-25% of survivors.
Embolic		
Men more than women	*Warning:* TIA (uncommon) *Onset:* Sudden onset, most likely to occur during activity	Single event, signs and symptoms develop quickly, usually some improvement, recurrence common without aggressive treatment of underlying disease.
Hemorrhagic		
Incidence: Accounts for 13% of strokes		
Intracerebral		
Slightly higher in women	*Warning:* Headache (25% of cases) *Onset:* Activity (often)	Progression over 24 hr. Poor prognosis, fatality more likely with presence of coma.
Subarachnoid		
Slightly higher in women Youngest median age	*Warning:* Headache (common) *Onset:* Activity (often), sudden onset, most commonly related to head trauma	Usually single sudden event, fatality more likely with presence of coma.

TIA, Transient ischemic attack.

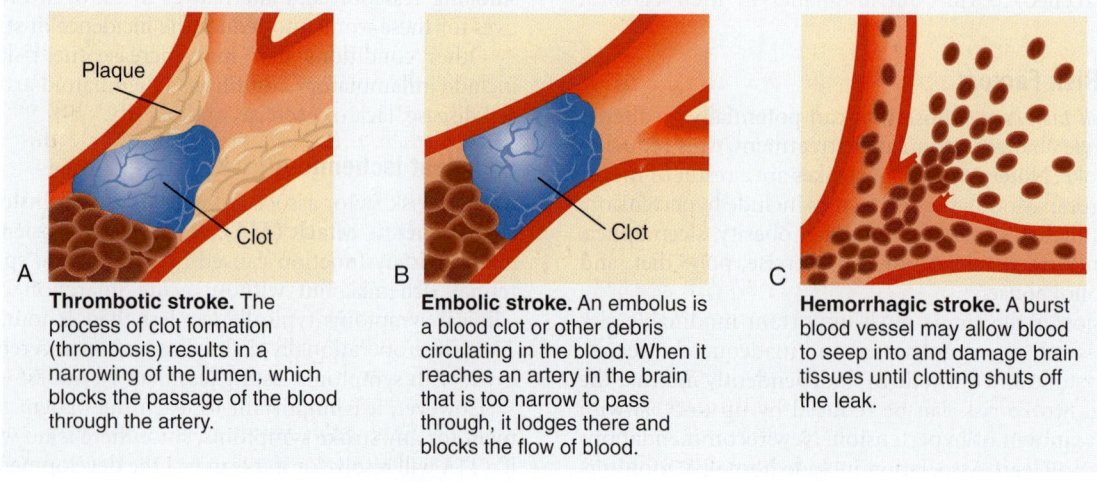

A **Thrombotic stroke.** The process of clot formation (thrombosis) results in a narrowing of the lumen, which blocks the passage of the blood through the artery.

B **Embolic stroke.** An embolus is a blood clot or other debris circulating in the blood. When it reaches an artery in the brain that is too narrow to pass through, it lodges there and blocks the flow of blood.

C **Hemorrhagic stroke.** A burst blood vessel may allow blood to seep into and damage brain tissues until clotting shuts off the leak.

FIG. 57-2 Major types of stroke.

majority of thrombotic strokes are associated with hypertension or diabetes mellitus, both of which accelerate atherosclerosis. Many times thrombotic strokes are preceded by a TIA.[8]

The extent of the stroke depends on rapidity of onset, size of the damaged area, and presence of collateral circulation. Most patients with ischemic stroke do not have a decreased level of consciousness in the first 24 hours, unless it is due to a brainstem stroke or other conditions such as seizures, increased ICP, or hemorrhage. Manifestations of ischemic stroke may progress in the first 72 hours as infarction and cerebral edema increase.

Embolic Stroke. Embolic stroke occurs when an embolus lodges in and occludes a cerebral artery, resulting in infarction and edema of the area supplied by the involved vessel (Fig. 57-2, B). Embolism is the second most common cause of stroke.[2] Most emboli originate in the endocardial (inside) layer of the heart, with plaque breaking off from the endocardium and entering the circulation. The embolus travels upward to the cerebral circulation and lodges where a vessel narrows or bifurcates (splits). Heart conditions, which account for most of embolic ischemic strokes, include atrial fibrillation, myocardial infarction, infective endocarditis, rheumatic heart disease, valvular heart prostheses, and atrial septal defects.[2] Less common causes of emboli include air and fat from long bone (e.g., femur) fractures.

The patient with an embolic stroke commonly has severe clinical manifestations that occur suddenly. Embolic strokes can affect any age group. Rheumatic heart disease is a cause of embolic stroke in young to middle-aged adults. An embolus arising from an atherosclerotic plaque is more common in older adults.

Warning signs are less common with embolic than with thrombotic stroke. The embolic stroke often occurs rapidly, giving little time to accommodate to an obstructed blood vessel with the development of collateral circulation. The patient usually remains conscious, although he or she may have a headache. The effects of the emboli are initially characterized by severe neurologic deficits, which can be temporary if the clot breaks up and allows blood to flow. Smaller emboli then continue to obstruct smaller vessels, which in turn involve smaller portions of the brain with fewer deficits noted.

The prognosis is related to the amount of brain tissue deprived of its blood supply. Recurrence of embolic stroke is common unless the underlying cause is aggressively treated.

Hemorrhagic Stroke

Hemorrhagic strokes result from bleeding into the brain tissue itself (intracerebral or intraparenchymal hemorrhage) or into the subarachnoid space or ventricles (subarachnoid hemorrhage or intraventricular hemorrhage).

Intracerebral Hemorrhage. Intracerebral hemorrhage is bleeding within the brain caused by a rupture of a vessel (usually in the basal ganglia) (Fig. 57-2, C). The prognosis of patients with intracerebral hemorrhage is poor, with the 30-day mortality rate at 40% to 80%. Fifty percent of the deaths occur within the first 48 hours.[2]

Hypertension is the most common cause of intracerebral hemorrhage (Fig. 57-3). Other causes include vascular malformations, coagulation disorders, anticoagulant and thrombolytic drugs, trauma, brain tumors, and ruptured aneurysms. Hemorrhage commonly occurs during periods of activity. Most

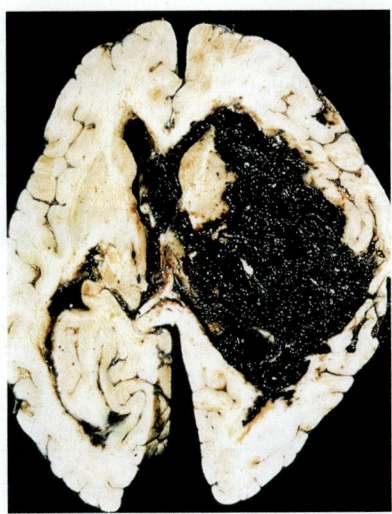

FIG. 57-3 Massive hypertensive hemorrhage rupturing into a lateral ventricle of the brain. (From Kumar V, Abbas AK, Aster JC, et al: *Robbins and Cotran pathologic basis of disease*, ed 8, Philadelphia, 2010, Saunders.)

often there is a sudden onset of symptoms, with progression over minutes to hours because of ongoing bleeding.

Manifestations include neurologic deficits, headache, nausea, vomiting, decreased level of consciousness, and hypertension. The extent of the symptoms varies depending on the amount, location, and duration of the bleeding. A blood clot within the closed skull can result in a mass that causes pressure on brain tissue, displaces brain tissue, and decreases cerebral blood flow, leading to ischemia and infarction.

Approximately half of intracerebral hemorrhages occur in the putamen and internal capsule, central white matter, thalamus, cerebellar hemispheres, and pons. Initially, patients experience a severe headache with nausea and vomiting. Clinical manifestations of putaminal and internal capsule bleeding include weakness of one side (including the face, arm, and leg), slurred speech, and deviation of the eyes. Progression of symptoms related to a severe hemorrhage includes hemiplegia, fixed and dilated pupils, abnormal body posturing, and coma. Thalamic hemorrhage results in hemiplegia with more sensory than motor loss. Bleeding into the subthalamic areas of the brain leads to problems with vision and eye movement. Cerebellar hemorrhages are characterized by severe headache, vomiting, loss of ability to walk, dysphagia, dysarthria, and eye movement disturbances.

Hemorrhage in the pons is the most serious because basic life functions (e.g., respiration) are rapidly affected. Hemorrhage in the pons can be characterized by hemiplegia leading to complete paralysis, coma, abnormal body posturing, fixed pupils (small in size), hyperthermia, and death.

Subarachnoid Hemorrhage. Subarachnoid hemorrhage (SAH) occurs when there is intracranial bleeding into the cerebrospinal fluid–filled space between the arachnoid and pia mater membranes on the surface of the brain. SAH is commonly caused by rupture of a cerebral aneurysm (congenital or acquired weakness and ballooning of vessels). Aneurysms may be saccular or berry aneurysms, ranging from a few millimeters to 20 to 30 mm in size, or fusiform atherosclerotic aneurysms. The majority of aneurysms are in the Circle of Willis. Other causes of SAH include trauma and illicit drug (cocaine) abuse. The incidence of SAH increases with age and is higher in women than men.

The patient may have warning signs and symptoms if the ballooning artery applies pressure to brain tissue, or minor warning symptoms may result from leaking of an aneurysm before major rupture. In general, cerebral aneurysms are viewed as a "silent killer," since individuals do not have warning signs or symptoms of an aneurysm until rupture has occurred.

> ### ❓ CHECK YOUR PRACTICE
>
> You are watching your husband's "for fun" soccer game. He leaves the game and is kneeling on the ground. When you try to assess what is going on he says, "I've got a terrible headache. It just started." Knowing that he sometimes gets headaches when he is stressed, you ask him if he is feeling stressed. He almost screams back at you, "NO! This is the worst headache of my life!"
> • What should you do?

Loss of consciousness may or may not occur. The patient's level of consciousness may range from alert to comatose, depending on the severity of the bleed. Other manifestations include focal neurologic deficits (including cranial nerve deficits), nausea, vomiting, seizures, and stiff neck.

Complications of aneurysmal SAH include rebleeding before surgery or other therapy is initiated and cerebral vasospasm (narrowing of the blood vessels), which can result in cerebral infarction. Cerebral vasospasm is most likely due to an interaction between the metabolites of blood and the vascular smooth muscle. This occurs when the subarachnoid blood clots break down or dissolve, releasing metabolites that can cause endothelial damage and vasoconstriction. In addition, release of endothelin (a potent vasoconstrictor) may play a major role in the induction of cerebral vasospasm after SAH. Patients with SAH who are at risk for vasospasm are often kept in the intensive care unit (up to 14 days) until the threat of vasospasm is reduced. Peak time for vasospasm occurs 6 to 10 days after the initial bleed.

Despite improvements in surgical techniques and management, many patients with SAH die. Some die almost immediately when a rupture occurs. Others die from subsequent bleeding. Survivors may be left with significant morbidity, including cognitive difficulties.

CLINICAL MANIFESTATIONS OF STROKE

Neurologic manifestations do not significantly differ between ischemic and hemorrhagic stroke. The reason for this is that destruction of neural tissue is the basis for neurologic dysfunction caused by both types of stroke. The clinical manifestations are related to the location of the stroke. Specific manifestations related to the type of stroke are discussed in the previous section. The general clinical manifestations of ischemic and hemorrhagic stroke are discussed together here.

A stroke can affect many body functions, including motor activity, bladder and bowel elimination, intellectual function, spatial-perceptual alterations, personality, affect, sensation, swallowing, and communication. The functions affected are directly related to the artery involved and area of the brain that it supplies (Table 57-3). Manifestations related to right- and left-brain damage differ somewhat and are shown in Fig. 57-4.

An additional assessment question that you need to ask is the time of the onset of symptoms. This is important for all types of stroke, especially ischemic strokes, since the time can affect treatment decisions.

Motor Function

Motor deficits are the most obvious effect of stroke. Motor deficits include impairment of (1) mobility, (2) respiratory function, (3) swallowing and speech, (4) gag reflex, and (5) self-care abilities. Symptoms are caused by the destruction of motor neurons in the pyramidal pathway (nerve fibers from the brain that pass through the spinal cord to the motor cells). The characteristic motor deficits include loss of skilled voluntary movement *(akinesia)*, impairment of integration of movements, alterations in muscle tone, and alterations in reflexes. The initial *hyporeflexia* (depressed reflexes) progresses to *hyperreflexia* (hyperactive reflexes) for most patients.

Motor deficits after a stroke follow certain specific patterns. Because the pyramidal pathway crosses at the level of the medulla, a lesion on one side of the brain affects motor function

TABLE 57-3   Stroke Manifestations Related to Artery Involvement

Artery	Manifestations
Anterior cerebral	Motor and/or sensory deficit (contralateral), sucking or rooting reflex, rigidity, gait problems, loss of proprioception and fine touch
Middle cerebral	*Dominant side:* Aphasia, motor and sensory deficit, hemianopsia
	Nondominant side: Neglect, motor and sensory deficit, hemianopsia
Posterior cerebral	Hemianopsia, visual hallucination, spontaneous pain, motor deficit
Vertebral	Cranial nerve deficits, diplopia, dizziness, nausea, vomiting, dysarthria, dysphagia, and/or coma

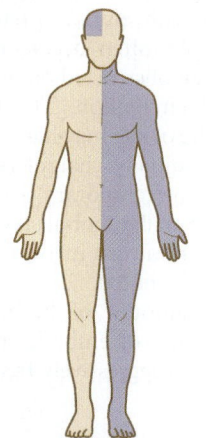
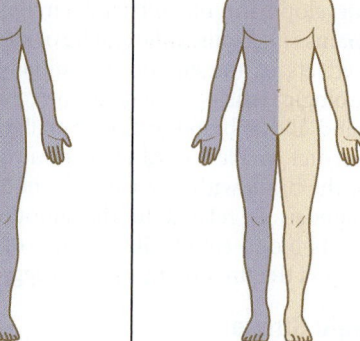

Right-brain damage (stroke on right side of the brain)	**Left-brain damage** (stroke on left side of the brain)
• Paralyzed left side: hemiplegia	• Paralyzed right side: hemiplegia
• Left-sided neglect	• Impaired speech/language aphasias
• Spatial-perceptual deficits	• Impaired right/left discrimination
• Tends to deny or minimize problems	• Slow performance, cautious
• Rapid performance, short attention span	• Aware of deficits: depression, anxiety
• Impulsive, safety problems	• Impaired comprehension related to language, math
• Impaired judgment	
• Impaired time concepts	

FIG. 57-4   Manifestations of right-brain and left-brain stroke.

on the opposite side of the body (contralateral). The arms and legs of the affected side may be weakened or paralyzed to different degrees depending on which part of and to what extent the cerebral circulation was compromised. A stroke affecting the middle cerebral artery leads to a greater weakness in the upper extremity than the lower extremity. The affected shoulder tends to rotate internally, and the hip rotates externally. The affected foot is plantar flexed and inverted. An initial period of flaccidity may last from days to several weeks and is related to nerve damage. Spasticity of the muscles, which follows the flaccid stage, is related to interruption of upper motor neuron influence.

Communication

The left hemisphere is dominant for language skills in right-handed persons and in most left-handed persons.[10] Language disorders involve expression and comprehension of written and spoken words. The patient may experience aphasia, which may be *receptive aphasia* (loss of comprehension), *expressive aphasia* (inability to produce language), or *global aphasia* (total inability to communicate). Aphasia occurs when a stroke damages the dominant hemisphere of the brain.

Dysphasia refers to impaired ability to communicate. However, in most settings the terms *aphasia* and *dysphasia* are used interchangeably, with aphasia often being the more common term used. (Dysphasia should not be confused with the similarly pronounced *dysphagia*, which is difficulty swallowing.)

Patterns of aphasia may differ, since the stroke affects different portions of the brain. Aphasia may be classified as *nonfluent* (minimal speech activity with slow speech that requires obvious effort) or *fluent* (speech is present but contains little meaningful communication) (Table 57-4). Most types of aphasia are mixed, with impairment in both expression and understanding. A massive stroke may result in global aphasia.

Many stroke patients also experience dysarthria, a disturbance in the muscular control of speech. Impairment may involve pronunciation, articulation, and phonation. Dysarthria does not affect the meaning of communication or the comprehension of language, but it does affect the mechanics of speech. Some patients experience a combination of aphasia and dysarthria.

Affect

Patients who have had a stroke may have difficulty controlling their emotions. Emotional responses may be exaggerated or unpredictable. Depression and feelings associated with changes in body image and loss of function can make this worse.[11] Patients may also be frustrated by mobility and communication problems.

CHECK YOUR PRACTICE

You are working in the outpatient stroke clinic and counseling with the family of one of your favorite patients. He is a well-respected 65-yr-old business man who has returned home following a stroke. His family tells you that during meals he becomes frustrated and begins to cry because of the difficulty getting food into his mouth and chewing. They tell you that this is something that he was able to do easily before his stroke. His family cannot understand why a previously very competent man is so emotional.
- How should you counsel the family and what teaching is needed?

TABLE 57-4   Types of Aphasia

Type	Characteristics
Broca's	• Type of nonfluent aphasia. • Damage to frontal lobe of brain. • Frequently speak in short phrases that make sense but are produced with great effort. • Often omit small words such as "is," "and," and "the." • May say, "Walk dog," meaning, "I will take the dog for a walk," or "book book two table," for "There are two books on the table." • Typically understand speech of others fairly well. • Often aware of their difficulties and can become easily frustrated.
Wernicke's	• Type of fluent aphasia. • Damage occurs in left temporal lobe, although it can result from damage to right lobe. • May speak in long sentences that have no meaning, add unnecessary words, and even create made-up words. • May say, "You know that smoodle pinkered and that I want to get him round and take care of him like you want before." • Often difficult to follow what person is trying to say. • Usually have great difficulty understanding speech. • Often unaware of their mistakes.
Global	• Type of nonfluent aphasia. • Results from damage to extensive portions of language areas of brain. • Have severe communication difficulties. • May be extremely limited in ability to speak or comprehend language.
Other	• Results from damage to different language areas in brain. • Some patients may have difficulty repeating words and sentences, even though they can speak and they understand the meaning of the word or sentence. • Other patients may have difficulty naming objects, even though they know what the object is and what its use is.

Intellectual Function

Both memory and judgment may be impaired as a result of stroke. These impairments can occur with strokes affecting either side of the brain. A left-brain stroke is more likely to result in memory problems related to language. Patients with a left-brain stroke often are cautious in making judgments. The patient with a right-brain stroke tends to be impulsive and to move quickly.

An example of behavior in people with right-brain stroke is that they try to rise quickly from a wheelchair without locking the wheels or raising the footrests. On the other hand, people with a left-brain stroke would move slowly and cautiously from the wheelchair. Patients with either type of stroke may have difficulty making generalizations, which interferes with their ability to learn.

Spatial-Perceptual Alterations

Individuals who have had a stroke on the right side of the brain are more likely to have problems with spatial-perceptual orientation. However, this can also occur in people with left-brain stroke.

Spatial-perceptual problems may be divided into four categories.

- The first is the result of damage of the parietal lobe and causes the patient to have an incorrect perception of self and illness. In this situation, patients may deny their illnesses or not recognize their own body parts.
- The second category occurs when the patient neglects all input from the affected side (erroneous perception of self in space). This may be worsened by *homonymous hemianopsia*, in which blindness occurs in the same half of the visual fields of both eyes. The patient also has difficulty with spatial orientation, such as judging distances.
- The third spatial-perceptual deficit is *agnosia*, the inability to recognize an object by sight, touch, or hearing.
- The fourth deficit is *apraxia*, the inability to carry out learned sequential movements on command. Because patients may or may not be aware of their spatial-perceptual alterations, you need to assess for this potential problem, since it will affect rehabilitation and recovery.

Elimination

Most problems with urinary and bowel elimination occur initially and are temporary. When a stroke affects one hemisphere of the brain, the prognosis for normal bladder function is excellent. At least partial sensation for bladder filling remains, and voluntary urination is present. Initially, the patient may experience frequency, urgency, and incontinence. Although motor control of the bowel is usually not a problem, patients are frequently constipated. Constipation is associated with immobility, weak abdominal muscles, dehydration, and diminished response to the defecation reflex. Urinary and bowel elimination problems may also be related to inability to verbalize the need to eliminate and difficulty with managing clothing (resulting in incontinence). Scheduled toileting and clothes that are easily removed may encourage independence.

DIAGNOSTIC STUDIES FOR STROKE

When manifestations of a stroke occur, diagnostic studies (Table 57-5) are done to (1) confirm that it is a stroke and not another type of brain lesion and (2) identify the likely cause of the stroke. Diagnostic study results also guide decisions about therapy.

Important diagnostic tools for patients who have experienced a stroke are an MRI or noncontrast CT scan.[12] These tests can rapidly distinguish between ischemic and hemorrhagic stroke and help determine the size and location of the stroke. Serial scans may be used to assess the effectiveness of treatment and to evaluate recovery. Once the individual suspected of TIA or stroke arrives in the emergency department, it is important to rapidly assess and diagnose the patient (usually through a noncontrast head CT or MRI). Rapid access to these diagnostic tools is important, since the results will determine treatment options for the patient. MRI is more effective in identifying ischemic stroke than CT scans. However, a CT scan is a rapid diagnostic tool to rule out hemorrhage.[12]

CT angiography (CTA) provides visualization of cerebral blood vessels. It can be performed after or at the same time as the noncontrast CT scan. CTA can provide an estimate of perfusion and detect filling defects in the cerebral arteries. Magnetic resonance angiography (MRA) can detect vascular lesions and blockages, similar to CTA. CT/MRI perfusion and diffusion imaging may also be done.

TABLE 57-5 **Diagnostic Studies**	
Stroke	

Diagnosis of Stroke (Including Extent of Involvement)	**Cardiac Assessment**
• CT scan • CT angiography (CTA) • MRI • Magnetic resonance angiography (MRA) • CT/MRI perfusion and diffusion imaging	• Electrocardiogram • Chest x-ray • Cardiac markers (troponin, creatine kinase-MB) • Echocardiography (transthoracic, transesophageal)
Cerebral Blood Flow	**Additional Studies**
• Cerebral angiography • Carotid angiography • Digital subtraction angiography • Transcranial Doppler ultrasonography • Carotid duplex scanning	• Complete blood count (including platelets) and glucose • Coagulation studies: prothrombin time, activated partial thromboplastin time • Electrolytes, blood glucose • Renal and hepatic studies • Lipid profile • Cerebrospinal fluid analysis*

*A lumbar puncture to obtain cerebrospinal fluid is avoided if increased intracranial pressure is suspected.

Cardiac imaging is also recommended because many strokes are caused by blood clots from the heart. Angiography can identify cervical and cerebrovascular occlusion, atherosclerotic plaques, and malformation of vessels. Cerebral angiography is a definitive study to identify the source of SAH. Risks of angiography include dislodging an embolus, causing vasospasm, inducing further hemorrhage, and provoking an allergic reaction to contrast media.

Intraarterial digital subtraction angiography (DSA) reduces the dose of contrast material, uses smaller catheters, and shortens the length of the procedure compared with conventional angiography. DSA involves the injection of a contrast agent to visualize blood vessels in the neck and the large vessels of the Circle of Willis. It is considered safer than cerebral angiography because less vascular manipulation is required.

Transcranial Doppler (TCD) ultrasonography is a noninvasive study that measures the velocity of blood flow in the major cerebral arteries. TCD is effective in detecting microemboli and vasospasm and is ideal for the patient suspected of having an SAH. Carotid duplex scanning is used not only to detect the cause of the stroke but also to stratify patients for either medical management or carotid intervention if they have carotid stenoses.

A lumbar puncture may be done to look for evidence of red blood cells in the cerebrospinal fluid if an SAH is suspected but the CT does not show hemorrhage. A lumbar puncture is avoided if the patient is suspected of having an obstruction in the foramen magnum or other signs of increased ICP because of the danger of herniation of the brain downward, leading to pressure on cardiac and respiratory centers in the brainstem and potentially death.

If the suspected cause of the stroke includes emboli from the heart, diagnostic cardiac tests should be done. Blood tests are also done to help identify conditions contributing to stroke and to guide treatment (Table 57-5).

The LICOX system may be used as a diagnostic tool to evaluate the progression of stroke. LICOX measures brain oxygenation and temperature (see discussion in Chapter 56 on pp. 1321-1322 and Fig. 56-10). Secondary brain injury adds significantly to mortality risk and poor functional outcome after a stroke.

INTERPROFESSIONAL CARE FOR STROKE

Preventive Therapy

Primary prevention is a priority for decreasing morbidity and mortality risk from stroke (Table 57-6). The goals of stroke prevention include health promotion for a healthy lifestyle and management of modifiable risk factors to prevent a stroke. Health promotion focuses on (1) healthy diet, (2) weight control, (3) regular exercise, (4) no smoking, (5) limiting alcohol consumption, (6) BP management, and (7) routine health assessments. Patients with known risk factors such as diabetes mellitus, hypertension, obesity, high serum lipids, or cardiac dysfunction require close management.

 HEALTHY PEOPLE

Prevention of Stroke

- Reduce salt and sodium intake.
- Maintain a normal body weight.
- Maintain a normal BP.
- Increase level of physical exercise.
- Avoid cigarette smoking or tobacco products.
- Limit consumption of alcohol to moderate levels.
- Follow a diet that is low in saturated fat, total fat, and dietary cholesterol and high in fruits and vegetables (e.g., Mediterranean diet).

Preventive Drug Therapy. Measures to prevent the development of a thrombus or an embolus are used in patients with TIAs, since they are at high risk for stroke. Antiplatelet drugs are usually the chosen treatment to prevent stroke in patients who have had a TIA. Aspirin is the most frequently used antiplatelet agent, commonly at a dose of 81 to 325 mg/day. Other drugs include ticlopidine, clopidogrel (Plavix), dipyridamole (Persantine), and combined dipyridamole and aspirin (Aggrenox).

 DRUG ALERT Ticlopidine and Clopidogrel (Plavix)
- All HCPs and dentists must be informed that the drug is being taken, especially before scheduling surgery or major dental procedures.
- Drug may have to be discontinued 10 to 14 days before surgery if antiplatelet effect is not desired.

For patients who have atrial fibrillation, oral anticoagulation can include warfarin (Coumadin) and the direct factor Xa inhibitors: rivaroxaban (Xarelto), dabigatran (Pradaxa), and apixaban (Eliquis). The primary advantage of direct factor Xa inhibitors (compared to warfarin) is that these drugs do not need close monitoring or dosage adjustments. Statins (simvastatin [Zocor], lovastatin) have also been shown to be effective in the prevention of stroke for individuals who have experienced a TIA in the past.[9]

Left Atrial Appendage Occlusion. The left atrial appendage (LAA) is a pouch that extends off the left atrium. The LAA is believed to be the source of a majority of stroke-causing emboli in patients with atrial fibrillation. LAA occlusion is a treatment strategy to prevent blood clot formation in patients who have atrial fibrillation. By removing or occluding the LAA, the incidence of strokes can be decreased.

A special stapler can be used to remove the LAA or sutures can be used to manually occlude the LAA. In addition, LAA occlusion

 TABLE 57-6 Interprofessional Care

Stroke

Diagnostic Assessment
- History and physical examination
- Diagnostic studies (Table 57-5)

Management

Prevention
- Control of hypertension
- Control of diabetes mellitus
- Treatment of underlying cardiac problem
- No smoking
- Limiting alcohol intake

Drug Therapy
- Platelet inhibitors (e.g., aspirin)
- Anticoagulation therapy for patients with atrial fibrillation

Surgical Therapy
- Carotid endarterectomy
- Stenting of carotid artery
- Transluminal angioplasty
- Surgical interventions for aneurysms at risk of bleeding

Acute Care
- Maintenance of airway
- Fluid therapy
- Treatment of cerebral edema
- Prevention of secondary injury

Ischemic Stroke
- Tissue plasminogen activator (tPA) IV or intraarterial
- Endovascular therapy

Hemorrhagic Stroke
- Surgical decompression if indicated
- Clipping or coiling of aneurysm

Rehabilitation
- Focus on helping patient achieve independence and functional recovery

devices (e.g., AtriClip, Watchman) are available. These devices are positioned around the LAA and then closed, similar to a clamp that is used to shut off the blood supply. This prevents blood from flowing into and out of the LAA. LAA occlusion can be used as an alternative for patients who cannot use oral anticoagulants such as warfarin. This procedure may reduce the risk of stroke, and patients may be able to stop taking anticoagulants.

Surgical/Endovascular Therapy for TIA and Stroke Prevention. Surgical interventions for the patient with TIAs due to carotid disease include carotid endarterectomy, transluminal angioplasty, and stenting. In a *carotid endarterectomy* (CEA), the atheromatous lesion is removed from the carotid artery to improve blood flow.[13]

Transluminal angioplasty is the insertion of a balloon to open a stenosed artery in the brain and improve blood flow. The balloon is threaded up to the carotid artery via a catheter inserted in the femoral artery.

Stenting involves intravascular placement of a stent in an attempt to maintain patency of the artery (Fig. 57-5). The stent can be inserted during an angioplasty. Once in place, the system can be used with a tiny filter that opens like an umbrella. The filter catches and removes the debris that is stirred up during the stenting procedure before it floats to the brain, where it can trigger a stroke. Stenting is a less invasive strategy for revascularization in patients unable to withstand the CEA because of coexisting medical conditions.

Postoperative nursing care for these patients consists of neurovascular assessment, BP management, assessment of stent occlusion or retroperitoneal hemorrhage as complications, and minimization of complications at the insertion site by keeping the patient's leg straight for the prescribed time.

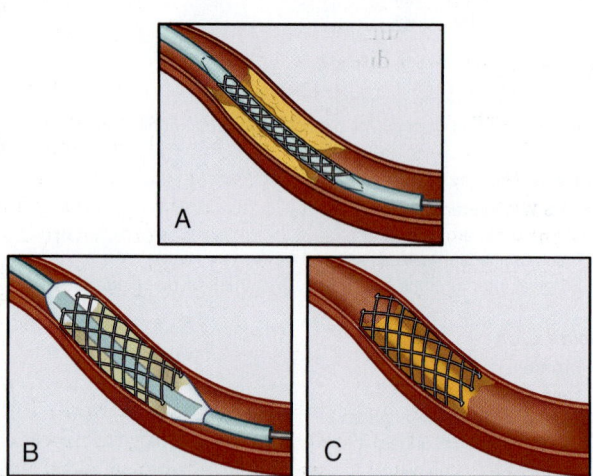

FIG. 57-5 Brain stent used to treat blockages in cerebral blood flow. **A,** A balloon catheter is used to implant the stent into an artery of the brain. **B,** The balloon catheter is moved to the blocked area of the artery and then inflated. The stent expands due to inflation of the balloon. **C,** The balloon is deflated and withdrawn, leaving the stent permanently in place holding the artery open and improving the flow of blood.

Acute Care for Ischemic Stroke

During initial evaluation, the single most important point in the patient's history is the time of onset of symptoms. Interprofessional goals during the acute phase are preserving life, preventing further brain damage, and reducing disability.

Table 57-7 outlines the emergency management of the patient with a stroke. In the unresponsive person, acute care begins with assessing circulation, airway, and breathing. Patients may have difficulty keeping an open and clear airway because of a decreased level of consciousness or decreased or absent gag and swallowing reflexes. Maintaining adequate oxygenation is important. O_2 administration, artificial airway insertion, intubation, and mechanical ventilation may be required. Baseline neurologic assessment is carried out, and patients are monitored closely for signs of increasing neurologic deficit. Many patients may worsen in the first 24 to 48 hours.

For emergency care, patients should be transported to the closest certified stroke center or, when such an institution is not available, the closest facility offering emergency stroke care. The American Heart Association recommends that acute care facilities have stroke teams in place. The stroke team generally consists of a registered nurse, neurologist, radiologist, and radiologic technician.[13]

Elevated BP is common immediately after a stroke and may be a protective response to maintain cerebral perfusion. However, it can also be detrimental. Immediately after an ischemic stroke in those patients who do not receive fibrinolytic therapy (discussed later), the use of drugs to lower BP is recommended only if BP is markedly increased (systolic BP greater than 220 mm Hg or diastolic greater than 120 mm Hg). In a patient who is going to have fibrinolytic therapy, the BP must be less than 185/110 mm Hg and then maintained at or below 180/105 mm Hg for at least 24 hours after fibrinolytic therapy. In an acute stroke, IV antihypertensives such as labetalol and

✚ TABLE 57-7   Emergency Management

Stroke

Etiology	Assessment Findings	Interventions
• Sudden vascular compromise causing disruption of blood flow to brain • Thrombosis • Trauma • Aneurysm • Embolism • Hemorrhage • Arteriovenous malformation	• Altered level of consciousness • Weakness, numbness, or paralysis of portion of body • Speech or visual disturbances • Severe headache • Heart rate ↑ or ↓ • Respiratory distress • Unequal pupils • Hypertension • Facial drooping on affected side • Difficulty swallowing • Seizures • Bladder or bowel incontinence • Nausea and vomiting • Vertigo	**Initial** • If unresponsive, assess circulation, airway, and breathing. • If responsive, monitor airway, breathing, and circulation. • Call stroke code or stroke team. • Remove dentures. • Perform pulse oximetry. • Maintain adequate oxygenation (SaO_2 >95%) with supplemental O_2, if necessary. • Establish IV access with normal saline. • Maintain BP according to guidelines (e.g., Cardiac Life Support).* • Remove clothing. • Obtain CT scan or MRI immediately. • Perform baseline laboratory tests (including blood glucose) immediately, and treat if hypoglycemic. • Position head in midline. • Elevate head of bed 30 degrees if no symptoms of shock or injury. • Institute seizure precautions. • Anticipate thrombolytic therapy for ischemic stroke. • Keep patient NPO until swallow reflex evaluated. **Ongoing Monitoring** • Monitor vital signs and neurologic status, including level of consciousness (NIH Stroke Scale), motor and sensory function, pupil size and reactivity, SaO_2, and cardiac rhythm. • Reassure patient and family.

NIH, National Institutes of Health; *SaO₂,* arterial O_2 saturation.
*See Appendix A.

nicardipine (Cardene) are preferred. Although low BP immediately after a stroke is uncommon, hypotension and hypovolemia should be corrected if present.

Fluid and electrolyte balance must be controlled carefully. Generally the goal is to keep the patient adequately hydrated to promote perfusion and decrease further brain injury. Overhydration may compromise perfusion by increasing cerebral edema. Adequate fluid intake during acute care via oral, IV, or tube feedings is a priority. Also monitor urine output to make sure the patient does not become dehydrated.

If secretion of antidiuretic hormone (ADH) increases in response to the stroke, urine output decreases and fluid is retained. Low serum sodium (hyponatremia) may occur. IV solutions with glucose and water are avoided because they are hypotonic and may further increase cerebral edema and ICP. Glycemic control should be maintained to avoid extreme hypo- or hyperglycemia. In general, decisions regarding individualized fluid and electrolyte replacement therapy are based on the extent of intracranial edema, manifestations of increased ICP, central venous pressure levels, electrolyte levels, and intake and output.

Increased ICP is more likely to occur with hemorrhagic strokes but can occur with ischemic strokes. Increased ICP from cerebral edema usually peaks in 72 hours and may cause brain herniation. Management of increased ICP includes practices that improve venous drainage, such as elevating the head of the bed, maintaining head and neck in alignment, and avoiding hip flexion. Additional measures for reducing ICP include management of hyperthermia (goal temperature of 96.8° to 98.6° F [36° to 37° C]), drug therapy to prevent seizures, pain management, avoidance of hypervolemia, and management of constipation. Cerebrospinal fluid drainage may be used in some patients to reduce ICP. (The specific management of increased ICP is discussed in Chapter 56.)

Drug Therapy for Ischemic Stroke. Fibrinolytic therapy should not be delayed. Recombinant tissue plasminogen activator (tPA) is used to produce localized fibrinolysis by binding to the fibrin in the thrombi. The fibrinolytic action of tPA occurs as the plasminogen is converted to plasmin, whose enzymatic action then digests fibrin and fibrinogen, thus breaking down the clot. Other fibrinolytic agents cannot be substituted for tPA. (Fibrinolytic [thrombolytic] therapy is discussed in Chapter 33.)

tPA is administered IV to reestablish blood flow through a blocked artery to prevent cell death in patients with the acute onset of ischemic stroke. tPA must be administered within 3 to 4½ hours of the onset of clinical signs of ischemic stroke.[9] Patients are screened carefully before tPA can be given. Screening includes a noncontrast CT scan or MRI to rule out hemorrhagic stroke; blood tests for glucose level and coagulation disorders; screening for recent history of gastrointestinal bleeding, stroke, or head trauma within the past 3 months; major surgery within 14 days; or recent active internal bleeding within 22 days.[14]

During infusion of the drug, closely monitor the patient's vital signs and neurologic status to assess for improvement or for potential deterioration related to intracerebral hemorrhage. Control of BP (SBP less than 185 mm Hg) is critical during treatment and for 24 hours following.

Intraarterial infusion of tPA may also be used for patients with an ischemic stroke when mechanical thrombectomy is not an option. To be effective, intraarterial tPA must be administered within 6 hours of the onset of stroke symptoms.

In the intraarterial tPA procedure, the neurovascular specialist inserts a thin, flexible catheter into an artery (usually the femoral artery) and guides the catheter (using angiogram) to the area of the clot. The tPA is administered through the catheter and immediately targets the clot. Less tPA is needed when it is delivered directly to the clot, which can reduce the possibility of intracranial hemorrhage.[15]

The use of anticoagulants (e.g., heparin) in the emergency phase after an ischemic stroke is generally not recommended because of the risk for intracranial hemorrhage. Acetylsalicylic acid (aspirin) at a dose of 325 mg may be initiated within 24 to 48 hours after the onset of an ischemic stroke. Complications of aspirin (with higher doses) include gastrointestinal bleeding. Aspirin should be administered cautiously if the patient has a history of peptic ulcer disease.

After the patient has stabilized and to prevent further clot formation, patients with strokes caused by thrombi and emboli may be treated with anticoagulants and platelet inhibitors (see discussion on prevention of stroke on pp. 1353-1354). For patients who have atrial fibrillation, oral anticoagulants include warfarin and the direct factor Xa inhibitors: rivaroxaban (Xarelto), dabigatran (Pradaxa), and apixaban (Eliquis). Platelet inhibitors include aspirin, ticlopidine, clopidogrel, and dipyridamole. Additionally, the use of statins has been shown to be effective for the patient with an ischemic stroke.[7]

Endovascular Therapy for Ischemic Stroke. Stent retrievers (e.g., Solitaire FR) are a way of opening blocked arteries in the brain by using a removable stent system.[16] During the procedure, a catheter is used to guide the small stent from the femoral artery in the groin area to the affected artery in the brain. The stent is guided (using neuroimaging) into the part of the artery where a blood clot has formed. The stent expands the interior walls of the artery and allows blood to get to the patient's brain immediately to prevent as much brain damage as possible. The clot seeps into the mesh of the stent. Then, after a few minutes the stent and clot are removed together. Stent retrievers are becoming the most effective way of managing ischemic stroke.[16,17]

The ENROUTE device accesses the carotid arteries through the neck, rather than the groin. The ENROUTE uses a blood flow reversal system to capture pieces of the blockage dislodged during stenting procedures, while also maintaining blood flow to the brain.[18]

Acute Care for Hemorrhagic Stroke

Drug Therapy for Hemorrhagic Stroke. Anticoagulants and platelet inhibitors are contraindicated in patients with hemorrhagic strokes. The main drug therapy for patients with hemorrhagic stroke is the management of hypertension. Oral and IV agents may be used to maintain BP within a normal to high-normal range (systolic BP less than 160 mm Hg). Seizure prophylaxis in the acute period after intracerebral and subarachnoid hemorrhages is situation specific and should be discussed with the interprofessional care team.[19]

Surgical Therapy for Hemorrhagic Stroke. Surgical interventions for hemorrhagic stroke include immediate evacuation of aneurysm-induced hematomas or cerebellar hematomas larger than 3 cm. Individuals who have an arteriovenous malformation (AVM) may experience a hemorrhagic stroke if the AVM ruptures. The treatment of AVM is surgical resection and/or radiosurgery (i.e., gamma knife). Both may be preceded by interventional neuroradiology to embolize the blood vessels that supply the AVM.

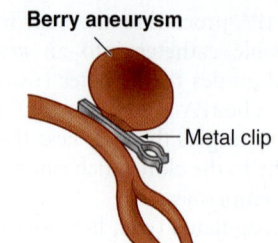

FIG. 57-6   Clipping of aneurysms.

In a subarachnoid hemorrhage, bleeding from a damaged vessel causes blood to accumulate between the brain and skull. The leaked blood can irritate, damage, or destroy the surrounding brain cells. When blood enters the subarachnoid space, it mixes with the cerebrospinal fluid (CSF). This can block CSF circulation, thus causing increased pressure on the brain. The open spaces in the brain (ventricles) may enlarge, resulting in hydrocephalus. This further increases ICP (due to the large accumulation of blood) and can result in further brain injury. Insertion of a ventriculostomy for CSF drainage can dramatically improve these situations by reducing the ICP.[20] Goals for managing ICP are the same for patients with SAH as they are for patients dealing with acute stroke. (The management of ICP is discussed in Chapter 56.)

SAH is usually caused by a ruptured aneurysm. Patients may have multiple aneurysms. Treatment of an aneurysm involves clipping or coiling the aneurysm to prevent rebleeding (Figs. 57-6 and 57-7). In *clipping* the aneurysm, the neurosurgeon places a metallic clip on the neck of the aneurysm to block blood flow and prevent rupture. The clip remains in place for life.

In the procedure known as *coiling*, a hydrogel-coated platinum coil is inserted into the lumen of the aneurysm via interventional neuroradiology (Fig. 57-7). Guglielmi detachable coils (GDCs) provide immediate protection against hemorrhage by reducing the blood pulsations within the aneurysm. Eventually, a thrombus forms within the aneurysm. Then the aneurysm becomes sealed off from the parent vessel by the formation of an endothelialized layer of connective tissue.

After aneurysmal occlusion via clipping or coiling, hyperdynamic therapy (hemodilution-induced hypertension using vasoconstricting agents such as phenylephrine or dopamine and hypervolemia) may be instituted in an effort to increase the mean arterial pressure and increase cerebral perfusion. Volume expansion is achieved via crystalloid or colloid solution.

Interventions to treat cerebral vasospasm either before or after aneurysm clipping or coiling include administration of the calcium channel blocker nimodipine, which is given to patients with SAH to decrease the effects of vasospasm and minimize cerebral damage. Nimodipine restricts the influx of calcium ions into cells by reducing the number of open calcium channels. Although nimodipine is a calcium channel blocker, its exact mechanism of action in reducing vasospasm is not well understood.

💊 **DRUG ALERT**   Nimodipine
- Assess BP and apical pulses before administration.
- If pulse is ≤60 beats/min or systolic BP is <90 mm Hg, hold medication and contact physician.

Rehabilitation Care

After the stroke patient has stabilized for 12 to 24 hours, interprofessional care shifts from preserving life to lessening

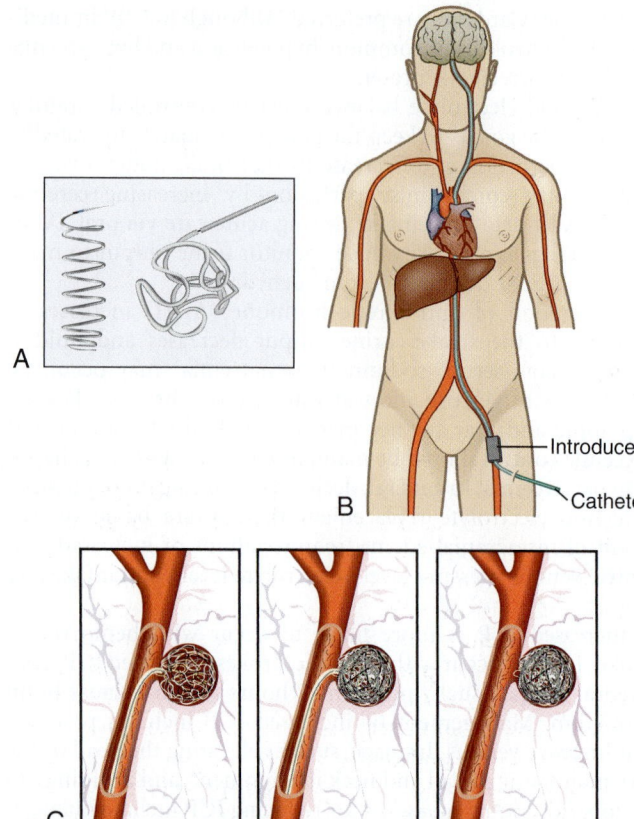

FIG. 57-7   Guglielmi detachable coil (GDC). **A,** A coil is used to occlude an aneurysm. Coils are made of soft, springlike platinum. The softness of the platinum allows the coil to assume the shape of irregularly shaped aneurysms while posing little threat of rupture of the aneurysm. **B,** A catheter is inserted through an introducer (small tube) in an artery in the leg. The catheter is threaded up to the cerebral blood vessels. **C,** Platinum coils attached to a thin wire are inserted into the catheter and then placed in the aneurysm until the aneurysm is filled with coils. Packing the aneurysm with coils prevents the blood from circulating through the aneurysm, reducing the risk of rupture.

disability and attaining optimal function. Many of the interventions discussed in the acute phase are maintained during this phase. The patient may be evaluated by a physiatrist (a physician who specializes in physical medicine and rehabilitation). Remember that some aspects of rehabilitation actually begin in the acute care phase as soon as the patient is stabilized. Specific measures related to rehabilitation are discussed in the section on Ambulatory Care on pp. 1362-1365.

Core Measures for Stroke

The stroke (STK) core measures (Table 57-8) were developed in partnership with the American Stroke Association (ASA) for use by primary stroke centers. These core measures are used by hospitals for accreditation and certification. Measures are implemented during the hospital admission and prior to discharge and align with guidelines supported by the AHA Get With The Guidelines (GWTG) stroke patient management tool and the Centers for Disease Control and Prevention (CDC) Paul Coverdell National Acute Stroke Registry (PCNASR).

❖ NURSING MANAGEMENT: STROKE

◆ Nursing Assessment

Subjective and objective data that should be obtained from a person who has had a stroke are presented in Table 57-9.

TABLE 57-8 Stroke (STK) Core Measure Set

Measure	Topic
STK-1	Venous thromboembolism (VTE) prophylaxis
STK-2	Discharged on antithrombotic therapy
STK-3	Anticoagulation therapy for atrial fibrillation/flutter
STK-4	Thrombolytic therapy
STK-5	Antithrombotic therapy by end of hospital day 2
STK-6	Discharged on statin medication
STK-8	Stroke education
STK-10	Assessed for rehabilitation

Source: The Joint Commission. Stroke Core Measures. Retrieved from *www.jointcommission.org/stroke.*

Primary assessment focuses on cardiac and respiratory status and neurologic assessment. If the patient is stable, the nursing history is obtained as follows: (1) description of the current illness with attention to initial symptoms, particularly symptom onset and duration, nature (intermittent or continuous), and changes; (2) history of similar symptoms previously experienced; (3) current medications; (4) history of risk factors and other illnesses such as hypertension; and (5) family history of stroke, aneurysm, or cardiovascular diseases. This information is gained through an interview of the patient, caregiver, family members, and/or significant others.

Secondary assessment includes a comprehensive neurologic examination of the patient. This includes (1) level of consciousness, including assessment using the National Institutes of Health (NIH) Stroke Scale (NIHSS) (Table 57-10); (2) cognition; (3) motor abilities; (4) cranial nerve function; (5) sensation; (6) proprioception; (7) cerebellar function; and (8) deep tendon reflexes. Clear documentation of initial and ongoing neurologic examinations is essential to note changes in the patient's status.

◆ Nursing Diagnoses

Nursing diagnoses for the person with a stroke may include, but are not limited to

- Decreased intracranial adaptive capacity *related to* decreased cerebral perfusion pressure of ≤50 to 60 mm Hg and sustained increase in ICP secondary to thrombus, embolus, or hemorrhage
- Risk for aspiration *related to* decreased level of consciousness and decreased or absent gag and swallowing reflexes
- Impaired physical mobility *related to* neuromuscular and cognitive impairment and decreased muscle strength and control
- Impaired verbal communication *related to* aphasia
- Unilateral neglect *related to* visual field cut and loss on one side of body (hemianopsia) and brain injury from cerebrovascular problems
- Impaired swallowing *related to* weakness or paralysis of affected muscles
- Situational low self-esteem *related to* actual or perceived loss of function and altered body image

Additional information on nursing diagnoses are presented in eNursing Care Plan 57-1 (available on the website for this chapter).

◆ Planning

Establish the goals of nursing care together with the patient, caregiver, and family. Typical goals are that the patient will (1) maintain a stable or improved level of consciousness,

TABLE 57-9 Nursing Assessment

Stroke

Subjective Data

Important Health Information

Past health history: Hypertension. Previous stroke, TIA, aneurysm, cardiac disease (including recent myocardial infarction), dysrhythmias, heart failure, valvular heart disease, infective endocarditis. Hyperlipidemia, polycythemia, diabetes, gout. Previous head injury, family history of hypertension, diabetes, stroke, or coronary artery disease

Family history: Neurologic disorders, aneurysms, stroke, or transient ischemic attack (TIA)

Medications: Oral contraceptives; use of and compliance with antihypertensive and anticoagulant therapy; illegal substances and drug use (cocaine)

Functional Health Patterns

Health perception–health management: Positive family history of stroke. Alcohol abuse, smoking, drug abuse

Nutritional-metabolic: Anorexia, nausea, vomiting. Dysphagia, altered sense of taste and smell

Elimination: Change in bowel and bladder patterns

Activity-exercise: Loss of movement and sensation. Syncope, weakness on one side, generalized weakness, easy fatigability

Cognitive-perceptual: Numbness, tingling of one side of the body, loss of memory. Alteration in speech, language, problem-solving ability. Pain, headache (possibly sudden and severe) (hemorrhage). Visual disturbances. Denial of illness

Objective Data

General

Emotional lability, lethargy, apathy or combativeness, fever

Respiratory

Loss of cough reflex, labored or irregular respirations, tachypnea, wheezes (aspiration), airway occlusion (tongue), apnea, coughing when eating or delayed coughing

Cardiovascular

Hypertension, tachycardia, carotid bruit

Gastrointestinal

Loss of gag reflex, bowel incontinence, decreased or absent bowel sounds, constipation

Urinary

Frequency, urgency, incontinence

Neurologic

Contralateral motor and sensory deficits, including weakness, paresis, paralysis, anesthesia. Unequal pupils, hand grasps. Akinesia, aphasia (expressive, receptive, global), dysarthria (slurred speech), agnosias, apraxia, visual deficits, perceptual or spatial disturbances, altered level of consciousness (drowsiness to deep coma) and Babinski's sign, ↓ followed by ↑ deep tendon reflexes, flaccidity followed by spasticity, amnesia, ataxia, personality change, nuchal rigidity, seizures

Possible Diagnostic Findings

Positive CT, CTA, MRI, MRA, or other neuroimaging scans showing size, location, and type of lesion. Positive Doppler ultrasonography and angiography indicating stenosis

CTA, Computed tomographic angiography; *MRA,* magnetic resonance angiography; *TIA,* transient ischemic attack.

TABLE 57-10 National Institutes of Health Stroke Scale (NIHSS)

Description

The National Institutes of Health Stroke Scale (NIHSS) is a 15-item neurologic examination used to evaluate the effect of an acute stroke. Total scores on the NIHSS range from 0-42, with higher values reflecting more severity.

Procedure for Use

A trained observer rates the patient's ability to answer questions and perform activities. Ratings for each item are scored and there is an allowance for untestable (UN) items. If an item is left untested, a detailed explanation must be clearly written on the form. Training can be completed free at *www.nihstrokescale.org.*

Item	Scale Definition
Level of consciousness	0 = Alert 1 = Not alert, but arousable by minor stimulation 2 = Not alert, requires repeated stimulation to get attention 3 = Responds only with reflex motor or autonomic effects or totally unresponsive, flaccid, areflexic
Level of consciousness questions	0 = Answers both questions correctly 1 = Answers one question correctly 2 = Answers neither question correctly
Level of consciousness commands	0 = Performs both tasks correctly 1 = Performs one task correctly 2 = Performs neither task correctly
Best gaze	0 = Normal 1 = Partial gaze palsy 2 = Forced deviation, or total gaze paresis
Visual	0 = No visual loss 1 = Partial hemianopsia 2 = Complete hemianopsia 3 = Bilateral hemianopsia or blind
Facial palsy	0 = Normal symmetric movement 1 = Minor paralysis 2 = Partial paralysis 3 = Complete paralysis of one or both sides
Motor and drift (for each extremity)	0 = No drift 1 = Drift 2 = Some effort against gravity 3 = No effort against gravity, limb falls 4 = No movement UN = Amputation
Limb ataxia	0 = Absent 1 = Present in one limb 2 = Present in two limbs
Sensory	0 = Normal 1 = Mild to moderate sensory loss 2 = Severe to total sensory loss
Best language	0 = No aphasia, normal 1 = Mild to moderate aphasia 2 = Severe aphasia 3 = Mute, no usable speech or auditory comprehension
Dysarthria	0 = Normal 1 = Mild to moderate 2 = Severe UN = Intubated or other physical barrier
Extinction or inattention	0 = No abnormality 1 = Inattention or extinction to bilateral stimulation 2 = Does not recognize own hand
Distal motor function	0 = Normal (no flexion after 5 sec) 1 = At least some extension but not fully extended 2 = No voluntary extension after 5 sec

Source: American Stroke Association: NIH stroke scale, 2009. Retrieved from *www.ninds.nih.gov/doctors/NIH_Stroke_Scale.pdf.*

(2) attain maximum physical functioning, (3) attain maximum self-care abilities and skills, (4) maintain stable body functions (e.g., bladder control), (5) maximize communication abilities, (6) maintain adequate nutrition, (7) avoid complications of stroke, and (8) maintain effective personal and family coping.

Nursing Implementation

Health Promotion. You have a major role in the promotion of a healthy lifestyle. Teaching should focus on stroke prevention, particularly for persons with known risk factors. As previously mentioned, most strokes are caused by modifiable risk factors. Nursing measures to reduce risk factors for stroke are similar to those for coronary artery disease (see Chapter 33, Table 33-2) and are discussed earlier in this chapter on pp. 1346-1348.

Uncontrolled or undiagnosed hypertension is the primary cause of stroke. Therefore you need to be involved in BP screening and ensuring that patients adhere to the use of their antihypertensive medications and home monitoring of BP. If a person is a diabetic, it is important that the diabetes is well controlled. If an individual has atrial fibrillation, an anticoagulant (see p. 1347) or aspirin may be used to reduce the risk of stroke. Because smoking is a major risk factor for stroke, you need to be actively involved in helping patients to stop smoking (see Chapter 10, Tables 10-4 to 10-6).

Another important aspect of health promotion is teaching patients and families about early symptoms associated with stroke or TIA. Table 57-1 presents information on when to seek health care for these symptoms.

Acute Care

Respiratory System. During the acute phase after a stroke, management of the respiratory system is a nursing priority.[21] Stroke patients are particularly vulnerable to respiratory problems. Advancing age and immobility increase the risk for atelectasis and pneumonia.

Risk for aspiration pneumonia is high because of impaired consciousness or dysphagia. Dysphagia after stroke is common. Airway obstruction can occur because of problems with chewing and swallowing, food pocketing (food remaining in the buccal cavity of the mouth), and the tongue falling back. Some stroke patients, especially those with brainstem or hemorrhagic stroke, may require endotracheal intubation and mechanical ventilation initially. Enteral tube feedings also place the patient at risk for aspiration pneumonia. All patients should be screened for their ability to swallow and kept on nothing-by-mouth (NPO) status until dysphagia has been ruled out.

Nursing interventions to support adequate respiratory function are individualized to meet the patient's needs. An oropharyngeal airway may be used in comatose patients to prevent the tongue from falling back and obstructing the airway and to provide access for suctioning. Alternatively, a nasopharyngeal airway may be used to provide airway protection and access. When an artificial airway is required for a prolonged time, a tracheostomy may be performed.

Nursing interventions include frequently assessing airway patency and function, providing oxygenation, suctioning, promoting patient mobility, positioning the patient to prevent aspiration, and encouraging deep breathing. In patients who are on mechanical ventilation, oral care at least every 2 hours reduces the occurrence of ventilator-assisted pneumonia.[21]

Patients who have an unclipped or uncoiled aneurysm may experience rebleeding and the possibility of increasing ICP further with coughing or suctioning, so nursing management is aimed at reducing these interventions while maintaining a proper airway.

Interventions related to maintenance of airway function are described in eNursing Care Plan 57-1.

◆ **Neurologic System.** The primary clinical assessment tool to evaluate and document neurologic status in acute stroke patients is the NIH Stroke Scale (NIHSS), which measures stroke severity[22] (Table 57-10). The NIHSS is a predictor of both short- and long-term outcomes of stroke patients. Additionally, it serves as a data collection tool for planning patient care and exchanging information among HCPs.

Additional neurologic assessment includes mental status, pupillary responses, and extremity movement and strength. Also closely monitor vital signs. A decreasing level of consciousness may indicate increasing ICP. Monitor ICP and cerebral perfusion pressure if the patient is in a critical care environment. Record your nursing assessment on flowsheets to communicate the patient's neurologic status to the stroke team.

◆ **Cardiovascular System.** Nursing goals for the cardiovascular system are aimed at maintaining homeostasis. Many patients with stroke have decreased cardiac reserves secondary to cardiac disease. Cardiac efficiency may be further compromised by fluid retention, overhydration, dehydration, or BP variations. Central venous pressure, pulmonary artery pressure, or hemodynamic monitoring may be used as indicators of fluid balance or cardiac function in the critical care unit.

Nursing interventions include (1) monitoring vital signs frequently; (2) monitoring cardiac rhythms; (3) calculating intake and output, noting imbalances; (4) regulating IV infusions; (5) adjusting fluid intake to individual patient needs; (6) monitoring lung sounds for crackles and wheezes, indicating pulmonary congestion; and (7) monitoring heart sounds for murmurs. Bedside monitors or telemetry may record cardiac rhythms.

Hypertension is sometimes seen after a stroke as the body attempts to increase cerebral blood flow. It is also important to monitor for orthostatic hypotension before ambulating the patient for the first time. Neurologic changes can occur with a sudden decrease in BP.

After a stroke, the patient is at risk for venous thromboembolism (VTE), especially in the weak or paralyzed lower extremity. VTE is related to immobility, loss of venous tone, and decreased muscle pumping activity in the leg. The most effective prevention is to keep the patient moving. Teach the patient active range-of-motion exercises if the patient has voluntary movement in the affected extremity. For the patient with hemiplegia, perform passive range-of-motion exercises several times a day. Additional measures to prevent VTE include positioning to minimize the effects of dependent edema and using sequential compression devices for bedridden patients. VTE prophylaxis may include low-molecular-weight heparin (e.g., enoxaparin [Lovenox]). The nursing assessment for VTE includes measuring the calf and thigh daily, observing for swelling of the lower extremities, noting unusual warmth of the leg, and asking the patient about pain in the calf.[23]

◆ **Musculoskeletal System.** The nursing goal for the musculoskeletal system is to maintain optimal function by preventing joint contractures and muscular atrophy. In the acute phase, range-of-motion exercises and positioning are important nursing interventions. Passive range-of-motion exercise is begun on the first day of hospitalization. Muscle atrophy secondary to lack of innervation and activity can develop after

TEAMWORK & COLLABORATION
Caring for the Patient With an Acute Stroke

During the first 48 hr after an acute stroke, some nursing activities may be delegated to licensed practical/vocational nurses (LPNs/LVNs) and unlicensed assistive personnel (UAP). The registered nurse (RN) should communicate frequently with these staff members to rapidly intervene based on changes in the patient status.

Role of Nursing Personnel
Registered Nurse (RN)
- Assess clinical manifestations of stroke and determine when clinical manifestations started.
- Screen patient for contraindications for tissue plasminogen activator (tPA) therapy.
- Infuse tPA for patients with ischemic stroke who meet the criteria for tPA administration.
- Assess respiratory status and initiate needed actions such as O_2, oropharyngeal or nasopharyngeal airways, suctioning, and patient positioning to prevent aspiration, obstruction, and atelectasis.
- Assess neurologic status, including intracranial pressure (ICP), if needed.
- Monitor cardiovascular status, including hemodynamic monitoring, if needed.
- Assess patient's ability to swallow (in conjunction with the speech therapist).

Licensed Practical/Vocational Nurse (LPN/LVN)
- Administer scheduled anticoagulant and antiplatelet medications.

Unlicensed Assistive Personnel (UAP)
- Obtain vital signs frequently and report these to RN.
- Measure and record urine output.
- Assist with positioning and turning patient at least every 2 hr (as directed by RN).
- Perform passive and active range-of-motion exercises (after being trained and evaluated in these procedures).
- Place equipment needed for seizure precautions in patient room.

Role of Other Team Members
Speech Therapy
- Assess swallowing reflex.
- Evaluate patient for communication defects (e.g., aphasia).

Physical Therapy
- Position patient in a functional position.
- Assess function and together with patient, plan a rehabilitation program.

stroke, so exercise is an important intervention for rehabilitation and recovery.

The paralyzed or weak side requires special attention when the patient is positioned. Position each joint higher than the joint proximal to it to prevent dependent edema. Specific deformities on the weak or paralyzed side that may be present in patients with stroke include internal rotation of the shoulder; flexion contractures of the hand, wrist, and elbow; external rotation of the hip; and plantar flexion of the foot. Subluxation of the shoulder on the affected side is common. Careful positioning and moving of the affected arm may prevent development of a painful shoulder condition. Immobilization of the affected upper extremity may precipitate a painful shoulder-hand syndrome.

Nursing interventions to optimize musculoskeletal function include (1) trochanter roll at the hip to prevent external rotation; (2) hand cones (not rolled washcloths) to prevent hand contractures; (3) arm supports with slings and lap boards to prevent shoulder displacement; (4) avoidance of pulling the patient by the arm to avoid shoulder displacement; (5) posterior leg splints, footboards, or high-top tennis shoes to prevent footdrop; and (6) hand splints to reduce spasticity.

Use of a footboard for the patient with spasticity is controversial. Rather than preventing plantar flexion (footdrop), the sensory stimulation of a footboard against the bottom of the foot increases plantar flexion. Likewise, experts disagree on whether hand splints facilitate or diminish spasticity. The decision regarding the use of footboards or hand splints is made on an individual patient basis.

◆ ***Integumentary System.*** The skin of the patient with stroke is particularly susceptible to breakdown related to loss of sensation, decreased circulation, and immobility. This is compounded by advanced age, poor nutrition, dehydration, edema, and incontinence.

The nursing plan for prevention of skin breakdown includes (1) pressure relief by position changes, special mattresses, or wheelchair cushions; (2) good skin hygiene; (3) emollients applied to dry skin; and (4) early mobility. An example of a position change schedule is side-back-side, with a maximum duration of 2 hours for any position. Position the patient on the weak or paralyzed side for only 30 minutes. If an area of redness develops and does not return to normal color within 15 minutes of pressure relief, the epidermis and dermis are damaged.

Do not massage the damaged area because this may cause additional damage. Control of pressure is the single most important factor in both the prevention and treatment of skin breakdown. Pillows can be used under lower extremities to reduce pressure on the heels. Vigilance and good nursing care are required to prevent pressure sores.

◆ ***Gastrointestinal System.*** The most common bowel problem for the stroke patient is constipation. Patients may be prophylactically placed on stool softeners and/or fiber (psyllium [Metamucil]). If a patient has liquid stools, check for stool impaction. Fluid and fiber intake goals should be discussed with the stroke team and are based on the patient's nutritional and fluid status.

Physical activity also promotes bowel function. Laxatives, suppositories, or additional stool softeners may be ordered if the patient does not respond to increased fluid and fiber. Enemas are used only if suppositories and digital stimulation are ineffective because they cause vagal stimulation and increase ICP.

Bowel retraining may be needed and continues into the rehabilitation phase. A bowel management program consists of placing the patient on the bedpan or bedside commode or taking the patient to the bathroom at a regular time daily to reestablish bowel regularity. A good time for the bowel program is 30 minutes after breakfast because eating stimulates the gastrocolic reflex and peristalsis, but timing may have to be adjusted, since individual bowel habits may vary.

◆ ***Urinary System.*** In the acute stage of stroke, the primary urinary problem is poor bladder control, resulting in incontinence. Take steps to promote normal bladder function and avoid the use of indwelling catheters. If an indwelling catheter must be used initially, remove it as soon as the patient is medically and neurologically stable. Long-term use of an indwelling catheter is associated with urinary tract infections and delayed bladder retraining.

Avoid bladder overdistention. An intermittent catheterization program may be used for patients with urinary retention because of the lower incidence of urinary infections. An alternative to intermittent catheterizations is the external catheter for male patients with urinary incontinence. External catheters do not alleviate the problem of urine retention.

Assist the patient with urinary difficulties or incontinence. Often the patient with stroke has functional incontinence, which is associated with communication difficulties, mobility problems, and dressing or undressing difficulties. A bladder retraining program consists of (1) adequate fluid intake with most of it given between 7:00 AM and 7:00 PM; (2) scheduled toileting every 2 hours using bedpan, commode, or bathroom while encouraging the usual position for urinating (standing for men and sitting for women); (3) observation for signs of restlessness, which may indicate the need for urination; and (4) assessment for bladder distention by palpation. Encourage patients to wear pants without drawstrings, buttons, or zippers, as these can be difficult to manage if motor or sensory deficits exist.

Assessment of postvoid residual volume is often done using bladder ultrasound. The ultrasound measures how much urine is in the bladder after voiding. If urine remains in the bladder, incomplete emptying is a problem and may cause urinary tract infections. A coordinated program by the entire nursing staff is needed to achieve urinary continence.

◆ ***Nutrition.*** The patient's nutritional needs require quick assessment and treatment. The patient may initially receive IV infusions to maintain fluid and electrolyte balance and to administer drugs. Patients with severe impairment may require enteral or parenteral nutrition support. Patients should have their nutritional needs addressed in the first 24 hours of admission to the hospital because nutrition is important for recovery and healing.[24]

⚠ SAFETY ALERT   Oral Feeding After Stroke
- The gag reflex may be impaired due to dysphagia and must be assessed.
- Therefore the first oral feeding should be carefully planned.

Speech therapists (if available) should perform a swallowing evaluation before a patient's oral intake is initiated. The majority of patients experience dysphagia after a stroke.[24] Before initiating feeding, assess the gag reflex by gently stimulating the back of the throat with a tongue blade. If a gag reflex is present, the patient will gag spontaneously. If it is absent, defer the feeding, and begin exercises to stimulate swallowing. The speech therapist or occupational therapist is usually responsible for designing this program. However, you may be involved in helping to develop the program in some clinical settings.

To assess swallowing ability, elevate the head of the bed to an upright position (unless contraindicated) and give the patient a small amount of crushed ice or ice water to swallow. If the gag reflex is present and the patient is able to swallow safely, you may proceed with feeding.

After careful assessment of swallowing, chewing, gag reflex, and pocketing, oral feedings can be initiated. Mouth care before feeding helps stimulate sensory awareness and salivation and can facilitate swallowing. The patient should remain in a high Fowler's position, preferably in a chair with the head flexed forward, for the feeding and for 30 minutes afterward.

The speech therapist may recommend various dietary items. Foods should be easy to swallow and provide enough texture,

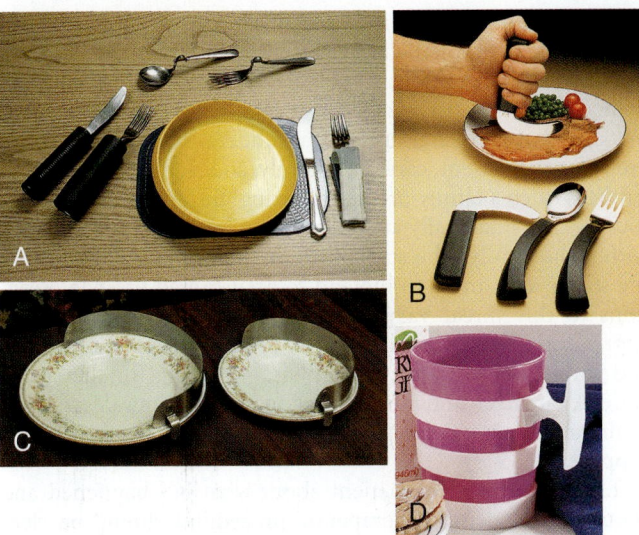

FIG. 57-8 Assistive devices for eating. **A,** The curved fork fits over the hand. The rounded plate helps keep food on the plate. Special grips and swivel handles are helpful for some persons. **B,** Knives with rounded blades are rocked back and forth to cut food. The person does not need a fork in one hand and a knife in the other. **C,** Plate guards help keep food on the plate. **D,** Cup with special handle. (Courtesy Sammons Preston, Bolingbrook, Ill.)

TABLE 57-11 **Communication With a Patient With Aphasia**
The following are guidelines for communicating with a patient with aphasia.
1. Decrease environmental stimuli that may be distracting and disrupting to communication efforts.
2. Treat the patient as an adult.
3. Speak with normal volume and tone.
4. Present one thought or idea at a time.
5. Keep questions simple or ask questions that can be answered with "yes" or "no."
6. Let the person speak. Do not interrupt. Allow time for the individual to complete thoughts.
7. Make use of gestures or demonstration as an acceptable alternative form of communication. Encourage this by saying, "Show me ..." or "Point to what you want."
8. Do not pretend to understand the person if you do not. Calmly say you do not understand and encourage the use of nonverbal communication, or ask the person to write out what he or she wants.
9. Give the patient time to process information and generate a response before repeating a question or statement.
10. Allow body contact (e.g., clasp of a hand, touching) as much as possible. Realize that touching may be the only way the patient can express feelings.
11. Organize the patient's day by preparing and following a schedule (the more familiar the routine, the easier it will be).
12. Do not push communication if the person is tired or upset. Aphasia worsens with fatigue and anxiety.
13. Teach communication techniques to caregiver and family members.

temperature (warm or cold), and flavor to stimulate a swallow reflex. Crushed ice can be used as a stimulant. Instruct the patient to swallow and then swallow again. Pureed foods are not usually the best choice because they are often bland and too smooth. Thin liquids are often difficult to swallow and may promote coughing. Thin liquids can be thickened with a commercially available thickening agent (e.g., Thick-It). Avoid milk products because they tend to increase the viscosity of mucus and increase salivation.

Place food on the unaffected side of the mouth. Feedings must be followed by scrupulous oral hygiene because food may collect on the affected side of the mouth. During the acute and rehabilitation phase of the stroke, a dietitian can assist in determining the appropriate daily caloric intake based on the patient's size, weight, and activity level. If the patient is unable to take in an adequate oral diet and dysphagia persists, a percutaneous endoscopic gastrostomy (PEG) tube (see Chapter 39, Fig. 39-7) may be used for nutritional support. Most commercially prepared formulas provide about 1 cal/mL. (Enteral feedings are described in Chapter 39.)

The inability to feed oneself can be frustrating and may result in malnutrition and dehydration. Interventions to promote self-feeding include using the unaffected upper extremity to eat; employing assistive devices such as rocker knives, plate guards, and nonslip pads for dishes (Fig. 57-8); removing unnecessary items from the tray or table, which can reduce spills; and providing a calm environment (e.g., turn off the television) to decrease sensory overload and distraction. The effectiveness of the dietary program is evaluated in terms of maintenance of weight, adequate hydration, and patient satisfaction. Introduce these interventions in the acute care setting so that maximum rehabilitation can occur once the patient is discharged.

Communication. During the acute stage of stroke, your role in meeting the patient's psychologic needs is primarily supportive. Speech, comprehension, and language deficits are the most difficult problems for the patient and caregiver. Assess the patient for both the ability to speak and the ability to understand. The patient's response to simple questions can guide you in structuring explanations and instructions. If the patient cannot understand words, use gestures to support verbal cues. Collaborate with the speech therapist to assess and formulate a plan of care to enhance communication.

Nursing interventions that support communication include (1) communicating frequently and meaningfully; (2) allowing time for the patient to comprehend and answer; (3) using simple, short sentences; (4) using visual cues; (5) structuring conversation so that it permits simple answers by the patient; and (6) praising the patient honestly for improvements with speech.[25]

An alert patient is usually anxious because of lack of understanding about what has happened and because of difficulty with communication or inability to communicate. The stroke patient with aphasia may easily be overwhelmed by verbal stimuli. Give the patient extra time to comprehend and respond to communication. (Guidelines for communicating with a patient who has aphasia are presented in Table 57-11.) A picture board may be helpful for communicating with the stroke patient. Further evaluation and treatment of language and communication deficits are often done by the speech therapist once the patient has stabilized. It is also important to teach the caregiver and family these communication strategies.

Sensory-Perceptual Alterations. Patients who have had a stroke frequently have perceptual deficits. Patients with a stroke on the right side of the brain usually have difficulty judging position, distance, and rate of movement. These patients are often impulsive and impatient and tend to deny problems related to strokes. They may fail to correlate spatial-perceptual problems with the inability to perform activities, such as guiding a wheelchair through the doorway. The patient with a right-brain stroke (left hemiplegia) is at higher risk for injury because

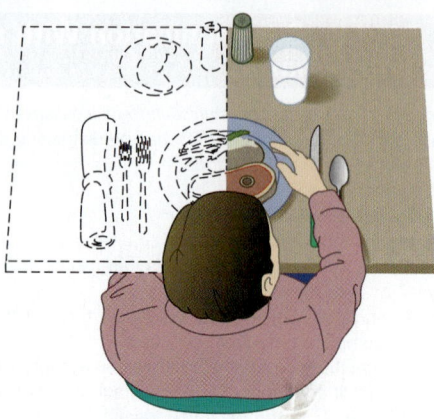

FIG. 57-9 Spatial and perceptual deficits in stroke. Perception of a patient with homonymous hemianopsia shows that food on the left side is not seen and thus is ignored. (Modified from Hoeman SP: *Rehabilitation nursing*, ed 2, St Louis, 1995, Mosby.)

of mobility difficulties. Directions for activities are best given verbally for comprehension. Break the task down into simple steps for ease of understanding. Environmental control, such as removing clutter and obstacles and using good lighting, aids in concentration and safer mobility. Provide nonslip socks at all times. One-sided neglect is common for people with right-brain stroke, so you may assist or remind the patient to dress the weak or paralyzed side or shave the forgotten side of the face.

Patients with a left-brain stroke (right hemiplegia) commonly are slower in organization and performance of tasks. They tend to have impaired spatial discrimination. These patients usually admit to deficits and have a fearful, anxious response to a stroke. Their behaviors are slow and cautious. Nonverbal cues and instructions are helpful for comprehension with patients who have had a left-brain stroke.

Homonymous hemianopsia (blindness in the same half of each visual field) is a common problem after a stroke. Persistent disregard of objects in part of the visual field should alert you to this possibility. Initially, help the patient to compensate by arranging the environment within the patient's perceptual field, such as arranging the food tray so that all foods are on the right side or the left side to accommodate for field of vision (Fig. 57-9). Later, the patient learns to compensate for the visual defect by consciously attending or by scanning the neglected side. The weak or paralyzed extremities are carefully checked for adequacy of dressing, hygiene, and trauma.

In the clinical situation, it is often difficult to distinguish between a visual field cut and a neglect syndrome. Both problems may occur with strokes affecting either the right or the left side of the brain. A person may be unfortunate enough to have both homonymous hemianopsia and a neglect syndrome, which increases the inattention to the weak or paralyzed side. A neglect syndrome results in decreased safety awareness and places the patient at high risk for injury. Immediately after the stroke, anticipate safety hazards and provide protection from injury. Safety measures can include closely observing the patient, elevating side rails, lowering the height of the bed, and using video monitors. Avoid the use of restraints and soft vests because this may agitate the patient.

Other visual problems may include *diplopia* (double vision), loss of the corneal reflex, and *ptosis* (drooping eyelid), especially if the stroke is in the vertebrobasilar distribution. Diplopia is often treated with an eye patch. If the corneal reflex is absent, the patient is at risk for corneal abrasion and should be observed

closely and protected against eye injuries. Corneal abrasion can be prevented with artificial tears or gel to keep the eyes moist and an eye shield (especially at night). Ptosis is generally not treated because it usually does not inhibit vision.

◆ *Coping.* A stroke is usually a sudden, extremely stressful event for the patient, caregiver, family, and significant others. A stroke is often a family disease, affecting the family emotionally, socially, and financially and changing roles and responsibilities within the family. The stroke patient and family may perceive the stroke as a threat to life and to accustomed lifestyle. Reactions to this threat vary considerably but may involve fear, apprehension, denial of the severity of stroke, depression, anger, and sorrow. During the acute phase of caring for the stroke patient, caregiver, and family, nursing interventions designed to facilitate coping involve providing information and emotional support.

Explanations to the patient about what has happened and about diagnostic and therapeutic procedures should be clear and understandable, with reinforcement as needed. Decision making and upholding the patient's wishes during this challenging time are of upmost importance. Advance directives should be honored, and family meetings or updates should be held daily about feeding tube placement or tracheostomy.

Give the caregiver and family a careful, detailed explanation of what has happened to the patient. However, if the family is extremely anxious and upset during the acute phase, explanations may have to be repeated at a later time. Because family members usually have not had time to prepare for the illness, they may need assistance in arranging care for family members or pets and for transportation and finances. A social services referral is often helpful.

It is particularly challenging to keep the patient with aphasia adequately informed. Use demeanor and touch to convey support. When communicating with a patient who has a communication deficit, speak in a normal volume and tone, keep questions simple, and present one thought or idea at a time. To decrease frustration, always let the patient speak without interruption and make use of gestures. Do not forget to use writing and communication boards.[25]

◆ **Ambulatory Care.** The patient is usually discharged from the acute care setting to home, an intermediate- or long-term care facility, or a rehabilitation facility. Ideally, discharge planning with the patient and caregiver starts early in the hospitalization and promotes a smooth transition from one care setting to another. The stroke team provides guidance for the appropriate care necessary after discharge. If the patient requires a short- or long-term health care facility, the team can make appropriate referrals that allow time to select and arrange for care. A critical factor in discharge planning is the patient's level of independence in performing ADLs.[26] If the patient is returning home, the team can make referrals for needed equipment and services in preparation for discharge.

You have an excellent opportunity to prepare the patient and caregiver for discharge through teaching, demonstration and return demonstration, practice, and evaluation of self-care skills. Total care is considered in discharge planning: medications, nutrition, mobility, exercises, hygiene, and toileting. Follow-up care is carefully planned to permit continuing nursing care; physical, occupational, and speech therapy; and medical care. Identify community resources to provide recreational activities, group support, spiritual assistance, respite care, adult day care, and home assistance based on the patient's needs.

◆ ***Rehabilitation.*** *Rehabilitation* is the process of maximizing the patient's capabilities and resources to promote optimal functioning related to physical, mental, and social well-being. The goals of rehabilitation are to prevent deformity and maintain and improve function. Regardless of the care setting, ongoing rehabilitation is essential to maximize the patient's abilities. Most patients recover in the first 6 months following a stroke, with maximum benefit 1 year after a stroke.[1]

Rehabilitation requires a team approach so that the patient and caregiver can benefit from the combined, expert care of a stroke interprofessional team. The team must communicate and coordinate care to achieve the patient's goals. As a nurse, you are in a good position to facilitate this process and are often the key to successful rehabilitation efforts. The stroke interprofessional team is composed of many members, including nurses, physicians, psychiatrist, physical therapist, occupational therapist, speech therapist, registered dietitian, respiratory therapist, vocational therapist, recreational therapist, social worker, psychologist, pharmacist, and chaplain.

Physical therapy focuses on mobility, progressive ambulation, transfer techniques, and equipment needed for mobility. Occupational therapy emphasizes retraining for skills of daily living such as eating, dressing, hygiene, and cooking. Occupational therapists are also skilled in cognitive and perceptual evaluation and training. Speech therapy focuses on speech, communication, cognition, and eating abilities.

INFORMATICS IN PRACTICE

Video Games for Stroke Recovery

- Patients dealing with the effects of a stroke often have difficulty performing activities of daily living.
- Playing active video games, such as Nintendo Wii or Xbox Kinect, brings some fun into stroke recovery and may get patients to spend more time in therapy.
- Gaming helps patients regain lost strength, improve motor skills, and improve problem solving and short- and long-term memory.
- Patients can play with their families, including children, making gaming a way to involve others in rehabilitation.

Many of the nursing interventions outlined in eNursing Care Plan 57-1 for the patient with a stroke are initiated in the acute phase of care and continue throughout rehabilitation. Some of the interventions are independent nursing actions, whereas others involve the entire team.

The rehabilitation nurse assesses the patient, caregiver, and family with attention to the (1) patient's rehabilitation potential, (2) physical status of all body systems, (3) complications caused by the stroke or other chronic conditions, (4) patient's cognitive status, (5) family resources and support, and (6) expectations of the patient and caregiver related to the rehabilitation program.

◆ ***Musculoskeletal Function.*** Initially emphasize the musculoskeletal functions of eating, toileting, and walking for rehabilitation of the patient. Initial assessment consists of determining the stage of recovery of muscle function. If the muscles are still flaccid several weeks after the stroke, the prognosis for regaining function is poor, and care focuses on preventing additional loss (Fig. 57-10).

Most patients begin to show signs of spasticity with exaggerated reflexes within 48 hours after the stroke. Spasticity at this phase of stroke denotes progress toward recovery. As improvement continues, small voluntary movements of the hip or shoulder may be accompanied by involuntary movements in

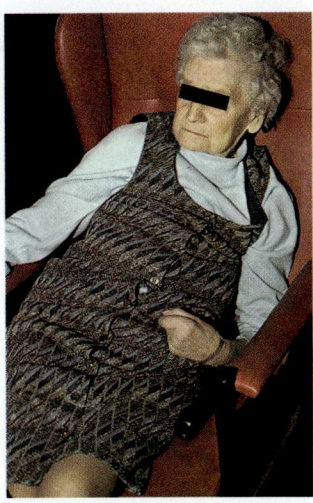

FIG. 57-10 Loss of postural stability is common after stroke. When the nondominant hemisphere is involved, walking apraxia and loss of postural control are usually apparent. The patient is unable to sit upright and tends to fall sideways. Provide appropriate support with pillows or cushions. (From Forbes CD, Jackson WF: *Colour atlas and text of clinical medicine,* ed 3, London, 2003, Mosby.)

EVIDENCE-BASED PRACTICE

Applying the Evidence

Virtual Reality and Stroke

You are a nurse working in an outpatient rehabilitation facility with C.W., a 70-yr-old female who was diagnosed with a stroke 3 months ago. You note she has right-sided weakness, especially in her arm. She tells you that she cannot write very well or use a computer, and she misses e-mailing her friends and family since her stroke.

Making Clinical Decisions

Best Available Evidence. Virtual reality and interactive video gaming may improve upper limb mobility and daily functioning in patients undergoing rehabilitation for stroke.

Clinician Expertise. You know the therapeutic use of interactive video games in rehabilitation helps patients to move the unaffected hand with the assistance of virtual mirror feedback. You also note the benefit of virtual reality for practicing daily tasks that may currently be unsafe in the home, such as showering and dressing.

Patient Preferences and Values. C.W. says, "It will be fun to play video games while I rehab."

Implications for Nursing Practice

1. What parameters will you use to assess C.W.'s progression with the virtual reality intervention?
2. Why is it important for you to determine with C.W. if virtual training translates into the actual performance of activities at home?
3. As you coordinate her rehabilitation care, how will you facilitate communication among interprofessional team members?

Reference for Evidence

Laver KE, George S, Thomas S, et al: Virtual reality for stroke rehabilitation, *Cochrane Database Syst Rev* 2:CD008349, 2015.

the rest of the extremity *(synergy)*. The final stage of recovery occurs when the patient has voluntary control of isolated muscle groups.

Interventions for the musculoskeletal system advance in a manner of progressive activity. Balance training is the initial step and begins with the patient sitting up in bed or dangling the legs over the edge of the bed. Evaluate tolerance by noting dizziness or syncope caused by vasomotor instability.

EVIDENCE-BASED PRACTICE
Applying the Evidence

Walking and Stroke

You are a nurse caring for S.F., a 68-yr-old male who had a stroke 7 months ago. S.F. is unhappy that he is not able to perform activities on his own because of difficulties with physical mobility. You note his gait remains unsteady when walking with assistance from his wife who is his caregiver. He tells you a physical therapist is coming to his home but not on a regular basis.

Making Clinical Decisions

Best Available Evidence. In the chronic stage of stroke (>6 months after stroke), high-frequency walking training can increase walking capacity including speed and walking distance. Training frequency should be at least 24 sessions over 7 weeks for effective improvements in walking.

Clinician Expertise. You know a consistent walking program is an important part of rehabilitation following stroke. You also know improvements in physical mobility reach their maximum potential in the first year following stroke.

Patient Preferences and Values. S.F. has a goal of being able to walk independently in the next 6 months.

Implications for Nursing Practice

1. In what ways will you collaborate with physical therapy to monitor the progress of S.F. in meeting his goal?
2. How will you determine S.F.'s motivation to stay engaged in a consistent supervised walking program?
3. Why is it important to assess caregiver needs and coping at every patient visit, and how will you assist in providing caregiver resources?

Reference for Evidence

Peurala S, Karttunen A, Sjögren T, et al: Evidence for the effectiveness of walking training on walking and self-care after stroke: A systematic review and meta-analysis of randomized controlled trials, *J Rehabil Med* 46:387, 2014.

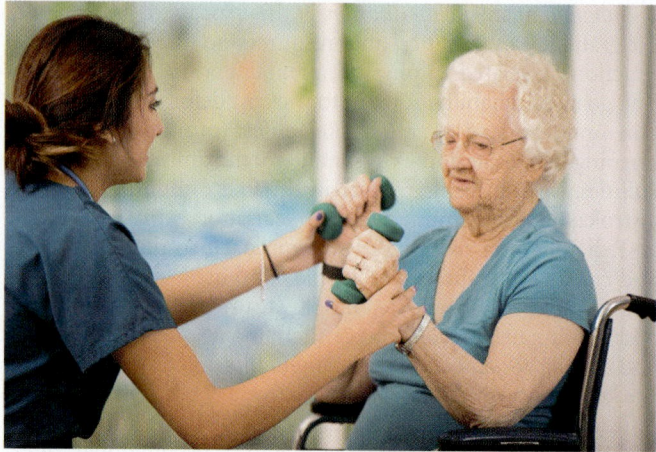

FIG. 57-11 A patient who had a stroke works with a physical therapist to improve arm strength. (©Thinkstock 78783452)

Also assess whether patients autocorrect their posture when sitting on the edge of the bed. If the patient can straighten his or her posture instead of leaning to the weaker side, the patient may be ready for the next step of transferring from bed to chair. Place the chair beside the bed so that the patient can lead with the stronger arm and leg. The patient sits on the side of the bed, stands, places the strong hand on the far wheelchair arm, and sits down. You may either supervise the transfer or provide minimal assistance by guiding the patient's strong hand to the wheelchair arm, standing in front of the patient while blocking the patient's knees with your knees to prevent knee buckling, and guiding the patient into a sitting position.

In some rehabilitation units, the Bobath method is used as an approach to mobility *(http://ibita.org)*. The goal of this approach is to help the patient gain control over patterns of spasticity by inhibiting abnormal reflex patterns. Therapists and nurses use the Bobath approach to encourage normal muscle tone, normal movement, and bilateral function of the body. An example is to have the patient transfer into the wheelchair using the weak or paralyzed side and the stronger side to facilitate more bilateral functioning.

Another approach to stroke rehabilitation is *constraint-induced movement therapy* (CIMT). CIMT encourages the patient to use the weakened extremity by restricting movement of the normal extremity. Complying with this approach can be challenging for patients and may limit its use. Movement training, skill acquisition, splinting, and exercise are additional therapies offered for rehabilitation of the stroke patient.[27]

Supportive or assistive equipment, such as canes, walkers, and leg braces, may be needed on a short- or long-term basis for mobility. The physical therapist usually selects the most appropriate supportive device(s) to meet individual needs and instructs the patient regarding use. Incorporate physical therapy activities into the patient's daily routine for additional practice and repetition of rehabilitation efforts (Fig. 57-11).

◆ **Stroke Survivorship and Coping.** Patients who have had strokes often exhibit emotional responses that are not appropriate or typical for the situation. Patients may appear apathetic, depressed, fearful, anxious, weepy, frustrated, and angry. Some patients, especially those with a stroke on the left side of the brain (right hemiplegia), have exaggerated mood swings. The patient may be unable to control emotions and may suddenly burst into tears or laughter. This behavior is out of context and often is unrelated to the patient's underlying emotional state. Nursing interventions for atypical emotional response are to (1) distract the patient who suddenly becomes emotional, (2) explain to the patient and family that emotional outbursts may occur after a stroke, (3) maintain a calm environment, and (4) avoid shaming or scolding the patient during emotional outbursts.

The patient with a stroke may experience many losses, including sensory, intellectual, communicative, functional, role behavior, emotional, social, and vocational losses. The patient, caregiver, and family often go through the process of grief and mourning associated with the losses. Some patients experience long-term depression with symptoms such as anxiety, weight loss, fatigue, poor appetite, and sleep disturbances. In addition, the time and energy required to perform previously simple tasks can result in anger and frustration.

The patient, caregiver, and family need help coping with the losses associated with stroke. Provide assistance by (1) supporting communication between the patient and family; (2) discussing lifestyle changes resulting from stroke deficits; (3) discussing changing roles and responsibilities within the family; (4) being an active listener to allow the expression of fear, frustration, and anxiety; (5) including the family and patient in short- and long-term goal planning and patient care; (6) supporting family conferences, and (7) identifying support groups and referrals as needed.

Maladjusted dependence with inadequate coping occurs when the patient does not maintain optimal functioning for self-care, family responsibilities, decision making, or socialization. This situation can cause resentment from both the patient and family with a negative cycle of interpersonal dependency and control. Caregivers and family members must cope with three aspects of the patient's behavior: (1) recognition of behavioral changes resulting from neurologic deficits that are not changeable, (2) responses to multiple losses by both the patient and family, and (3) behaviors that may have been reinforced during the early stages of stroke as continued dependency.

The patient, caregiver, and family may express guilt over not living healthy lifestyles or not seeking professional help sooner. Family therapy is a helpful adjunct to rehabilitation. Open communication, information regarding the total effects of stroke, teaching regarding stroke treatment, and therapy are helpful. Stroke support groups in rehabilitation facilities and in the community are helpful in terms of mutual sharing, education, coping skills, and understanding.

 Sexual Function. A patient who has had a stroke may be concerned about the loss of sexual function. Many patients are comfortable talking about their anxieties and fears regarding sexual function if you are comfortable and open to the topic. You may initiate a discussion about the topic with the patient and spouse or significant other. Common concerns regarding sexual activity are impotence and the occurrence of another stroke during sex. Nursing interventions for sexual activity include teaching about (1) optional positioning of partners, (2) timing for peak energy periods, and (3) patient and partner counseling.

Community Integration. Traditionally, successful community integration after stroke has been difficult for the patient because of persistent problems with cognition, coping, physical deficits, and emotional changes that interfere with functioning. Older patients who have had a stroke often have more severe deficits and frequently experience multiple health problems. Failure to continue the rehabilitation regimen at home may result in deterioration and further complications.

Community resources can be an asset to patients and their families. The National Stroke Association provides information, resources, referral services, and quarterly newsletters on stroke. The American Stroke Association, a division of the American Heart Association, has information regarding stroke, hypertension, diet, exercise, and assistive devices. This association sponsors self-help groups in many areas. Easter Seals provides wheelchairs and other assistive devices for stroke patients. Local groups can offer more daily assistance such as meals and transportation. These resources can be identified by nurse case managers, home health nurses, discharge planners, and clinical nurse specialists.

Gerontologic Considerations: Stroke

Stroke is a significant cause of death and disability. The majority (66%) of strokes that require hospitalization occur in adults over 65.[4] Stroke can result in a profound disruption in the life of an older person. The magnitude of disability and changes in total function can leave patients wondering if they can ever return to their "old self," and loss of independence may be a major concern. The ability to perform ADLs may require many adaptive changes because of physical, emotional, perceptual, and cognitive deficits. Home management may be a particular challenge if the patient has an older spouse caregiver who also has health problems. There may be limited family members (including adult children) living in close proximity to provide help.

The rehabilitative phase and helping the older patient deal with the residual deficits of stroke, as well as aging, can provide a challenging nursing experience. Patients may become fearful and depressed because they think they may have another stroke or die. The fear can become immobilizing and interfere with effective rehabilitation.

Changes may occur in the patient-spouse relationship. The dependency resulting from a stroke may threaten the relationship. The spouse may also have chronic medical problems that can affect the ability to take care of the stroke survivor. The patient may not want anyone other than the spouse to provide care, thus putting a significant burden on the spouse.

You have the opportunity to assist the patient and caregiver in the transition through acute hospitalization, rehabilitation, long-term care, and home care. The needs of the patient, caregiver, and family require ongoing nursing assessment and adaptation of interventions in response to changing needs to optimize quality of life for all of them.

 BECOMING A NURSE LEADER

Dealing With a Changing Environment

Situation

You have just gotten your first job after nursing school. You are so excited to be working at a rehabilitation center that has just moved into a new building and has new ownership. On your first day of work, you meet Evelyn and Martha, two older nurses who have worked for the center for over 20 years. In your first conversation with them Evelyn tells you, "The new management requires specialized computer training for all nursing staff. We are not going to do it and we will fight them on this issue and all the other changes they want to make." Martha adds, "Not only that, but we will threaten to quit if they do not listen to us and they better listen as we have been here for many years."

Points for Consideration

- Change is inevitable. Health care is constantly adapting and changing to new policies, technology, and medical advances.
- Resistance to change may be due to a variety of reasons. Deal with resistance by identifying the underlying fears that are causing it. Manage resistance by recognizing the benefits that change will bring. Reassure others that training will be provided for adapting to the new changes.
- Traditional practices are challenged with a changing environment. Nurses are put in positions of needing to do things that they have little experience with or have never done before.
- Integrating technology into nursing practice can improve health care, prevent medical errors, and decrease paperwork. However, technology can be very intimidating for nurses who have no or limited experience with it.
- Being leaders and responding to change is the responsibility of every nurse. Recognize that people will respond better to change if they are involved in the change process. Support other nurses as they adapt to and accept the changes.

Discussion Questions

1. Why are Evelyn and Martha resistant to the changes at the rehabilitation center?
2. How would you respond to Evelyn and Martha? Is there anything that you can do or say that would change their attitude about change?
3. As a new nurse, how can you take a leadership role to pave the way for the new changes at the center?

CASE STUDY

Stroke

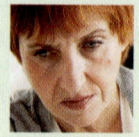

(©iStockphoto/ Thinkstock)

Patient Profile

J.K. is a 57-yr-old white woman who was is referred to the neurosurgery service for management of her temporal-parietal glioblastoma (see Assessment Case Study in Chapter 55 on pp. 1302, 1304, and 1307). She was diagnosed after presenting with persistent headaches, a seizure in her HCP's office, and left side upper visual field loss and neglect. Her MRI/MRA demonstrated a temporal-parietal glioblastoma that extends into the occipital lobes. She is scheduled for surgery to debulk the tumor. J.K. lives alone and holds a management position. She is concerned about her ability to return to work after her surgery.

J.K. returns from surgery to the neurosurgery unit drowsy but following commands. During the night J.K. is noted to have a pronator drift of the left arm, her pupils are equal and respond to light, but she has also developed left-sided weakness of both arm and leg and difficulty with answering questions.

Medications: dexamethasone 4 mg q6hr, famotidine, metoclopramide, ondansetron (Zofran), codeine, and levetiracetam (Keppra) since her admitting seizure

Subjective Data

- Left arm and leg are weak and feel numb
- She is trying to answer questions but looks confused and cannot follow commands

Objective Data

- BP 150/90 mm Hg
- Right gaze preference
- Left homonymous hemianopsia
- Left arm weakness (3/5) greater than leg weakness (4/5)

- Decreased sensation on both left arm and leg
- Has speech but not clear. Difficulty with word finding and following commands
- A diagnostic CT scan demonstrates a hemorrhagic stroke into the site of the tumor bed, and temporal-parietal and anterior occipital areas extending into the thalamus.

Discussion Questions

1. How does J.K.'s diagnosis (glioblastoma) put her at risk for a stroke?
2. **Priority Decisions:** What are the priority decisions that need to made regarding safety and self-care related to the left neglect and visual field cut?
3. **Patient-Centered Care:** What factors should you assess for related to rehabilitation for J.K.?
4. **Priority Decisions:** What are the priority nursing interventions for J.K.?
5. **Priority Decisions:** Based on the assessment data provided, what are the priority nursing diagnoses and are there any collaborative problems?
6. **Teamwork and Collaboration:** What nursing interventions for J.K. can the RN delegate to unlicensed assistive personnel ((UAP)?
7. **Teamwork and Collaboration:** How can you work together with the interprofessional team to develop and implement strategies to improve communication for J.K.?
8. **Safety:** How can you ensure safety for J.K. in light of her homonymous hemianopsia and left-sided neglect?
9. **Patient-Centered Care:** How can you address J.K.'s concerns about her finances and self-care?
10. **Patient-Centered Care:** J.K.'s family wants to know if her tumor surgery caused her hemorrhagic stroke and if so, what they should watch out for at home.

Answers available at *http://evolve.elsevier.com/Lewis/medsurg.*

BRIDGE TO NCLEX EXAMINATION

The number of the question corresponds to the same-numbered outcome at the beginning of the chapter.

1. Of the following patients, the nurse recognizes that the one with the highest risk for a stroke is a(n)
   a. obese 45-yr-old Native American.
   b. 35-yr-old Asian American woman who smokes.
   c. 32-yr-old white woman taking oral contraceptives.
   d. 65-yr-old African American man with hypertension.

2. The factor related to cerebral blood flow that *most* often determines the extent of cerebral damage from a stroke is the
   a. amount of cardiac output.
   b. O_2 content of the blood.
   c. degree of collateral circulation.
   d. level of CO_2 in the blood.

3. Information provided by the patient that would help differentiate a hemorrhagic stroke from a thrombotic stroke includes
   a. sensory disturbance.
   b. a history of hypertension.
   c. presence of motor weakness.
   d. sudden onset of severe headache.

4. A patient is exhibiting word finding difficulty and weakness in his right arm. What area of the brain is *most* likely involved?
   a. brainstem.
   b. vertebral artery.
   c. left middle cerebral artery.
   d. right middle cerebral artery.

5. The nurse explains to the patient with a stroke who is scheduled for angiography that this test is used to determine the
   a. presence of increased ICP.
   b. site and size of the infarction.
   c. patency of the cerebral blood vessels.
   d. presence of blood in the cerebrospinal fluid.

6. A patient experiencing TIAs is scheduled for a carotid endarterectomy. The nurse explains that this procedure is done to
   a. decrease cerebral edema.
   b. reduce the brain damage that occurs during a stroke in evolution.
   c. prevent a stroke by removing atherosclerotic plaques blocking cerebral blood flow.
   d. provide a circulatory bypass around thrombotic plaques obstructing cranial circulation.

7. For a patient who is suspected of having a stroke, one of the *most* important pieces of information that the nurse can obtain is
   a. time of the patient's last meal.
   b. time at which stroke symptoms first appeared.
   c. patient's hypertension history and management.
   d. family history of stroke and other cardiovascular diseases.

8. Bladder training in a male patient who has urinary incontinence after a stroke includes
   a. limiting fluid intake.
   b. keeping a urinal in place at all times.
   c. assisting the patient to stand to void.
   d. catheterizing the patient every 4 hours.

9. Common psychosocial reactions of the stroke patient to the stroke include *(select all that apply)*
   a. depression.
   b. disassociation.
   c. intellectualization.
   d. sleep disturbances.
   e. denial of severity of stroke.

1. d, 2, c, 3, d, 4, c, 5, c, 6, c, 7, b, 8, c, 9, a, d, e

For rationales to these answers and even more NCLEX review questions, visit *http://evolve.elsevier.com/Lewis/medsurg.*

ⓔ EVOLVE WEBSITE

http://evolve.elsevier.com/Lewis/medsurg
Review Questions (Online Only)
Key Points
Answer Keys for Questions
· Rationales for Bridge to NCLEX Examination Questions
· Answer Guidelines for Case Study on p. 1366
Student Case Studies
· Patient With Hypertension and Stroke
· Patient With Stroke
eNursing Care Plans
· eNursing Care Plan 57-1: Patient With Stroke
Conceptual Care Map Creator
· Conceptual Care Map for Case Study on p. 1366
Audio Glossary
Content Updates

REFERENCES

1. National Stroke Association: Stroke Survivors. Retrieved from *www.stroke.org/we-can-help/survivors.*
2. Center for Disease Control and Prevention: Stroke Facts. Retrieved from *www.cdc.gov/stroke/facts.htm.*
3. American Heart Association: Stroke falls to No. 5 Killer in US. Retrieved from *http://blog.heart.org/stroke-falls-no-5-killer-u-s.*
4. Vega C: Updated guidelines available for primary prevention of stroke CME/CE. Retrieved from *www.medscape.org/viewarticle/834329.*
*5. Kruithof W, Post M, Visser-Meily J: Measuring negative and positive caregiving experiences: A psychometric analysis of the Caregiver Strain Index Expanded, *Clin Rehabil* 29:1224, 2015.
*6. O'Donnell M and INTERSTROKE Study Team: Risk factors for ischaemic and intracerebral haemorrhagic stroke in 22 countries (the INTERSTROKE study): a case-control study, *Lancet Neurol* 376(9735):112, 2010.
7. Meschia J, Bushnel C, Boden-Albala B, et al: Guidelines for the primary prevention of stroke: A statement for healthcare professionals from the American Heart Association/American Stroke Association, *Stroke* 45(12):3754, 2014.
8. National Institute of Neurological Disorders and Stroke: Brain basics, preventing strokes. Retrieved from *www.ninds.nih.gov/disorders/stroke/preventing_stroke.htm#Risk%20Factors.*
9. American Heart Association/American Stroke Association: Transient ischemic attacks. Retrieved from *www.strokeassociation.org/STROKEORG/AboutStroke/TypesofStroke/TIA/TIA-Transient-Ischemic-Attack_UCM_310942_Article.jsp.*
10. American Heart Association/American Stroke Association: Ischemic Strokes (Clots). Retrieved from *www.strokeassociation.org/STROKEORG/AboutStroke/TypesofStroke/IschemicClots/Ischemic-Strokes-Clots_UCM_310939_Article.jsp.*
*11. Eriksen S, Gay C, Lerdal A: Acute phase factors associated with the course of depression during the first 18 months after first ever stroke, *Disability and Rehabilitation* 38:30, 2016.
*12. Schellinger P, Bryan R, Caplan L, et al: Evidence-based guideline: The role of diffusion and perfusion MRI for the diagnosis of acute ischemic stroke. Report of the Therapeutics and Technology Assessment Subcommittee of the American Academy of Neurology, *Neurology* 75(2):177, 2010.
13. Patel V, Gupta R, Horn C, et al: The neuro-critical care management of the endovascular stroke patient, *Curr Treat Options Neurol* 15(2):113, 2013.
*14. Hanselman C: Timing of tissue plasminogen activator for acute ischemic stroke: outcomes-based recommendations for practice, *J Neuroscience Nurs* 46(6): 314, 2014.
*15. Spiotta A, Chaudry M, Hui F, et al: Evolution of thrombectomy approaches and devices for acute stroke: A technical review, *J Neurointerv Surg* 7:12, 2015.
*16. Campbell BC, Mitchell PJ, Kleinig TJ, et al: Endovascular therapy for ischemic stroke with perfusion-imaging selection, *N Engl J Med* 372:1009, 2015.
17. Furlan AJ: Endovascular therapy for stroke—it's about time, *N Engl J Med* 2015; 150417035025009 DOI: 10.1056/NEJMe1503217.
18. U.S. Food and Drug Administration FDA: Clears system to reduce stroke during stent and angioplasty procedures. Retrieved from *www.fda.gov/NewsEvents/Newsroom/PressAnnouncements/ucm433482.htm?source=govdelivery&utm_medium=email&utm_source=govdelivery.*
19. Kirkman M, Citerio G, Smith M: The intensive care management of acute ischemic stroke: an overview, *Intens Care Med* 40(5):640, 2014.
20. Watson J: Subarachnoid hemorrhage surgery. Retrieved from *http://emedicine.medscape.com/article/247090-overview.*
21. Green T, Kelloway L, Davies-Schinkel C, et al: Nurses' accountability for stroke quality of care, part one: review of the literature on nursing-sensitive outcomes, *Can J Neurosci* 33(3):13, 2011.
22. American Stroke Association: NIH stroke scale international. Retrieved from *www.nihstrokescale.org.*
*23. CLOTS Trial Collaboration: Effect of intermittent pneumatic compression on disability, living circumstances, quality of life, and hospital costs after stroke: secondary analyses from CLOTS 3, *Lancet Neurol* 13(12):1186, 2014.
*24. Hutchinson E, Wilson N: Acute stroke, dysphagia, and nutritional support, *Br J Community Nurs* S26-29, 2013.
*25. Wallace S, Purdy M, Skidmore E: A multimodal communication program for aphasia during inpatient rehabilitation: a case study, *NeuroRehabilitation* 35(3):615, 2014.
*26. Van der Cruyssen K, Vereeck L, Saeys W, et al: Prognostic factors for discharge destinations after acute stroke: a comprehensive literature review, *Disabil Rehabil* 37:1214, 2015.
*27. Saunders DH, Sanderson M, Brazzelli M, et al: Physical fitness training for stroke patients, *Cochrane Database Syst Rev*, 2013. Issue 10. CD003316. DOI:10.1002/146518.CD003316.pub5.

*Evidence-based information for clinical practice.

58

Chronic Neurologic Problems

Dottie Roberts, Madona Plueger

If you don't like something, change it. If you can't change it, change your attitude.

Maya Angelou

http://evolve.elsevier.com/Lewis/medsurg/

LEARNING OUTCOMES

1. Compare and contrast the etiology, clinical manifestations, interprofessional care, and nursing management of tension-type, migraine, and cluster headaches.
2. Differentiate the etiology, clinical manifestations, diagnostic studies, interprofessional care, and nursing management of seizure disorders, multiple sclerosis, Parkinson's disease, and myasthenia gravis.
3. Describe the clinical manifestations and nursing and interprofessional management of restless legs syndrome, amyotrophic lateral sclerosis, and Huntington's disease.
4. Explain the potential impact of chronic neurologic disease on physical and psychologic well-being.
5. Outline the major goals of treatment for the patient with a chronic, progressive neurologic disease.

KEY TERMS

absence seizure, p. 1375
amyotrophic lateral sclerosis (ALS), p. 1395
aura, p. 1371
cluster headaches, p. 1371
epilepsy, p. 1374
focal seizures, p. 1376
generalized seizures, p. 1375

headache, p. 1368
Huntington's disease (HD), p. 1395
migraine headache, p. 1370
multiple sclerosis (MS), p. 1383
myasthenia gravis (MG), p. 1393
myasthenic crisis, p. 1393
Parkinson's disease (PD), p. 1387

restless legs syndrome (RLS), p. 1382
seizure, p. 1374
status epilepticus, p. 1376
tension-type headache, p. 1370
tonic seizure, p. 1376
tonic-clonic seizure, p. 1375

This chapter discusses headaches, chronic neurologic disorders, and degenerative neurologic disorders. Chronic neurologic disorders include seizure disorders and restless legs syndrome. Degenerative neurologic disorders include multiple sclerosis, Parkinson's disease, myasthenia gravis, amyotrophic lateral sclerosis, and Huntington's disease.

HEADACHES

Headache is probably the most common type of pain that humans experience. The majority of people have functional headaches, such as migraine or tension-type headaches. Others have organic headaches caused by intracranial or extracranial disease.

Pain-sensitive structures in the head include venous sinuses, dura, cranial blood vessels, three divisions of the trigeminal nerve (cranial nerve [CN] V), facial nerve (CN VII), glossopharyngeal nerve (CN IX), vagus nerve (CN X), and the first three cervical nerves. Because these nerves have both motor and sensory functions, increased pain intensity and symptoms can occur when a person moves.

Headaches are classified as primary or secondary headache. *Primary headache* classifications include tension-type, migraine, and cluster headaches. Primary headaches are not caused by a disease or another medical condition. The type of primary headache is determined using the International Headache Society (IHS) guidelines based on characteristics of the headache (Table 58-1). *Secondary headaches* are caused by another condition or disorder, such as sinus infection, neck injury, and brain tumor.

A patient may have more than one type of headache. The history and neurologic examination are diagnostic keys to determine the type of headache. The examination of a person with a headache is often normal. Unexplained abnormal findings require additional diagnostic studies to identify underlying causes and additional risk factors.

Reviewed by Sonya H. Blevins, RN, DNP, CMSRN, CNE, Assistant Professor of Nursing, Mary Black School of Nursing, University of South Carolina Upstate, Greenville, South Carolina; Regina Gonzalez-Lama, RN, MS, Lecturer, College of Staten Island–CUNY, Staten Island, New York; Linda Littlejohns, RN, MSN, CNRN, FAAN, Neuroscience Clinical Nursing Consultant, San Juan Capistrano, California; Pamela K. Newland, RN, PhD, CMSRN, Assistant Professor, Goldfarb School of Nursing at Barnes Jewish College, St. Louis, Missouri; and Daryle Wane, PhD, ARNP, FNP-BC, RN to BSN Coordinator, Professor of Nursing, Department of Health Occupations, Pasco-Hernando State College, New Port Richey, Florida.

TABLE 58-1 Interprofessional Care

Headaches

Tension-Type Headaches	Migraine Headache	Cluster Headache
Location		
Bilateral, band-like pressure at base of skull	Unilateral (in 60%), may switch sides, commonly anterior location	Unilateral, radiating up or down from one eye
Quality		
Constant, squeezing tightness	Throbbing, synchronous with pulse	Severe, bone crushing
Frequency		
Cycles for many years	Periodic, cycles of several months and years	May have months or years between attacks
		Attacks occur in clusters over a period of 2-12 wk
Duration		
30 min-7 days	4-72 hr	5 min-3 hr
Time and Mode of Onset		
Not related to time	May be preceded by premonitory symptoms or aura	Nocturnal, commonly awakens person from sleep
	Onset after awakening	
	Improves with sleep	
Associated Symptoms		
Palpable neck and shoulder muscle tension	Irritability, sweating	Facial flushing or pallor
Stiff neck	Nausea, vomiting	Unilateral lacrimation, ptosis, rhinitis
Tenderness	Photophobia	
	Phonophobia	
	Premonitory symptoms: sensory, motor, or psychic phenomena	
	Family history (in 65%)	
Treatment: Abortive and Symptomatic Drugs		
Non-opioid analgesics: aspirin, acetaminophen, NSAIDS	Non-opioid analgesics: aspirin, NSAIDs	α-Adrenergic blockers
Analgesic combinations	Serotonin receptor agonists	• ergotamine tartrate (Ergomar)
• butalbital/aspirin/caffeine (Fiorinal)	• almotriptan (Axert)	Serotonin receptor agonists
• butalbital/acetaminophen/caffeine	• eletriptan (Relpax)	• almotriptan
• dichloralphenazone/acetaminophen/ isomethepetene	• frovatriptan (Frova)	• eletriptan
Muscle relaxants	• naratriptan (Amerge)	• frovatriptan
	• rizatriptan (Maxalt)	• naratriptan
	• sumatriptan (Imitrex)	• rizatriptan
	• zolmitriptan (Zomig)	• sumatriptan
	• sumatriptan transdermal system (Zecuity)	• zolmitriptan
	Combination	O₂ 100% inhalation via mask
	• sumatriptan/naproxen (Treximet)	
	α-Adrenergic blockers	
	• ergotamine tartrate (Ergomar)	
	• dihydroergotamine nasal spray (Migranal)	
	Analgesic combinations	
	• acetaminophen/caffeine/aspirin	
	• acetaminophen/isomeptene/ dichloralphenazone	
	Corticosteroids	
	• dexamethasone	
Treatment: Preventive		
Tricyclic antidepressants	β-Adrenergic blocker	α-Adrenergic blockers
• amitriptyline	• propranolol	• ergotamine tartrate
• nortriptyline (Pamelor)	Antidepressants	Corticosteroid
• doxepin	• amitriptyline	• prednisone
Selective serotonin reuptake inhibitors	• imipramine (Tofranil)	Calcium channel blocker
• fluoxetine (Prozac)	Antiseizure drugs	• verapamil
• paroxetine (Paxil)	• valproic acid (Depakene)	Lithium
β-Adrenergic blocker:	• divalproex	Biofeedback
• propranolol (Inderal)	• topiramate	
Antiseizure drugs	• gabapentin (Neurontin)	
• topiramate (Topamax)	Calcium channel blocker	
• divalproex (Depakote)	• verapamil (Calan)	
Other drugs	• nifedipine (Procardia)	
• mirtazapine (Remeron)	Botulinum toxin A (Botox)	
Biofeedback	Biofeedback	
Psychotherapy	Relaxation therapy	
Muscle relaxation training	Cognitive-behavioral therapy	

TENSION-TYPE HEADACHE

Tension-type headache, also called *stress headache,* is the most common type of headache. These headaches are characterized by their bilateral location and pressing or tightening quality. Tension-type headaches are usually of mild or moderate intensity and can last from minutes to days. Tension-type headaches are divided by frequency into episodic and chronic types.[1]

Etiology and Pathophysiology

The cause of tension-type headache is not fully understood, but it may have a neurobiologic basis similar to migraine headaches. For some, episodic headaches evolve to chronic headaches. Increased frequency does not necessarily produce increased headache intensity. However, chronic tension-type headache can cause diminished quality of life and severe disability.[1]

Clinical Manifestations

Patients often have a bilateral frontal-occipital headache described as a constant, dull pressure, or band-like headache associated with neck pain and increased tone in the cervical and neck muscles. The headache may involve sensitivity to light *(photophobia)* or sound *(phonophobia)* but does not involve nausea or vomiting. There are no *premonitory symptoms* (warning symptoms of impending headache), and physical activity does not aggravate symptoms. The headaches may occur intermittently for weeks, months, or even years.

Many patients have a combination of migraine and tension-type headaches, with features of both occurring simultaneously. Patients with migraine headaches may experience tension-type headaches between migraine attacks. Fig. 58-1 shows the location of pain for common headache syndromes.

Diagnostic Studies

Careful history taking may be the most important tool for diagnosing tension-type headache (Table 58-2). If tension-type headache is present during physical examination, increased resistance to passive movement of the head and tenderness of the head and neck may be noted. Electromyography (EMG) may reveal sustained contraction of neck, scalp, or facial muscles. However, the patient may not show increased muscle tension with this test, even when it is done during an actual headache.

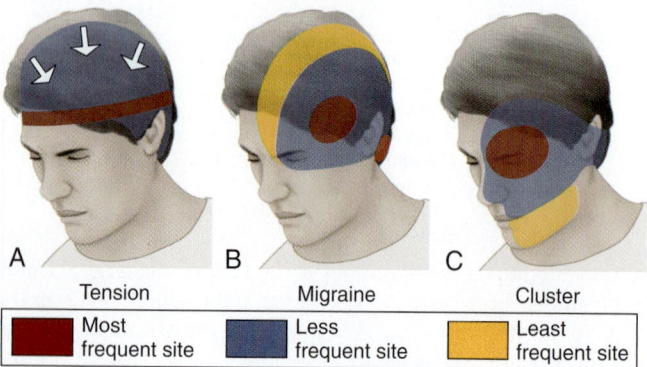

| Most frequent site | Less frequent site | Least frequent site |

FIG. 58-1 Location of pain for common headache syndromes. **A,** Tension headache is often described as feeling of a weight in or on the head or a band squeezing the head. **B,** Migraine headache is described as an intense throbbing or pounding pain that involves one temple. The pain usually is unilateral (on one side of the head), although it can be bilateral. **C,** Cluster headache pain is focused in and around one eye and is often described as sharp, penetrating, or burning.

MIGRAINE HEADACHE

Migraine headache is a recurring headache characterized by unilateral throbbing pain. Light, sound, and smell sensitivity and other environmental factors may be either premonitory symptoms or triggers for the migraine headache.[2] Manifestations of migraine are associated with neurologic and autonomic nervous system dysfunction. The most common age for onset of migraine is between 20 and 30 years. Migraine affects as many as 18% of females and 6% of males in the United States.[3] Migraines are more common in women than men (see Gender Differences box). Risk factors for migraine include family history, low level of education, low socioeconomic status, high workload, and frequent tension-type headaches.

GENDER DIFFERENCES
Headaches

Men	Women
• Cluster headaches are more common than in women (6:1).	• Migraine headaches are more common than in men (3:1).
• Exercise-induced headaches are more common than in women.	• Tension headaches are more common than in men.

The IHS subdivides migraines into categories. *Migraine without aura* (formerly called *common migraine*) is the most common type. *Migraine with aura* (formerly called *classic migraine*) occurs in only 10% of migraine headache episodes.[1]

Etiology and Pathophysiology

Although many theories have addressed the cause of migraine headaches, the exact etiology is not known. The current theory is that a complex series of neurovascular events initiates a migraine headache. People who have migraines have a state of neuronal hyperexcitability in the cerebral cortex, especially in the occipital cortex. Genetic factors may account for about 50% of an individual's risk for migraine headache.[3]

Migraine is associated with seizure disorders, ischemic stroke, asthma, depression, anxiety, myocardial infarction, Raynaud's syndrome, and irritable bowel syndrome. In many cases, migraine headaches have no known precipitating events. However, for some patients, specific factors may trigger a headache. These include foods, menstruation, head trauma, physical exertion,

TABLE 58-2 Diagnostic Studies
Headaches

History and Physical Examination
- Neurologic examination (often negative)
- Inspection for local infection
- Palpation of head for tenderness, bony swellings
- Auscultation for bruits over major arteries, especially neck

Routine Laboratory Studies
- Complete blood count (CBC) (may indicate anemia, infection)
- Electrolytes (may indicate dehydration, other illnesses)
- Urinalysis (may indicate infection, other medical diagnoses [e.g., diabetes])
- Other diagnostic studies to assess evidence of disease, deformity, or infection: angiography, EMG, EEG, MRA, MRI, lumbar puncture

EEG, Electroencephalography; *EMG,* electromyography; *MRA,* magnetic resonance angiography.

fatigue, stress, missed meals, weather, and drugs. Food triggers include chocolate, cheese, oranges, tomatoes, onions, monosodium glutamate, aspartame, and alcohol (particularly red wine).

Clinical Manifestations

Premonitory symptoms and an *aura* may precede the headache phase by several hours or several days. Premonitory symptoms may include neurologic (e.g., photophobia), psychologic (e.g., hyperactivity, irritability), and other (e.g., food craving) manifestations. An aura is a complex of neurologic symptoms that occur before a headache for some patients. It may be characterized by visual symptoms, such as bright lights, scotomas (patchy blindness), visual distortions, or zigzag lines. Sensory (voices or sounds that do not exist, strange smells), and/or motor (e.g., weakness, paralysis, feeling that limbs are moving) phenomena may also be part of an aura.

A migraine headache may last 4 to 72 hours. The headache is described as a steady, throbbing pain that is synchronous with the pulse. Although the headache is usually unilateral, it may switch to the opposite side in another episode. During the headache phase, some patients with migraine may tend to seek shelter from noise, light, odors, people, and problems.

The presentation of migraine varies in severity. Not all migraine headaches are disabling, and many patients who have migraines do not seek treatment for them. In some patients, migraine symptoms may become worse over time.

Diagnostic Studies

The diagnosis of migraine headache is usually based on the patient history. The neurologic and other diagnostic examinations are often normal (Table 58-2).

No specific laboratory or radiologic test can diagnose migraine headache. Neuroimaging techniques (e.g., head CT scan, with or without contrast, and MRI) are not recommended for routine evaluation of headache, unless the neurologic examination reveals abnormal findings. If atypical features are present, then additional testing is done to rule out a secondary headache.

CLUSTER HEADACHE

Cluster headaches are the most severe form of primary headache. Repeated headaches occur in clusters, generally at the same time of day or night. Age at onset is typically 20 to 45 years, but they can start at any age. Men are affected three times more often than women.[4]

Etiology and Pathophysiology

Neither the cause nor the pathophysiologic mechanism of cluster headache is fully known. The unilateral pain may occur with activation of neurons in the ophthalmic branch of the trigeminal nerve. Cluster headaches also involve the hypothalamus, with irregularities in melatonin and cortisol. This indicates a dysfunction of circadian rhythm. Imaging studies show hypothalamic activation at the onset of cluster headache.[5] Alcohol is a dietary trigger. Strong odors, weather changes, and napping are other triggers.

Clinical Manifestations

The cluster headache is one of the most severe forms of headache, with intense pain lasting from a few minutes to 3 hours. In contrast to the pulsing pain of migraine headache, the pain of cluster headache is sharp and stabbing. The pain is generally located around the eye, radiating to the temple, forehead, cheek, nose, or gums. Other manifestations may include swelling around the eye, lacrimation (tearing), facial flushing or pallor, nasal congestion, and miosis (constriction of the pupil). During the headache, the patient is often agitated and restless, unable to sit still or relax. A majority of patients have at least three of these symptoms. In addition, an aura similar to migraine may occur in 14% of patients up to 60 minutes before an attack.[5]

Cluster headaches can occur every other day and as often as eight times a day. A cluster typically lasts 2 weeks to 3 months, and then the patient goes into remission for months to years. Typically, two cluster periods a year may be separated by months without symptoms. Because cluster periods often occur seasonally, headaches may be mistaken for symptoms of allergies.

Diagnostic Studies

The diagnosis of cluster headache is based on the patient history according to IHS criteria. Asking patients to keep a headache diary can be useful. CT scan, MRI, or magnetic resonance angiography (MRA) may rule out an aneurysm, a tumor, or an infection. A lumbar puncture may rule out other disorders that may cause similar symptoms.

OTHER TYPES OF HEADACHES

Although tension, migraine, and cluster headaches are by far the most common types of headaches, other types can occur. These headaches may be the first symptom of a more serious illness. Headache can accompany subarachnoid hemorrhage; brain tumors; other intracranial masses; vascular abnormalities; trigeminal neuralgia (tic douloureux); diseases of the eyes, nose, and teeth; and systemic illness (e.g., bacteremia, carbon monoxide poisoning, altitude sickness, polycythemia vera). Because of the varied causes of headache, clinical evaluation must be thorough. It should include assessment of personality, life adjustment, environment, and family situation, as well as a comprehensive evaluation of neurologic and physical status.

INFORMATICS IN PRACTICE

Social Media Use for Patients With Migraine Headaches

- Many patients with migraine headaches believe their pain and its impact on their quality of life are poorly understood by others.
- Encourage patients to participate in a social media outlet (e.g., Twitter) where people who have migraines share their experiences.
- Using social media allows patients to describe their physical and emotional pain and can help them cope better with their condition and improve their quality of life.

INTERPROFESSIONAL CARE FOR HEADACHES

If no systemic underlying disease is the cause, the type of headache guides therapy. Table 58-2 outlines the general workup for a patient with headache to rule out any intracranial or extracranial disease. Table 58-1 summarizes current therapies for prevention and management of different types of headaches. These therapies include drugs, meditation, yoga, biofeedback, cognitive-behavioral therapy, and relaxation training.

Cognitive-behavioral therapy and relaxation therapy used alone or in conjunction with drug therapy may be beneficial to some patients. Biofeedback involves the use of physiologic monitoring equipment to give the patient information regarding muscle tension and peripheral blood flow (e.g., skin temperature of the fingers). The patient is trained to relax the muscles and raise the finger temperature and is given reinforcement (operant conditioning) in accomplishing these changes. Acupuncture, acupressure, and hypnosis also work well in some patients with headaches.

Drug Therapy

Tension-Type Headache. Drug therapy for tension-type headache usually involves aspirin, acetaminophen (Tylenol), or nonsteroidal antiinflammatory drugs (NSAIDs) used alone or in combination with a sedative, muscle relaxant, or tranquilizer. However, many of these drugs have serious side effects. Caution the patient about the long-term use of aspirin and aspirin-containing drugs because they can cause upper gastrointestinal (GI) bleeding and coagulation abnormalities in susceptible patients. Drugs containing acetaminophen can cause kidney damage with chronic use and liver damage when taken in large doses or when combined with alcohol. To decrease the recurrence of tension-type headache, the patient may receive preventive therapy with a tricyclic antidepressant (e.g., amitriptyline, nortriptyline) or mirtazapine (Remeron), a nonadrenergic serotonergic antidepressant (NaSSA). Antiseizure medications such as topiramate (Topamax) or divalproex (Depakote) may also be used.

Migraine Headache. The aim of drug treatment of an acute migraine attack is terminating or decreasing the symptoms. Many people with mild or moderate migraine can obtain relief with NSAIDs, aspirin, or caffeine-containing combination analgesics. For moderate to severe headaches, the triptans have become the first line of therapy. Triptans (e.g., sumatriptan [Imitrex]) affect selected serotonin receptors, thus reducing neurogenic inflammation of the cerebral blood vessels and producing vasoconstriction (Table 58-1). They are most effective when taken at the onset of migraine headache or during the aura. Sumatriptan is available in various forms: oral, subcutaneous, nasal spray, transdermal.

Some patients respond better to one triptan than to others, so HCPs need to be knowledgeable about all of them. Because these drugs cause vasoconstriction, patients with a history of heart disease or stroke should avoid their use. The combination drug sumatriptan/naproxen (Treximet) combines a triptan with an antiinflammatory drug. However, risk of serious cardiovascular events such as myocardial infarction, thromboembolic events, and stroke may increase over time with this drug.

 DRUG ALERT Sumatriptan (Imitrex)
- Should not be given to patients with the following:
  - History or manifestations of ischemic cardiac, cerebrovascular, or peripheral vascular problems.
  - Uncontrolled hypertension (may increase BP).
- Excess dosage may produce tremor and decrease respirations.

Zecuity (sumatriptan transdermal system) is the first skin patch indicated for the treatment of migraine headache and for intense nausea secondary to the headache itself. Zecuity is applied either to the upper arm or thigh. It should not be applied over red or irritated skin or over scars, tattoos, or broken skin. The patient pushes a button to deliver the drug through the skin over a course of 4 hours. Zecuity has similar contraindications to other triptans.[6] When triptans are contraindicated or ineffective, other drugs can be used (Table 58-1).

Preventive treatment is important in the management of migraine headaches. The decision to initiate preventive

treatment is individually determined based on frequency, severity, and any disability related to headaches. Several different classes of medications are used.

Topiramate, an antiseizure drug, may be taken daily for migraine prevention. Common side effects include hypoglycemia, paresthesia, weight loss, and cognitive changes. Usually these side effects are mild to moderate and transient. Topiramate must be used for 2 to 3 months to determine its effectiveness. Not all patients become pain free on this medication. HCPs must offer thorough teaching regarding topiramate to promote patient adherence.

 DRUG ALERT Topiramate (Topamax)
Instruct patient to do the following:
- Not abruptly discontinue because this may cause seizures.
- Avoid tasks that require alertness until response to drug is established.
- Take adequate fluids to decrease risk of renal stone development.

Botulinum toxin A (Botox) may be an effective prophylactic treatment for patients who have chronic migraines lasting for 4 hours or more at least 15 days each month, or migraines that do not respond to other medications. Botox is given by multiple injections around the head and neck. Effects last 2 to 4 months; the injections are repeated every 3 months. The most common adverse reactions are neck pain and headache. A slight risk exists for the toxin to migrate from the injection site to other areas of the face and neck, causing swallowing and breathing difficulties. Teach the patient to seek immediate medical attention if this occurs.

Gabapentin (Neurontin) is another antiseizure drug used for migraine prevention. Selective serotonin reuptake inhibitors (e.g., fluoxetine [Prozac]) may also be prescribed. Other drugs used for migraine headache prevention are listed in Table 58-1.

Cluster Headache. Triptans are a gold standard of treatment for occasional cluster headache. Either nasal administration or subcutaneous injection is appropriate. However, as noted in the discussion of migraine headache, triptans are vasoconstrictors. Thus they are contraindicated for patients with vascular risk factors.[5]

High-flow 100% O_2 by non-rebreather mask is well tolerated, safe, and effective as an alternative treatment. O_2 delivered at a rate of 6 to 8 L/min for 10 minutes may relieve headache by causing vasoconstriction and increasing synthesis of serotonin in the central nervous system. Treatment can be repeated after a 5-minute rest. However, a drawback to this treatment is that the patient must have continuous access to the O_2 supply.

For chronic cluster headache, preventive treatment is needed. High-dose verapamil is the first-choice drug. However, because of its effects on cardiac conduction, verapamil should be initiated only after careful consideration of the risks. Careful monitoring is needed during treatment. Other drug options may include lithium, ergotamine, antiseizure drugs (e.g., topiramate), and melatonin. Options for patients with refractory cluster headaches include invasive nerve blocks, deep brain stimulation, and ablative neurosurgical procedures (e.g., percutaneous radiofrequency).

Other Headaches. Patients with frequent headaches may overuse analgesics or other medications indicated for headache treatment. *Medication overuse headache* (MOH) is the term used to describe a new type of headache, or marked worsening of a preexisting headache condition. Drugs known to cause this problem are acetaminophen, aspirin, NSAIDs (e.g., ibuprofen), butalbital, triptans, ergotamine, and opioids.[1] Patients with daily headaches may complain of early awakening with decreased appetite, nausea, restlessness, decreased memory, and irritability. Treatment involves abrupt withdrawal of the offending drug (except for opioids, which must be tapered) and initiation of alternative drugs such as amitriptyline.

❖ NURSING MANAGEMENT: HEADACHES

◆ Nursing Assessment

Table 58-3 outlines subjective and objective data that you should obtain from a patient with headache. Because the history provides the key to assessment of headache, it should include specific details of the headache, such as the location and type of pain, onset, frequency, duration, relation to events (emotional, psychologic, physical), and time of day of the occurrence. Obtain information about previous illnesses, surgery, trauma, allergies, family history, and response to medication.

Suggest that the patient keep a diary of headache episodes with specific details. This record can be of great help in determining the type of headache and precipitating events. If the patient has a history of migraine, tension-type, or cluster headaches, ask the patient if the character, intensity, or location of the headache has changed. The answer may be an important clue about the cause of the headache.

◆ Nursing Diagnoses

Nursing diagnoses for the patient with headache may include, but are not limited to, the following:

- Acute pain *related to* headache
- Ineffective health management *related to* drug therapy and lifestyle adjustments

Additional information on nursing diagnoses is presented in eNursing Care Plan 58-1 for the patient with headache (available on the website for this chapter).

◆ Planning

The overall goals are that the patient with a headache will (1) have reduced or no pain, (2) demonstrate understanding of triggering events and treatment strategies, (3) use positive coping strategies to deal with pain, and (4) experience increased quality of life and decreased disability.

◆ Nursing Implementation

The patient with chronic headache presents a great challenge to HCPs. Because an inability to cope with daily stresses can cause headaches, an effective therapy may involve helping the patient examine the daily routine, recognize stressful situations, and develop more appropriate coping strategies. Help the patient identify precipitating factors and develop ways to avoid them. Encourage daily exercise, relaxation periods, and socialization because they can decrease the recurrence of headache. Suggest alternative ways to address headache pain through techniques, such as relaxation, meditation, and yoga.

In addition to using analgesics and analgesic combinations for symptomatic relief of headache, encourage the migraine sufferer to seek a quiet, dimly lit environment. Massage and moist hot packs to the neck and head can help a patient with tension-type headaches. The patient should learn about the drugs prescribed for preventive and abortive/symptomatic treatment of headache and should be able to describe the purpose, action, dosage, and side effects of the drugs. To prevent

---

TABLE 58-3	**Nursing Assessment**

Headaches

Subjective Data

Important Health Information

Past health history: Seizures, cancer, recent fall or trauma, cranial infection, stroke. Asthma or allergies. Relationship of headache to overwork, stress, menstruation, exercise, food, sexual activity, travel, bright lights, or noxious environmental stimuli

Medications: Hydralazine, bromides, nitroglycerin, ergotamine (withdrawal), NSAIDs (in high daily doses), estrogen preparations, oral contraceptives, over-the-counter or prescription remedies

Surgical interventions or other treatments: Craniotomy, sinus surgery, facial surgery

Functional Health Pattern

Health perception–health management: Positive family history. Malaise

Nutritional-metabolic: Ingestion of alcohol, caffeine, cheese, chocolate, monosodium glutamate, aspartame, lunch meats (nitrites in cured meats), sausage, hot dogs, onions, avocados. History of anorexia, nausea, vomiting (migraine premonitory symptom); unilateral lacrimation (cluster)

Activity, exercise: Vertigo, fatigue, weakness, paralysis, fainting

Sleep-rest: Insomnia

Cognitive-perceptual

- *Migraine:* Aura. Unilateral, severe, throbbing headache (possible switching of side). Visual disturbances, photophobia, phonophobia, dizziness, tingling or burning sensations
- *Cluster:* Unilateral and severe, nocturnal headache. Nasal stuffiness
- *Tension type:* Bilateral, band-like, dull and persistent, base-of-skull headache, neck tenderness.

Self-perception–self-concept: Depression

Coping–stress tolerance: Stress, anxiety, irritability, withdrawal

Objective Data

General

Anxiety, apprehension

Integumentary

Cluster: Forehead diaphoresis, pallor, unilateral facial flushing with cheek edema, conjunctivitis

Migraine: Generalized edema (premonitory symptom) pallor, diaphoresis

Neurologic

Horner's syndrome, restlessness (cluster), hemiparesis (migraine)

Musculoskeletal

Resistance of head and neck movement, nuchal rigidity (meningeal, tension type), palpable neck and shoulder muscle tension (tension type)

Possible Diagnostic Findings

Evidence of disease, deformity, or infection on brain imaging (CT, MRI, MRA), cerebral angiogram, lumbar puncture, EEG, EMG

EEG, Electroencephalography; *EMG,* electromyography; *MRA,* magnetic resonance angiography.

---

accidental overdose, the patient should make a written note of each dose of drug or headache remedy.

For the patient with headaches triggered by food, provide dietary counseling. Encourage the patient to eliminate foods that may provoke headaches, such as chocolate, cheese, oranges, tomatoes, onions, monosodium glutamate, aspartame, alcohol (particularly red wine), excessive caffeine, and fermented or

TABLE 58-4   Patient & Caregiver Teaching

Headaches

Include the following instructions when teaching the patient with a headache and the patient's caregiver.

1. Keep a diary or calendar of headaches and possible precipitating events.
2. Avoid possible triggers for a headache:
   - Foods containing amines (cheese, chocolate), nitrites (meats such as hot dogs), vinegar, onions, monosodium glutamate
   - Fermented or marinated foods
   - Caffeine
   - Oranges
   - Tomatoes
   - Aspartame
   - Nicotine
   - Ice cream
   - Alcohol (particularly red wine)
   - Emotional stress
   - Fatigue
   - Drugs such as ergot-containing preparations (ergotamine tartrate [Ergomar]) and monoamine oxidase inhibitors (e.g., rasagiline [Azilect])
3. Learn the purpose, action, dosage, and side effects of drugs taken.
4. Self-administer sumatriptan (Imitrex) subcutaneously if prescribed.
5. Self-administer sumatriptan transdermal patch (Zecuity) (if prescribed) and describe appropriate disposal method for used patch.
6. Use stress management techniques (Chapter 6).
7. Participate in regular exercise.
8. Contact HCP if any of the following occur:
   - Symptoms become more severe, last longer than usual, or are resistant to medication
   - Nausea and vomiting (if severe or not typical), change in vision, or fever occurs with the headache
   - Problems occur with any drugs

marinated foods. Active challenge and provocative testing (designed specifically to provoke symptoms) with suspect foods may help determine specific causative agents. However, teach the patient that food triggers may change over time.

Teach patients to avoid smoking and exposure to triggers, such as strong perfumes, volatile solvents, and gasoline fumes. Cluster headaches may occur at high altitudes with low O_2 levels during air travel. Ergotamine, taken before the plane takes off, may decrease the likelihood of these attacks. See Table 58-4 for a teaching guide for the patient with a headache.

◆ Evaluation

Expected outcomes are that the patient with headache will
- Report satisfaction with pain management
- Use drug and nondrug measures appropriately to manage pain

Additional information on expected outcomes for the patient with headache is presented in eNursing Care Plan 58-1 (available on the website for this chapter).

CHRONIC NEUROLOGIC DISORDERS

EPILEPSY AND SEIZURE DISORDERS

Epilepsy is a disease marked by a continuing predisposition to seizures, with neurobiologic, cognitive, psychologic, and social consequences.[7] It is the fourth most common neurologic disorder, with only migraine, stroke, and Alzheimer's disease occurring more frequently. In the United States, approximately 2.2

million people have active epilepsy, with 150,000 new cases diagnosed each year.[8] The incidence of epilepsy is higher in young children and older adults.

New cases of epilepsy are more common in African Americans and in socially disadvantaged populations. Males are slightly more likely to develop epilepsy than females. People with Alzheimer's disease or who have had a stroke are at high risk for developing epilepsy. The risk is slightly increased in the child of a person who has epilepsy. However, most children will not inherit epilepsy from a parent.

Seizure is a transient, uncontrolled electrical discharge of neurons in the brain that interrupts normal function. Seizures may accompany a variety of disorders, or they may occur spontaneously without any apparent cause. Seizures resulting from systemic and metabolic disturbances are not considered epilepsy if the seizures cease when the underlying problem is corrected. Metabolic disturbances that cause seizures include acidosis, electrolyte imbalances, hypoglycemia, hypoxia, alcohol and barbiturate withdrawal, dehydration, and water intoxication. Extracranial disorders that can cause seizures are heart, lung, liver, or kidney diseases; systemic lupus erythematosus; diabetes mellitus; hypertension; and septicemia.

Etiology and Pathophysiology

Seizure disorders have many possible causes, with the most common causes varying by age. The most common causes of seizure disorder during the first 6 months of life are severe birth injury, congenital defects involving the central nervous system (CNS), infections, and inborn errors of metabolism. In people between 2 and 20 years of age, primary causes are birth injury, infection, trauma, and genetic factors. In individuals between 20 and 30 years of age, seizure disorder usually occurs as the result of structural lesions, such as trauma, brain tumors, or vascular disease. After 50 years of age, the primary causes of seizure disorders are stroke and metastatic brain tumors. However, one third of all epilepsy cases are idiopathic, meaning they are not attributable to a specific cause. These cases are known as *idiopathic generalized epilepsy (IGE)*.

Epilepsy (recurring seizures) is caused by a group of abnormal neurons that seem to undergo spontaneous firing. This firing spreads by physiologic pathways to involve adjacent or distant areas of the brain. If this activity spreads to involve the whole brain, a generalized seizure occurs. The cause of this abnormal firing is not clear. Any stimulus that causes the neuron's cell membrane to depolarize induces a tendency for spontaneous firing. Localization of the *seizure focus* (the place where the seizure originates) is critical to the success of any anticipated surgical treatment.

Scar tissue *(gliosis)* is often found in the area of the brain from which the seizure activity arises. Scarring is believed to interfere with the normal chemical and structural environment of the brain neurons, making them more likely to fire abnormally.

In addition to neuronal alterations, changes in the function of astrocytes may play several key roles in recurring seizures. Activation of astrocytes by hyperactive neurons is one of the crucial factors that predisposes nearby neurons to generate an epileptic discharge.

Genetic Link

Genetic abnormalities may be the most important factor contributing to IGE. Some types of epilepsy tend to run in families, suggesting a genetic influence. Other types of IGE are related to abnormalities in specific genes that control the flow of ions in and out of cells and regulate neuron signaling or are involved with protein and carbohydrate metabolism. Many genetic mutations associated with epilepsy appear to be acquired (occurring after birth) rather than inherited mutations.[9] (Genetics is discussed in Chapter 12.)

The role of genetics in the etiology of seizure disorders has been difficult to determine because of the problem of separating genetic from environmental or acquired influences. In some forms of epilepsy, families carry a predisposition to seizure disorders in the form of an inherently low threshold to seizure-producing stimuli, such as trauma, disease, and high fever.

Abnormal genes may influence the disorder in subtle ways. For example, a person with epilepsy may have an abnormally active version of a gene that increases resistance to drugs. This may help explain why antiseizure drugs do not work for some people.

Clinical Manifestations

Specific clinical manifestations of a seizure are determined by the site of the electrical disturbance. The preferred method of classifying seizures is presented in Table 58-5. This system, which is based on the clinical and electroencephalographic manifestations of seizures, divides seizures into two major classes: *generalized* and *focal* (Fig. 58-2). Depending on the type, a seizure may occur in multiple phases: (1) *prodromal phase*, with sensations or behavior changes that precede a seizure; (2) *aural phase*, with a sensory warning that is similar each time a seizure occurs; (3) *ictal phase*, from first symptoms to the end of seizure activity; and (4) *postictal phase*, the recovery period after the seizure.

Generalized Seizures. Generalized seizures quickly involve both sides of the brain and are characterized by bilateral synchronous epileptic discharges in the brain from the onset of the seizure. In most cases, the patient loses consciousness for a few seconds to several minutes.

Tonic-Clonic Seizures. The most common generalized seizure is the tonic-clonic seizure. Tonic-clonic seizure (formerly known as *grand mal*) is characterized by losing consciousness and falling to the ground if the patient is upright, followed by

stiffening of the body (tonic phase) for 10 to 20 seconds and subsequent jerking of the extremities (clonic phase) for another 30 to 40 seconds. Cyanosis, excessive salivation, tongue or cheek biting, and incontinence may accompany the seizure.

In the postictal phase, the patient usually has muscle soreness, feels tired, and may sleep for several hours. Some patients may not feel normal for several hours or days after a seizure. The patient has no memory of the seizure.

Typical Absence Seizures. Absence seizure (formerly called *petit mal*) usually occurs only in children and rarely continues beyond adolescence. This type of seizure may cease altogether as the child matures, or it may evolve into another type of seizure. The typical clinical manifestation of a simple absence seizure is a brief staring spell resembling "daydreaming" that lasts less than 10 seconds, so it often goes unnoticed. In complex absence seizures, the blank stare is accompanied by some type of movement (e.g., blinking, chewing, hand gestures) and can last up to 20 seconds. When untreated, seizures may occur up to 100 times a day. An electroencephalogram (EEG) demonstrates a 3-Hz (cycles per second) spike-and-wave pattern that

TABLE 58-5	Classification of Seizure Disorders
Primary Generalized Seizures (Involve both hemispheres of brain) • Tonic-clonic seizures • Absence seizures (simple or complex) • Typical • Atypical • Absence with special features • Myoclonic seizures • Tonic seizures • Atonic seizures (akinetic) • Clonic seizures	**Focal Seizures** (Involve one hemisphere of brain) • Simple focal seizures (no impairment of awareness/ consciousness) • Complex focal seizures (impairment of awareness/ consciousness) • Focal seizures evolving to secondary generalized seizures **Unknown** (Events not clearly diagnosed into categories above)

Adapted from International League Against Epilepsy: ILAE revised terminology for organization of seizures and epilepsies 2011-2013. Retrieved from *www.ilae.org/ visitors/centre/documents/OrganizationEpilepsy-overview.pdf.*

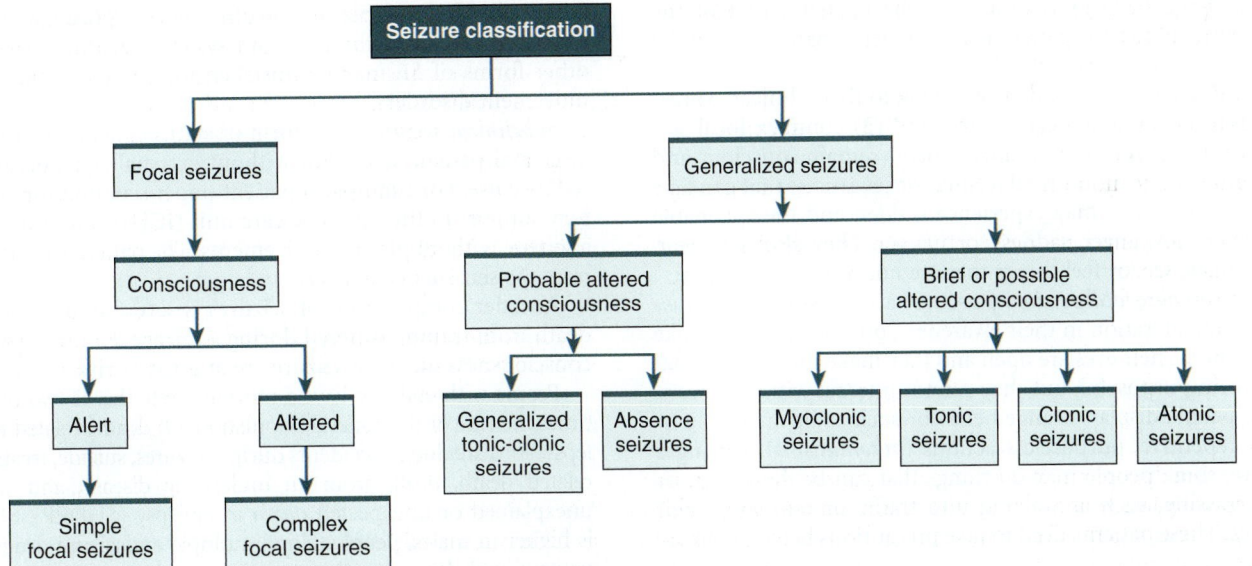

FIG. 58-2 Algorithm for classification of seizures.

is unique to this type of seizure. Hyperventilation and flashing lights can precipitate absence seizures.

Atypical Absence Seizures. In *atypical absence seizure,* the staring spell is accompanied by other signs and symptoms, such as eye blinking or jerking movements of the lips. The patient may be somewhat responsive during seizure activity. This type of seizure commonly lasts more than 10 seconds (as much as 30 seconds), with a gradual beginning and end. If the patient has cognitive impairment, seizure activity may be difficult to distinguish from usual behavior. Atypical absence seizures usually continue into adulthood. An EEG demonstrates atypical spike-and-wave patterns, usually greater or less than 3 Hz.

Other Types of Generalized Seizures. Other generalized seizures are myoclonic, atonic, tonic, and clonic seizures. A *myoclonic seizure* is characterized by a sudden, excessive jerk or twitch of the body or extremities. The jerk represents a muscle contraction and may be forceful enough to hurl the person to the ground. These seizures last no more than a few seconds, but they may occur in clusters.

An *atonic seizure* (akinetic seizure or drop attack) involves either a tonic episode or a paroxysmal loss of muscle tone and begins suddenly with the person falling to the ground. Seizures typically last less than 15 seconds. The person usually remains conscious, and normal activity can be resumed immediately. Patients with this type of seizure are at a great risk of head injury and often have to wear protective helmets.

A tonic seizure involves a sudden onset of increased tone in the extensor muscles, contributing to sudden stiff movements. Tonic seizures most often occur in sleep and affect both sides of the body. Patients will fall if they are standing when the seizure occurs. Tonic seizures usually last less than 20 seconds. The patient usually remains conscious.

Clonic seizures begin with loss of consciousness and sudden loss of muscle tone, followed by rhythmic limb jerking that may or may not be symmetric. Clonic seizures are relatively rare.

Focal Seizures. *Focal seizures,* also called *partial* or *partial focal seizures,* are the other major class of seizures (Table 58-5). Focal seizures begin in one hemisphere of the brain in a specific region of the cortex, as indicated by the EEG. They produce sensory, motor, cognitive, or emotional manifestations based on the function of the involved area of the brain. For example, if the discharging focus is located in the medial aspect of the postcentral gyrus, the patient may experience paresthesia in the leg on the side opposite the focus.

Focal seizures are divided according to their clinical expression into (1) simple focal seizures and (2) complex focal seizures.[10] In a *simple focal seizure,* patients remain conscious and alert but experience unusual feelings or sensations that can take many forms. They may experience sudden and unexplainable feelings of joy, anger, sadness, or nausea. They also may hear, smell, taste, see, or feel things that are not real.

In a *complex focal seizure,* patients have a loss of consciousness or an alteration in their awareness, producing a dreamlike experience. Their eyes are open and they make movements that may seem purposeful, but they cannot interact with observers. Some people display strange behavior such as lip smacking or other repetitive, purposeless actions *(automatisms).* During a seizure, some people may do things that can be dangerous or embarrassing, such as walking into traffic or removing their clothes. These patients need to take precautions before a seizure occurs.

Patients may continue an activity started before the seizure, such as counting coins or choosing items from a grocery shelf, but after the seizure they do not remember the activity performed during the seizure. These seizures usually last between 30 seconds and 2 minutes. Patients may be tired or confused following the seizure and may not return to normal activity for hours.

Focal seizures may be confined to one side of the brain and remain focal (partial) in nature, or they may spread to involve the entire brain, culminating in a generalized tonic-clonic seizure. Any tonic-clonic seizure that is preceded by an aura or warning is a focal seizure that generalizes secondarily. Many tonic-clonic seizures that appear to be generalized from the outset may actually be secondary generalized seizures. However, the preceding partial component may be so brief that it is undetected by the patient or the observer, or even on the EEG. Unlike the primary generalized tonic-clonic seizure, the secondary generalized seizure may result in a transient residual neurologic deficit postictally. This is called *Todd's paralysis* (focal weakness), which resolves after varying lengths of time.

Psychogenic Seizures. Because they closely resemble epileptic seizures, psychogenic seizures may be misdiagnosed as epilepsy. Proper diagnosis usually requires video-EEG monitoring to identify associated events. If the diagnosis of epilepsy is excluded, history of emotional or physical abuse or a specific traumatic event often emerges. Some patients may have both psychogenic seizures and epilepsy. Care provided by a specialist in epilepsy is essential.

Complications

Physical. Status epilepticus (SE) is a state of continuous seizure activity or a condition in which seizures recur in rapid succession without return to consciousness between seizures. It is defined as any seizure lasting longer than 5 minutes. The longer a seizure lasts, the less likely it is to stop without drug therapy.[11]

SE is a neurologic emergency that can occur with any type of seizure. The highest incidence occurs in children and older adults. During repeated seizures, the brain uses more energy than can be supplied. As neurons become exhausted and cease to function, permanent brain damage may result. *Convulsive status epilepticus* is the most dangerous type because it can cause potentially fatal ventilatory insufficiency, hypoxemia, cardiac dysrhythmias, hyperthermia, and systemic acidosis. However, other forms of SE may be mistaken for altered mentation or movement disorders.

Subclinical seizures are a form of status epilepticus in which a sedated patient seizes but without external signs because of sedative use. For example, a patient under sedation for ventilatory support in the intensive care unit (ICU) could experience a seizure without physical movements. The patient's HCP could miss the seizure occurrence.

Another complication of seizures is severe injury and even death from trauma suffered during a seizure. Patients who lose consciousness during a seizure are at greatest risk.

People with epilepsy have a mortality rate that is two or three times the rate of the general population. Of deaths related to epilepsy, 40% are due to accidents during seizures, suicide, treatment-related death, death from an underlying disease, and sudden unexplained or unexpected death in epilepsy (SUDEP). SUDEP is higher in males, people taking multiple antiseizure drugs, and patients with long-standing epilepsy who have poorly managed seizure activity. The direct cause of SUDEP is unknown but thought to be related to respiratory dysfunction, cardiac dysrhythmias, or cerebral depression.[12] Specific teaching about medication adherence and disease awareness is critical for at-risk people.

Psychosocial. Perhaps the most common complication of seizure disorders is its effect on a patient's lifestyle. Patients may develop ineffective coping methods because of psychosocial problems related to having a seizure disorder. In particular, an increased incidence of depression occurs in people who have seizures that are difficult to control. Antiseizure drugs and the continued need to manage a chronic disease also can contribute to depression.

Although attitudes have improved in recent years, a diagnosis of epilepsy still carries a social stigma. Patients with epilepsy may experience discrimination in employment and educational opportunities. Transportation may be difficult because of legal sanctions against driving. Screen patients frequently for depression, and encourage them to pursue available treatment options.

Diagnostic Studies

A diagnosis of epilepsy or seizure disorder has many socioeconomic, physical, and psychologic consequences for the patient. Thus accurate diagnosis is crucial. The most useful diagnostic tool is an accurate, comprehensive description of seizures and the patient's health history (Table 58-6).

The EEG is a useful diagnostic adjuvant to the history, but only if it shows abnormalities. Abnormal findings help determine the type of seizure and pinpoint the seizure focus. Ideally, an EEG should be done within 24 hours of a suspected seizure. Unfortunately, only a small percentage of patients with seizure disorders have abnormal EEG findings the first time the test is done. Either repeated EEGs or continuous EEG monitoring may be needed to detect abnormalities. An EEG is not a definitive test because some patients without seizure disorders have abnormal patterns on their EEGs, while many patients with seizure disorders have normal EEG results between seizures. If abnormal discharges do not occur during the 30 to 40 minutes of sampling during EEG, the test may not indicate an abnormality. Magnetoencephalography may be done in conjunction with the EEG. This test has greater sensitivity in detecting small magnetic fields generated by neuronal activity.

A complete blood count, serum chemistries, studies of liver and kidney function, and a urinalysis should be done to rule out metabolic disorders. A CT scan or MRI should be done in any new-onset seizure to rule out a structural lesion. Cerebral angiography, single-photon emission computed tomography (SPECT), magnetic resonance spectroscopy (MRS), MRA, and positron emission tomography (PET) may be used in selected clinical situations.

The International League Against Epilepsy has developed specific diagnostic criteria for each type of seizure, including conditions that resolve over time *(www.ilae.org)*. If a patient is diagnosed with a seizure disorder, the seizure type must be correctly identified (Fig. 58-2 and Table 58-6) to determine appropriate treatment.

Interprofessional Care

Most seizures do not require emergency medical care because they are self-limiting and rarely cause bodily injury. However, if status epilepticus or significant bodily harm occurs, or if the event is a first-time seizure, medical care should be sought immediately. Table 58-6 outlines the diagnostic studies and interprofessional care of seizure disorders. Table 58-7 summarizes emergency care of the patient with a generalized tonic-clonic seizure, the seizure most likely to warrant emergency medical care.

Drug Therapy. The primary treatment for seizure disorders is antiseizure drugs (Table 58-8). Because a cure is not possible, the goal of therapy is to prevent seizures with minimal toxic side effects from drug therapy. Drugs generally act by stabilizing nerve cell membranes and preventing spread of the epileptic discharge. Drug therapy should begin with a single drug based on the patient's age and weight and type, frequency, and cause of seizure. Dosage should be increased until seizures are controlled or toxic side effects occur.

If seizure control is not achieved with a single drug, dosage or timing of administration may be changed or a second drug may be added. About one third of patients require a combination regimen for adequate control. Patients should discuss emerging treatments with their HCPs to provide the best control with the least amount of medication.

The therapeutic range for each drug indicates the serum level above which most patients experience toxic side effects and below which most continue to have seizures. However, therapeutic drug ranges are only guides for therapy. If the patient's seizures are well controlled with a subtherapeutic level, the drug dosage does not have to be increased. Likewise, if a drug level is above the therapeutic range and the patient has good seizure control without toxic side effects, the drug dosage does not have to be decreased. Serum drug levels are monitored if seizures continue to occur, seizure frequency increases, or drug adherence is questioned. Because they have a very large therapeutic range, many newer drugs do not require drug-level monitoring.

The primary drugs to treat generalized tonic-clonic and focal seizures are phenytoin (Dilantin), carbamazepine (Tegretol), phenobarbital, divalproex, and primidone (Mysoline). The drugs used to treat absence and myoclonic seizures include ethosuximide (Zarontin), divalproex, and clonazepam (Klonopin).

TABLE 58-6   Interprofessional Care

Epilepsy and Seizure Disorders

Diagnostic Assessment
History and Physical Examination
- Birth and developmental history
- Significant illnesses and injuries
- Family history
- Febrile seizures
- Comprehensive neurologic assessment

Seizure History
- Precipitating factors
- Antecedent events
- Seizure description (including onset, duration, frequency, postictal state)

Diagnostic Studies
- CBC, urinalysis, electrolytes, creatinine, fasting blood glucose
- Lumbar puncture for CSF analysis
- CT, MRI, MRA, MRS, PET scan
- Electroencephalography (EEG)

Management
- Antiseizure drugs (Table 58-8)
- Surgery
- Vagal nerve stimulation
- Psychosocial counseling
- Physical therapy

MRA, Magnetic resonance angiography; *MRS,* magnetic resonance spectroscopy; *PET,* positron emission tomography.

✚ TABLE 58-7   Emergency Management
Tonic-Clonic Seizures

Etiology	Assessment Findings	Interventions
Head Trauma • Epidural hematoma • Subdural hematoma • Intracranial hematoma • Cerebral contusion • Traumatic birth injury	**Aural Phase** • Peculiar sensations that precede seizure • Loss of consciousness • Bowel and bladder incontinence • Tachycardia • Diaphoresis • Warm skin • Pallor, flushing, or cyanosis	**Initial** Ensure patent airway. Protect patient from injury during seizure. *Do not restrain.* Pad side rails. Remove or loosen tight clothing. Establish IV access. Stay with patient until seizure has passed. Anticipate administration of phenobarbital, phenytoin (Dilantin), or benzodiazepines (e.g., diazepam [Valium], midazolam [Versed], lorazepam [Ativan]) to attempt to abort seizures.
Drug-Related Processes • Overdose • Withdrawal of alcohol, opioids, antiseizure drugs • Ingestion, inhalation	**Tonic Phase** • Continuous muscle contractions	Suction as needed. Assist ventilations if patient does not breathe spontaneously after seizure. Anticipate need for intubation if gag reflex absent.
Infectious Processes • Meningitis • Septicemia • Encephalitis	**Hypertonic Phase** • Extreme muscular rigidity lasting 5-15 sec	
Intracranial Events • Brain tumor • Subarachnoid hemorrhage • Stroke • Hypertensive crisis • Increased ICP secondary to clogged shunt	**Clonic Phase** • Rigidity and relaxation alternating in rapid succession **Postictal Phase** • Lethargy, altered level of consciousness	**Ongoing Monitoring** Monitor vital signs, level of consciousness, O₂ saturation, Glasgow Coma Scale results, pupil size and reactivity. Reassure and orient patient after seizure.
Metabolic Imbalances • Fluid and electrolyte imbalance • Hypoglycemia	• Confusion and headache • Repeated tonic-clonic seizures for several min	Never force an airway between patient's clenched teeth. Give IV dextrose for hypoglycemia.
Medical Disorders • Heart, liver, lung, or kidney disease • Systemic lupus erythematosus		
Idiopathic		
Other • Cardiac arrest • Psychiatric disorders • High fever		

ICP, Intracranial pressure.

TABLE 58-8   Drug Therapy
Seizure Disorders

• brivaracetam (Briviact)	• levetiracetam (Keppra)
• carbamazepine (Tegretol)	• lorazepam (Ativan)
• clonazepam (Klonopin)	• oxcarbazepine (Trileptal)
• daclizumab (Zinbryta)	• perampanel (Fycompa)
• diazepam (Diastat)	• phenytoin (Dilantin)
• divalproex (Depakote)	• pregabalin (Lyrica)
• eslicarbazepine (Aptiom)	• primidone (Mysoline)
• ethosuximide (Zarontin)	• tiagabine (Gabitril)
• ezogabine (Potiga)	• topiramate (Topamax)
• felbamate (Felbatol)	• valproic acid (Depakene)
• gabapentin (Neurontin)	• vigabatrin (Sabril)
• lacosamide (Vimpat)	• zonisamide (Zonegran)
• lamotrigine (Lamictal)	

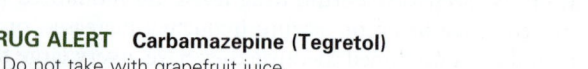

> **DRUG ALERT   Carbamazepine (Tegretol)**
> • Do not take with grapefruit juice.
> • Instruct patient to report visual abnormalities.
> • Abrupt withdrawal after long-term use may precipitate seizures.

Other antiseizure drugs include gabapentin, topiramate, lamotrigine (Lamictal), tiagabine (Gabitril), levetiracetam (Keppra), and zonisamide (Zonegran). Some of these drugs are broad spectrum and appear to be effective for multiple seizure types. Pregabalin (Lyrica) is used as an additional treatment for focal seizures not successfully controlled with a single medication.

Treatment of status epilepticus requires initiation of a rapid-acting IV antiseizure drug. The drugs most commonly used are lorazepam (Ativan) and diazepam (Valium). Because these are short-acting drugs, their administration is followed with long-acting drugs such as phenytoin or phenobarbital.

Because many of the antiseizure drugs (e.g., phenytoin, phenobarbital, ethosuximide, lamotrigine, topiramate) have a long half-life, they can be given in once- or twice-daily doses. This simplifies the drug regimen and increases the patient's adherence because the drug does not have to be taken at work or school. Unnecessary combination therapy should be avoided whenever possible. Medications should be reviewed routinely and the least effective medication discontinued by tapering.

> **DRUG ALERT   Antiseizure Drugs**
> • Abrupt withdrawal after long-term use may precipitate seizures.
> • If weaning is to occur, the patient must be seizure free for a prolonged period (e.g., 2 to 5 yr) and have a normal neurologic examination and EEG.

Side effects of antiseizure drugs involve the CNS and include diplopia, drowsiness, ataxia, and mental slowness. Neurologic assessment for dose-related toxicity involves testing the eyes for nystagmus and evaluating hand and gait coordination, cognitive functioning, and general alertness.

As a nurse, be knowledgeable about these side effects so that you can inform patients and institute proper treatment. Common side effects of phenytoin are gingival hyperplasia (excessive growth of gingival tissue) and hirsutism, especially in young adults. Good dental hygiene, including regular tooth brushing and flossing, can decrease gingival hyperplasia. If gingival hyperplasia is extensive, the hyperplastic tissue may have to be surgically removed (gingivectomy) and phenytoin replaced with another antiseizure drug.

Medication nonadherence can be a problem in people with a seizure disorder. Take measures to increase patient adherence to the prescribed drug regimens. If HCPs are aware of nonadherence issues, they can work with the patient to find an acceptable drug regimen. For example, using pregabalin as an adjunct medication in some cases may allow a decreased dose of the primary antiseizure drug, thus decreasing undesirable side effects.

Gerontologic Considerations: Drug Therapy for Seizure Disorders

Many older adults experience a first single seizure, and a large percentage of them do not have another seizure. To be considered for antiseizure drug therapy, older adults should have recurrent seizures, an obvious structural predisposition for seizures, or onset of epilepsy presenting as status epilepticus. Older adults are more responsive to antiseizure drugs than younger adults, but they also are more likely to experience side effects at lower serum drug concentrations.

In considering antiseizure drug therapy for older adults, you should recall the relationship between drug action and normal changes that occur with aging. For example, phenytoin is widely used to treat seizure disorders. However, because the liver metabolizes phenytoin, its use should be avoided in older patients with compromised liver function. Age-related changes in liver enzymes decrease the liver's ability to metabolize drugs. Because phenobarbital, carbamazepine, and primidone have potential effects on cognitive function, their use may also be less desirable for older adults. Use of carbamazepine, phenytoin, phenobarbital, primidone, topiramate, and oxcarbazepine can increase the risk of osteopenia and osteoporosis in older adults.[13]

Several newer antiseizure drugs offer greater treatment benefit to older adults. Compared with older drugs, gabapentin, lamotrigine, oxcarbazepine, and levetiracetam may be safer, have fewer effects on cognitive function, and have fewer interactions with other drugs.

Surgical Therapy. Despite availability of newer drugs with fewer side effects, no solution has been found for *medically refractory epilepsy* (unresponsive to drug therapy). If a patient's seizures fail to respond to the first two prescribed antiseizure medications, the likelihood of achieving a seizure-free life with further medication changes is only 5% to 10%.[14] However, a substantial number of patients with uncontrolled epilepsy are candidates for surgical therapy to remove the epileptic focus or prevent spread of epileptic activity in the brain. The classic surgical intervention has been an anterior temporal lobe resection. However, the current goal of neurosurgery is a careful resection of a precisely localized area within a lobe of the brain. Approximately 70% to 80% of patients become seizure free after surgery, and 10% to 20% experience a marked reduction in seizure activity.[14]

Not all types of epilepsy benefit from surgery. An extensive preoperative evaluation is important, including continuous EEG monitoring and other specific tests to ensure precise localization of the focal point. Surgical candidates must meet three requirements: (1) a confirmed diagnosis of epilepsy, (2) an adequate trial with drug therapy without satisfactory results, and (3) a defined electroclinical syndrome (type of seizure disorder).

Other Therapies. *Vagal nerve stimulation*, a form of neuromodulation, is used as an adjunct to drugs when an accessible focal point cannot be identified for surgical removal. The exact mechanism of action is unknown, but it is thought to interrupt the synchronization of epileptic brain wave activity and stop excessive discharge of neurons. In vagal nerve stimulation, a surgically implanted electrode in the neck is programmed to deliver the electrical impulse to the vagus nerve, usually on the left side. The patient can activate it with a magnet when he or she senses a seizure is imminent. Vagal nerve stimulation can cause adverse effects such as coughing, hoarseness, dyspnea, and tingling in the neck. Battery life is 5 to 10 years, and surgical replacement is required. Benefits of this therapy can be seen within 24 months after implantation.

A *ketogenic diet* is a special high-fat, low-carbohydrate diet that has been used to control seizures in some people with epilepsy. When a person is on this diet, ketones are produced and pass into the brain and replace glucose as an energy source. Meals must be carefully planned because the amount of protein and carbohydrate in the diet must be restricted. Patients on this diet who use anticoagulants need close monitoring for bleeding. Although HCPs are more likely to recommend the diet for children than adults, the diet can work equally well in both age groups. However, long-term effects of the diet are not clear.[15]

Biofeedback to control seizures is aimed at teaching the patient to maintain a certain brain wave frequency that is refractory to seizure activity. Further trials are needed to assess the effectiveness of biofeedback for seizure control.

❖ NURSING MANAGEMENT: SEIZURE DISORDERS AND EPILEPSY

◆ Nursing Assessment

Subjective and objective data to obtain from a patient with a seizure disorder are presented in Table 58-9. Obtain data related to a specific seizure episode from a witness.

◆ Nursing Diagnoses

Nursing diagnoses for the patient with seizure disorders and epilepsy may include, but are not limited to, the following:

- Ineffective breathing pattern *related to* neuromuscular impairment
- Ineffective health management *related to* drug therapy and lifestyle adjustments
- Risk for injury *related to* loss of consciousness during seizure activity and postictal physical weakness

Additional information on nursing diagnoses for the patient with a seizure disorder is presented in eNursing Care Plan 58-2 (available on the website for this chapter).

◆ Planning

The overall goals are that the patient with seizures will (1) be free from injury during a seizure, (2) have optimal mental and physical functioning while taking antiseizure drugs, and (3) have satisfactory psychosocial functioning.

TABLE 58-9 Nursing Assessment
Epilepsy and Seizure Disorders

Subjective Data

Important Health Information

Past health history: Previous seizures, birth defects or injuries, anoxic episodes. CNS trauma, tumors, or infections. Stroke, metabolic disorders, alcoholism, exposure to metals and carbon monoxide, hepatic or renal failure, fever, pregnancy, systemic lupus erythematosus

Medications: Adherence to antiseizure medication regimen. Barbiturate or alcohol withdrawal. Use and overdose of cocaine, amphetamines, lidocaine, theophylline, penicillin, lithium, phenothiazines, tricyclic antidepressants, benzodiazepines

Functional Health Patterns

Health perception–health management: Positive family history
Cognitive-perceptual: Headaches, aura, mood or behavioral changes before seizure. Mentation changes. Abdominal pain, muscle pain (postictal)
Self-perception–self-concept: Anxiety, depression. Loss of self-esteem, social isolation
Sexuality-reproductive: Decreased sexual drive, erectile dysfunction. Increased sexual drive (postictal)

Objective Data

General

Precipitating factors, including severe metabolic acidosis or alkalosis, hyperkalemia, hypoglycemia, dehydration, or water intoxication

Integumentary

Bitten tongue, soft tissue damage, cyanosis, diaphoresis (postictal)

Respiratory

Abnormal respiratory rate, rhythm, or depth. Apnea (ictal). Absent or abnormal breath sounds, possible airway occlusion

Cardiovascular

Hypertension, tachycardia or bradycardia (ictal)

Gastrointestinal

Bowel incontinence, excessive salivation

Urinary

Incontinence

Neurologic

Generalized

Tonic-clonic: Loss of consciousness, muscle tightening, then jerking. Dilated pupils. Hyperventilation, then apnea. Postictal somnolence
Absence: Altered consciousness (5-30 sec), minor facial motor activity

Focal

Simple: Aura. Focal sensory, motor, cognitive, or emotional phenomena (focal motor). Unilateral "marching" motor seizure (jacksonian)
Complex: Altered consciousness with inappropriate behaviors, automatisms, amnesia of event

Musculoskeletal

Weakness, paralysis, ataxia (postictal)

Possible Diagnostic Findings

Positive toxicology screen or blood alcohol level. Altered serum electrolytes, acidosis or alkalosis, very low blood glucose, ↑ blood urea nitrogen or serum creatinine, abnormal liver function tests, ammonia; abnormal CT scan or MRI of head, abnormal findings from lumbar puncture. Abnormal discharges on EEG

◆ Nursing Implementation

◆ **Health Promotion.** Some seizure disorders can be prevented by promoting general safety measures, such as wearing helmets in situations involving risk of head injury. Improved perinatal, labor, and delivery care have reduced fetal trauma and hypoxia and thus have reduced brain damage leading to seizure disorders.

The patient with a seizure disorder should practice good general health habits (e.g., maintain proper diet, get adequate rest, exercise). Help the patient identify events or situations that precipitate the seizures and provide suggestions for avoiding them or handling them better. Teach the patient to avoid excessive alcohol intake, fatigue, and loss of sleep. Help the patient handle stress constructively.

◆ **Acute Care.** Nursing care for a hospitalized patient with a seizure disorder or a patient who has had seizures secondary to other factors involves observation and treatment of the seizure, patient and caregiver teaching, and psychosocial intervention.

> **❓ CHECK YOUR PRACTICE**
>
> You are making your morning rounds and go to check your 34-yr-old male patient who was admitted the night before with increased seizure activity. When you go to his room, his roommate is yelling, "Help, help!" You notice that the patient is on the floor jerking and stiffening and does not respond to you.
> • What should you do?

When a seizure occurs, carefully observe and record details of the event because the diagnosis and subsequent treatment often rest solely on the seizure description. Note all aspects of the seizure. What events preceded the seizure? When did the seizure occur? How long did each phase (aural [if any], ictal, postictal) last? What occurred during each phase?

Both subjective data (usually the only type of data in the aural phase) and objective data are important. Note the exact onset of the seizure (which body part was affected first and how); the course and nature of the seizure activity (loss of consciousness, tongue biting, automatisms, stiffening, jerking, total lack of muscle tone); body parts involved and their sequence of involvement; and autonomic signs, such as dilated pupils, excessive salivation, altered breathing, cyanosis, flushing, diaphoresis, or incontinence. Assessment of the postictal period should include a detailed description of the level of consciousness, vital signs, pupil size and position of the eyes, memory loss, muscle soreness, speech disorders (aphasia, dysarthria), weakness or paralysis, sleep period, and the duration of each sign or symptom.

> **⚠ SAFETY ALERT** Seizure
> During a seizure, you should do the following:
> • Maintain a patent airway for the patient.
> • Protect the patient's head, turn the patient to the side, loosen constrictive clothing, ease patient to the floor (if seated).
> • Do not restrain the patient.
> • Do not place any objects in the patient's mouth.

After the seizure the patient may require repositioning (to open and maintain the airway), suctioning, and O_2. A seizure can be frightening for the patient and for others who witnessed it. Assess their level of understanding and provide information about how and why the event occurred. This is an excellent opportunity for you to dispel many common misconceptions about seizures.

TEAMWORK & COLLABORATION
Caring for the Patient With a Seizure Disorder

Because any nursing staff member may be present when a patient experiences a seizure, all staff members are responsible for maintaining patient safety.

Role of Nursing Personnel
Registered Nurse (RN)
- Teach patient about factors that increase risk for seizures, such as alcohol use, fatigue, inadequate sleep, and stress.
- Teach patient about prescribed antiseizure medications, including drug regimen, side effects, and required monitoring of drug levels.
- Assess and document details of seizure events, including events preceding the seizure; length of each phase of the seizure; course and nature of seizure activity; and level of consciousness, vital signs, and activity during the postictal period.
- Assess airway patency, and position patient to maintain airway during and after any seizures.
- Administer IV antiseizure medications to the patient experiencing status epilepticus.
- Make appropriate referrals to the Epilepsy Foundation and community agencies to assist patient with financial impact of the disorder, work training, employment, and living arrangements.
- Teach family members and caregivers about management of seizures and status epilepticus.
- In the ambulatory and home care setting, evaluate patient self-management of medications and lifestyle.

Licensed Practical/Vocational Nurse (LPN/LVN)
- Administer oral antiseizure medications as scheduled.
- In the ambulatory and home setting, monitor patient adherence to medications and lifestyle changes and report problems to the RN.

Unlicensed Assistive Personnel (UAP)
- Place suction equipment, bag valve mask, and O_2 at the patient's bedside.
- Remove potentially harmful objects from the bedside and pad side rails.
- Immediately report any seizure activity to the RN.
- Observe and report events of the seizure to the RN.
- Obtain vital signs during the postictal period.
- Provide oropharyngeal suctioning after a seizure (after being trained and evaluated in this procedure).

Role of Other Team Members
Physical, Occupational, or Respiratory Therapist
- Remove potentially harmful objects from the bedside and pad side rails.
- Assess airway patency and position patient to maintain airway during and after any seizures.
- Immediately report any seizure activity to the RN.
- Observe and report events of the seizure to the RN.

TABLE 58-10 Patient & Caregiver Teaching
Seizure Disorders

Include the following information in the teaching plan for the patient with a seizure disorder.
1. Take antiseizure medications as prescribed. Report any and all drug side effects to the HCP. When necessary, blood is drawn to ensure maintenance of therapeutic drug levels. Schedule regular communication with the HCP to explore additional treatment options.
2. Use nondrug techniques, such as relaxation therapy, to potentially reduce the number of seizures.
3. Be aware of community and online resources for education and help with tracking and explaining seizure activity.
4. Wear a medical alert bracelet or necklace, and carry an identification card.
5. Avoid excessive alcohol intake, fatigue, and loss of sleep.
6. Eat regular meals and snacks in between if feeling shaky, faint, or hungry.
7. Be knowledgeable as a woman of childbearing age regarding antiseizure medications and contraceptive use.

Caregivers should receive the following information.

Focal Seizures
1. Stay calm. Guide patient to safety to prevent injury but do not restrain.
2. Observe for asymmetry of activity and focus on specific actions, such as lip smacking and abnormal movements.
3. Assess patient's level of consciousness and ability to converse and respond appropriately
4. Observe the time the event started and stopped. Pay attention to the time of return to baseline.
5. Provide respect and explanation of occurrence.

Generalized Tonic-Clonic Seizures
1. When seizure occurs outside the hospital setting, activate ERS if (1) the duration is greater than 5 minutes; (2) events recur without the patient recovering to baseline; (3) the patient is unable to establish a normal breathing pattern, is injured or pregnant; or (4) you do not know if this is a first-time seizure event.
2. Maintain patient safety. Lower the patient to the floor or bed, remove glasses if on, and loosen restrictive clothing.
3. Do not place anything in the patient's mouth. Patient's teeth/dentures may be damaged, and caregiver may be bitten.
4. Position patient on side (if possible) to improve the patient's ability to release oral secretions.
5. Observe the time event started and stopped. Pay attention to the time of return to baseline.
6. Assess for possible injury or any lingering motor weakness.

◆ **Ambulatory Care.** Prevention of recurring seizures is the major goal in the treatment of epilepsy. For treatment to be effective, drugs must be taken regularly and continuously, often for a lifetime. Help the patient understand this and review details of the drug regimen and what to do if a dose is missed. Usually the dose is made up if the omission is remembered within 24 hours. Caution the patient not to adjust drug dosages without professional guidance because this can increase seizure frequency and even cause status epilepticus. Encourage the patient to report any medication side effects and to keep regular appointments with the HCP.

You have an important role in teaching the patient and caregiver. Review the guidelines for teaching presented in Table 58-10. Teach the caregiver, family members, and significant others the emergency management of tonic-clonic seizures (Table 58-7). Remind them that it is not necessary to call an ambulance or send a person to the hospital after a single seizure unless the seizure is prolonged, another seizure immediately follows, extensive injury has occurred, or if it is unknown if there was a first-time seizure.

Patients with a seizure disorder may experience concerns or fears related to recurrent seizures, incontinence, or loss of self-control. Support the patient through teaching and by helping him or her use effective coping mechanisms.

Perhaps the greatest challenge for a patient with a seizure disorder is adjusting to the personal and societal limitations imposed by the illness. Discrimination in employment is the most serious problem facing the person with a seizure disorder. For issues relating to job discrimination, refer patients to the state department of vocational rehabilitation or the U.S. Equal Employment Opportunity Commission (EEOC).

Assist the patient in finding appropriate resources. If you believe that associating with others who have a seizure disorder would be beneficial, refer the patient to the local chapter of the Epilepsy Foundation (EF), a volunteer agency that offers varied services to patients with epilepsy (www.epilepsy.com). Refer the patient who is an eligible veteran to a Department of Veterans Affairs medical center that provides comprehensive care. If intensive psychologic counseling is needed, refer the patient to a community mental health center.

Social workers and welfare agencies can help with financial implications and living arrangements. State agencies specializing in vocational rehabilitation services can provide vocational assessment, counseling, funding for training, and assistance with job placement for patients whose seizures are not well controlled. They can also offer financial assistance for transportation and medical costs related to vocational rehabilitation or job maintenance.

Driving laws for patients who have had a seizure vary from state to state. For example, some states require a 3-month seizure-free period before issuing or reissuing a driver's license, whereas others require up to 1 year. The EF provides current information on driving laws for each state.

Inform the patient that medical alert bracelets, necklaces, and identification cards are available through the EF, local pharmacies, or companies specializing in identification devices (e.g., Medic Alert). However, the use of these medical identification tags is optional. Some patients have found them beneficial, but others prefer not to be identified as having a seizure disorder.

Encourage the patient to learn more about epilepsy through self-education. The EF provides informational pamphlets, has an extensive website, and may facilitate support groups. Many agencies that offer services to patients with epilepsy also offer teaching aids and support.

◆ **Evaluation**

Expected outcomes are that the patient with seizures will
- Experience breathing pattern adequate to meet O_2 needs
- Experience no seizure-related injury
- Express acceptance of seizure disorder by admitting presence of epilepsy and adhering to recommended treatment regimen

Additional expected outcomes are presented in eNursing Care Plan 58-2 available on the website.

RESTLESS LEGS SYNDROME

Etiology and Pathophysiology

Restless legs syndrome (RLS), also called *Willis-Ekbom disease*, is a relatively common condition characterized by unpleasant sensory (paresthesia) and motor abnormalities of one or both legs. Up to 10% of the U.S. population may have RLS.[16] However, the numbers may be higher because the condition is underdiagnosed. RLS is more common in older adults. It is also more common in women than men, and women may have an earlier age of onset.

Two distinct types of RLS have been identified: primary (idiopathic) and secondary. The majority of cases are primary, and many patients with this type of RLS report a positive family history. Secondary RLS can occur with metabolic abnormalities associated with iron deficiency, renal failure, hypertension, diabetes mellitus, spinal disorders, or rheumatoid arthritis. Conditions such as anemia or pregnancy and certain medications can cause or worsen symptoms.

Although the exact pathophysiology of the primary disorder is unknown, RLS is believed to be related to a dysfunction in the brain's basal ganglia circuits that use the neurotransmitter dopamine, which controls movements. In RLS, this dysfunction causes the urge to move the legs. Abnormal iron metabolism or brain iron deficiencies reflected by low serum ferritin may also play a role in RLS.[16]

Clinical Manifestations

The severity of RLS sensory symptoms ranges from infrequent minor discomfort (paresthesia, including numbness, tingling, and "pins and needles" sensation) to severe pain. Sensory symptoms often appear first. Patients describe annoying and uncomfortable (but usually not painful) sensations in the legs. Some compare the sensations to bugs creeping or crawling on the legs. The leg pain is localized within the calf muscles. Patients can also experience pain in the upper extremities and trunk. The discomfort occurs when the patient is sedentary and is most common in the evening or at night.

The pain at night can disrupt sleep. Physical activity, such as walking, stretching, rocking, or kicking, often relieves the pain. In the most severe cases, patients sleep only a few hours at night, resulting in daytime fatigue and disruption of the daily routine. The motor abnormalities associated with RLS consist of voluntary restlessness and stereotyped, periodic, involuntary movements. The involuntary movements usually occur during sleep. Fatigue further aggravates symptoms. Over time, RLS advances to more frequent and severe episodes.

Diagnostic Studies

RLS is a clinical diagnosis, based in large part on the patient's history or the report of the bed partner related to nighttime activities. The diagnosis of RLS can be made when the patient meets all five specific criteria: (1) urge to move the legs, often accompanied by uncomfortable or unpleasant sensations in the legs; (2) any uncomfortable sensations begin or worsen with periods of inactivity; (3) any uncomfortable sensations are partially or totally relieved by movement, as long as the activity continues; (4) urge to move the legs and any accompanying sensations become worse in the evening or night; and (5) occurrence of these features is not primary to another medical or behavioral condition.[17]

The patient may undergo polysomnography studies during sleep to distinguish RLS from other clinical conditions that can disturb sleep (e.g., sleep apnea). However, periodic leg movements in sleep are a common feature in RLS patients. Blood tests, such as a complete blood count, serum ferritin, and renal function tests (e.g., serum creatinine), may help exclude secondary causes of RLS. A patient's history of diabetes mellitus and its management may provide information to determine if paresthesia is caused by peripheral neuropathy related to diabetes or RLS.

❖ NURSING AND INTERPROFESSIONAL MANAGEMENT: RESTLESS LEGS SYNDROME

The goal of interprofessional management is to reduce patient discomfort and distress and to improve sleep quality. When RLS is secondary to renal failure or iron deficiency, treatment of these conditions will decrease symptoms. Nondrug approaches to RLS management include establishing regular sleep habits; exercising; avoiding activities that cause symptoms; and eliminating aggravating factors, such as alcohol, caffeine, and certain drugs (neuroleptics, lithium, antihistamines, antidepressants). Yoga has been found to improve mood, sleep, and function in RLS.[18]

If nondrug measures fail to provide symptom relief, drug therapy is an option. No single medication effectively manages RLS for all patients. The main drugs used in RLS include dopamine precursors (e.g., carbidopa/levodopa) and dopamine agonists (e.g., ropinirole [Requip], pramipexole [Mirapex]) to increase the amount of dopamine in the brain. The antiseizure drug gabapentin enacarbil (Horizant) is used to decrease the sensory sensations. If the patient has iron deficiency or low serum ferritin, iron supplementation is considered.

Other drugs may relieve some symptoms of RLS. These include opioids and benzodiazepines. Low doses of opioids (e.g., oxycodone) are usually reserved for patients with severe symptoms who fail to respond to other drug therapies. The main side effect of opioids is constipation, so patients may need to take a stool softener or laxative. Clonidine (Catapres) and propranolol (Inderal) are also effective in some patients.

Relaxis is a device that produces vibration and provides a counterstimulation that competes with and diminishes the RLS sensations. The patient places the legs on the Relaxis pad, which provides 30 minutes of uninterrupted vibration after being activated and then slowly winds down over an additional 5 minutes to complete a 35-minute therapy cycle. If needed, it may be restarted one more time. The patient chooses the vibration intensity based on symptoms.[19]

DEGENERATIVE NEUROLOGIC DISORDERS

Degenerative nerve diseases lead to nerve damage that worsens as the diseases progress. These diseases affect many activities, including balance, movement, speech, and respiratory and heart function. Some diseases have no known cause, but many are known to have a genetic basis. Most degenerative nerve diseases have no cure. Treatment aims to reduce symptoms and help the patient maintain an optimal level of function.

Patients with these diseases have similar concerns and problems. They must deal with not only their disease but also the impact of the disease on their quality of life. Many patients have concerns regarding safety, mobility, self-care, and coping. Patients and their families often require psychosocial support, especially as the disease progresses and patients' disability gets worse.

MULTIPLE SCLEROSIS

Multiple sclerosis (MS) is a chronic, progressive, degenerative disorder of the CNS characterized by disseminated demyelination of nerve fibers of the brain and spinal cord. MS can affect people of any age. The onset of MS is usually between 20 and 50 years of age, with symptoms first appearing at an average of 30 to 35 years of age. People who are diagnosed at 50 years of age or older generally have more progressive disease. Women are affected two to three times more often than men. An estimated 400,000 people in the United States have MS, with approximately 10,000 new cases diagnosed annually.[20]

MS is more prevalent in temperate climates (between 45 and 65 degrees of latitude), such as those found in the northern United States, Canada, and Europe, as compared with tropical regions. People who are born in an area of high risk but migrate to an area of low risk before age 15 assume the risk of their new home. Researchers thus suspect that exposure to some environmental agent before puberty may predispose a person to develop MS later in life. MS is less common in Hispanics, Asians, and people of African descent. It rarely occurs in some ethnic groups, including Alaskan Natives and Aborigines.

Etiology and Pathophysiology

Although the cause of MS is unknown, it is unlikely to be related to a single cause. The disease develops in a genetically susceptible person as a result of environmental exposure, such as an infection. Multiple genes are believed to be involved in the inherited susceptibility to MS. Having a first-degree relative with MS increases a person's risk of developing the disease. Common genetic factors have also been found in families with more than one affected member.[21]

Possible precipitating factors include infection, smoking, physical injury, emotional stress, excessive fatigue, pregnancy, and a poor state of health. The role of precipitating factors such as exposure to pathogenic agents is controversial. More than a dozen viruses and bacteria have been investigated, but none has definitely been proven to cause MS.

Three pathologic processes characterize MS: chronic inflammation, demyelination, and gliosis in the CNS. The primary neuropathologic condition is an autoimmune process orchestrated by activated T cells. An unknown trigger in genetically susceptible individuals may initiate this process. The activated T cells in the systemic circulation migrate to the CNS, disrupting the blood-brain barrier. This is likely the initial event in the development of MS. Subsequent antigen-antibody reaction within the CNS activates the inflammatory response and leads to the demyelination of axons.

Initially, attacks on the myelin sheaths of the neurons in the brain and spinal cord result in damage to the myelin sheath (Fig. 58-3, *A* to *C*). However, the nerve fiber is not affected. Transmission of nerve impulses still occurs, but it is slowed. The patient may complain of a noticeable impairment of function (e.g., weakness). However, myelin can regenerate. When it does,

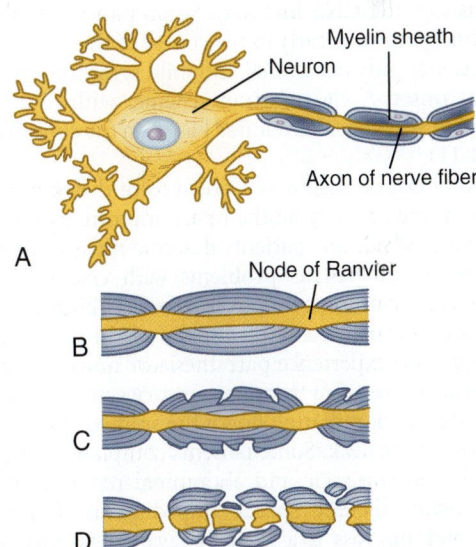

FIG. 58-3 Pathogenesis of multiple sclerosis. **A,** Normal nerve cell with myelin sheath. **B,** Normal axon. **C,** Myelin breakdown. **D,** Myelin totally disrupted; axon not functioning.

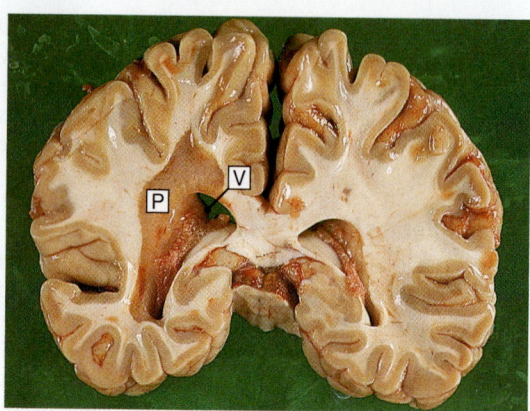

FIG. 58-4 Chronic multiple sclerosis. Demyelination plaque *(P)* at gray-white junction and adjacent partially remyelinated shadow plaque *(V).* (From Stevens A, Lowe J: *Pathology: illustrated review in colour,* ed 2, London, 2000, Mosby.)

TABLE 58-11	**Patterns of Multiple Sclerosis**
Category	**Characteristics**
Relapsing-remitting	• Clearly defined attacks of worsening neurologic function *(relapses)* with partial or complete recovery *(remission).* • Approximately 85% of people are initially diagnosed with this type of MS.
Primary-progressive	• Steadily worsening neurologic function from the beginning with minor improvements but no distinct relapses or remissions. • About 10% of people are diagnosed with this type of MS.
Secondary-progressive	• A relapsing-remitting initial course, followed by progression with or without occasional relapses, minor remissions, and plateaus. • New treatments may slow progression. • Most people initially diagnosed with relapsing-remitting MS eventually transition to this type.
Progressive-relapsing	• Progressive disease from onset, with clear acute relapses, with or without full recovery. Periods between relapses are characterized by continuing progression. • Only 5% of people experience this type of MS.

symptoms disappear. At that point, the patient experiences a remission.

As ongoing inflammation occurs, nearby oligodendrocytes are affected, and myelin loses the ability to regenerate. Eventually damage occurs to the underlying axon. Nerve impulse transmission is disrupted, resulting in permanent loss of nerve function (Fig. 58-3, *D*). As inflammation subsides, glial scar tissue replaces damaged tissue, leading to formation of hard, sclerotic plaques (Fig. 58-4). These plaques are found throughout the white matter of the CNS.

Clinical Manifestations

The onset of MS is often insidious and gradual, with vague symptoms occurring intermittently over months or years that do not prompt the patient to seek medical attention. Thus the disease may not be diagnosed until long after the onset of the first symptom. The disease is characterized by chronic, progressive deterioration in some patients, and remissions and exacerbations in others. With repeated exacerbations, the overall trend is progressive deterioration in neurologic function.

Because the disease process has a spotty distribution in the CNS, clinical manifestations vary with each patient according to the areas of the CNS involved. Some patients have severe, long-lasting symptoms early in the course of the disease. Others may experience only occasional and mild symptoms for several years after onset. A classification scheme, with four primary patterns of MS, has been developed based on the clinical course[22] (Table 58-11).

Blurred or double vision, red-green color distortion, or even blindness in one eye may be the first symptom experienced by a person with MS. Many patients describe muscle weakness in the extremities as well as problems with coordination and balance. Those symptoms may even affect walking or standing. MS can cause partial or complete paralysis in the worst cases. Most people also experience paresthesia or numbness and tingling. *Lhermitte's sign* is a transient sensory symptom described as an electric shock radiating down the spine or into the limbs with flexion of the neck. Some patients complain of pain, especially in the low thoracic and abdominal regions. Other frequent problems include speech impediments, tremors, and dizziness. Hearing loss is also an occasional finding. Possible cerebellar signs include nystagmus, ataxia, dysarthria, and dysphagia. Many patients have severe fatigue, sometimes with significant disability. The fatigue is aggravated by heat, humidity, deconditioning, and medication side effects.

Bowel and bladder function can be affected if the sclerotic plaque is located in areas of the CNS that control elimination. Problems with defecation usually involve constipation rather than fecal incontinence. Urinary problems are variable. A common problem in patients with MS is a *spastic* (uninhibited) bladder. As a result, the bladder has a small capacity for urine, and its contractions are unchecked. The result is urinary urgency and frequency, often accompanied by dribbling or incontinence.

A *flaccid* (hypotonic) bladder indicates a lesion in the reflex arc controlling bladder function. A flaccid bladder has a large capacity for urine because there is no sensation or desire to void, no pressure, and no pain. Generally, the patient has urinary retention, but urgency and frequency may also occur with this type of lesion. Another urinary problem is a combination of the previous two. Urinary problems cannot be adequately diagnosed and treated without urodynamic studies.

Sexual dysfunction occurs in many people with MS. Physiologic erectile dysfunction may result from spinal cord involvement in men. Women may experience decreased libido, difficulty with orgasmic response, painful intercourse, and decreased vaginal lubrication. Diminished sensation can prevent a normal sexual response in both men and women. The emotional effects of chronic illness and the loss of self-esteem also contribute to loss of sexual response.

Some women with MS who become pregnant experience remission or an improvement in their symptoms during the gestation period. Hormonal changes associated with pregnancy appear to affect the immune system. However, during the postpartum period, women are at greater risk for exacerbation of the disease.

About half of people with MS experience some problems with cognitive function. For most people, the problems are difficulties with short-term memory, attention, information processing, planning, visual perception, and word finding. General intellect remains unchanged and intact, including long-term memory, conversational skills, and reading comprehension. Symptoms can be mild and thus easily overlooked. However, cognitive changes are so severe in about 5% to 10% of patients with MS that they significantly impair the person's ability to perform activities of daily living. Most of the time, cognitive difficulties occur later in the course of the disease. However, they can occur much earlier in the disease process, and occasionally they are present at the onset of MS.

People with MS may also experience emotional changes such as anger, depression, or euphoria. Physical and emotional trauma, fatigue, and infection may aggravate or trigger signs and symptoms.

The average life expectancy after the onset of symptoms is more than 25 years. Death usually occurs due to infectious complications of immobility (e.g., pneumonia) or because of an unrelated disease.

Diagnostic Studies

Because there is no definitive diagnostic test for MS, factors considered are the history, clinical manifestations, and results of certain diagnostic tests (Table 58-12). An MRI of the brain and spinal cord may show plaques, inflammation, atrophy, and tissue breakdown and destruction. Cerebrospinal fluid (CSF) analysis may show an increase in immunoglobulin G and the presence of oligoclonal banding.[23] Evoked potential responses are often delayed in people with MS because of decreased nerve conduction from the eye and ear to the brain.

To be diagnosed with MS, the patient must have (1) evidence of at least two inflammatory demyelinating lesions in at least two different locations within the CNS, (2) damage or an attack occurring at different times (usually 1 month or more apart), and (3) all other possible diagnoses ruled out. If evidence exists for only one lesion, or only one clinical attack has occurred, the HCP will monitor the patient for another attack or for an attack at a different site in the CNS.[23]

Interprofessional Care

Drug Therapy. Because no cure currently exists for MS, interprofessional care is aimed at treating the disease process and providing symptomatic relief (Table 58-12). Because no two cases of MS are alike, therapy is tailored specifically to the disease pattern and manifestations experienced by each patient (Table 58-13). Disease-modifying therapy has been found to be more effective when initiated early in the course of MS. Delays in treatment have been associated with poor outcomes.

Treatment of MS begins with use of immunomodulator drugs to modify the disease progression and prevent relapses. These drugs include (1) interferon β-1a (Rebif, Plegridy [given subcutaneously]) and interferon β-1a (Avonex) (given IM), (2) interferon β-1b (Betaseron, Extavia) (given subcutaneously), and (3) glatiramer acetate (Copaxone) (given subcutaneously).

DRUG ALERT β-Interferon
- Rotate injection sites with each dose.
- Assess for depression and suicidal ideation.
- Instruct patient to wear sunscreen and protective clothing while exposed to sun.
- Inform the patient that flu-like symptoms are common after initiation of therapy.

Teriflunomide (Aubagio) is an immunomodulatory agent with antiinflammatory properties. The exact mechanism of action is unknown but may involve a reduction in the number

TABLE 58-12 Interprofessional Care
Multiple Sclerosis

Diagnostic Assessment	Management
• History and physical examination	• Drug therapy (Table 58-13)
• CSF analysis	• Surgical therapy
• CT scan	• Thalamotomy (unmanageable tremor)
• MRI, MRS	• Neurectomy, rhizotomy, cordotomy (unmanageable spasticity)
• Evoked potential testing	
• Somatosensory evoked potential (SSEP)	• Physical therapy
• Auditory evoked potential (AEP)	• Occupational therapy
• Visual evoked potential (VEP)	

MRS, Magnetic resonance spectroscopy.

TABLE 58-13 Drug Therapy
Multiple Sclerosis

Drug	Patient Teaching
Disease-Modifying Drugs *Immunomodulators*	
β-1a interferon (Rebif, Plegridy, Avonex) β-1b interferon (Betaseron, Extavia) glatiramer acetate (Copaxone)	• Perform self-injection techniques. • Report side effects. • Treat flu-like symptoms with an NSAID or acetaminophen.
teriflunomide (Aubagio)	• Because it may cause serious liver disease, monitor liver tests. • Avoid pregnancy.
Immunosuppressant mitoxantrone dimethyl fumarate (Tecfidera)	• Report side effects. • Avoid pregnancy. • Avoid contact with large crowds and people who have an infection.
Sphingosine 1-Phosphate Receptor Modulator fingolimod (Gilenya)	• Report side effects. • Monitor blood pressure regularly. • Avoid pregnancy.
Monoclonal Antibody natalizumab (Tysabri) alemtuzumab (Lemtrada) daclizumab (Zinbryta)	• Report side effects. • Avoid pregnancy.
Drugs for Managing Exacerbations *Corticosteroids* ACTH prednisone methylprednisolone	• Restrict salt intake. • Do not abruptly stop therapy. • Know drug interactions.
Drugs for Symptom Management *Cholinergics* bethanechol (Urecholine) neostigmine	• Consult with HCP before using other drugs, including over-the-counter drugs.
Anticholinergics propantheline oxybutynin (Ditropan XL)	• Consult HCP before using other drugs, especially sleeping aids, antihistamines (possibly leading to potentiated effect).
Muscle Relaxants diazepam (Valium) baclofen (Lioresal) dantrolene (Dantrium) tizanidine (Zanaflex)	• Avoid driving and similar activities because of sedative effects. • Do not abruptly stop therapy. • Avoid use with tranquilizers and alcohol.
Nerve Conduction Enhancer dalfampridine (Ampyra)	• Be aware that it may cause seizures, especially at higher doses. • Take the tablet whole. Do not take more than 2 in 24 hr.

ACTH, Adrenocorticotropic hormone.

of activated lymphocytes in the CNS. Fingolimod (Gilenya) reduces MS disease activity by preventing lymphocytes from reaching the CNS and causing damage. Both drugs are specifically indicated for treatment of relapsing forms of MS.

For more active and aggressive forms of MS, natalizumab (Tysabri), alemtuzumab (Lemtrada), mitoxantrone, and dimethyl fumarate (Tecfidera) may be used. Natalizumab is given when patients have had an inadequate response to other drugs. An adverse effect of natalizumab is the increased risk of progressive multifocal leukoencephalopathy, a potentially fatal viral infection of the brain. Because of its safety profile, alemtuzumab is generally reserved for patients who have an inadequate response to two or more drugs indicated for the treatment of MS.[24]

Mitoxantrone, an antineoplastic medication, has serious effects, including cardiotoxicity, leukemia, and infertility. Dimethyl fumarate provides a new approach to treating MS by activating the Nrf2 pathway. This pathway provides a way for cells in the body to defend themselves against the inflammation and oxidative stress caused by MS.

Corticosteroids (e.g., methylprednisolone, prednisone) are most helpful to treat acute exacerbations of MS. They reduce edema and acute inflammation at the site of demyelination. However, these drugs do not affect the ultimate outcome or the degree of residual neurologic impairment from the exacerbation. Therapeutic plasma exchange *(plasmapheresis)* and IV immunoglobulin G may be considered when treatment with corticosteroids alone does not achieve symptom improvement.

Many other drugs are used to treat the various symptoms of MS, which may include fatigue, spasticity, tremor, vertigo or dizziness, depression, pain, bowel problems, bladder problems, sexual dysfunction, and cognitive changes. For example, muscle relaxants are used for spasticity. Amantadine and CNS stimulants (pemoline, methylphenidate [Ritalin], and modafinil [Provigil]) are used to treat fatigue. Anticholinergics are used to treat bladder symptoms. Tricyclic antidepressants and anti-seizure drugs are used for chronic pain syndromes.

Dalfampridine (Ampyra) is used to improve walking speed in MS patients. It is a selective potassium channel blocker and improves nerve conduction in damaged nerve segments. It should not be used in patients with a history of seizure disorders or with moderate to severe kidney disease.

Other Therapies. Spasticity is treated primarily with muscle relaxants. However, surgery (e.g., neurectomy, rhizotomy, cordotomy), dorsal-column electrical stimulation, or intrathecal baclofen (Lioresal) delivered by pump may be required. Tremors that become unmanageable with drugs are sometimes treated by thalamotomy or deep brain stimulation.

Neurologic dysfunction sometimes improves with physical and speech therapies. Exercise improves the daily functioning for patients with MS not experiencing an exacerbation. Exercise decreases spasticity, increases coordination, and retrains unaffected muscles to substitute for impaired ones. An especially beneficial type of physical therapy is water exercise (Fig. 58-5). Water, which gives buoyancy to the body, allows the patient to have more control over the body and perform activities that would normally be impossible.

❖ NURSING MANAGEMENT: MULTIPLE SCLEROSIS

◆ Nursing Assessment

Subjective and objective data that should be obtained from a patient with MS are presented in Table 58-14.

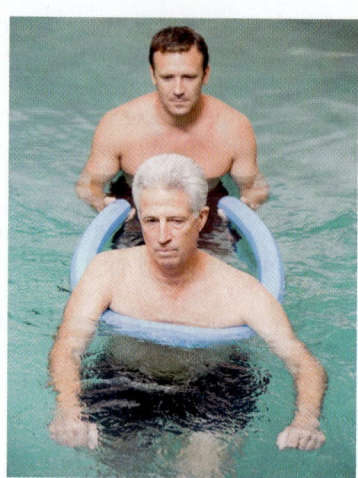

FIG. 58-5 Water therapy provides exercise and recreation for the patient with a chronic neurologic disease. (©Photos.com/AbleStock.com/Thinkstock)

TABLE 58-14	Nursing Assessment

Multiple Sclerosis

Subjective Data
Important Health Information
Past health history: Recent or past viral infections or vaccinations, other recent infections, residence in cold or temperate climates, recent physical or emotional stress, pregnancy, exposure to extremes of heat and cold
Medications: Adherence to regimen of corticosteroids, immunomodulators, immunosuppressants, cholinergics, anticholinergics, antispasmodics

Functional Health Patterns
Health perception–health management: Positive family history; malaise
Nutritional-metabolic: Weight loss; difficulty in chewing, dysphagia
Elimination: Urinary frequency, urgency, dribbling or incontinence, retention; constipation
Activity-exercise: Generalized muscle weakness, muscle fatigue; tingling and numbness; ataxia (clumsiness)
Cognitive-perceptual: Eye, back, leg, joint pain; painful muscle spasms; vertigo; blurred or lost vision; diplopia; tinnitus
Sexuality-reproductive: Impotence, decreased libido
Coping–stress tolerance: Anger, depression, euphoria, social isolation

Objective Data
General
Apathy, inattentiveness

Integumentary
Pressure ulcers

Neurologic
Scanning speech, nystagmus, ataxia, tremor, spasticity, hyperreflexia, decreased hearing

Musculoskeletal
Muscle weakness, paresis, paralysis, spasms, foot dragging, dysarthria

Possible Diagnostic Findings
↓ T suppressor cells, demyelinating lesions on MRI or MRS scans, ↑ IgG or oligoclonal banding in cerebrospinal fluid, delayed evoked potential responses

IgG, Immunoglobulin G; *MRS,* magnetic resonance spectroscopy.

◆ **Nursing Diagnoses**

Nursing diagnoses for the patient with MS may include, but are not limited to, the following:

- Impaired physical mobility *related to* muscle weakness or paralysis and muscle spasticity
- Impaired urinary elimination *related to* sensorimotor deficits
- Ineffective health management *related to* knowledge deficit regarding management of MS

Additional information on nursing diagnoses for the patient with MS is presented in the eNursing Care Plan 58-3 (available on the website for this chapter).

◆ **Planning**

The overall goals are that the patient with MS will (1) maximize neuromuscular function, (2) maintain independence in activities of daily living for as long as possible, (3) manage disabling fatigue, (4) optimize psychosocial well-being, (5) adjust to the illness, and (6) reduce factors that precipitate exacerbations.

◆ **Nursing Implementation**

The patient with MS should be aware of triggers that may cause exacerbations or worsening of the disease. Exacerbations of MS are triggered by infection (especially upper respiratory and urinary tract infections), trauma, immunization, childbirth, stress, and change in climate. Each person responds differently to these triggers. Assist the patient in identifying triggers and developing ways to avoid them or minimize their effects.

During the diagnostic phase, the patient needs reassurance that certain diagnostic studies must be done to rule out other neurologic disorders, even though a tentative diagnosis of MS has been made. Assist the patient in dealing with anxiety caused by a diagnosis of a disabling illness. The patient with recently diagnosed MS may need assistance with the grieving process.

During an acute exacerbation, the patient may be immobile and confined to bed. The focus of nursing interventions at this phase is to prevent major complications of immobility, such as respiratory and urinary tract infections and pressure ulcers.

Focus patient teaching on building general resistance to illness, including avoiding fatigue, extremes of heat and cold, and exposure to infection. Encourage vigorous and early treatment of infection when it occurs. Teach the patient to achieve a good balance of exercise and rest; minimize caffeine intake; and eat nutritious, well-balanced meals. A diet high in fiber may help relieve constipation. The patient should know the treatment regimens, drug side effects, how to identify and manage side effects, and drug interactions with over-the-counter medications. The patient should consult an HCP before taking nonprescription drugs.

Bladder control is a major problem for many patients with MS. Although anticholinergics may be beneficial for some patients to decrease spasticity, you may need to teach others self-catheterization (discussed in Chapter 45 on p. 1050). Bowel problems, particularly constipation, frequently occur in patients with MS. Increasing dietary fiber intake may help some patients achieve regularity in bowel elimination.

The patient with MS and the caregiver need to make many emotional adjustments because of the unpredictability of the disease, need for lifestyle changes, and challenge of avoiding or decreasing precipitating factors. The National Multiple Sclerosis Society and its local chapters can offer a variety of services to meet the needs of patients with MS.

◆ **Evaluation**

The expected outcomes are that the patient with MS will

- Maintain or improve muscle strength and mobility
- Use assistive devices appropriately for ambulation and mobility
- Maintain urinary continence
- Make decisions about health and lifestyle modifications necessary for management of MS

Additional information on expected outcomes for the patient with MS are presented in eNursing Care Plan 58-3 (available on the website for this chapter).

PARKINSON'S DISEASE

Parkinson's disease (PD) is a chronic, progressive neurodegenerative disorder characterized by slowness in the initiation and execution of movement *(bradykinesia)*, increased muscle tone *(rigidity)*, tremor at rest, and gait disturbance. It is the most common form of *parkinsonism* (a syndrome characterized by similar symptoms).

Up to 1 million Americans are believed to be living with PD, with approximately 60,000 diagnosed each year. Incidence of PD increases with age, but an estimated 4% of people with PD are diagnosed before 50 years of age. PD is more common in men by a ratio of 3:2.[25]

Etiology and Pathophysiology

The exact cause of PD is unknown. Although PD is not considered a hereditary condition, genetic risk factors should be evaluated for their interplay with environmental factors. About 15% of patients with PD have a positive family history for the disease *(familial cases)* that may be caused by mutations in specific genes. In other people, risk for PD may be increased by well water, pesticides, herbicides, industrial chemicals, and wood pulp mills. Rural residence is also considered a risk factor.[26]

Many forms of secondary *(atypical)* parkinsonism exist other than PD. Symptoms of parkinsonism have occurred after exposure to a variety of chemicals, including carbon monoxide and manganese (among copper miners) and the product of meperidine analog synthesis, MPTP. Drug-induced parkinsonism can also follow therapy with metoclopramide (Reglan), reserpine, methyldopa, lithium, haloperidol (Haldol), and chlorpromazine. Parkinsonism can be seen after the use of illicit drugs, including amphetamine and methamphetamine. After stopping these drugs, symptoms of parkinsonism generally disappear; one notable exception is irreversible parkinsonism following MTPT exposure. Other causes of parkinsonism include hydrocephalus, other neurodegenerative disorders, hypoparathyroidism, infections, stroke, tumor, and trauma.[27]

Many changes found in the brains of people with PD may play a role in development of the disease, including a lack of dopamine (DA). The pathologic process of PD involves degeneration of the DA-producing neurons in the substantia nigra of the midbrain (Figs. 58-6 to 58-8), which in turn disrupts the normal balance between DA and acetylcholine (ACh) in the basal ganglia. The neurotransmitter DA is essential for normal functioning of the extrapyramidal motor system, including control of posture, support, and voluntary motion. Manifestations of PD do not occur until 80% of neurons in the substantia nigra are lost.

Lewy bodies, unusual clumps of protein, are found in the brains of patients with PD. It is not known what causes these bodies to form, but their presence indicates abnormal functioning of the brain. Lewy body dementia is discussed in Chapter 59.

Genetic Link

Approximately 15% of patients with PD have a family history of PD. Many autosomal dominant and recessive genes have been linked to familial PD. The most common genetic contributor to PD is the *LRRK2* gene. Mutations in this gene also appear to have a role in sporadic, or noninherited, cases of PD. Other genes involved in familial PD are parkin (*PARK2, PARK7*), *PINK1*, and *SNCA*. Mutations in these genes are often associated with a younger age of onset and have additional manifestations than those typically seen with age-related PD.[26] *PINK1* mutations are related to a rare, early-onset form of PD. It is not fully understood how genetic changes cause PD or influence the risk of developing the disorder.

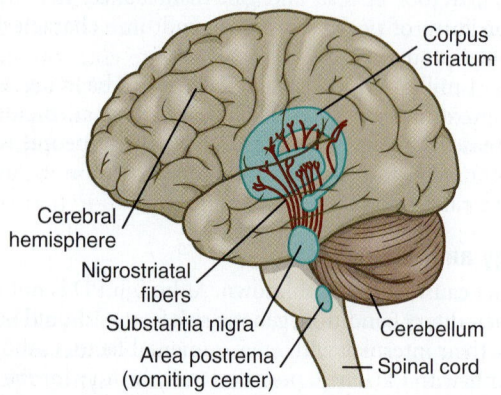

FIG. 58-6 Nigrostriatal disorders produce parkinsonism. Left-sided view of the human brain showing the substantia nigra and the corpus striatum *(shaded area)* lying deep within the cerebral hemisphere. Nerve fibers extend upward from the substantia nigra, divide into many branches, and carry dopamine to all regions of the corpus striatum.

Clinical Manifestations

The onset of PD is gradual and insidious, with an ongoing progression. Only one side of the body may be involved initially. Classic manifestations of PD are easily remembered by the mnemonic *TRAP* (**t**remor, **r**igidity, **a**kinesia, and **p**ostural instability).[26] In the beginning stages, only a mild tremor, a slight limp, or a decreased arm swing may be evident. Later in the disease, the patient may have a shuffling, propulsive gait with arms flexed, and show loss of postural reflexes. Up to 90% of patients also experience speech abnormalities *(hypokinetic dysarthria)* that can affect communication and quality of life.[28] None of these manifestations alone is sufficient evidence for a diagnosis of the disease.

Tremor. *Tremor* is often the first sign and may be minimal initially, so the patient is the only one who notices it. This tremor can affect handwriting, causing it to trail off, particularly toward the ends of words. Parkinsonian tremor is more prominent at rest and is aggravated by emotional stress or increased concentration. The hand tremor is described as "pill rolling"

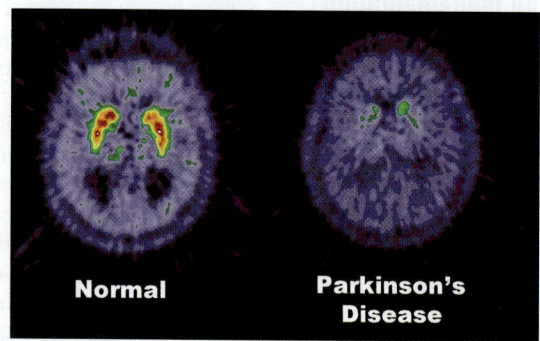

FIG. 58-8 In Parkinson's disease, positron emission tomography (PET) scan showing reduced fluorodopa uptake in the basal ganglia *(right)* compared with a normal control *(left)*. (From Aminoff MJ, Daroff RB: *Encyclopedia of the neurological sciences,* Waltham, Mass, 2003, Academic Press.)

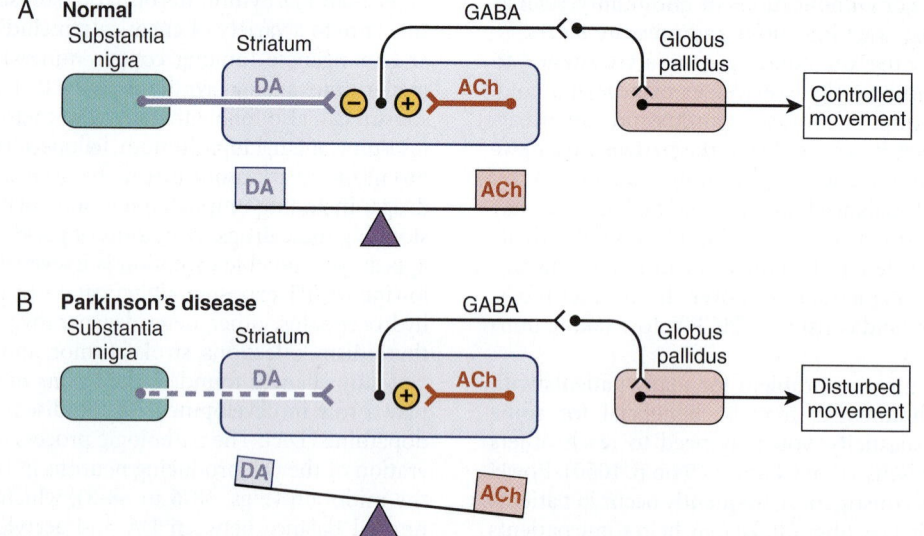

FIG. 58-7 A deficit in dopamine (DA) exists in Parkinson's disease. This deficit creates an imbalance between dopamine and the excitatory neurotransmitter acetylcholine. **A,** In a healthy person, dopamine released from neurons originating in the substantia nigra inhibits the firing of neurons in the striatum that release γ-aminobutyric acid *(GABA)*. Conversely, neurons located within the striatum, which release acetylcholine *(ACh)*, excite the GABAergic neurons. Under normal conditions, inhibitory actions of DA are balanced by excitatory actions of ACh, and controlled movement results. **B,** In Parkinson's disease, neurons in the substantia nigra that supply DA to the striatum degenerate. When a deficit of DA occurs, excitatory effects of ACh go unopposed and disturbed movements (tremor, rigidity) result. (From Lehne RA: *Pharmacology for nursing care,* ed 8, St Louis, 2013, Saunders.)

because the thumb and forefinger appear to move in a rotary fashion as if rolling a pill, coin, or other small object. Tremor can also involve the diaphragm, tongue, lips, and jaw but rarely causes shaking of the head.

Unfortunately, in many people a benign *essential tremor* is mistakenly diagnosed as PD. Essential tremor occurs during voluntary movement, has a more rapid frequency than parkinsonian tremor, and is often familial.

Rigidity. *Rigidity* is the increased resistance to passive motion when the limbs are moved through their range of motion. Parkinsonian rigidity is typified by a jerky quality *(cogwheel rigidity)*, as if there were intermittent catches in the passive movement of a joint. Sustained muscle contraction causes the rigidity and consequently elicits complaints of muscle soreness; feeling tired and achy; or pain in the head, upper body, spine, or legs. Slowness of movement is another consequence of rigidity because it inhibits the alternating contraction and relaxation in opposing muscle groups (e.g., biceps and triceps).

Akinesia. *Akinesia* is the absence or loss of control of voluntary muscle movements. In PD *bradykinesia* (slowness of movement) is particularly evident in the loss of automatic movements. This occurs because of the physical and chemical alteration of the basal ganglia and related structures in the extrapyramidal portion of the CNS. In the unaffected patient, automatic movements are involuntary and occur subconsciously. They include blinking of the eyelids, swinging of the arms while walking, swallowing of saliva, using facial and hand movements for self-expression, and making minor movements for postural adjustment.

The patient with PD does not execute these movements and lacks spontaneous activity. This accounts for the stooped posture, masked face (deadpan expression), drooling of saliva, and shuffling gait *(festination)* that are characteristic of a person with this disease. The posture is that of a slowed "old man" image, with the head and trunk bent forward and the legs constantly flexed (Fig. 58-9).

Postural Instability. *Postural instability* is common. Patients may complain of being unable to stop themselves from going forward *(propulsion)* or backward *(retropulsion)*. Assessment of postural instability includes the "pull test." The examiner stands behind the patient and gives a tug backward on the shoulder, causing the patient to lose his or her balance and fall backward.

In addition to the motor signs of PD, many nonmotor symptoms are common. They include depression, anxiety, apathy, fatigue, pain, urinary retention and constipation, erectile dysfunction, and memory changes. Sleep problems are common and include difficulty staying asleep at night, restless sleep, nightmares, and drowsiness or sudden sleep onset during the day. In particular, rapid eye movement (REM) behavior disorder is a preparkinsonian state that occurs in about one third of patients with PD. It is characterized by violent dreams and potentially dangerous motor activity during REM sleep.[26]

Complications

As the disease progresses, complications increase. These include motor symptoms (e.g., dyskinesias [spontaneous, involuntary movements], weakness, neurologic problems (e.g., dementia), and neuropsychiatric problems (e.g., depression, hallucinations, psychosis). As PD progresses, it often results in dementia, which is associated with an increase in mortality.

As swallowing becomes more difficult (dysphagia), malnutrition or aspiration may result. General debilitation may lead to pneumonia, urinary tract infections, and skin breakdown. Orthostatic hypotension occurs commonly and, along with loss of postural reflexes, may result in falls or other injury. The patient's increased fall risk increases the need for the primary caregiver to be aware of environmental conditions that may also contribute to falls.

Diagnostic Studies

Because no specific diagnostic test exists for PD, diagnosis is based on the patient's history and clinical features. Clinical diagnosis requires the presence of TRAP and asymmetric onset. Confirmation of PD is a positive response to antiparkinsonian drugs (levodopa or dopamine agonist). MRI and CT have a limited role in diagnosis of PD because they do not show a specific pathologic finding. However, they can rule out a stroke or brain tumor.

Interprofessional Care

Because PD has no cure, interprofessional care focuses on symptom management (Table 58-15).

Drug Therapy. Drug therapy for PD is aimed at correcting the imbalance of neurotransmitters within the CNS. Antiparkinsonian drugs either enhance the release or the supply of DA (dopaminergic) or antagonize or block the effects of the overactive cholinergic neurons in the striatum (anticholinergic) (Fig. 58-7). Levodopa with carbidopa (Sinemet) is the primary treatment for symptomatic patients. Levodopa is a chemical

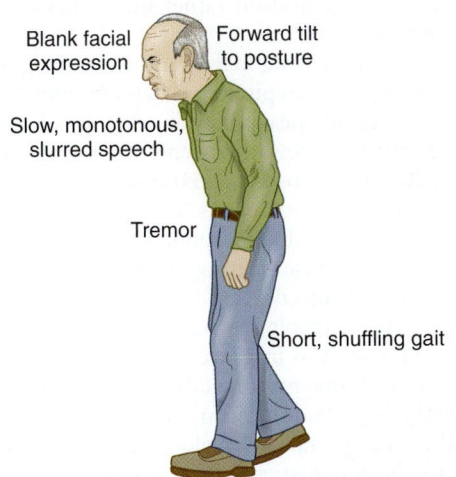

Blank facial expression

Forward tilt to posture

Slow, monotonous, slurred speech

Tremor

Short, shuffling gait

FIG. 58-9 Characteristic appearance of a patient with Parkinson's disease.

TABLE 58-15	**Interprofessional Care**

Parkinson's Disease

Diagnostic Assessment	Management
• History and physical examination	• Antiparkinsonian drugs (Table 58-16)
• TRAP (tremor, rigidity, akinesia and postural instability)	• Surgical therapy
• Positive response to antiparkinsonian drugs	• Deep brain stimulation
• MRI	• Ablation surgery
• Rule out side effects of phenothiazines, reserpine, benzodiazepines, haloperidol	• Physical therapy
	• Occupational therapy
	• Dietitian consult for nutritional therapy

precursor of DA and can cross the blood-brain barrier. It is converted to DA in the basal ganglia. Sinemet is the preferred drug because it also contains carbidopa, an agent that inhibits the enzyme dopa-decarboxylase in the peripheral tissues. Dopa-decarboxylase breaks down levodopa before it reaches the brain. The net result of the combination of levodopa and carbidopa is that more levodopa reaches the brain, and therefore less drug is needed. Levodopa has many side effects and drug interactions. Prolonged use often results in dyskinesias and "off/on" periods when the medication will unpredictably start or stop working.

 DRUG ALERT   **Carbidopa/Levodopa (Sinemet)**
- Monitor for signs of dyskinesia.
- Effects may be delayed for several weeks to months.
- Instruct patient or caregiver to report any uncontrolled movement of face, eyelids, mouth, tongue, arms, hands, or legs; mental changes; palpitations; severe nausea and vomiting; and difficulty urinating.

Many patients are given Sinemet early in the disease course for the management of motor symptoms. However, some HCPs believe that, after a few years of therapy, the effectiveness of Sinemet wears off. Therefore they prefer to start therapy with a DA receptor agonist, a drug that directly stimulates DA receptors. Ropinirole (Requip) and pramipexole (Mirapex) may be used alone or in combination with Sinemet. Bromocriptine (Parlodel) should not be used as first-line treatment because of possible serious side effects (e.g., high blood pressure, seizure, heart attack, stroke). Many of these medications are available in extended-release forms that improve patients' ability to adhere to treatment regimens. Rotigotine (Neupro), another DA receptor agonist, is available a transdermal patch applied once daily as an adjunctive therapy for patients taking Sinemet.

 DRUG ALERT   **Bromocriptine (Parlodel)**
- Patient may become dizzy or faint due to orthostatic hypotension, especially after the first dose.
- Notify physician immediately if a severe headache develops that does not improve or continues to get worse.

The antiviral agent amantadine is a weak antagonist of NMDA-type glutamate receptors, increases dopamine release, and blocks dopamine reuptake. Thus it provides only mild relief and is seldom used in early stages of PD.[29] In addition, withdrawal of amantadine even after extended therapy can worsen dyskinesia.

Anticholinergic drugs such as trihexyphenidyl and benztropine (Cogentin) are also used to manage PD. These drugs decrease the activity of ACh, thus providing balance between cholinergic and dopaminergic actions. Antihistamines (e.g., diphenhydramine) with anticholinergic properties may be used to manage tremors.

Selegiline (Eldepryl) and rasagiline (Azilect) are monoamine oxidase type B (MAO-B) inhibitors that may be used in combination with Sinemet. By inhibiting MAO-B, the degradative enzyme for DA, these agents increase the levels of DA and prolong the half-life of levodopa. Rasagiline can also be used alone as therapy in early PD. However, MAO-B inhibitors are less effective at treating motor symptoms than DA receptor agonists.

Entacapone (Comtan) and tolcapone (Tasmar) block the enzyme catechol *O*-methyltransferase (COMT), which breaks down levodopa in the peripheral circulation, and thus prolong the effect of Sinemet. These drugs are used only as adjuncts to levodopa; both drugs can exacerbate adverse effects of levodopa. Tolcapone is rarely prescribed because it has been associated with fatal hepatotoxicity.[26]

Rivastigmine (Exelon) or donepezil (Aricept) is used to treat dementia. Amitriptyline may be used to treat depression.

Table 58-16 summarizes the drugs commonly used in PD. The use of only one drug is preferred because fewer side effects occur and the drug dosage is easier to adjust than when several drugs are used. However, as the disease progresses, combination therapy is often required. Excessive amounts of dopaminergic drugs can lead to aggravation rather than relief of symptoms (*paradoxic intoxication*).

Within 3 to 5 years of standard Parkinson's drug treatments, many patients experience episodes of hypomobility (e.g., inability to rise from chair, speak, or walk; also called *off episodes*). The episodes can occur toward the end of a dosing interval with standard medications (so-called *end-of-dose wearing off*) or at unpredictable times (spontaneous "on/off"). A combination of carbidopa, levodopa, and entacapone (Stalevo) is available for patients with end-of-dose wearing off. It is typically prescribed for patients with advanced PD with evidence of intense motor fluctuations. The injectable DA receptor agonist apomorphine (Apokyn) is also used to improve movement in hypomobility episodes. Apomorphine must be taken with an antiemetic drug (e.g., trimethobenzamide [Tigan]) because it causes severe nausea and vomiting when taken alone. Apomorphine must not be taken with the antiemetics in the serotonin (5-HT3) receptor

TABLE 58-16 Drug Therapy
Parkinson's Disease

Drug	Mechanism of Action
Dopaminergics	
Dopamine Precursors	
levodopa (L-dopa)	Converted to dopamine in
levodopa/carbidopa (Sinemet)	basal ganglia
Dopamine Receptor Agonists	
bromocriptine (Parlodel)	Stimulate dopamine receptors
cabergoline	
pramipexole (Mirapex)	
ropinirole (Requip, Requip XL)	
rotigotine (Neupro [transdermal patch])	
Dopamine Agonists	
amantadine	Blocks NMDA-type glutamate receptors, increases dopamine release, and blocks dopamine reuptake
apomorphine (Apokyn)	Stimulates postsynaptic dopamine receptors
Anticholinergics	
trihexyphenidyl	Block cholinergic receptors, thus helping to balance cholinergic and dopaminergic activity
benztropine (Cogentin)	
Antihistamine	
diphenhydramine	Has anticholinergic effect
Monoamine Oxidase Inhibitors	
selegiline (Eldepryl)	Block breakdown of
rasagiline (Azilect)	dopamine
Catechol *O*-Methyltransferase (COMT) Inhibitors	
entacapone (Comtan)	Block COMT and slow the breakdown of levodopa, thus prolonging the action of levodopa
tolcapone (Tasmar)	

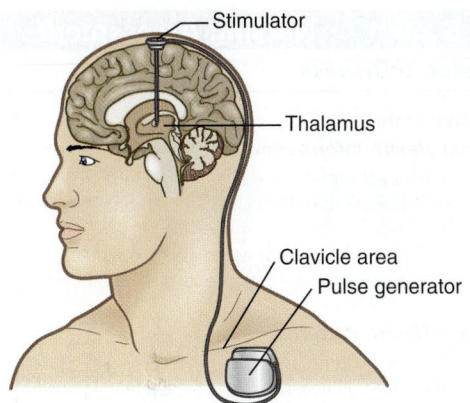

FIG. 58-10 Deep brain stimulation (DBS) can be used to treat tremors and uncontrolled movements of Parkinson's disease. Electrodes are surgically placed in the brain and connected to a neurostimulator (pacemaker device) in the chest.

antagonist class (e.g., ondansetron [Zofran]) because this drug combination can lead to very low blood pressure and loss of consciousness.

Surgical Therapy. Surgical procedures aimed at relieving symptoms of PD are usually used in patients who are unresponsive to drug therapy or who have developed severe motor complications. Surgical procedures fall into three categories: deep brain stimulation (DBS), ablation (destruction), and transplantation. The most common surgical treatment is DBS, which involves placing an electrode in the thalamus, globus pallidus, or subthalamic nucleus and connecting it to a generator placed in the upper chest (similar to a pacemaker) (Fig. 58-10). The device is programmed to deliver a specific current to the targeted brain location. DBS is preferred to ablation procedures because it is reversible and programmable and can be safely performed bilaterally. DBS procedures reduce the increased neuronal activity produced by DA depletion. It has been shown to improve motor function and reduce dyskinesia and medication usage. DBS is most effective when candidates are carefully selected and screened.[30]

Ablation surgery involves locating, targeting, and destroying an area of the brain affected by PD. The goal is to destroy tissue that produces abnormal chemical or electrical impulses leading to tremors or other symptoms. Typical targets of ablation are the thalamus *(thalamotomy)*, globus pallidus *(pallidotomy)*, and subthalamic nucleus *(subthalamic nucleotomy)*.

Transplantation of fetal neural tissue into the basal ganglia is designed to provide DA-producing cells in the brains of patients with PD. Research and clinical trials of this form of therapy are ongoing.

Nutritional Therapy. Diet is of major importance to patients with PD because malnutrition and constipation can be serious consequences of inadequate nutrition. Patients who have dysphagia and bradykinesia need appetizing foods that are easily chewed and swallowed. The diet should contain adequate fiber and fruit to avoid constipation. Cut food into bite-sized pieces before it is served, and serve it on a warmed plate to preserve its appeal.

Eating six small meals a day may be less exhausting than eating three large meals a day. Plan ample time for eating to avoid frustration. The absorption of levodopa can be impaired by protein ingestion and vitamin B_6. Therefore some patients are advised to limit their protein intake to the evening meal to decrease this problem. They also need to consult with their HCP regarding possible inclusion of vitamin B_6 in their multivitamins and fortified cereals.

❖ NURSING MANAGEMENT: PARKINSON'S DISEASE

◆ Nursing Assessment
Subjective and objective data that should be obtained from a patient with PD are presented in Table 58-17.

◆ Nursing Diagnoses
Nursing diagnoses for the patient with PD may include, but are not limited to, the following:
- Impaired physical mobility *related to* rigidity, bradykinesia, akinesia, and postural instability
- Imbalanced nutrition: less than body requirements *related to* inability to ingest food
- Impaired swallowing *related to* neuromuscular impairment (e.g., decreased or absent gag reflex)
- Impaired verbal communication *related to* dysarthria, tremor, and bradykinesia

Additional information on nursing diagnoses for the patient with PD is presented in eNursing Care Plan 58-4 (available on the website for this chapter).

TABLE 58-17 Nursing Assessment

Parkinson's Disease

Subjective Data

Important Health Information

Past health history: Central nervous system trauma, cerebrovascular disorders, exposure to metals and carbon monoxide, encephalitis or other infections

Medications: Major tranquilizers, especially haloperidol (Haldol), and phenothiazines, reserpine, methyldopa, amphetamines

Functional Health Patterns

Health perception–health management: Fatigue

Nutritional-metabolic: Excessive salivation, dysphagia, weight loss

Elimination: Constipation, incontinence, excessive sweating

Activity-exercise: Difficulty in initiating movements, frequent falls, loss of dexterity, micrographia (handwriting deterioration)

Sleep-rest: Insomnia, nightmares, daytime sleepiness

Cognitive-perceptual: Diffuse pain in head, shoulders, neck, back, legs, and hips. Muscle soreness and cramping

Self-perception–self-concept: Depression, mood swings, hallucinations

Objective Data

General

Blank (masked) facial expression, slow and monotonous speech, infrequent blinking

Integumentary

Seborrhea, dandruff; ankle edema

Cardiovascular

Postural hypotension

Gastrointestinal

Drooling

Neurologic

Tremor at rest, first in hands (pill rolling), later in legs, arms, face, and tongue. Aggravation of tremor with anxiety, absence in sleep. Poor coordination, cognitive impairment and dementia, impaired postural reflexes

Musculoskeletal

Cogwheel rigidity, dysarthria, bradykinesia, contractures, stooped posture, shuffling gait

Possible Diagnostic Findings

No specific tests. Diagnosis based on history and physical findings and ruling out of other diseases

---

? CHECK YOUR PRACTICE

You are working in a rehabilitation facility where one of your patients is a 78-yr-old man with Parkinson's disease. Six months ago he was also at your facility with a fractured hip after falling in his yard. The family has asked to talk with you about their fear of taking him for a walk in the hallways because he is so unstable.
• What advice would you provide to the family?

Promotion of physical exercise and a well-balanced diet are major concerns for nursing care. Exercise can limit the consequences of decreased mobility, such as muscle atrophy, contractures, and constipation. The American Parkinson Disease Association *(www.apdaparkinson.org)* publishes a series of booklets and videotapes with helpful exercises that can be used by family members and health care professionals.

A physical therapist may be consulted to design a personal exercise program aimed at strengthening and stretching specific muscles. Overall muscle tone and specific exercises to strengthen the muscles involved with speaking and swallowing should be included. Although exercise will not halt the progress of the disease, it will enhance the patient's functional ability. An occupational therapist can also assist the patient with strategies to increase self-care measures, including eating and dressing.

! SAFETY ALERT   Preventing Falls

Have patients who are at risk for falling and tend to "freeze" while walking do the following:
• Consciously think about stepping over imaginary or real lines on the floor.
• Drop rice kernels and step over them.
• Rock from side to side.
• Lift the toes when stepping.
• Take one step backward and two steps forward.

Work closely with the patient's caregiver and family in exploring creative adaptations that allow maximum independence and self-care. The patient can get out of a chair better by using an upright chair with arms and placing the back legs of the chair on small (2-inch) blocks. Encourage environmental alterations, such as removing rugs and excess furniture to avoid stumbling, using an elevated toilet seat to facilitate getting on and off the toilet, and elevating the legs on an ottoman to decrease dependent ankle edema. Clothing can be simplified by the use of slip-on shoes and Velcro hook-and-loop fasteners or zippers on clothing, instead of buttons and hooks.

Effective management of sleep problems can greatly improve the quality of life for patients with PD. Some patients find the use of satin nightwear or satin sheets beneficial. Information on teaching regarding sleep hygiene practices is presented in Chapter 7.

In the early stages of PD, many patients experience depression and anxiety. Patients need to adjust their lifestyle, including work and home responsibilities. As the disease progresses, the impact on the patient's psychologic well-being also increases. Assist the patient by listening, providing teaching, challenging distorted thoughts, and encouraging social interactions. Psychologic therapy and counseling can be helpful. Also ensure that patients with PD receives prescribed medications on time to avoid on-off effects.

In the early stage of the disease, the patient has subtle changes in cognitive function that can progress to dementia. This results in increased caregiver burden and the potential for long-term

◆ Planning

The overall goals are that the patient with PD will (1) maximize neurologic function, (2) maintain independence in activities of daily living for as long as possible, and (3) optimize psychosocial well-being.

◆ Nursing Implementation

Because PD is a chronic degenerative disorder with no acute exacerbations, teaching and nursing care are directed toward maintenance of good health, encouragement of independence, and avoidance of complications such as contractures and falls. Problems secondary to bradykinesia can be alleviated by relatively simple measures.

care placement. Information on care of the patient with dementia is provided in Chapter 59.

Family members (e.g., spouse, children) care for the majority of patients with PD. As the disease progresses, the caregiver burden increases, often while the caregiver's physical and mental health decline. Strategies to reduce caregiver burden are described in Chapter 4. Other interventions for patients with PD are presented in eNursing Care Plan 58-4 (available on the website for this chapter).

◆ **Evaluation**

The expected outcomes are that the patient with PD will
• Perform physical exercise to deter muscle atrophy and joint contractures
• Use assistive devices appropriately for ambulation and mobility
• Maintain nutritional intake adequate for metabolic needs
• Experience safe passage of fluids and/or solids from the mouth to the stomach
• Use methods of communication that meet needs for interaction with others

Additional information on expected outcomes for the patient with PD is presented in eNursing Care Plan 58-4 (available on the website).

MYASTHENIA GRAVIS

Myasthenia gravis (MG) is an autoimmune disease of the neuromuscular junction characterized by the fluctuating weakness of certain skeletal muscle groups. This weakness increases with muscle use. MG occurs in either gender and in people of any ethnicity. The prevalence rate is approximately 20 per 100,000; currently an estimated 60,000 people have MG in the United States. The mean age at onset in women is 28 years; in men the mean age at onset of MG is 42 years. Women are affected more often than men (3:2). In older adults, both men and women are equally affected.[31]

Etiology and Pathophysiology

MG is caused by an autoimmune process in which antibodies attack acetylcholine (ACh) receptors. This results in a decreased number of ACh receptor (AChR) sites at the neuromuscular junction. This prevents ACh molecules from attaching to receptors and stimulating muscle contraction. Anti-AChR antibodies are detectable in the serum of 90% of patients with generalized MG. In the 10% of patients who lack autoantibodies to AChR, their muscular weakness may be related to autoantibodies to muscle-specific tyrosine kinase or to other unknown antigens.[31] Thymic hyperplasia and tumors are common in patients with MG, suggesting autoantibody production occurs in the thymus.

Clinical Manifestations and Complications

The primary feature of MG is fluctuating weakness of skeletal muscles. The condition usually affects multiple muscle groups, including muscles used to move the eyes and eyelids, chew, swallow, speak, and breathe. These muscles are generally strongest in the morning and become exhausted with continued activity. By the end of the day muscle weakness is prominent. A period of rest usually restores strength.

At onset, only the ocular muscles are involved for about 50% of patients; bilateral ptosis and constant or transient diplopia result (Fig. 58-11). The disease does not progress beyond the

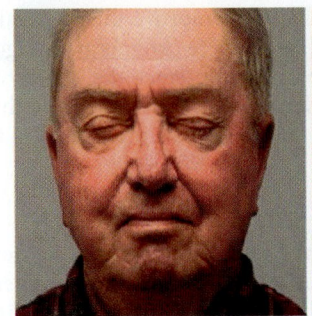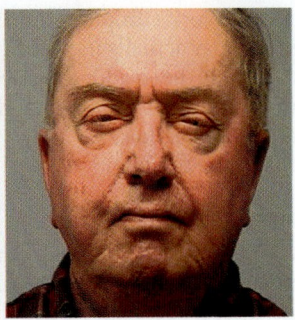

FIG. 58-11 "Peek" sign in myasthenia gravis. During sustained forced eyelid closure he is unable to bury his eyelashes *(left)* and, after 30 sec, he is unable to keep the lids fully closed *(right)*. (From Sanders DB, Massey JM: Clinical features of myasthenia gravis. In AG Engel, editor: *Neuromuscular junction disorders: handbook of clinical neurology*, New York, 2008, Elsevier.)

ocular muscles in about 20% of patients.[32] When facial muscles are affected, facial mobility and expression can be impaired. Patients may have difficulty chewing and swallowing food. Speech is affected, and the voice often fades after a long conversation. The muscles of the trunk and limbs are less often affected. Of these, the proximal muscles of the neck, shoulder, and hip are more often affected than the distal muscles. No other signs of neural disorder accompany MG. No sensory loss occurs, reflexes are normal, and muscle atrophy is rare.

The course of this disease is highly variable. Some patients may have short-term remissions, others may stabilize, and others may have severe, progressive involvement. Exacerbations of MG can be precipitated by emotional stress, pregnancy, menses, another illness, trauma, temperature extremes, and hypokalemia. Ingestion of drugs, including aminoglycoside antibiotics, β-adrenergic blockers, procainamide, quinidine, and phenytoin, can aggravate MG.[32] Psychotropic drugs (e.g., lithium carbonate, phenothiazines, benzodiazepines, tricyclic antidepressants) have also been associated with worsening of myasthenia, as have neuromuscular blocking agents (tubocurarine chloride, pancuronium, succinylcholine [Anectine]).

Myasthenic crisis is an acute exacerbation of muscle weakness triggered by respiratory infection, surgery, emotional distress, pregnancy, exposure to drugs that may increase myasthenic weakness, or beginning treatment with corticosteroids. The major complications of MG result from muscle weakness in areas that affect swallowing and breathing. This results in aspiration, respiratory insufficiency, and respiratory tract infection.

Diagnostic Studies

The diagnosis of MG can be made based on history and physical examination. However, other tests may be used to confirm a diagnosis. EMG may show a decreased response to repeated stimulation of the hand muscles, indicative of muscle fatigue. Single-fiber EMG is sensitive in confirming the diagnosis of MG. Use of drugs may also aid in the diagnosis. In addition, serologic testing for specific antibodies is useful.

The Tensilon test in a patient with MG reveals improved muscle contractility after IV injection of edrophonium chloride (Tensilon), which is an anticholinesterase agent. (Anticholinesterase blocks the enzyme acetylcholinesterase.) This test also aids in the diagnosis of cholinergic crisis (secondary to overdose of anticholinesterase drug), which occurs due to excessive cholinesterase inhibition. Clinical features include muscle fasciculation, sweating, excessive salivation, and constricted pupils. In this condition, edrophonium does not improve muscle weakness but may actually increase it. Atropine, a cholinergic antagonist, should be readily available to counteract the effects of edrophonium when it is used diagnostically. In patients with a confirmed diagnosis of MG, a chest CT scan may be done to evaluate the thymus.

Interprofessional Care

Drug Therapy. Drug therapy for MG includes anticholinesterase drugs, alternate-day corticosteroids, and immunosuppressants (Table 58-18). Anticholinesterase drugs are given to enhance transmission at the neuromuscular junction. Acetylcholinesterase is the enzyme that breaks down ACh. Thus inhibition of this enzyme by an anticholinesterase inhibitor will prolong the action of ACh and facilitate transmission of impulses at the neuromuscular junction. Pyridostigmine (Mestinon) is the most successful drug of this group in the long-term treatment of MG.

Tailoring the dose to avoid a myasthenic or cholinergic crisis often presents a clinical challenge. Corticosteroids (specifically prednisone) are used to suppress the immune response. Drugs such as azathioprine (Imuran), mycophenolate (CellCept), and cyclosporine (Sandimmune) may also be used for immunosuppression.

Many drugs are contraindicated or must be used with caution in patients with MG. Classes of drugs that should be cautiously evaluated before use include anesthetics, antidysrhythmics, antibiotics, quinine, antipsychotics, barbiturates and sedative-hypnotics, cathartics, diuretics, opioids, muscle relaxants, thyroid preparations, and tranquilizers.

Surgical Therapy. Because the presence of the thymus gland in the patient with MG appears to enhance the production of AChR antibodies, removal of the thymus gland results in improvement in a majority of patients. Thymectomy is indicated for almost all patients with thymoma, for patients with generalized MG between the ages of puberty and about 65 years, and for patients with purely ocular MG.

Other Therapies. Plasmapheresis and IV immunoglobulin G can yield short-term improvement in symptoms. They are indicated for patients in myasthenic crisis or in preparation for surgery when corticosteroids must be avoided. Plasmapheresis directly removes circulating AChR antibodies, leading to a decrease in symptoms. (Plasmapheresis is discussed in Chapter 13.) It is not certain how IV immunoglobulin works, but it is probably related to a decrease in antibody production.[32]

TABLE 58-18   Interprofessional Care
Myasthenia Gravis

Diagnostic Assessment	Management
• History and physical examination	• Drug therapy
• Fatigability with prolonged upward gaze (2-3 min)	• Anticholinesterase agents
• Muscle weakness	• Corticosteroids
• EMG	• Immunosuppressive agents
• Tensilon test	• Surgery (thymectomy)
• Acetylcholine receptor antibodies	• Plasmapheresis
• Chest x-ray	• IV immunoglobulin G

EMG, Electromyography.

❖ NURSING MANAGEMENT: MYASTHENIA GRAVIS

◆ Nursing Assessment

Assess the severity of MG by asking the patient about fatigability, what body parts are affected, and how severely they are affected. Some patients become so fatigued that they are no longer able to work or even walk. Assess the patient's coping abilities and strategies as well as understanding of the disorder.

Objective data should include respiratory rate and depth, O_2 saturation, arterial blood gas analyses, pulmonary function tests, and any evidence of respiratory distress in patients with acute myasthenic crisis. Assess muscle strength of all face and limb muscles, swallowing, speech (volume and clarity), and cough and gag reflexes.

◆ Nursing Diagnoses

Nursing diagnoses for the patient with MG may include, but are not limited to, the following:

• Ineffective airway clearance *related to* intercostal muscle weakness and impaired cough and gag reflex
• Impaired verbal communication *related to* weakness of the larynx, lips, mouth, pharynx, and jaw
• Activity intolerance *related to* muscle weakness and fatigability
• Disturbed body image *related to* inability to maintain usual lifestyle and role responsibilities

◆ Planning

The overall goals are that the patient with MG will (1) have a return of normal muscle endurance, (2) manage fatigue, (3) avoid complications, and (4) maintain a quality of life appropriate to the disease course.

◆ Nursing Implementation

The patient with MG who is admitted to the hospital usually has a respiratory tract infection or is in an acute myasthenic crisis. Nursing care is aimed at maintaining adequate ventilation, continuing drug therapy, and watching for side effects of therapy. Be able to distinguish cholinergic from myasthenic crisis (Table 58-19) because the causes and treatment of the two conditions differ greatly.

As with other chronic illnesses, focus care on the neurologic deficits and their impact on daily living. Teach the patient about a balanced diet that can easily be chewed and swallowed. Semisolid foods may be easier to eat than solids or liquids. Scheduling doses of drugs so that peak action is reached at mealtime may make eating less difficult. Arrange diversional activities that require little physical effort and match the patient's interests. Help the patient plan activities of daily living to avoid fatigue. Teaching should focus on adherence to the medical regimen, complications of the disease, potential adverse reactions to specific drugs, and complications of therapy (crisis conditions), and what to do about them. Explore community resources such as the Myasthenia Gravis Foundation of America and MG support groups.

◆ Evaluation

The expected outcomes are that the patient with MG will
• Maintain optimal muscle function
• Be free from side effects of drugs
• Not experience complications (myasthenic or cholinergic crises) from the disease
• Maintain a quality of life appropriate to the disease course

TABLE 58-19 Comparison of Myasthenic and Cholinergic Crises

Myasthenic Crisis	Cholinergic Crisis
Causes	
Exacerbation of myasthenia following precipitating factors or failure to take drug as prescribed or drug dose too low	Overdose of anticholinesterase drugs resulting in increased ACh at the receptor sites, remission (spontaneous or after thymectomy)
Differential Diagnosis	
Improved strength after IV administration of anticholinesterase drugs	Weakness within 1 hr after ingestion of anticholinesterase drugs
Increased weakness of skeletal muscles manifesting as ptosis, bulbar signs (e.g., difficulty swallowing, difficulty articulating words), or dyspnea	Increased weakness of skeletal muscles manifesting as ptosis, bulbar signs, dyspnea
	Effects on smooth muscle include pupillary miosis, salivation, diarrhea, nausea or vomiting, abdominal cramps, increased bronchial secretions, sweating, or lacrimation

ACh, Acetylcholine.

AMYOTROPHIC LATERAL SCLEROSIS

Amyotrophic lateral sclerosis (ALS) is a rare progressive neuromuscular disorder characterized by loss of motor neurons. ALS usually leads to death 2 to 5 years after diagnosis, but a few patients may survive for more than 10 years. This disease became known as *Lou Gehrig's disease* after the famous baseball player was stricken with it in 1939. Perhaps the best known patient with ALS is British theoretical physicist Stephen Hawking, diagnosed at age 21 years and now in his mid 70s. The typical onset is between 55 and 75 years of age. ALS is more common in men than women by a ratio of 2:1. Prevalence is approximately 3.9 cases of ALS per 100,000 people.[33,34]

In ALS, motor neurons in the brainstem and spinal cord gradually degenerate for unknown reasons. Dead motor neurons cannot produce or transport signals to muscles. Consequently, electrical and chemical messages originating in the brain do not reach the muscles to activate them.

Progressive muscle weakness, a classic sign of ALS, occurs in approximately 60% of diagnosed people. Early symptoms of weakness vary, but they often include tripping, dropping things, abnormal fatigue of the extremities, slurred speech, and muscle cramps and twitches. Muscle wasting and fasciculations result from the denervation of the muscles and lack of stimulation and use. Other symptoms include pain, sleep disorders, spasticity and hyperreflexia, drooling, emotional lability, constipation, and esophageal reflux. ALS does not affect a patient's intelligence, but affected people may experience depression and have alterations in decision making and memory. Death often results from respiratory tract infection secondary to compromised respiratory function.[34]

Unfortunately, there is no cure for ALS. Riluzole (Rilutek) slows the progression of ALS. This drug reduces damage to motor neurons by decreasing the release of glutamate (an excitatory neurotransmitter) in the brain.[34]

The illness trajectory for ALS is devastating because the patient remains cognitively intact while wasting away. Guide the patient in the use of moderate-intensity, endurance-type

INFORMATICS IN PRACTICE

Voice Banking Applications in Amyotrophic Lateral Sclerosis

- For patients with amyotrophic lateral sclerosis (ALS), the loss of voice and the ability to communicate can be isolating.
- Speech pathologists encourage patients to participate in voice banking programs to record key words and phrases in their own voices.
- Voice banking is intended to be used as an alternative communication tool when patients may not be able to speak.

exercises for the trunk and limbs because this may help to reduce ALS spasticity. Nursing interventions include (1) facilitating communication, (2) reducing risk of aspiration, (3) facilitating early identification of respiratory insufficiency, (4) decreasing pain secondary to muscle weakness, (5) decreasing risk of injury related to falls, and (6) providing diversional activities such as reading and companionship.

Support the patient's cognitive and emotional functions. Help the patient and family manage the disease process, including grieving related to the loss of motor function and ultimately death. Discuss advance directives and artificial methods of ventilation with the patient and caregiver.

HUNTINGTON'S DISEASE

Huntington's disease (HD) is a genetically transmitted, autosomal dominant disorder that affects men and women equally across races. The offspring of a person with this disease have a 50% risk of inheriting it (see Genetics in Clinical Practice box). The onset of HD is usually between 35 and 45 years of age. Often the diagnosis is made after the affected individual has had children. About 25,000 to 30,000 Americans are symptomatic and 150,000 or more are at risk for HD.[35]

The diagnostic process begins with a review of the family history and clinical symptoms. Genetic testing confirms the disease in a person with symptoms. People who are asymptomatic but who have a positive family history of HD face the dilemma of whether to be genetically tested. If the test is positive, the person will develop HD, but when and to what extent the disease develops cannot be determined.

Similar to PD, the pathologic process of HD involves the basal ganglia and the extrapyramidal motor system. However, instead of a deficiency of DA, HD involves a deficiency of the neurotransmitters ACh and γ-aminobutyric acid (GABA). The net effect is an excess of DA, which leads to symptoms that are the opposite of those of parkinsonism.

The clinical manifestations include a movement disorder and cognitive and psychiatric manifestations. The movement disorder is characterized by abnormal and excessive involuntary movements *(chorea)*. These are writhing, twisting movements of the face, limbs, and body. The movements get worse as the disease progresses. Because facial movements involving speech, chewing, and swallowing are affected, aspiration and malnutrition are likely. The gait deteriorates, and ambulation eventually becomes impossible.

Psychiatric symptoms are frequently present in the early stage of the disease, often before the onset of motor symptoms. Depression is common. Other psychiatric symptoms include anxiety, agitation, impulsivity, apathy, social withdrawal, and obsessiveness. Cognitive deterioration is more variable and

GENETICS IN CLINICAL PRACTICE

Huntington's Disease (HD)

Genetic Basis
- Autosomal dominant disorder.
- Caused by mutation in *HTT* gene located on chromosome 4.

Incidence
- 3 to 7 in 100,000 people of European ancestry.
- Less common in other populations, including people of Japanese, Chinese, and African descent.
- Offspring of a person with a pathogenic variant have a 50% chance of inheriting the disease-causing allele.

Genetic Testing
- DNA testing is available.
- DNA testing can be done on fetal cells obtained by amniocentesis or chorionic villus sampling.
- Preimplantation genetic diagnosis can be done on embryos before implantation and pregnancy.
- One copy of altered gene (heterozygous) is sufficient to cause HD.
- No test is available to predict when symptoms will develop.

Clinical Implications
- HD is a progressive, degenerative brain disorder.
- Onset of disease usually occurs at 30-50 yr of age. No cure is available.
- Drugs are available to control movements and behavioral problems.
- Genetic counseling may be considered if there is a family history of HD.
- Because HD is an autosomal dominant disorder, individuals who are at risk have a strong motivation to seek genetic testing.
- A positive result is not considered a diagnosis because it may be obtained decades before symptoms begin.
- A negative test means the individual does not carry the mutated gene and will not develop HD.

involves perception, memory, attention, and learning. Eventually all psychomotor processes, including the ability to eat and talk, are impaired.

Death usually occurs 10 to 20 years after the onset of symptoms.[36] The most common cause of death is pneumonia, followed by suicide. Other causes of death include injuries related to a fall and other complications.

Because HD has no cure, interprofessional care is palliative. Tetrabenazine (Xenazine) is used to treat the chorea by decreasing the amount of DA available at synapses in the brain and thus reducing the involuntary movements of chorea. If chorea is accompanied by other symptoms, tetrabenazine may not be the treatment of choice. For example, depression can be exacerbated by tetrabenazine, so aripripazole (Abilify) may be a better treatment option.[35]

Other medications used for the movement disorder include neuroleptics such as haloperidol and risperidone (Risperdal), benzodiazepines such as diazepam and clonazepam, and DA-depleting agents such as reserpine. Cognitive disorders are treated as needed with nondrug therapies (e.g., counseling, memory books). Psychiatric disorders can be treated with selective serotonin reuptake inhibitors such as sertraline (Zoloft) and paroxetine (Paxil). Antipsychotic medication, such as haloperidol or risperidone, may also be needed. HD presents a great challenge to health care professionals. The goal of nursing management is to provide the most comfortable environment possible for the patient and caregiver by maintaining physical safety, treating physical symptoms, and providing emotional and psychologic support.

Because of the choreic movements, caloric requirements are high. The patient may require as many as 4000 to 5000 cal/day to maintain body weight. As the disease progresses, meeting caloric needs becomes a greater challenge when the patient has difficulty swallowing and holding the head still. Depression and mental deterioration can also compromise nutritional intake. Alternative sources of nutrition may be indicated as the disease progresses.

End-of-life issues need to be discussed with the patient and caregiver. These include care in the home or long-term care facility, artificial methods of feeding, advance directives and cardiopulmonary resuscitation (CPR), use of antibiotics to treat infections, and guardianship. These topics should be addressed throughout the course of the disease as the patient and caregiver adapt to increasing disability.

CASE STUDY

Epilepsy With Headache

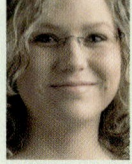

(©Purestock/ Thinkstock)

Patient Profile

J.P. is a 24-yr-old woman who was diagnosed with epilepsy at age 15. At that time, she had a tonic-clonic seizure and was given a prescription for valproate (Depakote). She had a second witnessed seizure 4 mo later but has since been seizure free. J.P. now has complaints of headaches and says she is afraid her seizures are going to return. She is single, lives alone, and describes her job as stressful.

Subjective Data
- Describes headache pain on the left side of her forehead as throbbing
- Has vomited with headache
- Describes changes in vision, including flashing lights
- Headache occurs nearly every month on a regular cycle

Objective Data
- Alert and oriented to person
- Neurologic examination negative
- Serum valproate levels within normal limits
- EEG normal
- CT of head normal

Discussion Questions
1. What is epilepsy?
2. What is the pathophysiology of epilepsy?
3. What is the significance of the laboratory and diagnostic findings?
4. Is the headache related to seizure activity?
5. ***Safety:*** To ensure J.P.'s safety, what nursing interventions are necessary?
6. ***Patient-Centered Care:*** What teaching will you include in the plan of care for J.P. regarding the course of the disease?
7. ***Priority Decision:*** Based on the assessment data, what are the priority nursing diagnoses?
8. ***Evidence-Based Practice:*** Based on current treatment guidelines, what medication may be effective in managing both J.P.'s epilepsy and her migraine headaches?

BRIDGE TO NCLEX EXAMINATION

The number of the question corresponds to the same-numbered outcome at the beginning of the chapter.

1. A 50-yr-old man complains of recurring headaches. He describes these as sharp, stabbing, and located around his left eye. He also reports that his left eye seems to swell and get teary when these headaches occur. Based on this history, you suspect that he has
   a. cluster headaches.
   b. tension headaches.
   c. migraine headaches.
   d. medication overuse headaches.

2. A 65-yr-old woman was just diagnosed with Parkinson's disease. The priority nursing intervention is
   a. searching the Internet for educational videos.
   b. evaluating the home for environmental safety.
   c. promoting physical exercise and a well-balanced diet.
   d. designing an exercise program to strengthen and stretch specific muscles.

3. The nurse finds an 87-yr-old woman with Alzheimer's disease is continually rubbing, flexing, and kicking her legs throughout the day. The night shift reports this same behavior escalates at night, preventing her from obtaining her required sleep. The next step the nurse should take is to
   a. ask the physician for a daytime sedative for the patient.
   b. request soft restraints to prevent her from falling out of her bed.
   c. ask the physician for a nighttime sleep medication for the patient.
   d. assess the patient more closely, suspecting a disorder such as restless legs syndrome.

4. Social effects of a chronic neurologic disease include (select all that apply)
   a. divorce.
   b. job loss.
   c. depression.
   d. role changes.
   e. loss of self-esteem.

5. The nurse is reinforcing teaching with a patient newly diagnosed with amyotrophic lateral sclerosis (ALS). Which statement would be appropriate to include in the teaching?
   a. "ALS results from an excess chemical in the brain, and the symptoms can be controlled with medication."
   b. "Even though the symptoms you are experiencing are severe, most people recover with treatment."
   c. "You need to consider advance directives now, because you will lose cognitive function as the disease progresses."
   d. "This is a progressing disease that eventually results in permanent paralysis, though you will not lose any cognitive function."

1. a, 2. c, 3. d, 4. a, b, c, d, e, 5. d

For rationales to these answers and even more NCLEX review questions, visit *http://evolve.elsevier.com/Lewis/medsurg*.

ⓔ EVOLVE WEBSITE

http://evolve.elsevier.com/Lewis/medsurg
Review Questions (Online Only)
Key Points
Answer Keys for Questions
- Rationales for Bridge to NCLEX Examination Questions
- Answer Guidelines for Case Study on p. 1396
Student Case Studies
- Patient With Parkinson's Disease and Hip Fracture
- Patient With Seizures
Nursing Care Plans
- eNursing Care Plan 58-1: Patient With Headache
- eNursing Care Plan 58-2: Patient With Seizure Disorder or Epilepsy
- eNursing Care Plan 58-3: Patient With Multiple Sclerosis
- eNursing Care Plan 58-4: Patient With Parkinson's Disease
Conceptual Care Map Creator
- Conceptual Care Map for Case Study on p. 1396
Audio Glossary
Content Updates

REFERENCES

1. Headache Classification Committee of the International Headache Society. The international classification of headache disorders, ed 3, *Cephalgia* 33:629, 2013.
*2. Charles A: The evolution of a migraine attack: a review of recent evidence, *Headache* 53:413, 2013.
3. Lipton RB, Silberstein SD: Episodic and chronic migraine headache: breaking down barriers to optimal treatment and prevention, *Headache* 55:S2, 2015.
4. National Institute of Neurological Disorders and Stroke: Headache: hope through research. 2015. Retrieved from *www.ninds.nih.gov/disorders/headache/detail_headache.htm*.
5. Braine ME: Cluster headache, *Br J Neuro Nurs* 9:8, 2013.
6. Zecuity (package insert). North Wales, Penn, Teva Pharmaceuticals USA, Inc. 2014.
7. Fisher RS: International League Against Epilepsy announces epilepsy: a new definition. 2014. Retrieved from *www.epilepsy.com/article/2014/4/revised-definition-epilepsy*.
8. Epilepsy Foundation: Epilepsy statistics. 2014. Retrieved from *www.epilepsy.com/learn/epilepsy-statistics*.
9. National Institute of Neurological Disorders and Stroke: NIH-funded study discovers new genes for childhood epilepsies. 2013. Retrieved from *http://www.ninds.nih.gov/news_and_events/news_articles/pressrelease_childhood_epilepsy_genes_08112013.htm*.
10. Epilepsy Foundation: Types of seizures. 2013. Retrieved from *www.epilepsy.com/learn/types-seizures*.
11. Epilepsy Foundation: Status epilepticus. 2015. Retrieved from *www.epilepsy.com/information/professionals/about-epilepsy-seizures/classifying-seizures/status-epilepticus*.
12. Epilepsy Foundation: How SUDEP occurs. 2013. Retrieved from *http://www.epilepsy.com/learn/impact/mortality/sudep/how-sudep-occurs*.
13. Tatum WO, Sirven JI, Cascino GD: *Epilepsy case studies: pearls for patient care*, New York, 2014, Springer.
14. Schulze-Bonhage A, Zentner J: The preoperative evaluation and surgical treatment of epilepsy, *Dtsch Arztebl Int* 111:313, 2014.
15. Epilepsy Foundation: Ketogenic diet. 2014. Retrieved from *http://www.epilepsy.com/learn/treating-seizures-and-epilepsy/dietary-therapies/ketogenic-diet*.
16. National Institute of Neurological Disorders and Stroke: Restless legs syndrome fact sheet. Retrieved from *www.ninds.nih.gov/disorders/restless_legs/detail_restless_legs.htm*.
17. Allen RP, Picchietti D, Garcia-Borreguero D, et al: Restless legs syndrome/Willis-Ekbom disease diagnostic criteria: updated International Restless Legs Study Group (IRLSG) consensus criteria—history, rationale, description, and significance, *Sleep Med* 15:860, 2014.

*18. Innes KE, Selfe TK, Agarwal P, et al: Efficacy of an eight-week yoga intervention on symptoms of restless legs syndrome (RLS): a pilot study, *J Alt Comp Med* 19:527, 2013.

19. Sleep Review: FDA clears non-pharmacological device for restless legs syndrome. 2014. Retrieved from *www.sleepreviewmag.com/2014/05/fda-clears-non-pharmacological-device-restless-legs-syndrome*.

20. Multiplesclerosis.net: MS statistics. 2013. Retrieved from *http://multiplesclerosis.net/what-is-ms/statistics*.

21. National Multiple Sclerosis Society: What causes MS? Retrieved from *www.nationalmssociety.org/What-is-MS/What-Causes-MS*.

22. National Multiple Sclerosis Society: Types of MS. Retrieved from *www.nationalmssociety.org/What-is-MS/Types-of-MS*.

23. Polman CH, Reingold SC, Banwell B, et al: Diagnostic criteria for multiple sclerosis: 2010 revisions to the McDonald Criteria, *Ann Neurol* 69:292, 2011.

24. National Multiple Sclerosis Society: FDA approves Lemtrada (alemtuzumab) for relapsing MS—update. 2014. Retrieved from *www.nationalmssociety.org/About-the-Society/News/FDA-Approves-Lemtrada%E2%84%A2-%28alemtuzumab%29-for-Relapsing*.

25. Parkinson's Disease Foundation: Statistics on Parkinson's, 2015. Retrieved from *www.pdf.org/en/parkinson_statistics*.

26. Nolden LF, Tartavoulle T, Porche DJ: Parkinson's disease: assessment, diagnosis, and management, *J Nurs Pract* 10:500, 2014.

27. Merck Manual: Parkinson disease. 2013. Retrieved from *http://www.merckmanuals.com/professional/neurologic-disorders/movement-and-cerebellar-disorders/parkinson-disease*.

28. Sapir S: Multiple factors are involved in the dysarthria associated with Parkinson's disease: a review with implications for clinical practice and research, *J Speech Lang Hear Res* 57:1330, 2014.

29. National Parkinson Foundation: Amantadine (Symmetrel). 2015. Retrieved from *www.parkinson.org/Parkinson-s-Disease/Treatment/Medications-for-Motor-Symptoms-of-PD/Amantadine-%28Symmetrel%29.aspx*.

30. Shukla AW, Okun MS: Surgical treatment of Parkinson's disease: patients, targets, devices, and approaches, *Neurother* 11:47, 2014.

31. Schub T, Buckley L, Pravicoff D: Myasthenia gravis. *CINAHL Information Systems*, 2014.

32. Mestecky AM: Myasthenia gravis, *Br J Neuro Nurs* 9:110, 2013.

33. Mehta P, Antao V, Kaye W, et al: Prevalence of amyotrophic lateral sclerosis—United States, 2010-2011, *MMWR* 63:1, 2014.

34. National Institute of Neurological Disorders and Stroke: Amyotrophic lateral sclerosis (ALS) fact sheet. Retrieved from *www.ninds.nih.gov/disorders/amyotrophiclateralsclerosis/detail_ALS.htm*.

35. Frank S: Treatment of Huntington's disease, *Neurother* 11:153, 2014.

*36. Scerri R: Living with advanced stage Huntington's disease: an exploration of the experiences of Maltese family caregivers, *Br J Neuro Nurse* 11:20, 2015.

*Evidence-based information for clinical practice.

59

Dementia and Delirium

Sharon L. Lewis

I am going to make the rest of my life the best of my life.

Unknown

e http://evolve.elsevier.com/Lewis/medsurg/

LEARNING OUTCOMES

1. Define dementia and describe its impact on society.
2. Compare and contrast different etiologies of dementia.
3. Describe the clinical manifestations, diagnostic studies, and interprofessional care of dementia.
4. Differentiate among neurodegenerative disorders associated with dementia, including dementia with Lewy bodies, frontotemporal lobar degeneration, and Down syndrome.
5. Describe the clinical manifestations of mild cognitive impairment.
6. Describe the clinical manifestations, diagnostic studies, and interprofessional care of Alzheimer's disease.
7. Describe the nursing management of the patient with Alzheimer's disease.
8. Describe the etiology, pathophysiology, clinical manifestations, diagnostic studies, and nursing and interprofessional management of delirium.

KEY TERMS

Alzheimer's disease (AD), p. 1401
delirium, p. 1414
dementia, p. 1399
dementia with Lewy bodies (DLB), Table 59-3, p. 1401

familial Alzheimer's disease (FAD), p. 1402
frontotemporal lobar degeneration (FTLD), Table 59-3, p. 1401
mild cognitive impairment (MCI), p. 1405
mixed dementia, p. 1400

neurofibrillary tangles, p. 1403
normal pressure hydrocephalus, p. 1400
retrogenesis, p. 1403
sundowning, p. 1411
vascular dementia, p. 1400

This chapter discusses the cognitive disorders of dementia and delirium, with a focus on the nursing management of patients with Alzheimer's disease. The etiology and pathophysiology of dementia and delirium are differentiated, and interprofessional and nursing management of patients with these cognitive disorders are described.

The three most common cognitive problems in adults are dementia, delirium (acute confusion), and depression (Table 59-1). Although this chapter focuses on dementia and delirium, depression is often associated with these conditions.

Depression is often mistaken for dementia in older adults, and, conversely, dementia for depression. Manifestations of depression (especially in the older adult) include sadness, difficulty thinking and concentrating, fatigue, apathy, feelings of despair, and inactivity. When depression is severe, poor concentration and attention may result, causing memory and functional impairment. When dementia and depression occur together (as happens in many patients with dementia), the intellectual deterioration can be extreme. Depression, alone or in combination with dementia, is treatable. The challenge is to make an accurate and early assessment and diagnosis (Table 59-1).

DEMENTIA

Dementia is a neurocognitive disorder characterized by dysfunction or loss of memory, orientation, attention, language, judgment, and reasoning. Personality changes and behavioral problems such as agitation, delusions, and hallucinations may occur. Ultimately, these problems result in alterations in the individual's ability to work, fulfill social and family responsibilities, and perform activities of daily living.

Fifteen percent of older Americans have dementia. As the average life span increases, the number of those affected with dementia is growing. There are about 100 causes of dementia, with about 60% to 80% of the patients with dementia having a diagnosis of Alzheimer's disease (AD) (Fig. 59-1). In the United States, about half of all patients in long-term care facilities have AD or a related dementia.[1]

Etiology and Pathophysiology

Dementia is due to both treatable and untreatable conditions. Treatable causes may initially be reversible (Table 59-2). However, with prolonged exposure or disease, irreversible changes may occur.

Reviewed by Abimbola Farinde, PharmD, MS, Professor, Columbia Southern University, Orange Beach, Alabama; Shari Gould, RN, MSN, Associate Professor of Nursing, Victoria College, Victoria, Texas; and Linda Littlejohns, MSN, RN, CNRN, FAAN, Vice President of Clinical Development Integra LifeSciences, Irvine, California.

TABLE 59-1	**Comparison of Dementia, Delirium, and Depression**		
Feature	**Dementia**	**Delirium**	**Depression**
Onset	Usually insidious.	Abrupt, although initially can be subtle.	Often coincides with life changes. Often abrupt.
Progression	Slow.	Abrupt. Can fluctuate from day to day.	Variable, rapid to slow but may be uneven.
Duration	Years (average of 8 yr but can be much longer).	Hours to days to weeks. Can be prolonged in some.	Can be several months to years, especially if not treated.
Thinking	Difficulty with abstract thinking, impaired judgment, words difficult to find.	Disorganized, distorted. Slow or accelerated incoherent speech.	Intact but with apathy, fatigue. May be indecisive. Feels sense of hopelessness. May not want to live.
Perception	Misperceptions often present. Delusions and hallucinations.	Distorted. Delusions and hallucinations.	May deny or be unaware of depression. May have feelings of guilt.
Psychomotor behavior	May pace or be hyperactive. As disease progresses, may not be able to perform tasks or movements when asked.	Variable. Can be hyperactive or hypoactive, or mixed.	Often withdrawn and hypoactive.
Sleep-wake cycle	Sleeps during day. Frequent awakenings at night. Fragmented sleep.	Disturbed sleep. Reversed sleep-wake cycle.	Disturbed, often with early morning awakening.

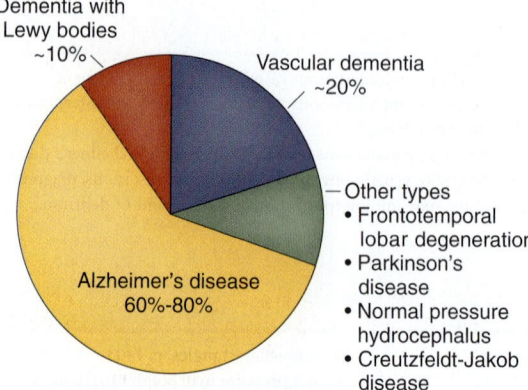

FIG. 59-1 Causes of dementia.

TABLE 59-2	**Causes of Dementia**
Type of Dementia	**Cause**
Neurodegenerative disorders	• Alzheimer's disease • Dementia with Lewy bodies (DLB) • Frontotemporal lobar degeneration (FTLD) • Down syndrome • Parkinson's disease • Huntington's disease • Amyotrophic lateral sclerosis (ALS)
Vascular diseases	• Vascular (multiinfarct) dementia • Subarachnoid hemorrhage* • Chronic subdural hematoma*
Toxic, metabolic, or nutritional diseases	• Alcoholism • Thiamine (vitamin B$_1$) deficiency* • Cobalamin (vitamin B$_{12}$) deficiency* • Folate deficiency* • Hyperthyroidism* • Hypothyroidism*
Immunologic diseases or infections	• Multiple sclerosis • Systemic exertion intolerance disease • Infections (e.g., Creutzfeldt-Jakob disease) • Acquired immunodeficiency syndrome (AIDS) • Meningitis* • Encephalitis* • Neurosyphilis* • Systemic lupus erythematosus*
Systemic diseases	• Uremic encephalopathy* • Dialysis dementia* • Hepatic encephalopathy* • Wilson's disease
Trauma	• Head injury*
Tumors	• Brain tumors (primary)* • Metastatic tumors*
Ventricular disorders	• Hydrocephalus*
Drugs†	• Anticholinergics • phenytoin (Dilantin) • Opioids • Hypnotics • Tranquilizers • Antiparkinsonian drugs • Cardiac drugs: digoxin, methyldopa • Cocaine • Heroin

*Potentially reversible.
†These are examples of drugs that may cause cognitive impairment that is potentially reversible.

The most common causes of dementia are neurodegenerative conditions, with the majority of cases being Alzheimer's disease (Table 59-3). Vascular conditions are the second most common cause of dementia.[1] **Vascular dementia**, also called *multiinfarct dementia*, is loss of cognitive function resulting from ischemic or hemorrhagic brain lesions caused by cardiovascular disease. This type of dementia is the result of decreased blood supply from narrowing and blocking of arteries that supply the brain. Vascular dementia may be caused by a single stroke (infarct) or by multiple strokes.

Mixed dementia occurs when two or more types of dementia are present at the same time. It is characterized by the hallmark abnormalities of Alzheimer's disease and another type of dementia. Usually the other type of dementia is vascular dementia, but it can be other types.

Normal pressure hydrocephalus is an uncommon disorder characterized by an obstruction in the flow of CSF, causing a buildup of CSF in the brain. Manifestations include dementia, urinary incontinence, and difficulty walking. Meningitis, encephalitis, or head injury may cause the condition. If diagnosed early, normal pressure hydrocephalus is treatable by surgery in which a shunt is inserted to divert the fluid away from the brain.

Clinical Manifestations

Depending on the cause of the dementia, the onset of manifestations may be insidious and gradual or more abrupt. Often dementia associated with neurologic degeneration is gradual

TABLE 59-3 Neurodegenerative Causes of Dementia*

Neurodegenerative Disorder	Characteristics	Management

Dementia With Lewy Bodies (DLB)
• Characterized by presence of Lewy bodies (abnormal deposits of protein α-synuclein) in brainstem and cortex
• Has features of both AD and Parkinson's disease.
• Imperative that a correct diagnosis is made
	• Typically have manifestations of parkinsonism, hallucinations, short-term memory loss, unpredictable cognitive shifts, and sleep disturbances
	• Diagnosis of LBD is based on clinical manifestations:
	  • Extrapyramidal signs (bradykinesia, rigidity, and postural instability, but not always a tremor)
	  • Fluctuating cognitive ability
	  • Hallucinations
	• Pneumonia is a common complication
		• Drugs may include levodopa/carbidopa and acetylcholinesterase inhibitors.
		• Manage dementia and problems related to dysphagia and immobility
		• Swallowing problems can lead to impaired nutrition
		• At risk for falls from impaired mobility and balance.

Frontotemporal Lobar Degeneration (FTLD) • Associated with atrophy of frontal and temporal lobes of brain • In Pick's disease, one type of FTLD, brain may have abnormal microscopic deposits called *Pick bodies* • Often misdiagnosed as a psychiatric problem because of strange behaviors	• Characterized by disturbances in behavior, sleep, personality, and eventually memory • Progresses relentlessly and may ultimately include language impairment, erratic behavior, and dementia. • Tends to occur at a younger age than does AD, typically about age 60	• No specific treatment • Antidepressants and antipsychotics to treat behavioral manifestations
Down Syndrome • Genetic disorder caused by presence of all or part of a third copy of chromosome 21	• Typically associated with physical growth delays, characteristic facial features, and mild to moderate intellectual disability	• Much higher risk of developing dementia • Estimated 80% will develop dementia
Parkinson's Disease, Huntington's Disease, and Amyotrophic Lateral Sclerosis • Chronic, progressive, and incurable diseases	• Associated with development of dementia in the later stages of disease	See Chapter 58

*Alzheimer's disease is the most common neurodegenerative disorder causing dementia. It is the focus of this chapter.

and progressive over time. Causes of vascular dementia often result in symptoms that appear suddenly or progress in a step-wise pattern. However, it is difficult to distinguish the etiology of dementia (vascular versus neurodegenerative) based on symptom progression alone.

An acute (days to weeks) or subacute (weeks to months) pattern of change may be indicative of an infectious or metabolic cause of dementia, including encephalitis, meningitis, hypothyroidism, or drug-related dementia. The manifestations of different types of dementia overlap and can be further complicated by coexisting medical conditions.

Other clinical manifestations of dementia are discussed in the section on clinical manifestations of AD on pp. 1403-1404.

Diagnostic Studies

The diagnosis of dementia is focused on determining the cause (e.g., reversible versus irreversible factors). An important first step is a thorough medical, neurologic, and psychologic history. A thorough physical examination is performed to rule out other potential medical conditions. Screening for cobalamin (vitamin B$_{12}$) deficiency and hypothyroidism is often performed. Based on patient history, testing for neurosyphilis (see Chapter 52) may be performed. Neuroimaging techniques (CT or MRI) may be used to rule out or confirm causes of dementia. (Diagnostic studies for Alzheimer's disease are discussed later in this chapter on pp. 1405-1408.)

❖ NURSING AND INTERPROFESSIONAL MANAGEMENT: DEMENTIA

In many ways, management of the patient with dementia is similar to management of the patient with AD (described later in this chapter). One form of dementia, vascular dementia, can often be prevented. Preventive measures include treatment of

risk factors such as hypertension, diabetes, smoking, hypercholesterolemia, and cardiac dysrhythmias. (Stroke is discussed in Chapter 57.) Drugs that are used for patients with AD are also useful in patients with vascular dementia. Drug therapy is discussed on p. 1408 later in this chapter.

ALZHEIMER'S DISEASE

Alzheimer's disease (AD) is a chronic, progressive, neurodegenerative disease of the brain. It is the most common form of dementia, accounting for 60% to 80% of all cases of dementia.[1] AD is named after Alois Alzheimer, a German physician who in 1906 described changes in the brain tissue of a 55-year-old woman who had died of an unusual mental illness.

Approximately 5.4 million Americans suffer from AD. It is estimated that 11% of people age 65 and older, and nearly one third of those over age 85, have AD. Ultimately the disease is fatal, with death typically occurring 4 to 8 years after diagnosis, although some patients live for 20 years. AD is the sixth leading cause of death in the United States.[1]

AD is the only cause of death among the top 10 in United States that cannot be prevented or cured, or its progression even slowed. The burden of care for the patient with AD on the family, caregivers, and society is staggering. AD has often been referred to as the "long good-bye" or "death in slow motion."

The incidence of AD is higher in African Americans and Hispanics than in whites. AD has been associated with lower socioeconomic status and education level and poor access to health care.[1] Women are more likely than men to develop AD, primarily because they live longer (see the Gender Differences box).

Etiology

The exact etiology of AD is unknown but is likely a combination of multiple factors. These factors are discussed in this section.

GENDER DIFFERENCES
Alzheimer's Disease and Dementia

Men	Women
• Men have a higher incidence of vascular dementia than women.	• Nearly two thirds of people with Alzheimer's disease are women. • Women are more likely to develop Alzheimer's disease than men, primarily because they live longer. • About twice as many women as men die each year from Alzheimer's disease.

CULTURAL & ETHNIC HEALTH DISPARITIES
Alzheimer's Disease and Dementia

- Older African Americans are about twice as likely to have Alzheimer's and other dementias as older whites.
- Older Hispanics are about one and one-half times as likely to have Alzheimer's and other dementias as older whites.
- Variations in health, lifestyle, and socioeconomic risk factors across ethnic groups account for most of the differences in risk of Alzheimer's disease and other dementias.
- Health conditions such as cardiovascular disease and diabetes, which increase risk for Alzheimer's disease and other dementias, account for differences as they are more prevalent in African American and Hispanic people.
- Lower levels of education and other socioeconomic characteristics may also increase risk.

Source: Alzheimer's Association: 2015 Alzheimer's Association facts and figures report. Retrieved from *www.alz.org/facts/downloads/facts_figures_2015.pdf*.

Aging. The greatest risk factor for AD is age. Most people with AD are diagnosed at age 65 or older. While age is the greatest risk factor, AD is not a normal part of aging, and age alone is not sufficient to cause the disease.[1]

Family History. Family history is also an important risk factor, since those with a first-degree relative with dementia are more likely to develop the disease. Those who have more than one first-degree relative (parent, brother, sister) with dementia are even at higher risk of developing the disease. However, a family history is not necessary for an individual to develop AD.[1]

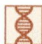

Genetic Link

Only a small percentage of people younger than 60 years old develop AD. When AD develops in someone younger than 60 years old, it is referred to as *early-onset AD*. AD that becomes evident in individuals more than 60 years old is called *late-onset AD* (see the Genetics in Clinical Practice box).

Individuals with a clear pattern of inheritance within a family have **familial Alzheimer's disease (FAD)**. Other cases in which no familial connection can be made are termed *sporadic*. FAD is associated with an early onset (before 60 years of age) and a more rapid disease course. In both FAD and sporadic AD, the pathogenesis of AD is similar.

In patients with early-onset AD, three genes have been identified as important in the etiology (see the Genetics in Clinical Practice box). When the *presenilin-1, presenilin-2,* and *amyloid precursor protein (APP)* genes are mutated, they cause brain cells to overproduce β-amyloid.[2]

The first gene associated with AD was the *epsilon (E)-4* allele of the *apolipoprotein E (ApoE)* gene on chromosome 19. *ApoE* comes in several different alleles or forms, but three alleles occur

GENETICS IN CLINICAL PRACTICE
Alzheimer's Disease (AD)

Genetic Basis
Early Onset (Familial) (<60 Yr Old at Onset)
- Autosomal dominant disorder.
- Various mutations in the following genes:
  - Amyloid precursor protein *(APP)* gene on chromosome 21
  - Presenilin-1 *(PSEN1)* gene on chromosome 14
  - Presenilin-2 *(PSEN2)* gene on chromosome 1

Late Onset (Sporadic) (>60 Yr Old at Onset)
- Genetically more complex than early-onset form.
- Apolipoprotein E-4 *(ApoE-4)* allele on chromosome 19 increases the likelihood of developing AD.
- Presence of *ApoE-2* allele is associated with a lower risk of AD.

Incidence
Early Onset
- Rare form of AD, accounting for <5% of cases.
- Fifty percent risk of disease for children of affected parents.
- May occur in people as young as 30 yr old.

Late Onset
- *ApoE-4* is present in about 40% of people with late-onset AD. (It is present in 25%-30% of normal population.)
- Many *ApoE-4*-positive people do not develop AD, and many *ApoE-4*-negative people do.

Genetic Testing
Early Onset
- Genetic screening is available for mutations on chromosomes 1, 14, and 21.

Late Onset
- Blood test can identify which *ApoE* allele a person has but cannot predict who will develop disease.
- *ApoE* testing is mainly used in research to identify people who may have an increased risk of developing AD.*

Clinical Implications
- AD is the most common cause of dementia.
- Genetic testing and counseling for family members of patients with early-onset AD may be appropriate.
- If person tests positive for *ApoE-4,* it does not mean that the person will develop AD.

*ApoE testing is useful for studying AD risk in large groups of people, but not for determining an individual's specific risk.

most commonly. People inherit one allele (i.e., *ApoE-2, ApoE-3,* or *ApoE-4*) from each parent. *ApoE* contains the instructions to make a protein that helps to carry cholesterol and other types of fat in the bloodstream. *ApoE* may have a role in clearing amyloid plaques. Mutations in this gene result in greater amyloid deposition. The presence of *ApoE-4,* which is a risk-factor gene, increases the risk of a person developing late-onset AD. However, the presence of the gene alone is not adequate to account for AD, since many people with *ApoE-4* do not develop AD.

Cardiovascular Factors. The health of the brain is closely linked to the health of the heart and blood vessels. The functioning of the brain is dependent on a good blood supply and nutrients delivered to it by that blood supply.

Many factors increase the risk of cardiovascular disease. These include diabetes mellitus, hypertension, obesity, hypercholesterolemia, and smoking. Diabetes dramatically increases a person's risk of developing AD or other types of dementia. Diabetes can contribute to dementia in several ways. Chronic high levels of insulin and glucose may be directly toxic to brain cells. Insulin resistance, which causes high blood glucose and in some cases leads to type 2 diabetes, may interfere with the body's ability to break down amyloid, a protein that forms brain plaques in AD. In addition, high blood glucose along with high cholesterol has a role in atherosclerosis, which contributes to vascular dementia.[3,4]

Diabetes may contribute to poor memory and diminished mental function in various other ways. The disease causes microangiopathy, which damages small blood vessels throughout the body. Ongoing damage to blood vessels in the brain may be one reason why people with diabetes are at a higher risk of cognitive problems as they grow older. People with diabetes may lose brain volume (especially gray matter) as the disease progresses.[3,4]

Head Trauma. Head trauma is also a risk factor for dementia. Professional football players and military veterans who had traumatic brain injury or posttraumatic stress disorder have an increased risk for AD and other types of dementia.[5,6]

Pathophysiology

Characteristic findings of AD relate to changes in the brain's structure and function: (1) amyloid plaques, (2) neurofibrillary tangles, (3) loss of connections between neurons, and (4) neuron death. Fig. 59-2 shows the pathologic changes in AD.

As part of aging, people develop some plaques in their brain tissue, but in AD more plaques appear in certain parts of the brain. These plaques consist of clusters of insoluble deposits of a protein called *β-amyloid*, other proteins, remnants of neurons, non-nerve cells such as microglia (cells that surround and digest damaged cells or foreign substances), and other cells such as astrocytes.

β-Amyloid is cleaved from amyloid precursor protein (APP), which is associated with the cell membrane (Fig. 59-3). The normal function of APP is unknown. Genetic factors may play a critical role in how the brain processes the β-amyloid protein. Overproduction of β-amyloid appears to be an important risk factor for AD. Abnormally high levels of β-amyloid cause cell damage either directly or by eliciting an inflammatory response and ultimately neuron death.

In AD, plaques develop first in areas of the brain used for memory and cognitive function, including the hippocampus (a structure that is important in forming and storing short-term memories). Eventually AD attacks the cerebral cortex, especially the areas responsible for language and reasoning.

Neurofibrillary tangles are abnormal collections of twisted protein threads inside nerve cells. The main component of these structures is a protein called *tau.* Tau proteins in the central nervous system (CNS) are involved in providing support for intracellular structure through their support of microtubules. Tau proteins hold the microtubules together like railroad ties hold railroad tracks together. In AD the tau protein is altered, and as a result, the microtubules twist together in a helical fashion (Fig. 59-3). This ultimately forms the neurofibrillary tangles found in the neurons of people with AD.

Plaques and neurofibrillary tangles are not unique to patients with AD or dementia. They are also found in the brains of individuals without evidence of cognitive impairment. However, they are more abundant in the brains of individuals with AD.

The other feature of AD is the loss of connections between neurons and neuron death. These processes result in structural damage. Affected parts of the brain begin to shrink in a process called brain atrophy. By the final stage of AD, brain tissue has shrunk significantly (Fig. 59-4).

Clinical Manifestations

Pathologic changes often precede clinical manifestations of dementia by anywhere from 5 to 20 years. The Alzheimer's Association has developed a list of 10 warning signs that are common manifestations of AD (Table 59-4). The stages of AD can be categorized as mild, moderate, and severe (Table 59-5). The rate of progression from mild to severe is highly variable and ranges from 3 to 20 years.

The initial manifestations are usually related to changes in cognitive functioning. Patients may have complaints of memory loss, mild disorientation, or trouble with words and numbers. Often it is a family member, in particular the spouse, who reports the patient's declining memory to the HCP.

Normal age-related memory decline is characterized by mild changes that do not interfere with activities of daily living (Table 59-6). In AD the memory loss initially relates to recent events, with remote memories still intact. With time and progression of AD, memory loss includes both recent and remote memory and ultimately affects the ability to perform self-care.

As AD progresses, personal hygiene deteriorates, as does the ability to concentrate and maintain attention. Ongoing loss of neurons in AD can cause a person to act in altered or unpredictable ways. Behavioral manifestations of AD (e.g., agitation, aggression) result from changes that take place within the brain. They are neither intentional nor controllable by the individual with the disease. Some patients develop delusions and hallucinations.

With progression of AD, additional cognitive impairments are noted. These include *dysphasia* (difficulty comprehending language and oral communication), *apraxia* (inability to manipulate objects or perform purposeful acts), *visual agnosia* (inability to recognize objects by sight), and *dysgraphia* (difficulty communicating via writing). Eventually long-term memories cannot be recalled, and patients lose the ability to recognize family members and friends. Other problems include aggression and a tendency to wander.

Later in the disease, the ability to communicate and perform activities of daily living is lost. In the late stages of AD, the patient is unresponsive and incontinent and requires total care.

Retrogenesis. Retrogenesis is the process in AD patients in which degenerative changes occur in the reverse order in which

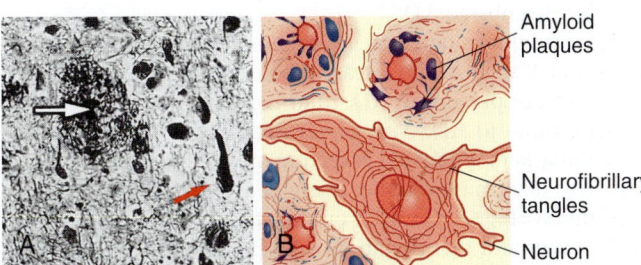

FIG. 59-2 Pathologic changes in Alzheimer's disease **A,** Plaque with central amyloid core *(white arrow)* next to a neurofibrillary tangle *(red arrow)* on the histologic specimen from a brain autopsy. **B,** Schematic representation of amyloid plaque and neurofibrillary tangle.

Amyloid plaques

Neurofibrillary tangles

Neuron

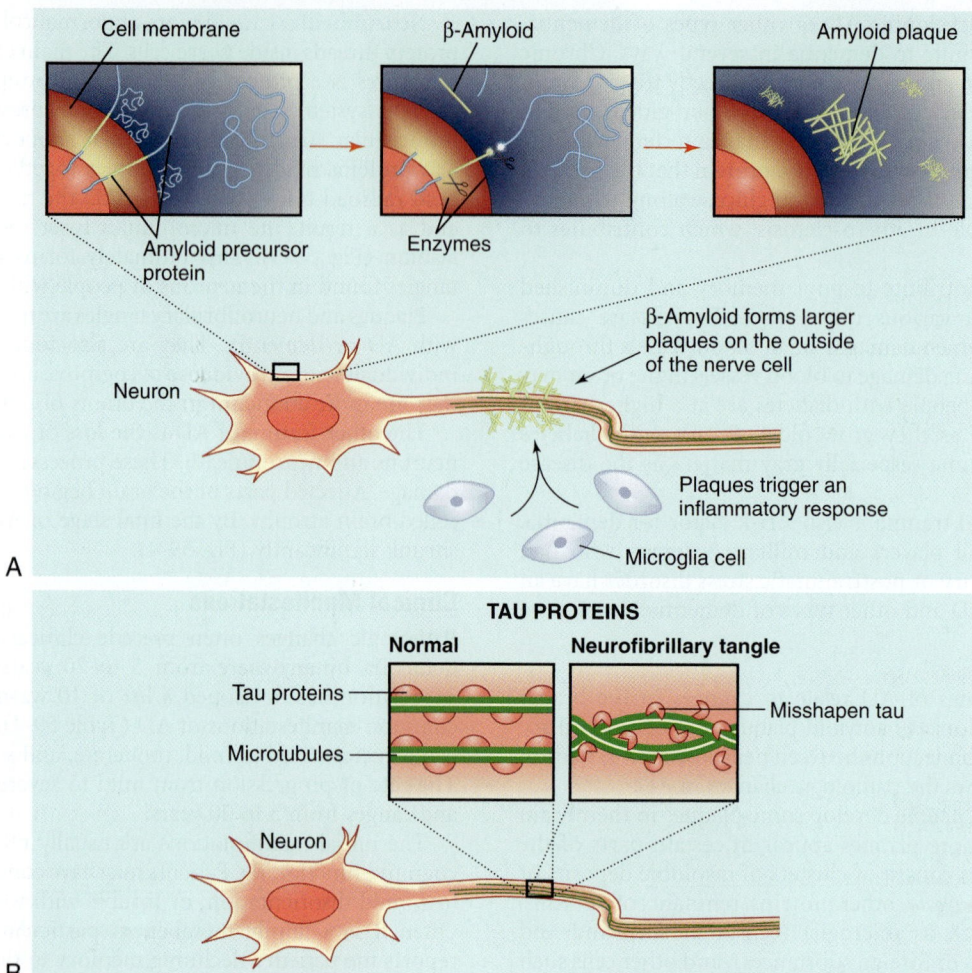

FIG. 59-3   Current etiologic theories for the development of Alzheimer's disease. **A,** Abnormal amounts of β-amyloid are cleaved from the amyloid precursor protein *(APP)* and released into the circulation. The β-amyloid fragments come together in clumps to form plaques that attach to the neuron. Microglia react to the plaque, and an inflammatory response results. **B,** Tau proteins provide structural support for the neuron microtubules. Chemical changes in the neuron produce structural changes in tau proteins. This results in twisting and tangling (neurofibrillary tangles).

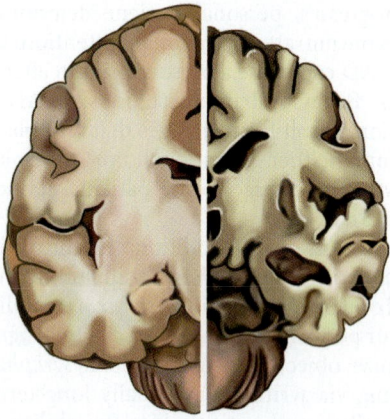

FIG. 59-4   Effects of Alzheimer's disease on the brain. This figure compares a normal brain *(left)* with a brain that has been affected by Alzheimer's disease *(right).*

they were acquired.[7] This theory compares the developmental stages in children with the deterioration in AD patients. As seen in Fig. 59-5, a relationship exists between the developmental stage and deterioration of function. For example, it is appropriate for a person with AD in the moderate stage to feel good about putting together puzzles that belong to his 3-year-old grandson. In fact, they may play well together on the same task or project.

Diagnostic Criteria for Alzheimer's Disease

AD may cause changes in the brain many years before symptoms appear. In addition, symptoms do not always directly relate to abnormal changes in the brain caused by AD. Based on these findings, in 2011 the National Institute on Aging and the Alzheimer's Association proposed revised criteria and guidelines for diagnosing AD.[8,9]

AD is now considered on a spectrum, where dementia marks the terminal stage of the disease (Table 59-7). The stages in this spectrum are preclinical AD, mild cognitive impairment, and dementia due to AD.[8] Guidelines address the use of imaging and biomarkers (discussed in section on diagnostic studies) that may help determine whether changes are due to AD.[9]

Preclinical Stage.   A long lag exists between pathologic changes in the brain and manifestations of AD. The future goal would be to modify the disease process of AD before it becomes symptomatic. Once plaques and tangles have formed in sufficient quantity, it may be too late to intervene to prevent the disease or its progression. Although currently all attempts at modifying

TABLE 59-4 Patient & Caregiver Teaching

Early Warning Signs of Alzheimer's Disease

Include the following information in the teaching plan for the patient with Alzheimer's disease.

1. **Memory loss that affects job skills**
   - Frequent forgetfulness or unexplainable confusion at home or in the workplace may signal that something is wrong.
   - This type of memory loss goes beyond forgetting an assignment, colleague's name, deadline, or phone number.

2. **Difficulty performing familiar tasks**
   - It is normal for most people to become distracted and to forget something (e.g., leave something on the stove too long).
   - People with AD may cook a meal but then forget not only to serve it but also that they made it.

3. **Problems with language**
   - Most people have trouble finding the "right" word from time to time.
   - People with AD may forget simple words or substitute inappropriate words, making their speech difficult to understand.

4. **Disorientation to time and place**
   - Most individuals occasionally forget the day of the week or what they need from the store.
   - People with AD can become lost on their own street, not knowing where they are, how they got there, or how to get back home.

5. **Poor or decreased judgment**
   - Many individuals from time to time may choose not to dress appropriately for the weather (e.g., not bringing a coat or sweater on a cold evening).
   - The person with AD may dress inappropriately in more noticeable ways, such as wearing a bathrobe to the store or a sweater on a hot day.

6. **Problems with abstract thinking**
   - For the person with AD, this goes beyond challenges such as balancing a checkbook.
   - The person with AD may have difficulty recognizing numbers or doing even basic calculations.

7. **Misplacing things**
   - For many individuals, temporarily misplacing keys, purses, or wallets is a normal, albeit frustrating, event.
   - The person with AD may put items in inappropriate places (e.g., eating utensils in clothing drawers) but have no memory of how they got there.

8. **Changes in mood or behavior**
   - Most individuals experience mood changes.
   - The person with AD tends to exhibit more rapid mood swings for no apparent reason.

9. **Changes in personality**
   - As most individuals age, they may demonstrate some change in personality (e.g., become less tolerant).
   - The person with AD can change dramatically, either suddenly or over time. For example, someone who is generally easygoing may become angry, suspicious, or fearful.

10. **Loss of initiative**
    - The person with AD may become and remain uninterested and uninvolved in many or all of his or her usual pursuits.

Adapted from Alzheimer's Association: *Early warning signs*, Chicago, The Association. www.alz.org/alzheimers_disease_know_the_10_signs.asp.

the disease process have failed, research is ongoing. The model for early intervention is seen in other diseases, such as removing polyps to prevent colon cancer, controlling blood glucose in diabetes before the disease progresses to heart and kidney disease, and treating cardiac risk factors before a person has a myocardial infarction.

Mild Cognitive Impairment. Mild cognitive impairment (MCI), the second stage in the AD spectrum, is a state of cognitive function in which individuals have problems with memory, language, or another essential cognitive function that are severe enough to be noticeable to others and show up on tests. However, these manifestations may not be severe enough to interfere with activities of daily living. Because the problems do not interfere with daily activities, the person does not meet the criteria for being diagnosed with dementia.[10]

To the casual observer, an individual with MCI may seem fairly normal. However, the person with MCI is often aware of a significant change in memory, and family members may observe changes in the individual's abilities (Table 59-6).

Between 10% and 20% of people 65 years old and older have MCI and are at high risk of developing AD. Some individuals with MCI show no progression and do not go on to develop AD, but an estimated 15% of people with MCI eventually do.[1]

No drugs have been approved for the treatment of MCI. There is little evidence that medications used in AD (e.g., cholinesterase inhibitors) affect progression to dementia or cognitive test scores in people with MCI.[11]

Currently the primary treatment of MCI consists of ongoing monitoring. Recognize the importance of monitoring the patient with MCI for changes in memory and thinking skills that would indicate a worsening of symptoms or a progression to dementia. It is critical that you understand the 10 early warning signs of AD (Table 59-4).

Diagnostic Studies

No definitive diagnostic test exists for AD. The diagnosis of AD is primarily a diagnosis of exclusion. In patients with cognitive impairment, there is increased emphasis on early and careful evaluation. As indicated earlier in this chapter, many conditions can cause manifestations of dementia, some of which are treatable or reversible (Table 59-2).

When all other possible conditions that can cause cognitive impairment have been ruled out, a clinical diagnosis of AD can be made. A comprehensive patient evaluation includes a complete health history, physical examination, neurologic and mental status assessments, and laboratory tests (Table 59-8). Brain imaging tests (e.g., CT or MRI) may show brain atrophy in the later stages of the disease, although this finding occurs in other diseases and can also be seen in people without cognitive impairment. Positron emission tomography (PET) scanning can be used to differentiate AD from other forms of dementia (Fig. 59-6). Neuroimaging techniques allow for detection of changes early in the disease and monitoring of treatment response. A definitive diagnosis of AD usually requires examination of brain tissue at autopsy and findings of neurofibrillary tangles and plaques.

The new criteria and guidelines identify two biomarker categories: (1) biomarkers showing the level of β-amyloid accumulation in the brain and (2) biomarkers showing that nerve cells in the brain are injured or actually degenerating. Biomarkers include (1) cerebrospinal fluid (CSF) neurochemical markers: β-amyloid and tau proteins and (2) imaging biomarkers: volumetric MRI and PET. The level of tau in the CSF is an indication of neurodegeneration. (Plasma levels of tau or β-amyloid are not of any value in diagnosing AD.) In AD, multiple brain structures atrophy and the volume of the brain correlates with neurodegeneration. PET determines brain metabolism using glucose tracers (Fig. 59-6). PET can also be used to detect amyloid.

Some imaging biomarkers are used in specialized clinical settings. CSF biomarkers are mainly used for research.

TABLE 59-5   Stages of Alzheimer's Disease

Mild	Moderate	Severe
• Forgetfulness beyond what is seen in a normal person • Short-term memory impairment, especially for new learning • Loss of initiative and interests • May forget recent events or the names of people or things • Small personality changes • May no longer be able to solve simple math problems • Slowly loses the ability to plan and organize	• Memory loss and confusion become more obvious • Has more trouble organizing, planning, and following directions • May need help getting dressed • May start having episodes of incontinence • Trouble recognizing family members and friends • Agitation, restlessness • May lack judgment and begin to wander, gets lost • May have trouble sleeping • Delusions, hallucinations, paranoia • Behavioral problems	• Severe impairment of all cognitive functions • Little memory, unable to process new information • Unable to perform self-care activities • Often needs help with daily needs • May not be able to talk • Cannot understand words • May have difficulty eating, swallowing • May not be able to walk or sit up without help • Immobility • Incontinence

TABLE 59-6   Comparison of Normal Forgetfulness and Memory Loss

Normal Forgetfulness	Memory Loss in Mild Cognitive Impairment	Memory Loss in Alzheimer's Disease
• Sometimes misplaces keys, eyeglasses, or other items • Momentarily forgets an acquaintance's name • Occasionally has to search for a word • Occasionally forgets to run an errand • May forget an event from the distant past • When driving, may momentarily forget where to turn, but quickly orients self • Jokes about memory loss	• Frequently misplaces items • Frequently forgets people's names and is slow to recall them • Has increasing difficulty finding desired words • Begins to forget important events and appointments • May forget recent events or newly learned information • Becomes temporarily lost more often, may have trouble understanding and following a map • Worries about memory loss, family and friends notice lapses	• Forgets what an item is used for or puts it in an inappropriate place • May not remember knowing a person • Begins to lose language skills and may withdraw from social interaction • Loses sense of time, does not know what day it is • Has seriously impaired recent memory and difficulty learning and remembering new information • Becomes easily disoriented or lost in familiar places, sometimes for hours • May have little or no awareness of cognitive problems

Adapted from Rabins P: Memory. In *The Johns Hopkins white papers*, Baltimore, 2007, Johns Hopkins University.

TABLE 59-7   Diagnostic Criteria for Alzheimer's Disease*

	Stage and Description	Recommendations for Biomarkers
Preclinical Alzheimer's disease (AD)	• Brain changes, including amyloid buildup and other early neuron changes, may already be in process • At this point, significant clinical symptoms are not yet evident • In some people, amyloid buildup can be detected with positron emission tomography (PET) scans and cerebrospinal fluid (CSF) analysis	• Use of imaging and biomarker tests at this stage are recommended only for research • Biomarkers are still being developed and standardized, and are not used by clinicians in general practice
Mild cognitive impairment (MCI) due to Alzheimer's disease	• MCI stage is marked by symptoms of memory problems, enough to be noticed and measured, but not compromising a person's independence • People with MCI may or may not progress to Alzheimer's dementia	• Used primarily by researchers • May be used in specialized clinical settings to supplement standard clinical tests to help determine possible causes of MCI • May help confirm that the person's impairment is related to AD
Dementia due to Alzheimer's disease	• Characterized by memory, thinking, and behavioral symptoms that impair a person's ability to function in daily life • Dementia marks the terminal stage of AD • Encompasses all stages presented in Table 59-5	• May be used in some cases to increase the level of certainty about a diagnosis of AD • Also may be used to distinguish AD from other dementias

Source: Jack CR, Albert MS, Knopman DS, et al: Introduction to the recommendations from the National Institute on Aging–Alzheimer's Association workgroups on diagnostic guidelines for Alzheimer's disease, *Alzheimers Dement* 7:257, 2011.
*Note that these are recommended criteria and guidelines. More research is needed, especially biomarker research, before the new criteria and guidelines can be used in clinical settings.

Stage	Alzheimer's Disease	Reisberg Stage*	Developmental Age	Diversion/Distraction Activities
Mild	No difficulty at all	1		
	Some memory trouble begins to affect job/home. Forgets familiar names.	2		
	Much difficulty maintaining job performance. Withdrawal from difficult situations.	3	12+ yr	Can function with understanding. Enjoy things previously enjoyed—watch TV, play and listen to music, play games.
	Can no longer hold a job, plan and prepare meals, handle personal finances, etc. Driving becomes difficult although can drive to familiar places.	4	8-12 yr	Can still enjoy simple games, watch TV and videos. Enjoys family photos and memories.
Moderate	Can no longer select proper clothing for occasion or season. Needs help to remain safe in home. Forgets to bathe.	5	5-7 yr	Needs age appropriate toys and games.
	Requires assistance with dressing.	6a	4-5 yr	Enjoy many of the same activities as preschoolers.
	Requires assistance with bathing.	6b	4-5 yr	
	Can no longer use toilet without assistance.	6c	4 yr	
	Urinary incontinence	6d	3-4.5 yr	
	Fecal incontinence	6e	2-3 yr	
Severe	Speech now limited to about words per day.	7a	15 mo	Enjoys infant toys, mobiles, dangling ribbons.
	Speech now limited to one word per day.	7b	1 yr	
	Can no longer walk without assistance.	7c	1 yr	
	Can no longer sit up without assistance.	7d	6-10 mo	
	Can no longer smile.	7e	2-4 mo	
	Can no longer hold up head.	7f	1-3 mo	

FIG. 59-5   Retrogenesis (back to birth) in Alzheimer's disease. (*These stages are based on Functional Assessment Staging. Reisberg B: Functional assessment staging [FAST], *Psychopharmacol Bull* 24:653, 1988.)

TABLE 59-8   Interprofessional Care

Alzheimer's Disease

Diagnostic Assessment
- History and physical examination, including psychologic evaluation
- Neuropsychologic testing, including Mini-Cog (Table 59-9), Mini-Mental State Examination (Table 59-10)
- Brain imaging tests: CT, MRI, MRS, PET
- Complete blood count
- Electrocardiogram
- Serum glucose, creatinine, BUN
- Serum levels of vitamins B_1, B_6, B_{12}
- Thyroid function tests
- Liver function tests
- Screening for depression

Management
- Drug therapy for cognitive problems (Table 59-11)
- Behavioral modification
- Moderate exercise
- Assistance with functional independence
- Assistance and support for caregiver

MRS, Magnetic resonance spectroscopy; *PET*, positron emission tomography.

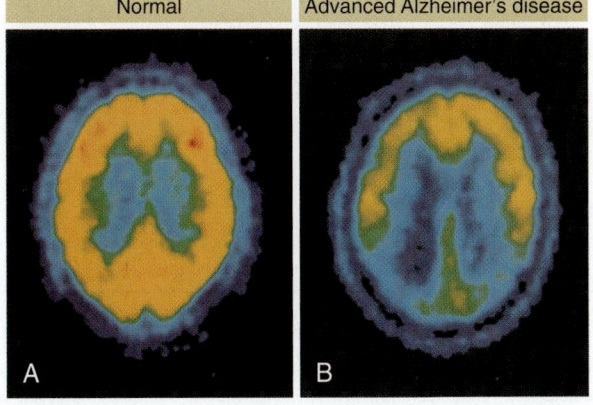

Normal	Advanced Alzheimer's disease
A	B

FIG. 59-6   Positron emission tomography (PET) scan can be used to assist in the diagnosis of Alzheimer's disease (AD). Radioactive fluorine is applied to glucose (fluorodeoxyglucose), and the yellow areas indicate metabolically active cells. **A,** A normal brain. **B,** Advanced AD is recognized by hypometabolism in many areas of the brain. (From Roberts GS: *Neuropsychiatric disorders*, London, 1993, Mosby-Wolfe.)

<table>
<tr><td colspan="2">

| TABLE 59-9 | The Mini-Cog |
</td></tr>
</table>

TABLE 59-9 The Mini-Cog

Introduction

The Mini-Cog is used as a brief assessment tool for cognitive impairment. It can be quickly administered and can guide the need for further evaluation.

Administration

1. Instruct the patient to listen carefully to and remember three unrelated words and then to repeat the words. *Example:* apple, table, penny. (This initial step is not scored.) The same three words may be repeated to the patient up to three tries to register all three words.
2. Instruct the patient to draw the face of a clock, either on a blank sheet of paper or on a sheet with the clock circle already drawn on the page. After the patient puts the numbers on the clock face, ask him or her to draw the hands of the clock to read a specific time (11:10). The test is considered normal if all numbers are present in the correct sequence and position, and the hands readably display the requested time.
3. Ask the patient to repeat the three previously stated words.

Scoring (out of total of 5 points)

Give 1 point for each recalled word after the clock drawing test.
- Patients recalling none of the three words are classified as cognitively impaired (score = 0).
- Patients recalling all three words are classified as not cognitively impaired (score = 3).
- Patients with intermediate word recall of one or two words are classified on the clock drawing test:
  The clock drawing test is scored 2 if normal and 0 if abnormal.
  Interpretation of results
  0-2: Positive screen for dementia
  3-5: Negative screen for dementia

Source: Borson S, Scanlan J, Brush M, et al: The Mini-Cog: a cognitive "vital signs" measure for dementia screening in multi-lingual elderly, *Intern J Geriatr Psychiatry* 15(11):1021, 2000.

TABLE 59-10 Mini-Mental State Examination (MMSE)

Sample Items

Orientation to Time

"What is the date?"

Registration

"Listen carefully, I am going to say three words. You say them back after I stop. Ready? Here they are . . . HOUSE (pause), CAR (pause), LAKE (pause). Now repeat those words back to me." (Repeat up to five times, but score only the first trial.)

Naming

"What is this?" (Point to a pencil or pen.)

Reading

"Please read this and do what it says." (Show examinee the words CLOSE YOUR EYES on the stimulus form.)

Reproduced by special permission of the Publisher, Psychological Assessment Resource, Inc., 16204 North Florida Avenue, Lutz, Fla. 33549, from the Mini-Mental State Examination, by Marshal Folstein and Susan Folstein, Copyright 1975, 1998, 2001 by Mini-Mental, LLC, Inc. Published 2001 by Psychological Assessment Resources, Inc. Further reproduction is prohibited without permission from PAR, Inc. The MMSE can be purchased from PAR, Inc., by calling 813-968-3003.

Biomarkers may be used in some cases to increase the level of certainty about a diagnosis of Alzheimer's dementia and to distinguish Alzheimer's dementia from other dementias. However, more research is needed with biomarkers before they are used routinely in clinical practice.

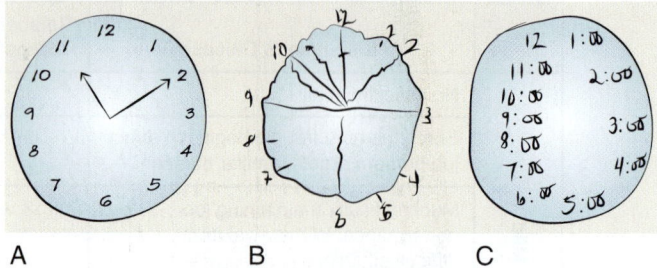

FIG. 59-7 Clock drawing is a simple test that can be used as an assessment technique in dementia. The person undergoing testing is asked to draw a clock, put in all of the numbers, and set the hands at 10 past 11. **A,** Shows a clock drawn by a person with no dementia. **B** and **C** show clocks drawn by people with dementia. (Modified from Stern TA: *Massachusetts General Hospital comprehensive clinical psychiatry*, Philadelphia, 2008, Mosby.)

TABLE 59-11 Drug Therapy

Alzheimer's Disease

Problem	Drugs
Decreased memory and cognition	Cholinesterase inhibitors • donepezil (Aricept) • rivastigmine (Exelon) • galantamine (Razadyne) *N*-methyl-D-aspartate (NMDA) receptor antagonist • memantine (Namenda)
Depression	Selective serotonin reuptake inhibitors (SSRIs) • sertraline (Zoloft) • fluvoxamine (Luvox) • citalopram (Celexa) • fluoxetine (Prozac) Atypical antidepressants • mirtazapine (Remeron) • trazodone
Behavioral problems (e.g., agitation, physical aggression, disinhibition)	Antipsychotics* • haloperidol (Haldol) • risperidone (Risperdal) • olanzapine (Zyprexa) • quetiapine (Seroquel) • aripiprazole (Abilify) Benzodiazepines • lorazepam (Ativan) • clonazepam (Klonopin)
Sleep disturbances	• zolpidem (Ambien)

*The use of these drugs in older patients with dementia is associated with an increased risk of death.

Neuropsychologic testing with tools such as the Mini-Cog (Table 59-9) and the Mini-Mental State Examination (Table 59-10) can help document the degree of cognitive impairment.[12] The clock drawing test can be used as part of the Mini-Cog or by itself to assess cognitive function (Fig. 59-7). Neuropsychologic testing is important not only for diagnostic purposes but also to establish a baseline for evaluating changes over time.

Interprofessional Care

At this time there is no cure for AD. No treatment is available to stop the deterioration of brain cells in AD. Nothing stops or really slows the progression of the disease.

The interprofessional care of AD is aimed at (1) controlling the undesirable behavioral manifestations that the patient may exhibit and (2) providing support for the family caregiver.

Drug Therapy. Although drug therapy for AD is available (Table 59-11), these drugs do not cure or reverse the progression of the disease. Drugs help many people, but not for very long and

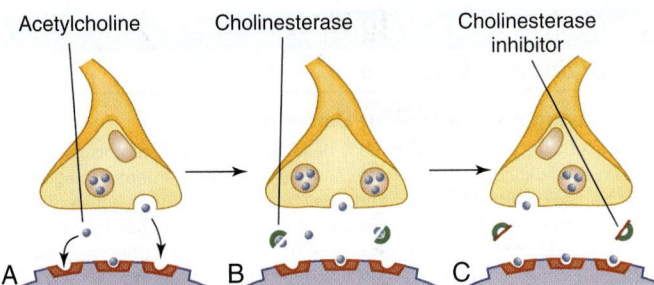

FIG. 59-8 Mechanism of action of cholinesterase inhibitors. **A,** Acetylcholine is released from the nerve synapses and carries a message across the synapse. **B,** Cholinesterase breaks down acetylcholine. **C,** Cholinesterase inhibitors block cholinesterase, thus giving acetylcholine more time to transmit the message.

not very well. The use of drugs may lead to a modest decrease in the rate of decline of cognitive function. However, the drugs have no effect on overall disease progression.[1]

Cholinesterase inhibitors block cholinesterase, the enzyme responsible for the breakdown of acetylcholine in the synaptic cleft (Fig. 59-8). Cholinesterase inhibitors include donepezil (Aricept), rivastigmine (Exelon), and galantamine (Razadyne). Rivastigmine is available as a patch.

Memantine (Namenda) protects the brain's nerve cells against excess amounts of glutamate, which is released in large amounts by cells damaged by AD. The attachment of glutamate to *N*-methyl-D-aspartate (NMDA) receptors permits calcium to flow freely into the cell, which in turn may lead to cell degeneration. Memantine may prevent this destructive sequence by blocking the action of glutamate.

Treating the depression that is often associated with AD may improve cognitive ability. Depression is often treated with selective serotonin reuptake inhibitors, including fluoxetine (Prozac), sertraline (Zoloft), fluvoxamine (Luvox), and citalopram (Celexa). The antidepressant trazodone may help with problems related to sleep.

Although antipsychotic drugs are approved for treating psychotic conditions (e.g., schizophrenia), they have been used for the management of behavioral problems (e.g., agitation, aggressive behavior) that occur in patients with AD. However, these drugs have been shown to increase the risk of death in older dementia patients. The Food and Drug Administration (FDA) has warned that antipsychotics are not indicated for the treatment of dementia-related psychosis. However, the warning does not mean that the drugs cannot be used for these patients with dementia.[13]

❖ NURSING MANAGEMENT: ALZHEIMER'S DISEASE

◆ Nursing Assessment

Subjective and objective data that should be obtained from a person with AD are presented in Table 59-12. Useful questions for the patient and caregiver are, "When did you first notice the memory loss?" and "How has the memory loss progressed since then?"

◆ Nursing Diagnoses

Nursing diagnoses for AD may include, but are not limited to, the following:
- Impaired memory *related to* the effects of dementia
- Self-neglect *related to* memory deficit, cognitive impairment, and neuromuscular impairment

TABLE 59-12 Nursing Assessment

Alzheimer's Disease

Subjective Data
Important Health Information
Past health history: Repeated head trauma, stroke, previous CNS infection, family history of dementia
Medications: Use of any drug to decrease symptoms (e.g., tranquilizers, hypnotics, antidepressants, antipsychotics)

Functional Health Patterns
Health perception–health management: Positive family history. Emotional lability
Nutritional-metabolic: Anorexia, malnutrition, weight loss
Elimination: Incontinence
Activity-exercise: Poor personal hygiene, gait instability, weakness, inability to perform activities of daily living
Sleep-rest: Frequent nighttime awakening, daytime napping
Cognitive-perceptual: Forgetfulness, inability to cope with complex situations, difficulty with problem solving (early signs), depression, withdrawal, suicidal ideation (early)

Objective Data
General
Disheveled appearance, agitation

Neurologic
Mild: Loss of recent memory, disorientation to date and time, flat affect, lack of spontaneity. Impaired abstraction, cognition, and judgment
Moderate: Agitation, impaired ability to recognize close family and friends, loss of remote memory, confusion, apraxia, agnosia, alexia (inability to understand written language); aphasia, inability to do simple tasks
Severe: Inability to do self-care, incontinence, immobility, limb rigidity, flexor posturing

Possible Diagnostic Findings
Diagnosis by exclusion, cerebral cortical atrophy on CT scan, poor scores on mental status tests, hippocampal atrophy on MRI scan, abnormal changes on PET

- Risk for injury *related to* impaired judgment, gait instability, muscle weakness, and sensory/perceptual alteration
- Wandering *related to* cognitive impairment

Additional information on nursing diagnoses for the patient with AD is presented in eNursing Care Plan 59-1 (available on the website for this chapter).

◆ Planning

The overall goals are that the patient with AD will (1) maintain functional ability for as long as possible, (2) be maintained in a safe environment with a minimum of injuries, (3) have personal care needs met, and (4) have dignity maintained. The overall goals for the caregiver of a patient with AD are to (1) reduce caregiver stress; (2) maintain personal, emotional, and physical health; and (3) cope with the long-term effects of caregiving.

◆ Nursing Implementation

Health Promotion. Can AD be prevented? Although there is no known definitive way to prevent AD, there are several things that you can do to keep your brain healthy and modify your risks for developing dementia[14] (Table 59-13).

Early recognition and treatment of AD are important. You have a responsibility to inform patients and their families regarding the early signs of AD (Table 59-4).

TABLE 59-13   Decreasing Risk of Cognitive Decline

The following are tips to reduce the risk of cognitive decline and dementia.

1. **Avoid harmful substances**
   Excessive drinking and drug abuse can damage brain cells. Stop smoking because it increases the risk of cognitive decline.
2. **Challenge your mind**
   Read frequently, do crossword puzzles. Keep mentally active. Learn new skills. Go back to school. This strengthens the brain connections and promotes new ones.
3. **Exercise regularly**
   Even low to moderate level activity such as walking or gardening three to five times per week can make you feel better. Daily physical activity, even in older adults, can decrease the risk for cognitive decline.
4. **Stay socially active**
   Pursue social activities that have meaning to you. Family, friends, church, and a sense of community may all contribute to better brain health.
5. **Avoid trauma to the brain**
   Because traumatic brain injury may be a risk factor for developing AD, promote safety in physical activities and driving. Use the car seat belt. Wear a helmet when playing contact sports or riding a bike. Fall proof your home.
6. **Take care of mental health**
   Recognize and treat depression early. Depression may cause or worsen memory loss and other cognitive impairment.
7. **Treat diabetes.**
   Better blood glucose control can help to prevent the cognitive decline associated with diabetes.
8. **Take care of your heart**
   Risk factors for cardiovascular disease and stroke (hypertension, obesity) negatively affect your cognitive health. Heart health is linked to brain health.
9. **Get enough sleep**
   Not getting enough sleep may result in problems with memory and thinking.
10. **Get the right fuel**
    A healthy and balanced diet low in fats and high in vegetables and fruits helps to reduce the risk of cognitive decline.

Adapted from Alzheimer's Association: 10 Ways to love your brain. Retrieved from *www.alz.org/northcentraltexas/in_my_community_101405.asp*; and Baumgart M, Snyder HM, Carrillo MC, et al: Summary of evidence on modifiable risk factors for cognitive decline and dementia: a population-based perspective, *Alzheimers Dement* 11:718, 2015.

EVIDENCE-BASED PRACTICE
Applying the Evidence

Modifying Risk Factors for Dementia

G.C., a 63-yr-old woman with early-onset dementia, is being discharged from the hospital tomorrow after surgery to repair ligament damage in her left ankle. She had wandered away from her daughter's house (with whom she lives) and had fallen off the curb, injuring her left ankle. Healing has been impaired because of her diabetes. V.Z., her daughter, is very upset with her mother's declining cognitive abilities and asks you what she can do to help her mother. She also asks you what she personally can do to prevent getting this "awful" disease.

Making Clinical Decisions

Best Available Evidence. Regular physical activity and management of cardiovascular risk factors (diabetes, obesity, smoking, and hypertension) reduce the risk of cognitive decline and may reduce the risk of dementia. A healthy diet and lifelong learning/cognitive training may also reduce the risk of cognitive decline.

Clinician Expertise. Good nutrition and physical exercise can improve both a person's physical as well as emotional health. G.C. and V.Z. can exercise (e.g., walking) together, and that may also decrease G.C's wandering.

Patient Preferences and Values. V.Z. recognizes that her meal planning for the family is very haphazard and they eat a lot of fast foods. She also recognizes that sitting in front of the TV has become a refuge and they get very little exercise.

Implications for Nursing Practice

1. How will you assess the risk factors for dementia and cognitive decline in both G.C. and V.Z.?
2. What strategies can you discuss with V.Z. that she can personally implement in her life to decrease her risk for dementia?
3. How can you engage G.C. in activities to prevent further cognitive decline?

Reference for Evidence

Baumgart M, Snyder HM, Carrillo MC, et al: Summary of evidence on modifiable risk factors for cognitive decline and dementia: a population-based perspective, *Alzheimers Dement* 11:718, 2015.

◆ **Acute Care.** The diagnosis of AD is traumatic for both the patient and family. It is not unusual for the patient to respond with depression, denial, anxiety, fear, withdrawal, and feelings of loss.[15] In the early stages of AD, patients are often aware that their memory is faulty and do things to cover up or mask the problem. *What Happens Next?* is a free booklet specifically for people dealing with the beginning stages of dementia (available at *www.alzheimers.nia.nih.gov*).

You are in an important position to assess for depression. Antidepressant drugs and counseling may be indicated. Family caregivers may also be in denial and may not seek medical attention early in the disease. Along with patient assessment, assess family caregivers and their ability to accept and cope with the diagnosis.

Although no current treatment is available for reversing AD, there is a need for ongoing monitoring of both the patient with AD and the patient's caregiver. An important nursing responsibility is to work collaboratively with the caregiver to manage clinical manifestations effectively as they change over time.[16] You are often responsible for teaching the caregiver to perform the many tasks that are required to manage the patient's care.

Consider both the patient with AD and the caregiver as patients with overlapping but unique problems.[17]

Patients with AD may be hospitalized for other health problems. Patients with AD have other illnesses (both acute and chronic) and may require surgical interventions. Their inability to communicate symptoms of health problems places the responsibility for assessment and diagnosis on caregivers and health care professionals. Hospitalization of the patient with AD can be a traumatic event for both the patient and caregiver and can precipitate a worsening of dementia or development of delirium. Patients with AD in the acute care setting need to be observed more closely because of concerns for safety, frequently oriented to place and time, and given reassurance. Anxiety or disruptive behavior may be reduced with using consistent nursing staff.

◆ **Ambulatory Care.** Currently, family members and friends care for most individuals with AD in their homes. Others with AD reside in various facilities, including long-term care and assisted living facilities. A facility that is good for one person may not be suitable for another. Also, what is helpful for a person at one point in the disease process may be completely different from what is best when the disease progresses.

Patients with AD move through the stages at variable rates. The nursing care required by the patient with AD changes as the disease progresses, which emphasizes the need for regular assessment and support. Regardless of the setting, the severity of the problems and amount of nursing care required intensify over time. The specific manifestations of the disease depend on the area of the brain involved. Nursing care focuses on decreasing clinical manifestations, preventing harm, and supporting the patient and caregiver throughout the disease process.

In the early stages of AD, memory aids (e.g., calendars) may be beneficial. Patients often develop depression during this phase. Depression may be related to the diagnosis of an incurable disorder and the impact of the disease on activities of daily living (e.g., driving, socializing with friends, participating in hobbies or recreational activities).

After the initial diagnosis, patients need to be aware that the progression of the disease is variable. Effective management of the disease may slow the progress of the disease and decrease the burden on the patient, caregiver, and family. However, decisions related to care should be made with the patient, family members, and interprofessional care team early in the disease. You have a role in advising the patient and caregiver to initiate health care decisions, including advance directives, while the patient has the capacity to do so. This can ease the burden for the caregiver as the disease progresses.

Adult day care is one of the options available to the person with AD. Although programs vary in size, structure, physical environment, and staff experience, the common goals of all day care programs are to provide respite for the family and a protective environment for the patient. During the early and moderate stages of AD, the person can still benefit from stimulating activities that encourage independence and decision making in a protective environment. The patient returns home tired, content, less frustrated, and ready to be with the family. The respite from the demands of care allows the caregiver to be more responsive to the patient's needs.

As the disease progresses, the demands on the caregiver eventually exceed the resources, and the person with AD may need to be placed in a long-term care facility. Special dementia units are becoming increasingly common. The dementia unit is designed with an emphasis on safety. For example, many facilities have designated areas that allow the patient to walk freely within the unit, while the unit is secured so that the patient cannot wander outside of it.

As the patient with AD progresses to the late stages (severe impairment) of AD, he or she has increased difficulty with the most basic functions, including walking and talking. Total care is required.

Specific problems relate to the care of the patient with AD in all phases of the disease. These problems are described below.

Behavioral Problems. Behavioral problems occur in about 90% of patients with AD. These problems include repetitiveness (asking the same question repeatedly), delusions (false beliefs), hallucinations, agitation, aggression, altered sleeping patterns, wandering, hoarding, and resisting care. Many times these behaviors are unpredictable and may challenge caregivers. Caregivers must be aware that these behaviors are not intentional and are often difficult to control. Behavioral problems are often the reason that patients are placed in institutional care settings.

These behaviors are often the patient's way of responding to a precipitating factor (e.g., pain, frustration, temperature extremes, anxiety). When these behaviors become problematic, you must plan interventions carefully. Initially assess the patient's physical status. Check the patient for changes in vital signs, urinary and bowel patterns, and pain that could account for behavioral problems. Then assess the environment to identify factors that may trigger behavior disruptions. Extremes in

temperature or excessive noise may lead to behavior changes. When a patient is agitated by the environment, either move the patient or remove the stimulus.

When a patient resists or pulls tubes or dressings, cover these items with stretch tube gauze or remove them from the visual field. Reassure the patient that you are present to keep him or her safe. Do not ask the confused or agitated patient challenging "why" questions. The person with AD cannot think logically. If the patient cannot verbalize distress, validate his or her mood. Rephrase the patient's statement to validate its meaning. Closely observe the patient's emotional state.

Nursing strategies that address difficult behavior include redirection, distraction, and reassurance. For the patient who is restless or agitated, redirecting involves changing the patient's focus (e.g., having the patient perform activities such as sweeping, raking, or dusting). Ways to distract the agitated patient may include providing snacks, taking a car ride, sitting on a porch swing or rocker, listening to favorite music, watching videotapes, looking at family photographs, or walking. Reassurance involves communicating to the patient that he or she will be protected from danger, harm, or embarrassment. Use of repetitive activities, songs, poems, music, massage, aromas, or a favorite object can be soothing to patients.

When dealing with the difficult patient, do not threaten to restrain the patient or call the HCP. A calming family member can be asked to stay with the patient until the patient becomes calmer. Monitor the patient frequently, and document all interventions. As verbal skills decline, you and the caregiver must rely more on the patient's body language to communicate care needs. The use of positive nurse actions can reduce the use of chemical (drug therapy) restraints.

Disruptive behaviors have been treated with antipsychotic drugs (Table 59-11). However, as discussed on p. 1409, these drugs have adverse side effects. Before these drugs are used, all other measures of treating behavioral issues should be exhausted.

> **? CHECK YOUR PRACTICE**
>
> You are working in a secure Alzheimer's unit. Today while making rounds at 4 PM you observe Dan, one of the assistants, screaming and yelling at an 84-yr-old man who has been a resident in the facility for 6 months. When you approach Dan and the resident, you ask what is going on. Dan responds, "Every day about this time he gets so agitated and starts yelling at me so I yell back."
> • How would you handle the situation, and what teaching is needed for Dan?

A specific type of agitation, termed **sundowning,** is when the patient becomes more confused and agitated in the late afternoon or evening. Behaviors related to sundowning include agitation, aggressiveness, wandering, resistance to redirection, and increased verbal activity such as yelling. The cause of sundowning is unclear, but it may be due to a disruption of circadian rhythms. Other possible causes include fatigue, unfamiliar environment and noise (especially in an acute care setting), medications, reduced lighting, and sleep fragmentation.

When a patient has sundowning, remain calm and avoid confrontation. Assess the situation for possible causes of the agitation. Nursing interventions that may be helpful include (1) creating a quiet, calm environment; (2) maximizing exposure to daylight (open blinds and turn on lights during the day); (3) evaluating medications to determine if any could cause sleep disturbance; (4) limiting naps and caffeine; and

Caring for the Patient With Alzheimer's Disease

All staff members who care for a patient with Alzheimer's disease (AD) are responsible for ensuring the patient's physiologic and psychosocial safety. The registered nurse (RN) is responsible for ongoing assessments of the patient's level of function and for development of the plan of care. Since most patients with AD are cared for at home or in long-term care settings, many routine nursing activities are delegated to licensed practical/vocational nurses (LPN/LVNs), unlicensed assistive personnel (UAP), or family caregivers.

Role of Nursing Personnel
Registered Nurse (RN)
- Assess patient memory and level of function.
- Teach patient and caregivers memory enhancement aids (e.g., calendars, notes).
- Monitor for physiologic problems associated with AD, such as pain, swallowing difficulties, urinary tract infection, pneumonia, skin breakdown, and constipation.
- Assess patient's nutritional and fluid intake and develop a plan to ensure adequate intake.
- Evaluate patient's safety risk factors.
- Determine possible precipitating factors for behavioral changes and develop strategies to address difficult behavior.
- Assess the family caregiver's stress level and coping strategies.
- Make referrals for community services such as adult day care and respite care.

Licensed Practical/Vocational Nurse (LPN/LVN)
- Monitor for behavioral changes that may indicate physiologic problems.
- Check patient environment for potential safety hazards.
- Administer enteral feedings to patients who are unable to swallow (if ordered).
- Administer ordered drug therapy.

Unlicensed Assistive Personnel (UAP)
- Assist patient to use the toilet, commode, or bedpan at frequent intervals.
- Provide personal hygiene, skin care, oral care.
- Help patients with eating.
- Assist patients with daily activities.
- Use bed alarms and surveillance to decrease risk for falls.

(5) consulting with the HCP regarding drug therapy. Management of sundowning can be challenging for you, the patient, and the family.

Safety. The person with AD is at risk for problems related to personal safety. Potential hazards include falling, ingesting dangerous substances, wandering, injuring others and self with sharp objects, being burned, and being unable to respond to crisis situations. These concerns require careful attention to the home environment to minimize risk. Supervision is also required. As the patient's cognitive function declines over time, the patient may have difficulty navigating physical spaces and interpreting environmental cues. Assist the caregiver in assessing the home environment for safety risks.

 SAFETY ALERT **Preventing Falls**
Teach the caregiver to take the following steps:
- Have stairwells well lit.
- Make sure the patient can grasp the handrails.
- Tack down carpet edges.
- Remove throw rugs and extension cords.
- Use nonskid mats in tub or shower.
- Install handrails in the bath and by the commode.

Wandering is a major concern for caregivers. Wandering may be related to loss of memory or to side effects of drugs, or it may be an expression of a physical or emotional need, restlessness, curiosity, or stimuli that trigger memories of earlier routines. As with other behaviors, observe for factors or events that may precipitate wandering. For example, the patient may be sensitive to stress and tension in the environment. In such cases, wandering may reflect an attempt to leave.

When someone with AD is discovered missing, every second counts. To assist caregivers with locating them, the Alzheimer's Association and the MedicAlert Foundation have created an alliance called MedicAlert + Alzheimer's Association Safe Return.[18] This program includes identification products (e.g., bracelet, necklace, wallet cards), a national photo and information database, a 24-hour toll-free emergency crisis line, local chapter support, and wandering behavior education and training for caregivers and families.

Tracking devices such as a global positioning system (GPS) can also be used to detect and find people who wander. These devices can be placed in shoes, sewn into pockets, worn as a bracelet or pendant, or clipped to a belt.

Pain Management. Because of difficulties with oral and written language, AD patients may have difficulty expressing physical complaints, including pain. You need to rely on other clues such as the patient's behavior. Pain can result in alterations in the patient's behavior, such as increased vocalization, agitation, withdrawal, and changes in function. Pain should be recognized and treated promptly and the patient's response monitored.

Eating and Swallowing Difficulties. Undernutrition is a problem in the moderate and severe stages of AD. Loss of interest in food and decreased ability to self-feed (*feeding apraxia*), as well as co-morbid conditions, can result in significant nutritional deficiencies in the patient with AD. In long-term care facilities, inadequate assistance with feeding may add to the problem.

Use pureed foods, thickened liquids, and nutritional supplements when chewing and swallowing become problematic for the patient. Patients may need reminders to chew their food and to swallow. Patients need a quiet and unhurried environment for eating. Avoid distractions at mealtimes, including the television. Low lighting, music, and simulated nature sounds may improve eating behaviors. Easy-grip eating utensils and finger foods may allow the patient to self-feed. Offer liquids frequently.

When oral feeding is not possible, explore alternative routes. Nasogastric (NG) feeding may be used for short periods. However, for the long term the NG tube is uncomfortable and may add to the patient's agitation. A percutaneous endoscopic gastrostomy (PEG) tube provides another option (see Fig. 39-7). However, PEG tubes can be problematic, since patients with AD are particularly vulnerable to aspiration of feeding formula and tube dislodgment. The potential positive outcomes to be gained from nutritional therapies are considered in light of overall outcome goals and potential adverse effects of the specific therapy. Nutritional support therapies are described in Chapter 39.

Oral Care. In the late stages of AD, the patient is unable to perform oral self-care. With decreased tooth brushing and flossing, dental problems are likely to occur. Because of swallowing difficulties, patients may retain food in the mouth, adding to the potential for tooth decay. Dental caries and tooth abscess can add to patient discomfort or pain and subsequently may increase agitation. Inspect the mouth regularly and provide mouth care to those patients unable to do self-care.

◆ *Infection Prevention.* Urinary tract infection and pneumonia are the most common infections in patients with AD. Such infections are ultimately the cause of death in many patients with AD. Because of feeding and swallowing problems, the patient is at risk for aspiration pneumonia. Immobility can also predispose the patient to pneumonia.

Reduced fluid intake, prostate enlargement in men, poor hygiene, and urinary drainage devices (e.g., catheters) can predispose patients to bladder infection. Any manifestations of infection, such as a change in behavior, fever, cough (pneumonia), or pain on urination (bladder), need prompt evaluation and treatment.

◆ *Skin Care.* It is important to monitor the patient's skin over time. Note and treat rashes, areas of redness, and skin breakdown. In the late stages, incontinence along with immobility and undernutrition can place the patient at risk for skin breakdown. Keep the skin dry and clean, and change the patient's position regularly to avoid areas of pressure over bony prominences.

◆ *Elimination Problems.* During the moderate and severe stages of AD, urinary and fecal incontinence lead to increased need for nursing care. When possible, behavioral retraining of bladder and bowel function (e.g., scheduled toileting) may help decrease episodes of incontinence.

Another common elimination problem is constipation. Causes may relate to immobility, dietary intake (e.g., reduced fiber intake), and decreased fluid intake. Increased dietary fiber, fiber supplements, and stool softeners are the first lines of management. The combination of aging, other health problems, and swallowing difficulties may increase the risk of complications associated with the use of mineral oil, stimulants, osmotic agents, and enemas. Management of constipation is discussed in Chapter 42.

◆ *Caregiver Support.* More than 15 million Americans provide unpaid care for people with AD or other dementias.[1] The majority of these are family members providing care in the home (Fig. 59-9). AD is a disease that disrupts all aspects of personal and family life. Caregivers for people with AD describe it as very stressful (see Table 4-5). These caregivers also exhibit adverse consequences relating to their own emotional and physical health.

The chronic and often severe stress associated with dementia caregiving increases the risk for the development of dementia in spouse caregivers.[19] One mechanism proposed is that the detrimental effects of the chronic stress of caregiving can affect the hippocampus, a region of the brain responsible for memory.

As the disease progresses, the relationship of the caregiver to the patient changes. Family roles may be altered or reversed (e.g., son caring for father). Decisions must be made, including when to tell the patient about the diagnosis, when to have the patient stop driving or doing activities that may be dangerous, when to ask for assistance, and when to place the patient in adult day care or a long-term care facility. With early-onset AD, the patient is affected during his or her most productive years in terms of career and family. The consequences can be devastating for the patient and family.

Sexual relations for couples are also seriously affected by AD. As the disease progresses, sexual interest may decline for both the patient and partner. A number of reasons account for this, including fatigue, memory impairment, and episodes of incontinence. The patient may also become sexually driven as the disease progresses and the patient becomes more uninhibited.

Work with the caregiver to assess stressors (see Table 4-4) and to identify coping strategies to reduce the burden of caregiving. For example, ask which behaviors are most disruptive to family life at a given time, while remembering that this is likely to change as the disease progresses. Determining what the caregiver views as most disruptive or distressful can help to establish priorities for care.

Safety of the patient is a high priority. It is also important to assess what the caregiver's expectations are regarding the patient's behavior. Are the expectations reasonable given the progression of the disease? A family and caregiver teaching guide based on the disease stages is provided in Table 59-14. Other tips for caregivers are listed in Table 59-15. A nursing care plan for the family caregiver (eNursing Care Plan 59-2) is available on the website for this chapter.

Support groups for caregivers and family members (Fig. 59-10) can provide an atmosphere of understanding and give current information about the disease itself and related topics such as safety, legal, ethical, and financial issues. The needs of family caregivers are discussed in Chapter 4 on pp. 49-50. Strategies related to stress management are discussed in Chapter 6.

The Alzheimer's Association has many educational and support systems available to help family caregivers (*www.alz.org*).

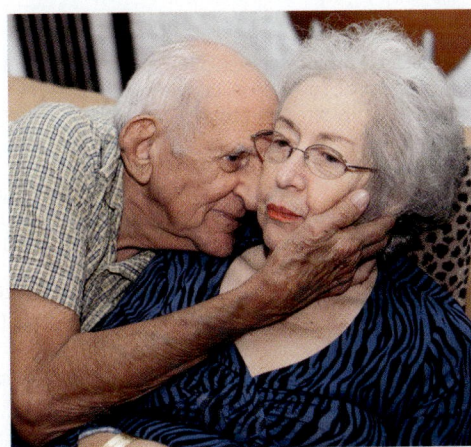

FIG. 59-9 Caregivers of patients with dementia face an incredible challenge that often causes deterioration in their own physical and emotional health. (©iStock/Thinkstock)

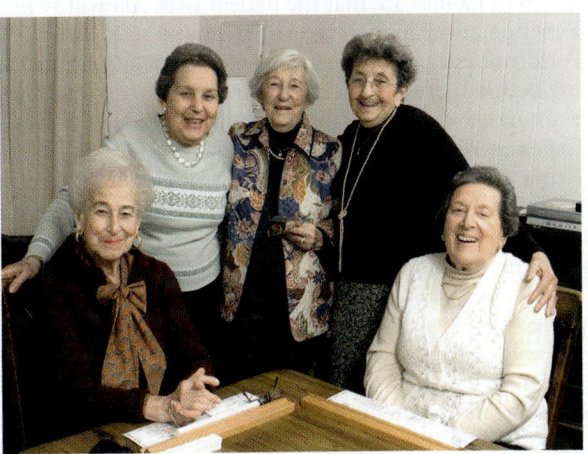

FIG. 59-10 Support groups are an effective way to help caregivers cope. (©iStockphoto/Thinkstock)

TABLE 59-14 Family & Caregiver Teaching
Alzheimer's Disease

Include the following instructions when teaching families and caregivers the management of the patient with Alzheimer's disease.

Mild Stage

- Many treatable (and potentially reversible) conditions can mimic dementia (Table 59-2). Try to get a definitive diagnosis.
- Get the person to stop driving. Confusion and poor judgment can impair driving skills and potentially put others at risk.
- Encourage activities such as visiting with friends and family, listening to music, participating in hobbies, and exercising.
- Provide cues in the home, establish a routine, and determine a specific location where essential items (e.g., glasses) must be kept.
- Do not correct misstatements or faulty memory.
- Register with MedicAlert + Alzheimer's Association Safe Return, a program established by the MedicAlert Foundation and the Alzheimer's Association to locate individuals who wander from their homes.
- Make plans for the future in terms of advance directives, care options, financial concerns, and personal preference for care.

Moderate Stage

- Install door locks for patient safety.
- Provide protective wear for urinary and fecal incontinence.
- Ensure that the home has good lighting, install handrails in stairways and bathroom, and remove area rugs.
- Label drawers and faucets (hot and cold) to ensure safety.
- Develop strategies such as distraction and diversion to cope with behavioral problems. Identify and reduce potential triggers (e.g., reduce stress, extremes in temperature) for disruptive behavior.
- Provide memory triggers, such as pictures of family and friends.

Severe Stage

- Provide a regular schedule for toileting to reduce incontinence.
- Provide care to meet needs, including oral care and skin care.
- Monitor diet and fluid intake to ensure their adequacy.
- Continue communication through talking and touching.
- Consider placement in a long-term care facility when providing total care becomes too difficult.

A booklet for caregivers, *Caring for a Person With Alzheimer's Disease*, is available at *www.nia.nih.gov/sites/default/files/caring_for_a_person_with_alzheimers_disease_0.pdf.*

◆ Evaluation

Expected outcomes are that the patient with AD will
- Function at the highest level of cognitive ability
- Perform basic personal care activities of daily living, including bathing, dressing, feeding, and toileting by self or with assistance as needed
- Experience no injury
- Remain in a restricted area during ambulation and activity
Additional information on the expected outcomes for the patient with AD is addressed in eNursing Care Plan 59-1 (available on the website for this chapter).

DELIRIUM

Delirium, a state of temporary but acute mental confusion, is a common, life-threatening syndrome. Delirium affects as many as 50% of people older than 65 years who are hospitalized, and as many as 80% of patients in an ICU.[20,21] In many cases, delirium is preventable and/or reversible.

TABLE 59-15 Guidelines for Dealing With Dementia Patients

Do

- Treat them like adults, with respect and dignity, even when their behavior is childlike.
- Use gentle touch and direct eye contact.
- Remain patient, flexible, calm, and understanding.
- Anticipate challenging behaviors, since the patient's ability to think logically has been affected.
- Give directions using gestures or pictures.
- Simplify tasks. Focus on one thing at a time.
- Avoid questions or topics that require extensive thought, memory, or words.
- Be flexible. If one approach does not work, try another.
- Use distraction, changing the subject, redirecting to another activity.
- Provide reassurance. Praise sincerely for success.

Do Not

- Criticize, correct, or argue.
- Rush or hurry the patient.
- Force participation in activities or events.
- Talk about the patient as if he or she is not there.
- Blame the person with AD. Instead, blame the disease.
- Take challenging behaviors personally. These behaviors are due to the patient's disease.
- Use condescending terms, such as "honey" or "sweetie."
- Use threatening gestures.
- Overreact to the person with AD.
- Try to explain "why" or rationalize.

✳ BECOMING A NURSE LEADER
Elder Abuse

Situation

While attending nursing school, you are working as a patient care technician in a long-term care facility. You are in charge of feeding five patients their dinner, including Mrs. Talbot, who is confused and has difficulty swallowing. You are approached by Joan, the LPN, who berates you for feeding Mrs. Talbot so slowly. Joan takes the spoon from your hand and feeds Mrs. Talbot a huge mouthful of food, which causes her to choke and cough. Joan then gives her a push and says, "Calm down." You are stunned and resume feeding Mrs. Talbot smaller bites. Joan then returns and says to you, "You will never get done at the rate you are going!"

Points for Consideration

- Elder abuse occurs in community settings, such as private homes as well as long-term care facilities.
- Types of abuse can include physical, sexual, emotional, neglect, self-neglect, and financial/exploitation.
- Elder mistreatment is often unrecognized, hidden, and underreported.
- People with dementia are at great risk of abuse.
- Health care professionals, including nurses, are frequently unaware of the various forms of elder abuse that take place and the proper course of action to pursue when mistreatment is suspected.

Discussion Questions

1. What responsibility do you have to Mrs. Talbot?
2. What should you say to Joan?
3. What role can you have to prevent this abuse from occurring again?

Reference

National Center on Elder Abuse. Administration on Aging: Retrieved from *www.ncea.aoa.gov.*

Etiology and Pathophysiology

The pathophysiologic mechanism of delirium is poorly understood. A main contributing factor is impairment of cerebral oxidative metabolism (brain gets less oxygen and has problems using it). Multiple neurotransmitter abnormalities may also be involved. Cholinergic deficiency, excess release of dopamine, and both increased and decreased serotonergic activity may contribute to delirium. Proinflammatory cytokines, including interleukin-1, interleukin-2, interleukin-6, tumor necrosis factor–α (TNF-α), and interferon, appear to play a role.

Dementia is the leading risk factor for delirium. Furthermore, delirium is a risk factor for the subsequent development of dementia. Delirium may cause permanent neuronal damage and lead to dementia.[22]

Clinically, delirium is rarely caused by a single factor. Stress, surgery, and sleep deprivation have been linked to the onset of delirium. Pain and depression also contribute to delirium, especially in postoperative older patients.[21]

Delirium is often the result of the interaction of the patient's underlying condition with a precipitating event. Delirium can occur after a relatively minor insult in a vulnerable patient. For example, a patient with underlying health problems such as heart failure, cancer, cognitive impairment, or sensory limitations may develop delirium in response to a relatively minor change (e.g., use of a sleeping medication). In other less vulnerable patients, it may take a combination of factors (e.g., anesthesia, major surgery, mechanical ventilation, infection, prolonged sleep deprivation) to precipitate delirium. Delirium can also be a symptom of a serious medical illness such as bacterial meningitis.

Understanding factors that can lead to delirium can help in determining effective interventions. Several factors that can precipitate or cause delirium are listed in Tables 59-16 and 59-17. Many of these factors are more common in older patients. In addition, older patients have limited compensatory mechanisms to deal with physiologic insults such as hypoxia, hypoglycemia, and dehydration. Older adults are more susceptible to drug-induced delirium, in part because of their increased use of multiple drugs. Many medications, including sedative-hypnotics, opioids (especially meperidine [Demerol]), benzodiazepines, and drugs with anticholinergic properties, can cause or contribute to delirium, especially in older or vulnerable patients.[23]

Clinical Manifestations

Patients with delirium can have a variety of manifestations ranging from hypoactivity and lethargy to hyperactivity, agitation, and hallucinations. Patients can also have mixed delirium, manifesting both hypoactive and hyperactive symptoms. Delirium can develop over the course of hours to days. In most patients, delirium usually develops over a 2- to 3-day period. The early manifestations often include inability to concentrate, disorganized thinking, irritability, insomnia, loss of appetite, restlessness, and confusion. Later manifestations may include agitation, misperception, misinterpretation, and hallucinations.

Delirium can last from 1 to 7 days. However, some delirium manifestations may persist up for months or years. Some patients do not completely recover.

Manifestations of delirium are sometimes confused with those of dementia. A key distinction between delirium and dementia is that the person who exhibits sudden cognitive impairment, disorientation, or clouded sensorium is more likely to have delirium rather than dementia. (A comparison of delirium and dementia is presented in Table 59-1.)

TABLE 59-16 Factors That Precipitate Delirium

Demographic Characteristics
- Age 65 yr or older
- Male gender

Cognitive Status
- Cognitive impairment
- Dementia
- Depression
- History of delirium

Environmental
- Admission to ICU
- Emotional stress
- Pain (especially untreated)
- Sleep deprivation
- Use of physical restraints

Functional Status
- Functional dependence
- History of falls
- Immobility

Sensory
- Sensory deprivation
- Sensory overload
- Visual or hearing impairment

Decreased Oral Intake
- Dehydration
- Malnutrition

Drugs
- Alcohol or drug abuse or withdrawal
- Aminoglycosides
- Anticholinergics
- Opioids
- Sedative-hypnotics
- Treatment with multiple drugs

Coexisting Medical Conditions
- Acute infection, sepsis, fever
- Chronic kidney or liver disease
- Electrolyte imbalances
- Fracture or trauma
- History of stroke
- Neurologic disease
- Severe acute illness
- Terminal illness

Surgery
- Cardiac surgery
- Noncardiac surgery
- Orthopedic surgery
- Prolonged cardiopulmonary bypass

TABLE 59-17 Mnemonic for Causes of Delirium

Dementia, dehydration
Electrolyte imbalances, emotional stress
Lung, liver, heart, kidney, brain
Infection, intensive care unit
Rx drugs
Injury, immobility
Untreated pain, unfamiliar environment
Metabolic disorders

Diagnostic Studies

Diagnosing delirium is complicated because many critically ill patients cannot communicate their needs. A careful medical and psychologic history and physical examination are the first steps in diagnosing delirium. This includes careful attention to medications, both prescription and over-the-counter drugs. The Confusion Assessment Method (CAM) has been extensively studied and is a reliable tool for assessing delirium (Table 59-18). It is important to distinguish whether the delirium is part of an underlying problem of dementia.

Once delirium has been diagnosed, explore potential causes. Carefully review the patient's health history and medication record. Laboratory tests include complete blood count, serum electrolytes, blood urea nitrogen, and creatinine levels; ECG; urinalysis; liver and thyroid function tests; and oxygen saturation level. Drug and alcohol levels may be obtained. If unexplained fever or nuchal rigidity is present and meningitis or encephalitis is suspected, a lumbar puncture may be performed. CSF is examined for glucose, protein, and bacteria. If the

TABLE 59-18   Confusion Assessment Method (CAM)

Delirium is diagnosed with the presence of features 1 and 2, and either 3 or 4.

Feature 1

Acute Onset and Fluctuating Course

Data usually obtained from a family member or nurse.

Shown by positive responses to following questions:

- Is there evidence of an acute change in mental status from the patient's baseline?
- Did the (abnormal) behavior fluctuate during the day (i.e., tend to come and go, or increase and decrease in severity)?

Feature 2

Inattention

Shown by positive response to following question:

- Did the patient have difficulty focusing attention (e.g., being easily distractible, or having difficulty keeping track of what was being said)?

Feature 3

Disorganized Thinking

Shown by a positive response to following question:

- Was the patient's thinking disorganized or incoherent, such as rambling or irrelevant conversation, unclear or illogical flow of ideas, or unpredictable switching from subject to subject?

Feature 4

Altered Level of Consciousness

Shown by any answer other than "alert" to the following question:

- Overall, how would you rate this patient's level of consciousness (alert [normal], vigilant [hyperalert], lethargic [drowsy, easily aroused], stupor [difficult to arouse], or coma [unarousable])?

Adapted from Inouye S, van Dyck C, Alessi C, et al: Clarifying confusion: the Confusion Assessment Method, *Ann Intern Med* 113(12):941, 1990.

patient's history includes head injury, appropriate x-rays or scans may be ordered. In general, brain imaging studies such as CT and MRI are used only in situations in which head injury is known or suspected.

❖ NURSING AND INTERPROFESSIONAL MANAGEMENT: DELIRIUM

Treatment is important as many cases of delirium are potentially reversible. In caring for the patient with delirium, your roles include prevention, early recognition, and treatment. Prevention of delirium involves recognition of high-risk patients.[24] Patient groups at risk include those with neurologic disorders (e.g., dementia, stroke, CNS infection, Parkinson's disease), sensory impairment, and older age. Other risk factors, including surgery, hospitalization in an ICU, and untreated pain, are listed in Table 59-16.

Care of the patient with delirium focuses on eliminating precipitating factors. If it is drug induced, medications are discontinued. Keep in mind that delirium can also accompany drug and alcohol withdrawal. Depending on patient history, drug screening may be performed. Fluid and electrolyte imbalances and nutritional deficiencies (e.g., thiamine) are corrected if appropriate. If the problem is related to environmental conditions (e.g., an overstimulating or understimulating environment), changes should be made. If delirium is secondary to infection, appropriate antibiotic therapy is started. Similarly, if delirium is secondary to chronic illness such as chronic kidney disease or heart failure, treatment focuses on these conditions.

Care of the patient experiencing delirium includes protecting the patient from harm. Give priority to creating a calm

ETHICAL/LEGAL DILEMMAS

Board of Nursing Disciplinary Action

Situation

The State Board of Nursing has received multiple complaints about J.R., a registered nurse (RN) who works in a long-term care facility. J.R. has signed off on three controlled substances count sheets that have been determined to be inaccurate. During an investigation it was discovered that several members of the nursing staff knew about J.R.'s reported behavior, but they did not report their observations to the unit administrator. After the investigation, the board of nursing subpoenas J.R. to a meeting to discuss charges in preparation for a disciplinary hearing.

Ethical/Legal Points for Consideration

- Regulation of professional nursing practice is the right of each of the 50 states, most of which have separate regulatory agencies charged with writing regulations and rules to implement the State Nurse Practice Act. The regulations approved by these agencies carry the weight of law. Failure to behave accordingly places a nurse at risk for disciplinary action.
- The RN who is charged with unprofessional behavior has been charged with an offense and is entitled to the same legal rights as any other individual, including a fair and timely hearing, opportunity to confront the accusers, right to be represented by an attorney, and right to prepare a defense.
- Possible disciplinary actions include temporary suspension of the nursing license, revocation of the nursing license, mandatory rehabilitation for substance abuse, and mandated supervision and evaluation of practice. Sometimes the disciplinary action includes fines and requires reeducation. In addition, the State Board of Nursing may report the action to the state attorney general if evidence suggests that a crime has been committed. The RN who has been found guilty of unprofessional practice must report this action on all future applications for nursing positions.
- All RNs should be familiar with their state's nurse practice act and regulations, as well as the composition and actions of the State Board of Nursing. Nurses should pay particular attention to the regulation that lists examples of actionable behavior and disciplinary actions sanctioned by the state.
- RNs have a legal and ethical obligation to report suspected illegal behavior to their administrators and to continue reporting until the situation is resolved. By failing to report, the RN may be charged as an accessory to the act or aiding and abetting the behavior. This RN may be charged with unprofessional behavior and risks losing his or her nursing license. Shifting the obligation to someone else to report or failure to continue reporting each incident does not satisfy this duty.

Discussion Questions

1. How would you handle a situation where retaliation for reporting unprofessional behavior is likely?
2. What would you do if the nurse suspected of illegal behavior is related to someone in the administrative hierarchy?

and safe environment. This may include encouraging family members to stay at the bedside, providing familiar objects and family photos, transferring the patient to a private room or one closer to the nurses' station, and planning for consistent nursing staff if possible. Use reorientation and behavioral interventions in patients with delirium. Provide the patient with reassurance and reorienting information as to place, time, and procedures. Clocks, calendars, and lists of the patient's scheduled activities are also useful in reducing confusion. Reduce environmental stimuli, including noise and light levels.[25]

Personal contact through touch and verbal communication can be an important reorienting strategy. If the patient uses eyeglasses or a hearing aid, they should be readily available because sensory deprivation can precipitate delirium. Avoid the use of restraints. Other interventions, including relaxation techniques, music therapy, and massage, may also be appropriate for some patients with delirium.

Comprehensive, multicomponent interventions to prevent delirium are the most effective and should be implemented by the interprofessional care team.[26] This team may also address issues related to polypharmacy, pain, nutritional status, and potential for incontinence. The patient experiencing delirium is also at risk for the adverse consequences of immobility, including skin breakdown. Give attention to increasing physical activity or providing range-of-motion exercises, when appropriate, and maintaining skin integrity.

Also focus on supporting the family and caregivers during episodes of delirium. Family members need to understand factors that may have precipitated the delirium, as well as the potential outcomes. Patient education materials are available at *www.ICUdelirium.org*.

◆ Drug Therapy

Drug therapy is reserved for patients with severe agitation, especially when it interferes with needed medical therapy (e.g., fluid replacement, intubation, dialysis). Agitation can put the patient at risk for falls and injury. Drug therapy is used cautiously because many of the drugs used to manage agitation have psychoactive properties. Drugs should be used only when nonpharmacologic interventions have failed.

Dexmedetomidine (Precedex), an α-adrenergic receptor agonist, has been used in ICU settings for sedation. In addition, low-dose antipsychotics (neuroleptics) may be used, such as haloperidol (Haldol), risperidone (Risperdal), olanzapine (Zyprexa), and quetiapine (Seroquel). Haloperidol can be administered IV, IM, or orally and will produce sedation. In addition to sedation, other side effects of antipsychotics include hypotension; extrapyramidal side effects, including *tardive dyskinesia* (involuntary muscle movements of face, trunk, and arms) and *athetosis* (involuntary writhing movements of the limbs); muscle tone changes; and anticholinergic effects. Carefully monitor older patients receiving antipsychotic agents.

Short-acting benzodiazepines (e.g., lorazepam [Ativan]) can be used to treat delirium associated with sedative and alcohol withdrawal or in conjunction with antipsychotics to reduce extrapyramidal side effects. However, these drugs may worsen delirium caused by other factors and must be used cautiously.

CASE STUDY

Alzheimer's Disease

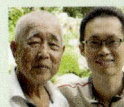
(©iStock/Thinkstock)

Patient Profile
M.Y., a 78-yr-old Asian American man, was diagnosed with Alzheimer's disease (AD) 3 yr ago shortly after his wife died. Today his 45-yr-old son brings him to the emergency department because he wandered from his son's home, fell, and injured his left hip.

Subjective Data
• Can state his name, confused as to place and time
• Denies memory of wandering or falling
• Agitated, trying to get up
• Denies pain

Objective Data
Physical Examination
• Left leg shorter than right leg
• Tense and anxious

Diagnostic Studies
• X-ray of left hip indicates a fracture
• Mini-Cog testing indicates cognitive impairment

Discussion Questions
1. What is the pathogenesis of AD?
2. What precipitating factors may have resulted in M.Y.'s fall?
3. *Safety:* What safety precautions need to be taken regarding the inpatient care of M.Y.?
4. *Patient-Centered Care:* What is the priority nursing intervention for M.Y.?
5. *Patient-Centered Care:* What teaching plan should you develop for M.Y. and his son?
6. Surgery is planned to repair his fractured hip. Why is he at risk for delirium?
7. *Priority Decision:* Based on the assessment data, what are the priority nursing diagnoses? Are there any collaborative problems?
8. *Teamwork and Collaboration:* What nursing activities can the RN delegate to unlicensed assistive personnel (UAP)?
9. *Evidence-Based Practice:* M.Y.'s son asks you if he should give his father ginkgo to help his memory. How would you respond?

Answers available at http://evolve.elsevier.com/Lewis/medsurg.

BRIDGE TO NCLEX EXAMINATION

The number of the question corresponds to the same-numbered outcome at the beginning of the chapter.

1. Dementia is defined as a
   a. syndrome that results only in memory loss.
   b. disease associated with abrupt changes in behavior.
   c. disease that is always due to reduced blood flow to the brain.
   d. syndrome characterized by cognitive dysfunction and loss of memory.

2. Vascular dementia is associated with
   a. transient ischemic attacks.
   b. bacterial or viral infection of neuronal tissue.
   c. cognitive changes secondary to cerebral ischemia.
   d. abrupt changes in cognitive function that are irreversible.

3. The clinical diagnosis of dementia is based on
   a. CT or MRS.
   b. brain biopsy.
   c. electroencephalogram.
   d. patient history and cognitive assessment.

4. Dementia with Lewy bodies (DLB) is characterized by
   a. remissions and exacerbations over many years.
   b. memory impairment, muscle jerks, and blindness.
   c. parkinsonian symptoms, including muscle rigidity.
   d. increased intracranial pressure secondary to decreased CSF drainage.

5. Which statement(s) accurately describe(s) mild cognitive impairment (select all that apply)?
   a. Always progresses to AD
   b. Caused by variety of factors and may progress to AD
   c. Should be aggressively treated with acetylcholinesterase drugs
   d. Caused by vascular infarcts that, if treated, will delay progression to AD
   e. Patient is usually not aware that there is a problem with his or her memory

6. The early stage of AD is characterized by
   a. no noticeable change in behavior.
   b. memory problems and mild confusion.
   c. increased time spent sleeping or in bed.
   d. incontinence, agitation, and wandering behavior.

7. A *priority* goal of treatment for the patient with AD is to
   a. maintain patient safety.
   b. maintain or increase body weight.
   c. return to a higher level of self-care.
   d. enhance functional ability over time.

8. Which patient is *most* at risk for developing delirium?
   a. A 50-yr-old woman with cholecystitis
   b. A 19-yr-old man with a fractured femur
   c. A 42-yr-old woman having an elective hysterectomy
   d. A 78-yr-old man admitted to the medical unit with complications related to heart failure

1. d, 2, c, 3. d, 4. c, 5. b, 6. b, 7. a, 8. d

For rationales to these answers and even more NCLEX review questions, visit *http://evolve.elsevier.com/Lewis/medsurg.*

EVOLVE WEBSITE

http://evolve.elsevier.com/Lewis/medsurg
Review Questions (Online Only)
Key Points
Answer Keys for Questions
* Rationales for Bridge to NCLEX Examination Questions
* Answer Guidelines for Case Study on p. 1417
Student Case Study
* Patient With Alzheimer's Disease
eNursing Care Plans
* eNursing Care Plan 59-1: Patient With Alzheimer's Disease
* eNursing Care Plan 59-2: Family Caregivers
Conceptual Care Map Creator
Audio Glossary
Content Updates

REFERENCES

1. Alzheimer's Association: 2016 Alzheimer's Association facts and figures report. Retrieved from *www.alz.org/documents_custom/2016-facts-and-figures.pdf.*
2. Alzheimer's Disease Education and Referral Center: Alzheimer's disease genetics: facts sheet. Retrieved from *www.nia.nih.gov/alzheimers/publication/alzheimers-disease-genetics-fact-sheet.*
*3. Chiu WC, Ho WC, Liao DL, et al: Progress of diabetic severity and risk of dementia, *J Clin Endocrinol Metab* 100(8):2899, 2015.
*4. Bryan RN, Bilello M, Davatzikos C, et al. Effect of diabetes on brain structure: the action to control cardiovascular risk in diabetes MRI imaging baseline data, *Radiology* 272(1):210, 2014.
5. List J, Ott S, Bukowski M, et al: Cognitive function and brain structure after recurrent mild traumatic brain injuries in young-to-middle-aged adults, *Front Hum Neurosci* 9:228, 2015.
6. Barnes DE, Kaup A, Kirby KA, et al: Traumatic brain injury and risk of dementia in older veterans, *Neurology* 83(4):312, 2014.
*7. Reisberg B, Franssen EH, Souren LE, et al: Evidence and mechanisms of retrogenesis in Alzheimer's and other dementias: management and treatment import, *Am J Alzheimers Dis Other Demen* 17(4):202, 2002. (Classic)
*8. Jack CR, Albert MS, Knopman DS, et al: Introduction to the recommendations from the National Institute on Aging—Alzheimer's Association workgroups on diagnostic guidelines for Alzheimer's disease, *Alzheimers Dement* 7:257, 2011.
*9. McKhann GM, Knopman DS, Chertkow H, et al: The diagnosis of dementia due to Alzheimer's disease: recommendations from the National Institute on Aging and the Alzheimer's Association workgroup, *Alzheimers Dement* 7:263, 2011.
*10. Breitner JCS: Mild cognitive impairment and progression to dementia: new findings, *Neurology* 82:e34, 2014.
*11. Russ TC, Morling JR: Cholinesterase inhibitors for mild cognitive impairment, *Cochrane Database Syst Rev* 9:CD009132, 2012.
*12. Tsoi KK, Chan JY, Hirai HW, et al. Cognitive tests to detect dementia: a systematic review and meta-analysis, *JAMA Intern Med* 175(9):1450, 2015.
*13. Tan L, Tan L, Wang HF, et al: Efficacy and safety of atypical antipsychotic drug treatment for dementia: a systematic review and meta-analysis, *Alzheimers Res Ther* 7(1):20, 2015.
14. Baumgart M, Snyder HM, Carrillo MC, et al: Summary of evidence on modifiable risk factors for cognitive decline and dementia: a population-based perspective, *Alzheimers Dement* 11:718, 2015.
15. Volland J, Fisher A: Best practices for engaging patients with dementia, *Nursing* 44(11):44, 2014.
16. Brandon IL: Easing the burden on family caregivers, *Nursing* 43(8):36, 2013.
17. Beach PR, White BE: Applying the evidence to help caregivers torn in two, *Nursing* 45(6):30, 2015.
18. Alzheimer's Association: MedicAlert + Alzheimer's Association Safe Return. Retrieved from *www.alz.org/care/dementia-medic-alert-safe-return.asp.*
*19. Pertl MM, Lawlor BA, Robertson IH, et al: Risk of cognitive and functional impairment in spouses of people with dementia: evidence from the health and retirement study, *J Geriatr Psychiatry Neurol* 28(4):260, 2015.
20. Inouye SK, Westendorp RG, Saczynski JS: Delirium in elderly people, *Lancet* 83(9920):911, 2014.
21. Kosar CM, Tabloski PA, Travison TG, et al: Effect of preoperative pain and depressive symptoms on the development of postoperative delirium, *Lancet Psychiatry* 1(6):431, 2014.
22. Fong TG, Davis D, Growdon ME, et al: The interface between delirium and dementia in elderly adults, *Lancet Neurol* 14(8):823, 2015.
*23. American Geriatrics Society Expert Panel on Postoperative Delirium in Older Adults: Postoperative delirium in older adults: best practice statement from the American Geriatrics Society, *J Am Coll Surg* 220(2):136, 2015.
24. Delirium Prevention and Safety: Starting with the ABCDEF's. Retrieved from *www.icudelirium.org/medicalprofessionals.html.*
25. ICU Delirium and Cognitive Impairment Study Group: Delirium in the ICU. Retrieved from *www.icudelirium.org/docs/delirium_education_brochure.pdf*
*26. Hshieh TT, Yue J, Oh E, et al: Effectiveness of multicomponent nonpharmacological delirium interventions: a meta-analysis, *JAMA Intern Med* 175(4):512, 2015.

*Evidence-based information for clinical practice.

60

Spinal Cord and Peripheral Nerve Problems

Cindy M. Sullivan

I think a hero is an ordinary individual who finds strength to persevere and endure in spite of overwhelming obstacles.

Christopher Reeve

e http://evolve.elsevier.com/Lewis/medsurg/

LEARNING OUTCOMES

1. Describe the classification of spinal cord injuries and associated clinical manifestations.
2. Describe the clinical manifestations, interprofessional care, and nursing management of neurogenic and spinal shock.
3. Relate the clinical manifestations of spinal cord injury to the level of disruption and rehabilitation potential.
4. Describe the nursing management of the major physical and psychologic problems of the patient with a spinal cord injury.
5. Describe the effects of spinal cord injury on the older adult.
6. Explain the types, clinical manifestations, interprofessional care, and nursing management of spinal cord tumors.
7. Explain the etiology, clinical manifestations, interprofessional care, and nursing management of trigeminal neuralgia and Bell's palsy.
8. Explain the etiology, clinical manifestations, interprofessional care, and nursing management of Guillain-Barré syndrome/acute inflammatory demyelinating polyneuropathy.
9. Explain the etiology, clinical manifestations, interprofessional care, and nursing management of chronic inflammatory demyelinating polyneuropathy.

KEY TERMS

acute inflammatory demyelinating polyneuropathy (AIDP), p. 1440
anterior cord syndrome, Table 60-1, p. 1422
autonomic hyperreflexia, p. 1431
Bell's palsy, p. 1439
botulism, p. 1442
Brown-Séquard syndrome, Table 60-1, p. 1422
cauda equina syndrome, Table 60-1, p. 1422

central cord syndrome, Table 60-1, p. 1422
chronic inflammatory demyelinating polyneuropathy (CIDP), p. 1441
conus medullaris syndrome, Table 60-1, p. 1422
Guillain-Barré syndrome (GBS), p. 1440
neurogenic bladder, p. 1423
neurogenic bowel, p. 1423
neurogenic shock, p. 1420

paraplegia, p. 1420
spinal cord injury (SCI), p. 1419
spinal shock, p. 1420
tetanus, p. 1442
tetraplegia, p. 1420
trigeminal neuralgia (TN), p. 1437

This chapter discusses spinal cord and peripheral nerve problems, including spinal cord injuries, spinal cord tumors, cranial nerve disorders, and polyneuropathies. A focus of this chapter is the nursing management of the many problems encountered by the patient with a spinal cord injury.

SPINAL CORD PROBLEMS

SPINAL CORD INJURY

Spinal cord injury (SCI) is caused by trauma or damage to the spinal cord. It can result in temporary or permanent alteration in the function of the spinal cord. About 12,500 Americans experience SCI each year. Approximately 276,000 people in the

United States are living with SCI. Young adult men ages 16 to 30 years have the greatest risk for SCI. With improved treatment strategies, even the very young patient with SCI can anticipate a long life.[1]

The number of older adults with SCI has increased. This increase is related to people with SCI living longer and older age at the time of injury.[1]

The potential for disruption of individual growth and development, altered family dynamics, economic loss in terms of employment, and the high cost of rehabilitation and long-term health care make SCI a major problem. Although many people with SCI can care for themselves independently, those with the highest level of injury may require around-the-clock care at home or in a long-term care facility.

Reviewed by Linda Littlejohns, RN, MSN, CNRN, FAAN, Neuroscience Clinical Nursing Consultant, San Juan Capistrano, California; Jessica Pastor, MSN, DNP(c), ACNP-BC, SANE-A, TNCC, Clinical Nursing Instructor, Wayne State University, Detroit, Michigan, and Nurse Practitioner, Infectious Diseases and Emergency Medicine, Troy Beaumont, Troy, Michigan; Crystal R. Sherman, DNP, CNP, FNP-BC, APHN-BC, Assistant Professor of Nursing, Shawnee State University, Portsmouth, Ohio; and Olga Van Dyke, RN, MSN, CAGS, Assistant Professor, School of Nursing, MCPHS University, Boston, Massachusetts.

Etiology and Pathophysiology

SCI is usually a result of trauma. The most common causes are motor vehicle collisions (38%), falls (30%), violence (14%), sports injuries (9%), and other miscellaneous causes (9%).[1]

Types of Injury. The extent of neurologic damage caused by SCI results from primary injury (initial physical disruption of the spinal cord) and secondary injury (from processes such as ischemia, hypoxia, hemorrhage, and edema).

Primary Injury. SCI can result from cord compression by bone displacement, interruption of blood supply to the cord, or traction from pulling on the cord. Penetrating trauma, such as gunshot and stab wounds, can cause tearing and transection. The initial mechanical disruption of axons as a result of stretch or laceration is referred to as the *primary injury*.

Secondary Injury. Secondary injury refers to the ongoing, progressive damage that occurs after the primary injury. Several theories exist on what causes this ongoing damage. Possible causes include vascular changes due to hemorrhage, vasospasm, thrombosis, loss of autoregulation, breakdown of the blood-brain barrier, and infiltration of inflammatory cells that cause ischemia, edema, and cellular necrosis. Free radical formation, lipid peroxidation, release of glutamate, and disruption of the ionic balance of potassium, sodium, and calcium lead to neuronal cell death and reduced spinal cord blood flow. *Apoptosis* (programmed cell death) may continue for weeks after injury and contribute to postinjury demyelination.[2] These processes lead to scar tissue formation, irreversible nerve damage, and permanent neurologic deficit.

Fig. 60-1 illustrates the cascade of events causing secondary injury after traumatic SCI. The resulting hypoxia reduces O_2 levels below the metabolic needs of the spinal cord. Lactate metabolites accumulate, and an increase in vasoactive substances, including norepinephrine, serotonin, and dopamine occurs. High levels of these vasoactive substances cause vasospasms and hypoxia with subsequent necrosis. Unfortunately, the spinal cord has minimal ability to adapt to vasospasm.

Within 24 hours, permanent damage may occur because of edema. Edema secondary to the inflammatory response is particularly harmful because of limited space for tissue expansion. Thus compression of the spinal cord occurs. Edema extends above and below the injury, increasing ischemic damage. Because secondary injury progresses over time, the extent of the injury and prognosis for recovery are most accurately determined 72 hours or more after injury. Important signs of improvement include muscular strength and pinprick sensation below the level of injury. The greatest improvement occurs in the first 3 to 6 months following injury and can continue over years in 20% of cases.[3]

Spinal and Neurogenic Shock. **Spinal shock** may occur following acute SCI. This temporary shock is characterized by decreased reflexes, loss of sensation, absent thermoregulation, and flaccid paralysis below the level of injury. This syndrome lasts days to weeks and may mask postinjury neurologic function.

In contrast to spinal shock, **neurogenic shock** results from the loss of vasomotor tone caused by injury and is characterized by hypotension and bradycardia. Loss of sympathetic nervous system innervation causes peripheral vasodilation, venous pooling, and decreased cardiac output. These effects are generally associated with a cervical or high thoracic injury.[4]

Classification of Spinal Cord Injury. SCI is classified by the (1) mechanism of injury, (2) level of injury, and (3) degree of injury.

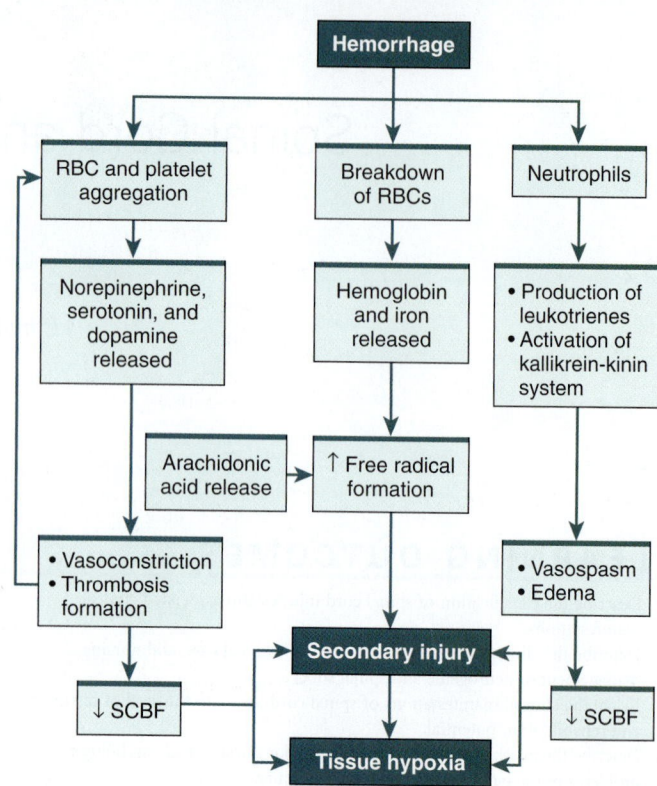

FIG. 60-1 Cascade of metabolic and cellular events that leads to spinal cord ischemia and hypoxia of secondary injury. *RBCs,* Red blood cells; *SCBF,* spinal cord blood flow. (Modified from Marciano FF, Greene KA, Apostolides PJ, et al: Pharmacologic management of spinal cord injury: review of the literature, *BNI Q* 11[2]:11, 1995. In McCance KL, Huether SE, editors: *Pathophysiology: the biologic basis for disease in adults and children,* ed 5, St Louis, 2006, Mosby.)

Mechanisms of Injury. The major mechanisms of injury are flexion, hyperextension, flexion-rotation, extension-rotation, and compression[5] (Fig. 60-2). The flexion-rotation injury is the most unstable because ligaments that stabilize the spine are torn. This injury most often contributes to severe neurologic deficits.

Level of Injury. *Skeletal level of injury* is the vertebral level with the most damage to vertebral bones and ligaments. *Neurologic level* is the lowest segment of the spinal cord with normal sensory and motor function on both sides of the body. The level of injury may be cervical, thoracic, lumbar, or sacral. Cervical and lumbar injuries are most common because they are associated with the greatest flexibility and movement. If the cervical cord is involved, paralysis of all four extremities occurs, resulting in **tetraplegia** (formerly termed *quadriplegia*). The degree of impairment in the arms following cervical injury depends on the level of injury. The lower the level, the more function is retained in the arms.

If the thoracic, lumbar, or sacral spinal cord is damaged, the result is **paraplegia** (paralysis and loss of sensation in the legs). Fig. 60-3 shows affected structures and functions at different levels of cord injury.

Degree of Injury. The degree of spinal cord involvement may be complete or incomplete (partial). *Complete cord involvement* results in total loss of sensory and motor function below the level of injury. *Incomplete cord involvement* results in a mixed

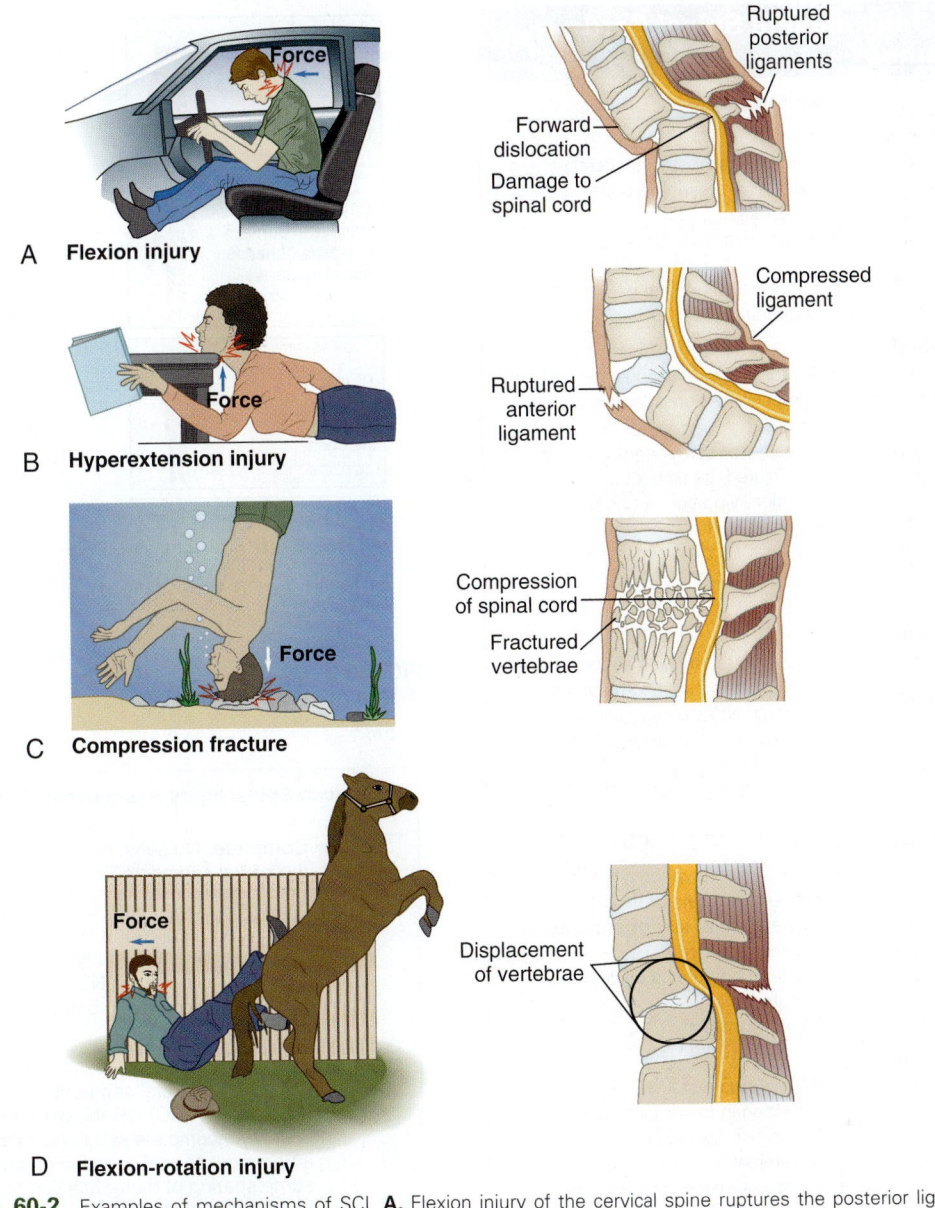

FIG. 60-2 Examples of mechanisms of SCI. **A,** Flexion injury of the cervical spine ruptures the posterior ligaments. **B,** Hyperextension injury of the cervical spine ruptures the anterior ligaments. **C,** Compression fractures
crush the vertebrae and force bony fragments into the spinal canal. **D,** Flexion-rotation injury of the cervical spine
often results in tearing of ligamentous structures that normally stabilize the spine. (*A, B, C,* From Copstead-Kirkhorn
LC, Banasik JL: *Pathophysiology,* ed 5, St Louis, 2014, Mosby.)

loss of voluntary motor activity and sensation and leaves some
tracts intact. The degree of sensory and motor loss depends on
the level of injury and reflects specific damaged nerve tracts.

Five major syndromes are associated with incomplete injuries: central cord syndrome, anterior cord syndrome, Brown-
Séquard syndrome, cauda equina syndrome, and conus
medullaris syndrome (Table 60-1).

Clinical Manifestations

Manifestations of SCI are generally related to the direct result
of trauma that causes cord compression, ischemia, edema, and
possible cord transection. These manifestations are also related
to the level and degree of injury. The patient with an incomplete
injury may demonstrate a mixture of manifestations.

Motor and Sensory Effects. The American Spinal Injury Association (ASIA) Impairment Scale is recommended for classifying

the severity of impairment from SCI. It combines assessments of
motor and sensory function to determine neurologic level and
completeness of injury[5] (Fig. 60-4).

The sensory regions are called *dermatomes,* with each
segment of the spinal cord innervating a particular area of skin.
Each dermatome has a specific point recommended for testing.
A dermatome map is shown in Fig. 55-7 on p. 1299.

The ASIA Impairment Scale is useful for recording changes
in neurologic status and identifying appropriate rehabilitation
goals. Movement and rehabilitation potential related to specific
locations of SCI are described in Table 60-2. In general, sensory
function closely parallels motor function at all levels.

Respiratory System. Respiratory complications closely correspond to the level of injury. Cervical injuries above C4 present
special problems because of the total loss of respiratory muscle
function. Injury or fracture below C4 results in diaphragmatic

TABLE 60-1   Incomplete Spinal Cord Injury Syndromes

Description	Manifestations
Central Cord Syndrome • Caused by damage to central spinal cord • Occurs most commonly in cervical cord region • More common in older adults	• Motor weakness and altered sensation present in upper extremities • Lower extremities not usually affected • Dysesthetic burning pain in upper extremities
Anterior Cord Syndrome • Caused by damage to anterior spinal artery • Results in compromised blood flow to anterior spinal cord • Typically results from acute compression of anterior portion of the spinal cord, often due to flexion injury	• Motor paralysis and loss of pain and temperature sensation below level of injury • Because posterior cord tracts are not injured, sensations of touch, position, vibration, and motion remain intact
Brown-Séquard Syndrome • Results from damage to one half of the spinal cord • Typically results from penetrating injury to spinal cord	• *Ipsilateral* (same side as injury): Loss of motor function and pressure, position, and vibratory sense • *Contralateral* (opposite side of injury): Loss of light touch, pain, and temperature sensation below level of injury
Conus Medullaris Syndrome • Results from damage to the conus medullaris (lowest portion of spinal cord)	• Motor function in legs may be preserved, weak, or flaccid • Decrease in or loss of sensation in perianal area • Areflexic bowel and bladder • Impotence • Pain uncommon
Cauda Equina Syndrome • Results from damage to cauda equina (lumbar and sacral nerve roots)	• Asymmetric distal weakness, patchy sensation in lower extremities • May cause flaccid paralysis of lower extremities • Complete loss of sensation between legs and over buttocks, inner thighs, and backs of legs *(saddle area)* • Areflexic (flaccid) bladder and bowel • Severe, radicular, asymmetric pain

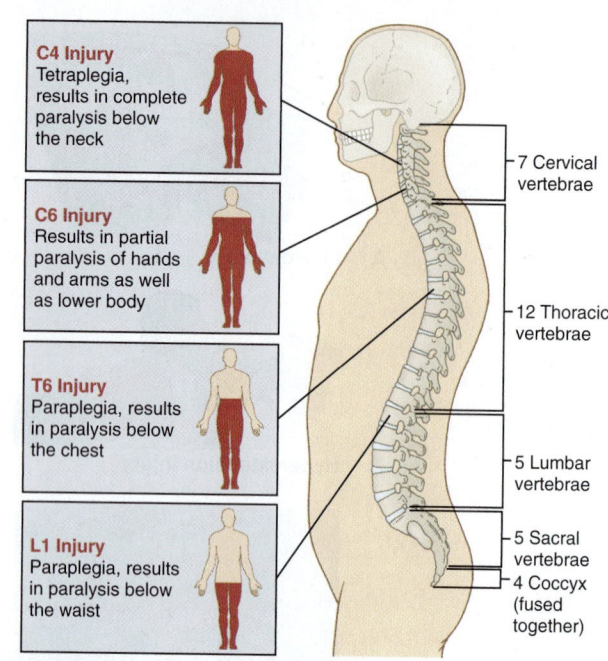

C4 Injury Tetraplegia, results in complete paralysis below the neck

C6 Injury Results in partial paralysis of hands and arms as well as lower body

T6 Injury Paraplegia, results in paralysis below the chest

L1 Injury Paraplegia, results in paralysis below the waist

7 Cervical vertebrae

12 Thoracic vertebrae

5 Lumbar vertebrae

5 Sacral vertebrae

4 Coccyx (fused together)

FIG. 60-3   Symptoms, degree of paralysis, and potential for rehabilitation depend on level of spinal injury.

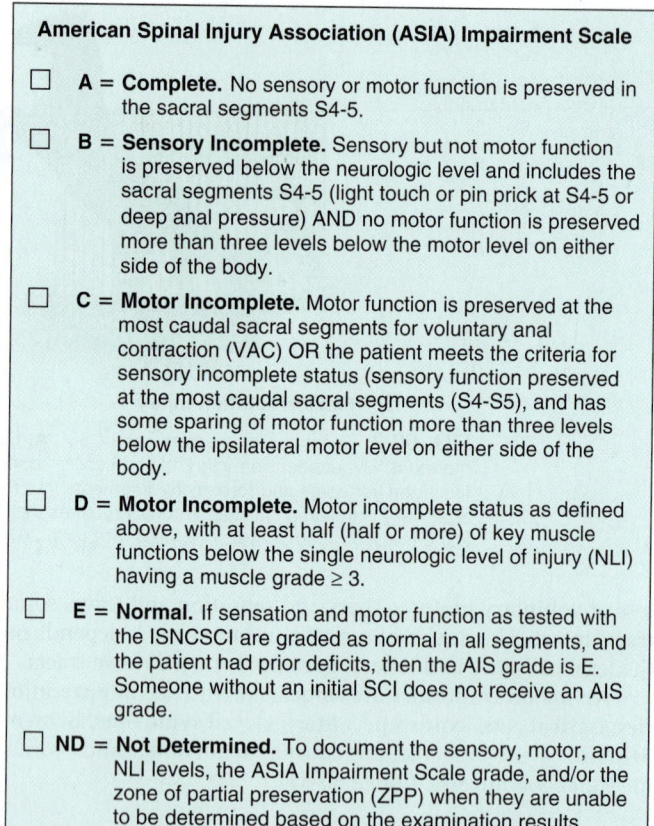

American Spinal Injury Association (ASIA) Impairment Scale

☐ **A = Complete.** No sensory or motor function is preserved in the sacral segments S4-5.

☐ **B = Sensory Incomplete.** Sensory but not motor function is preserved below the neurologic level and includes the sacral segments S4-5 (light touch or pin prick at S4-5 or deep anal pressure) AND no motor function is preserved more than three levels below the motor level on either side of the body.

☐ **C = Motor Incomplete.** Motor function is preserved at the most caudal sacral segments for voluntary anal contraction (VAC) OR the patient meets the criteria for sensory incomplete status (sensory function preserved at the most caudal sacral segments (S4-S5), and has some sparing of motor function more than three levels below the ipsilateral motor level on either side of the body.

☐ **D = Motor Incomplete.** Motor incomplete status as defined above, with at least half (half or more) of key muscle functions below the single neurologic level of injury (NLI) having a muscle grade ≥ 3.

☐ **E = Normal.** If sensation and motor function as tested with the ISNCSCI are graded as normal in all segments, and the patient had prior deficits, then the AIS grade is E. Someone without an initial SCI does not receive an AIS grade.

☐ **ND = Not Determined.** To document the sensory, motor, and NLI levels, the ASIA Impairment Scale grade, and/or the zone of partial preservation (ZPP) when they are unable to be determined based on the examination results.

FIG. 60-4   The American Spinal Injury Association Impairment Scale. The worksheet for determining the classification is the International Standards for Neurologic Classification of Spinal Cord Injury (ISNCSCI) and is available at *www.asia-spinalinjury.org/elearning/isncsci_worksheet_2015_web.pdf.* (From American Spinal Injury Association.)

breathing if the phrenic nerve is functioning. Even if the injury is below C4, spinal cord edema and hemorrhage can affect the function of the phrenic nerve and cause respiratory insufficiency. Hypoventilation and impairment of the intercostal muscles lead to a decrease in vital capacity and tidal volume.[6]

Cervical and thoracic injuries cause paralysis of abdominal muscles and often the intercostal muscles. Thus the patient cannot cough effectively enough to remove secretions, increasing the risk for aspiration, atelectasis, and pneumonia. Neurogenic pulmonary edema may occur secondary to a dramatic increase in sympathetic nervous system activity at the time of injury, which shunts blood to the lungs. In addition, pulmonary edema may occur in response to fluid overload. To improve respiratory function for patients with SCI, resistive inspiratory muscle training may be effective.[7]

TABLE 60-2 Level of Spinal Cord Injury and Rehabilitation Potential

Movement Remaining	Rehabilitation Potential	Movement Remaining	Rehabilitation Potential
Tetraplegia		**C7-8**	
C1-3		• All triceps to elbow extension, finger extensors and flexors	• Able to transfer self to wheelchair
• Often fatal injury	• Able to drive electric wheelchair equipped with portable ventilator by using chin control or mouth stick, headrest to stabilize head	• Good grasp with some decreased strength	• Able to roll over and sit up in bed
• Movement in neck and above, loss of innervation to diaphragm, absence of independent respiratory function	• Able to use computer with mouth stick, head wand, or noise control	• Decreased respiratory reserve	• Able to push self on most surfaces
	• Attendant care 24 hr/day. Able to instruct others		• Able to perform most self-care
			• Independent use of wheelchair
			• Able to drive car with powered hand controls (in some patients)
			• Attendant care 0-6 hr/day
C4		**Paraplegia**	
• Sensation and movement in neck and above	• Same as C1-3	**T1-6**	
• May be able to breathe without a ventilator		• Full innervation of upper extremities.	• Full independence in self-care and in wheelchair
C5		• Back, essential intrinsic muscles of hand. Full strength and dexterity of grasp.	• Able to drive car with hand controls (in most patients)
• Full neck, partial shoulder, back, biceps	• Able to drive electric wheelchair with mobile hand supports	• Decreased trunk stability, decreased respiratory reserve	• Independent standing in standing frame
• Gross elbow, inability to roll over or use hands	• Indoor mobility in manual wheelchair	**T6-12**	
• Decreased respiratory reserve	• Able to feed self with setup and adaptive equipment	• Full, stable thoracic muscles and upper back	• Full independent use of wheelchair
	• Attendant care 10 hr/day	• Functional intercostal muscles, resulting in increased respiratory reserve	• Able to stand erect with full leg brace, ambulate on crutches with swing (although gait difficult)
C6			• Unable to climb stairs
• Shoulder and upper back abduction and rotation at shoulder	• Able to assist with transfer and perform some self-care	**L1-2**	
• Full biceps to elbow flexion, wrist extension, weak grasp of thumb	• Able to feed self with hand devices	• Varying control of legs and pelvis	• Good sitting balance
• Decreased respiratory reserve	• Able to push wheelchair on smooth, flat surface	• Instability of lower back	• Full use of wheelchair
	• Able to drive adapted van from wheelchair		• Able to ambulate with long leg braces
	• Independent computer use with adaptive equipment	**L3-4**	
	• Attendant care 6 hr/day	• Quadriceps and hip flexors	• Completely independent ambulation with short leg braces and canes
		• Absence of hamstring function, flail ankles	• Unable to stand for long periods

Cardiovascular System. Any cord injury above T6 leads to dysfunction of the sympathetic nervous system. The result may be bradycardia, peripheral vasodilation, and hypotension (neurogenic shock). Peripheral vasodilation causes a relative hypovolemia because of the increase in the capacity of the dilated veins. It also reduces venous return of blood to the heart. Cardiac output then decreases, leading to hypotension. Other injuries can also cause hemorrhagic shock and further reduce BP. It is important to identify all causes of hypotension in the person with SCI.

Urinary System. Urinary dysfunction occurs in the majority of patients following SCI. Neurogenic bladder describes any type of bladder dysfunction related to abnormal or absent bladder innervation. After spinal cord shock resolves, depending on the completeness of the SCI, patients usually have some degree of neurogenic bladder. Normal voiding requires nervous system coordination of urethral and pelvic floor relaxation, with simultaneous contraction of the detrusor muscle.

Depending on the injury, a neurogenic bladder may (1) have no reflex detrusor contractions (*flaccid, hypotonic*), (2) have hyperactive reflex detrusor contractions (*spastic*), or (3) lack coordination between detrusor contraction and urethral relaxation (*dyssynergia*). Common problems with a neurogenic bladder include urgency, frequency, incontinence, inability to void, and high bladder pressures resulting in reflux of urine into the kidneys.[8]

Urinary retention is a common development in acute SCI and spinal shock. While the patient is in spinal shock, the bladder is atonic, becomes overdistended, and fails to empty. In the postacute phase of SCI, the bladder may become hyperirritable. A loss of inhibition from the brain results in reflex emptying and failure to store urine (*urinary incontinence*).[9]

Gastrointestinal System. Decreased GI motor activity contributes to gastric distention and development of paralytic ileus. Gastric emptying may be delayed, especially in patients with higher level SCI. Excessive release of HCl acid in the stomach may cause stress ulcers. Dysphagia may also be present in patients who require mechanical ventilation, tracheostomy, and anterior spine surgery.

Intraabdominal bleeding may be difficult to diagnose because the person with SCI may not experience pain or tenderness. Continued hypotension and decreases in hemoglobin and hematocrit may indicate bleeding. Expanding abdominal girth may also be noted.

Loss of voluntary control of the bowel following SCI results in neurogenic bowel. SCI above the level of the conus medullaris causes the anal sphincter to remain tight, and the ability to sense a full rectum is lost. Bowel movement occurs on a reflex basis when the rectum is full (*incontinence*). SCI at or below the conus medullaris causes the bowel to be *areflexic*. Peristalsis is impaired and stool propulsion is slow. The defecation reflex may be damaged and anal sphincter tone relaxed (*retention*).

ETHICAL/LEGAL DILEMMAS
Right to Refuse Treatment

Situation

R.D., a 25-yr-old man, suffered a spinal cord injury (SCI) to C7-8 following a motorcycle accident. He was diagnosed with anterior cord syndrome and has motor paralysis, which may prevent him from riding motorcycles again. He has become extremely depressed and states he no longer wishes to live. Because of his emotional state, R.D. is now refusing to eat. Can he be forced to receive enteral nutrition (tube feeding)?

Ethical/Legal Points for Consideration

- Withholding treatment in a newly injured but otherwise healthy young adult may present an ethical dilemma for some nurses. They may consider it assisted suicide and believe that it violates the ethical principles of beneficence and nonmaleficence.
- A competent adult has the right to consent to or refuse medical treatment under the right to privacy, the Fourteenth Amendment of the Constitution, and case law.*
- Case law has also supported the concept that forced treatment constitutes battery (unlawful use of force). Furthermore, a mentally competent, physically incapacitated adult can refuse feeding by nasogastric tube and compel the health facility to follow the patient's wishes.†
- To be competent to participate in informed consent or refusal, an adult must be able to understand the information provided about the procedure or treatment, consider choices between alternatives available, and make a choice based on his values and preferences. Depression may not be a determinant in competency to make informed treatment choices.
- If, after adequate evaluation and treatment for pain, depression, or other medical conditions, the patient persists in his refusal, his wishes must be respected.
- Refusal to eat or drink has never been upheld as illegal, and the alternative—forced eating and drinking—is clearly a criminal act of battery and a violation of patient rights.

Discussion Questions

1. What are your feelings about requests to withhold treatment in a young person with a newly acquired disability?
2. What resources are available to help R.D., his family, and nursing staff deal with this emotionally charged and ethically complex situation?

*Cruzan v. Director, Missouri Department of Health, 497 U.S. 261, 1990. Retrieved from *http://supreme.justia.com/cases/federal/us/497/261*.
†Bouvia v. Superior Court, 1986. Retrieved from *http://law.justia.com/cases/california/calapp3d/179/1127.html*.

This leads to constipation, increased risk of incontinence, and possible impaction, ileus, or megacolon. Hemorrhoids can occur over time.

Integumentary System. The risk for skin breakdown over bony prominences in areas of decreased or absent sensation is a major consequence of immobility related to SCI. Pressure ulcers can occur quickly and lead to major infection and sepsis.

Thermoregulation. *Poikilothermism* is the adjustment of body temperature to room temperature. It occurs in SCI because interruption of the sympathetic nervous system prevents peripheral temperature sensations from reaching the hypothalamus. Spinal cord disruption is also marked by decreased ability to sweat or shiver below the level of injury, which affects the ability to regulate body temperature. The degree of poikilothermism depends on the level of injury. High cervical injuries are associated with a greater loss of ability to regulate temperature than are thoracic or lumbar injuries.

Metabolic Needs. Nasogastric suctioning may lead to metabolic alkalosis. It is especially important to monitor sodium and potassium until suctioning is discontinued and a normal diet is resumed.

The person with SCI has increased nutritional needs due to increased metabolism and more protein breakdown. Lean body mass is lost and muscle atrophy leads to weight loss. Nutritional support should focus on a diet that addresses the person's caloric and nitrogen needs.[10] Adequate nutrition helps to prevent skin breakdown, reduce infection, and decrease the rate of muscle atrophy.

Peripheral Vascular Problems. Venous thromboembolism (VTE) is a common problem accompanying SCI during the first 3 months.[11] Detecting deep venous thrombosis (DVT) may be difficult in a person with SCI because usual signs and symptoms, such as pain and tenderness, are not present. Pulmonary embolism is a leading cause of death in patients with SCI.[1]

Pain. Pain following SCI differs in type and severity, and is influenced by the patient's physical functioning and emotions. The pain can be nociceptive or neuropathic.

Nociceptive pain in SCI can develop from musculoskeletal, visceral, and/or other types of injury (e.g., skin ulceration, headache). Patients often describe musculoskeletal pain as dull or aching. It starts or worsens with movement. Visceral pain is located in the thorax, abdomen, and/or pelvis, and may be dull, tender, or cramping.

Neuropathic pain in SCI occurs from damage to the spinal cord or nerve roots. The pain can be located at or below the level of injury. Patients often identify neuropathic pain as hot, burning, tingling, pins and needles, cold, and/or shooting. They may be extremely sensitive to stimuli and even light touch can cause significant pain.[12] (Pain is discussed in Chapter 8.)

Diagnostic Studies

CT scan is the preferred imaging study to diagnose the location and degree of injury as well as the degree of spinal canal compromise. Cervical x-rays are obtained when CT scan is not readily available. However, visualizing C7 and T1 on cervical x-rays is often difficult, and the ability to fully evaluate cervical spine injury is compromised.

MRI is used to assess soft tissue injury, neurologic changes, unexplained neurologic deficits, or worsening neurologic condition.[13] Perform a comprehensive neurologic examination with assessment of the head, chest, and abdomen for additional injuries or trauma. Patients with cervical injuries who demonstrate altered mental status may also need a CT angiogram to rule out vertebral artery damage. Duplex Doppler ultrasound, impedance plethysmography, venous occlusion plethysmography, venography, and clinical examination are used to diagnose DVT.

Interprofessional Care

Prehospital. Immediate postinjury goals include maintaining a patent *airway*, adequate ventilation/*breathing*, and adequate *circulating* blood volume (ABCs) as well as preventing extension of spinal cord damage (secondary injury). Table 60-3 outlines emergency management of the patient with SCI. Recommended immobilization includes a combination of a rigid cervical collar and supportive blocks on a backboard with straps. Spinal immobilization with sandbags and tape is insufficient and is not recommended. Spinal immobilization in patients with penetrating trauma is also not recommended because of increased mortality. The concern during initial management of patients with potential cervical spinal injuries is impairment of neurologic function due to movement of the injured vertebrae.[14]

✚ TABLE 60-3 Emergency Management

Spinal Cord Injury

Etiology	Assessment Findings	Interventions
Blunt Trauma	• Respiratory distress/difficulty breathing	**Initial**
• Compression, flexion, extension, or rotation injuries to spinal column	• Neurogenic shock: hypotension, bradycardia, cool or warm dry skin	• Ensure patent airway and adequate respirations.
	• Spinal shock	• Maintain SaO_2 > 90%: Administer O_2 via nasal cannula, non-rebreather mask, or endotracheal tube.
• Motor vehicle crash	• Muscle weakness, paralysis, or flaccidity	• Maintain SBP > 90 mm Hg.
• Pedestrian accidents	• Alterations in sensation: temperature, light touch, deep pressure, proprioception	• Establish IV access with two large-bore catheters to infuse normal saline or lactated Ringer's solution as appropriate.
• Falls	• Numbness, paresthesia	• Immobilize and stabilize cervical spine.*
• Diving	• Pain, tenderness, deformities, or muscle spasms adjacent to vertebral column	• Assess for other injuries.
• Sports injuries		• Control external bleeding.
Penetrating Trauma	• Cuts; bruises; open wounds on head, face, neck, or back	• Obtain appropriate imaging.
• Stretched, torn, crushed, or lacerated spinal cord	• Bowel and bladder incontinence	**Ongoing Monitoring**
	• Urinary retention	• Monitor vital signs, level of consciousness (neurologic status), O_2 saturation, cardiac rhythm, urine output.
• Gunshot wounds	• Priapism	• Anticipate need for intubation if in respiratory distress or gag reflex absent.
• Stab wounds	• Diminished rectal sphincter tone	• Keep warm.

*Spinal immobilization is not recommended in patients with penetrating trauma.

Systemic and neurogenic shock must be treated to maintain systolic BP greater than 90 mm Hg. Following cervical injury, all body systems must be maintained until the full extent of the damage can be evaluated. After stabilization at the injury scene, the person should be transferred by the most appropriate mode of transportation available to the nearest medical facility, preferably one that specializes in acute SCI care.[15] A thorough assessment allows evaluation of the degree of deficit and establishes the level and degree of injury.

Acute Care. Interprofessional care during the acute phase for a patient with a cervical injury is described in Table 60-4. Compared to cervical injury, patients with SCI of the thoracic and lumbar vertebrae require less intense support. At this level of injury, respiratory compromise is not as severe and bradycardia is usually not a problem. Other problems are treated symptomatically.

Obtain a history, with emphasis on how the incident occurred. Assess the extent of injury perceived by the patient or by the emergency response system (ERS) personnel immediately after the event. Initial assessment (which usually occurs in the emergency department) includes managing the person's ABCs and vital signs to ensure the airway is secure, oxygenation saturation (SaO_2) is greater than 90%, and SBP is greater than 90 mm Hg. Appropriate medical interventions and diagnostics are implemented to ensure the patient is hemodynamically stable.

A complete neurologic assessment is completed using the ASIA tool (Fig. 60-4). The International Standards for Neurologic Classification of Spinal Cord Injury is available at www.asia-spinalinjury.org/elearning/isncsci_worksheet_2015_web.pdf.

Muscle groups are tested with and against gravity, alone and against resistance, on both sides of the body. Ask the patient to move legs and then hands, spread fingers, extend wrists, and shrug shoulders. Record symmetry and spontaneous movement. After assessing motor status, complete a sensory examination, including touch and pain as tested by pinprick, starting at the toes and working upward toward the head. Assess rectal tone. Voluntary anal contraction indicates incomplete SCI. If time and conditions permit, also assess position sense and vibration.

Mechanisms of injury that cause spinal cord trauma, especially involving the cervical cord, may also result in brain injury and/or vertebral artery injury. Assess for a history of unconsciousness, signs of concussion, and increased intracranial pressure (see Chapter 56). In addition, perform a careful assessment for musculoskeletal injuries and trauma to internal organs. Because the patient has no muscle, bone, or visceral sensations, the only clue to internal trauma with hemorrhage may be a rapidly decreasing BP and increasing pulse. Examine urine for hematuria, which also indicates internal injuries.

Move the patient in alignment as a unit (logroll) during transfers and when repositioning to prevent further injury. Monitor respiratory, cardiac, urinary, and GI functions. The patient may go directly to surgery after initial immobilization or to the intensive care unit (ICU) for monitoring and management.

Nonoperative Stabilization. Nonoperative treatments involve stabilization of the injured spinal segment and decompression, either through traction or realignment. Stabilization eliminates damaging motion at the injury site. It is intended to prevent secondary spinal cord damage caused by narrowing of the spinal canal, or continued contusion or compression of the spinal cord at the level of the injury. Early realignment of an unstable fracture-dislocation injury by closed reduction through craniocervical traction has been found to be effective and safe.

Surgical Therapy. Surgical treatment is used following acute SCI to address the instability and decompress the spinal cord. The type of surgery depends on the severity and level of the injury, mechanism of injury, and location and degree of compression. Early spinal cord decompression may reduce secondary injury and thus improve the patient's outcome. Surgery within the first 24 hours after SCI is safe and associated with improved neurologic outcome.

Surgery to stabilize the spine can be performed from the back of the spine (posterior approach) or from the front of the spine (anterior approach). In some cases, both approaches may be needed. Fusion involves attaching metal screws, plates, or other devices to the bones of the spine to keep them aligned. This procedure is usually done when two or more vertebrae have been injured. Small pieces of bone may also be attached to

TABLE 60-4 Interprofessional Care
Cervical Cord Injury

Diagnostic Assessment
- History and physical examination, including complete neurologic examination
- Arterial blood gases
- Electrolytes, serum glucose, coagulation profile, hemoglobin and hematocrit
- Urinalysis
- CT scan, MRI, EMG (measure evoked potentials)
- Anteroposterior, lateral, and odontoid spinal x-rays
- Serial bedside PFTs
- Duplex Doppler ultrasound, impedance plethysmography

Management
Acute Care
- Immobilization and stabilization of vertebral column
- ABCs (airway, breathing, circulation)
- O_2 by high-humidity mask (PaO_2 >60 mm Hg)
- Intubation (if indicated by ABGs and PFTs)
- Maintenance of heart rate (e.g., atropine) and BP (e.g., dopamine) (SBP >90 mm Hg, MAP >85)
- Administration of IV fluids
- Insertion of nasogastric tube and attach to suction.
- Assessment and management of nutrition
- Maintenance of normal body temperature (*normothermia*)
- Indwelling urinary catheter
- Pain management
- VTE prophylaxis
- Pressure ulcer prevention
- Stress ulcer prophylaxis
- Bowel and bladder care and training
- Mobilization once spine stabilized
- Physical, occupational, speech therapy and physiatrist consults

Rehabilitation and Home Care
- Physical therapy (ROM, mobility, strength, equipment)
- Occupational therapy (splints, ADLs training)
- Speech therapy (swallow and cognition)
- Pain management
- Spasticity management
- Bowel and bladder training
- Autonomic hyperreflexia prevention
- Pressure ulcer prevention
- Recreational therapy
- Patient and caregiver teaching

ADL, Activities of daily living; *PFT*, pulmonary function test; *VTE*, venous thromboembolism.

the injured bones to help them fuse into one solid piece. The bone used for this procedure can be obtained from the patient's spinal bone harvested during surgery, from another bone in the patient's body (*autologous*), or from donor bone (*allograft*). (Specific surgical and nursing interventions for these techniques are discussed in Chapter 63 on pp. 1506-1507.)

Drug Therapy. Methylprednisolone (MP), which was used for many years to treat acute SCI, is no longer approved by the Food and Drug Administration (FDA) for this use. No evidence suggests clinical benefit of MP to treat acute SCI. High-dose MP is associated with harmful side effects, including immunosuppression with increased risk of infection, increased frequency of upper GI bleeding, sepsis, longer stays in the ICU, and even death.[16]

Low-molecular-weight heparin (e.g., enoxaparin [Lovenox]) is used to prevent VTE unless contraindicated. Contraindications include internal bleeding, abnormal kidney function, and

recent surgery. Oral anticoagulation alone is not recommended as a prophylactic treatment strategy.

Vasopressor agents, such as phenylephrine or norepinephrine (Levophed), are used in the acute phase as adjuvants to treatment. These agents maintain the mean arterial pressure (MAP) at greater than 85 to 90 mm Hg to improve perfusion to the spinal cord. Use of vasopressors has significant risk of complications, including ventricular tachycardia, troponin elevation, metabolic acidosis, and atrial fibrillation. Dopamine has been shown to have more complications than phenylephrine in SCI.[17] Because drug metabolism is altered in patients with SCI, drug interactions may occur. Differences in drug metabolism correlate with level and completeness of injury, with greater change apparent following cervical cord injury than injury at lower spinal levels.

❖ NURSING MANAGEMENT: SPINAL CORD INJURY

◆ Nursing Assessment

Subjective and objective data that should be obtained from a patient with recent SCI are presented in Table 60-5.

◆ Nursing Diagnoses

Nursing diagnoses for the patient with SCI depend on the severity of the injury and level of dysfunction. Nursing diagnoses for a patient with SCI may include, but are not limited to, the following:

- Ineffective breathing pattern *related to* respiratory muscle fatigue, neuromuscular paralysis, and/or retained secretions
- Imbalanced nutrition: less than body requirements *related to* paralytic ileus and metabolic demands of body
- Ineffective peripheral tissue perfusion *related to* hypotension and lack of mobility
- Impaired skin integrity *related to* immobility and/or poor tissue perfusion
- Impaired urinary elimination *related to* spinal injury and/or limited fluid intake
- Constipation *related to* neurogenic bowel, inadequate fluid intake, and/or immobility
- Risk for autonomic hyperreflexia (dysreflexia) *related to* reflex stimulation of sympathetic nervous system

Additional information on nursing diagnoses for the patient with SCI is presented in eNursing Care Plan 60-1 (available on the website for this chapter). The care plan is for a patient with a complete cervical cord injury.

◆ Planning

Overall goals are that the patient with SCI will (1) maintain an optimal level of neurologic functioning; (2) have minimal or no complications of immobility; (3) learn new skills, gain new knowledge, and acquire new behaviors to be able to care for self or successfully direct others to do so; and (4) return home at an optimal level of functioning.

◆ Nursing Implementation

◆ **Health Promotion.** Nursing interventions for prevention of SCI include identifying high-risk populations, counseling, and teaching. Support legislation to prohibit texting while driving and to mandate use of seat belts in cars, helmets for motorcyclists and bicyclists, and child safety seats. Also recommend tougher penalties for drunk-driving offenses.

Emphasize the importance of other health promotion and health screening following SCI. Health-promoting behaviors

TABLE 60-5 Nursing Assessment

Spinal Cord Injury

Subjective Data

Important Health Information

Health history: Motor vehicle crash, sports injury, industrial incident, gunshot or stabbing injury, falls

Functional Health Patterns

Health perception–health management: Use of alcohol or recreational drugs. Risk-taking behaviors

Activity-exercise: Loss of strength, movement, and sensation below level of injury. Dyspnea, inability to breathe adequately ("air hunger")

Cognitive-perceptual: Tenderness, pain at or above level of injury. Numbness, tingling, burning, twitching of extremities

Coping–stress tolerance: Fear, denial, anger, depression

Objective Data

General

Poikilothermism (unable to regulate body heat)

Integumentary

Warm, dry skin below level of injury (neurogenic shock)

Respiratory

Injury at C1-3: Apnea, inability to cough

Injury at C4: Poor cough, diaphragmatic breathing, hypoventilation

Injury at C5-T6: Decreased respiratory reserve

Cardiovascular

Injury above T6: Bradycardia, hypotension, postural hypotension, absence of vasomotor tone

Gastrointestinal

Decreased or absent bowel sounds (paralytic ileus in injuries above T5), abdominal distention, constipation, fecal incontinence, fecal impaction

Urinary

Retention (for injuries at T1-L2), flaccid bladder (acute stages), spasticity with reflex bladder emptying (later stages)

Reproductive

Priapism, altered sexual function

Neurologic

Complete: Areflexic, flaccid paralysis and anesthesia below level of injury resulting in tetraplegia (injuries above C8) or paraplegia (injuries below C8), hyperactive deep tendon reflexes and bilaterally positive Babinski test (after resolution of spinal shock)

Incomplete: Mixed loss of voluntary motor activity and sensation

Musculoskeletal

Muscle atony (in flaccid state), contractures (in spastic state)

Pain

Neuropathic, musculoskeletal, and/or visceral

Possible Diagnostic Findings

Location of level and type of bony involvement on spinal x-ray. Injury, edema, compression on CT scan and MRI; positive finding on myelogram

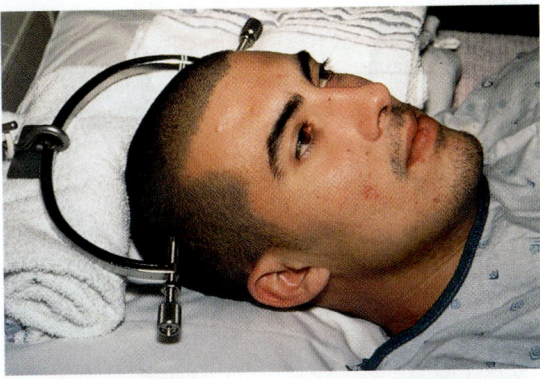

FIG. 60-5 Cervical traction is attached to tongs inserted in the skull. (Courtesy Michael S. Clement, MD, Mesa, Ariz.)

after injury can have significant impact on the general health and well-being of the individual with SCI. Nursing interventions include (1) teaching and counseling; (2) referring to programs such as smoking cessation classes, recreation and exercise programs, and alcohol treatment programs; and (3) performing routine physical examinations for non-neurologic problems. Screening and prevention programs must be accessible to and accommodate people with SCI. Nurses in these clinical settings should advocate for wheelchair-accessible examination rooms, adjustable-height examination tables, and appointment scheduling that allows extra time if needed.

◆ **Acute Care.** High cervical cord injury caused by flexion-rotation is the most complex SCI and is discussed in this section. Interventions for this type of injury can be modified for patients with less severe injuries.

◆ ***Immobilization.*** Proper immobilization of the neck involves the maintenance of a neutral position.

> ⚠ **SAFETY ALERT** **Cervical Spine Injuries**
> - Use a hard cervical collar and a backboard to stabilize the neck to prevent lateral rotation of the cervical spine.
> - Always keep the patient's body in correct alignment.
> - Turn the patient as a unit (logrolling) to prevent movement of the spine.

For cervical injuries, closed reduction with skeletal traction is used for early realignment (*reduction*) of the injury. Crutchfield (Fig. 60-5) or Gardner-Wells tongs or halo (halo ring) can provide this type of traction, using a rope that extends from the center of the device over a pulley to weights attached at the end. Traction must be maintained at all times. Possible displacement of the skull pins is a disadvantage of tongs. If displacement occurs, hold the head in a neutral position and get help. Immobilize the head while the surgeon reinserts the tongs.

No specific recommendations are available regarding maximum weight for traction. The surgeon may start with 10 pounds and add 5 pounds for each level to the injury. The goal is spinal reduction. Awake patients are monitored with x-ray as well as neurologic and pain assessment. Comatose patients require serial x-rays to evaluate the effects of traction.

The need for surgery is determined after the spine is reduced. After cervical fusion or other stabilization surgery, the patient may wear a hard cervical collar or sternal-occipital-mandibular immobilizer brace (Fig. 60-6).

When a patient can begin to mobilize after a stable injury (for which surgery is not needed), the halo frame can be attached to a special vest (*Halo vest*) (Fig. 60-7). This allows the patient to mobilize and ambulate while cervical bones fuse.

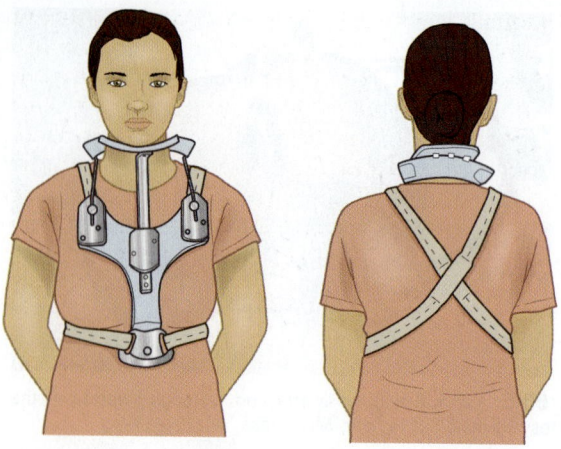

FIG. 60-6 Sternal-occipital-mandibular immobilizer brace.

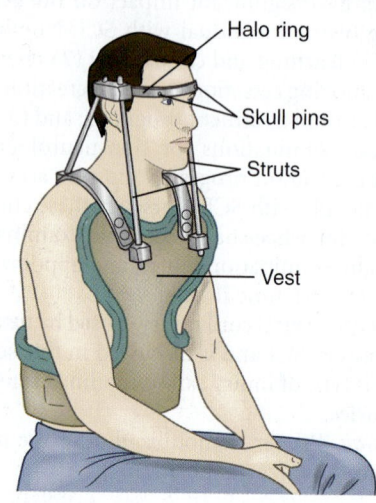

Halo ring
Skull pins
Struts
Vest

FIG. 60-7 Halo vest. The halo traction brace immobilizes the cervical spine, which allows the patient to ambulate and participate in self-care. (Modified from Urden LD, Stacy KM, Lough ME: *Priorities in critical care nursing,* ed 6, St Louis, 2012, Mosby.)

However, the halo is not indicated if the patient has ligament instability from the injury. That patient will require surgery. Infection at the sites of tong or halo pin insertion is another potential problem. Preventive care is based on hospital protocol. A common protocol involves cleansing sites twice a day with half strength peroxide and normal saline solution and applying an antibiotic ointment to act as a mechanical barrier to the entrance of bacteria. Patient and caregiver teaching for a patient with a halo vest is presented in Table 60-6.

Special beds are often used in the management of the patient with SCI (Fig. 60-8). Kinetic therapy involves continuous side-to-side rotation of a patient to 40 degrees or more to help prevent pulmonary complications. This lateral rotation also redistributes pressure, helping prevent pressure ulcers.

Patients with stable thoracic or lumbar spine injuries may be immobilized with a custom thoracolumbar orthosis (TLSO or body jacket) to inhibit spinal flexion, extension, and rotation. Alternately, a Jewett brace may be used to restrict forward flexion. Unstable injuries may require surgical decompression and fusion in addition to the TLSO or lumbosacral orthotic (LSO).

Immobilization of the neck of the patient with SCI prevents further injury, but the effects of immobility are profound. Meticulous skin care is critical because decreased sensation and

TABLE 60-6 Patient & Caregiver Teaching

Halo Vest Care

Include the following instructions when teaching the patient and caregiver management of a halo vest.

1. Inspect the pins on the halo traction ring. Report to HCP if pins are loose or signs of infection are present, including redness, tenderness, swelling, or drainage at insertion sites.
2. Clean around pin sites carefully with half-strength hydrogen peroxide, water, or alcohol on a cotton swab as directed.
3. Apply antibiotic ointment as prescribed.
4. To receive skin care, have patient lie down with the head resting on a pillow to reduce pressure on the brace. Loosen one side of the vest. Gently wash the skin under the vest with soap and water, rinse area, and then dry it thoroughly. At the same time, check the skin for pressure points, redness, swelling, bruising, or chafing. Close the open side and repeat the procedure on the opposite side.
5. If the vest becomes wet or damp, carefully dry it with a blow dryer.
6. Encourage patient to use assistive device (e.g., cane, walker) to improve balance; encourage use of flat shoes.
7. Remind patient to turn the entire body, not just the head and neck, when trying to look sideways.
8. In case of an emergency, keep a set of wrenches close to the halo vest at all times.
9. Mark the vest strap to maintain consistent buckling and fit.
10. Avoid grabbing bars or vest to assist the patient.
11. Keep sheepskin pad under vest. Change and wash pad at least weekly.
12. If perspiration or itching is a problem, encourage patient to wear a cotton T shirt under the sheepskin. The T-shirt can be modified with a Velcro seam closure on one side.

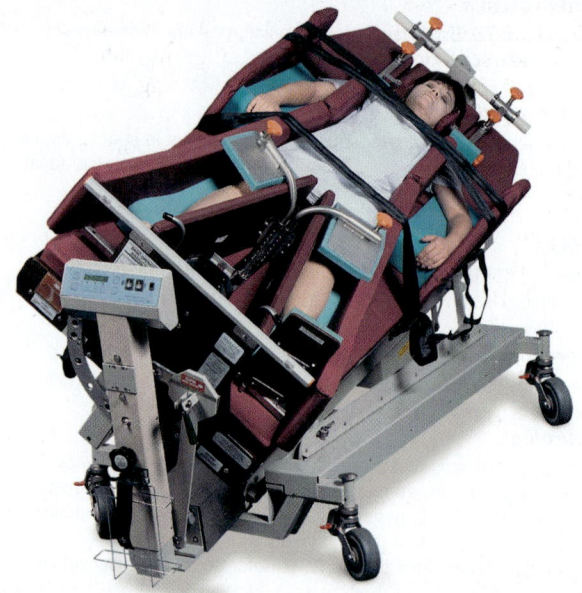

FIG. 60-8 The RotoRest Therapy System helps prevent and treat pulmonary complications for immobile patients, including those with unstable cervical, thoracic, and lumbar fractures. Kinetic therapy, the continual side-to-side bilateral rotation of the patient, redistributes pulmonary blood flow and mobilizes secretions to improve ventilation and perfusion matching. The therapy system also helps to prevent pressure ulcers. (Courtesy Arjo Huntleigh, Addison, Ill.)

circulation make the patient more susceptible to skin breakdown. Remove the patient's backboard as soon as possible and replace it with other forms of immobilization to prevent skin breakdown in the coccygeal and occipital areas. Fit cervical collars properly. Inspect areas under the halo vest or jacket or under braces or orthoses to assess the skin.

◆ *Respiratory Dysfunction.* Respiratory complications are the leading cause of death in people with SCI.[18] During the first 48 hours after injury, spinal cord edema may increase the level of dysfunction, and respiratory distress may occur. Patients with acute cervical SCI are initially managed in a monitored unit or ICU.[9] If the injury is at or above C4, the phrenic nerve leading to the diaphragm may be affected and breathing can stop. If the patient is exhausted from labored breathing or ABGs indicate inadequate oxygenation or ventilation, endotracheal intubation or tracheostomy and mechanical ventilation are needed. Monitor the patient carefully for respiratory compromise and be prepared for quick action if arrest occurs. Pneumonia and atelectasis may occur due to reduced vital capacity and loss of intercostal and abdominal muscle function, resulting in diaphragmatic breathing, pooled secretions, and ineffective cough.

Regularly assess (1) breath sounds, (2) ABGs, (3) tidal volume, (4) vital capacity, (5) skin color, (6) breathing patterns (especially use of accessory muscles), (7) subjective comments about the ability to breathe, and (8) amount and color of sputum. A PaO_2 (partial pressure of O_2 in arterial blood) greater than 60 mm Hg and a $PaCO_2$ (partial pressure of CO_2 in arterial blood) less than 45 mm Hg are acceptable values in a patient with uncomplicated tetraplegia. A patient who is unable to count to 10 aloud without taking a breath needs immediate attention.

In addition to ongoing assessment, intervene to maintain ventilation. Administer O_2 and provide ventilatory support until ABGs stabilize. Patients who experienced chest trauma or have difficulty weaning from the ventilator may require a tracheostomy for airway management.

Chest physiotherapy and assisted (augmented) coughing help to clear secretions. Assisted coughing simulates the action of the ineffective abdominal muscles during the expiratory phase of a cough. Place the heels of both hands just below the xiphoid process and exert firm upward pressure to the area timed with the patient's efforts to cough (see Fig. 67-7).

Perform tracheal suctioning if crackles or coarse breath sounds are present. Incentive spirometry can also be used to improve the patient's respiratory status. The older adult has more difficulty responding to hypoxia and hypercapnia. Thus aggressive chest physiotherapy, adequate oxygenation, and appropriate pain management are essential to maximize respiratory function and gas exchange. Other respiratory problems include nasal stuffiness and bronchospasm.

◆ *Cardiovascular Instability.* Because of unopposed vagal response, heart rate is slowed, often to less than 60 beats/minute. Any increase in vagal stimulation, as occurs with turning or suctioning, can cause cardiac arrest. Loss of sympathetic nervous system tone in peripheral vessels results in chronic low BP with potential postural hypotension. The lack of muscle tone to aid venous return can cause sluggish blood flow and predispose the patient to VTE. Dysrhythmias may also occur.

Frequently assess vital signs. If bradycardia is symptomatic, administer an anticholinergic drug such as atropine. A temporary or permanent pacemaker may be inserted. Maintain SBP greater than 90 mm Hg at all times and keep MAP between 85 and 90 mm Hg for the first 7 days following SCI. Manage hypotension with fluid replacement and a vasopressor agent, such as phenylephrine or norepinephrine.

If blood loss has occurred from other injuries, monitor hemoglobin and hematocrit and administer blood according to protocol. Also assess the patient for indications of hypovolemic shock secondary to hemorrhage.

Orthostatic hypotension is likely to occur in the patient with injury at T6 and above. The patient may complain of lightheadedness, dizziness, and nausea, and lose consciousness when moved from a bed to a chair. Assess orthostatic BP when mobilizing the patient. For symptomatic patients, use an abdominal binder and graduated compression stockings to promote venous return. Drugs used to increase intravascular volume include salt tablets and fludrocortisone. Midodrine may be given to promote blood vessel contraction and increase venous return.

Consider the effects of aging on the cardiovascular system of the older adult. The older patient is less able to manage the stress of traumatic injury because heart contractions weaken and cardiac output is reduced. Maximum heart rate is also reduced. In addition to the effects of aging, the older person may have cardiovascular disease.

Use low-molecular-weight heparin or low-dose heparin in combination, sequential compression devices (SCDs), or graduated compression stockings to promote venous return and prevent VTE.[11] Venous duplex studies may be performed before applying compression devices. Remove stockings every 8 hours for skin care. Also assess thighs and calves every shift for signs of DVT (e.g., deep reddish color, edema). Regularly perform range of motion (ROM) exercises and stretching. Continue VTE prophylaxis for 3 months following injury.

◆ *Fluid and Nutritional Management.* During the first 48 to 72 hours after the injury, the GI tract may stop functioning (*paralytic ileus*). A nasogastric tube must be inserted if ileus occurs. Because the patient cannot have oral intake, carefully monitor fluid and electrolyte status.

Nutrition should be started within the first 72 hours following injury. Specific solutions and additives are ordered based on individual requirements. Due to severe catabolism, a high-protein, high-calorie diet is needed for energy and tissue repair. If the patient cannot be fed through the GI system, either orally or through a feeding tube placed into the duodenum, parenteral nutrition should be initiated to reduce nitrogen losses that occur during the hypermetabolic state.

Once bowel sounds are present or flatus is passed, and the patient is not receiving mechanical ventilation, a formal swallow evaluation should be done. If no risk of aspiration is identified, gradually introduce oral food and fluids. If the patient fails the swallow evaluation or is unable to eat due to an endotracheal tube or tracheostomy, a more secure feeding tube may be placed in the stomach or jejunum (see Chapter 39).

❓ CHECK YOUR PRACTICE

You are working in the spinal cord unit. Today your 28-yr-old male patient with SCI at T6 weighs 168 pounds. When he was admitted 3 weeks ago, he weighed 186 pounds. He asks you, "Well, what is my weight? Are you gonna make me eat now? You know you can't do that."

• What assessment data are important for you to obtain?
• What interventions would help him avoid further weight loss and regain lean body mass?

Patients may experience anorexia due to depression, boredom with institutional food, or discomfort at being fed (often by a hurried nurse). Some patients have a normally small appetite. Occasionally refusal to eat is a means of maintaining control over the environment because of diminished or absent body control. If the patient is not eating adequately, assess the cause.

Based on assessment findings, make a contract with the patient with mutual goal setting for the diet. This contract gives the patient increased control and often results in improved nutritional intake. General measures may also be effective, such as providing a pleasant eating environment, allowing adequate time to eat (including any self-feeding the patient can achieve), encouraging the family to bring in special foods, and planning social rewards for eating.

Keep a calorie count and record the patient's daily weight to evaluate progress. If feasible, the patient should participate in recording calorie intake. Dietary supplements may be needed to meet nutritional goals. Include increased dietary fiber to promote bowel function. Avoid allowing the patient's nutritional intake to become a basis for a power struggle.

◆ *Bladder and Bowel Management.* Immediately after the injury, urine is retained because of the loss of autonomic and reflex control of the bladder and sphincter *(neurogenic bladder).* Because there is no sensation of fullness, overdistention of the bladder can result in reflux into the kidney and cause renal failure. Bladder overdistention may even result in rupture of the bladder. Thus an indwelling catheter may be inserted as soon as possible after injury. Ensure patency of the catheter by frequent inspection and irrigation if necessary. In some institutions, an HCP's order is required for this procedure. Strict aseptic technique for catheter care is essential to prevent infection. During the period of indwelling catheterization, encourage a large fluid intake. Check the catheter to prevent kinking and ensure free flow of urine.

Catheter-acquired urinary tract infection (CAUTI) is a common problem. The best method for preventing UTI is regular and complete bladder drainage. After the patient is stabilized, assess the best means of managing long-term urinary function. Usually the patient is started on an intermittent catheterization program. (CAUTI and intermittent catheterization are discussed in Chapter 45.)

Intermittent catheterization should be done four to six times daily to prevent bacterial overgrowth from urinary stasis. Keep urine residuals under 500 mL to prevent bladder distention. If the urine is cloudy or has a strong, or if the patient develops symptoms of a UTI (e.g., chills, fever, malaise), send a specimen for culture.

Consider age-related changes in renal function. Older adults are more likely to develop renal calculi. Older men may have benign prostatic hyperplasia, which may interfere with urinary flow and complicate management of urinary problems.

Constipation is generally a problem during spinal shock because no voluntary or involuntary *(reflex)* evacuation of the bowel occurs *(neurogenic bowel).* Start a bowel program during acute care. This involves choosing a rectal stimulant (suppository or small-volume enema) to be inserted daily at a regular time, followed by gentle digital stimulation or manual evacuation until evacuation is complete. Initially the program may be done in bed with the patient in the side-lying position. However, as soon as the patient has resumed sitting, the patient should be in the upright position on a padded bedside commode chair. These programs typically require 30 to 60 minutes to complete. Constipation can be reduced with adequate fluid intake, a healthy diet of fiber and vegetables, and increased activity and exercise.[19]

◆ *Temperature Control.* Because the patient has no vasoconstriction, piloerection (erection of body hair), or heat loss through perspiration below the level of injury, temperature control is largely external. Monitor the environment closely to maintain an appropriate temperature. Also regularly monitor the patient's body temperature. Do not use excessive covers or unduly expose the patient (such as during bathing). If an infection with high fever develops, more aggressive methods for temperature control may be needed (e.g., a cooling blanket).

◆ *Stress Ulcers.* Stress ulcers can occur in the patient with SCI because of the physiologic response to severe trauma and psychologic stress. Peak incidence of stress ulcers is 6 to 14 days after injury. Test stool and gastric contents daily for blood, and monitor the hematocrit for a slow drop. Histamine (H_2)-receptor blockers (e.g., ranitidine [Zantac], famotidine [Pepcid]) or proton pump inhibitors (e.g., pantoprazole [Protonix], omeprazole [Prilosec]) may be given prophylactically to decrease the secretion of HCl acid and prevent ulcers during the initial phase.

◆ *Sensory Deprivation.* To prevent sensory deprivation, compensate for the patient's absent sensations by stimulating the patient above the level of injury. Conversation, music, and interesting foods can be part of the nursing care plan. If the head of the bed must remain flat, provide prism glasses to help the patient read and watch television.

Help the patient avoid withdrawing from the environment. Promote adequate rest and sleep and assess for changes in mood. Depression is a common problem (discussed later in chapter on p. 1435).

◆ *Pain Management.* Musculoskeletal nociceptive pain can develop secondary to injuries to bones, muscles, and ligaments. This pain is aggravated with movement or palpation. Antiinflammatory drugs such as ibuprofen may help with pain. Opioids may also be used to manage nociceptive pain.

Visceral nociceptive pain is a dull, tender, or cramping pain in the thorax, abdomen, or pelvis. This type of pain may result from the bladder and bowel. Assess the patient's bowel and bladder function to avoid bladder distention or constipation. Other causes of nociceptive pain include UTI and ureteral calculus. Notify the HCP if the patient experiences persistent pain despite treatment. Diagnostic imaging may be needed to fully evaluate its cause.

Neuropathic pain in the initial phase is usually at the level of SCI. It may occur on one or both sides of the body within the affected dermatome, and up to three levels below. The patient will complain of hot, burning, tingling, shooting, electric pain. Gabapentin (Neurontin) or pregabalin (Lyrica) may be used to reduce pain. Neuropathic pain can occur months or years after SCI and become chronic and permanent. The patient's mood can affect the pain, as can sudden noise, constipation, or infections. Teach the patient and caregiver about possible pain triggers and offer relaxation therapy. Other modes of treatment may include tricyclic antidepressants, intrathecal medication, antiseizure drugs, epidural stimulation, and destructive surgical intervention.

◆ *Skin Care.* Healthy skin requires adequate blood circulation. Constant pressure in one position can compress blood vessels and limit blood supply, causing cell death and pressure ulcers. The most common location of pressure ulcers, which occur in about 25% of all patients with SCI, is the sacrum.[20]

Pressure ulcers are preventable with diligent nursing care. Perform a comprehensive visual and tactile examination of the skin at least once daily, with special attention to areas over bony prominences. Areas most vulnerable to breakdown include the sacrum, ischia, trochanters, and heels. Assess surgical incisions for healing and integrity of the skin under collars and braces.

Carefully position and reposition the patient at least every 2 hours, with gradual increases in the times between turns if no redness over bony prominences is seen at the time of turning. While the patient is supine in bed, float the heels to reduce pressure. Move the patient carefully during turns and transfers to avoid stretching and folding of soft tissues (*shear*) or abrasion.

Specialty mattresses are used to reduce the incidence of pressure ulcers. When the patient is moved to a chair or wheelchair, use pressure-relieving cushions. Pressure relief should be performed every 15 to 20 minutes when the patient is in a chair and should last 30 to 60 seconds each time.

Regularly assess nutritional status. Both weight loss and gain can contribute to skin breakdown. Adequate intake of protein is essential for skin health. Evaluation of prealbumin, total protein, and albumin can help identify inadequate protein intake. Stress the importance of nutrition for skin health.

◆ *Reflexes.* Once spinal shock is resolved, return of reflexes may complicate rehabilitation. Lacking control from the higher brain centers, reflexes are often hyperactive and produce exaggerated responses. Penile erection can occur from a variety of stimuli, causing embarrassment and discomfort. Spasms ranging from mild twitches to convulsive movements below the level of injury may also occur. The patient or caregiver may interpret this reflex activity as a return of function. Tactfully explain the reason for the activity. Inform the patient of the positive use of these reflexes in sexual, bowel, and bladder retraining. Spasms may be controlled with the use of antispasmodic drugs such as baclofen, dantrolene (Dantrium), and tizanidine (Zanaflex). Botulism toxin injections may also be given to treat severe spasticity.

◆ *Autonomic Hyperreflexia.* The return of reflexes after the resolution of spinal shock means patients with injury at T6 or higher may develop autonomic hyperreflexia. Autonomic hyperreflexia (also known as *autonomic dysreflexia*) is a massive uncompensated cardiovascular reaction mediated by the sympathetic nervous system. It involves stimulation of sensory receptors below the level of the SCI. The intact sympathetic nervous system below the level of injury responds to the stimulation with a reflex arteriolar vasoconstriction that increases BP, but the parasympathetic nervous system is unable to directly counteract these responses via the injured spinal cord. Baroreceptors in the carotid sinus and aorta sense the hypertension and stimulate the parasympathetic system. This results in a decrease in heart rate, but visceral and peripheral vessels do not dilate because efferent impulses cannot pass through the injured spinal cord.

The most common precipitating cause of autonomic hyperreflexia is a distended bladder or rectum. However, autonomic hyperreflexia can be caused by any sensory stimulation, including contraction of the bladder or rectum, stimulation of the skin, or stimulation of pain receptors.

Manifestations include hypertension (up to 300 mm Hg SBP), throbbing headache, marked diaphoresis above the level of injury, bradycardia (30 to 40 beats/minute), piloerection as a result of pilomotor spasm, flushing of the skin above the level of injury, blurred vision or spots in the visual fields, nasal congestion, anxiety, and nausea. Measure BP when a patient with SCI complains of a headache.

Autonomic hyperreflexia is a life-threatening condition that requires immediate resolution. If uncorrected, it can lead to status epilepticus, stroke, myocardial infarction, and even death.

Nursing interventions in this serious emergency include elevating the head of the bed 45 degrees or sitting the patient upright, determining the cause, and notifying the HCP. The most common cause is bladder irritation. Immediate catheterization to relieve bladder distention may be necessary. Instill lidocaine jelly in the urethra before catheterization. If a catheter is already in place, check it for kinks or folds. If it is plugged, perform small-volume irrigation slowly and gently to open the catheter, or insert a new catheter.

Stool impaction can also cause autonomic hyperreflexia. Perform a digital rectal examination (if trained) only after application of an anesthetic ointment to decrease rectal stimulation and avoid increasing symptoms. Remove all skin stimuli, such as constrictive clothing and tight shoes. Monitor BP frequently during the episode. If symptoms persist after the source has been relieved, administer a rapid onset and short duration agent such as nitroglycerin, nitroprusside, or hydralazine. Continue careful monitoring until vital signs stabilize.

Teach the patient and caregiver to recognize causes and symptoms of autonomic hyperreflexia (Table 60-7). They must understand the life-threatening nature of this dysfunction, know how to relieve the cause, and activate the ERS if needed.

◆ **Rehabilitation and Home Care.** Rehabilitation of the person with SCI is complex. With physical and psychologic care and intensive and specialized rehabilitation, the patient with SCI can learn to function at the highest level of wellness. All patients with new SCI should receive comprehensive inpatient rehabilitation in a rehabilitation unit or center that specializes in spinal cord rehabilitation.

Many of the problems identified in the acute period become chronic and continue throughout life. Rehabilitation focuses on retraining physiologic processes as well as extensive patient, caregiver, and family teaching about how to manage the physiologic and life changes resulting from the injury (Fig. 60-9).

TABLE 60-7 Patient & Caregiver Teaching

Autonomic Hyperreflexia

For a patient at risk for autonomic hyperreflexia, include the following information in the teaching plan for the patient and caregiver.

1. Signs and symptoms
   - Sudden onset of acute headache
   - Elevation in BP and/or reduction in pulse rate
   - Flushed face and upper chest (above level of injury) and pale extremities (below level of injury)
   - Sweating above level of injury
   - Nasal congestion
   - Feeling of apprehension
2. Immediate interventions
   - Raise the person to a sitting position.
   - Remove the noxious stimulus (fecal impaction, kinked urinary catheter, tight clothing).
   - Call the HCP if above actions do not relieve the signs and symptoms.
3. Measures to decrease the incidence of autonomic hyperreflexia
   - Maintain regular bowel function.
   - Use a local anesthetic to prevent autonomic hyperreflexia if manual rectal stimulation is used to promote bowel function.
   - Monitor urine output.
   - Encourage the patient to wear a Medic Alert bracelet indicating a history of risk for autonomic hyperreflexia.

Rehabilitation is an interprofessional team effort. Team members include rehabilitation nurses, HCPs, physical therapists, occupational therapists, speech therapists, vocational counselors, psychologists, therapeutic recreation specialists, prosthetists, orthotists, case managers, social workers, and dietitians.

Rehabilitation care is organized around the patient's goals and needs. The patient is expected to be involved in therapies and learn self-care for several hours each day. Such intensive work at a time when the patient is dealing with the sudden change in health and function can be stressful. Progress may be slow. The rehabilitation nurse has a pivotal role in providing encouragement, specialized nursing care, and patient and caregiver teaching, and in helping to coordinate efforts of the rehabilitation team.

Respiratory Rehabilitation. The patient with cervical injury above C3 requires mechanical ventilation because the phrenic nerve is not stimulated and thus the diaphragm is not functional. The patient will need around-the-clock caregivers who are knowledgeable about respiratory hygiene and tracheostomy care.[21] The rehabilitation nurse and respiratory therapist provide teaching on removing secretions through suctioning and assisted (augmented) coughing (see Fig. 67-7). The patient may also require chest percussion or postural drainage to manage secretions.

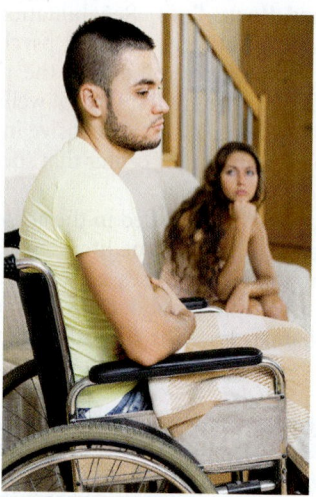

FIG. 60-9 A spinal cord injury has a major effect on a person's physical, emotional, and psychologic health. (©JackF/iStock/Thinkstock)

Some patients with high cervical SCI may have greatly increased mobility with phrenic nerve stimulators or electronic diaphragmatic pacemakers. These devices are not appropriate for all ventilator-dependent patients but may be helpful for those with an intact phrenic nerve. Some ventilators are also portable, allowing ventilator-dependent patients with tetraplegia to be mobile and less dependent. Patients and caregivers should be taught home ventilator and tracheostomy care, with referrals to appropriate community agencies as needed.

If the patient was successfully weaned from the ventilator during hospitalization, downsizing (gradual decrease in size) and removal of the tracheostomy will be done during rehabilitation. Teach assisted coughing, regular use of incentive spirometry, and breathing exercises to the patient with cervical injury who is not ventilator dependent. Limit exposure to people with fever, cold, and cough. Adhere to swallowing precautions (e.g., proper positioning of head and neck) and diet recommendations to prevent aspiration.

Neurogenic Bladder. Types of neurogenic bladder are presented in Table 60-8. Diagnostic and interprofessional care of neurogenic bladder is described in Table 60-9. The patient with SCI and a neurogenic bladder requires a comprehensive program to manage bladder function.

After the patient's overall condition is stable and assessment indicates return of neurologic reflexes, urodynamic testing (see Table 44-8) and a urine culture may be done. Many factors are considered when selecting a bladder management strategy. These include patient preference, upper extremity function, and availability of a caregiver. The type of bladder dysfunction (Table 60-8) also determines management options.

Various drugs can be used to treat the patient with a neurogenic bladder. Anticholinergic drugs (oxybutynin [Ditropan XL], tolterodine [Detrol]) may be used to suppress bladder contraction. α-Adrenergic blockers (e.g., terazosin, doxazosin [Cardura]) may be used to relax the urethral sphincter. Antispasmodic drugs (e.g., baclofen) may be used to decrease spasticity of pelvic floor muscles.

Numerous drainage methods are possible, including bladder reflex retraining if partial voiding control remains, indwelling catheter, intermittent catheterization, and external catheter (condom catheter). Evaluate long-term use of an indwelling catheter because of the associated high incidence of CAUTI, fistula formation, and diverticula. However, for some patients

TABLE 60-8 Types of Neurogenic Bladder

Type	Characteristics	Causes	Manifestations
Uninhibited bladder (reflexic)	• No inhibitions influence time and place of voiding • Bladder empties in response to stretching of bladder wall	• Results from lesions above the pons • Observed in stroke, brain tumor, brain trauma	• Incontinence, frequency, urgency • Voiding is unpredictable and incomplete

Upper motor neuron bladder (mixed areflexic or hyperactive)	• *Mixed A type* (most common):
	  • Bladder is flaccid and external sphincter is spastic, leading to urinary retention
	• *Mixed B type*:
	  • Bladder is spastic with flaccid external sphincter leading to urinary incontinence.
		• Results from lesions between pons and sacral spinal cord
		• Observed in SCI or multiple sclerosis involving the cervicothoracic spinal cord
			• Detrusor-sphincter dyssynergia
			• Can lead to high bladder pressures and kidney damage from urinary reflux
			• Sensory function impaired

Lower motor neuron bladder (areflexic)	• Bladder acts as if all motor functions were paralyzed • Bladder fills without emptying	• Results from lower motor neuron injury caused by trauma involving S2-4 • Lesions of cauda equina, pelvic nerves	• If sensory function intact, patient feels bladder distention and hesitancy. • No control of micturition, resulting in over distention of bladder, overflow incontinence, and UTI

TABLE 60-9 Interprofessional Care
Neurogenic Bladder

Diagnostic Assessment
- History and physical examination, including neurologic examination
- Laboratory: Urinalysis, urine culture and sensitivity, blood urea nitrogen, serum creatinine, creatinine clearance
- Urodynamic testing (postvoid residual, cystometric testing, electromyography, urethral pressure profile)

Management
- Patient teaching
- Bladder retraining: time voiding, manual expression, intermittent catheterization
- Fluid schedule: intake of 1800-2000 mL/day
- Indwelling urinary catheter

Drug Therapy
- Tricyclic antidepressants
- Anticholinergic drugs
- α-Adrenergic blockers
- Antispasmodics
- Botulinum toxin injection into bladder wall

Bladder and/or Urethral Surgical Therapy
- Bladder augmentation
- Sphincter resection or removal (sphincterotomy)
- Electrode placement for electrical stimulation
- Urinary diversion
- Urethral stents and balloon dilation
- Artificial urinary sphincter

TABLE 60-10 Patient & Caregiver Teaching
Bowel Management After Spinal Cord Injury

For the patient with a spinal cord injury, include the following information about bowel management in the teaching plan for the patient and caregiver.
1. Optimal nutritional intake includes the following:
   - Three well-balanced meals each day
   - Two servings from the milk group
   - Two or more servings from the meat group, including beef, pork, poultry, eggs, fish
   - Four or more servings from the vegetable and fruit groups
   - Four or more servings from the bread and cereal group
2. Fiber intake should be approximately 20-30 g/day. Increase the amount of fiber eaten gradually over 1-2 wk.
3. At least 2 to 3 L of fluid should be consumed per day unless contraindicated. Water or fruit juices should be used (fluid softens hard stools). Caffeinated beverages such as coffee, tea, and cola should be limited (caffeine stimulates fluid loss through urination).
4. Avoid foods that produce gas (e.g., beans) or upper GI upset (e.g., spicy foods).
5. *Timing:* Establish a regular schedule for bowel evacuation. A good time is 30 min after the first meal of the day.
6. *Position:* If possible, an upright position with feet flat on the floor or on a step stool enhances bowel evacuation. Staying on the toilet, commode, or bedpan for longer than 20-30 min may cause skin breakdown. Based on stability, someone may need to stay with the patient.
7. *Activity:* Exercise is important for bowel function. In addition to improving muscle tone, it increases appetite and GI transit time. Exercise muscles, including stretching, ROM, position changing, and functional movement.
8. *Drug treatment:* Suppositories may be needed to stimulate a bowel movement. Manual stimulation of the rectum may also be helpful in initiating defecation. Use stool softeners as needed to regulate stool consistency. Use oral laxatives only if necessary.

this may be the best option. Patients with indwelling catheters need to have adequate fluid intake (at least 3 to 4 L/day). Regularly check the patency of the indwelling catheter. Frequency of routine catheter changes ranges widely depending on the type of catheter used and agency policy.

Intermittent catheterization is the most commonly recommended method of bladder management (see Chapter 45). Nursing assessment is important in selecting the time interval between catheterizations. Initially, catheterization is done every 4 hours. Bladder volume can be assessed before catheterization using a portable bladder ultrasound machine. If less than 200 mL of urine is measured, the time interval until catheterization may be extended. If more than 500 mL of urine is measured, the time interval is shortened. Intermittent catheterization is usually done four to six times daily.

Urinary diversion surgery may be needed if the patient has repeated UTI with renal involvement or repeated stones, or if therapeutic interventions have been unsuccessful. Surgical treatment of neurogenic bladder includes bladder neck revision (sphincterotomy), bladder augmentation (augmentation cystoplasty), penile prosthesis, artificial sphincter, perineal ureterostomy, cystotomy, vesicotomy, and anterior urethral transplantation. (Urinary diversion procedures are discussed in Chapter 45.)

No matter which bladder management strategy is selected, teach the patient, caregiver, and family successful self-management. Inform them about the various management techniques, how to obtain necessary supplies, care of supplies and equipment, and when to seek health care.

Neurogenic Bowel. Careful management of bowel evacuation is necessary in the patient with SCI because voluntary control of this function may be lost. Usual measures for

preventing constipation include high-fiber diet and adequate fluid intake (see Table 42-7). Patient and caregiver teaching guidelines related to bowel management are presented in Table 60-10. However, these measures alone may not be adequate to stimulate evacuation. In addition, suppositories (bisacodyl or glycerin) or small-volume enemas and digital stimulation (performed 20 to 30 minutes after suppository insertion) by the nurse or patient may be needed. In the patient with an upper motor neuron injury, digital stimulation is needed to relax the external sphincter to promote defecation. A stool softener such as docusate sodium can be used to regulate stool consistency. Oral stimulant laxatives should be used only if absolutely necessary and not on a regular basis.

Valsalva maneuver and manual stimulation are useful in patients with lower motor neuron injuries. Because the Valsalva maneuver requires intact abdominal muscles, it is used in patients with injuries below T12. In general, a bowel movement every other day is considered adequate. However, consider preinjury patterns. Fecal incontinence can result from too much stool softener or a fecal impaction.

Record all bowel movements, including amount, time, and consistency. Timing of defecation may also be important. Planning bowel evacuation for 30 to 60 minutes after the first meal of the day may enhance success by taking advantage of the gastrocolic reflex induced by eating. This reflex may also be stimulated by drinking a warm beverage immediately after the meal. Patient, caregiver, and family teaching is required to promote successful independent bowel management. Timing of the bowel program should also be discussed among the inter-professional team so there are no interruptions when the patient is doing therapy (e.g., swimming pool therapy).

◆ *Spasticity.* Weeks after the initial SCI, the patient may start to have involuntary spasms of the muscles below the level of injury. This indicates resolution of the spinal shock or flaccid stage of SCI. Spasticity can be both beneficial and undesirable. It aids with mobility, especially for the patient with incomplete SCI. Spasticity improves circulation by promoting venous return and decreases orthostatic hypotension and the risk of VTE. Unfortunately, the patient with marked spasticity and tone may have difficulty with positioning and mobility second-ary to the spasms. Spasms can cause significant pain and make activities of daily living (ADLs) difficult for the patient.

The Ashworth and modified Ashworth scales are used to evaluate spasticity (www.scireproject.com/outcome-measures-new/ashworth-and-modified-ashworth-scale-mas). Treatment strategies include ROM exercises to prevent muscle and joint tightness and reduce the risk of contracture. Antispasmodic medications such as baclofen or tizanidine may be adminis-tered. Botulinum toxin injection is useful for specific muscle involvement.

◆ *Skin Care.* Prevention of pressure ulcers is part of the life-long treatment plan following SCI. Nurses in rehabilitation are responsible for teaching the patient and caregiver about daily skin care. A comprehensive visual and tactile examination should be performed daily with special attention to bony prom-inences. Teach the patient and caregiver to carefully move the patient to prevent injury and to reposition at least every 2 hours while in bed and every 15 to 20 minutes when in a chair or wheelchair. Also include information on the importance of adequate nutrition and how it affects the skin.

Protect the skin by avoiding thermal injury. Burns can be caused by hot food or liquids, bath or shower water that is too warm, radiators, heating pads, and uninsulated plumbing. Thermal injury also can result from extreme cold (*frostbite*). Injuries may not be noticed until severe damage has occurred. Anticipatory guidance about potential risks is essential. Patient and caregiver teaching related to skin care is provided in Table 60-11.

◆ *Pain Management.* The acute pain of the initial injury may persist during the first few weeks of rehabilitation. Assess, evalu-ate, and treat pain routinely. Use analgesics and interventions

such as massage and repositioning to help the patient during therapy.

Chronic pain can also result from overuse of muscles in the shoulders and arms for movement and repositioning. Sleep may be disrupted due to pain. The patient may benefit from referral to an HCP who specializes in pain management.

◆ *Sexuality.* Sexuality is an important issue regardless of the patient's age or sex. To provide accurate and sensitive coun-seling and teaching about sexuality, be aware of your own sexuality and understand the human sexual responses. When discussing sexual potential, use scientific terminology rather than slang whenever possible. Knowledge of the level and com-pleteness of injury is needed to understand the male patient's potential for orgasm, erection, and fertility, and the patient's capacity for sexual satisfaction.

Men normally have two types of erections: psychogenic and reflex. The process of *psychogenic erection* begins in the brain with sexual thoughts. Signals from the brain are sent through the nerves of the spinal cord to the T10-L2 levels. The signals are then relayed to the penis and trigger an erection. Men with low-level incomplete injuries are more likely to have psycho-genic erection than men with higher-level incomplete injuries. Men with complete injuries are less likely to experience psycho-genic erection.

A *reflex erection* occurs with direct physical contact to the penis or other erotic areas. A reflex erection is involuntary and can occur without sexually stimulating thoughts. These reflex erections are often short lived and uncontrolled and cannot be maintained or summoned at the time of coitus. The nerves that control a man's ability to have a reflex erection are located in the sacral nerves (S2-4) of the spinal cord. Most men with SCI are able to have a reflex erection with physical stimulation regardless of the extent of the injury if the S2-4 nerve pathways are not damaged.

Treatment for erectile dysfunction includes drugs, vacuum devices, and surgical procedures. Phosphodiesterase inhibitors such as sildenafil (Viagra) have become the first-line treat-ment in men with SCI. Sexual stimulation is required to get an erection after taking the medication. Penile injection of vasoactive substances (papaverine, prostaglandin E) is another medical treatment. Risks include prolonged penile erection (*priapism*) and scarring, so these substances should be con-sidered only after failure of sildenafil. Vacuum suction devices use negative pressure to encourage blood flow into the penis. Erection is maintained by a constriction band placed at the base of the penis. The main surgical option is implantation of a penile prosthesis.[22] (Erectile dysfunction is discussed in Chapter 54.)

SCI affects male fertility, causing poor sperm quality and ejaculatory dysfunction. Recent advances in methods of sperm retrieval include penile vibratory stimulation and electroejacu-lation. Combined with ovulation induction and intrauterine insemination of the female partner, these techniques have changed the prognosis for men with SCI to father children from unlikely to a reasonable possibility of successful outcomes.

The effect of SCI on female sexual response is less clear. A woman of childbearing age with SCI usually remains fertile. The injury does not affect the ability to become pregnant or to deliver normally through the birth canal. Menses may cease for as long as 6 months after injury. If sexual activity is resumed, protection against unplanned pregnancy is needed. A normal pregnancy may be complicated by UTI, anemia, and autonomic

---

TABLE 60-11 Patient & Caregiver Teaching
Skin Care After Spinal Cord Injury

To prevent skin breakdown in a patient with spinal cord injury, include the following instructions when teaching the patient and caregiver.

Change Position Frequently
- If in a wheelchair, lift self and shift weight every 15-30 min.
- If in bed, change position with a regular turning schedule (at least every 2 hr) that includes sides, back, and abdomen.
- Use pressure-reducing mattresses and wheelchair cushions (not eggcrate).
- Use pillows to protect bony prominences when in bed.

Monitor Skin Condition
- Inspect skin frequently for areas of redness, swelling, and breakdown.
- Keep fingernails trimmed to avoid scratches and abrasions.
- If a wound develops, follow standard wound care procedures.

hyperreflexia. Because uterine contractions are not felt, precipitous delivery is always a danger.[23]

Care should be taken not to dislodge an indwelling catheter during sexual activity. If an external catheter is used, instruct the patient to refrain from fluids and remove the catheter before sexual activity. The bowel program should include evacuation the morning of sexual activity. Encourage the patient to inform the partner that incontinence is always possible. The woman may need a water-soluble lubricant to supplement diminished vaginal secretions and facilitate vaginal penetration.

Open discussion with the patient regarding sexual rehabilitation is essential. This important aspect of rehabilitation should be addressed by a professional trained in sexual counseling. A nurse or other rehabilitation professional with such expertise provides support for the patient and partner, with an emphasis on open communication. Alternative methods of obtaining sexual satisfaction, such as oral-genital sex (cunnilingus and fellatio), may be suggested. Explicit films may also be used, such as a film demonstrating the sexual activities of a patient with paraplegia and a nondisabled partner. Use graphics cautiously because they may focus too much on the mechanics of sex rather than on the relationship.

Grief and Depression. Depression after SCI is common and disabling.[24] Patients with SCI may feel an overwhelming sense of loss. They may temporarily lose control over everyday activities as they depend on others for ADLs and for life-sustaining measures. Patients may believe they are useless and burdens to their families. At a life stage when independence is of great importance, they may be totally dependent on others.

Working through grief is a difficult, lifelong process for which the patient needs support and encouragement. Table 60-12 summarizes the grief response to SCI and appropriate nursing interventions. With recent advances in rehabilitation, the patient is often independent physically and discharged from the rehabilitation center before completing the grief process.

The goal of recovery is related more to adjustment than to acceptance. *Adjustment* implies the ability to go on with living with certain limitations. Although the patient who is cooperative and accepting is easier to treat, expect a wide fluctuation of emotions from a patient with SCI. Your role in grief work is to allow mourning as part of the rehabilitation process. Maintaining hope is important during the grieving process and should not be interpreted as denial.

When the patient is depressed, sympathy is not helpful. Treat the patient as an adult and encourage participation in care planning. A primary nurse relationship is helpful. Staff planning and sessions in which staff members can express their feelings help to provide consistency of care. To adjust, the patient needs continual support throughout the rehabilitation process in the form of acceptance, affection, and caring. Be attentive when the patient needs to talk and sensitive to needs at various stages of the grief process.

Although depression during the grief process usually lasts days to weeks, some individuals may become clinically depressed and require treatment for depression. Evaluation by a psychiatric nurse or psychiatrist is recommended. Treatment may include drugs and therapy. Treatment is maximized when the patient's personal preferences are identified and care is tailored to individual needs.

The patient's caregiver and family also require counseling to avoid promoting dependency in the patient through guilt or misplaced sympathy. The family also experiences intense grieving. A support group of family members and friends of patients

TABLE 60-12	**Grief Response in Spinal Cord Injury**
Patient Behavior	**Nursing Intervention**
Shock and Denial	
Struggle for survival, complete dependence, excessive sleep, withdrawal, fantasies, unrealistic expectations	• Provide honest information. • Use simple diagrams to explain injury. • Encourage patient to begin road to recovery. • Establish agreement to use and improve all current abilities while not denying the possibility of future improvement.
Anger	
Refusal to discuss paralysis, decreased self-esteem, manipulation, hostile and abusive language	• Coordinate care with patient and encourage self-care. • Support family members. • Use humor appropriately. • Allow patient outbursts of emotions. • Do not allow fixation on injury.
Depression	
Sadness, pessimism, anorexia, nightmares, insomnia, agitation, "blues," suicidal preoccupation, refusal to participate in any self-care activities	• Encourage family involvement and use of community resources. • Plan graded steps in rehabilitation to give success with minimal opportunity for frustration. • Give cheerful and willing assistance with ADLs. • Avoid sympathy. • Use firm kindness.
Adjustment and Acceptance	
Planning for future, actively participating in therapy, finding personal meaning in experience and continuation of growth, returning to premorbid personality.	• Remember patients have unique personalities. • Balance support systems to encourage independence. • Set goals with patient input. • Emphasize potential.

with SCI can help family members increase their participation and knowledge of the grieving process, physical difficulties, rehabilitation plan, and meaning of the disability.

Evaluation

Expected outcomes are that the patient with SCI will:
- Maintain adequate ventilation and have no signs of respiratory distress
- Maintain adequate circulation and BP
- Maintain intact skin over bony prominences
- Maintain adequate nutrition
- Establish a bowel management program based on neurologic function and personal preference
- Establish a bladder management program based on neurologic function, caregiver status, and lifestyle choices
- Experience no episodes of autonomic hyperreflexia

Additional information on expected outcomes for the patient with SCI is addressed in eNursing Care Plan 60-1 available on the website for this chapter.

Gerontologic Considerations: Spinal Cord Injury

Because of the aging population and increased work and recreational activities among older adults, more of them experience SCI (Fig. 60-10). Falls are the leading cause of SCI for people age 65 years and older. Older adults with traumatic injuries experience more complications than younger patients, are hospitalized longer, and have higher mortality rates.

Demographics of people living with SCI are changing. Given their longer life spans, an increasing number of older adults are now living with SCI. Chronic illnesses associated with aging can also have a serious impact on these older adults. As patients with SCI age, both individual aging changes and length of time since injury can affect functional ability. For example, bowel and bladder dysfunction can increase with the duration and severity of SCI.

Health promotion and screening are important for the older patient with SCI. Daily skin inspections and UTI prevention measures are critical. Regular breast examinations for women and prostate cancer screening for men are recommended. Cardiovascular disease is the most common cause of morbidity and mortality among older adults with SCI. The lack of sensation, including chest pain, in people with high-level injuries may mask acute myocardial ischemia. Altered autonomic nervous system function and decreases in physical activity can place patients at risk for cardiovascular problems, including hypertension.

To decrease the risk of injury, instruct patients and caregivers on fall prevention strategies. For example, remove loose rugs from the floor, use a step stool or a long-handled reacher to access high shelves, and install handrails on stairs.

Rehabilitation for the older person with SCI may take longer because of preexisting conditions and poorer health status at the time of initial injury. An interprofessional team approach to rehabilitation is essential in preventing secondary complications associated with SCI, especially in older adults.

SPINAL CORD TUMORS

Spinal cord tumors can have a devastating impact due to spinal compression and neurologic dysfunction. Tumors are classified as *primary* (arising from some component of spinal cord, dura, nerves, or vessels) or *secondary* (from primary growths in other places in the body that have metastasized to the spinal cord).[25,26]

Etiology and Pathophysiology

Spinal cord tumors are further classified as *extradural* (outside the dura), *intradural extramedullary* (between the spinal cord and dura), and *intramedullary* (within the substance of spinal cord itself) (Fig. 60-11, Table 60-13).

Extradural tumors account for about 60% of all spinal tumors. They include metastatic cancer and benign schwannomas. Many patients with cancer have metastasis to the spine.[27] These metastatic lesions can invade intradurally and compress the spinal cord. Tumors that commonly metastasize to the spinal epidural space are those that spread to bone, such as prostate, breast, lung, and kidney cancer.

Because many spinal cord tumors are slow growing, their symptoms are due to the mechanical effects of slow compression

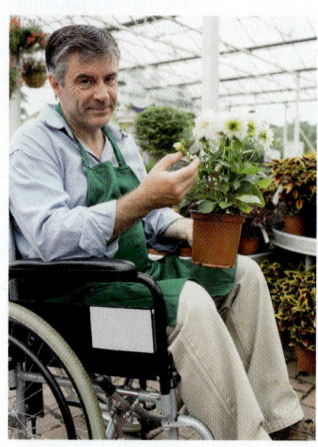

FIG. 60-10 An increasing number of older adults are living with a chronic spinal cord injury. (©WavebreakmediaLtd/WavebreakMedia/Thinkstock)

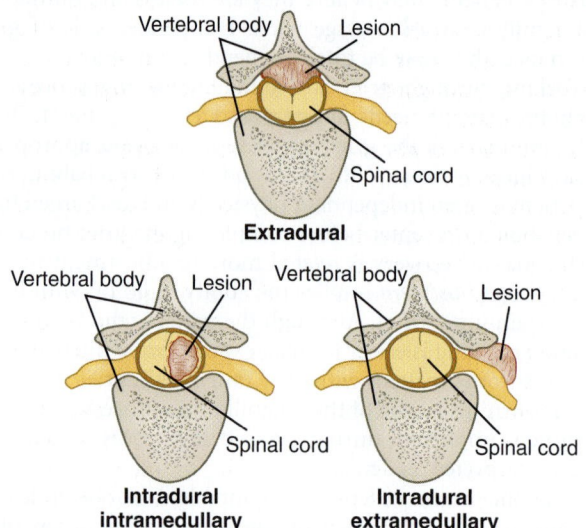

FIG. 60-11 Types of spinal cord tumors.

TABLE 60-13	**Classification of Spinal Cord Tumors**		
Type	**Incidence**	**Treatment**	**Prognosis**
Extradural Outside spinal cord in extradural space	Metastatic lesions and benign schwannomas	Relief of cord pressure by surgical laminectomy, radiation, chemotherapy, or combination approach.	*Benign:* Excellent with resection. *Metastatic:* Poor. Treatment usually palliative.
Intradural Extramedullary Within dura mater but outside spinal cord	Mostly benign. Meningiomas, neurofibromas, and schwannomas	Complete surgical removal of tumor (if possible). Partial removal followed by radiation.	Usually very good if no damage to cord from compression.
Intramedullary Within spinal cord	Mostly benign Astrocytomas, ependymomas	Complete surgical removal of tumor (if possible). Partial removal followed by radiation.	Usually very good if no damage to cord from compression. Complete surgical resection of astrocytomas difficult.

and irritation of nerve roots, displacement of the spinal cord, or gradual obstruction of the vascular supply. The slowness of growth does not cause autodestruction (secondary injury) as in traumatic SCI. Thus complete functional restoration may be possible when the tumor is removed.

Clinical Manifestations

Both sensory and motor problems may result, with the location and extent of the tumor determining the severity and extent of the problem. The most common early symptom of a spinal cord tumor is back pain or pain radiating along the compressed nerve route. Location of the pain depends on the level of compression. Pain may worsen with activity, coughing, straining, and/or lying down. Motor disturbance may also occur as slowly increasing clumsiness, weakness, and spasticity. Paralysis can develop. Sensory disruption is later marked by coldness, numbness, and tingling in one or more extremities. Bladder disturbances are marked by urgency with difficulty in starting the flow, progressing to retention with overflow incontinence.

❖ NURSING AND INTERPROFESSIONAL MANAGEMENT: SPINAL CORD TUMORS

Extradural tumors can be seen on routine spinal x-rays, whereas intradural extramedullary and intramedullary tumors require MRI, CT scan, or CT myelogram for detection. Cerebrospinal fluid (CSF) analysis may reveal tumor cells. Patients with tumors suspicious for metastatic disease will require an oncology referral and further diagnostic testing to identify the primary cancer.

Compression of the spinal cord is an emergency. Relief of ischemia related to compression is the goal of therapy. Corticosteroids are generally prescribed immediately to relieve tumor-related edema. Dexamethasone, often in large doses, may also be administered to treat edema.

Indications for surgery depend on the type of tumor and neurologic deficit. Emergency surgery may be needed to decompress the spinal cord, obtain tissue for pathology, and help to determine appropriate adjunctive treatment.[28] Primary spinal tumors may be removed with the goal of cure. In patients with metastatic tumors, treatment is primarily palliative, with the goal of restoring or preserving neurologic function, stabilizing the spine, and alleviating pain. Radiation and/or chemotherapy may be used to treat the tumor.

Relieving pain and maximizing neurologic function are the ultimate goals of treatment. Assess the patient's neurologic status before and after treatment. Administering analgesia as needed is an important nursing responsibility. Depending on the amount of neurologic dysfunction, care of the patient may be similar to that of a patient recovering from SCI.

CRANIAL NERVE DISORDERS

Cranial nerve disorders are commonly classified as peripheral neuropathies. The 12 pairs of cranial nerves are considered the peripheral nerves of the brain. The disorders usually involve the motor and/or sensory branches of a single nerve (*mononeuropathies*). Causes of cranial nerve problems include tumors, trauma, infection, inflammatory processes, and unknown (*idiopathic*) causes. Two cranial nerve disorders discussed in this chapter are trigeminal neuralgia and Bell's palsy.

TRIGEMINAL NEURALGIA

Trigeminal neuralgia (TN) (*tic douloureux*) is characterized by sudden, usually unilateral, severe, brief, stabbing, recurrent episodes of pain in the distribution of the trigeminal nerve. It is diagnosed in about 12 per 100,000 Americans each year and occurs approximately twice as often in women as in men. More than 90% of cases are diagnosed in people over the age of 50 years.[29]

TN is classified as *classic* (TN 1) or *atypical* (TN 2). Patients may experience both types. Although this condition is considered benign, pain intensity and lifestyle disruption can cause marked physical and psychologic dysfunction (even suicide).

Etiology and Pathophysiology

The trigeminal nerve (CN V) has both motor and sensory branches. The sensory (afferent) branches of the second and third division (maxillary and mandibular branches) of CN V are most often affected in TN[30] (Fig. 60-12).

The majority of cases result from vascular compression of the trigeminal nerve root by an abnormal loop of the superior cerebellar artery. This artery compresses the nerve as it exits the brainstem. Constant compression of the blood vessel appears to lead to chronic injury, causing demyelination of the nerve and impairment of the nociceptive system.[31] In some cases, TN may be secondary to underlying pathology, such as multiple sclerosis, shingles, or masses in the cerebellum or brainstem.

Clinical Manifestations

The first episode of TN is sudden with a memorable onset. Diagnosis is based almost entirely on history. In TN 1, the patient experiences an abrupt onset of paroxysms of excruciating pain described as a burning, knifelike, or lightning-like

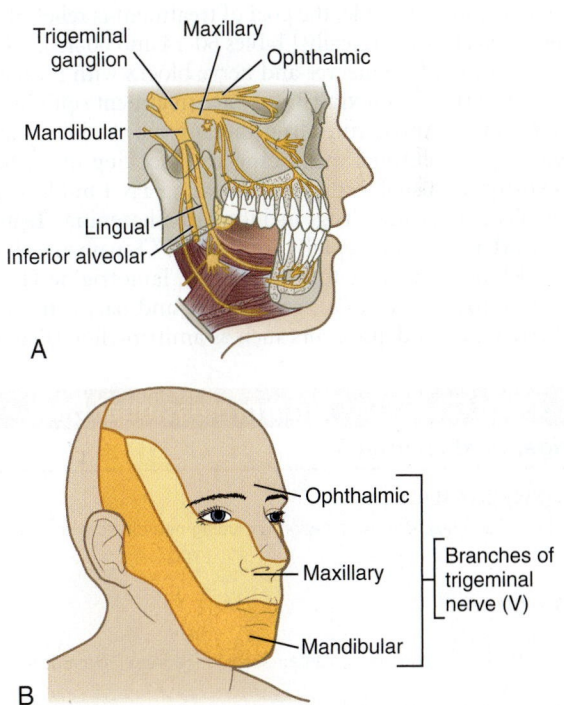

FIG. 60-12   A, Trigeminal nerve (CNV) and its three main divisions: ophthalmic, maxillary, and mandibular nerves. **B,** Cutaneous innervation of the head. (Modified from Patton KT, Thibodeau GA: *Anatomy and physiology,* ed 8, St Louis, 2013, Mosby.)

shock in the lips, upper or lower gums, cheek, forehead, or side of the nose. Intense pain, facial twitching, grimacing, and frequent blinking and tearing of the eye occur during the acute attack (giving rise to the term *tic douloureux*). Some patients may also experience facial sensory loss. Attacks are usually brief, lasting only seconds to 2 or 3 minutes, and are unilateral.

Recurrences are unpredictable and may occur several times a day, or weeks or months apart. After the pain-free *(refractory)* period, a phenomenon known as *clustering* can occur. Clustering is characterized by a cycle of pain and refractoriness that continues for hours.

Painful episodes are usually initiated by a triggering mechanism of light touch at a specific point *(trigger zone)* along the distribution of the nerve branches. Precipitating stimuli include chewing, brushing the teeth, feeling a hot or cold blast of air on the face, washing the face, yawning, or even talking. As a result, the patient may eat improperly, neglect hygienic practices, wear a cloth over the face, and withdraw from interaction with others. The patient may sleep excessively as a means of coping with pain.

TN 2 is distinguished by constant aching, burning, crushing, or stabbing pain. The pain has a lower intensity and does not subside completely. The distinct attacks associated with TN 1 do not occur in TN 2.

Diagnostic Studies

MRI with or without contrast is used to rule out other causes of pain, such as sinusitis, extracranial and cavernous sinus masses, cancer, multiple sclerosis, brain lesions in the thalamus or brainstem, or masses in the cerebellopontine angle.[32] A complete neurologic assessment is done, including audiologic evaluation. Results are usually normal.

Interprofessional Care

Once a diagnosis is made, the goal of treatment is relief of pain either medically or surgically (Tables 60-14 and 60-15). Electrical stimulation of the nerves and nerve blocks with local anesthetics or botulinum toxin (Botox) are treatment options.

Drug Therapy. Antiseizure drug therapy may reduce pain by stabilizing the neuronal membrane and blocking nerve firing. These drugs are usually effective in treating TN 1 but less effective in TN 2. First-line drugs include carbamazepine (Tegretol) and oxcarbazepine (Trileptal). Topiramate (Topamax), clonazepam (Klonopin), phenytoin (Dilantin), lamotrigine (Lamictal), divalproex (Depakote), gabapentin, and baclofen may be used. Tricyclic antidepressants such as amitriptyline (Elavil) or nortriptyline (Pamelor) can be used to treat constant burning or aching pain. Analgesics or opioids are usually not effective in controlling pain in TN1 but may help with pain in TN2.

Surgical Therapy. If a conservative approach is ineffective or the patient is unable to tolerate adverse effects of medications, surgical therapy is available (Table 60-15). In percutaneous procedures, affected nerve fibers are damaged to eliminate pain. Although most patients are pain free after any of the procedures, pain relief lasts longer with microvascular decompression. Recurrence rates are about 50% at 1 year.[30-32]

❖ NURSING MANAGEMENT: TRIGEMINAL NEURALGIA

The patient with trigeminal neuralgia is primarily treated as an outpatient. Assess the attacks in detail, including triggering factors, characteristics, frequency, and pain management techniques. This information helps you to plan patient care. Include

TABLE 60-14	**Interprofessional Care**

Trigeminal Neuralgia

Diagnostic Assessment
- History and physical examination (including neurologic examination)
- MRI

Management
- Drug therapy
  - Antiseizure drugs (e.g., carbamazepine [Tegretol], oxcarbazepine [Trileptal])
  - gabapentin (Neurontin)
  - Tricyclic antidepressants (e.g., amitriptyline)
- Local nerve block
- Surgical therapy (Table 60-15)

TABLE 60-15	**Surgical Therapy for Trigeminal Neuralgia**

Procedure	Description
Percutaneous Procedures	
Glycerol rhizotomy (injection into one or more branches of trigeminal nerve) (Fig. 60-13)	• Thin needle inserted through puncture in cheek and guided through natural opening in base of skull. • Glycerol injected into trigeminal ganglion. • Procedure can be repeated multiple times.
Percutaneous radiofrequency rhizotomy	• Needle passed through cheek thorough a natural opening in base of skull. • Patient is awakened and a small electric current is passed through the needled causing tingling. • When the needle is positioned so the tingling occurs in the same area of pain, patient is sedated again and radiofrequency current is used to destroy part of the nerve. • Can result in facial numbness (although some degree of sensation may be retained), corneal anesthesia, and trigeminal motor weakness
Balloon compression	• Cannula is inserted through cheek and guided to a natural opening in the base of skull. • Soft catheter with a balloon tip is threaded through cannula. • Balloon is inflated and mechanical compression damages trigeminal nerve
Surgical Procedures	
Microvascular decompression (open surgery)	• Small craniotomy is first performed behind the ear (suboccipital craniotomy). • Blood vessels that appear to be compressing the nerve at the root entry zone where it exits the pons are then displaced and repositioned.
Gamma knife radiosurgery	• Uses stereotactic localization to focus high doses of radiation to area where trigeminal nerve exits the brainstem. • Radiation causes slow formation of a lesion on nerve and disrupts transmission of pain signals to brain. • Pain relief from this procedure may take several months. (Radiosurgery is discussed in Chapter 56.)

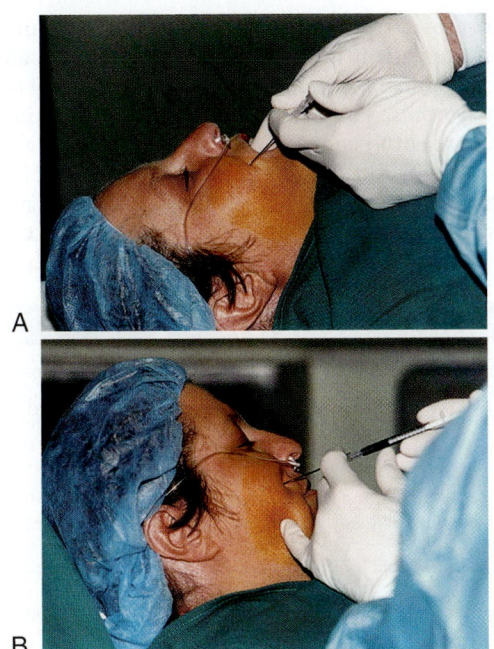

FIG. 60-13 Glycerol rhizotomy for the treatment of trigeminal neuralgia. **A,** Patient with trigeminal neuralgia having needle placed. **B,** Physician injecting glycerol. (Courtesy Joe Rothrock, Media, Pa.)

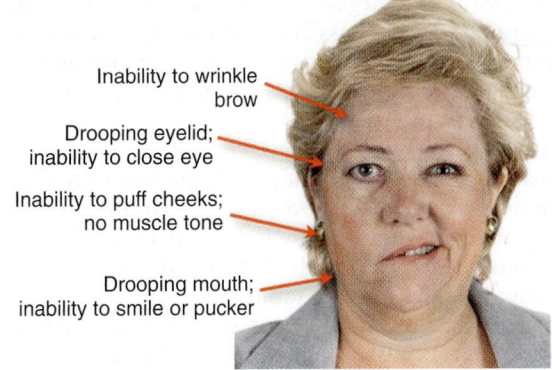

Inability to wrinkle brow
Drooping eyelid; inability to close eye
Inability to puff cheeks; no muscle tone
Drooping mouth; inability to smile or pucker

FIG. 60-14 Facial characteristics of a person with Bell's palsy. (©Jo Ann Snover/123RF Stock Photo/123rf.com)

the patient's nutritional status, hygiene (especially oral), and behavior (including withdrawal). Evaluate the degree of pain and its effects on the patient's lifestyle, drug use, emotional state, and suicidal tendencies.

Monitor the patient's response to drug therapy and note any side effects. Discuss alternative pain management measures, such as acupuncture, biofeedback, and yoga. Environmental assessment is essential during an acute period to decrease triggering stimuli. The room should be kept at an even, moderate temperature and free of drafts. The patient may prefer to complete all self-care activities, fearing someone else will inadvertently cause injury.

Teach the patient about the importance of nutrition, hygiene, and oral care, and convey understanding if previous oral neglect is apparent. A small, soft-bristled toothbrush or a warm mouthwash assists in promoting oral care. Hygiene activities are best performed when analgesia is at its peak.

Encourage food that is high in protein and calories and easy to chew. It should be served lukewarm and offered frequently. If oral intake is sharply reduced and the patient's nutritional status is compromised, a nasogastric tube can be inserted on the unaffected side for enteral feedings.

Appropriate teaching related to surgical procedures depends on the type of procedure planned (e.g., percutaneous). The patient needs to know he or she will be awake during local procedures in order to cooperate when corneal and ciliary reflexes and facial sensations are checked. After the procedure, compare the patient's pain with the preoperative intensity. Evaluate the corneal reflex, extraocular muscles, hearing, sensation, and facial nerve function frequently (see Chapter 55). If the corneal reflex is impaired, take special care to protect the eyes. This includes using artificial tears or eye shields.

After a percutaneous radiofrequency procedure, apply an ice pack to the jaw on the operative side for 3 to 5 hours. To avoid injuring the mouth, the patient should not chew on the operative side until sensation has returned.

If intracranial surgery is performed, general postoperative nursing care after a craniotomy is appropriate. (Nursing care related to craniotomy is discussed in Chapter 56 on pp. 1337-1338.)

Plan for regular follow-up care, and instruct the patient on the dosage and side effects of medications. Although pain may be relieved, encourage the patient to keep environmental stimuli to a moderate level and to use stress management techniques. Long-term management after surgical intervention depends on residual effects of the procedure. If anesthesia is present or the corneal reflex is altered, teach the patient to (1) chew on the unaffected side; (2) avoid hot foods or beverages, which can burn the mucous membranes; (3) check the oral cavity after meals to remove food particles; (4) practice meticulous oral hygiene and continue with semiannual dental visits; (5) protect the face against extremes of temperature; (6) use an electric razor; (7) wear a protective eye shield and avoid rubbing eyes; and (8) examine eye regularly for symptoms of infection or irritation.

BELL'S PALSY

Bell's palsy is an acute peripheral facial paresis of unknown cause. As the most common facial nerve disorder, it is characterized by inflammation of the facial nerve (CN VII) on one side of the face in the absence of any other disease (e.g., stroke).

Each year about 40,000 Americans are diagnosed with Bell's palsy. It is evenly distributed between men and women and can affect any age group, with peak incidence usually between ages 15 and 50 years.[33] Susceptible groups include women in the third trimester of pregnancy and early postpartum, older adults, and people with diabetes or hypothyroidism.

Bell's palsy is considered benign, and most patients recover spontaneously within 3 weeks to 9 months. One third of patients may have residual effects of facial weakness, involuntary movements, and persistent tearing of the eye on the affected side.[34]

Etiology and Pathophysiology

Although the exact etiology is not known, several theories exist as to the underlying cause. One suggested mechanism is acute demyelination similar to Guillain-Barré disease. The most strongly supported cause is reactivation of herpes simplex virus isoform (HSV-1) and/or herpes zoster virus (HZV). The viral infection causes inflammation, leading to nerve compression and clinical features such as facial paralysis (Fig. 60-14). Other known documented infectious causes include adenovirus,

Coxsackie virus, cytomegalovirus, Epstein-Barr virus, influenza, mumps, and rubella. Possible noninfectious causes include Hashimoto's encephalopathy, atherosclerosis (causing ischemia and edema of the facial nerve), and genetic factors.

Clinical Manifestations

The onset of Bell's palsy is sudden with a rapid onset of unilateral facial weakness that can occur in a few hours. Maximum facial weakness is seen within 2 days. Many patients have a history of a recent viral illness. Patients may complain of pain around and behind the ear. Additional manifestations include numbness of the face, tongue, and ear; tinnitus; headache; and hearing deficit. Paralysis of the motor branches of the facial nerve typically results in flaccidity of the affected side of the face, with drooping of the mouth accompanied by drooling.

Bell's phenomenon, an inability to close the eyelid with an upward movement of the eyeball when closure is attempted, is a hallmark sign of Bell's palsy. Other manifestations include a widened *palpebral fissure* (opening between the eyelids); flattening of the nasolabial fold; and inability to smile, frown, or whistle. Unilateral loss of taste is common. Decreased muscle movement may alter chewing ability. Although some patients experience a loss of tearing, many patients complain of excessive tearing. Muscle weakness causes the lower lid to turn out, allowing overflow of normal tear production. Pain may occur behind the ear on the affected side, especially before onset of paralysis.

Complications include psychologic withdrawal because of changes in appearance, malnutrition, dehydration, mucous membrane trauma, corneal abrasions, muscle stretching, and facial spasms and contractures.

Diagnostic Studies

Diagnosis of Bell's palsy is by exclusion. No definitive diagnostic test exists. The diagnosis and prognosis are indicated by observing the typical pattern of onset and signs, and testing percutaneous nerve excitability by electromyography (EMG). MRI and CT can eliminate other causes for facial paralysis. Blood tests can be used to diagnose infections or other diseases. Patients should be referred to a neurologist or otolaryngologist as soon as possible to exclude other neurologic conditions.

Interprofessional Care

Treatment of Bell's palsy includes moist heat, gentle massage, electrical stimulation of the nerve, and prescribed exercises. Stimulation may maintain muscle tone and prevent atrophy. Care is primarily focused on relief of symptoms, prevention of complications, and protection of the eye on the affected side.

Corticosteroids are started immediately, with best results if they are initiated before paralysis is complete. When the patient improves to the point that corticosteroids are no longer necessary, the drug should be tapered over a 2-week period. Treatment with antivirals, such as acyclovir (Zovirax), valacyclovir (Valtrex), and famciclovir (Famvir), has not been effective in the management of Bell's palsy. Surgical decompression of the facial nerve remains controversial and is considered in refractory cases.

❖ NURSING MANAGEMENT: BELL'S PALSY

The patient with Bell's palsy is treated as an outpatient. Mild analgesics can relieve pain. Hot wet packs can reduce the discomfort of herpetic lesions, aid circulation, and relieve pain. Tell the patient to protect the face from cold and drafts because trigeminal *hyperesthesia* (extreme sensitivity to pain or touch) may occur. Maintenance of good nutrition is important. Teach the patient to chew on the unaffected side of the mouth to avoid trapping food and to enjoy the taste of food. Thorough oral hygiene must be performed after each meal to prevent parotitis, caries, and periodontal disease from accumulated residual food.

🅠 CHECK YOUR PRACTICE

You are working in the outpatient neurology clinic. Your patient is a 68-yr-old woman who has been diagnosed with Bell's palsy. Her primary complaint today is dry eyes. When you are doing an assessment, she tells you, "I hate the way I look. I cannot go anywhere and I am afraid to leave the house. I am ugly and scary looking."
• How can you help her cope with her disorder?
• What will you suggest to decrease moisture loss in the eye on the affected side?

The patient may wear dark glasses for protective and cosmetic reasons. Artificial tears (methylcellulose) should be instilled frequently during the day to prevent drying of the cornea. Ointment and an impermeable eye shield can be used at night to retain moisture. Taping the lids closed at night may be needed to provide protection. Instruct the patient to report ocular pain, drainage, or discharge.

A facial sling may be helpful to support affected muscles, improve lip alignment, and facilitate eating. The facial sling is usually made and fitted by a physical or occupational therapist. When function begins to return, active facial muscle exercises should be performed several times a day.

The change in physical appearance as a result of Bell's palsy can be devastating. Reassure the patient that a stroke did not occur and that chances for a full recovery are good. Enlisting support from family and friends is important. Tell the patient most people recover within 3 to 6 months after onset of symptoms.

▌ POLYNEUROPATHIES

GUILLAIN-BARRÉ SYNDROME

Guillain-Barré syndrome (GBS) is characterized by an autoimmune process that occurs a few days or weeks following a viral or bacterial infection.[35] GBS is a collection of clinical syndromes that manifest as acute inflammatory polyneuropathy. The most common type of GBS diagnosed in the United States is **acute inflammatory demyelinating polyneuropathy (AIDP)**. GBS is rare, affecting approximately 1 person in every 100,000.[36,37]

The main features of GBS include acute, ascending, rapidly progressive, symmetric weakness of the limbs. Maximal weakness is reached in 4 weeks. Reflexes in the affected limbs are weak or absent. Respiratory muscles may also be affected and some patients require mechanical ventilation.

Etiology and Pathophysiology

The etiology of this syndrome is unknown. Both cellular and humoral immune mechanisms play a role in the immune reaction directed at the nerves. The result is segmental loss of myelin with edema and inflammation of affected nerves. As demyelination occurs, transmission of nerve impulses is stopped or slowed. Muscles innervated by the damaged peripheral nerves undergo denervation and atrophy. In the recovery phase, remyelination occurs slowly, and neurologic function returns in a proximal-to-distal pattern.

Most cases of GBS follow viral or bacterial infection of the gastrointestinal or upper respiratory tract. Cytomegalovirus is the most common viral cause. *Campylobacter jejuni* gastroenteritis is the most common bacterial cause. Surgery and trauma may also trigger GBS.

Clinical Manifestations and Complications

GBS is a heterogeneous condition with manifestations ranging from mild to severe. The first symptoms are pain, *paresthesia* (numbness and tingling) and *hypotonia* (reduced muscle tone) of the limbs. *Areflexia* (lack of reflexes), and weakness or paralysis of the limbs usually peak within 4 weeks. Autonomic nervous system dysfunction results, with manifestations of orthostatic hypotension, hypertension, and abnormal vagal responses (bradycardia, heart block, asystole).

Other autonomic dysfunctions include bowel and bladder dysfunction, facial flushing, and diaphoresis. Cranial nerve involvement is manifested as facial weakness and paresthesia, extraocular eye movement difficulties, and dysphagia.

Pain is a common symptom in the patient with GBS. It can include paresthesia, muscular aches and cramps, and hyperesthesia, and appears to be worse at night. Pain may contribute to decreased appetite and may interfere with sleep.

The most serious complication of GBS is respiratory failure, which occurs as the paralysis progresses to nerves that innervate the thoracic area. Assess the respiratory system frequently by checking respiratory rate and depth to determine the need for immediate intervention, including intubation and mechanical ventilation. Respiratory infection or UTI may occur. Immobility from paralysis can cause paralytic ileus, muscle atrophy, VTE, pressure ulcers, orthostatic hypotension, and nutritional deficiencies.

Diagnostic Studies

Diagnosis is based primarily on the patient's history and clinical signs. Clinical features required for diagnosis include progressive weakness of more than one limb and diminished or absent reflexes. CSF analysis is helpful in excluding other causes. In GBS, the CSF has more protein than normal. EMG and nerve conduction studies are used to confirm the diagnosis.

❖ NURSING AND PROFESSIONAL MANAGEMENT: GUILLAIN-BARRÉ SYNDROME

Management of GBS is interprofessional and is aimed at supportive care. Ventilatory support is critical during the acute phase, as 30% of GBS cases progress to respiratory failure.[35] Patients are admitted to ICU for hemodynamic monitoring.

Immunomodulating treatments such as plasma exchange (*plasmapheresis*) or high-dose IV immunoglobulin (*IV Ig*) are most effective if administered to patients within the first 2 weeks of symptom onset. They are equally effective. Plasmapheresis removes antibodies and other immune factors. It is used five times either daily or every other day in the first 2 weeks. (Plasmapheresis is discussed in Chapter 13.) IV Ig interferes with antigen presentation and is given over 5 days. Because it is more readily available, it has replaced plasmapheresis as the preferred treatment in many centers.[37] Beyond 4 weeks after disease onset, plasmapheresis and

IV Ig therapies have little value. Corticosteroids appear to have little effect on the prognosis or duration of the disease.

Assessment of the patient is the most important aspect of nursing care during the acute phase. During the neurologic assessment, evaluate motor and sensory function. Report changes in motor function (e.g., ascending paralysis), reflexes, cranial nerve function (e.g., gag, cornea, swallow), and level of consciousness.

Carefully assess respiratory and cardiac function. Monitor arterial blood gases (ABGs) and vital capacity. Closely monitor BP and cardiac rate and rhythm during the acute phase because dysrhythmias may occur. Autonomic dysfunction commonly occurs, including tachycardia, bradycardia, hypertension, hypotension, abnormal sweating, and paralytic ileus.[37] Orthostatic hypotension secondary to muscle atony may occur in severe cases. Vasopressor agents and volume expanders may be needed to treat low BP. If fever develops, obtain sputum and blood cultures to identify the pathogen. Appropriate antibiotic therapy is then initiated.

Nutritional needs must be met in spite of possible problems associated with delayed gastric emptying, paralytic ileus, and potential for aspiration if the gag reflex is lost. In addition to testing for the gag reflex, note drooling and other difficulties with secretions that may indicate an inadequate gag reflex. Initially, enteral or parenteral nutrition may be used to ensure adequate caloric intake. Because of delayed gastric emptying, assess residual volumes of the feedings at regular intervals or before feedings (see Chapter 39).

Throughout the course of the illness, provide support and encouragement to the patient, caregiver, and family. Early referral should be made to physical, occupational, and speech therapists. Counseling may help the patient adjust to the sudden disabling syndrome and dependence on others.

Most patients with GBS will start to recover spontaneously at about 28 days. Although 80% of patients almost completely recover, the process is slow and takes months or years. About 65% of patients have minor residual signs or symptoms.[35] Older age, rapid onset, and mechanical ventilation are associated with poor prognosis.

CHRONIC INFLAMMATORY DEMYELINATING POLYNEUROPATHY (CIDP)

Chronic inflammatory demyelinating polyneuropathy (CIDP) is a motor and sensory neuropathy. CIDP is a rare autoimmune disorder with a prevalence of 1.5 to 3.6 in a million people.[38] Similar to GBS, there are different types of CIDP. It occurs more than twice as often in men as is women and develops primarily when people are in their 60s and 70s.[39]

CIDP differs from GBS as the symptoms gradually occur over 8 weeks and there is not an acute onset. Also unlike GBS, CIDP is not self-limiting (with an end to the acute phase). If untreated, 30% of CIDP patients will progress to wheelchair dependence.[38] Early recognition and treatment can help the patient avoid significant disability.

Etiology and Pathophysiology

The cause of CIDP is unclear. Although it is considered an autoimmune disease, no causative antigens have been found. It is unclear if CIDP is associated with a previous illness. It may be associated with infection, HIV, hepatitis C, Sjögren's syndrome, inflammatory bowel disease, melanoma, lymphoma, diabetes mellitus, and types of monoclonal gammopathy.

Clinical Manifestations and Diagnostic Studies

Patients with CIDP have a similar clinical presentation to GBS, with symmetric weakness in the arms and legs, impaired sensation, paresthesia, and absent or diminished reflexes. However, development of CIDP symptoms occurs gradually over a period of at least 8 weeks. This is an important difference as patients may be diagnosed with GBS and the confusion may lead to incorrect or delayed treatment. Unlike GBS, CIDP does not automatically resolve. Most patients with GBS can walk without help within three months. Patients with CIDP require maintenance therapy to prevent relapse.[40]

CIDP assessment and diagnosis are similar to GBD. CSF demonstrates elevated protein levels. MRI may show changes. Key identifying features of CIDP include nerve conduction block and slowed conduction velocity, suggestive of demyelination.[41] Nerve biopsy shows unequivocal evidence of demyelination or remyelination.

❖ NURSING AND INTERPROFESSIONAL MANAGEMENT: CIDP

Early recognition and diagnosis of the syndrome are key to reducing permanent disability. The goal of treatment is to halt the immune response and stop nerve inflammation and demyelination. Unlike GBS, corticosteroids are recommended for all patients with CIDP and considered standard therapy. Additionally, IV Ig or plasmapheresis may be used. They have been shown to be equally effective, so the treatment decision is based on personal preference, cost, and availability.[37] Chemotherapy and immunosuppressive agents have also been used to treat CIDP.

Regardless of the treatment, patients continue on therapy until maximum clinical improvement is achieved or until they reach a clinical plateau. Patients will require maintenance therapy to prevent relapse or progression.[41] Appropriate referrals to rehabilitation should be made early to promote maximum recovery.

TETANUS

Tetanus (lockjaw) is a severe infection of the nervous system affecting spinal and cranial nerves. It results from the effects of a potent neurotoxin released by the anaerobic bacillus *Clostridium tetani*. The spores of the bacillus are present in soil, garden mold, and manure. *C. tetani* enters the body through a wound that provides an appropriate low-O_2 environment for organisms to mature and produce toxin. Examples of possible wounds include IV drug use injection sites, human and animal bites, cuts from stepping on nails, gardening injuries, burns, frostbite, open fractures, and gunshot wounds.

Initial manifestations of tetanus include stiffness in the jaw *(trismus)* and neck and signs of infection (e.g., fever). As the disease progresses, the neck muscles, back, abdomen, and extremities become progressively rigid. In severe forms, continuous tonic seizures may occur with *opisthotonos* (extreme arching of the back and retraction of the head). Laryngeal and respiratory spasms cause apnea and anoxia. The slightest noise,

jarring motion, or bright light can cause a seizure. These seizures are agonizingly painful. Mortality rate is almost 100% in the severe form.[42]

Tetanus prevention and immunizations, which are the most important factors influencing the incidence of this disease, are summarized in Table 68-6. Adults should receive a tetanus and diphtheria toxoid booster every 10 years. Teach the patient that immediate, thorough cleansing of all wounds with soap and water is important to prevent tetanus. If an open wound occurs and the patient has not been immunized within 5 years, the HCP should be contacted so that a tetanus booster can be given.

The management of tetanus includes administration of a tetanus toxoid, diphtheria toxoid, and pertussis (Tdap) booster and tetanus immune globulin (TIG) in different sites before the onset of symptoms to neutralize circulating toxins (see Table 68-6). A much larger dose of TIG is administered to patients with clinical manifestations of tetanus.

Control of spasms is essential and is managed by sedation and skeletal muscle relaxation, usually with diazepam (Valium), barbiturates, and, in severe cases, neuromuscular blocking agents that act to paralyze skeletal muscles. Opioid analgesics such as morphine or fentanyl are also indicated for pain management. A 10-14 day course of penicillin, metronidazole, tetracycline, or doxycycline is recommended to inhibit further growth of *C. tetani*.

Because of laryngospasm and the potential need for neuromuscular-blocking drugs, a tracheostomy is usually performed early and the patient is maintained on mechanical ventilation. Sedative agents and opioid analgesics are given concomitantly to all patients who are pharmacologically paralyzed. Any recognized wound should be debrided or an abscess drained. Antibiotics may be given to prevent secondary infections.

BOTULISM

Botulism is rare but the most serious type of food poisoning. It is caused by gastrointestinal (GI) absorption of the neurotoxin produced by *Clostridium botulinum*. This organism is found in the soil, and the spores are difficult to destroy. It can grow in any food contaminated with the spores.

Improper home canning of foods is often the cause. It is thought that the neurotoxin destroys or inhibits the neurotransmission of acetylcholine at the myoneural junction, resulting in disturbed muscle innervation.

Neurologic manifestations can develop rapidly or evolve over several days. They include a descending paralysis with muscle incoordination and weakness, difficulty swallowing, seizures, and respiratory muscle weakness that can rapidly deteriorate to respiratory and/or cardiac arrest.

The clinical manifestations, prevention, and treatment are presented in Table 41-24. Patient and caregiving teaching related to food poisoning is presented in Table 41-25. Nursing care during the acute illness is similar to that for GBS. Supportive nursing interventions include rest, activities to maintain respiratory function, adequate nutrition, and prevention of loss of muscle mass.

CASE STUDY
Spinal Cord Injury

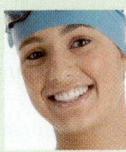

Patient Profile
Acute Phase

S.W., an 18-yr-old white woman, is admitted to the emergency department with the diagnosis of a cervical SCI. S.W. was swimming at a neighbor's backyard pool. She dove into the shallow end, striking her head on the bottom of the pool. Her friends noticed she did not resurface. They rescued her and brought her to the side of the pool. They maintained neck immobilization until rescue crews arrived.

(©Comstock-Images/Stockbyte/Thinkstock)

Subjective Data
- Awake and alert
- Complaining of neck pain
- Anxious and asking why she cannot move her legs
- Asking to see her family

Objective Data
Physical Examination
- Weak biceps movement bilaterally
- No triceps movement bilaterally
- Gross elbow movement present bilaterally
- No movement in bilateral lower extremities
- Decreased sensation from the shoulders down
- No bladder or bowel control
- BP 85/50 mm Hg; pulse 56 beats/min; respirations 32 breaths/min and labored

Diagnostic Studies
- CT C-spine shows C5 subluxation and compression fracture
- MRI C-spine shows severe spinal cord compression at C5-6

Interprofessional Care
- Intubated in the emergency department
- Started on mechanical ventilation
- Placed in tongs and traction on arrival to the ICU

Discussion Questions (Acute Phase)
1. *Priority Decision:* What nursing activities would be a priority on S.W.'s arrival in the ICU?
2. What physiologic problems are causing S.W. to have hypotension and bradycardia?
3. What would be the initial treatment for S.W.'s hypotension and bradycardia?

4. *Safety:* What signs and symptoms would indicate respiratory distress? What physiologic problem would cause respiratory distress in S.W.'s injury state?
5. *Teamwork and Collaboration:* What can the interprofessional team do to decrease S.W.'s anxiety?
6. *Priority Decision:* Based on the assessment data provided, what are the priority nursing diagnoses? What are the collaborative problems?
7. *Teamwork and Collaboration:* Identify activities that can be delegated to unlicensed assistive personnel (UAP).

Patient Profile
Rehabilitation Phase

S.W. is now 1 month postinjury and has been admitted to a local inpatient SCI rehabilitation facility. She has been extubated and uses a wheelchair to mobilize. She eats three meals a day with assistance and is on a strict bowel and bladder program.

Subjective Data
- Awake and alert but anxious
- Complaining of severe headache, blurred vision, and nausea

Objective Data
Physical Examination
- Flushed and diaphoretic above the level of injury
- No bowel movement for 2 days
- BP 235/106 mm Hg, pulse 32 beats/min, respirations 30 breaths/min and labored

Discussion Questions (Rehabilitation Phase)
1. *Priority Decision:* What initial priority nursing interventions would be appropriate?
2. What physiologic problem is causing S.W.'s hypertension and bradycardia?
3. Once the HCP has been notified, what other interventions would be appropriate?
4. *Quality Improvement:* What outcomes would indicate that nursing interventions were successful?
5. *Priority Decision:* Based on the assessment data provided, what are the priority nursing diagnoses?
6. *Patient-Centered Care:* Patient and family involvement in the rehabilitation process is vital. What teaching will you provide about bowel management?
7. *Evidence-Based Practice:* S.W. and her family are concerned about the risk of autonomic hyperreflexia. What effective strategies to prevent autonomic hyperreflexia would you discuss with the patient and family?

Answers available at *http://evolve.elsevier.com/Lewis/medsurg.*

◼ BRIDGE TO NCLEX EXAMINATION

The number of the question corresponds to the same-numbered outcome at the beginning of the chapter.

1. During rehabilitation, a patient with spinal cord injury begins to ambulate with long leg braces. Which level of injury does the nurse associate with this degree of recovery?
   a. L1-2
   b. T6-7
   c. T1-2
   d. C7-8

2. A patient with a T4 spinal cord injury experiences neurogenic shock as a result of sympathetic nervous system dysfunction. What would the nurse recognize as characteristic of this condition?
   a. Tachycardia
   b. Hypotension
   c. Increased cardiac output
   d. Peripheral vasoconstriction

3. A patient with spinal cord injury is experiencing severe neurologic deficits. What is the *most* likely mechanism of injury for this patient?
   a. Compression
   b. Hyperextension
   c. Flexion-rotation
   d. Extension-rotation

4. A patient with a C7 spinal cord injury undergoing rehabilitation tells the nurse he must have the flu because he has a bad headache and nausea. The nurse's *first priority* is to
   a. call the HCP.
   b. check the patient's temperature.
   c. take the patient's blood pressure.
   d. elevate the head of the bed to 90 degrees.

5. For a 65-year-old woman who has lived with a T1 spinal cord injury for 20 years, which health teaching instructions should the nurse emphasize?
   a. A mammogram is needed every year.
   b. Bladder function tends to improve with age.
   c. Heart disease is not common in people with spinal cord injury.
   d. As a person ages, the need to change body position is less important.

6. The most common early symptom of a spinal cord tumor is
   a. urinary incontinence.
   b. back pain that worsens with activity.
   c. paralysis below the level of involvement.
   d. impaired sensation of pain, temperature, and light touch.

7. During assessment of the patient with trigeminal neuralgia, the nurse should *(select all that apply)*
   a. inspect all aspects of the mouth and teeth.
   b. assess the gag reflex and respiratory rate and depth.
   c. lightly palpate the affected side of the face for edema.
   d. test for temperature and sensation perception on the face.
   e. ask the patient to describe factors that initiate an episode.

8. During routine assessment of a patient with Guillain-Barré syndrome, the nurse finds the patient is short of breath. The patient's respiratory distress is caused by
   a. elevated protein in the CSF.
   b. immobility resulting from ascending paralysis.
   c. degeneration of motor neurons in the brainstem and spinal cord.
   d. paralysis ascending to the nerves that stimulate the thoracic area.

9. A nurse is caring for a patient newly diagnosed with chronic inflammatory demyelinating polyneuropathy (CIDP). Which statement can the nurse accurately use to teach the patient about CIDP?
   a. "Corticosteroids have little effect on this disease."
   b. "Maintenance therapy will be needed to prevent relapse."
   c. "You will go into remission in approximately eight weeks."
   d. "You should be able to walk without help within three months."

1. a, 2. b, 3. c, 4. c, 5. a, 6. b, 7. a, d, e, 8. d, 9. b.

For rationales to these answers and even more NCLEX review questions, visit *http://evolve.elsevier.com/Lewis/medsurg.*

EVOLVE WEBSITE

http://evolve.elsevier.com/Lewis/medsurg
Review Questions (Online Only)
Key Points
Answer Keys for Questions
• Rationales for Bridge to NCLEX Examination Questions
• Answer Guidelines for Case Study on p. 1443
Student Case Study
• Patient With Spinal Cord Injury
Nursing Care Plan
• eNursing Care Plan 60-1: Patient With a Spinal Cord Injury
Conceptual Care Map Creator
Audio Glossary
Content Updates

REFERENCES

1. The National SCI Statistical Center: Spinal cord injury (SCI) facts and figures at a glance. Retrieved from *www.nscisc.uab.edu/PublicDocuments/fact_figures_docs/Facts%202015.pdf.*
2. Silva NA, Sousa N, Reis RL, et al: From basics to clinical: a comprehensive review on spinal cord injury, *Prog Neurobiol* 114:25, 2014.
3. Grafman J, Salazar A: Traumatic Brain Injury, Part I. In Aminoff MJ, Boller F, Swaab DF: *Handbook of clinical neurology,* St Louis, 2015, Elsevier.
4. Fox A: Assessment and treatment of spinal cord injuries and neurogenic shock. *JEMS* Retrieved from *http://www.jems.com/articles/print/volume-39/issue-11/patient-care/assessment-and-treatment-spinal-cord-inj.html,* 2014.
5. International Standards for Neurologic Classification of Spinal Cord Injury (ISNCSCI). Retrieved from *www.asia-spinalinjury.org/elearning/isncsci_worksheet_2015_web.pdf.*
6. Vazquez RG, Sedes PR, Farina MM, et al: Respiratory management in the patient with spinal cord injury, *BioMed Res Internat* 2013:168757, 2013.

*7. Postma K, Haisma JA, Hopman MTE, et al: Resistive inspiratory muscle training in people with spinal cord injury during inpatient rehabilitation: a randomized controlled trial, *Phys Ther* 94:1709, 2014.
8. Merck Manual: Neurogenic bladder. Retrieved from *www.merckmanuals.com/professional/genitourinary-disorders/voiding-disorders/neurogenic-bladder.*
9. Christopher & Dana Reeve Foundation Paralysis Resource Center: Bladder management. Retrieved from *http://www.christopherreeve.org/atf/cf/%7B173bca02-3665-49ab-9378-be009c58a5d3%7D/BLADDERMGMT713.PDF.*
10. Dhall SS, Hadley MN, Bizhan A, et al: Nutritional support after spinal cord injury, *Neurosurg* 72(suppl 2):255, 2013.
11. Dhall SS, Hadley MN, Bizhan A, et al: Deep venous thrombosis and thromboembolism in patients with cervical spinal cord injuries, *Neurosurg* 72(suppl 2):244, 2013.
12. Widerstrom-Noga E, Biering-Sroensen F, Bryce TN, et al: The international spinal cord injury pain basic data set (version 2.0), *Spinal Cord* 52:282, 2014.
13. Ryken TC, Hadley MN, Walters BC, et al: Radiographic assessment. *Neurosurg* 72(suppl):3, 2013.
14. Theodore N, Hadley MN, Aarabi B, et al: Prehospital cervical spinal immobilization after trauma, *Neurosurg* 72(suppl):3, 2013.
15. Theodore N, Aarabi B, Dhall SS, et al: Transportation of patients with acute traumatic cervical spine injuries, *Neurosurg* 72(suppl):3, 2013.
16. Hurlbert RJ, Hadley MN, Walters B, et al: Pharmacological therapy for acute spinal cord injury, *Neurosurg* 72(suppl):93, 2013.
17. Inoue T, Manley GT, Patel N, et al: Medical and surgical management after spinal cord injury: vasopressor usage, early surgeries, and complications, *J Neurotraum* 31:284, 2014.
18. National Institute of Neurological Disorders and Stroke: Spinal cord injury hope through research. Retrieved from *www.ninds.nih.gov/disorders/sci/detail_sci.htm.*
19. Christopher & Dana Reeve Foundation Paralysis Resource Center: Bowel management. Retrieved from *www.christopherreeve.org/atf/cf/%7B173bca02-3665-49ab-9378-be009c58a5d3%7D/Bowel914.pdf.*

20. Saulino MF, Goldstein JA: Rehabilitation of persons with spinal cord injuries. Retrieved from *http://emedicine.Medscape.com/article/1265209-overview*, 2014.

21. Christopher & Dana Reeve Foundation Paralysis Resource Center: Respirator, ventilator, and trach resources. Retrieved from *www.christopherreeve.org/atf/cf/%7B173bca02-3665-49ab-9378-be009c58a5d3%7D/VENT-TRACH%20_RESPIRATORY_%208-10.PDF*.

22. Sexual function in men with SCI. Retrieved from *http://images.main.uab.edu/spinalcord/SCI%20Infosheets%20in%20PDF/Sexual%20Function%20for%20Men%20with%20SCI.pdf*.

23. Sexuality for women with spinal cord injury. Retrieved from *http://images.main.uab.edu/spinalcord/SCI%20Infosheets%20in%20PDF/Sexuality%20for%20Women%20with%20SCI.pdf*.

24. Fann JR, Crane DA, Graves DE, et al: Depression treatment preferences after acute traumatic spinal cord injury, *Arch Phys Med Rehab* 94:2389, 2013.

25. Huff JS, Brenner BE: Spinal cord neoplasms: epidemiology. Retrieved from *http://emedicine.medscape.com/article/779872-overview#a6*.

26. Mechtler LL: Spinal cord tumors: new views and future directions, *Neuro Clinic* 31:241, 2013.

27. American Association of Neurological Surgeons: Spinal tumors. Retrieved from *www.aans.org/Patient%20Information/conditions%20and%20Treatments/Spinal%20Tumor.aspx*.

*28. Sharma M, Sonig A, Ambekar S, et al: Discharge dispositions, complications, and costs of hospitalization in spinal cord tumor surgery: analysis of data from the United States nationwide inpatient sample, 2003-2010, *J Neurosurg Spine* 20:125, 2014.

29. Trigeminal neuralgia fact sheet. Retrieved from *www.ninds.nih.gov/disorders/trigeminal_neuralgia/detail_trigeminal_neuralgia.htm*.

30. Trigeminal neuralgia. Retrieved from *http://ihs-classification.org/en/02_klassifikation/04_teil3/13.01.01_facialpain.html*.

31. Zakrzewska JM, Linskey JE: Trigeminal neuralgia, *BMJ* 348:g474, 2014.

32. Lettmair S: Radiosurgery in trigeminal neuralgia, *Phys Med* 30:592, 2014.

33. National Institute of Neurological Disorders and Stroke: Bell's palsy fact sheet. Retrieved from *www.ninds.nih.gov/disorders/bells/detail_bells.htm*.

34. Zandian A, Osiro S, Hudson R, et al: The neurologist's dilemma: a comprehensive clinical review of Bell's palsy, with emphasis on current management trends, *Med Sci Mon* 20:83, 2014.

35. Dimachkie MM, Barohn RJ: Guillain-Barré syndrome, *Curr Treat Options Neurol* 15:338, 2013.

36. Van Doorn PA: Diagnosis, treatment, and prognosis of Guillain-Barré syndrome (GBS), *Presse Med* 42(6 Pt 2):e193, 2013.

37. Eldar AH, Chapman J: Guillain Barré syndrome and other immune mediated neuropathies: diagnosis and classification, *Autoimmune Rev* 13:525, 2014.

38. GBS/CIDP Foundation International: All about CIDP. Retrieved from *www.gbs-cidp.org/cidp/all-about-cidp*.

39. American Association of Neuromuscular and Electrodiagnostic Medicine: Chronic inflammatory demyelinating polyneuropathy. Retrieved from *http://aanem.org/Education/Patient-Resources/Disorders/Chronic-Inflammatory-Demyelinating-Polyradiculoneu.aspx*.

40. Sung JY, Tani J, Park SB, et al: Early identification of acute-onset chronic inflammatory demyelinating polyneuropathy, *Brain* 137:2155, 2014.

41. Taylor T: Chronic inflammatory demyelinating polyradiculoneuropathy: in a remote northern Ontario hospital, *Can Fam Phys* 59:368, 2013.

42. Centers for Disease Control and Prevention: Make sure your family is fully immunized. Retrieved from *www.cdc.gov/Features/Tetanus*.

*Evidence-based information for clinical practice.

61

Assessment of Musculoskeletal System

Michael E. Zychowicz

I think self-discipline is something, it's like a muscle. The more you exercise it, the stronger it gets.

Daniel Goldstein

e http://evolve.elsevier.com/Lewis/medsurg/

LEARNING OUTCOMES

1. Describe the gross and microscopic anatomy of bone.
2. Explain the classification system for joints and movements at synovial joints.
3. Compare and contrast the types and structure of muscle tissue.
4. Describe the functions of cartilage, muscles, ligaments, tendons, fascia, and bursae.
5. Link age-related changes in the musculoskeletal system to the differences in assessment findings.
6. Obtain significant subjective and objective assessment data related to the musculoskeletal system from a patient.
7. Perform a physical assessment of the musculoskeletal system using appropriate techniques.
8. Differentiate normal from abnormal findings of a physical assessment of the musculoskeletal system.
9. Describe the purpose, significance of results, and nursing responsibilities related to diagnostic studies of the musculoskeletal system.

KEY TERMS

ankylosis, Table 61-6, p. 1456
arthrocentesis, Table 61-7, p. 1459
arthroscopy, Table 61-7, p. 1458
atrophy, Table 61-6, p. 1456
contracture, Table 61-6, p. 1456

crepitation, Table 61-6, p. 1456
isometric contractions, p. 1449
isotonic contractions, p. 1449
kyphosis, Table 61-6, p. 1456
lordosis, Table 61-6, p. 1456

osteons, p. 1446
range of motion, p. 1454
scoliosis, p. 1455
x-ray, p. 1455

This chapter provides a review of the structure and function of the musculoskeletal system to facilitate nursing assessment and evaluation of the assessment findings for this system. The musculoskeletal system is composed of voluntary muscle and six types of connective tissue: bone, cartilage, ligaments, tendons, fascia, and bursae. The purpose of the musculoskeletal system is to protect body organs, provide support and stability for the body, and allow coordinated movement.

STRUCTURES AND FUNCTIONS OF MUSCULOSKELETAL SYSTEM

Bone

Function. The main functions of bone are support, protection of internal organs, voluntary movement, blood cell production, and mineral storage.[1] Bones provide the supporting framework that keeps the body from collapsing and also allows the body to bear weight. Bones also protect underlying vital organs and tissues. For example, the skull encloses the brain, vertebrae surround the spinal cord, and rib cage protects the lungs and heart.

Bones serve as a point of attachment for muscles, which are connected to bones by tendons. Bones act as a lever for muscles, and movement occurs as a result of muscle contractions applied to these levers. Bones also serve as a point of attachment for ligaments, which provide stability to joints. Bones contain hematopoietic tissue for the production of red and white blood cells. Bones also serve as a storage site for inorganic minerals such as calcium and phosphorus.

Bone is a dynamic tissue that continuously changes form and composition. It contains both organic material (collagen) and inorganic material (calcium, phosphate). The internal and external growth and remodeling of bone are ongoing processes.

Microscopic Structure. Bone is classified according to structure as *cortical* (compact and dense) or *cancellous* (spongy). In *cortical bone*, cylindrical structural units called **osteons** *(Haversian systems)* fit closely together, creating a dense bone structure (Fig. 61-1, *A*). Within the systems, the Haversian canals run parallel to the bone's long axis and contain the blood vessels that travel to the bone's interior from the periosteum. Surrounding each osteon are concentric rings known as *lamellae*,

Reviewed by Judy Carlyle, RN, MNSc, ARNEC Faculty, Clinical Liaison, Arkansas Rural Education Consortium, Nashville, Arkansas; and Colleen R. Walsh, RN, DNP, ONC, ONP-C, CNS, ACNP-BC, Contract Clinical Assistant Professor, Graduate Nursing, University of Southern Indiana, College of Nursing and Health Professions, Evansville, Indiana.

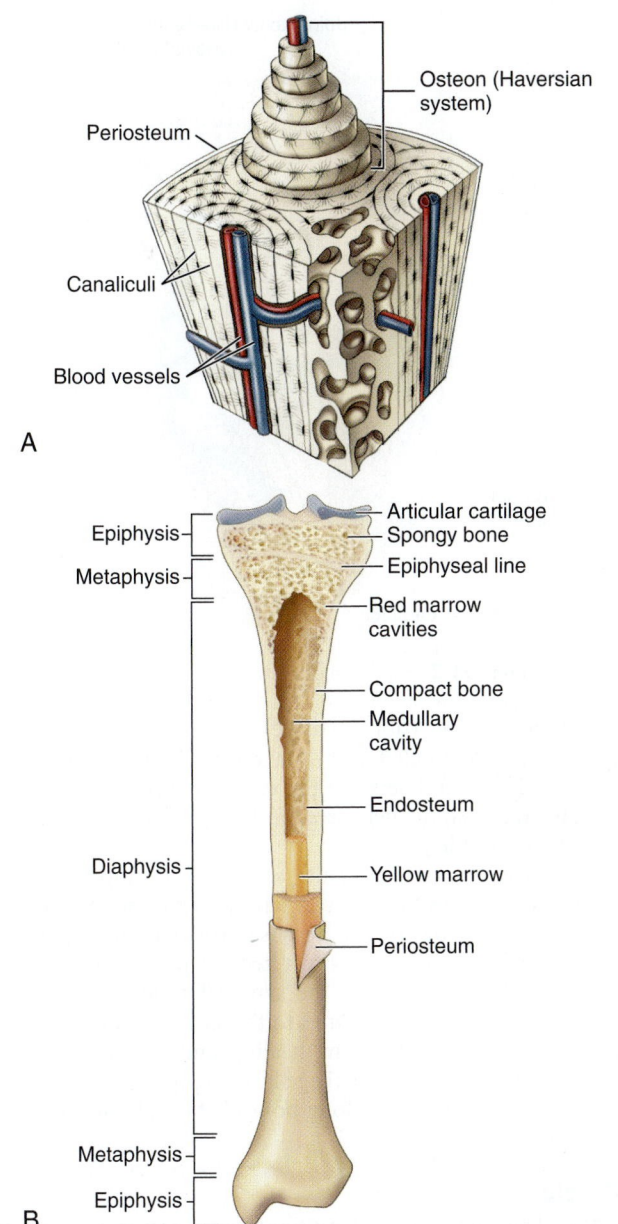

A

Osteon (Haversian system)
Periosteum
Canaliculi
Blood vessels

Epiphysis — Articular cartilage / Spongy bone
Metaphysis — Epiphyseal line
— Red marrow cavities
— Compact bone
— Medullary cavity
— Endosteum
Diaphysis — Yellow marrow
— Periosteum
Metaphysis
Epiphysis
B

FIG. 61-1 Bone structure. **A,** Cortical bone showing numerous structural units called osteons. **B,** Anatomy of a long bone (tibia) showing cancellous and compact bone. (*A,* From Herlihy B, Maebius N: *The human body in health and illness,* ed 4, Philadelphia, 2011, Saunders. *B,* From Patton KT, Thibodeau GA: *Anatomy and physiology,* ed 8, St Louis, 2013, Mosby.)

which characterize mature bone. Smaller canals *(canaliculi)* extend from the Haversian canals to the *lacunae,* where mature bone cells are embedded.

Cancellous bone has a different structure than cortical bone. The lamellae are not arranged in concentric rings but rather along the lines of maximum stress placed on the bone. Cancellous bone is filled with red or yellow marrow, and blood reaches the bone cells by passing through spaces in the marrow.

The three types of bone cells are osteoblasts, osteocytes, and osteoclasts.[2] *Osteoblasts* synthesize organic bone matrix (collagen) and are the basic bone-forming cells. *Osteocytes* are mature bone cells. *Osteoclasts* participate in bone remodeling by assisting in the breakdown of bone tissue. *Bone remodeling* is the removal of old bone by osteoclasts *(resorption)* and the

deposition of new bone by osteoblasts *(ossification).* The inner layer of bone is composed primarily of osteoblasts with a few osteoclasts.

Gross Structure. The anatomic structure of bone is best represented by a typical long bone such as the tibia (Fig. 61-1, *B*). Each long bone consists of the epiphysis, diaphysis, and metaphysis. The *epiphysis,* the widened area at each end of a long bone, is composed primarily of cancellous bone. The wide epiphysis allows for greater weight distribution and provides stability for the joint. The epiphysis is also a primary location of muscle attachment. Articular cartilage covers the ends of the epiphysis to provide a smooth, low-friction surface for joint movement.

The *diaphysis* is the main shaft of the long bone. It provides structural support and is composed of cortical bone. The tubular structure of the diaphysis allows it to more easily withstand bending and twisting forces.

The *metaphysis* is the flared area between the epiphysis and diaphysis. Like the epiphysis, it is composed of cancellous bone.

The *epiphyseal plate* (physis or growth plate) is the cartilaginous area between the epiphysis and metaphysis. In skeletally immature children who still have open growth plates, the epiphyseal plate actively produces chondrocytes that become mature bone. Division of the chondrocytes causes longitudinal bone growth in children. Injury to the epiphyseal plate in a growing child can cause cessation of new bone formation at the growth plate. This leads to a shorter extremity and may contribute to significant functional problems. In the adult, the metaphysis and epiphysis become joined when chondrocyte formation at the growth plate ceases and the plate becomes fully ossified.

The *periosteum* is composed of fibrous connective tissue that covers the bone. Tiny blood vessels penetrate the periosteum to provide nutrition to underlying bone. Musculotendinous fibers attach to the outer layer of the periosteum. The inner layer of the periosteum is attached to the bone by collagen bundles. No periosteum exists on the articular surfaces of long bones. These bone ends are covered by articular cartilage.

The medullary *(marrow)* cavity in the center of the diaphysis contains either red or yellow bone marrow.[3] In the growing child, red bone marrow is actively involved in blood cell production (hematopoiesis). In the adult, the medullary cavity of long bones contains yellow bone marrow, which is mainly adipose tissue. Yellow marrow is involved in hematopoiesis only in times of great blood cell need. In adults, red marrow is found mainly in the *flat bones,* such as the pelvis, skull, sternum, cranium, ribs, vertebrae, and scapulae, and in the *cancellous* ("spongy") bone at the epiphyseal ends of long bones such as the femur and humerus.

Types. The skeleton consists of 206 bones, which are classified according to shape as long, short, flat, or irregular.

Long bones are characterized by a central shaft *(diaphysis)* and two widened ends *(epiphyses)* (Fig. 61-1, *B*). Examples include the femur, humerus, and tibia. *Short bones* are composed of cancellous bone covered by a thin layer of compact bone. Examples include the carpals in the hand and tarsals in the foot.

Flat bones have two layers of compact bone separated by a layer of cancellous bone. Examples include the ribs, skull, scapula, and sternum. The spaces in the cancellous bone contain bone marrow. *Irregular bones* appear in a variety of shapes

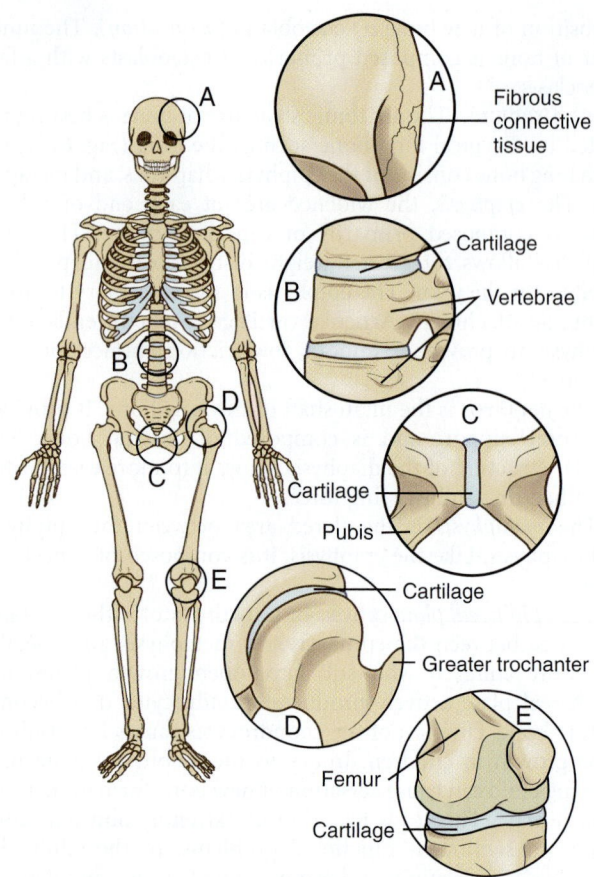

FIG. 61-2 Classification of joints. **A** to **C,** Synarthrotic (immovable) and amphiarthrotic (slightly movable) joints. **D** and **E,** Diarthrodial (*freely* movable) joints.

and sizes. Examples include the sacrum, mandible, and ear ossicles.

Joints

A *joint* (articulation) is a place where the ends of two bones are in proximity and move in relation to each other. Joints are classified by the degree of movement that they allow (Fig. 61-2).

The most common joint is the freely movable *diarthrodial* (synovial) type. Each joint is enclosed in a capsule of fibrous connective tissue, which joins the two bones together to form a cavity (Fig. 61-3). The capsule is lined by a synovial membrane, which secretes thick synovial fluid to lubricate the joint, reduce friction, and allow opposing surfaces to slide smoothly over each other. The end of each bone is covered with articular (hyaline) cartilage. Supporting structures (e.g., ligaments, tendons) reinforce the joint capsule and provide limits and stability to joint movement. Types of diarthrodial joints are shown in Fig. 61-4.

Cartilage

The three types of *cartilage* are hyaline, elastic, and fibrous. *Hyaline cartilage,* the most common, contains a moderate amount of collagen fibers. It is found in the trachea, bronchi, nose, epiphyseal plate, and articular surfaces of bones.

Elastic cartilage, which contains both collagen and elastic fibers, is more flexible than hyaline cartilage. It is found in the ear, epiglottis, and larynx.

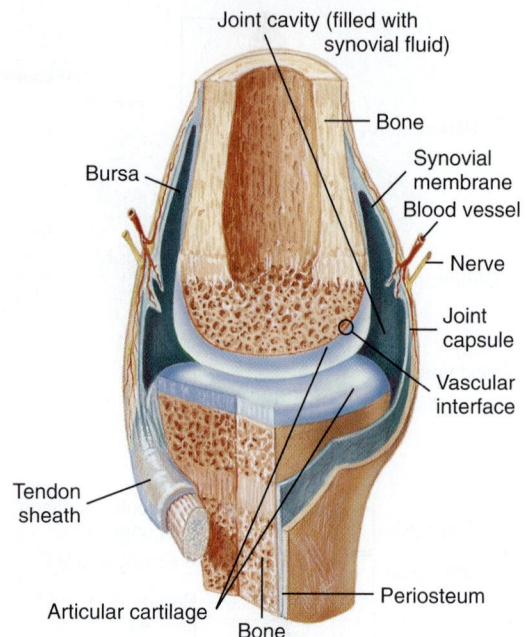

FIG. 61-3 Structure of diarthrodial (synovial) joint.

Fibrous cartilage (fibrocartilage) consists mostly of collagen fibers and is a tough tissue that often functions as a shock absorber. It is found between the vertebral discs and also forms a protective cushion between the bones of the pelvic girdle, knee, and shoulder.

Cartilage in synovial joints serves as a support for soft tissue and provides the articular surface for joint movement. It protects underlying tissues. Because articular cartilage is considered to be avascular, it must receive nourishment by the diffusion of material from the synovial fluid. The lack of a direct blood supply contributes to the slow metabolism of cartilage cells and explains why healing and repair of cartilage tissue occur slowly. The cartilage in the epiphyseal plate is also involved in the growth of long bones before physical maturity is reached.

Muscle

Types. The three types of muscle tissue are cardiac (striated, involuntary), smooth (nonstriated, involuntary), and skeletal (striated, voluntary) muscle. *Cardiac muscle* occurs only in the heart. Its spontaneous contractions propel blood through the circulatory system. *Smooth muscle* is found in the walls of hollow structures such as airways, arteries, gastrointestinal (GI) tract, urinary bladder, and uterus. Smooth muscle contraction is modulated by neuronal and hormonal influences. *Skeletal muscle,* which requires neuronal stimulation for contraction, accounts for about half of a human's body weight. It is the focus of the following discussion.

Structure. The skeletal muscle is enclosed by the *epimysium,* a continuous layer of deep fascia. The epimysium helps muscles slide over nearby structures. Connective tissue surrounding and extending into the muscle can be subdivided into fiber bundles, or *fasciculi.* These bundles are covered by *perimysium* and an innermost connective tissue layer called the *endomysium* that surrounds each fiber (Fig. 61-5).

The structural unit of skeletal muscle is the muscle cell or muscle fiber, which is highly specialized for contraction. Skeletal muscle fibers are long, multinucleated cylinders that contain

Joint	Movement	Examples	Illustration
Hinge joint	Flexion, extension	Elbow joint (shown), interphalangeal joints, knee joint	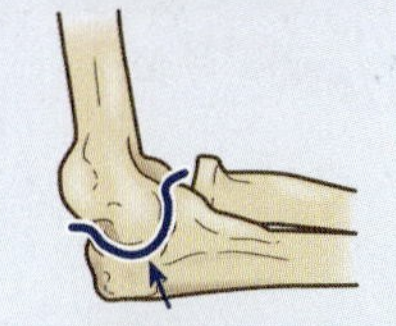
Ball and socket (spheroidal)	Flexion, extension; adduction, abduction; circumduction	Shoulder (shown), hip	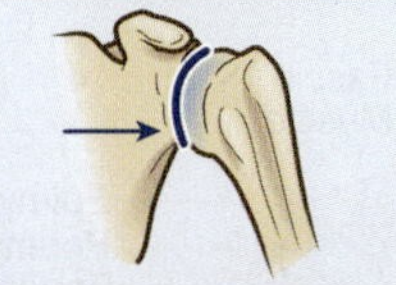
Pivot (rotary)	Rotation	Atlas-axis, proximal radioulnar joint (shown)	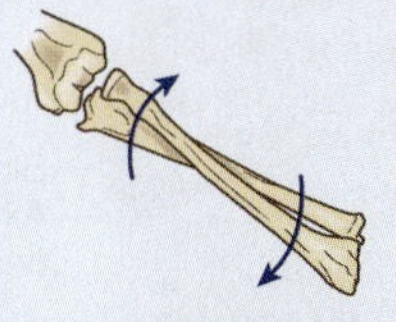
Condyloid	Flexion, extension; abduction, adduction; circumduction	Wrist joint (between radial and carpals) (shown)	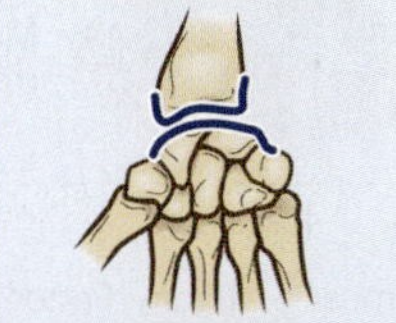
Saddle	Flexion, extension; abduction, adduction; circumduction, thumb-finger opposition	Carpometacarpal joint of thumb (shown)	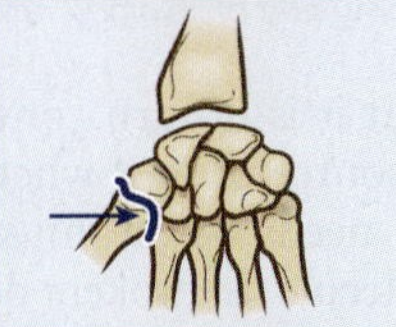
Gliding	One surface moves over another surface	Between tarsal bones, sacroiliac joint, between articular processes of vertebrae, between carpal bones (shown)	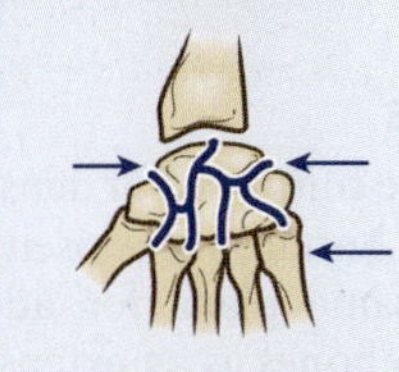

FIG. 61-4 Types of diarthrodial (synovial) joints.

many mitochondria to support their high metabolic activity. Muscle fibers are composed of myofibrils, which in turn are made up of protein contractile filaments. The *sarcomere* is the contractile unit of the myofibrils. Each sarcomere consists of *myosin* (thick) filaments and *actin* (thin) filaments. The arrangement of the thin and thick filaments accounts for the characteristic banding of muscle when it is seen under a microscope. Muscle contraction occurs as thick and thin filaments slide past each other, causing the sarcomeres to shorten.

Contractions. Skeletal muscle contractions allow posture maintenance, body movement, and facial expressions. **Isometric contractions** increase the tension within a muscle but do not produce movement. **Isotonic contractions** shorten a muscle to produce movement. Most contractions are a combination of tension generation *(isometric)* and shortening *(isotonic)*. Repeated isometric and/or isotonic contractions provide stress to stimulate muscle growth. Muscular *atrophy* (decrease in size) occurs with the absence of contraction that results from immobility or decreased neuronal stimulation. Increased muscular activity leads to *hypertrophy* (increase in size).

Skeletal muscle fibers are divided into two groups based on the type of activity they demonstrate. *Slow-twitch muscle fibers* support prolonged muscle activity such as marathon running. Because they also support the body against gravity, they assist in posture maintenance. *Fast-twitch muscle fibers* are used for rapid muscle contraction required for activities such as blinking the eye, jumping, or sprinting. Fast-twitch fibers tend to tire more quickly than slow-twitch fibers.

Neuromuscular Junction. Skeletal muscle fibers require a nerve impulse to contract. A nerve fiber and the skeletal muscle fibers it stimulates are called a *motor endplate*. The junction between the axon of the nerve cell and the adjacent muscle cell is called the *myoneural* or *neuromuscular junction* (Fig. 61-6).

Acetylcholine is released from the presynaptic neuron and diffuses across the neuromuscular junction to bind with receptors on the motor endplate of the muscle. In response to this stimulation, the sarcoplasmic reticulum releases calcium ions into the cytoplasm. The presence of calcium triggers the contraction in the myofibrils. When calcium is low, *tetany* (involuntary contractions of skeletal muscle) can occur.

Energy Source. The direct energy source for muscle fiber contractions is adenosine triphosphate (ATP). ATP is synthesized by cellular oxidative metabolism in numerous mitochondria located close to the myofibrils. It is rapidly depleted through conversion to adenosine diphosphate (ADP) and must be rephosphorylated. Phosphocreatine provides a rapid source for

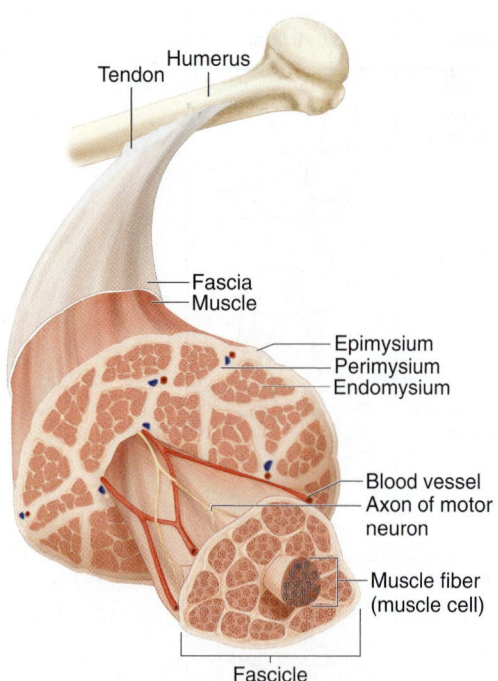

FIG. 61-5 Structure of a muscle. (From Patton KT, Thibodeau GA, Douglas M: *Essentials of anatomy and physiology,* St Louis, 2012, Mosby.)

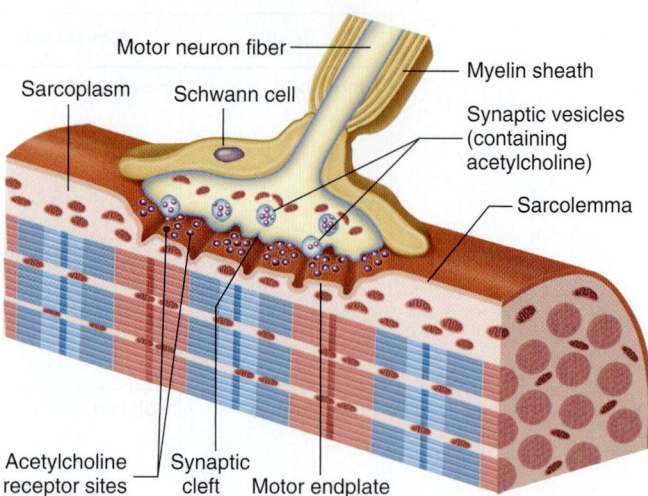

FIG. 61-6 Neuromuscular junction. (From Patton KT, Thibodeau GA: *Anatomy and physiology,* ed 8, St Louis, 2013, Mosby.)

the resynthesis of ATP, but it is in turn converted to creatine. Glycolysis can serve as a source of ATP when the O_2 supply is inadequate for metabolic needs of the muscle tissue. In this process, one glucose molecule is broken down to two ATP molecules.

Ligaments and Tendons

Ligaments and tendons are composed of dense, fibrous connective tissue that contains bundles of closely packed collagen fibers arranged in the same plane for additional strength. *Tendons* attach muscles to bones as an extension of the muscle sheath that adheres to the periosteum. *Ligaments* connect bones to bones (e.g., tibia to femur at knee joint). They have a higher elastic content than tendons.[4] Ligaments provide stability while permitting controlled movement at joints.

Ligaments and tendons have a relatively poor blood supply, usually making tissue repair a slow process after injury. For example, the stretching or tearing of ligaments that occurs with a sprain may require a long time to mend.

Fascia

Fascia refers to layers of connective tissue with intermeshed fibers that can withstand limited stretching. Superficial fascia lies immediately under the skin. Deep fascia is a dense, fibrous tissue that surrounds muscle bundles, nerves, and blood vessels. It also encloses individual muscles, allowing them to act independently and to glide over each other during contraction. In addition, fascia provides strength to muscle tissues.

Bursae

Bursae are small sacs of connective tissue lined with synovial membrane and containing viscous synovial fluid. They are typically located at bony prominences or joints to relieve pressure and decrease friction between moving parts.[5] For example, bursae are found between the (1) patella and skin (prepatellar bursae), (2) olecranon process of the elbow and skin (olecranon bursae), (3) head of the humerus and acromion process of the scapula (subacromial bursae), and (4) greater trochanter of the proximal femur and skin (trochanteric bursae). *Bursitis* is an inflammation of a bursa sac. The inflammation may be acute or chronic.

Gerontologic Considerations: Effects of Aging on Musculoskeletal System

Many functional problems experienced by the older adult are related to changes of the musculoskeletal system. Although some changes begin in early adulthood, obvious signs of musculoskeletal impairment may not appear until later adult years. Alterations may affect the older adult's ability to complete self-care tasks and pursue other usual activities. Effects of musculoskeletal changes may range from mild discomfort and decreased ability to perform ADLs to severe, chronic pain and immobility.

The risk for falls also increases in the older adult due in part to a loss of strength. Aging can also bring changes in the patient's balance, thus making the person unsteady, and *proprioception* (awareness of self in relation to the environment) may be altered.

The bone remodeling process is altered in the aging adult. Increased bone resorption and decreased bone formation cause a loss of bone density, contributing to the development of osteopenia and osteoporosis (see Chapter 63). Muscle mass and strength also decrease with aging. Almost 30% of muscle mass is lost by age 70. A loss of motor neurons can cause additional problems with skeletal muscle movement. Tendons and ligaments become less flexible, and movement becomes more rigid. Joints in the aging adult are also more likely to be affected by osteoarthritis[6] (see Chapter 64).

Perform a musculoskeletal assessment with particular emphasis on exercise practices. Obtain information on the type of exercise performed, including frequency and warm-up activities. Determine the impact of age-related changes of the musculoskeletal system on the older adult's functional status. Specifically inquire about changes in self-care habits and ability to be self-sufficient in the home environment.

Identify any musculoskeletal changes that increase the patient's risk for falls, and discuss fall prevention strategies. Functional limitations that are accepted by the older adult as a

TABLE 61-1   Gerontologic Assessment Differences

Musculoskeletal System

Changes	Differences in Assessment Findings
Muscle	
• Decreased number and diameter of muscle cells. Replacement of muscle cells by fibrous connective tissue. • Loss of elasticity and deterioration of cartilage. • Reduced ability to store glycogen. Decreased ability to release glycogen as quick energy during stress. • Decreased basal metabolic rate.	• Decreased muscle strength and mass. Abdominal protrusion. • Increased rigidity in neck, shoulders, back, hips, and knees. • Decreased fine motor dexterity, decreased agility. • Slowed reaction times and reflexes as a result of slowed conduction of nerve impulses along motor units. Earlier fatigue with activity.
Joints	
• Increased risk for cartilage erosion that leads to direct contact between bone ends and overgrowth of bone around joint margins. • Loss of water from discs between vertebrae, decreased height of intervertebral spaces.	• Joint stiffness, decreased mobility, limited ROM, possible crepitation on movement. • Pain with motion and/or weight bearing. • Loss of height and shortening of trunk from disc compression. Posture change.
Bone	
• Decreased bone density and strength. • Slowed remodeling process.	• Loss of height and deformity such as dowager's hump (kyphosis) from vertebral compression and degeneration. • Back pain, stiffness. • Bony prominences more pronounced. • Increased risk of osteopenia and osteoporosis.

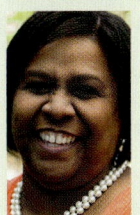
normal part of aging can often be halted or reversed with appropriate preventive strategies (see Table 62-1).

Diseases such as osteoarthritis and osteoporosis are not a normal part of growing older. These metabolic bone diseases involve the deterioration of bone tissue (osteoporosis) and destruction of cartilage (osteoarthritis). Carefully differentiate between expected changes and the effects of disease in the aging adult. Symptoms of disease can be treated in many cases, helping the older adult to return to a higher functional level. Age-related changes in the musculoskeletal system and differences in assessment findings are presented in Table 61-1.

ASSESSMENT OF MUSCULOSKELETAL SYSTEM

Subjective Data

Important Health Information. The most common manifestations of musculoskeletal impairment include pain, weakness, deformity, limitation of movement, stiffness, and joint crepitation (crackling sound). Ask the patient about changes in sensation or in the size of a muscle.

Past Health History. Because certain illnesses are known to affect the musculoskeletal system directly or indirectly, question the patient about past medical problems, including tuberculosis, poliomyelitis, diabetes mellitus, parathyroid problems, hemophilia, rickets, soft tissue infection, and neuromuscular

disability. In addition, past or developing musculoskeletal problems can affect the patient's overall health. Trauma to the musculoskeletal system is a common reason for seeking medical evaluation.

Questions should also focus on symptoms of arthritic and connective tissue diseases (e.g., gout, psoriatic arthritis, systemic lupus erythematosus), osteomalacia, osteomyelitis, and fungal infection of bones or joints. Ask the patient about possible sources of a secondary bacterial infection, such as ears, tonsils, teeth, sinuses, lungs, or genitourinary tract. These infections can enter the bones, resulting in osteomyelitis or joint destruction. Obtain a detailed account of the course and treatment of any of these problems.

Medications. Question the patient regarding prescription and over-the-counter drugs, herbal products, and nutritional supplements (see the Complementary & Alternative Therapies box in Chapter 3 on p. 38). Obtain detailed information about each treatment, including its name, the dose and frequency, length of time it was taken, reason for use, and any possible side effects. Inquire about the use of skeletal muscle relaxants, opioids, nonsteroidal antiinflammatory drugs, and systemic and topical corticosteroids. Question the patient who has taken antiinflammatory drugs about GI distress or signs of bleeding.

In addition to drugs taken for treatment of a musculoskeletal problem, ask the patient about drugs that can have detrimental effects on the musculoskeletal system. Some of these drugs and their potential side effects include antiseizure drugs (osteomalacia), phenothiazines (gait disturbances), corticosteroids (avascular necrosis, decreased bone and muscle mass), and potassium-depleting diuretics (muscle cramps and weakness). Question women about their menstrual history. Episodes of premenopausal amenorrhea can contribute to the development of osteoporosis.[7] Ask postmenopausal women about their use of hormone therapy. Inquire about calcium and vitamin D supplements for women and men.

Surgery or Other Treatments. Obtain information about past hospitalizations related to a musculoskeletal problem. Document the reason for hospitalization; the date and duration; and the treatment, including ongoing rehabilitation. Also record details of emergency treatment for musculoskeletal injuries. Obtain specific information regarding any surgical procedure, postoperative course, and complications. If the patient experienced a period of prolonged immobilization, consider the possible development of osteoporosis and muscle atrophy.

TABLE 61-2   Health History

Musculoskeletal System

Health Perception–Health Management Pattern

- Describe your usual daily activities.
- Do you experience any difficulties performing these activities?* Describe what you do if you experience difficulty in dressing, preparing meals and feeding yourself, performing basic hygiene, writing or using the phone, or maintaining your home.
- Do you have to lift heavy objects? Do your work or exercise habits require repetitive motion or joint stress? Describe any specialized equipment you use or wear when you work or exercise that helps protect you from injury.
- Do you take any drugs or herbal products to manage your musculoskeletal problem? If so, what are their names and what are the expected effects?

Nutritional-Metabolic Pattern

- What is your usual daily intake of food and snacks?
- Do you have difficulties preparing your food?
- What dietary supplements do you take? (Ask specifically about calcium, vitamin D supplements, and herbal products.)
- What is your weight? Describe any recent weight loss or gain.

Elimination Pattern

- Does your musculoskeletal problem make it difficult for you to reach the toilet in time?*
- Do you need any assistive devices or equipment to achieve satisfactory toileting?*
- Do you experience constipation related to decreased mobility or drugs taken for your musculoskeletal problem?*

Activity-Exercise Pattern

- Do you require assistance in completing your usual daily activities because of a musculoskeletal problem?*
- Describe your usual exercise pattern. Do you experience musculoskeletal symptoms before, during, or after exercising?*
- Are you able to move all your joints comfortably through full range of motion?
- Do you use any prosthetic or orthotic devices?*

Sleep-Rest Pattern

- Do you experience any difficulty sleeping because of a musculoskeletal problem?*
- Do you require frequent position changes at night?*
- Do you wake up at night because of musculoskeletal pain?*
- Do you use complementary and alternative therapies to help you sleep at night?*

Cognitive-Perceptual Pattern

- Describe any musculoskeletal pain you experience. How do you manage your pain? (Ask specifically about adjunctive therapies such as heat and cold or complementary and alternative therapies such as acupuncture.)

Self-Perception–Self-Concept Pattern

- Describe how changes in your musculoskeletal system (posture, walking, muscle strength) and decreased ability to do certain things may affect how you feel about yourself.
- Have these changes affected your lifestyle?*

Role-Relationship Pattern

- Do you live alone?
- Describe how family, friends, or others assist you with your musculoskeletal problem.
- Describe the effect of your musculoskeletal problem on your work and on your social relationships.

Sexuality-Reproductive Pattern

- Describe any sexual concerns related to your musculoskeletal problem.

Coping–Stress Tolerance Pattern

- Describe how you deal with problems such as pain, weakness, or immobility that have resulted from your musculoskeletal problem.

Value-Belief Pattern

- Describe any cultural practices or religious beliefs that may influence the treatment of your musculoskeletal problem.

*If yes, describe.

Functional Health Patterns. The use of functional health patterns assists in organizing assessment data. Table 61-2 summarizes specific questions to ask in relation to functional health patterns.

Health Perception–Health Management Pattern. Ask about the patient's health practices related to the musculoskeletal system, such as maintenance of normal body weight, avoidance of excessive stress on muscles and joints, and use of proper body mechanics when lifting objects. Question the patient specifically about tetanus and polio immunizations. Obtain the most current date and reaction to a tuberculin skin test.

The patient who is a good historian can recount numerous minor and major injuries of the musculoskeletal system. Record information chronologically and include the following:

- Mechanism and circumstances of the injury (e.g., twist, crush, stretch)
- Methods and duration of treatment
- Current status related to the injury
- Need for assistive devices
- Interference with activities of daily living

Safety practices can affect the patient's predisposition for certain injuries and illnesses. Therefore ask the patient about safety practices related to the work environment, home life, recreation, and exercise. For example, if the patient is a computer programmer, ask about ergonomic adaptations in the office that decrease the risk of carpal tunnel syndrome or low back pain. Identification of problems in this area will direct your plan for patient teaching.

Obtain a family history related to rheumatoid arthritis, systemic lupus erythematosus, ankylosing spondylitis, osteoarthritis, gout, osteoporosis, and scoliosis because a patient may have a genetic predisposition to these or other musculoskeletal disorders.

Nutritional-Metabolic Pattern. The patient's description of a typical day's diet provides clues to areas of nutritional concern that can affect the musculoskeletal system. Adequate intake of vitamins C and D, calcium, and protein is essential for a healthy, intact musculoskeletal system. Abnormal nutritional patterns can predispose individuals to problems such as osteomalacia and osteoporosis. In addition, maintenance of normal weight is an important nutritional goal. Obesity places additional stress on weight-bearing joints such as the knees, hips, and spine, predisposing individuals to cartilage deterioration and ligament instability.

Elimination Pattern. Questions about the patient's mobility may reveal difficulty with ambulating to the toilet. Ask the

---

⚕ **GENETIC RISK ALERT**

Autoimmune Diseases
- Many autoimmune diseases of the musculoskeletal system have a genetic basis involving human leukocyte antigens (HLAs).
- These diseases include ankylosing spondylitis, rheumatoid arthritis, and systemic lupus erythematosus.

Osteoporosis
- Genetic factors contribute to osteoporosis by influencing not only bone mineral density but also bone size, bone quality, and bone turnover.

Osteoarthritis, Gout, and Scoliosis
- A genetic predisposition is a contributing risk factor in all these diseases.

Muscular Dystrophy
- The most common types of muscular dystrophy are X-linked recessive disorders.

---

patient if an assistive device such as an elevated toilet seat or a grab bar is necessary to accomplish toileting. Decreased mobility secondary to a musculoskeletal problem can lead to constipation. In addition, musculoskeletal problems can contribute to bowel or bladder incontinence when ambulation is a problem.

Activity-Exercise Pattern. Obtain a detailed account of the type, duration, and frequency of exercise and recreational activities. Compare daily, weekend, and seasonal patterns because occasional or sporadic exercise can be more problematic than regular exercise. Many musculoskeletal problems can affect the patient's activity-exercise pattern. Question the patient about clumsiness or limitations in movement, pain, weakness, crepitus, or any change in bones or joints that interferes with daily activities.

Extremes of activity related to occupation can also affect the musculoskeletal system. A sedentary occupation can negatively affect muscle flexibility and strength. Jobs that require extreme effort through heavy lifting or pushing can lead to damage of joints and supporting structures. Specifically question the patient about work-related injuries to the musculoskeletal system, including treatment and time lost from work.

Sleep-Rest Pattern. The discomfort caused by musculoskeletal disorders can interfere with the patient's normal sleep pattern. Ask the patient about possible alterations in sleep patterns. If the patient describes sleep interference related to a musculoskeletal problem, inquire further about the type of bedding and pillows used, bedtime routine, sleeping partner, and sleeping positions.

Cognitive-Perceptual Pattern. Fully explore and document any pain experienced by the patient as a result of a musculoskeletal problem. To provide a baseline for later reassessment, ask the patient to describe the intensity of the pain on a numeric scale from 0 to 10 (0 = no pain, 10 = most severe pain imaginable).[8] Reassessments over time assist in determining the effectiveness of any treatment plan. Question the patient about measures used at home for managing pain. Ask about related problems such as joint swelling or muscle weakness and any accommodations that help with the problem. (Pain is discussed in Chapter 8.)

Self-Perception–Self-Concept Pattern. Many chronic musculoskeletal problems lead to deformities and a reduction in activities that can have a serious negative impact on the patient's body image and sense of personal worth. Assess the patient's feelings about these changes and the effect they may have on interactions with family and friends.

Role-Relationship Pattern. Impaired mobility and chronic pain from musculoskeletal problems can negatively affect the patient's ability to perform in roles of spouse, parent, and/or employee. The ability to pursue and maintain meaningful social and personal relationships can also be affected by musculoskeletal problems. Carefully question the patient about role performance and relationships.

If the patient lives alone, the current musculoskeletal problem and rehabilitation may make it difficult or impossible to continue this arrangement. Determine the degree of assistance available from family, friends, and other caregivers. Find out if additional resources are needed such as physical therapy and home health care.

Sexuality-Reproductive Pattern. The pain of musculoskeletal problems can impede the patient's ability to obtain sexual satisfaction. Explore this area with a sensitive and nonjudgmental attitude. Help the patient feel comfortable discussing any sexual problems related to pain, movement, and positioning. Additional information on obtaining patient data in this area is presented in Chapter 50.

Coping–Stress Tolerance Pattern. Mobility limitations and pain (acute or chronic) are serious potential stressors that challenge the patient's coping resources. Recognize the potential for ineffective coping in the patient and family or significant other. Additional questioning will help to determine if a musculoskeletal problem is causing difficulties in coping and adjusting.

Value-Belief Pattern. Ask the patient about cultural or religious beliefs that may influence the patient's acceptance of treatment for the musculoskeletal problem. These may include recommendations for diet, exercise, medication, and lifestyle modifications.

Objective Data

Physical Examination. The basic musculoskeletal physical examination involves inspection, palpation, range of motion, strength testing, reflexes, and neurovascular assessment. Other special tests can be used to further assess for specific conditions. Conduct a general overview. While obtaining a careful health history, choose areas to concentrate on during the local examination. Take specific measurements as indicated by the local examination.

Inspection. A systematic inspection is performed starting at the head and neck and proceeding to the upper extremities, lower extremities, and trunk. The regular use of a systematic approach is important to avoid missing important aspects of the examination. Inspect the skin for general color, scars, or other overt signs of previous injury or surgery. Certain cutaneous lesions require additional investigation because they can indicate underlying disorders. For example, butterfly rash over the cheeks and nose is characteristic of systemic lupus erythematosus.

Note the patient's general posture and body build, muscle size and symmetry, and symmetry and contour of joints. Observe for any swelling, deformity, nodules or masses, and discrepancies in limb length or muscle size. Use the patient's opposite body part for comparison when an abnormality is suspected.

Palpation. As with inspection, palpation usually proceeds in a head to toe fashion, examining the neck, shoulders, elbows,

Subjective Data

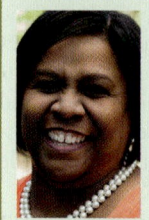

(©pixelhead-photo/iStock/Thinkstock)

A focused subjective assessment of G.A. revealed the following information:

PMH: Hypertension for 6 years. Type 2 diabetes for 11 yr. 40-pack-yr smoking history.

Medications: Metformin (Glucophage) 500 mg PO bid; glyburide (DiaBeta) 5 mg/day PO; hydrochlorothiazide 50 mg PO bid.

Health Perception–Health Management: Currently smokes 1 pack of cigarettes per day. Is trying to quit but finding it difficult. Drinks alcohol at night.

Nutritional-Metabolic: G.A. is 5 ft 2 in tall and weighs 160 lb (BMI 29.3 kg/m^2). Does not take any nutritional supplements and avoids milk and other dairy products because they make her "gassy."

Activity-Exercise: Leads a very sedentary lifestyle. Able to perform ADLs without assistance. Denies any history of musculoskeletal problems.

Cognitive-Perceptual: Rates toe pain at 8 on a scale of 0-10. Describes sharp, burning pain that increases in intensity with any movement.

Coping–Stress Tolerance: Is asking for pain medicine "as strong as you can give me."

Discussion Questions

1. What type of assessment would be most appropriate for G.A.: comprehensive, focused, or emergency? On what basis would you make that decision?
2. What assessment questions will you ask G.A.?
3. How will you individualize the assessment based on her age, ethnic/cultural background, and condition?
4. What subjective assessment findings are of most concern to you?
5. Is this an appropriate time to talk with G.A. about her weight?
6. Based on these subjective findings, what type of physical assessment should be performed?

You will learn more about the physical assessment of the musculoskeletal system in the next section.

See p. 1457 for more information on G.A.

Answers available at *http://evolve.elsevier.com/Lewis/medsurg*.

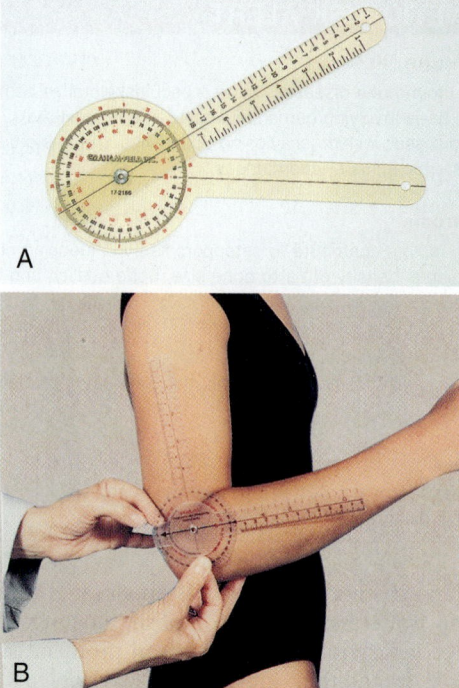

FIG. 61-7 **A,** Goniometer. **B,** Measurement of joint range of motion using a goniometer. (*A,* From Wilson SF, Giddens JF: *Health assessment for nursing practice,* ed 5, St Louis, 2013, Mosby. *B,* From Barkauskas V, Baumann L, Stoltenberg-Allen K, et al: *Health and physical assessment,* ed 2, St Louis, 1998, Mosby.)

wrists, hands, back, hips, knees, ankles, and feet. Warm your hands to prevent muscle spasm, which can interfere with identification of essential landmarks or soft tissue structures. Carefully palpate any specific areas of concern because of a subjective complaint or abnormal appearance on inspection.

Both superficial and deep palpation are usually performed consecutively. Consider the underlying anatomy structures and landmarks that are being palpated. Purposefully palpate both muscles and joints to allow evaluation of skin temperature, local tenderness, swelling, and crepitation. Establish the relationship of adjacent structures, and evaluate the general contour, abnormal prominences, and local landmarks. Make note of the specific anatomic location of any abnormal findings.

Motion. When assessing the patient's joint mobility, carefully evaluate active and passive **range of motion** (full movement potential of a joint). Measurements should be similar for both active and passive maneuvers. *Active range of motion* means the patient takes his or her own joints through all movements without assistance. *Passive range of motion* occurs when someone else moves the patient's joints without his or her assistance through the full range of motion. Be careful in performing passive range of motion because of the risk of injury to underlying structures. If pain or resistance is encountered, stop manipulation immediately.

If you note deficits in active or passive range of motion, also assess functional range of motion to determine if performance of ADLs has been affected by joint changes. This is done by asking the patient if activities such as eating, grooming, dressing, and bathing must be performed with assistance or cannot be done at all.

Range of motion is most accurately assessed with a goniometer, which measures the angle of the joint (Fig. 61-7). Specific degrees of range of motion of all joints are usually not measured. If a specific musculoskeletal problem has been identified, measure range of motion of the affected joint. A less exact but valuable assessment method is simply to compare the range of motion of one extremity with that on the opposite side. Common movements that occur at the synovial joints, including *abduction, adduction, flexion,* and *extension,* are described in Table 61-3.

Muscle-Strength Testing. Grade the strength of individual muscles or groups of muscles during contraction on a 5-point scale (Table 61-4). Grade normal muscle strength with full resistance to opposition as a 5/5 bilaterally. To test resistance to opposition, have the patient apply resistance against a force you are exerting. For example, have the patient try to extend the elbow while you attempt to flex it. Compare muscle strength with the strength of the opposite extremity. Note any subtle variations in muscle strength when comparing the patient's dominant and nondominant sides. Variations in strength also exist when comparing individuals.

Measurement. When limb length discrepancies or subjective problems are noted, obtain limb length and circumferential muscle mass measurements. For example, when gait disorders are observed, measure leg length between the anterosuperior iliac crest and the bottom of the medial malleolus. Then compare it with the similar measurement of the opposite extremity. Measure muscle mass circumferentially at the largest area of the muscle. When recording measurements, document the exact location at which the measurements were obtained (e.g., the left quadriceps muscle was measured 15 cm above the patella). This informs the next examiner of the exact area to measure and ensures consistency during reassessment.

Other. Note the patient's use of an assistive device such as a walker or cane. Assess the patient for proper fit while reviewing the safe and correct technique for using these devices. Regularly review with the patient the use of the assistive device to ensure it remains appropriate and safe.[9]

If the patient is able to move independently, assess posture and gait by watching the patient walk, stand, and sit. Musculoskeletal and neurologic problems can result in abnormal gait patterns.

Scoliosis is a lateral S-shaped curvature of the thoracic and lumbar spine. Unequal shoulder and scapula height is usually noted when the patient is observed from the back (Fig. 61-8). Ask the patient to place the hands together above the head as if diving into a swimming pool and slowly bend forward at the waist, allowing for assessment of thoracic rib prominence or paravertebral muscle prominence in the lumbar spine. Lung and cardiac function may be impaired with advancing scoliosis deformity.

The *straight-leg-raising test* is performed on the supine patient with sciatica or leg pain. Passively raise the patient's leg 60 degrees or less. The test is positive if the patient complains of pain along the distribution of the sciatic nerve. A positive test indicates nerve root irritation from intervertebral disc prolapse and herniation, particularly at the level of L4-5 or L5-S1.

Assessment of reflexes is discussed in Chapter 55. Table 61-5 is an example of how to record a normal physical assessment of the musculoskeletal system. Abnormal assessment findings of the musculoskeletal system are presented in Table 61-6.

A *focused assessment* is used to evaluate the status of previously identified musculoskeletal problems and to monitor for signs of new problems (see Table 3-7). A focused assessment of the musculoskeletal system is presented in the box.

DIAGNOSTIC STUDIES OF MUSCULOSKELETAL SYSTEM

Numerous diagnostic studies are available to assess the musculoskeletal system. Table 61-7 presents the most common studies, and select studies are described in more detail below.

The use of studies such as x-rays, MRI, and bone scans has greatly improved orthopedic care. The x-ray is the most common diagnostic study used to assess musculoskeletal problems and to monitor the effectiveness of treatment. Because bones are denser than other tissues and contain calcium, most x-rays are absorbed by the bone tissue and do not penetrate it. Dense areas

TABLE 61-3	**Synovial Joint Movements**
Movement	**Description**
Abduction	Movement of part away from midline of body
Adduction	Movement of part toward midline of body
Circumduction	Circular motion of a body part resulting from a combination of flexion, abduction, extension, and adduction
Dorsiflexion	Flexion of the ankle and toes toward the shin
Eversion	Turning of sole outward away from midline of body
Extension	Straightening of joint that increases angle between two bones
External rotation	Movement along longitudinal axis away from midline of body
Flexion	Bending of joint as a result of muscle contraction that causes decreased angle between two bones
Hyperextension	Extension in which angle exceeds 180 degrees
Internal rotation	Movement along longitudinal axis toward midline of body
Inversion	Turning of sole inward toward midline of body
Opposition	Moving the first and fifth metacarpals anteriorly from a flattened palm ("cupping position"); makes it possible to hold objects between the thumb and fingers
Plantar flexion	Flexion of the ankle and toes toward the plantar surface of the foot ("toes pointed")
Pronation	Turning of palm downward
Supination	Turning of palm upward

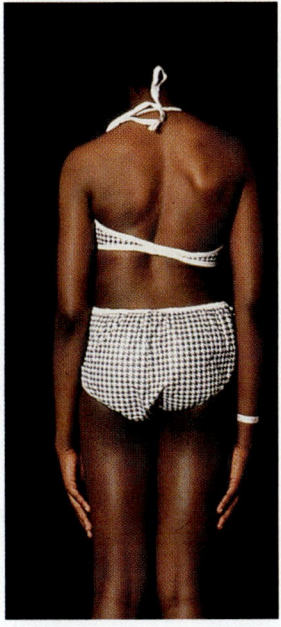

FIG. 61-8 Scoliosis in a standing erect posture. (From Zitelli BJ, McIntire SC, Nowalk AJ: *Zitelli and Davis' atlas of pediatric physical diagnosis*, ed 6, St Louis, 2012, Mosby.)

TABLE 61-4	**Muscle Strength Scale**
0/5	No detection of muscular contraction
1/5	A barely detectable flicker or trace of contraction with observation or palpation
2/5	Active movement of body part with elimination of gravity
3/5	Active movement against gravity only and not against resistance
4/5	Active movement against gravity and some resistance
5/5	Active movement against full resistance without evident fatigue (normal muscle strength)

TABLE 61-5   **Normal Physical Assessment of the Musculoskeletal System**

- Normal spinal curvatures
- No muscle atrophy or asymmetry
- No joint swelling, deformity, or crepitation
- No tenderness on palpation of spine, joints, or muscles
- Full range of motion of all joints without pain or laxity
- Muscle strength of 5/5

TABLE 61-6   Assessment Abnormalities

Musculoskeletal System

Finding	Description	Possible Etiology and Significance
Achilles tendonitis	Pain in ankle and posterior calf, initially when running or walking. Can progress to pain at rest.	Cumulative stress on Achilles tendon resulting in inflammation.
Ankylosis	Stiffness and fixation of a joint.	Chronic joint inflammation and destruction (e.g., rheumatoid arthritis).
Antalgic gait	Shortened stride with minimal weight bearing on the affected side, resulting in a limp.	Pain or discomfort in the lower extremity on weight bearing. Can be related to trauma or other disorders.
Ataxic gait	Staggering, uncoordinated gait often with sway.	Neurogenic disorders (e.g., spinal cord lesion).
Atrophy	Decreased size and strength of muscle leading to decreased function and tone.	Muscle denervation, contracture, prolonged disuse as a result of immobilization.
Boutonnière deformity	Finger abnormality, flexion of proximal interphalangeal (PIP) joint and hyperextension of the distal interphalangeal (DIP) joint of the fingers (see Fig. 64-4, *B*).	Typical deformity of rheumatoid and psoriatic arthritis caused by disruption of extensor tendons over the fingers.
Contracture	Resistance of movement of muscle or joint as a result of fibrosis of supporting soft tissues.	Shortening of muscle or ligaments, tightness of soft tissue, incorrect positioning of immobilized extremity.
Crepitation (crepitus)	Frequent, audible crackling sound with palpable grating that accompanies movement.	Fracture, dislocation, temporomandibular joint dysfunction, osteoarthritis.
Dislocation	Separation of two bones from their normal position within a joint.	Trauma, disorders of surrounding soft tissues.
Festinating gait	While walking, neck, trunk, and knees flex and the body is rigid. Delayed start with short, quick, shuffling steps. Speed may increase as if patient is unable to stop (festination).	Neurogenic disorders (e.g., Parkinson's disease).
Ganglion cyst	Small fluid-filled mass over a tendon sheath or joint, usually on dorsal surface of wrist or foot.	Inflammation of tissues around a joint, which can increase in size or disappear.
Kyphosis (dowager's hump)	Exaggerated thoracic curvature.	Poor posture, tuberculosis, arthritis, osteoporosis, growth disturbance of vertebral epiphyses.
Lateral epicondylitis (tennis elbow)	Dull ache along outer aspect of elbow, worsens with twisting and grasping motions.	Injury, inflammation, and/or partial tearing of tendon at its insertion on epicondyle.
Limited range of motion (ROM)	Joint does not achieve expected degrees of motion.	Injury, inflammation, contracture.
Lordosis (swayback)	Exaggerated lumbar curvature.	Secondary to other spinal deformities, muscular dystrophy, obesity, flexion contracture of hip, congenital dislocation of hip.
Muscle spasticity	Increased muscle tone (rigidity) with sustained muscle contractions (spasms); stiffness or tightness may interfere with gait, movement, speech.	Neuromuscular disorders such as multiple sclerosis (MS) or cerebral palsy.
Myalgia	General muscle tenderness and pain.	Chronic pain syndromes (e.g., fibromyalgia). Overuse, injury, or strain.
Paresthesia	Numbness and tingling, often described as a "pins and needles" sensation.	Compromised sensory nerves, often due to edema in a closed space such as a cast or bulky dressing. May also result from spinal stenosis.
Pes planus (flatfoot)	Abnormal flatness of the sole and arch of the foot.	Hereditary, muscle paralysis, mild cerebral palsy, early muscular dystrophy, injury to posterior tibial tendon.
Plantar fasciitis	Burning, sharp pain on heel and sole of foot. Worse in the morning with first step out of bed.	Chronic degenerative/reparative cycle resulting in inflammation.
Scoliosis	Asymmetric elevation of shoulders, scapulae, and iliac crests with lateral spine curvature (Fig. 61-8).	Idiopathic or congenital condition, fracture or dislocation, osteomalacia.
Short-leg gait	A limp, unless corrective footwear used.	Leg length discrepancy ≥1 in, generally of structural origin (arthritis, fracture).
Spastic gait	Short steps with dragging of foot. Jerky, uncoordinated, cross-knee (scissor) movement.	Neurogenic (e.g., cerebral palsy, hemiplegia).
Steppage gait	Increased hip and knee flexion to clear the foot from the floor. Footdrop is evident, foot slaps down and along walking surface.	Neurogenic disorders (e.g., peroneal nerve injury, paralyzed dorsiflexor muscles).
Subluxation	Partial dislocation of joint.	Instability of joint capsule and supporting ligaments (e.g., trauma, arthritis).
Swan neck deformity	Hyperextension of the PIP joint with flexion of the metacarpophalangeal (MCP) and DIP joints of the fingers (see Fig. 64-4, *D*).	Typical deformity of rheumatoid and psoriatic arthritis caused by contracture of muscles and tendons.
Swelling	Enlargement, often of a joint due to fluid collection. Generally leads to pain, stiffness.	Trauma or inflammation.
Tenosynovitis	Superficial swelling, pain, and tenderness along a tendon sheath.	Inflammation that often occurs with infection, injury, or overuse.
Torticollis (wryneck)	Neck is rotated and laterally bent in unusual position to one side.	Prolonged contraction of neck muscles (congenital or acquired).
Ulnar deviation (ulnar drift)	Fingers drift to ulnar side of forearm (see Fig. 64-4, *A*).	Typical deformity of rheumatoid arthritis due to tendon contracture.
Valgum deformity (knock-knees)	When knees are together and there is >1 in (2.5 cm) between the medial malleoli.	Poliomyelitis, congenital deformity, arthritis.
Varum deformity (bowlegs)	When knees are apart and the medial malleoli are together, a space of >1 in (2.5 cm) exists.	Arthritis, congenital deformity.

show as white on the standard x-ray. X-rays provide information about bone deformity, joint congruity, bone density, and calcification in soft tissue. X-rays are useful for diagnosing fractures and evaluating genetic, developmental, infectious, inflammatory, neoplastic, metabolic, and degenerative disorders.

Visualization and analysis of aspirated synovial fluid allows assessment of volume, color, clarity, viscosity, and mucin clot formation. Normal synovial fluid is transparent and colorless or straw colored. It should be scant in amount and of low viscosity. Fluid from an infected joint may be purulent and thick or gray and thin. In gout, the fluid may be whitish yellow. Blood may be aspirated if there is hemarthrosis due to injury or a bleeding disorder.

The mucin clot test indicates the character of the protein portion of the synovial fluid. Normally a white, ropelike mucin clot is formed. In the presence of inflammation, the clot fragments easily. The fluid is examined grossly for floating fat globules, which indicate bone injury. In septic arthritis, protein content is elevated and glucose is considerably decreased. Presence of uric acid crystals suggests a diagnosis of gout. A Gram stain and culture may also be done to assess for the presence and type of infection.

CASE STUDY–cont'd
Objective Data: Physical Examination

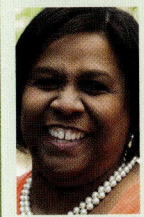

(©pixelhead-photo/iStock/Thinkstock)

A focused assessment of G.A. reveals the following: BP 128/94, heart rate 88, respiratory rate 26, temp 96.8° F, O₂ saturation 98%. Alert and oriented × 3. Lungs are clear bilaterally. Left great toe is red and swollen. No open wounds. Tremendous pain on palpation and with any movement of the left great toe. +1 Pedal pulses bilaterally.

Discussion Questions

1. What should be included in the physical assessment?
   What findings would be of most concern to you?
2. Based on results of the subjective and physical assessment, what diagnostic studies might you expect to be included for G.A.?
   You will learn more about diagnostic studies related to the musculoskeletal system in the next section.
   See p. 1460 for more information on G.A.

Answers available at *http://evolve.elsevier.com/Lewis/medsurg.*

FOCUSED ASSESSMENT
Musculoskeletal System

Use this checklist to be sure key assessment steps have been done.

Subjective
Ask the patient about any of the following and note responses.

Joint pain or stiffness	Y	N
Muscle weakness	Y	N
Bone pain	Y	N

Objective: Diagnostic
Check the results of the following diagnostic studies.

X-ray	✓
MRI or CT scan	✓
Bone scan	✓

Objective: Physical Examination
Inspect and Palpate

Spine and extremities (compare sides) for alignment, contour, symmetry, size, gross deformities	✓
Joints for range of motion, tenderness or pain, heat, crepitus, swelling	✓
Muscles (compare sides) for size, symmetry, tone, tenderness or pain	✓
Bones for tenderness or pain	✓

TABLE 61-7   Diagnostic Studies
Musculoskeletal System

Study	Description and Purpose	Nursing Responsibility
Radiologic Studies		
Standard x-ray	Evaluates structural or functional changes of bones and joints. Can give a general impression of bone density. In anteroposterior view, x-ray beam passes from front to back, allowing one-dimensional view. Lateral position provides two-dimensional view.	*Before:* Remove any radiopaque objects that can interfere with results. Explain procedure to patient. *During:* Avoid excessive exposure of patient and self.
Diskogram	X-ray of cervical or lumbar intervertebral disc is done after injection of contrast media into nucleus pulposus. Permits visualization of intervertebral disc abnormalities.	*Before:* Assess patient for possible allergy to contrast medium. Explain procedure.
Computed tomography (CT) scan	X-ray beam used with a computer to provide a 3D picture. Used to identify soft tissue abnormalities, bony abnormalities, and various types of musculoskeletal trauma.	*Before:* Inform patient that procedure is painless. Inform patient of importance of remaining still during procedure. If contrast medium is being used, verify that patient does not have shellfish allergy.
Myelogram with or without CT	Involves injecting a radiographic contrast medium into sac around nerve roots. CT scan may follow to show how the bone is affecting the nerve roots. Sensitive test for nerve impingement and can detect subtle lesions and injuries.	*Before:* Inform patient that headache may occur after procedure but should resolve in 1-2 days with rest and fluids, but should be reported to HCP.
MRI	Radio waves and magnetic field are used to view soft tissue. Especially useful in the diagnosis of avascular necrosis, disc disease, tumors, osteomyelitis, ligament tears, and cartilage tears. Patient is placed inside scanning chamber. Gadolinium may be injected IV to enhance visualization of structures. Open MRI (patient not placed in chamber) may be indicated for obese patient or patient with large chest and abdominal girth or severe claustrophobia. Contraindicated in patient with aneurysm clips, metallic implants, pacemakers, electronic devices, hearing aids, and shrapnel.	*Before:* Inform patient that procedure is painless. Explain that the machine will make loud tapping noises intermittently and there is no cause for alarm. Ear plugs can be requested or music to listen to. Ensure that patient has no metal on clothing (e.g., snaps, zippers), jewelry, credit cards. Inform patient to remain still throughout procedure. Inform patients who are claustrophobic that they may experience symptoms during examination. Administer antianxiety agent if indicated and ordered.

Continued

TABLE 61-7 Diagnostic Studies

Musculoskeletal System—cont'd

Study	Description and Purpose	Nursing Responsibility
Bone Mineral Density (BMD) Measurements		
Dual energy x-ray absorptiometry (DXA)	Measures bone mineral density of spine, femur, forearm, and total body. Allows assessment of bone density with minimal radiation exposure. Used to diagnose metabolic bone disease (e.g., osteoporosis) and monitor changes in bone density with treatment.	*Before:* Inform patient that procedure is painless.
Quantitative ultrasound (QUS)	Evaluates density, elasticity, and strength of bone using ultrasound rather than radiation. Common area assessed is calcaneus (heel).	Same as above.
Radioisotope Studies		
Bone scan	Involves injection of radioisotope (usually technetium [Tc]-99m) that is taken up by bone. Uniform uptake of the isotope is normal. Increased uptake is seen in osteomyelitis, primary and metastatic cancer of bone, and certain fractures. Decreased uptake is seen in areas of avascular necrosis.	*Before:* Explain that radioisotope is given 2 hr before procedure. Ensure that bladder is emptied before scan. Inform patient that procedure requires 1 hr while patient lies supine and that no pain or harm will result from isotopes. *After:* Increase fluids after scan.
Endoscopy		
Arthroscopy	Involves insertion of arthroscope into joint for visualization of interior of joint cavity. Can be used for surgery (removal of loose bodies, biopsy); repair of joint structures; and diagnosis of abnormalities of meniscus, articular cartilage, ligaments, or joint capsule. Structures that can be visualized through an arthroscope include knee, shoulder, elbow, wrist, jaw, hip, and ankle (Fig. 61-9).	*Before:* Inform patient that procedure can be performed in outpatient setting and that local or general anesthesia may be used. *After:* Cover wound with sterile dressing. Explain any postprocedure activity restrictions.
Mineral Metabolism		
Alkaline phosphatase	This enzyme is produced by osteoblasts and is needed for mineralization of organic bone matrix. Elevated levels are found in healing fractures, bone cancers, osteoporosis, osteomalacia, and Paget's disease. *Reference interval:* 38-126 U/L (0.65-2.14 µkat/L)	*During:* Obtain blood samples by venipuncture. Observe venipuncture site for bleeding or hematoma formation. Inform patient that procedure does not require fasting.
Calcium	Bone is primary organ for calcium storage. Calcium provides bone with rigid structure. Decreased serum level is found in osteomalacia, kidney disease, and hypoparathyroidism. Increased level is found in hyperparathyroidism and some bone tumors. *Reference interval:* 8.6-10.2 mg/dL (2.20-2.55 mmol/L)	Same as above.
Phosphorus	Amount present is indirectly related to calcium metabolism. Decreased level is found in osteomalacia. Increased level is found in chronic kidney disease, healing fractures, and osteolytic metastatic tumor. *Reference interval:* 2.4-4.4 mg/dL (0.78-1.42 mmol/L)	Same as above.
Serologic Studies		
Rheumatoid factor (RF)	Assesses presence of autoantibody (rheumatoid factor) in serum. Factor is not specific for rheumatoid arthritis and is seen in other connective tissue diseases and in a small percentage of normal population. *Reference interval:* Negative or titer <1:17	Same as above.
Anticyclic citrullinated peptide (anti-CCP)	Assesses presence of CCP antibodies. More specific for rheumatoid arthritis than rheumatoid factor. Positive result indicates high likelihood of RA. *Reference interval:* Negative or <20.0 U	Same as above.
Antinuclear antibody (ANA)	Assesses presence of antibodies capable of destroying nucleus of body's tissue cells. Finding is positive in 95% of patients with systemic lupus erythematosus and may also be positive in individuals with scleroderma or rheumatoid arthritis and in a small percentage of normal population. *Reference interval:* Negative at 1:40 dilution	Same as above.
Anti-DNA antibody	Detects serum antibodies that react with DNA. Most specific test for systemic lupus erythematosus. *Reference interval:* <70 IU/mL	Same as above.

TABLE 61-7 **Diagnostic Studies**

Musculoskeletal System—cont'd

Study	Description and Purpose	Nursing Responsibility
Complement, total hemolytic (CH$_{50}$)	Complement, a normal body protein, is essential to immune and inflammatory reactions. Complement components used in these reactions are depleted. Complement depletions may be found in patients with rheumatoid arthritis or systemic lupus erythematosus. *Reference interval:* 75-160 U/mL (75-160 kU/L)	Same as above.
Uric acid	End product of purine metabolism normally excreted in urine. Although not specific, levels are usually elevated in gout. *Male:* 4.4-7.6 mg/dL (262-452 μmol/L) *Female:* 2.3-6.6 mg/dL (137-393 μmol/L)	Same as above.
C-reactive protein (CRP)	Used to diagnose inflammatory diseases, infections, and active widespread malignancy. Synthesized by the liver and is present in large amounts in serum 18-24 hr after onset of tissue damage. *Reference interval:* 6.8-820 mcg/dL (68-8200 mcg/L)	Same as above.
Human leukocyte antigen (HLA)–B27	Antigen often present in autoimmune disorders such as ankylosing spondylitis and rheumatoid arthritis.	Same as above.
Markers of Muscle Injury		
Creatine kinase (CK)	Highest concentration found in skeletal muscle. Increased serum CK found in progressive muscular dystrophy, polymyositis, and traumatic injuries. *Male:* 20-200 U/L *Female:* 20-180 U/L	Same as above.
Potassium	Increased in muscle trauma as cell destruction releases this electrolyte into serum. Cardiac dysrhythmias can be caused by hyperkalemia or hypokalemia. *Reference interval:* 3.5-5.0 mEq/L (3.5-5.0 mmol/L)	Same as above.
Aldolase	Useful in monitoring muscular dystrophy and dermatomyositis. *Reference interval:* 1.5-8.1 U/L	Same as above.
Invasive Procedures		
Arthrocentesis	Incision or puncture of joint capsule to obtain samples of synovial fluid or to remove excess fluid. Local anesthesia and aseptic preparation are used before needle is inserted into joint and fluid aspirated. Useful in diagnosis of joint inflammation, infection, meniscal tears, and subtle fractures.	*Before:* Inform patient that procedure is usually done at bedside or in examination room. *After:* Send samples of synovial fluid to laboratory for examination (if indicated). Apply compression dressing. Observe for leakage of blood or fluid on dressing.
Electromyogram (EMG)	Evaluates electrical potential associated with skeletal muscle contraction. Small-gauge needles are inserted into certain muscles. Needle probes are attached to leads that send information to EMG machine. Recordings of electrical activity of muscle are traced on audio transmitter and on oscilloscope and recording paper. Useful in providing information related to lower motor neuron dysfunction and primary muscle disease.	*Before:* Inform patient that procedure is usually done in EMG laboratory while patient lies supine on special table. Inform patient that procedure involves some discomfort from needle insertion. Avoid stimulants, including caffeine, and sedatives 24 hr before procedure.
Miscellaneous		
Duplex venous Doppler	Ultrasound of the veins, usually of the lower extremities, to detect blood flow abnormalities that could indicate DVT.	*Before:* Inform patient that procedure is painless and noninvasive.
Thermography	Uses infrared detector to measure degree of heat radiating from skin surface. Useful in investigating cause of inflamed joint and in determining patient response to antiinflammatory drug therapy.	Same as above.
Plethysmography	Records variations in volume and pressure of blood passing through tissues. Test is nonspecific.	Same as above.
Somatosensory evoked potential (SSEP)	Evaluates evoked potential of muscle contractions. Electrodes are placed on skin and provide recordings of electrical activity of muscle. Useful in identifying subtle dysfunction of lower motor neuron and primary muscle disease. Measures nerve conduction along pathways not accessible by EMG. Transcutaneous or percutaneous electrodes are applied to the skin to help identify neuropathy and myopathy. Often used during spinal surgery for scoliosis to detect neurologic compromise when patient is under anesthesia.	*Before:* Inform patient that procedure is similar to EMG but does not involve needles. Electrodes are applied to the skin.

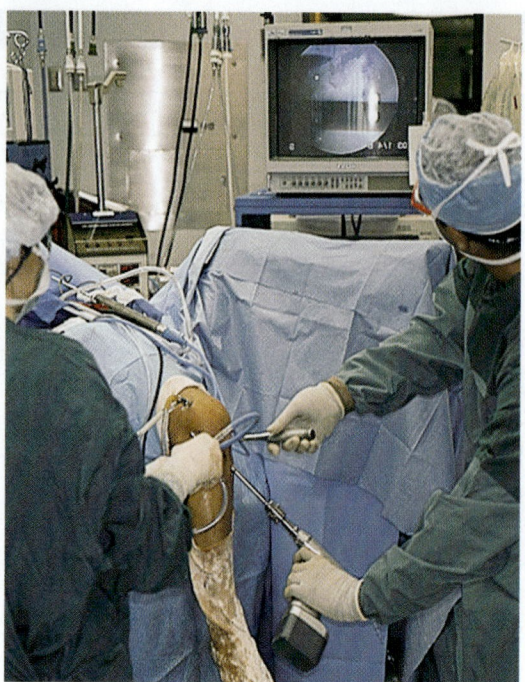

FIG. 61-9   Knee arthroscopy in progress. Notice the monitor in the background. (From Miller MD, Howard RF, Plancher KD: *Surgical atlas of sports medicine,* Philadelphia, 2003, Saunders.)

CASE STUDY—cont'd

Objective Data: Diagnostic Studies

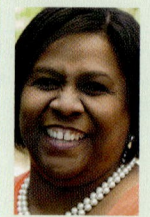

(©pixelhead-photo/iStock/Thinkstock)

The HCP in the ED immediately orders the following diagnostic studies:
- X-ray of left foot
- CBC, electrolytes
- Aspiration of the great toe

The x-ray of the foot reveals minor soft tissue swelling but no evidence of fracture. Very mild arthritis is noted at the interphalangeal joint of the great toe. CBC and electrolytes are within normal limits.

Aspiration of the interphalangeal joint shows clear synovial fluid. Protein and glucose are within normal limits. Microscopic analysis of the synovial fluid shows urate crystals.

Discussion Questions

1. Which diagnostic results are abnormal?
2. What diagnostic study results are of most concern to you?

Answers available at *http://evolve.elsevier.com/Lewis/medsurg.*

BRIDGE TO NCLEX EXAMINATION

The number of the question corresponds to the same-numbered outcome at the beginning of the chapter.

1. The bone cells that function in the resorption of bone tissue are called
   a. osteoids.
   b. osteocytes.
   c. osteoclasts.
   d. osteoblasts.

2. While performing passive range of motion for a patient, the nurse puts the ankle joint through the movements of *(select all that apply)*
   a. flexion and extension.
   b. inversion and eversion.
   c. pronation and supination.
   d. flexion, extension, abduction, and adduction.
   e. pronation, supination, rotation, and circumduction.

3. To prevent muscle atrophy, the nurse teaches the patient with a leg immobilized in traction to perform *(select all that apply)*
   a. flexion contractions.
   b. tetanic contractions.
   c. isotonic contractions.
   d. isometric contractions.
   e. extension contractions.

4. A patient with tendonitis asks what the tendon does. The nurse's response is based on the knowledge that tendons
   a. connect bone to muscle.
   b. provide strength to muscle.
   c. lubricate joints with synovial fluid.
   d. relieve friction between moving parts.

5. The increased risk for falls in the older adult is *most* likely due to
   a. changes in balance.
   b. decrease in bone mass.
   c. loss of ligament elasticity.
   d. erosion of articular cartilage.

6. While obtaining subjective assessment data related to the musculoskeletal system, the nurse must ask a patient about other medical problems such as
   a. hypertension.
   b. thyroid problems.
   c. diabetes mellitus.
   d. chronic bronchitis.

7. When grading muscle strength, the nurse records a score of 3/5, which indicates
   a. no detection of muscular contraction.
   b. a barely detectable flicker of contraction.
   c. active movement against full resistance without fatigue.
   d. active movement against gravity but not against resistance.

8. A normal assessment finding of the musculoskeletal system is
   a. no deformity or crepitation.
   b. muscle and bone strength of 4.
   c. ulnar deviation and subluxation.
   d. angulation of bone toward midline.

9. A patient is scheduled for an electromyogram (EMG). The nurse explains that this diagnostic test involves
   a. incision or puncture of the joint capsule.
   b. insertion of small needles into certain muscles.
   c. administration of a radioisotope before the procedure.
   d. placement of skin electrodes to record muscle activity.

10. What would the nurse recognize as a possible difference in the assessment of a gerontologic patient?
    a. Slowed reaction time
    b. Quicker reflex response
    c. Decreased joint stiffness
    d. Increased fine motor dexterity

1. c, 2. a, b, 3. d, 4. a, 5. a, 6. c, 7. d, 8. a, 9. b, 10. a

For rationales to these answers and even more NCLEX review questions, visit *http://evolve.elsevier.com/Lewis/medsurg.*

ⓔ EVOLVE WEBSITE

http://evolve.elsevier.com/Lewis/medsurg

Review Questions (Online Only)
Key Points
Answer Keys for Questions
- Rationales for Bridge to NCLEX Examination Questions
- Answer Guidelines for Case Study on pp. 1451, 1454, 1457, and 1460
Conceptual Care Map Creator
Audio Glossary
Supporting Media
- Animation
  - Overview of the Musculoskeletal System
Content Updates

REFERENCES

1. Moore KL, Anne MR, Dailey AF: *Essential clinical anatomy*, ed 5, Philadelphia, 2015, Wolters Kluwer Health.
2. Crowther-Radulewicz CL: The musculoskeletal system. In McCance KL, Heuther SE, editors: *Pathophysiology: the biologic basis for disease in adults and children*, ed 7, St Louis, 2014, Mosby.
3. Martini FH, Nath JL, Bartholomew EF: *Fundamentals of anatomy and physiology*, ed 10, New York, 2014, Pearson.
4. Patton KT, Thibodeau GA: *Anatomy & physiology*, ed 8, St Louis, 2013, Mosby.
5. Zychowicz ME, Ballard PC: Musculoskeletal system. In Estes MEZ, editor: *Health assessment & physical examination*, ed 5, Clifton Park, NY, 2014, Cengage.
6. Stoppiello LA, Mapp PI, Wilson D, et al: Structural associations of symptomatic knee osteoarthritis, *Arthr Rheum* 66:3018, 2014.
7. Zychowicz ME, South T, Martin-Plank L, et al: Musculoskeletal problems. In Dunphy LM, Winland-Brown JE, Porter BO, et al, editors: *Primary care: the art and science of advanced practice nursing*, ed 4, Philadelphia, 2015, FA Davis.
8. Ward CW: Procedure-specific postoperative pain management, *MEDSURG* 23:107, 2014.
*9. Fischer J, Nüesch C, Göpfert B, et al: Forearm pressure distribution during ambulation with elbow crutches: a cross-sectional study, *J Neuroeng Rehab* 11:61, 2014.

*Evidence-based information for clinical practice.

62

Musculoskeletal Trauma and Orthopedic Surgery

Mary K. Wollan

With the new day comes new strength and new thoughts.

Eleanor Roosevelt

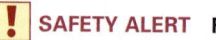 http://evolve.elsevier.com/Lewis/medsurg/

LEARNING OUTCOMES

1. Differentiate among the etiology, pathophysiology, clinical manifestations, and interprofessional care of soft tissue injuries, including strains, sprains, dislocations, subluxations, bursitis, repetitive strain injury, carpal tunnel syndrome, and injuries to the rotator cuff, meniscus, and anterior cruciate ligament.
2. Relate the sequential events involved in fracture healing.
3. Compare closed reduction, cast immobilization, open reduction, and traction in terms of purpose, complications, and nursing management.
4. Assess the neurovascular condition of an injured extremity.

5. Explain common complications associated with a fracture and fracture healing.
6. Describe the interprofessional care and nursing management of patients with various kinds of fractures.
7. Describe indications for and interprofessional care and nursing management of the patient with an amputation.
8. Describe types of joint replacement surgery for arthritis and other disorders.
9. Prioritize preoperative and postoperative management of the patient having joint replacement surgery.

KEY TERMS

amputation, p. 1487
arthrodesis, p. 1492
arthroplasty, p. 1491
bursitis, p. 1468
carpal tunnel syndrome (CTS), p. 1465
compartment syndrome, p. 1479

debridement, p. 1491
dislocation, p. 1464
fat embolism syndrome (FES), p. 1480
fracture, p. 1468
osteotomy, p. 1490
phantom limb sensation, p. 1488

repetitive strain injury (RSI), p. 1465
sprain, p. 1463
strain, p. 1463
subluxation, p. 1464
synovectomy, p. 1490
traction, p. 1470

Musculoskeletal problems resulting from trauma and common orthopedic surgical procedures are discussed in this chapter. The nurse's role in prevention of complications and promotion of function in patients with fractures and orthopedic surgery is emphasized.

The most common cause of musculoskeletal injury is a traumatic event resulting in fracture, dislocation, and/or soft tissue injury. Although most of these injuries are not fatal, the cost in terms of pain, disability, medical expense, and lost wages is enormous. Accidents are one of the top three causes of death for persons ages 1 to 64 years. Accidental injuries (e.g., motor vehicle collisions, drowning, burns) are the leading cause of death in children and young adults in the United States.[1]

Teaching the public about basic principles of safety and accident prevention is important. The morbidity associated with accidents can be significantly reduced if people are aware of environmental hazards, use appropriate safety equipment, and apply safety and traffic rules. In the occupational and industrial setting, teach employees and employers about use of proper safety equipment and avoidance of hazardous working situations.

> ! **SAFETY ALERT** **Falls**
> - Falls account for many musculoskeletal injuries in the home.
> - Provide preventive teaching to high-risk individuals (e.g., people with gait instability, visual or cognitive impairment).
> - Stress the importance of wearing shoes with functional, stable soles and heels; avoiding wet or slippery surfaces; and removing throw rugs in the home.

Ways to prevent common musculoskeletal problems in the older adult are listed in Table 62-1.

SOFT TISSUE INJURIES

Soft tissue injuries, including sprains, strains, dislocations, and subluxations, usually result from trauma. The increasing number of people involved in a fitness program or participating in sports has contributed to the increased incidence of soft

Reviewed by Judy Carlyle, RN, MNSc, Faculty/Clinical Liaison, Arkansas Rural Nursing Education Consortium (ARNEC), Nashville, Arkansas; Roberta Goff, RN, MSN Ed, ACNS-BC, RN-BC, ONC, Clinical Nurse Specialist, Munson Medical Center, Traverse City, Michigan; Matthew C. Price, RN, MSN, CNP, ONP-C, RNFA, Manager, Orthopedic Advanced Practice Providers, Riverside Methodist Hospital, Columbus, Ohio; and Laura C. Williams, RN, MSN, CNS, ONC, CCNS, Orthopedic Clinical Nurse Specialist, Orlando Health, Orlando, Florida.

tissue injuries. Common sports-related injuries are summarized in Table 62-2. The most common sports injuries that result in a visit to the emergency department for younger patients are sprains and strains, growth plate injuries, and repetitive motion injuries.[2]

SPRAINS AND STRAINS

Sprains and strains commonly occur during vigorous activities from abnormal stretching or twisting forces. These injuries tend to occur around joints and in the spinal musculature.

A **sprain** is an injury to the ligaments surrounding a joint, usually caused by a wrenching or twisting motion. Most sprains occur in the ankle, wrist, and knee joints.[3] A sprain is classified

TABLE 62-1 Patient & Caregiver Teaching
Prevention of Musculoskeletal Problems in Older Adults

To prevent musculoskeletal problems, include the following instructions when teaching older adults and their caregivers.
1. Use ramps in buildings and at street corners instead of steps to prevent falls.
2. Eliminate scatter rugs in the home.
3. Treat pain and discomfort from osteoarthritis.
   - Rest in positions that decrease discomfort.
   - Use medication as prescribed for pain.
4. Use a walker or cane to help prevent falls.
5. Eat the amount and kind of foods needed to prevent excessive weight gain. Obesity adds stress to joints, which may predispose to osteoarthritis.
6. Get regular and frequent exercise.
   - Activities of daily living provide range-of-motion exercises. Tai Chi may also be helpful.
   - Hobbies (e.g., jigsaw puzzles, needlework, model building) exercise finger joints and prevent stiffness.
   - Weight-bearing exercise (e.g., walking) should be done on a daily basis to improve bone health.
7. Use shoes with good support for safety and comfort.
8. Avoid sudden change in position. Rise slowly to a standing position to prevent dizziness, falls, and fractures.
9. Avoid walking on uneven surfaces and wet floors.

according to the degree of ligament damage. A *first-degree (mild) sprain* involves tears in only a few fibers, resulting in mild tenderness and minimal swelling. A *second-degree (moderate) sprain* is partial disruption of the involved tissue with more swelling and tenderness. A *third-degree (severe) sprain* is complete tearing of the ligament in association with moderate to severe swelling. A gap in the muscle may be apparent or palpated through the skin if the muscle is torn. Because areas around joints are rich in nerve endings, the injury can be extremely painful.

A **strain** is an excessive stretching of a muscle, its fascial sheath, or a tendon. Most strains occur in the large muscle groups, including the lower back, calf, and hamstrings. Strains may also be classified as first degree (mild or slightly pulled muscle), second degree (moderate or moderately torn muscle), and third degree (severely torn or ruptured muscle).

Clinical manifestations of sprains and strains are similar and include pain, edema, decreased function, and contusion. Pain aggravated by continued use of the joint, tendon, or ligament is common. Edema develops in the injured area because of the local inflammatory response.

Mild sprains and strains are usually self-limiting, with full function returning within 3 to 6 weeks. X-rays of the affected part may be taken to rule out a fracture. A severe sprain can result in a concomitant *avulsion fracture,* in which the ligament pulls loose a fragment of bone. Alternatively, the joint structure may become unstable and result in subluxation or dislocation. At the time of injury, *hemarthrosis* (bleeding into a joint space or cavity) or disruption of the synovial lining may occur. Severe strains may require surgical repair of the muscle, tendon, or surrounding fascia.[4]

❖ NURSING MANAGEMENT: SPRAINS AND STRAINS

◆ Nursing Implementation

◆ **Health Promotion.** Warming up muscles before exercising and vigorous activity, followed by stretching, may significantly reduce the risk of sprains and strains. Strength, balance, and endurance exercises are also important. Strengthening exercises

TABLE 62-2 Sports-Related Injuries

Injury	Description	Treatment
Impingement syndrome	Entrapment of soft tissues and nerves under coracoacromial arch of shoulder.	NSAIDs. Rest until symptoms decrease and then gradual ROM and strengthening exercises.
Rotator cuff tear	Tear within muscle, tendons, or ligaments around shoulder.	*If minor tear:* Rest, NSAIDs, and gradual mobilization with ROM and strengthening exercises. *If major tear:* Surgical repair.
Shin splints	Inflammation of periosteal bone (*periostitis*) along anterior calf caused by improper shoes, overuse, or running on hard pavement.	Rest, ice, NSAIDs, proper shoes. Gradual increase in activity. If pain persists, x-ray to rule out tibial stress fracture.
Tendonitis	Inflammation of tendon as a result of overuse or incorrect use.	Rest, ice, NSAIDs. Gradual return to sport activity. Protective brace (*orthosis*) may be necessary if symptoms recur.
Ligament injury	Tearing or stretching of ligament. Usually occurs as a result of inversion, eversion, shearing, or torque applied to a joint. Characterized by sudden pain, swelling, and instability.	Rest, ice, elevation of extremity if possible, NSAIDs. Protect affected extremity by use of brace. If symptoms persist, surgical repair may be needed.
Meniscus injury	Injury to fibrocartilage discs in knee characterized by popping, clicking, tearing sensation, effusion, and/or swelling.	Rest, ice, elevation of extremity if possible, NSAIDs. Gradual return to regular activities. If symptoms persist, MRI to assess meniscus injury. Possible arthroscopic surgery.
Anterior cruciate ligament tear	Tearing of ligament by deceleration forces with pivoting or odd positions of the knee or leg.	Physical therapy with rehabilitation, knee brace. If knee instability or additional injury, reconstructive surgery may be done.

that involve working against resistance build muscle strength and bone density. Balance exercises, which may overlap with some strengthening exercises, help to prevent falls. Endurance exercises should start at a low level of effort and progress gradually to a moderate level.

HEALTHY PEOPLE

Health Impact of Regular Physical Activity

- Assists in weight management.
- Helps maintain and improve bone mass.
- Helps prevent high BP.
- Increases lean muscle and decreases body fat.
- Increases muscle strength, flexibility, and endurance.
- Appears to reduce symptoms of depression and anxiety.
- Reduces the risk of heart disease, diabetes, and colon cancer.
- Enhances sense of well-being and may reduce risk of depression.

◆ **Acute Care.** If an injury occurs, immediate care focuses on (1) stopping the activity and limiting movement, (2) applying ice packs to the injured area, (3) compressing the involved area, (4) elevating the extremity, and (5) providing analgesia as needed (Table 62-3).

RICE (*R*est, *I*ce, *C*ompression, *E*levation) may decrease local inflammation and pain for most musculoskeletal injuries. Movement should be restricted and the extremity rested as soon as pain is felt. Unless the injury is severe, prolonged rest is usually not indicated.

Cold *(cryotherapy)* in several forms can be used to produce hypothermia in the involved part. The cold induces physiologic changes in soft tissue, including vasoconstriction and a reduction in the transmission and perception of nerve pain impulses. In addition to pain relief, these changes reduce muscle spasms, inflammation, and edema. Cold is most useful when applied immediately after the injury has occurred. Apply ice no more than 20 to 30 minutes at a time; avoid applying ice directly to the skin.

An elastic compression bandage can be wrapped around the injured part. To prevent edema and encourage fluid return, wrap the bandage starting distally (at the point farthest from the trunk of the body) and progress proximally (toward the trunk of the body). The bandage is too tight if numbness or tingling is felt below the area of compression or additional pain or swelling occurs beyond the edge of the bandage. Leave the bandage in place for 30 minutes and then remove it for 15 minutes. However, some elastic wraps are left on during training, athletic, and occupational activities.

Elevate the injured part above heart level, even during sleep, to help mobilize excess fluid from the area and prevent further edema. Mild analgesics and nonsteroidal antiinflammatory drugs (NSAIDs) may be used to manage patient discomfort.

After the acute phase (usually 24 to 48 hours), apply warm, moist heat to the affected part to reduce swelling and provide comfort. Heat applications should not exceed 20 to 30 minutes, allowing a "cool-down" time between applications. Encourage the patient to use the limb if the joint is protected by means of casting, bracing, taping, or splinting. Joint movement maintains nutrition to the cartilage, and muscle contraction improves circulation and resolution of contusion and swelling.

◆ **Ambulatory Care.** Most sprains and strains are treated in the outpatient setting. Instruct the patient to use ice and elevate for 24 to 48 hours after the injury to reduce edema. Encourage the use of mild analgesics to promote comfort. Use of an elastic wrap may provide additional support during activity. Emphasize to the patient the importance of strengthening and conditioning exercises to prevent reinjury.[5]

The physical therapist may help provide pain relief by modalities such as ultrasound. The therapist may also teach the patient exercises to improve flexibility and strength.

DISLOCATION AND SUBLUXATION

A **dislocation** is the complete displacement or separation of the articular surfaces of the joint. It results from severe injury of the ligaments surrounding the joint. A **subluxation** is a partial or incomplete displacement of the joint surface. The clinical manifestations of a subluxation are similar to those of a dislocation but are less severe.

Dislocations characteristically result from forces transmitted to the joint that disrupt the soft tissue support structures

✚ TABLE 62-3 Emergency Management
Acute Soft Tissue Injury

Etiology	Assessment Findings	Interventions
• Falls • Direct blows • Crush injury • Motor vehicle crashes • Sports injuries	• Edema • Bruising (contusion) • Pain, tenderness • Decreased sensation with severe edema • Decreased pulse, coolness, capillary refill >2 sec • Decreased movement • Pallor • Shortening or rotation of extremity • Inability to bear weight with lower extremity involvement • Limited or decreased function with upper extremity involvement • Muscle spasms	**Initial** • Ensure airway, breathing, and circulation. • Perform neurovascular assessment of involved limb. • Elevate involved limb. • Apply compression bandage unless dislocation present. • Apply ice packs to affected area. • Immobilize affected extremity in the position found. Do *not* attempt to realign or reinsert protruding bones. • Anticipate x-rays of injured extremity. • Give analgesia as necessary. • Administer tetanus and diphtheria prophylaxis if there is an open fracture. • Administer antibiotic prophylaxis for open fracture, large tissue defects, or mangled extremity injury. **Ongoing Monitoring** • Monitor for changes in neurovascular condition. • Implement weight-bearing restrictions as ordered for lower extremity involvement. • Anticipate compartment pressure monitoring if neurovascular assessment changes and compartment syndrome suspected.

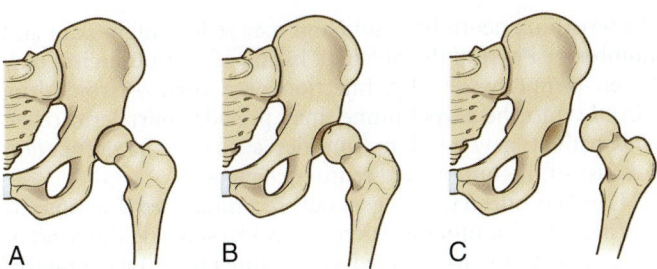

FIG. 62-1 Soft tissue injury of the hip. **A,** Normal. **B,** Subluxation (partial dislocation). **C,** Dislocation.

surrounding it. The joints most frequently dislocated in the upper extremity include the thumb, elbow, and shoulder. In the lower extremity, the hip is vulnerable to dislocation as a result of severe trauma, often associated with motor vehicle crashes (Fig. 62-1). The kneecap (patella) may dislocate because of a sharp, direct blow or after a sudden twisting inward motion while the planted foot is pointed outward.[6]

The most obvious clinical manifestation of a dislocation is deformity. For example, if a hip is dislocated in a posterior (or backward) direction, the affected limb may be shorter and internally rotated. Additional manifestations include local pain, tenderness, loss of function of the injured part, and swelling of soft tissues near the joint. Major complications of a dislocated joint are open joint injuries, fractures within the joint (intraarticular), avascular necrosis (bone cell death due to inadequate blood supply), and damage to adjacent nerves and blood vessels.

X-rays are performed to determine the extent of displacement. The joint may also be aspirated to assess for hemarthrosis or fat cells. Fat cells in the aspirate indicate a probable intraarticular fracture.

❖ NURSING AND INTERPROFESSIONAL MANAGEMENT: DISLOCATION

A dislocation requires prompt attention. It is often considered an orthopedic emergency because it may be associated with significant vascular injury. The longer the joint remains unreduced, the greater the possibility of avascular necrosis. The femoral head of the hip joint is particularly susceptible to avascular necrosis. Compartment syndrome (discussed on p. 1479) may also occur after dislocation due to vascular injury and resulting ischemia. Neurovascular assessment is critical (see pp. 1474-1475).

The first goal of management of a dislocation is to realign the dislocated portion of the joint to its original anatomic position. Closed reduction (no incision) may be performed under local or general anesthesia or IV moderate to deep sedation (formerly called conscious sedation). Anesthesia is often needed to relax the muscle so that the bones can be manipulated. In some situations, open reduction (joint visualized through surgical incision) may be needed. After reduction, the extremity is immobilized by a brace, splint, or sling, or by taping to allow torn ligaments and surrounding tissue to heal.

Nursing management of subluxation or dislocation is directed toward pain management and support and protection of the injured joint. After the joint has been reduced and immobilized, motion is usually restricted. A carefully monitored rehabilitation program can prevent fracture instability and joint dysfunction. Gentle range-of-motion (ROM) exercises may be

recommended if the joint is stable and well supported. An exercise program slowly restores the joint to its original ROM without causing another dislocation. The patient should gradually return to normal activities.

A patient who has dislocated a joint may be at greater risk for repeated dislocations because of loose ligaments. Activity restrictions may be imposed on the affected joint to decrease the risk of repeated dislocations.

REPETITIVE STRAIN INJURY

Repetitive strain injury (RSI) and cumulative trauma disorder are terms used to describe injuries resulting from prolonged force or repetitive movements and awkward postures. RSI is also referred to as repetitive trauma disorder, nontraumatic musculoskeletal injury, overuse syndrome (sports medicine), regional musculoskeletal disorder, and work-related musculoskeletal disorder. Repeated movements strain the tendons, ligaments, and muscles, causing tiny tears that become inflamed. The exact cause of these disorders is unknown. No specific diagnostic tests exist, and diagnosis is often difficult.

Persons at risk for RSI include musicians, dancers, butchers, grocery clerks, vibratory tool workers, and those who frequently use a computer mouse and keyboard. Competitive athletes and poorly trained athletes may also develop RSI. Swimming, overhead throwing (e.g., baseball), weight lifting, gymnastics, tennis, skiing, and kicking sports (e.g., soccer) require repetitive motion. Overtraining compounds the effects of RSI.

In addition to repetitive movements, other factors related to RSI include poor posture and positioning, poor workspace ergonomics, badly designed workplace equipment (e.g., computer keyboard), and repetitive lifting of heavy objects without sufficient muscle rest. Inflammation, swelling, and pain in the muscles, tendons, and nerves of the neck, spine, shoulder, forearm, and hand may result. Symptoms of RSI include pain, weakness, numbness, or impaired motor function.

RSI can be prevented through education and ergonomics (the science that promotes efficiency and safety in the interaction of humans and their work environment). Ergonomic considerations for persons who work at a desk and use a computer include keeping the hips and knees flexed to 90 degrees with the feet flat, keeping the wrist straight to type, having the top of the computer monitor even with the forehead, and taking at least hourly stretch breaks.

Once RSI is diagnosed, treatment consists of (1) identification of the precipitating activity, (2) modification of equipment or activity, (3) pain management, including heat or cold application and NSAIDs, (4) rest, (5) physical therapy for strengthening and conditioning exercises, and (6) lifestyle changes.

CARPAL TUNNEL SYNDROME

Carpal tunnel syndrome (CTS) is caused by compression of the median nerve, which enters the hand at the wrist through the narrow carpal tunnel (Fig. 62-2). The carpal tunnel is formed by ligaments and bones. CTS is the most common compression neuropathy in the upper extremity. It is associated with hobbies or occupations that require continuous wrist movement (e.g., musicians, carpenters, computer operators).

This condition is often caused by pressure from trauma or edema (secondary to inflammation of a tendon [tenosynovitis]), neoplasm, rheumatoid arthritis, or soft tissue masses such as

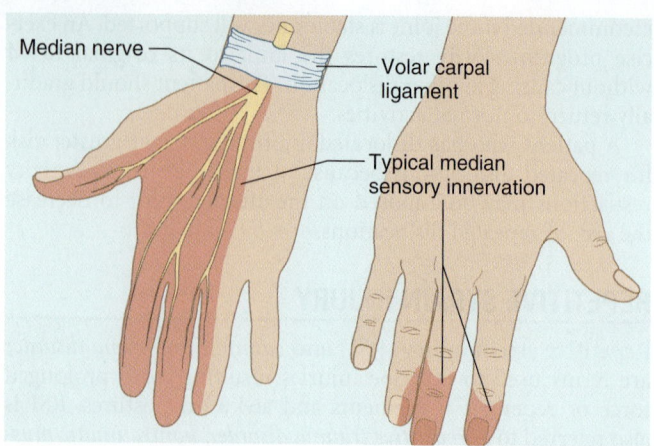

FIG. 62-2 Wrist structures involved in carpal tunnel syndrome. Median nerve distribution. Shaded areas depict the locations of pain in carpal tunnel syndrome. (From Buttaravoli P: *Minor emergencies*, ed 3, Philadelphia, Saunders, 2012.)

ganglia. Hormones may be involved because initial manifestations of CTS often occur during the premenstrual period, pregnancy, and menopause. Persons with diabetes mellitus, peripheral vascular disease, and rheumatoid arthritis have a higher incidence of CTS because of swelling that changes blood flow to the nerve and narrows the carpal tunnel.[7] Women are more likely than men to develop CTS, possibly because of a smaller carpal tunnel.

Clinical manifestations of CTS are weakness, pain, numbness, or impaired sensation in the distribution of the median nerve (Fig. 62-2). Numbness and tingling may awaken the patient at night. Shaking the hands often relieves these symptoms. Clumsiness in performing fine hand movements is also common.

Manifestations of CTS include a positive Tinel's sign and Phalen's sign. *Tinel's sign* can be elicited by tapping over the median nerve as it passes through the carpal tunnel in the wrist. A positive response is a sensation of tingling in the distribution of the median nerve over the hand. *Phalen's sign* can be elicited by allowing the wrists to fall freely into maximum flexion and maintain the position for longer than 60 seconds. A positive response is a sensation of tingling in the distribution of the median nerve over the hand. In late stages, atrophy of the thenar muscles around the base of the thumb results in recurrent pain and eventual dysfunction of the hand.

❖ NURSING AND INTERPROFESSIONAL MANAGEMENT: CARPAL TUNNEL SYNDROME

To prevent CTS, teach employees and employers to identify risk factors. Adaptive devices such as wrist splints may be worn to hold the wrist in a slight extension and relieve pressure on the median nerve. Special keyboard pads and computer mice that help prevent repetitive pressure on the median nerve are available for computer users. Other ergonomic changes include workstation modifications, change in body positions, and frequent breaks from work-related activities.

Interprofessional care of the patient with CTS is directed toward relieving the underlying cause of the nerve compression. Early symptoms of CTS can usually be relieved by stopping the aggravating movement and by resting the hand and wrist by immobilization in a hand splint. Splints worn at night help keep the wrist in a neutral position and may reduce night pain and numbness. Physical therapy with hand and wrist exercises may lessen symptom severity. Injection of a corticosteroid drug directly into the carpal tunnel may provide short-term relief. The patient may need to consider a change in occupation because of discomfort and sensory changes.

Carpal tunnel release is generally recommended if symptoms last more than 6 months. Surgery involves severing the band of tissue around the wrist to reduce pressure on the median nerve (Fig. 62-2). Surgery is performed in the outpatient setting using local anesthesia. The types of carpal tunnel release surgery include open release and endoscopic surgery. In *open release surgery*, an incision is made in the wrist and then the carpal ligament is cut to enlarge the carpal tunnel. *Endoscopic carpal tunnel release* is performed through one or more small puncture incisions in the wrist and palm. A camera is attached to a tube, and the carpal ligament is cut. The endoscopic approach may allow a faster recovery and cause less postoperative discomfort than traditional open release surgery.

Although symptoms may be relieved immediately after surgery, full recovery may take months. After surgery, assess the hand's neurovascular status. Instruct the patient about wound care and appropriate assessments to perform at home.

ROTATOR CUFF INJURY

The rotator cuff is a complex of four muscles in the shoulder: the supraspinatus, infraspinatus, teres minor, and subscapularis muscles. These muscles stabilize the humeral head in the glenoid fossa while assisting with ROM of the shoulder joint and rotation of the humerus.

A tear in the rotator cuff may occur as a gradual, degenerative process due to aging, repetitive stress (especially overhead arm motions), or injury to the shoulder while falling. The rotator cuff can also tear as a result of sudden adduction forces applied to the cuff while the arm is held in abduction. In sports, repetitive overhead motions, such as in swimming, weight lifting, and swinging a racquet (tennis, racquetball), often cause injury. Other causes include (1) falling onto an outstretched arm and hand, (2) a blow to the upper arm, (3) heavy lifting, or (4) repetitive work motions.

Manifestations of rotator cuff injury include shoulder weakness, pain, and decreased ROM. The patient usually experiences severe pain when the arm is abducted between 60 and 120 degrees (the painful arc). A positive *drop arm test* is another sign of rotator cuff injury. In this test, the arm is abducted 90 degrees, and the patient is asked to slowly lower the arm to the side. If the arm falls suddenly, rotator cuff injury is suspected. An x-ray alone is not beneficial in the diagnosis. A tear can usually be confirmed by MRI.

The patient with a partial tear or cuff inflammation may be treated conservatively with rest, ice and heat, NSAIDs, corticosteroid injections into the joint, ultrasound, and physical therapy.[8] If the patient does not respond to conservative treatment or if a complete tear is present, surgical repair may be needed. Most surgical repairs are performed as outpatient procedures through an arthroscope (Fig. 62-3). If the tear is extensive, part of the acromion may be surgically removed (*acromioplasty*) to relieve compression of the rotator cuff during movement. A sling and swathe or a shoulder immobilizer may be used immediately after surgery to limit shoulder movement. However, the shoulder should not be immobilized for too long

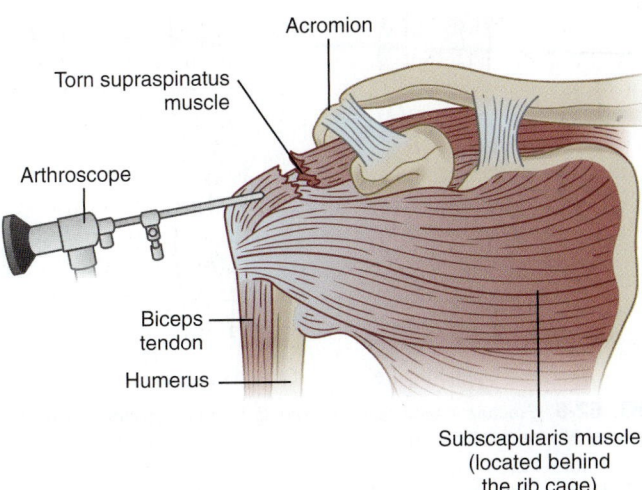

FIG. 62-3 A torn rotator cuff is repaired using arthroscopic surgery.

because "frozen" shoulder (*arthrofibrosis*) may occur. Pendulum exercises and physical therapy begin the first postoperative day. Weight restrictions for lifting are usually given. Full recovery often takes up to 6 months.

MENISCUS INJURY

The menisci are crescent-shaped pieces of fibrocartilage in the knee. Menisci are also found in other joints, including the acromioclavicular (AC), sternoclavicular, and temporomandibular joints. Meniscus injuries are closely associated with ligament sprains common among athletes in sports such as basketball, football, soccer, and hockey. These activities produce rotational stress when the knee is in varying degrees of flexion and the foot is planted or fixed. A blow to the knee can cause shearing of the meniscus between the femoral condyles and tibial plateau, resulting in a torn meniscus. Older patients and people who work in occupations that require squatting or kneeling may be at risk for degenerative tears.

Meniscus injuries alone do not usually cause significant edema because most of the cartilage is avascular. However, an acutely torn meniscus may be suspected when localized tenderness, pain, and effusion occur (Fig. 62-4). Pain is elicited by flexion, internal rotation, and then extension of the knee (*McMurray's test*). The patient may feel that the knee is unstable and often reports that the knee "clicks," "pops," "locks," or "gives way." Quadriceps atrophy is usually evident if the injury has been present for some time. Traumatic arthritis may occur from repeated meniscus injury and chronic inflammation.

MRI is beneficial in confirming the diagnosis before arthroscopy. The degree of knee pain and dysfunction, occupation, sport activities, and age may affect the patient's decision to have or postpone surgery.

❖ NURSING AND INTERPROFESSIONAL MANAGEMENT: MENISCUS INJURY

Because meniscus injuries are commonly caused by sports-related activity, teach athletes to do warm-up exercises. The acutely injured knee should be examined within 24 hours of injury. Initial care of this injury involves ice application, immobilization, and use of crutches with weight bearing as tolerated. Most meniscus injuries are treated in an outpatient setting.

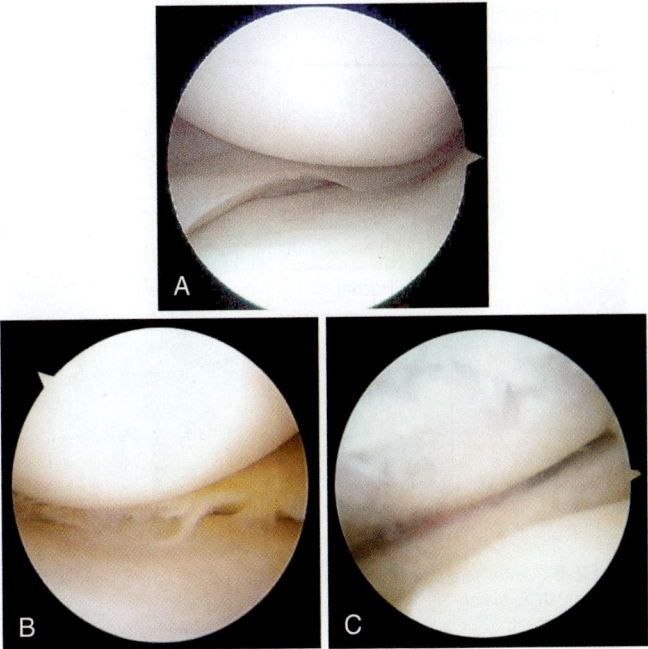

FIG. 62-4 Arthroscopic views of the meniscus. **A,** Normal meniscus. **B,** Torn meniscus. **C,** Surgically repaired meniscus. (*A,* From David Lintner, MD, Houston, Tex., *www.drlintner.com. B* and *C,* Courtesy Peter Bonner, Placitas, N. Mex.)

Using a knee brace or immobilizer during the first few days after the injury protects the knee and offers some pain relief.

After acute pain has decreased, physical therapy can help the patient regain knee flexion and muscle strength to assist in returning to full function. In older adults with degenerative meniscus tears, progressive exercise therapy may improve neuromuscular function and muscle strength.[9]

Surgical repair or excision of part of the meniscus (*meniscectomy*) may be necessary (Fig. 62-4). Meniscal surgery is performed by arthroscopy. Pain relief may include NSAIDs or other analgesics. Rehabilitation starts soon after surgery, including quadriceps and hamstring strengthening exercises and ROM. When the patient's strength is back to its preinjury level, normal activities may be resumed.

ANTERIOR CRUCIATE LIGAMENT INJURY

Knee injuries account for more than 50% of all sport injuries.[10] The most commonly injured knee ligament is the anterior cruciate ligament (ACL). ACL injuries are usually noncontact injuries that occur when the athlete pivots, lands from a jump, or slows down when running. Patients often report coming down on the knee, twisting, and hearing a pop, followed by acute knee pain and swelling. Athletes usually cannot continue playing, and the knee may feel unstable. Injury to the ACL can result in a partial tear, a complete tear, or an *avulsion* (tearing away) from the bones that form the knee (Fig. 62-5).

During examination of the affected knee, a positive *Lachman's test* will suggest an ACL tear.[10] This test is performed by flexing the knee 15 to 30 degrees and pulling the tibia forward while the femur is stabilized. The test is considered positive for an ACL tear if forward motion of the tibia occurs with the feeling of a soft or indistinct endpoint. MRI is often used to diagnose an ACL tear and coexisting conditions, including a fracture, meniscus tearing, and collateral ligament injuries.

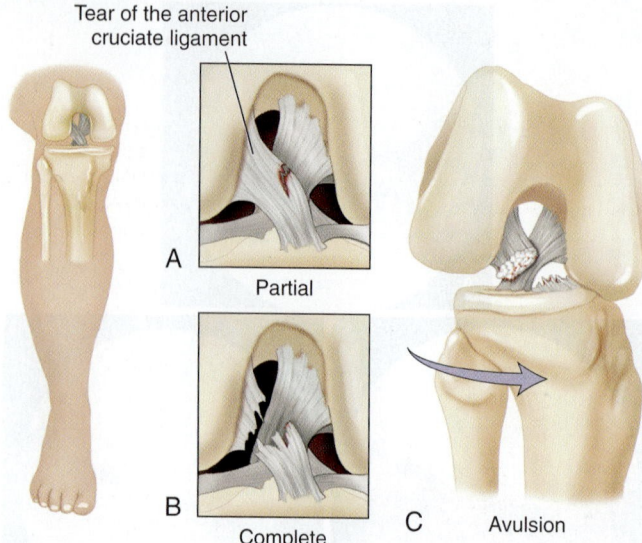

FIG. 62-5   Anterior cruciate ligament (ACL) injury. **A,** Partial tear. **B,** Complete tear. **C,** Avulsion.

❖ NURSING AND INTERPROFESSIONAL MANAGEMENT: ANTERIOR CRUCIATE LIGAMENT INJURY

Prevention programs have been shown to significantly reduce ACL injuries in athletes. Conservative treatment for an intact ACL injury includes rest, ice, NSAIDs, elevation, and ambulation as tolerated with crutches. If present, a tight, painful effusion may be aspirated. A knee immobilizer or hinged knee brace may provide support. Physical therapy often assists the patient in maintaining knee joint motion and muscle tone.

Reconstructive surgery is usually recommended for physically active patients who have sustained severe injury to the ACL and meniscus. In reconstruction, the torn ACL tissue is removed and replaced with autologous or allograft tissue. ROM is encouraged soon after surgery, and the knee is placed in a brace or immobilizer. Rehabilitation with physical therapy is critical, with progressive weight bearing determined by the degree of surgical repair. A safe return to the patient's prior level of physical functioning may take 6 to 8 months.

BURSITIS

Bursae are closed sacs that are lined with synovial membrane and contain a small amount of synovial fluid. They are located at sites of friction, such as between tendons and bones and near the joints. Bursitis (inflammation of the bursa) results from repeated or excessive trauma or friction, gout, rheumatoid arthritis, or infection.

Clinical manifestations of bursitis are warmth, pain, swelling, and limited ROM in the affected part. Common sites of bursitis include the hands, elbows, shoulders, knees, and greater trochanters of the hip. Improper body mechanics, repetitive kneeling (carpet layers, coal miners, and gardeners), jogging in worn-out shoes, and prolonged sitting with crossed legs are common precipitating activities.

Try to determine and correct the cause of the bursitis. Rest is often the only treatment needed. The affected part may be immobilized in a compression dressing or splint. Ice and

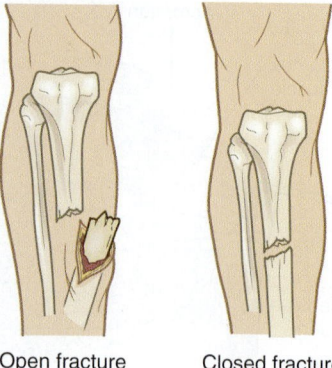

FIG. 62-6   Fracture classification according to communication with the external environment.

NSAIDs may be used to reduce pain and inflammation.[11] Aspiration of the bursal fluid and intraarticular corticosteroid injection may be needed. If the bursal wall has become thickened and continues to interfere with normal joint function, surgical excision *(bursectomy)* is often done. Septic bursae usually require surgical incision and drainage.

FRACTURES

Classification

A fracture is a disruption or break in the continuity of bone. Although traumatic injuries account for the majority of fractures, some fractures are secondary to a disease process such as cancer or osteoporosis *(pathologic fracture).*

Fractures can be classified as *open* or *closed* based on possible communication with the external environment (Fig. 62-6). In an *open fracture,* the skin is broken and bone exposed, causing soft tissue injury. In a *closed fracture,* the skin remains intact.

Fractures can also be classified as complete or incomplete. A fracture is termed *complete* if the break goes completely through the bone. An *incomplete* fracture occurs partly across a bone shaft but the bone is still intact. An incomplete fracture is often the result of bending or crushing forces applied to a bone.

Fractures are also identified according to the direction of the fracture line. Types include linear, oblique, transverse, longitudinal, and spiral fractures (Fig. 62-7).

Fractures can be classified as displaced or nondisplaced. In a *displaced* fracture, the two ends of the broken bone are separated from one another and out of their normal positions. Displaced fractures are often *comminuted* (more than two fragments) or *oblique* (Fig. 62-7). In a *nondisplaced* fracture, the periosteum is intact across the fracture and the bone fragments are still in alignment. Nondisplaced fractures are usually transverse, spiral, or greenstick (Fig. 62-7).

Clinical Manifestations

Clinical manifestations of fracture include immediate localized pain, decreased function, and inability to bear weight or use the affected part (Table 62-4). The patient guards and protects the extremity against movement. Obvious bone deformity may not be present. If a fracture is suspected, the extremity is immobilized in the position in which it is found. Unnecessary movement increases soft tissue damage. It may also convert a closed fracture to an open fracture or create further injury to adjacent nerves and blood vessels.

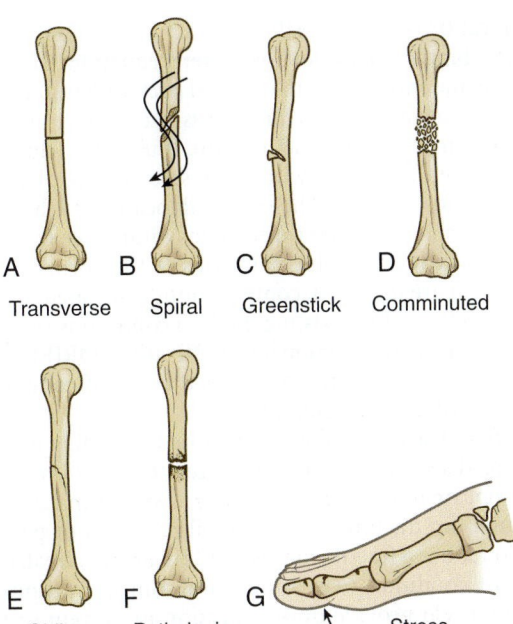

FIG. 62-7 Types of fractures. **A,** Transverse fracture: the line of the fracture extends across the bone shaft at a right angle to the longitudinal axis. **B,** Spiral fracture: the line of the fracture extends in a spiral direction along the bone shaft. **C,** Greenstick fracture: an incomplete fracture with one side splintered and the other side bent. **D,** Comminuted fracture: a fracture with more than two fragments. The smaller fragments appear to be floating. **E,** Oblique fracture: the line of the fracture extends across and down the bone. **F,** Pathologic fracture: a spontaneous fracture at the site of a diseased bone. **G,** Stress fracture: occurs in normal or abnormal bone that is subject to repeated stress, such as from jogging or running.

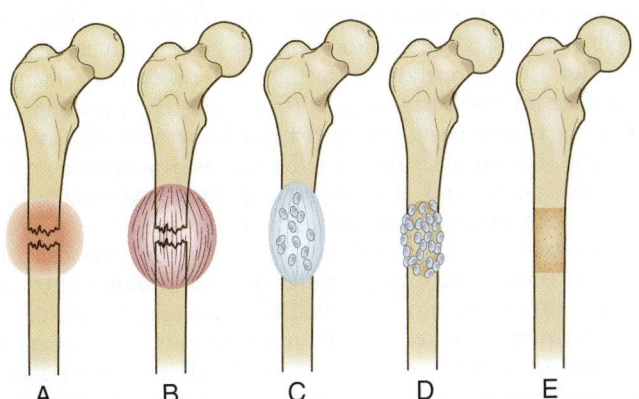

FIG. 62-8 Bone healing (schematic representation). **A,** Bleeding at fractured ends of the bone with subsequent hematoma formation. **B,** Organization of hematoma into fibrous network. **C,** Invasion of osteoblasts, lengthening of collagen strands, and deposition of calcium. **D,** Callus formation: new bone is built up as osteoclasts destroy dead bone. **E,** Remodeling is accomplished as excess callus is resorbed and trabecular bone is laid down.

Fracture Healing

Knowledge of the stages of fracture healing (Fig. 62-8) is needed to provide appropriate interventions. Bone goes through a complex multistage healing process *(union)* that occurs in the following stages[12]:

1. *Fracture hematoma:* When a fracture occurs, bleeding creates a hematoma that surrounds the ends of the bone fragments. The hematoma is extravasated blood that changes from a liquid to a semisolid clot. This occurs in the first 72 hours after injury.

TABLE 62-4	**Manifestations of Fracture**
Manifestation	**Significance**
Edema and Swelling Disruption or penetration of skin or soft tissues by bone fragments, or bleeding into surrounding tissues.	Unchecked bleeding and swelling in closed space can occlude blood vessels and damage nerves (e.g., increased risk of compartment syndrome).
Pain and Tenderness Muscle spasm due to involuntary reflex action of muscle, direct tissue trauma, increased pressure on nerves, movement of fracture fragments.	Pain and tenderness encourage the patient to splint muscle around fracture and reduce motion of injured area.
Muscle Spasm Irritation of tissues and protective response to injury and fracture.	Muscle spasms may displace nondisplaced fracture or prevent it from reducing spontaneously.
Deformity Abnormal position of extremity or part as result of original forces of injury and action of muscles pulling fragment into abnormal position. Seen as a loss of normal bony contours.	Deformity is cardinal sign of fracture. If uncorrected, it may result in problems with bony union and restoration of function of injured part.
Contusion Discoloration of skin (bruising) as a result of extravasation of blood in subcutaneous tissues.	Bruising may appear immediately after injury and may appear distal to injury. Reassure patient that process is normal and discoloration will eventually resolve.
Loss of Function Disruption of bone or joint, preventing functional use of limb or part.	Fracture must be managed properly to ensure restoration of function to limb or part.
Crepitation Grating or crunching of bony fragments, producing palpable or audible crunching or popping sensation.	Crepitation may increase chance for nonunion if bone ends are allowed to move excessively. Micromovement of fragments (postfracture) assists in osteogenesis (new bone growth).

2. *Granulation tissue:* During this stage, active phagocytosis absorbs the products of local necrosis. The hematoma converts to granulation tissue. Granulation tissue (consisting of new blood vessels, fibroblasts, and osteoblasts) forms the basis for new bone substance *(osteoid)* during days 3 to 14 after injury.

3. *Callus formation:* As minerals (calcium, phosphorus, and magnesium) and new bone matrix are deposited in the osteoid, an unorganized network of bone is formed and woven about the fracture parts. *Callus* is primarily composed of cartilage, osteoblasts, calcium, and phosphorus. It usually appears by the end of the second week after injury. Evidence of callus formation can be verified by x-ray.

4. *Ossification:* Ossification of the callus occurs from 3 weeks to 6 months after the fracture and continues until the fracture has healed. Callus ossification is sufficient to prevent

movement at the fracture site when the bones are gently stressed. However, the fracture is still evident on x-ray. During this stage of *clinical union,* the patient may be allowed limited mobility or the cast may be removed.

5. *Consolidation:* As callus continues to develop, the distance between bone fragments decreases and eventually closes. Ossification continues and can be equated with *radiologic union,* which occurs when an x-ray shows complete bony union. This phase can occur up to 1 year after injury.

6. *Remodeling:* Excess bone tissue is resorbed in the final stage of bone healing, and union is complete. Gradual return of the injured bone to its preinjury structural strength and shape occurs. Bone remodels in response to physical loading stress (Wolff's law). Initially, stress is provided through exercise. Weight bearing is gradually introduced. New bone is deposited in sites subjected to stress and resorbed at areas of little stress.

Many factors influence the time required for complete fracture healing, including displacement and site of the fracture, blood supply to the area, immobilization, and use of internal fixation devices (e.g., screws, pins). The ossification process may be slowed or even stopped by inadequate reduction and immobilization, excessive movement of fracture fragments, infection, poor nutrition, and systemic disease. Healing time for fractures increases with age. For example, an uncomplicated midshaft femur fracture heals in 3 weeks in a newborn and in 20 weeks in an adult. Smoking also increases fracture healing time. Fracture healing may not occur in the expected time *(delayed union)* or may not occur at all *(nonunion).* Table 62-5 summarizes complications of fracture healing.

Interprofessional Care

The overall goals of fracture treatment are (1) anatomic realignment of bone fragments through reduction, (2) immobilization to maintain realignment, and (3) restoration of normal or near-normal function of the injured part. Table 62-6 summarizes the interprofessional care of fractures.

Fracture Reduction

Closed Reduction. *Closed reduction* is nonsurgical, manual realignment of bone fragments to their previous anatomic position. Traction and countertraction are manually applied to the bone fragments to restore position, length, and alignment. Closed reduction is usually performed while the patient is under local or general anesthesia. Traction, casting, splints, or orthoses (braces) may be used after reduction to maintain alignment and immobilize the injured part until healing occurs.

Open Reduction. *Open reduction* is the correction of bone alignment through a surgical incision. It usually includes internal fixation of the fracture with wires, screws, pins, plates, intramedullary rods, or nails. The type and location of the fracture, patient age, and concurrent disease may influence the decision to use open reduction. The main risks of this form of fracture management are infection, complications associated with anesthesia, and effect of preexisting medical conditions (e.g., diabetes). However, open reduction internal fixation (ORIF) facilitates early ambulation and thus decreases the risk of complications related to prolonged immobility.

Traction. Traction is the application of a pulling force to an injured or diseased body part or extremity. Traction is used to (1) prevent or reduce pain and muscle spasm (e.g., whiplash, unrepaired hip fracture), (2) immobilize a joint or part of the body, (3) reduce a fracture or dislocation, and (4) treat a pathologic joint condition (e.g., tumor, infection). Traction is also indicated to (1) provide immobilization to prevent soft tissue damage, (2) promote active and passive exercise, (3) expand a joint space during arthroscopic procedures, and (4) expand a joint space before major joint reconstruction.

Traction devices apply a pulling force on a fractured extremity to attain realignment while *countertraction* pulls in the opposite direction. The most common types of traction are skin traction and skeletal traction. *Skin traction* is generally used for short-term treatment (48 to 72 hours) until skeletal traction or surgery is possible. Tape, boots, or splints are applied directly to the skin, primarily to help diminish muscle spasms in the injured extremity. Traction weights are usually limited to 5 to 10 lb (2.3 to 4.5 kg). A *Buck's traction* boot is a type of skin traction used preoperatively for the patient with a hip fracture to reduce muscle spasms (Fig. 62-9). Pelvic or cervical skin traction may require heavier weights applied intermittently. In skin traction, regular assessment of the skin is a priority because pressure points and skin breakdown may develop quickly. Assess key pressure points every 2 to 4 hours.

Skeletal traction, generally in place for longer periods than skin traction, is used to align injured bones and joints or to treat joint contractures and congenital hip dysplasia. It provides a long-term pull that keeps the injured bones and joints aligned. To apply skeletal traction, the surgeon inserts a pin or wire into the bone, and weights are attached to align and immobilize the injured body part. Weight for skeletal traction ranges from 5 to

TABLE 62-5	**Complications of Fracture Healing**
Complication	**Description**
Delayed union	Fracture healing progresses more slowly than expected. Healing eventually occurs.
Nonunion	Fracture fails to heal despite treatment. No x-ray evidence of callus formation.
Malunion	Fracture heals in expected time but in unsatisfactory position, possibly resulting in deformity or dysfunction.
Angulation	Fracture heals in abnormal position in relation to midline of structure (type of malunion).
Pseudoarthrosis	Type of nonunion occurring at fracture site in which a false joint is formed with abnormal movement at site.
Refracture	New fracture occurs at original fracture site.
Myositis ossificans	Deposition of calcium in muscle tissue at site of significant blunt muscle trauma or repeated muscle injury.

TABLE 62-6 Interprofessional Care
Fractures

Diagnostic Assessment
- History and physical examination
- X-ray
- CT scan, MRI

Management
Fracture Reduction
- Manual traction
- Closed reduction
- Skeletal traction
- Open reduction

Fracture Immobilization
- Casting or splinting
- Skeletal traction
- External fixation
- Internal fixation

Open Fractures
- Surgical debridement and irrigation
- Tetanus and diphtheria immunization
- Prophylactic antibiotic therapy
- Immobilization

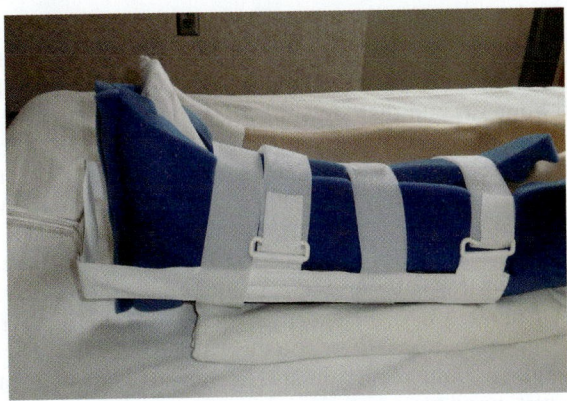

FIG. 62-9 Buck's traction is most commonly used for fractures of the hip and femur. (Courtesy Mary Wollan, RN, BAN, ONC, Spring Park, Minn.)

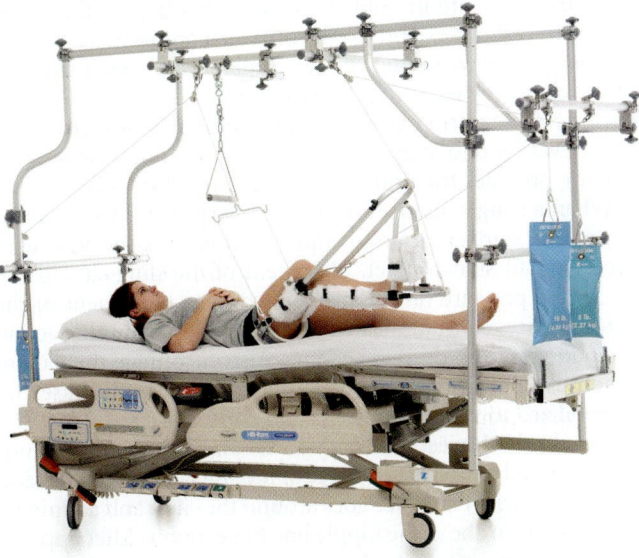

FIG. 62-10 Balanced suspension skeletal traction. Most commonly used for fractures of the femur, hip, and lower leg. (Courtesy Zimmer, Inc.)

45 lb (2.3 to 20.4 kg). The use of too much weight can result in delayed union or nonunion. The major complications of skeletal traction are infection at the pin insertion site and the effects of prolonged immobility.[13]

When traction is used to treat fractures, the forces are usually exerted on the distal bone fragment to align it with the proximal fragment. Several types of traction are used for this purpose. One of the more common types of skeletal traction is balanced suspension traction (Fig. 62-10). Fracture alignment depends on the correct positioning and alignment of the patient while the traction forces remain constant. For extremity traction to be effective, forces must be pulling in the opposite direction *(countertraction)*. Countertraction is commonly supplied by the patient's body weight or by weights pulling in the opposite direction, and it may be augmented by elevating the end of the bed. Traction must be maintained continuously. Keep the weights off the floor and moving freely through the pulleys.

Fracture Immobilization. Fracture immobilization can be done using casts, braces, splints, immobilizers, and external and internal fixation devices.

Casts. A *cast* is a temporary circumferential immobilization device. Casting is a common treatment following closed reduction. It allows the patient to perform many normal activities of

daily living while providing sufficient immobilization to ensure stability. Cast materials are natural (plaster of Paris), synthetic acrylic, fiberglass-free, latex-free polymer, or a hybrid of materials. Synthetic casting materials are commonly used because they are lighter and dry more quickly than plaster of Paris. Plaster of Paris is now used primarily for contact casting in the

---

TEAMWORK & COLLABORATION

Caring for the Patient With a Cast or Traction

Role of Nursing Personnel

Registered Nurse (RN)
- Perform neurovascular assessment on the affected extremity.
- Assess for manifestations of compartment syndrome.
- Monitor cast during drying for denting or flattening.
- Teach patient and caregiver about cast care and complications of casting.
- Determine correct body alignment to enhance traction.
- Instruct patient and caregiver about traction and correct body positioning.
- Teach patient and caregiver ROM exercises.
- Assess for complications associated with immobility or fracture (e.g., wound infection, constipation, VTE, renal calculi, atelectasis).
- Develop plan to minimize complications associated with immobility or fracture.

Licensed Practical/Vocational Nurse (LPN/LVN)
- Check color, temperature, capillary refill, and pulses distal to the cast.
- Mark circumference of any drainage on the cast.
- Monitor skin integrity around cast and at traction pin sites.
- Pad cast edges and traction connections to prevent skin irritation.
- Monitor pain intensity and administer prescribed analgesics.
- Notify RN of changes in pain or if pain persists after prescribed analgesics are administered.

Unlicensed Assistive Personnel (UAP)
- Position casted extremity above heart level as directed by RN.
- Apply ice to cast as directed by RN.
- Maintain body position and integrity of traction (after being trained and evaluated in this procedure).
- Assist patient with passive and active ROM exercises.
- Notify RN about patient complaints of pain, tingling, or decreased sensation in the affected extremity.

Role of Other Team Members

Physical Therapist
- Assess patient's current mobility and need for assistance.
- Teach safe ambulation with assistive device based on patient's weight-bearing restrictions.
- Establish exercise regimen and teach patient to perform exercises safely.
- Coordinate physical therapy with RN so that patient can receive timely analgesia.
- Discuss home environment with patient and identify possible modifications to facilitate recovery (e.g., stair training if allowed by patient's weight-bearing restrictions, bed placement on first level to avoid stairs).

Occupational Therapist
- Assess impact of patient's condition on ability to perform ADLs.
- Instruct patient in use of assistive devices (e.g., long-handled reacher, shoe donner) to facilitate self-care while maintaining activity restrictions.
- Discuss home environment with patient and identify possible modifications to facilitate recovery (e.g., bed placement on first level for access to bathroom).

treatment of diabetic foot ulcers.[14] A cast generally incorporates the joints above and below a fracture. Immobilization above and below a joint restricts tendon and ligament movement, thus assisting with joint stabilization while the fracture heals.

To apply a cast on an extremity, first cover the affected part with stockinette that is cut longer than the extremity. Then place cotton padding over the stockinette, with extra padding for bony prominences. If plaster of Paris casting material is used, immerse it in warm water and then wrap and mold it around the affected part. The number of layers of plaster bandage and the technique of application determine the strength of the cast. The plaster sets within 15 minutes, so the patient may move around without difficulty. However, it is not strong enough for weight bearing until about 24 to 72 hours after application. The final decision about the patient's weight bearing is made by the surgeon.

A fresh plaster cast should never be covered because air cannot circulate. Heat then builds up in the cast and may cause a burn, and drying is delayed. Avoid direct pressure on the cast during the drying period. Handle the cast gently with an open palm to avoid denting the cast. Once the cast is thoroughly dry, the rough edges may be *petaled* to minimize skin irritation. Petaling also prevents plaster of Paris debris from falling into the cast and causing irritation or pressure necrosis. Place several strips (petals) of tape over the rough areas to ensure a smooth cast edge.

Casts made of synthetic materials are used more than plaster because they are lightweight, stronger, and relatively waterproof and provide for early weight bearing. The synthetic casting materials (thermolabile plastic, thermoplastic resins, polyurethane, fiberglass) are activated by submersion in cool or tepid water. Then they are molded to fit the torso or extremity.

Upper extremity injuries. Immobilization of an acute fracture or soft tissue injury of the upper extremity is often accomplished by use of a (1) sugar-tong splint, (2) posterior splint, (3) short arm cast, or (4) long arm cast (Fig. 62-11). The *sugar-tong splint* is typically used for acute wrist injuries or injuries that may result in significant swelling. Splints are applied over a well-padded forearm, beginning at the phalangeal joints of the hand, extending up the dorsal aspect of the forearm around the distal humerus and then down the volar aspect of the forearm to the distal palmar crease. The splinting material is wrapped with either elastic bandage or bias stockinette. The sugar-tong posterior splint accommodates early swelling in the fractured extremity.

The *short arm cast* is often used for the treatment of stable wrist or metacarpal fractures. An aluminum finger splint can be incorporated into the short arm cast for concurrent treatment of phalangeal injuries. The short arm cast is a circular cast extending from the distal palmar crease to the proximal forearm. This cast provides wrist immobilization and permits unrestricted elbow motion.

The *long arm cast* is commonly used for stable forearm or elbow fractures and unstable wrist fractures. It is similar to the short arm cast but extends to the proximal humerus, restricting motion at the wrist and elbow. Support the extremity and reduce edema by elevating the extremity with a sling. However, when a hanging arm cast is used for a proximal humerus fracture, elevation or a supportive sling is contraindicated because hanging provides traction and maintains fracture alignment.

When a sling is used, ensure the axillary area is well padded to prevent skin excoriation and maceration associated with direct skin-to-skin contact. Placement of the sling should not put undue pressure on the neck. Encourage movement of the fingers (unless contraindicated) to enhance the pumping action of blood vessels to decrease edema. Also encourage the patient to actively move joints of the upper extremity that are not immobilized to prevent stiffness and contractures.

Vertebral injuries. The *body jacket brace* is used for immobilization and support for stable spine injuries of the thoracic or lumbar spine. The brace goes around the chest and abdomen, extending from above the nipple line to the pubis. After application of the brace, assess the patient for the development of superior mesenteric artery syndrome *(cast syndrome)*. This condition occurs if the brace is applied too tightly, compressing the superior mesenteric artery against the duodenum. The patient generally complains of abdominal pain, abdominal pressure, nausea, and vomiting. Assess the abdomen for decreased bowel sounds (a window in the brace may be left over the umbilicus). Treatment of cast syndrome includes gastric decompression with a nasogastric (NG) tube and suction. Also assess respiratory status, bowel and bladder function, and areas of pressure over the bony prominences, especially the iliac crest. The brace may have to be adjusted or removed if any complications occur.

Lower extremity injuries. Injuries to the lower extremity are often immobilized by long leg cast, short leg cast, cylinder cast, or prefabricated splint or immobilizer. The usual indications for a long leg cast are an unstable ankle fracture, soft tissue injuries, a fractured tibia, and knee injuries. The cast usually extends from the base of the toes to the groin and gluteal crease. The short leg cast is used primarily for stable ankle and foot injuries. A cylinder cast, which is used for knee injuries or fractures, extends from the groin to the malleoli of the ankle. A Robert Jones dressing may be used temporarily to limit mobility of a joint. It is composed of soft padding materials (absorption dressing and cotton sheet wadding), splints, and an elastic wrap or bias-cut stockinette.

After application of a lower extremity cast or dressing, the extremity should be elevated on pillows above heart level for

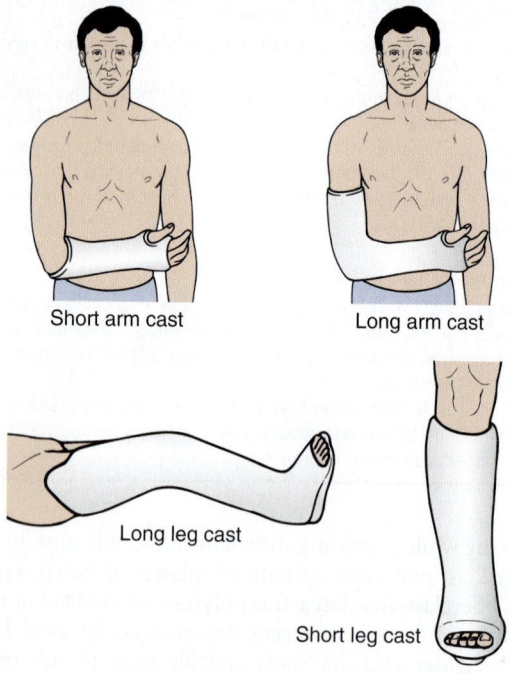

Short arm cast   Long arm cast

Long leg cast

Short leg cast

FIG. 62-11   Common types of casts.

the first 24 hours. After the initial phase, a casted extremity should not be placed in a dependent position because of the possibility of excessive edema. After cast application, observe for signs of compartment syndrome (discussed on p. 1479) and increased pressure, especially in the heel, anterior tibia, head of the fibula, and malleoli. This increased pressure is manifested by pain or a burning feeling in these areas.

Prefabricated knee and ankle splints and immobilizers are used in many settings. This type of immobilization is easy to apply and remove, which permits close observation of the affected joint for swelling and skin breakdown (Fig. 62-12). Depending on the injury, removal of the splint or immobilizer facilitates ROM of the affected joint and faster return to function.

The *hip spica cast* is now mainly used for femur fractures in children to immobilize the affected extremity and trunk. It extends from above the nipple line to the base of the foot (single spica) and may include the opposite extremity up to an area above the knee (spica and a half) or both extremities (double spica). Assess the patient with a hip spica cast for the same problems associated with the body jacket brace.

External Fixation. An *external fixator* is a device composed of metal pins that are inserted into the bone and attached to external rods to stabilize the fracture while it heals. It can be used to apply traction or to compress fracture fragments and immobilize reduced fragments when the use of a cast or other traction is not appropriate. The external device holds fracture fragments in place similar to a surgically implanted internal device. The external fixator is attached directly to the bones by percutaneous transfixing pins or wires (Fig. 62-13). External fixation is indicated primarily for complex fractures with extensive soft tissue damage, correction of congenital bony defects, nonunion or malunion, and limb lengthening.

External fixation is often used in an attempt to salvage extremities that otherwise may require amputation. Because the use of an external device is a long-term process, ongoing assessment for pin loosening and infection is critical. Infection (indicated by exudate, erythema, tenderness, and pain) may require removal of the device. Instruct the patient and caregiver about meticulous pin care. Although each surgeon has a protocol for pin care cleaning, chlorhexidine 2 mg/mL is often used.[15] Hydrogen peroxide may be cytotoxic to osteoblasts and may not be bactericidal.

Internal Fixation. Internal fixation devices (pins, plates, intramedullary rods, metal and bioabsorbable screws) are surgically inserted to realign and maintain position of bony fragments (Fig. 62-14). These metal devices are biologically inert and made from stainless steel, vitallium, or titanium. Proper alignment and bone healing are evaluated regularly by x-rays.

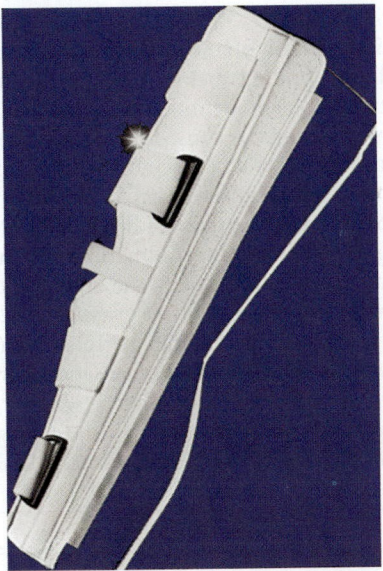

FIG. 62-12 Knee immobilizer. (From Maher AB, Salmond SW, Pellino T, editors: *Orthopaedic nursing*, ed 3, Philadelphia, 2002, Saunders.)

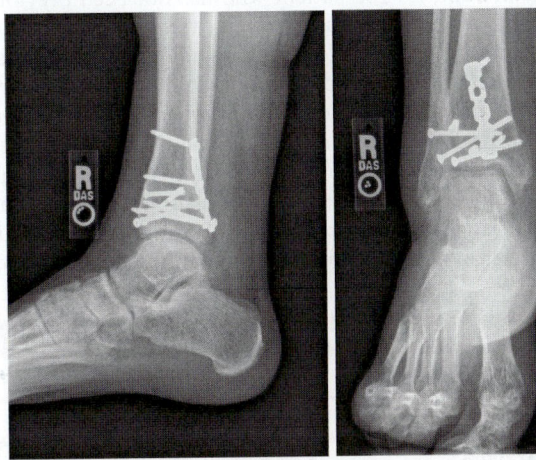

FIG. 62-14 Views of internal fixation devices to stabilize a fractured tibia and fibula. (From Jeremy Lewis, MD, Albuquerque, N. Mex.)

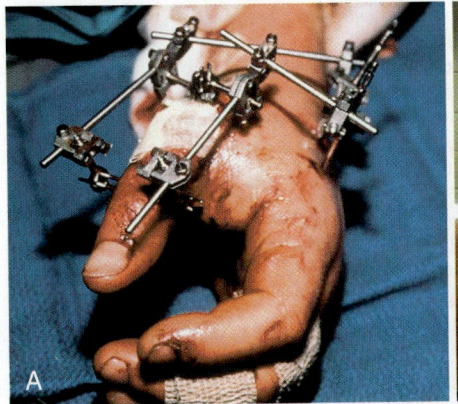
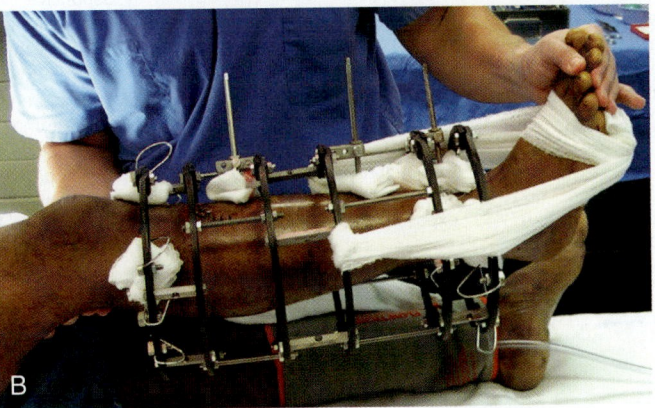

FIG. 62-13 External fixators. **A,** Stabilization of hand injury. **B,** Stabilization of a tibial fracture. (*A,* Courtesy Howmedica, Inc, Allendale, Pa. *B,* From Canale ST, Beaty JH: *Campbell's operative orthopaedics,* ed 12, Philadelphia, 2013, Mosby.)

Electrical Bone Growth Stimulation. Electrical bone growth stimulation is used to facilitate the healing process, especially for fracture nonunion or delayed union. The mechanism of action of electrical bone growth stimulation may include (1) increasing the calcium uptake of bone, (2) activating intracellular calcium stores, and (3) increasing the production of bone growth factors (e.g., bone morphogenic protein).

Noninvasive, semi-invasive, and invasive methods of electrical bone growth stimulation are used. Noninvasive stimulators use direct current or pulsed electromagnetic fields (PEMFs) to generate a weak electrical current. Electrodes are typically in a band applied over the patient's skin or cast and worn 10 to 12 hours each day, usually while the patient is sleeping. Semi-invasive or percutaneous bone growth stimulators use an external power supply and electrodes that are inserted through the skin and into the bone. Invasive stimulators require surgical implantation of a current generator in an IM or subcutaneous space. An electrode is implanted in the bone fragments.

Drug Therapy. Patients with fractures experience varying degrees of pain associated with muscle spasms. Central and peripheral muscle relaxants, such as carisoprodol (Soma), cyclobenzaprine, or methocarbamol (Robaxin), may be prescribed for management of pain associated with muscle spasms.[16]

The threat of tetanus from an open fracture can be reduced by administering tetanus and diphtheria toxoid or tetanus immunoglobulin for the patient who has not been previously immunized or whose immunization is expired (see Table 68-6). Bone-penetrating antibiotics, such as a cephalosporin (e.g., cefazolin [Kefzol]), are used prophylactically before surgery.

Nutritional Therapy. Proper nutrition is an essential component of the healing process in injured tissue. An adequate energy source is needed to promote muscle strength and tone, build endurance, and provide energy for ambulation and gait-training skills. The patient's dietary requirements must include adequate protein (e.g., 1 g/kg of body weight), vitamins (especially B, C,

and D), calcium, phosphorus, and magnesium to ensure optimal soft tissue and bone healing. Low serum protein and vitamin C deficiencies interfere with tissue healing. Immobility and bone healing increase calcium needs.

Three well-balanced meals a day usually provide the necessary nutrients. A well-balanced diet should be supplemented by fluid intake of 2000 to 3000 mL/day to promote optimal bladder and bowel function. Adequate fluid and a high-fiber diet with fruits and vegetables prevent constipation. If immobilized in bed with skeletal traction or in a body jacket brace, the patient should eat six small meals to avoid overeating that can contribute to abdominal pressure and cramping.

❖ NURSING MANAGEMENT: FRACTURES

◆ Nursing Assessment

A brief history of the traumatic episode, mechanism of injury, and position in which the victim was found can be obtained from the patient or witnesses. As soon as possible, the patient should be transported to an emergency department, where thorough assessment can be performed and treatment initiated (Table 62-7). Subjective and objective data that should be obtained from an individual with a fracture are presented in Table 62-8.

Place special emphasis on the region distal to the site of injury. Document clinical findings before fracture treatment to avoid doubts about if a problem identified later was missed during the original examination or was caused by the treatment.

◆ **Neurovascular Assessment.** Musculoskeletal injuries may cause changes in the neurovascular status of an injured extremity. Application of a cast or constrictive dressing, poor positioning, and physiologic responses to the traumatic injury can cause nerve or vascular damage, usually distal to the injury. The neurovascular assessment should consist of *peripheral vascular assessment* (color, temperature, capillary refill, peripheral pulses, edema) and *peripheral neurologic assessment* (sensation, motor function,

---

✚ TABLE 62-7   Emergency Management

Fractured Extremity

Etiology	Assessment Findings	Interventions
Blunt Trauma	• Deformity (loss of normal bony contours) or unnatural position of affected limb	**Initial**
• Motor vehicle crash	• Edema, contusion	• Treat life-threatening injuries first.
• Pedestrian event	• Muscle spasm	• If unresponsive, assess circulation, airway, and breathing.
• Fall	• Tenderness, pain	• If responsive, monitor airway, breathing, and circulation.
• Direct blow	• Warmth at site	• Control external bleeding with direct pressure or sterile pressure dressing and elevation of the extremity.
• Forced flexion or hyperextension	• Loss of function	• Assess neurovascular condition distal to injury before and after splinting.
• Twisting force	• Numbness, tingling, decreased distal pulses	• Elevate injured limb if possible.
	• Grating (crepitus)	• Do *not* attempt to straighten fractured or dislocated joints.
Penetrating Trauma	• Open wound over injured site, exposure of bone	• Do *not* manipulate protruding bone ends.
• Gunshot		• Apply ice packs to affected area.
• Blast		• Obtain x-rays of affected limb.
		• Administer tetanus and diphtheria prophylaxis if there is a break in skin integrity.
Other		• Mark location of pulses to facilitate repeat assessment.
• Pathologic condition		• Splint fracture site, including joints above and below fracture site.
• Violent muscle contraction (seizures)		**Ongoing Monitoring**
• Crush injury		• Assess vital signs, level of consciousness, O₂ saturation, neurovascular condition, pain.
		• Assess for compartment syndrome characterized by excessive pain, pain with passive stretch of the affected extremity muscles, pallor, paresthesia (with late signs of paralysis and pulselessness).
		• Assess for fat embolism (dyspnea, chest pain, temperature elevation).

TABLE 62-8 Nursing Assessment

Fracture

Subjective Data

Important Health Information

Past health history: Traumatic injury, long-term repetitive forces (stress fracture), bone or systemic diseases, prolonged immobility, osteopenia, osteoporosis

Medications: Corticosteroids (osteoporotic fractures); analgesics

Surgery or other treatments: First aid treatment of fracture, previous musculoskeletal surgeries

Functional Health Patterns

Health perception–health management: Calcium and vitamin D supplementation

Activity-exercise: Loss of motion or weakness of affected part, muscle spasms

Cognitive-perceptual: Sudden and severe pain in affected area; numbness, tingling, loss of sensation distal to injury; ongoing pain that increases with activity (stress fracture)

Objective Data

General

Apprehension, guarding of injured site

Integumentary

Skin lacerations, pallor and cool skin or bluish and warm skin distal to injury; bruising, edema at fracture site

Cardiovascular

Reduced or absent pulse distal to injury, ↓ skin temperature, delayed capillary refill

Neurovascular

Paresthesia, absent or ↓ sensation, hypersensation

Musculoskeletal

Restricted or lost function of affected part; local bony deformities, abnormal angulation; shortening, rotation, or crepitation of affected part; muscle weakness

Possible Diagnostic Findings

Identification and extent of fracture on x-ray, bone scan, CT scan, or MRI

---

pain). Throughout the neurovascular assessment, compare both extremities to obtain an accurate assessment.

Assess an extremity's color (pink, pale, cyanotic) and temperature (hot, warm, cool, cold) in the area of the injury. Pallor or a cool-to-cold extremity below the injury could indicate arterial insufficiency. A warm, cyanotic extremity could indicate poor venous return. Next assess capillary refill (blanching of the nail bed). A compressed nail bed should return to its original color within 3 seconds.

Compare pulses on the unaffected and injured extremity to identify differences in rate or quality. This contralateral evaluation is critical. Pulses are described as strong, diminished, audible by Doppler, or absent. A diminished or absent pulse distal to the injury can indicate vascular dysfunction and insufficiency. Also assess peripheral edema. Pitting edema may be present with severe injury.

Assess ulnar, median, and radial nerve function to evaluate sensation and motor innervation in the upper extremity. Assess motor function by asking the patient to (1) abduct the fingers (ulnar nerve), (2) oppose the thumb and small finger (median

nerve), and (3) flex and extend the wrist (or the fingers, if in a cast) (radial nerve). In the lower extremity, assess the patient's ability to perform dorsiflexion (peroneal nerve) and plantar flexion (tibial nerve). Evaluate sensory function of the peroneal nerve by touching the web space between the great and second toes. Stroke the plantar surface (sole) of the foot to assess sensory function of the tibial nerve.[17]

Paresthesia (abnormal sensation [e.g., numbness, tingling]) and hypersensation or hyperesthesia may be reported by the patient. Partial or full loss of sensation (paresis or paralysis) may be a late sign of neurovascular damage. Instruct patients to immediately report any changes in sensation or the ability to move the digits in the affected extremity.

◆ Nursing Diagnoses

Nursing diagnoses for the patient with a fracture may include, but are not limited to, the following:

- Impaired physical mobility *related to* loss of integrity of bone structures, movement of bone fragments, and prescribed movement restrictions
- Risk for peripheral neurovascular dysfunction *related to* vascular insufficiency and nerve compression secondary to edema and/or mechanical compression by traction, splints, or casts
- Acute pain *related to* edema, movement of bone fragments, and muscle spasms
- Readiness for enhanced self–health management

Additional information on nursing diagnoses for the patient with a fracture is presented in eNursing Care Plan 62-1 (on the website for this chapter).

◆ Planning

The overall goals are that the patient with a fracture will (1) have healing with no associated complications, (2) obtain satisfactory pain relief, and (3) achieve maximal rehabilitation potential.

◆ Nursing Implementation

◆ **Health Promotion.** Teach people in the community to take appropriate safety precautions to prevent injuries while at home or work, when driving, or when participating in sports. Be an advocate for personal actions known to reduce injuries, such as (1) regularly using seat belts, (2) driving within posted speed limits, (3) avoiding distracted driving (e.g., not texting on a cell phone) or driving under the influence of alcohol or drugs (prescribed or illicit) that may affect response times, (4) warming up muscles before exercise, (5) using protective athletic equipment (helmets and knee, wrist, and elbow pads), and (6) using safety equipment at work.

Encourage individuals, especially older adults, to participate in moderate exercise to help maintain muscle strength and balance. To reduce risk for falls, also urge them to wear nonskid, hard-soled footwear and assess their living environment for safety risks (e.g., remove scatter rugs, ensure adequate lighting, maintain clear paths to the bathroom for nighttime use) (Table 62-1). Also stress the importance of adequate calcium and vitamin D intake for bone health.

◆ **Acute Care.** Patients with fractures may be treated in an emergency department or a physician's office and released to home care, or they may require hospitalization for varying amounts of time. Specific nursing measures depend on the setting and type of treatment.

EVIDENCE-BASED PRACTICE
Translating Research Into Practice

Do Physical Activity Exercises Decrease Sport Injuries?
Clinical Question

Among physically active adults and adolescents (P), what is the effect of stretching, strength training, and proprioception exercises (I) versus control group (C) on acute and overuse sport injuries (O)?

Synthesis of Best Available Evidence

- Systematic review and meta-analysis of randomized controlled trials (RCTs).
- 25 RCTs of adults and adolescents (*n* = 26,610) with acute and overuse sport injuries (*n* = 3464). Intervention was physical activity exercises including strength training, stretching, and/or proprioception exercises that improve joint mobility.
- Sport injuries were not prevented by stretching before or after the sport activity.
- Strength training and/or proprioception exercises showed a positive effect in reducing sport injuries.
- Strength training reduced sports injuries by 30% with overuse injuries decreased by almost 50%.
- A trend was noted for strength training to have a greater preventive effect against injury compared to proprioception training.

Conclusion

- Participation in strength training and/or proprioception exercises decreases the incidence of acute and overuse sport injuries.

Implications for Nursing Practice

1. What would you advise a person who participates in sports and solely commits to stretching for physical activity exercise?
2. Why is it important for you to discuss the benefits of adherence to strength training when persons are involved in multiple extensive physical activity programs?

Reference for Evidence

Lauersen JB, Bertelsen DM, Andersen LB: The effectiveness of exercise interventions to prevent sports injuries: a systematic review and meta-analysis of randomised controlled trials, *Br J Sports Med* 48:871, 2014.

P, Patient population of interest; *I*, intervention or area of interest; *C*, comparison of interest or comparison group; *O*, outcomes of interest; *T*, timing (see p. 15).

Preoperative Care. If surgical intervention is required to treat a fracture, patients need preoperative preparation. In addition to the usual preoperative nursing measures (see Chapter 17), inform patients of the type of immobilization and assistive devices that will be used and the expected activity limitations after surgery. Assure patients that nursing staff will help meet their personal needs until they can resume self-care. Remind patients that pain medication will be available if needed.

Postoperative Care. In general, postoperative nursing care and management are directed toward monitoring vital signs and applying general principles of postoperative nursing care (see Chapter 19). Frequent neurovascular assessment of the affected extremity is necessary to detect early and subtle changes. Closely monitor any limitations related to turning, positioning, and extremity support. Minimize pain and discomfort through proper alignment and positioning. Carefully observe dressings or casts for any signs of bleeding or drainage. Report a significant increase in size of the drainage area. If a wound drainage system is in place, regularly measure the volume of drainage and assess its character (e.g., bloody, purulent). Report increased or purulent drainage immediately to the surgeon. Also assess the patency of the drainage system, using aseptic technique to avoid contamination.

Additional nursing responsibilities depend on the type of immobilization used. A blood salvage and reinfusion system may be used to allow recovery and reinfusion of the patient's own blood. The blood is retrieved from a joint space or cavity, and the patient receives this blood in the form of an autotransfusion. (Autotransfusion is discussed in Chapter 30.) Additional nursing measures for the patient who has had orthopedic surgery are discussed in eNursing Care Plan 62-2 (on the website for this chapter).

Other Measures. Patients often have reduced mobility as a result of a fracture. Plan care to decrease risk for the many complications associated with immobility. Prevent constipation by increasing patient activity and maintaining high fluid intake (more than 2500 mL/day unless contraindicated by the patient's health status) and a diet high in bulk and roughage (fresh fruits and vegetables). If these measures are not effective in maintaining the patient's normal bowel elimination pattern, administer stool softeners, laxatives, or suppositories. Maintain a regular time for elimination to promote bowel regularity.

Renal calculi can develop from bone demineralization related to reduced mobility. Hypercalcemia from demineralization causes a rise in urine pH and stone formation from the precipitation of calcium. Unless contraindicated, fluid intake of 2500 mL/day is recommended to decrease the risk of calculi formation. (Renal calculi are discussed in Chapter 45.)

Rapid deconditioning of the cardiopulmonary system can occur as a result of prolonged bed rest, resulting in orthostatic hypotension and decreased lung capacity. Unless contraindicated, these effects can be diminished by having the patient sit on the side of the bed, allowing the patient's lower limbs to dangle over the bedside, and having the patient perform standing transfers. When the patient is allowed to increase activity, assess for orthostatic hypotension. Also assess patients for venous thromboembolism (VTE) (VTE is discussed in Chapter 37.)

Traction. When slings are used with traction, regularly inspect exposed skin areas. Pressure over a bony prominence created by wrinkled sheets or blankets may cause pressure necrosis. Persistent skin pressure may impair blood flow and cause injury to peripheral nerves and blood vessels. Observe skeletal traction or external fixation pin sites for signs of infection. Pin site care may vary but often includes regularly cleansing with chlorhexidine, rinsing pin sites with sterile saline, and drying the area with sterile gauze.

External rotation of the affected extremity is a classic assessment finding for a patient with unrepaired hip fracture. If skin traction is ordered preoperatively, apply traction without attempting to reposition or realign the extremity. Movement of fracture fragments can occur during repositioning, causing increased pain and possible nerve impingement. Keep the patient in the center of the bed in a supine position to provide adequate countertraction.

To offset possible problems associated with prolonged immobility, discuss specific patient activity with the HCP. If exercise is permitted, encourage patient participation in a simple exercise regimen based on activity restrictions. Encourage the patient to participate in frequent position changes, ROM exercises of unaffected joints, deep-breathing exercises, isometric exercises, and use of the trapeze bar (if permitted) to raise the body off the bed for linen changes and placement of the bedpan. These activities should be performed several times

INFORMATICS IN PRACTICE

Web-Based Knee and Hip Replacement Community

- Many hospitals provide preoperative classes for patients undergoing joint replacement surgery, but fewer resources are available for postdischarge support.
- With careful research, the patient can locate online knee and hip replacement communities to share experiences and receive social support. The patient is likely to feel relieved knowing that others have similar experiences.
- Encourage patients to validate any advice with their surgeons before taking action.

each day. Encourage and help the hospitalized patient to stay connected with friends and family by telephone or through social media resources (see Informatics in Practice box).

◆ **Ambulatory Care**

◆ *Cast Care.* Because uncomplicated fractures are treated in an outpatient setting, the patient may require only a short hospitalization or none at all. Regardless of the type of cast material, a cast can interfere with circulation and nerve function if it is applied too tightly or excessive edema occurs after application. Frequent neurovascular assessment of the immobilized extremity is critical. Teach the patient to recognize and promptly report the signs of cast complications. Explain the importance of elevating the extremity above heart level to promote venous return and applying ice to control or prevent edema during the initial phase. However, if compartment syndrome is suspected, do not elevate the extremity above the heart.

Instruct the patient to exercise joints above and below the cast. Instruct the patient to avoid scratching or placing foreign objects inside the cast because this may cause skin breakdown and infection. For itching, suggest the use of a hair dryer on a cool setting to be directed under the cast.

Patient and caregiver teaching is important to prevent complications. In addition to specific instructions for cast care and recognition of complications, encourage the patient to contact the HCP with any questions. Table 62-9 summarizes patient and caregiver instructions for cast care. Validate the patient's and caregiver's understanding of these instructions before discharge. A follow-up phone call is appropriate. Home care nursing visits may be warranted, especially for the patient with a body jacket brace.

The cast is typically removed in the outpatient setting. Patients often fear being cut by the oscillating blade of the cast saw. Reassure the patient that damage to the skin is unlikely.[18] Teach the patient about possible alterations in the appearance of the extremity beneath the cast (e.g., dry, wrinkled skin; atrophied muscle). The patient may also have anxiety related to using the injured extremity after cast removal.

◆ *Psychosocial Problems.* Short-term rehabilitative goals address the transition from dependence to independence in performing simple ADLs and preserving or increasing strength and endurance. Long-term rehabilitative goals are aimed at preventing problems associated with musculoskeletal injury (Table 62-10). During the rehabilitative phase, help the patient adjust to any problems caused by the injury (e.g., separation from family, financial impact of medical care, loss of income from inability to work, potential for lifetime disability). Offer support and encouragement while actively listening to the patient's and caregiver's concerns.

TABLE 62-9 Patient & Caregiver Teaching

Cast Care

After a cast is applied, include the following instructions when teaching the patient and the caregiver.

Do

1. Apply ice directly over fracture site for first 24 hr (avoid getting cast wet by keeping ice in plastic bag and protecting cast with cloth).
2. Check with HCP before getting fiberglass cast wet.
3. Dry cast thoroughly if inadvertently exposed to water.
   - Blot dry with towel.
   - Use hair dryer on low setting until cast is thoroughly dry.
4. Elevate extremity above level of heart for first 48 hr.
5. Regularly move joints above and below cast.
6. Use hair dryer on cool setting for itching inside the cast.
7. Report signs of possible problems to HCP:
   - Increasing pain despite elevation, ice, analgesia.
   - Swelling associated with pain and discoloration of toes or fingers.
   - Pain during movement.
   - Burning or tingling under cast.
   - Sores or foul odor under cast.
8. Keep appointment to have fracture and cast checked.

Do Not

1. Get cast wet.
2. Remove any padding.
3. Insert any objects inside cast.
4. Bear weight on new cast for 48 hr (not all casts are made for weight bearing; check with HCP when unsure).
5. Cover cast with plastic for prolonged periods.

◆ *Ambulation.* Know the overall goals of physical therapy in relation to the patient's abilities, needs, and tolerance. Mobility training and instruction in the use of assistive aids (cane, crutches, walker) are major areas of responsibility for the physical therapist. Reinforce these instructions to the patient. The patient with lower extremity dysfunction usually starts mobility training when able to sit in bed and dangle the feet over the side. Collaborate with the physical therapist to administer analgesia before a physical therapy session.

When the patient begins to ambulate, know the patient's weight-bearing status and the correct technique if the patient is using an assistive device. Ambulation occurs in different degrees of weight-bearing: (1) non–weight bearing (no weight on the involved extremity), (2) touch-down/toe-touch weight bearing (contact with floor for balance but no weight borne), (3) partial–weight-bearing ambulation (25% to 50% of patient's weight borne), (4) weight bearing as tolerated (based on patient's pain and tolerance), and (5) full–weight-bearing ambulation (no limitations).

◆ *Assistive Devices.* Devices for ambulation range from a cane (can relieve up to 40% of the weight normally borne by a lower limb) to a walker or crutches (may allow for complete non–weight-bearing ambulation). The HCP decides which device is appropriate, balancing the need for maximum stability and safety with the need for maneuverabiliy in small spaces such as bathrooms. Discuss with the patient his or her lifestyle requirements and select a device that allows each patient to feel most secure and independent. The technique for using assistive ambulation devices varies. The involved limb is usually advanced at the same time or immediately after advance of the device. The uninvolved limb is advanced last. In almost all cases, canes are held in the hand opposite the involved extremity.

TABLE 62-10 Problems Associated With Musculoskeletal Injuries

Problem	Description	Nursing Considerations
Muscle atrophy	• Decreased muscle mass occurs as a result of disuse after prolonged immobilization. • Loss of nerve function can precipitate muscle atrophy.	• Isometric muscle-strengthening exercises as able with immobilization device assists in reducing amount of atrophy. • Muscle atrophy interferes with and prolongs rehabilitation process.
Contracture	• Abnormal condition of joint characterized by flexion and fixation. • Caused by atrophy and shortening of muscle fibers and ligaments, or by loss of normal elasticity of skin over joint.	• Can be prevented by frequent position change, correct body alignment, active-passive ROM exercises several times a day. • Intervention requires gradual progressive stretching of muscles or ligaments in region of joint.
Footdrop	• Plantar-flexed position of the foot occurs when Achilles tendon in ankle shortens because it has been allowed to assume an unsupported position. • Peroneal nerve palsy (a compression neuropathy) can cause footdrop and spinal nerve compression.	• For patient with long-term injuries, support foot in neutral position to decrease risk of footdrop. • Once footdrop has developed, ambulation and gait training may be significantly hindered. • May require splint to keep feet in neutral position. • High-top athletic shoes may also help. Apply at scheduled times to keep feet in neutral position.
Pain	• Frequently associated with fractures, edema, muscle spasm. • Pain may be mild to severe and is described as aching, dull, burning, throbbing, sharp, or deep.	• Causes of pain include incorrect positioning and alignment of extremity, incorrect support of extremity, sudden movement of extremity, immobilization device that is applied too tightly or incorrectly, constrictive dressings, motion at fracture site. • Determine causes of pain so that corrective action can be taken.
Muscle spasms	• Caused by involuntary muscle contraction after fracture, muscle strain, or nerve injury. • May last several weeks. • Pain associated with muscle spasms is often intense and can last from several seconds to several minutes.	• Measures to reduce intensity of muscle spasms are similar to actions for pain management. • Do not massage muscle spasms. Massage may stimulate muscle tissue contraction that increases spasm and pain. • Thermotherapy, especially heat, may reduce muscle spasm.

Place a transfer belt (gait belt) around the patient's waist to provide stability while he or she is learning to use an assistive device. Discourage the patient from reaching for furniture or relying on another person for support. If the patient has inadequate upper limb strength or poorly fitted crutches, he or she bears weight at the axilla rather than at the hands, endangering the neurovascular bundle that passes across the axilla. If verbal coaching does not correct the problem, instruct the patient in another form of ambulation (e.g., walker) until strength is adequate.

Patients who must ambulate without weight bearing require sufficient upper limb strength to lift their own weight at each step. Because the muscles of the shoulder girdle and upper arm may not be accustomed to this work, patients require vigorous and diligent training for this task. Push-ups, pull-ups using the overhead trapeze bar, and weight lifting develop the triceps and biceps muscles. Straight-leg raises and quadriceps-setting exercises strengthen the quadriceps muscles.

Counseling and Referrals. During the rehabilitative process, the patient's caregiver assumes an important role in the provision of long-term care. Instruct the caregiver in strength and endurance exercises, assistance with mobility training, and promotion of activities that enhance the quality of daily living. Also evaluate patients for posttraumatic stress disorder. This is especially important if significant injury to others or fatalities were associated with the patient's injuries.

Evaluation

The expected outcomes are that the patient with a fracture will
• Report satisfactory pain management
• Demonstrate appropriate care of cast or immobilizer
• Experience no peripheral neurovascular dysfunction
• Experience uncomplicated bone healing

COMPLICATIONS OF FRACTURES

The majority of fractures heal without complications. Death after a fracture is usually the result of damage to underlying organs and vascular structures or from complications of the fracture or immobility. Complications of fractures may be direct or indirect. *Direct complications* include problems with bone infection, bone union, and avascular necrosis. *Indirect complications* are associated with blood vessel and nerve damage resulting in conditions such as compartment syndrome, VTE, fat embolism syndrome (FES), breakdown of skeletal muscle *(rhabdomyolysis),* and hypovolemic shock. Most musculoskeletal injuries are not life threatening. However, open fractures, fractures accompanied by severe blood loss, and fractures that damage vital organs (e.g., lung, heart) are medical emergencies requiring immediate attention.

Infection

Open fractures and soft tissue injuries have a high incidence of infection. An open fracture usually results from severe external forces. Massive or blunt soft tissue injury often has more serious consequences than the fracture. Devitalized and contaminated tissue is an ideal medium for many common pathogens, including gas-forming (anaerobic) bacilli such as *Clostridium tetani.* Treatment of infection is costly in terms of extended nursing and medical care, time for treatment, and loss of patient income. Delayed or ineffective treatment can lead to the development of chronic osteomyelitis[19] (see Chapter 63).

Open fractures require aggressive surgical debridement. The wound is initially cleaned by pulsating saline lavage in the operating room. Gross contaminants are irrigated and mechanically removed. Contused, contaminated, and devitalized tissue (muscle, subcutaneous fat, skin, and bone fragments) are surgically excised *(debridement).* The extent of soft tissue damage determines if the wound is closed at the time of surgery and if it requires repeat debridement, closed suction drainage, and/or skin grafting. Depending on the location and extent of the fracture, reduction may be maintained by external fixation or traction. During surgery, the open wound may be irrigated with antibiotic solution. Antibiotic-impregnated beads may also be placed in the surgical site. The patient may have antibiotics administered IV for 3 to 7 days during the postoperative phase of care. In conjunction with aggressive surgical management, antibiotics have greatly reduced the occurrence of infection.

Compartment Syndrome

Compartment syndrome is a condition in which swelling causes increased pressure within a limited space (muscle compartment). Because the fascia surrounding the muscle has limited ability to stretch, continued swelling can cause pressure that compromises the function of blood vessels and nerves in the compartment. Capillary perfusion is reduced below a level needed for tissue viability. Compartment syndrome usually involves the leg but can also occur in any muscle group (e.g., arm, shoulder, buttock, abdomen).

Thirty-eight compartments are located in the upper and lower extremities. Two basic causes of compartment syndrome are (1) decreased compartment size resulting from restrictive dressings, splints, casts, excessive traction, or premature closure of fascia; and (2) increased compartment contents related to bleeding, inflammation, edema, or IV infiltration.

Edema can create sufficient pressure to obstruct circulation and cause venous occlusion, which further increases edema. Arterial flow is eventually compromised, causing ischemia in the extremity. As ischemia continues, muscle and nerve cells are destroyed. Fibrotic tissue eventually replaces healthy tissue. Contracture, disability, and loss of function can occur. Delays in diagnosis and treatment result in irreversible muscle and nerve ischemia. The extremity may become functionally useless or severely impaired.

Compartment syndrome is usually associated with trauma, fractures (especially of long bones), extensive soft tissue damage, and crush injury. Fractures of the distal humerus and proximal tibia are the most common fractures associated with compartment syndrome. Compartment injury can also occur after knee or leg surgery. Prolonged pressure on a muscle compartment may result when someone is trapped under a heavy object or a person's limb is trapped beneath the body because of response to drugs or alcohol.

❓ CHECK YOUR PRACTICE

Your 32-yr-old male patient had a skiing injury. He returned from surgery 8 hours ago with a long leg cast placed for open fractures of the femur and tibia. He continually complains of pain and IV morphine does not seem to help.

- How will you assess his neurovascular condition? What signs and symptoms would suggest the development of compartment syndrome?
- What is the most likely intervention if compartment syndrome is developing?

Clinical Manifestations. Compartment syndrome may occur initially from the body's physiologic response to the injury, or it may be delayed for several days after the original insult or injury. Ischemia can occur within 4 to 8 hours after the onset of compartment syndrome.

One or more of the following six *P*s are characteristic of compartment syndrome: (1) *pain* out of proportion to the injury that is not managed by opioid analgesics, and *pain* on passive stretch of muscle traveling through the compartment; (2) increasing *pressure* in the compartment; (3) *paresthesia* (numbness and tingling); (4) *pallor*, coolness, and loss of normal color of the extremity; (5) *paralysis* or loss of function; and (6) *pulselessness* (diminished or absent peripheral pulses).

Interprofessional Care. Prompt, accurate diagnosis of compartment syndrome is critical.[20] Perform and document regular neurovascular assessment on all patients with fractures, especially those with injury of the extremities or soft tissue in these areas. Early recognition and effective treatment of compartment syndrome are essential to avoid permanent damage to muscles and nerves.

Carefully assess the location, quality, and intensity of the pain (see Chapter 8). Evaluate the patient's level of pain on a scale of 0 to 10. Pain unrelieved by drugs and out of proportion to the level of injury is one of the *first* indications of impending compartment syndrome. Paresthesia is also an early sign. Notify the HCP immediately of these changes in the patient's condition. If the source of pressure is relieved (e.g., cast is cut [bivalve] or dressing loosened by order of the HCP), pain and paresthesia typically decrease and compartment syndrome is avoided. Reducing traction weight may also decrease external pressures on the extremity. Pulselessness and paralysis are later signs of compartment syndrome. Do not wait until these late signs occur to contact the HCP, as the limb may require amputation if pressure progresses to this state.

Because of the possibility of muscle damage, assess urine output. Myoglobin released from damaged muscle cells precipitates and causes obstruction in renal tubules. This condition results in acute tubular necrosis and acute kidney injury (AKI). Common signs are dark reddish brown urine and clinical manifestations associated with AKI (see Chapter 46).

Elevation of the extremity may lower venous pressure and slow arterial perfusion. With suspected compartment syndrome, the extremity should not be elevated above the heart level. Similarly, application of cold compresses should be avoided because they may cause vasoconstriction and exacerbate compartment syndrome.

Surgical decompression (e.g., fasciotomy) of the involved compartment may be necessary (Fig. 62-15). The fasciotomy site is left open for several days to ensure adequate soft tissue decompression. Infection resulting from delayed wound closure is a potential problem after fasciotomy. In severe cases of compartment syndrome, amputation may be required.

Venous Thromboembolism

Veins of the lower extremities and pelvis are highly susceptible to thrombus formation after a fracture, especially a hip fracture. VTE may also occur after total hip or total knee replacement surgery. In patients with limited mobility, venous stasis is aggravated by inactivity of muscles that normally assist in pumping venous blood from the extremities to the heart.

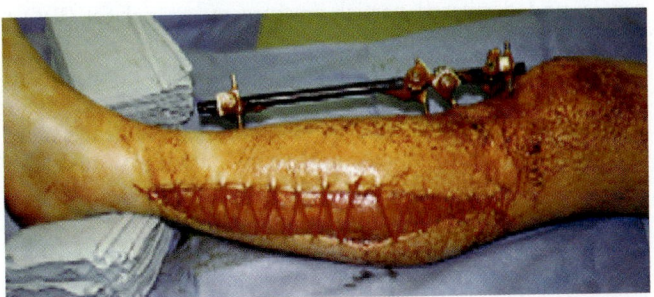

FIG. 62-15 Fasciotomy associated with compartment syndrome. Stabilization of fracture with external fixator. (From Browner BD, Jupiter JB, Levine AM, Trafton P: *Skeletal trauma: fractures, dislocations, ligamentous injuries*, ed 4, Philadelphia, 2009, Saunders.)

Because of the high risk of VTE in the orthopedic surgical patient, prophylactic anticoagulant drugs may be ordered: (1) warfarin (Coumadin), (2) low-molecular-weight heparin (LMWH) (e.g., enoxaparin [Lovenox], dalteparin [Fragmin]), or (3) a factor Xa inhibitor (fondaparinux [Arixtra], rivaroxaban [Xarelto], apixaban [Eliquis]). In addition to wearing compression gradient stockings (antiembolism hose) or using sequential compression devices, the patient should dorsiflex and plantar flex the ankle of an affected lower extremity against resistance and perform ROM exercises on the unaffected leg. For upper extremity injuries, the patient should flex and extend the wrist if not immobilized by a cast or splint and perform ROM exercises on the unaffected arm. (Assessment and management of VTE are discussed in Chapter 37.)

> **⚠ SAFETY ALERT   Anticoagulant Therapy**
> - Monitor for signs of external bleeding (e.g., nosebleeds) or internal bleeding (e.g., tea-colored urine).
> - Teach patient about signs of bleeding and what to do if excessive bleeding occurs (i.e., apply pressure for 10 minutes, seek medical attention if bleeding does not stop).
> - Teach patient safe self-injection if taking an injectable anticoagulant after discharge.
> - Encourage patient to keep all follow-up appointments for laboratory testing to monitor effects of warfarin (if prescribed).

Fat Embolism Syndrome

Fat embolism syndrome (FES) is characterized by systemic fat globules from fractures that are distributed into tissues, lungs, and other organs after a traumatic skeletal injury. FES is a contributory factor in mortality associated with fractures. The fractures that most often are associated with FES include those of the long bones, ribs, tibia, and pelvis. FES can also occur after total joint replacement, spinal fusion, liposuction, crush injuries, and bone marrow transplantation.

Two theories about FES exist. According to the mechanical theory, fat emboli may originate from fat released from the marrow of injured bone. The fat then enters systemic circulation, where it embolizes to other organs such as the brain.[21] As fat droplets lodge in small blood vessels, local ischemia and inflammation occur. The biochemical theory suggests hormonal changes caused by trauma or sepsis stimulate the systemic release of free fatty acids (e.g., chylomicrons) that form the fat emboli.

Clinical Manifestations. Early recognition of FES is crucial to prevent a potentially lethal course. Most patients manifest symptoms within 24 to 48 hours after injury. Severe forms have occurred within hours of injury. Fat emboli in the lungs cause a hemorrhagic interstitial pneumonitis with signs and symptoms of acute respiratory distress syndrome (ARDS), such as chest pain, tachypnea, cyanosis, dyspnea, apprehension, tachycardia, and decreased partial pressure of arterial O_2 (PaO_2). These symptoms are caused by poor oxygen exchange. Changes in mental status (a result of hypoxemia) are also part of the classic triad of signs and symptoms. Investigate memory loss, restlessness, confusion, elevated temperature, and headache so that central nervous system involvement is not mistaken for alcohol withdrawal or acute head injury. Petechiae located on the neck, anterior chest wall, axilla, buccal membrane, and conjunctiva of the eye may help distinguish fat emboli from other problems. They may appear due to intravascular thromboses caused by decreased oxygenation. However, petechiae are only seen in 25% to 50% of cases of FES and may fade before noticed.[21]

The clinical course of a fat embolus may be rapid and acute. Frequently the patient expresses a feeling of impending disaster. In a short time, skin color changes from pallor to cyanosis, and the patient may become comatose. No specific laboratory examinations are available to aid in the diagnosis. However, certain abnormalities may be present. These include fat cells in blood, urine, or sputum; a decrease of PaO_2 to less than 60 mm Hg; ST segment and T-wave changes on ECG; a decrease in the platelet count and hematocrit; and an elevated erythrocyte sedimentation rate (ESR). A chest x-ray may show bilateral pulmonary infiltrates.

> **❓ CHECK YOUR PRACTICE**
>
> You are caring for a 24-yr-old male patient who had a femur fracture in a motorcycle accident last night. He is scheduled for ORIF later today. While doing your assessment, you notice that he seems very restless. You also observe some axillary petechiae.
> - What complication would you suspect is occurring?
> - Why is this patient particularly at risk for this complication?
> - What is the most important intervention for a patient with this complication?

Interprofessional Care. Treatment of fat embolism is directed at prevention. Careful immobilization and handling of a long bone fracture are probably the most important factors in prevention of fat embolism. Reposition the patient as little as possible before fracture immobilization or stabilization because of the danger of dislodging fat droplets into the general circulation. Management of FES is mostly supportive and related to management of symptoms. Treatment includes fluid resuscitation to prevent hypovolemic shock, correction of acidosis, and blood transfusion. Use of corticosteroids to prevent or treat fat embolism is controversial.

Encourage coughing and deep breathing. Administer O_2 to treat hypoxia. Intubation or intermittent positive pressure ventilation may be considered if satisfactory PaO_2 cannot be obtained with supplemental oxygen alone. Some patients may develop pulmonary edema and/or ARDS leading to increased mortality. Most persons survive FES with few sequelae.

TYPES OF FRACTURES

COLLES' FRACTURE

A *Colles' fracture* is a fracture of the distal radius and is one of the most common fractures in adults (Fig. 62-16). The styloid process of the ulna may be involved as well. The injury usually occurs when the patient falls on an outstretched arm and hand. This type of fracture most often occurs in patients over 50 years old whose bones are osteoporotic (*fragility fracture*). A younger person with a Colles' fracture caused by a low-energy force should be referred for an osteoporosis evaluation.

Clinical manifestations of Colles' fracture are pain in the immediate area of injury, pronounced swelling, and dorsal displacement of the distal fragment (silver-fork deformity). This displacement appears as an obvious deformity of the wrist. The major complication associated with a Colles' fracture is vascular insufficiency secondary to edema. Carpal tunnel syndrome can be a later complication.

A Colles' fracture is usually managed with closed reduction of the fracture and immobilization by a splint or cast. If displaced, the fracture is typically managed with open reduction

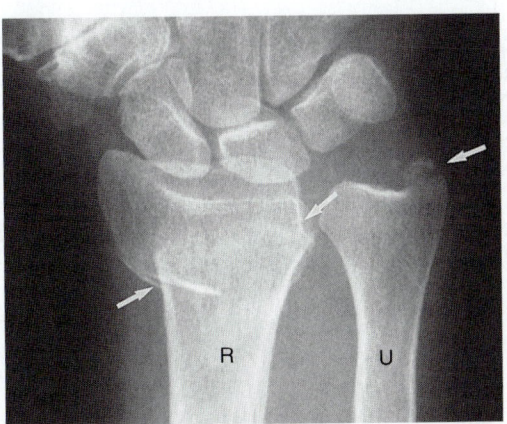

FIG. 62-16 Colles' fracture. Fracture of the distal radius *(R)* and ulnar *(U)* styloid from patient falling on the outstretched hand. (From Mettler FA: *Essentials of radiology,* ed 2, Philadelphia, 2005, Saunders.)

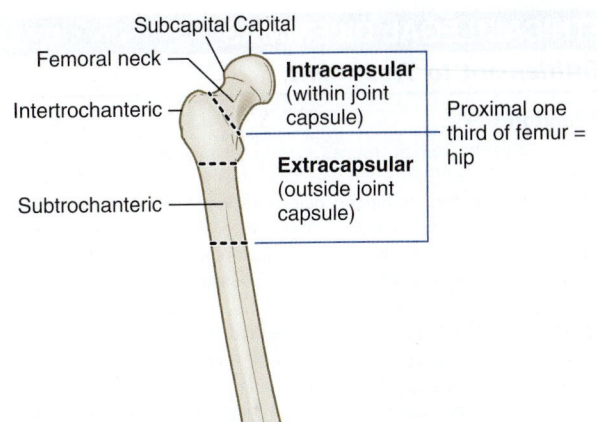

FIG. 62-17 Femur with location of various types of fracture.

and internal or external fixation. Nursing management includes frequent neurovascular assessment and measures to reduce edema. Provide support and protect the extremity. Encourage active movement of the thumb and fingers to reduce edema and increase venous return. Also instruct the patient to perform active movements of the shoulder to prevent stiffness or contracture.

HUMERAL SHAFT FRACTURE

Fractures involving the shaft of the humerus are common among young and middle-aged adults. The most common clinical manifestations are an obvious displacement of the humeral shaft, shortened extremity, abnormal mobility, and pain. Major complications associated with a humeral shaft fracture are radial nerve injury and injury to the brachial artery as a result of laceration, transection, or muscle spasm.

The treatment for a humeral shaft fracture depends on the location and displacement of the fracture. Nonoperative treatment may include a hanging arm cast; shoulder immobilizer; or sling and swathe (a type of immobilizer that prevents glenohumeral movement). The swathe encircles the trunk and humerus as an additional binder. It is often used after surgical repairs (e.g., rotator cuff repair) and shoulder dislocation.

When these devices are used, elevate the head of the bed to assist gravity in reducing the fracture. Allow the arm to hang freely when the patient is sitting or standing. Include measures to protect the axilla and prevent skin breakdown. Carefully place absorbable composite dressing pads (i.e., ABD pads) in the axilla and change them twice daily or as needed. Skin or skeletal traction may be used for reduction and immobilization.

During the rehabilitative phase, an exercise program to improve strength and motion of the injured extremity is extremely important. Exercises should include assisted motion of the hand and fingers. The shoulder can also be exercised if the fracture is stable. This helps prevent stiffness secondary to frozen shoulder or fibrosis of the shoulder capsule.

PELVIC FRACTURE

Pelvic fractures range from relatively minor to life threatening, depending on the mechanism of injury and associated vascular damage. Although only a small percentage of all fractures are pelvic fractures, this type of injury is associated with a high

mortality rate. Preoccupation with more obvious injuries at the time of a traumatic event may result in oversight of pelvic injuries.

Pelvic fractures may cause serious intraabdominal injury, including laceration and hemorrhage of the urethra, bladder, or colon. Pelvic fractures can cause acute pelvic compartment syndrome. Paralytic ileus may also occur following pelvic fracture. Patients may survive the initial pelvic injury, only to die from sepsis, FES, or VTE.

Physical examination of the abdomen may identify local swelling, tenderness, deformity, unusual pelvic movement, and ecchymosis. Assess the neurovascular condition of the lower extremities and determine associated injuries. Pelvic fractures are diagnosed by x-ray and CT scan.

Treatment of a pelvic fracture depends on the severity of the injury. Stable, nondisplaced fractures require limited intervention. Bed rest, sometimes with the use of a pelvic sling, is typically maintained for a few days. Progressive ambulation with guarded weight bearing is then encouraged. Complex or displaced fractures (e.g., open book fracture) require external fixation alone or combined with ORIF, often performed emergently. Use extreme care in handling or moving the patient to prevent additional injury. Turn the patient only when ordered by the HCP. Because a pelvic fracture can damage other organs, assess bowel and urinary elimination. Regularly perform distal neurovascular assessment. Provide back care while the patient is raised from the bed by independent use of the trapeze or with adequate assistance.

HIP FRACTURE

Hip fractures are common in older adults, with 95% of these fractures resulting from a fall.[22] More than 320,000 patients are admitted to hospitals annually because of a hip fracture. By age 90, approximately 33% of all women and 17% of all men will have sustained a hip fracture. In adults more than 65 years old, hip fracture occurs more frequently in women than in men because of osteoporosis. Many older adults with a hip fracture develop disabilities that require long-term care. One in five people experiencing a hip fracture will die within 1 year of injury.[23]

Hip fracture (Fig. 62-17) refers to a fracture of the proximal (upper) third of the femur, which extends 5 cm below the lesser trochanter. Fractures that occur within the hip joint capsule are called *intracapsular fractures.* Intracapsular fractures are further identified by their specific locations: (1) *capital* (fracture of the

ETHICAL/LEGAL DILEMMAS
Entitlement to Treatment

Situation

H.Z., a 35-yr-old German tourist, was in a hang-gliding accident while touring the United States. He was taken to the regional trauma center for treatment of internal injuries, blood loss, and severe pelvic fractures. He has become septic, is now in renal failure, and has acute respiratory distress syndrome. He has no health insurance. Despite a poor chance of survival, his wife and parents want all possible measures to be taken.

Ethical/Legal Points for Consideration

- Federal law requires hospitals receiving federal funds through Medicare and Medicaid to provide emergency evaluation and treatment to stabilize patients (Emergency Medical Treatment and Active Labor Act [EMTALA]). They are under no obligation to continue treatment and may transfer the patient to another facility.
- In addition, the Hill-Burton Act requires states to have sufficient hospitals to provide necessary services for those unable to pay.
- Discussions with the family must occur to clarify treatment goals (e.g., recovery, survival, continued biologic existence, nonabandonment of the patient) and what they mean by wanting "everything done." There is no legal or ethical obligation to continue medical treatment when treatment goals cannot be met.
- Contact with the German consulate may result in collaboration to stabilize the patient and transport him to Germany.
- Neither HCPs nor hospitals are required to provide medically futile care (care that provides no benefit to the patient).
- Although his home country (Germany) offers universal health care, H.Z. assumed the risk when engaging in a potentially dangerous activity and did not obtain international health insurance coverage for his visit to a foreign country.

Discussion Questions

1. How can the nurse facilitate discussions with the family regarding treatment goals for H.Z.? Are family members able to verbalize H.Z.'s wishes for his own care in such a situation?
2. If a person engages in risky behavior, is withholding treatment an option because of the behavior?

❓ CHECK YOUR PRACTICE

You are taking care of an 83-yr-old patient who fell down the steps outside her house while getting her mail. She was diagnosed with a femoral neck fracture and Colles' fracture. She is returning to the clinical unit following surgery. She had an ORIF of the femoral neck fracture and closed reduction of the Colles' fracture.

- Based on these injuries, what do you think are possible complications?
- How will the interprofessional team mobilize a patient with these injuries?
- What are your postdischarge concerns for this patient?

---

head of the femur), (2) *subcapital* (fracture just below the head of the femur), and (3) *transcervical* (fracture of the femoral neck). These fractures are often associated with osteoporosis and minor trauma and are identified as *fragility fractures.*

Extracapsular fractures occur outside the joint capsule. They are termed (1) *intertrochanteric* (in a region between the greater and lesser trochanter) or (2) *subtrochanteric* (below the lesser trochanter). Extracapsular fractures are usually caused by severe direct trauma or a fall.

Clinical Manifestations

Clinical manifestations of hip fractures are external rotation, muscle spasm, shortening of the affected extremity, and severe pain and tenderness around the fracture site. Displaced femoral

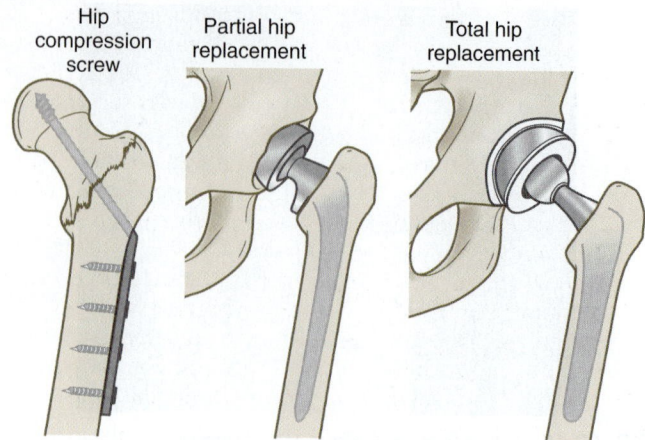

FIG. 62-18   Types of surgical repair for a hip fracture.

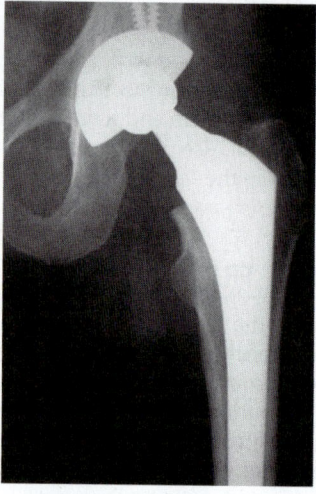

FIG. 62-19   Total hip replacement (arthroplasty) with cementless femoral prosthesis of metal alloy with plastic acetabular socket.

neck fractures may cause serious disruption of blood supply to the femoral head, which can result in avascular necrosis of the femoral head.

Interprofessional Care

Initially the affected extremity may be temporarily immobilized by Buck's traction (Fig. 62-9) until the patient's physical condition is stabilized and surgery can be performed. Buck's traction relieves painful muscle spasms and can be used for 24 to 48 hours.

Surgical treatment of hip fractures permits early mobilization and decreases the risk of major complications. The type of surgery depends on the location and severity of the fracture and the person's age. Surgical options include (1) repair with internal fixation devices (e.g., hip compression screw, intramedullary devices) (Fig. 62-18), (2) replacement of the femoral head with a prosthesis (partial hip replacement or *hemiarthroplasty,* often used for fracture of the femoral neck) (Fig. 62-18), and (3) total hip replacement (involves both the femur and acetabulum) (Figs. 62-18 and 62-19).

❖ NURSING MANAGEMENT: HIP FRACTURE

◆ Nursing Implementation

◆ **Preoperative Care.** The majority of people who have hip fractures are older adults. When planning treatment of the hip fracture, consider the patient's chronic health problems (e.g., diabetes mellitus, cardiac and pulmonary disease). Surgery may be delayed for a brief time until the patient's general health is stabilized, but better outcomes are associated with surgery performed within 24 hours of injury.[24]

Before surgery, severe muscle spasms can increase pain. Appropriate analgesics or muscle relaxants, comfortable positioning (unless contraindicated), and properly applied traction (if used) can help to manage the spasms.

Teaching is often done in the emergency department because quick surgical intervention is the standard of care. Most patients are medically stable and thus do not have an overnight preoperative period in which to receive instructions. The patient also may not have the cognitive ability to retain this important patient teaching.

When possible, teach the patient the method for exercising the unaffected leg and both arms. Plans for discharge begin as soon as the patient enters the hospital because the length of stay postoperatively will only be a few days.

◆ **Postoperative Care.** Similar principles of patient care apply to any of the surgical procedures for hip fractures. In the initial postoperative period, assess vital signs, intake, and output; monitor respiratory function and encourage deep breathing and coughing; administer pain medication; and observe the dressing and incision for signs of bleeding. (eNursing Care Plan 62-2 for the orthopedic surgical patient is presented on the website for this chapter.)

Neurovascular impairment is possible. Assess the patient's extremity for (1) color, (2) temperature, (3) capillary refill, (4) distal pulses, (5) edema, (6) sensation, (7) motor function, and (8) pain. Edema is alleviated by elevating the leg when the patient is in bed or in a chair. The pain resulting from surgical repair of the affected extremity can be reduced by maintaining limb alignment with pillows between the patient's knees when turning the patient to the nonoperative side.

Encourage the patient to use the overhead trapeze bar and the opposite side rail to assist in changing positions. Avoid turning the patient to the affected side unless approved by the surgeon. A physical therapist can teach the patient how to perform out-of-bed and chair transfers.

If the hip fracture has been repaired with hemiarthroplasty or total joint replacement by a *posterior approach* (incision posterior to the midline of the greater trochanter down the femoral shaft), measures to prevent dislocation must be used (Table 62-11). Inform the patient and caregiver about positions and activities that place the patient at risk for dislocation (more than 90 degrees of flexion, adduction across the midline [crossing of legs and ankles], internal rotation of hip). Many daily activities may reproduce these positions: (1) putting on shoes and socks, (2) crossing the legs or feet while seated, (3) assuming the side-lying position incorrectly, (4) standing up or sitting down while the hip is flexed more than 90 degrees relative to the chair, and (5) sitting on low seats, especially low toilet seats. Teach the patient to avoid these activities until the soft tissue capsule around the hip has healed enough to stabilize the prosthesis (usually at least 6 weeks).

Elevated toilet seats and chair alterations (e.g., raising the seat with a folded blanket, maintaining a straight back) are necessary. Avoid placing a soft pillow in the patient's seat because sitting on it can cause internal rotation. If a foam abduction wedge is ordered to prevent joint dislocation, place it between the patient's legs (Fig. 62-20). Apply the top straps above the knee to avoid placing pressure on the peroneal nerve

TABLE 62-11   Patient & Caregiver Teaching

Hip Replacement*

After a hip replacement by posterior surgical approach, include the following instructions when teaching a patient and caregiver.

Do

- Use an elevated toilet seat.
- Place chair inside shower or tub and remain seated while washing.
- Use pillow between legs for first 6 wk after surgery when lying on nonoperative side or when supine.
- Keep hip in neutral, straight position when sitting, walking, or lying.
- Notify surgeon immediately if severe pain, deformity, or loss of function occurs.
- Discuss personal risk factors for prosthetic joint infection with surgeon and dentist before dental work.

Do Not

- Flex hip greater than 90 degrees (e.g., sitting in low chairs or toilet seats).
- Adduct hip (i.e., bring legs together at knees).
- Internally rotate hip (i.e., turn toward planted foot on affected side).
- Cross legs at knees or ankles.
- Put on own shoes or stockings without adaptive device (e.g., long-handled shoehorn or stocking-helper) until 4-6 wk after surgery.
- Sit on chairs without arms. The arms of chairs will help the patient rise to a standing position.

*For patients having surgery by a posterior approach.

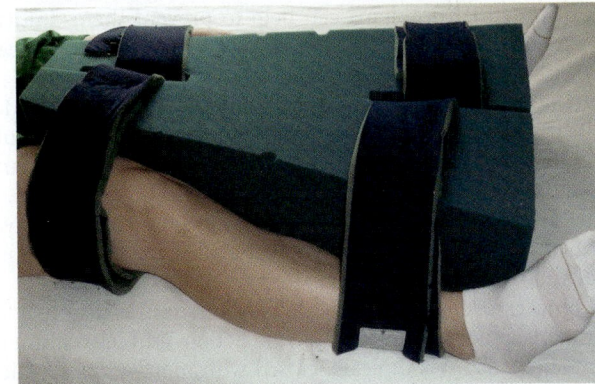

FIG. 62-20 Maintaining postoperative abduction following total hip replacement. (Courtesy Mary Wollan, RN, BAN, ONC, Spring Park, Minn.)

at the lateral tibial tubercle. Some HCPs prefer that the patient keep the abductor wedge in place except when bathing or walking.

If the hip fracture has been repaired with hemiarthroplasty or total joint replacement by an *anterior approach* (incision is made in the front of the hip with patient lying on the back), the hip muscles are left intact. This approach generally results in a more stable hip in the postoperative period with a lower rate of complications. Patient precautions related to motion and weight bearing are few but typically include instructions to avoid hyperextension.

Weight bearing on the involved extremity varies. Limited weight bearing is typically the only restriction for the patient who had ORIF of the hip fracture. Complete weight bearing following ORIF is generally restricted until x-ray examination indicates adequate healing, usually 6 to 12 weeks. Inform the caregiver about the patient's weight-bearing status after surgery.

Taking a tub bath and driving a car are not allowed for 4 to 6 weeks. An occupational therapist may teach the patient to use assistive devices such as reachers or grabbers to avoid bending over to pick up something on the floor, long-handled shoe-horns, or sock assists. The knees must be kept apart. Instruct the patient to never cross the legs or twist to reach behind.

The physical therapist usually supervises exercises for the affected extremity and ambulation when the surgeon permits it. The patient is usually out of bed by the first postoperative day. In collaboration with the physical therapist, monitor the patient's ambulation for proper use of crutches or a walker. To be discharged home, the patient must demonstrate the proper use of crutches or a walker over a functional distance (approximately 150 feet), and the ability to transfer to and from a chair and bed and to go up and down stairs.

Complications associated with femoral neck fracture include nonunion, avascular necrosis, dislocation, and osteoarthritis (OA). The affected leg may be shortened if the patient had an intertrochanteric fracture. A cane or shoe lift may be required for safe ambulation.

Sudden severe pain, a lump in the buttock, limb shortening, and external rotation indicate prosthesis dislocation. This requires a closed reduction with moderate to deep sedation or open reduction under general anesthesia to realign the femoral head in the acetabulum. If any of these manifestations occur, (regardless of the setting), keep the patient NPO in anticipation of surgical intervention.

Assist the patient and caregiver in adjusting to restrictions and dependence imposed by the hip fracture. Anxiety and depression can easily occur, but creative nursing care and awareness of potential problems can help to prevent them. Inform the patient and caregiver about community services that can help with rehabilitation after hospital discharge.

◆ **Ambulatory Care.** Hospitalization averages 3 or 4 days. Older adults or patients who live alone may require care in a subacute rehabilitation unit, at a skilled nursing facility, or in an acute rehabilitation facility for a few weeks before returning home. If the patient has skilled nursing needs or is homebound for physical therapy after discharge from post-acute care, the HCP may order follow-up home health care.

Home care considerations include ongoing assessment of pain management, monitoring for infection, and prevention of VTE. The incision is typically closed with metal staples, which are removed at the surgeon's office. If warfarin is used to decrease the high risk for VTE, inform the patient and caregiver of required testing for the international normalized ratio (INR), which is the standardized system of reporting prothrombin times. Adjust anticoagulation based on HCP order. Alternatives to warfarin include LMWH or factor Xa inhibitors. These newer anticoagulants require less monitoring than warfarin. Teach the patient who is receiving an anticoagulant to immediately report signs of bleeding to the HCP (see Chapter 37).

Exercises designed to restore strength and tone in the quadriceps and muscles around the hip are essential to improve function and ROM. These include quadriceps setting (e.g., pressing the kneecap down), gluteal muscle setting (e.g., tightening the buttocks), leg raises in supine and prone positions, and abduction exercises from the supine and standing positions (e.g., swinging the leg out but never crossing midline). The patient continues these exercises for many months after discharge. Teach the exercise program to the caregiver who will be encouraging the patient at home.

A physical therapist assesses ROM, ambulation, and adherence to the exercise program. The patient gradually increases the number of repetitions of exercises and may add ankle weights. Swimming and stationary cycling may also tone quadriceps and improve cardiovascular fitness. Instruct the patient to avoid high-impact exercises and sports, such as jogging and tennis, because they may loosen the implant. A physical therapist may also perform a home assessment to identify hazards that may cause the patient to fall again.

◆ **Evaluation**

The expected outcomes are that the patient with a hip fracture will
- Report satisfactory pain management
- Participate in exercise therapy
- Understand prescribed treatment plan

Gerontologic Considerations: Hip Fracture

Factors that increase the risk of a hip fracture in older adults include (1) a tendency to fall due to an altered center of gravity and the inability to correct a postural imbalance, (2) decreased fat and muscle to act as local tissue shock absorbers, and (3) reduced skeletal strength. Other factors that increase the older adult's risk of falling include (1) gait and balance problems, (2) altered vision and hearing, (3) slowed reflexes, (4) orthostatic hypotension, and (5) medication use. Homes can be made safer by (1) eliminating tripping hazards (e.g., loose rugs, uneven surfaces), (2) adding grab bars inside and outside the tub or shower, and beside the toilet, (3) adding railings on both sides of the stairs, and (4) installing better lighting.[25]

Many falls are associated with getting in or out of a chair or bed. Falls to the side, the most common type seen in frail older adults, are more likely to result in a hip fracture than a forward fall. External hip protectors may help prevent hip fractures in the frail older patient.[26] Older adults may have low bone density (*osteopenia*) or osteoporosis, which increases their risk of fragility fractures.

Calcium and vitamin D supplementation is indicated for anyone with osteopenia or osteoporosis. A bisphosphonate drug (e.g., alendronate [Fosamax]) or teriparatide (Forteo, a form of parathyroid hormone) may also be prescribed to decrease bone loss or increase bone density and thus reduce the likelihood of fracture. (Osteoporosis is discussed in Chapter 63.)

FEMORAL SHAFT FRACTURE

Because the femur can bend slightly to absorb stress, femoral shaft fracture occurs from a severe direct force. The force exerted to cause the fracture (e.g., from a motor vehicle crash or gunshot wound) frequently also damages the adjacent soft tissue. These injuries may be more serious than the bone injury. Young adults have a higher incidence of this type of fracture.

Displacement of fracture fragments often causes increased soft tissue damage. Considerable blood loss (1 to 1.5 L) can occur. The most common types of femoral shaft fracture include transverse, spiral, comminuted, oblique, and open (Figs. 62-6 and 62-7).

Clinical manifestations of a femoral shaft fracture are usually obvious. They include pain, marked deformity and angulation, shortening of the extremity, and inability to move the hip or knee. Common complications associated with femoral shaft fracture include FES; nerve and vascular injury; and problems associated with bone union, open fracture, and soft tissue damage.

Initial management of a femoral shaft fracture is directed toward stabilization of the patient and immobilization of the fracture. Traction may be used as a temporary measure before surgical treatment or in the patient unable to undergo surgery. Placement of an *intramedullary rod* is the most common surgical treatment for femoral shaft fracture. A metal rod is placed into the marrow canal of the femur. The rod passes across the fracture to keep it in position. Plates and screws may also be used. Internal fixation is preferred because it reduces the hospital stay and complications associated with prolonged bed rest. External fixation would be used for an open fracture.

After surgery, gluteal and quadriceps isometric exercises will promote and maintain strength in the affected extremity. Encourage the patient to perform ROM and strengthening exercises for all uninvolved extremities in preparation for ambulation. The patient may be allowed to begin non–weight-bearing activities with an ambulatory assistive device (e.g., walker, crutches). Full weight bearing is usually restricted until x-rays show union of fracture fragments. Teach the patient to carefully follow the HCP's instructions for weight bearing.

TIBIAL FRACTURE

Although the tibia is vulnerable to injury because it lacks a covering of anterior muscle, strong force is required to cause a tibial fracture. As a result, soft tissue damage, devascularization, and open fracture are frequent. The tibia is a common site for stress fracture. Complications associated with tibial fracture are compartment syndrome, FES, delayed union or nonunion, and possible infection with an open fracture.

The recommended management for closed tibial fracture is closed reduction followed by immobilization in a long leg cast. ORIF with intramedullary rods, plate fixation, or external fixation is indicated for complex tibial fractures and those with extensive soft tissue damage. Locking plates (screw and plate system) may also be used for surgical repair. Emphasis for either type of reduction is on maintaining quadriceps strength.

Assess the neurovascular condition of the affected extremity at least every 2 hours during the first 48 hours. Instruct patients to perform active ROM exercises with the uninvolved leg and the upper extremities to build the strength required for crutch walking. When the HCP has determined the patient is ready for gait training, reinforce the principles of crutch walking introduced by the physical therapist. The patient may be non–weight bearing for 6 to 12 weeks, depending on healing. Home nursing visits may be initiated to monitor the patient's progress if the patient is homebound.

STABLE VERTEBRAL FRACTURE

Stable fractures of the vertebral column are usually caused by motor vehicle crashes, falls, diving, or sports injuries. Patients with osteoporosis experience more than 700,000 vertebral compression fractures annually, many of which are stable. In a stable fracture, the fracture fragments are unlikely to move or cause spinal cord damage. This type of injury is frequently confined to the vertebral body (anterior element of the spinal column) in the lumbar region and less frequently involves the cervical and thoracic regions. Vertebral bodies are usually protected from displacement by intact spinal ligaments.

Most patients with stable spinal fractures experience only brief periods of disability. However, if spinal ligaments are significantly disrupted, dislocation of the vertebrae may occur. Instability and injury to the spinal cord may result (unstable fracture). These injuries generally require surgery. The most serious complication of vertebral fractures is fracture displacement, which can cause damage to the spinal cord (see Chapter 60). Although stable vertebral fractures are not associated with abnormal spinal cord pathology, all spinal injuries should be considered unstable and potentially serious until diagnostic tests determine the fracture to be stable.

The patient usually complains of pain and tenderness in the affected region of the spine. Sudden loss of function below the fracture indicates spinal cord impingement and paraplegia. Stable compression fractures are associated with a kyphotic deformity (flexion angulation of thoracic vertebrae) known as a *dowager's hump*. This deformity is readily identified during the physical examination (see Fig. 63-9). *Lordosis* (extreme inward curve of lumbar spine) and cervical spine involvement are also possible. Bowel and bladder dysfunction may indicate an interruption of the autonomic nervous system nerves or injury to the spinal cord.

The overall goal in management of stable vertebral fractures is to keep the spine in good alignment until union has been accomplished. Many nursing interventions are aimed at assessing for the possibility of spinal cord trauma. Regularly evaluate vital signs and bowel and bladder function. Also monitor the motor and sensory function of peripheral nerves distal to the injured region. Promptly report any deterioration in the patient's neurovascular condition.

Treatment includes pain medication followed by early mobilization and bracing. The patient's mattress should offer firm support to support the spinal column, relax muscles, decrease edema, and prevent potential compression on nerve roots. Teach the patient to keep the spine straight when turning by moving the shoulders and pelvis together. The patient will need nursing assistance to learn the technique of logrolling. Several days after the initial injury, the HCP may apply a specially constructed orthotic device (e.g., thoracolumbar sacral orthosis [TLSO]), a jacket cast, or a removable corset if there is no evidence of neurologic deficit. The device provides extra support during healing and is used for a short period of time.

Lightweight bracing (e.g., Jewett or Bähler-Vogt brace) may be used for patients with stable vertebral compression fractures due to osteoporosis. Patients with osteoporosis may also be treated with two outpatient procedures: vertebroplasty or balloon kyphoplasty. *Vertebroplasty* uses radioimaging to guide the injection of bone cement into a fractured vertebral body. When hardened, the cement stabilizes the vertebra and prevents further compression. *Balloon kyphoplasty* involves first inserting a balloon into the vertebral body and then inflating it. This creates a cavity that is filled with bone cement under low pressure to restore the height of the vertebral body. Kyphoplasty is now the surgical treatment of choice for compression fractures. This is due largely to the decreased incidence of bone cement leakage into nearby structures (e.g., colon, lung) compared to vertebroplasty. Patients experience decreased pain almost immediately with these procedures. However, later compression fractures of adjacent vertebrae are a risk.

If the fracture is in the cervical spine, the patient may wear a hard cervical collar. Some cervical fractures are immobilized by use of a halo vest (see Fig. 60-7). This consists of a plastic jacket or cast fitted about the chest and attached to a halo that is held in place by skeletal pins inserted into the cranium. These devices immobilize the spine in the fracture area but allow the patient to ambulate.

The patient with a stable vertebral fracture is discharged after (1) demonstrating safe ambulation, (2) learning care of the cast or orthotic device, and (3) verbalizing strategies to address safety and security concerns related to the injury and treatment. Unstable vertebral fractures and spinal cord injuries are discussed in Chapter 60.

FACIAL FRACTURE

Any bone of the face can be fractured as a result of trauma, such as a motor vehicle crash, an assault, or a fall.[27] It is critically important after facial injury to establish and maintain a patent airway and provide adequate ventilation. Suctioning may be needed to remove foreign material and blood. A surgically created airway (tracheostomy) may be needed if a patent airway cannot be maintained.

Facial fractures and cervical spine injuries commonly occur together. All patients with facial injuries should be treated as if they have a cervical injury until proven otherwise by examination and CT scan or x-ray. Table 62-12 describes clinical manifestations of common facial fractures.

Related soft tissue injury often makes assessment of facial injury difficult. Perform oral and facial examinations after any life-threatening situations have been treated. Carefully assess ocular muscles and cranial nerves III, IV, and VI.[28] X-rays are used to determine the extent of the injury. CT scanning helps differentiate between bone and soft tissue.

Suspect injury to the eye when facial injury occurs, particularly if the injury is near the orbit. If an eye-globe rupture is suspected, stop the examination and place a protective shield over the eye. Signs of rupture include vitreous humor forced out of the eye, or brown tissue (iris or ciliary body) on the surface of the globe or penetrating through a laceration with an off-center or teardrop-shaped pupil.

Specific treatment depends on the site and extent of the facial fracture and associated soft tissue injury. Immobilization or surgical stabilization may be necessary. Maintain a patent airway and adequate nutrition throughout the recovery period.

Be sensitive about alterations in appearance that may occur after facial fracture. Changes in appearance may be drastic. Edema and discoloration subside with time, but concurrent soft tissue injuries may result in permanent scarring.

Mandibular Fracture

Mandibular fracture may result from trauma to the face or jaw. Maxillary fractures may also occur, but they are less common than mandibular fractures. The mandibular fracture may be simple, with no bone displacement, or may involve loss of tissue and bone. The fracture may require immediate treatment to ensure the patient's survival. Long-term treatment is sometimes needed to restore satisfactory appearance and function.

Mandibular fractures may also be therapeutically performed to correct an underlying alignment problem (malocclusion) that cannot be adjusted by orthodontics alone. The mandible is resected during surgery and manipulated forward or backward to correct the occlusion problem.

Surgery for a mandibular fracture includes immobilization, usually by wiring the jaws (intermaxillary fixation). Internal fixation may be done with screws and plates. In a simple fracture with no loss of teeth, the lower jaw is wired to the upper jaw. Wires are placed around the teeth, and then cross-wires or rubber bands are used to hold the lower jaw tight against the upper jaw (Fig. 62-21). Arch bars may be placed on the maxillary and mandibular arches of the teeth. Vertical wires are placed between the arch bars, holding the jaws together. If teeth are missing or bone is displaced, other forms of fixation may be needed (e.g., metal arch bars in the mouth or insertion of a pin in the bone). Bone grafting may also be required. Immobilization is usually necessary for only 4 to 6 weeks because the fractures often heal rapidly.

❖ NURSING MANAGEMENT: MANDIBULAR FRACTURE

Inform the patient preoperatively about what is involved in the surgical procedure, how the face will look afterward, and alterations caused by the surgery. Reassure the patient about the ability to breathe normally, speak, and swallow liquids. Hospitalization for respiratory monitoring is brief unless there are other injuries or problems.

Postoperative care focuses on a patent airway, oral hygiene, communication, pain management, and adequate nutrition. Two potential problems in the immediate postoperative period are airway obstruction and aspiration of vomitus. Because the patient cannot open the jaws, an airway must be maintained. Observe for signs of respiratory distress (e.g., dyspnea; alterations in rate, quality, and depth of respirations). After surgery place the patient on the side with the head slightly elevated immediately.

Tape a wire cutter or scissors (for rubber bands) to the head of the bed and send it with the patient to all appointments and examinations away from the bedside. The wire cutter or scissors

TABLE 62-12	Manifestations of Facial Fractures
Fracture	**Manifestation**
Frontal bone	Rapid edema that may mask underlying fractures
Periorbital bone	Possible frontal sinus involvement, entrapment of ocular muscles
Nasal bone	Displacement of nasal bones, nosebleed (epistaxis)
Zygomatic arch	Depression of cheek bone (zygomatic arch) and entrapment of ocular muscles
Maxilla	Segmental motion (instability) of maxilla and tooth fracture at socket
Mandible	Tooth fractures, bleeding, limited motion of mandible

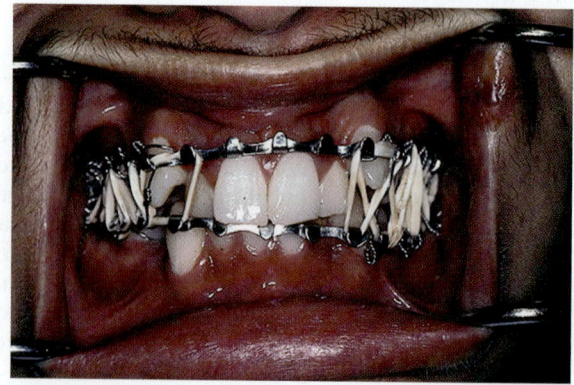

FIG. 62-21   Intermaxillary fixation. (Courtesy R.A. Weinstein, Denver, Colo.)

may be used to cut the wires or elastic bands in case of an emergency requiring access to the pharynx or lungs (e.g., cardiac arrest or respiratory distress). In the care plan include a picture with the appropriate wires to cut in an emergency. In some cases, cutting the wires may cause the entire facial and upper jaw structure to shift or collapse and worsen the problem. A tracheostomy or endotracheal tray should always be available.

If the patient begins to vomit or choke, try to clear the mouth and airway. Suctioning may be done by the nasopharyngeal or oral route, depending on the extent of injury and type of repair. An NG tube may be used for decompression to remove fluids and gas from the stomach to help prevent aspiration. An NG tube also helps prevent vomiting. Antiemetics may also be used. The NG tube can later be used as a feeding tube. Teach the patient to clear secretions and vomitus.

Oral hygiene is extremely important. Teach the patient to remove food debris by rinsing the mouth often, particularly after meals and snacks. Warm normal saline solution, water, or alkaline mouthwashes may be used. A syringe and soft irrigation catheter or a Water Pik may be effective for thorough oral cleansing. Inspect the mouth several times a day to see that it is clean. Use a tongue depressor to retract the cheeks. Keep the lips, corners of the mouth, and buccal mucosa moist. Cover any sharp edges of the wires with dental wax to prevent irritation of the buccal mucosa.

Communication may be a problem, particularly in the early postoperative period. Establish an effective way of communicating preoperatively (e.g., use of dry erase board, pad and pencil). Usually the patient can speak well enough to be understood, especially a few days after surgery.

Intake of adequate nutrients poses a challenge because the diet must be liquid. The patient easily tires of sucking through a straw or laboriously using a spoon. Work with the dietitian and patient to plan a diet with adequate calories, protein, and fluids. Liquid protein supplements may help the patient improve the nutritional status. A low-bulk, high-carbohydrate diet and intake of air through the straw contribute to constipation and gas. Ambulation, prune juice, and bulk-forming laxatives may help relieve these problems.

The patient is usually discharged with the wires in place. Encourage the patient to verbalize feelings about the altered appearance. Discharge teaching should include oral care, diet, techniques for handling secretions, how and when to use wire cutters or scissors, and when to notify the HCP about concerns and problems.

AMPUTATION

An amputation is the removal of a body extremity by trauma or surgery. About 2 million people in the United States are living with limb loss.[29] Older people have the highest incidence of amputation due to peripheral vascular disease (PVD), atherosclerosis, and vascular changes related to diabetes mellitus. Amputation in young people is usually secondary to trauma (e.g., motor vehicle crashes, land mines, farm-related injury). More than 1700 American military personnel have undergone a service-related amputation as part of the U.S. combat mission in Iraq.[30]

Clinical Indications

Most amputations are performed due to PVD, especially in older patients with diabetes mellitus. These patients often

TABLE 62-13 Interprofessional Care

Amputation

Diagnostic Assessment	Management
• History and physical examination	**Medical**
• Physical appearance of soft tissues	• Appropriate management of underlying disease
• Skin temperature	• Stabilization of trauma victim
• Sensory function	
• Quality of peripheral pulses	**Surgical**
• Arteriography	• Residual limb management
• Venography	• Immediate or delayed prosthesis fitting
• Plethysmography	
• Transcutaneous ultrasonic Doppler recordings	**Rehabilitation**
	• Coordination of prosthesis-fitting and gait-training activities
	• Coordination of muscle-strengthening and physical therapy regimens

experience peripheral neuropathy that progresses to trophic ulcers and gangrene. Other common reasons for amputation are trauma, thermal injuries, tumors, osteomyelitis, and congenital limb disorders. Although pain is often present, it is not usually the primary reason for amputation.

Diagnostic Studies

Diagnostic studies depend on the underlying problem that makes the amputation necessary (Table 62-13). An elevated white blood cell (WBC) count with abnormal differential may indicate infection. Vascular tests such as arteriography, Doppler studies, and venography provide information about the circulation of the extremity.

Interprofessional Care

If amputation is planned or elective, as for the patient with PVD, carefully assess the patient's general health. Chronic illnesses and infection must be managed before an amputation is performed. Help the patient and caregiver understand the need for the amputation and assure them that rehabilitation can help with postoperative quality of life. If the amputation is performed emergently after trauma, patient management is physically and emotionally more complicated.

The goal of surgery is to preserve the greatest extremity length and function while removing all infected, pathologic, or ischemic tissue. (Levels of amputation of upper and lower extremities are illustrated in Fig. 62-22.) The type of amputation depends on the reason for the surgery. A closed amputation is performed to create a weight-bearing *residual limb* (or stump). An anterior skin flap with dissected soft tissue padding covers the bony part of the residual limb. The skin flap is sutured posteriorly so that the suture line will not be in a weight-bearing area. Special care is needed to prevent accumulation of drainage, which can produce pressure and harbor bacteria that may cause infection.

Disarticulation is an amputation performed through a joint. A *Syme's amputation* is a form of disarticulation at the ankle. After an open amputation (*guillotine amputation*), the surface of the residual limb is left uncovered with skin. This type of surgery is generally indicated to control actual or potential infection. The wound is usually closed later by a second surgical procedure or closed by skin traction surrounding the residual limb.

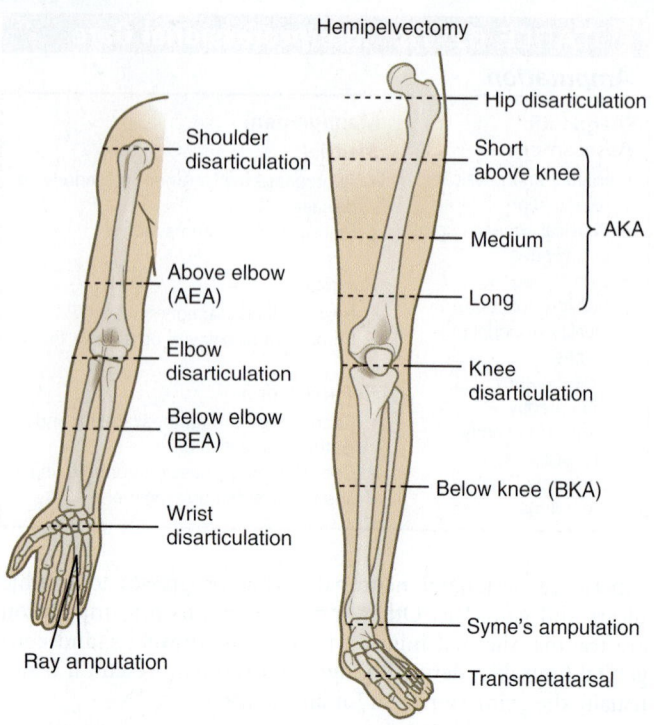

FIG. 62-22 Location and description of amputation sites of the upper and lower extremities. *AKA,* Above-the-knee amputation.

❖ NURSING MANAGEMENT: AMPUTATION

◆ Nursing Assessment

Assess any preexisting illnesses. Because most amputations are performed for vascular problems, assessment of vascular and neurologic condition is especially important (see Chapters 31 and 55).

◆ Nursing Diagnoses

Nursing diagnoses for the patient with an amputation may include, but are not limited to, the following:

- Disturbed body image *related to* loss of body part and impaired mobility
- Impaired skin integrity *related to* immobility and improperly fitted prosthesis
- Chronic pain *related to* phantom limb sensation or residual limb pain
- Impaired physical mobility *related to* amputation of lower limb

◆ Planning

The overall goals are that the patient with an amputation will (1) have adequate relief from the underlying health problem, (2) have satisfactory pain management, (3) reach maximum rehabilitation potential (with the use of a prosthesis, if indicated), (4) cope with the body image changes, and (5) make satisfying lifestyle adjustments.

◆ Nursing Implementation

◆ **Health Promotion.** Control of causative illnesses such as PVD, diabetes mellitus, chronic osteomyelitis, and pressure ulcers can eliminate or delay the need for amputation. Teach patients with these problems to carefully examine their lower extremities daily for signs of infection or skin breakdown. If the patient

cannot do this, the caregiver should help. Instruct the patient and caregiver to report changes in the feet or toes to the HCP, including changes in skin color or temperature, decreased or absent sensation, tingling, burning pain, cuts, or abrasions.

Instruct people in safety precautions for recreational activities and potentially hazardous work. This responsibility is especially critical for the occupational health nurse.

◆ **Acute Care.** Reasons for amputation and the rehabilitation potential depend on a person's age, diagnosis, occupation, personality, resources, and support system. Be aware of the tremendous psychologic and social implications of amputation. The disruption in body image caused by amputation often causes a patient to go through the grieving process. Use therapeutic communication to assist the patient and caregiver through this process to develop a realistic attitude about the future.

◆ *Preoperative Care.* Before surgery, reinforce information that the patient and caregiver have received about reasons for the amputation, proposed prosthesis, and mobility-training program. To meet the patient's educational needs, know the level of amputation, type of postsurgical dressings to be applied, and type of prosthesis to be used. Teach the patient to perform upper extremity exercises such as push-ups in bed or the wheelchair to promote arm strength essential for crutch walking and gait training. Discuss general postoperative nursing care, including positioning, support, and residual limb care. If a compression bandage is to be used after surgery, instruct the patient about its purpose and how it will be applied. If immediate prosthesis use is planned, discuss general ambulation expectations.

Tell the patient that the amputated limb may feel like it is still present after surgery. This phenomenon, termed phantom limb sensation, occurs in many amputees. (Nursing management of phantom limb sensation is discussed in the next section.)

◆ *Postoperative Care.* General postoperative care for the patient who has had an amputation depends largely on the patient's age and general state of health, and the reason for the amputation. Monitor individuals who undergo amputation as a result of a traumatic injury for posttraumatic stress disorder because they have had no time to prepare or perhaps even to participate in the decision to have a limb amputated.

Prevention and detection of complications are important after surgery. Carefully monitor the patient's vital signs. Assess dressings for hemorrhage in the operative area. Use sterile technique during dressing changes to reduce the risk for wound infection.

If an *immediate* postoperative prosthesis has been applied, carefully observe the surgical site. If excessive bleeding occurs, notify the surgeon immediately. A surgical tourniquet must always be available for emergency use.

The *delayed* prosthetic fitting may be the best choice for patients who have had amputations above the knee or below the elbow, older adults, and those with infection (Fig. 62-23). Appropriate timing for the use of a prosthesis depends on satisfactory healing of the residual limb and the patient's general condition. A temporary prosthesis may be used for partial weight bearing after sutures are removed. If there are no problems, the patient can bear full weight on a permanent prosthesis approximately 3 months after amputation.

Not all patients are candidates for prostheses. The seriously ill or debilitated patient may not have the upper body strength and energy needed to use a lower extremity prosthesis. Mobility with a wheelchair may be the most realistic goal for this patient.

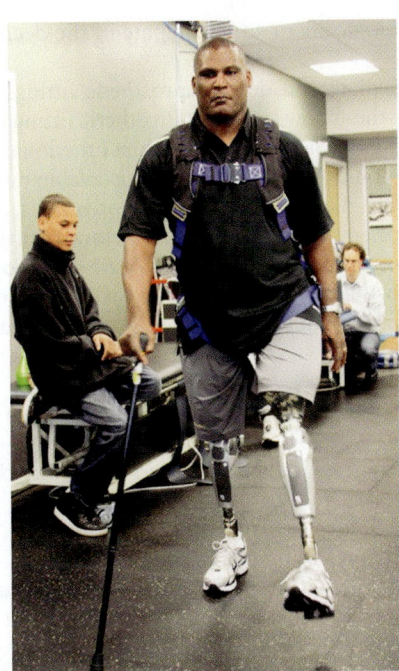

FIG. 62-23   A double amputee fitted with prostheses. (Photo courtesy U.S. Army.)

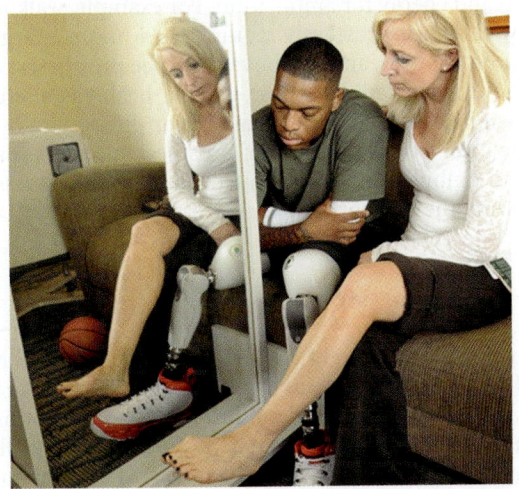

FIG. 62-24   Mirror therapy, a type of treatment that may reduce phantom limb sensation and pain. (U.S. Navy photo courtesy Mass Communication Specialist Seaman Joseph A. Boomhower.)

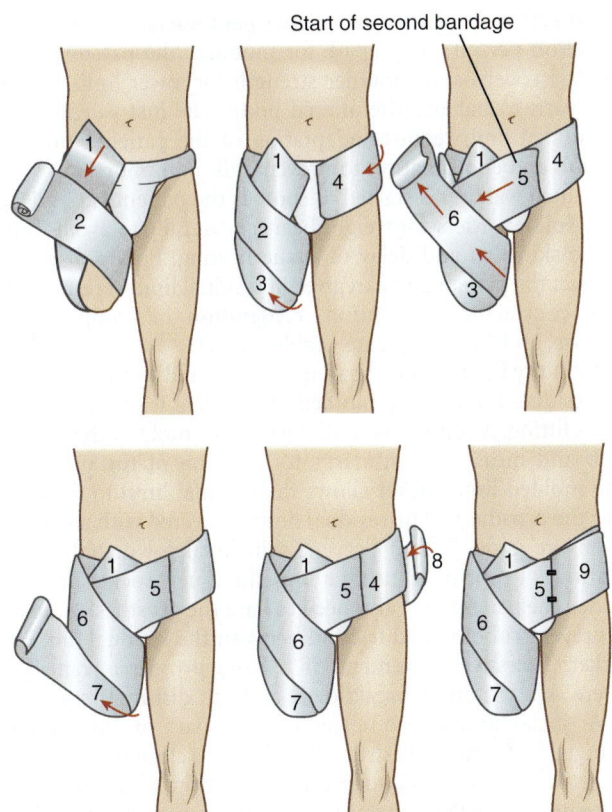

Start of second bandage

FIG. 62-25   Bandaging for the above-the-knee amputation residual limb. Figure-eight style covers progressive areas of the residual limb. Two elastic wraps are required.

Patients are often extremely worried about phantom limb sensation because they still perceive pain in the missing portion of the limb. As recovery and ambulation progress, phantom limb sensation and pain usually subside. However, the pain may become chronic. The patient may complain of shooting, burning, or crushing pain as well as feelings of coldness, heaviness, and cramping,

Mirror therapy reduces phantom limb sensation and pain in some patients[31] (Fig. 62-24). The mirror is thought to provide visual information to the brain, replacing sensory feedback expected from the missing limb. However, it is unknown why looking in the mirror at the remaining limb would decrease phantom limb sensation and pain. Mirror therapy may also improve patient functioning after a stroke.

Success of the rehabilitation program depends on the patient's physical and emotional health. Chronic illness and deconditioning can complicate rehabilitation. Physical and occupational therapy must be an integral component of the patient's overall plan of care.

Flexion contractures may delay rehabilitation. The most common and debilitating contracture is hip flexion. Hip adduction contracture is rare. To prevent flexion contractures, have patients avoid sitting in a chair for more than 1 hour with hips flexed or having pillows under the surgical extremity. Unless specifically contraindicated, patients should lie on their abdomen for 30 minutes three or four times each day and position the hip in extension while prone.

Proper bandaging ensures the residual limb is shaped and molded for eventual prosthesis fitting (Fig. 62-25). The surgeon usually orders a compression bandage to be applied immediately after surgery to support soft tissues, reduce edema, hasten healing, minimize pain, and promote residual limb shrinkage and maturation. This bandage may be an elastic roll applied to the residual limb or a residual limb shrinker, which is an elastic stocking that fits tightly over the residual limb.

The patient initially wears the compression bandage at all times except during physical therapy and bathing. Remove and reapply the bandage several times daily. Take care to apply it snugly but not so tight as to interfere with circulation. Wash and change shrinker bandages daily. After the residual limb is healed, bandage it only when the patient is not wearing the prosthesis. Instruct the patient to avoid dangling the residual limb over the bedside to decrease edema.

As the patient's overall condition improves, the HCP and physical therapist generally start and supervise an exercise regimen. Active ROM exercises for all joints should be started as soon after surgery as the patient's pain intensity and medical condition permit. To prepare for mobility, the patient should increase triceps and shoulder strength for lower limb support and learn to balance the altered body. The lost weight of an amputated limb requires adaptation of the patient's proprioception and coordination to prevent falls and injury.

Crutch walking is started as soon as the patient is physically able. Follow orders for weight bearing carefully to avoid injury to the skin flap and delay of tissue healing. Before discharge, instruct the patient and caregiver in residual limb care, ambulation, contracture prevention, recognition of complications, exercise, and follow-up care (Table 62-14).

◆ **Ambulatory Care.** When healing has occurred satisfactorily and the residual limb is well molded, the patient is ready for prosthesis fitting. A prosthetist initially makes a mold of the residual limb and measures landmarks for creation of the prosthesis. The molded limb socket allows the residual limb to fit snugly into the prosthesis. The residual limb is covered with a stocking to ensure good fit and prevent skin breakdown. If the limb continues to shrink, causing a loose fit, a new socket has to be made. The patient may also need to have the prosthesis adjusted to prevent rubbing and friction between the residual limb and socket. Excessive movement of a loose prosthesis can cause severe skin irritation, breakdown, and gait disturbances.

Artificial limbs become an integral part of the patient's changed body image. Instruct the patient to clean the prosthesis socket daily with mild soap and rinse thoroughly to remove irritants. Leather and metal parts of the prosthesis should not get wet. Encourage the patient to have regular maintenance on the prosthesis. Also consider the condition of the patient's shoe. A badly worn shoe alters the gait and may damage the prosthesis.

◆ **Special Considerations in Upper Limb Amputation.** Emotional implications of an upper limb amputation are often more devastating than for lower limb amputation. The enforced dependency due to one-handedness may be depressing and frustrating to the patient. Because most upper extremity amputations result from trauma, the patient has likely had little time to adjust psychologically or to participate in the decision-making process.

Both immediate and delayed prosthetic fittings are possible for the below-the-elbow amputee. Prosthetic fitting is delayed for the above-the-elbow amputee. The usual functional prosthesis is the arm and hook. A cosmetic hand is available but has limited functional value. As with the lower limb prosthesis, patient motivation and perseverance are major factors contributing to a satisfactory outcome. Recent technologic advances in upper extremity prostheses have led to increased functionality, with movements and capabilities that are closer to the natural arm.[32]

◆ **Evaluation**

The expected outcomes are that the patient with an amputation will

- Accept changed body image and integrate changes into lifestyle
- Have no evidence of skin breakdown
- Have reduction or absence of pain
- Become mobile within limitations imposed by amputation

Gerontologic Considerations: Amputation

If a lower limb amputation has been performed on an older adult, the patient's previous ability to ambulate may affect the extent of recovery. Use of a prosthesis requires significant strength and energy for ambulation. For example, walking with a below-the-knee prosthesis requires 40% more energy than walking on two legs, and an above-the-knee prosthesis requires 60% more. Older adults whose general health is altered and weakened by disorders such as cardiac or pulmonary dysfunction may not be candidates for prosthesis use. The patient's ability to ambulate may be limited. If possible, discuss these issues with the patient and caregiver before surgery so that realistic expectations can be set.

COMMON JOINT SURGICAL PROCEDURES

Surgery plays an important role in the treatment and rehabilitation of patients with various types of joint disease. Surgery is aimed at relieving chronic pain, improving joint motion, correcting deformity and misalignment, and removing diseased cartilage. If the joint problem is not corrected, contraction with permanent limitation of motion may occur. Limited joint motion can be demonstrated on physical examination. Joint-space narrowing is also apparent on x-rays.

TYPES OF JOINT SURGERIES

Synovectomy

Synovectomy (removal of synovial membrane) is performed to remove inflamed tissue that is causing unacceptable pain or limiting ROM in rheumatoid arthritis (RA). A synovectomy is best performed early in the disease process when there is minimal bone or cartilage destruction. Removal of the thickened synovium does not cure the disease but may relieve symptoms temporarily. Common sites for this surgery include the elbow, wrist, and fingers. Synovectomy in the knee is done less frequently because knee joint replacement is usually performed.

Osteotomy

An osteotomy involves removing a wedge or slice of bone to restore alignment (joint and vertebral) and to shift weight

---

TABLE 62-14   Patient & Caregiver Teaching

Following Lower Extremity Amputation

After lower extremity amputation, include the following instructions when teaching the patient and caregiver.

1. Inspect the residual limb daily for signs of skin irritation, especially redness, abrasion, and odor. Pay particular attention to areas prone to pressure.
2. Discontinue use of the prosthesis if irritation develops. Have the area checked before resuming use of the prosthesis.
3. Wash the residual limb thoroughly each night with warm water and bacteriostatic soap. Rinse thoroughly and dry gently. Expose the residual limb to air for 20 min.
4. Do not use lotions, alcohol, powders, or oil on residual limb unless prescribed by the HCP.
5. Wear only a residual limb sock in good condition and supplied by the prosthetist.
6. Change residual limb sock daily. Launder in mild soap, squeeze, lay flat to dry.
7. Use prescribed pain management techniques.
8. Perform ROM to all joints daily. Perform general strengthening exercises (including for upper extremities) daily.
9. Do not elevate residual limb on a pillow.
10. Lay prone with hip in extension for 30 min three or four times daily.

bearing, thus relieving pain. Cervical osteotomy may be used to correct a kyphotic deformity in some patients with ankylosing spondylitis. Halo vests and body jacket braces are worn until fusion occurs (3 to 4 months). Osteotomy has proven ineffective in patients with inflammatory joint disease. However, femoral osteotomy may provide some pain relief and improve motion in selected patients with hip osteoarthritis (OA). Tibial osteotomy also provides pain relief in selected patients, but a majority of patients require later knee replacement surgery.

Care of a patient who has undergone osteotomy is similar to that of a patient with ORIF of a fracture at a comparable site (see pp. 1474-1478). Internal wires, screws and plates, bone grafts, or an external fixator usually fixes the bone in place.

Debridement

Debridement is the removal of degenerative debris such as pieces of bone or cartilage (*loose bodies)* or osteophytes from a joint using a fiberoptic arthroscope. This procedure is usually performed on an outpatient basis on the knee or shoulder. A compression dressing is applied postoperatively. Weight bearing is permitted following knee arthroscopy. Patient teaching includes monitoring for signs of infection, managing pain, and restricting excessive activity for 24 to 48 hours.

Arthroplasty

Arthroplasty is the reconstruction or replacement of a joint to relieve pain, improve or maintain ROM, and correct deformity. Arthroplasty is most commonly performed on patients with OA, RA, avascular necrosis, congenital deformities or dislocations, and other systemic problems. There are several types of arthroplasty, including surgical reshaping of the bones of the joints, replacement of part of a joint (hemiarthroplasty), and total joint replacement. Replacement arthroplasty is available for elbows, shoulders, phalangeal joints of the fingers, wrists, hips, knees, ankles, and feet. More than 1 million Americans have knee and hip replacement surgery annually.[33]

Total Hip Arthroplasty. Total hip arthroplasty (THA) (total hip replacement) provides significant relief of pain and improved function for patients with joint deterioration from OA, RA, and other conditions. Partial and total hip replacements are also used to treat hip fractures.

In THA, the prosthesis (implant) replaces the ball-and-socket joint and upper shaft of the femur (Fig. 62-19). The socket can be cemented in place with polymethyl methacrylate, which bonds to the bone. The socket may also be inserted without cement (cementless). Cementless THA may provide longer-term prosthesis stability by enabling biologic ingrowth of new bone tissue into the porous surface coating of the prosthesis. Cementless devices are most often recommended for younger, more active patients and patients with good bone quality so that bone ingrowth into the components can be readily achieved.

The nursing care for a patient who has THA is discussed in the section on nursing management of a patient with a hip fracture on pp. 1482-1484.

Hip Resurfacing Arthroplasty. An alternative to hip replacement is hip resurfacing arthroplasty, which allows the femoral head (ball) to be preserved and reshaped rather than replaced as in THA. The resurfaced femoral head is then capped by a metal prosthesis. Hip resurfacing is a more favorable option for patients younger than age 60 with larger frames. A small percentage of patients will experience femoral neck fracture after hip resurfacing; this is not possible with THA. In addition,

metal ions may be released into the bloodstream from the prosthesis. Patients may develop sensitivity or allergy to these particles.[34] Patients receiving a smaller femoral head (including many women) have a higher failure rate with a resurfaced implant when compared with patients receiving THA.

Knee Arthroplasty. Unremitting pain and instability as a result of severe deterioration of the knee joint are the main indications for total knee arthroplasty (TKA). Partial (*unicompartmental)* arthroplasty can be performed on a patient with osteoarthritis limited to one part (compartment) of the knee.

Immediately after knee arthroplasty a compression dressing may be used to immobilize the knee in extension. This dressing is removed before discharge. If the patient is unable to perform a straight leg raise, a knee immobilizer or posterior plastic shell to maintain extension may be used during ambulation and at rest for about 4 weeks.

After surgery, an emphasis is placed on pain management and physical therapy. Because postoperative pain can significantly reduce the patient's ability to participate in therapy, effective pain management is a primary nursing care goal.[35] Physical therapy begins early with isometric quadriceps setting. Therapy progresses to straight-leg raises and gentle ROM to increase muscle strength and obtain 90-degree knee flexion. Active flexion exercises or passive flexion exercises with a continuous passive motion (CPM) machine may promote joint mobility. Ambulation is also begun early and typically progresses to full weight bearing before discharge. An active home exercise program involves progressive ROM with muscle strengthening and flexibility exercises.

Adequate analgesia should be ordered at discharge to allow the patient to continue with the exercise program. Effective pain management is key to achieving positive rehabilitation outcomes. After TKA, many older patients with advanced OA show significant improvement in mobility, motor function tests, and ability to complete daily tasks.

Finger Joint Arthroplasty. A silicone rubber arthroplastic device is used to restore function in the fingers of the patient with RA. Ulnar deviation often causes severe functional limitations of the hand. The goal of hand surgery is primarily to restore function related to grasp, pinch, stability, and strength rather than to correct cosmetic deformity. Before surgery the patient is instructed in hand exercises, including flexion, extension, abduction, and adduction of the fingers.

Postoperatively, a bulk dressing is placed and the hand is kept elevated. Perform regular neurovascular assessment and monitor for signs of infection. Success of the surgery depends largely on the postoperative treatment plan, which is usually implemented by an occupational therapist. After the dressing is removed, a guided splinting program is initiated. The patient is discharged with splints to use while sleeping and hand exercises to perform at least three or four times a day for 10 to 12 weeks. Instruct the patient to avoid lifting heavy objects.

Elbow and Shoulder Arthroplasty. Although available, total replacement of elbow and shoulder joints is not as common as other forms of arthroplasty. Shoulder replacements are performed in patients with severe pain because of RA, OA, avascular necrosis, or previous trauma. The shoulder replacement is usually considered if the patient has adequate surrounding muscle strength and bone density. If joint replacement is needed for both elbow and shoulder, the elbow is usually done first because a severely painful elbow interferes with the shoulder rehabilitation program.

Significant pain relief has been achieved after elbow and shoulder arthroplasty, with most patients having no pain at rest or minimal pain with activity. Functional improvements have also contributed to better hygiene and increased ability to perform activities of daily living. However, rehabilitation is longer and more difficult than with other joint surgeries.

Ankle Arthroplasty. Total ankle arthroplasty (TAA) is indicated for RA, OA, trauma, and avascular necrosis. Although use of TAA is not widespread, it is a viable alternative to fusion for treatment of severe ankle arthritis in certain patients. Available devices include several fixed-bearing devices and a mobile-bearing cementless prosthesis. This device more closely imitates natural ankle function.

Ankle fusion is often selected over arthroplasty because the result is more durable. However, the patient is left with a stiff foot and the inability to change heel height. TAA achieves a more normal gait pattern. Postoperatively, the patient may not bear weight for 6 weeks. Teach the patient to elevate the extremity to reduce and prevent edema, take steps to prevent postoperative infection, and maintain immobilization as directed by the surgeon.

Arthrodesis

Arthrodesis is the surgical fusion of a joint. This procedure is indicated only if articular surfaces are too severely damaged or infected to allow joint replacement or if reconstructive surgery fails. Arthrodesis relieves pain and provides a stable but immobile joint. The fusion is usually accomplished by removing the articular hyaline cartilage and adding bone grafts across the joint surface. The affected joint must be immobilized until bone healing has occurred. Common areas of fusion are wrist, ankle, cervical spine, lumbar spine, and metatarsophalangeal (MTP) joint of the great toe.

Complications of Joint Surgery

Infection is a serious complication of joint surgery, particularly joint replacement surgery. The most common causative organisms are gram-positive aerobic streptococci and staphylococci. Infection may lead to pain and loosening of the prosthesis, generally requiring additional surgery. Efforts to reduce the incidence of infection include the use of specially designed self-contained operating suites, operating rooms with laminar airflow, and prophylactic antibiotic administration.

VTE is another potentially serious complication after joint surgeries, particularly those involving the lower extremities. Prophylactic measures such as anticoagulant medications, sequential compression devices, and early ambulation are usually instituted. Patients may be assessed postoperatively with venous Doppler ultrasound to detect DVT, the source of most pulmonary emboli.

Interprofessional Care

Preoperative Management. The primary goal of preoperative assessment is to identify risk factors for postoperative complications so nursing strategies can be implemented to promote optimal outcomes. A careful history includes (1) previous medical diagnoses and complications such as diabetes and VTE, (2) pain tolerance and management preferences, (3) current functional level and expectations following surgery, (4) current social support, and (5) home care needs after discharge. The patient should be free from infection and acute joint inflammation.

If lower extremity surgery is planned, assess upper extremity muscle strength and joint function to determine the type of assistive devices needed postoperatively for ambulation and ADL performance. Preoperative teaching about the expected hospital course and postoperative management at home is important for the patient and caregiver. Discuss ways to maximize the usefulness and longevity of the prosthesis. Patients also need to realize that recovery does not occur rapidly. Talking with other people who have had total joint arthroplasty may help the patient better understand the reality of rehabilitation.

Postoperative Management. Postoperatively, regularly perform neurovascular assessment. Administer anticoagulant medication, analgesia, and parenteral antibiotics. Pain management strategies may include epidural or intrathecal analgesia, femoral nerve block, patient-controlled IV analgesia, and oral opioids or NSAIDs. Assess patient comfort frequently during the postoperative period.

In general, the affected joint is exercised and ambulation is encouraged as early as possible to prevent complications of immobility. Specific protocols vary according to the patient, type of prosthesis, and surgeon preference. Depending upon the surgical approach, an abduction pillow may be used after THA. CPM machines may be used after TKA.

The hospital stay after arthroplasty is 3 to 5 days depending on the patient's course and need for physical therapy. Some patients are discharged in 1 to 2 days. Physical therapy and ambulation enhance mobility, build muscle strength, and reduce the risk of VTE. If the patient is taking warfarin, therapy starts on the day of surgery and the INR and prothrombin times are measured daily. With LMWH (e.g., enoxaparin), therapy starts 12 to 24 hours after surgery and continues for 7 to 10 days postoperatively. Fondaparinux is started no earlier than 6 hours after surgery, with the usual duration of therapy 5 to 9 days. Apixaban is generally taken for 12 days. Daily monitoring of the patient's coagulation status is not necessary when the patient is taking LMWH or a factor Xa inhibitor.

❖ NURSING MANAGEMENT: JOINT SURGERY

The nursing management of the patient undergoing joint surgery begins with preoperative teaching and realistic goal setting. Help the patient understand and accept limitations of the proposed surgery and realize surgery may not remove or cure the underlying disease. Explain postoperative procedures such as turning, deep breathing, use of bedpan and bedside commode, and use of an abductor pillow. Reassure the patient that analgesia will be available. A preoperative visit from a physical therapist allows practice of postoperative exercises and measurement for crutches or other assistive devices. Provide opportunities for practice with assistive devices.

Discharge planning begins immediately. Discuss the duration of the hospital stay and the expected postoperative events so that the patient and caregiver can prepare. Teach them to assess the home environment for safety (e.g., scatter rugs, electric cords) and accessibility. Are the bathroom and bedroom on the first floor? Are door frames wide enough to accommodate a walker? Assess the patient's social support. Is a friend or family member available to assist the patient in the home? Will the patient require homemaker or meal services? The older patient may need to be discharged to a subacute or extended care facility for a few weeks to progressively regain independent living skills. Nursing interventions for the patient having orthopedic surgery are presented in eNursing Care Plan 62-2 (on the website for this chapter).

Instruct the patient on reporting complications, including infection (e.g., fever, increased pain, drainage) and dislocation of the prosthesis (e.g., pain, loss of function, shortening or malalignment of an extremity). Act as the liaison between the patient and surgeon, while monitoring for postoperative complications. Also assess the patient's comfort level and ROM at regular intervals to facilitate the goal of improved functional performance.

CASE STUDY

Periprosthetic Hip Fracture and Revision Arthroplasty

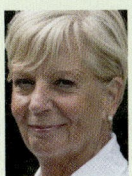

Patient Profile

M.C. is a 58-yr-old white woman who has had both hips replaced (left 10 yr ago, right 5 yr ago). She had a total hysterectomy 3 yr ago and stopping taking hormone replacement therapy at that time. She also has a history of hypothyroidism. She was admitted to emergency department after tripping over a short retaining wall in her backyard while gardening. She landed on her right side.

(©iStockphoto/Thinkstock)

Subjective Data

- Acute, severe pain in right hip, unable to bear weight on right leg
- Taking levothyroxine (Synthroid) 125 mcg every morning
- Taking cholecalciferol (vitamin D₃) 1000 IU every day without calcium supplement. States calcium upsets her stomach
- Reports loss of approximately 30 lb in the last year through diet and exercise. Continues to exercise three times a week
- Lives in multilevel house with her husband. Bedrooms are on the second level
- Nonsmoker, identifies herself as "a very light social drinker"

Objective Data

- 5 ft 6 in tall, 155 lb

Diagnostic Studies

- X-rays reveal periprosthetic right femoral fracture at the greater trochanter with resulting loss of fixation in the femoral component of the right total hip replacement
- Normal CBC, chest x-ray
- Serum calcium 8.1 mg/dL

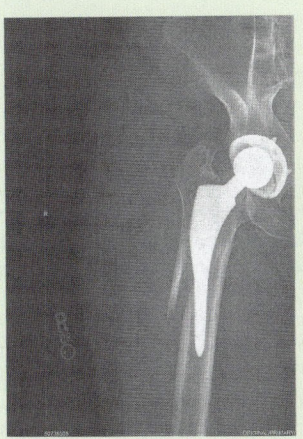

Interprofessional Care

- Revision of femoral component of her right total hip replacement with open reduction of the femoral fracture and fixation with three wires
- Pain management, transitioning from IV hydromorphone (Dilaudid) to oral oxycodone (Roxicodone) as tolerated
- Cefazolin 1 g IV every 8 hours for 24 hours
- Enoxaparin (Lovenox) 40 mg subcutaneous every day for 4 weeks
- Calcium citrate (Citracal) 600 mg plus 800 IU vitamin D PO every day with food
- Physical therapy for transfers, gait, and stair training
- Occupational therapy for ADL training
Discharge planning based on mobility limitations and need for continued PT and OT

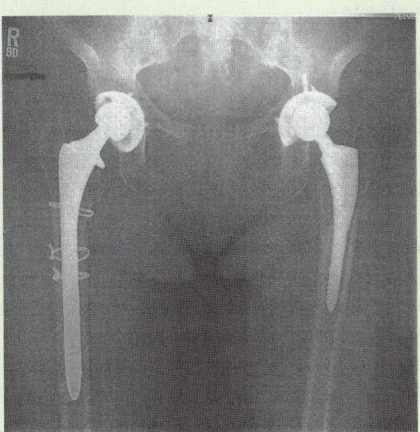

Discussion Questions

1. ***Patient-Centered Care:*** How do M.C.'s previous total joint surgeries affect her recovery following this surgery?
2. ***Priority Decision:*** As you plan care for M.C., what are the perioperative priority nursing interventions?
3. What are the most likely postoperative complications M.C. could develop?
4. In considering M.C.'s patient profile, what issues can you identify that may affect her bone healing?
5. ***Priority Decision:*** What are the priority assessments that should be done prior to discharge?
6. ***Teamwork and Collaboration:*** What is the interprofessional team's top priority at this time for M.C.?
7. ***Quality Improvement:*** What outcomes would indicate interprofessional care was effective?
8. ***Safety:*** What safety precautions should be considered for M.C.?
9. ***Evidence-Based Practice:*** Why is satisfactory pain management an important postoperative nursing goal for M.C.?

Answers available at *http://evolve.elsevier.com/Lewis/medsurg.*

BRIDGE TO NCLEX EXAMINATION

The number of the question corresponds to the same-numbered outcome at the beginning of the chapter.

1. The nurse suspects an ankle sprain when a patient at the urgent care center describes
   a. being hit by another soccer player during a game.
   b. having ankle pain after sprinting around the track.
   c. dropping a 10-lb weight on his lower leg at the health club.
   d. twisting his ankle while running bases during a baseball game.

2. A patient with a humeral fracture is returning for a 4-week checkup. The nurse explains that initial evidence of healing on x-ray is indicated by
   a. formation of callus.
   b. complete bony union.
   c. hematoma at the fracture site.
   d. presence of granulation tissue.

3. A patient with a comminuted fracture of the tibia is to have an open reduction with internal fixation (ORIF) of the fracture. The nurse explains that ORIF is indicated when
   a. the patient is unable to tolerate prolonged immobilization.
   b. the patient cannot tolerate the surgery for a closed reduction.
   c. a temporary cast would be too unstable to provide normal mobility.
   d. adequate alignment cannot be obtained by other nonsurgical methods.

4. The nurse suspects a neurovascular problem based on assessment of
   a. exaggerated strength with movement.
   b. increased redness and heat below the injury.
   c. decreased sensation distal to the fracture site.
   d. purulent drainage at the site of an open fracture.

5. A patient with a stable, closed humeral fracture has a temporary splint with bulky padding applied with an elastic bandage. The nurse notifies the surgeon of possible early compartment syndrome when the patient experiences
   a. increasing edema of the limb.
   b. muscle spasms of the lower arm.
   c. bounding pulse at the fracture site.
   d. pain when passively extending the fingers.

6. A patient with a pelvic fracture should be monitored for
   a. changes in urine output.
   b. petechiae on the abdomen.
   c. a palpable lump in the buttock.
   d. sudden increase in blood pressure.

7. The nurse instructs the patient with an above-the-knee amputation that the residual limb should not be routinely elevated because this position promotes
   a. hip flexion contracture.
   b. clot formation at the incision.
   c. skin irritation and breakdown.
   d. increased risk of wound dehiscence.

8. A patient with osteoarthritis is scheduled for a total hip arthroplasty. The nurse explains the purpose of this procedure is to (select all that apply)
   a. fuse the joint.
   b. replace the joint.
   c. prevent further damage.
   d. improve or maintain ROM.
   e. decrease the amount of destruction in the joint.

9. A patient is scheduled for total ankle replacement. The nurse should tell the patient that after surgery he should avoid
   a. lifting heavy objects.
   b. sleeping on the back.
   c. abduction exercises of the affected ankle.
   d. bearing weight on the affected leg for 6 weeks.

1. d, 2. a, 3. d, 4. c, 5. d, 6. a, 7. a, 8. b, d, 9. d

For rationales to these answers and even more NCLEX review questions, visit *http://evolve.elsevier.com/Lewis/medsurg*.

ⓔ EVOLVE WEBSITE

http://evolve.elsevier.com/Lewis/medsurg
Review Questions (Online Only)
Key Points
Answer Keys for Questions
• Rationales for Bridge to NCLEX Examination Questions
• Answer Guidelines for Case Study on p. 1493
Student Case Studies
• Patient With Musculoskeletal Trauma
• Patient With Parkinson's Disease and Hip Fracture
Nursing Care Plans
• eNursing Care Plan 62-1: Patient With a Fracture
• eNursing Care Plan 62-2: Patient Having Orthopedic Surgery
Concept Map Creator
Audio Glossary
Supporting Media
• Animations
   • ORIF Ankle
   • Total Knee Replacement
Content Updates

REFERENCES

1. Centers for Disease Control and Prevention: Death in the United States, 2011. Retrieved from *http://www.cdc.gov/nchs/data/databriefs/db115.htm*.
2. National Institute of Arthritis and Musculoskeletal and Skin Diseases: Preventing sports injuries in youth: a guide for parents. Retrieved from *www.niams.nih.gov/Health_Info/Sports_Injuries/child_sports_injuries.asp*.
3. American Academy of Orthopaedic Surgeons: Sprains, strains, and other soft-tissue injuries. Retrieved from *www.orthoinfo.org/topic.cfm?topic=A00111*.
4. Myrick K: Clinical assessment and management of ankle sprains, *Orthop Nurs* 33:244, 2014.
*5. Lewis J: A systematic literature review of the relationship between stretching and athletic injury prevention, *Orthop Nurs* 33:321, 2014.
6. American Academy of Orthopaedic Surgeons: Common knee injuries. Retrieved from *http://orthoinfo.aaos.org/topic.cfm?topic=A00325*.
7. Mayo Clinic: Carpal tunnel syndrome. Retrieved from *www.mayoclinic.org/diseases-conditions/carpal-tunnel-syndrome/basics/definition/con-20030332*.

8. Agency for Healthcare Research and Quality: Comparative effectiveness of interventions for rotator cuff tears in adults: clinician guide. Retrieved from *http://effectivehealthcare.ahrq.gov/ehc/index.cfm/ search-for-guides-reviews-and-reports/?pageAction=displayProduct&p roductID=544.*

9. National Institute of Arthritis and Musculoskeletal and Skin Diseases: Spotlight on research: Physical therapy to treat torn meniscus comparable to surgery for many patients. Retrieved from *www.niams.nih.gov/News_and_Events/Spotlight_on_Research/2013/ pt_surgery_meniscus.asp.*

10. Atkinson Smith M, Smith WT: Anterior cruciate ligament tears reconstruction and rehabilitation, *Orthop Nurs* 33:25, 2015.

11. Mayo Clinic: Bursitis. Retrieved from *www.mayoclinic.org/diseases -conditions/bursitis/basics/definition/con-20015102.*

12. McDevitt KA: Orthopaedic trauma. In Schoenly L, editor: *Core curriculum for orthopaedic nursing*, ed 7, Chicago, 2013, National Association of Orthopaedic Nurses.

*13. Austin D, Donegan D, Mehta S: Low complication rates associated with the application of lower extremity traction pins, *J Orthop Trauma* 29:e259, 2015.

14. American Orthopaedic Foot and Ankle Society: Foot ulcers and the total contact cast. Retrieved from *www.aofas.org/footcaremd/conditions/ diabetic-foot/Pages/Foot-Ulcers-and-the-Total-Contact-Cast.aspx.*

15. Royal College of Nursing: Guidance on pin site care. Retrieved from *www.rcn.org.uk/__data/assets/pdf_file/0009/413982/004137.pdf.*

16. *Saunders nursing drug handbook*, St Louis, 2016, Elsevier.

17. The Royal Children's Hospital Melbourne: Neurovascular observations. Retrieved from *www.rch.org.au/rchcpg/hospital_clinical_guideline_index/ Neurovascular_observations.*

18. Abu-Ghanem Y, Abu-Ghanem N, Albagly A, et al: Limb position significantly affects safety distance during cast removal, *Orthop Nurs* 34:110, 2015.

19. Greene LR: Orthopaedic infections. In Schoenly L, editor: *Core curriculum for orthopaedic nursing*, ed 7, Chicago, 2013, National Association of Orthopaedic Nurses.

20. Azar F: Traumatic disorders. In Canale S, Beaty J, editors: *Canale and Beaty: Campbell's operative orthopaedics*, ed 12, St Louis, 2013, Mosby.

21. Parker R: Orthopaedic complications. In Schoenly L, editor: *Core curriculum for orthopaedic nursing*, ed 7, Chicago, 2013, National Association of Orthopaedic Nurses.

22. Centers for Disease Control and Prevention: Hip fractures among older adults. Retrieved from *www.cdc.gov/HomeandRecreationalSafety/Falls/ adulthipfx.html.*

23. Abel LE: Metabolic bone conditions. In Schoenly L, editor: *Core curriculum for orthopaedic nursing*, ed 7, Chicago, 2013, National Association of Orthopaedic Nurses.

24. Kahn-Kastell B: The hip, femur, and pelvis. In Schoenly L, editor: *Core curriculum for orthopaedic nursing*, ed 7, Chicago, 2013, National Association of Orthopaedic Nurses.

25. Center for Disease Control and Prevention: Preventing falls among older adults. Retrieved from *www.cdc.gov/Features/OlderAmericans.*

*26. Santesso N, Carrasco-Labra A, Brignardello-Petersen R: Hip protectors for preventing hip fracture in older people. Retrieved from *www.cochrane.org/CD001255/MUSKINJ_hip-protectors-for-preventing -hip-fractures-in-older-people.*

*27. Motamedi MHK, Dadgar E, Ebrahimi A, et al: Pattern of maxillofacial fractures: a 5-year analysis of 8,818 patients, *J Trauma Acute Care Surg* 77:630, 2014.

28. Anthony A, Ranzer M, Cohen M: Assessment of the trauma patient. In Taub P, Patel P, Buchman S, et al, editors: *Ferraro's fundamentals of maxillofacial surgery*, New York, 2015, Springer.

29. Amputee Coalition: Limb loss statistics. Retrieved from *www.amputee -coalition.org/limb-loss-resource-center/resources-by-topic/limb-loss -statistics/limb-loss-statistics.*

30. Fischer H: U.S. military casualty statistics: Operation New Dawn, Operation Iraqi Freedom, and Operation Enduring Freedom. Retrieved from *http://journalistsresource.org/wp-content/uploads/2013/02/ RS22452.pdf.*

*31. Kiabi FS, Habibi MR, Soleimani A, et al: Mirror therapy as an alternative treatment for phantom limb pain: a short literature review, *Korean J Pain* 26:309, 2013.

32. Gonzalez-Fernandez M: Development of upper limb prostheses: current progress and areas for growth, *Arch Phys Med and Rehab* 95:1013, 2014.

33. National Institute of Arthritis and Musculoskeletal and Skin Diseases: Joint replacement surgery: health information basics for you and your family. Retrieved from *www.niams.nih.gov/health_info/joint_replacement/#4.*

34. American Academy of Orthopaedic Surgeons: Hip resurfacing. Retrieved from *http://orthoinfo.aaos.org/topic.cfm?topic=A00586.*

*35. Wittig-Wells D, Shapiro S, Higgins M: Patients' experience of pain in the 48 hours following total knee arthroplasty, *Orthop Nurs* 32:39, 2013.

*Evidence-based information for clinical practice.

63

Musculoskeletal Problems

Matthew C. Price

Toughness is in the soul and spirit, not in muscles.

Alex Karras

ℯ http://evolve.elsevier.com/Lewis/medsurg/

LEARNING OUTCOMES

1. Describe the pathophysiology, clinical manifestations, interprofessional care, and nursing management of osteomyelitis.
2. Differentiate among the types, pathophysiology, clinical manifestations, and interprofessional care of bone cancer.
3. Differentiate between the causes and characteristics of acute and chronic low back pain.
4. Explain the conservative and surgical treatment of intervertebral disc damage.
5. Describe the postoperative nursing management of a patient who has undergone vertebral disc surgery.
6. Specify the etiology and nursing management of common foot disorders.
7. Describe the etiology, pathophysiology, clinical manifestations, and nursing and interprofessional management of osteomalacia, osteoporosis, and Paget's disease.

KEY TERMS

degenerative disc disease (DDD), p. 1504
hallux valgus, p. 1508
herniated disc, p. 1505
low back pain, p. 1502
muscular dystrophy (MD), p. 1501

osteochondroma, p. 1500
osteomalacia, p. 1510
osteomyelitis, p. 1496
osteopenia, p. 1511
osteoporosis, p. 1510

osteosarcoma, p. 1500
Paget's disease, p. 1514
sarcoma, p. 1500

Acute and chronic musculoskeletal problems are a common source of pain and disability. A variety of problems unrelated to trauma that affect the musculoskeletal system are presented in this chapter, including osteomyelitis, bone cancer, muscular dystrophy, foot disorders, and metabolic bone diseases. Management of the patient with acute and chronic low back pain is addressed, and spinal vertebral disc surgery is discussed. The nurse's role in prevention of injury and maintenance of mobility is emphasized.

OSTEOMYELITIS

Etiology and Pathophysiology

Osteomyelitis is a severe infection of the bone, bone marrow, and surrounding soft tissue. Although *Staphylococcus aureus* is a common cause of infection, a variety of microorganisms may cause osteomyelitis[1] (Table 63-1).

Infecting microorganisms can invade by indirect or direct entry. *Indirect entry* (hematogenous) of microorganisms most frequently affects growing bone in boys younger than 12 years old and is associated with their higher incidence of blunt trauma. Adults with genitourinary and respiratory tract infections or disorders marked by vascular insufficiency (e.g., diabetes mellitus) are at high risk for the spread of a primary infection via the blood to the bone. As highly vascular bones, the pelvis, tibia, and vertebrae are the most common sites of infection.

Direct entry osteomyelitis can occur at any age when an open wound (e.g., penetrating wounds, fractures) allows microorganisms to enter the body. Osteomyelitis may also be related to a foreign body such as an implant or an orthopedic prosthetic device (e.g., plate, total joint prosthesis).

After gaining entry into the blood, microorganisms grow and pressure increases because of the nonexpanding nature of most bone. This increasing pressure eventually leads to ischemia and vascular compromise of the periosteum. The infection spreads through the bone cortex and marrow cavity, causing cortical devascularization and necrosis.

Bone death occurs as a result of ischemia. The area of dead bone eventually separates from the surrounding living bone, forming *sequestra*. The part of the periosteum that continues to have a blood supply forms new bone called *involucrum* (Fig. 63-1). Antibiotics or white blood cells (WBCs) have difficulty

Reviewed by Judy Carlyle, RN, MNSc, ARNEC Faculty/Clinical Liaison, Arkansas Rural Nursing Education Consortium (ARNEC), Nashville, Arkansas; Monica L. Johnson, RN, MSN, MBA-HCM, CMSRN, ONC, LNC, Acute Care Division Clinical Educator, East Jefferson General Hospital, and Adjunct Clinical Faculty, Delgado Community College Charity School of Nursing, New Orleans, Louisiana; Rebecca Liebert, RN, MSN, FNP-C, ONP-C, Nurse Practitioner, Tomah Memorial Hospital and Specialty Clinic/Orthopedics, Tomah, Wisconsin; and Laura C. Williams, RN, MSN, CNS, ONC, CCNS, Orthopedic Clinical Nurse Specialist, Orlando Health, Orlando, Florida.

TABLE 63-1	Organisms Causing Osteomyelitis
Organism	**Predisposing Problem**
Staphylococcus aureus	Pressure ulcer, penetrating wound, open fracture, orthopedic surgery, disorders with vascular insufficiency (e.g., diabetes, atherosclerosis)
Staphylococcus epidermidis	Indwelling prosthetic devices (e.g., joint replacements, fracture fixation devices)
Streptococcus viridans	Abscessed tooth, gingival disease
Escherichia coli	Urinary tract infection
Mycobacterium tuberculosis	Tuberculosis
Neisseria gonorrhoeae	Gonorrhea
Pseudomonas	Puncture wounds, IV drug use
Salmonella	Sickle cell disease
Fungi, mycobacteria	Immunocompromised host

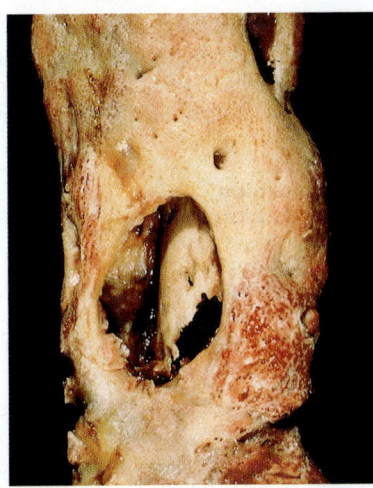

FIG. 63-2 Resection of femur due to osteomyelitis. (From Thibodeau GA, Patton KT: *The human body in health and disease*, ed 5, St Louis, 2010, Mosby.)

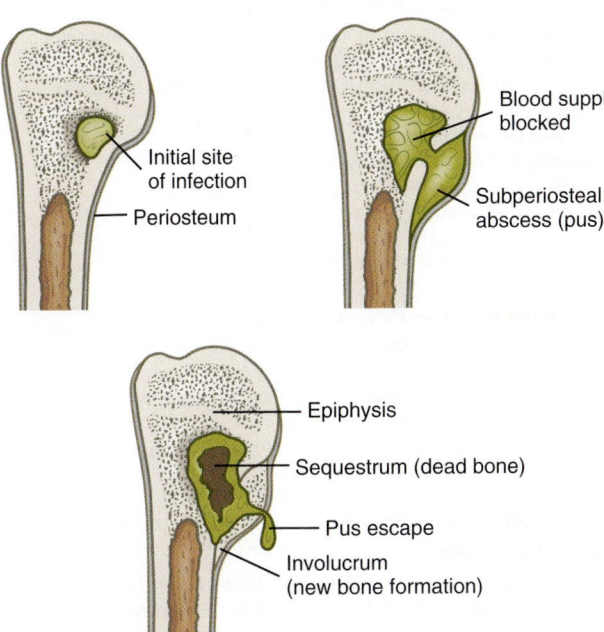

FIG. 63-1 Development of osteomyelitis infection with involucrum and sequestrum.

reaching the sequestrum through the blood. Thus sequestrum may become a reservoir for microorganisms that spread to other sites, including the lungs and brain. If the sequestrum does not resolve or is not debrided surgically, a sinus tract may develop. Chronic, purulent cutaneous drainage from the tract results.

Clinical Manifestations and Complications

Acute osteomyelitis refers to the initial infection or an infection of less than 1 month in duration. Clinical manifestations of acute osteomyelitis are local and systemic. Local manifestations include constant bone pain that worsens with activity and is unrelieved by rest; swelling, tenderness, and warmth at the infection site; and restricted movement of the affected part. Systemic manifestations include fever, night sweats, chills, restlessness, nausea, and malaise. Later signs include drainage from cutaneous sinus tracts or the fracture site.

Chronic osteomyelitis refers to a bone infection that lasts longer than 1 month or an infection that has failed to respond

to initial antibiotic treatment. Chronic osteomyelitis may be a continuous, persistent problem (a result of inadequate acute treatment) or a process of exacerbations and remissions (Fig. 63-2). Systemic manifestations may be reduced. Local signs of infection become more common, including constant bone pain as well as swelling and warmth at the infection site. Over time, granulation tissue turns to scar tissue. The avascular scar tissue provides an ideal site for continued microorganism growth because it cannot be penetrated by antibiotics.

Long-term and mostly rare complications of osteomyelitis include septicemia, septic arthritis, pathologic fractures, and amyloidosis.

Diagnostic Studies

Bone or soft tissue biopsy is the definitive way to identify the causative microorganism. The patient's blood and wound cultures are frequently positive for microorganisms.[2] Elevated WBC count and erythrocyte sedimentation rate (ESR) may also be found. While elevated ESR is usually seen in chronic infective processes, elevated C-reactive protein (CRP) may also suggest acute infection. Signs of osteomyelitis usually do not appear on x-rays until 10 days to weeks after the initial clinical symptoms. By this time, the disease will have progressed. Compared to x-rays, CT scan may be more helpful in assessing the extent of infection. Especially in the acute phase, MRI may be more sensitive than CT in detecting bone marrow edema, which is an early indication of osteomyelitis.[3] Radionuclide bone scans (gallium and indium) are helpful in diagnosis and are usually positive in the area of infection.

Interprofessional Care

Aggressive, prolonged IV antibiotic therapy is the treatment of choice for acute osteomyelitis if bone ischemia has not yet occurred. Cultures or a bone biopsy should be done if possible before initiating drug therapy. If antibiotic therapy is delayed, surgical debridement and decompression are often needed.

Patients are often discharged to home care or a skilled nursing facility with IV antibiotics delivered via a central venous access device (CVAD). These include centrally inserted catheters, peripherally inserted central catheters (PICCs), and implanted ports. (CVADs are discussed in Chapter 16.) IV antibiotic therapy may be started in the hospital and continued at home for 4 to 6 weeks or as long as 3 to 6 months. A variety of antibiotics may be prescribed depending on the microorganism. These drugs include penicillin, nafcillin, neomycin, vancomycin, cephalexin, cefazolin, cefoxitin, gentamicin, and tobramycin.

 DRUG ALERT Gentamicin
- Assess patient for dehydration before starting therapy.
- Ensure renal function testing is done before starting therapy, especially in older patients.
- Monitor peak and trough blood levels to achieve therapeutic effect and minimize renal and inner ear toxicity.[4]
- Instruct patient to notify HCP if any visual, hearing, or urinary problems develop.

In adults with chronic osteomyelitis, oral therapy with a fluoroquinolone (e.g., ciprofloxacin [Cipro]) for 6 to 8 weeks may be prescribed instead of IV antibiotics. Oral antibiotics may also be given after acute IV therapy is completed to ensure the infection is resolved. The patient's response to drug therapy is monitored through bone scans and ESR testing.

Treatment of chronic osteomyelitis includes (1) surgical removal of the poorly perfused tissue and dead bone and (2) extended use of antibiotics.[5] Acrylic bead chains containing antibiotics may also be implanted to help combat the infection. After debridement of the dead, infected tissue, a suction irrigation system may be inserted and the wound closed. Intermittent or constant irrigation of the area with antibiotics may also be initiated. The limb or the surgical site is often protected with casts or braces. Postoperatively, negative-pressure wound therapy may be used (discussed in Chapter 11 on pp. 169-170).

Hyperbaric O_2 may be given as an adjunct therapy in refractory cases of chronic osteomyelitis. It stimulates new blood growth and healing in the infected tissue (see p. 170 in Chapter 11).

If orthopedic prosthetic devices are a source of chronic infection, they must be removed. Muscle flaps or skin grafts provide wound coverage over the dead space (cavity) in the bone. Bone grafts may help to restore blood flow. However, flaps or grafts should never be placed in the presence of active or suspected infection.

Amputation of the extremity may be needed if bone destruction is extensive. Amputation should improve quality of life and may save the patient's life if systemic complications are developing.

❖ NURSING MANAGEMENT: OSTEOMYELITIS

◆ Nursing Assessment

Subjective and objective data that should be obtained from an individual with osteomyelitis are presented in Table 63-2.

◆ Nursing Diagnoses

Nursing diagnoses for the patient with osteomyelitis may include, but are not limited to, the following:
- Acute pain *related to* inflammatory process secondary to infection
- Ineffective health maintenance *related to* lack of knowledge regarding long-term management of osteomyelitis
- Impaired physical mobility *related to* pain, immobilization devices, and weight-bearing limitations

Additional information on nursing diagnoses for the patient with osteomyelitis is available in eNursing Care Plan 63-1 (on the website for this chapter).

TEAMWORK & COLLABORATION
Caring for the Patient With Osteomyelitis

Role of Nursing Personnel
Registered Nurse (RN)
- Administer IV antibiotics as ordered.
- Assess wound for signs of worsening infection.
- Teach patient and caregiver about antibiotic side effects and length of treatment, signs and symptoms of worsening infection, and use of hyperbaric O_2 if ordered.
- Assess for muscle spasms and administer muscle relaxant as ordered.
- Assess pain intensity and administer analgesics as ordered. Assess patient response.
- Handle affected limb carefully to decrease pain and additional injury.
- Assess neurovascular condition of affected limb and immediately inform HCP of significant changes.

Licensed Practical/Vocational Nurse (LPN/LVN)
- Monitor color, temperature, capillary refill, and pulses of affected limb and immediately inform RN of significant changes.
- Handle affected limb carefully to decrease pain and additional injury.
- Administer muscle relaxants as ordered. Notify RN if muscle spasms persist after muscle relaxants are administered.
- Reinforce teaching related to antibiotic therapy.
- Monitor pain intensity and administer prescribed analgesics.
- Notify RN of changes in pain or if pain persists after prescribed analgesics are administered.

Unlicensed Assistive Personnel (UAP)
- Handle affected limb carefully (based on RN instruction) to decrease pain and additional injury.
- Assist patient with passive ROM of adjacent joints and active ROM exercises of unaffected limb.
- Notify RN about patient complaints of pain, tingling, or decreased sensation in the affected extremity.

Role of Other Team Members
Physical Therapist
- Assess patient's current mobility and need for assistance.
- Teach safe ambulation with assistive device based on patient's weight-bearing restrictions.
- Establish exercise regimen and teach patient to perform exercises safely.
- Coordinate PT with RN so that patient can receive timely analgesia.
- Discuss home environment with patient and identify possible modifications to facilitate recovery (e.g., stair training if allowed by patient's weight-bearing restrictions, bed placement on first level to avoid stairs).

Occupational Therapist
- Assess impact of patient's condition on ability to perform activities of daily living.
- Instruct patient in use of assistive devices (e.g., long-handled reacher, shoe donner) to facilitate self-care while maintaining activity restrictions.
- Discuss home environment with patient and identify possible modifications to facilitate recovery (e.g., bed placement on first level for access to bathroom).

◆ Planning

The overall goals are that the patient with osteomyelitis will (1) have satisfactory pain and fever management, (2) not experience any complications associated with osteomyelitis, (3) adhere to the treatment plan, and (4) maintain a positive outlook on the outcome of the disease.

TABLE 63-2   Nursing Assessment
Osteomyelitis

Subjective Data

Important Health Information

Past health history: Bone trauma, open fracture, open or puncture wounds, other infections (e.g., streptococcal sore throat, bacterial pneumonia, sinusitis, skin or tooth infection, chronic urinary tract infection)

Medications: Analgesics or antibiotics

Surgery or other treatments: Bone surgery

Functional Health Patterns

Health perception–health management: IV drug and alcohol abuse. Malaise

Nutritional-metabolic: Anorexia, weight loss. Chills

Activity-exercise: Weakness, paralysis, muscle spasms around affected area

Cognitive-perceptual: Local tenderness over affected area, increased pain with movement of affected area

Coping–stress tolerance: Irritability, withdrawal, dependency, anger

Objective Data

General

Restlessness. High, spiking temperature. Night sweats

Integumentary

Diaphoresis. Erythema, warmth, edema at site of infection

Musculoskeletal

Restricted movement; wound drainage. Spontaneous fracture

Possible Diagnostic Findings

Leukocytosis, positive blood and/or wound cultures, ↑ erythrocyte sedimentation rate. Presence of sequestrum and involucrum on x-rays, radionuclide bone scans, CT, and MRI

◆ Nursing Implementation

◆ **Health Promotion.** Control of other current infections (e.g., urinary or respiratory tract, pressure ulcers) is important in preventing osteomyelitis. Persons especially at risk for osteomyelitis are those who are immunocompromised, or who have diabetes, orthopedic prosthetic devices, or vascular insufficiency. Instruct the at-risk patient about the local and systemic signs of osteomyelitis. Encourage the patient to immediately tell the HCP about bone pain, fever, swelling, and restricted limb movement so that treatment can be started. Also teach family members about their role in monitoring the patient's health.

◆ **Acute Care.** Some immobilization of the affected limb (e.g., splint, traction) is usually needed to decrease pain and reduce risk of additional injury. Carefully handle the limb and avoid undue manipulation, which may increase pain and cause a pathologic fracture. Assess the patient's pain. Muscle spasms may cause minor to severe pain. Nonsteroidal antiinflammatory drugs (NSAIDs), opioid analgesics, and muscle relaxants may be prescribed for patient comfort. Encourage nondrug approaches to pain management (e.g., guided imagery, relaxation breathing) (see Chapter 6).

Dressings are used to absorb drainage from wounds and debride dead tissue from the wound bed. These include dry, sterile dressings; dressings saturated in saline or antibiotic solution; wet-to-dry dressings; and dressings applied with negative-pressure wound therapy. Sterile technique is essential when changing the dressing. Handle soiled dressings carefully to prevent transfer of bacteria to other areas of the wound. Discard dressings appropriately to prevent spread of infection to other patients. The patient is frequently placed on bed rest in the early stages of acute infection. Good body alignment and frequent position changes promote comfort and prevent complications related to immobility. Flexion contracture of the affected lower extremity is common as the patient frequently positions the leg in a flexed position to promote comfort. Footdrop can develop quickly due to Achilles tendon contracture if the foot is not correctly supported in a neutral position by a splint or boot. A tight splint or dressing may also compress and injure the peroneal nerve.

Teach the patient the possible adverse and toxic reactions associated with prolonged high-dose antibiotic therapy (e.g., tobramycin, neomycin). These reactions include hearing deficit, impaired renal function, and neurotoxicity (e.g., limb weakness or numbness, cognitive changes or loss of memory, vision changes, headache, behavioral problems). Reactions associated with cephalosporins (e.g., cefazolin) include hives, severe or watery diarrhea, blood in stools, and throat or mouth sores.

Tendonitis or tendon rupture (especially the Achilles tendon) can occur with use of fluoroquinolones (e.g., ciprofloxacin, levofloxacin [Levaquin]). Peak and trough blood levels of most antibiotics should be monitored to avoid adverse effects. Lengthy antibiotic therapy can also cause an overgrowth of *Candida albicans* and *Clostridium difficile* in the genitourinary and gastrointestinal (GI) tracts, especially in immunosuppressed and older patients. Instruct the patient to report any changes in the oral cavity (e.g., whitish yellow, curdlike lesions) or the genitourinary cavity (e.g., perianal itching or diarrhea).

❓ CHECK YOUR PRACTICE

Your patient on the orthopedic unit is a 22-yr-old man who was involved in an all-terrain vehicle accident in a remote area 4 days ago. He was airlifted to your hospital because he was unconscious when he was found. He is now slowly recovering from his head injury and surgical repair of an open fracture of the femur. Yesterday he was diagnosed with acute osteomyelitis. He is very angry and at times disoriented. When you try to assess his leg, he yells at you, "It hurts. Leave it alone!"

- What are your priorities of care?
- What signs and symptoms would suggest the patient's condition is worsening?

The patient, caregiver, and family may be anxious and discouraged because of the serious nature of osteomyelitis, the uncertainty of the outcome, and the long, costly treatment. Continued psychologic and emotional support is an integral part of nursing management. A nursing care plan for the patient with osteomyelitis (eNursing Care Plan 63-1) is available on the website for this chapter.

◆ **Ambulatory Care.** IV antibiotics can be administered to the patient in a skilled nursing facility or home setting. If at home, instruct the patient and caregiver how to manage the CVAD. Also teach them how to administer the antibiotic when scheduled and reinforce the need for follow-up laboratory testing. Stress the importance of continuing to take antibiotics after symptoms have improved.

Dressing changes are often required if the patient has an open wound. The patient and caregiver may need supplies and instruction for completing the dressing change. If the osteomyelitis becomes chronic, the patient needs continued physical and psychologic support.

◆ **Evaluation**

The expected outcomes are that the patient with osteomyelitis will:

- Have satisfactory pain management
- Adhere to the recommended treatment regimen
- Verbalize confidence in ability to implement treatment regimen at home
- Demonstrate a consistent increase in mobility and range of motion

BONE TUMORS

Primary bone tumors, both benign and malignant, are relatively rare in adults. They account for only about 3% of all tumors. Metastatic bone cancer in which cancer has spread from another site is a more common problem.

BENIGN BONE TUMORS

Bone tumors are relatively rare when compared to other types of tumors. However, benign bone tumors are more common than primary malignant tumors. The main types of benign bone tumors are osteochondroma, osteoclastoma, and enchondroma (Table 63-3). These types of tumors are often removed by surgery.

Osteochondroma

Osteochondroma is the most common primary benign bone tumor. It is characterized by an overgrowth of cartilage and bone near the end of the bone at the growth plate. It is more commonly found in the pelvis, scapula, or long bones of the leg.

Clinical manifestations include a painless, hard, immobile mass; lower-than-normal height for age; soreness of muscles close to the tumor; one leg or arm longer than the other; and pressure or irritation with exercise. Patients may also be asymptomatic. Diagnosis is confirmed using x-ray, CT scan, and MRI.

No treatment is necessary for asymptomatic osteochondroma. If the tumor is causing pain or neurologic manifestations because of compression, surgical removal is usually done. Patients should have regular screening examinations to detect progression to malignancy as soon as possible.

MALIGNANT BONE TUMORS

A sarcoma is a malignant tumor that develops in bone, muscle, fat, nerve, or cartilage. The most common types of malignant bone tumors are osteosarcoma, chondrosarcoma, and Ewing's sarcoma (Table 63-3). About 2970 new cases of bone and joint cancer occur annually in the United States, with an estimated 1500 deaths.[6] Primary malignant tumors occur most often during childhood and young adulthood. They are characterized by their rapid metastasis and bone destruction.

Osteosarcoma

Osteosarcoma is an extremely aggressive primary malignant bone tumor that rapidly spreads to distant sites. It usually occurs in the pelvis or metaphyseal region of the long bones of extremities, particularly in the distal femur, proximal tibia, and proximal humerus (Fig. 63-3, A). Osteosarcoma is the most common malignant bone tumor affecting children and young adults. It can also occur in older adults, but not as commonly.

TABLE 63-3	Types of Primary Bone Tumors
Types	**Description**
Benign	
Osteochondroma	• Most common benign bone tumor
	• Frequently located in pelvis, scapula, or metaphyseal portion of long bones
	• Occurs most often in people ages 10-25 years
	• May transform to malignancy (chondrosarcoma)
Osteoclastoma (giant cell tumor)	• Arises in cancellous ends of arm and leg bones
	• About 10% are locally aggressive and may spread to lungs
	• High rate of local recurrence after surgery and chemotherapy
Enchondroma	• Intramedullary cartilage tumor usually found in cavity of a single hand or foot bone
	• Rarely transforms to malignancy
	• If tumor becomes painful, surgical resection is done
	• Peak incidence in people ages 10-20
Malignant	
Osteosarcoma	• Most common primary bone cancer
	• Occurs mostly in males ages 10-25
	• Most often in pelvis or bones of arms, legs (Fig. 63-3, A)
Chondrosarcoma	• Occurs in cartilage most commonly in arm, leg, and pelvic bones of adults ages 50-70
	• Can also arise from benign bone tumors (osteochondromas)
	• Wide surgical resection is typically done as tumor rarely responds to radiation and chemotherapy
	• Survival rate depends on stage, size, and grade of tumor (Fig. 63-3, B)
Ewing's sarcoma	• Develops in medullary cavity of pelvis and long bones, especially femur, humerus, and tibia
	• Usually occurs in children and teenagers
	• Use of wide surgical resection, radiation, and chemotherapy has improved 5-yr survival rate to 60%

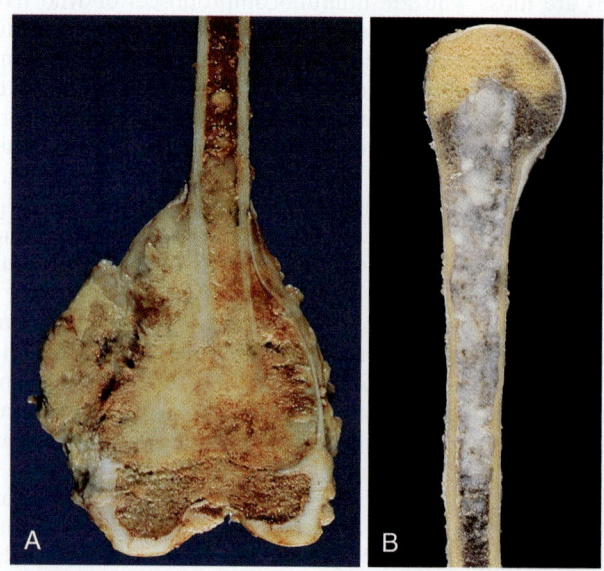

FIG. 63-3 **A,** Osteosarcoma. **B,** Chondrosarcoma. (From Damjanov I, Linder J: *Anderson's pathology,* ed 10, St Louis, 1996, Mosby.)

It is most often associated with Paget's disease (discussed on p. 1514) and prior radiation.

Clinical manifestations of osteosarcoma are usually associated with the gradual onset of pain and swelling, especially around the knee. A minor injury does not cause the neoplasm but may bring the preexisting condition to medical attention. Metastasis is present in 10% to 20% of individuals when they are diagnosed with osteosarcoma.

Diagnosis is confirmed from tissue biopsy, elevation of serum alkaline phosphatase and calcium, x-ray, CT or positron emission tomography (PET) scans, and MRI.

Preoperative (neoadjuvant) chemotherapy may be used to decrease tumor size before surgery. Limb salvage procedures are usually considered if a clear (no cancer present) 6- to 7-cm margin surrounds the lesion. Limb salvage is usually contraindicated if the patient has major neurovascular involvement, pathologic fracture, infection, or extensive muscle involvement.

The use of adjunct chemotherapy after amputation or limb salvage has increased the 5-year survival rate to 70% in people without metastasis. Chemotherapy includes methotrexate, doxorubicin, cisplatin, cyclophosphamide, and etoposide.[7]

Metastatic Bone Cancer

The most common type of malignant bone tumor occurs as a result of spread *(metastasis)* from a primary tumor at another site. Common primary sites include breast, prostate, lungs, kidney, and thyroid. Metastatic cancer cells travel from the primary tumor to the bone via the lymph and blood supply. Metastatic bone lesions are commonly found in vertebrae, pelvis, femur, humerus, or ribs.[8] Pathologic fractures at the site of metastasis are common because the bone has weakened. High serum calcium occurs as calcium is released from damaged bones.

Once a primary lesion has been identified, radionuclide bone scans are often done to detect metastatic lesions before they are visible on x-ray. Metastatic bone lesions may occur at any time (even years later) following diagnosis and treatment of the primary tumor. Metastasis to the bone should be suspected in any patient who has local bone pain and a past history of cancer. Surgical stabilization of the bone may be indicated for fracture or to prevent fracture in a high-risk patient. Prognosis depends on the primary type of cancer and any other sites of metastasis. Possible palliative treatment consists of radiation and pain management (see Chapter 15).

❖ NURSING MANAGEMENT: BONE CANCER

Assess the patient with bone cancer for the location and severity of pain. Also note weakness caused by anemia and decreased mobility. Monitor the tumor site for swelling; changes in circulation; and decreased movement, sensation, or joint function.

Nursing care of the patient with a malignant bone tumor does not differ significantly from the care provided to the patient with cancer of any other body system (see Chapter 15). However, use special care to prevent pathologic fractures or reduce the complications associated with them. Prevent fractures by careful handling and support of the affected extremity and logrolling for the patient on bed rest.

Treatment for hypercalcemia may be initiated if bone decalcification occurs (see Table 15-19, p. 263). The patient may be unwilling to participate in exercise or therapeutic activities because of weakness from the disease and treatment, fear of falling and fracturing a bone, and fear of pain. Provide regular rest periods between activities.

The pain associated with bone cancer can be severe. It is often caused by the tumor pressing against nerves and other organs near the bone. New onset or changes in severity of pain may also indicate pathologic fracture. Carefully assess the patient's pain and ensure adequate pain medication is provided. Sometimes radiation therapy is used as a palliative therapy to shrink the tumor and decrease pain.

Assist the patient and caregiver in accepting the poor prognosis associated with bone malignancy. General principles related to cancer nursing are applicable (see Chapter 15). Special attention is needed for problems of pain and disability, side effects of chemotherapy, and postoperative care (e.g., after spinal cord decompression or amputation). As with all types of cancer, stress the importance of follow-up examinations.

MUSCULAR DYSTROPHY

Muscular dystrophy (MD) is a group of genetic diseases characterized by progressive symmetric wasting of skeletal muscles without evidence of neurologic involvement. A gradual loss of strength with increasing disability and deformity occurs with all forms of MD. The types of MD differ in the groups of muscles affected, age of onset, rate of progression, and mode of genetic inheritance (Table 63-4). Duchenne MD is the most common type.

TABLE 63-4	**Types of Muscular Dystrophy**	
Type*	**Genetic Basis**	**Manifestations**
Duchenne	• X-linked • Mutation of dystrophin gene	• Most common form of MD • Primarily affects boys • Onset before age 5 • Progressive weakness of pelvic and shoulder muscles • Unable to walk by age 12 • Cardiomyopathy • Respiratory failure in 20s • Mental impairment
Becker	• X-linked • Mutation of dystrophin gene	• Very similar but less severe than Duchenne MD • Onset ages 5-15 • Slower course of pelvic and shoulder muscle wasting than Duchenne • Cardiomyopathy • Respiratory failure • May survive into 40s
Facioscapulohumeral	• Autosomal dominant • Deletion of chromosome 4q35	• Onset before age 20 • Slowly progressive weakness of face, shoulder muscles, and upper arms and lower legs • Can affect vision and hearing
Limb-girdle	• Autosomal recessive or autosomal dominant • Mutation in any of at least 15 genes affecting proteins needed for muscle function	• Group of disorders affecting voluntary muscles, especially those of hips and shoulders • Onset ranges from early childhood to early adulthood or later • Slow progressive weakness of hip and shoulder muscles

*List is not all-inclusive.

Genetic Link

Duchenne and Becker MD are X-linked recessive disorders usually seen only in males. (X-linked recessive disorders are discussed in Chapter 12.) These disorders are characterized by a mutation of the dystrophin *(DMD)* gene. Dystrophin is a protein that helps keep skeletal muscle fibers intact. Abnormal dystrophin can cause defects in the muscle fiber and results in muscle fiber degeneration.

A family history can be used to obtain a family pedigree. Family pedigrees for X-linked recessive disorders are shown in Figs. 12-4 and 12-5.

Diagnostic studies for MD include muscle serum enzymes (especially creatine kinase), electromyogram (EMG) testing, muscle fiber biopsy, and electrocardiogram for abnormalities that suggest cardiomyopathy. Muscle biopsy confirms the diagnosis with classic findings of fat and connective tissue deposits, muscle fiber degeneration and necrosis, and a deficiency of dystrophin.

No definitive therapy is available to stop the progressive wasting of MD. Primary treatment goals are to preserve mobility and independence through exercise, physical therapy, and use of assistive devices. Progressive muscle weakening around the trunk can cause spinal collapse. The patient may be fitted early with an orthotic jacket to provide stability and prevent further deformity or injury.

Cardiomyopathy often occurs and causes heart failure. Dysrhythmias are a frequent cause of death.[9] Gradual decreases in respiratory function often lead to the use of continuous positive airway pressure (CPAP). Eventually tracheostomy and mechanical ventilation are needed to support respiratory function. Corticosteroid therapy may slow disease progression for up to 2 years.[10]

Encourage communication between the patient and family to cope with the emotional and physical demands of MD. Teach the patient and caregiver range-of-motion (ROM) exercises, principles of good nutrition, and signs of disease progression. Genetic testing and counseling may be recommended for persons with a family history of MD.

Focus care on keeping the patient active as long as possible. Prolonged bed rest should be avoided because immobility can cause more muscle wasting. As the disease progresses, teach the patient to limit sedentary periods to prevent skin breakdown and respiratory complications. Ongoing medical and nursing care is required throughout the patient's life. The Muscular Dystrophy Association *(www.mda.org)* is an important resource and provides information on support services for the patient, caregiver, and family.

> **⚠ SAFETY ALERT** **Muscular Dystrophy**
> - Support respiratory function as needed.
> - Fit patient with an orthotic jacket or brace to prevent deformity or injury.
> - Teach patient, caregiver, and family the signs of disease progression.

LOW BACK PAIN

Low back pain is most often due to a musculoskeletal problem. It may be experienced as localized or diffuse. In *localized pain,* patients feel soreness or discomfort when a specific area of the lower back is palpated or pressed. *Diffuse pain* occurs over a larger area and comes from deep tissue.

Low back pain may be radicular or referred. *Radicular pain* is caused by irritation of a nerve root. Radicular pain is not

GENETICS IN CLINICAL PRACTICE
Duchenne and Becker Muscular Dystrophy (MD)

Genetic Basis
- Caused by mutations in the dystrophin *(DMD)* gene. Many mutations have been identified.
- Gene provides instructions for making dystrophin (protein that helps to keep muscle cells intact) located primarily in skeletal and cardiac muscle.
- Inherited in an X-linked recessive pattern.

Incidence
- Between 400 and 600 boys are born with MD each year in the United States.
- Together these disorders affect 1 in 3500 to 5000 newborn males worldwide.
- Females in these families have a 50% chance of inheriting and passing the defective gene to their children.

Genetic Testing
- DNA testing for mutations in dystrophin gene is available.
- Genetic testing and counseling should be considered in individuals with a family history of MD.

Clinical Implications
- Muscular dystrophies are a group of genetic conditions characterized by progressive muscle weakness and atrophy.
- These conditions differ in their severity, age of onset, and rate of progression (Table 63-4).
- Males with Duchenne MD typically live into their 20s, whereas those with Becker MD may live into their 40s or beyond.
- Because there are many types of MD with different genetic bases, establishing the type of MD is important to determine treatment and possible genetic counseling recommendations.

typically isolated to a single location but instead radiates or moves along a nerve distribution. Sciatica is an example of radicular pain. *Referred pain* is felt in the lower back, but the source of the pain is another location (e.g., kidneys, lower abdomen).

Low back pain has affected about 80% of adults in the United States at least once during their lives. Backache is second only to headache as the most common pain complaint. Low back pain is the leading cause of job-related disability and a major contributor to missed work days.[11]

Low back pain is a common problem because the lumbar region (1) bears most of the weight of the body, (2) is the most flexible region of the spinal column, (3) contains nerve roots that are at risk for injury or disease, and (4) has a naturally poor biomechanical structure. Risk factors associated with low back pain include lack of muscle tone, excess body weight, stress, poor posture, cigarette smoking, pregnancy, prior compression fracture of the spine, spinal problems since birth, and a family history of back pain. Jobs that require repetitive heavy lifting, vibration (such as a jackhammer operator), and extended periods of sitting are also associated with low back pain.

The causes of low back pain of musculoskeletal origin include (1) acute lumbosacral strain, (2) instability of the lumbosacral bony mechanism, (3) osteoarthritis of the lumbosacral vertebrae, (4) degenerative disc disease, and (5) herniation of an intervertebral disc.

Health care personnel who perform direct patient care activities are at high risk for development of low back pain.[12] Lifting and moving patients, excessive bending or leaning forward, and frequent twisting can result in low back pain that causes lost time and productivity and disability.

ACUTE LOW BACK PAIN

Acute low back pain lasts 4 weeks or less. Most acute low back pain is caused by trauma or an activity that produces undue stress (often hyperflexion) on the lower back. Examples of trauma or activity that could cause acute back pain are heavy lifting, overuse of back muscles during yard work, a sports injury, or a sudden jolt as in a motor vehicle crash.

Often symptoms do not appear at the time of injury. They develop later (usually within 24 hours) because of a gradual increase in pressure on the nerve from an intervertebral disc and/or associated edema. Symptoms may range from muscle ache to shooting or stabbing pain, limited flexibility or ROM, or an inability to stand upright.

Few definitive diagnostic abnormalities are present with nerve irritation and muscle strain. One test is the straight-leg–raising test (see Chapter 61, p. 1455). MRI and CT scans are generally not done unless trauma or systemic disease (e.g., cancer, spinal infection) is suspected. MRI findings may also be limited in the acute phase of an injury due to increased edema near the injury.

❖ NURSING AND INTERPROFESSIONAL MANAGEMENT: ACUTE LOW BACK PAIN

◆ Nursing Assessment

Subjective and objective data that should be obtained from the patient with low back pain are summarized in Table 63-5.

◆ Nursing Implementation
◆ **Health Promotion.** Use proper body mechanics at all times to serve as a role model. This includes increasing the patient's bed height, bending at the knees, asking for help in lifting and moving patients, and using lifting devices.

Assess the patient's use of body mechanics and offer advice when the person does activities that could produce back strain (Table 63-6). Some HCPs refer patients with back pain to a program called "Back School." This formal program is usually taught by health care professionals such as HCPs, nurses, and physical therapists. It is designed to teach the patient how to minimize back pain and avoid repeat episodes of low back pain. Tips for prevention of back injury are listed in Table 63-6. Referral to a physical therapist or personal trainer to address posture as well as core and abdomen strength may also be appropriate. Recommend flat shoes or shoes with low heels and shock-absorbing shoe inserts for women.

Advise patients to maintain a healthy body weight. Excess body weight places additional stress on the lower back. It also weakens abdominal muscles that support the lower back. The position assumed while sleeping is also important in preventing low back pain. Advise patients to avoid sleeping in a prone position because it produces excessive lumbar lordosis, placing excessive stress on the lower back. Encourage the patient to sleep in a supine or side-lying position with knees and hips flexed to prevent unnecessary pressure on support muscles, ligaments, and lumbosacral joints. Recommend use of a firm mattress.

TABLE 63-5   Nursing Assessment
Low Back Pain
Subjective Data ***Important Health Information*** *Past health history:* Acute or chronic lumbosacral strain/trauma, osteoarthritis, degenerative disc disease, obesity *Medications:* Opioid analgesics and NSAIDs, muscle relaxants, corticosteroids, over-the-counter remedies (e.g., topical ointments, patches) *Surgery or other treatments:* Previous back surgery, epidural corticosteroid injections ***Functional Health Patterns*** *Health perception–health management:* Smoking, lack of exercise *Nutritional-metabolic:* Obesity *Activity-exercise:* Poor posture, muscle spasms, activity intolerance *Elimination:* Constipation *Sleep-rest:* Interrupted sleep *Cognitive-perceptual:* Pain in back, buttocks, or leg associated with walking, turning, straining, coughing, leg raising. Numbness or tingling of legs, feet, toes *Role-relationship:* Occupations requiring heavy lifting, vibrations, or extended driving. Change in role within family structure due to inability to work and provide income **Objective Data** ***General*** Guarded movement ***Neurologic*** Depressed or absent Achilles tendon reflex or patellar tendon reflex. Positive straight-leg-raising test, positive crossover straight-leg-raising test, positive Trendelenburg test ***Musculoskeletal*** Tense, tight paravertebral muscles on palpation, ↓ range of motion in spine ***Possible Diagnostic Findings*** Localization of site of lesion or disorder on myelogram, CT scan, or MRI. Determination of nerve root impingement on electromyography (EMG)

Teach patients the importance of smoking cessation. Tobacco use impairs circulation to the intervertebral discs and may contribute to low back pain.

◆ **Acute Care.** If acute muscle spasms and accompanying pain are not severe and unbearable, the patient may be treated as an outpatient with NSAIDs and muscle relaxants (e.g., cyclobenzaprine). Massage and back manipulation, acupuncture, and the application of cold and hot compresses may help some patients.[13] Severe pain may require a brief course of corticosteroids or opioid analgesics.

Some people may need a brief period (1 to 2 days) of rest at home but should avoid prolonged bed rest.[14] Most patients do better if they continue their regular activities. Patients should refrain from activities that increase the pain, including lifting, bending, twisting, and prolonged sitting. Symptoms of acute low back pain generally improve within 2 weeks and often resolve without treatment.

Teach the patient about the cause of the pain and ways to prevent additional episodes. Muscle stretching and strengthening exercises may be part of the management plan. Although

TABLE 63-6   Patient & Caregiver Teaching

Low Back Problems

Include the following instructions when teaching the patient and caregiver how to manage low back problems.

Do

- Maintain healthy body weight.
- Maintain a neutral pelvic position if standing. Place one foot on a low stool if standing for long periods.
- Choose a seat with good lower back support, armrests, and a swivel base. Place a pillow at the lumbar spine to maintain normal curvature. Keep knees and hips level.
- Sleep in a side-lying position with knees and hips bent, and a pillow between the knees for support.
- Sleep on back with a lift under knees and legs or on back with 10-in–high pillow under knees to flex hips and knees.
- Use proper body mechanics when lifting heavy objects. Bend at the knees, not at the waist, and stand up slowly while holding object close to your body.
- Participate in regular strength and flexibility training and low-impact aerobic exercise.
- Use local heat and cold application to relieve muscle tension.

Do Not

- Lean forward without bending knees.
- Lift anything above level of elbows.
- Stand unmoving for prolonged time.
- Sleep on abdomen or on back or side with legs out straight.
- Exercise without consulting HCP if having severe pain.
- Exceed prescribed amount and type of exercises without consulting HCP.
- Smoke or use tobacco products.

exercises are often taught by a physical therapist, reinforce the type and frequency of prescribed exercise and the rationale for the program.

Other nursing interventions for the patient with low back pain are summarized in eNursing Care Plan 63-2 (on the website for this chapter).

◆ **Ambulatory Care.** The goal of management is to make an episode of acute low back pain an isolated incident. If the lumbosacral area is unstable, repeated episodes are likely. Obesity, poor posture, poor muscle support, older age, or trauma may weaken the lumbosacral spine, so it is unable to meet the demands placed on it without strain. Exercise is aimed at strengthening the supporting muscles (see earlier).

Persistent use of poor body mechanics may also result in repeated episodes of low back pain. If the strain is work related, occupational counseling may be needed. Low back pain can cause frustration, pain, and disability. Provide emotional support and understanding care of the patient.

CHRONIC LOW BACK PAIN

Chronic low back pain lasts more than 3 months or involves a repeated incapacitating episode. It is often progressive, and the cause can be difficult to determine. Causes include (1) degenerative conditions such as arthritis or disc disease; (2) osteoporosis or other metabolic bone diseases; (3) weakness from the scar tissue of prior injury; (4) chronic strain on lower back muscles from obesity, pregnancy, or stressful postures on the job; and (5) congenital spine problems.

Spinal Stenosis

Spinal stenosis is a narrowing of the spinal canal (contains the spinal cord). Stenosis in the lumbar spine is a common cause of chronic low back pain. Spinal stenosis can be caused by acquired or inherited conditions. A common acquired cause is osteoarthritis. Arthritic changes (bone spurs, calcification of spinal ligaments, disc degeneration) narrow the space around the spinal canal and nerve roots, eventually leading to compression. Inflammation caused by the compression results in pain, weakness, and numbness.

Other acquired conditions that may cause spinal stenosis include rheumatoid arthritis, spinal tumors, Paget's disease, and traumatic damage to the vertebral column. Inherited conditions that lead to spinal stenosis include congenital spinal stenosis and scoliosis.

The pain associated with lumbar spinal stenosis often starts in the lower back and then radiates to the buttock and leg. It is worse with walking or prolonged standing. Numbness, tingling, weakness, and heaviness in the legs and buttocks may also be present. History of decreased pain when the patient bends forward or sits is often a sign of spinal stenosis. In most cases, stenosis slowly progresses.

❖ **NURSING AND INTERPROFESSIONAL MANAGEMENT: CHRONIC LOW BACK PAIN**

Nursing management and treatment of chronic low back pain are similar to acute low back pain. Manage the patient's pain and stiffness with mild analgesics, such as NSAIDs, for daily comfort. Antidepressants (e.g., duloxetine [Cymbalta]) may help with pain management and sleep problems. The antiseizure drug gabapentin (Neurontin) may improve walking and relieve leg symptoms.

Weight reduction, sufficient rest periods, local heat or cold application, physical therapy, and exercise and activity throughout the day assist in keeping the muscles and joints mobilized. Cold, damp weather aggravates the back pain, which can be decreased with rest and local heat application. Complementary and alternative therapies such as biofeedback, acupuncture, and yoga may also help reduce the pain. "Back School" (discussed on p. 1503) can significantly reduce pain and improve body posture.[15]

Minimally invasive treatments, such as epidural corticosteroid injections and implanted devices that deliver pain medication, may be used for patients with chronic low back pain that fails to respond to the usual therapeutic options. Surgical intervention may be indicated in patients with severe chronic low back pain who receive no benefit from conservative care and/or have continued neurologic deficits. (Surgery for low back pain is discussed on p. 1506.)

INTERVERTEBRAL DISC DISEASE

Intervertebral discs separate the vertebrae and help absorb shock for the spine. *Intervertebral disc disease* involves the deterioration, herniation, or other dysfunction of the intervertebral discs. Disc disorders can affect the cervical, thoracic, and lumbar spine.

Etiology and Pathophysiology

Degenerative disc disease (DDD) results from loss of fluid in the intervertebral discs with aging. The discs lose their elasticity, flexibility, and shock-absorbing abilities. Unless it is accompanied by pain, this condition is a normal process.[16] The discs become thinner as the *nucleus pulposus* (gelatinous center of the disc) starts to dry out and shrink. This change limits the disc's ability to distribute pressure between vertebrae. The pressure is then transferred to the *annulus fibrosus* (strong outside portion of the disc), causing progressive destruction. When the disc is damaged, the nucleus pulposus may seep through a torn or stretched annulus. This is called a **herniated disc** *(slipped disc)*, a condition in which a spinal disc bulges outward between the vertebrae (Fig. 63-4).

A herniated disc can result from degeneration with age or repeated stress and trauma to the spine. The most common sites of herniation are the lumbosacral discs, specifically L4-5 and L5-S1. Disc herniation may also occur at C5-6 and C6-7. Disc herniation may be the result of spinal stenosis, in which narrowing of the spinal canal forces the intervertebral disc to bulge.

The spinal nerves emerge from the spinal column through an opening *(intervertebral foramen)* between adjacent vertebrae. Herniated discs can press against these nerves ("pinched nerve") causing *radiculopathy* (radiating pain, numbness, tingling, and diminished strength and/or range of motion).

Osteoarthritis (OA) of the spine is associated with DDD and the stresses placed on the vertebrae. As the poorly lubricated joints rub against each other, the protective cartilage is damaged and painful bone spurs occur as one of the changes found in OA.

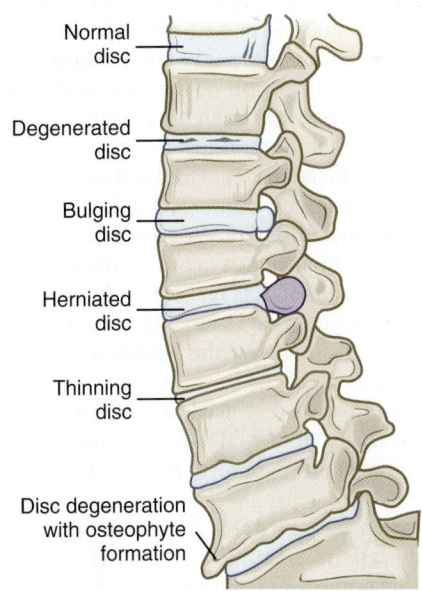

Normal disc

Degenerated disc

Bulging disc

Herniated disc

Thinning disc

Disc degeneration with osteophyte formation

FIG. 63-4   Common causes of degenerative disc damage.

Clinical Manifestations

In *lumbar disc disease*, the most common manifestation is low back pain. Radicular pain that radiates down the buttock and below the knee, along the distribution of the sciatic nerve, generally indicates disc herniation. (Specific manifestations of lumbar disc herniation are summarized in Table 63-7.) A positive straight-leg-raising test may indicate nerve root irritation (see Chapter 61, p. 1455). Back or leg pain may be reproduced by raising the leg.

Low back pain from other causes may not be accompanied by leg pain. Reflexes may be depressed or absent, depending on the spinal nerve root involved. Numbness and tingling *(paresthesia)* or muscle weakness in the legs, feet, or toes may occur.

Multiple nerve root compressions *(cauda equina syndrome)* from a herniated disc, tumor, or an epidural abscess may be marked by (1) severe low back pain, (2) progressive weakness, (3) increased pain, and (4) bowel and bladder incontinence.[17] This condition is a medical emergency that requires surgical decompression to reduce pressure on the nerves.

In *cervical disc disease*, pain radiates into the arms and hands, following the pattern of the involved nerve. Similar to lumbar disc disease, reflexes may or may not be present. The handgrip is often weak. Because manifestations of cervical disc disease may include shoulder pain and dysfunction, the HCP must rule out shoulder disorders as part of the diagnosis.

Diagnostic Studies

X-rays are done to detect any structural defects. A myelogram, MRI, or CT scan is helpful in localizing the damaged site. An epidural venogram or diskogram may be needed if other diagnostic studies are inconclusive. An EMG of the extremities can be performed to determine the severity of nerve irritation or to rule out other conditions such as peripheral neuropathy.

Interprofessional Care

The patient with suspected disc damage is usually managed with conservative therapy (Table 63-8). This includes limitation of extremes of spinal movement (brace, corset, or belt), local heat or ice, ultrasound and massage, traction, and transcutaneous electrical nerve stimulation (TENS). Drug therapy to manage pain includes NSAIDs, short-term use of oral corticosteroids, opioid analgesics, muscle relaxants, antiseizure drugs, and antidepressants.[18] Epidural corticosteroid injections may reduce inflammation and relieve acute pain. However, if the underlying cause remains, pain tends to recur.

When symptoms subside, the patient should begin back-strengthening exercises twice a day and continue for life. Teach the patient the principles of good body mechanics. Discourage extremes of flexion and torsion. With a conservative treatment plan, most patients heal after 6 months.

TABLE 63-7	**Manifestations of Lumbar Disc Herniation***			
Intervertebral Level	Pain	Affected Reflex	Motor Function	Sensation
L3-4	Back to buttocks to posterior thigh to inner calf	Patellar	Quadriceps, anterior tibialis	Inner aspect of lower leg, anterior part of thigh
L4-5	Back to buttocks to dorsum of foot and big toe	None	Anterior tibialis, extensor hallucis longus, gluteus medius	Dorsum of foot and big toe
L5-S1	Back to buttocks to sole of foot and heel	Achilles	Gastrocnemius, hamstring, gluteus maximus	Heel and lateral foot

*A disc herniation can involve pressure on more than one nerve root.

TABLE 63-8 Interprofessional Care
Intervertebral Disc Disease

Diagnostic Assessment
- History and physical examination
- X-ray
- CT scan
- MRI
- Myelogram
- Diskogram
- Electromyogram (EMG)

Management
Conservative Therapy
- Restricted activity for several days, limited total bed rest
- Local ice or heat
- Physical therapy
- Analgesics (e.g., tramadol [Ultram])
- Nonsteroidal antiinflammatory drugs
- Muscle relaxants (e.g., cyclobenzaprine)
- Antiseizure drugs (e.g., gabapentin)
- Antidepressants (e.g., pregabalin [Lyrica])
- Epidural corticosteroid injections

Surgical Therapy
- Intradiscal electrothermoplasty (IDET)
- Radiofrequency discal nucleoplasty
- Interspinous process decompression system (X-Stop)
- Laminectomy with or without spinal fusion
- Discectomy
- Percutaneous laser discectomy
- Artificial disc replacement (e.g., Charité disc)
- Spinal fusion with instrumentation (e.g., plates, screws) or without instrumentation

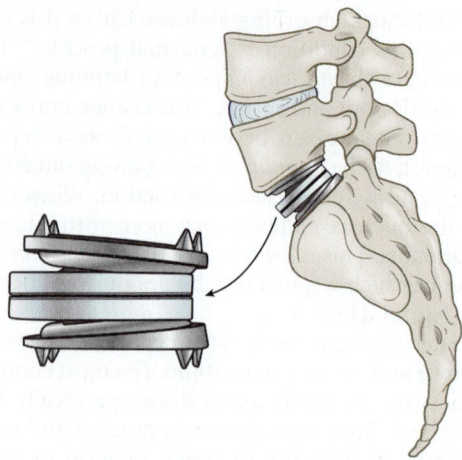

FIG. 63-5 The Charité artificial disc, used to replace a damaged intervertebral disc in degenerative disc disease of the lumbar spine. A movable high-density plastic core is sandwiched between two cobalt-chromium alloy endplates. The disc's design helps realign the spine and preserve movement.

Surgical Therapy. If conservative treatment is unsuccessful, radiculopathy becomes worse, or loss of bowel or bladder control (cauda equina syndrome) occurs, surgery may be considered. Surgery for a damaged disc is generally performed if the patient is in constant pain and/or has a persistent neurologic deficit.

Intradiscal electrothermoplasty (IDET) is a minimally invasive outpatient procedure for treatment of back and sciatic pain. A needle is inserted into the affected disc with x-ray guidance. A wire is then threaded through the needle and into the disc. As the wire is heated, small nerve fibers that have invaded the degenerating disc are destroyed. The heat also partially melts the annulus fibrosus. This causes the body to generate new reinforcing proteins in the fibers of the annulus.

Another outpatient technique is *radiofrequency discal nucleoplasty* (coblation nucleoplasty). A needle is inserted into the disc similar to IDET. Instead of a heated wire, a special radiofrequency probe is used. The probe generates energy that breaks the molecular bonds of the gel in the nucleus pulposus. Up to 20% of the nucleus is removed. This decompresses the disc and reduces pressure on the disc and surrounding nerve roots. Subsequent pain relief varies.

A third procedure involves use of an *interspinous process decompression system* (X-Stop). This titanium device fits onto a mount that is placed on vertebrae in the lower back. The X-Stop is used in patients with pain due to lumbar spinal stenosis. The device works by lifting vertebrae off the pinched nerve.

Laminectomy is a common, traditional surgical procedure for lumbar disc disease. It involves surgical excision of part of the vertebra (referred to as the *lamina*) to access and remove the protruding disc. Laminectomy is often performed as an outpatient procedure, but a hospital stay of 1 to 3 days is not uncommon.

Discectomy can also be performed to decompress the nerve root.[11] Microsurgical discectomy is a version of the standard procedure. The surgeon uses a microscope for better visualization of the disc and disc space to aid in removal of the damaged portion. This helps maintain bony stability of the spine.

Percutaneous discectomy is a safe and effective outpatient surgical procedure. A tube is passed through the retroperitoneal soft tissues to the disc with the aid of fluoroscopy. A laser is then used on the damaged portion of the disc. Minimal blood loss occurs because of access through small stab wounds. The procedure decreases rehabilitation time.

The goals of artificial disc replacement surgery are to restore movement and eliminate pain. The *Charité disc* is used in patients with lumbar disc damage associated with DDD. This artificial disc has a high-density core sandwiched between two cobalt-chromium endplates (Fig. 63-5). After the damaged disc is removed, this device is surgically placed in the spine (usually through a small incision below the umbilicus). The disc restores movement at the level of the implant. The *ProDisc-L* is another type of artificial lumbar disc used to treat DDD.[19]

Options for treatment of DDD of the cervical spine include the *Prestige cervical disc, Mobi-C disc,* and *Secure-C artificial cervical disc.*

A *spinal fusion* may be needed if the spine is unstable. The spine is stabilized by creating *ankylosis* (fusion) of adjacent vertebrae with a bone graft from the patient's fibula or iliac crest (*autograft*) or from donated cadaver bone (*allograft*). Metal fixation with rods, plates, or screws may also be placed at the time of spinal surgery to provide more stability and decrease vertebral motion. A posterior lumbar fusion may be performed in patients to provide extra support for bone grafting or a prosthetic device.

Bone morphogenetic protein (BMP), a genetically engineered protein, may be used to stimulate bone growth of the graft in spinal fusions.[20] A dissolvable sponge soaked with BMP is implanted into the spine. The protein on the sponge stimulates the body's cells to become active and produce bone. BMP begins the process of fusion, which continues after the protein and sponge dissolve to leave living bone behind.

❖ NURSING MANAGEMENT: VERTEBRAL DISC SURGERY

After vertebral disc surgery, postoperative nursing interventions mainly focus on maintaining proper alignment of the spine until it has healed. Depending on the type and extent of surgery and the surgeon's preference, the patient may be able to dangle the legs at the side of the bed, stand, or even ambulate the day of surgery.

After lumbar fusion, place pillows under the patient's thighs when supine and between the legs when in the side-lying position to provide comfort and ensure alignment. The patient often fears turning or any movement that may increase pain by stressing the surgical area. Reassure the patient that proper technique is being used to maintain body alignment. Enough staff should be available to move the patient without undue pain or strain for the patient or staff.

Postoperatively, most patients require opioids such as morphine IV for 24 to 48 hours. Patient-controlled analgesia (PCA) allows maintenance of optimal analgesic levels and is the preferred method of continuous pain management. Once the patient receives oral fluids, oral drugs such as acetaminophen with codeine, hydrocodone, or oxycodone (Percocet) may be used. Diazepam (Valium) may be prescribed for muscle relaxation. Assess and document pain intensity and pain management effectiveness.

Because the spinal canal may be entered during surgery, cerebrospinal fluid (CSF) leakage is possible. Immediately report leakage of CSF on the dressing or if the patient complains of severe headache. CSF appears as clear or slightly yellow drainage on the dressing. It has a high glucose concentration and is positive for glucose when tested with a dipstick. Note the amount, color, and characteristics of drainage.

Frequently assess the patient's peripheral neurologic condition after spinal surgery. Movement of the arms and legs and assessment of sensation should at least equal the preoperative status. Repeat these assessments every 2 to 4 hours during the first 48 hours after surgery and compare with the preoperative assessment. Paresthesia may not be relieved immediately after surgery. Report any new muscle weakness or paresthesia immediately to the surgeon and document this finding in the patient's medical record. Assess extremity circulation using skin temperature, capillary refill, and pulses.

Paralytic ileus and interference with bowel function may occur for several days and may manifest as nausea, abdominal distention, and constipation. Opioids can also slow bowel elimination. Assess if the patient is passing gas, has bowel sounds in all quadrants, and has a flat, soft abdomen. Stool softeners (e.g., docusate [Colace]) and laxatives may prevent and relieve constipation.

Emptying the bladder may be difficult due to activity restrictions, opioids, or anesthesia. Encourage men to dangle the legs over the side of the bed or stand to urinate if allowed by the surgeon. Urge patients to use a bedside commode or ambulate to the bathroom when allowed to promote bladder emptying. Ensure that privacy is maintained. Intermittent catheterization or an indwelling urinary catheter may be needed by patients who have difficulty urinating.

Loss of sphincter tone or bladder tone may indicate nerve damage. Monitor for incontinence or difficulty with bowel or bladder elimination, and immediately report problems to the surgeon.

In addition to nursing care appropriate for a patient who had a laminectomy, other nursing activities are indicated if the patient has also had a spinal fusion. Because a bone graft is usually involved, the postoperative healing time is prolonged compared with a laminectomy. Activity limitations may be needed for an extended time. A rigid orthosis (thoracic-lumbar-sacral orthosis [TLSO] or chairback brace) is often used during this period. Some surgeons want patients to be taught to apply and remove the brace by logrolling in bed. Others allow their patients to apply the brace in a sitting or standing position. Verify the surgeon's preferred method before starting this activity.

If surgery is done on the cervical spine, be alert for indications of spinal cord edema such as respiratory distress and a worsening neurologic condition of the upper extremities. After surgery, the patient's neck may be immobilized in a soft or hard cervical collar.

In addition to the primary surgical site, regularly assess the bone graft donor site. The posterior iliac crest is the most commonly used donor site, although the fibula may also be used. The donor site usually causes greater pain than the spinal fusion area. The donor site is bandaged with a pressure dressing to prevent excessive bleeding. If the donor site is the fibula, frequent neurovascular assessment of the extremity is a postoperative nursing responsibility.

After spinal fusion, the patient may experience some immobility of the spine at the fusion site. Instruct the patient to use proper body mechanics and avoid sitting or standing for prolonged periods. Encourage activities that include walking, lying down, and shifting weight from one foot to the other when standing. Instruct the patient on any lifting restrictions after spinal surgery. Encourage the patient to think through an activity before starting any potentially injurious task such as bending or stooping. Any twisting movement of the spine is contraindicated. Teach the patient to use the thighs and knees, rather than the back, to absorb the shock of activity and movement. A firm mattress or bed board is essential.

NECK PAIN

Neck pain occurs almost as frequently as low back pain, affecting up to 10% of adults at any point in time. Neck pain may result from many different conditions, including benign (e.g., poor posture) and serious (e.g., herniated cervical disc)[21] (Table 63-9).

Cervical neck sprains and strains occur from hyperflexion and hyperextension injuries. Patients complain of stiffness and neck pain with possible radicular pain into the arm and hand. Pain may also radiate to the head, anterior chest, thoracic spine region, and shoulders. Weakness or paresthesia of the arm and hand may suggest cervical nerve root compression from stenosis, DDD, or herniation.

The cause of neck pain is diagnosed by history, physical examination, x-ray, MRI, CT scan, and myelogram. An EMG of the upper extremities may diagnose cervical radiculopathy.

TABLE 63-9   Causes of Neck Pain

• Poor posture	• Spondylosis
• Strain or sprain	• Rheumatoid arthritis
• Degenerative disc disease, including herniation	• Tumor
• Trauma (e.g., fractures, subluxation)	• Osteoporosis
	• Osteomyelitis
	• Meningitis

TABLE 63-10	Patient & Caregiver Teaching

Neck Exercises

When teaching the patient exercises for neck pain, include the following instructions for the patient and caregiver.

- Bend your head backward until you are looking up at the ceiling. Repeat slowly five times. Stop if experiencing dizziness.
- Bring your head forward so that your chin touches your chest and your face is looking down at the floor. Repeat slowly five times.
- With your head facing forward, bend your ear down toward one shoulder. Alternate this movement with your other ear. Repeat slowly five times on each side.
- Turn your head slowly around to one side as far as it will go. Repeat toward the other side. Repeat exercise five times on each side.

Conservative treatment for neck pain in patients without an underlying disorder includes head support using a soft cervical collar, gentle traction, heat and ice applications, massage, rest until symptoms subside, ultrasound, and NSAIDs. Therapeutic neck exercises and acupuncture may also be used for pain relief.[22] Most neck pain resolves without surgical intervention.

Preventing neck pain that occurs with everyday activities such as prolonged sitting at a computer or television, sleeping in nonaligned spinal positions, or making jarring movements during exercise is important. Encourage patients to practice good posture and maintain neck flexibility (Table 63-10).

FOOT DISORDERS

The foot is the platform that supports the weight of the body and absorbs shock when the person ambulates. It is a complicated structure composed of bony structures, muscles, tendons, and ligaments that can be affected by (1) congenital conditions, (2) structural weakness, (3) traumatic and stress injuries, and (4) systemic conditions such as diabetes mellitus and rheumatoid arthritis. A great deal of the pain, deformity, and disability of foot disorders can be directly attributed to or worsened by poorly fitting shoes. Shoes may cause crowding and angulation of the toes and inhibit normal movement of foot muscles.

Footwear is used to (1) provide support, foot stability, protection, shock absorption, and a foundation for orthoses; (2) increase friction with the walking surface; and (3) treat foot abnormalities. (Table 63-11 summarizes common foot disorders.)

❖ NURSING MANAGEMENT: FOOT DISORDERS

◆ Nursing Implementation

◆ **Health Promotion.** Well-made and properly fitted shoes are essential for healthy, pain-free feet. Women's footwear is often influenced by current styles instead of comfort and support. Stress the importance of having a shoe that conforms to the foot rather than to fashion trends. The shoe must be long enough and wide enough to avoid crowding the toes and forcing the great toe into a position of hallux valgus (Fig. 63-6). At the metatarsal head, the shoe should be wide enough to allow foot muscles to move freely and toes to bend. The shank (narrow part of sole under the instep) of the shoe should be rigid enough to give good support. The height of the heel should be realistic in relation to the shoe's purpose. Ideally, the heel of the shoe should not rise more than 1 inch higher than the forefoot

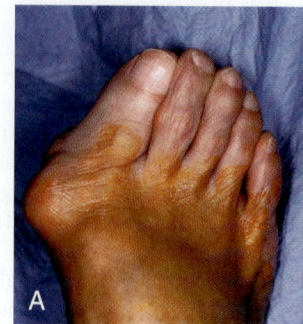
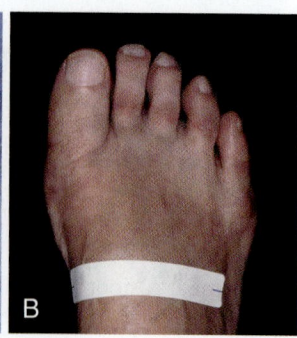

FIG. 63-6 A, Severe hallux valgus with bursa formation. **B,** Postoperative correction. (From Canale ST, Beaty JH: *Campbell's operative orthopaedics,* ed 12, Philadelphia, 2013, Mosby.)

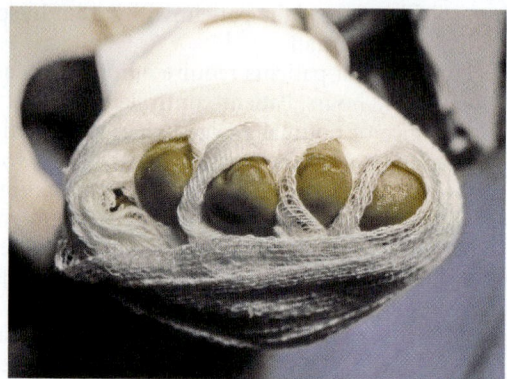

FIG. 63-7 Postoperative supportive dressing for treatment of moderate forefoot deformity. Dressing must be conforming and binding enough to hold toe in exact position. (From Canale ST, Beaty JH: *Campbell's operative orthopaedics,* ed 12, Philadelphia, 2013, Mosby.)

support. Wearing higher-heeled shoes with a narrow toe box will cause hammertoes and corns over time.

Prolonged use of this type of footwear can also result in a *Morton's neuroma* (compression of an intermetatarsal plantar nerve, usually between the third and fourth toes, resulting in paresthesia). Initially, patients with Morton's neuroma may complain of feeling as if a sock is rolled up under their toes.[23]

◆ **Acute Care.** Many foot problems require referral to a podiatrist. Depending on the problem, conservative therapies are tried first (Table 63-11). These therapies include NSAIDs, shock-wave therapy, ice, physical therapy, footwear alterations, stretching, warm soaks, orthotics, ultrasound, and corticosteroid injections. If these methods do not help, surgery may be recommended.

Depending on the type of surgery, pins or wires may extend through the toes, or a protective splint may be placed over the end of the foot. Postoperatively, the foot is usually immobilized by a bulky dressing (Fig. 63-7), short leg cast, slipper (plaster)

❓ CHECK YOUR PRACTICE

A 52-yr-old woman is scheduled for surgical correction of a bunion after a diagnosis of hallux valgus. You are doing her preoperative assessment. She asks you, "Do you think I caused this problem? I have been so vain all my life and had to wear only fancy shoes. Now I have to wear an ugly bunion shoe. I am not sure I can handle taking care of myself after surgery."

- How will you respond when the patient asks about the cause of this disorder?
- What teaching will you provide her about her postoperative care?

TABLE 63-11	**Common Foot Disorders**	
Disorder	**Description**	**Treatment**
Forefoot		
Hallux valgus (bunion)	Painful deformity of great toe with lateral angulation of great toe toward second toe, bony enlargement of medial side of first metatarsal head, swelling of bursa and formation of callus over bony enlargement (Fig. 63-6).	• Conservative treatment includes wearing shoes with wide forefoot or "bunion pocket" and use of bunion pads to relieve pressure on bursal sac. • Surgical treatment involves removal of bursal sac and bony enlargement and correction of lateral angulation of great toe. • May include temporary or permanent internal fixation.
Hallux rigidus	Painful stiffness of first MTP joint caused by osteoarthritis or local trauma.	• Conservative treatment includes intraarticular corticosteroids and passive manual stretching of first MTP joint. • Shoe with a stiff sole decreases pain in the joint during walking. • Surgical treatment is joint fusion or arthroplasty with silicone rubber implant.
Hammer and claw toes	Hammer toe is a deformity of PIP joint on 2nd to 5th toes causing toe to be permanently bent, resembling a hammer. Mallet toe is a similar condition affecting the DIP joint. Claw toe is a similar deformity with dorsiflexion of the proximal phalanx on the MTP joint combined with flexion of both PIP and DIP joints. Complaints include burning on bottom of foot and pain and difficulty walking when wearing shoes.	• Conservative treatment includes passive manual stretching of PIP joint and use of metatarsal arch support. • Surgical correction consists of resection of base of middle phalanx and head of proximal phalanx, bringing raw bone ends together. • Kirschner wire maintains straight position.
Morton's neuroma (Morton's toe or plantar neuroma)	Neuroma in web space between third and fourth metatarsal heads, causing sharp, sudden attacks of pain and burning sensations.	• Surgical excision is the usual treatment.
Midfoot		
Pes planus (flatfoot)	Loss of metatarsal arch causing pain in foot or leg.	• Symptoms are relieved by use of resilient longitudinal arch supports. • Surgical treatment consists of triple arthrodesis or fusion of subtalar joint.
Pes cavus	Elevation of longitudinal arch of foot resulting from contracture of plantar fascia or bony deformity of arch.	• Surgical correction is needed if condition interferes with ambulation.
Hindfoot		
Painful heels	Complaint of heel pain with weight bearing. Common causes are plantar bursitis, plantar fasciitis, or bone spur.	• Corticosteroids are injected locally into inflamed bursa, and sponge-rubber heel cup is used. • Surgical excision of bursa or spur is performed. • Stretching exercises, ice, shoe heel cup, shock-wave therapy, NSAIDs, and corticosteroids are used for plantar fasciitis.
Calcaneus stress fracture	Complaint of heel pain after moderate walking. Common causes are overtraining, running on hard surfaces, or osteoporosis.	• Rest, ice, shoe heel pad, and NSAIDs are used. • See HCP to assess for osteoporosis.
Other Problems		
Corn	Localized thickening of skin caused by continual pressure over bony prominences, especially metatarsal head, frequently causing localized pain.	• Corn is softened with warm water or preparations containing salicylic acid and trimmed with razor blade or scalpel. • Pressure on bony prominences caused by shoes is relieved.
Soft corn	Painful lesion caused by bony prominence of one toe pressing against adjacent toe. Usual location is web space between toes. Softness caused by secretions keeping web space relatively moist.	• Pain is relieved by placing cotton or spacers between toes to separate them. • Surgical treatment is excision of projecting bone spur (if present).
Callus	Similar formation to corn but covering wider area and usually located on weight-bearing part of foot.	• Same as for corn.
Plantar wart	Painful papillomatous growth caused by virus that may occur on any part of skin on sole of foot. Warts tend to cluster on pressure points.	• Remedies containing salicylic acid (e.g., Compound W), excision with electrocoagulation, or surgical removal. • Laser treatments may also be used. • May disappear without treatment.

DIP, Distal interphalangeal; *MTP,* metatarsophalangeal; *PIP,* proximal interphalangeal.

cast, or a platform shoe that fits over the dressing and has a rigid sole (also known as a *bunion shoe*).

Elevate the foot with the heel off the bed to reduce discomfort and prevent edema. Assess neurovascular condition frequently during the immediate postoperative period. Inserted devices may interfere with assessment for movement. Also be aware that evaluating sensation may be difficult because the patient may be unable to differentiate surgical pain from pain caused by nerve pressure or circulatory impairment.

The type and extent of surgery determine the orders for ambulation. Crutches, a walker, or a cane may be needed. The patient may experience pain or a throbbing sensation when lowering the affected leg. Reinforce instructions from the physical therapist. Remind the patient of the importance of walking with an erect posture with proper weight distribution. Report gait problems or continued pain to the surgeon. Instruct the patient about the importance of frequent rest periods with the foot elevated.

◆ **Ambulatory Care.** Instruct the patient to perform daily hygienic foot care and wear clean stockings. Stockings should be long enough to avoid wrinkling and causing pressure areas. Trimming toenails straight across helps prevent ingrown toenails and reduces the risk of infection. Provide detailed instruction to patients with impaired circulation or diabetes mellitus to prevent serious complications from blisters, pressure areas, and infection. (See Table 48-21 for guidelines on foot care.)

Gerontologic Considerations: Foot Problems

The older adult is prone to foot problems because of poor circulation, atherosclerosis, and decreased sensation in the lower extremities. This is especially true for older patients with diabetes mellitus.[24] A patient may develop an open wound but not feel it because of altered sensation from peripheral vascular disease or diabetic neuropathy. Instruct older adults to inspect their feet daily and report any open wounds or breaks in the skin to their HCP.[25]

Untreated wounds may become infected, lead to osteomyelitis, and require surgical debridement. If the infection becomes widespread, lower limb amputation may be necessary. Teach the caregiver of the older adult who needs assistance with hygiene practices the importance of carefully assessing the feet at regular intervals.

METABOLIC BONE DISEASES

Normal bone metabolism is affected by hormones, nutrition, and genetics. When dysfunction occurs in any of these factors, generalized reduction in bone mass and strength may result. Metabolic bone diseases include osteomalacia, osteoporosis, and Paget's disease.

OSTEOMALACIA

Osteomalacia is caused by a vitamin D deficiency that causes bone to lose calcium and become soft. The disease is uncommon in the United States. It is the same disorder as rickets in children, except the epiphyseal growth plates are closed in adults. Vitamin D is required for the absorption of calcium from the intestine. Insufficient vitamin D intake can interfere with normal bone mineralization; with little or no calcification, bones become soft.

Causes of osteomalacia include limited sun exposure (ultraviolet rays needed for vitamin D synthesis), GI malabsorption, extensive burns, chronic diarrhea, pregnancy, kidney disease, and use of drugs such as phenytoin (Dilantin). Residents of long-term care settings may have inadequate sun exposure and thus poor synthesis of vitamin D. Persons with dark skin also do not synthesize vitamin D as easily as persons with fair skin. Obese persons are at higher risk for osteomalacia because of decreased physical activity and poor diet (i.e., inadequate calcium and vitamin D intake). Chronic diseases of the liver, kidneys, and small intestine may also contribute to vitamin D deficiency. Long-term use of antiseizure drugs, phosphate-binding antacids (e.g., Maalox), sedatives, and muscle relaxants may decrease calcium and vitamin D absorption.[26]

Common manifestations of osteomalacia are bone pain and difficulty walking or rising from a chair.[27] Other manifestations include muscle weakness, especially in the pelvic girdle, weight loss, and progressive deformity of weight-bearing bones (e.g., spine, extremities). Fractures are common and indicate delayed bone healing.

Laboratory findings commonly include decreased serum calcium or phosphorus, decreased serum 25-hydroxyvitamin D, and elevated serum alkaline phosphatase. X-rays may show

effects of generalized bone demineralization, especially loss of calcium in the bones of the pelvis and associated bone deformity. *Looser's transformation zones* (ribbons of decalcification in bone found on x-ray) are diagnostic of osteomalacia. However, significant osteomalacia may exist without changes on x-ray.

Interprofessional care of osteomalacia is directed toward correction of vitamin D deficiency. The patient often shows a dramatic response when vitamin D_3 (cholecalciferol) and vitamin D_2 (ergocalciferol) supplements are used. Calcium or phosphorus supplements may also be prescribed. Encourage dietary intake of eggs, meat, and oily fish (e.g., salmon, tuna). Milk and breakfast cereals fortified with calcium and vitamin D should also be included in the diet. Exposure to sunlight and weight-bearing exercise are valuable as well.

Patients who have bariatric surgery to treat obesity should be assessed for osteomalacia. Any vitamin D deficiencies should be corrected before surgery.[26]

OSTEOPOROSIS

Osteoporosis is a chronic, progressive metabolic bone disease marked by low bone mass and deterioration of bone tissue, leading to increased bone fragility (Fig. 63-8). More than 54 million persons in the United States have decreased bone density or osteoporosis.[28] One in two women and one in four men over age 50 will sustain an osteoporosis-related fracture during their lifetime. Osteoporosis is known as the "silent thief" because it slowly robs the skeleton of its banked resources. Bones eventually become so fragile that they cannot withstand normal mechanical stress.

Osteoporosis is more common in women than in men for several reasons: (1) women tend to have lower calcium intake than men throughout their lives (men between 15 and 50 years of age consume twice as much calcium as women); (2) women have less bone mass because of their generally smaller frames; (3) bone resorption begins at an earlier age in women and becomes more rapid at menopause; (4) pregnancy and breastfeeding deplete a woman's skeletal reserve unless calcium intake is adequate; and (5) longevity increases the likelihood of osteoporosis.

Current guidelines recommend an initial bone density test in all women over age 65 years. Women who are younger than

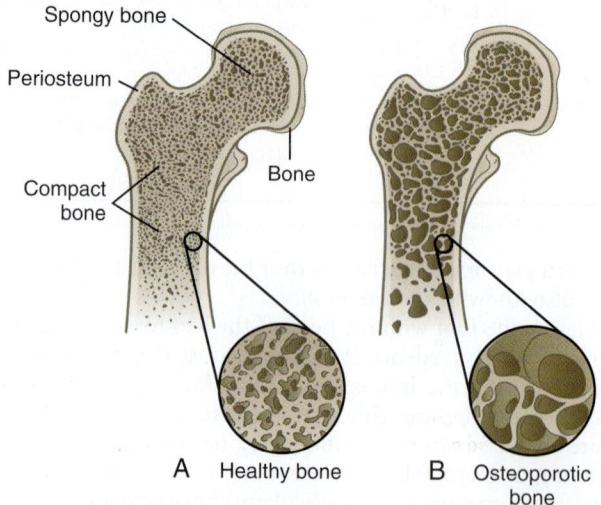

FIG. 63-8 A, Normal bone. **B,** Osteoporotic bone.

65 and at high risk (e.g., low body weight, smoker, prior fractures) should also have a bone density test. If results are normal and the person is at low risk for osteoporosis, another test is not needed for 15 years. Testing should start earlier and be done more frequently if a person is at high risk for fractures. Currently there is not sufficient evidence to demonstrate significant benefit for osteoporosis screening in men.[29]

⊕ CULTURAL & ETHNIC HEALTH DISPARITIES

Osteoporosis

- White and Asian American women have a higher incidence of osteoporosis than Native American, Hispanic, and African American women.
- African American women begin menopause with more bone mass and have a lower rate of bone loss after menopause than non–African American women.
- Risk of fracture in white women is higher than in nonwhite women of the same age.

Etiology and Pathophysiology

Risk factors for osteoporosis are listed in Table 63-12. Decreased risk is associated with regular weight-bearing exercise and adequate intake of fluoride, calcium, and vitamin D. Low testosterone is a major risk factor in men.

Peak bone mass (maximum bone tissue) is typically achieved before age 20. It is largely determined by four factors: heredity, nutrition, exercise, and hormone function. Heredity may be responsible for up to 70% of a person's peak bone mass. Bone loss from midlife (ages 35 to 40 years) onward is inevitable, but the rate of loss varies. At menopause, women experience rapid bone loss when the decline in estrogen production is the greatest. The rate of loss then slows and eventually matches the rate of bone lost by men ages 65 to 70 years. Genetic factors influence not only bone mineral density but also bone size, quality, and turnover.

Bone is continuously being deposited by osteoblasts and resorbed by osteoclasts, a process called *remodeling*. Rates of bone deposition and resorption are normally equal, so total bone mass remains constant.[30] In osteoporosis, bone resorption exceeds bone deposition.

Specific diseases associated with osteoporosis include inflammatory bowel disease, intestinal malabsorption, kidney disease, rheumatoid arthritis, hyperthyroidism, alcoholism, cirrhosis of the liver, hypogonadism, and diabetes mellitus. Many drugs can interfere with bone metabolism, including corticosteroids, antiseizure drugs (e.g., divalproex sodium [Depakote], phenytoin), aluminum-containing antacids, heparin, some chemotherapy drugs, and excessive thyroid hormones. When one of these drugs is prescribed, inform the patient of this possible side effect. Long-term corticosteroid use is a major contributor to osteoporosis.

GENDER DIFFERENCES

Osteoporosis

Men	Women
• Men are underdiagnosed and undertreated for osteoporosis as compared to women. • One in four men over age 50 will have an osteoporosis-related fracture in his lifetime.	• Osteoporosis is eight times more common in women than in men. • One in two women over age 50 years will have an osteoporosis-related fracture in her lifetime.

Clinical Manifestations

Osteoporosis occurs most commonly in bones of the spine, hips, and wrists. Typical early manifestations are back pain or spontaneous fractures. The loss of bone mass causes the bone to become mechanically weaker and prone to spontaneous fractures or fractures from minimal trauma. A person who has one vertebral fracture due to osteoporosis has an increased risk of having a second vertebral fracture within 1 year. Over time, vertebral fractures and wedging cause gradual loss of height and a humped thoracic spine (*kyphosis*, or "dowager's hump") (Fig. 63-9).

Diagnostic Studies

Osteoporosis often goes unnoticed because it cannot be detected by conventional x-ray until 25% to 40% of calcium in the bone is lost. Serum calcium, phosphorus, and alkaline phosphatase levels usually are normal, although alkaline phosphatase may be elevated after a fracture.

Bone mineral density (BMD) measurements are typically expressed as grams of mineral per unit volume.[31] BMD is determined by peak bone mass and amount of bone loss. (Procedures for BMD measurement are presented in Table 61-7.) BMD may be measured by quantitative ultrasound (QUS) and dual-energy x-ray absorptiometry (DXA). QUS uses sound waves to measure bone density in the heel, kneecap, or shin. DXA (considered the gold standard of BMD studies by the World Health Organization) measures bone density in the spine, hips, and forearm. These represent the most common sites of fragility fractures from osteoporosis. DXA studies are also useful to evaluate changes in bone density over time and assess effectiveness of osteoporosis treatment.

The BMD test results are compared to the ideal or peak bone mineral density of a healthy 30-year-old adult, and reported as T-scores. A T-score of 0 means the BMD is equal to the norm for a healthy young adult. Differences between the BMD and that of the healthy young adult norm are measured in units called *standard deviations (SDs)*. The more standard deviations below 0 (indicated as negative numbers), the lower the BMD and the higher the risk of fracture.

A T-score between +1 and −1 is considered normal. A T-score between −1 and −2.5 indicates osteopenia (bone loss that is more than normal, but not yet at the level for a diagnosis of osteoporosis). A T-score of −2.5 or lower indicates osteoporosis. The greater the negative number, the more severe the osteoporosis.

TABLE 63-12   Risk Factors for Osteoporosis

- Advancing age (>65 yr)
- Female gender
- Low body weight
- White or Asian ethnicity
- Current cigarette smoking
- Sedentary lifestyle
- Estrogen deficiency in women (surgical or age-related menopause)
- Family history of osteoporosis
- Diet low in calcium or vitamin D deficiency
- Excessive use of alcohol (>2 drinks/day)
- Low testosterone in men
- Long-term use of corticosteroids, thyroid replacement, heparin, long-acting sedatives, or antiseizure drugs

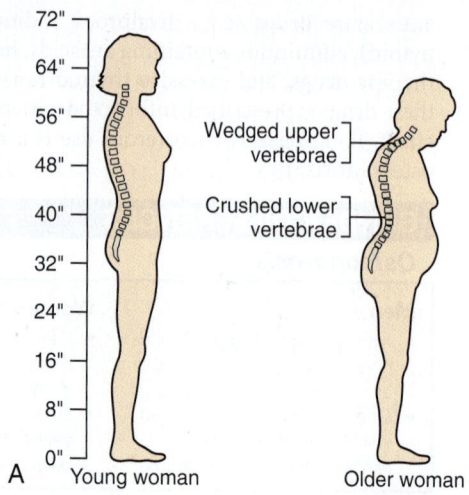

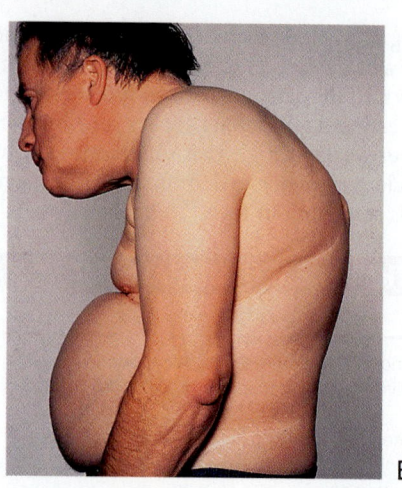

FIG. 63-9 The effects of osteoporosis. **A,** Comparison of young woman with an older woman. **B,** Severe fixed kyphosis producing a question-mark appearance. (*A,* From Phillips N: *Berry & Kohn's operating room technique,* ed 12, St Louis, 2013, Mosby. *B,* Courtesy MA Mir. In Kanski JJ: *Clinical diagnosis in ophthalmology,* St Louis, 2006, Mosby.)

Sometimes the HCP asks for a Z-score instead of a T-score. In this case, a person is compared with someone his or her own age, gender, and/or ethnic group instead of a healthy 30-year-old. Among older adults, Z-scores can be misleading because decreased bone density is common. If the Z-score is −2 or lower, it may suggest that something other than aging is causing abnormal bone loss.

❖ NURSING AND INTERPROFESSIONAL MANAGEMENT: OSTEOPOROSIS

Interprofessional care for osteoporosis focuses on proper nutrition, calcium supplementation, exercise, prevention of falls and fractures, and drugs (Table 63-13). The National Osteoporosis Foundation (*www.nof.org*) recommends treatment for osteoporosis for postmenopausal women with (1) a T-score of less than −2.5, (2) a T-score between −1 and −2.5 with additional risk factors (Table 63-12), or (3) prior history of a hip or vertebral fracture.

A patient's risk of fracture from osteoporosis can also be calculated with the Fracture Risk Assessment (FRAX) tool (*www.shef.ac.uk/FRAX*). The FRAX takes into account BMD and additional clinical factors when assessing fracture risk.[32]

Prevention and treatment of osteoporosis focus on adequate calcium intake (1000 mg/day for women ages 19 to 50 years and men ages 19 to 70 years; 1200 mg/day in women age 51 years or older and men 71 years or older). Foods high in calcium include milk, yogurt, turnip greens, cottage cheese, ice cream, sardines, and spinach (Table 63-14). If dietary intake of calcium is inadequate, supplemental calcium may be recommended.

Calcium is difficult to absorb in single doses greater than 500 mg.[33] Teach the patient the importance of taking calcium supplements as divided doses to increase absorption. The amount of elemental calcium varies in different calcium preparations. Calcium carbonate has 40% elemental calcium. It should be taken with meals because stomach acid is needed to dissolve and absorb this supplement. Calcium citrate offers about 20% elemental calcium but is less dependent on stomach acid for absorption. It is also better absorbed by patients taking a proton pump inhibitor (e.g., esomeprazole [Nexium]) or histamine receptor blocker (e.g., cimetidine) for acid reflux.[33]

TABLE 63-13   Interprofessional Care
Osteoporosis

Diagnostic Assessment
- History and physical examination
- Serum calcium, phosphorus, alkaline phosphatase, vitamin D
- Bone mineral densitometry
- Dual-energy x-ray absorptiometry (DXA)

Management
- Adequate dietary calcium (Table 63-14)
- Calcium supplements
- Sun exposure or vitamin D supplements
- Exercise program

Drug Therapy
- Bisphosphonates
  - alendronate (Fosamax, Binosto)
  - etidronate (Didronel)
  - ibandronate (Boniva)
  - pamidronate (Aredia)
  - risedronate (Actonel)
  - zoledronic acid (Reclast)
- Salmon calcitonin
- Selective estrogen receptor modulator (e.g., raloxifene [Evista])
- Recombinant parathyroid hormone (e.g., teriparatide [Forteo])
- Monoclonal antibody (e.g., denosumab [Prolia])

Minimally Invasive Procedures
- Vertebroplasty
- Kyphoplasty

Calcium lactate and calcium gluconate are not recommended because they have small amounts of elemental calcium.

Vitamin D is important in calcium absorption and function and may also have a role in bone formation. Most people get enough vitamin D from their diet or naturally through synthesis in the skin from exposure to sunlight. Being in the sun for 20 minutes a day is generally enough. However, supplemental vitamin D (800 IU) is recommended for postmenopausal women, older men, persons who are homebound or in long-term care settings, and those in northern climates due to decreased sun exposure.

TABLE 63-14 Nutritional Therapy

Sources of Calcium

Food	Calcium (mg)	Food	Calcium (mg)
Good Sources		**Good Sources—cont'd**	
1 cup milk		3 oz seafood	
• Whole	279	• Salmon	181
• Skim	299	• Sardines	325
6 oz calcium-fortified	261	1 cup almonds	304
orange juice		**Poor Sources**	
1 oz cheese		Egg	28
• Mozzarella	222	3 oz beef, pork, poultry	10
• Cheddar	214	Apple, banana	10
• Cottage	138	1 med potato	14
8 oz yogurt	313-384	1 med carrot	14
• Soft serve frozen	206	¼ head lettuce	27
1 cup ice cream	168		

Regular physical activity is important to build and maintain bone mass.[34] Exercise also increases muscle strength, coordination, and balance. The best exercises are weight-bearing exercises that force an individual to work against gravity. These exercises include walking, hiking, weight training, stair climbing, tennis, and dancing. Walking is preferred to high-impact aerobics or running, both of which may put too much stress on the bones and may cause stress fractures. Encourage patients to walk 30 minutes three times a week. Instruct patients to quit smoking and decrease alcohol intake to minimize negative effects on bone mass.

Although loss of bone cannot be significantly reversed, further loss can be prevented if the patient follows a regimen of calcium and vitamin D supplementation, exercise, and drugs (Table 63-13) as indicated. Encourage patients with osteoporosis to remain ambulatory to prevent further loss of bone density due to immobility.

Treatment may also involve the use of a gait aid to walk safely and protect areas of potential pathologic fractures. For example, a thoracolumbar sacral orthosis (TLSO) may be used to maintain the spine in proper alignment after fracture or treatment of a vertebral fracture. (Fractures are discussed in Chapter 62.)

Vertebroplasty and *kyphoplasty* are minimally invasive procedures used to treat osteoporotic vertebral fractures[35] (see Chapter 62). In vertebroplasty, bone cement is injected into the collapsed vertebra to stabilize the spine and improve the patient's pain. However, this procedure does not restore vertebral height or correct deformity. In kyphoplasty, a small balloon is inserted into the collapsed vertebra and inflated to restore vertebral body height before injection of bone cement. Kyphoplasty is now the preferred surgical treatment for vertebral compression fractures.

◆ Drug Therapy

Estrogen replacement therapy and estrogen with progesterone are no longer routinely given after menopause to prevent osteoporosis because they are associated with increased risk of heart disease as well as breast and uterine cancer. If a woman is taking short-term estrogen therapy to treat menopausal symptoms such as hot flashes, she may also receive some protection against bone loss and fractures of the hip and vertebrae.[36] Estrogen is believed to inhibit osteoclast activity, leading to decreased bone resorption and preventing loss of cortical and trabecular bone.

Bisphosphonates inhibit osteoclast-mediated bone resorption and slow the cycle of bone remodeling. Although a modest increase in BMD is typical, bone remodeling may be suppressed to the extent that normal bone formation is impaired and fracture risk increases. These drugs are widely used in the prevention and treatment of osteoporosis[37] (Table 63-13). Common side effects are anorexia, weight loss, and gastritis. Teach the patient to take the medication correctly to improve its absorption (see Drug Alert). These precautions have also been shown to decrease GI side effects (especially esophageal irritation). A rare and serious side effect of bisphosphonates is *osteonecrosis* (bone death) of the jaw. Its etiology is unknown. However, patients with dental disease, cancer, Paget's disease, or renal disease are most at risk for this complication. Patients should be evaluated by a dentist before beginning treatment and then annually to ensure good oral health.

 DRUG ALERT Bisphosphonates

Instruct patient to:
- Take with full glass of water.
- Take 30 min before food or other medications.
- Remain upright for at least 30 min after taking.

Alendronate (Fosamax) is available as a daily or weekly oral tablet. Ibandronate (Boniva) is available as a once-per-month oral tablet or can be given every 3 months by IV infusion. The immediate-release form of risedronate (Actonel) is given daily, weekly, or monthly based on the dose. Zoledronic acid (Reclast) is approved as a once-yearly IV infusion to treat osteoporosis, or is given every 2 years to prevent the disease. Renal function tests and serum calcium must be assessed before administration of the drug. Other bisphosphonates are identified in Table 63-13.

Calcitonin is secreted by the thyroid gland and inhibits bone resorption by directly interacting with active osteoclasts. Salmon calcitonin is available in IM, subcutaneous, and intranasal forms. Administration of the IM or subcutaneous form of the drug at night has been shown to decrease associated side effects of nausea and facial flushing. Nausea does not occur with the nasal spray. If patients are using the nasal form, teach them to alternate nostrils daily. Nasal dryness and irritation are the most frequent side effects. Calcium supplementation is needed to prevent secondary hyperparathyroidism.

Raloxifene (Evista) is a selective estrogen receptor modulator (SERM). This drug mimics the effect of estrogen on bone by reducing bone resorption without stimulating the tissues of the breast or uterus. Raloxifene in postmenopausal women significantly increases BMD. Side effects included leg cramps, hot flashes, and blood clots. Raloxifene may decrease breast cancer risk. Similar to tamoxifen, it blocks the estrogen receptor sites.

Teriparatide (Forteo) is a recombinant form of human parathyroid hormone (PTH) that increases the action of osteoblasts. This drug is used to treat osteoporosis in men and postmenopausal women at high risk for fractures, including risk related to long-term corticosteroid use. Side effects include leg cramps and dizziness. Teriparatide is the first drug approved to stimulate new bone formation in osteoporosis; most drugs only prevent further bone loss. It is self-administered daily by subcutaneous injection from a preloaded pen.

Denosumab (Prolia) may be used for postmenopausal women with osteoporosis who are at high risk for fractures. It is a monoclonal antibody that binds to a protein (RANKL) involved in the formation and function of osteoclasts. Denosumab is given by a health care professional as a subcutaneous injection every 6 months.

Medical management of patients receiving corticosteroids includes prescribing the lowest effective dose for the shortest possible time. Ensure an adequate intake of calcium and vitamin D, including supplementation when osteoporosis drugs are prescribed. If osteopenia is evident on bone densitometry in people who are taking corticosteroids, treatment with bisphosphonates may be considered.

PAGET'S DISEASE

Paget's disease (*osteitis deformans*) is a chronic skeletal bone disorder in which excessive bone resorption is followed by replacement of normal marrow by vascular, fibrous connective tissue. The new bone is larger, disorganized, and weaker. Commonly affected areas of the skeleton include pelvis, long bones, spine, ribs, sternum, and cranium. Up to 5% of adults in the United States are affected by Paget's disease.[38] The etiology is unknown, although a viral cause has been proposed. Up to 40% of all patients with Paget's disease have at least one relative with the disorder. Men are affected twice as often as women.

In milder forms of Paget's disease, patients may remain free of symptoms. The disease may be discovered incidentally through x-ray or serum chemistry findings of high alkaline phosphatase.[39] Bone pain may develop gradually and progress to severe intractable pain. Other early manifestations include fatigue and progressive development of a waddling gait. Patients may complain they are becoming shorter or their heads are becoming larger. Headaches, dementia, visual deficits, and loss of hearing can result from an enlarged, thickened skull. Increased bone volume in the spine can cause spinal cord or nerve root compression.

Pathologic fracture is the most common complication and may be the first indication of Paget's disease. Other complications include osteosarcoma, fibrosarcoma, and osteoclastoma (giant cell) tumors.

Serum alkaline phosphatase is markedly elevated in advanced disease, indicating high bone turnover.[40] X-rays may show curvature of an affected bone. The bone cortex becomes thicker and irregular, especially in weight-bearing bones and the cranium. Bone scans using a radiolabeled bisphosphonate demonstrate increased uptake in the affected skeletal areas.

Interprofessional care of Paget's disease is usually limited to symptomatic and supportive care with correction of secondary deformities by surgical intervention or braces. Bisphosphonate drugs (Table 63-13) are used to retard bone resorption. Zoledronic acid may be given specifically to build bone. Calcium and vitamin D are often given to decrease hypocalcemia, a common side effect with these drugs. Monitor drug effectiveness by regular assessment of serum alkaline phosphatase.

Calcitonin is recommended for patients who cannot tolerate bisphosphonates. Human calcitonin inhibits osteoclastic activity, prevents bone resorption, relieves acute symptoms, and lowers serum alkaline phosphatase. This drug is available as a subcutaneous injection. Salmon calcitonin can also be used to treat Paget's disease. It has a longer half-life and greater milligram potency than human calcitonin. Response to calcitonin therapy is not permanent and often stops when therapy is discontinued.

Pain is usually managed by NSAIDs. Orthopedic surgery for fractures, hip and knee replacement, and knee realignment may be needed.

A firm mattress should be used to provide back support and relieve pain. The patient may need to wear a corset or light brace to relieve back pain and provide support when upright. Teach the patient to correctly apply the device and regularly examine the skin for friction damage. Discourage lifting and twisting. Good body mechanics are essential. Physical therapy may increase muscle strength. A well-balanced diet is important in management of metabolic bone disorders. Vitamin D, calcium, and protein are especially important to ensure available components for bone formation. To decrease risk for falls and related fractures, teach the patient to use an assistive device and make environmental changes (e.g., eliminate throw rugs).

 SAFETY ALERT   **Paget's Disease**

To reduce the risk of patient harm from falls:
- Evaluate environmental fall risk factors.
- Identify personal risk factors for falls, including drugs and uncorrected vision.
- Take action to address any identified risks.

 Gerontologic Considerations: Metabolic Bone Diseases

Osteoporosis and Paget's disease are common in older adults. Instruct patients in proper nutrition to decrease risk for further bone loss. Keep the patient as active as possible to slow demineralization of bone from disuse or extended immobilization.

Because metabolic bone disorders increase the possibility of pathologic fractures, use extreme caution when turning or moving the patient. Hip fractures in particular may decrease quality of life and lead to admission to a long-term care facility. A supervised exercise program is essential to osteoporosis treatment. Encourage ambulation if the patient's condition permits.

CASE STUDY

Metastatic Bone Tumor/Pathologic Fracture

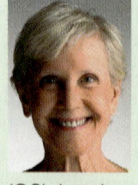

(©Christopher-Robbins/ Photodisc/ Thinkstock)

Patient Profile

L.R. is a 60-yr-old white woman with a history of hypertension, hypothyroidism, and osteoporosis. Four years ago she was diagnosed with Stage 3a breast cancer and treated with surgery, radiation therapy, and chemotherapy. Today she was admitted to the emergency department after a fall down two stairs.

Subjective Data

- Denies hitting her head or loss of consciousness
- States she was able to bear weight on her lower extremities but complains of significant left thigh pain after the fall
- Describes recent insidious onset of generalized weakness and fatigue

- Denies alcohol or tobacco use
- Takes levothyroxine (Synthroid) and atenolol (Tenormin) every morning. Takes ibandronate (Boniva) once a month

Objective Data

- Left lower extremity slightly shorter and externally rotated compared to right lower extremity
- Moderate edema with associated ecchymosis on left thigh
- Thigh soft, compressible to palpation
- Complains of pain with axial loading and internal/external rotation of left lower extremity
- Palpable dorsalis pedis and posterior tibialis pulses bilaterally
- Gross motor/sensation intact in all distributions in distal affected extremity

CASE STUDY

Metastatic Bone Tumor/Pathologic Fracture—cont'd

Diagnostic Studies

- X-ray reveals oblique mid-shaft left femur fracture with lytic lesion in the femoral neck
- Normal CBC and blood chemistry results, slightly elevated liver function tests
- CT scans of the chest, abdomen, and pelvis demonstrate multiple bony metastases throughout the pelvis as well as lesions of the liver and spleen, widespread abdominal cancer, compression fractures with lesions of T11 vertebral body, and bilateral rib fractures with associated lesions.
- Whole body bone scan consistent with findings from x-ray and CT
- CT-guided biopsy of femur fracture site showed poorly differentiated cells consistent with breast cancer

Interprofessional Care

- Diagnosed with stage IV breast cancer
- Intramedullary (IM) nail for femur fracture
- Pain management
- Postoperative chemotherapy and hormone therapy
- High-protein, high-calcium, nutrient-rich diet
- Depression assessment and management
- Ambulation evaluation with gait aids as needed

Discussion Questions

1. Why did a relatively low-energy injury cause L.R's fracture?
2. *Patient-Centered Care:* What factors could result in inadequate caloric intake postoperatively? How could you help L.R. increase her intake of protein and calcium?
3. What factors increase L.R.'s risk for delayed union or nonunion of the fracture?
4. *Priority Decision:* What are the priority teaching needs for L.R.?
5. *Teamwork and Collaboration:* Which personnel on the interprofessional team should be responsible for L.R.'s postoperative home care instructions? Who should be responsible for ambulation and home safety teaching and assessments? Who should assist L.R. with transfers and ambulation during her hospital stay?
6. *Priority Decision:* Based on the assessment data, what are the priority nursing diagnoses?
7. *Quality Improvement:* What outcomes would indicate that interprofessional care was effective?
8. *Safety:* What safety precautions should be considered for this patient?
9. *Evidence-Based Practice:* L.R asks why it is important for her to have daily injections of enoxaparin after surgery. How do you respond?

Answers available at *http://evolve.elsevier.com/Lewis/medsurg*.

BRIDGE TO NCLEX EXAMINATION

The number of the question corresponds to the same-numbered outcome at the beginning of the chapter.

1. A patient with osteomyelitis undergoes surgical debridement with implantation of antibiotic beads. When the patient asks why the beads are used, the nurse answers *(select all that apply)*
   a. "Oral or IV antibiotics are not effective in most cases of bone infection."
   b. "The beads are an adjunct to debridement and antibiotics for deep infections."
   c. "The beads are used to deliver antibiotics directly to the site of the infection."
   d. "This is the safest method to deliver long-term antibiotic therapy for bone infection."
   e. "Ischemia and bone death related to osteomyelitis are impenetrable to IV antibiotics."

2. A patient diagnosed with osteosarcoma of the humerus demonstrates understanding of his treatment options when he states
   a. "I accept that I have to lose my arm with surgery."
   b. "The chemotherapy before surgery will shrink the tumor."
   c. "This tumor is related to the melanoma I had 3 years ago."
   d. "I'm glad they can take out the cancer with such a small scar."

3. Which individuals would be at high risk for low back pain *(select all that apply)*?
   a. A 63-year-old man who is a long-distance truck driver
   b. A 36-year-old construction worker who is 6 ft 2 in and weighs 260 lb
   c. A 44-year-old female chef with prior compression fracture of the spine
   d. A 30-year-old nurse who works on an orthopedic unit and smokes
   e. A 28-year-old female yoga instructor who is 5 ft 6 in and weighs 130 lb

4. A patient with suspected disc herniation is experiencing acute pain and muscle spasms. The nurse's responsibility is to
   a. encourage total bed rest for several days.
   b. teach principles of back strengthening exercises.
   c. stress the importance of straight-leg raises to decrease pain.
   d. promote use of cold and hot compresses and pain medication.

5. In caring for a patient after a spinal fusion, the nurse would immediately report which of the following to the surgeon?
   a. The patient experiences a single episode of emesis.
   b. The patient is unable to move the lower extremities.
   c. The patient is nauseated and has not voided in 4 hours.
   d. The patient complains of pain at the bone graft donor site.

6. A patient who has had surgical correction of bilateral hallux valgus is being discharged from the same-day surgery unit. The nurse will instruct the patient to
   a. expect continued pain in the feet.
   b. rest frequently with the feet elevated.
   c. soak the feet in warm water several times a day.
   d. expect the feet to be numb for the next few days.

7. What is important to include in the teaching plan for a patient with osteopenia?
   a. Lose weight.
   b. Stop smoking.
   c. Eat a high-protein diet.
   d. Start swimming for exercise.

1. b, c, 2. b, 3. a, b, c, d, 4. d, 5. b, 6. b, 7. b

For rationales to these answers and even more NCLEX review questions, visit *http://evolve.elsevier.com/Lewis/medsurg*.

REFERENCES

1. Huether S, McCance K: *Understanding pathophysiology*, ed 5, St Louis, 2012, Mosby.

2. Beck-Broichsitter BE, Smeets R, Heiland M: Current concepts in pathogenesis of acute and chronic osteomyelitis, *Curr Opin Infect Dis* 28(3):240, 2015.

3. Schmitt S: Osteomyelitis. Retrieved from *www.merckmanuals.com/ professional/musculoskeletal-and-connective-tissue-disorders/infections-of- joints-and-bones/osteomyelitis#*.

4. Lehne R: *Pharmacology for nursing care*, ed 8, St Louis, 2013, Saunders.

5. Lima ALL, Oliveira PR, Carvalho VC, et al: Recommendations for the treatment of osteomyelitis, *Braz J Infect Dis* 18:526, 2014.

6. Siegel R, Naishadham D, Jemal A: Cancer statistics, *CA Cancer J Clin* 63:11, 2013.

7. Luetke A, Meyers PA, Lewis I, et al: Osteosarcoma treatment—Where do we stand? A state of the art review, *Canc Treat Rev* 40:523, 2014.

8. American Cancer Society: What is metastasis? Retrieved from *www.cancer.org/treatment/understandingyourdiagnosis/bonemetastasis/ bone-metastasis-what-is-bone-mets*.

9. Leung DG, Herzka DA, Thompson WR, et al: Sildenafil does not improve cardiomyopathy in Duchenne/Becker muscular dystrophy, *Ann Neur* 76:541, 2014.

10. Ruegg UT: Pharmacological prospects in the treatment of Duchenne muscular dystrophy, *Curr Op Neur* 26:577, 2013.

11. National Institute of Neurological Disorders and Stroke: Low back pain fact sheet. Retrieved from *www.ninds.nih.gov/disorders/backpain/ detail_backpain.htm*.

12. Lee S-J, Faucett J, Gillen M, et al: Musculoskeletal pain among critical-care nurses by availability and use of patient lifting equipment: an analysis of cross-sectional survey data, *Internat J Nurs Stud* 50:1648, 2013.

13. Knight CL, Deyo RA, Staiger TO, et al: Treatment of acute low back pain. Retrieved from *www.uptodate.com/contents/treatment-of-acute -low-back-pain?source=search_result&search=acute+back+pain&selectedTi tle=2~145*.

14. Becker JA, Stumbo JR: Back pain in adults, *Prim Care Clin Office Pract* 40:271, 2013.

15. Webster LR, Markman J: Medical management of chronic low back pain: efficacy and outcomes, *Neuromodulation* 17(Suppl 2):18, 2014.

16. Cleveland Clinic: Degenerative back conditions. Retrieved from *http://my.clevelandclinic.org/services/orthopaedics-rheumatology/ diseases-conditions/degenerative-back-conditions*.

17. American Academy of Orthopaedic Surgeons: Cauda equina syndrome. Retrieved from *http://orthoinfo.aaos.org/topic.cfm?topic=A00362&grpwebi d=20DEEB*.

18. Mayo Clinic: Herniated disc: Treatment and drugs. Retrieved from *www.mayoclinic.org/diseases-conditions/herniated-disk/basics/treatment/ con-20029957*.

*19. Phillips FM, Lee JYB, Geisler FH, et al: A prospective, randomized, controlled clinical investigation comparing PCM cervical disc arthroplasty with anterior cervical discectomy and fusion: 2-year results from the US FDA IDE Clinical Trial, *Spine* 38:E907, 2013.

20. Bae HW, Rajaee SS, Kanim LE: Nationwide trends in the surgical management of lumbar spinal stenosis, *Spine* 38:916, 2013.

21. Isaac Z: Evaluation of the patient with neck pain and cervical spine disorders. Retrieved from *www.uptodate.com/contents/evaluation-of-the -patient-with-neck-pain-and-cervical-spine-disorders?source=search_result &search=neck+pain&selectedTitle=1~150*.

*22. Gross A, Kay TM, Paquin JP, et al: Exercises for mechanical neck disorders, *Cochrane Library* Pub No. 10.1002/14651858.CD004250. pub5, 2015.

23. Fields KB: Evaluation and diagnosis of common causes of foot pain in adults. Retrieved from *www.uptodate.com/contents/evaluation-and -diagnosis-of-common-causes-of-foot-pain-in-adults?source=search_result &search=hammer+toe&selectedTitle=1~8*.

24. Edmonds ME, Foster AVM: *Managing the diabetic foot*, West Sussex, UK, 2014, Wiley Blackwell.

25. Stolt M, Suhonen R, Puukka P et al: Nurses' foot care activities in home health care, *Geriatric Nurs* 34:491, 2013.

26. Liu C, Wu D, Zhang J-F, et al: Changes in bone metabolism in morbidly obese patients after bariatric surgery: a meta-analysis, *Obes Surg* 26(1):91, 2016.

27. Blann A: An update on vitamin D deficiency and at risk groups, *J Fam Health* 25(3):16, 2015.

28. National Osteoporosis Foundation: Debunking the myths. Retrieved from *http://nof.org/OPmyths*.

*29. US Preventive Services Task Force: Screening for osteoporosis: systematic review to update the 2002 US Preventive Services Task Force recommendations. Retrieved from *www.ncbi.nlm.nih.gov/books/ NBK45201*.

30. Cleveland Clinic: Osteoporosis. Retrieved from *http://my.clevelandclinic .org/health/diseases_conditions/hic_Osteoporosis*.

31. Adams JE: Advances in bone imaging for osteoporosis, *Nat Rev Endocrinol* 9:28, 2013.

32. Lewiecki EM: Osteoporotic fracture risk assessment. Retrieved from *www.uptodate.com/contents/osteoporotic-fracture-risk-assessment?source =machineLearning&search=frax&selectedTitle=1~19&sectionRank=3&anc hor=H17#*.

33. Florence R, Allen S, Benedict L, et al: Diagnosis and treatment of osteoporosis. Retrieved from *www.guideline.gov/content.aspx?id=47543& search=osteoporosis*.

34. Golob AL, Laya MB: Osteoporosis: screening, prevention, and management, *Med Clin North Am* 99(3):587, 2015.

35. Wong CC, McGirt MJ: Vertebral compression fractures: a review of current management and multimodal therapy, *J Multidisc Health* 6:205, 2013.

36. Schmidt P: The 2012 hormone therapy position statement of the North American Menopause Society, *Menopause* 19:257, 2012.

37. Gatti D, Adami S, Viapiana O, et al: The use of bisphosphonates in women: when to use and when to stop, *Expert Opin Pharmacother* 11:1, 2015.

38. Ralston SH: Paget's disease of bone, *NEJM* 368:644, 2013.

39. White G, Rushbrook J: Paget's disease of bone, *Orthop Trauma* 27:254, 2013.

40. Pagana KD, Pagana TJ: *Mosby's manual of diagnostic and laboratory tests*, ed 5, St Louis, 2014, Mosby.

*Evidence-based information for clinical practice.

64

Arthritis and Connective Tissue Diseases

Dottie Roberts

Failure will never overtake me if my determination to succeed is strong enough.

Og Mandino

e http://evolve.elsevier.com/Lewis/medsurg/

LEARNING OUTCOMES

1. Compare and contrast the sequence of events leading to joint destruction in osteoarthritis and rheumatoid arthritis.
2. Detail the clinical manifestations, interprofessional care, and nursing management of osteoarthritis and rheumatoid arthritis.
3. Describe the pathophysiology, clinical manifestations, and interprofessional care of gout, Lyme disease, and septic arthritis.
4. Summarize the pathophysiology, clinical manifestations, interprofessional care, and nursing management of ankylosing spondylitis, psoriatic arthritis, and reactive arthritis.

5. Differentiate the pathophysiology, clinical manifestations, interprofessional care, and nursing management of systemic lupus erythematosus, scleroderma, polymyositis, dermatomyositis, and Sjögren's syndrome.
6. Explain the drug therapy and related nursing management associated with arthritis and connective tissue diseases.
7. Compare and contrast possible etiologies, clinical manifestations, and interprofessional and nursing management of fibromyalgia and systemic exertion tolerance disease.

KEY TERMS

ankylosing spondylitis (AS), p. 1536
arthritis, p. 1517
CREST syndrome, p. 1542
dermatomyositis (DM), p. 1544
fibromyalgia, p. 1546
gout, p. 1532
Lyme disease, p. 1534

myofascial pain syndrome, p. 1546
osteoarthritis (OA), p. 1517
polymyositis (PM), p. 1544
psoriatic arthritis (PsA), p. 1537
Raynaud's phenomenon, p. 1543
rheumatoid arthritis (RA), p. 1525
septic arthritis, p. 1535

scleroderma, p. 1542
Sjögren's syndrome, p. 1546
spondyloarthropathies, p. 1536
systemic exertion intolerance disease
(SEID), p. 1548
systemic lupus erythematosus (SLE), p. 1538

This chapter discusses *rheumatic diseases,* which primarily affect body joints, tendons, ligaments, muscles, and bones. These diseases are often characterized by inflammation and loss of function in one or more of the body's connecting or supporting structures. More than 100 kinds of rheumatic diseases have been identified.[1] An estimated 52.5 million people in the United States have rheumatic conditions.[2]

ARTHRITIS

Arthritis, a type of rheumatic disease, involves inflammation of a joint or joints. Most forms of arthritis affect women more frequently than men in every age group.[2] Osteoarthritis is the most common form of joint disease in the world.[3] Other forms that occur often include rheumatoid arthritis, fibromyalgia, systemic lupus erythematosus, and gout.

OSTEOARTHRITIS

Osteoarthritis (OA) is a slowly progressive noninflammatory disorder of the diarthrodial *(synovial)* joints. Currently 27 million Americans are affected by OA, with the numbers expected to greatly increase as the population ages.[4]

Etiology and Pathophysiology

OA involves the gradual loss of articular cartilage with formation of bony outgrowths *(osteophytes)* at the joint margins.[3] OA is not considered a normal part of the aging process, but aging is one risk factor for disease development.[4] Cartilage destruction may actually begin between ages 20 and 30, and the majority of adults are affected by age 40. Few patients experience symptoms until after age 50 or 60, but more than half of those over age 65 have x-ray evidence of OA in at least

Reviewed by Judy Carlyle, RN, MNSc, Faculty/Clinical Liaison, Arkansas Rural Nursing Education Consortium (ARNEC), Nashville, Arkansas; Kim Clevenger, RN, EdD, BC, Associate Professor of Nursing and BSN Program Coordinator, Morehead State University, Morehead, Kentucky; Michele M. Hughes, RN, MSN, ACNP, ONP-C, Nurse Practitioner, Bon Secours Memorial Regional Medical Center, Mechanicsville, Virginia; and Diane Ryzner, MSN, APN, CNS, OCNS-C, Advanced Practice Nurse, Northwest Community Hospital, Arlington Heights, Illinois.

TABLE 64-1 Causes of Osteoarthritis

Cause	Effects on Joint Cartilage
Trauma	Dislocations or fractures may lead to avascular necrosis or uneven stress on cartilage.
Mechanical stress	Repetitive physical activities (e.g., sports) cause cartilage deterioration.
Inflammation	Release of enzymes in response to local inflammation can affect cartilage health.
Joint instability	Damage to supporting structures causes instability, placing uneven stress on joint cartilage.
Neurologic disorders	Pain and loss of reflexes from neurologic disorders, such as diabetic neuropathy and Charcot joint, cause abnormal movements that contribute to cartilage deterioration.
Skeletal deformities	Congenital or acquired conditions such as Legg-Calvé-Perthes disease or dislocated hip contribute to cartilage deterioration.
Hematologic or endocrine disorders	Chronic hemarthrosis (e.g., from hemophilia) contributes to cartilage deterioration.
Drugs	Drugs such as indomethacin (Indocin), colchicine, and corticosteroids can stimulate collagen-digesting enzymes in joint synovium.

one joint. After age 50 years, women are affected by OA more often than men.[5]

OA may be caused by a known event or condition that directly damages cartilage or causes joint instability (Table 64-1). However, many persons with OA cannot identify a single cause. In these situations, subtle congenital or genetic cartilage defects may be present.

Decreased estrogen at menopause may contribute to the increased incidence of OA in aging women. Obesity is a modifiable risk factor that contributes to hip and knee OA by increasing the mechanical stress on the joints. Regular moderate exercise, which also helps with weight management, decreases the risk for disease development and progression. Anterior cruciate ligament injury from quick stops and pivoting, as in football and soccer, has been linked to an increased risk for knee OA.[6] Occupations that require frequent kneeling and stooping also increase the risk for knee OA.

The development of OA is complex. Genetic, metabolic, and local factors interact to cause cartilage deterioration from damage at the level of the chondrocytes (Fig. 64-1). The normally smooth, white, translucent articular cartilage becomes dull, yellow, and granular as the disease progresses. Affected

GENDER DIFFERENCES

Osteoarthritis (OA)

Men
- Except for traumatic arthritis, men do not experience OA as often as women until age 70 or 80 years.
- Hip OA is more common in men than in women.

Women
- Women are affected more often than men.
- Hand OA (interphalangeal joints and thumb base) is more common in women than in men.
- Knee OA is more common in women than in men, especially after menopause, and is likely to be more severe.

cartilage steadily becomes softer and less elastic. It is less able to resist wear with heavy use.

The body's attempts at cartilage repair cannot keep up with the destruction of OA. As the collagen structure of the cartilage changes, articular surfaces become cracked and worn. While central cartilage becomes thinner, cartilage at the joint edges becomes thicker and osteophytes form. Joint surfaces become uneven, affecting the distribution of stress across the joint and causing reduced motion.

Although inflammation is not typical of OA, secondary synovitis may occur when phagocytes try to rid the joint of small pieces of cartilage torn from the joint surface. These changes cause the early pain and stiffness of OA. Pain in later disease occurs when articular cartilage is lost and bony joint surfaces rub on each other.

Clinical Manifestations

Systemic. Fatigue, fever, and organ involvement are not present in OA. This is an important distinction between OA and inflammatory joint disorders such as rheumatoid arthritis.

Joints. Manifestations of OA range from mild discomfort to significant disability. Joint pain is the primary symptom and the typical reason the patient seeks medical attention. Pain generally gets worse with joint use. In early stages of OA, joint pain is relieved by rest. However, the patient with advanced disease may complain of pain at rest or have trouble sleeping due to increased joint pain. Pain may also worsen as the barometric pressure falls before the onset of severe weather.

As OA progresses, increasing pain can contribute greatly to disability and loss of function. The pain of OA may be referred to the groin, buttock, or the outside of the thigh or knee. Sitting down becomes difficult, as does rising from a chair when the hips are lower than the knees. As OA develops in the intervertebral *(apophyseal)* joints of the spine, local pain and stiffness are common.

Unlike pain, which typically worsens with activity, joint stiffness occurs after periods of rest or an unchanged position. Early morning stiffness is common but generally resolves within 30 minutes. This factor distinguishes OA from inflammatory arthritic disorders such as rheumatoid arthritis. Overactivity can cause a mild joint swelling that temporarily increases stiffness. *Crepitation,* a grating sensation caused by loose cartilage particles in the joint cavity, can also cause stiffness. Crepitation is common in patients with knee OA.

OA usually affects joints on one side of the body *(asymmetrically)* rather than in pairs. For example, the left knee may be affected and the right knee unchanged. The distal interphalangeal (DIP) and proximal interphalangeal (PIP) joints of the fingers, and the metacarpophalangeal (MCP) joint of the thumb are often affected. Weight-bearing joints (hips, knees), the metatarsophalangeal (MTP) joint of the foot, and the cervical and lower lumbar vertebrae are also commonly involved (Fig. 64-2).

Deformity. Deformity or instability associated with OA is specific to the involved joint. For example, *Heberden's nodes* occur on the DIP joints due to osteophyte formation and loss of joint space (Fig. 64-1, *D*). They can appear as early as age 40 and tend to be seen in family members. *Bouchard's nodes* on the PIP joints indicate similar disease involvement. Heberden's and Bouchard's nodes are often red, swollen, and tender. Although they usually do not cause significant loss of function, the patient may be bothered by the visible deformity.

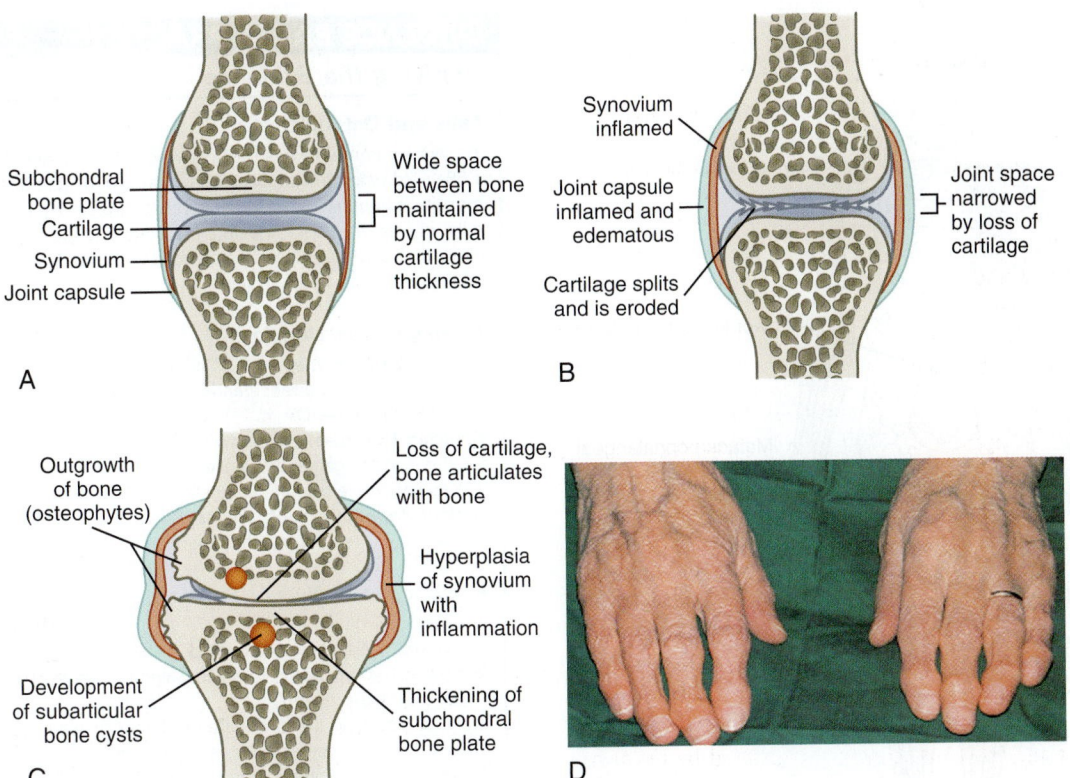

FIG. 64-1 Pathologic changes in osteoarthritis. **A,** Normal synovial joint. **B,** Early change in osteoarthritis is destruction of articular cartilage and narrowing of the joint space. There is inflammation and thickening of the joint capsule and synovium. **C,** With time, thickening of subarticular bone occurs, caused by constant friction of the two bone surfaces. Osteophytes form around the periphery of the joint by irregular overgrowths of bone. **D,** In osteoarthritis of the hands, osteophytes on the distal interphalangeal joints of the fingers, termed *Heberden's nodes,* appear as small nodules. (*D,* From Forbes CD, Jackson WF: *Color atlas and text of clinical medicine,* ed 3, London, 2003, Mosby.)

Knee OA often leads to obvious joint deformity as a result of cartilage loss in one joint compartment. For example, the patient becomes bowlegged *(varus deformity)* in response to medial joint arthritis. Lateral joint arthritis causes a knock-kneed appearance *(valgus deformity)*. In advanced hip OA, one of the patient's legs may become shorter as the joint space narrows.

Diagnostic Studies

A bone scan, CT scan, or MRI may be used to diagnose OA. These tests are able to detect early joint changes. X-rays are helpful in confirming disease and staging joint damage. As OA progresses, x-rays often show joint space narrowing and increasingly dense bone. Osteophytes are also visible. However, these changes do not always reflect the degree of pain the patient experiences. Despite strong x-ray evidence of disease, the patient may be relatively free of symptoms. On the other hand, another patient may have severe pain with only slight x-ray changes.

No laboratory tests or biomarkers can be used to diagnose OA. The erythrocyte sedimentation rate (ESR) is normal except during acute inflammation, when slight elevations may be seen. Other routine blood tests (e.g., complete blood count [CBC], renal and liver function tests) are useful only in screening for related conditions or for establishing baseline values before starting treatment. Synovial fluid analysis helps distinguish between OA and types of inflammatory arthritis. In OA, the fluid remains clear yellow with little or no sign of inflammation.

Interprofessional Care

Because OA has no cure, interprofessional care focuses on managing pain and inflammation, preventing disability, and maintaining and improving joint function (Table 64-2). Nondrug interventions are the basis for OA management. They should be maintained throughout the patient's treatment. Drug therapy supplements nondrug treatments.

Rest and Joint Protection. Teach the patient with OA to balance rest and activity. Rest the affected joint during any periods of acute inflammation. Keep it in a functional position with splints or braces if needed. However, avoid immobilization of more than 1 week because of the risk of joint stiffness with inactivity. Modify usual activities to decrease stress on affected joints. Teach the patient with knee OA to avoid standing, kneeling, or squatting for long periods of time. Using an assistive device such as a cane, walker, or crutches can also decrease joint stress.

Heat and Cold Applications. Apply heat and cold to help reduce pain and stiffness. Ice is not used as often as heat in OA treatment, but it can be helpful if the patient has acute inflammation. Heat therapy is especially useful for stiffness. Treatments include hot packs, whirlpool baths, ultrasound, and paraffin wax baths.

Nutritional Therapy and Exercise. If the patient is overweight, a weight-reduction program is a critical part of the treatment plan. Help the patient evaluate the current diet to make needed changes. (Chapter 40 discusses ways to assist the patient in attaining and maintaining a healthy body weight.) Because

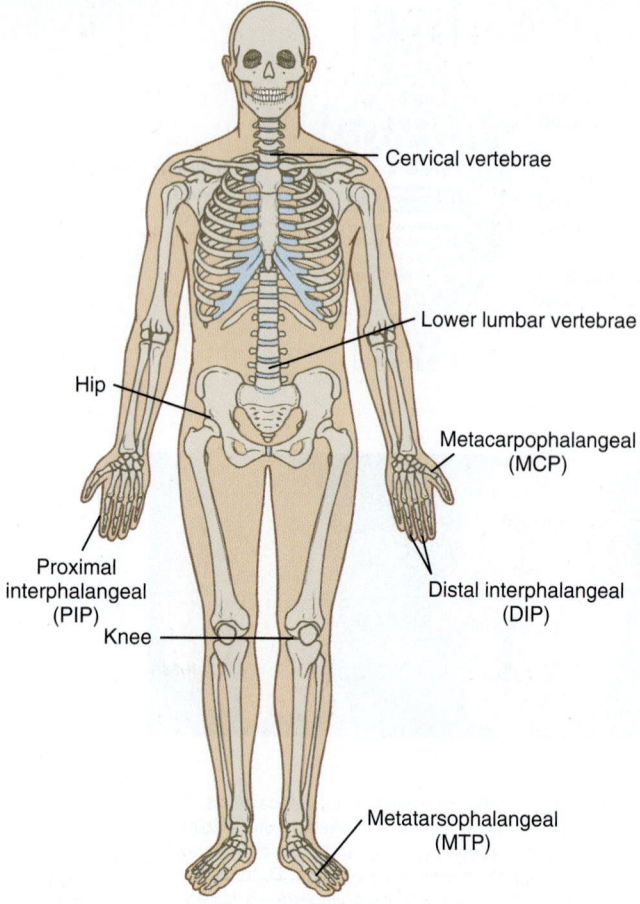

Cervical vertebrae

Lower lumbar vertebrae

Hip

Metacarpophalangeal
(MCP)

Proximal
interphalangeal
(PIP)

Distal interphalangeal
(DIP)

Knee

Metatarsophalangeal
(MTP)

FIG. 64-2 Joints most frequently involved in osteoarthritis.

TABLE 64-2   Interprofessional Care

Osteoarthritis

Diagnostic Assessment
- History and physical examination
- Radiologic studies of involved joints (e.g., x-ray, CT scan, MRI, bone scan)
- Synovial fluid analysis

Management
- Nutritional and weight management counseling
- Rest and joint protection, use of assistive devices
- Therapeutic exercise
- Heat and cold applications
- Complementary and alternative therapies
  - Herbs and nutritional supplements (e.g., fish oil, ginger, Sam-e)
  - Movement therapies (e.g., yoga, Tai Chi)
  - Acupuncture
  - Massage
- Transcutaneous electrical nerve stimulation (TENS)
- Reconstructive joint surgery

Drug Therapy *(Table 64-3)*
- acetaminophen
- Nonsteroidal antiinflammatory drugs
- Intraarticular corticosteroids

loading and mobilizing the joint are needed to preserve articular cartilage health, exercise is an important part of OA management.[7] Aerobic conditioning, range-of-motion (ROM) exercises, and programs for quadriceps strengthening have been helpful for many patients with knee OA.

EVIDENCE-BASED PRACTICE
Applying the Evidence

Falls and Osteoarthritis

You are a community health nurse who is starting home visits with R.F., a 68-yr-old woman with OA. Today during your visit she states that her mobility is becoming more limited due to worsening knee pain. R.F. also tells you that her pain is being "somewhat controlled" by acetaminophen and capsaicin cream. She misses physical activity and is now concerned about falling in her home.

Making Clinical Decisions

Best Available Evidence. Tai Chi, aerobic exercise, and strength training improve balance and reduce the risk of falling in older adults with knee OA.

Clinician Expertise. You know that arthritic knee pain can cause alterations in gait and balance that may increase the risk of falling. You know exercise and education are important in reducing falls.

Patient Preferences and Values. R.F. is interested in learning what she can do to decrease her chances of falling.

Implications for Nursing Practice

1. What information will you share with her about physical activities that may help to reduce her risk of falling?
2. How will you assist R.F. in accessing resources that will increase her physical activity?
3. What factors in the home are important to assess on your initial visit that may increase her risk of falling?
4. How will you facilitate ongoing communication with R.F's HCP to ensure satisfactory pain relief?

References for Evidence

Mat S, Tan M, Kamaruzzaman SB, et al: Physical therapies for improving balance and reducing falls risk in osteoarthritis of the knee: a systematic review, *Age Ageing* 44:16, 2015.
National Arthritis Foundation: Retrieved from *www.arthritistoday.org/about-arthritis/types-of-arthritis/osteoarthritis/daily-life/osteoarthritis-and-falls.php*.

Complementary and Alternative Therapies. Complementary and alternative therapies for OA symptom management are popular with patients who have not found relief through traditional medical care. Teach the patient to carefully research any alternative therapies and avoid replacing conventional OA treatments with unproven complementary approaches.[8] Acupuncture may reduce arthritis pain and improve joint mobility. Massage and Tai Chi may also reduce pain and improve function. Some nutritional supplements may have antiinflammatory effects (e.g., fish oil, ginger, Sam-e). However, results of studies on glucosamine and chondroitin are mixed. The American College of Rheumatology conditionally recommends that patients do not use glucosamine or chondroitin sulfate[7] (see the Complementary & Alternative Therapies boxes). Instruct patients to discuss any supplement use with their HCPs to identify possible interactions with prescribed medications.

Drug Therapy. Drug therapy is based on the severity of the patient's symptoms (Table 64-3). The patient with mild to moderate joint pain may get relief from acetaminophen (Tylenol).

A topical agent such as capsaicin cream may also be helpful, alone or with acetaminophen. It blocks pain by locally interfering with substance P, which is responsible for the transmission of pain impulses. A concentrated product is available by prescription, but creams of 0.025% to 0.075% capsaicin are available over the counter (OTC). Other OTC products that contain camphor, eucalyptus oil, and menthol (e.g., Bengay, Arthricare) may also provide temporary pain relief. Topical salicylates (e.g.,

TABLE 64-3   Drug Therapy
Arthritis and Connective Tissue Diseases

Drug	Mechanism of Action	Nursing Considerations
Salicylate aspirin, salicylate (salsalate)	Antiinflammatory Analgesic Fever reducer (antipyretic) Act by inhibiting prostaglandin synthesis	Administer with food, milk, antacids (as prescribed), or full glass of water. May use enteric-coated aspirin. Report signs of bleeding (e.g., tarry stools, bruising, petechiae, nosebleeds).
Nonsteroidal Antiinflammatory Drugs (NSAIDs) ibuprofen (Advil) naproxen (Aleve) ketoprofen piroxicam (Feldene) indomethacin (Indocin) sulindac tolmetin diclofenac meclofenamate nabumetone oxaprozin (Daypro) meloxicam (Mobic) celecoxib (Celebrex)	Antiinflammatory Analgesic Fever reducer (antipyretic) Act by inhibiting prostaglandin synthesis	Administer drug with food, milk, or antacids (as prescribed). Report signs of bleeding (e.g., tarry stools, bruising, petechiae, nosebleeds), edema, skin rashes, persistent headaches, visual disturbances. Monitor BP for elevations related to fluid retention. Must be used regularly for maximal effect.
Antibiotics doxycycline (Vibramycin) minocycline (Minocin)	Decreases action of enzymes on cartilage degradation Antirheumatic effect possibly related to immunomodulatory/antiinflammatory properties	Possible treatment alternative for mild disease.
Topical Analgesics capsaicin cream diclofenac sodium (Voltaren gel)	Depletes substance P from nerve endings, interrupting pain signals to the brain Antiinflammatory Analgesic	Must be used at regular intervals for maximal effect. Aloe vera cream may decrease burning sensation. Advise patient not to use cream with external heat source (heating pad) because of risk of burns. Available in OTC and prescriptive strengths. Advise patient to avoid sun and ultraviolet (UV) light exposure. Should not be used in combination with other oral NSAIDs or aspirin due to potential for increased side effects.
Corticosteroids *Intraarticular Injections* methylprednisolone acetate (Depo-Medrol) triamcinolone (Aristospan)	Antiinflammatory Analgesic Act by inhibiting synthesis and/or release of inflammatory mediators	Use strict aseptic technique for corticosteroid injection. Inform patient that joint may temporarily feel worse right after injection. Advise patient to avoid overusing affected joint immediately after injection. Inform patient improvement lasts weeks to months after injection.
Systemic hydrocortisone (Solu-Cortef) methylprednisolone (Solu-Medrol) dexamethasone prednisone triamcinolone	Antiinflammatory Analgesic Act by inhibiting synthesis and/or release of inflammatory mediators	Use only in life-threatening exacerbation or when symptoms persist after treatment with less potent antiinflammatory drugs. Administer for limited time only, tapering dose slowly. Be aware that exacerbation of symptoms occurs with abrupt withdrawal of drug. Monitor BP, weight, CBC, and serum potassium. Limit sodium intake. Report signs of infection.
Disease-Modifying Antirheumatic Drugs (DMARDs) methotrexate (Trexall) sulfasalazine (Azulfidine) leflunomide (Arava)	Antimetabolite Inhibits DNA, RNA, protein synthesis Sulfonamide Antiinflammatory Blocks prostaglandin synthesis Antiinflammatory Immunomodulatory agent that inhibits proliferation of lymphocytes	Monitor CBC and hepatic and renal function. Advise patient to report signs of anemia (fatigue, weakness). Keep patient well hydrated. Due to teratogenic effects, instruct female patient to use effective contraception during and 3 mo after treatment. Advise patient drug may cause orange-yellow discoloration of urine or skin. Space doses evenly around the clock, taking drug after food with 8 oz water. Treatment may be continued even after symptoms are relieved. Monitor CBC. Monitor hepatic function. Assess for decreased pain, swelling, stiffness, and increase in joint mobility. Advise women of childbearing age to avoid pregnancy.

Continued

TABLE 64-3 Drug Therapy
Arthritis and Connective Tissue Diseases—cont'd

Drug	Mechanism of Action	Nursing Considerations
Disease-Modifying Antirheumatic Drugs (DMARDs)—cont'd		
penicillamine (Cuprimine, Depen)	Antiinflammatory Exact mechanism unknown but may suppress cell-mediated immune response	Monitor WBC count, platelets, urinalysis. Advise patient to take medication 1 hr before or 2 hr after meals, and at least 1 hr away from any other drug, food, or milk.
Gold Compounds *Parenteral:* gold sodium thiomalate, aurothioglucose *Oral:* auranofin (Ridaura)	Alter immune responses, suppressing synovitis of active RA	Rule out pregnancy before beginning treatment. Monitor CBC, urinalysis, and hepatic and renal function. Advise patient therapeutic response may not occur for 3-6 mo. Advise patient to immediately report pruritus, rash, sore mouth, indigestion, or metallic taste.
Antimalarial hydroxychloroquine (Plaquenil)	Exact mechanism unknown but may suppress formation of antigens	Monitor CBC and hepatic function. Advise patient therapeutic response may not occur for up to 6 mo. Advise patient to immediately report visual difficulties, muscular weakness, and decreased hearing or tinnitus.
Immunosuppressants azathioprine (Imuran) cyclophosphamide	Inhibit DNA, RNA, protein synthesis	Assess for decreased pain, swelling, stiffness, and increase in joint mobility. Advise patient to immediately report unusual bleeding or bruising. Advise patient therapeutic response may take up to 12 wk. Advise women of childbearing age to avoid pregnancy. Encourage increased fluid intake to decrease risk of hemorrhagic cystitis.
mycophenolate mofetil (CellCept)	Inhibits DNA synthesis	Monitor blood count and liver function tests every 2-4 wk for first 3 mo of treatment, thereafter every 1-3 mo. Inform patient of increased infection risk. Instruct patients not to take antacids at same time because they may interfere with drug absorption.
JAK (Janus Kinase) Inhibitor tofacitinib (Xeljanz)	Inhibits action of JAK enzymes, signaling pathways inside the cell with an important role in inflammation of RA	Inform patient of increased infection risk, including opportunistic infections. Monitor patient for any sign or symptom of infection for early treatment.
Biologic Response Modifiers (Biologics, Immunotherapy)		
Tumor Necrosis Factor (TNF) Inhibitors etanercept (Enbrel) infliximab (Remicade) adalimumab (Humira) certolizumab (Cimzia) golimumab (Simponi)	Bind to TNF, thus blocking its interaction with cell surface receptors. Decrease inflammatory and immune responses	Assess for decreased pain, swelling, stiffness, and increase in joint mobility. Advise patient of increased risk for tuberculosis. Instruct patient to have yearly PPD. Monitor for infection, bleeding, and emergence of malignancies. Advise patient injection site reaction generally occurs in first month of treatment and decreases with continued therapy. Advise patient to not receive live virus vaccines during treatment.
Interleukin-1 Receptor Antagonist anakinra (Kineret)	Blocks the action of interleukin-1, decreasing inflammatory response	Assess for decreased pain, swelling, stiffness, and increase in joint mobility. Advise patient injection site reaction generally occurs in first month of treatment and decreases with continued therapy. Evaluate renal function. Monitor for infection. Inform patient to not take drug with TNF inhibitors.
Interleukin-6 Receptor Antagonist tocilizumab (Actemra)	Blocks action of interleukin-6, thus decreasing inflammatory response	Given to patients with RA for whom other therapies have failed. Monitor BP and for infection. Advise patient of GI effects (e.g., perforation). Monitor liver enzyme and serum low-density lipoprotein (LDL).
T Cell Activation Inhibitor abatacept (Orencia)	Inhibits T cell activation, thus suppressing immune response	Not recommended for concomitant use with TNF inhibitors. Assess for decreased pain, swelling, stiffness, and increase in joint mobility.
B Cell Depleting Agent rituximab (Rituxan)	Monoclonal antibody that binds to CD20, an antigen on B cells, destroying B cells and suppressing immune response	Monitor for infection and bleeding. Advise patient to not receive live virus vaccines with treatment. Monitor for low BP if also taking BP medication. Advise patient fatigue is common with this medication.

Acupuncture

Acupuncture is a traditional Chinese medical practice of inserting very fine needles into the skin to stimulate specific anatomic points in the body (called *acupoints*) for therapeutic purposes.

Scientific Evidence*

Acupuncture is associated with significant reduction in OA pain intensity, improved functional ability, and improved health-related quality of life.

Nursing Implications

- Research supports the use of acupuncture as an alternative for traditional analgesics in patients with OA.
- Refer interested patients to a practitioner who is appropriately trained and licensed.

*Source: Manyanga T, Froese M, Zarychanski R, et al: Pain management with acupuncture in osteoarthritis: a systematic review and meta-analysis, *BMC Comp Altern Med* 14:312, 2014.

Glucosamine and Chondroitin

Scientific Evidence*

- Combination of glucosamine plus chondroitin sulfate did not provide significant relief from OA pain among all participants.
- However, a smaller subgroup of study participants with moderate-to-severe pain showed significant relief with the combined supplements.
- Pain outcomes over 2 yr were similar to those of patients taking celecoxib (Celebrex) or placebo.
- Adverse reactions were mild. Serious adverse reactions were rare.

Nursing Implications

- Can be suggested to patients who are unable to take celecoxib or other NSAIDs.
- Discontinue if no effects after consistent use over 90-120 days.
- May decrease effectiveness of insulin or other drugs used to manage blood glucose.
- May increase the risk of bleeding.

*Source: National Center for Complementary and Alternative Medicine: Glucosamine/Chondroitin Arthritis Intervention Trial (GAIT): primary and ancillary study results. Retrieved from *https://nccih.nih.gov/research/results/gait*.

Aspercreme) may be an option for patients who are not able to take aspirin-containing medication. Several applications may be needed daily because topical agents have short-acting effects.

If a patient does not get adequate pain management with acetaminophen or has moderate to severe OA pain or signs of joint inflammation, a nonsteroidal antiinflammatory drug (NSAID) may be more effective. NSAID therapy typically is initiated in low-dose OTC strengths (e.g., ibuprofen) 200 mg up to four times daily). The dose may be increased if needed. If the patient is at risk for or develops gastrointestinal (GI) side effects with an NSAID, additional treatment with a protective agent such as misoprostol (Cytotec) may be needed. Arthrotec, a combination of misoprostol and the NSAID diclofenac, is also available. Diclofenac gel may be applied to the affected joint.

Because traditional NSAIDs block the production of prostaglandins from arachidonic acid by inhibiting the production of cyclooxygenase-1 (COX-1) and cyclooxygenase-2 (COX-2) (see Fig. 11-2), the risk for GI erosion and bleeding is increased.

Traditional NSAIDs affect platelet aggregation, leading to a prolonged bleeding time. Patients taking an anticoagulant (e.g., warfarin [Coumadin]) and an NSAID are at high risk for bleeding. Long-term NSAID treatment may also affect cartilage metabolism, especially in older patients who may have poor cartilage integrity. As an alternative to traditional NSAIDs, the COX-2 inhibitor celecoxib (Celebrex) may be considered in selected patients. However, all NSAIDs carry the same risk for GI effects.[9]

 HEALTHY PEOPLE

Prevention of Osteoarthritis

- Avoid cigarette smoking.
- Promptly treat any joint injury.
- Maintain healthy weight and eat a balanced diet.
- Use safety measures to protect and decrease risk of joint injury.
- Exercise regularly, including strength and endurance training.

When given in equivalent doses, all NSAIDs are comparably effective but vary widely in cost. Individual responses to the NSAIDs also vary. Some patients still prefer aspirin, but it is no longer a common treatment. It should be used cautiously with NSAIDs because both inhibit platelet function and prolong bleeding time. Intraarticular injections of corticosteroids may be suitable for the patient with local inflammation and swelling. Four or more injections without relief suggest the need for additional intervention. Systemic use of corticosteroids is not needed and may actually hasten the disease process.

Injection of hyaluronic acid (*viscosupplementation*) has been a common treatment for knee OA. However, its effectiveness in treating arthritis is not clear. Neither the American College of Rheumatology nor the American Academy of Orthopaedic Surgeons recommends using viscosupplementation with hyaluronates.[7,10] Research on the long-term effects of viscosupplementation continues.

Medications thought to slow the progression of OA or support joint healing are known as *disease-modifying osteoarthritis drugs (DMOADs)*. To date, no drugs have been approved to modify OA progression despite numerous clinical trials. Strontium ranelate is being evaluated in a variety of studies. Because of its potential ability to stimulate cartilage matrix, it may be helpful in OA treatment.[11]

Surgical Therapy. Symptoms of disease are often managed conservatively for many years. However, the patient's loss of joint function, unmanaged pain, and decreased independence in self-care may prompt a recommendation for surgery. Arthroscopy has been commonly performed for patients with knee OA. For most patients, however, this procedure provides no additional benefit over physical therapy and medical treatment.[12] Reconstructive surgical procedures (e.g., hip and knee replacements) are discussed in Chapter 62.

❖ NURSING MANAGEMENT: OSTEOARTHRITIS

◆ Nursing Assessment

Carefully assess and document the type, location, severity, frequency, and duration of the patient's joint pain and stiffness. Determine what makes the pain better or worse. Also ask the patient how these symptoms affect the ability to perform activities of daily living (ADLs). Identify the patient's pain management practices, and ask about success of each treatment.

Assess tenderness, swelling, limitation of movement, and crepitation of affected joints. Compare an involved joint with the opposite joint if it is not affected.

◆ Nursing Diagnoses

Nursing diagnoses for the patient with OA may include, but are not limited to, the following:

- Acute and chronic pain *related to* physical activity and lack of knowledge of pain self-management techniques
- Impaired physical mobility *related to* weakness, stiffness, or pain with ambulation
- Overweight or obesity *related to* intake in excess of energy output
- Depression *related to* chronic pain, changing physical appearance, and impaired social and work roles

◆ Planning

Overall goals are that the patient with OA will (1) maintain or improve joint function through a balance of rest and activity, (2) use joint protection measures (Table 64-4) to improve activity tolerance, (3) achieve independence in self-care and maintain optimal role function, and (4) use drug and nondrug strategies to manage pain satisfactorily.

◆ Nursing Implementation

◆ **Health Promotion.** Prevention of OA is possible in many cases. Focus community education on altering modifiable risk factors. For example, encourage the patient to lose weight and reduce occupational or recreational hazards. For athletic instruction and physical fitness programs, include safety measures that protect and reduce trauma to the joints. Traumatic joint injuries should be treated promptly to decrease the risk of OA.

◆ **Acute Care.** The person with OA most often complains of pain, stiffness, and limitation of function. In addition, the patient may experience daily frustration in coping with these physical difficulties. The older adult may believe OA is an inevitable part of aging and nothing can be done to decrease the discomfort and related disability.

The patient with OA is usually treated as an outpatient by an interprofessional team that may include an internal medicine physician or family HCP, a rheumatologist, a nurse, an occupational therapist, and a physical therapist. Health assessment questionnaires are often used to pinpoint areas of decreased function. Questionnaires are completed at regular intervals to document disease and treatment progression. Treatment goals can be based on data from the questionnaires and physical examination, with specific interventions for identified

problems. The patient is usually hospitalized only if joint surgery is planned (see Chapter 62).

Drugs are administered for the treatment of pain and inflammation. Nondrug strategies to decrease pain and disability may include massage, use of heat (thermal packs) or cold (ice packs), meditation, and yoga.[13] Splints may be prescribed to rest and stabilize painful or inflamed joints.

Once an acute flare has subsided, a physical therapist can provide valuable assistance in planning an exercise program. The therapist may recommend Tai Chi as a low-impact form of exercise. Tai Chi can be performed by patients of all ages and may be done in a wheelchair. Stress the importance of warming up before any exercise to decrease risk for injury.

Patient and caregiver teaching related to OA is an important nursing responsibility. Provide information about the nature and treatment of the disease, pain management, body mechanics, correct use of assistive devices (e.g., cane, walker), principles of joint protection and energy conservation (Table 64-4), nutritional choices, weight and stress management, and an exercise program.

Assure the patient that OA is a localized disease and severe deforming arthritis is not the usual course. The patient can also gain support and understanding of the disease process through community resources such as the Arthritis Foundation's self-help course (*www.arthritis.org*).

◆ **Ambulatory Care.** Adjust home management goals to meet the patient's needs. Include the caregiver, family members, and significant others in goal setting and teaching. Discuss home and work environment modification for patient safety, accessibility, and self-care. Measures include removing scatter rugs, providing rails at the stairs and bathtub, using night-lights, and wearing well-fitting supportive shoes. Assistive devices such as canes, walkers, elevated toilet seats, and grab bars also reduce the load on an affected joint and promote safety. Urge the patient to continue all prescribed therapies at home and be open to new approaches to symptom management.

Sexual counseling may help the patient and significant other to enjoy physical closeness by introducing the idea of alternate positions and timing for sexual activity. Discussion also increases awareness of each partner's needs. Encourage the patient to take analgesics or a warm bath to decrease joint stiffness before sexual activity.

◆ Evaluation

The expected outcomes are that the patient with OA will
- Experience adequate rest and activity
- Achieve satisfactory pain management
- Maintain joint flexibility and muscle strength through joint protection and therapeutic exercise
- Verbalize acceptance of OA as a chronic disease, collaborating with HCPs in disease management

---

TABLE 64-4 Patient & Caregiver Teaching

Joint Protection and Energy Conservation

Include the following instructions when teaching patients with arthritis to protect joints and conserve energy.
- Maintain healthy weight.
- Use assistive devices, if indicated.
- Avoid forceful repetitive movements.
- Avoid awkward positions that stress joints.
- Use good posture and body mechanics.
- Seek help with needed tasks that may cause pain.
- Organize routine tasks and pace yourself to decrease fatigue and joint pain.
- Modify home and work environment to perform tasks in less stressful ways.

❓ CHECK YOUR PRACTICE

A 54-yr-old woman is diagnosed with osteoarthritis of the left knee. X-rays show joint space narrowing in the medial compartment with several bone spurs. She receives an intraarticular corticosteroid injection in the left knee. She also receives a prescription for physical therapy.
- What information will you provide about diclofenac to ensure the patient's safe, effective use?
- What type of exercises will be appropriate for this patient?
- The patient asks about complementary and alternative therapies for osteoarthritis. What will you tell her?

RHEUMATOID ARTHRITIS

Rheumatoid arthritis (RA) is a chronic, systemic autoimmune disease characterized by inflammation of connective tissue in the diarthrodial (synovial) joints. RA is typically marked by periods of remission and exacerbation. RA often has extraarticular manifestations.

RA occurs globally, affecting all ethnic groups. It can occur at any time of life. However, incidence increases with age, peaking between ages 30 and 50 years. An estimated 1.5 million adult Americans are affected by RA. Almost three times as many women have the disease as men.[14]

Etiology and Pathophysiology

The exact cause of RA is unknown. However, it probably results from a combination of genetics and environmental triggers. An autoimmune etiology is currently the most widely accepted theory, suggesting changes of RA begin when a genetically susceptible person has an initial immune response to an antigen. Although a bacterium or virus has been proposed as a possible antigen, no infection or organism has been identified to date.

The antigen, which is probably not the same in all patients, triggers formation of an abnormal immunoglobulin G (IgG). RA is marked by autoantibodies to this abnormal IgG. The autoantibodies are known as *rheumatoid factor (RF)*. They combine with IgG to form immune complexes that initially deposit on synovial membranes or superficial articular cartilage in the joints. Immune complex formation leads to the activation of complement and an inflammatory response results. (Complement activation is discussed in Chapter 11, and immune complex formation is discussed in Chapter 13.)

Neutrophils are attracted to the site of inflammation, where they release proteolytic enzymes that damage articular cartilage and cause the synovial lining to thicken (Fig. 64-3). Other inflammatory cells include T helper (CD4) cells, which stimulate cell-mediated immune responses. Activated CD4 cells cause

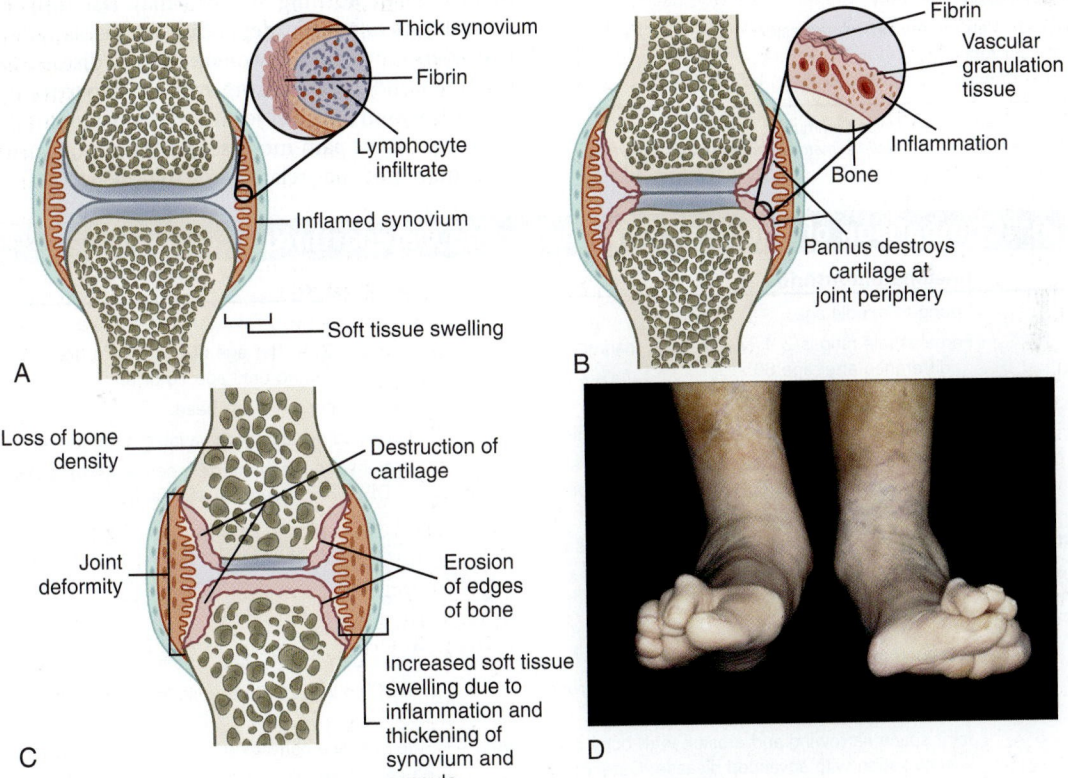

FIG. 64-3 Rheumatoid arthritis. **A,** Early pathologic change is rheumatoid synovitis. Synovium becomes inflamed. Lymphocytes and plasma cells increase greatly. **B,** Over time, articular cartilage destruction occurs and vascular granulation tissue grows across the cartilage surface (pannus) from the edges of the joint. Joint surface shows loss of cartilage beneath the extending pannus, most marked at joint margins. **C,** Inflammatory pannus causes focal destruction of bone. Osteolytic destruction of bone occurs at joint edges, causing erosions seen on x-rays. This phase is associated with joint deformity. **D,** Multiple deformities of the foot from rheumatoid arthritis. (*D,* From Canale ST, Beaty JH: *Campbell's operative orthopaedics,* ed 12, Philadelphia, 2013, Mosby.)

monocytes, macrophages, and synovial fibroblasts to secrete the proinflammatory cytokines interleukin-1 (IL-1), interleukin-6 (IL-6), and tumor necrosis factor (TNF). These cytokines drive the inflammatory response in RA.

Without adequate treatment, more than 60% of patients with RA may develop marked functional impairment within 20 years of diagnosis.[15] This includes the need for mobility aids, loss of self-care ability, and need for joint reconstruction. By end-stage disease, patients experience loss of independence and require daily care (Table 64-5).

 Genetic Link

Genetic predisposition is important in the development of RA. The strongest evidence for a genetic influence is the role of human leukocyte antigens (HLA), especially the HLA-DR4 and HLA-DR1 antigens. (HLA is discussed in Chapter 13.) Smoking increases the risk of RA for persons who are genetically predisposed to the disease and may interfere with treatment for diagnosed persons.[16]

Clinical Manifestations

Joints. The onset of RA is typically insidious. Nonspecific manifestations such as fatigue, anorexia, weight loss, and generalized stiffness may precede the onset of joint symptoms. Stiffness becomes more localized in the following weeks to months. Some patients report a precipitating stressful event such as infection, work stress, physical exertion, childbirth, surgery, or emotional upset. However, research has been unable to directly correlate such events with RA onset.

Specific joint involvement is marked by pain, stiffness, limited motion, and signs of inflammation (e.g., heat, swelling, tenderness). Joint symptoms occur symmetrically and often affect the small joints of the hands (PIP and MCP) and feet (MTP). Larger peripheral joints such as wrists, elbows, shoulders, knees, hips, ankles, and jaw may also be involved. The cervical spine may be affected, but the axial skeleton (spine and bones connected to it) is generally spared. Table 64-6 compares RA and OA.

The patient typically experiences joint stiffness after periods of inactivity. Morning stiffness may last from 60 minutes to several hours or more, depending on disease activity. MCP and PIP joints are typically swollen. In early disease, the fingers may become spindle shaped from synovial hypertrophy and thickening of the joint capsule. Joints are tender, painful, and warm to the touch. Joint pain increases with motion, varies in intensity, and may not be related to the degree of inflammation.

TABLE 64-5 Stages of Rheumatoid Arthritis

Stage	Characteristics
I	• Synovitis marked by: • Synovial membrane swelling with excess blood • Membrane containing small areas of lymphocyte infiltration • High WBC counts in synovial fluid (5000-60,000/μL) • X-ray results: soft tissue swelling, possible osteoporosis, but no evidence of joint destruction
II	• Increased joint inflammation, spreading across cartilage into joint cavity • Signs of gradual destruction in joint cartilage • Narrowing joint space from loss of cartilage
III	• Formation of synovial pannus • Joint cartilage becomes eroded, bone exposed • X-ray results: extensive cartilage loss, erosion at joint margins, possible deformity
IV	• End-stage: inflammatory process subsides • Loss of joint function • Formation of subcutaneous nodules

Source: Rheumatoid Arthritis.net: a Health Union Community: Understanding RA stages and progressions. Retrieved from *http://rheumatoidarthritis.net/what-is-ra/stages-and-progression*.

TABLE 64-6 Comparison of Rheumatoid Arthritis and Osteoarthritis

Parameter	Rheumatoid Arthritis	Osteoarthritis
Age at onset	Young to middle age.	Usually >40 yr.
Gender	Female/male ratio is 2:1 or 3:1. Less marked sex difference after age 60.	Females 2:1 after age 60; except for traumatic arthritis, men less affected until age 70 or 80.
Weight	Lost or maintained weight.	Often overweight or obese.
Disease	Systemic disease with exacerbations and remissions.	Localized disease with variable, progressive course.
Affected joints	Small joints typically affected first (PIPs, MCPs, MTPs), wrists, elbows, shoulders, knees. Usually bilateral, symmetric joint involvement.	Weight-bearing joints of knees and hips, small joints (MCPs, DIPs, PIPs), cervical and lumbar spine. Often asymmetric.
Pain characteristics	Stiffness lasts 1 hr to all day and may decrease with use. Pain is variable, may disrupt sleep.	Stiffness occurs on arising but usually subsides after 30 min. Pain gradually worsens with joint use and disease progression, relieved with joint rest but may disrupt sleep.
Effusions	Common.	Uncommon.
Nodules	Present, especially on extensor surfaces.	Heberden's (DIPs) and Bouchard's (PIPs) nodes.
Synovial fluid	WBC count 5000-60,000/μL with mostly neutrophils; decreased viscosity.	WBC count <2000/μL (mild leukocytosis); normal viscosity.
X-rays	Joint space narrowing and erosion with bony overgrowths, subluxation with advanced disease. Osteoporosis related to decreased activity, corticosteroid use.	Joint space narrowing, osteophytes, subchondral cysts, sclerosis.
Laboratory findings	RF positive in 70%-90% of patients; negative titers in early disease for about 25% of patients. ANA positive in 20%-30% of patients Positive anti-CCP in more than 80% of patients Elevated ESR, CRP indicative of active inflammation.	RF negative. ANA negative. Anti-CCP negative. Transient elevation in ESR related to synovitis.

ANA, Antinuclear antibodies; *anti-CCP*, anti-citrullinated peptide; *CRP*, C-reactive protein; *DIPs*, distal interphalangeal; *ESR*, erythrocyte sedimentation rate; *MCPs*, metacarpophalangeals; *MTPs*, metatarsophalangeals; *PIPs*, proximal interphalangeals; *RF*, rheumatoid factor.

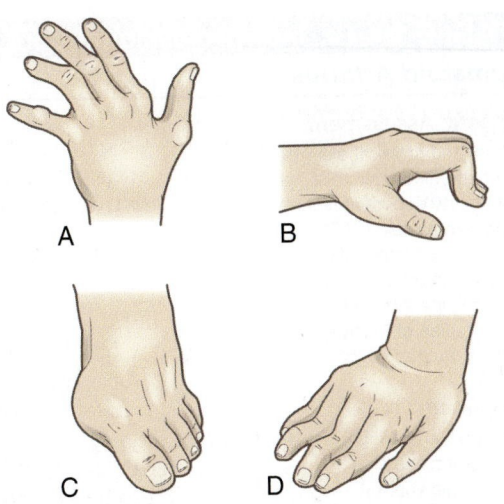

FIG. 64-4 Typical deformities of RA. **A,** Ulnar drift. **B,** Boutonnière deformity. **C,** Hallux valgus. **D,** Swan neck deformity.

Tenosynovitis frequently affects the extensor and flexor tendons around the wrists, producing symptoms of carpal tunnel syndrome and making it difficult for the patient to grasp objects.

As the disease progresses, inflammation and fibrosis of the joint capsule and supporting structures may cause deformity and disability. Muscle atrophy and tendon destruction cause one joint surface to slip past the other (*subluxation*). Metatarsal head dislocation and subluxation in the feet may cause pain and walking disability (Fig. 64-3, *D*). Ulnar drift ("zig-zag deformity"), swan neck, and boutonnière deformities are common in the hands (Fig. 64-4).

Extraarticular Manifestations. RA can affect nearly every body system (Fig. 64-5). Extraarticular manifestations are more likely to occur in the person with high levels of biomarkers such as RF.

Rheumatoid nodules develop in about half the patients with RA.[17] Rheumatoid nodules appear subcutaneously as firm, non-tender, granuloma-type masses. They are often located on bony areas exposed to pressure, such as the fingers and elbows. Nodules at the base of the spine and back of the head are common in older adults. Treatment is usually not needed. However, these nodules can break down, similar to pressure ulcers. Cataracts and vision loss can result from scleral nodules. Nodular myositis and muscle fiber degeneration can cause pain similar to that of vascular insufficiency. In later disease, nodules in the heart and lungs can cause pleurisy, pleural effusion, pericarditis, pericardial effusion, and cardiomyopathy.

Sjögren's syndrome can occur by itself or in conjunction with other arthritic disorders, such as RA and SLE. Affected patients have diminished lacrimal and salivary gland secretion, leading to a dry mouth; burning, itchy eyes with decreased tearing; and photosensitivity. (Sjögren's syndrome is discussed later in this chapter on p. 1546.)

Felty syndrome is rare but can occur in patients with long-standing RA. It is characterized by an enlarged spleen and low white blood cell (WBC) count. Patients with Felty syndrome are at increased risk of infection and lymphoma.

Flexion contractures and hand deformities cause diminished grasp strength and affect the patient's ability to perform self-care tasks. Depression also may occur. However, it is unclear if the patient becomes depressed from struggling with chronic pain and disability, or if depression is part of the autoimmune disease process.[18]

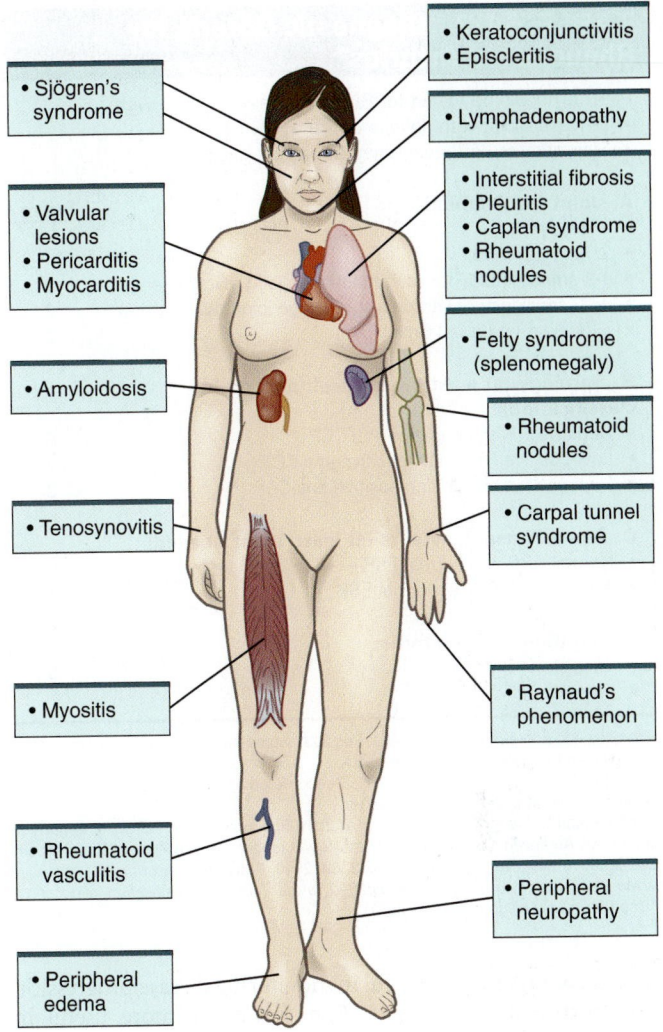

FIG. 64-5 Extraarticular manifestations of RA.

Diagnostic Studies

Accurate diagnosis is needed to start appropriate treatment and decrease the risk of disability. A diagnosis is often made based on history and physical findings. Some laboratory tests are also useful to confirm diagnosis and monitor disease progression (Tables 64-7 and 64-8).

Positive RF occurs in approximately 80% of adults with RA, and titers rise during active disease. ESR and C-reactive protein (CRP) are general indicators of active inflammation. An increase in antinuclear antibody (ANA) titers is also seen in 20% to 30% of patients with RA.[3] Testing for the antibodies to citrullinated peptide (anti-CCP) is also important in the diagnosis of RA. Levels of anti-CCP are more specific than RF for RA. In some cases, testing may allow an early, accurate diagnosis.[3]

Synovial fluid analysis in early disease often shows slightly cloudy, straw-colored fluid with many fibrin flecks. The enzyme MMP-3 is increased in the synovial fluid of the patient with RA, and it may be a marker of progressive joint damage. The WBC count of synovial fluid is elevated. Tissue biopsy can confirm inflammatory changes in the synovial membrane.

X-rays alone are not diagnostic of RA. They may show only soft tissue swelling and possible bone demineralization in early disease. A narrowed joint space, articular cartilage destruction, erosion, subluxation, and deformity are seen in later disease. Malalignment and ankylosis may be noted in advanced disease.

TABLE 64-7   Diagnostic Criteria for Rheumatoid Arthritis*

Patients should be tested for RA who initially are seen with:
- At least 1 joint with definite clinical synovitis
- Synovitis not better explained by another disease

A. Joint Involvement	Score
• 1 large joint	0
• 2-10 large joints	1
• 1-3 small joints (with or without large joint involvement)	2
• 4-10 small joints (with or without large joint involvement)	3
• >10 joints (at least 1 small joint)	5

B. Serology (at least 1 test result needed for classification)
• Negative RF *and* negative anti-CCP	0
• Low-positive RF *or* low-positive anti-CCP	2
• High-positive RF *or* high-positive anti-CCP	3

C. Acute Phase Reactants (at least 1 test needed)
• Normal CRP *and* normal ESR	0
• Abnormal CRP *or* abnormal ESR	1

D. Duration of Symptoms
• <6 wk	0
• ≥6 wk	1

SCORING: Add score of categories A-D. Possible scores range from 0-10. A score of ≥6 indicates the definitive presence of RA.
Anti-CCP, Anti-citrullinated peptide; *CRP*, C-reactive protein; *ESR*, erythrocyte sedimentation rate; *RF*, rheumatoid factor.
From Aletaha D, Neogi T, Silman AJ, et al: 2010 Rheumatoid arthritis classification criteria: an American College of Rheumatology/European League Against Rheumatism Collaborative Initiative, *Arthr Rheum* 62:2569, 2010. Retrieved from *http://www.rheumatology.org/Portals/0/Files/2010_revised_criteria_classification_ra.pdf*.
*Used for newly diagnosed patients.

TABLE 64-8   Interprofessional Care
Rheumatoid Arthritis

Diagnostic Assessment
- History and physical examination
- Complete blood cell (CBC) count
- Erythrocyte sedimentation rate (ESR)
- C-reactive protein (CRP)
- Rheumatoid factor (RF)
- Antibody to citrullinated peptide (anti-CCP)
- Antinuclear antibody (ANA)
- X-ray studies of involved joints
- Synovial fluid analysis

Management
- Nutritional and weight management counseling
- Therapeutic exercise
- Psychologic support
- Rest and joint protection, use of assistive devices
- Heat and cold applications
- Complementary and alternative therapies
  - Herbal products and nutritional supplements
  - Acupuncture
- Reconstructive surgery

Drug Therapy (Table 64-3)
- Disease-modifying antirheumatic drugs (DMARDs)
- Intraarticular or systemic corticosteroids
- Nonsteroidal antiinflammatory drugs (NSAIDs)
- Biologic response modifiers (BRMs)

Baseline x-rays may be useful in monitoring disease progression and treatment effectiveness. Bone scans are more useful in detecting early joint changes and confirming diagnosis so that RA treatment can be initiated.

Criteria for diagnosis of RA in a newly presenting patient are described in Table 64-7.

Interprofessional Care

Care of the patient with RA begins with a thorough program of education and drug therapy. Include information on correct administration, the need to report side effects, and medical and laboratory follow-up visits. Teach the patient and caregiver about the disease process and home management strategies. The physical therapist helps the patient maintain joint motion and muscle strength. An occupational therapist helps the patient maintain upper extremity function and encourages use of splints or other assistive devices for joint protection. A balance of rest and activity is also encouraged.

An individualized treatment plan considers disease activity, joint function, age, sex, family and social roles, and response to previous treatment (Table 64-8). A caring, long-term relationship with an interprofessional health care team can promote the patient's self-esteem and positive coping.

Drug Therapy

Disease-Modifying Antirheumatic Drugs. Drugs are the cornerstone of RA treatment (Table 64-3). Because irreversible joint changes can occur as early as the first year of RA, HCPs aggressively prescribe disease-modifying antirheumatic drugs (DMARDs). These drugs may slow disease progression and decrease risk of joint erosion and deformity. The choice of drug is based on disease activity; the patient's functional level; and lifestyle considerations, such as the wish to become pregnant.

Methotrexate is preferred for early treatment of patients diagnosed with RA. It has a lower risk of toxicity than other drugs. Rare but serious side effects include bone marrow suppression and hepatotoxicity. The patient begins to experience therapeutic effects within 4 to 6 weeks. Methotrexate therapy requires frequent laboratory monitoring, including CBC and blood chemistry.

Sulfasalazine (Azulfidine) and the antimalarial drug hydroxychloroquine (Plaquenil) may be effective DMARDs for mild to moderate disease. They are rapidly absorbed, relatively safe, and well-tolerated medications. A baseline eye exam with yearly follow up is recommended for the patient taking hydroxychloroquine because of the risk of vision loss.

The synthetic DMARD leflunomide (Arava) blocks immune cell overproduction. Its efficacy and side effects are similar to those of methotrexate and sulfasalazine. Because the drug is teratogenic, the possibility of pregnancy in women of childbearing age must be excluded before therapy is initiated. Adequate contraception is needed during treatment.

Tofacitinib (Xeljanz), a JAK (Janus kinase) inhibitor, is used to treat moderate-to-severe active RA. The drug interferes with JAK enzymes that contribute to joint inflammation in RA.

Biologic Response Modifiers. Biologic response modifiers (BRMs) (also called *biologics* or *immunotherapy*) are also used to slow disease progression in RA. These drugs are classified based on their mechanism of action (Table 64-3). They can be used to treat patients with moderate-to-severe who have not responded to DMARDs. They can also be used alone or in combination therapy with a DMARD such as methotrexate.

TEAMWORK & COLLABORATION
Caring for the Patient With Rheumatoid Arthritis

Role of Nursing Personnel
Registered Nurse (RN)
- Administer drug therapy as ordered.
- Teach patient and caregiver about medications, including increased risk of infection with disease-modifying agents.
- Assess disease impact on quality of life and joint function.
- Assess pain intensity and administer analgesics as ordered. Assess patient response.
- Develop program for rehabilitation and education with the interprofessional team.
- Teach patient about need for balance of rest and activity, with use of joint protective strategies.

Licensed Practical/Vocational Nurse (LPN/LVN)
- Reinforce teaching related to medication use and disease management strategies.
- Monitor pain intensity and administer prescribed analgesics.
- Notify RN of changes in pain or if pain persists after prescribed analgesics are administered.

Unlicensed Assistive Personnel (UAP)
- Assist patient with passive ROM of affected joints.
- Notify RN about patient complaints of pain.
- Assist patient with self-care needs.

Role of Other Team Members
Physical Therapist
- Assess patient's current mobility and need for assistance.
- Establish exercise regimen and teach patient to perform exercises safely.
- Coordinate PT with RN so that patient can receive timely analgesia.
- Discuss home environment with patient and identify possible modifications to facilitate disease management (e.g., bathroom on first level to avoid stairs).

Occupational Therapist
- Assess impact of patient's condition on ability to perform ADLs.
- Instruct patient in use of assistive devices (e.g., long-handled reacher, long-handled shoe horn) to facilitate self-care without increasing stress on joints.
- Discuss home environment with patient and identify possible modifications to facilitate role performance (e.g., kitchen modifications for meal preparation).

Social Worker
- Assess need for durable medical equipment (e.g., walker).
- Assess psychosocial and financial impact of disease. Arrange vocational retraining if needed.

TNF inhibitors include etanercept (Enbrel), infliximab (Remicade), adalimumab (Humira), certolizumab (Cimzia), and golimumab (Simponi). Etanercept is a biologically engineered copy of the TNF cell receptor. It binds to TNF in circulation before TNF can bind to the cell surface receptor. Thus etanercept inhibits the inflammatory response. This drug is given as a subcutaneous injection.

Infliximab and adalimumab are monoclonal antibodies that also bind to TNF, preventing it from binding to TNF receptors on cells. Infliximab is given IV in combination with methotrexate. Adalimumab is given subcutaneously.

Certolizumab and golimumab are TNF inhibitors that improve symptoms in patients with moderate-to-severe RA. Both drugs are given in combination with methotrexate.

 DRUG ALERT   Tumor Necrosis Factor Inhibitors
- Administer tuberculin test and perform chest x-ray before starting therapy.
- Monitor for signs of infection. Stop drug temporarily and notify HCP if acute infection develops.
- Instruct patients to avoid live vaccination while taking drug.
- Report bruising, bleeding, or persistent fever and other signs of infection.

Anakinra (Kineret) is an IL-1 receptor antagonist (IL-1Ra) created from new combinations of genetic material. It blocks the biologic activity of IL-1 by competitively inhibiting its ability to bind to the IL-1 receptor. Anakinra is given as a subcutaneous injection. It is used to reduce pain and swelling of moderate-to-severe RA. It can be used in combination with DMARDs but not with TNF inhibitors. Using these agents together can cause serious infection and neutropenia.

Tocilizumab (Actemra) blocks the action of IL-6, a cytokine that contributes to inflammation. It is used to treat patients with moderate-to-severe RA who have not adequately responded to or cannot tolerate other drugs for the disease.

Abatacept (Orencia) blocks T cell activation. It is recommended for patients who have inadequate response to DMARDs or TNF inhibitors. It is given IV. Similar to anakinra, it should not be used with TNF inhibitors.

Rituximab (Rituxan) is a monoclonal antibody that targets B cells (see Fig. 15-16). It may be used in combination with methotrexate for patients with moderate to severe RA not responding to TNF inhibitors. It is given IV.

Other Drug Therapy. Other medications for treating RA include antibiotics (minocycline [Minocin]), immunosuppressants (azathioprine [Imuran]), penicillamine (Cuprimine), and gold preparations (auranofin [Ridaura], gold sodium thiomalate [Myochrysine]). However, these medications are not commonly used.

Corticosteroid therapy can be used to manage symptoms during disease flares. Intraarticular injections may temporarily reduce acute pain and inflammation. Low-dose oral corticosteroids may be used for a limited time to decrease disease activity until the effects of DMARD therapy are seen. However, they are inadequate as a sole therapy, and their long-term use should not be a mainstay of RA treatment. Possible complications include osteoporosis and avascular necrosis.

Various NSAIDs and salicylates are used to treat arthritic pain and inflammation. Aspirin may be used in dosages of 3 to 4 g/day in three to four doses. Blood salicylate levels should be monitored in a patient taking more than 3600 mg daily.[19] NSAIDs have antiinflammatory and analgesic effects. Some relief may be noted within days of starting treatment with NSAIDs, but full effect may take 2 to 3 weeks. NSAIDs may be used when the patient cannot tolerate aspirin. The patient may be able to better follow the treatment regimen if using an antiinflammatory drug that can be taken only once or twice a day (Table 64-3). Celecoxib (Celebrex), the only available COX-2 inhibitor, is effective in RA as well as OA.

Nutritional Therapy. Although no special diet is needed for RA, balanced nutrition is important. Fatigue, pain, and depression may cause a loss of appetite. In addition, limited endurance and mobility deficits may interfere with the patient's ability to shop for and prepare food. Weight loss may result. The occupational therapist may help the patient modify the home environment and use assistive devices for easier food preparation.

Corticosteroid therapy or decreased mobility due to pain may cause unwanted weight gain. Corticosteroids increase the appetite, leading to higher caloric intake. A sensible weight loss program with balanced nutrition and exercise reduces stress on affected joints. In addition, the patient taking corticosteroids may become distressed as signs and symptoms of Cushing syndrome (e.g., moon face, redistribution of fatty tissue to the trunk) change the physical appearance. Encourage the patient not to change the dose or stop therapy abruptly. Weight will return to normal several months after treatment ends. Remind the patient to continue to eat a balanced diet.

Surgical Therapy. Surgery may be needed to relieve severe pain and improve the function of severely deformed joints. Removal of the joint lining (*synovectomy*) is one type of surgery. Total joint replacement (*arthroplasty*) can be done for many different joints in the body. Joint surgery is discussed in Chapter 62.

❖ NURSING MANAGEMENT: RHEUMATOID ARTHRITIS

◆ Nursing Assessment

Subjective and objective data that should be obtained from the patient with RA are presented in Table 64-9.

◆ Nursing Diagnoses

Nursing diagnoses for the patient with RA may include, but are not limited to, the following:

- Impaired physical mobility *related to* joint pain, stiffness, and deformity
- Chronic pain *related to* joint inflammation, overuse of joints, and ineffective pain and/or comfort measures
- Disturbed body image *related to* chronic disease activity, long-term treatment, deformities, stiffness, and inability to perform usual activities

Additional information on nursing diagnoses for the patient with RA is provided in eNursing Care Plan 64-1 (on the website for this chapter).

◆ Planning

The overall goals are that the patient with RA will (1) have satisfactory pain management, (2) have minimal loss of function of affected joints, (3) participate in planning and implementing the therapeutic regimen, (4) maintain a positive self-image, and (5) perform self-care to the maximum amount possible.

◆ Nursing Implementation

◆ **Health Promotion.** Prevention of RA is not possible at this time. However, early treatment can help prevent further joint damage. Community education programs should focus on symptom recognition to promote early diagnosis and treatment. The Arthritis Foundation offers many publications, classes, and support activities to help persons with RA.

◆ **Acute Care.** Primary goals in RA management are reduction of inflammation, management of pain, maintenance of joint function, and prevention or minimization of joint deformity. Goals may be met through a broad program of drug therapy, balance of rest and activity with joint protection, use of heat and cold applications, exercise, and patient and caregiver teaching. Work closely with the HCP, physical and occupational therapists, and social worker to help the patient regain function and adjust to chronic illness.

TABLE 64-9 **Nursing Assessment**
Rheumatoid Arthritis

Subjective Data

Important Health Information

Past health history: Recent infections. Precipitating factors such as emotional upset, infections, overwork, childbirth, surgery. Pattern of remissions and exacerbations

Medications: Aspirin, NSAIDs, corticosteroids, DMARDs, BRMs

Surgery or other treatments: Any joint surgery

Functional Health Patterns

Health perception–health management: Positive family history for rheumatoid arthritis or other autoimmune disorders. Malaise, ability to participate in therapeutic regimen. Impact of disease on functional ability

Nutritional-metabolic: Anorexia, weight loss, dry mucous membranes of mouth and pharynx

Activity-exercise: Stiffness and joint swelling, muscle weakness, difficulty walking, fatigue

Cognitive-perceptual: Paresthesia of hands and feet, loss of sensation; symmetric joint pain and aching that increases with motion or stress on joint, may interfere with rest

Objective Data

General

Lymphadenopathy, fever

Integumentary

Scleritis, uveitis, Sjögren's syndrome. Subcutaneous rheumatoid nodules on forearms, elbows. Skin ulcers. Shiny, taut skin over involved joints. Peripheral edema

Cardiovascular

Symmetric pallor and cyanosis of fingers (Raynaud's phenomenon). Distant heart sounds, murmurs, dysrhythmias

Respiratory

Bronchiectasis, pleural effusion, tuberculosis, interstitial lung disease

Gastrointestinal

Splenomegaly (Felty syndrome)

Musculoskeletal

Symmetric joint involvement with swelling, erythema, heat, tenderness. Deformities (with later disease). Enlargement of PIP and MCP joints. Limitation of joint movement, muscle contractures, muscle atrophy

Possible Diagnostic Findings

Positive RF, ANA, Anti-CCP. ↑ ESR; anemia. ↑ WBCs in synovial fluid. On x-ray evidence of joint space narrowing, bony erosion, deformity, possible osteoporosis

ANA, Antinuclear antibody; *anti-CCP,* anti-citrullinated peptide; *BRMs,* biologic response modifiers; *DMARDs,* disease-modifying antirheumatic drugs; *ESR,* erythrocyte sedimentation rate; *MCP,* metacarpophalangeal; *NSAIDs,* nonsteroidal antiinflammatory drugs; *PIP,* proximal interphalangeal; *RF,* rheumatoid factor.

The patient newly diagnosed with RA is usually treated on an outpatient basis. Hospitalization may be needed for the patient who has systemic complications or requires surgery for disabling deformities.

Intervention begins with a careful physical assessment (e.g., joint pain, swelling, ROM, general health status). Also evaluate psychosocial needs (e.g., family support, sexual satisfaction, emotional stress, financial constraints, vocational and career limitations) and environmental concerns (e.g., transportation, home or work modifications). After identifying the patient's problems, carefully plan a program for rehabilitation and education with the interprofessional care team.

Inflammation may be effectively treated through administration of NSAIDs, DMARDs, and BRMs. Careful timing of drug administration is critical to maintain a therapeutic drug level and reduce early morning stiffness. Discuss the action and side effects of each prescribed drug and the importance of laboratory monitoring. Many patients with RA take several different drugs, so make the drug regimen as understandable as possible. Encourage patients to develop a way to remember to take their medications (e.g., pill containers).

Nondrug management may include the use of therapeutic heat and cold, rest, relaxation techniques, joint protection (Tables 64-4 and 64-10), biofeedback, transcutaneous electrical nerve stimulation (see Chapter 8), and hypnosis. Allow the patient and caregiver to choose therapies that promote optimal comfort and fit their lifestyle.

Lightweight splints may be prescribed to rest an inflamed joint and prevent deformity from muscle spasms and contractures. Remove the splints regularly to assess skin and perform ROM exercises. After assessment and supportive care, reapply splints as prescribed. The occupational therapist may identify additional self-help devices for ADLs.

Plan care and procedures around the patient's morning stiffness. Sitting or standing in a warm shower, sitting in a tub with warm towels around the shoulders, or simply soaking the hands in a basin of warm water may relieve joint stiffness and allow the patient to perform ADLs more comfortably.

◆ **Ambulatory Care**

◆ *Rest.* Alternating scheduled rest periods with activity throughout the day helps relieve fatigue and pain. The amount of rest needed varies based on disease severity and the patient's limitations. The patient should rest before becoming exhausted. Total bed rest is rarely necessary and should be avoided to prevent stiffness and other effects of immobility. However, even a patient with mild disease may require daytime rest in addition to 8 to 10 hours of sleep at night. Help the patient identify ways to modify daily activities to avoid overexertion and fatigue, which can worsen disease activity. For example, the patient may be able to prepare meals more easily while sitting on a high stool in front of the sink.

Teach the patient to maintain good body alignment during rest through use of a firm mattress or bed board. Encourage positions of extension, and teach the patient to avoid positions of flexion. To decrease the risk of joint contracture, never place pillows under the knees. Use a small, flat pillow under the head and shoulders if needed.

◆ *Joint Protection.* Protecting joints from stress is important. Help the patient identify ways to alter routine tasks to put less stress on joints (Table 64-10). Energy conservation requires careful planning. The emphasis is on work simplification. Work for short periods with scheduled rest breaks to avoid fatigue (pacing). Organize activities to avoid going up and down stairs repeatedly. Use carts to carry supplies, or store frequently used materials in a convenient, easy-to-reach area. Use joint-protective devices (e.g., electric can opener) whenever possible. Also teach patients to delegate tasks to other family members.

Occupational therapy training may increase patient independence with assistive devices that simplify tasks (e.g., built-up utensils, buttonhooks, modified drawer handles, lightweight plastic dishes, raised toilet seats). Encourage the patient to make dressing easier by wearing shoes with Velcro fasteners and clothing with buttons or a zipper in the front instead of the back. Use a cane or a walker for support and decreased pain when walking.

◆ *Heat and Cold Therapy and Exercise.* Heat and cold applications can help relieve stiffness, pain, and muscle spasm. Ice is especially helpful during periods of increased disease activity, while moist heat seems to offer better relief for chronic stiffness. Heating pads, moist hot packs, paraffin baths, and warm baths or showers can relieve stiffness to allow the patient to participate in therapeutic exercise. Plastic bags of small frozen vegetables (peas or kernel corn) can easily mold around the shoulder, wrists, or knees to be an effective home treatment. The patient can also use ice cubes or small paper cups of frozen water to massage areas on either side of a painful joint. Heat and cold can be used several times a day as needed. However, heat application should not exceed 20 minutes at one time. Cold application should not exceed 10 to 15 minutes at one time. Alert the patient to the risk of a burn and the need to avoid using a heat-producing cream (e.g., capsaicin) with an external heat device.

Individualized exercise is an important part of the treatment plan. A physical therapist may develop a therapeutic exercise program to improve flexibility and strength of affected joints and increase the patient's endurance. Encourage program participation and reinforce correct performance of the exercises. Progressive joint immobility and muscle weakness can occur if the patient does not move the joints. Overaggressive exercise can cause increased pain, inflammation, and joint damage. Emphasize that participating in a recreational exercise program (e.g., walking, swimming) or performing usual daily activities does not take the place of therapeutic exercise to maintain adequate joint motion.

Gentle ROM exercises are usually done daily to keep joints functional. The patient should practice exercises with supervision. Aquatic exercises in warm water (78° to 86°F [25° to 30°C]) allow easier joint movement because of the buoyancy and warmth of the water. Although movement seems easier, water also provides two-way resistance that makes muscles

---

TABLE 64-10 Patient & Caregiver Teaching

Protection of Small Joints

Include the following instructions when teaching the patient with arthritis how to protect small joints.

1. Maintain joint in neutral position to minimize deformity.
   - Press water from a sponge instead of wringing.
2. Use strongest joint available for any task.
   - When rising from chair, push with palms rather than fingers.
   - Carry laundry basket in both arms rather than with fingers.
3. Distribute weight over many joints instead of stressing a few.
   - Slide objects instead of lifting them.
   - Hold packages close to body for support.
4. Change positions frequently.
   - Do not hold book or grip steering wheel for long periods without resting.
   - Avoid grasping pencil or cutting vegetables with knife for extended periods.
5. Avoid repetitive movements.
   - Do not knit or sew for long periods.
   - Rest between rooms when vacuuming.
   - Modify home environment to include faucets and doorknobs that are pushed rather than turned.
6. Modify chores to avoid stress on joints.
   - Avoid heavy lifting.
   - Sit on stool instead of standing during meal preparation.

work harder than they would on land. During acute inflammation, limit exercise to one or two repetitions.

◆   *Psychologic Support.* For effective self-management and adherence to an individualized home treatment program, help the patient understand the nature and course of RA and the goals of therapy. Also consider the patient's value system and perception of the disease.

The patient is challenged constantly by problems of limited function and fatigue, loss of self-esteem, altered body image, and fear of disability and deformity. Discuss alterations in sexuality. Chronic pain or loss of function may make the patient vulnerable to claims of false advertising about unproven or even dangerous remedies. Help the patient recognize fears and concerns faced by all people who live with chronic illness.

Evaluate the family support system. Financial planning may be necessary. Consider community resources such as a home care nurse, homemaker services, and vocational rehabilitation. Self-help groups are helpful for some patients.

Living with chronic pain may lead to depression. To decrease depressive symptoms, suggest activities such as listening to music, reading, exercising, and counseling. Hypnosis and biofeedback may also be useful.

 ## Gerontologic Considerations: Arthritis

The prevalence of arthritis in older adults is high. The disease is also accompanied by problems unique to this age group. Areas of concern for older adults include the following:
- The high incidence of OA in older adults often keeps the HCP from considering other types of arthritis.
- Age alone causes changes in blood testing, making interpretation of laboratory values such as RF and ESR more difficult. Drugs taken for co-morbid conditions can also affect laboratory values.
- Polypharmacy in older adults can also cause arthritis.
- Musculoskeletal pain syndromes and weakness may have no physical cause. Instead, they may be related to depression and physical inactivity.
- Diseases such as SLE, which commonly occurs in younger adults, can develop in a milder form in older adults.

Physical and metabolic changes of aging may increase the older patient's sensitivity to both therapeutic and toxic effects of some drugs. The older adult who takes NSAIDs has an increased risk for side effects, especially GI bleeding and renal toxicity. Using NSAIDs with a shorter half-life may require more frequent dosing but may also produce fewer side effects in the older patient with altered drug metabolism.

The common occurrence of polypharmacy in the older adult is a concern. Use of additional drugs in RA treatment may increase the likelihood of unexpected drug interactions. The drug regimen should be as simple as possible to increase adherence (e.g., limited number of drugs with decreased frequency of administration). This is especially important for the patient who lacks regular assistance.

Osteopenia from corticosteroid use can worsen the problem of decreased bone density from aging and inactivity. The risk of pathologic fractures is increased, especially vertebral compression fractures. Myopathy related to corticosteroid use can be minimized or prevented by an age-appropriate exercise program. An adequate support system for the older adult is critical to the ability to follow a treatment regimen that includes nutritional planning, exercise, general health maintenance, and appropriate therapy.

GOUT

Gout is a type of acute arthritis characterized by elevation of uric acid *(hyperuricemia)* and the deposit of uric acid crystals in one or more joints. Sodium urate crystals may be found in articular, periarticular, and subcutaneous tissues. Unlike chronic forms of arthritis, gout is marked by painful flares lasting days to weeks followed by long periods without symptoms. More than 8 million Americans are affected by gout, with men affected three times as often as women. The incidence among African American men is nearly twice that of white men.[20]

Hyperuricemia may be classified as primary or secondary.[21] In *primary hyperuricemia*, a hereditary error of purine metabolism leads to the overproduction or retention of uric acid. *Secondary hyperuricemia* may be related to another acquired disorder (Table 64-11) or may be caused by drugs known to inhibit uric acid excretion (e.g., thiazide diuretics, β-blockers, angiotensin-converting enzyme [ACE] inhibitors). Postmenopausal women and organ transplant recipients receiving immunosuppressive agents are also at risk for hyperuricemia.

Etiology and Pathophysiology

Uric acid is the major end product of purine catabolism and is primarily excreted by the kidneys. Gout is caused by (1) an increase in uric acid production; (2) reduced excretion of uric acid by the kidneys; or (3) increased intake of foods containing purines (e.g., red and organ meat, shellfish, fructose drinks), which are metabolized to uric acid by the body. Increased uric acid production is most commonly linked to obesity. Excessive alcohol consumption is also a risk factor.

High dietary intake of purine alone has relatively little effect on uric acid. Hyperuricemia may result from prolonged fasting or excessive alcohol drinking because of the increased production of keto acids, which then inhibit uric acid excretion. Reduced uric acid excretion can occur with chronic kidney disease or metabolic syndrome.

Clinical Manifestations and Complications

Gouty arthritis may occur acutely in one or more joints but usually less than four. Affected joints may appear dusky or cyanotic and are extremely tender. Inflammation of the great toe *(podagra)* is the most common initial problem. Other affected joints may include wrists, knees, ankles, and the midfoot. Olecranon bursae may also be involved. Acute gouty arthritis is usually triggered by events such as trauma, surgery, alcohol ingestion, or systemic infection. Symptom onset typically occurs at night with sudden swelling and severe pain peaking within several hours. Patients often indicate the painful

TABLE 64-11	Causes of Hyperuricemia
• Acidosis or ketosis	• Malignant disease
• Alcohol use	• Myeloproliferative disorders
• Atherosclerosis	• Obesity or starvation
• Chemotherapy drugs	• Renal insufficiency
• Diabetes mellitus	• Sickle cell anemia
• Drug-induced renal impairment	• Use of certain common drugs (aspirin, thiazide, diuretics, niacin)
• Exposure to lead	
• Hyperlipidemia	
• Hypertension	

area is highly sensitive to light touch. Low-grade fever is common.

Individual attacks usually end in 2 to 10 days with or without treatment. The affected joint returns to normal and patients have no symptoms between attacks.

Chronic gout is characterized by multiple joint involvement and visible deposits of sodium urate crystals (tophi). These are typically seen in the synovium, subchondral bone, olecranon bursae, and vertebrae; along tendons; and in the skin and cartilage (Fig. 64-6). Tophi are generally only noted many years after the onset of disease.

The severity of gouty arthritis varies. The clinical course may involve infrequent mild attacks or multiple severe episodes (up to 12 per year) marked by slowly progressive disability. In general, tophi appear earlier and the patient is prone to more frequent, severe episodes of gout if serum uric acid remains high. Chronic inflammation may cause joint deformity, and cartilage destruction may lead to secondary OA. Large urate crystal deposits may pierce overlying skin, producing draining sinuses that often become infected.

Excessive uric acid excretion may lead to stone formation in the kidneys or urinary tract. Pyelonephritis related to sodium urate deposits and obstruction may contribute to kidney disease.

Diagnostic Studies

In gout, serum uric acid is usually elevated above 6 mg/dL. However, hyperuricemia is not specifically diagnostic of gout because values may be normal during an acute gouty attack.[22] Increased uric acid may also be related to various drugs or may exist as an asymptomatic abnormality in the general population. Specimens may be obtained for 24-hour urine uric acid to determine if the disease is caused by decreased renal excretion or overproduction of uric acid.

The gold standard for diagnosis of gout is synovial fluid aspiration. Affected fluid characteristically contains needle-like monosodium urate crystals. This procedure is done in only about 11% of patients because diagnosis can typically be made on clinical symptoms alone.[21]

However, it is the only reliable way to distinguish gout from septic arthritis or *pseudogout* (calcium phosphate crystal formation). Aspiration also may have therapeutic value by decompressing a swollen joint capsule.

X-rays appear normal in the early stages of gout. In chronic disease, tophi may appear as eroded areas in the bone.

Interprofessional Care

Goals for the care of the patient with gout (Table 64-12) include ending an acute attack with an antiinflammatory agent such as colchicine. Drug therapy is the primary way to treat acute and chronic gout. Also recommend weight reduction as needed and possible avoidance of alcohol and foods high in purine.

Drug Therapy. Acute gout is treated with colchicine and NSAIDs. Because colchicine has antiinflammatory effects but is not an analgesic, an NSAID is added for pain management. Oral administration of colchicine generally produces dramatic pain relief when given within 12 to 24 hours of an attack.[23] Colchicine also helps in diagnosis because good response to this drug is further evidence of gout.

Future attacks of gout are prevented in part by a maintenance dose of a drug that lowers urate such as a xanthine oxidase inhibitor (allopurinol [Zyloprim, Aloprim]), or a drug that increases the excretion of uric acid in the urine (*uricosuric*) (probenecid). Febuxostat (Uloric), a selective inhibitor of xanthine oxidase, is used for long-term management of hyperuricemia in people with chronic gout.

Patients who cannot take or do not respond to drugs that lower serum uric acid may be given pegloticase (Krystexxa).

GENDER DIFFERENCES

Gout

Men
- Occurs three times more often in men than in women until age 60.
- Occurs predominantly in men ages 30 to 50.

Women
- Low occurrence in premenopausal women.

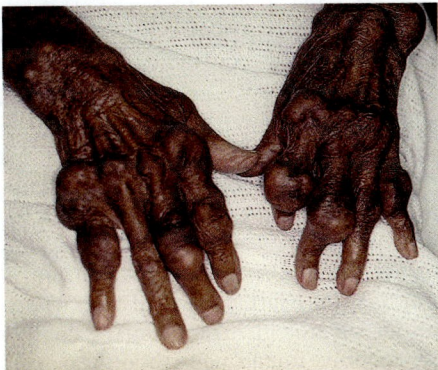

FIG. 64-6 Tophi associated with chronic gout. Painless nodules are filled with uric acid crystals. (Courtesy John Cook, MD. From Goldstein BG, Goldstein AE: *Practical dermatology*, ed 2, St Louis, 1997, Mosby.)

TABLE 64-12 Interprofessional Care

Gout

Diagnostic Asessment
- History and physical examination
- Family history of gout
- Sodium urate crystals in synovial fluid
- Elevated serum uric acid
- Elevated 24-hr urine for uric acid
- X-ray of affected joints

Management
- Joint immobilization
- Local application of heat and cold
- Joint aspiration and intraarticular corticosteroids
- Avoidance of food and fluids with high purine content (e.g., anchovies, liver, wine, beer)

Drug Therapy
- colchicine
- Nonsteroidal antiinflammatory drugs (e.g., naproxen [Naprosyn])
- allopurinol (Zyloprim)
- probenecid
- febuxostat (Uloric)
- pegloticase (Krystexxa)
- Corticosteroids (prednisone)
- Intraarticular corticosteroids (methylprednisolone)
- Adrenocorticotropic hormone (ACTH)

This drug is an enzyme that metabolizes uric acid into a harmless chemical excreted in the urine. The drug is given IV. Corticosteroids given orally or by intraarticular injection also can be helpful in treating acute attacks of gout. Systemic corticosteroids may be used only if routine therapies are contraindicated or ineffective. In addition, adrenocorticotropic hormone (ACTH) may be used for treating acute gout.

For many years, the standard therapy for hyperuricemia caused by decreased urate excretion has been uricosuric drugs such as probenecid. These drugs inhibit renal tubular reabsorption of urates. However, they are ineffective when creatinine clearance is reduced, as can occur in patients over age 60 years or with renal impairment. Aspirin inactivates the effect of these drugs, resulting in urate retention, and should be avoided during treatment. Acetaminophen can be used safely if analgesia is required.

Adequate urine volume with normal renal function (2 to 3 L/day) must be maintained to prevent precipitation of uric acid in the renal tubules. Allopurinol, which blocks the production of uric acid, is especially useful for patients with uric acid stones or renal impairment. Uricosuric drugs may be ineffective or dangerous for these patients. For patients who cannot tolerate allopurinol because of side effects, oxypurinol can be prescribed. Oxypurinol is the active metabolite of allopurinol. The angiotensin II receptor antagonist losartan (Cozaar) may be effective for treatment of older patients with gout and hypertension. Losartan promotes urate diuresis and may normalize serum urate. Combination therapy with losartan and allopurinol may also be used. Whatever drugs are prescribed, serum uric acid must be checked regularly to monitor treatment effectiveness.

Nutritional Therapy.   Dietary restrictions that limit alcohol and foods high in purine help minimize uric acid production (see Table 45-12). Instruct obese patients in a carefully planned weight-reduction program.

❖ NURSING MANAGEMENT: GOUT

Nursing interventions for the patient with acute gout include supportive care of the inflamed joints. Avoid causing pain by careless handling of an inflamed joint. Bed rest may be appropriate to immobilize affected joints as needed. Use a cradle or footboard to protect a painful lower extremity from the weight of bed linens. Assess limitation of motion and degree of pain. Document treatment effectiveness.

Hyperuricemia and gout are chronic problems that can be controlled with effective patient education and careful adherence to a treatment program.[22] Explain the importance of drug therapy and the need for regular assessment of serum uric acid. Teach the patient about factors that may cause an attack: (1) excessive caloric intake or overindulgence in purine-containing foods and alcohol, (2) starvation (fasting), (3) drug use (e.g., diuretics), and (4) major medical events (e.g., surgery, myocardial infarction).

LYME DISEASE

Lyme disease is an infection caused by the spirochete *Borrelia burgdorferi* and transmitted by the bite of an infected deer tick. It was first identified in 1975 in Lyme, Connecticut, after an unusual occurrence of arthritis in children. It is the most common vector-borne disease in the United States. The tick

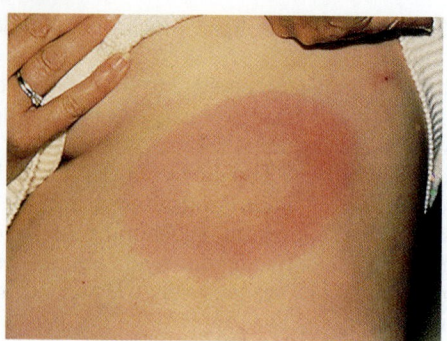

FIG. 64-7   Erythema migrans. Typical skin lesion of Lyme disease occurs at the site of tick bite. (From Marx J, Hockberger R, Walls R: *Rosen's emergency medicine*, ed 7, Philadelphia, 2009, Mosby.)

❓ CHECK YOUR PRACTICE

A patient is admitted to the medical unit with acute gout. The right great toe is swollen, red, and painful. He is prescribed colchicine.
- What nursing interventions will you use to protect the right foot and decrease pain?
- What information will you provide about the patient's medication?
- How will you explain the role of hyperuricemia in development of acute gout?
- What will you discuss with the patient concerning possible dietary changes to decrease risk of future attacks?

---

typically feeds on mice, dogs, cats, cows, horses, deer, and humans. Wild animals do not exhibit the illness, but clinical Lyme disease does occur in domestic animals. Person-to-person transmission does not occur.

The summer months are the peak season for human infection. Most U.S. cases occur in three areas: along the northeastern states from Virginia to Maine, in the Midwestern states of Wisconsin and Minnesota, and along the northwestern coast of California and Oregon. More than 30,000 cases are reported annually in the United States.[24] Reinfection is not uncommon.

Symptoms of Lyme disease can mimic those of other diseases such as multiple sclerosis, mononucleosis, and meningitis. The most characteristic clinical symptom of early localized disease is *erythema migrans* (EM). This "bull's eye rash" occurs in 70% to 80% of infected persons at the site of the tick bite within 3 to 30 days after exposure (Fig. 64-7). It may also appear anywhere else on the body as the disease progresses. The EM lesion begins as a central red macule or papule that slowly expands to include a red outer ring of up to 12 in, resembling a bull's eye. It may be warm to the touch but is not itchy or painful. The rash often occurs with acute flu-like symptoms: (1) low-grade fever, (2) chills, (3) headache, (4) stiff neck, (5) fatigue, (6) swollen lymph nodes, and (7) migratory joint and muscle pain. Loss of tone in facial muscles can appear as Bell's palsy. Symptoms usually occur in a week but may be delayed up to 30 days. Flu-like symptoms generally resolve over weeks or months, even if untreated.

If not treated, the spirochete can disseminate within several weeks or months to the heart, joints, and central nervous system (CNS). Chronic neurologic complaints include short-term memory loss, cognitive impairment, shooting pains, and numbness and tingling in the feet. Cardiac symptoms such as heart block and myocarditis may require hospitalization.[24] About 60% of persons with untreated infection develop chronic arthritic pain and swelling in the large joints, primarily the knee.

Diagnosis of Lyme disease is often based on clinical manifestations, in particular EM, and a history of exposure in one of the at-risk areas. CBC and ESR are usually normal. A two-step laboratory testing process is recommended by the Centers for Disease Control and Prevention (CDC) to confirm the diagnosis.[25] The first step is the enzyme immunoassay (EIA), which will have positive results for most people with Lyme disease. If the EIA is positive or inconclusive, a Western blot test is done. Results are diagnostic of Lyme disease only if both tests are positive. The CDC does not recommend completing the Western blot test alone as false-positive results lead to incorrect diagnosis and treatment. In individuals with neurologic involvement, cerebrospinal fluid should also be examined.

Active lesions can be treated with oral antibiotics. Doxycycline (Vibramycin), cefuroxime (Ceftin), and amoxicillin are often effective in treating early stage infection and preventing later stages of the disease. Doxycycline is preferred because it treats both Lyme disease and human granulocytic anaplasmosis, which can be transmitted as a co-infection with a single tick bite. Short-term therapy of 14 days is usually effective for solitary EM, but patients with neurologic or cardiac complications may require IV therapy with ceftriaxone (Rocephin) or penicillin G for 2 to 4 weeks.

Approximately 10% to 20% of persons treated with antibiotics for Lyme disease may experience lingering fatigue or joint and muscle pain. The International Lyme and Associated Diseases Society supports a definition of chronic Lyme disease in these cases, rather than posttreatment Lyme disease syndrome, and recommends extended antibiotic treatment until the patient shows subjective improvement.[25]

Reducing exposure to ticks is the best way to prevent Lyme disease. Patient and caregiver teaching for people living in endemic areas is outlined in Table 64-13. No vaccine is available for Lyme disease.

SEPTIC ARTHRITIS

Septic arthritis (infectious or bacterial arthritis) is caused by microorganisms invading the joint cavity. Bacteria can travel through the bloodstream from another site of active infection, resulting in hematogenous seeding of the joint. Organisms can also be introduced directly through trauma or surgical incision.

Any bacteria can cause the infection—even nonpathogenic bacteria in the immunocompromised patient. *Staphylococcus aureus* is the most common causative organism. Gonococcal infection was a common cause of septic arthritis in young sexually active adults, but its incidence is decreasing.[26] Factors that increase the risk of infection include (1) diseases with decreased host resistance (e.g., leukemia, diabetes mellitus), (2) treatment with corticosteroids or immunosuppressive drugs, and (3) debilitating chronic illness.

In septic arthritis, large joints such as the knee and hip are most frequently involved. Inflammation of the joint cavity causes severe pain, redness, and swelling. Septic arthritis of the hip can contribute to development of avascular necrosis. Because infection has often spread from a primary site elsewhere in the body, fever or shaking chills often accompany joint complaints. Diagnosis may be made by joint aspiration

TABLE 64-13 Patient & Caregiver Teaching

Prevention and Early Treatment of Lyme Disease

Include the following instructions when teaching patients how to prevent Lyme disease.
- Avoid walking through tall grasses and low brush, and sitting on logs.
- Mow grass. Remove brush around paths, buildings, and campsites to create tick-safe zones.
- Move woodpiles and bird feeders away from house. Discourage deer (main source of food for adult ticks) from being in the area.
- Wear long pants or nylon tights of tightly woven, light-colored fabric so that ticks can be easily seen.
- Tuck pants into boots or long socks, wear long-sleeved shirts tucked into pants, and wear closed shoes when hiking.
- Check often for ticks crawling from pant legs to open skin.
- Thoroughly inspect and wash clothes. Placing clothing in dryer on high heat kills ticks.
- Spray insect repellent containing DEET sparingly on skin or clothing, or apply permethrin to clothing and camping gear; protects for several hours.
- Have pets wear tick collars, inspect them often, and do not allow pets on furniture or beds.

Include the following instructions when teaching patients and caregivers living in endemic areas.
- Remove attached ticks with fine-tipped tweezers (not fingers). Grasp tick's mouth parts as close to skin as possible and pull straight out with steady, even pressure. Do not twist or jerk. Avoid folk solutions such as painting the tick with nail polish or petroleum jelly.
- Save the tick in a bottle of alcohol (if you need it later for identification). Never crush a tick with your fingers.
- Wash bitten area with soap and water, iodine scrub, or rubbing alcohol. Apply antiseptic. Wash hands.
- See an HCP immediately if flu-like symptoms or a bull's-eye rash appears within 2-30 days after removal of tick.

Adapted from Centers for Disease Control and Prevention: Prevent Lyme disease. Retrieved from *www.cdc.gov/features/lymedisease*; and Centers for Disease Control and Prevention: Tick removal. Retrieved from *www.cdc.gov/lyme/removal/index.html*. DEET, N,N-diethyl-m-toluamide.

(arthrocentesis) and synovial fluid culture. WBC counts may be low early in the infectious process, especially in persons who are immunosuppressed, so diagnosis is not possible solely based on WBC counts. Blood cultures for aerobic and anaerobic organisms should also be obtained.

Septic arthritis is an emergency that requires prompt treatment to prevent joint destruction and bone loss.[26] Broad-spectrum antibiotics against gram-negative organisms, pneumococci, and staphylococci are often started before the causative organism is identified. Once the organism is identified, specific treatment can be determined. Infections may respond to treatment within 2 weeks or may take as long as 4 to 6 weeks, depending on the causative organism.

Local aspiration or surgical drainage may be needed. If diagnosis and treatment are delayed, articular cartilage can be destroyed and loss of joint function occur. Chronic infection can also develop.

Assess and monitor joint inflammation, pain, and fever. To manage pain, use resting splints or traction to immobilize affected joints. Local hot compresses can also decrease pain. Initiate gentle ROM exercises as soon as tolerated to prevent muscle atrophy and joint contractures. Explain the need for antibiotics and the importance of their continued use until the infection is resolved. Offer support to the patient who requires joint drainage. Use strict aseptic technique when assisting with joint aspiration.

SPONDYLOARTHROPATHIES

The spondyloarthropathies are a group of multisystem inflammatory disorders that affect the spine, peripheral joints, and periarticular structures. These disorders are all negative for rheumatoid factor (RF) and thus are often referred to as *seronegative arthropathies.*

Inheritance of HLA-B27 is strongly associated with these diseases. Both genetic and environmental factors play a role in the development of this group of diseases, which includes ankylosing spondylitis, psoriatic arthritis, and reactive arthritis. (HLAs and their relationship to autoimmune diseases are discussed in Chapter 13.)

The spondyloarthropathies share clinical and laboratory characteristics that may make it difficult to distinguish among them in early disease. These characteristics include absence of antibodies in the serum, peripheral joint involvement predominantly of the lower extremities, low back pain *(sacroiliitis),* pain, and redness of the eyes *(uveitis),* intestinal inflammation, and skin lesions.[27]

ANKYLOSING SPONDYLITIS

Ankylosing spondylitis (AS) is a chronic inflammatory disease that primarily affects the axial skeleton, including the sacroiliac joints, intervertebral disc spaces, and costovertebral articulations. HLA-B27 antigen is found in 90% to 95% of people with AS.[3] Onset of AS is usually in the third decade of life, but onset in adolescence is fairly common. Men are three times more likely to develop AS than women. The disease also may go undetected in women because of a milder course.

Etiology and Pathophysiology

Genetic predisposition appears to play an important role in the pathogenesis of AS. However, the precise cause of the disease is unknown. Inflammation in the joints and adjacent tissue causes the formation of granulation tissue *(pannus)* and dense fibrous scars that can lead to joint fusions. Inflammation can affect the eyes, lungs, heart, kidneys, and peripheral nervous system.

Clinical Manifestations and Complications

AS is characterized by symmetric sacroiliitis and progressive inflammatory arthritis of the axial skeleton. Symptoms of inflammatory spine pain are the first clues to diagnosis of AS. The patient typically complains of low back pain, stiffness, and limitation of motion that is worse during the night and in the morning but improves with mild activity. In women, early symptoms may include pain and stiffness in the neck rather than the lower back. General symptoms such as fever, fatigue, anorexia, and weight loss are rarely present. Uveitis is the most common non-skeletal symptom. It can appear as an initial presentation of the disease years before arthritic symptoms develop. Patients with AS may also experience distressing chest pain and sternal/costal cartilage tenderness.

Severe postural abnormalities and deformity can cause significant disability for the patient with AS (Fig. 64-8). Impaired spinal ROM and fusion contribute to altered vision, raising concerns about safe ambulation. Aortic insufficiency and pulmonary fibrosis are frequent complications. Cauda equina syndrome (compression of the nerves at the end of the spinal cord)

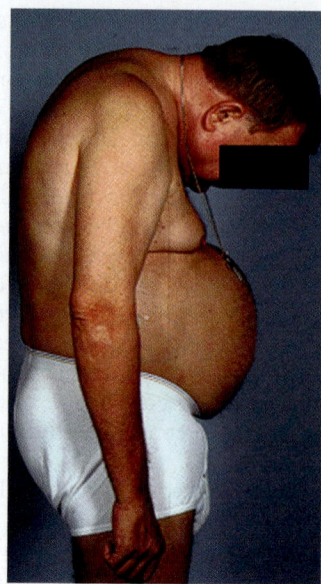

FIG. 64-8 Advanced ankylosing spondylitis. Kyphotic posture causes many patients to have a bulging abdomen due to pulmonary restriction. (From Kim DH, Henn J, Vaccaro AR, Dickman C: *Surgical anatomy and techniques to the spine,* Philadelphia, 2006, Saunders.)

GENETICS IN CLINICAL PRACTICE
Ankylosing Spondylitis

Genetic Basis
- Inheritance of human leukocyte antigen (HLA)-B27 increases susceptibility to development of ankylosing spondylitis (AS). It is not known how HLA-B27 increases the risk of AS.

Incidence
- About 90% to 95% of people with AS have HLA-B27 antigen.
- Inheriting HLA-B27 does not mean a person will develop AS. Of children who inherit HLA-B27 from a parent with AS, 80% do not develop the disease.
- AS is three times more common in men than in women. The disease may go undetected in women because of a milder course.
- It occurs more often in whites than in other ethnic groups.

Genetic Testing
- Testing for HLA-B27 antigen is available.

Clinical Implications
- Diagnosis of AS usually occurs in the third decade of life, but adolescents can also be affected.
- Multiple genetic and environmental factors play a role in pathogenesis of disease.
- Inflammation can affect the eyes, lungs, heart, kidneys, and peripheral nervous system.
- Severe postural abnormalities and deformity can cause significant disability for the patient with AS.

can also result, contributing to lower-extremity weakness and bladder dysfunction. In addition, the patient is at risk for spinal fracture because of associated osteoporosis.

Diagnostic Studies

X-rays are the most important radiographic technique for the diagnosis and follow up of AS. However, x-rays are limited in detecting early sacroiliitis or subtle changes in posterior vertebrae. MRI is useful in assessing early cartilage abnormalities, while CT scan is appropriate in specific situations (e.g., cases with subtle x-ray changes). Changes on later spinal films include the appearance of "bamboo spine," the result of calcifications *(syndesmophytes)* that bridge from one vertebra to another.

Laboratory testing is not specific, but an elevated ESR and mild anemia may be seen. When the suspicion of AS is high, the presence of the HLA-B27 antigen improves the likelihood of this diagnosis.

Interprofessional Care

Prevention of AS is not possible. However, families with other diagnosed HLA-B27-positive rheumatic diseases (e.g., psoriatic arthritis, juvenile spondyloarthritis) should be alert to signs of low back pain for early identification and treatment of AS.

Care of the patient with AS is aimed at maintaining maximal skeletal mobility while decreasing pain and inflammation. Heat applications can help relieve local symptoms. NSAIDs and salicylates are commonly prescribed. DMARDs such as sulfasalazine or methotrexate have little effect on spinal disease but may help with peripheral joint disease. Local corticosteroid injections may be helpful in relieving symptoms.

TNF, which promotes inflammation, is elevated in the blood and certain tissues of patients with AS. Etanercept, a BRM, binds TNF and inhibits its action. Etanercept reduces active inflammation and improves spinal mobility. Additional anti-TNF inhibitors (infliximab, adalimumab, golimumab) may also be effective.

Once pain and stiffness are managed, exercise is essential. Good posture is important to minimize spinal deformity. The exercise regimen should include back, neck, and chest stretches. Hydrotherapy (e.g., sauna, steam bath) has also been shown to decrease pain and facilitate spinal extension. Surgery may be needed for severe deformity and mobility impairment. Spinal osteotomy and total joint replacement are the most commonly performed procedures (see Chapter 62).

NURSING MANAGEMENT: ANKYLOSING SPONDYLITIS

A key nursing responsibility is to teach the patient with AS about the disease and principles of therapy. The home management program should include regular exercise and attention to posture, local moist heat applications, and knowledgeable use of drugs.

Baseline ROM assessment includes chest expansion (using breathing exercises). Encourage smoking cessation to decrease the risk for lung complications in persons with reduced chest expansion. Ongoing physical therapy includes gentle, graded stretching and strengthening exercises to preserve ROM and improve thoracolumbar flexion and extension.

Discourage excessive physical exertion during periods of increased disease activity. Proper positioning at rest is essential. Encourage the patient to use a firm mattress and sleep on the back with a flat pillow, avoiding positions that encourage flexion deformity. Postural training emphasizes avoiding spinal flexion (e.g., leaning over a desk); heavy lifting; and prolonged walking, standing, or sitting. Encourage sports that facilitate natural stretching, such as swimming and racquet games. Family counseling and vocational rehabilitation are important.

PSORIATIC ARTHRITIS

Psoriatic arthritis (PsA) is a progressive inflammatory disease that affects about 30% people with psoriasis.[28] *Psoriasis* is a

common, benign, inflammatory skin disorder characterized by red, irritated, and scaly patches. Both PsA and psoriasis appear to have a genetic link with the HLA antigens in many patients. Although the exact cause of PsA is unknown, a combination of immune, genetic, and environmental factors is suspected. Most people develop psoriasis first and later are diagnosed with PsA.

PsA can occur in different forms. *Distal arthritis* primarily involves the ends of the fingers and toes, with pitting and color changes in the fingernails and toenails. *Asymmetric arthritis* involves different joints between the extremities. *Symmetric psoriatic arthritis* resembles RA and affects joints on both sides of the body at the same time. It accounts for about 50% of cases. *Psoriatic spondylitis* is marked by pain and stiffness in the spine and neck. *Arthritis mutilans* is the most severe form of the disease, affecting only 5% of people with psoriatic arthritis but causing complete destruction of small joints.[28]

On x-ray, the cartilage loss and erosion are similar to RA. Advanced cases of PsA often reveal widened joint spaces. A "pencil in cup" deformity is common in the DIP joints as a result of thinning, weakened bone. In this deformity, the narrowed ends of the metacarpals or phalanges insert into the expanded end of the other bone sharing the joint. Elevated ESR, mild anemia, and elevated serum uric acid can be seen in some patients. Thus the diagnosis of gout must be excluded.

Treatment includes splinting, joint protection, and physical therapy. NSAIDs given early in the course of the disease may help with inflammation. Drug therapy also includes the DMARDs such as methotrexate, which is effective for both articular and cutaneous manifestations. Sulfasalazine, cyclosporine, and BRMs (e.g., etanercept, golimumab, adalimumab, infliximab) may also be used. Apremilast (Otezla), an inhibitor of the enzyme phosphodiesterase-4, can also be used to decrease inflammation.

REACTIVE ARTHRITIS

Reactive arthritis (Reiter's syndrome) occurs more commonly in young men than in young women. It is associated with a symptom complex that includes urethritis, conjunctivitis, and mucocutaneous lesions. Although the exact etiology is unknown, reactive arthritis appears to be a reaction triggered in the body after exposure to specific genitourinary or GI tract infections. *Chlamydia trachomatis* is most often implicated in sexually transmitted reactive arthritis.[3] Reactive arthritis is also associated with GI infections from *Shigella*, *Salmonella*, *Campylobacter*, or *Yersinia* species and other microorganisms.

Individuals who are positive for HLA-B27 are at increased risk of developing reactive arthritis after sexual contact or exposure to certain enteric pathogens. This finding supports the suggestion of genetic predisposition.

Urethritis develops within 1 to 2 weeks after sexual contact or GI infection. In women, symptoms include cervicitis. Low-grade fever, conjunctivitis, and arthritis may occur over the next several weeks. This type of arthritis tends to be asymmetric, frequently involving the large joints of the lower extremities and toes. Lower back pain may occur with severe disease. Lesions involving the skin and mucous membranes commonly occur as small, painless, superficial ulcerations on the tongue, oral mucosa, and glans penis. Soft tissue manifestations commonly include Achilles tendinitis or plantar fasciitis. Few laboratory abnormalities occur, although the ESR may be elevated.

Most patients recover in 2 to 16 weeks. Because reactive arthritis is often associated with *C. trachomatis* infection, treatment with doxycycline is widely recommended for patients and their sexual partners. Antibiotics have no effect on arthritis or other symptoms. Topical ophthalmic corticosteroids may be prescribed for treatment of uveitis, but conjunctivitis and lesions generally require no treatment. Drug therapy may also include NSAIDs and DMARDs (e.g., methotrexate, sulfasalazine). Physical therapy may be helpful during recovery.

Most patients have complete remission with return of full joint function. About 20% of patients may develop chronic arthritis, but the condition is often mild.[3] X-ray changes in chronic reactive arthritis closely resemble those of AS. Treatment is based on symptoms.

SYSTEMIC LUPUS ERYTHEMATOSUS

Systemic lupus erythematosus (SLE) is a multisystem inflammatory autoimmune disease. It is a complex disorder of multifactorial origin resulting from interactions among genetic, hormonal, environmental, and immunologic factors. SLE typically affects the skin, joints, and serous membranes (pleura, pericardium), along with the renal, hematologic, and neurologic systems. SLE is marked by a chronic unpredictable course with alternating periods of remission and exacerbation.

About 250,000 people in the United States have SLE. Most cases occur in women in their childbearing years. Women are 6 to 10 times more likely than men to develop SLE. African Americans, Asian Americans, Hispanics, and Native Americans are more likely than whites to develop the disease.[3]

Etiology and Pathophysiology

The etiology of the abnormal immune response in SLE is unknown. Based on the high prevalence of SLE among family members, a genetic influence is suspected. Multiple genes from the HLA complex, including *HLA-DR2* and *HLA-DR3,* show associations with SLE.

Hormones are also known to play a role in the etiology of SLE. Onset or worsening of disease symptoms sometimes occurs after the start of menses, with the use of oral contraceptives, and during and after pregnancy. The disease also tends to become worse in the immediate postpartum period.

Environmental factors are believed to contribute to the occurrence of SLE. These include sun or ultraviolet light exposure, stress, and exposure to some chemicals and toxins. Infectious agents such as viruses also may stimulate immune hyperactivity. In addition, at least 40 medications currently in use may trigger SLE. The most frequently identified drugs include procainamide, hydralazine, and quinidine. Drug-induced SLE should not be confused with medication side effects, which typically occur within a few hours or days of short-term drug use. SLE generally occurs months to years after continuous therapy with a causative drug.[29]

In SLE, varied autoantibodies are produced against nucleic acids (e.g., single- and double-stranded DNA), erythrocytes, coagulation proteins, lymphocytes, platelets, and many other self-proteins. Autoimmune reactions (antinuclear antibodies [ANA]) are typically directed against constituents of the cell nucleus, especially DNA.

Circulating immune complexes with antibody against DNA are deposited in the basement membranes of capillaries in the kidneys, heart, skin, brain, and joints. These complexes trigger inflammation that causes tissue destruction. Overaggressive autoimmune responses are also related to activation of B and T

cells. Specific disease effects depend on the involved cell types or organs. (SLE is a type III hypersensitivity response [see Chapter 13].)

Clinical Manifestations and Complications

Severity of SLE is extremely variable. It ranges from a relatively mild disorder to a rapidly progressive disease affecting many body systems (Fig. 64-9). No characteristic pattern occurs in the progressive involvement of SLE. Any organ can be affected by the circulating immune complexes. The most commonly affected tissues are the skin and muscle, lining of the lungs, heart, nervous tissue, and kidneys. General complaints such as fever, weight loss, joint pain (arthralgia), and excessive fatigue may precede worsened disease activity.

Dermatologic Problems. Vascular skin lesions can appear anywhere but are most likely to develop on sun-exposed areas. Severe skin reactions can occur in people who are sensitive to sunlight (photosensitivity). The classic butterfly rash over the cheeks and bridge of the nose occurs in 55% to 85% of patients at some time during the disease[3] (Fig. 64-10). About 20% of patients have discoid (round, coin-shaped) lesions. A small number of patients have persistent lesions, photosensitivity, and mild systemic disease in a syndrome known as subacute cutaneous lupus.

Oral or nasopharyngeal ulcers occur in up to one third of patients with SLE. Alopecia is also common, with or without related scalp lesions. The hair may grow back during remission, but hair loss may be permanent over lesions. The scalp becomes dry, scaly, and atrophied.

Musculoskeletal Problems. Arthritis occurs in about 95% of patients with SLE.[3] Pain in multiple joints (polyarthralgia) with morning stiffness is often the first complaint. It may precede the onset of multisystem disease by many years. Diffuse swelling occurs with joint and muscle pain and some stiffness. Lupus-related arthritis is generally nonerosive but may cause deformities (e.g., swan neck deformity of the fingers [Fig. 64-4, *D*], ulnar deviation, subluxation with joint laxity). Patients with SLE also have increased risk of bone loss and fracture.

Cardiopulmonary Problems. Tachypnea and cough in patients with SLE suggest presence of lung disease. Pleurisy is also possible. Cardiac involvement may include dysrhythmias due to fibrosis of the sinoatrial and atrioventricular nodes. This indicates advanced disease, contributing greatly to the morbidity and mortality of SLE. Pericarditis can also occur. Clinical factors such as hypertension and hypercholesterolemia require aggressive treatment and careful monitoring. In addition, people with SLE are at risk for secondary antiphospholipid syndrome. This disorder of coagulation leads to clots in the arteries and veins with related risk of stroke, gangrene, and heart attack.

Renal Problems. About 75% of persons with SLE experience kidney damage. Renal involvement is usually evident within the first 2 years after diagnosis.[3] Manifestations of renal involvement vary from mild proteinuria to rapidly progressive glomerulonephritis. Scarring and permanent damage can lead to end-stage renal disease (ESRD).

The primary goal is to slow the progression of nephropathy and preserve renal function by managing the underlying disease. The importance of obtaining a renal biopsy is controversial, but findings can help guide treatment. Although renal failure is the leading cause of death for patients with SLE, effective

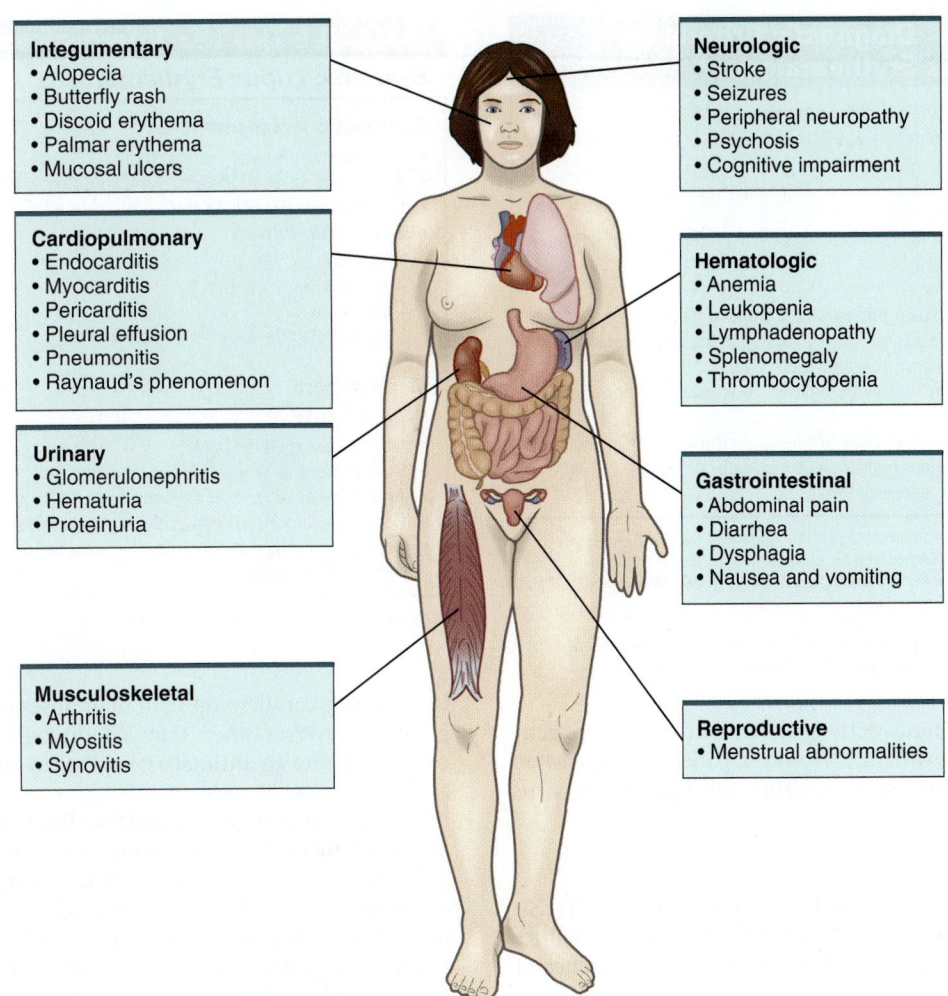

Integumentary
- Alopecia
- Butterfly rash
- Discoid erythema
- Palmar erythema
- Mucosal ulcers

Cardiopulmonary
- Endocarditis
- Myocarditis
- Pericarditis
- Pleural effusion
- Pneumonitis
- Raynaud's phenomenon

Urinary
- Glomerulonephritis
- Hematuria
- Proteinuria

Musculoskeletal
- Arthritis
- Myositis
- Synovitis

Neurologic
- Stroke
- Seizures
- Peripheral neuropathy
- Psychosis
- Cognitive impairment

Hematologic
- Anemia
- Leukopenia
- Lymphadenopathy
- Splenomegaly
- Thrombocytopenia

Gastrointestinal
- Abdominal pain
- Diarrhea
- Dysphagia
- Nausea and vomiting

Reproductive
- Menstrual abnormalities

FIG. 64-9 Multisystem involvement in systemic lupus erythematosus.

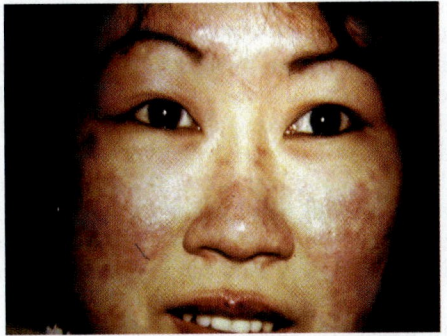

FIG. 64-10 Butterfly rash of systemic lupus erythematosus. (From Firestein GS, Budd RC, Gabriel SE, McInnes IB: *Kelley's textbook of rheumatology*, ed 9, Philadelphia, 2012, Saunders.)

treatments are available. These typically include corticosteroids, cytotoxic agents (cyclophosphamide), and immunosuppressive agents (azathioprine, cyclosporine, mycophenolate mofetil [CellCept]). Rituximab and eculizumab (Soliris) are being studied as possible treatments.[30] Oral prednisone or pulsed IV methylprednisolone may also be used, especially in the initial treatment period when cytotoxic agents have not yet taken effect.

Nervous System Problems. Along with renal involvement, neuropsychiatric manifestations are prevalent in SLE. Generalized or focal seizures of the CNS occur in as many as 15% of patients with SLE by the time of diagnosis. Seizures are generally controlled by corticosteroids or antiseizure drugs. Peripheral neuropathy can also occur, leading to sensory and motor deficits.

Cognitive dysfunction may result from the deposit of immune complexes within the brain. It is marked by disordered thinking, disorientation, and memory deficits. Various psychiatric disorders are reported in SLE, including depression, mood disorders, anxiety, and psychosis. However, they may be related to the stress of having a major illness or to associated drug therapies. Occasionally SLE may cause a stroke or aseptic meningitis. Headaches are also common and can become severe during a disease flare.

Hematologic Problems. Abnormal blood conditions are common in SLE due to formation of antibodies against blood cells. Anemia, leukopenia, thrombocytopenia, and coagulation disorders (excessive bleeding or clotting) are often present.[31] Many patients with SLE benefit from high-intensity treatment with warfarin.

Infection. Patients with SLE appear to have increased susceptibility to infection. Risk may be due to impaired ability to phagocytize invading bacteria, deficient production of antibodies, and immunosuppressive effects of many antiinflammatory drugs. Infection is a major cause of death, and pneumonia is the most common infection. Fever may indicate an underlying

TABLE 64-14 Diagnostic Criteria for Systemic Lupus Erythematosus*

- *Malar rash:* fixed erythema, flat or raised (butterfly rash)
- *Discoid rash:* raised patches with scaling follicular plugging; scarring in older lesions
- *Photosensitivity:* skin rash as unusual reaction to light
- *Oral ulcers:* usually painless
- *Nonerosive arthritis:* two or more peripheral joints with tenderness, swelling, effusion
- Pleuritis or pericarditis
- *Renal disorder:* persistent proteinuria or cellular casts in urine
- *Neurologic disorder:* seizures or psychosis (in the absence of causative drugs or known metabolic disorders)
- *Hematologic disorder:* hemolytic anemia, leukopenia, lymphopenia, or thrombocytopenia
- *Immunologic disorder:* anti-DNA antibody or antibody to Sm nuclear antigen or positive antiphospholipid antibodies
- *Antinuclear antibody:* abnormal titer

Source: American College of Rheumatology: 1997 update of the 1982 American College of Rheumatology revised criteria for classification of systemic lupus erythematosus. Retrieved from *http://www.rheumatology.org/Portals/0/Files/1997%20 Update%20of%201982%20Revised.pdf.*
Sm, Smith.
*A person is classified as having SLE if four or more of the criteria are present, serially or simultaneously, during any interval of observation.

TABLE 64-15 Interprofessional Care
Systemic Lupus Erythematosus

Diagnostic Assessment
- History and physical examination
- Antibodies (e.g., ANA, anti-DNA, anti-Sm, antiphospholipid)
- Complete blood cell count
- Serum complement
- Urinalysis
- X-ray of affected joints
- Chest x-ray
- ECG to determine cardiac involvement

Management
Drug Therapy
- NSAIDs for mild disease
- Steroid-sparing drugs (e.g., methotrexate)
- Antimalarials (e.g., hydroxychloroquine [Plaquenil])
- Corticosteroids for flares and severe disease
- Immunosuppressive drugs (e.g., cyclophosphamide, mycophenolate mofetil [CellCept])

ANA, Antinuclear antibody; *anti-Sm,* Smith.

infection rather than lupus activity alone. Vaccinations are generally safe for patients with SLE. However, patients being treated with corticosteroids or cytotoxic drugs must avoid live virus vaccines.

Diagnostic Studies

Diagnosis of SLE is based on distinct criteria (Table 64-14). No specific test is diagnostic for SLE, but a variety of abnormalities may be present in the blood. SLE is marked by the presence of ANA in 97% of persons with the disease.[32]

Anti-DNA antibodies are found in half the persons with SLE, but lupus can still be present if these antibodies are not identified. The anti-Smith (Sm) antibodies are found in 30% to 40% of persons with lupus and are almost always considered diagnostic. Nearly 30% of people with lupus will have antiphospholipid antibodies. Antibodies to histone are most often seen in people with drug-induced SLE. Elevated ESR and CRP are not diagnostic of SLE but may be used to monitor disease activity and effectiveness of therapy.

Interprofessional Care

A major challenge in the treatment of SLE is managing active disease while preventing complications of treatment. Survival is influenced by several factors, including age, race, sex, socioeconomic status, co-morbid conditions, and disease severity. Prognosis can be improved with early diagnosis, ongoing assessment and prompt recognition of serious organ involvement, and effective therapeutic regimens.

Drug Therapy. NSAIDs continue to be an important intervention, especially for patients with mild arthralgia or arthritis. Careful patient monitoring during long-term NSAID use must include potential GI and renal effects.

Antimalarial agents such as hydroxychloroquine and chloroquine are often used to treat fatigue and skin and joint problems. They modulate the immune system but do not cause immunosuppression. These drugs may also reduce occurrence of flares. Patients taking hydroxychloroquine should have eye examinations by an ophthalmologist every 6 to 12 months.

Retinopathy can develop with high doses of these drugs, but it generally reverses when they are discontinued. If the patient cannot tolerate an antimalarial agent, an antileprosy drug such as dapsone may be used.

Use of corticosteroids should be limited. However, tapering doses of IV methylprednisolone may manage severe flares of polyarthritis. Steroid-sparing immunosuppressants such as methotrexate can serve as an alternative treatment. They are prescribed with folic acid to decrease corticosteroid side effects. However, high doses of corticosteroids may be especially appropriate for the patient with severe cutaneous SLE.

Immunosuppressive drugs such as azathioprine and cyclophosphamide may be used to reduce the need for long-term corticosteroid therapy. Either drug is also an appropriate treatment for severe organ-system disease, especially renal problems. Close monitoring is needed to decrease the risk of drug toxicity and side effects. Because blood clots can be a life-threatening complication of SLE, anticoagulants such as warfarin may be prescribed.

Topical immunomodulators can be used instead of corticosteroids to treat serious skin conditions. Tacrolimus (Protopic, Prograf) and pimecrolimus (Elidel) suppress immune activity in the skin, affecting the butterfly rash and possibly discoid lesions.

Clinical trials are currently investigating the effect of various medications on SLE management. These include agents that interfere with the immune response such as abatacept, and hormones (prasterone) to combat corticosteroid-induced osteoporosis. Lenalidomide, a chemical derivative of thalidomide, can improve cutaneous lupus without adverse neurologic effects.

When teaching patients about their prescribed drugs, include indications for use, proper administration, and possible side effects. Help patients understand that abruptly stopping a medication may worsen disease activity.

Disease management is most appropriately monitored by serial anti-DNA titers and serum complement (Table 64-15). Simpler, less costly tests such as ESR or CRP may also be helpful.

❖ NURSING MANAGEMENT: SYSTEMIC LUPUS ERYTHEMATOSUS

◆ Nursing Assessment

Subjective and objective data that should be obtained from the patient with SLE are presented in Table 64-16. In particular, evaluate the effect of pain and fatigue on ability to perform ADLs.

◆ Nursing Diagnoses

Nursing diagnoses for the patient with SLE may include, but are not limited to, the following:

- Fatigue *related to* chronic inflammation and altered immunity
- Impaired skin integrity *related to* photosensitivity, skin rash, and alopecia
- Impaired comfort *related to* symptoms of illness, treatment side effects, and potential variable and unpredictable disease progression

Additional information on nursing diagnoses for the patient with SLE is presented in eNursing Care Plan 64-2 (on the website for this chapter).

◆ Planning

Overall goals are that the patient with SLE will (1) have satisfactory pain management, (2) adhere to the therapeutic regimen to achieve maximum symptom management, (3) demonstrate awareness of and avoid activities that worsen the disease, and (4) maintain optimal role function and positive self-image.

◆ Nursing Implementation

◆ **Health Promotion.** Prevention of SLE is not currently possible. Education for health professionals and the community should create a clear understanding of the disease and the need for early diagnosis and treatment.

◆ **Acute Care.** As in most rheumatic diseases, the unpredictable nature of SLE presents many challenges for the patient and caregiver. Physical, psychologic, and sociocultural problems linked to long-term management of SLE require varied approaches and skills from an interprofessional health care team.

During a disease flare, the patient may quickly become very ill. Nursing interventions include accurately recording the severity of symptoms and documenting the response to therapy. Specifically assess fever pattern, joint inflammation, limitation of motion, location and degree of discomfort, and fatigue. Monitor the patient's weight and fluid intake and output. This is especially important if corticosteroids are prescribed because of related fluid retention and possible renal failure. Collect 24-hour urine samples for protein and creatinine clearance as ordered. Observe for signs of bleeding due to drug therapy (e.g., pallor, skin bruising, petechiae, tarry stools).

Carefully assess neurologic function. Observe for vision problems, headaches, personality changes, seizures, and memory loss. Psychosis may result from CNS disease or be an effect of corticosteroid therapy. Nerve irritation of the extremities *(peripheral neuropathy)* may cause numbness, tingling, and weakness of the hands and feet.

Explain the nature of the disease, types of therapy, and all diagnostic procedures. Provide emotional support for the patient and family, especially during a disease flare.

TABLE 64-16 Nursing Assessment
Systemic Lupus Erythematosus

Subjective Data

Important Health Information

Past health history: Exposure to ultraviolet light, drugs, chemicals, viral infections. Physical or psychologic stress. States of increased estrogen activity, including early onset of menses, pregnancy, and postpartum period. Pattern of remissions and flares

Medications: Oral contraceptives, procainamide (Pronestyl), hydralazine, isoniazid, antiseizure drugs, antibiotics (possibly causing symptoms of SLE), corticosteroids, NSAIDs

Functional Health Patterns

Health perception–health management: Family history of autoimmune disorders, frequent infections, malaise, impact of disease on functional ability

Nutritional-metabolic: Weight loss, oral and nasal ulcers, nausea and vomiting, dry mouth *(xerostomia)*, dysphagia, photosensitivity with rash, frequent infections

Elimination: Decreased urine output, diarrhea or constipation

Activity-exercise: Morning stiffness, joint swelling and deformity, shortness of breath *(dyspnea)*, excessive fatigue

Sleep-rest: Insomnia

Cognitive-perceptual: Vision problems, vertigo, headache, arthralgia, chest pain (pericardial, pleuritic), abdominal pain. Painful, throbbing, cold fingers with numbness and tingling

Sexuality-reproductive: Amenorrhea, irregular menstrual periods

Coping–stress tolerance: Depression, withdrawal

Objective Data

General

Fever, lymphadenopathy, periorbital edema

Integumentary

Alopecia. Dry, scaly scalp. Keratoconjunctivitis, malar butterfly rash, palmar or discoid erythema, hives (urticaria), erythema at fingernails or toenails, purpura, or petechiae. Leg ulcers

Respiratory

Pleural friction rub, decreased breath sounds

Cardiovascular

Vasculitis, pericardial friction rub, hypertension, edema, dysrhythmias, murmurs. Bilateral, symmetric pallor and cyanosis of fingers (Raynaud's phenomenon)

Gastrointestinal

Oral and pharyngeal ulcers; splenomegaly

Neurologic

Facial weakness, peripheral neuropathies, papilledema, dysarthria, confusion, hallucination, disorientation, psychosis, seizures, aphasia, hemiparesis

Musculoskeletal

Myopathy, myositis, arthritis

Urinary

Proteinuria

Possible Diagnostic Findings

Presence of anti-DNA, anti-Sm, and antinuclear antibodies. Anemia, leukopenia, thrombocytopenia. ↑ Erythrocyte sedimentation rate (ESR), ↑ serum creatinine. Microscopic hematuria, cellular casts in urine. Pericarditis or pleural effusion on chest x-ray

Sm, Smith.

TABLE 64-17 Patient & Caregiver Teaching

Systemic Lupus Erythematosus

Include the following information in the teaching plan for a patient with systemic lupus erythematosus and the caregiver.
- Disease process
- Names of drugs, actions, side effects, dosage, administration
- Pain management strategies
- Energy conservation and pacing techniques
- Therapeutic exercise, use of heat therapy (for arthralgia)
- Relaxation therapy
- Avoidance of physical and emotional stress
- Avoidance of exposure to individuals with infection
- Avoidance of drying soaps, powders, household chemicals
- Use of sunscreen protection (at least SPF 15) and protective clothing, with minimal sun exposure from 11:00 AM to 3:00 PM
- Regular medical and laboratory follow-up
- Marital and pregnancy counseling as needed
- Community resources and health care agencies

SPF, Sun protection factor.

◆ **Ambulatory Care.** Emphasize the importance of patient involvement for successful home management. Help the patient understand that even strong adherence to the treatment plan is no guarantee against flares due to the unpredictable disease course. Various factors may increase disease activity, such as fatigue, sun exposure, emotional stress, infection, drugs, and surgery. Help the patient and caregiver eliminate or reduce exposure to such factors (Table 64-17).

◆ *Lupus and Pregnancy.* Because SLE is most common in women of childbearing age, treatment during pregnancy must be considered. The woman's primary HCP (or rheumatologist) and obstetrician should thoroughly discuss with the woman her desire to become pregnant. Infertility may have resulted from renal involvement and previous use of high-dose corticosteroid and immunosuppressive drugs. The patient should understand spontaneous abortion, stillbirth, and intrauterine growth retardation are common problems with pregnancy. They occur because immune complexes are deposited in the placenta and inflammation occurs in placental blood vessels.

Renal, cardiovascular, pulmonary, and central nervous systems may be affected during pregnancy. Women who already show serious effects in these systems should be counseled against pregnancy. For the best outcome, pregnancy should be planned when disease activity is minimal. Flares are common during the postpartum period. Therapeutic abortion offers the same risk of postdelivery exacerbation as carrying the fetus to term.

◆ *Psychosocial Issues.* The patient with SLE faces many psychosocial issues.[33] Disease onset and symptoms may be vague, and SLE may be undiagnosed for a long time. Supportive therapies may be as important as medical treatment in helping the patient cope with the disease. Inform the patient and caregiver that SLE has a good prognosis for most people.

Stress the importance of planning both recreational and occupational activities. The young adult may find sun restrictions and physical limitations difficult to follow. Help the patient develop and accomplish reasonable goals for improving or maintaining mobility, energy, and self-esteem.

Families worry about hereditary aspects and want to know if their children will also have SLE. Many couples require pregnancy and sexual counseling. Individuals making decisions about marriage and careers worry how SLE will interfere with

their plans. Teach teachers, employers, and co-workers as needed about the impact of SLE.

◆ **Evaluation**

The expected outcomes are that the patient with SLE will
- Use energy-conservation techniques
- Adapt lifestyle to current energy
- Maintain skin integrity with use of topical treatments
- Prevent disease flare with use of sunscreens and limited sun exposure

Additional information on expected outcomes for the patient with SLE is presented in eNursing Care Plan 64-2 (on the website for this chapter).

SCLERODERMA

Scleroderma (*systemic sclerosis*) is a disorder of connective tissue characterized by fibrotic, degenerative, and occasionally inflammatory changes in the skin, blood vessels, synovium, skeletal muscle, and internal organs.

Scleroderma occurs in all ethnic groups but is more common in African Americans than whites. Native Americans and persons of Japanese descent may also be at higher risk than whites. Although symptoms may begin at any time, the usual age at onset is between 30 and 50 years. Scleroderma is relatively rare, with approximately 20 adults per 1 million in the United States affected. Incidence in women is four times more common than in men.[3]

Two types of disease exist: *localized scleroderma*, which is the more common form, and *diffuse systemic scleroderma*. Skin changes of localized disease are usually limited to the face, fingers, and distal extremities without involvement of the trunk or internal organs. The prognosis of patients with limited disease is generally better than for those with diffuse disease. Skin changes are rapidly progressive during the first months of diffuse scleroderma, which is associated with internal organ involvement.

Etiology and Pathophysiology

The exact cause of scleroderma is unknown. Immunologic dysfunction and vascular abnormalities are believed to play a role in the development of widespread systemic disease. Other risk factors for skin thickening include environmental or occupational exposure to coal, plastics, and silica dust.

In scleroderma, collagen (protein that gives normal skin its strength and elasticity) is overproduced (Fig. 64-11). This leads to progressive tissue fibrosis and occlusion of blood vessels. Proliferation of collagen also disrupts normal function of internal organs, such as the lungs, kidney, heart, and GI tract.

Vascular alterations, which primarily involve the small arteries and arterioles, are almost always present. These changes are some of the earliest changes in scleroderma.

Clinical Manifestations

Manifestations of scleroderma range from diffuse cutaneous thickening with rapidly progressive and widespread organ involvement to the more benign limited cutaneous form. Localized disease is often marked by the **CREST syndrome**:

Calcinosis: painful deposits of calcium in skin of fingers, forearms, pressure points

Raynaud's phenomenon: intermittent vasospasm of fingertips in response to cold or stress

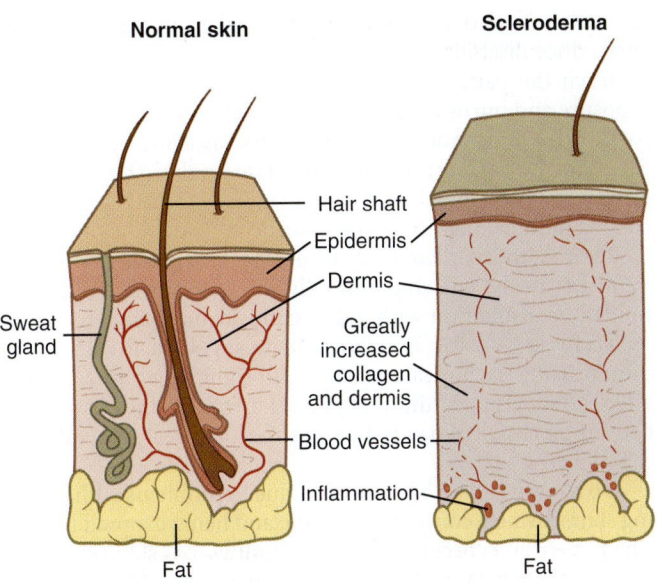

FIG. 64-11 Skin changes in scleroderma.

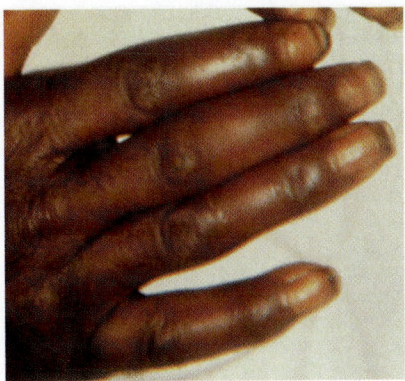

FIG. 64-12 Sclerodactyly in the hand of a patient with scleroderma. (From Zitelli BJ, Davis HW: *Atlas of pediatric physical diagnosis*, ed 4, St Louis, 2002, Mosby.)

Esophageal dysfunction: difficulty swallowing due to internal scarring

Sclerodactyly: tightening of skin on fingers and toes

Telangiectasia: red spots on hands, forearms, palms, face, and lips from capillary dilation

Raynaud's Phenomenon. Raynaud's phenomenon (sudden vasospasm of the digits) is the most common initial complaint in localized scleroderma. Patients have diminished blood flow to the fingers and toes on exposure to cold (*blanching or white phase*), followed by cyanosis as hemoglobin releases O_2 to the tissues (*blue phase*), and then erythema during rewarming (*red phase*). Color changes often occur with numbness and tingling. Raynaud's phenomenon may precede the onset of systemic disease by months, years, or even decades. (Raynaud's phenomenon is described in more detail in Chapter 37.)

Skin and Joint Changes. Symmetric painless swelling or thickening of the skin of the fingers and hands may progress to diffuse scleroderma of the trunk. In localized disease, skin thickening generally does not extend above the elbow or knee, although the face may be affected. In diffuse disease, the skin loses elasticity and becomes taut and shiny. This produces the typical expressionless face with tightly pursed lips. Skin changes in the face may also contribute to reduced ROM in the temporomandibular joint. The fingers may remain in a semi-flexed position (*sclerodactyly*), with tightened skin to the wrist (Fig. 64-12). Reduced peripheral joint function may occur as an early symptom of arthritis.

Internal Organ Involvement. About 20% of people with scleroderma develop secondary Sjögren's syndrome, a condition associated with dry eyes and dry mouth. Dysphagia, gum disease, and dental decay can result. Frequent reflux of gastric acid can also occur due to esophageal fibrosis. If swallowing becomes difficult, the patient is likely to decrease food intake and lose weight. Additional GI effects include constipation from colonic hypomotility and diarrhea due to malabsorption from bacterial overgrowth.

Lung involvement includes pleural thickening, pulmonary fibrosis, and abnormal pulmonary function. The patient develops a cough and dyspnea. Pulmonary arterial hypertension and interstitial lung disease may occur. (These disorders are discussed in Chapter 27.) Lung disease is the main cause of death in scleroderma.

Primary heart disease consists of pericarditis, pericardial effusion, and dysrhythmias. Heart failure from myocardial fibrosis occurs most often in patients with diffuse disease.

Renal disease was previously a major cause of death in diffuse scleroderma. Because malignant hypertension associated with rapidly progressive, irreversible renal insufficiency can occur, early recognition of renal involvement and initiation of therapy are critical. Recent improvements in dialysis, bilateral nephrectomy in patients with uncontrollable hypertension, and kidney transplant have offered hope to patients with renal failure. In particular, use of angiotensin-converting enzyme (ACE) inhibitors (e.g., lisinopril [Prinivil]) has had a marked effect on the ability to treat renal disease.

Diagnostic Studies

Laboratory results in scleroderma are relatively normal. Blood studies may reveal mild hemolytic anemia as a result of RBC damage in diseased small vessels. Anticentromere antibodies related to CREST syndrome are found in about 60% to 80% of people with localized scleroderma. Antibodies to topoisomerase-1 are present in about 30% of people with diffuse disease. Presence of either antibody is highly specific for diagnosis. If renal involvement is present, urinalysis may show proteinuria, microscopic hematuria, and casts. Serum creatinine may be elevated. X-ray evidence of subcutaneous calcification, distal esophageal hypomotility, or bibasilar pulmonary fibrosis is diagnostic of scleroderma. Pulmonary function studies reveal decreased vital capacity and lung compliance.

Interprofessional Care

Interprofessional care of scleroderma (Table 64-18) offers no specific treatment. Supportive care is directed toward preventing or treating secondary complications of involved organs. Physical therapy helps to maintain joint mobility and preserve muscle strength. Occupational therapy assists the patient in maintaining functional abilities.

Drug Therapy. No specific drug or combination of drugs has proven effective for treatment of scleroderma. Vasoactive agents are often prescribed in early disease. Calcium channel blockers (nifedipine [Procardia], diltiazem [Cardizem]) and the angiotensin II blocker losartan are common treatments for Raynaud's phenomenon. Reserpine, an α-adrenergic blocking agent, increases blood flow to the fingers. Bosentan (Tracleer), an

TABLE 64-18 **Interprofessional Care**

Scleroderma

Diagnostic Assessment
- History and physical examination
- Antibodies to topoisomerase-1
- Anticentromere antibody
- Nail bed capillary microscopy
- Chest x-ray
- Skin or organ biopsy
- Urinalysis (proteinuria, hematuria, casts)
- Pulmonary function tests
- ECG

Management
- Physical therapy
- Occupational therapy

Drug Therapy
- *Vasoactive agents:* reserpine, bosentan, epoprostenol
- *Calcium channel blockers:* diltiazem, nifedipine
- *Angiotensin-converting enzyme inhibitors:* lisinopril (Prinivil)
- *Immunosuppressive drugs:* cyclophosphamide, mycophenolate mofetil (CellCept)

endothelin-receptor antagonist, and the vasodilator epoprostenol (Flolan) may help prevent and treat digital ulcers. They also improve exercise capacity and heart and lung dynamics.

Corticosteroids may have little effect on scleroderma and may actually cause a renal crisis. Topical agents may provide some relief from joint pain. Capsaicin cream may be useful, not only as a local analgesic but also as a vasodilator. Other therapies prescribed to treat specific systemic problems include (1) tetracycline for diarrhea caused by bacterial overgrowth, (2) histamine (H_2) receptor blockers (e.g., cimetidine) and proton pump inhibitors (e.g., omeprazole [Prilosec]) for esophageal symptoms, (3) antihypertensive agent (e.g., captopril, propranolol [Inderal], methyldopa) for hypertension with renal involvement, and (4) immunosuppressive drugs (e.g., cyclophosphamide, mycophenolate mofetil).

❖ NURSING MANAGEMENT: SCLERODERMA

Prevention of scleroderma is not possible. Nursing interventions often begin during a hospitalization for diagnosis. Assess vital signs, weight, intake and output, respiratory and bowel function, and joint ROM regularly as indicated by specific symptoms to plan appropriate care. Emotional stress and cold ambient temperatures may aggravate Raynaud's phenomenon. Instruct patients with scleroderma to avoid finger-stick blood testing because of compromised circulation and poor healing of the fingers.

Teaching is an important nursing intervention as the patient and family begin to live with this disease. Obvious changes in the face and hands often lead to poor self-image and loss of mobility and function. The patient must regularly participate in therapeutic exercises at home to prevent skin retraction and promote vascularization. Mouth excursion (yawning with an open mouth) is a good exercise to help with temporomandibular joint function. Isometric exercises are best if the patient has arthropathy because no joint movement occurs. Encourage the use of moist heat applications or paraffin baths to promote skin flexibility in the hands and feet. Teach the patient to use assistive devices as needed and organize activities to preserve strength and reduce disability.

Teach the patient to protect the hands and feet from cold exposure and burns or cuts that may heal slowly. Encourage the patient to avoid smoking because of its vasoconstricting effect. Report signs of infection promptly. Use alcohol-free lotions to improve skin dryness and cracking. However, they must be rubbed in for a long time to be absorbed through the thick skin.

Remind the patient to reduce dysphagia by eating small, frequent meals; chewing carefully and slowly; and drinking fluids. A consultation with a dietitian is beneficial.

Decrease risk for heartburn by using antacids 45 to 60 minutes after each meal and sitting upright for at least 2 hours after eating. Using additional pillows or raising the head of the bed on blocks also may reduce gastroesophageal reflux during the night.

Job alterations are often needed due to problems with climbing stairs, using a computer, writing, and being exposed to cold. The patient may become socially withdrawn as skin tightening changes the appearance of the face and hands. Dining out may become socially embarrassing because of the patient's small mouth, swallowing difficulty, and reflux. Some persons with scleroderma wear gloves to protect fingertip ulcers and provide extra warmth. Emphasize daily oral hygiene because neglect may lead to increased tooth and gum problems. The patient needs a dentist who is familiar with scleroderma and able to adapt care to a small mouth.

Psychologic support, biofeedback training, and relaxation can reduce stress and improve sleeping habits. Sexual dysfunction from body changes, pain, muscular weakness, limited mobility, decreased self-esteem, erectile dysfunction, and decreased vaginal secretions may require sensitive counseling.

❓ CHECK YOUR PRACTICE

A 34-yr-old woman hospitalized for aspiration pneumonia also has a 5-year history of scleroderma.
- How could scleroderma have contributed to the aspiration pneumonia?
- What strategies will you suggest to decrease the risk of pneumonia recurrence?
- What other self-care strategies will you reinforce with this patient?

POLYMYOSITIS AND DERMATOMYOSITIS

Polymyositis (PM) is diffuse, idiopathic, inflammatory myopathy of striated muscle that produces bilateral weakness, usually most severe in the proximal or limb girdle muscles. When muscle changes associated with PM are accompanied by distinctive skin changes, the disorder is called **dermatomyositis (DM)**.

These relatively rare disorders can be similar in signs, symptoms, and treatment, but they are two distinct diseases. They typically affect adults ages 40 to 60 years. Both PM and DM occur twice as often in women as in men. Patients with PM generally have more severe disease than those with DM.

Etiology and Pathophysiology

The exact cause of PM and DM is unknown, but evidence suggests an autoimmune origin involving HLA immune response genes.[34] Environmental factors are also likely, including viral and bacterial infection; certain drugs, supplements, and vaccines; medical implants; and occupational exposures.

Clinical Manifestations and Complications

Muscular. The patient with PM and DM experiences weight loss and increasing fatigue, with a gradually developing weakness of muscles that leads to difficulty performing routine activities. The most commonly affected muscles are in the shoulders, legs, arms, and pelvic girdle. The patient may have difficulty rising from a chair or bathtub, climbing stairs, combing hair, or reaching into a high cupboard. Repetitive movements are more likely to cause trouble than a single strength exercise. The patient may also be unable to raise the head from a pillow as neck muscles weaken. Muscle discomfort or tenderness is uncommon. Muscle examination reveals an inability to move against resistance or even gravity. Weak pharyngeal muscles may produce dysphagia and dysphonia (nasal or hoarse voice).

Dermal. Skin changes of DM include a classic red or purple symmetric rash *(heliotrope)* with edema around the eyelids. The typical skin rash is not commonly found with other disorders. An additional scaly, smooth, or raised rash may be seen on the knuckles and sides of the hands *(Gottron's papules)* (Fig. 64-13).

These skin changes usually prompt earlier recognition of DM than PM, which has no rash. Reddened, smooth, or scaly patches appear with the same symmetric distribution but sparing the interphalangeal spaces *(Gottron's sign)*. The rash can be confused with psoriasis or seborrheic dermatitis. A red, scaling rash *(poikiloderma)* may develop as a late finding on the back, buttocks, and a V-shaped area of the anterior neck and chest. Hyperemia and telangiectasia are often present at the nail beds. Calcium nodules *(calcinosis cutis)* can develop throughout the skin and are especially common in long-standing DM.

Other Manifestations. Joint redness, pain, and inflammation often occur and contribute to limited joint ROM in PM and DM. Contractures and muscle atrophy may occur with advanced disease. Weakened pharyngeal muscles can lead to poor cough effort, difficulty swallowing, and increased risk for aspiration pneumonia in both disorders. Interstitial lung disease is a frequent complication. All patients with PM or DM should be evaluated routinely with a chest x-ray and pulmonary function tests. People with DM also have an increased risk of cancer and should receive age- and gender-appropriate screenings. PM and DM may be associated with other connective tissue disorders (e.g., scleroderma).

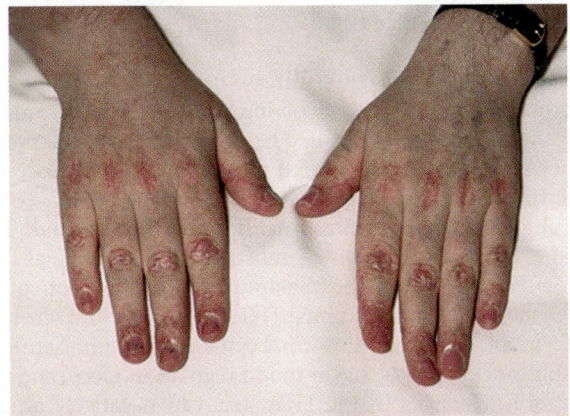

FIG. 64-13 Dermatomyositis skin changes indicating Gottron's papules. (From Firestein GS, Budd RC, Gabriel SE, McInnes IB: *Kelley's textbook of rheumatology*, ed 9, Philadelphia, 2012, Saunders.)

Diagnostic Studies

Biopsy is the gold standard for diagnosis of PM or DM after other neuromuscular diseases have been excluded. Muscle biopsy reveals necrosis, degeneration, regeneration, and fibrosis with pathologic findings distinct for DM or PM. MRI can be used to identify areas of inflammation and guide the biopsy site selection. Laboratory tests are helpful, but not diagnostic of either disease. Increased muscle enzymes (e.g., creatine kinase, myoglobin) reflect muscle damage but will decrease to normal or near normal with treatment. An electromyogram (EMG) suggestive of PM shows bizarre high-frequency discharges and spontaneous fibrillation, with positive spikes at rest. Elevation of the ESR or CRP occurs with active disease.

❖ NURSING AND INTERPROFESSIONAL MANAGEMENT: POLYMYOSITIS AND DERMATOMYOSITIS

PM and DM are treated initially with high-dose oral corticosteroids. Improvement generally occurs if corticosteroid therapy is instituted promptly. Dosage can be reduced as the patient improves until the lowest possible dose associated with symptom management is reached. Long-term corticosteroid therapy may be required because relapses are common when the drug is withdrawn.

For patients who do not respond to corticosteroids, immunosuppressive drugs (methotrexate, azathioprine, tacrolimus, cyclophosphamide) may be used. IV immunoglobulin (IV Ig) may also be administered with corticosteroids or immunosuppressants, but it is not a first-line treatment.

💊 DRUG ALERT   IV Immunoglobulin (IV Ig)

- Administer by slow infusion to decrease risk of thromboembolic complications.
- Hydrate patient well during infusion to decrease risk of renal failure.
- Treat transient adverse effects such as headache.

The role of newer drugs such as TNF inhibitors remains unclear. The most promising BRM for treatment of PM and DM is rituximab.[35]

Physical therapy can be helpful and should be tailored to disease activity. Massage and passive movement are appropriate during active disease. Delay more aggressive exercises until disease activity is minimal, as evidenced by low serum muscle enzymes.

Teach the patient about the disease, prescribed therapies, diagnostic tests, and the need for regular medical care. Help the patient understand that the benefits of therapy are often delayed. For example, weakness may increase during the first few weeks of corticosteroid therapy. Pay special attention to patient safety. Encourage the use of assistive devices to decrease risk of falls. To prevent aspiration, encourage the patient to rest before meals, maintain an upright position when eating, and choose easily swallowed foods.

Assist the patient to organize activities and use pacing techniques to conserve energy. Encourage daily ROM exercises to prevent contractures. When inflammation is decreased, start muscle-strengthening (repetitive) exercises. Home care and bed rest may be needed during acute PM because the patient may not be able to complete ADLs because of profound muscle weakness.

MIXED CONNECTIVE TISSUE DISEASE

Patients having a combination of clinical features of several rheumatic diseases are described as having *mixed connective tissue disease.* The term describes a disorder with features primarily of SLE, scleroderma, and PM. This disease occurs most often in women in their 20s and 30s.

About 25% of persons with a connective tissue disease develop another related disease over the course of several years, which is known as *overlap syndrome.*[36]

SJÖGREN'S SYNDROME

Sjögren's syndrome is a relatively common autoimmune disease that targets the moisture-producing exocrine glands, which leads to *xerostomia* (dry mouth) and *keratoconjunctivitis sicca* (dry eyes).[37] The nose, throat, airways, and skin can also become dry. The disease may affect other glands as well, including those in the stomach, pancreas, and intestines (extraglandular involvement). The disease is usually diagnosed in people over age 40 but can be found in all age groups. Women are 10 times more likely than men to have Sjögren's syndrome.

In primary Sjögren's syndrome, symptoms can be traced to problems with lacrimal and salivary glands. About half the cases of Sjögren's syndrome develop alone as primary disease.[37] The patient with secondary Sjögren's syndrome typically had another autoimmune disease (e.g., RA, SLE) before Sjögren's developed.

Sjögren's syndrome appears to be caused by genetic and environmental factors. Several genes seem to be involved. One gene predisposes whites to the disease, whereas other genes are linked to the disease in people of Japanese, Chinese, and African-American heritage. The trigger may be a viral or bacterial infection that adversely stimulates the immune system. In Sjögren's syndrome, lymphocytes attack and damage the lacrimal and salivary glands.

Decreased tearing causes dry eyes, which leads to a gritty sensation in the eyes, burning, blurred vision, and photosensitivity. Dry mouth produces buccal membrane fissures, altered sense of taste, dysphagia, and increased mouth infection or dental decay. Dry skin and rashes, joint and muscle pain, and thyroid problems may be present. Other exocrine glands can also be affected. For example, vaginal dryness may lead to painful intercourse (*dyspareunia*).

Autoimmune thyroid disorders, including Graves' disease and Hashimoto's thyroiditis, are common with Sjögren's syndrome. Histologic study reveals lymphocyte infiltration of salivary and lacrimal glands. The disease may become more generalized and involve the lymph nodes, bone marrow, and visceral organs (pseudolymphoma). Persons with Sjögren's syndrome have an increased risk of developing non-Hodgkin's lymphoma.[38]

Ophthalmologic examination (Schirmer's test for tear production), measures of salivary gland function, and lower lip biopsy of minor salivary glands aid in diagnosis. The treatment of Sjögren's syndrome is symptomatic, including (1) instillation of preservative-free artificial tears or ophthalmic antiinflammatory drops (e.g., cyclosporine [Restasis]) as needed for adequate hydration and lubrication, (2) surgical punctal occlusion, and (3) increased fluids with meals. Dental hygiene is important.

Pilocarpine (Salagen) and cevimeline (Evoxac) can be used to treat symptoms of dry mouth. Increased humidity at home may reduce respiratory tract infections. Vaginal lubrication with a water-soluble product such as K-Y jelly may increase comfort during intercourse.

> ⚠ **SAFETY ALERT** Sjögren's Syndrome
> To help with chewing and swallowing:
> - Moisten food with mayonnaise, sauces, gravy, or yogurt.
> - Thin foods with skim milk or broth.
> - Use a food processor or blender to finely chop or liquefy foods.
> - Try soft, creamy foods (e.g., mashed potatoes, macaroni and cheese).
> - Drink high-calorie cold liquids (e.g., breakfast drinks).
> - Avoid salty, acidic, or spicy foods.

MYOFASCIAL PAIN SYNDROME

Myofascial pain syndrome is a chronic form of muscle pain. It is marked by musculoskeletal pain and tenderness, typically in the chest, neck, shoulders, hips, and lower back. Referred pain from these muscle groups can also travel to the buttocks, hands, and head, causing severe headaches. Temporomandibular joint pain may also originate in myofascial pain. Regions of pain are often within the connective tissue (*fascia*) that covers skeletal muscles. Trigger or tender points are thought to activate a characteristic pattern of pain that worsens with activity or stress.

Myofascial pain syndrome occurs more often in middle-aged adults and in women rather than men. Patients complain of deep, aching pain accompanied by a sensation of burning, stinging, and stiffness.

Physical therapy is one treatment used for myofascial pain syndrome. A typical treatment is the "spray and stretch" method, in which the painful area is iced or sprayed with a coolant such as ethyl chloride and then stretched. Positive results have been seen with topical patches and injection of the trigger points with a local anesthetic (e.g., 1% lidocaine). Massage, acupuncture, biofeedback, and ultrasound therapy have also benefited some patients.[39]

FIBROMYALGIA

Fibromyalgia is a chronic central pain syndrome marked by widespread, nonarticular musculoskeletal pain and fatigue with multiple tender points. People with fibromyalgia may also experience nonrestorative sleep, morning stiffness, irritable bowel syndrome, and anxiety. Fibromyalgia is a commonly diagnosed musculoskeletal disorder and a major cause of disability. It affects an estimated 2% of the general U.S. population. The disease is 4 to 10 times more common in women than men.[3] Fibromyalgia and systemic exertion intolerance disease (SEID) (formerly called chronic fatigue syndrome) share many common features (Table 64-19).

Etiology and Pathophysiology

Fibromyalgia is a disorder involving abnormal central processing of nociceptive pain input. The increased pain experienced by the affected patient is due to abnormal sensory processing in the CNS.

Multiple physiologic abnormalities have been found. They include (1) increased levels of substance P in the spinal fluid, (2) low blood flow to the thalamus, (3) dysfunction of the hypothalamic-pituitary-adrenal (HPA) axis, (4) low serotonin and tryptophan, and (5) abnormal cytokine function. Serotonin and substance P play a role in mood regulation, sleep, and pain perception. Changes in the HPA axis can negatively affect a person's physical and mental health. An increased incidence of depression and decreased response to stress occur. Genetic factors also contribute to the development of fibromyalgia, as

TABLE 64-19 Common Features of Fibromyalgia and Systemic Exertion Intolerance Disease (SEID)

Occurrence
Previously healthy, young and middle-aged women.

Etiology (theories)
Infectious trigger, dysfunction in HPA axis, alteration in CNS.

Clinical Manifestations
Generalized musculoskeletal pain, malaise and fatigue, cognitive dysfunction, headaches, sleep disturbances, depression, anxiety, fever.

Disease Course
Variable intensity of symptoms, fluctuates over time.

Diagnosis
No definitive laboratory tests or joint and muscle examinations. Mainly a diagnosis of exclusion.

Management
Symptomatic treatment may include antidepressant drugs such as amitriptyline and fluoxetine (Prozac). Other measures are heat, massage, regular stretching, biofeedback, stress management, and relaxation training. Patient and caregiver teaching is essential.

HPA, Hypothalamic-pituitary-adrenal.

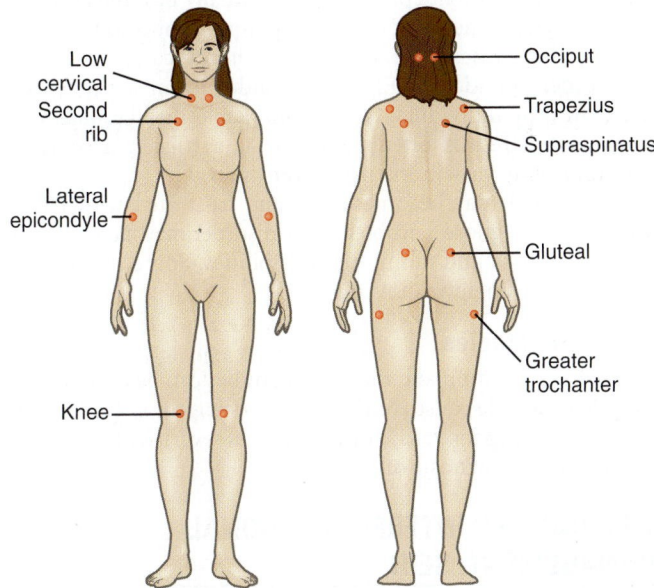

FIG. 64-14 Tender points in fibromyalgia.

a familial tendency exists. Recent illness or trauma may be a trigger in susceptible people.

Clinical Manifestations and Complications

The patient complains of a widespread burning pain that worsens and improves through the course of a day. The patient often has trouble determining if pain occurs in the muscles, joints, or soft tissues. Head or facial pain often results from stiff or painful neck and shoulder muscles. The pain can accompany temporomandibular joint dysfunction, which affects an estimated one third of patients with fibromyalgia.

Physical examination typically reveals point tenderness at 11 or more of 18 identified sites (Fig. 64-14). Patients with fibromyalgia are sensitive to painful stimuli throughout the body, not just at the identified tender sites. They may also experience pain in response to a stimulus that does not typically cause pain *(allodynia)*. In addition, point tenderness can vary from day to day. Sometimes, the patient may respond to fewer than 11 tender points. At other times, palpation of all sites may cause pain.

Cognitive effects range from difficulty concentrating to memory lapses and a feeling of being overwhelmed when dealing with multiple tasks. Many individuals report migraine headaches. Depression and anxiety often occur and may require drug therapy. Stiffness, nonrefreshing sleep, fatigue, and numbness or tingling in the hands or feet often accompany fibromyalgia. Restless legs syndrome is also typical, with patients describing an irresistible urge to move the legs when at rest or lying down.

Irritable bowel syndrome with manifestations of constipation and/or diarrhea, abdominal pain, and bloating is common. Patients may also experience difficulty swallowing, perhaps because of problems in esophageal smooth muscle function. Increased frequency of urination and urinary urgency, in the absence of a bladder infection, are typical complaints. Women with fibromyalgia may experience more difficult menstruation with a worsening of disease symptoms during this time.

Diagnostic Studies

A definitive diagnosis of fibromyalgia is often difficult to establish. Lack of knowledge about the disease and its manifestations among HCPs may also cause delays in diagnosis and treatment.

Laboratory results in most cases help rule out other suspected disorders. Muscle biopsy may reveal a nonspecific moth-eaten appearance or fiber atrophy.

The American College of Rheumatology (ACR) classifies an individual as having fibromyalgia if two criteria are met: (1) pain is experienced in 11 of the 18 tender points on palpation (Fig. 64-14) and (2) a history of widespread pain is noted for at least 3 months.[40] Widespread pain is defined as pain that occurs on both sides of the body and above and below the waist. In addition, fatigue, cognitive symptoms, and extensive somatic symptoms are considered in establishing a diagnosis.

A subsequent classification by the ACR used non–tender point diagnostic criteria as an alternative method of diagnosis, using a symptom severity scale and a widespread pain index to identify disease characteristics.[41] It is suggested this classification be used with the previous ACR criteria.

Interprofessional Care

Treatment of fibromyalgia is symptomatic and requires a high level of patient motivation. Teach the patient to be an active participant in the therapeutic regimen. Rest can help the pain, aching, and tenderness.

Drug therapy for the chronic widespread pain associated with fibromyalgia includes pregabalin (Lyrica), duloxetine (Cymbalta), and milnacipran (Savella). Low-dose tricyclic antidepressants, selective serotonin reuptake inhibitors (SSRIs), or benzodiazepines (e.g., diazepam [Valium]) may also be prescribed. If the tricyclic antidepressant amitriptyline is not well tolerated, similar drugs can be substituted (e.g., doxepin, imipramine [Tofranil], trazodone). SSRI antidepressants (e.g., sertraline [Zoloft] or paroxetine [Paxil]) tend to be reserved for patients who also have depression. SSRIs may have to be prescribed at higher doses than when used to treat depression. Both antidepressants and muscle relaxants (e.g., baclofen [Lioresal]) have sedative effects that can improve nighttime rest for the patient with fibromyalgia.

Long-acting opioids generally are not recommended unless other therapies are unsuccessful. In some patients, pain may be managed with OTC analgesics such as acetaminophen, ibuprofen, or naproxen (Aleve) used in combination with a TCA. Nonopioids such as tramadol (Ultram) may also be used. In addition, zolpidem (Ambien) or trazodone is sometimes prescribed for short-term intervention in patients with severe sleep problems.

❖ NURSING MANAGEMENT: FIBROMYALGIA

Because of the chronic nature of fibromyalgia, the patient needs consistent support from interprofessional team members. Massage is often combined with ultrasound or the application of alternating heat and cold packs to soothe tense, sore muscles and increase blood circulation. Gentle stretching to relieve muscle tension and spasm can be performed by a physical therapist or practiced by the patient at home. Yoga and Tai Chi are often helpful. Low-impact aerobic exercise, such as walking, can help prevent muscle atrophy.

Patients with fibromyalgia may consider limiting the consumption of sugar, caffeine, and alcohol because these substances may be muscle irritants. Vitamin and mineral supplements may help combat stress, correct deficiencies, and support the immune system. However, unproven miracle diets or supplements should be carefully investigated by the patient and discussed with the HCP before using them. Inform the patient that some foods and supplements can cause serious or even dangerous side effects when mixed with certain drugs.

Pain and the related symptoms of fibromyalgia can cause significant stress. Patients with fibromyalgia may not cope well with stress. Effective relaxation strategies include biofeedback, imagery, meditation, and cognitive behavioral therapy. Patients need to receive initial training for these interventions, but they can then continue to practice in their own homes. (Stress management is discussed in Chapter 6.) Psychologic counseling (individual or group) and a support group may also be beneficial for the patient with fibromyalgia.

SYSTEMIC EXERTION INTOLERANCE DISEASE (SEID)

Systemic exertion intolerance disease (SEID), formerly called *chronic fatigue syndrome,* is a serious, complex, multisystem disease in which exertion of any sort (physical, emotional, cognitive) can adversely affect multiple organs in a person.[42] SEID is a poorly understood condition that can have a devastating impact on the lives of patients and their families.

SEID affects 83,000 to 2.5 million people in the United States. Women are affected more often than men. SEID occurs in all ethnic and socioeconomic groups. The true prevalence of SEID is unknown because many people with the disease have not been diagnosed.[42]

Etiology and Pathophysiology

Despite efforts to determine the etiology and pathology of SEID, precise mechanisms remain unknown. However, many theories exist about the cause of SEID. Neuroendocrine abnormalities have been implicated involving a hypofunction of the HPA axis and hypothalamic-pituitary-gonadal (HPG) axis,

which together regulate the stress response and reproductive hormone levels. Several microorganisms have been investigated as causative agents, including herpes viruses (e.g., Epstein-Barr virus [EBV], cytomegalovirus [CMV]), retroviruses, enteroviruses, *Candida albicans,* and mycoplasma. Because many patients have cognitive deficits (e.g., decreased memory, attention, concentration), changes in the CNS have been suggested as the cause of SEID.

Clinical Manifestations

Diagnosis of SEID requires that the patient have the following three symptoms:
1. Profound fatigue lasting at least 6 months
2. Postexertional malaise: total exhaustion after even minor physical or mental exertion that the patient sometimes describes as a "crash"
3. Unrefreshing sleep
   At least one of the following manifestations is also required:
1. Cognitive impairment ("brain fog")
2. Worsening of symptoms upon standing (*orthostatic intolerance*)

SEID is often difficult to distinguish from fibromyalgia because many clinical features are similar (Table 64-19). In about half the cases, SEID develops insidiously, or the patient may have intermittent episodes that gradually become chronic. Severe fatigue is the most common symptom of SEID and the problem that causes the patient to seek health care.

In other situations, SEID arises suddenly in a previously active, healthy individual. An unremarkable flu-like illness or other acute stress is often identified as a trigger. Associated symptoms may vary in intensity over time.

The patient may become angry and frustrated with HCPs who cannot diagnose a problem. The disorder may have a major impact on work and family responsibilities. Some individuals may even need help with ADLs.

Diagnostic Studies

Physical examination and diagnostic studies can be used to rule out other possible causes of the patient's symptoms. No laboratory test can diagnose SEID or measure its severity. SEID generally remains a diagnosis of exclusion.

NURSING AND INTERPROFESSIONAL MANAGEMENT: SEID

Because no definitive treatment exists for SEID, supportive management is essential. Tell the patient what is known about the disease. Take all complaints seriously.

NSAIDs can be used to treat headaches, muscle and joint aches, and fever. Because many patients with SEID also have allergies and sinusitis, antihistamines and decongestants can be used to treat allergic symptoms. Tricyclic antidepressants (e.g., doxepin, amitriptyline) and SSRIs (e.g., fluoxetine, paroxetine) can improve mood and sleep problems. Clonazepam (Klonopin) can also be used to treat sleep disturbances and panic disorders. Use of low-dose hydrocortisone to decrease fatigue and disability is being studied.

Advise the patient to avoid total rest because it can contribute to the self-image of the patient as an invalid. On the other hand, strenuous exertion can exacerbate the exhaustion. Urge the patient to plan a carefully graduated exercise program. Also encourage a well-balanced diet, including fiber and fresh dark-colored fruits and vegetables for antioxidant action. Behavioral therapy may be used to promote a positive outlook and improve overall disability, fatigue, and other symptoms.

One of the major problems facing many patients with SEID is loss of livelihood and economic security. When the illness strikes, they cannot work or must decrease the amount of time working. Loss of a job often leads to loss of medical insurance. Obtaining disability benefits can be frustrating because of the difficulty of establishing a definitive diagnosis of SEID. Patients with SEID may experience substantial occupational and psychosocial loss, including the social pressure and isolation from being characterized as lazy or crazy.

SEID does not appear to progress. Although most patients recover or at least gradually improve, some do not show substantial improvement. Recovery is more common in persons with a sudden onset of SEID.

EVIDENCE-BASED PRACTICE

Translating Research Into Practice

Does Exercise Reduce Fatigue in Chronic Fatigue Syndrome?*

Clinical Question

For individuals with chronic fatigue syndrome (P), what is the effect of exercise therapy (I) versus control group (C) on fatigue, sleep, physical function, and self-perceived health (O) after 12 to 26 weeks of therapy (T)?

Synthesis of Best Available Evidence

- Systematic review of randomized controlled trials (RCTs).
- 8 RCTs of individuals (n = 1518) with chronic fatigue syndrome (CFS). Intervention was anaerobic and aerobic exercise including cycling, dancing, and walking. Length of exercise therapy was 12 to 26 weeks. Control groups included usual, relaxation, cognitive behavior therapy (CBT), supportive listening, and pharmacologic treatment. Outcomes were fatigue, sleep, physical function, self-perceived health, quality of life, depression, anxiety, and pain.
- Reduction in fatigue following exercise therapy.
- Positive effects of exercise on sleep, physical function, and self-perceived changes in health.
- Unable to determine effect of exercise on pain, quality of life, anxiety, and depression.
- CBT appeared equally effective as exercise in reducing fatigue.

Conclusions

- Reductions in fatigue occurred following exercise therapy.
- Sleep, physical function, and self-reported health also improved with exercise.

Implications for Nursing Practice

1. Why is it important to discuss positive effects of exercise for patients with CFS who are sedentary and experience sleep difficulties?
2. What would you advise a patient who is interested in learning about CBT to improve physical functioning? How would you help this person access resources?

Reference for Evidence

Larun L, Brurberg KG, Odgaard-Jensen J, et al: Exercise therapy for chronic fatigue syndrome. *Cochrane Database Syst Rev* 2:CD003200, 2015.

P, Patient population of interest; *I,* intervention or area of interest; *C,* comparison of interest or comparison group; *O,* outcomes of interest; *T,* timing (see p. 15).
*Chronic fatigue syndrome is now referred to as systemic exertion intolerance disease.

CASE STUDY

Rheumatoid Arthritis

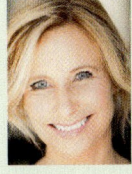

(©iStockphoto/ Thinkstock)

Patient Profile

K.R., a 42-yr-old married white woman, is seen at the rheumatology clinic with complaints of tenderness and pain in the small joints of her hands.

Subjective Data

- Complains of tenderness, joint pain, and stiffness in her hands for the last 3 mo
- Experiencing fatigue, anorexia, and morning stiffness
- Mother diagnosed with ankylosing spondylitis 8 yr ago
- Expresses doubt about her ability to manage disease

Objective Data

Physical Examination

- Swelling, warmth, and tenderness of third and fourth metacarpophalangeal joints of both hands
- Mild pain with neck motion
- Tenosynovitis

Diagnostic Studies

- Positive ESR, RF, and anti-CCP
- Mild bone demineralization evident bilaterally in hand x-rays

Interprofessional Care

- Diagnosed with RA
- Started on methotrexate 7.5 mg PO once per week, etanercept (Enbrel) 50 mg subcutaneously once per week, prednisone 10 mg/day

Discussion Questions

1. How will you explain the pathophysiology of RA to K.R.?
2. K.R. asks you if genetic factors are related to a diagnosis of RA. How will you respond?
3. **Safety:** What are some home and work modifications you can suggest to K.R. to reduce her symptoms?
4. **Patient-Centered Care:** What suggestions can you make to K.R. about coping with fatigue?
5. **Teamwork and Collaboration:** What referrals may be needed for K.R.?
6. **Priority Decision:** Based on the assessment data presented, what are the priority nursing diagnoses? Are there any interprofessional problems?
7. **Quality Improvement**: What outcomes would indicate interprofessional care was effective?
8. **Evidence-Based Practice:** Why is an exercise program important in the treatment plan for K.R.?

Answers and a corresponding conceptual care map are available at *http://evolve.elsevier.com/Lewis/medsurg.*

BRIDGE TO NCLEX EXAMINATION

The number of the question corresponds to the same-numbered outcome at the beginning of the chapter.

1. In assessing the joints of a patient with osteoarthritis, the nurse understands that Bouchard's nodes
   a. are often red, swollen, and tender.
   b. indicate osteophyte formation at the PIP joints.
   c. are the result of pannus formation at the DIP joints.
   d. occur from deterioration of cartilage by proteolytic enzymes.

2. A patient with rheumatoid arthritis is experiencing articular involvement. The nurse recognizes these characteristic changes include (*select all that apply*)
   a. bamboo-shaped fingers.
   b. metatarsal head dislocation in feet.
   c. noninflammatory pain in large joints.
   d. asymmetric involvement of small joints.
   e. morning stiffness lasting 60 minutes or more.

3. When administering medications to the patient with chronic gout, the nurse would recognize which drug is used as a treatment for this disease?
   a. Colchicine
   b. Febuxostat
   c. Sulfasalazine
   d. Cyclosporine

4. The nurse should teach the patient with ankylosing spondylitis the importance of
   a. regularly exercising and maintaining proper posture.
   b. avoiding extremes in environmental temperatures.
   c. maintaining patient's usual physical activity during flares.
   d. applying hot and cool compresses for relief of local symptoms.

5. In teaching a patient with SLE about the disorder, the nurse knows the pathophysiology of SLE includes
   a. circulating immune complexes formed from IgG autoantibodies reacting with IgG.
   b. an autoimmune T-cell reaction that results in destruction of the deep dermal skin layer.
   c. immunologic dysfunction leading to chronic inflammation in the cartilage and muscles.
   d. the production of a variety of autoantibodies directed against components of the cell nucleus.

6. In teaching a patient with Sjögren's syndrome about drug therapy for this disorder, the nurse includes instruction on use of which drug?
   a. Pregabalin (Lyrica)
   b. Etanercept (Enbrel)
   c. Cyclosporine (Restasis)
   d. Cyclobenzaprine (Flexeril)

7. Teach the patient with fibromyalgia the importance of limiting intake of which foods (*select all that apply*)?
   a. Sugar
   b. Alcohol
   c. Caffeine
   d. Red meat
   e. Root vegetables

1. b, 2. b, e, 3. b, 4. a, 5. d, 6. c, 7. a, b, c

For rationales to these answers and even more NCLEX review questions, visit *http://evolve.elsevier.com/Lewis/medsurg*.

(e) EVOLVE WEBSITE

http://evolve.elsevier.com/Lewis/medsurg

Review Questions (Online Only)
Key Points
Answer Keys for Questions
- Rationales for Bridge to NCLEX Examination Questions
- Answer Guidelines for Case Study on p. 1549
- Answer Guidelines for Managing Care of Multiple Patients Case Study (Section 11 on p. 1552)

Students Case Studies
- Patient With Obesity and Osteoarthritis
- Patient With Rheumatoid Arthritis
- Patient With Systemic Lupus Erythematosus

Nursing Care Plans
- eNursing Care Plan 64-1: Patient With Rheumatoid Arthritis
- eNursing Care Plan 64-2: Patient With Systemic Lupus Erythematosus

Conceptual Care Map Creator
- Conceptual Care Map for Case Study on p. 1549

Audio Glossary
Content Updates

REFERENCES

1. National Institute of Arthritis and Musculoskeletal and Skin Disease: Arthritis and rheumatic diseases. Retrieved from *www.niams.nih.gov/health_info/Arthritis/arthritis_rheumatic.asp*.
2. Centers for Disease Control and Prevention: Arthritis: meeting the challenge of living well. Retrieved from *www.cdc.gov/chronicdisease/resources/publications/aag/pdf/2014/arthritis-aag-2014.pdf*.
3. Roberts D: Arthritis and connective tissue disorders. In Schoenly L, editor: *NAON core curriculum for orthopaedic nursing*, ed 7, Chicago, 2013, National Association of Orthopaedic Nurses.
4. Arthritis Foundation: What is osteoarthritis? Retrieved from *www.arthritis.org/about-arthritis/types/osteoarthritis/what-is-osteoarthritis.php*.
5. Centers for Disease Control and Prevention: Osteoarthritis. Retrieved from *www.cdc.gov/arthritis/basics/osteoarthritis.htm*.
*6. Barenius B, Ponzer S, Shalabi A, et al: Increased risk of osteoarthritis after anterior cruciate ligament reconstruction: a 14-year follow-up study of a randomized controlled trial, *Am J Sports Med* 42:1049, 2014.
*7. *www.tylenol.com/safety-dosing/usage/dosage-for-adults*.
8. National Center for Complementary and Integrative Health: Osteoarthritis and complementary health approaches. Retrieved from *https://nccih.nih.gov/health/arthritis/osteoarthritis*.
9. RxList: Celebrex. Retrieved from *www.rxlist.com/celebrex-drug/warnings-precautions.htm*.
10. American Academy of Orthopaedic Surgeons: Viscosupplementation treatment for knee arthritis. Retrieved from *http://orthoinfo.aaos.org/topic.cfm?topic=A00217*.
*11. Reginster JY, Badurski J, Bellamy N, et al: Efficacy and safety of strontium ranelate in the treatment of knee osteoarthritis: results of a double-blind, randomized placebo-controlled trial, *Ann Rheum Dis* 72:179, 2013.
12. Arthritis Foundation: Arthroscopic knee surgery little help for arthritis. Retrieved from *www.arthritis.org/living-with-arthritis/treatments/joint-surgery/types/knee/arthroscopic-knee-surgery.php*.
13. Arthritis Foundation: Other natural therapies for osteoarthritis. Retrieved from *www.arthritis.org/living-with-arthritis/treatments/natural/other-therapies*.

14. Arthritis Foundation: What is rheumatoid arthritis? Retrieved from *www.arthritis.org/about-arthritis/types/rheumatoid-arthritis/what-is-rheumatoid-arthritis.php*.

15. Health Union: Understanding RA changes and progression. Retrieved from *http://rheumatoidarthritis.net/what-is-ra/stages-and-progression*.

16. Harrison P: Rheumatoid arthritis: smoking exacerbates disease activity. Retrieved from *http://www.medscape.com/viewarticle/821446*.

17. Arthritis Foundation: More than just joints: how rheumatoid arthritis affects the rest of your body. Retrieved from *www.arthritis.org/about-arthritis/types/rheumatoid-arthritis/articles/rheumatoid-arthritis-affects-body.php*.

18. Arthritis Foundation: Depression common in rheumatoid arthritis. Retrieved from *www.arthritis.org/living-with-arthritis/comorbidities/depression-and-arthritis/depression-rheumatoid-arthritis.php*.

19. Arthritis Foundation: Arthritis Today drug guide. Retrieved from *www.arthritis.org/living-with-arthritis/treatments/medication/drug-guide*.

20. Centers for Disease Control and Prevention: Gout. Retrieved from *www.cdc.gov/arthritis/basics/gout.html*.

21. Burbage G: Gout: clinical presentation and management, *Nurs Standard* 29:50, 2014.

22. Finney D: Managing gout: not a trivial matter, *Practice Nurs* 24;179, 2013.

23. Rees F, Doherty M: Patient with gout can be cured in primary care, *Practitioner* 258:15, 2014.

24. Moore KS: Lyme disease: diagnosis, treatment guidelines, and controversy, *J Nurse Pract* 11:64, 2015.

25. Centers for Disease Control and Prevention: Two-step laboratory testing process. Retrieved from *www.cdc.gov/lyme/diagnosistesting/labtest/twostep/index.html*.

26. Sharff KA, Richards EP, Townes JM: Clinical management of septic arthritis, *Curr Rheum Rep* 15:332, 2013.

27. Arthritis Foundation: Spondyloarthritis. Retrieved from *www.arthritis.org/about-arthritis/types/spondyloarthritis*.

28. Arthritis Foundation: What is psoriatic arthritis? Retrieved from *www.arthritis.org/about-arthritis/types/psoriatic-arthritis/what-is-psoriatic-arthritis.php*.

29. Lupus Foundation of America: Which medications cause drug-induced lupus? Retrieved from *www.lupus.org/answers/entry/which-medications-cause-drug-induced-lupus*.

30. Lupus Foundation of America: How does lupus affect the renal (kidney) system? Retrieved from *www.lupus.org/answers/entry/lupus-and-kidneys*.

31. Arthritis Foundation: Lupus symptoms. Retrieved from *www.arthritis.org/about-arthritis/types/lupus/symptoms.php*.

32. Lupus Foundation of America: What are the laboratory tests for lupus? Retrieved from *www.lupus.org/answers/entry/lupus-tests*.

*33. Sutanto B, Singh-Grewal D, McNeil HP, et al: Experiences and perspectives of adults living with systemic lupus erythematosus: thematic synthesis of qualitative studies, *Arthr Care Res* 65:1752, 2013.

34. Hylland TL, Doerner J: Polymyositis: essential information for primary care providers, *J Nurse Pract* 10:560, 2014.

35. Lundberg IE, Vencovsky J, Alexanderson H: Therapy of myositis: biological and physical, *Curr Opin Rheum* 26:704, 2014.

36. Cleveland Clinic: Mixed connective tissue disease. Retrieved from *http://my.clevelandclinic.org/health/diseases_conditions/hic_Mixed_Connective_Tissue_Disease*.

37. Catanzaro J, Dinkel S: Sjögren's syndrome: the hidden disease, *MED SURG Nurs* 23:219, 2014.

38. Arthritis Foundation: Sjögren's syndrome and lymphoma risk. Retrieved from *www.arthritis.org/about-arthritis/types/sjogrens-syndrome/articles/lymphoma-risk-and-sjogrens-syndrome-230.php*.

39. Mayo Clinic: Myofascial pain syndrome. Retrieved from *www.mayoclinic.org/diseases-conditions/myofascial-pain-syndrome/basics/treatment/con-20033195*.

40. Wolfe F, Smythe HA, Yunus MB, et al: The American College of Rheumatology 1990 criteria for the classification of fibromyalgia, *Arthr Rheum* 33:160, 1990. (Classic)

41. Wolfe F, Clauw DJ, Fitzcharles M-A, et al: The American College of Rheumatology preliminary diagnostic criteria for fibromyalgia and measurement of symptom severity, *Arthr Care Res* 62:600, 2010. (Classic)

42. Institute of Medicine: Beyond myalgic encephalopathy/chronic fatigue syndrome: redefining an illness. Retrieved from *http://iom.nationalacademies.org/~/media/Files/Report%20Files/2015/MECFS/MECFScliniciansguide.pdf*.

*Evidence-based information for clinical practice.

CASE STUDY

Managing Care of Multiple Patients

You are working on the medical-surgical unit and have been assigned to care for the following five patients. You have one LPN/LVN and one UAP on your team to help you.

Patients

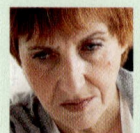

(©iStockphoto/ Thinkstock)

J.K. is a 57-yr-old white woman who had debulking surgery for a temporal-parietal glioblastoma. She was diagnosed after presenting with persistent headaches, a seizure in her HCP's office, and left side upper visual field loss. Her MRI/MRA demonstrated a temporal-parietal glioblastoma that extended into the occipital lobes. Four days ago she developed a hemorrhagic stroke into the site of the tumor bed extending into the thalamus. She now has left homonymous hemianopsia and left-sided weakness.

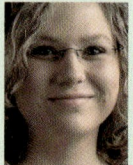

(©Purestock/ Thinkstock)

J.P. is a 24-yr-old woman who fell and hit her head after experiencing a tonic-clonic seizure. Her boyfriend found her lying semiconscious on the floor of her apartment. She had an emergency evacuation of a subdural hematoma and was initially admitted to the ICU. She was transferred to the medical-surgical unit yesterday and is scheduled for a rehabilitation evaluation. She is oriented to person only and is somewhat restless. A safety sitter is at the bedside at all times.

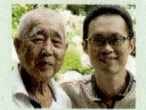

(©iStockphoto/ Thinkstock)

M.Y., an 78-yr-old Asian American man, had an ORIF 2 days ago for a fractured left hip. He has a 3-yr history of Alzheimer's disease and is confused to place and time. Although he has a history of agitation, he has been pleasant and cooperative. He has a personal alarm and bed alarm on for safety. His hip dressing is dry and intact and the drainage in the Hemovac drain is minimal.

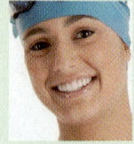

(©iStockphoto/ Thinkstock)

S.W., an 18-yr-old woman, sustained a C5 cervical spinal cord injury when she dove into the shallow end of a neighbor's backyard pool and struck her head on the bottom. She was initially placed in cervical traction, intubated, and mechanically ventilated. She has since undergone surgical stabilization and the traction was removed. After spending 1 week in an inpatient SCI rehabilitation facility, she was transferred to the medical-surgical unit this morning with severe headache, blurred vision, and nausea.

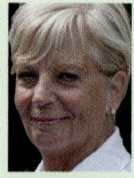

(©iStockphoto/ Thinkstock)

M.C. is a 58-yr-old white woman who suffered a right femoral fracture of the greater trochanter after falling over a wall while gardening. She previously has had both hips replaced. She had surgery 4 days ago to repair the femoral component of her right total hip replacement. She is planning to be discharged home today.

Discussion Questions

1. **Priority Decision:** After receiving report, which patient should you see first? Provide a rationale.
2. **Teamwork and Collaboration:** Which tasks could you delegate to UAP (select all that apply)?
   a. Explain discharge instructions to M.C.
   b. Change the dressing on M.Y.'s left hip.
   c. Obtain vital signs on M.C. before discharge.
   d. Sit with J.P. while the safety sitter takes a break.
   e. Assess J.K.'s ability to swallow before feeding her breakfast.

3. **Priority and Teamwork and Collaboration:** When you enter the room to assess S.W., you find her diaphoretic with a flushed face and pale extremities. Her BP is 200/102 mm Hg. Which two initial actions would be *most* appropriate?
   a. Ask the UAP to obtain a stat bladder scan.
   b. Have the LPN administer her oral antihypertensive meds stat.
   c. Elevate the head of the bed while assessing for any noxious stimuli.
   d. Ask the LPN to stay with S.W. while you call S.W.'s health care provider.
   e. Insert rectal suppository after applying lidocaine to the area around the rectum.

Case Study Progression

S.W.'s bladder scan revealed 700 mL of urine. After you have the LPN catheterize her using a local anesthetic gel, her symptoms subside. You take this time to further teach S.W. about the clinical manifestations of autonomic dysreflexia and the need to report any symptom as soon as it appears. You also take the time to discuss bladder training strategies and how to avoid bladder distention in the future. S.W. is grateful for the information and your caring attitude. Just as you are finishing, the UAP informs you that M.Y. has pulled out his Hemovac drain.

4. What should be your *initial* intervention for M.Y.?
   a. Reinsert the Hemovac drain.
   b. Assess the incision site for a hematoma.
   c. Notify M.Y.'s surgeon that the drain was removed.
   d. Apply pressure to the incisional site where the drain had been placed.
5. Which intervention would be *most* appropriate in caring for J.K.?
   a. Place her left arm in a sling for support.
   b. Arrange the food tray so that all foods are on the right side.
   c. Position her left leg so that the ankle is lower than the knee to prevent contractures.
   d. Call the health care provider to get an order of warfarin to prevent deep vein thrombosis.
6. When teaching J.P.'s boyfriend about what to expect during recovery from a head injury, which statement is *most* accurate?
   a. "You can tell by how great she looks physically that she will ultimately function well at the home."
   b. "One good thing that will come out of this injury is that her seizures should occur less frequently."
   c. "Most patients are transferred out of the hospital for acute rehabilitation management to prepare them for going home."
   d. "She can expect a full recovery without any chronic problems, but it may take a few months to achieve that goal."
7. **Priority and Management Decision:** As you enter M.C.'s room to discuss her discharge plans, you find her all packed up and ready to go. She tells you the UAP already told her what she needed to do. What is your *best* initial action?
   a. Ask M.C. if she has any further questions.
   b. Call the UAP to M.C's room to find out what she told her.
   c. Review discharge instructions with M.C. to ascertain correct understanding.
   d. Give M.C. a telephone number to call in case she has any concerns when she gets home.

Nursing Care in Critical Care Settings

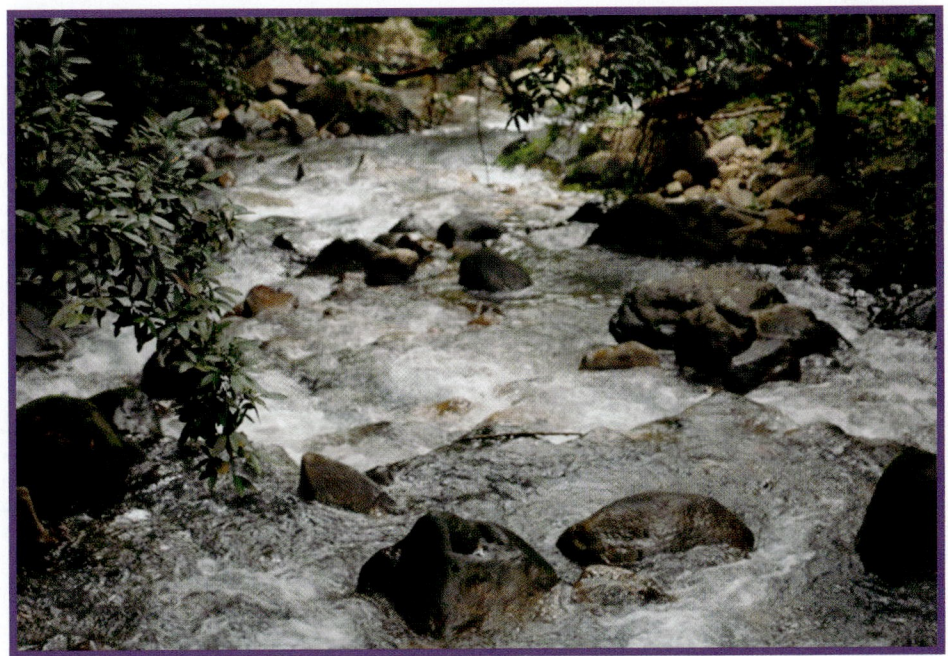

Peter Bonner

Rivers have what man most respects and longs for in his own life—a capacity for renewal and replenishment, continual energy, creativity, cleansing.

John Kaufman

65

Critical Care

Maureen A. Seckel, Linda Bucher

Health is not valued till sickness comes.

Thomas Fuller

http://evolve.elsevier.com/Lewis/medsurg/

LEARNING OUTCOMES

1. Differentiate the various certification opportunities for critical care nurses.
2. Select appropriate nursing interventions to manage common problems and needs of critically ill patients.
3. Develop strategies to manage issues related to caregivers of critically ill patients.
4. Apply the principles of hemodynamic monitoring to the nursing and interprofessional management of patients receiving this intervention.
5. Differentiate the purpose of, indications for, and function of circulatory assist devices and related nursing and interprofessional management.
6. Differentiate the indications for and modes of mechanical ventilation.
7. Select appropriate nursing interventions related to the care of an intubated patient.
8. Relate the principles of mechanical ventilation to the nursing and interprofessional management of patients receiving this intervention.

KEY TERMS

arterial pressure–based cardiac output (APCO), p. 1562
assist-control ventilation (ACV), p. 1575
circulatory assist devices (CADs), p. 1566
continuous positive airway pressure (CPAP), p. 1577
endotracheal (ET) intubation, p. 1569

hemodynamic monitoring, p. 1558
high-frequency oscillatory ventilation (HFOV), p. 1578
intraaortic balloon pump (IABP), p. 1566
mechanical ventilation, p. 1574
negative pressure ventilation, p. 1574

positive end-expiratory pressure (PEEP), p. 1577
positive pressure ventilation (PPV), p. 1574
pressure support ventilation (PSV), p. 1576
ventricular assist device (VAD), p. 1568
volume ventilation, p. 1574
weaning, p. 1582

This chapter focuses on the role of the critical care nurse in the management of critically ill patients in an intensive care setting. The chapter reviews the concepts related to cardiovascular and respiratory dynamics. It emphasizes the interprofessional care and nursing management of patients needing aspects of critical care not addressed in other chapters. These include hemodynamic monitoring, circulatory assist devices, artificial airways, and mechanical ventilation.

CRITICAL CARE NURSING

The American Association of Critical-Care Nurses (AACN) defines *critical care nursing* as that specialty dealing with human responses to life-threatening problems.[1] Critical care nurses care for patients with acute and unstable physiologic problems and their caregivers. This involves assessing life-threatening conditions, starting appropriate interventions, evaluating the outcomes of the interventions, and providing teaching and emotional support to caregivers.

Critical Care Units

Critical care units (CCUs) or *intensive care units* (ICUs) are designed to meet the special needs of acutely and critically ill patients. In many hospitals, the concept of ICU care has expanded from delivering care in a standard unit to bringing ICU care to patients wherever they may be. For example, the *electronic* or *teleICU* assists the bedside ICU team by monitoring the patient from a remote location (Fig. 65-1).

Similarly, the development of *rapid response teams* (RRTs) provides for the delivery of advanced care by an interprofessional team usually composed of a critical care nurse, respiratory therapist, and critical care physician or an advanced practice registered nurse (APRN). RRTs bring rapid and immediate care to unstable patients in noncritical care settings. Patients often exhibit early and subtle signs of deterioration (e.g., mild confusion, tachypnea) 6 to 8 hours before cardiac or respiratory arrest. Early critical care intervention has made significant contributions to reducing mortality rates in these patients.[2]

Reviewed by Donna C. Bond, RN, DNP, CCNS, AE-C, CTTS, Pulmonary Clinical Nursing Specialist, Carilion Clinic, Roanoke, Virginia; Melissa Hutchinson, RN, MN, CCNS, CCRN, Clinical Nurse Specialist, MICU/CU VA Puget Sound Health Care System, Seattle, Washington; Patricia Lea, RN, DNP, CCRN, Assistant Professor, University of Texas Medical Branch School of Nursing, Galveston, Texas; and Eugene E. Mondor, RN, MN, CNCC(C), Clinical Nurse Educator, Adult Critical Care, Royal Alexandra Hospital, Edmonton, Alberta, Canada.

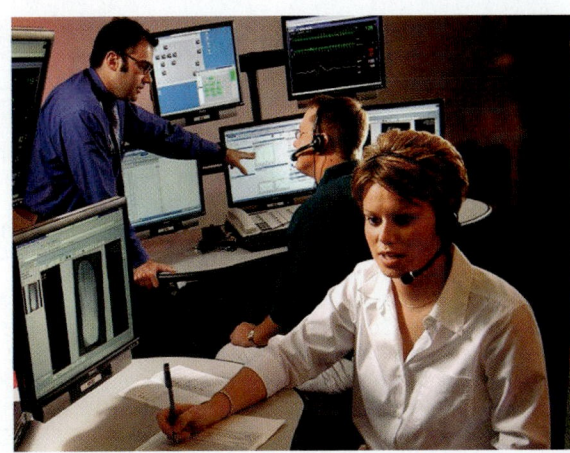

FIG. 65-1 Tele-intensive care unit control room. (From Avera Health, Sioux Falls, S. Dak.)

The technology available in the ICU is extensive and always evolving. It is possible to continuously monitor the electrocardiogram (ECG), BP, O_2 saturation, cardiac output (CO), intracranial pressure, and temperature. More advanced monitoring devices measure cardiac index (CI), stroke volume (SV), stroke volume variation (SVV), ejection fraction (EF), end-tidal carbon dioxide (CO_2), and tissue O_2 consumption. Patients may receive ongoing support from mechanical ventilators, intraaortic balloon pumps (IABPs), circulatory assist devices (CADs), or dialysis machines.

Progressive care units (PCUs), also called *intermediate care* or *step-down units,* provide a transition between the ICU and the general care unit or discharge. Generally, PCU patients are at risk for serious complications, but their risk is lower than that of ICU patients. Examples of patients in PCUs include those scheduled for interventional cardiac procedures (e.g., stent placement), awaiting heart transplant, receiving stable doses of vasoactive IV drugs (e.g., diltiazem [Cardizem]), or being weaned from prolonged mechanical ventilation. Monitoring capabilities in these units may include continuous ECG, arterial BP, O_2 saturation, and end-tidal CO_2. The use of PCUs provides critical care nursing for an at-risk patient population in a more cost-effective environment.

Critical Care Nurse

A critical care nurse has in-depth knowledge of anatomy, physiology, pathophysiology, pharmacology, and advanced assessment skills, as well as the ability to use advanced technology. As a critical care nurse, you perform frequent assessments to monitor trends (patterns) in the patient's physiologic parameters (e.g., BP, ECG). This allows you to rapidly recognize and manage complications while aiding healing and recovery. You must also provide psychologic support to the patient and caregiver. To be effective, you must be able to communicate and collaborate with all interprofessional team members (e.g., physician, dietitian, social worker, respiratory therapist, APRN).

As a critical care nurse, you will face ethical dilemmas related to the care of your patients. Moral distress over perceived issues of delivering futile or nonbeneficial care can lead to emotional exhaustion or burnout. Consequently, it is important that all members of the interprofessional care team coexist in a healthy work environment.

Specialization in critical care nursing requires formal education combined with a preceptored clinical orientation, often over several months. The AACN Certification Corporation offers (1) critical care certification (CCRN) in direct care adult, pediatric, and neonatal critical care nursing; (2) critical care certification knowledge (CCRN-K) for adult, pediatric, and neonatal critical care nurses who do not provide direct care but affect acute and critically ill patients and families in their role; (3) progressive care certification (PCCN); and (4) teleICU certification (CCRN-E). Additional certifications are available in cardiac medicine (CMC) and cardiac surgery (CSC). Certification requires registered nurse (RN) licensure, practice experience in the related area, and successful completion of a written test. It validates basic knowledge of critical or progressive care nursing. Certification is not the same as advanced practice.

APRNs have a graduate (master's or doctorate) degree.[3] These nurses function in a variety of roles: patient and staff educators, consultants, administrators, researchers, or expert practitioners. The APRN who is a clinical nurse specialist (CNS) typically provides advanced nursing care to meet the needs of adult-gerontology, pediatric, or neonatal patient populations. Certification for the CNS in acute and critical care (ACCNS) is available through the AACN.

Another APRN role is the acute care nurse practitioner (ACNP). This APRN provides comprehensive care to select critically ill patients and their caregivers. The ACNP conducts comprehensive assessments, orders and interprets diagnostic tests, manages health problems and disease-related symptoms, prescribes treatments, and coordinates care during transitions in settings. Certification as an ACNP in adult gerontology (ACNPC-AG) is available through the AACN. Prescriptive authority and licensure regulations for APRNs vary by state.

Critical Care Patient

AACN defines a *critically ill patient* as one who is at high risk for actual or potential life-threatening health problems and who requires intense and vigilant nursing care.[1] A patient is generally admitted to the ICU for one of three reasons. First, the patient may be physiologically unstable, requiring advanced clinical judgments by you and the HCP. Second, the patient may be at risk for serious complications and need frequent assessments and often invasive interventions. Third, the patient may need intensive and complicated nursing support related to the use of IV polypharmacy (e.g., sedation, thrombolytics, drugs requiring titration [e.g., vasopressors]) and advanced technology (e.g., mechanical ventilation, intracranial pressure monitoring, continuous renal replacement therapy, hemodynamic monitoring).

ICU patients can be clustered by disease condition (e.g., neurology, pulmonary) or age-group (e.g., neonatal, pediatrics). ICU patients are sometimes clustered by acuity (e.g., acute and unstable versus chronic but technology dependent and stable). Patients commonly treated in the ICU include those with respiratory distress, myocardial infarction, or acute neurologic impairment or those receiving care after heart surgery or other major surgical procedures (e.g., organ transplantation). Trauma and burn ICUs care for critically injured patients. Patients with medical emergencies (e.g., sepsis, diabetic ketoacidosis, drug overdoses, thyroid crisis) are treated in a medical ICU. Fig. 65-2 shows a typical ICU.

The patient who is not expected to recover from an illness is usually not admitted to an ICU. For example, the ICU is not

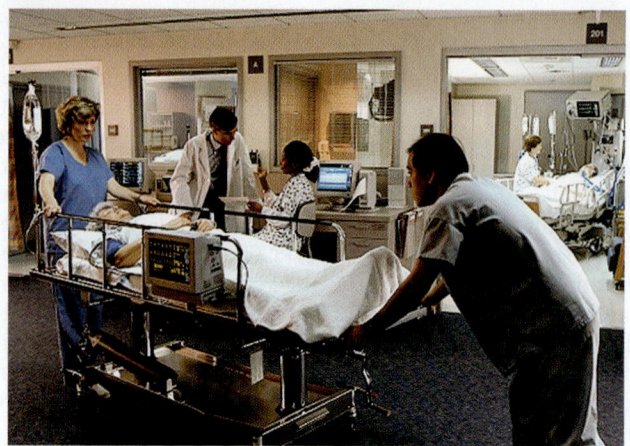

FIG. 65-2 Typical intensive care unit. (Courtesy Spacelabs Medical, Snoquaime, Wash.)

used to manage the patient in a persistent, vegetative state or to prolong the natural process of death.

Despite the emphasis on caring for patients who are expected to survive, the incidence of death is higher in ICU patients than in non-ICU patients. In general, nonsurvivors are older, have co-morbidities (e.g., liver disease, obesity), and experience longer ICU stays.[4] Consequently, it is important that you are skilled in palliative and end-of-life care (see Chapter 9).

Common Problems of Critical Care Patients. The patient admitted to the ICU is at risk for numerous complications and special problems. Critically ill patients are often intubated and mechanically ventilated, immobile, and at high risk for skin problems (see Chapter 23) and venous thromboembolism (see Chapter 37). The use of multiple, invasive devices predisposes the patient to health care–associated infections (HAIs). Sepsis and multiple organ dysfunction syndrome (MODS) may follow (see Chapter 66). Other special problems relate to anxiety, pain, impaired communication, sensory-perceptual problems, sleep, and nutrition.

Anxiety. Anxiety is a common problem for ICU patients. The primary sources of anxiety include the perceived or anticipated threat to health or life, loss of control of body functions, and an environment that is foreign. Many patients and caregivers feel uncomfortable in the ICU with its complex equipment, high noise and light levels, and intense pace of activity. Pain, impaired communication, sleeplessness, immobilization, and loss of control all enhance anxiety.

To help reduce anxiety, teach patients and caregivers to express concerns, ask questions, and state their needs. Include the patient and caregiver in all conversations and explain the purpose of equipment and procedures. Be sure to structure the patient's environment in a way that decreases anxiety. For example, encourage caregivers to bring in photographs and personal items. Appropriate use of antianxiety drugs (e.g., lorazepam [Ativan]) and relaxation techniques (e.g., music therapy) may reduce the stress response that can be triggered by anxiety.[5]

Pain. The control of pain in the ICU patient is very important. As many as 70% of ICU patients report moderate to severe unrelieved pain.[6] Inadequate pain control is often linked with agitation and anxiety and is known to add to the stress response. ICU patients at high risk for pain include those who (1) have medical conditions that include ischemic, infectious, or inflammatory processes; (2) are immobilized; (3) have invasive monitoring devices, including endotracheal tubes; and (4) require invasive or noninvasive procedures.

For many critically ill patients (e.g., those intubated), continuous IV sedation (e.g., propofol [Diprivan]) and an analgesic agent (e.g., fentanyl [Sublimaze]) are used for sedation and pain control. However, patients getting deep sedation are often unresponsive. This prevents you and other HCPs from fully assessing the patient's neurologic status. To address this issue, guidelines should include a daily, scheduled interruption of sedation, or "sedation holiday" for select patients. These daily interruptions allow you to awaken the patient to conduct a neurologic examination.[6] (Pain management is discussed in Chapter 8.)

Impaired Communication. Inability to communicate is distressing for patients who cannot speak because of the use of sedative and paralyzing drugs or an endotracheal tube. As part of every procedure, explain what will happen or is happening to the patient. When the patient cannot speak, explore other methods of communication, such as picture boards, notepads, magic slates, or computer keyboards. When speaking with the patient, look directly at the patient and use hand gestures when appropriate. For patients and caregivers who do not speak English, an approved interpreter or interpreter phone service must be provided (see Chapter 2).

Nonverbal communication is important. High levels of procedure-related touch and lower levels of comfort-related touch often characterize the ICU environment. Patients have different levels of tolerance for being touched, usually related to culture and personal history. If appropriate, use comforting touch with ongoing evaluation of the patient's response. Similarly, encourage caregivers to touch and talk with the patient even if the patient is unresponsive.

Sleep. Nearly all ICU patients have sleep disturbances. Patients may have difficulty falling asleep or have disrupted sleep because of noise, anxiety, pain, frequent monitoring, or treatment procedures. Sleep disturbance has been associated with delirium and delayed recovery.[6]

Arrange the environment to promote the patient's sleep-wake cycle. Strategies include scheduling rest periods, dimming lights at nighttime, providing eye masks/ear plugs, opening curtains during the daytime, getting physiologic measurements without disturbing the patient, limiting noise, and providing comfort measures (e.g., massage).[7] If necessary, use benzodiazepines (e.g., temazepam [Restoril]) and benzodiazepine-like drugs (e.g., zolpidem [Ambien]) to aid and maintain sleep. (Sleep and sleep disorders are discussed in Chapter 7.)

Sensory-Perceptual Problems. Acute and reversible sensory-perceptual changes are common in ICU patients. The combination of alterations in mentation (e.g., delusions, short attention span, loss of recent memory), psychomotor behavior (e.g., restlessness, lethargy), and sleep-wake cycle (e.g., daytime sleepiness, nighttime agitation) has been inappropriately called *ICU psychosis.* The patient experiencing these changes is not psychotic but is suffering from *delirium.* It is estimated that the prevalence of delirium in ICU patients is as high as 80%.[8]

Significant risk factors for delirium include preexisting dementia, history of baseline hypertension or alcohol abuse, and severe illness on admission. Environmental factors that can contribute to delirium include sleep deprivation, anxiety, sensory overload, and immobilization. Physical conditions such as hemodynamic instability, hypoxemia, hypercarbia, electrolyte disturbances, and severe infections can lead to delirium. Last, certain drugs (e.g., sedatives [benzodiazepines], analgesics [opioids], and antimicrobials [aminoglycosides]) have been linked with the development of delirium.[8] (Chapter 59 discusses delirium.)

Monitor all ICU patients for delirium. Assessment tools include the Confusion Assessment Method (see Table 59-15) and the Intensive Care Delirium Screening Checklist[7] (both available at *www.icudelirium.org/delirium/monitoring.html*). It is critical to address physiologic factors (e.g., correction of oxygenation, perfusion, and electrolyte problems). The use of clocks and calendars can help orient the patient. If the patient has hyperactivity, insomnia, or delusions, treatment with sedative drugs with anxiolytic effects (e.g., dexmedetomidine [Precedex]) can be used.[8] In addition, the presence of a caregiver may help orient the patient and reduce agitation. Last, the introduction of early mobility protocols has also helped to reduce agitation and delirium in ICU patients.[9]

Sensory overload can also result in patient distress and anxiety. Environmental noise levels are particularly high in the ICU. You can limit noise and assist the patient in understanding noises that cannot be prevented. Conversation is a particularly stressful noise, especially when the discussion concerns the patient and is held in the presence of, but without participation from, the patient.[7] Reduce this source of stress by finding suitable places for patient-related discussions. Whenever possible, include the patient and caregiver in the discussion.

You can also limit noise levels by muting phones, setting alarms based on the patient's condition, and reducing unnecessary alarms. For example, silence the BP alarm when handling invasive lines and then reset the alarm when done. Similarly, silence ventilator alarms when suctioning. Last, limit overhead paging and all unnecessary noise in patient care areas.

Nutrition. Patients often arrive at ICUs with conditions that result in either hypermetabolic states (e.g., burns, sepsis) or catabolic states (e.g., acute kidney injury). Other times, patients are in severely malnourished states (e.g., chronic heart, pulmonary, or liver disease). In general, inadequate nutrition is linked to increased mortality and morbidity rates. One contributing factor to underfeeding patients is the frequent interruptions in enteral feedings to give drugs and for tests and procedures. Determining whom to feed, what to feed, when to feed, and how to feed (e.g., route of administration) is crucial when caring for critically ill patients.[10] Collaborate with the HCP and dietitian to determine how best to meet the nutritional needs of ICU patients.

The primary goal of nutritional support is to prevent or correct nutritional deficiencies. This is usually done by the early provision of enteral nutrition (i.e., delivery of calories via the gastrointestinal [GI] tract) or parenteral nutrition (i.e., IV delivery of calories). Enteral nutrition preserves the structure and function of the gut mucosa and stops the movement of gut bacteria across the intestinal wall and into the bloodstream. In addition, early enteral nutrition is associated with fewer complications and shorter hospital stays and is less expensive than parenteral nutrition.[10] (Enteral and parenteral nutrition are discussed in Chapter 39.)

Parenteral nutrition is used when the enteral route cannot provide adequate nutrition or is contraindicated.[10] Examples of these conditions are paralytic ileus, diffuse peritonitis, intestinal obstruction, pancreatitis, GI ischemia, abdominal trauma or surgery, and severe diarrhea.

Issues Related to Caregivers

When someone becomes critically ill, care extends beyond the patient to the patient's caregivers. Caregivers play a valuable role in the patient's recovery and are members of the interprofessional care team. They contribute to the patient's well-being by
- Advising the patient in health care decisions or serving as the decision maker when the patient cannot
- Helping with activities of daily living (e.g., bathing, oral care)
- Providing positive, loving, and caring support
- Providing a link to the patient's personal life (e.g., news of family, job)

To be effective in caring for their loved one, caregivers need your guidance and support. The experience of having a friend or relative in the ICU is physically and emotionally difficult, often to the point of exhaustion. Anxiety and concerns regarding the patient's condition, prognosis, and pain are some of the issues that caregivers have. In addition, caregivers commonly experience anxiety over the financial issues related to the provision of care during a critical illness. Consulting with the case manager or social worker is helpful in these instances.

Caregivers often disrupt their daily routines to support the patient. They may be far from their own home, friends, and relatives. Ultimately, caregivers of the critically ill are in crisis, and family-centered care is essential.[11] To provide family-centered care effectively, you must be skilled in crisis intervention. Conduct a family assessment and intervene as necessary. Strategies include active listening, reduction of anxiety, and support of those who become upset or angry. Recognize the caregivers' feelings, listen to them openly and without being judgmental, and acknowledge their decisions. Consult other team members (e.g., chaplains, psychologists, patient representatives) as necessary to help caregivers cope.

The major needs of caregivers of critically ill patients include information, reassurance, and access.[12] Lack of information is a major source of anxiety for the caregivers. Assess the caregiver's understanding of the patient's status, treatment plan, and prognosis and provide information as appropriate. Identify a spokesperson for the family to help coordinate information exchange between the interprofessional care team and family.

The caregiver needs reassurance regarding the way in which the patient's care is managed and decisions are made. Invite the caregiver to meet the interprofessional care team. Evaluate the appropriateness of including caregivers in rounds and patient care conferences. It helps caregivers accept and cope with problems when they see that the team is caring and competent, decisions are deliberate, and their input is valued. If the patient has an advance directive, the caregiver needs to see that the patient's wishes are followed. If the patient has a durable power of attorney for health care, this person must be involved in the patient's plan of care.

Caregivers of critically ill patients need access to the patient. Limiting visitation does not protect the patient from adverse physiologic consequences. AACN strongly recommends less restrictive, individualized visiting policies. This is accomplished by assessing the patient's and caregiver's needs and preferences and incorporating these into the plan of care.[13]

ETHICAL/LEGAL DILEMMAS
Family Presence and Visitation in the Adult ICU

Situation
B.W., a new nurse, is undergoing orientation in the surgical intensive care unit (ICU). He asks his preceptor why the patients' families are permitted on the unit throughout the day and even the night. B.W. states that, in his last position, visiting hours in the ICU were 10 AM to noon and 4 to 6 PM. He adds that families make him nervous when they watch what he is doing and ask him multiple questions. B.W. states that he intends to tell the visitors to leave the patient's room when he is providing care.

Ethical/Legal Points for Consideration
- The majority of nurses in adult ICUs prefer unrestricted visiting policies, but most ICU policies limit visitation.
- Family visitation was thought to cause the patient physiologic stress and interfere with care. Additionally, it was believed that family visitation was mentally exhausting to patients and families and even contributed to increased infection rates. Evidence does not support any of these beliefs.[1,2]
- Evidence suggests several positive benefits of flexible family visitation for the patient: decreases in anxiety, confusion, and agitation; reductions in cardiovascular complications; decreases in length of ICU stay; and reports that patients feel more secure and satisfied with care.[1]
- Similar evidence exists for the benefits of flexible visitation for family members: increases in satisfaction, decreases in anxiety, promotion of better communication, and increases in opportunities for patient and family teaching as the family becomes more involved in care.[1]
- Some conditions may require restricting visitation: a legal reason is documented in the chart; visitor behavior presents a risk to the patient, family, staff, or others; visitor behavior disrupts the functioning of the unit; visitor has a contagious illness or has been exposed to a contagious disease that could endanger the patient's health; or the patient requests fewer or no visitors.

Discussion Questions
1. How should the preceptor respond to B.W.'s statement of his intentions?
2. Does B.W. have an ethical or legal obligation to permit family visitation regardless of his personal concerns? Defend your position.

References
1. American Association of Critical-Care Nurses: AACN practice alert: family presence: visitation in the adult ICU. Retrieved from *www.aacn.org/WD/practice/docs/practicealerts/family-visitation-adult-icu-practicealert.pdf.*
2. American Association of Critical-Care Nurses: AACN practice alert: family presence during resuscitation and invasive procedures. Retrieved from *www.aacn.org/wd/practice/docs/practicealerts/family-presence-during-resuscitation-invasive-procedures.pdf.*

The first time that caregivers visit it is important for you to prepare them for the experience. Briefly describe the patient's appearance and physical environment (e.g., equipment, noise).[14] Join caregivers as they enter the room. Observe the responses of the patient and caregivers. Invite the caregivers to participate in the patient's care if they desire. In some ICUs, visitation includes animal-assisted therapy or pet visitation. The positive benefits of these interventions (e.g., decreases in BP and anxiety) far outweigh the risks (e.g., transmission of infection from animal to patient). They should be a part of the visitation policy.

In addition to traditional visiting, caregivers of patients undergoing invasive procedures (e.g., central line insertion) and cardiopulmonary resuscitation (CPR) want the option of being present at the bedside during these events. Even when the outcomes are not favorable, being present helps caregivers to (1) overcome doubts about the patient's condition, (2) reduce their anxiety and fear, (3) meet their need to be together with and to support their loved one, and (4) begin the grief process if death occurs. AACN encourages critical care nurses to develop policies and procedures that provide for the option of family presence during invasive procedures and CPR.[15]

Culturally Competent Care: Critical Care Patients
Providing culturally competent care to critically ill patients and caregivers is challenging. Often, meeting the patient's physiologic needs is a priority and overshadows the influence of the patient's culture on the illness experience. It remains important to consider the cultural aspects of the meaning of sickness and health, pain, dying and death, and grief when caring for critically ill patients and their caregivers (see Chapter 2).

Cultural perspectives on dying and death are complex. Telling some patients that they are dying as a way of letting them prepare for death may impose on the family's role. Others view a discussion about advance directives as a legal way to withhold, withdraw, or deny care.

Customs surrounding dying and death vary. Caregiver requests may range from asking you to leave a window open so that the spirit of the deceased can leave, to providing the final bath for the deceased. Ask the caregivers about their cultural traditions when caring for the dying patient.

Several variables influence the expressions of grief that follow the loss of a loved one. These include the relationship between the grieving person and the deceased, whether the loss is sudden or anticipated, the support systems available to the grieving person, past experiences with loss, and the person's religious and cultural beliefs. Proceed cautiously when approaching patients facing death and their caregivers. Asking patients, "What do you want to know?" and "Who do you want with you when discussing options?" are good starting points.[16] (Chapter 9 provides additional information about end-of-life care.)

HEMODYNAMIC MONITORING

Hemodynamic monitoring is the measurement of pressure, flow, and oxygenation within the cardiovascular system. The purpose of hemodynamic monitoring is to assess heart function, fluid balance, and the effects of fluids and drugs on CO. Both invasive (internally placed devices) and noninvasive (external devices) hemodynamic parameters (values) are obtained. These include systemic and pulmonary arterial pressures, central venous pressure (CVP), pulmonary artery wedge pressure

(PAWP) (also known as *pulmonary artery occlusive pressure [PAOP]*), CO/CI, SV/SV index [SVI], SVV, O_2 saturation of the hemoglobin of arterial blood (SaO_2), and mixed venous O_2 saturation (SvO_2).

From these measurements you can calculate several values, including the resistance of the systemic and pulmonary arterial vasculature and O_2 content, delivery, and consumption. When you combine these data, you get a picture of the patient's hemodynamic status and the effect of therapy over time (trends). Make all measurements with attention to accuracy. Inaccurate data can result in unnecessary or inappropriate treatment.

Hemodynamic Terminology

Cardiac Output and Cardiac Index. *Cardiac output* (CO) is the volume of blood in liters pumped by the heart in 1 minute. *Cardiac index* (CI) is the measurement of the CO adjusted for body surface area (BSA). It is a more precise measurement of the efficiency of the heart's pumping action. Although minor beat-to-beat variations may occur, the left and right ventricles pump the same volume. The volume ejected with each heartbeat is the *stroke volume* (SV). Like CI, *stroke volume index* (SVI) is the measurement of SV adjusted for BSA.

CO and the forces opposing blood flow determine BP. *Systemic vascular resistance* (SVR) (opposition encountered by the left ventricle) or *pulmonary vascular resistance* (PVR) (opposition encountered by the right ventricle) is the resistance to blood flow by the vessels. Preload, afterload, and contractility (see Chapter 31) determine SV (and thus CO and BP). It is essential that you understand these concepts and relationships. In addition, you must understand the physiologic effects of manipulating each of these variables. Table 65-1 presents the formulas and values for common hemodynamic parameters.

Preload. *Preload* is the volume within the ventricle at the end of diastole. Unfortunately, chamber volume measurements are difficult to obtain. Instead, various pressures are used to estimate the volume. Left ventricular preload is called *left ventricular end-diastolic pressure.* PAWP, a measurement of pulmonary capillary pressure, reflects left ventricular end-diastolic pressure under normal conditions (i.e., when there is no mitral valve dysfunction, intracardiac defect, or dysrhythmia). CVP,

TABLE 65-1   Resting Hemodynamic Parameters

Indicators	Normal Range
Preload	
Right atrial pressure (RAP) or central venous pressure (CVP)	2-8 mm Hg
Pulmonary artery wedge pressure (PAWP) or left atrial pressure (LAP)	6-12 mm Hg
Pulmonary artery diastolic pressure (PADP)	4-12 mm Hg
Right ventricular end-diastolic volume $(RVEDV) = \dfrac{\text{Stroke volume (SV)}}{\text{Right ventricular ejection fraction (RVEF)}}$	100-160 mL
Afterload	
Pulmonary vascular resistance $(PVR) = \dfrac{(\text{Pulmonary artery mean pressure [PAMP]} - \text{PAWP}) \times 80}{\text{Cardiac output (CO)}}$	<250 dynes/sec/cm^{-5}
Pulmonary vascular resistance index $(PVRI) = \dfrac{(\text{PAMP} - \text{PAWP}) \times 80}{\text{Cardiac index (CI)}}$	160-380 dynes/sec/cm^{-5}/m^2
Systemic vascular resistance $(SVR) = \dfrac{(\text{Mean arterial pressure [MAP]} - \text{CVP}) \times 80}{\text{CO}}$	800-1200 dynes/sec/cm^{-5}
Systemic vascular resistance index $(SVRI) = \dfrac{(\text{MAP} - \text{CVP}) \times 80}{\text{CI}}$	1970-2390 dynes/sec/cm^{-5}/m^2
$MAP = \dfrac{\text{Systolic blood pressure} + 2\,(\text{Diastolic blood pressure})}{3^*}$	70-105 mm Hg
$PAMP = \dfrac{\text{Pulmonary artery systolic pressure (PASP)} + 2\,\text{PADP}}{3^*}$	10-20 mm Hg
Other	
Stroke volume $= \dfrac{\text{CO}}{\text{Heart rate}}$	60-150 mL/beat
Stroke volume index $(SVI) = \dfrac{\text{CI}}{\text{Heart rate}}$	30-65 mL/beat/m^2
Stroke volume variation $(SVV) = \dfrac{SV_{max} - SV_{min}}{SV_{mean}}$	<13%
Heart rate (HR)	60-100 beats/min
$CO = SV \times HR$	4-8 L/min
$CI = \dfrac{\text{CO}}{\text{Body surface area (BSA)}}$	2.2-4 L/min/m^2
$RVEF = \dfrac{\text{SV}}{\text{RVEDV}} \times 100$	40%-60%
Arterial hemoglobin O_2 saturation	95%-100%
Mixed venous hemoglobin O_2 saturation	60%-80%
Venous hemoglobin O_2 saturation	70%

*This formula is an approximation because it does not take into consideration the heart rate. The monitor looks at the area under the pressure curve, as well as the heart rate, to calculate MAP and PAMP.

measured in the right atrium or in the vena cava close to the heart, is the right ventricular preload or right ventricular end-diastolic pressure when there is no tricuspid valve dysfunction, intracardiac defect, or dysrhythmia.

Frank-Starling's law explains the effects of preload. It states that the more a myocardial fiber is stretched during filling, the more it shortens during systole and the greater the force of the contraction. As preload increases, force generated in the subsequent contraction increases, and thus SV and CO increase. The greater the preload, the greater the myocardial stretch and the greater the O_2 requirement of the myocardium. Thus increases in CO via increased preload require increased delivery of O_2 to the myocardium. However, the clinical measurement made is not a direct measurement of the muscle length. The measurement is of the pressure at the time of the peak stretch (end diastole) (Table 65-1). This pressure indirectly indicates the amount of stretch and the volume. This pressure is also important because it indicates pressure in the blood vessels of the lungs or in the blood returning to the heart. Diuresis and vasodilation decrease preload, and fluid administration increases preload.

Afterload. *Afterload* refers to the forces opposing ventricular ejection. These forces include systemic arterial pressure, the resistance offered by the aortic valve, and the mass and density of the blood to be moved. Clinically, although the measures fail to include all the components of afterload, SVR and arterial pressure are indices of left ventricular afterload. Similarly, PVR and pulmonary arterial pressure are indices of right ventricular afterload. Increased afterload often results in a decreased CO and increased O_2 demand. CO can be restored and myocardial O_2 needs reduced by decreasing afterload (i.e., decreasing forces opposing contraction). For example, vasodilator drug therapy (e.g., milrinone) can reduce afterload.

Vascular Resistance. *Systemic vascular resistance* (SVR) is the resistance of the systemic vascular bed. *Pulmonary vascular resistance* (PVR) is the resistance of the pulmonary vascular bed. Both these measures reflect afterload as described earlier and can be adjusted for body size (Table 65-1).

Contractility. *Contractility* describes the strength of contraction. Contractility is said to increase when preload is unchanged yet the heart contracts more forcefully. Epinephrine, norepinephrine (Levophed), isoproterenol (Isuprel), dopamine, dobutamine, digitalis-like drugs, calcium, and milrinone increase or improve contractility. These drugs are termed *positive inotropes.* Contractility is reduced by *negative inotropes.* Examples include certain drugs (e.g., calcium channel blockers, β-adrenergic blockers [β-blockers]) and clinical conditions (e.g., acidosis). Increased contractility results in increased SV and increased myocardial O_2 requirements.

There are no direct clinical measures of cardiac contractility. Measuring the patient's preload (PAWP) and CO and graphing the results indirectly indicate contractility. If preload, heart rate (HR), and afterload remain constant yet CO changes, contractility is changed. Contractility is reduced in the failing heart.

Principles of Invasive Pressure Monitoring

Invasive lines are used in the ICU to measure systemic and pulmonary BPs. Fig. 65-3 shows the components of a typical invasive arterial BP monitoring system. The catheter, pressure tubing, flush system, and transducer are disposable.

Pressure monitoring equipment is referenced and zero balanced to the environment and dynamic response characteristics

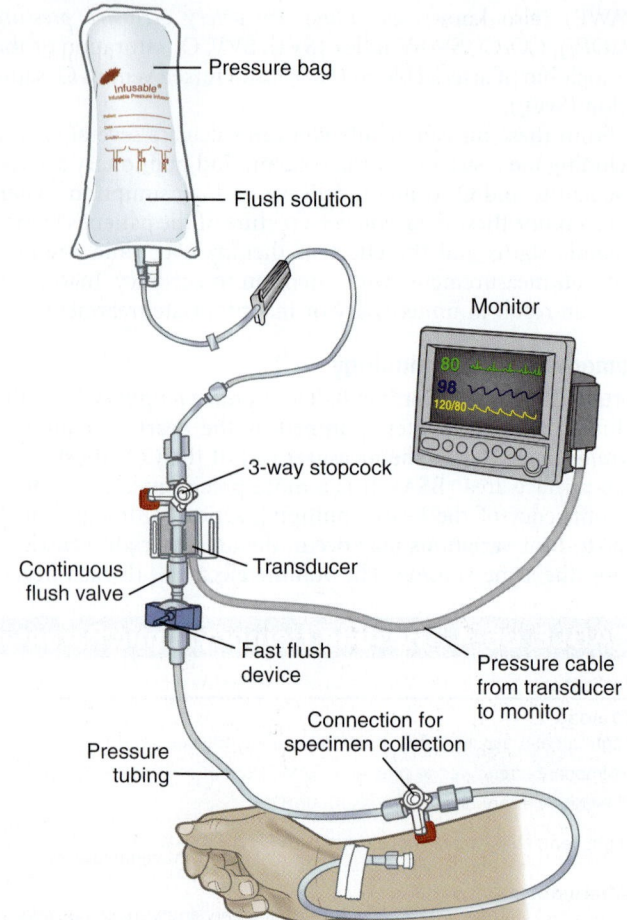

FIG. 65-3 Components of a pressure monitoring system. The cannula, shown entering the radial artery, is connected via pressure (nondistensible) tubing to the transducer. The transducer converts the pressure wave into an electronic signal. The transducer is wired to the electronic monitoring system, which amplifies, conditions, displays, and records the signal. Stopcocks are inserted into the line for specimen withdrawal and for referencing and zero-balancing procedures. A flush system, consisting of a pressurized bag of IV fluid, tubing, and a flush device, is connected to the system. The flush system provides continuous slow (approximately 3 mL/hr) flushing and provides a mechanism for fast flushing of lines.

optimized for accuracy. *Referencing* means placing the transducer so that the zero reference point is at the level of the atria of the heart. The stopcock nearest the transducer is used for the zero reference. To place this level with the atria, use an external landmark, the phlebostatic axis. To identify the *phlebostatic axis,* draw two imaginary lines with the patient supine (Fig. 65-4, *A*). Draw a horizontal line down from the axilla, midway between the anterior and posterior chest walls. Draw a vertical line laterally through the fourth intercostal space along the chest wall. The phlebostatic axis is the intersection of the two imaginary lines. Mark this location on the patient's chest with a permanent marker. Position the port of the stopcock nearest the transducer level at the phlebostatic axis. Tape the transducer to the patient's chest at the phlebostatic axis or mount it on a bedside pole (Fig. 65-4, *B*).

Zeroing confirms that when pressure within the system is zero, the monitor reads zero. To do this, open the reference stopcock to room air (off to the patient) and observe the monitor for a reading of zero. This allows the monitor to use the atmospheric pressure as a reference for zero. Zero the transducer

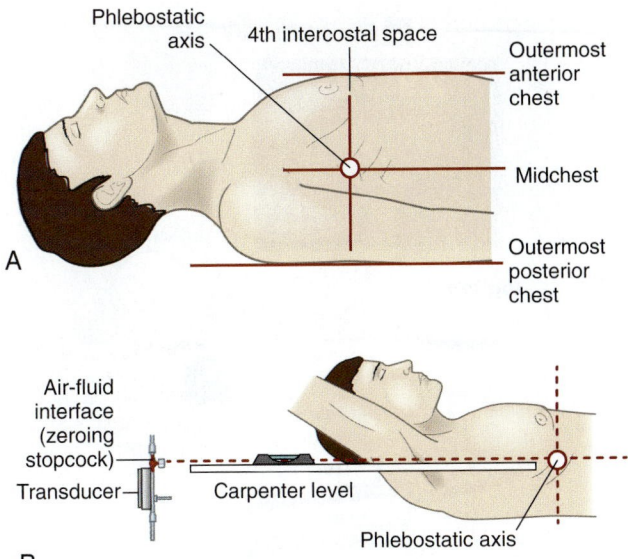

FIG. 65-4   Identification of the phlebostatic axis. **A,** Phlebostatic axis is an external landmark used to identify the level of the atria in the supine patient. It is defined as the intersection of two imaginary lines: one drawn horizontally from the axilla, midway between the anterior and posterior chest walls, and the other drawn vertically through the fourth intercostal space along the lateral chest wall. **B,** Air-fluid interface (zeroing the stopcock) is level with the phlebostatic axis using a carpenter's or laser level.

TABLE 65-2   Invasive Arterial Blood Pressure Measurement

1. Explain the procedure to the patient.
2. Position the patient supine and flat or (if appropriate) with the head of the bed less than 45 degrees or prone.
3. Confirm that the zero reference (port of the stopcock nearest the transducer) is placed at the level of the phlebostatic axis (Fig. 65-4). If the reference stopcock is not taped to the patient's chest, use a leveling device to position the stopcock on a bedside pole at the point level with the phlebostatic axis.
4. Observe the monitor tracing and assess the quality of the tracing. Perform a dynamic response test (Fig. 65-5).
5. Obtain an analog printout (if available) and measure the systolic and diastolic pressures at end expiration (Fig. 65-6). If no printout is available, freeze the tracing on the oscilloscope screen and use the cursor to measure the pressures at end expiration.
6. Record the pressure measurements promptly, including (if available) the printout marked to identify the points read.

during the initial setup, immediately after insertion of the arterial line, when the transducer has been disconnected from the pressure cable or the pressure cable has been disconnected from the monitor, and when the accuracy of the measurements is questioned. Always follow the manufacturer's guidelines.

Optimizing dynamic response characteristics involves checking that the equipment reproduces, without distortion, a signal that changes rapidly. Perform a *dynamic response test (square wave test)* every 8 to 12 hours and when the system is opened to air or the accuracy of the measurements is questioned. It involves activating the fast flush and checking that the equipment reproduces a distortion-free signal (Fig. 65-5).

Table 65-2 outlines the steps in obtaining BP measurements with an invasive line. Obtain measurements from both digital and printed analog outputs. Readings from a printed pressure tracing at the end of expiration (to limit the effect of the respiratory cycle on arterial BP) are most accurate. Position the

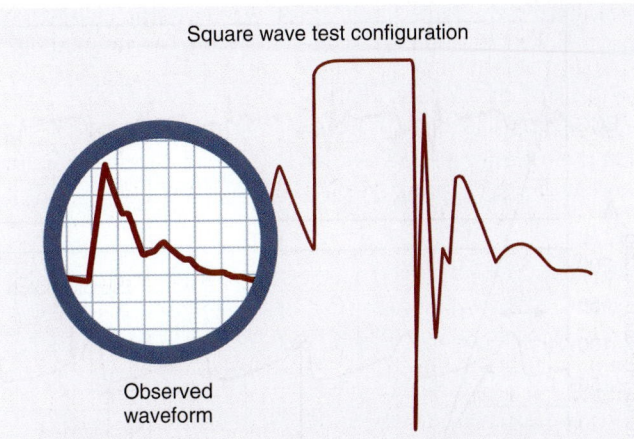

Square wave test configuration

Observed waveform

When the fast flush of the continuous flush system is activated and quickly released, a sharp upstroke terminates in a flat line at the maximal indicator on the monitor and hard copy. This is then followed by an immediate rapid downstroke extending below baseline with just 1 or 2 oscillations within 0.12 second (minimal ringing) and a quick return to a baseline. The patient's pressure waveform is also clearly defined with all components of the waveform, such as the dicrotic notch on an arterial waveform, clearly visible.

FIG. 65-5   Optimally damped system. Dynamic response test (square wave test) using the fast flush system: normal response. No adjustment in the monitoring system is required. (From Darovic GO, Vanriper S, Vanriper J: Fluid-filled monitoring systems. In Darovic GO: *Hemodynamic monitoring,* ed 2, Philadelphia, 1995, Saunders.)

patient supine for initial readings. Values with head of bed (HOB) elevation (up to 45 degrees) are generally equal to measurements with the patient supine, unless the patient's BP is extremely sensitive to orthostatic changes. Additionally, readings in the prone position are generally accurate. However, there is little support for the accuracy of readings in the lateral positions.[17] It is not necessary to reposition the patient for each pressure reading. However, it is important to keep the zero reference stopcock level with the phlebostatic axis.

!   SAFETY ALERT   Positioning the Zero Reference Stopcock
* Mark the location of the phlebostatic axis on the patient's chest with a permanent marker.
* Recheck the leveling of the zero reference stopcock to the phlebostatic axis with any change in the patient's position before obtaining a reading.
* Transducers placed higher than the phlebostatic axis will produce falsely low BP readings.
* Transducers placed lower than the phlebostatic axis will produce falsely high BP readings.

Types of Invasive Pressure Monitoring

Arterial Blood Pressure.   Continuous arterial BP monitoring is indicated for patients in many situations, including acute hypertension and hypotension, respiratory failure, shock, neurologic injury, coronary interventional procedures, continuous infusion of vasoactive drugs (e.g., sodium nitroprusside), and frequent arterial blood gas (ABG) sampling. A nontapered Teflon catheter is typically used to cannulate an artery (e.g., radial, femoral) using a percutaneous approach. After insertion, the catheter is usually sutured in place. You must immobilize the insertion site to prevent dislodging or kinking the catheter line.

Measurements.   Use the arterial line to obtain systolic, diastolic, and mean arterial pressure (MAP) (Fig. 65-6). The

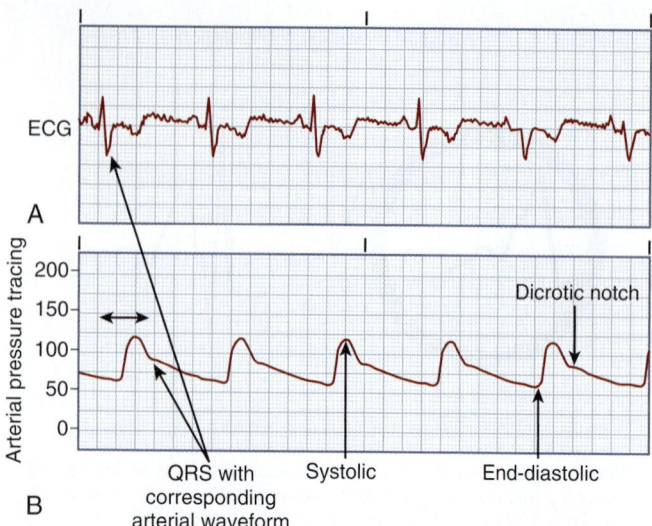

FIG. 65-6   **A,** Simultaneously recorded electrocardiogram (ECG) tracing. **B,** Systemic arterial pressure tracing. Systolic pressure is the peak pressure. The *dicrotic notch* indicates aortic valve closure. Diastolic pressure is the lowest value before contraction. Mean pressure is the average pressure over time calculated by the monitoring equipment. (Modified from Urden LD, Stacy KM, Lough ME: *Critical care nursing: diagnosis and management,* ed 6, St Louis, 2010, Mosby.)

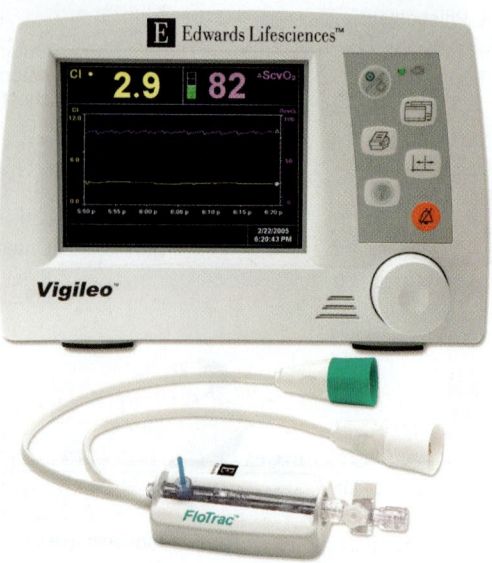

FIG. 65-7   FloTrac sensor and Vigileo monitor. (Courtesy Edwards Lifesciences, Irvine, Calif.)

high- and low-pressure alarms are set based on the patient's current status and then activated. Various patient conditions will change the pressure tracings. In heart failure, the systolic upstroke may be slower. In volume depletion, systolic pressure varies greatly with mechanical ventilation, decreasing during inspiration. Observe simultaneous ECG and pressure tracings with dysrhythmias. Dysrhythmias that significantly diminish arterial BP are more urgent than those that cause only a slight decrease in systolic amplitude.

Complications. Arterial lines carry the risk of hemorrhage, infection, thrombus formation, neurovascular impairment, and loss of limb. Hemorrhage is most likely to occur when the catheter dislodges or the line disconnects. To avoid this serious complication, use Luer-Lok connections, always check the arterial waveform, and activate alarms. If the pressure in the line falls (e.g., when the line is disconnected), the low-pressure alarm sounds immediately, allowing you to promptly correct the problem.

Infection is a risk with any invasive line. To limit the risk of catheter-related infection, inspect the insertion site for local signs of inflammation and monitor the patient for signs of systemic infection. Change the pressure tubing, flush bag, and transducer every 96 hours or according to agency policy. If infection is suspected, notify the HCP, remove the catheter, and replace the equipment.

Circulatory impairment can result from formation of a thrombus around the catheter, release of an embolus, spasm, or occlusion of the circulation by the catheter. Before inserting a line into the radial artery, perform an *Allen test* to confirm that ulnar circulation to the hand is adequate. In this test, apply pressure to the radial and ulnar arteries simultaneously. Ask the patient to open and close the hand repeatedly. The hand should blanch. Release the pressure on the ulnar artery while maintaining pressure on the radial artery. If pinkness fails to return within 6 seconds, the ulnar artery is inadequate and you should not use the radial artery for line insertion.

To maintain line patency and limit thrombus formation, assess the flush system every 1 to 4 hours to determine that the (1) pressure bag is inflated to 300 mm Hg, (2) flush bag contains fluid, and (3) system is delivering a continuous slow (approximately 3 mL/hr) flush. Because of the risk of heparin-induced thrombocytopenia (HIT), use normal saline for the flush solution.[17] (HIT is discussed in Chapter 30.)

Once the catheter is inserted, evaluate the neurovascular status distal to the arterial insertion site hourly. The limb with compromised arterial flow will be cool and pale, with capillary refill time longer than 3 seconds. The patient may have symptoms of neurologic impairment (e.g., paresthesia, pain, paralysis). Neurovascular impairment, which can result in the loss of a limb, is an emergency and must be reported to the HCP immediately.

Arterial Pressure–Based Cardiac Output.   Arterial pressure–based cardiac output (APCO) monitoring is a minimally invasive technique to determine *continuous CO (CCO)/continuous CI (CCI).* In addition to measuring CCO, APCO is used to assess a patient's ability to respond to fluids by increasing SV (*preload responsiveness*). This is determined by using *stroke volume variation* (SVV) or by measuring the percent increase in SV after a fluid bolus[18] (Table 65-1). This technology uses a specialized sensor that attaches to a standard arterial pressure line and a monitor (Fig. 65-7).

SVV is the variation of the arterial pulsation caused by the heart-lung interaction. It is a sensitive indicator of preload responsiveness when used on select patients. SVV helps predict whether or not a patient would benefit from an IV fluid challenge that may help optimize hemodynamic status. SVV is only used for patients on controlled mechanical ventilation with a fixed respiratory rate and a tidal volume (V_T) greater than 8 mL/kg. Also, the APCO monitor may not be able to filter certain dysrhythmias, specifically atrial fibrillation, thus limiting the use of SVV in these patients.[18] These limitations only apply to SVV, not to the use of APCO for CO monitoring.

Measurements. Arterial pressure is the force generated by the ejection of blood from the left ventricle into the arterial circulation. Pulsatile pressure waves are produced by the heart's contractions (systole). The specialized sensor measures the arterial pulse pressure, which is proportional to SV. APCO monitoring uses the arterial waveform characteristics along with patient demographic data (i.e., gender, age, height, and weight) to calculate SV and pulse rate (PR) to calculate CCO/CCI and SV/SVI every 20 seconds. CO is calculated by multiplying the PR and calculated SV and is displayed on a continuous basis.[19]

APCO monitoring is frequently used in conjunction with a central venous oximetry catheter. Together, these allow for continuous monitoring of central venous O_2 saturation ($ScvO_2$) and SVR that is derived from the CVP. APCO is indicated only in adult patients and cannot be used in patients who are on IABP therapy.[19]

Pulmonary Artery Flow-Directed Catheter. Pulmonary artery (PA) pressure monitoring guides the management of patients with select complicated heart and lung problems (Table 65-3). PA diastolic (PAD) pressure and PAWP are sensitive indicators of heart function and fluid volume status. PAD pressure and PAWP increase in heart failure and fluid volume overload. They decrease with volume depletion. Fluid therapy based on PA pressures can restore fluid balance while limiting overcorrection or undercorrection of the problem. Monitoring PA pressures permits precise therapeutic manipulation of preload. This allows CO to be maintained without placing the patient at risk for pulmonary edema.

A PA flow-directed catheter (e.g., Swan-Ganz) is used to measure PA pressures, including PAWP. The standard PA catheter has multiple lumens (Fig. 65-8). When properly positioned, the distal lumen port (catheter tip) is within the PA. This port is used to monitor PA pressures and sample mixed venous blood (e.g., to evaluate O_2 saturation).

A balloon connected to an external valve surrounds the distal lumen port. Balloon inflation has two purposes: (1) to allow blood to "float" the catheter forward and (2) to allow PAWP measurement. The catheter has one or two proximal lumens,

TABLE 65-3	Indications and Contraindications for Pulmonary Artery Catheterization*

Indications
- Assessment of response to therapy in patients with pulmonary hypertension and mixed types of shock
- Cardiogenic shock
- Differential diagnosis of pulmonary hypertension
- Myocardial infarction with complications (e.g., heart failure, cardiogenic shock)
- Potentially reversible systolic heart failure (e.g., fulminant myocarditis)
- Severe chronic heart failure requiring inotropic, vasopressor, and vasodilator therapy
- Transplantation work-up

Contraindications
- Coagulopathy (may be overlooked in emergency situations)
- Endocardial pacemaker
- Endocarditis
- Right heart mass (e.g., thrombus, tumor)
- Mechanical tricuspid or pulmonic valve

*List is not all-inclusive.

with exit ports in the right atrium or right atrium and right ventricle (if two). The right atrium port is used for measurement of CVP, injection of fluid for CO determination, and withdrawal of blood specimens. The second proximal port (if available) is used for infusion of fluids and drugs or blood sampling. A thermistor (temperature sensor) is located near the distal tip and is wired to an external connector. This is used to monitor core temperature and for the thermodilution method of measuring CO.[20]

In addition to providing most of the same functions as the standard PA catheter, the advanced technology PA catheter

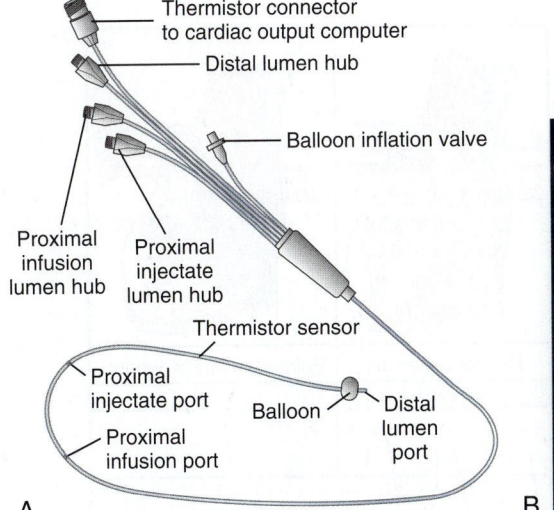
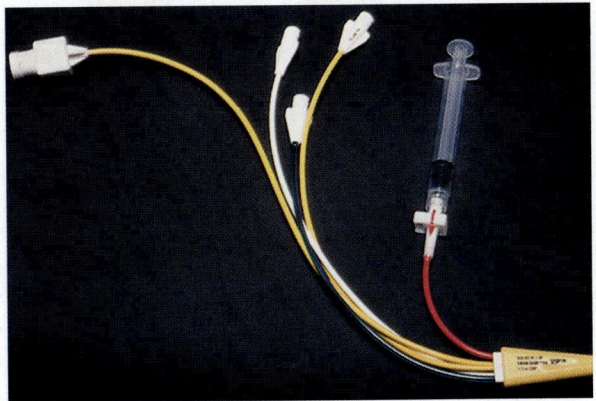

FIG. 65-8 Pulmonary artery (PA) catheter. **A,** Illustrated catheter has five lumens. When properly positioned, the distal lumen exit port is in the PA and the proximal lumen ports are in the right atrium and right ventricle. The distal and one of the proximal ports are used to measure PA and central venous pressures, respectively. A balloon surrounds the catheter near the distal end. The balloon inflation valve is used to inflate the balloon with air to allow reading of the pulmonary artery wedge pressure. A thermistor located near the distal tip senses PA temperature and is used to measure thermodilution cardiac output when solution cooler than body temperature is injected into a proximal port. **B,** Photo of an actual catheter. (*B,* Courtesy Edwards Critical Care Division, Baxter Healthcare Corporation, Santa Ana, Calif.)

Labels for Figure A:
- Thermistor connector to cardiac output computer
- Distal lumen hub
- Balloon inflation valve
- Proximal infusion lumen hub
- Proximal injectate lumen hub
- Thermistor sensor
- Proximal injectate port
- Balloon
- Distal lumen port
- Proximal infusion port

can continuously monitor the patient's SvO_2. This provides a global indicator of the balance between O_2 delivery and O_2 consumption. CCO and right ventricular EF (RVEF) also can be measured using advanced thermodilution technology. RVEF provides information regarding RV function and helps to assess right heart contractility. RV end-diastolic volume is continuously measured by dividing SV by RVEF (Table 65-1). This serves as a key indicator of preload.

Pulmonary Artery Catheter Insertion. Before PA catheter insertion, note the patient's electrolyte, acid-base, oxygenation, and coagulation status. Imbalances such as hypokalemia, hypomagnesemia, hypoxemia, or acidosis can make the heart more irritable. This can increase the risk of ventricular dysrhythmia during catheter insertion. Coagulopathy increases the risk of hemorrhage. Preparation for the procedure includes arranging the monitor, cables, and infusion and pressurized flush solutions. The system is leveled and zero referenced to the phlebostatic axis.

The HCP explains the procedure to the patient and obtains informed consent. The patient is positioned supine and flat. The PA catheter is inserted percutaneously through a sheath (introducer) into the internal jugular, subclavian, antecubital, or femoral vein using surgical asepsis. Most catheters have a plastic "sleeve" connected to the sheath. This allows the catheter to be advanced or pulled back while maintaining sterility. Most catheters also have a side port that serves as a large-bore IV line. Venous cut-down is rarely needed. The catheter is advanced through the venous system to the right side of the heart. The HCP (e.g., ACNP) usually positions the PA catheter, but this practice varies by agency and state.

Continuously observe the characteristic waveforms on the monitor as the catheter is moved through the heart to the PA (Fig. 65-9). When the tip reaches the right atrium, the balloon is inflated. Inflation of the balloon should not exceed the balloon's capacity (1.5 mL of air). The catheter is then "floated" through the tricuspid valve into the right ventricle and then through the pulmonic valve to the PA. Monitor the ECG continuously during insertion because of the risk for dysrhythmias, particularly when the catheter reaches the right ventricle. Once a typical PAWP tracing is observed, the balloon is deflated, and the PA waveform should return on the monitor.

After insertion and before the PA catheter is used, a chest x-ray must confirm the catheter's position. To maintain the catheter in its proper place, secure it at the point of entry into the skin. Note and record the measurement at the exit point. Finally, apply an occlusive dressing and change it according to agency policy.

Recently, the use of PA pressure monitoring has decreased dramatically. This is due, in part, to risks associated with this invasive technology (e.g., dysrhythmias, infection) and the development of less invasive techniques (e.g., APCO monitoring, bedside echocardiography).

Central Venous or Right Atrial Pressure Measurement. CVP is a measurement of right ventricular preload and reflects fluid volume status. It is most often measured with a central venous catheter placed in the internal jugular or subclavian vein. It can be measured with a PA catheter using the proximal lumen located in the right atrium. CVP waveforms (Fig. 65-10) are similar to PAWP waveforms. CVP is measured as a mean pressure at the end of expiration. An elevated CVP indicates right ventricular failure or volume overload. A low CVP indicates hypovolemia.

Venous Oxygen Saturation Monitoring. In critically ill patients, measurement of the O_2 saturation of hemoglobin in venous blood helps to determine the adequacy of tissue oxygenation. The O_2 saturation of venous blood from the CVP catheter is termed *central venous O_2 saturation* ($ScvO_2$). Similarly, the O_2 saturation of blood from the PA catheter is termed *mixed venous*

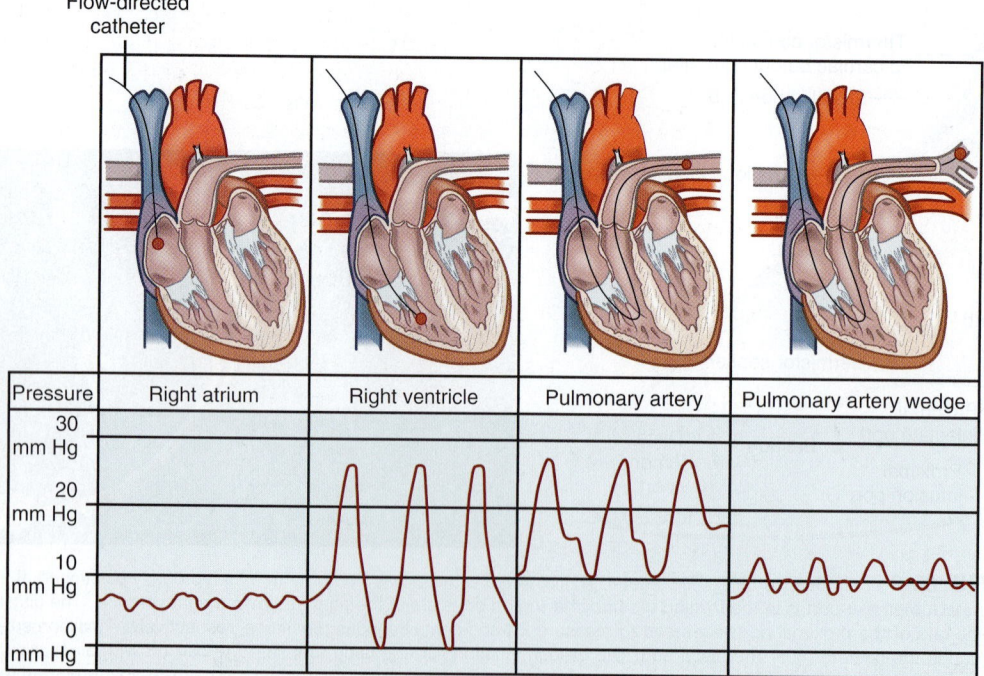

FIG. 65-9   Position of the pulmonary artery flow-directed catheter during progressive stages of insertion with corresponding pressure waveforms. (Modified from Urden LD, Stacy KM, Lough ME: *Critical care nursing: diagnosis and management,* ed 6, St Louis, 2010, Mosby.)

TABLE 65-4   Interpreting ScvO₂ and SvO₂* Measurements

ScvO₂ and SvO₂ Measurement	Physiologic Basis for Change in ScvO₂ or SvO₂	Clinical Diagnosis and Rationale
High ScvO₂ or SvO₂ (80%-95%)	Increased O₂ supply Decreased O₂ demand	• Patient receiving more O₂ than required by clinical condition • Anesthesia, which causes sedation and decreased muscle movement • Hypothermia, which lowers metabolic demand (e.g., with cardiopulmonary bypass) • Sepsis caused by decreased ability of tissues to use O₂ at the cellular level • False high positive because pulmonary artery catheter is wedged in a pulmonary capillary (SvO₂ only)
Normal ScvO₂ or SvO₂ (60%-80%)	Normal O₂ supply and metabolic demand	• Balanced O₂ supply and demand
Low ScvO₂ or SvO₂ (<60%)	Decreased O₂ supply caused by • Low hemoglobin • Low arterial saturation (SaO₂) • Low cardiac output • Increased O₂ demand	• Anemia or bleeding with compromised cardiopulmonary system • Hypoxemia resulting from decreased O₂ supply or lung disease • Cardiogenic shock caused by left ventricular pump failure • Metabolic demand exceeds O₂ supply in conditions that increase muscle movement and metabolic rate. These include physiologic states such as shivering, seizures, and hyperthermia and nursing interventions such as being weighed on a bedside scale and turning

*ScvO₂ values are generally slightly higher than SvO₂ values.
Source: Urden LD, Lough ME, Stacy KM: *Critical care nursing: diagnosis and management,* ed 6, St Louis, 2010, Mosby.

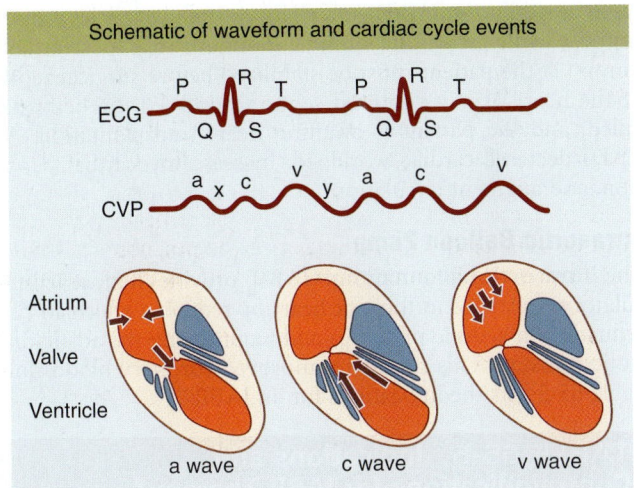

FIG. 65-10 Cardiac events that produce the central venous pressure (CVP) waveform with *a, c,* and *v* waves. The *a* wave represents atrial contraction. The *x* descent represents atrial relaxation. The *c* wave represents the bulging of the closed tricuspid valve into the right atrium during ventricular systole. The *v* wave represents atrial filling. The *y* descent represents opening of the tricuspid valve and filling of the ventricle. (Modified from Urden LD, Stacy KM, Lough ME: *Critical care nursing: diagnosis and management,* ed 6, St Louis, 2010, Mosby.)

oxygen saturation (SvO₂). The measurements of ScvO₂ and SvO₂ reflect the balance among oxygenation of the arterial blood, tissue perfusion, and tissue O₂ consumption. ScvO₂ and SvO₂ are useful in assessing hemodynamic status and response to treatments or activities when considered in conjunction with arterial O₂ saturation (Table 65-4). Normal ScvO₂ or SvO₂ at rest is 60% to 80%.

Carefully review sustained decreases and increases in ScvO₂ or SvO₂. Decreased ScvO₂ or SvO₂ may indicate decreased arterial oxygenation, low CO, low hemoglobin level, or increased O₂ consumption or extraction. If the ScvO₂ or SvO₂ falls below 60%, determine which of these factors has changed. Observe for changes in arterial oxygenation (e.g., monitor pulse oximetry or ABGs) and indirectly assess CO and tissue perfusion. This is done by noting any changes in mental status, strength and quality of peripheral pulses, capillary refill, urine output, and

skin color and temperature. If arterial oxygenation, CO, and hemoglobin level are unchanged, a fall in ScvO₂ or SvO₂ indicates increased O₂ consumption or extraction. This could represent an increased metabolic rate, pain, movement, or fever. If O₂ consumption increases without a comparable increase in O₂ delivery, more O₂ is extracted from the blood, and ScvO₂ and SvO₂ will continue to fall.[21]

Increased ScvO₂ or SvO₂ is also clinically significant. It may indicate a clinical improvement (e.g., increased arterial O₂ saturation, improved perfusion, decreased metabolic rate) or problem (e.g., sepsis). In sepsis, O₂ is not extracted properly at the tissue level, resulting in increased ScvO₂ or SvO₂.

Your interventions are guided by changes in ScvO₂ or SvO₂. For example, you may note that the patient's HR increased slightly during repositioning but that the ScvO₂ or SvO₂ remained stable. In this case, you would conclude that the patient tolerated the position change. If the ScvO₂ or SvO₂ dropped, this would be a sign to stop the activity until the ScvO₂ or SvO₂ returns to baseline.

In many cases, as activity or metabolism increases, HR and CO increase, and ScvO₂ or SvO₂ remains constant or varies slightly. However, critically ill patients often have conditions (e.g., heart failure, shock) that prevent substantial increases in CO. In these cases, ScvO₂ or SvO₂ can be a useful indicator of the balance between O₂ delivery and consumption.

CHECK YOUR PRACTICE

You are caring for a 38-yr-old woman admitted with sepsis secondary to a ruptured ectopic pregnancy. She has CVP and ScvO₂ monitoring in place. Trends in ScvO₂ have shown a slow, steady decline with the most recent reading being 55%.

• What additional assessment data would you explore to explain this drop in readings?

Noninvasive Arterial Oxygenation Monitoring

Pulse oximetry is a noninvasive and continuous method of determining the O₂ saturation of hemoglobin (SpO₂). Monitoring SpO₂ may reduce the frequency of ABG sampling (see Chapter 25). SpO₂ is normally 95% to 100%. Accurate SpO₂ measurements may be difficult to obtain on patients who are hypothermic, receiving IV vasopressor therapy (e.g., norepinephrine), or experiencing hypoperfusion and vasoconstriction (e.g., shock). Consider alternative locations for placement of the pulse oximetry probe (e.g., forehead, earlobe).

A common use for pulse oximetry is to evaluate the effectiveness of O_2 therapy. Decreased SpO_2 indicates inadequate oxygenation of the blood in the pulmonary capillaries. You can correct this by increasing the fraction of inspired O_2 (FIO_2) and evaluating the patient's response. Similarly, use SpO_2 to monitor how the patient tolerates decreases in FIO_2 and responds to interventions. For example, if SpO_2 falls when you position the patient in a left lateral recumbent position, plan position changes that pose less risk for the patient.

Noninvasive Hemodynamic Monitoring: Impedance Cardiography

Impedance cardiography (ICG) is a continuous or intermittent, noninvasive method of obtaining CO and assessing thoracic fluid status. Based on the concepts of *impedance* (the resistance to the flow of electric current [Ω]), ICG uses four sets of external electrodes to deliver a high-frequency, low-amplitude current that is similar to that used in apnea monitors. Blood is an excellent conductor of electricity (lower impedance), and pulsatile blood flow generates electrical impedance changes. ICG measures the change in impedance (dΩ) in the ascending aorta and left ventricle over time (dt) and is represented as dΩ/dt. Ωo is the measurement of the average impedance of the fluid in the thorax. Impedance-based hemodynamic parameters (CO, SV, and SVR) are calculated from Ωo, dΩ/dt, mean arterial pressure (MAP), CVP, and ECG.

Major indications for ICG include (1) early signs and symptoms of pulmonary or cardiac dysfunction, (2) differentiation of cardiac or pulmonary cause of shortness of breath, (3) evaluation of etiology and management of hypotension, (4) monitoring after discontinuing a PA catheter or justification for insertion of a PA catheter, (5) evaluation of drug therapy, and (6) diagnosis of rejection after heart transplantation. ICG is not recommended in patients who have generalized edema or third spacing because the excess volume interferes with accurate signals.

❖ NURSING AND INTERPROFESSIONAL MANAGEMENT: HEMODYNAMIC MONITORING

Assessment of hemodynamic status requires integrating data from many sources and trending these data over time. Comprehensive nursing observations provide important clues about the patient's hemodynamic status.

Begin by obtaining baseline data regarding the patient's general appearance, level of consciousness, skin color and temperature, vital signs, peripheral pulses, capillary refill, and urine output. Does the patient appear tired, weak, exhausted? There may be too little cardiac reserve to sustain even minimum activity. Pallor, cool skin, and diminished pulses may indicate decreased CO. Changes in mental status may reflect problems with cerebral perfusion or oxygenation. Monitor urine output to determine the adequacy of perfusion to the kidneys. The patient with diminished perfusion to the GI tract may develop hypoactive or absent bowel sounds. If the patient is bleeding and developing shock, BP may initially be relatively stable, yet the patient may become increasingly pale and cool from peripheral vasoconstriction. Conversely, the patient experiencing

septic shock may remain warm and pink yet develop tachycardia and BP instability. Elevated HRs are common in stressed, compromised, critically ill patients. However, sustained tachycardia increases myocardial O_2 demand and can result in decreased CO.

Always correlate observational data with data obtained from technology (e.g., ECG, arterial and PA pressures, $ScvO_2$ or SvO_2). Single hemodynamic values are rarely helpful. You must monitor trends in these values over time and evaluate the whole clinical picture with the goals of recognizing early clues and intervening before problems escalate.

CIRCULATORY ASSIST DEVICES

Mechanical **circulatory assist devices (CADs)** are used to decrease cardiac work and improve organ perfusion in patients with heart failure when conventional drug therapy is no longer adequate. CADs include intraaortic balloon pump (IABP) and left or right ventricular assist device (VAD).

The type of device used depends on the extent and nature of the heart problem. CADs provide interim support in three types of situations: (1) the left, right, or both ventricles require support while recovering from acute injury (e.g., postcardiotomy); (2) the patient must be stabilized before surgical repair of the heart (e.g., a ruptured septum); and (3) the heart has failed, and the patient is awaiting heart transplantation. All CADs decrease cardiac workload, increase myocardial perfusion, and augment circulation.

Intraaortic Balloon Pump

The **intraaortic balloon pump (IABP)** provides temporary circulatory assistance to the sick heart by reducing afterload (via reduction in systolic pressure) and augmenting the aortic diastolic pressure. This results in improved coronary blood flow. Table 65-5 lists the indications for an IABP.

TABLE 65-5 Indications and Contraindications for IABP Therapy*

Indications
- Refractory unstable angina (when drugs have failed)
- Short-term bridge to heart transplantation
- Acute myocardial infarction with any of the following:†
  - Ventricular aneurysm accompanied by ventricular dysrhythmias
  - Acute ventricular septal defect
  - Acute mitral valve dysfunction
  - Cardiogenic shock
  - Refractory chest pain with or without ventricular dysrhythmias
- Preoperative, intraoperative, and postoperative cardiac surgery (e.g., prophylaxis before surgery, failure to wean from cardiopulmonary bypass, left ventricular failure after cardiopulmonary bypass)
- High-risk interventional cardiology procedures

Contraindications
- Irreversible brain damage
- Major coagulopathy (e.g., disseminated intravascular coagulation [DIC])
- Terminal or untreatable diseases of any major organ system
- Abdominal aortic and thoracic aneurysms
- Moderate to severe aortic insufficiency
- Generalized peripheral vascular disease (e.g., aortoiliac disease)‡

*List is not all-inclusive.
†Allows time for emergent angiography and corrective heart surgery to be done.
‡May inhibit placement of balloon and is considered a relative contraindication; sheathless insertion may be used.

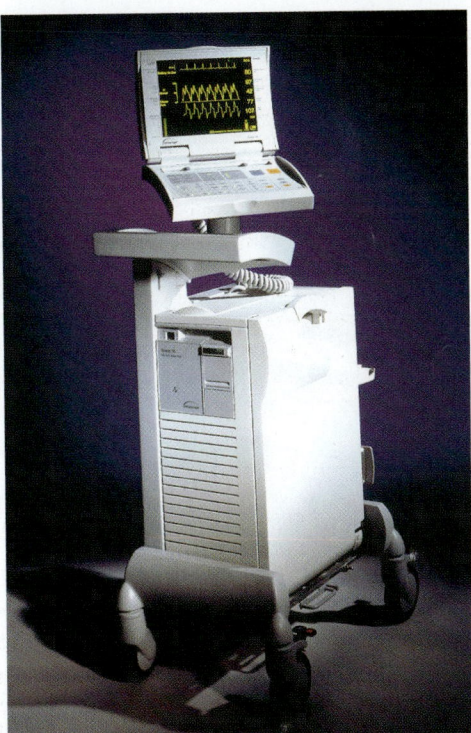

FIG. 65-11   Intraaortic balloon pump machine. (Courtesy Datascope Corp, Fairfield, NJ.)

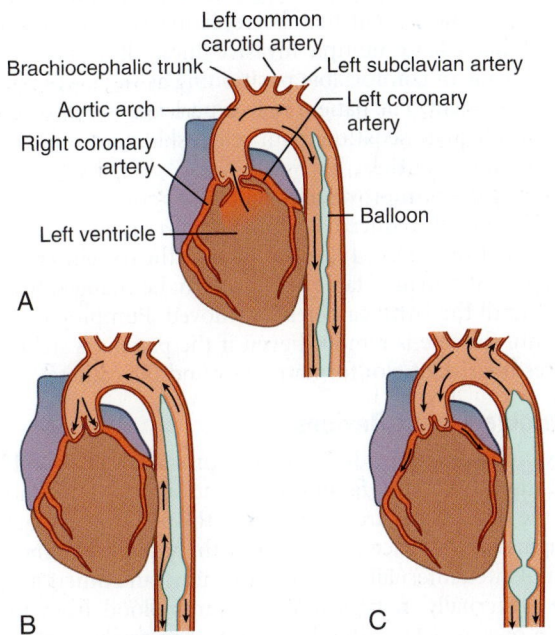

FIG. 65-12   Intraaortic balloon pump. **A,** During systole the balloon is deflated, which facilitates ejection of blood into the periphery. **B,** In early diastole, the balloon begins to inflate. **C,** In late diastole, the balloon is totally inflated, which augments aortic pressure and increases the coronary perfusion pressure with the end result of increased coronary and cerebral blood flow.

The IABP consists of a sausage-shaped balloon, a pump that inflates and deflates the balloon, a control panel for synchronizing the balloon inflation to the cardiac cycle, and failsafe features (Fig. 65-11). The balloon is inserted percutaneously or surgically into the femoral artery. It is moved toward the heart and placed in the descending thoracic aorta just below the

TABLE 65-6   Hemodynamic Effects of Counterpulsation

Effects of Inflation During Diastole
- Increased diastolic pressure (may exceed systolic pressure)
- Increased pressure in the aortic root during diastole
- Increased coronary artery perfusion pressure
- Improved O₂ delivery to the myocardium
  - Decreased angina
  - Decreased ECG evidence of ischemia
  - Decreased ventricular ectopy

Effects of Deflation During Systole
- Decreased afterload
- Decreased peak systolic pressure
- Decreased myocardial O₂ consumption
- Increased stroke volume, possibly associated with
  - Improved mentation
  - Warm skin
  - Increased urine output
  - Decreased heart rate
- Increased forward flow of blood, decreasing preload
  - Decreased PA pressures, including PAWP
  - Decreased crackles

PA, Pulmonary artery; *PAWP,* PA wedge pressure.

left subclavian artery and above the renal arteries (Fig. 65-12). After placement, an x-ray confirms the position.

A pneumatic device fills the balloon with helium at the start of diastole (immediately after aortic valve closure) and deflates it just before the next systole. The ECG is the trigger used to start the deflation on the upstroke of the R wave (of the QRS) and inflation on the T wave. The dicrotic notch of the arterial pressure tracing is used to refine timing.

IABP therapy is known as *counterpulsation* because the timing of balloon inflation is opposite to ventricular contraction. The IABP assist ratio is 1:1 in the acute phase of treatment, meaning that one IABP cycle of inflation and deflation occurs for every heartbeat.

Effects of Counterpulsation. In late diastole when the balloon is totally inflated, blood is forcibly displaced distal to the extremities and proximal to the coronary arteries and main branches of the aortic arch. Diastolic arterial pressure rises (diastolic augmentation), increasing coronary artery perfusion pressure and perfusion of vital organs. The rise in coronary artery perfusion pressure causes an increase in blood flow to the myocardium. The balloon is rapidly deflated just before systole. This creates a vacuum that causes aortic pressure to drop. When aortic resistance to left ventricular ejection is reduced (reduced afterload), the left ventricle empties more easily and completely. As with other types of afterload reduction, the SV increases, yet the myocardial O₂ consumption decreases. Table 65-6 summarizes the hemodynamic effects of IABP therapy.

Complications With IABP Therapy. Vascular injuries such as dislodgment of plaque, aortic dissection, and compromised distal circulation are common with IABP therapy. Thrombus and embolus formation add to the risk of circulatory compromise to the extremity. The action of the IABP can also destroy platelets and cause thrombocytopenia. Movement of the balloon can block the left subclavian, renal, or mesenteric arteries. This can result in a weak or absent radial pulse, decreased urine output, and reduced or absent bowel sounds. Patients receiving IABP therapy are prone to infection. Local or systemic

TABLE 65-7   Managing Complications of IABP Therapy

Potential Complications	Nursing Interventions
Site infection from invasive lines	• Use strict aseptic technique for insertion and dressing changes for all lines. • Cover all insertion sites with occlusive dressings. • Give prescribed prophylactic antibiotic for entire course of therapy.
Issues related to immobilization (e.g., pressure ulcers, pneumonia)	• Reposition patient at least q2hr, being careful not to displace balloon. • If patient requires chest physiotherapy, avoid introducing ECG artifact.
Arterial trauma caused by insertion or displacement of balloon	• Evaluate and mark peripheral pulses before insertion of balloon to use as baseline for assessing pulses after insertion. • After insertion of balloon, evaluate perfusion to both upper and lower extremities at least every hour. • Measure urine output at least every hour (occlusion of renal arteries causes severe decrease in urine output). • Observe arterial waveforms for sudden changes. • Keep head of bed no higher than 45 degrees. • Do not flex cannulated leg at the hip. • Immobilize cannulated leg to prevent flexion using a draw sheet tucked under the mattress, soft ankle restraint, or knee immobilizer.
Thromboembolism caused by trauma, balloon obstruction of blood flow distal to catheter	• Give prophylactic heparin therapy (if ordered). • Evaluate pulses, urine output, and level of consciousness at least every hour. • Check circulation, sensation, and movement in both legs at least every hour.
Hematologic complications caused by platelet aggregation along the balloon (e.g., thrombocytopenia)	• Monitor coagulation profiles, hematocrit, and platelet count.
Hemorrhage from insertion site	• Check site for bleeding at least every hour. • Monitor vital signs for signs of hypovolemia with each check.
Balloon leak or rupture	• Prepare for emergent removal and possible reinsertion.

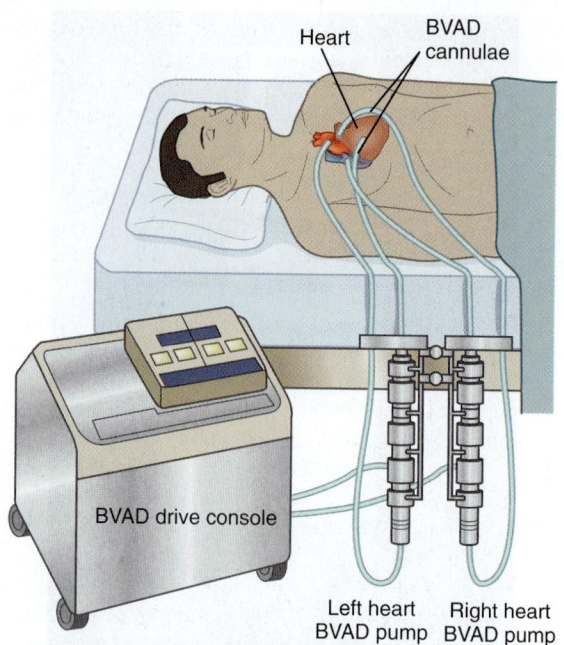

FIG. 65-13 Schematic diagram of a biventricular assist device (BVAD).

signs of infection require catheter removal.[22] To reduce these complications, perform cardiovascular, neurovascular, and hemodynamic assessments every 15 to 60 minutes, depending on the patient's status (Table 65-7).

Mechanical complications from IABP are rare but can occur. Improper timing of balloon inflation may cause increased afterload, decreased CO, myocardial ischemia, and increased myocardial O_2 demand. These complications must be recognized immediately and reported to the HCP. If the balloon develops a leak, the pump will automatically stop. The catheter is promptly removed to avoid an embolus. Signs of a leak include less effective augmentation, repeated alarms for gas loss, and blood backing up into the catheter. A malfunction of the balloon

or console triggers fail-safe alarms and automatically shuts down the unit.

The patient with an IABP is relatively immobile, limited to side-lying or supine positions with the HOB elevated less than 45 degrees. The patient may be receiving ventilatory support and will likely have multiple invasive lines. All of this increases the challenge of comfortable positioning as well as the risk for skin impairment. The patient may experience sleeplessness and anxiety. Adequate sedation, pain relief, skin care, and comfort measures are essential.

As the patient improves, circulatory support provided by the IABP is gradually reduced. Weaning involves reducing the IABP assist ratio from 1:1 to 1:2 and assessing the patient's response. If the patient remains stable, the ratio can be changed from 1:2 to 1:3 until the IABP catheter is removed. Pumping is continued until the line is removed even if the patient is stable. This reduces the risk of clot formation around the catheter.

Ventricular Assist Devices

The **ventricular assist device (VAD)** provides short- and long-term support for the failing heart and allows more mobility than the IABP. VADs are inserted into the path of flowing blood to augment or replace the action of the ventricle. Some VADs are implanted internally (e.g., peritoneum), and others are positioned externally. A typical VAD shunts blood from the left atrium or ventricle to the device and then to the aorta. Some VADs provide right or biventricular support (Fig. 65-13).

Failure to wean from cardiopulmonary bypass (CPB) after surgery is a primary indicator for VAD support. VADs are also used to support patients with heart failure caused by myocardial infarction and patients awaiting heart transplantation. A VAD is a temporary device that can partially or totally support circulation until the heart recovers or a donor heart is found.

Appropriate patient selection for VAD therapy is critical. Indications include (1) failure to wean from CPB or postcardiotomy cardiogenic shock, (2) a bridge to recovery or heart transplantation, and (3) patients with New York Heart Association Class IV heart disease (see Table 34-3) who have failed medical therapy. Relative contraindications for VAD therapy include (1) body surface area (BSA) less than manufacturer's limit (e.g., 1.3 m^2), (2) renal or liver failure unrelated to a cardiac event, and (3) co-morbidities that would limit life expectancy to less than 3 years.[23]

Implantable Artificial Heart

Every year about 2200 patients receive heart transplants, yet the demand for donor hearts far exceeds the supply. Research on mechanical CADs has led to the development of a fully implantable artificial heart that can sustain the body's circulatory system. This device is used to replace the hearts of patients who are not eligible for a transplant and have no other treatment options. One major advantage of the artificial heart compared with heart transplantation is decreased costs for implantation and drug therapies. Patients do not require immunosuppression therapy and thus do not experience its inevitable, long-term effects. However, patients do require lifelong anticoagulation.[24]

❖ NURSING AND INTERPROFESSIONAL MANAGEMENT: CIRCULATORY ASSIST DEVICES

The patient with an IABP requires highly skilled care. Perform frequent and thorough cardiovascular assessments. These include measurement of hemodynamic parameters (e.g., arterial BP, CO/CI, SVR), auscultation of the heart and lungs, and evaluation of the ECG (e.g., rate, rhythm). Assess for adequate tissue perfusion (e.g., skin color and temperature, mental status, capillary refill, peripheral pulses, urine output, bowel sounds) at regular intervals. It is expected that IABP therapy will improve these findings.

Nursing care of the patient with a VAD is similar to that of the patient with an IABP. Observe the patient for bleeding, cardiac tamponade, ventricular failure, infection, dysrhythmias, renal failure, hemolysis, and thromboembolism. Unlike the patient with an IABP, who must remain in bed with limited position change, the patient with VAD may be mobile and require an activity plan. In some cases, patients with VADs may go home. Preparation for discharge is complex and requires

in-depth teaching about the device and support equipment (e.g., battery chargers). A competent caregiver must be present at all times.

Ideally, patients with CADs will recover, undergo heart transplantation, or receive an artificial heart. However, many patients die, or the decision to terminate the device is made and death follows. Both the patient and caregiver require emotional support. Consult other team members, such as social workers or clergy, as appropriate.

ARTIFICIAL AIRWAYS

Patients in the ICU often need mechanical assistance to maintain airway patency. Inserting a tube into the trachea, bypassing upper airway and laryngeal structures, creates an artificial airway. The tube is placed into the trachea via the mouth or nose past the larynx (**endotracheal [ET] intubation**) or through a stoma in the neck (*tracheostomy*). ET intubation is more common in ICU patients than a tracheostomy. It is performed quickly and safely at the bedside. Indications for ET intubation include (1) upper airway obstruction (e.g., secondary to burns, tumor, bleeding), (2) apnea, (3) high risk for aspiration, (4) ineffective clearance of secretions, and (5) respiratory distress. Fig. 65-14 shows the parts of an ET tube.

A *tracheotomy* is a surgical procedure that is performed when the need for an artificial airway is expected to be long term. There is ongoing debate regarding the timing of a tracheotomy in the patient requiring an ET tube. Research suggests that early tracheotomy (2 to 10 days) may have advantages over delayed tracheotomy, particularly when mechanical ventilation is predicted to be needed for longer than 10 to 14 days.[25] The situation varies with the patient, HCP, and agency. Chapter 26 discusses tracheostomy tubes and related nursing management.

Endotracheal Tubes

In *oral intubation*, the ET tube is passed through the mouth and vocal cords and into the trachea with the aid of a laryngoscope or a bronchoscope. In *nasal ET intubation*, the ET is placed blindly (i.e., without seeing the larynx) through the nose,

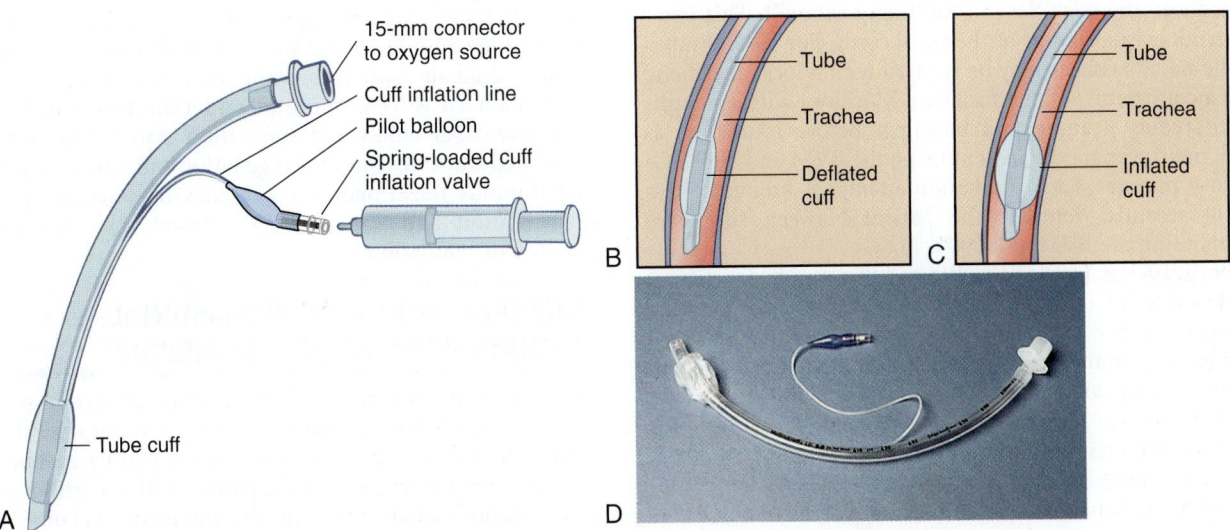

FIG. 65-14   Endotracheal tube. **A,** Parts of an endotracheal tube. **B,** Tube in place with cuff deflated. **C,** Tube in place with the cuff inflated. **D,** Photo of tube before placement. (*A,* From Beare PG, Myers JL: *Adult health nursing,* ed 3, St Louis, 1998, Mosby.)

nasopharynx, and vocal cords. Oral ET intubation is preferred for most emergencies because the airway can be secured rapidly and a larger-diameter tube is used. A larger-bore ET tube reduces the *work of breathing* (WOB) because of less airway resistance. It is easier to remove secretions and perform bronchoscopy if needed. Nasal ET intubation is rarely used but may be needed when oral intubation is not possible (e.g., unstable cervical spine injury, dental abscess, epiglottitis).

There are risks associated with oral ET intubation. It is difficult to place an oral tube if head and neck mobility are limited (e.g., suspected spinal cord injury). Teeth can be chipped or accidentally removed during the procedure. Salivation is increased and swallowing is difficult. Patients can obstruct the ET tube by biting down on it. Sedation along with a bite block or oropharyngeal airway may be used to prevent this. The ET tube and bite block (if used) should be secured (separately) to the face. Mouth care is a challenge because of limited space in the oral cavity. Manage this by using smaller or pediatric-sized oral products for tooth brushing, cleaning, and suctioning.

Endotracheal Intubation Procedure

Unless ET intubation is emergent, consent for the procedure is obtained. Tell the patient and caregiver the reason for ET intubation, steps in the procedure, and patient's role in the procedure (if indicated). Also explain that, while intubated, the patient will not be able to speak, but that you will provide other means of communication. Tell them that the patient's hands may have removable mitts placed to remind him or her not to touch the airway.

Have a self-inflating *bag-valve-mask* (BVM) (e.g., *Ambu bag*) attached to O_2, suctioning equipment ready at the bedside, and IV access. The BVM contains a reservoir that is filled with O_2 so that concentrations of 90% to 95% are delivered. The slower the bag is deflated and inflated, the higher the O_2 concentration that is delivered. Assemble and check the equipment to be used, remove the patient's dentures or partial plates (for oral intubation), and give drugs as ordered. Premedication varies depending on the patient's level of consciousness (e.g., awake, obtunded), nature of the procedure (e.g., emergent, nonemergent), and the HCP's preferences.

For oral intubation, place the patient supine with the head extended and the neck flexed ("sniffing position"). This position permits visualization of the vocal cords. For nasal intubation, the nasal passages may be sprayed with a local anesthetic and vasoconstrictor (e.g., lidocaine [Xylocaine] with epinephrine) to reduce trauma and bleeding. Before intubation is started, preoxygenate the patient using the BVM and 100% O_2 for 3 to 5 minutes. Each intubation attempt is limited to less than 30 seconds. Ventilate the patient between successive attempts using the BVM and 100% O_2.

Rapid-sequence intubation (RSI) is the rapid, concurrent administration of both a sedative and paralytic drug during emergency airway management to decrease the risks of aspiration and injury to the patient. RSI is not indicated in patients who are in cardiac arrest or have a known difficult airway.[26] A sedative-hypnotic-amnesic (e.g., midazolam, etomidate [Amidate]) is used to induce unconsciousness, along with a rapid-onset opioid (e.g., fentanyl) to blunt the pain of the procedure. A paralytic drug (e.g., succinylcholine [Anectine]) is then given to produce skeletal muscle paralysis. Monitor the patient's O_2 status during the procedure with pulse oximetry.

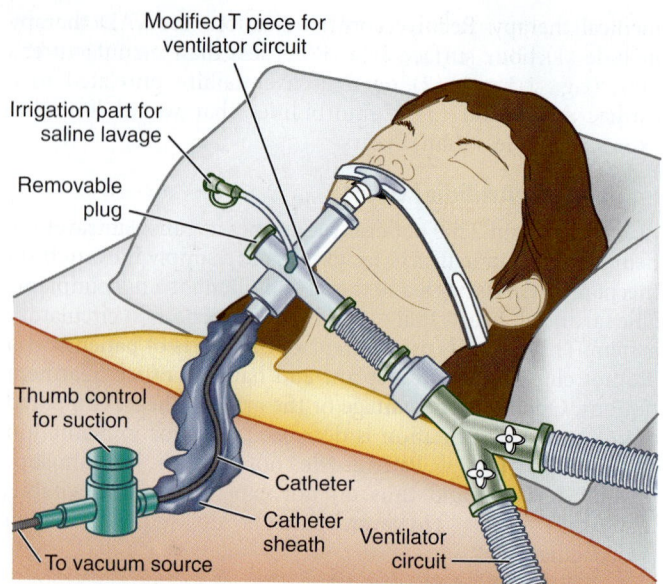

FIG. 65-15 Closed tracheal suction system.

After intubation, inflate the cuff and confirm the placement of the ET tube while the patient is manually ventilated using the BVM with 100% O_2. Use an end-tidal CO_2 detector to confirm proper placement by noting the presence of exhaled CO_2 from the lungs. Place the detector between the BVM and ET tube and look for a color change (indicating the presence of CO_2) or a number. If no CO_2 is detected, the tube is in the esophagus and must be reinserted.[27] Auscultate the lungs for bilateral breath sounds and the epigastrium for the absence of air sounds. Observe the chest for symmetric chest wall movement. In addition, SpO_2 should be stable or improved.

If the findings support proper ET tube placement, connect the tube to a mechanical ventilator and secure per agency policy (Fig. 65-15). Suction the ET tube and pharynx, and insert a bite block if needed. Obtain a chest x-ray immediately to confirm tube location (2 to 6 cm above the carina in the adult). This position allows the patient to move the neck without moving the tube or causing it to enter the right mainstem bronchus. Once proper positioning is confirmed with x-ray, record and mark the position of the tube at the lip or teeth (usually 21 cm for women and 23 cm for men) or nose. Cut excess tubing to reduce dead air space (according to agency policy).

Obtain ABGs 15 to 30 minutes after intubation to determine baseline oxygenation and ventilation status. ABG values are reviewed and used to guide oxygenation and ventilation changes. Continuous pulse oximetry provides data regarding arterial oxygenation and end-tidal CO_2 monitoring provides data related to ventilation.

❖ NURSING AND INTERPROFESSIONAL MANAGEMENT: ARTIFICIAL AIRWAY

Management of a patient with an artificial airway is often a shared responsibility between you and the respiratory therapist, with specific management tasks determined by agency policy. Nursing responsibilities for the patient with an artificial airway may include some or all of the following: (1) maintaining correct tube placement, (2) maintaining proper cuff inflation, (3) monitoring oxygenation and ventilation, (4) maintaining tube patency, (5) providing oral care and maintaining skin integrity, (6) fostering comfort and communication, and (7) assessing for complications. eNursing Care Plan 65-1 for the patient on a mechanical ventilator is available on the website for this chapter.

◆ Maintaining Correct Tube Placement

Continuously monitor the patient with an ET tube for proper placement. If the tube moves or is dislodged, it could end up in the pharynx or enter the esophagus or the right mainstem bronchus (thus ventilating only the right lung).

> ⚠ **SAFETY ALERT** **Endotracheal Tube Placement**
> • Maintain proper ET tube position by placing an "exit mark" on the tube.
> • Confirm that the mark remains constant while at rest and during patient care, repositioning, and transport.

Observe for symmetric chest wall movement and auscultate to confirm bilateral breath sounds. If the ET tube is not positioned properly, it is an airway emergency. Stay with the patient, maintain the airway, support ventilation with a BVM and 100% O_2, and call for the appropriate help to immediately reposition the tube. If a dislodged tube is not repositioned, minimal or no O_2 is delivered to the lungs or the entire V_T is delivered to one lung. This places the patient at risk for pneumothorax.

◆ Maintaining Proper Cuff Inflation

The cuff is an inflatable, pliable sleeve encircling the lower, outer wall of the ET tube (Fig. 65-14). The high-volume, low-pressure cuff stabilizes and "seals" the ET tube within the trachea and prevents escape of ventilating gases. However, excess volume in the cuff can damage the tracheal mucosa. To prevent this, inflate the cuff with air, and measure and monitor the cuff pressure. To ensure adequate tracheal perfusion, maintain cuff pressure at 20 to 25 cm H_2O.[28] Measure and record cuff pressure after intubation and on a routine basis (e.g., every 8 hours) using the *minimal occluding volume* (MOV) *technique* or *the minimal leak technique* (MLT).

The steps in the MOV technique for cuff inflation are as follows: (1) for the mechanically ventilated patient, place a stethoscope over the trachea and inflate the cuff to MOV by adding air until no air leak is heard at peak inspiratory pressure (end of ventilator inspiration); (2) for the spontaneously breathing intubated patient, inflate until no sound is heard after a deep breath or after inhalation with a BVM; (3) use a manometer to verify that cuff pressure is between 20 and 25 cm H_2O; and (4) record cuff pressure in the chart. If adequate cuff pressure cannot be maintained or larger volumes of air are needed to keep the cuff inflated, there could be a leak in the cuff or tracheal dilation at the cuff site. In these situations, notify the HCP.

The procedure for MLT is similar with one exception. Remove a small amount of air from the cuff until a slight air leak is auscultated at peak inflation. Both techniques aim to prevent the risks of tracheal damage from high cuff pressures.

◆ Monitoring Oxygenation and Ventilation

Closely monitor the patient with an ET tube for adequate oxygenation by assessing clinical findings, ABGs, SpO_2, and, if available, $ScvO_2$ or SvO_2. Assess for signs of hypoxemia such as a change in mental status (e.g., confusion), anxiety, dusky skin, and dysrhythmias. Periodic ABGs and continuous SpO_2 provide objective data regarding oxygenation. Lower PaO_2 values are expected in patients with some disease states, such as chronic

obstructive pulmonary disease (COPD). CVP or PA catheters with $ScvO_2$ or SvO_2 capability provide an indirect indication of the patient's tissue oxygenation status (Table 65-4).

Indicators of ventilation include clinical findings, $PaCO_2$, and continuous partial pressure of end-tidal CO_2 ($PETCO_2$). Assess the patient's respirations for rate, rhythm, and use of accessory muscles. The patient who is hyperventilating will be breathing rapidly and deeply and may experience circumoral and peripheral numbness and tingling. The patient who is hypoventilating will be breathing shallowly or slowly and may appear dusky. $PaCO_2$ is the best indicator of alveolar hyperventilation (e.g., decreased $PaCO_2$, increased pH indicate respiratory alkalosis) or hypoventilation (e.g., increased $PaCO_2$, decreased pH indicate respiratory acidosis).

$PETCO_2$ monitoring (*capnography*) is done by analyzing exhaled gas directly at the patient-ventilator circuit (*mainstream sampling*) or by transporting a sample of gas via a small-bore tubing to a bedside monitor (*sidestream sampling*). Continuous $PETCO_2$ monitoring can assess the patency of the airway and presence of breathing. In addition, gradual changes in $PETCO_2$ values may accompany an increase in CO_2 production (e.g., sepsis, hypoventilation, neuromuscular blockade) or a decrease in CO_2 production (e.g., hypothermia, decreased CO, metabolic acidosis). In patients with normal ventilation-to-perfusion ratios (see Chapter 67), $PETCO_2$ can be used as an estimate of $PaCO_2$, with $PETCO_2$ generally 1 to 5 mm Hg lower than $PaCO_2$. However, in patients with unusually large dead air space or serious mismatch between ventilation and perfusion, $PETCO_2$ is not a reliable estimate of $PaCO_2$.[27]

◆ Maintaining Tube Patency

Do not routinely suction a patient. Regularly assess the patient to determine if suctioning is needed. Indications for suctioning include (1) visible secretions in the ET tube, (2) sudden onset of respiratory distress, (3) suspected aspiration of secretions, (4) increase in respiratory rate with or without sustained coughing, and (5) sudden decrease in SpO_2. Other signs that may indicate the patient needs suctioning include an increase in peak airway pressure and auscultation of adventitious breath sounds over the trachea or bronchi.

Table 65-8 describes two recommended suctioning methods, the *closed-suction technique* (CST) and the *open-suction technique* (OST). The CST uses a suction catheter that is enclosed in a plastic sleeve connected directly to the patient-ventilator circuit (Fig. 65-15). With the CST, oxygenation and ventilation are maintained during suctioning, and exposure to the patient's secretions and possible infection is reduced for the patient's and HCP's safety. The CST should be used for patients who (1) require high levels of positive end-expiratory pressure (PEEP) (greater than 10 cm H_2O), (2) have high levels of FIO_2, (3) have bloody or infected pulmonary secretions, (4) require frequent suctioning, and (5) experience clinical instability with the OST.[29]

Potential complications associated with suctioning include hypoxemia, bronchospasm, increased intracranial pressure, dysrhythmias, hypertension, hypotension, mucosal damage, pulmonary bleeding, pain, and infection. Closely assess the patient before, during, and after the suctioning procedure. If the patient does not tolerate suctioning (e.g., decreased SpO_2, increased or decreased BP, sustained coughing, development of dysrhythmias), immediately stop the procedure. Hyperoxygenate the patient. Continue to reassess the patient

TABLE 65-8   Suctioning Procedures for Patient on Mechanical Ventilator

General Measures for Open- and Closed-Suction Techniques

1. Gather all equipment.
2. Wash hands and don personal protective equipment.
3. Explain procedure and patient's role in assisting with secretion removal by coughing.
4. Monitor patient's cardiopulmonary status (e.g., vital signs, SpO$_2$, SvO$_2$ or ScvO$_2$, ECG, level of consciousness) before, during, and after the procedure.
5. Turn on suction and set vacuum to 100-120 mm Hg.
6. Pause ventilator alarms.

Open-Suction Technique

7. Open sterile catheter package using the inside of the package as a sterile field. NOTE: Suction catheter should be no wider than half the diameter of the ET tube (e.g., for a 7-mm ET tube, select a 10F suction catheter).
8. Fill the sterile solution container with sterile normal saline or water.
9. Don sterile gloves.
10. Pick up sterile suction catheter with dominant hand. Using nondominant hand, secure the connecting tube (to suction) to the suction catheter.
11. Check equipment for proper functioning by suctioning a small volume of sterile saline solution from the container. **(Go to step 13.)**

Closed-Suction Technique

12. Connect the suction tubing to the closed suction port.
13. Hyperoxygenate the patient for 30 sec using one of the following methods:
    - Activate the suction hyperoxygenation setting on the ventilator using nondominant hand.
    - Increase FIO$_2$ to 100%. NOTE: Remember to return FIO$_2$ to baseline level at the completion of the procedure if not done automatically after preset time by ventilator.
    - Disconnect the ventilator tubing from the ET tube and manually ventilate the patient with 100% O$_2$ using a BVM device.* Administer five or six breaths over 30 sec. NOTE: Use of a second person to deliver the manual breaths significantly increases the V$_T$ delivered.
14. With suction off, gently and quickly insert the catheter using the dominant hand. When you meet resistance, pull back ½ in.
15. Apply continuous or intermittent suction using the nondominant thumb. Withdraw the catheter over 10 sec or less.
16. Hyperoxygenate for 30 sec as described in step 13.
17. If secretions remain and the patient has tolerated the procedure, perform two or three suction passes as described in steps 14 and 15. NOTE: Rinse the suction catheter with sterile saline solution between suctioning passes as needed.
18. Reconnect patient to ventilator (open-suction technique).
19. At the completion of ET tube suctioning, rinse the catheter and connecting tubing with the sterile saline solution.
20. Suction oral pharynx. NOTE: Use a separate catheter for this step when using the closed-suction technique.
21. Discard the suction catheter and rinse the connecting tubing with the sterile saline solution (open-suction technique).
22. Reset FIO$_2$ (if necessary) and ventilator alarms.
23. Reassess patient for signs of effective suctioning.

BVM, Bag-valve-mask; *ECG*, electrocardiogram; *ET*, endotracheal; *FIO$_2$*, fraction of inspired O$_2$; *PEEP*, positive end-expiratory pressure; *V$_T$*, tidal volume.
*Attach a PEEP valve to the BVM for patients on >5 cm H$_2$O PEEP.
Adapted from Seckel MA: Suctioning: endotracheal or tracheostomy tube. In Wiegand DL-M, editor: *AACN procedure manual for critical care*, ed 7, St Louis, 2017, Elsevier. (in press)

until hemodynamic stability is achieved, the patient recovers, and/or the situation resolves before attempting another suction pass. Prevent hypoxemia by hyperoxygenating the patient before and after each suctioning pass and limiting each pass to 10 seconds or less (Table 65-8). Assess both the ECG and SpO$_2$ before, during, and after the suctioning procedure.

Causes of dysrhythmias during suctioning include (1) hypoxemia resulting in myocardial ischemia; (2) vagal stimulation caused by tracheal irritation; and (3) sympathetic nervous system stimulation caused by anxiety, discomfort, or pain. Dysrhythmias include tachydysrhythmias and bradydysrhythmias, premature beats, and asystole. Stop suctioning if any new dysrhythmias develop. Avoid excessive suctioning in patients with severe hypoxemia or bradycardia.

Tracheal mucosal damage may occur due to excessive suction pressures (greater than 120 mm Hg), overly vigorous catheter insertion, and the suction catheter itself. Blood streaks or tissue shreds in aspirated secretions may indicate mucosal damage. This increases the risk of infection and bleeding, particularly if the patient is receiving anticoagulants.[29] Trauma to the mucosa can be prevented by following the steps described in Table 65-8.

Secretions may be thick and difficult to suction because of inadequate hydration or humidification, infection, or inaccessibility of the lower airways. Adequately hydrate the patient (e.g., oral or IV fluids) and provide supplemental humidification of inspired gases to help thin secretions. Do not instill normal saline into the ET tube as it may be harmful. If infection is the cause of thick secretions, give the patient appropriate antibiotics. Mobilize and turn the patient (e.g., every 2 hours) to help move secretions into larger airways.

◆ Providing Oral Care and Maintaining Skin Integrity

When an oral ET tube is in place, the patient's mouth is always open. Moisten the lips, tongue, and gums with saline or water swabs to prevent mucosal drying. Proper oral care provides comfort and prevents injury to the gums and plaque formation (Table 65-9).

TABLE 65-9   Oral Care for Patient on Mechanical Ventilator

General Measures

1. Gather all equipment.
2. Wash hands and don personal protective equipment.
3. Explain procedure to the patient and caregiver (if present).
4. Perform oral care using pediatric or adult soft toothbrushes at least twice a day by gently brushing to clean and remove plaque.
5. Use oral swabs with a 1.5% hydrogen peroxide solution every 2-4 hr.
6. Use 0.12% chlorhexidine oral rinse twice daily.
7. Apply a mouth moisturizer to oral mucosa and lips with each cleaning.
8. Suction oral cavity and pharynx frequently. Fig. 65-16 is an example of an endotracheal tube that can provide continuous or intermittent subglottic suctioning.

NOTE:
- Change all oral suction equipment and suction tubing every 24 hr.
- Rinse nondisposable oral suction apparatus with sterile normal saline after each use and place on a dry paper towel.

Adapted from Vollman KM, Sole ML: Endotracheal tube and oral care. In Wiegand DL-M, editor: *AACN procedure manual for critical care*, ed 6, St Louis, 2011, Saunders; and Institute for Healthcare Improvement: How-to guide: prevent ventilator-associated pneumonia. Retrieved from *www.ihi.org/resources/Pages/Tools/HowtoGuidePreventVAP.aspx*.

Frequent assessment and meticulous care are required to prevent skin breakdown on the face, lips, tongue, and nares because of pressure from the ET tube or bite block or the method used to secure the ET tube to the patient's face. Reposition and retape the ET tube (per agency policy) and as needed to prevent skin breakdown.

For the nasally intubated patient, remove the old tape and clean the skin around the ET tube with saline-soaked gauze or cotton swabs. For the orally intubated patient, remove the bite block (if present) and the old tape. Provide oral hygiene and then reposition the ET tube to the opposite side of the mouth. Replace the bite block (if appropriate) and reconfirm proper cuff inflation and tube placement. Secure the ET tube again (per agency policy).

Commercial ET holders are often used. These may increase the risk for skin breakdown compared to tape.[30] If a commercial ET holder is used, follow the manufacturer's directions for maintaining tube position, providing skin care, and preventing skin breakdown.

Ongoing assessment is shared between nursing and respiratory therapy. Repositioning the ET tube may be limited to respiratory therapy. Two staff members should always perform the repositioning procedure to prevent accidental ET tube dislodgment. Monitor the patient for any signs of respiratory distress throughout the procedure.

◆ Fostering Comfort and Communication

Intubation is a major stressor for the patient.[31] The intubated patient may experience anxiety from not being able to talk or not knowing what to expect. Communicating with the intubated patient can be frustrating for the patient, caregiver, and interprofessional care team. To communicate more effectively, use a variety of methods.[32] (See Common Problems of Critical Care Patients earlier in this chapter on pp. 1556-1557.)

The physical discomfort associated with ET intubation and mechanical ventilation often requires sedating the patient and giving an analgesic until the ET tube is no longer needed. The patient may need fentanyl, midazolam, propofol, or other sedatives to blunt the anxiety and discomfort related to intubation. Evaluate the drugs' effectiveness in achieving an acceptable level of patient comfort by using a valid pain scale, sedation scale (e.g., Ramsey Sedation Scale), and/or delirium scale.[6] In addition, consider using relaxation techniques (e.g., music therapy) to complement drug therapy.

◆ Complications of Endotracheal Intubation

Two major complications of ET intubation are unplanned extubation and aspiration. Unplanned *extubation* (i.e., removal of the ET tube from the trachea) can be a catastrophic event and may complicate the patient's recovery. Unplanned extubations can be due to patient removal of the ET tube or accidental removal during movement or a procedure. Usually the unplanned extubation is obvious (i.e., the patient is holding the ET tube). Other times, the tip of the ET tube is in the hypopharynx or esophagus, and the extubation is not so obvious.

> **⚠ SAFETY ALERT   Unplanned Extubation**
> Observe for signs of unplanned extubation, which can be a life-threatening event:
> - Patient talking
> - Activation of the low-pressure ventilator alarm
> - Diminished or absent breath sounds
> - Respiratory distress

You are responsible for preventing unplanned extubation by ensuring that the ET tube is secured and observing and supporting the ET tube during repositioning, procedures, and patient transfers. Additionally, giving adequate sedation and analgesia and using standardized weaning protocols decrease the incidence of self-extubation.[33]

The use of soft wrist restraints to immobilize the patient's hands is not an absolute deterrent to self-extubation.[34] Be sure to explain to the patient and caregiver when you use short-term restraints for patient safety and discuss the use of alternatives. Reassess for the continued need of restraints (per agency policy).

Should an unplanned extubation occur, stay with the patient and call for help. Interventions are aimed at maintaining the patient's airway, supporting ventilation (e.g., manually ventilating the patient with a BVM and 100% O_2), securing the appropriate assistance to immediately reintubate the patient (if necessary), and providing psychologic support to the patient.

Aspiration is another potential hazard for the patient with an ET tube. The ET tube passes through the epiglottis, splinting it in an open position. Thus the intubated patient cannot protect the airway from aspiration. The high-volume, low-pressure ET or tracheal cuff cannot totally prevent the trickle of oral or gastric secretions into the trachea. Further, secretions collect above the cuff. When the cuff is deflated, those secretions can move into the lungs. Some ET tubes provide continuous suctioning of secretions above the cuff (Fig. 65-16).

Oral intubation increases salivation, yet swallowing is difficult, so suction the patient's mouth frequently. Use a Yankauer (tonsil-tip) suction catheter or a sterile single-use catheter. Other factors contributing to aspiration include improper cuff inflation, patient positioning, and decreased gastric mobility and bowel function if receiving tube feedings. The patient with an ET tube is at risk for aspiration of gastric contents. Even when the cuff is properly inflated, take precautions to prevent vomiting, which can lead to aspiration.[35]

Often, a nasogastric (NG) or an orogastric (OG) tube is inserted and connected to low, intermittent suction when a patient is first intubated. An OG tube is preferred over an NG tube to reduce the risk of sinusitis. All patients who are intubated or receiving enteral feedings must have the HOB elevated a minimum of 30 to 45 degrees unless medically contraindicated.

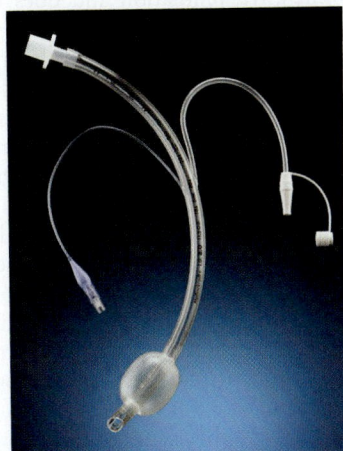

FIG. 65-16   Continuous subglottal suctioning can be provided by the Hi Lo Evac Tube. A dorsal lumen above the cuff allows for suctioning of secretions from the subglottic area. (Reprinted by permission of Nellcor Puritan Bennett Inc, Pleasanton, Calif.)

MECHANICAL VENTILATION

Mechanical ventilation is the process by which the FIO_2 (21% [room air] or more) is moved in and out of the lungs by a mechanical ventilator. Mechanical ventilation is not curative. It is a means of supporting patients until they recover the ability to breathe independently. It can also serve as a bridge to long-term mechanical ventilation, or until a decision is made to withdraw ventilatory support.

Indications for mechanical ventilation include (1) apnea or impending inability to breathe or protect the airway, (2) acute respiratory failure (see Chapter 67), (3) severe hypoxia, and (4) respiratory muscle fatigue.[36] Patients with chronic pulmonary disease and their caregivers should be given the opportunity to discuss mechanical ventilation before end-stage respiratory disease develops. Encourage all patients, particularly those with chronic illnesses, to discuss the subject with their families and HCPs. They should record and place the results of these discussions in an advance directive.

The decision to use, withhold, or withdraw mechanical ventilation must be made carefully, respecting the wishes of the patient and caregiver. When the interprofessional care team, patient, and/or caregiver disagree over the treatment plan, family conferences are essential to keep the lines of communication open and discuss options. You may need to consult the agency's ethics committee for assistance.

Types of Mechanical Ventilation

The two major types of mechanical ventilation are negative pressure and positive pressure ventilation.

Negative Pressure Ventilation. Negative pressure ventilation involves the use of chambers that encase the chest or body and surround it with intermittent subatmospheric (or negative) pressure. The "iron lung" was the first form of negative pressure ventilation, developed during the polio epidemic. Intermittent negative pressure around the chest wall causes the chest to be pulled outward, reducing intrathoracic pressure. Air rushes in via the upper airway, which is outside the sealed chamber. Expiration is passive. The machine cycles off, allowing chest retraction. This type of ventilation is similar to normal ventilation in that decreased intrathoracic pressures produce inspiration, and expiration is passive. Negative pressure ventilation is delivered by noninvasive ventilation and does not require an artificial airway.

Several portable negative pressure ventilators are available for home use for patients with neuromuscular diseases, central nervous system disorders, diseases and injuries of the spinal cord, and severe COPD (Fig. 65-17). Negative pressure ventilators are not routinely used for acutely ill patients.

Positive Pressure Ventilation. Positive pressure ventilation (PPV) is the primary method used with acutely ill patients (Fig. 65-18). During inspiration the ventilator pushes air into the lungs under positive pressure. Unlike spontaneous ventilation, intrathoracic pressure is raised during lung inflation rather than lowered. Expiration occurs passively as in normal expiration. Modes of PPV are categorized into two groups: volume and pressure ventilation.[36]

Volume Ventilation. With volume ventilation a predetermined tidal volume (V_T) is delivered with each inspiration, and the amount of pressure needed to deliver the breath varies based on compliance and resistance factors of the patient-ventilator

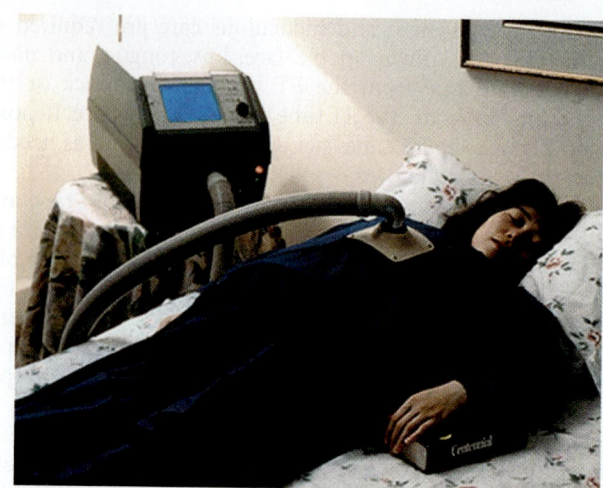

FIG. 65-17 Negative pressure ventilator. (Courtesy Lifecare, Westminster, Colo.)

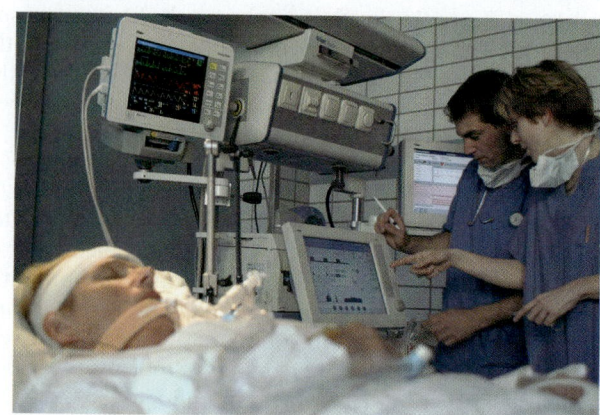

FIG. 65-18 Patient receiving mechanical ventilation. (Courtesy Draeger Medical.)

system. Consequently, the V_T is consistent from breath to breath, but airway pressures vary.

Pressure Ventilation. With *pressure ventilation* the peak inspiratory pressure is predetermined, and the V_T delivered to the patient varies based on the selected pressure and compliance and resistance factors of the patient-ventilator system. With this understanding, careful attention must be given to the V_T to prevent unplanned hyperventilation or hypoventilation. For example, when the patient breathes out of synchrony with the ventilator, the pressure limit may be reached quickly, and the volume of gas delivered may be small. Initially, pressure ventilation was used only in stable patients being weaned from the ventilator. Today, pressure ventilation is frequently used to treat critically ill patients.

Settings of Mechanical Ventilators

Mechanical ventilator settings regulate rate, V_T, O_2 concentration, and other characteristics of ventilation (Table 65-10). Settings are based on the patient's status (e.g., ABGs, ideal body weight, current physiologic state, level of consciousness, respiratory muscle strength). Settings are evaluated and adjusted until oxygenation and ventilation targets have been reached.

TABLE 65-10 Settings of Mechanical Ventilation

Parameter	Description
Respiratory rate (f)	Number of breaths the ventilator delivers per minute. *Usual setting:* 6-20 breaths/min
Tidal volume (V_T)	Volume of gas delivered to patient during each ventilator breath. *Usual volume:* 6-10 mL/kg
O_2 concentration (FIO_2)	Fraction of inspired O_2 (FIO_2) delivered to patient. May be set between 21% (essentially room air) and 100%. *Usually adjusted* to maintain PaO_2 level >60 mm Hg or SpO_2 level >90%
Positive end-expiratory pressure (PEEP)	Positive pressure applied at the end of expiration of ventilator breaths. *Usual setting:* 5 cm H_2O
Pressure support	Positive pressure used to augment patient's inspiratory pressure. *Usual setting:* 6-18 cm H_2O
I:E ratio	Duration of inspiration (I) to duration of expiration (E). *Usual setting:* 1:2 to 1:1.5 unless IRV is desired
Inspiratory flow rate and time	Speed with which the V_T is delivered. *Usual setting:* 40-80 L/min and time is 0.8-1.2 sec
Sensitivity	Determines the amount of effort the patient must generate to initiate a ventilator breath. It may be set for pressure triggering or flow triggering. *Usual setting:* A pressure trigger is set 0.5-1.5 cm H_2O below baseline pressure and a flow trigger is set 1-3 L/min below baseline flow
High-pressure limit	Regulates the maximal pressure the ventilator can generate to deliver the V_T. When the pressure limit is reached, the ventilator terminates the breath and spills the undelivered volume into the atmosphere. *Usual setting:* 10-20 cm H_2O above peak inspiratory pressure

IRV, Inverse ratio ventilation.
Adapted from Urden LD, Lough ME, Stacy KM: *Critical care nursing: diagnosis and management,* ed 6, St Louis, 2010, Mosby.

It is important that you check that all ventilator alarms are always on. Alarms alert the staff to potentially dangerous situations such as mechanical malfunction, apnea, unplanned extubation, or patient asynchrony with the ventilator[37] (Table 65-11). On many ventilators the alarms can be temporarily suspended or silenced for up to 2 minutes for suctioning or testing while a staff member is in the room. After that time, the alarm system automatically turns back on.

⚠ SAFETY ALERT   Alarm Fatigue
- Alarm fatigue can develop in those who are exposed to an excessive number of alarms and results in sensory overload.
- This can cause a delayed response to alarms or dismissing them altogether and can lead to serious adverse events (e.g., patient death).
- One alarm management strategy to reduce alarm fatigue includes customizing alarm parameters based on individual patient needs.[37]

TABLE 65-11 Mechanical Ventilation Alarms

Alarm	Possible Causes
High-pressure limit	- Secretions, coughing, or gagging - Patient fighting ventilator (ventilator asynchrony) - Condensate (water) in tubing - Kinked or compressed tubing (e.g., patient biting on endotracheal tube [ET] tube) - Increased resistance (e.g., bronchospasm) - Decreased compliance (e.g., pulmonary edema, pneumothorax)
Low-pressure limit	- Total or partial ventilator disconnect - Loss of airway (e.g., total or partial extubation) - ET tube or tracheotomy cuff leak (e.g., patient speaking, grunting)
Apnea	- Respiratory arrest - Oversedation - Change in patient condition - Loss of airway (e.g., total or partial extubation)
High V_T, minute ventilation, or respiratory rate	- Pain, anxiety - Change in patient condition - Excess condensate in tubing (i.e., false reading)
Low V_T or minute ventilation	- Change in patient's breathing efforts (e.g., rate and volume) - Patient disconnection, loose connection, or leak in circuit - ET tube or tracheotomy cuff leak (e.g., patient speaking, grunting) - Insufficient gas flow
Ventilator inoperative or low battery	- Machine malfunction - Unplugged, power failure, or internal battery not charged

V_T, Tidal volume.
Adapted from Pierce LN: *Management of the mechanically ventilated patient,* ed 2, St Louis, 2007, Saunders.

Modes of Volume Ventilation

The methods by which the patient and ventilator interact to deliver effective ventilation are called *ventilator modes.* The selected ventilator mode is based on how much WOB the patient should or can perform. WOB refers to inspiratory effort needed to overcome the elasticity and viscosity of the lungs along with the airway resistance. The mode is determined by the patient's ventilatory status, respiratory drive, and ABGs. Generally, ventilator modes are controlled or assisted.

With controlled ventilatory support, the ventilator does all of the WOB. With assisted ventilatory support, the ventilator and patient share the WOB. Historically, volume modes such as controlled mandatory ventilation (CMV), assist-control ventilation (ACV), and synchronized intermittent mandatory ventilation (SIMV) have been used to treat critically ill patients. Currently, pressure modes such as pressure support ventilation (PSV), pressure-control ventilation (PCV), and inverse ratio ventilation (PC-IRV) are more common.[36] Table 65-12 describes these ventilator modes.

Assist-Control Ventilation. With assist-control ventilation (ACV), the ventilator delivers a preset V_T at a preset frequency. When the patient initiates a spontaneous breath, the ventilator senses a decrease in intrathoracic pressure and then delivers the

TABLE 65-12 Modes of Mechanical Ventilation

Volume Modes

Assist-Control (AC) or Assisted Mandatory Ventilation (AMV)

- Requires that rate, V_T, inspiratory time, and PEEP be set for the patient.
- The ventilator sensitivity is also set, and when the patient initiates a spontaneous breath, a full-volume breath is delivered.

Intermittent Mandatory Ventilation (IMV) and Synchronized Intermittent Mandatory Ventilation (SIMV)

- Requires that rate, V_T, inspiratory time, sensitivity, and PEEP are set for the patient.
- In between "mandatory breaths," patients spontaneously breathe at their own rates and V_T. With SIMV, the ventilator synchronizes the mandatory breaths with the patient's own inspirations.

Pressure Modes

Pressure Support Ventilation (PSV)

- Provides an augmented inspiration to a spontaneously breathing patient.
- The clinician selects an inspiratory pressure level, PEEP, and sensitivity.
- When the patient initiates a breath, a high flow of gas is delivered to the preselected pressure level, and pressure is maintained throughout inspiration.
- The patient determines the parameters of V_T, rate, and inspiratory time.

Pressure-Control Inverse Ratio Ventilation (PC-IRV)

- Combines pressure-limited ventilation with an inverse ratio of inspiration to expiration.
- The clinician selects the pressure level, rate, inspiratory time (1:1, 2:1, 3:1, 4:1), and the PEEP level.
- With the prolonged inspiratory times, auto-PEEP may result.
- The auto-PEEP may be a desirable outcome of the inverse ratios.
- Some clinicians use PC without IRV.
- Conventional inspiratory times are used and rate, pressure level, and PEEP are selected.

Airway Pressure Release Ventilation (APRV)

- Provides two levels of continuous positive airway pressure (CPAP) with timed releases, and permits spontaneous breathing throughout the respiratory cycle.
- The clinician selects both pressure high and pressure low along with time high and time low. V_T is not a set variable and depends on the CPAP level, the patient's compliance and resistance, and spontaneous breathing effort.

Positive End-Expiratory Pressure (PEEP) and Continuous Positive Airway Pressure (CPAP)

PEEP

- Creates positive pressure at end exhalation and restores functional residual capacity (FRC).
- The term *PEEP* is used when end-expiratory pressure is provided during ventilator positive pressure breaths.

CPAP

- Similar to PEEP, CPAP restores FRC.
- This pressure is continuous during spontaneous breathing; no positive pressure breaths are present.

Modified from Burns SM: Invasive mechanical ventilation (through an artificial airway) volume and pressure modes. In Wiegand DL-M, editor: *AACN procedure manual for critical care*, ed 6, St Louis, 2011, Saunders.

preset V_T. The patient can breathe faster than the preset rate but not slower. This mode has the advantage of allowing the patient some control over ventilation while providing some assistance. ACV is used in patients with a variety of conditions, including neuromuscular disorders (e.g., Guillain-Barré syndrome), pulmonary edema, and acute respiratory failure.

In the ACV mode, the patient has the potential for hyperventilation. The spontaneously breathing patient can easily be overventilated, resulting in hyperventilation. If the volume or minimum rate is set too low and the patient is apneic or weak, the patient can be hypoventilated. Thus these patients require vigilant assessment and monitoring of ventilatory status, including respiratory rate, ABGs, SpO_2, and $ScvO_2$ or SvO_2. It is also important that the sensitivity or amount of negative pressure required to start a breath is appropriate to the patient's condition. For example, if it is too difficult for the patient to begin a breath, the WOB is increased and the patient may tire (i.e., the patient "rides" the ventilator) or develop ventilator asynchrony (i.e., the patient "fights" the ventilator).

Synchronized Intermittent Mandatory Ventilation. With *synchronized intermittent mandatory ventilation* (SIMV), the ventilator delivers a preset V_T at a preset frequency in synchrony with the patient's spontaneous breathing. Between ventilator-delivered breaths, the patient is able to breathe spontaneously through the ventilator circuit. Thus the patient receives the preset FIO_2 during the spontaneous breaths but self-regulates the rate and V_T of those breaths. This mode of ventilation differs from ACV, in which all breaths are of the same preset volume. It is used during continuous ventilation and during weaning from the ventilator. SIMV may also be combined with PSV (described later). Potential benefits of SIMV include improved patient-ventilator synchrony, lower mean airway pressure, and prevention of muscle atrophy as the patient takes on more of the WOB.

SIMV also has disadvantages. If spontaneous breathing decreases when the preset rate is low, ventilation may not be adequately supported. Only patients with regular, spontaneous breathing should use low-rate SIMV. Weaning with SIMV demands close monitoring and may take longer because the rate of breathing is gradually reduced. Patients being weaned with SIMV may also have increased muscle fatigue associated with spontaneous breathing efforts.

Modes of Pressure Ventilation

Pressure Support Ventilation. With **pressure support ventilation (PSV)**, positive pressure is applied to the airway only during inspiration and is used with the patient's spontaneous respirations. The patient must be able to initiate a breath in this modality. The level of positive airway pressure is preset so that the gas flow rate is greater than the patient's inspiratory flow rate. As the patient starts a breath, the machine senses the spontaneous effort and supplies a rapid flow of gas at the initiation of the breath and variable flow throughout the breath. With PSV the patient determines inspiratory length, V_T, and respiratory rate. V_T depends on the pressure level and airway compliance.

PSV is used with continuous ventilation and during weaning. PSV may also be used with SIMV during weaning. PSV is not often used as ventilatory support during acute respiratory failure because of the risk of hypoventilation and apnea. Advantages of PSV include increased patient comfort, decreased WOB (because inspiratory efforts are augmented), decreased O_2 consumption (because inspiratory work is reduced), and increased endurance conditioning (because the patient is exercising respiratory muscles).

Pressure-Control and Pressure-Control Inverse Ratio Ventilation. *Pressure-control ventilation* (PCV) provides a pressure-limited breath delivered at a set rate and may permit spontaneous breathing. The V_T is not set. It is determined by the pressure limit set. *Pressure-control inverse ratio ventilation* (PC-IRV) combines pressure-limited ventilation with an inverse ratio of inspiration (I) to expiration (E). Some HCPs use PC without IRV.

The *I/E ratio* is the ratio of duration of inspiration to the duration of expiration. This ratio is normally 1:2 or 1:3. With IRV, the I/E ratio begins at 1:1 and may progress to 4:1. Prolonged positive pressure is applied, increasing inspiratory time. IRV gradually expands collapsed alveoli. The short expiratory time has a PEEP-like effect, preventing alveolar collapse. Because IRV imposes a nonphysiologic breathing pattern, the patient needs sedation and often paralysis.

PC-IRV is indicated for patients with acute respiratory distress syndrome (ARDS) who continue to have refractory hypoxemia despite high levels of PEEP. Not all patients with poor oxygenation respond to PC-IRV.

Airway Pressure Release Ventilation. *Airway pressure release ventilation* (APRV) permits spontaneous breathing at any point during the respiratory cycle with a preset continuous positive airway pressure (CPAP) with short timed pressure releases. The CPAP level (pressure high, pressure low) is adjusted to keep oxygenation goals while the timed releases (time high, time low) are increased or decreased to meet ventilation goals. V_T is not a set variable and depends on the CPAP level, the patient's compliance and resistance, and spontaneous breathing effort. The mode is designed for patients who need high pressure levels for alveolar recruitment (open collapsed alveoli). One advantage of this mode is the ability to permit spontaneous respirations. This may reduce the need for deep sedation or paralytics.

Other Modes. Advances in ventilator technology have led to the development of additional pressure modes. However, because of the nonstandardization of these options, the names and features are manufacturer specific. The superiority of these modes has not been established. Some examples include *volume-assured pressure ventilation* and *adaptive support ventilation*.

Other Ventilatory Maneuvers

Positive End-Expiratory Pressure. Positive end-expiratory pressure (PEEP) is a ventilatory maneuver in which positive pressure is applied to the airway during exhalation. Normally during exhalation, airway pressure drops to near zero, and exhalation occurs passively. With PEEP, exhalation remains passive, but pressure falls to a preset level, often 3 to 20 cm H_2O. Lung volume during expiration and between breaths is greater than normal with PEEP. This increases functional residual capacity (FRC) and often improves oxygenation with restoration of lung volume that normally remains at the end of passive exhalation. The mechanisms by which PEEP increases FRC and oxygenation include increased aeration of patent alveoli, aeration of previously collapsed alveoli, and prevention of alveolar collapse throughout the respiratory cycle.

PEEP is titrated to the point that oxygenation improves without compromising hemodynamics. This is termed *optimal PEEP*. Often 5 cm H_2O PEEP (referred to as *physiologic PEEP*) is used prophylactically to replace the glottic mechanism, help maintain a normal FRC, and prevent alveolar collapse. PEEP of 5 cm H_2O is also used for patients with a history of alveolar collapse during weaning. PEEP improves gas exchange, vital capacity, and inspiratory force when used during weaning.

In contrast, *auto-PEEP* is not purposely set on the ventilator but is a result of inadequate exhalation time. Auto-PEEP is additional PEEP over what is set by the HCP. This additional PEEP may result in increased WOB, barotrauma, and hemodynamic instability. Interventions to limit auto-PEEP include sedation and analgesia, large-diameter ET tube, bronchodilators, short inspiratory times, and decreased respiratory rates. Reducing water accumulation in the ventilator circuit by frequent emptying or use of heated circuits also limits auto-PEEP. In patients with short exhalation times and early airway closure (e.g., asthma), setting PEEP above auto-PEEP can offset auto-PEEP effects by splinting the airway open during exhalation and preventing "air trapping."

In general, the major purpose of PEEP is to maintain or improve oxygenation while limiting risk of O_2 toxicity. FIO_2 can often be reduced when PEEP is used. PEEP is generally indicated in all patients who are mechanically ventilated. The classic indication for PEEP therapy is ARDS (see Chapter 67). PEEP is used with caution in patients with increased intracranial pressure, low cardiac output, and hypovolemia. In these cases the adverse effects of PEEP may outweigh any benefits.

? CHECK YOUR PRACTICE

You are caring for a 75-yr-old woman who was orally intubated yesterday for respiratory distress secondary to pneumonia and placed on ACV. Her ventilator settings are: FIO_2 40%, V_T 400, RR 14 (set), PEEP 5. You respond to the ventilator alarm sounding and note that she is speaking. The alarm panel shows "low exhaled tidal volume." She appears confused with the following vital signs: HR 102, RR 24, and SpO_2 89%.
• What would be your next steps?

Continuous Positive Airway Pressure. Continuous positive airway pressure (CPAP) restores FRC and is similar to PEEP. However, the pressure in CPAP is delivered continuously during spontaneous breathing, thus preventing the patient's airway pressure from falling to zero. For example, if CPAP is 5 cm H_2O, airway pressure during expiration is 5 cm H_2O. During inspiration, 1 to 2 cm H_2O of negative pressure is generated, thus reducing airway pressure to 3 or 4 cm H_2O. CPAP is commonly used in the treatment of obstructive sleep apnea.[36] CPAP can be administered with a tight-fitting mask or an ET or tracheal tube. CPAP increases WOB because the patient must forcibly exhale against the CPAP. Therefore it must be used with caution in patients with myocardial compromise.

Automatic Tube Compensation. *Automatic tube compensation* (ATC) is an adjunct designed to overcome WOB through an artificial airway. It is currently available on many ventilators. ATC is increased during inspiration and decreased during expiration. It is set by entering the internal diameter of the patient's airway along with the desired percentage of compensation. ATC may become less effective in patients with excessive secretions and who require longer-term ventilation.[38]

Bilevel Positive Airway Pressure. In addition to O_2, *bilevel positive airway pressure* (BiPAP) provides two levels of positive pressure support: higher inspiratory positive airway pressure and lower expiratory positive airway pressure. It is a noninvasive modality and is delivered through a tight-fitting face mask, nasal mask, or nasal pillows. The patient must be able to spontaneously breathe and cooperate with this treatment.[36]

BiPAP is used for COPD patients with heart failure and acute respiratory failure and for patients with sleep apnea. BiPAP may also be used after extubation to prevent reintubation. Patients with shock, altered mental status, or increased airway secretions are not candidates for BiPAP because of the risk of aspiration and the inability to remove the mask.

High-Frequency Oscillatory Ventilation. High-frequency oscillatory ventilation (HFOV) involves delivery of a small V_T (usually 1 to 5 mL/kg of body weight) at rapid respiratory rates (100 to 300 breaths/minute) in an effort to recruit and maintain lung volume and reduce intrapulmonary shunting. While HFOV may be a useful mode for patients with life-threatening hypoxia, it has not improved survival or provided lung protection in patients with ARDS.[39] Patients receiving HFOV must be sedated and may be paralyzed to suppress spontaneous respiration. All patients must receive concurrent sedation and analgesia if using a paralytic drug (see Chapter 67).

Nitric Oxide. *Nitric oxide* (NO) is a gaseous molecule that is made intravascularly and participates in the regulation of pulmonary vascular tone. Inhibition of NO production results in pulmonary vasoconstriction, and administration of continuous inhaled NO results in pulmonary vasodilation. NO may be administered via an ET tube, a tracheostomy, or a face mask. Currently, NO is used as a diagnostic screening tool for pulmonary hypertension and to improve oxygenation during mechanical ventilation in this patient population. Although the use of NO does not reduce mortality in patients with ARDS, it may be used in patients with life-threatening hypoxia.[40]

Prone Positioning. *Prone positioning* is the repositioning of a patient from a supine or lateral position to a prone (on the stomach, face down) position. This repositioning improves lung recruitment (i.e., alveolar expansion) through various mechanisms. Gravity reverses the effects of fluid in the dependent parts of the lungs as the patient is moved from supine to prone. The heart rests on the sternum, away from the lungs, contributing to an overall uniformity of pleural pressures. The prone position is a relatively safe (although nurse-intensive), supportive therapy used in critically ill patients with severe ARDS to improve oxygenation.[41]

Extracorporeal Membrane Oxygenation. *Extracorporeal membrane oxygenation* (ECMO) is an alternative form of pulmonary support for the patient with severe respiratory failure. It is used more frequently in the pediatric and neonatal populations but is increasingly being used in adults. ECMO is a modification of cardiac bypass and involves partially removing blood from a patient with large-bore catheters, infusing O_2, removing CO_2, and returning the blood to the patient. This intensive therapy requires systemic anticoagulation and is a time-limited intervention. A skilled team of specialists, including a perfusionist, is required continuously at the bedside.[42]

INFORMATICS IN PRACTICE

Importing Monitor and Ventilator Data

- In many ICUs, the monitor data (e.g., vital signs, hemodynamic pressures, core temperature, pulse oximetry) are directly imported into the electronic health record (EHR). Ventilator data may also be sent to the EHR.
- Depending on the agency's information technology system, this connectivity of monitoring devices and ventilators can help drive evidence-based practice. Trends can be readily noted and prompts can link the user to protocols.
- Some systems have the capability of sending alarms or notifications to the HCP from the EHR.
- Always verify that accurate patient data are imported when documenting. Check to ensure that artifact or false data are deleted and confirm the procedure according to your agency's policy.

Complications of Positive Pressure Ventilation

Although PPV may be essential to maintain ventilation and oxygenation, it can cause adverse effects. It is often difficult to distinguish complications of mechanical ventilation from the underlying disease.

Cardiovascular System. PPV can affect circulation because of the transmission of increased mean airway pressure to various structures in the thorax. With increased intrathoracic pressure, thoracic vessels are compressed. The compression causes decreased venous return to the heart, left ventricular end-diastolic volume (preload), and CO, and results in hypotension. Mean airway pressure is further increased if PEEP is being titrated (greater than 5 cm H_2O) to improve oxygenation.

If the lungs are noncompliant (e.g., ARDS), airway pressures are not as easily transmitted to the heart and blood vessels. Thus effects of PPV on CO are reduced. Conversely, with compliant lungs (e.g., COPD), there is increased danger of transmission of high airway pressures and negative effects on hemodynamics.

Compromised venous return by PPV is worsened by hypovolemia (e.g., hemorrhage) and decreased venous tone (e.g., sepsis, spinal shock). Restoration and maintenance of the circulating blood volume are important in minimizing cardiovascular complications.

Pulmonary System

Barotrauma. As lung inflation pressures increase, risk of *barotrauma* increases. Patients with compliant lungs (e.g., COPD) are at greater risk for barotrauma. This results when the increased airway pressure distends the lungs and possibly ruptures fragile alveoli or emphysematous blebs. Patients with stiff lungs (e.g., ARDS) who are given high inspiratory pressures and high levels of PEEP (greater than 5 cm H_2O) and patients with lung abscesses resulting from necrotizing organisms (e.g., staphylococci) are also susceptible to barotrauma.

Air can escape into the pleural space from alveoli or interstitium and become trapped. Pleural pressure increases and collapses the lung, causing pneumothorax. (Chapter 27 discusses the clinical manifestations of pneumothorax.) The lungs receive air during inspiration but cannot expel it during expiration. Respiratory bronchioles are larger on inspiration than expiration. They may close on expiration, and air becomes trapped. With PPV, a simple pneumothorax can become a life-threatening tension pneumothorax. The mediastinum and contralateral lung are compressed, reducing CO. Immediate treatment of the pneumothorax is required.

Pneumomediastinum usually begins with rupture of alveoli into the lung interstitium. Progressive air movement occurs into the mediastinum and subcutaneous neck tissue, and a pneumothorax often follows. New, unexplained subcutaneous emphysema is an indication for immediate chest x-ray. Pneumomediastinum and subcutaneous emphysema may be too small to detect on x-ray or clinically before the development of a pneumothorax.

Volutrauma. The concept of *volutrauma* in PPV relates to the lung injury that occurs when a large V_T is used to ventilate noncompliant lungs. Volutrauma results in alveolar fractures and movement of fluids and proteins into the alveolar spaces. Low-volume ventilation rather than pressure ventilation should be used in ARDS patients to protect the lungs.

Alveolar Hypoventilation. *Alveolar hypoventilation* can be caused by inappropriate ventilator settings, leakage of air from the ventilator tubing or around the ET tube or tracheostomy cuff, lung secretions or obstruction, and low ventilation/perfusion ratio. A low V_T or respiratory rate decreases minute ventilation. This results in hypoventilation, atelectasis, and respiratory acidosis. A leaking cuff or tubing that is not secured may cause air leakage and lower V_T. Lung secretions can cause hypoventilation. Mobilizing the patient, turning the patient at least every 2 hours, encouraging deep breathing and coughing, and suctioning (as needed) may limit this. Increasing the V_T, adding small increments of PEEP, and adding a preset number of *sighs* to the ventilator settings (i.e., a deeper than normal breath incorporated into the respiratory cycle) can help reduce the risk of atelectasis.

Alveolar Hyperventilation. Respiratory alkalosis can occur if the respiratory rate or V_T is set too high (*mechanical overventilation*) or if the patient receiving assisted ventilation is *hyperventilating*. It is easy to overventilate a patient on PPV. Particularly at risk are patients with chronic alveolar hypoventilation and CO_2 retention. For example, the patient with COPD may have a chronic $PaCO_2$ elevation (acidosis) and compensatory bicarbonate retention by the kidneys. When the patient is ventilated, the patient's "normal baseline" rather than the standard normal values is the therapeutic goal. If the COPD patient is returned to a standard normal $PaCO_2$, the patient will develop alkalosis because of the retained bicarbonate. Such a patient could move from compensated respiratory acidosis to serious metabolic alkalosis.

The presence of alkalosis makes weaning from the ventilator difficult. Alkalosis, especially if the onset is abrupt, can have additional serious consequences, including hypokalemia, hypocalcemia, and dysrhythmias. Usually the patient with COPD who is supported on the ventilator does better with a short inspiratory and longer expiratory time.

If hyperventilation is spontaneous, it is important to determine the cause and treat it. Possible causes include hypoxemia, pain, fear, anxiety, or compensation for metabolic acidosis. Patients who fight the ventilator or breathe out of synchrony may be anxious or in pain. If the patient is anxious and fearful, sitting with the patient and verbally coaching the patient to breathe with the ventilator may help. If these measures fail, manually ventilating the patient slowly with a BVM and 100% O_2 may slow breathing enough to bring it in synchrony with the ventilator.

Ventilator-Associated Pneumonia. The risk for health care–associated pneumonia is highest in patients requiring mechanical ventilation because the ET or tracheostomy tube bypasses normal upper airway defenses. In addition, a poor nutritional state, immobility, and the underlying disease process (e.g., immunosuppression, organ failure) make the patient more prone to infection. *Ventilator-associated pneumonia* (VAP) is pneumonia that occurs 48 hours or more after ET intubation.[43] It occurs in as many as 27% of all intubated patients, with half of the cases developing within the first 4 days of mechanical ventilation. In addition, patients who develop VAP have significantly longer hospital stays and higher mortality rates than those who do not.

In patients with early VAP (within 96 hours of mechanical ventilation), sputum cultures often grow gram-negative bacteria (e.g., *Escherichia coli, Klebsiella, Streptococcus pneumoniae, Haemophilus influenzae*). Organisms associated with late VAP include antibiotic-resistant organisms such as *Pseudomonas aeruginosa* and oxacillin-resistant *Staphylococcus aureus*. These organisms are abundant in the hospital environment and the

patient's GI tract. They can spread in a number of ways, including contaminated respiratory equipment, inadequate hand washing, adverse environmental factors such as poor room ventilation and high traffic flow, and decreased patient ability to cough and clear secretions. Colonization of the oropharynx tract by gram-negative organisms predisposes the patient to gram-negative pneumonia.

Clinical evidence suggesting VAP includes fever, elevated white blood cell count, purulent or odorous sputum, crackles or wheezes on auscultation, and pulmonary infiltrates noted on chest x-ray. The patient is given antibiotics after appropriate cultures are taken by tracheal suctioning or bronchoscopy and when infection is evident.

Guidelines on VAP prevention include (1) minimizing sedation including daily spontaneous awakening trials (SATs) and daily spontaneous breathing trials (SBTs), (2) early exercise and mobilization, (3) use of ET tubes with subglottic secretion drainage ports for patients likely to be intubated greater than 48 to 72 hours, (4) HOB elevation at a minimum of 30 to 45 degrees unless medically contraindicated, and (5) no routine changes of the patient's ventilator circuit tubing[44] (Fig. 65-16).

Prevention also includes strict hand washing before and after suctioning, whenever ventilator equipment is touched, and after contact with any respiratory secretions (see Nursing Management: Artificial Airway earlier in this chapter). Always wear gloves when in contact with the patient and change gloves between activities (e.g., emptying urinary catheter drainage, hanging an IV drug). Last, always drain the water that collects in the ventilator tubing away from the patient as it collects.

💊 DRUG ALERT   Oxygen

- O_2 is considered a drug and overexposure can lead to O_2 toxicity.
- Mechanically ventilated patients receiving high levels of FIO_2 for prolonged periods of time (e.g., 40% FIO_2 for >24 hours) are at risk for O_2 toxicity.
- Target FIO_2 levels are to maintain SpO_2 >90% and PaO_2 between 60 and 90 mm Hg.
- Assess ABGs for evidence of excess O_2.
- Monitor patient for signs of O_2 toxicity: uncontrolled coughing, chest pain, and dyspnea.

Sodium and Water Imbalance. Progressive fluid retention often occurs after 48 to 72 hours of PPV, especially PPV with PEEP. Fluid retention is associated with decreased urine output and increased sodium retention. Fluid balance changes may be due to decreased CO, which in turn results in diminished renal perfusion. Consequently, renin release is stimulated with subsequent production of angiotensin and aldosterone (see Chapter 44, Fig. 44-4). This results in sodium and water retention. It is also possible that pressure changes within the thorax are associated with decreased release of atrial natriuretic peptide, which also causes sodium retention. Mild water retention is also associated with PPV. Less insensible water loss occurs via the airway because ventilated delivered gases are humidified with body-temperature water. In addition, as a part of the stress response, release of antidiuretic hormone and cortisol contributes to sodium and water retention.

Neurologic System. In patients with head injury, PPV (especially with PEEP) can impair cerebral blood flow. The increased intrathoracic positive pressure impedes venous drainage from the head. This results in jugular venous distention. The patient may have increases in intracranial pressure due to the impaired venous return and subsequent increase in cerebral volume.

Elevating the HOB and keeping the patient's head in alignment may reduce the harmful effects of PPV on intracranial pressure.

Gastrointestinal System. Patients receiving PPV are stressed because of the serious illness, immobility, or discomforts associated with the ventilator. This places the ventilated patient at risk for developing stress ulcers and GI bleeding. Patients with a preexisting ulcer or those receiving corticosteroids are at an increased risk. Any kind of circulatory compromise, including reduction of CO caused by PPV, may contribute to ischemia of the gastric and intestinal mucosa and possibly increase the risk of translocation of GI bacteria.

Stress ulcer prophylaxis includes giving histamine (H_2)-receptor blockers (e.g., ranitidine [Zantac]), proton pump inhibitors (PPIs) (e.g., esomeprazole [Nexium]), or enteral nutrition to decrease gastric acidity and reduce the risk of stress ulcer and hemorrhage. The use of PPIs may be linked to an increase in the development of *Clostridium difficile*–associated diarrhea.[45] (This is discussed in Chapter 41 on p. 902.)

Gastric and bowel dilation may occur because of gas accumulation in the GI tract from swallowed air. The irritation of an artificial airway may cause excessive air swallowing and subsequent gastric dilation. Gastric or bowel dilation may put pressure on the vena cava, decrease CO, and prohibit adequate diaphragmatic excursion during spontaneous breathing. Elevation of the diaphragm as a result of paralytic ileus or bowel dilation leads to compression of the lower lobes of the lungs. This may cause atelectasis and compromise respiratory function. Decompression of the stomach is done by inserting an OG or NG tube.[46]

Immobility, sedation, circulatory impairment, decreased oral intake, use of opioid pain medications, and stress contribute to decreased peristalsis. The patient's inability to exhale against a closed glottis may make defecation difficult. As a result, the ventilated patient is at risk for constipation, and a bowel regimen should be started.

Musculoskeletal System. Maintenance of muscle strength and prevention of the problems linked with immobility are important. Adequate analgesia and nutrition can enhance exercise tolerance. Plan for early and progressive mobility of appropriate patients receiving PPV.[9,47] In collaboration with physical and occupational therapy, perform passive and active exercises to maintain muscle tone in the upper and lower extremities. Simple maneuvers such as leg lifts, knee bends, quadriceps setting, or arm circles are appropriate. Prevent contractures, pressure ulcers, foot drop, and external rotation of the hip and legs by proper positioning and the use of specialized mattresses or beds. Use a portable ventilator or manually ventilate the patient with a BVM and 100% O_2 when ambulating.

Psychosocial Needs. The patient receiving mechanical ventilation often experiences physical and emotional stress. In addition to the problems related to critical care patients discussed at the beginning of this chapter, the patient supported by a mechanical ventilator is unable to speak, eat, move, or breathe normally. Tubes and machines cause pain, fear, and anxiety. Usual activities of daily living such as eating, elimination, and coughing are extremely complicated.

Feeling safe is an overpowering need of patients on mechanical ventilation. In addition, four related needs include the need to know (information), the need to regain control, the need to hope, and the need to trust. When patients' needs are met, they feel safe. Work to strengthen the various factors that affect feeling safe. Encourage hope, as appropriate, and build trusting relationships with both the patient and caregiver. Involve patients and caregivers in decision making as much as possible.[14,15]

Patients receiving PPV may require sedation (e.g., propofol) and/or analgesia (e.g., fentanyl) to facilitate optimal ventilation. Before starting sedation or analgesia in the mechanically ventilated patient who is agitated or anxious, identify the cause of distress. Common problems that can result in patient agitation or anxiety include PPV, nutritional deficits, pain, hypoxemia, hypercapnia, drugs, and environmental stressors (e.g., sleep deprivation).

Delirium is an acute change in mental status. It is a marker of cerebral insufficiency and associated with longer hospital stays and higher mortality rates. ICU patients are particularly vulnerable to delirium. Assess for delirium using a valid tool, initiate prevention strategies, and recognize and treat delirium when it occurs.[6,8]

At times, the decision is made to paralyze the patient with a neuromuscular blocking agent (e.g., cisatracurium [Nimbex]) to provide more effective synchrony with the ventilator and improve oxygenation. Remember that the paralyzed patient can hear, see, and feel. It is essential to give IV sedation and analgesia concurrently when the patient is paralyzed. Monitoring patients receiving these drugs is challenging. Assess the patient using train-of-four (TOF) peripheral nerve stimulation, physiologic signs of pain or anxiety (e.g., changes in HR and BP), and ventilator synchrony. The TOF assessment involves using a peripheral nerve stimulator to deliver four successive stimulating currents to elicit muscle twitches (Fig. 65-19). The number of twitches varies with the percentage of neuromuscular blockade. The usual goal is one or two twitches out of four.

Noninvasive electroencephalogram technology (e.g., bispectral index monitoring [BIS]) may be useful and can help guide sedative and analgesic therapy in these patients.[6] Excessive administration of neuromuscular blocking agents may predispose the patient to prolonged paralysis and muscle weakness even after these agents are stopped.

Many patients have few memories of their time in the ICU, whereas others remember vivid details. Although appearing to be asleep, sedated, or paralyzed, patients may be aware of their

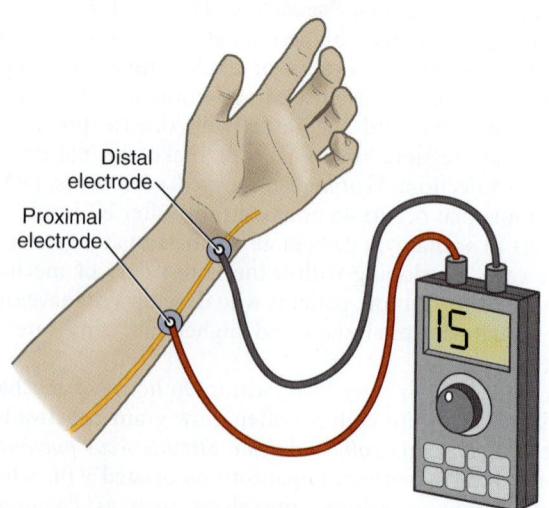

FIG. 65-19 Placement of electrodes along ulnar nerve.

Distal electrode

Proximal electrode

surroundings, and you should always address them as if they were awake and alert.[48]

Ventilator Disconnection or Malfunction. Mechanical ventilators may become disconnected or malfunction. When turned on and operative, alarms alert you to problems (Table 65-11). Most deaths from accidental ventilator disconnection occur while the alarm is off. Most accidental disconnections in critical care settings are discovered by low-pressure alarms. The most frequent site for disconnection is between the tracheal tube and the adapter. Push connections together and then twist to secure more tightly. Be certain that alarms are set and activated at all times, and chart that this is the case. You can pause alarms (not inactivate) during suctioning or removal from the ventilator, but you must reactivate them before leaving the patient's bedside.

Ventilator malfunction may also occur due to several factors. Although most agencies have emergency generators in the event of a power failure and newer ventilators may have battery backup, power failure is always a possibility. Have a plan for manually ventilating all patients who depend on a ventilator. If, at any time, you determine that the ventilator is malfunctioning (e.g., failure of O_2 supply), disconnect the patient from the machine and manually ventilate with a BVM and 100% O_2 until the ventilator is fixed or replaced.

Nutritional Therapy: Patient Receiving Positive Pressure Ventilation

PPV and the hypermetabolism associated with critical illness can contribute to inadequate nutrition. The presence of an ET tube eliminates the normal route for eating. Patients with a long-term tracheostomy may be able to eat normally once the stoma heals. Swallowing studies and a consultation with a speech therapist are done to assess the patient's readiness. When eating with a tracheostomy tube in place, the patient should tilt the head slightly forward to facilitate swallowing and to prevent aspiration. Diet may be restricted to soft foods (e.g., puddings, ice cream) and thickened liquids.

Patients unlikely to be able to eat for 3 to 5 days should have a nutritional assessment and enteral feeding started within 24 to 48 hours of admission.[10,49] Inadequate nutrition makes the patient receiving prolonged mechanical ventilation prone to poor O_2 transport secondary to anemia and to poor tolerance of minimal exercise. Critically ill patients have frequent interruptions of enteral feedings because of problems with residuals, transportation to and during tests, and routine nursing care. Poor nutrition and the disuse of respiratory muscles contribute to decreased respiratory muscle strength. In addition, critical illness, trauma, and surgery are associated with

---

TEAMWORK & COLLABORATION

Caring for the Patient Requiring Mechanical Ventilation

In the critically ill patient who requires mechanical ventilation the registered nurse (RN) and respiratory therapist provide most of the care. Some patients who require chronic mechanical ventilation may be in long-term care settings or at home. In these settings, the RN and respiratory therapist assess the patient and plan and evaluate care, but implementation of some activities may be delegated.

Role of Nursing Personnel
Registered Nurse (RN)
- Develop plan for communication with the patient who has a tracheostomy or an ET tube.
- Give sedatives, analgesics, and paralytic drugs as needed.
- Teach patient and caregiver about mechanical ventilation and weaning procedures.
- Auscultate breath sounds and respiratory effort, assessing for decreased ventilation or adventitious sounds.
- Monitor ventilator settings and alarms.
- Determine need for ET tube suctioning and suction patients as needed.
- Reposition and secure ET tube (based on agency policy).
- Monitor oxygenation level and signs of respiratory fatigue during weaning procedure.

Licensed Practical/Vocational Nurse (LPN/LVN)
- Suction tracheostomy or ET tube for stable patients as directed by RN.
- Give routinely scheduled drugs (based on state Nurse Practice Act and agency policy).
- Assist RN or respiratory therapist with repositioning and securing ET tube.
- Administer enteral nutrition to stable patients as directed by RN.

Unlicensed Assistive Personnel (UAP)
- Obtain vital signs and report these to the RN.
- Perform bedside glucose testing, if needed and according to agency policy.
- Provide personal hygiene, skin care, and oral care, as directed by RN.
- Assist with frequent position changes, including ambulation, as directed by the RN.
- Help to perform passive or active range-of-motion exercises.
- Measure urine output and report information to RN.

Role of Other Team Members
Respiratory Therapist*
- Auscultate breath sounds and respiratory effort, assessing for decreased ventilation or adventitious sounds.
- Monitor ventilator settings and alarms.
- Change ventilator settings as needed or ordered.
- Maintain appropriate cuff inflation on ET tube.
- Determine need for ET tube suctioning and suction patients as needed.
- Reposition and secure ET tube (based on agency policy).
- Monitor oxygenation level and signs of respiratory fatigue during weaning procedure.

Physical/Occupational Therapist
- Assist with range of motion exercises.
- Assist with early and progressive ambulation as directed by the RN.

Dietitian
- Assess and monitor patient's nutritional status.
- Recommend formulations for enteral and/or parenteral nutrition as needed.

Speech Therapist
- Perform swallowing studies as appropriate.
- Provide teaching for patient with a long-term tracheostomy.

*Some of these activities are often shared by RNs.

hypermetabolism, anxiety, pain, and increased WOB, which greatly increase caloric expenditure. Serum protein levels (e.g., albumin, prealbumin, transferrin, total protein) are usually decreased. Inadequate nutrition can delay weaning, decrease resistance to infection, and slow down recovery. Enteral gastric or small bowel feeding is the preferred method to meet caloric needs of ventilated patients (see Chapter 39 for discussion of enteral feeding).

Verification of feeding tube placement includes (1) x-ray confirmation before initial use, (2) marking and ongoing assessment of the tube's exit site, and (3) ongoing review of routine x-rays and aspirate.[46] The auscultatory method of assessment (i.e., listening for air after injection) is not a reliable method for verifying the placement of feeding tubes.

A concern regarding the nutritional support of patients receiving PPV is the carbohydrate content of the diet. Metabolism of carbohydrates may increase the serum CO_2 levels. This can result in a higher required minute ventilation and increased WOB. Limiting carbohydrate content in the diet may lower CO_2 production.[10] Consult the dietitian to determine the caloric and nutrient needs of these patients.

Weaning From Positive Pressure Ventilation and Extubation

Weaning is the process of reducing ventilator support and resuming spontaneous breathing. The weaning process differs for patients requiring short-term ventilation (up to 3 days) versus long-term ventilation (longer than 3 days). Patients requiring short-term ventilation (e.g., after heart surgery) experience a linear weaning process. Patients likely to require prolonged PPV (e.g., patients with COPD who develop respiratory failure) often experience a weaning process that consists of alternating gains and losses. Preparation for weaning begins when PPV is started and involves a team approach (e.g., nurse, HCP, patient, caregiver, dietitian, respiratory therapist).

Weaning generally consists of three phases: the *preweaning phase*, the *weaning process*, and the *outcome phase*. The preweaning or assessment phase determines the patient's ability to breathe spontaneously. Assessment in this phase depends on a combination of respiratory (Table 65-13) and nonrespiratory factors. Note the resolution of the primary problem that prompted patient admission to the ICU. In addition, the patient's lungs should be reasonably clear on auscultation and chest x-ray. Weaning assessment parameters should include criteria to assess muscle strength (negative inspiratory force) and endurance (spontaneous V_T, vital capacity, minute ventilation, and rapid shallow breathing index).

Nonrespiratory factors include the patient's neurologic status; hemodynamics; fluid, electrolytes, and acid-base balance; nutrition; and hemoglobin. It is important to have an alert, well-rested, and well-informed patient relatively free from pain and anxiety who can cooperate with the weaning plan. This does not mean complete withdrawal from sedatives or analgesics. Instead, drugs should be titrated to achieve comfort without causing excessive drowsiness.

A *spontaneous awakening trial* (SAT) and a *spontaneous breathing trial* (SBT) are recommended in patients who meet a daily safety screen. This is part of what is known as the *Awakening and Breathing Trial Coordination, Daily Delirium Monitoring and Management, and Early Exercise and Mobility (ABCDE) bundle* for ventilator management.[50] An SAT should be done by stopping all sedatives and, in patients without active pain, all opioids.

Sedation should be restarted at 50% the previous dose in patients who "fail" the SAT and remain off in patients who "pass."

An SBT should last at least 30 minutes but no more than 120 minutes. It may be done with low levels of CPAP, low levels of PSV, or a T piece. Tolerance of the trial may lead to extubation. Failure to tolerate an SBT should prompt a search for reversible or complicating factors and a return to a nonfatiguing ventilator modality for the patient. The SBT should be reattempted the next day.

The use of a weaning protocol decreases ventilator days. The ventilator settings are not as important as the use of a daily protocol to prevent delays in weaning. The patient receiving SIMV can have the ventilator breaths gradually reduced as his or her ventilatory status permits. CPAP or PSV can be added to SIMV. PSV is thought to provide gentle, slow respiratory muscle conditioning. It may be especially beneficial for patients who are deconditioned or have heart problems. Some patients may be weaned by simply providing humidified O_2 (T-piece or flow-by method).

Weaning may be tried at any time of day, although it is usually done during the day, with the patient ventilated at night in a rest mode. The rest mode should be a stable, nonfatiguing, and comfortable form of support for the patient. Regardless of the weaning mode selected, all health care team members should be familiar with the weaning plan. Additionally, it is important to permit the patient's respiratory muscles to rest between weaning trials. Once the respiratory muscles become fatigued, they may require 12 to 24 hours to recover.

The patient being weaned and the caregiver need ongoing emotional support. Explain the weaning process to them and keep them informed of progress. Place the patient in a comfortable sitting or semirecumbent position. Obtain baseline vital signs and respiratory parameters. During the weaning trial, closely monitor the patient for signs and symptoms that may signal a need to end the trial (e.g., tachypnea, dyspnea, tachycardia, dysrhythmias, sustained desaturation [SpO_2 less than 90%], hypertension or hypotension, agitation, diaphoresis, anxiety, sustained V_T less than 5 mL/kg, changes in mentation). Record the patient's tolerance throughout the weaning process and include statements regarding the patient's and the caregiver's perceptions.

The weaning outcome phase is the period when the patient is extubated or weaning is stopped because no further progress is being made. The patient who is ready for extubation should receive hyperoxygenation and suctioning (e.g., oropharynx, ET tube). Loosen the ET tapes or commercial holder or the tracheostomy ties. Instruct the patient to take a deep breath, and at the peak of inspiration, deflate the cuff and remove the tube in one motion. After removal, encourage the patient to deep breathe and cough, and suction the oropharynx as needed. Give supplemental O_2 and provide naso-oral care. Carefully monitor the patient's vital signs, respiratory status, and oxygenation immediately after extubation, within 1 hour, and per agency policy. If the patient does not tolerate extubation (e.g., decreased level of consciousness, tachycardia, tachypnea or bradypnea, decrease in PaO_2, increase in $PaCO_2$, decreased SpO_2 levels), immediate reintubation or a trial of noninvasive ventilation may be needed.

Chronic Mechanical Ventilation

Mechanical ventilators are no longer limited to the ICU but are now a part of long-term and home care. In some instances, terminally ill, ventilated patients may be discharged to hospice.

TABLE 65-13   Indicators for Weaning

Weaning Readiness

Patients receiving mechanical ventilation for respiratory failure should undergo a formal assessment of weaning potential if the following are satisfied:*

1. Reversal of the underlying cause of respiratory failure
2. Adequate oxygenation
   - PaO_2/FIO_2 >150-200
   - SpO_2 ≥90%
   - PEEP ≤5-8 cm H_2O
   - FIO_2 ≤40%-50%
   - pH ≥7.25

3. Hemodynamic stability
   - Absence of myocardial ischemia
   - Absence of clinically significant hypotension (no vasopressor therapy or low dose)
4. Patient ability to initiate an inspiratory effort
5. Optional criteria
   - Hemoglobin ≥7-10 g/dL
   - Core temperature ≤100.4° F (38° C) to 101.3° F (38.5° C)
   - Mental status awake and alert or easily arousable

WEANING ASSESSMENT

Measurement	Significance	Normal Values	Indices for Weaning
Spontaneous respiratory rate (f)	Respiratory rate/frequency over 1 min.	12-20 min	<35 min
Spontaneous tidal volume (V_T)	Amount of air exchanged during normal breathing at rest. Measure of muscle endurance.	7-9 mL/kg	≥5 mL/kg
Minute ventilation (V_E)	V_T multiplied by respiratory rate over 1 min. *For example:* 0.350 (V_T) × 28 (f) = 9.8 L/min	5-10 L/min	≤10 L/min
Negative inspiratory force or pressure (NIF, NIP)	Amount of negative pressure that a patient is able to generate to initiate spontaneous respirations. *Measured by clinician:* After complete occlusion of inspiratory valve, a pressure manometer is attached to airway or mouth for 10-20 sec while negative inspiratory efforts are noted.	–75 to –100 cm H_2O	>–20 cm H_2O The more negative the number, the better indication for weaning.
Positive expiratory pressure (PEP)	Measure of expiratory muscle strength and ability to cough. *Measured by clinician:* After complete occlusion of expiratory valve, a pressure manometer is attached to the airway or mouth for 10-20 sec while positive expiratory efforts are noted.	60-85 cm H_2O	≥30 cm H_2O
Compliance, rate, oxygenation, and pressure (CROP) index	Combined index that is complex to calculate. $C_{Dyn} \times NIF \times (PaO_2/PAO_2)/f$ C_{Dyn} = Compliance PaO_2/PAO_2 = Oxygenation ratio of arterial O_2/alveolar O_2	Not applicable	>13
Rapid shallow breathing index (f/V_T)	Spontaneous respiratory rate over 1 min divided by V_T (in liters). *For example:* 30 (f)/0.400 (V_T) = 75/L	60-105/L	<105/L
Vital capacity (VC)	Maximum inspiration and then measurement of air during maximal forced expiration. Measure of respiratory muscle endurance or reserve or both. Requires patient cooperation.	65-75 mL/kg	≥10-15 mL/kg
Spontaneous breathing trial (SBT)	If patient passes daily weaning screen, assess patient during spontaneous breathing with little or no ventilator assistance. Trial should be at least 30 min to a maximum of 120 min.		Successful completion of trial is based on an integrated patient assessment.

*The decision to use these criteria must be individualized to the patient.
Adapted from A Collective Task Force Facilitated by the American College of Chest Physicians, the American Association for Respiratory Care, and the American College of Critical Care Medicine: Evidence-based guidelines for weaning and discontinuing ventilatory support, *Resp Care* 47:69, 2002; and Burns SM: Weaning process. In Wiegand DL-M, editor: *AACN procedure manual for critical care*, ed 6, St Louis, 2011, Saunders.

The emphasis on controlling hospital costs has increased the early discharge of patients and the need to provide highly technical care such as mechanical ventilation in home settings. The success of home mechanical ventilation depends, in part, on careful predischarge assessment and planning for both the patient and caregivers.

Both negative pressure and positive pressure ventilators are used in the home. Negative pressure ventilators do not require an artificial airway and are less complicated to use. Several types of small, portable (battery-powered) positive pressure ventilators are available and can be attached to a wheelchair or placed on a bedside table. Settings and alarms on these ventilators are simpler to use than on the standard ICU ventilators.

Home mechanical ventilation has advantages and disadvantages. Having the patient in the home eliminates the strain that the hospital setting imposes on family dynamics. Caregivers may feel helpless when they first hear about the necessity for long-term mechanical ventilation. However, these feelings are frequently balanced by the opportunity to participate in the patient's care in the home setting. At home the patient may be able to take part in more activities of daily living around an individualized schedule and, because of the smaller size of the home ventilator, be more mobile. Another advantage of home mechanical ventilation is the reduced risk of HAIs.

Disadvantages of home mechanical ventilation include problems related to equipment, reimbursement, caregiver stress and fatigue, and the patient's complex needs. Ventilated patients are usually dependent, requiring extensive nursing care, at least initially. Disposable products may not be reimbursable. Financial resources must be carefully assessed when arranging home mechanical ventilation. Schedule a meeting with the interprofessional care team (e.g., social worker, home health care nurse, respiratory therapist) before starting a discharge teaching plan.

Another disadvantage of home mechanical ventilation is its potential impact on the family. Caregivers may seem enthusiastic about caring for their loved one in the home but may be motivated by numerous, complex factors. They may not understand the sacrifices they may have to make financially and in personal time and commitment. Encourage caregivers to consider respite care to periodically relieve their stress and fatigue.

❖ NURSING MANAGEMENT: MECHANICAL VENTILATION

eNursing Care Plan 65-1 for the patient receiving mechanical ventilation is available on the website for this chapter.

OTHER CRITICAL CARE CONTENT

Table 65-14 lists additional critical care content presented in other chapters of this book.

TABLE 65-14 Cross-References to Critical Care Content

Topic	Discussed in Chapter	Topic	Discussed in Chapter
Acute coronary syndrome (ACS)	33	Enteral nutrition (EN)	39
Acute heart failure	34	Head injury, including ICP monitoring	56
Acute respiratory distress syndrome (ARDS)	67	Multiple organ dysfunction syndrome (MODS)	66
Acute respiratory failure	67	Myocardial infarction (MI)	33
Basic life support and CPR	Appendix A	Oxygen delivery	28
Burns	24	Pain management	8
Cardiac dysrhythmias	35	Parenteral nutrition (PN)	39
Cardiac pacemakers	35	Pulmonary edema	34
Cardiac surgery	33	Renal dialysis	46
Central venous access device (CVAD)	16	Shock	66
Continuous renal replacement therapy (CRRT)	46	Stroke	57
Delirium	59	Systemic inflammatory response syndrome (SIRS)	66
Emergencies	68	Tracheostomy	26
End-of-life (EOL) care	9	Trauma	68

CPR, Cardiopulmonary resuscitation; *ICP,* intracranial pressure.

CASE STUDY

Critical Care and Mechanical Ventilation

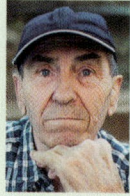
(©Thinkstock)

Patient Profile
R.K. is a 72-yr-old white man who collapsed in his home. He was found by his daughter, and she activated the emergency response system. He was unresponsive on admission to the emergency department and remains unresponsive on arrival to the ICU. He has an oral ET tube in place and is receiving mechanical ventilation. A large-bore, peripheral IV has been placed and fluids are infusing.

Subjective Data
None. Patient is unresponsive to painful stimuli.

Objective Data
Physical Examination
- Noninvasive BP 100/75 mm Hg; apical-radial heart rate 128; temperature 102°F (38.8°C); SpO₂ is 98%
- ECG: atrial fibrillation with a rapid ventricular response
- Purulent secretions suctioned from ET tube
- Breath sounds: coarse crackles bilaterally, decreased breath sounds on the right
- Weight: 168 lb (76 kg)

Diagnostic Studies
- Chest x-ray reveals right lower lung consolidation
- ABGs: pH 7.48; PaO₂ 94 mm Hg; PaCO₂ 30 mm Hg; HCO₃ 34 mEq/L
- CT scan is positive for a hemorrhagic stroke

Interprofessional Care
- Positive pressure ventilation settings: assist-control mode
- Settings: FIO₂ 70%, V_T 700 mL, respiratory rate 16 breaths/min, PEEP 5 cm H₂O
- Orogastric tube to low, intermittent suction
- Enteral feeding at 25 mL/hr to start on day 2

- External condom catheter for urinary drainage and measurement
- HOB elevated at 40 degrees
- Reposition at least every 2 hr
- Azithromycin (Zithromax) 500 mg IV q24hr
- Cefotaxime (Claforan) 2 g IV q6hr
- NS with KCl 20 mEq/L at 100 mL/hr

Discussion Questions
1. Identify two reasons for intubating and providing mechanical ventilation for R.K.
2. What do R.K.'s ABGs indicate, and which ventilator setting(s) should be changed?
3. What is his PaO₂/FIO₂ ratio, and what does it indicate?
4. R.K.'s BP drops to 80 mm Hg. Despite increasing doses of vasopressors and fluid challenges, his BP remains low. A central venous catheter and an arterial line are inserted. APCO monitoring is started. What would be the purpose of hemodynamic monitoring in this patient?
5. **Priority Decision:** What are two priority nursing considerations for a patient with invasive monitoring?
6. R.K.'s pulmonary condition deteriorates. PaO₂ drops to 70 mm Hg, and SpO₂ is 89%. PEEP is increased to 7.5 cm H₂O. What implications does this have for R.K. given his hemodynamic status?
7. **Priority Decision:** Based on the data presented, what are the priority nursing diagnoses? Are there any collaborative problems?
8. **Teamwork and Collaboration:** What patient care activities can you delegate to unlicensed assistive personnel?
9. **Evidence-Based Practice:** R.K.'s family wants to know why he is to receive tube feedings. What would you tell the family? What is the evidence to support the use of tube feedings?
10. **Patient-Centered Care:** After 4 days, R.K. remains unresponsive and has developed renal failure. The HCP believes the patient will not recover from his neurologic injury and wishes to discuss goals of care with the patient's caregiver. What would be your role in this meeting?

Answers available at *http://evolve.elsevier.com/Lewis/medsurg.*

BRIDGE TO NCLEX EXAMINATION

The number of the question corresponds to the same-numbered outcome at the beginning of the chapter.

1. Certification in critical care nursing (CCRN) by the American Association of Critical-Care Nurses indicates that the nurse
   a. is an advanced practice nurse who cares for acutely and critically ill patients.
   b. may practice independently to provide symptom management for the critically ill.
   c. has earned a master's degree in the field of advanced acute and critical care nursing.
   d. has practiced in critical care and successfully completed a test of critical care knowledge.

2. What are the appropriate nursing interventions for the patient with delirium in the ICU (select all that apply)?
   a. Use clocks and calendars to maintain orientation.
   b. Encourage round-the-clock presence of caregivers at the bedside.
   c. Silence all alarms, reduce overhead paging, and avoid conversations around the patient.
   d. Sedate the patient with appropriate drugs to protect the patient from harmful behaviors.
   e. Identify physiologic factors that may be contributing to the patient's confusion and irritability.

3. The critical care nurse recognizes that an ideal plan for caregiver involvement includes
   a. a caregiver at the bedside at all times.
   b. allowing caregivers at the bedside at preset, brief intervals.
   c. an individually devised plan to involve caregivers with care and comfort measures.
   d. restriction of visiting in the ICU because the environment is overwhelming to caregivers.

4. To establish hemodynamic monitoring for a patient, the nurse zeros the
   a. cardiac output monitoring system to the level of the left ventricle.
   b. pressure monitoring system to the level of the catheter tip located in the patient.
   c. pressure monitoring system to the level of the atrium, identified as the phlebostatic axis.
   d. pressure monitoring system to the level of the atrium, identified as the midclavicular line.

5. The hemodynamic changes the nurse expects to find after successful initiation of intraaortic balloon pump therapy in a patient with cardiogenic shock include (select all that apply)
   a. decreased SV.
   b. decreased SVR.
   c. decreased PAWP.
   d. increased diastolic BP.
   e. decreased myocardial O_2 consumption.

6. The purpose of adding PEEP to positive pressure ventilation is to
   a. increase functional residual capacity and improve oxygenation.
   b. increase FIO_2 in an attempt to wean the patient and avoid O_2 toxicity.
   c. determine if the patient is in synchrony with the ventilator or needs to be paralyzed.
   d. determine if the patient is able to be weaned and avoid the risk of pneumomediastinum.

7. The nursing management of a patient with an artificial airway includes
   a. maintaining ET tube cuff pressure at 30 cm H_2O.
   b. routine suctioning of the tube at least every 2 hours.
   c. observing for cardiac dysrhythmias during suctioning.
   d. preventing tube dislodgment by limiting mouth care to lubrication of the lips.

8. The nurse monitors the patient with positive pressure mechanical ventilation for
   a. paralytic ileus because pressure on the abdominal contents affects bowel motility.
   b. diuresis and sodium depletion because of increased release of atrial natriuretic peptide.
   c. signs of cardiovascular insufficiency because pressure in the chest impedes venous return.
   d. respiratory acidosis in a patient with COPD because of alveolar hyperventilation and increased PaO_2 levels.

1. d, 2, a, d, e, 3, c, 4, c, 5, b, c, d, e, 6, a, 7, c, 8, c

For rationales to these answers and even more NCLEX review questions, visit *http://evolve.elsevier.com/Lewis/medsurg*.

ⓔ EVOLVE WEBSITE

http://evolve.elsevier.com/Lewis/medsurg
Review Questions (Online Only)
Key Points
Answer Keys to Questions
• Rationales for Bridge to NCLEX Examination Questions
• Answer Guidelines for Case Study on p. 1584
Student Case Study
• Patient With Pulmonary Embolism and Respiratory Failure
Nursing Care Plan
• eNursing Care Plan 65-1: Patient on Mechanical Ventilation
Conceptual Care Map Creator
Audio Glossary
Supporting Media
• Animation
  • Endotracheal Intubation
Content Updates

REFERENCES

1. American Association of Critical-Care Nurses: About critical care nursing. Retrieved from *www.aacn.org/wd/publishing/content/pressroom/aboutcriticalcarenursing.pcms?menu=.*
*2. Maharaj R, Raffaele I, Wendon J: Rapid response systems: a systematic review and meta-analysis, *Crit Care* 19:254, 2015.
3. American Association of Critical-Care Nurses: Frequently asked questions about APRN Consensus Model—for nurse practitioners. Retrieved from *www.aacn.org/wd/certifications/content/aprn-nurses-np-faqs.pcms?menu=certification.*
4. Society of Critical Care Medicine: Critical care statistics. Retrieved from *www.sccm.org/Communications/Pages/CriticalCareStats.aspx.*
*5. Woods S: Spiritual and complementary therapies to promote healing and reduce stress. In Molter NC, editor: *Protocols for practice: creating healing environments*, ed 2, Sudbury, Mass, 2007, Jones & Bartlett. (Classic)

*6. Barr J, Fraser GL, Puntillo K, et al: Clinical practice guidelines for the management of pain, agitation, and delirium in adult patients in the intensive care unit, *Crit Care Med* 41:263, 2013.

7. Stafford A, Haverland A, Bridges E: Noise in the ICU—what we know and what we can do about it, *AJN* 114:57, 2014.

*8. American Association of Critical-Care Nurses: Delirium assessment and management. Retrieved from *www.aacn.org/wd/practice/content/practicealerts/delirium-practice-alert.pcms?menu=practice.*

*9. American Association of Critical-Care Nurses: ABCDE tool kit, AACN PEARL: early progressive mobility protocol. Retrieved from *www.aacn.org/wd/practice/docs/tool%20kits/early-progressive-mobility-protocol.pdf.*

*10. McClave SA, Taylor BE, Martindale RG, et al: Guidelines for the provision and assessment of nutrition support therapy in the adult critically ill patient: Society of Critical Care Medicine (SCCM) and American Society for Parenteral and Enteral Nutrition (A.S.P.E.N.), *J Parenter Enteral Nutr* 40:159, 2016.

11. Bell L: Patient care page: patient-centered care, *Am J Crit Care* 23:325, 2014.

*12. Leske JS, Pasquale MA: Family needs, interventions and presence. In Molter NC, editor: *Protocols for practice: creating healing environments,* ed 2, Sudbury, Mass, 2007, Jones & Bartlett. (Classic)

*13. American Association of Critical-Care Nurses: AACN practice alert: family presence: visitation in the adult ICU. Retrieved from *www.aacn.org/wd/practice/content/practicealerts/family-visitation-icu-practice-alert.pcms?menu=practice.*

14. Society of Critical Care Medicine: Patient and family resources: ICU issues and answers brochures. Retrieved from *http://store.sccm.org/SearchResults.aspx?Category=BROC.*

*15. American Association of Critical-Care Nurses: AACN practice alert: family presence during CPR and invasive procedures. Retrieved from *www.aacn.org/wd/practice/docs/practicealerts/family-presence-during-resuscitation-invasive-procedures.pdf.*

*16. Medina J, Puntillo K, editors: *AACN protocols for practice: palliative care and end-of-life issues in critical care,* Sudbury, Mass, 2006, Jones & Bartlett. (Classic)

*17. Shaffer RB: Arterial catheter insertion (assist). In Wiegand DL-M, editor: *AACN procedure manual for critical care,* ed 6, St Louis, 2011, Saunders.

18. Edwards Lifesciences: Advanced hemodynamic monitoring. Retrieved from *www.edwards.com/products/mininvasive/Pages/strokevolumevariationwp.aspx.*

*19. Kern ME: Arterial pressure-based cardiac output monitoring. In Wiegand DL-M, editor: *AACN procedure manual for critical care,* ed 6, St Louis, 2011, Saunders.

*20. Klein DG: Cardiac output measurement techniques (invasive). In Wiegand DL-M, editor: *AACN procedure manual for critical care,* ed 6, St Louis, 2011, Saunders.

*21. Headley JM, Giuliano KK: Continuous venous oxygenation monitoring. In Wiegand DL-M, editor: *AACN procedure manual for critical care,* ed 6, St Louis, 2011, Saunders.

*22. Castelluci D: Intraaortic balloon pump management. In Wiegand DL-M, editor: *AACN procedure manual for critical care,* ed 6, St Louis, 2011, Saunders.

*23. Puhlman M, Hargraves J: Ventricular assist devices. In Wiegand DL-M, editor: *AACN procedure manual for critical care,* ed 6, St Louis, 2011, Saunders.

24. Abiomed: Frequently asked questions. Retrieved from *www.abiomed.com/assets/2010/11/AbioCor-FAQ-FINAL.pdf.*

25. Villwock JA, Jones K: Outcomes of early versus late tracheostomy: 2008-2010, *Laryngoscope* 124:1801, 2014.

26. Stollings JL, Diedrich DA, Oyen LJ, et al: Rapid-sequence intubation: a review of the process and considerations when choosing medications, *Ann Pharmacother* 48:62, 2014.

27. Walsh BK, Crotwell DN, Restrepo RD: Capnography/capnometry during mechanical ventilation, *Respir Care* 56:503, 2011.

*28. American Association of Respiratory Care: AARC clinical practice guidelines: endotracheal suctioning of mechanically ventilated patients with artificial airways, *Respir Care* 55:758, 2010.

*29. Seckel MA: Suctioning: endotracheal or tracheostomy tube. In Wiegand DL-M, editor: *AACN procedure manual for critical care,* ed 7, St Louis, 2017, Elsevier. *(in press)*

*30. Fisher DF, Chenelle CT, Marchese AD, et al: Comparison of commercial and noncommercial endotracheal tube-securing devices, *Respir Care* 59:1315, 2014.

*31. Wade D, Hardy R, Howell D, et al: Identifying clinical and acute psychological risk factors for PTSD after critical care: a systematic review, *Minerva Anestesiol* 79:944, 2013.

*32. Happ MB: Communicating with mechanically ventilated patients: state of the science, *AACN Clin Issues* 12:247, 2001. (Classic)

33. Jarachovic M, Mason M, Kerber K, et al: The role of standardized protocols in unplanned extubations in a medical intensive care unit, *Am J Crit Care* 20:304, 2011.

*34. Chang L, Wang KK, Yann-Fen C: Influence of physical restraint of unplanned extubation of adult intensive care patient: a case control study, *Am J Crit Care* 17:408, 2008. (Classic)

*35. American Association of Critical-Care Nurses: AACN practice alert: prevention of aspiration. Retrieved from *www.aacn.org/wd/practice/docs/practicealerts/prevention-aspiration-practice-alert.pdf?menu=aboutus.*

*36. Gallagher J: Mechanical ventilation (through an artificial airway): volume and pressure modes. In Wiegand DL-M, editor: *AACN procedure manual for critical care,* ed 7, St Louis, 2017, Elsevier. *(in press)*

*37. American Association of Critical-Care Nurses: Alarm management. Retrieved from *www.aacn.org/wd/practice/content/practicealerts/alarm-management-practice-alert.pcms?menu=practice.*

38. Oto J, Imanaka H, Nakataki E, et al: Potential inadequacy of automatic tube compensation to decrease inspiratory work load after at least 48 hours of endotracheal tube use in the clinical setting, *Respir Care* 57:697, 2012.

*39. Huang C, Lin H, Ruan S, et al: Efficacy and adverse events of high-frequency oscillatory ventilation in adult patients with acute respiratory distress syndrome: a meta-analysis, *Crit Care* 18:R102, 2014.

*40. Adhikari NK, Dellinger RP, Lundin S, et al: Inhaled nitric oxide does not reduce mortality in patients with acute respiratory distress syndrome regardless of severity: systematic review and meta-analysis, *Crit Care Med* 42:404, 2013.

*41. Lee JM, Bae W, Lee YJ, et al: The efficacy and safety of prone positional ventilation in acute respiratory distress syndrome: updated study-level meta-analysis of 11 randomized controlled trials, *Crit Care Med* 42:1252, 2014.

*42. Combes A, Brodie D, Bartlett R, et al: Position paper for the organization of extracorporeal membrane oxygenation programs for acute respiratory failure in adult patients, *Am J Respir Crit Care Med* 190:488, 2014.

43. Kalanuria AA, Zai W, Mirski M: Ventilator-associated pneumonia in the ICU, *Crit Care* 18:208, 2014.

*44. Klompas M, Branson R, Eichenwald EC, et al: Strategies to prevent ventilator-associated pneumonia in acute care hospitals: a 2014 update, *Infect Cont Hosp Epidemiol* 35:915, 2014.

*45. Dubberke ER, Carling P, Carrico R, et al: Strategies to prevent *Clostridium difficile* infections in acute care hospitals: 2014 update, *Infect Cont Hosp Epidemiol* 35:628, 2014.

*46. American Association of Critical-Care Nurses: AACN practice alert: verification of feeding tube placement. Retrieved from *www.aacn.org/WD/Practice/Docs/Verification_of_Feeding_Tube_Placement_05-2005.pdf*

47. Campbell MR, Fisher J, Anderson L, et al: Implementation of early exercise and mobility–steps to success, *Crit Care Nurs* 35:82, 2015.

48. Desai SV, Law TJ, Needham DM: Long-term complications of critical care, *Crit Care Med* 39:371, 2011.

49. Casaer MP, Van den Berghe G: Nutrition in the acute phase of critical illness, *NEJM* 370:1227, 2014.

50. Balas MC, Vasilevskis EE, Burke WJ, et al: Critical care nurses' role in implementing the "ABCDE bundle" into practice, *Crit Care Nurs* 32:35, 2012.

*Evidence-based information for clinical practice.

66

Shock, Sepsis, and Multiple Organ Dysfunction Syndrome

Maureen A. Seckel

In order for you to shine, you have to get through the darkness.

Mario Tomasello

http://evolve.elsevier.com/Lewis/medsurg/

LEARNING OUTCOMES

1. Relate the pathophysiology to the clinical manifestations of the different types of shock: cardiogenic, hypovolemic, distributive, and obstructive.
2. Compare the effects of shock, systemic inflammatory response syndrome, sepsis, and multiple organ dysfunction syndrome on the major body systems.
3. Compare the interprofessional care, drug therapy, and nursing management of patients experiencing different types of shock.
4. Describe the interprofessional care and nursing management of a patient experiencing multiple organ dysfunction syndrome.

KEY TERMS

anaphylactic shock, p. 1590
cardiogenic shock, p. 1587
hypovolemic shock, p. 1589
multiple organ dysfunction syndrome (MODS), p. 1605

neurogenic shock, p. 1590
obstructive shock, p. 1593
sepsis, p. 1592
septic shock, p. 1592

shock, p. 1587
systemic inflammatory response syndrome (SIRS), p. 1604

Shock, systemic inflammatory response syndrome (SIRS), sepsis, and multiple organ dysfunction syndrome (MODS) are serious and interrelated problems (Fig. 66-1). This chapter provides an overview of the different types of shock, SIRS, sepsis, and MODS, and the related management of each.

SHOCK

Shock is a syndrome characterized by decreased tissue perfusion and impaired cellular metabolism. This results in an imbalance between the supply of and demand for O_2 and nutrients. The exchange of O_2 and nutrients at the cellular level is essential to life. When cells experience hypoperfusion, the demand for O_2 and nutrients exceeds the supply at the microcirculatory level.

Classification of Shock

The four main categories of shock are cardiogenic, hypovolemic, distributive, and obstructive[1,2] (Table 66-1). Although the cause, initial presentation, and management strategies vary for each type of shock, the physiologic responses of the cells to hypoperfusion are similar.

Cardiogenic Shock. Cardiogenic shock occurs when either systolic or diastolic dysfunction of the heart's pumping action results in reduced cardiac output (CO). Causes of cardiogenic

shock are listed in Table 66-1. Mortality rates for patients with cardiogenic shock approach 60%.[3] Decreased filling of the heart results in decreased stroke volume (SV).

The heart's inability to pump the blood forward is called *systolic dysfunction.* Systolic dysfunction primarily affects the left ventricle, since systolic pressure is greater on the left side of the heart. When systolic dysfunction affects the right side of the heart, blood flow through the pulmonary circulation is reduced. The most common cause of systolic dysfunction is acute myocardial infarction (MI). Cardiogenic shock is the leading cause of death from acute MI.[4] Causes of diastolic dysfunction are listed in Table 66-1.

Fig. 66-2 describes the pathophysiology of cardiogenic shock. Whether the first event is myocardial ischemia, a structural problem (e.g., valvular disorder, ventricular septal rupture), or dysrhythmias, the physiologic responses are similar: the patient experiences impaired tissue perfusion and cellular metabolism.

The early clinical presentation of a patient with cardiogenic shock is similar to that of a patient with acute decompensated heart failure (see Chapter 34). The patient may have tachycardia and hypotension. Pulse pressure may be narrowed due to the heart's inability to pump blood forward during systole and increased volume during diastole. An increase in systemic vascular resistance (SVR) increases the workload of the heart, thus

Reviewed by Carla V. Hannon, MS, APRN, CCRN, CCNS, Clinical Nurse Specialist, Medical Intensive Care Unit, Yale–New Haven Hospital, New Haven, Connecticut; Patricia Lea, RN, DNP, CCRN, Assistant Professor, University of Texas Medical Branch School of Nursing, Galveston, Texas; and Anna P. Moore, RN, MS, Associate Professor, School of Nursing and Allied Health, J. Sargeant Reynolds Community College, Richmond, Virginia.

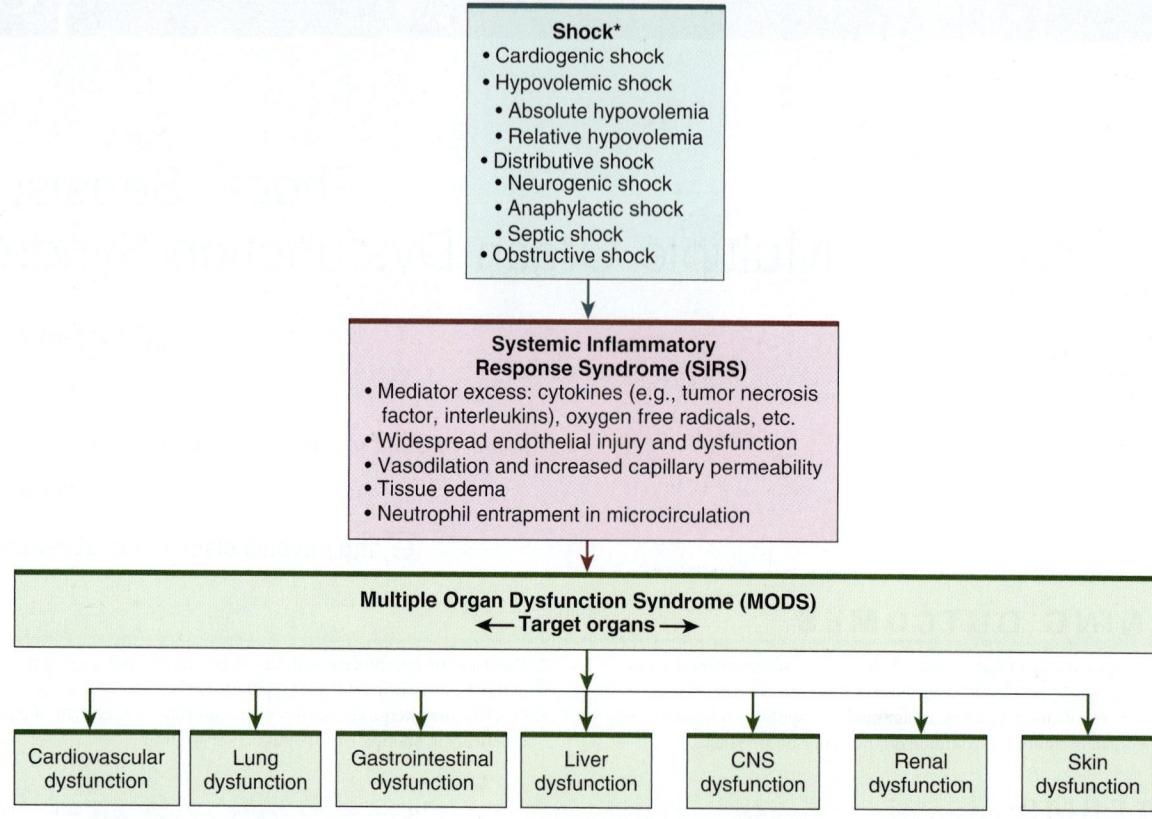

FIG. 66-1 Relationship of shock, systemic inflammatory response syndrome, and multiple organ dysfunction syndrome. *CNS,* Central nervous system. (*See Table 66-1 for causes of shock states.)

TABLE 66-1 Classification of Shock States

Types and Causes	Examples	Types and Causes	Examples
Cardiogenic Shock		**Distributive Shock**	
• Systolic dysfunction: inability of the heart to pump blood forward	Myocardial infarction, cardiomyopathy, blunt cardiac injury, severe systemic or pulmonary hypertension, myocardial depression from metabolic problems	**Neurogenic Shock**	
		• Hemodynamic consequence of spinal cord injury and/or disease at or above T5	Severe pain, drugs, hypoglycemia, injury
• Diastolic dysfunction: inability of the heart to fill	Cardiac tamponade, ventricular hypertrophy, cardiomyopathy	• Spinal anesthesia	
• Dysrhythmias	Bradydysrhythmias, tachydysrhythmias	• Vasomotor center depression	
• Structural factors	Valvular stenosis or regurgitation, ventricular septal rupture, tension pneumothorax	**Anaphylactic Shock**	
		• Hypersensitivity (allergic) reaction to a sensitizing substance	Contrast media, blood or blood products, drugs, insect bites, anesthetic agents, food or food additives, vaccines, environmental agents, latex
Hypovolemic Shock			
Absolute Hypovolemia			
• External loss of whole blood	Hemorrhage from trauma, surgery, GI bleeding	**Septic Shock**	
• Loss of other body fluids	Vomiting, diarrhea, excessive diuresis, diabetes insipidus, diabetes mellitus	• Infection	Pneumonia, peritonitis, urinary tract, invasive procedures, indwelling lines and catheters
Relative Hypovolemia		• At-risk patients	Older adults, patients with chronic diseases (e.g., diabetes mellitus, chronic kidney disease, heart failure), patients receiving immunosuppressive therapy or who are malnourished or debilitated
• Pooling of blood or fluids	Bowel obstruction		
• Fluid shifts	Burn injuries, ascites		
• Internal bleeding	Fracture of long bones, ruptured spleen, hemothorax, severe pancreatitis		
• Massive vasodilation	Sepsis	**Obstructive Shock**	
		• Physical obstruction impeding the filling or outflow of blood resulting in reduced cardiac output	Cardiac tamponade, tension pneumothorax, superior vena cava syndrome, abdominal compartment syndrome, pulmonary embolism

PATHOPHYSIOLOGY MAP

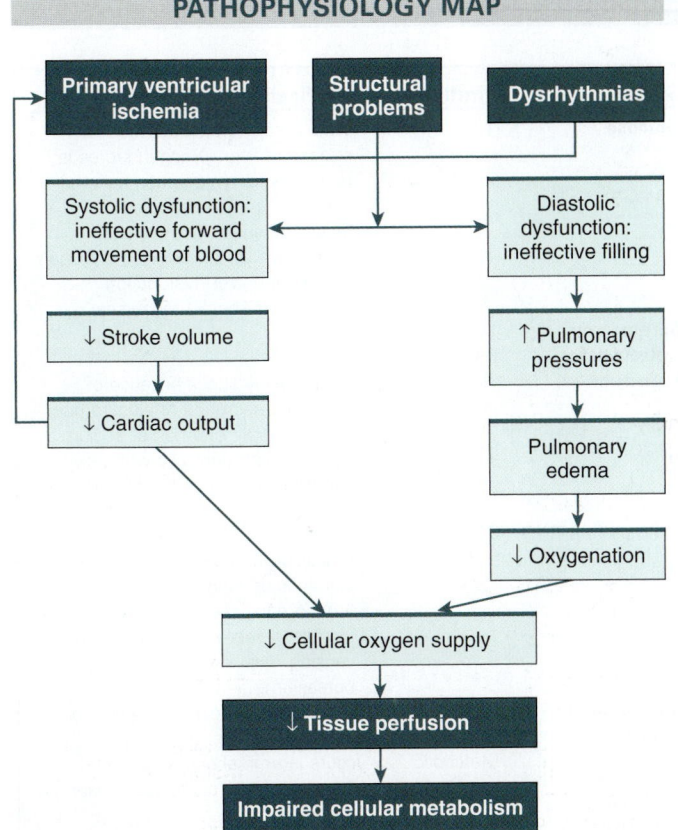

FIG. 66-2 The pathophysiology of cardiogenic shock. (Modified from Urden LD, Stacy KM, Lough ME: *Critical care nursing: diagnosis and management,* ed 6, St Louis, 2010, Mosby.)

PATHOPHYSIOLOGY MAP

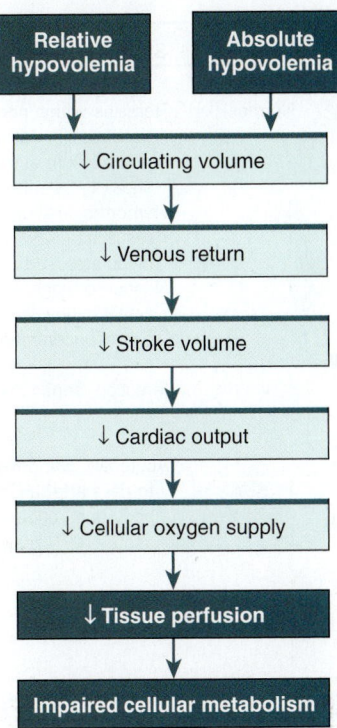

FIG. 66-3 The pathophysiology of hypovolemic shock. (Modified from Urden LD, Stacy KM, Lough ME: *Critical care nursing: diagnosis and management,* ed 6, St Louis, 2010, Mosby.)

increasing the myocardial O_2 consumption. The heart's inability to pump blood forward also results in a low CO (less than 4 L/minute) and *cardiac index* (less than 2.5 L/minute/m^2).

On assessment, the patient is tachypneic and has crackles on auscultation of breath sounds because of pulmonary congestion. The hemodynamic profile demonstrates an increase in the pulmonary artery wedge pressure (PAWP), stroke volume variation (SVV), and pulmonary vascular resistance.

Signs of peripheral hypoperfusion (e.g., cyanosis, pallor, diaphoresis, weak peripheral pulses, cool and clammy skin, delayed capillary refill) are seen. Decreased renal blood flow results in sodium and water retention and decreased urine output. Anxiety, confusion, and agitation may develop as cerebral perfusion is impaired. Tables 66-2 and 66-3 describe the laboratory findings and clinical presentation of a patient with cardiogenic shock.

Hypovolemic Shock. **Hypovolemic shock** occurs after a loss of intravascular fluid volume (Table 66-1). The volume is inadequate to fill the vascular space. The volume loss may be either an absolute or a relative volume loss. *Absolute hypovolemia* results when fluid is lost through hemorrhage, gastrointestinal (GI) loss (e.g., vomiting, diarrhea), fistula drainage, diabetes insipidus, or diuresis. In *relative hypovolemia,* fluid volume moves out of the vascular space into the extravascular space (e.g., intracavitary space). This type of fluid shift is called *third spacing.* One example of relative volume loss is leakage of fluid from the vascular space to the interstitial space from increased capillary permeability, as seen in burns (see Chapter 24).

In hypovolemic shock the size of the vascular compartment remains unchanged while the volume of blood or plasma

decreases. Whether the loss of intravascular volume is absolute or relative, the physiologic consequences are similar. A reduction in intravascular volume results in a decreased venous return to the heart, decreased preload, decreased SV, and decreased CO. A cascade of events results in decreased tissue perfusion and impaired cellular metabolism, the hallmarks of shock (Fig. 66-3).

The patient's response to acute volume loss depends on a number of factors, including extent of injury, age, and general state of health. However, the clinical presentation of hypovolemic shock is consistent (Table 66-3). An overall assessment of physiologic reserves may indicate the patient's ability to compensate. A patient may compensate for a loss of up to 15% of the total blood volume (approximately 750 mL). Further loss of volume (15% to 30%) results in a sympathetic nervous system (SNS)–mediated response. This response results in an increase in heart rate, CO, and respiratory rate and depth. The SV, central venous pressure (CVP), and PAWP are decreased because of the decreased circulating blood volume.

The patient may appear anxious, and urine output begins to decrease. If hypovolemia is corrected by crystalloid fluid replacement at this time, tissue dysfunction is generally reversible. If volume loss is greater than 30%, compensatory mechanisms may fail and immediate replacement with blood products should be started. Loss of autoregulation in the microcirculation and irreversible tissue destruction occur with loss of more than 40% of the total blood volume.[5] Common laboratory studies and assessments that are done include serial measurements of hemoglobin and hematocrit levels, electrolytes, lactate, blood gases, mixed central venous O_2 saturation (SvO_2), and hourly urine outputs (Table 66-2).

TABLE 66-2 Diagnostic Studies

Shock

Study	Finding	Significance of Finding	Study	Finding	Significance of Finding
Red blood cells			**Glucose**	↑	Found in early shock because of release of liver glycogen stores in response to sympathetic nervous system stimulation and cortisol. Insulin insensitivity develops.
RBC count, hematocrit, hemoglobin	Normal	Remains within normal limits in shock because of relative hypovolemia and pump failure and in hemorrhagic shock before fluid resuscitation.		↓	Occurs because of depleted glycogen stores with liver dysfunction possible as shock progresses.
	↓	Hemorrhagic shock after fluid resuscitation when fluids other than blood are used.	**Serum electrolytes**		
	↑	Nonhemorrhagic shock caused by actual hypovolemia and hemoconcentration.	• Sodium	↑	Found in early shock because of increased secretion of aldosterone, causing renal retention of sodium.
White blood cells				↓	May occur iatrogenically when excess hypotonic fluid is administered after fluid loss.
WBC count, presence of bands	↑, ↓	Infection, septic shock.	• Potassium	↑	Results when dead cells release potassium. Also occurs in acute kidney injury and acidosis.
DIC screen		Acute DIC can develop within hours to days after an initial assault on the body (e.g., shock).		↓	Found in early shock because of increased secretion of aldosterone, causing renal excretion of potassium.
• Fibrin split products (FSP)	↑		**Arterial blood gases**	Respiratory alkalosis	Found in early shock secondary to hyperventilation.
• Fibrinogen level	↓			Metabolic acidosis	Occurs later in shock when lactate accumulates in blood from anaerobic metabolism.
• Platelet count	↓				
• PTT and PT	↑				
• INR	↑		**Base deficit**	>−6	Indicates acid production secondary to hypoxia.
• Thrombin time	↑		**Blood cultures**	Growth of organisms	May grow organisms in patients who are in septic shock.
• D-dimer	↑		**Lactate level**	↑	Usually increases once significant hypoperfusion and impaired O$_2$ utilization at the cellular level have occurred. By-product of anaerobic metabolism.
Creatine kinase	↑	Trauma, myocardial infarction in response to cellular damage and/or hypoxia.			
Troponin	↑	Increases in myocardial infarction.			
BUN	↑	Indicates impaired kidney function caused by hypoperfusion as a result of severe vasoconstriction, or occurs secondary to catabolism of cells (e.g., trauma, infection).			
Creatinine	↑	Indicates impaired kidney function caused by hypoperfusion as a result of severe vasoconstriction. Is more sensitive indicator of renal function than BUN.	**Liver enzymes (ALT, AST, GGT)**	↑	Elevations indicate liver cell destruction in progressive stage of shock.
Procalcitonin (PCT)	↑	Biomarker that is released in response to bacterial infections.			

ALT, Alanine aminotransferase; *AST*, aspartate aminotransferase; *BUN*, blood urea nitrogen; *DIC*, disseminated intravascular coagulation; *GGT*, γ-glutamyl transferase; *INR*, international normalized ratio; *PT*, prothrombin time; *PTT*, partial thromboplastin time.

Distributive Shock

Neurogenic Shock. **Neurogenic shock** is a hemodynamic phenomenon that can occur within 30 minutes of a spinal cord injury and can last up to 6 weeks. Neurogenic shock related to spinal cord injuries is generally associated with a cervical or high thoracic injury. The injury results in a massive vasodilation without compensation because of the loss of SNS vasoconstrictor tone. This massive vasodilation leads to a pooling of blood in the blood vessels, tissue hypoperfusion, and ultimately impaired cellular metabolism (Fig. 66-4).

In addition to spinal cord injury, spinal anesthesia can block transmission of impulses from the SNS. Depression of the vasomotor center of the medulla from drugs (e.g., opioids, benzodiazepines) also can decrease the vasoconstrictor tone of the peripheral blood vessels, resulting in neurogenic shock (Table 66-1).

The most important clinical manifestations in neurogenic shock are hypotension (from the massive vasodilation) and bradycardia (from unopposed parasympathetic stimulation).[6] The patient may not be able to regulate body temperature.

Combined with massive vasodilation, the inability to regulate temperature promotes heat loss. Initially, the patient's skin is warm due to the massive vasodilation. As the heat disperses, the patient is at risk for hypothermia. Later, the patient's skin may be cool or warm depending on the ambient temperature (*poikilothermia*, taking on the temperature of the environment). In either case, the skin is usually dry. Tables 66-2 and 66-3 further describe the laboratory findings and clinical presentation of a patient with neurogenic shock.

Although spinal shock and neurogenic shock often occur in the same patient, they are not the same disorder. *Spinal shock* is a transient condition that is present after an acute spinal cord injury (see Chapter 60). The patient with spinal shock experiences the absence of all voluntary and reflex neurologic activity below the level of the injury.

Anaphylactic Shock. **Anaphylactic shock** is an acute, life-threatening hypersensitivity (allergic) reaction to a sensitizing substance (e.g., drug, chemical, vaccine, food, insect venom). The reaction quickly causes massive vasodilation, release of vasoactive mediators, and an increase in capillary permeability.

TABLE 66-3   Clinical Presentation of Types of Shock

Cardiogenic Shock	Hypovolemic Shock	Neurogenic Shock	Anaphylactic Shock	Septic Shock	Obstructive Shock
		DISTRIBUTIVE SHOCK			
Cardiovascular System					
Tachycardia	↓ Preload	↓ BP	Chest pain	↓/↑ Temperature	↓ BP
↓ BP	↓ Stroke volume	↓/↑ Temperature	Third spacing of fluid	Myocardial dysfunction	↓ Preload
↓ Capillary refill	↓ Capillary refill	Bradycardia		Biventricular dilation	
Chest pain may or may not be present				↓ Ejection fraction	
Respiratory System					
Tachypnea	Tachypnea → bradypnea (late)	Dysfunction related to level of injury	Shortness of breath	Hyperventilation	Tachypnea → bradypnea (late)
Crackles			Edema of larynx and epiglottis	Crackles	Shortness of breath
Cyanosis			Wheezing	Respiratory alkalosis → respiratory acidosis	
			Stridor	Hypoxemia	
			Rhinitis	Respiratory failure	
				ARDS	
				Pulmonary hypertension	
Renal System					
↑ Na⁺ and H₂O retention	↓ Urine output	Bladder dysfunction	Incontinence	↓ Urine output	↓ Urine output
↓ Renal blood flow					
↓ Urine output					
Skin					
Pallor	Pallor	↓ Skin perfusion	Flushing	Warm and flushed → cool and mottled (late)	Pallor
Cool, clammy	Cool, clammy	Cool or warm	Pruritus		Cool, clammy
		Dry	Urticaria		
			Angioedema		
Neurologic System					
↓ Cerebral perfusion:	↓ Cerebral perfusion:	Flaccid paralysis below the level of the lesion	Anxiety	Alteration in mental status (e.g., confusion)	↓ Cerebral perfusion:
• Anxiety	• Anxiety	Loss of reflex activity	Feeling of impending doom	Agitation	• Anxiety
• Confusion	• Confusion		Confusion	Coma (late)	• Confusion
• Agitation	• Agitation		↓ LOC		• Agitation
			Metallic taste		
Gastrointestinal System					
↓ Bowel sounds	Absent bowel sounds	Bowel dysfunction	Cramping	GI bleeding	↓ to absent bowel sounds
Nausea, vomiting			Abdominal pain	Paralytic ileus	
			Nausea		
			Vomiting		
			Diarrhea		
Diagnostic Findings*					
↑ Cardiac biomarkers	↓ Hematocrit		Sudden onset	↑/↓ WBC	Specific to cause of obstruction
↑ b-Type natriuretic peptide (BNP)	↓ Hemoglobin		History of allergies	↓ Platelets	
↑ Blood glucose	↑ Lactate		Exposure to contrast media	↑ Lactate	
↑ BUN	↑ Urine specific gravity			↑ Blood glucose	
ECG (e.g., dysrhythmias)	Changes in electrolytes			↑ Procalcitonin	
Echocardiogram (e.g., left ventricular dysfunction)				↑ Urine specific gravity	
Chest x-ray (e.g., pulmonary infiltrates)				↓ Urine Na⁺	
				Positive blood cultures	

ARDS, Acute respiratory distress syndrome; *BUN,* blood urea nitrogen; *LOC,* level of consciousness.
*Also see Table 66-2.

As capillary permeability increases, fluid leaks from the vascular space into the interstitial space.

Anaphylactic shock can lead to respiratory distress due to laryngeal edema or severe bronchospasm, and circulatory failure from the massive vasodilation.[7,8] The patient has a sudden onset of symptoms, including dizziness, chest pain, incontinence, swelling of the lips and tongue, wheezing, and stridor. Skin changes include flushing, pruritus, urticaria, and angioedema. In addition, the patient may be anxious and confused and have a sense of impending doom.

A patient can have a severe allergic reaction, possibly leading to anaphylactic shock, after contact, inhalation, ingestion, or injection with an antigen (allergen) to which the individual has previously been sensitized (Table 66-1). Parenteral administration of the antigen (allergen) is the route most likely to cause anaphylaxis. However, oral, topical, and inhalation routes can also cause anaphylactic reactions. Tables 66-2 and 66-3 describe the laboratory findings and clinical presentation of a patient in anaphylactic shock. Quick and decisive action is critical to prevent the progression of an

PATHOPHYSIOLOGY MAP

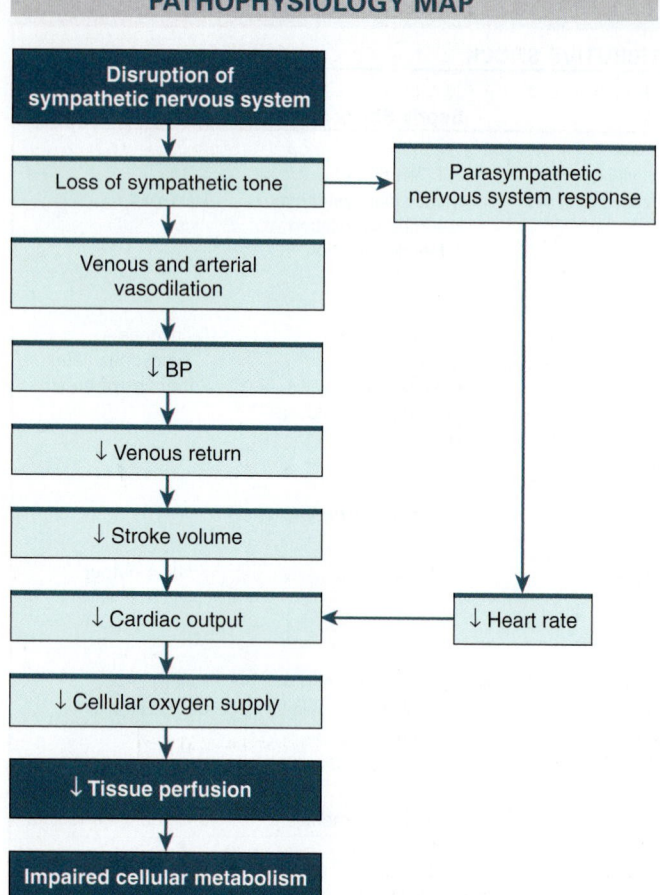

FIG. 66-4 The pathophysiology of neurogenic shock. (Modified from Urden LD, Stacy KM, Lough ME: *Critical care nursing: diagnosis and management,* ed 6, St Louis, 2010, Mosby.)

TABLE 66-4 Diagnostic Criteria for Sepsis

Infection, documented or suspected, and some of the following:

General Variables
- Fever (temperature >100.9° F [38.3° C])
- Hypothermia (core temperature <97.0° F [36° C])
- Heart rate >90 beats/min
- Tachypnea (respiratory rate ≥ 22/min)
- SBP ≤ 100 mm Hg
- Altered mental status
- Significant edema or positive fluid balance (>20 mL/kg over 24 hr)
- Hyperglycemia (blood glucose >140 mg/dL) in the absence of diabetes

Inflammatory Variables
- Leukocytosis (WBC count >12,000/μL)
- Leukopenia (WBC count <4000/μL)
- Normal WBC count with >10% immature forms (bands)
- Elevated C-reactive protein
- Elevated procalcitonin

Hemodynamic Variables
- Arterial hypotension (SBP <90 mm Hg, MAP <70 mm Hg, or a decrease in SBP >40 mm Hg)

Organ Dysfunction Variables
- Arterial hypoxemia (PaO_2/FIO_2 <300)
- Acute oliguria (urine output <0.5 mL/kg/hr for at least 2 hr despite adequate fluid resuscitation)
- Serum creatinine increase >0.5 mg/dL
- Coagulation abnormalities (INR >1.5 or PTT >60 sec)
- Ileus (absent bowel sounds)
- Thrombocytopenia (platelet count <100,000/μL)
- Hyperbilirubinemia (total bilirubin >4 mg/dL)

Tissue Perfusion Variables
- Hyperlactatemia (>1 mmol/L)
- Decreased capillary refill or mottling

Sources: Dellinger RP, Levy MM, Rhodes A, et al: Surviving sepsis campaign: international guidelines for management of severe sepsis and septic shock: 2012, *Crit Care Med* 41:580, 2013; and Singer M, Deutschman CS, Seymour CW, et al: The third international consensus definitions for sepsis and septic shock (Sepsis-3), *JAMA* 315:801, 2016..
FIO$_2$, Fraction of inspired O$_2$; *INR*, international normalized ratio; *MAP*, mean arterial pressure; *PaO$_2$*, partial pressure of arterial O$_2$; *PTT*, partial thromboplastin time; *SBP*, systolic blood pressure.

allergic reaction to anaphylactic shock. (Anaphylaxis is discussed in Chapter 13.)

Septic Shock. **Sepsis** is defined as a constellation of symptoms or syndrome in response to an infection. It is characterized by a dysregulated patient response along with new organ dysfunction related to the infection[9] (Table 66-4). In as many as 10% to 30% of patients with sepsis, the causative organism is not identified. Sepsis and septic shock have a high incidence worldwide with a mortality rate of 25% or higher.[10]

Septic shock is a subset of sepsis with an increased mortality risk due to profound circulatory, cellular, and metabolic abnormalities. Septic shock is characterized by persistent hypotension despite adequate fluid resuscitation requiring vasopressors, along with inadequate tissue perfusion resulting in tissue hypoxia.[9] The main organisms that cause sepsis are gramnegative and gram-positive bacteria. Parasites, fungi, and viruses can also cause sepsis and septic shock.[9] Fig. 66-5 presents the pathophysiology of septic shock.

When a microorganism enters the body, the normal immune or inflammatory responses are triggered. However, in sepsis and septic shock the body's response to the microorganism is exaggerated. Both proinflammatory and antiinflammatory responses are activated, coagulation increases, and fibrinolysis decreases.[9] Endotoxins from the microorganism cell wall stimulate the release of cytokines, including tumor necrosis factor (TNF), interleukin-1 (IL-1), and other proinflammatory mediators that

act through secondary mediators such as platelet-activating factor, IL-6, and IL-8.[9] (See Chapter 11 for discussion of the inflammatory response.) The release of platelet-activating factor results in the formation of microthrombi and obstruction of the microvasculature. The combined effects of the mediators result in damage to the endothelium, vasodilation, increased capillary permeability, and neutrophil and platelet aggregation and adhesion to the endothelium.

Septic shock has three major pathophysiologic effects: vasodilation, maldistribution of blood flow, and myocardial depression. Patients may be euvolemic, but because of acute vasodilation, relative hypovolemia and hypotension occur. In addition, blood flow in the microcirculation is decreased, causing poor O$_2$ delivery and tissue hypoxia. The combination of TNF and IL-1 is thought to have a role in sepsis-induced myocardial dysfunction. The ejection fraction is decreased for the first few days after the initial insult. Because of a decreased ejection fraction, the ventricles dilate to maintain the SV. The ejection fraction typically improves, and ventricular dilation

PATHOPHYSIOLOGY MAP

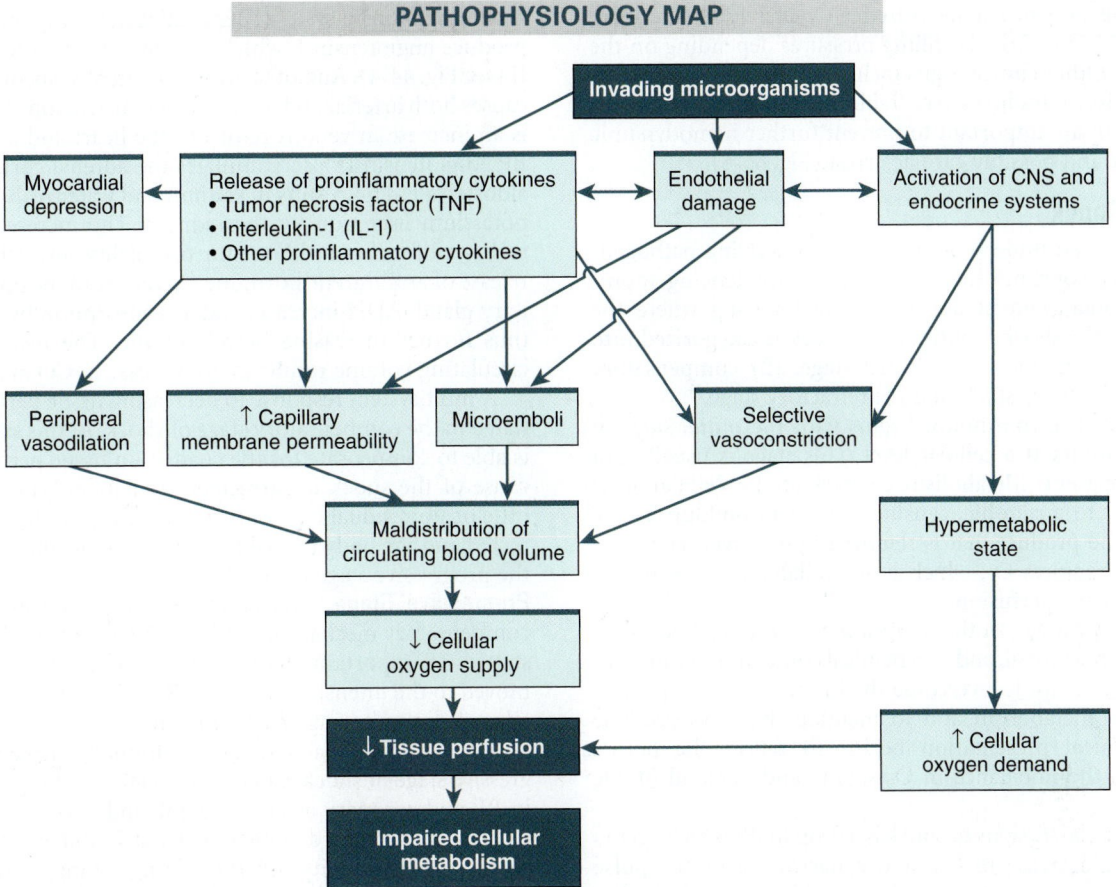

FIG. 66-5   The pathophysiology of septic shock. *CNS,* Central nervous system. (Modified from Urden LD, Stacy KM, Lough ME: *Critical care nursing: diagnosis and management,* ed 6, St Louis, 2010, Mosby.)

resolves over 7 to 10 days. Persistence of a high CO and a low SVR beyond 24 hours is an ominous finding and is often associated with an increased development of hypotension and MODS. Coronary artery perfusion and myocardial O_2 metabolism are not primarily altered in septic shock.

In addition to the cardiovascular dysfunction that accompanies sepsis, respiratory failure is common. The patient initially hyperventilates as a compensatory mechanism, resulting in respiratory alkalosis. Once the patient can no longer compensate, respiratory acidosis develops. Respiratory failure develops in 85% of patients with sepsis, and 40% develop acute respiratory distress syndrome (ARDS) (see Chapter 67). These patients may need to be intubated and mechanically ventilated.

Other clinical signs of septic shock include alteration in neurologic status; decreased urine output; and GI dysfunction, such as GI bleeding and paralytic ileus. Table 66-3 gives the clinical presentation of a patient with septic shock.

Obstructive Shock. Obstructive shock develops when a physical obstruction to blood flow occurs with a decreased CO (Fig. 66-6). This can be caused by restricted diastolic filling of the right ventricle from compression (e.g., cardiac tamponade, tension pneumothorax, superior vena cava syndrome). Other causes include *abdominal compartment syndrome,* in which increased abdominal pressures compress the inferior vena cava, thus decreasing venous return to the heart (see Chapter 42). Pulmonary embolism and right ventricular thrombi cause an outflow obstruction as blood leaves the right ventricle through the pulmonary artery. This leads to decreased blood flow to the lungs and decreased blood return to the left atrium.

PATHOPHYSIOLOGY MAP

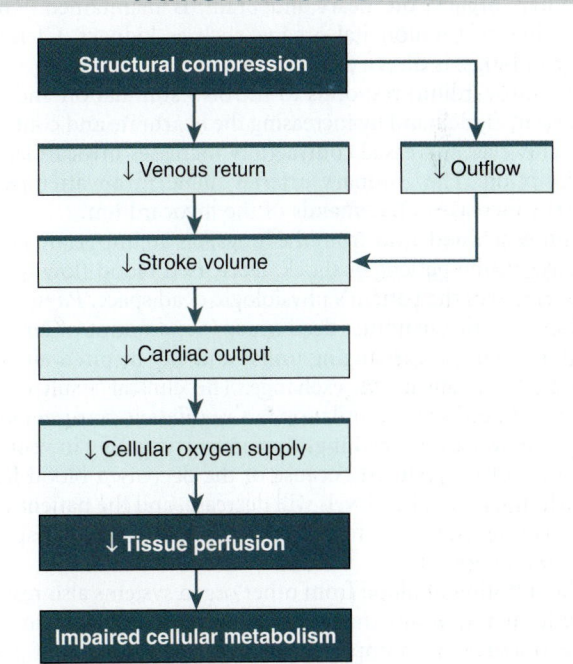

FIG. 66-6   The pathophysiology of obstructive shock.

Patients experience a decreased CO, increased afterload, and variable left ventricular filling pressures depending on the obstruction. Other clinical signs include jugular venous distention and pulsus paradoxus (see Table 36-5). Rapid assessment and treatment are important to prevent further hemodynamic compromise and possibly cardiac arrest (Fig. 66-6).

Stages of Shock

In addition to an understanding of the underlying pathogenesis of the type of shock that the patient is experiencing, monitoring and management are guided by knowing where the patient is on the shock "continuum." Shock is categorized into four overlapping stages: (1) initial stage, (2) compensatory stage, (3) progressive stage, and (4) refractory stage.[11]

Initial Stage. The continuum begins with the *initial stage* of shock that occurs at a cellular level. This stage is usually not clinically apparent. Metabolism changes at the cellular level from aerobic to anaerobic, causing lactic acid buildup. Lactic acid is a waste product that is removed by the liver. However, this process requires O_2, which is unavailable because of the decrease in tissue perfusion.

Compensatory Stage. In the *compensatory stage* the body activates neural, hormonal, and biochemical compensatory mechanisms in an attempt to overcome the increasing consequences of anaerobic metabolism and to maintain homeostasis. The patient's clinical presentation begins to reflect the body's responses to the imbalance in O_2 supply and demand (Table 66-5).

One of the classic signs of shock is a drop in BP, which occurs because of a decrease in CO and a narrowing of the pulse pressure. The baroreceptors in the carotid and aortic bodies immediately respond by activating the SNS. The SNS stimulates vasoconstriction and the release of the potent vasoconstrictors epinephrine and norepinephrine. Blood flow to the most essential (vital) organs, the heart and brain, is maintained, while blood flow to the nonvital organs, such as kidneys, GI tract, skin, and lungs, is diverted or shunted.

The myocardium responds to the SNS stimulation and the increase in O_2 demand by increasing the heart rate and contractility. However, increased contractility increases myocardial O_2 consumption. The coronary arteries dilate in an attempt to meet the increased O_2 demands of the myocardium.

Shunting blood away from the lungs has an important clinical effect in the patient in shock. Decreased blood flow to the lungs increases the patient's physiologic dead space. *Physiologic dead space* is the anatomic dead space (the amount of air that will not reach gas-exchanging units) and any inspired air that cannot participate in gas exchange. The clinical result of an increase in dead space ventilation is a *ventilation-perfusion mismatch*. Some areas of the lungs that are participating in ventilation will not be perfused because of the decreased blood flow to the lungs. Arterial O_2 levels will decrease, and the patient will have a compensatory increase in the rate and depth of respirations (see Chapter 67).

The shunting of blood from other organ systems also results in clinically important changes. The decrease in blood flow to the GI tract results in impaired motility and a slowing of peristalsis. This increases the risk for the development of a paralytic ileus.

Decreased blood flow to the skin results in the patient feeling cool and clammy. The exception is the patient in early septic shock who may feel warm and flushed because of a hyperdynamic state. Decreased blood flow to the kidneys activates the renin-angiotensin system. Renin stimulates angiotensinogen to produce angiotensin I, which is then converted to angiotensin II (see Fig. 44-4). Angiotensin II is a potent vasoconstrictor that causes both arterial and venous vasoconstriction. The net result is an increase in venous return to the heart and an increase in BP. Angiotensin II also stimulates the adrenal cortex to release aldosterone. This results in sodium and water reabsorption and potassium excretion by the kidneys. The increase in sodium reabsorption raises the serum osmolality and stimulates the release of antidiuretic hormone (ADH) from the posterior pituitary gland. ADH increases water reabsorption by the kidneys, thus further increasing blood volume. The increase in total circulating volume results in an increase in CO and BP.

A multisystem response to decreasing tissue perfusion is initiated in the compensatory stage of shock. At this stage the body is able to compensate for the changes in tissue perfusion. If the cause of the shock is corrected, the patient will recover with little or no residual effects. If the cause of the shock is not corrected and the body is unable to compensate, the patient enters the progressive stage of shock.

Progressive Stage. The *progressive stage* of shock begins as compensatory mechanisms fail. Changes in the patient's mental status are important findings in this stage. Patients must be moved to the intensive care unit (ICU), if not already there, for advanced monitoring and treatment.

The cardiovascular system is profoundly affected in the progressive stage of shock. CO begins to fall, resulting in a decrease in BP and coronary artery, cerebral, and peripheral perfusion. Continued decreased cellular perfusion and resulting altered capillary permeability are the distinguishing features of this stage. Altered capillary permeability allows leakage of fluid and protein out of the vascular space into the surrounding interstitial space. In addition to the decrease in circulating volume, there is an increase in systemic interstitial edema. The patient may have *anasarca* (diffuse profound edema). Fluid leakage from the vascular space also affects the solid organs (e.g., liver, spleen, GI tract, lungs) and peripheral tissues by further decreasing perfusion.

Sustained hypoperfusion results in weak peripheral pulses, and ischemia of the distal extremities eventually occurs. Myocardial dysfunction from decreased perfusion results in dysrhythmias, myocardial ischemia, and possibly MI. The end result is a complete deterioration of the cardiovascular system.

The pulmonary system is often the first system to display signs of critical dysfunction. During the compensatory stage, blood flow to the lungs is already reduced. In response to the decreased blood flow and the SNS stimulation, the pulmonary arterioles constrict, resulting in increased pulmonary artery (PA) pressure. As the pressure within the pulmonary vasculature increases, blood flow to the pulmonary capillaries decreases and ventilation-perfusion mismatch worsens.

Another key response in the lungs is the movement of fluid from the pulmonary vasculature into the interstitial space. As capillary permeability increases, the movement of fluid to the interstitial spaces results in interstitial edema, bronchoconstriction, and a decrease in functional residual capacity. With further increases in capillary permeability, the fluid moves to the alveoli, with resultant alveolar edema and a decrease in surfactant production. The combined effects of pulmonary vasoconstriction and bronchoconstriction are impaired gas exchange, decreased compliance, and worsening ventilation-perfusion mismatch. Clinically, the patient has tachypnea, crackles, and an overall increased work of breathing.

TABLE 66-5   Manifestations of Stages of Shock*

Compensatory Stage	Progressive Stage	Refractory Stage
Neurologic System		
Oriented to person, place, time	↓ Cerebral perfusion pressure	Unresponsive
Restless, apprehensive, confused	↓ Cerebral blood flow	Areflexia (loss of reflexes)
Change in level of consciousness	↓ Responsiveness to stimuli	Pupils nonreactive and dilated
	Delirium	
Cardiovascular System		
Sympathetic nervous system response:	↑ Capillary permeability → systemic interstitial edema	Profound hypotension
• Release of epinephrine/	↓ Cardiac output → ↓ BP and ↑ HR	↓ Cardiac output
norepinephrine (vasoconstriction)	MAP <60 mm Hg (or 40 mm Hg drop in BP from baseline)	Bradycardia, irregular rhythm
• ↑ MVO_2	↓ Coronary perfusion → dysrhythmias, myocardial	↓ BP inadequate to perfuse vital organs
• ↑ Contractility	ischemia, myocardial infarction	
• ↑ HR	↓ Peripheral perfusion → ischemia of distal extremities,	
Coronary artery dilation	diminished pulses, ↓ capillary refill	
Narrowed pulse pressure		
↓ BP		
Respiratory System		
↓ Blood flow to the lungs:	Acute respiratory distress syndrome (ARDS):	Severe refractory hypoxemia
• ↑ Physiologic dead space	• ↑ Capillary permeability	Respiratory failure
• ↑ Ventilation-perfusion mismatch	• Pulmonary vasoconstriction	
• Hyperventilation	• Pulmonary interstitial edema	
• ↑ Minute ventilation (V_E)	• Alveolar edema	
• Tachypnea	• Diffuse infiltrates	
	• Tachypnea	
	• ↓ Compliance	
	• Moist crackles	
Gastrointestinal System		
↓ Blood supply	Vasoconstriction and ↓ perfusion → ischemic gut (e.g.,	Ischemic gut
↓ GI motility	stomach, small and large intestines, gallbladder,	
Hypoactive bowel sounds	pancreas)	
↑ Risk for paralytic ileus	• Erosive ulcers	
	• GI bleeding	
	• Translocation of GI bacteria	
	• Impaired absorption of nutrients	
Renal System		
↓ Renal blood flow	Renal tubules become ischemic → acute tubular necrosis	Anuria
↑ Renin resulting in release of	↓ Urine output	
angiotensin (vasoconstrictor)	↑ BUN/creatinine ratio	
↑ Aldosterone resulting in Na^+ and H_2O	↑ Urine sodium	
reabsorption	↓ Urine osmolality and specific gravity	
↑ Antidiuretic hormone resulting in H_2O	↓ Urine potassium	
reabsorption	Metabolic acidosis	
Hepatic System		
	Failure to metabolize drugs and waste products	Metabolic changes from accumulation of
	Cell death (↑ liver enzymes)	waste products (e.g., NH_3, lactate, CO_2)
	Jaundice (decreased clearance of bilirubin)	
	↑ NH_3 and lactate	
Hematologic System		
	DIC	DIC progresses
	• Thrombin clots in microcirculation	
	• Consumption of platelets and clotting factors	
Temperature		
Normal or abnormal	Hypothermia or hyperthermia	Hypothermia
Skin		
Pale and cool	Cold and clammy	Mottled, cyanotic
Warm and flushed		

DIC, Disseminated intravascular coagulation; *MAP,* mean arterial pressure; *MVO_2,* myocardial O_2 consumption; *NH_3,* ammonia.
*The shock continuum begins with the *initial stage* of shock. This stage occurs at the cellular level and is usually not clinically apparent. Also see Table 66-2 and Table 66-3.

The GI system is also affected by prolonged decreased tissue perfusion. As the blood supply to the GI tract is decreased, the normally protective mucosal barrier becomes ischemic. This ischemia predisposes the patient to ulcers and GI bleeding (see Chapter 41). It also increases the risk of bacterial migration from the GI tract to the blood. The decreased perfusion to the GI tract also leads to a decreased ability to absorb nutrients.

The effect of prolonged hypoperfusion on the kidneys is renal tubular ischemia. The resulting acute tubular necrosis may lead to acute kidney injury. This can be worsened by nephrotoxic drugs (e.g., certain antibiotics, anesthetics, diuretics) (see

Chapter 46). The patient has decreased urine output and elevated blood urea nitrogen (BUN) and serum creatinine. Metabolic acidosis occurs from the kidneys' inability to excrete acids (especially lactic acid) and reabsorb bicarbonate.

Other organ systems are also affected by the sustained hypoperfusion in the progressive stage of shock. The loss of the functional ability of the liver leads to a failure of the liver to metabolize drugs and waste products (e.g., lactate, ammonia). Jaundice results from an accumulation of bilirubin. As the liver cells die, enzymes become elevated (e.g., alanine aminotransferase [ALT], aspartate aminotransferase [AST], γ-glutamyl transferase [GGT]). The liver also loses its ability to function as an immune organ. Bacteria that may move from the GI tract are no longer destroyed by the Kupffer cells. Instead, they are released into the bloodstream, thus increasing the possibility of bacteremia.

Dysfunction of the hematologic system adds to the complexity of the clinical picture. The patient is at risk for disseminated intravascular coagulation (DIC). The consumption of the platelets and clotting factors with secondary fibrinolysis results in clinically significant bleeding from many orifices. These include, but are not limited to, the GI tract, lungs, and puncture sites (see Chapter 30). Altered laboratory values in DIC are presented in Table 66-3.

In this stage, aggressive interventions are necessary to prevent the development of MODS.

Refractory Stage. In the final stage of shock, the *refractory stage*, decreased perfusion from peripheral vasoconstriction and decreased CO exacerbate anaerobic metabolism. The accumulation of lactic acid contributes to increased capillary permeability and dilation. Increased capillary permeability allows fluid and plasma proteins to leave the vascular space and move to the interstitial space. Blood pools in the capillary beds secondary to the constricted venules and dilated arterioles. The loss of intravascular volume worsens hypotension and tachycardia and decreases coronary blood flow. Decreased coronary blood flow leads to worsening myocardial depression and a further decline in CO. Cerebral blood flow cannot be maintained and cerebral ischemia results.

The patient in this stage of shock demonstrates profound hypotension and hypoxemia. The failure of the liver, lungs, and kidneys results in an accumulation of waste products, such as lactate, urea, ammonia, and CO_2. The failure of one organ system affects several other organ systems. Recovery is unlikely in this stage. The organs are in failure and the body's compensatory mechanisms are overwhelmed (Table 66-5).

Diagnostic Studies

There is no single diagnostic study to determine whether a patient is in shock. The diagnosis starts with a history and physical examination. Obtaining a thorough medical and surgical history, and a history of recent events (e.g., surgery, chest pain, trauma), provides valuable data.

Decreased tissue perfusion in shock leads to an elevation of lactate and a base deficit (the amount needed to bring the pH back to normal). These laboratory changes may reflect an increase in anaerobic metabolism. Table 66-2 summarizes other laboratory findings seen in shock.

Additional diagnostic studies include a 12-lead electrocardiogram (ECG), continuous ECG monitoring, chest x-ray, continuous pulse oximetry, and invasive and noninvasive hemodynamic monitoring. (Chapter 65 discusses hemodynamic monitoring.)

Interprofessional Care: General Measures

Critical factors in the successful management of a patient experiencing shock relate to the early recognition and treatment of the shock state. Prompt intervention in the early stages of shock may prevent the decline to the progressive or irreversible stage. Successful management of the patient in shock includes the following:

1. Identification of patients at risk for developing shock
2. Integration of the patient's history, physical examination, and clinical findings to establish a diagnosis
3. Interventions to control or eliminate the cause of the decreased perfusion
4. Protection of target and distal organs from dysfunction
5. Provision of multisystem supportive care

Table 66-6 provides an overview of the initial assessment findings and interventions for the emergency care of patients in shock.[12] General management strategies begin with ensuring that the patient is responsive and has a patent airway. Once the airway is established, either naturally or with an endotracheal tube, O_2 delivery must be optimized. Supplemental O_2 and mechanical ventilation may be necessary to maintain an arterial O_2 saturation of 90% or more (PaO_2 greater than 60 mm Hg) to avoid hypoxemia (see Chapter 65). The mean arterial pressure (MAP) and circulating blood volume are optimized with fluid replacement and drug therapy.

Oxygen and Ventilation. O_2 delivery depends on CO, available hemoglobin, and arterial O_2 saturation (SaO_2). Methods to optimize O_2 delivery are directed at increasing supply and decreasing demand. Supply is increased by (1) optimizing the CO with fluid replacement or drug therapy, (2) increasing the hemoglobin through transfusion of whole blood or packed red blood cells (RBCs), and/or (3) increasing the arterial O_2 saturation with supplemental O_2 and mechanical ventilation.

Plan care to avoid disrupting the balance of O_2 supply and demand. Space activities that increase O_2 consumption (e.g., endotracheal suctioning, position changes) appropriately for O_2 conservation. Intermittent or continuous monitoring of $ScvO_2$ by a central venous catheter or mixed venous O_2 saturation (SvO_2) may be helpful. Both reflect the dynamic balance between O_2 supply and demand. Assess these values along with related hemodynamic measures (e.g., arterial pressure–based cardiac output [APCO], O_2 consumption, hemoglobin) to evaluate the patient's response to treatments or activities (see Chapter 65).

Fluid Resuscitation. The cornerstone of therapy for septic, hypovolemic, and anaphylactic shock is volume expansion with administration of the appropriate fluid. Fluid resuscitation should start using one or two large-bore (e.g., 14- to 16-gauge) IV catheters; an intraosseous (IO) access device; or a central venous catheter. Both crystalloids (e.g., normal saline, lactated Ringer's) and colloids (e.g., albumin) have a role in fluid resuscitation (Table 66-7; see Table 16-17).

⚠️ **SAFETY ALERT** **Intraosseous (IO) Access**
- Use an IO access device for emergency resuscitation when IV access cannot be obtained.
- Insertion sites include sternum, proximal and distal tibia, and proximal and distal humerus.
- Remove IO devices within 24 hours of insertion or as soon as possible after peripheral or central IV access is obtained.
- Monitor for complications: extravasation of drugs and fluids into the soft tissue, fractures caused during insertion, and osteomyelitis.

✚ TABLE 66-6 Emergency Management

Shock

Etiology*	Assessment Findings	Interventions
Surgical • Postoperative bleeding • Ruptured organ or vessel • Gastrointestinal bleeding • Aortic dissection • Vaginal bleeding • Ruptured ectopic pregnancy or ovarian cyst **Medical** • Myocardial infarction • Dehydration • Addisonian crisis • Diabetes insipidus • Sepsis • Diabetes mellitus • Pulmonary embolus **Trauma** • Ruptured or lacerated vessel or organ (e.g., spleen) • Fractures, spinal injury • Multiorgan injury	• Restlessness • Confusion • Anxiety • Feeling of impending doom • Decreased level of consciousness • Weakness • Rapid, weak, thready pulses • Dysrhythmias • Hypotension • Narrowed pulse pressure • Cool, clammy skin (warm skin in early onset of septic and neurogenic shock) • Tachypnea, dyspnea, or shallow, irregular respirations • Decreased O₂ saturation • Extreme thirst • Nausea and vomiting • Chills • Pallor • Cyanosis • Obvious hemorrhage or injury • Temperature dysregulation	**Initial** • If unresponsive, assess circulation, airway, and breathing (CAB). • If responsive, monitor airway, breathing, and circulation (ABC). • Stabilize cervical spine as appropriate. • Control any external bleeding with direct pressure or pressure dressing. • Give high-flow O₂ (100%) by non-rebreather mask or bag-valve-mask. • Anticipate need for intubation and mechanical ventilation. • Establish IV access with two large-bore catheters (14- to 16-gauge) or an intraosseous access device, or assist with insertion of central line. • Begin fluid resuscitation with crystalloids (e.g., 30 mL/kg repeated until hemodynamic improvement is noted). • Draw blood for laboratory studies (e.g., blood cultures, lactate, WBC). • Assess for life-threatening injuries (e.g., cardiac tamponade, liver laceration, tension pneumothorax). • Consider vasopressor therapy if hypotension persists after fluid resuscitation. • Insert an indwelling urinary catheter and nasogastric tube. • Start antibiotic therapy after blood cultures if sepsis is suspected. • Obtain 12-lead ECG and treat dysrhythmias. **Ongoing Monitoring** • ABCs • Level of consciousness • Vital signs, including pulse oximetry; peripheral pulses, capillary refill, skin color and temperature • Respiratory status • Heart rate and rhythm • Urine output

*See Table 66-1 for additional causes of shock.

TABLE 66-7 Fluid Therapy in Shock

Fluid Type	Mechanism of Action	Type of Shock	Nursing Implications
Crystalloids **Isotonic** • 0.9% NaCl (NSS) • Lactated Ringer's (LR)	Fluid primarily remains in the intravascular space, increasing intravascular volume.	Used for initial volume replacement in most types of shock.	Monitor patient closely for circulatory overload. Do not use LR in patients with liver failure. LR may be used if hyperchloremic acidosis develops from use of NSS in fluid resuscitation.
Hypertonic • 1.8%, 3%, 5% NaCl	Fluid remains in the intravascular space, increases serum osmolarity, shifts fluid volume from intracellular space to extracellular space to intravascular space.	May be used for initial volume expansion in hypovolemic shock.	Monitor patient closely for signs of hypernatremia (e.g., disorientation, convulsions). Central line preferred for infusing saline solutions ≥3%, since these may damage veins.
Blood or Blood Products Packed red blood cells	Replaces blood loss, increases O₂-carrying capability.	All types of shock.	Same precautions as any blood administration (see Chapter 30).
Fresh frozen plasma	Replaces coagulation factors.		
Platelets	Helps control bleeding caused by thrombocytopenia.		
Colloids Human serum albumin (5% or 25%)	Can increase plasma colloid osmotic pressure. Rapid volume expansion.	All types of shock except cardiogenic and neurogenic shock.	Use 5% solution in hypovolemic patients. Use 25% solution in patients with fluid and sodium restrictions. Monitor for circulatory overload. Mild side effects of chills, fever, and urticaria may develop. More expensive than crystalloids.
dextran (dextran 40)	Hyperosmotic glucose polymer.	Limited use because of side effects, including reducing platelet adhesion, diluting clotting factors.	Increases risk of bleeding. Important to monitor patient for allergic reactions and acute kidney injury. Has maximum volume recommendations per manufacturer.

NSS, Normal saline solution.

The ideal choice of fluid for resuscitation remains controversial. Currently, normal saline is most often used in the initial resuscitation of shock. While large volume resuscitation with normal saline can lead to hyperchloremic metabolic acidosis, lactated Ringer's solution may also cause serum lactate levels to increase because the failing liver cannot convert lactate to bicarbonate.[13] In some cases, hypertonic saline may be considered to expand plasma volume.

Colloids (4% to 5%) are effective volume expanders because the size of their molecules keeps them in the vascular space for a longer time. However, colloids are costly. Studies have shown that they are safe to use, but none have shown that using colloids versus crystalloids for resuscitation improves patient outcomes.[14]

The choice of resuscitation fluid is also based on the type and volume of fluid lost and the patient's clinical status. *Fluid responsiveness* is determined by clinical assessment. This includes vital signs, cerebral and abdominal perfusion pressures, capillary refill, skin temperature and urine output. Hemodynamic parameters, such as SVV or CO, are also used.[15] Monitor trends in BP with an automatic BP cuff or an arterial catheter to assess the patient's response. Use an indwelling urinary catheter to monitor urine output during resuscitation.

When large amounts of fluids are required, you must protect the patient against two major complications: hypothermia and coagulopathy. If the patient has persistent hypotension after adequate fluid resuscitation, a vasopressor (e.g., norepinephrine [Levophed], dopamine) and/or an inotrope (e.g., dobutamine) may be added. The goal for fluid resuscitation is restoration of tissue perfusion. Thus decisions on which drug to use should be based on the physiologic goal. Although BP helps determine whether the patient's CO is adequate, an assessment of end-organ perfusion (e.g., urine output, neurologic function, peripheral pulses) provides more relevant data.

⚠ **SAFETY ALERT** **Fluid Resuscitation**
- Warm crystalloid and colloid solutions during massive fluid resuscitation.
- When administering large volumes of packed RBCs, remember that they do not contain clotting factors. Replace these factors based on the clinical situation and laboratory studies.

Drug Therapy. The primary goal of drug therapy for shock is the correction of decreased tissue perfusion. Drugs used to improve perfusion in shock are given IV via an infusion pump and central venous line. Many of these drugs have vasoconstrictor properties that are harmful if the drug extravasates while being infused peripherally (Table 66-8).

Sympathomimetic Drugs. Many of the drugs used in the treatment of shock have an effect on the SNS. Drugs that mimic the action of the SNS are termed *sympathomimetic*. The effects of these drugs are mediated through their binding to α- or β-adrenergic receptors. The various drugs differ in their relative α- and β-adrenergic effects. (See Chapter 32 and Table 32-7.)

Many of the sympathomimetic drugs cause peripheral vasoconstriction and are called *vasopressor drugs* (e.g., norepinephrine, dopamine, phenylephrine). These drugs can cause severe peripheral vasoconstriction and an increase in SVR, further risking tissue perfusion. The increased SVR increases the workload of the heart and can harm a patient in cardiogenic shock by causing further myocardial damage. Use of vasopressor drugs is limited to patients who do not respond to fluid resuscitation. Adequate fluid resuscitation must be achieved

before starting vasopressors because the vasoconstrictor effects in patients with low blood volume will cause further reduction in tissue perfusion.

The goal of vasopressor therapy is to achieve and maintain a MAP of greater than 65 mm Hg.[10] Continuously monitor end-organ perfusion (e.g., urine output, level of consciousness) and serum lactate levels (e.g., every 3 hours for the first 6 hours) to ensure that tissue perfusion is adequate.

Vasodilator Drugs. Patients in cardiogenic shock have decreased myocardial contractility, and vasodilators may be needed to decrease afterload. This reduces myocardial workload and O_2 requirements. Although generalized sympathetic vasoconstriction is a useful compensatory mechanism for maintaining BP, excessive constriction can reduce tissue blood flow and increase the workload of the heart. The rationale for using vasodilator therapy for a patient in shock is to break the harmful cycle of widespread vasoconstriction causing a decrease in CO and BP, resulting in further sympathetic-induced vasoconstriction.

The goal of vasodilator therapy, as in vasopressor therapy, is to maintain the MAP greater than 65 mm Hg. Monitor hemodynamic parameters (e.g., CVP, CO, $ScvO_2$/SvO_2, SV, PA pressures) along with physical assessment so that fluids can be increased or vasodilator therapy decreased if a serious fall in CO or BP occurs. The vasodilator agent most often used for the patient in cardiogenic shock is nitroglycerin. Vasodilation may be enhanced with nitroprusside or nitroglycerin in noncardiogenic shock.

Nutritional Therapy. Protein-calorie malnutrition is one of the main manifestations of hypermetabolism in shock. Nutrition is vital to reducing mortality. Enteral nutrition should be started within the first 24 hours. However, full calorie replacement is not recommended for previously well-nourished adults early on in critical illness.[16] Generally, parenteral nutrition is used only if enteral feedings are contraindicated. (Chapter 39 discusses parenteral and enteral nutrition.)

Start the patient on a *trophic feeding*. This is defined as a slow drip of small amounts of enteral nutrition (e.g., 10 mL/hr). Early enteral feedings enhance the perfusion of the GI tract and help maintain the integrity of the gut mucosa. Advance feedings as tolerated and as prescribed.

Weigh the patient daily on the same scale (usually the bed scale) at the same time of day. If the patient has a significant weight loss, rule out dehydration before adding more calories. Large weight gains are common because of third spacing of fluids. Therefore daily weights serve as a better indicator of fluid status than caloric needs. Serum protein, total albumin, prealbumin, BUN, serum glucose, and serum electrolytes are all used to assess nutritional status.

Interprofessional Care: Specific Measures

Cardiogenic Shock. For a patient in cardiogenic shock, the overall goal is to restore blood flow to the myocardium by restoring the balance between O_2 supply and demand. Cardiac catheterization is performed as soon as possible after the initial insult. Specific measures to restore blood flow include angioplasty with stenting, emergency revascularization, and valve replacement (see Chapter 33). Until these interventions are done, the heart must be supported to optimize SV and CO to achieve optimal perfusion (Tables 66-8 and 66-9).

Hemodynamic management of a patient in cardiogenic shock aims to reduce the workload of the heart through drug

TABLE 66-8 Drug Therapy

Shock

Drug*	Mechanism of Action	Type of Shock	Nursing Implications
dobutamine	↑ Myocardial contractility ↓ Ventricular filling pressures ↓ SVR, PAWP ↑ CO, stroke volume, CVP ↑/↓ HR	Used in cardiogenic shock with severe systolic dysfunction Used in septic shock to increase O₂ delivery and raise ScvO₂ or SvO₂ to 70% if Hgb >7 g/dL or Hct ≥30%	Administration via central line is recommended (infiltration leads to tissue sloughing). Do not administer in same line with NaHCO₃. Monitor HR, BP (hypotension may worsen, requiring addition of a vasopressor). Stop infusion if tachydysrhythmias develop.

dopamine	Positive inotropic effects:
	  ↑ Myocardial contractility
	  ↑ Automaticity
	  ↑ Atrioventricular conduction
	  ↑ HR, CO
	  ↑ BP, ↑ MAP
	  ↑ MVO₂
	Can cause progressive vasoconstriction at high doses
		Cardiogenic shock	Administration via central line is recommended (infiltration leads to tissue sloughing).
			Do not give in same line with NaHCO₃.
			Monitor for tachydysrhythmias.
			Monitor for peripheral vasoconstriction (e.g., paresthesias, coldness in extremities) at moderate to high doses.

epinephrine (Adrenalin)	*Low doses:* β-Adrenergic agonist (cardiac stimulation, bronchodilation, peripheral vasodilation) ↑ HR, contractility, CO ↓ SVR *High doses:* α-Adrenergic agonist (peripheral vasoconstriction) ↑ Stroke volume, SVR ↑ Systolic/↓ diastolic BP, widened pulse pressure ↑ CVP, PAWP	Cardiogenic shock Anaphylactic shock Septic shock requiring additional agent after norepinephrine Cardiac arrest, pulseless ventricular tachycardia, ventricular fibrillation, asystole	Monitor for HR >110 beats/min. Monitor for dyspnea, pulmonary edema. Monitor for chest pain, dysrhythmias secondary to ↑ MVO₂. Monitor for renal failure secondary to ischemia.
hydrocortisone (Solu-Cortef)	Decreases inflammation, reverses increased capillary permeability ↑ BP, HR	Septic shock requiring vasopressor therapy (despite fluid resuscitation) to maintain adequate BP Anaphylactic shock if hypotension persists after initial therapy	Monitor for hypokalemia, hyperglycemia. Consider use as continuous infusion.
norepinephrine (Levophed)	β₁-Adrenergic agonist (cardiac stimulation) α-Adrenergic agonist (peripheral vasoconstriction) Renal and splanchnic vasoconstriction ↑ BP, MAP, CVP, PAWP, SVR ↑/↓ CO	Cardiogenic shock after myocardial infarction Septic shock—first drug of choice for BP unresponsive to adequate fluid resuscitation	Administration via central line is required (infiltration leads to tissue sloughing). Monitor for dysrhythmias secondary to ↑ MVO₂ requirements.
phenylephrine	α-Adrenergic agonist (peripheral vasoconstriction) Renal, mesenteric, splanchnic, cutaneous, and pulmonary blood vessel constriction ↑ HR, BP, SVR ↑/↓ CO	Neurogenic shock	Monitor for reflex bradycardia, headache, restlessness. Monitor for renal failure secondary to ↓ renal blood flow. Administration via central line is recommended (infiltration leads to tissue sloughing).
nitroglycerin	Venodilation Dilates coronary arteries ↓ Preload, MVO₂, SVR, BP	Cardiogenic shock	Continuously monitor BP and HR, since reflex tachycardia may occur. Glass bottle recommended for infusion.
sodium nitroprusside	Arterial and venous vasodilation ↓ Preload, afterload ↓ CVP, PAWP ↑/↓ CO ↓ BP	Cardiogenic shock with ↑ SVR	Continuously monitor BP. Protect solution from light. Wrap infusion bottle with opaque covering. Give with D₅W only. Monitor serum cyanide levels and for signs of cyanide toxicity (e.g., metabolic acidosis, tachycardia, altered level of consciousness, seizures, coma, almond smell on breath).
vasopressin	Antidiuretic hormone Nonadrenergic vasoconstrictor ↑ MAP ↑ Urine output	Shock states (most commonly septic shock) refractory to other vasopressors	Administered with norepinephrine and in low doses. Infusions are not titrated. Monitor hemodynamic pressures and urine output.

CO, Cardiac output; *CVP,* central venous pressure; *MAP,* mean arterial pressure; *MVO₂,* myocardial O₂ consumption; *PAWP,* pulmonary artery wedge pressure; *PT,* prothrombin time; *PTT,* partial thromboplastin time; *SVR,* systemic vascular resistance.

*Consult agency guidelines, pharmacist, pharmacology references, and drug manufacturer's administration materials for additional information and dosing recommendations.

TABLE 66-9   Interprofessional Care

Shock

Oxygenation	Circulation	Drug Therapies	Supportive Therapies
Cardiogenic Shock			
• Provide supplemental O$_2$ (e.g., nasal cannula, non-rebreather mask) • Intubation and mechanical ventilation, if necessary • Monitor ScvO$_2$ or SvO$_2$	• Restore blood flow with thrombolytics, angioplasty with stenting, emergent coronary revascularization • Reduce workload of heart with circulatory assist devices: IABP, VAD	• Nitrates (e.g., nitroglycerin) • Inotropes (e.g., dobutamine) • Diuretics (e.g., furosemide) • β-Adrenergic blockers (contraindicated with ↓ ejection fraction)	• Treat dysrhythmias
Hypovolemic Shock			

• Provide supplemental O$_2$
• Monitor ScvO$_2$ or ScvO$_2$
	• Rapid fluid replacement using two large-bore (14-16 gauge) peripheral IV lines, an intraosseous access device, or central venous catheter
	• Restore fluid volume (e.g., blood or blood products, crystalloids)
	• End points of fluid resuscitation:
	  • CVP 15 mm Hg
	  • PAWP 10-12 mm Hg
		• No specific drug therapy	• Correct the cause (e.g., stop bleeding, GI losses)
			• Use warmed IV fluids, including blood products (if appropriate)

Septic Shock			

• Provide supplemental O$_2$
• Intubation and mechanical ventilation, if necessary
• Monitor ScvO$_2$ or SvO$_2$
	• Aggressive fluid resuscitation (e.g., 30 mL/kg of crystalloids repeated as long as hemodynamic improvement is noted)
	• End points of fluid resuscitation are based on:
	  1. Focused physical examination including vital signs, cardiopulmonary assessment, capillary refill, peripheral pulses, and skin or any 2 of the following:
	    • ScvO$_2$ >70 or SvO$_2$ >65
	    • CVP 8-12 mm Hg
	    • Cardiovascular ultrasound
	  2. Assessment of fluid responsiveness with passive leg raise or fluid challenge
		• Antibiotics as ordered
		• Vasopressors (e.g., norepinephrine)
		• Inotropes (e.g., dobutamine)
		• Anticoagulants (e.g., low-molecular-weight heparin)
			• Obtain cultures (e.g., blood, wound) before beginning antibiotics
			• Monitor temperature
			• Control blood glucose
			• Stress ulcer prophylaxis

Neurogenic Shock			
• Maintain patent airway • Provide supplemental O$_2$ • Intubation and mechanical ventilation (if necessary)	• Cautious administration of fluids	• Vasopressors (e.g., phenylephrine) • Atropine (for bradycardia)	• Minimize spinal cord trauma with stabilization • Monitor temperature
Anaphylactic Shock			
• Maintain patent airway • Optimize oxygenation with supplemental O$_2$ • Intubation and mechanical ventilation, if necessary	• Aggressive fluid resuscitation with colloids	• Epinephrine (IM or IV) • Antihistamines (e.g., diphenhydramine) • Histamine (H$_2$)-receptor blockers (e.g., ranitidine [Zantac]) • Bronchodilators: nebulized (e.g., albuterol) • Corticosteroids (if hypotension persists)	• Identify and remove offending cause • Prevent via avoidance of known allergens • Premedicate with history of prior sensitivity (e.g., contrast media)
Obstructive Shock			
• Maintain patent airway • Provide supplemental O$_2$ • Intubation and mechanical ventilation, if necessary	• Restore circulation by treating cause of obstruction • Fluid resuscitation may provide temporary improvement in CO and BP	• No specific drug therapy	• Treat cause of obstruction (e.g., pericardiocentesis for cardiac tamponade, needle decompression or chest tube insertion for tension pneumothorax, embolectomy for pulmonary embolism)

CO, Cardiac output; *CVP,* central venous pressure; *IABP,* intraaortic balloon pump; *PAWP,* pulmonary artery wedge pressure; *VAD,* ventricular assist device.

therapy and/or mechanical interventions. Drug selection is based on the clinical goal and a thorough understanding of each drug's mechanism of action. Drugs can be used to decrease the workload of the heart by dilating coronary arteries (e.g., nitrates), reducing preload (e.g., diuretics), reducing afterload (e.g., vasodilators), and reducing heart rate and contractility (e.g., β-adrenergic blockers).

The patient may also benefit from a circulatory assist device (e.g., intraaortic balloon pump, ventricular assist device [VAD])[4,17] (see Chapter 65). The goals of this intervention are to decrease the SVR and the left ventricular workload so that the heart can heal. A VAD may be used as a temporary measure for the patient in cardiogenic shock who is awaiting heart transplantation. Heart transplantation is an option for a small, select group of patients with cardiogenic shock.

Hypovolemic Shock. The underlying principles of managing patients with hypovolemic shock focus on stopping the loss of fluid and restoring the circulating volume. Fluid resuscitation in hypovolemic shock initially is calculated using a 3:1 rule (3 mL of isotonic crystalloid for every 1 mL of estimated blood loss). Table 66-7 delineates the different types of fluid used for volume resuscitation, the mechanisms of action, and specific nursing implications for each fluid type.

Septic Shock. Patients in septic shock require large amounts of fluid replacement. Volume resuscitation of 30 to 50 mL/kg is usually done with isotonic crystalloids to achieve adequate fluid resuscitation. Albumin 4% to 5% may be added when patients require substantial volumes.

A fluid challenge technique (e.g., to achieve a minimum of 30 mL/kg of crystalloids) is used and repeated until hemodynamic improvement (e.g., increase in MAP and/or CVP, change in SVV) is noted.[18] Table 66-9 presents predetermined end points of fluid resuscitation along with methods to reassess volume status.

One of these methods is a *passive leg raise* (PLR) challenge along with hemodynamic measures to monitor response.[15] A PLR challenge provides a transient increase in fluid volume of 150 to 500 mL by placing the patient supine and raising the legs to 45 degrees. Response is monitored within 1 to 2 minutes by measuring CO, CI, SV, SVV, or other parameters for improvement. If the response is positive, then the patient is fluid responsive and should receive additional fluids. To optimize and evaluate large-volume fluid resuscitation, hemodynamic monitoring with various noninvasive or invasive monitors is necessary. The overall goal of fluid resuscitation is to restore the intravascular volume and organ perfusion.

If the patient remains hypotensive after initial volume resuscitation with minimally 30 mL/kg and the patient is no longer fluid responsive, vasopressors may be added. The first drug of choice is norepinephrine. Vasodilation and low CO, or vasodilation alone, can cause low BP in spite of adequate fluid resuscitation. Vasopressin may be added for patients refractory to initial vasopressor therapy. Exogenous vasopressin is used to replace the stores of physiologic vasopressin that are often depleted in septic shock.

🔔 DRUG ALERT Vasopressin
- Given along with norepinephrine.
- Infuse at low doses (e.g., 0.03 U/min) using an IV pump.
- Do not titrate infusion.
- Use cautiously in patients with coronary artery disease.

Vasopressor drugs may increase BP but may also decrease SV. An inotropic agent (e.g., dobutamine) may be added to offset the decrease in SV and increase tissue perfusion (Table 66-8). IV corticosteroids may be considered for patients in septic shock who cannot maintain an adequate BP with vasopressor therapy despite fluid resuscitation. In an attempt to meet the increasing tissue demands coupled with a low SVR, the patient initially demonstrates a normal or high CO. If the patient is unable to achieve and maintain an adequate CO and has unmet tissue O_2 demands, the CO may have to be increased using drug therapy (e.g., dopamine). $ScvO_2$ or SvO_2 monitoring is used to assess the balance between O_2 delivery and consumption, and the adequacy of the CO (see Chapter 65). If balance is maintained, the tissue demands will be met.

Antibiotics are an important and early component of therapy. They should be started within the first hour of severe sepsis or septic shock. Every hour delay has shown to significantly decrease survival.[19] Obtain cultures (e.g., blood, wound exudate, urine, stool, sputum) before antibiotics are started. However, this should not delay the start of antibiotics within the first hour. Broad-spectrum antibiotics are given first. More specific antibiotics may be ordered once the organism has been identified.

Glucose levels should be maintained below 180 mg/dL (10.0 mmol/L) for patients in shock. Intensive glucose control (81 to 108 mg/dL) actually increases mortality.[20] Monitor glucose levels in all patients in septic shock according to agency policy.

Stress ulcer prophylaxis with proton pump inhibitors (e.g., pantoprazole) for patients with bleeding risk factors and venous thromboembolism prophylaxis (e.g., heparin, enoxaparin [Lovenox]) are also recommended for these patients.[10]

Neurogenic Shock. The specific treatment of neurogenic shock is based on the cause. If the cause is spinal cord injury, general measures to promote spinal stability (e.g., spinal precautions, cervical stabilization with a collar) are initially used. Once the spine is stabilized, definitive treatment of the hypotension and bradycardia is essential to prevent further spinal cord damage. Hypotension, which occurs as a result of a loss of sympathetic tone, is associated with peripheral vasodilation and decreased venous return. Treatment involves the use of vasopressors (e.g., phenylephrine) to maintain BP and organ perfusion (Table 66-8). Bradycardia may be treated with atropine. Infuse fluids cautiously as the cause of the hypotension is not related to fluid loss.

The patient with a spinal cord injury also needs to be monitored for hypothermia caused by hypothalamic dysfunction (Table 66-9). Corticosteroids do not have an effect in neurogenic shock, and current guidelines no longer recommend the use of methylprednisolone (Solu-Medrol) for patients with a spinal cord injury.[21] (see Chapter 60).

Anaphylactic Shock. The first strategy in managing patients at risk for anaphylactic shock is prevention. A thorough history is key to avoiding the risk factors for anaphylaxis (Table 66-1). The clinical presentation of anaphylactic shock is dramatic, and immediate intervention is required. IM epinephrine is the first drug of choice to treat anaphylactic shock.[7,8] It causes peripheral vasoconstriction and bronchodilation and opposes the effect of histamine. Diphenhydramine and ranitidine (Zantac) are given as adjunctive therapies to block the ongoing release of histamine from the allergic reaction.

Maintaining a patent airway is important because the patient can quickly develop airway compromise from laryngeal edema or bronchoconstriction. Nebulized bronchodilators are highly effective. Aerosolized epinephrine can also be used to treat laryngeal edema. Endotracheal intubation or cricothyroidotomy may be necessary to secure and maintain a patent airway.

Hypotension results from leakage of fluid out of the intravascular space into the interstitial space as a result of increased vascular permeability and vasodilation. Aggressive fluid resuscitation, usually with crystalloids, is necessary. IV corticosteroids may be helpful in anaphylactic shock if significant hypotension persists after 1 to 2 hours of aggressive therapy (Tables 66-8 and 66-9).

Obstructive Shock. The primary strategy in treating obstructive shock is early recognition and treatment to relieve or manage the obstruction (Table 66-1). Mechanical decompression for pericardial tamponade, tension pneumothorax, and hemopneumothorax may be done by needle or tube insertion. Obstructive shock from a pulmonary embolism may require thrombolytic therapy. Superior vena cava syndrome, a compression or obstruction of the outflow tract of the mediastinum, may be treated by radiation, debulking, or removal of the mass or cause. A decompressive laparotomy may be indicated for abdominal compartment syndrome for patients with high intraabdominal pressures and hemodynamic instability.

❖ NURSING MANAGEMENT: SHOCK

◆ Nursing Assessment

Your role is vital in caring for patients who are at risk for developing shock or are in a state of shock. Focus your assessment on the ABCs: airway, breathing, and circulation. Next, assess for tissue perfusion. This includes evaluating vital signs, level of consciousness, peripheral pulses, capillary refill, skin (e.g., temperature, color, moisture), and urine output. As shock progresses, the patient's neurologic status declines, urine output decreases, skin becomes cooler and mottled, and peripheral pulses diminish.

To understand the complexity of the patient's clinical status, integrate all of the assessment data. It is essential to obtain a brief history from the patient or caregiver, including a description of the events leading to the shock condition, time of onset and duration of symptoms, and a health history (e.g., medications, allergies, date of last tetanus vaccination, recent travel). In addition, obtain details regarding any care that the patient received before hospitalization.

◆ Nursing Diagnoses

Nursing diagnoses for the patient in shock may include, but are not limited to, the following:

- Ineffective peripheral tissue perfusion and risk for decreased cardiac tissue perfusion, ineffective cerebral tissue perfusion, ineffective renal perfusion, impaired liver function, and ineffective GI perfusion *related to* low blood flow or maldistribution of blood
- Anxiety *related to* severity of condition and hypoxemia

Additional information on nursing diagnoses for the patient with shock is presented in eNursing Care Plan 66-1 (available on the website for this chapter).

◆ Planning

The overall goals for a patient in shock include (1) evidence of adequate tissue perfusion, (2) restoration of normal or baseline BP, (3) recovery of organ function, (4) avoidance of complications from prolonged states of hypoperfusion, and

(5) prevention of health care–associated complications of disease management and care.

◆ Nursing Implementation

◆ Health Promotion.
You have an important role in the prevention of shock, beginning with the identification of patients at risk. In general, patients who are older, are immunocompromised, or have chronic illnesses are at an increased risk. Any person who has surgery or trauma is at risk for shock resulting from hemorrhage, spinal cord injury, sepsis, and other conditions (Table 66-1).

Planning is essential to help prevent shock after you identify an at-risk person. For example, a person with an acute anterior wall MI is at high risk for cardiogenic shock.[22] The primary goal for this patient is to limit the infarct size. This is done by restoring coronary blood flow through percutaneous coronary intervention, thrombolytic therapy, or surgical revascularization. Rest, analgesics, and sedation can reduce the myocardial demand for O_2. Modify the ICU environment to provide care at intervals that will not increase the patient's O_2 demand. For example, if the patient becomes tired with bathing, perform this care at a time that does not interfere with tests or other activities that may also increase O_2 demand.

A person with a severe allergy to things such as drugs, shellfish, insect bites, and latex is at increased risk for anaphylactic shock. This risk can be decreased if the patient is carefully questioned about allergies.

> ⚠ **SAFETY ALERT**   **Preventing Allergic Reactions**
> - Always confirm the patient's allergies before giving drugs or starting diagnostic procedures (e.g., CT scan with contrast media).
> - Premedicate (e.g., diphenhydramine, methylprednisolone) patients who need a drug to which they are at high risk for an allergic reaction (e.g., contrast media).
> - Encourage patients with allergies to obtain and wear a medical alert device and report their allergies to their HCPs.
> - Tell patients about the availability of kits that contain equipment and drugs (e.g., epinephrine [EpiPen]) for the treatment of acute allergic reactions.

Careful monitoring of fluid balance can help prevent hypovolemic shock. Ongoing monitoring of intake and output and daily weights is important. In addition, monitoring the patient's clinical status is essential because trends in clinical findings are more meaningful than any one piece of clinical information.

Carefully monitor all patients for the development of infection. Progression from an infection to sepsis and septic shock depends on the patient's defense mechanisms. Patients who are immunocompromised are at high risk for opportunistic infections. Strategies to decrease the risk of health care–associated infections (HAIs) include decreasing the number of invasive catheters (e.g., central lines, bladder catheters), using aseptic technique during invasive procedures, and paying strict attention to hand washing. In addition, all equipment must be changed per agency policy and thoroughly cleaned or discarded (if disposable) between patient use.

Evidence-based guidelines are available to reduce the risk of HAIs (e.g., ventilator-associated pneumonia, central line infections, catheter-associated urinary tract infections). These guidelines, called *care bundles,* outline key interventions aimed at reducing infections (see *http://www.ihi.org/topics/Bundles/Pages/default.aspx*).

◆ Acute Care.
Your role in shock involves (1) monitoring the patient's ongoing physical and emotional status, (2) identifying

trends to detect changes in the patient's condition, (3) planning and implementing nursing interventions and therapy, (4) evaluating the patient's response to therapy, (5) providing emotional support to the patient and caregiver, and (6) collaborating with other members of the interprofessional team to coordinate care (see Chapter 65).

◆ *Neurologic Status.* Assess the patient's neurologic status, including orientation and level of consciousness using a valid tool, at least every 1 to 2 hours. The patient's neurologic status is the best indicator of cerebral blood flow. Be aware of the clinical manifestations of neurologic involvement (e.g., changes in behavior, restlessness, hyperalertness, blurred vision, confusion, paresthesias). Note and report any subtle changes in the patient's mental status (e.g., mild agitation).

Orient the patient to person, place, time, and events on a regular basis. Orientation to the ICU environment is particularly important. Reduce noise and light levels to control sensory input. Keep a day-night cycle of activity and rest as much as possible. Sensory overload and disruption of the patient's diurnal cycle may contribute to delirium (see Chapter 65).

◆ *Cardiovascular Status.* Most of the therapy for shock is based on information about the patient's cardiovascular status. If the patient is unstable, continuously assess heart rate and rhythm, BP, CVP, and PA pressures, including CO, SVR, SV, and SVV (if available). (Chapter 65 discusses hemodynamic monitoring.) Monitoring trends in hemodynamic parameters provides more important information than single values. Integration of hemodynamic data with physical assessment data is essential in planning strategies to manage the patient with shock.

Patients in shock often have hypotension. The Trendelenburg (head-down) position should not be used to treat hypotension. Patients in this position may experience compromised pulmonary function and increased intracranial pressure.[23]

Continuously monitor the patient's ECG to detect dysrhythmias that may result from the cardiovascular and metabolic abnormalities associated with shock. Assess heart sounds for an S_3 or S_4 sound or new murmurs. An S_3 sound usually indicates heart failure.

In addition to monitoring the patient's cardiovascular status, give the prescribed therapy to correct the dysfunctions of the cardiovascular system. Assess the patient's response to fluid and drug administration as often as every 10 to 15 minutes. Make appropriate adjustments (e.g., drug titration) as needed. Once tissue perfusion is restored and the patient is stabilized, you can decrease the frequency of monitoring and slowly wean the patient off drugs to support BP and tissue perfusion.

❓ CHECK YOUR PRACTICE

A 69-yr-old male patient has just been transferred to the ICU from the emergency department with a diagnosis of sepsis. Your assessment indicates that he is confused with weak peripheral pulses and a BP of 84/50.
- What fluids would you expect to be ordered and what volume (amount) would you expect to be initially infused to improve his BP?
- In spite of aggressive fluid resuscitation, the patient remains hypotensive. What drug would you expect to be ordered to improve tissue perfusion?

◆ *Respiratory Status.* Frequently assess the respiratory status of the patient in shock to ensure adequate oxygenation, detect complications early, and provide data regarding the patient's acid-base status. Initially monitor the rate, depth, and rhythm of respirations as frequently as every 15 to 30 minutes. Increased rate and depth provide information regarding the patient's attempts to correct metabolic acidosis. Assess breath sounds every 1 to 2 hours and as needed for any changes that may indicate fluid overload or accumulation of secretions.

Use pulse oximetry to continuously monitor O_2 saturation. Pulse oximetry using a patient's finger may not be accurate in a shock state because of poor peripheral circulation. Instead, attach the probe to the ear, nose, or forehead (according to the manufacturer's guidelines). Arterial blood gases (ABGs) provide definitive information on ventilation and oxygenation status and acid-base balance. Initial interpretation of ABGs is often your responsibility. A PaO_2 below 60 mm Hg (in the absence of chronic lung disease) indicates hypoxemia and the need for higher O_2 concentrations or for a different mode of O_2 administration. Low $PaCO_2$ with a low pH and low bicarbonate level may indicate that the patient is attempting to compensate for metabolic acidosis from increasing lactate levels.

A rising $PaCO_2$ with a persistently low pH and PaO_2 indicates the need for advanced pulmonary management. Many patients in shock are intubated and on mechanical ventilation. Maintaining a patent airway and monitoring for ventilator-related complications are critical. (Chapter 65 discusses artificial airways and mechanical ventilation.)

◆ *Renal Status.* Initially, measure urine output every 1 to 2 hours to assess the adequacy of renal perfusion. Inserting an indwelling urinary catheter facilitates measurements during resuscitation. Urine output below 0.5 mL/kg/hr may indicate inadequate perfusion of the kidneys. Also use trends in serum creatinine values to assess renal function. Serum creatinine is a better indicator of renal function than BUN levels, since BUN is affected by the patient's catabolic state.

◆ *Body Temperature and Skin Changes.* Monitor temperature every 4 hours if normal. In the presence of an elevated or subnormal temperature, obtain hourly core temperatures (e.g., urinary, esophageal, or PA catheter). Use light covers and control the room temperature to keep the patient comfortably warm. If the patient's temperature rises above 101.5° F (38.6° C) and the patient becomes uncomfortable or experiences cardiovascular compromise, treat the fever with antipyretic drugs (e.g., ibuprofen, acetaminophen [Tylenol]) and remove some of the patient's covers. Consider a cooling device if fever persists despite treatment.

Monitor the patient's skin (e.g., upper and lower extremities) for signs of adequate perfusion. Changes in temperature, pallor, flushing, cyanosis, diaphoresis, and piloerection may indicate hypoperfusion.

◆ *Gastrointestinal Status.* Auscultate bowel sounds at least every 4 hours, and monitor for abdominal distention. If a nasogastric tube is present, measure drainage and check for occult blood. Similarly, check all stools for occult blood.

◆ *Personal Hygiene.* Hygiene is especially important for the patient in shock because impaired tissue perfusion predisposes the patient to skin breakdown and infection. Perform bathing and other nursing measures carefully because a patient in shock is experiencing problems with O_2 delivery to tissues. The increased O_2 demand that occurs during bathing and repositioning of patients with limited O_2 reserves makes the prevention of health care–associated pressure ulcers challenging. Turn the patient at least every 1 to 2 hours and maintain good body alignment to help prevent pressure ulcers. Use a pressure-relieving or pressure-reducing mattress or a specialty bed as needed.

Oral care for the patient in shock is essential because mucous membranes may become dry and fragile in the volume-depleted patient. In addition, the intubated patient usually has difficulty swallowing, resulting in pooled secretions in the mouth. Apply a water-soluble lubricant to the lips to prevent drying and cracking. Brush the patient's teeth or gums with a soft toothbrush every 12 hours, and swab the lips and oral mucosa with a moisturizing solution every 2 to 4 hours.[24] Perform passive range of motion three or four times a day to maintain joint mobility. Use good clinical judgment in determining priorities of care to limit the demands for increased O_2. Monitor trends in O_2 consumption (e.g., SpO_2, $ScvO_2/SvO_2$) during all nursing interventions to assess the patient's tolerance of activity.

Emotional Support and Comfort. Do not underestimate the effects of fear and anxiety when the patient and caregiver are faced with a critical, life-threatening situation (see Chapter 65). Fear, anxiety, and pain may aggravate respiratory distress and increase the release of catecholamines. When implementing care, monitor the patient's mental state and level of pain using valid assessment tools. Provide drugs to decrease anxiety and pain as appropriate. Continuous infusions of a benzodiazepine (e.g., lorazepam [Ativan]) and an opioid or sedative (e.g., morphine, propofol [Diprivan]) are extremely helpful in decreasing anxiety and pain.

Talk to the patient and encourage the caregiver to talk to the patient, even if the patient is intubated, is sedated, or appears comatose. Hearing is often the last sense to decrease. Even if the patient cannot respond, he or she may still be able to hear. If the intubated patient is capable of writing, provide a "magic slate" or a pencil and paper. Alphabet boards or signboards with common requests (e.g., turn, fan, lights) are also useful.

Give the patient simple explanations of all procedures before you carry them out, as well as information regarding the current plan of care. If the patient or caregiver asks questions about progress and prognosis, provide simple and honest answers.

Do not overlook the patient's spiritual needs. Patients may desire a visit from a chaplain, priest, rabbi, or minister. One way to provide support is to offer to call a member of the clergy rather than wait for the patient or caregiver to express a wish for spiritual counseling.

Caregivers can have a therapeutic effect on the patient by providing support and comfort. Caregivers (1) link the patient to the outside world; (2) facilitate decision making and advise the patient; (3) assist with activities of daily living; (4) act as liaisons to advise the health care team of the patient's wishes for care; and (5) provide safe, caring, familiar relationships for the patient.[25,26]

Most important, caregivers wish to be kept informed of the patient's condition. If possible, the same nurses should continually care for the patient to decrease anxiety, limit conflicting information, and increase trust. If the prognosis becomes grave, support the patient's caregiver when making difficult decisions such as withdrawing life support. The interprofessional care team must promote realistic expectations and outcomes. Remember, compassion is as essential as scientific and technical expertise in the total care of the patient and caregiver.

Ensure that the caregiver is able to spend time with the patient, provided the patient perceives this time as comforting. Explain in simple terms the purpose of any tubes and equipment attached to or surrounding the patient. Inform the caregivers of what they may and may not touch. If possible, place

---

CHECK YOUR PRACTICE

Your patient is a 74-yr-old man recovering from septic shock secondary to a perforated diverticulum. He has been in the ICU for 7 days, and his condition has finally stabilized. His wife has been at his bedside for the duration of his ICU stay. While caring for him, you suggest that she could take a brief walk and get some coffee. She bursts out with tears, "I can't leave him. You know that he almost died."

• How can you support this caregiver?

---

the patient's hands and arms outside the sheets to encourage therapeutic touch. Encourage caregivers to perform simple comfort measures if desired. Provide privacy as much as possible, but assure the patient and caregiver that assistance is readily available should it be needed. Position the call bell in reach of the patient or caregiver at all times.

Ambulatory Care. Rehabilitation of the patient who has experienced critical illness requires (1) correction of the precipitating cause, (2) prevention or early treatment of complications, and (3) teaching focused on disease management or prevention of recurrence based on the initial cause of shock. Continue to monitor the patient for indications of complications throughout the recovery period. These may include decreased range of motion, muscle weakness, decreased physical endurance, acute kidney injury (acute tubular necrosis) (see Chapter 46), and fibrotic lung disease (from ARDS) (see Chapter 67). Patients recovering from shock often require diverse services after discharge. These can include admission to transitional care units (e.g., for mechanical ventilation weaning), rehabilitation centers (inpatient or outpatient), or home health care agencies. Start planning for a safe transition from hospital to home as soon as the patient is admitted to the hospital.

Evaluation

The expected outcomes are that the patient who experiences shock will have:

• Adequate tissue perfusion with restoration of normal or baseline BP
• Normal organ function with no complications from hypoperfusion
• Decreased fear and anxiety and increased psychologic comfort

Additional information on expected outcomes for the patient with shock is presented in eNursing Care Plan 66-1 (available on the website for this chapter).

SYSTEMIC INFLAMMATORY RESPONSE SYNDROME AND MULTIPLE ORGAN DYSFUNCTION SYNDROME

Etiology and Pathophysiology

Systemic inflammatory response syndrome (SIRS) is a systemic inflammatory response to a variety of insults, including infection (referred to as *sepsis*), ischemia, infarction, and injury (Table 66-4). Generalized inflammation in organs remote from the initial insult characterizes SIRS.[10] A systemic inflammatory response can be triggered by many different mechanisms, including the following:

• Mechanical tissue trauma: Burns, crush injuries, surgical procedures
• Abscess formation: Intraabdominal, extremities
• Ischemic or necrotic tissue: Pancreatitis, vascular disease, MI

- Microbial invasion: Bacteria, viruses, fungi, parasites
- Endotoxin release: Gram-negative and gram-positive bacteria
- Global perfusion deficits: Postcardiac resuscitation, shock states
- Regional perfusion deficits: Distal perfusion deficits

Multiple organ dysfunction syndrome (MODS) is the failure of two or more organ systems in an acutely ill patient such that homeostasis cannot be maintained without intervention. MODS results from SIRS. These two syndromes represent the ends of a continuum. Transition from SIRS to MODS does not occur in a clear-cut manner[10] (Fig. 66-1).

Organ and Metabolic Dysfunction. When the inflammatory response is activated, consequences include the release of mediators, direct damage to the endothelium, and hypermetabolism. In addition, vascular permeability increases. This allows mediators and protein to leak out of the endothelium and into the interstitial space. White blood cells begin to digest the foreign debris, and the coagulation cascade is activated (see Chapter 29). Hypotension, decreased perfusion, microemboli, and redistributed or shunted blood flow eventually compromise organ perfusion.

The respiratory system is often the first system to show signs of dysfunction in SIRS and MODS.[10] Inflammatory mediators have a direct effect on the pulmonary vasculature. The endothelial damage from the release of inflammatory mediators causes increased capillary permeability. This causes movement of fluid from the pulmonary vasculature into the pulmonary interstitial spaces. The fluid then moves to the alveoli, causing alveolar edema. Type I pneumocytes (alveolar cells) are destroyed. Type II pneumocytes are damaged, and surfactant production is decreased. The alveoli collapse. This creates an increase in *shunt* (blood flow to the lungs that does not participate in gas exchange) and worsening ventilation-perfusion mismatch. The end result is ARDS. Patients with ARDS need aggressive pulmonary management with mechanical ventilation. (See Chapter 67 for a complete discussion of ARDS.)

Cardiovascular changes include myocardial depression and massive vasodilation in response to increasing tissue demands. Vasodilation results in decreased SVR and BP. The baroreceptor reflex causes release of *inotropic* (increasing force of contraction) and *chronotropic* (increasing heart rate) factors that enhance CO. To compensate for hypotension, CO increases by an increase in heart rate and SV. Increases in capillary permeability cause a shift of albumin and fluid out of the vascular space, further reducing venous return and thus preload. The patient becomes warm and tachycardic with a high CO and a low SVR. Other signs include decreased capillary refill, skin mottling, increased CVP and PAWP, and dysrhythmias. ScvO$_2$ or SvO$_2$ may be abnormally high because the patient is perfusing areas not consuming much O$_2$ (e.g., skin, nonworking muscle) while other areas may have blood shunted away from them. Eventually, either perfusion of vital organs becomes insufficient or the cells are unable to use O$_2$ and their function is further compromised.

Neurologic dysfunction commonly presents as mental status changes with SIRS and MODS. These acute changes can be an early sign of SIRS or MODS. The patient may become confused and agitated, combative, disoriented, lethargic, or comatose. These mental status changes may be due to hypoxemia, the effects of inflammatory mediators, or impaired perfusion.

Acute kidney injury (AKI) is frequently seen in SIRS and MODS. Hypoperfusion and the effects of the mediators can cause AKI. Decreased perfusion to the kidneys activates the SNS and the renin-angiotensin system. The stimulation of the renin-angiotensin system results in systemic vasoconstriction and aldosterone-mediated sodium and water reabsorption. Another risk factor for the development of AKI is the use of nephrotoxic drugs. Antibiotics commonly used to treat gram-negative bacteria (e.g., aminoglycosides) can be nephrotoxic. Careful monitoring of drug levels is essential to avoid the nephrotoxic effects.

The GI tract also plays a key role in the development of MODS. GI motility is often decreased in critical illness, causing abdominal distention and paralytic ileus. In the early stages of SIRS and MODS, blood is also shunted away from the GI mucosa, making it highly vulnerable to ischemic injury. Decreased perfusion leads to a breakdown of this normally protective mucosal barrier, thus increasing the risk for ulceration, GI bleeding, and bacterial movement from the GI tract into circulation.

Metabolic changes are pronounced in SIRS and MODS. Both syndromes trigger a hypermetabolic response. Glycogen stores are rapidly converted to glucose (glycogenolysis). Once glycogen is depleted, amino acids are converted to glucose (gluconeogenesis), reducing protein stores. Fatty acids are mobilized for fuel. Catecholamines and glucocorticoids are released and result in hyperglycemia and insulin resistance. The net result is a catabolic state, and lean body mass (muscle) is lost.

The hypermetabolism associated with SIRS and MODS may last for several days and results in liver dysfunction. Liver dysfunction in MODS may begin long before clinical evidence of it is present. Protein synthesis is impaired. The liver cannot make albumin, one of the key proteins in maintaining plasma oncotic pressure. Consequently, plasma oncotic pressure is altered, and fluid and protein leak from the vascular spaces to the interstitial space. Administration of albumin does not normalize oncotic pressure in these patients at this point.

As the state of hypermetabolism persists, the patient cannot convert lactate to glucose, and lactate accumulates (lactic acidosis). Despite increases in glycogenolysis and gluconeogenesis, eventually the liver is unable to maintain an adequate glucose level and the patient becomes hypoglycemic. Hypoglycemia can also develop due to acute adrenal insufficiency.

DIC may result from dysfunction of the coagulation system. DIC causes simultaneous microvascular clotting and bleeding because of the depletion of clotting factors and platelets in addition to excessive fibrinolysis. (Chapter 30 discusses DIC.)

Electrolyte imbalances are common and result from the hormonal and metabolic changes and fluid shifts. These changes worsen mental status changes, neuromuscular dysfunction, and dysrhythmias. The release of ADH and aldosterone results in sodium and water retention. Aldosterone increases urinary potassium loss, and catecholamines cause potassium to move into the cell, resulting in hypokalemia. Hypokalemia is associated with dysrhythmias and muscle weakness. Metabolic acidosis results from impaired tissue perfusion, hypoxia, and a shift to anaerobic metabolism with a resultant increase in lactate levels. Progressive renal dysfunction also contributes to metabolic acidosis. Hypocalcemia, hypomagnesemia, and hypophosphatemia are common.

Clinical Manifestations of SIRS and MODS

The clinical manifestations of SIRS and MODS are presented in Table 66-10.

TABLE 66-10   Manifestations and Management of SIRS and MODS

Manifestations	Management	Manifestations	Management
Respiratory System		**Renal System**	
Development of ARDS (see Chapter 67): • Severe dyspnea • Tachypnea • PaO_2/FIO_2 ratio <200 • Bilateral fluffy infiltrates on chest x-ray • PAWP <18 mm Hg • Ventilation-perfusion (V/Q) mismatch • Pulmonary hypertension • Increased minute ventilation • Decreased compliance • Refractory hypoxemia	Prevention Optimize O_2 delivery and minimize O_2 consumption Mechanical ventilation (see Chapter 65) • Positive end-expiratory pressure • Lung protective modes (e.g., pressure-control inverse ratio ventilation, low tidal volumes) • Permissive hypercapnia • Positioning (e.g., continuous lateral rotation therapy, prone positioning)	*Prerenal:* Renal hypoperfusion • BUN/creatinine ratio >20:1 • ↓ Urine Na^+ <20 mEq/L • ↑ Urine specific gravity >1.020 • ↑ Urine osmolality *Intrarenal:* Acute tubular necrosis • BUN/creatinine ratio <10:1-15:1 • ↑ Urine Na^+ >20 mEq/L • ↓ Urine osmolality • Urine specific gravity ~1.010	Diuretics • Loop diuretics (e.g., furosemide [Lasix]) • May need to increase dosage due to ↓ glomerular filtration rate Continuous renal replacement therapy (see Chapter 46)
Cardiovascular System		**Gastrointestinal System**	
Myocardial depression Massive vasodilation ↓ SVR, BP ↓ MAP ↑ HR, stroke volume ↑ CO Systolic, diastolic dysfunction Biventricular failure	Volume management • Central venous or PA catheter for hemodynamic monitoring • Minimally invasive hemodynamic monitoring • ↑ Preload via volume replacement • Arterial pressure monitoring • Maintain MAP >65 mm Hg Vasopressors Intermittent or continuous $ScvO_2$ or SvO_2 monitoring Balance O_2 supply and demand Continuous ECG monitoring Circulatory assist devices Venous thromboembolism prophylaxis	Mucosal ischemia • ↓ Intramucosal pH • Potential translocation of gut bacteria • Potential abdominal compartment syndrome Hypoperfusion → ↓ peristalsis, paralytic ileus Mucosal ulceration on endoscopy GI bleeding	Stress ulcer prophylaxis • Antacids (e.g., Maalox) • Proton pump inhibitors (e.g., omeprazole [Prilosec]) • sucralfate (Carafate) • Monitor abdominal distention, intraabdominal pressures • Dietary consultation • Enteral feedings • Stimulate mucosal activity • Provide essential nutrients and optimal calories
		Hepatic System	
		Bilirubin >2 mg/dL (34 µmol/L) ↑ Liver enzymes (ALT, AST, GGT) ↑ Serum NH_3 ↓ Serum albumin, prealbumin, transferrin Jaundice Hepatic encephalopathy	Maintain adequate tissue perfusion Provide nutritional support (e.g., enteral feedings) Careful use of drugs metabolized by liver
Central Nervous System		**Hematologic System**	
Acute change in neurologic status Fever Hepatic encephalopathy Seizures Confusion, disorientation, delirium Failure to wean, prolonged rehabilitation	Evaluate for hepatic or metabolic encephalopathy Optimize cerebral blood flow ↓ Cerebral O_2 requirements Prevent secondary tissue ischemia Calcium channel blockers (reduce cerebral vasospasm)	↑ Bleeding times, ↑ PT, ↑ PTT ↓ Platelet count (thrombocytopenia) ↑ Fibrin split products ↑ D-dimer	Observe for bleeding from obvious and/or occult sites Replace factors being lost (e.g., platelets) Minimize traumatic interventions (e.g., IM injections, multiple venipunctures)
Endocrine System			
Hyperglycemia → hypoglycemia	Provide continuous infusion of insulin and glucose to maintain blood glucose 140-180 mg/dL (7.77-10.0 mmol/L)		

ALT, Alanine aminotransferase; *APCO,* arterial pressure–based cardiac output; *ARDS,* acute respiratory distress syndrome; *AST,* aspartate aminotransferase; *BUN,* blood urea nitrogen; *CO,* cardiac output; *GGT,* γ-glutamyl transferase; *MAP,* mean arterial pressure; *NH₃,* ammonia; *PA,* pulmonary artery; *PAWP,* pulmonary artery wedge pressure; *PT,* prothrombin time; *PTT,* partial thromboplastin time; *ScvO₂,* O_2 saturation in venous blood; *SvO₂,* O_2 saturation in mixed venous blood; *SVR,* systemic vascular resistance.

❖ NURSING AND INTERPROFESSIONAL MANAGEMENT: SIRS AND MODS

The prognosis for the patient with MODS is poor, with mortality rates of 70% to 80% when three or more organ systems fail.[10] The most common cause of death continues to be sepsis. Survival improves with *early, goal-directed therapy.*[10] Therefore the most important goal is to prevent the progression of SIRS to MODS.

A critical part of your role is vigilant assessment and ongoing monitoring to detect early signs of deterioration or organ dysfunction. Interprofessional care for patients with SIRS and MODS focuses on (1) prevention and treatment of infection, (2) maintenance of tissue oxygenation, (3) nutritional and metabolic support, and (4) appropriate support of individual failing organs. Table 66-10 summarizes the management for patients with SIRS and MODS.

◆ Prevention and Treatment of Infection

Aggressive infection control strategies are essential to decrease the risk for HAIs. Early, aggressive surgery is recommended to remove necrotic tissue (e.g., early debridement of burn tissue) that can provide a culture medium for microorganisms. Aggressive pulmonary management, including early mobilization, can reduce the risk of infection. Strict asepsis can decrease infections related to intraarterial lines, endotracheal tubes, indwelling urinary catheters, IV lines, and other invasive devices or procedures. Daily assessment of the ongoing need for invasive lines and other devices is an important strategy to prevent or limit HAIs.

Despite aggressive strategies, infection may develop. Once an infection is suspected, begin interventions to treat the cause. Send appropriate cultures and start broad-spectrum antibiotic therapy, as ordered. Adjust therapy based on the culture results, if needed.

◆ Maintenance of Tissue Oxygenation

Hypoxemia frequently occurs in patients with SIRS and MODS. These patients have greater O_2 needs and decreased O_2 supply to the tissues. Interventions that decrease O_2 demand and increase O_2 delivery are essential. Sedation, mechanical ventilation, analgesia, and rest may decrease O_2 demand and should be considered. O_2 delivery may be optimized by using individualized tidal volumes with positive end-expiratory pressure, increasing preload (e.g., fluids) or myocardial contractility to enhance CO, or reducing afterload to increase CO.

◆ Nutritional and Metabolic Needs

Hypermetabolism in SIRS or MODS can result in profound weight loss, cachexia, and further organ failure. Protein-calorie malnutrition is one of the primary signs of hypermetabolism in SIRS and MODS. Total energy expenditure is often increased 1.5 to 2.0 times the normal metabolic rate. Because of their relatively short half-life, monitor plasma transferrin and prealbumin levels to assess hepatic protein synthesis.

The goal of nutritional support is to preserve organ function. Providing early and optimal nutrition decreases morbidity and mortality rates in patients with SIRS and MODS. The enteral route is preferred. If it cannot be used, parenteral nutrition should be considered.[16] (Chapter 39 discusses enteral and parenteral nutrition.) Provide glycemic control with a goal of 140 to 180 mg/dL with insulin infusions in these patients.[10,16]

◆ Support of Failing Organs

Support of any failing organ is a primary goal of therapy. For example, the patient with ARDS requires aggressive O_2 therapy and mechanical ventilation (see Chapter 67). DIC should be treated appropriately (e.g., blood products) (see Chapter 30). Renal failure may require dialysis. Continuous renal replacement therapy is better tolerated than hemodialysis, especially in a patient with hemodynamic instability (see Chapter 46).

A final consideration may be that further interventions are futile. It is important to maintain communication between the health care team and the patient's caregiver regarding realistic goals and likely outcomes for the patient with MODS. Withdrawal of life support and starting end-of-life care may be the best options for the patient.

CASE STUDY

Shock

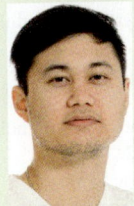
(©Thinkstock)

Patient Profile

K.L., a 25-yr-old Korean American, was not wearing his seat belt when he was the driver involved in a motor vehicle crash. The windshield was broken and K.L. was found 10 ft from his car. He was face down, conscious, and moaning. His wife and daughter were found in the car with their seat belts on. They sustained minor injuries and were very frightened and upset. All passengers were taken to the emergency department (ED). The following information pertains to K.L.

Subjective Data

- States, "I can't breathe"
- Cries out when abdomen is palpated

Objective Data

Physical Examination

- *Cardiovascular:* BP 80/56 mm Hg; apical pulse 138 but no palpable radial or pedal pulses; carotid pulse present but weak
  - ECG as follows:

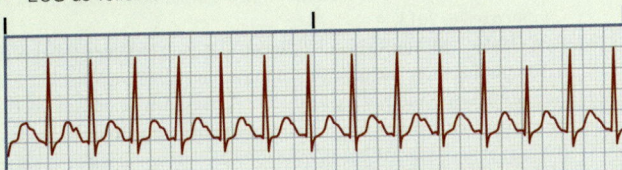

- *Respiratory:* respiratory rate 35 breaths/minute; labored breathing with shallow respirations; asymmetric chest wall movement; absence of breath sounds on left side
  - Trachea deviated slightly to the right
- *Abdomen:* slightly distended and left upper quadrant painful on palpation
- *Musculoskeletal:* open compound fracture of the lower left leg

Diagnostic Studies

- Chest x-ray: Hemothorax and six rib fractures on left side
- Hematocrit: 28%

Interprofessional Care (in the ED)

- Intraosseous access in right proximal tibia placed prehospital
- Left chest tube placed, draining bright red blood
- Fluid resuscitation started with crystalloids
- High-flow O_2 via non-rebreather mask

Emergency Surgical Procedures

- Splenectomy
- Repair of torn intercostal artery
- Repair of compound fracture

Discussion Questions

1. What types of shock is K.L. experiencing? What clinical manifestations did he display that support your answer?
2. What were the causes of K.L.'s shock states? What are other causes of these types of shock?
3. **Priority Decision:** What are the priority nursing responsibilities for K.L.?
4. **Priority Decision:** What ongoing nursing assessment parameters are essential for this patient?
5. What are his potential complications?
6. **Patient-Centered Care:** K.L.'s parents arrive. English is their second language. They are very anxious and asking about their son. What can you do to provide culturally competent family-centered care?
7. **Priority Decision:** Based on the assessment data presented, what are the priority nursing diagnoses?
8. **Teamwork and Collaboration:** Identify the tasks that could be delegated to unlicensed assistive personnel (UAP).
9. **Evidence-Based Practice:** You are orienting a new graduate RN. He asks you why crystalloids are used instead of colloids for fluid resuscitation. What is your response?

Answers available at *http://evolve.elsevier.com/Lewis/medsurg.*

BRIDGE TO NCLEX EXAMINATION

The number of the question corresponds to the same-numbered outcome at the beginning of the chapter.

1. A patient has a spinal cord injury at T4. Vital signs include falling blood pressure with bradycardia. The nurse recognizes that the patient is experiencing
   a. a relative hypervolemia.
   b. an absolute hypovolemia.
   c. neurogenic shock from low blood flow.
   d. neurogenic shock from massive vasodilation.

2. A 78-yr-old man has confusion and temperature of 104°F (40°C). He is a diabetic with purulent drainage from his right heel. After an infusion of 3 L of normal saline solution, his assessment findings are BP 84/40 mm Hg; heart rate 110; respiratory rate 42 and shallow; CO 8 L/minute; and PAWP 4 mm Hg. This patient's symptoms are *most* likely indicative of
   a. sepsis.
   b. septic shock.
   c. multiple organ dysfunction syndrome.
   d. systemic inflammatory response syndrome.

3. Appropriate treatment modalities for the management of cardiogenic shock include *(select all that apply)*
   a. dobutamine to increase myocardial contractility.
   b. vasopressors to increase systemic vascular resistance.
   c. circulatory assist devices such as an intraaortic balloon pump.
   d. corticosteroids to stabilize the cell wall in the infarcted myocardium.
   e. Trendelenburg positioning to facilitate venous return and increase preload.

4. The *most* accurate assessment parameters for the nurse to use to determine adequate tissue perfusion in the patient with MODS are
   a. blood pressure, pulse, and respirations.
   b. breath sounds, blood pressure, and body temperature.
   c. pulse pressure, level of consciousness, and pupillary response.
   d. level of consciousness, urine output, and skin color and temperature.

1. d, 2. b, 3. a, c, 4. d

For rationales to these answers and even more NCLEX review questions, visit *http://evolve.elsevier.com/Lewis/medsurg*.

EVOLVE WEBSITE

http://evolve.elsevier.com/Lewis/medsurg
Review Questions (Online Only)
Key Points
Answer Keys to Questions
- Rationales for Bridge to NCLEX Examination Questions
- Answer Guidelines for Case Study on p. 1607
Student Case Studies
- Patient With Acute Pancreatitis and Septic Shock
- Patient With Cardiogenic Shock
- Patient With Sepsis
Nursing Care Plan
- eNursing Care Plan 66-1: Patient in Shock
Conceptual Care Map Creator
Audio Glossary
Content Updates

REFERENCES

1. Dries D, Sarani B: Diagnosis and management of shock. In Dries DJ, editor: *Guide for fundamental critical care support*, ed 5, Mount Pleasant, Ill, 2012, Society of Critical Care Medicine.
2. Galeski DF: Definition, classification, etiology, and pathophysiology of shock in adults. 2015. Retrieved from *www.uptodate.com+definition-classification-etiology-and-pathophysiology-of-shock-in-adults*.
3. Patel AK, Hollenberg SM: Cardiovascular failure and cardiogenic shock, *Semin Respir Crit Care Med* 22:598, 2011.
4. Shabana A, Moustafa M, El-Menyar A, et al: Cardiogenic shock complicating myocardial infarction: an updated review, *Br J Med Res* 3:622, 2013.
5. Mandel J, Palevsky PM: Treatment of severe hypovolemia or hypovolemic shock in adults, 2015. Retrieved from *www.uptodate.com/contents/treatment-of-severe-hypovolemia-or-hypovolemic-shock-in-adults*.
*6. Casha S, Christie S: A systematic review of intensive cardiopulmonary management after spinal cord injury, *J Neurotrauma* 28:1479, 2011.
*7. Simons FF, Ardusso LR, Dimov V, et al: World Allergy Organization Anaphylaxis Guidelines: 2013 update of the evidence base, *Int Arch Allergy Immunol* 162:193, 2013.
8. Zilberstein J, McCurdy MT, Winters ME: Anaphylaxis, *J Emerg Med* 47:182, 2014.
*9. Singer M, Deutschman CS, Seymour CW, et al: The third international consensus definitions for sepsis and septic shock (Sepsis-3), *JAMA* 315:801, 2016.
*10. Dellinger RP, Levy MM, Rhodes A, et al: Surviving sepsis campaign: international guidelines for management of severe sepsis and septic shock: 2012, *Crit Care Med* 41:50, 2013.

11. Leeper B: Cardiovascular system. In Burns S, editor: *AACN essentials of critical care nursing*, ed 3, New York, 2014, McGraw-Hill Education.
12. Strickler J: Halt the downward spiral of traumatic hypovolemic shock, *Nurs Crit Care* 7:42, 2012.
13. Finfer SR, Vincent JL: Resuscitation fluids, *N Engl J Med* 369:1243, 2013.
*14. Patel A, Laffan MA, Waheed U, et al: Randomized trials of albumin for adults with sepsis: systematic review and meta-analysis with trial sequential analysis of all-cause mortality, *BMJ* 349:g4561, 2014.
15. Marik PE, Monnet X, Teboul J: Hemodynamic parameters to guide fluid therapy, *Ann Intensive Care* 1:1, 2011.
16. Casaer MP, Van den Berghe G: Nutrition in the acute phase of critical illness, *N Engl J Med* 370:1227, 2014.
17. Myers TJ: Temporary ventricular assist devices in the intensive care unit as a bridge to decision, *AACN Adv Crit Care* 23:55, 2012.
*18. Surviving Sepsis Campaign: Updated bundles in response to new evidence, 2015. Retrieved from *www.survivingsepsis.org/SiteCollectionDocuments/SSC_Bundle.pdf*.
*19. Ferrer R, Martin-Loeches I, Phillips G, et al: Empiric antibiotic treatment reduces mortality in severe sepsis and septic shock from the first hour: results from a guideline-based performance improvement program, *Crit Care Med* 42:1749, 2014.
*20. Finfer S, Blair D, Bellomo R, et al: Intensive versus conventional glucose control in critically ill patients, *N Engl J Med* 360:1283, 2009. (Classic)
21. Hurlbert RJ, Hadley MN, Walters BC, et al: Pharmacological therapy for acute spinal cord injury, *Neurosurgery* 72:93, 2013.
*22. O'Gara PT, Kushner FG, Ascheim DD, et al: 2013 ACCF/AHA guideline for the management of ST-elevation myocardial infarction, *J Am Coll Cardiol* 61:e78, 2013.
23. Flynn Makic MB, VonRueden KT, Rauen CA, et al: Evidence-based practice habits: putting more sacred cows out to pasture, *Crit Care Nurse* 31:31, 2011.
*24. American Association of Critical-Care Nurses: AACN practice alert: oral care for patients at risk for ventilator-associated pneumonia. Retrieved from *www.aacn.org/wd/practice/docs/practicealerts/oral-care-patients-at-risk-vap.pdf*.
*25. American Association of Critical-Care Nurses: AACN practice alert: family presence during resuscitation and invasive procedures. Retrieved from *www.aacn.org/wd/practice/docs/practicealerts/family-presence-during-resuscitation-invasive-procedures.pdf*.
*26. American Association of Critical-Care Nurses: AACN practice alert: family presence: visitation in the adult ICU. Retrieved from *www.aacn.org/WD/practice/docs/practicealerts/family-visitation-adult-icu-practicealert.pdf*

*Evidence-based information for clinical practice.

67

Acute Respiratory Failure and Acute Respiratory Distress Syndrome

Richard Arbour

> *Hope lies in dreams, in imagination, and in the courage of those who dare to make dreams into reality.*
>
> *Jonas Salk*

http://evolve.elsevier.com/Lewis/medsurg/

LEARNING OUTCOMES

1. Compare the pathophysiologic mechanisms and clinical manifestations that result in hypoxemic and hypercapnic respiratory failure.
2. Differentiate between the nursing and interprofessional management of the patient with hypoxemic or hypercapnic respiratory failure.
3. Relate the pathophysiologic mechanisms and clinical manifestations associated with acute respiratory failure and acute respiratory distress syndrome (ARDS).
4. Select appropriate nursing and interprofessional interventions for the patient with ARDS.
5. Prioritize measures to prevent or reverse complications that can result from acute respiratory failure or ARDS.

KEY TERMS

acute respiratory distress syndrome (ARDS), p. 1620
acute respiratory failure, p. 1609
alveolar hypoventilation, p. 1612

hypercapnia, p. 1609
hypercapnic respiratory failure, p. 1610
hypoxemia, p. 1609
hypoxemic respiratory failure, p. 1609

hypoxia, p. 1613
refractory hypoxemia, p. 1621
shunt, p. 1611
work of breathing (WOB), p. 1613

This chapter discusses the etiology, pathophysiology, and clinical manifestations of acute respiratory failure and acute respiratory distress syndrome (ARDS). Nursing and interprofessional management of patients with acute respiratory failure and ARDS focus on interventions to promote adequate oxygenation and ventilation while addressing the underlying causes.

ACUTE RESPIRATORY FAILURE

The major function of the respiratory system is gas exchange. This involves the transfer of O_2 and CO_2 between atmospheric air and circulating blood within the pulmonary capillary bed (Fig. 67-1). **Acute respiratory failure** results when one or both of these gas-exchanging functions are inadequate (e.g., insufficient O_2 is transferred to the blood or inadequate CO_2 is removed from the lungs).

Conditions that interfere with adequate O_2 transfer result in **hypoxemia**. This causes a decrease in arterial O_2 (PaO_2) and saturation (SaO_2). Insufficient CO_2 removal results in **hypercapnia**. This causes an increase in arterial CO_2 ($PaCO_2$).[1]

Arterial blood gases (ABGs) are used to assess changes in pH, PaO_2, $PaCO_2$, bicarbonate, and SaO_2. Pulse oximetry is used intermittently or continuously to assess arterial O_2 saturation (SpO_2).

Acute respiratory failure is not a disease but a symptom of underlying pathology affecting lung function. When respiratory function is insufficient, O_2 delivery, cardiac output (CO), clinical assessment findings, and/or baseline metabolic state may exhibit abnormalities specific to the affected body system(s). It is a condition that occurs because of one or more disorders involving the lungs or other body systems (Table 67-1).

Respiratory failure is classified as hypoxemic or hypercapnic (Fig. 67-2). Hypoxemic respiratory failure is also referred to as *oxygenation failure* because the primary problem is inadequate O_2 transfer between the alveoli and pulmonary capillaries. Although no universal definition exists, **hypoxemic respiratory failure** is commonly defined as a PaO_2 less than 60 mm Hg when the patient is receiving an inspired O_2 concentration of 60% or more. This definition incorporates two important concepts: (1) the PaO_2 level indicates inadequate O_2 saturation of

Reviewed by Susan J. Eisel, RN, MSEd, Associate Professor of Nursing, Mercy College of Ohio, Toledo, Ohio; Eugene E. Mondor, RN, MN, CNCC(C), Clinical Nurse Educator, Royal Alexandra Hospital, Edmonton, Alberta, Canada; and Julie Rogan, RN, MSN, ACCNS-AG, AOCNS, CCRN, Clinical Nurse Specialist, Medical Intensive Care Unit, Thomas Jefferson University Hospital, Philadelphia, Pennsylvania.

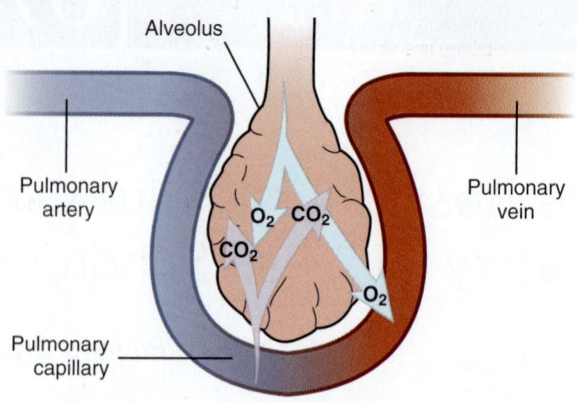

FIG. 67-1 Normal gas exchange unit in the lung.

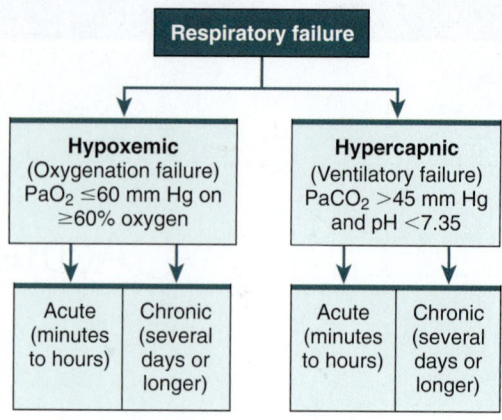

FIG. 67-2 Classification of respiratory failure.

TABLE 67-1 Causes of Hypoxemic and Hypercapnic Respiratory Failure*	
Hypoxemic Respiratory Failure	**Hypercapnic Respiratory Failure**
Respiratory System	**Respiratory System**
• Acute respiratory distress syndrome (ARDS)	• Asthma
• Pneumonia	• COPD
• Toxic inhalation (e.g., smoke inhalation)	• Cystic fibrosis
• Hepatopulmonary syndrome (e.g., low-resistance flow state, V/Q mismatch)	**Central Nervous System**
	• Brainstem injury or infarction
	• Sedative and opioid overdose
• Massive pulmonary embolism (e.g., thrombus emboli, fat emboli)	• Spinal cord injury
	• Severe head injury
• Pulmonary artery laceration and hemorrhage	**Chest Wall**
	• Thoracic trauma (e.g., flail chest)
• Inflammatory state and related alveolar injury	• Kyphoscoliosis
	• Pain
Cardiac System	• Severe obesity
• Anatomic shunt (e.g., ventricular septal defect)	**Neuromuscular System**
	• Myasthenia gravis
• Cardiogenic pulmonary edema	• Critical illness polyneuropathy
	• Acute myopathy
• Shock (decreasing blood flow through pulmonary vasculature)	• Toxin exposure or ingestion (e.g., tree tobacco, acetylcholinesterase inhibitors, carbamate or organophosphate poisoning)
• High cardiac output states: diffusion limitation	• Amyotrophic lateral sclerosis
	• Phrenic nerve injury
	• Guillain-Barré syndrome
	• Poliomyelitis
	• Muscular dystrophy
	• Multiple sclerosis

*List is not all-inclusive.

hemoglobin and (2) this PaO₂ level exists despite giving supplemental O₂ at a percentage (60%) that is about three times that in room air (21%).

Hypercapnic respiratory failure is also referred to as *ventilatory failure* because the primary problem is insufficient CO_2 removal. Hypercapnic respiratory failure is commonly defined as a $PaCO_2$ greater than 45 mm Hg in combination with acidemia (arterial pH less than 7.35). This definition incorporates three important concepts: (1) the $PaCO_2$ is higher than normal, (2) there is evidence of the body's inability to compensate for this increase (acidemia), and (3) the pH is at a level where a further decrease may lead to severe acid-base imbalance. (See Chapter 16 for a discussion of acid-base balance.) Numerous

disorders can compromise lung ventilation and subsequent CO_2 removal[2] (Table 67-1).

Patients may experience both hypoxemic and hypercapnic respiratory failure at the same time.[3] For example, a patient with chronic obstructive pulmonary disease (COPD) who develops pulmonary edema could be experiencing both acute and chronic respiratory failure. Always interpret patient-specific data within the context of your assessment findings and the patient's baseline (when known). A person with COPD who develops pneumonia may have a higher baseline $PaCO_2$. This information should be used for interpreting ABGs and other patient data.

Etiology and Pathophysiology

Hypoxemic Respiratory Failure. Four physiologic mechanisms may cause hypoxemia and subsequent hypoxemic respiratory failure: (1) mismatch between ventilation (V) and perfusion (Q), commonly referred to as V/Q mismatch; (2) shunt; (3) diffusion limitation; and (4) alveolar hypoventilation. The most common causes are V/Q mismatch and shunt.

Ventilation-Perfusion Mismatch. In normal lungs the volume of blood perfusing the lungs each minute (4 to 5 L) is approximately equal to the amount of gas that reaches the alveoli each minute (4 to 5 L). In a perfectly matched system, each portion of the lung would receive 1 mL of air (ventilation) for each 1 mL of blood flow (perfusion). This match of ventilation and perfusion would result in a V/Q ratio of 1:1, which is expressed as V/Q = 1. When the match is not 1:1, a *V/Q mismatch* occurs.

Although this example implies that ventilation and perfusion are ideally matched in all areas of the lung, this situation does not normally exist. In reality, some regional mismatch occurs. At the lung apex, V/Q ratios are greater than 1 (more ventilation than perfusion). At the lung base, V/Q ratios are less than 1 (less ventilation than perfusion). Because changes at the lung apex balance changes at the base, the net effect is a close overall match (Fig. 67-3).

Many diseases and conditions cause V/Q mismatch (Fig. 67-4). The most common are those in which increased secretions are present in the airways (e.g., COPD) or alveoli (e.g., pneumonia), and in which bronchospasm is present (e.g., asthma).[2] V/Q mismatch may also result from alveolar collapse (*atelectasis*) or as a result of pain.

Pain interferes with chest and abdominal wall movement, increases muscle tension, and produces generalized muscle rigidity. This often compromises ventilation. Pain also activates

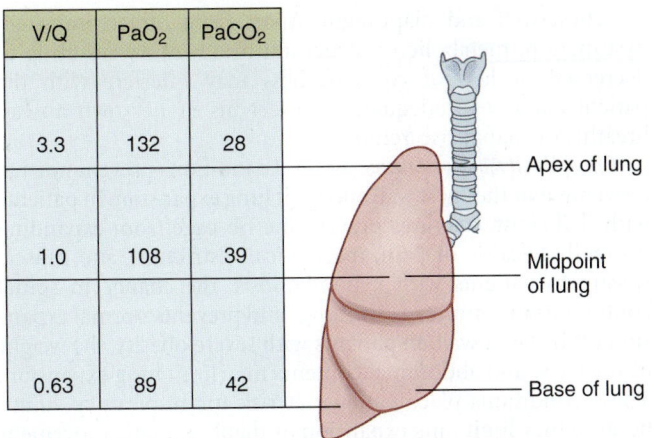

V/Q	PaO$_2$	PaCO$_2$
3.3	132	28
1.0	108	39
0.63	89	42

- Apex of lung
- Midpoint of lung
- Base of lung

FIG. 67-3 Regional V/Q differences in the normal lung. This difference causes the PaO$_2$ to be higher at the apex of the lung and lower at the base. Values for PaCO$_2$ are the opposite (i.e., lower at the apex and higher at the base). Blood that exits the lung is a mixture of these values.

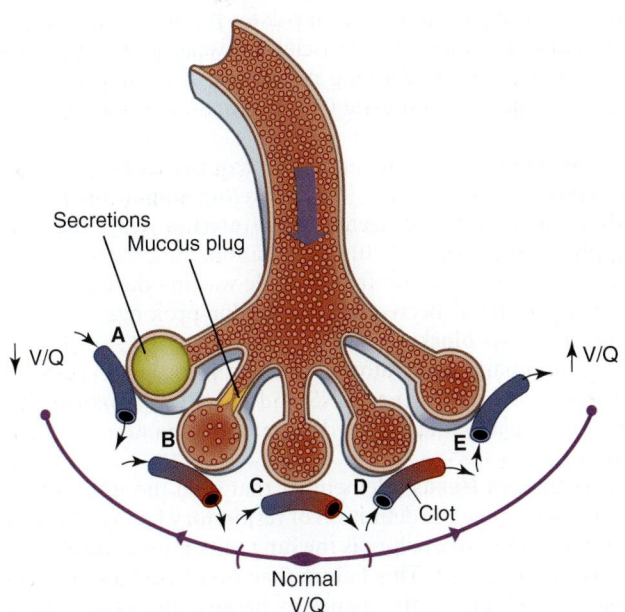

Secretions
Mucous plug
↓ V/Q
A
B
C
D
E
Clot
↑ V/Q
Normal V/Q

FIG. 67-4 Range of ventilation-to-perfusion (V/Q) relationships. *A*, Absolute shunt, no ventilation because of fluid filling the alveoli. *B*, V/Q mismatch, ventilation partially compromised by secretions in the airway. *C*, Normal lung unit. *D*, V/Q mismatch, perfusion partially compromised by emboli obstructing blood flow. *E*, Dead space, no perfusion because of obstruction of the pulmonary capillary.

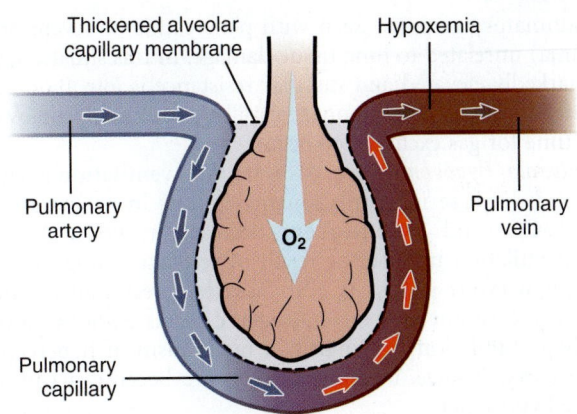

Thickened alveolar capillary membrane
Hypoxemia
Pulmonary artery
Pulmonary vein
Pulmonary capillary
O$_2$

FIG. 67-5 Diffusion limitation. Exchange of CO$_2$ and O$_2$ cannot occur because of the thickened alveolar-capillary membrane.

the stress response, increasing baseline metabolic state. It may increase O$_2$ consumption and CO$_2$ production.[4] With a significant increase in metabolic rate, O$_2$ is consumed and CO$_2$ (as a by-product of cell/tissue metabolism) is increased. In this case, increased O$_2$ demand and CO$_2$ production may increase ventilation demands. All these conditions result in limited airflow *(ventilation)* to alveoli but have no effect on blood flow *(perfusion)* to the gas exchange units (Fig. 67-1). The consequence of the imbalance is V/Q mismatch.

A pulmonary embolus affects the perfusion portion of the V/Q relationship. The embolus limits blood flow distal to the occlusion. When a pulmonary embolus occurs, areas of normal lung ventilation remain but have significantly decreased perfusion resulting from the vessel occlusion. This results in a V/Q

mismatch[5] (Fig. 67-4). If large enough, the embolus can cause hemodynamic compromise due to the blockage of a large pulmonary artery.

O$_2$ therapy is an appropriate first step to reverse hypoxemia caused by V/Q mismatch, even though not all gas exchange units are affected equally. O$_2$ therapy increases the PaO$_2$ in blood leaving normal gas exchange units, thus causing a higher-than-normal PaO$_2$. The well-oxygenated blood mixes with poorly oxygenated blood, raising the overall PaO$_2$ of blood leaving the lungs. The best approach to treat hypoxemia caused by a V/Q mismatch is aimed at the cause.

Shunt. A **shunt** occurs when blood exits the heart without having participated in gas exchange. A shunt can be viewed as an extreme V/Q mismatch (Fig. 67-4). There are two types of shunt: anatomic and intrapulmonary. An *anatomic shunt* occurs when blood passes through an anatomic channel in the heart (e.g., a ventricular septal defect) and bypasses the lungs. An *intrapulmonary shunt* occurs when blood flows through the pulmonary capillaries without participating in gas exchange. An intrapulmonary shunt is seen in conditions in which the alveoli fill with fluid (e.g., acute respiratory distress syndrome [ARDS], pneumonia) and gas exchange is limited at the alveolar-capillary membrane.

O$_2$ therapy alone is often ineffective at increasing the PaO$_2$ if hypoxemia is due to a shunt. Patients with a shunt are usually more hypoxemic than patients with V/Q mismatch. They often require mechanical ventilation and a high fraction of inspired O$_2$ (FIO$_2$) to improve gas exchange.

Diffusion Limitation. *Diffusion limitation* occurs when gas exchange across the alveolar-capillary membrane is compromised by a process that thickens, damages, or destroys the alveolar membrane or affects blood flow through the pulmonary capillaries (Fig. 67-5). Diffusion limitation is worsened by disease states affecting the pulmonary vascular bed, such as severe COPD or recurrent pulmonary emboli. Some disease states cause the alveolar-capillary membrane to become thicker (fibrotic), which slows gas transport. These include pulmonary fibrosis, interstitial lung disease, and ARDS.

The classic sign of diffusion limitation is hypoxemia that is present during exercise but not at rest. During exercise, blood moves more rapidly through the lungs. This decreases the time for diffusion of O$_2$ across the alveolar-capillary membrane. Diffusion limitation may also occur in a high CO state (e.g., hepatopulmonary syndrome) or other disease states (e.g., inflammatory response seen with pancreatitis or severe brain trauma) unrelated to lung tissue damage. In this situation, CO is markedly elevated and vascular resistance is low. Blood circulates through the pulmonary capillary bed rapidly, allowing less time for gas exchange to occur.[6]

Alveolar Hypoventilation. **Alveolar hypoventilation** is a generalized decrease in ventilation that results in an increase in the $PaCO_2$ and a consequent decrease in PaO_2. Alveolar hypoventilation may be the result of restrictive lung diseases, central nervous system (CNS) diseases, chest wall dysfunction, acute asthma, or neuromuscular diseases. Although alveolar hypoventilation is primarily a mechanism of hypercapnic respiratory failure, it is mentioned here because it can also cause hypoxemia.

Interrelationship of Mechanisms. Frequently, hypoxemic respiratory failure is caused by a combination of two or more of the following: V/Q mismatch, shunt, diffusion limitation, and alveolar hypoventilation. For example, the patient with acute respiratory failure secondary to pneumonia may have a combination of V/Q mismatch and shunt. In this case, inflammation, edema, and hypersecretion of exudate within the bronchioles and gas exchange units obstruct the airways (V/Q mismatch) and fill the alveoli with exudate (shunt). Additional contributing factors to hypoxemic respiratory failure include increases in O_2 demand such as with anxiety or agitation and unrelieved pain.

Hypercapnic Respiratory Failure.
Hypercapnic respiratory failure is sometimes called *ventilatory failure*. When CO_2 levels cannot be maintained within normal limits by the respiratory system, one of two primary problems exists: (1) an increase in CO_2 production or (2) a decrease in alveolar ventilation. Hypercapnic respiratory failure may also be acute or chronic in nature. For example, a patient who experiences sudden onset of decreased level of consciousness due to drug overdose may not ventilate appropriately, producing an acute increase in CO_2 levels. Overall, hypercapnia often reflects substantial lung dysfunction.

Many different conditions can cause a limitation in ventilatory supply (Table 67-1). These can be grouped into four categories: (1) abnormalities of the airways and alveoli, (2) abnormalities of the CNS, (3) abnormalities of the chest wall, and (4) neuromuscular conditions.

Airway and Alveoli Abnormalities. Patients with asthma, COPD, and cystic fibrosis are at high risk for hypercapnic respiratory failure because the underlying pathophysiology of these conditions results in airflow obstruction and air trapping. Ultimately respiratory muscle fatigue and ventilatory failure occur due to the additional work needed to inspire adequate tidal volumes against increased airway resistance and air trapped within the alveoli.[7]

Central Nervous System Abnormalities. A variety of CNS problems may suppress the drive to breathe. A common example is an overdose of a respiratory depressant drug (e.g., opioids, benzodiazepines). In a dose-related manner, CNS depressants decrease CO_2 reactivity in the brainstem. This allows arterial CO_2 levels to rise. A brainstem infarction or severe head injury may also interfere with normal function of the respiratory center in the medulla. Patients with these conditions are at risk for respiratory failure because the medulla does not alter the respiratory rate in response to a change in $PaCO_2$.

CNS dysfunction may also include high-level spinal cord injuries that limit nerve supply to the respiratory muscles of the chest wall and diaphragm. Apart from direct brainstem dysfunction, metabolic or structural brain injury resulting in decreased or loss of consciousness may interfere with the patient's ability to adequately protect his or her own airway, breathe, or manage secretions.

Chest Wall Abnormalities. Several conditions prevent normal movement of the chest wall and limit lung expansion. In patients with flail chest, fractures prevent the rib cage from expanding normally because of pain, mechanical restriction, and muscle spasm. In patients with kyphoscoliosis, the change in spinal configuration compresses the lungs and prevents normal expansion of the chest wall. In patients with severe obesity, the weight of the chest and abdominal contents may limit lung expansion. These conditions place patients at risk for respiratory failure because they limit lung expansion or diaphragmatic movement and consequently gas exchange.

Neuromuscular Conditions. Various types of neuromuscular diseases may result in respiratory muscle weakness or paralysis (Table 67-1). For example, patients with Guillain-Barré syndrome, muscular dystrophy, myasthenia gravis (acute exacerbation), or multiple sclerosis are at risk for respiratory failure. This is because the respiratory muscles are weakened or paralyzed as a result of the underlying neuromuscular condition. Thus they are unable to eliminate CO_2 and maintain normal $PaCO_2$ levels.[8]

Neuromuscular disorders may be acquired as a consequence of exposure to toxins (e.g., carbamate/organophosphate pesticides, chemical nerve agents) that interfere with the nerve supply to muscles and lung ventilation. Respiratory muscle weakness may also result from muscle wasting during a critical illness, peripheral nerve damage, and/or prolonged effects of neuromuscular blocking agents.

In summary, respiratory failure can occur in three of these four categories (i.e., CNS and chest wall abnormalities, neuromuscular conditions) despite the presence of normal lungs.

Tissue Oxygen Needs.
Remember that even though PaO_2 and $PaCO_2$ determine the definition of respiratory failure, the major cause of respiratory failure is the lung's inability to meet the O_2 needs of the tissues. This failure may occur because of inadequate O_2 delivery to the tissues or because the tissues cannot use the O_2 delivered to them. It may also occur as a result of the stress response and a demand for O_2 greater than what can be supplied to the tissues. Tissue O_2 delivery is determined by cardiac output and the amount of O_2 carried in hemoglobin. Therefore respiratory failure places the patient at greater risk if there are coexisting heart problems or anemia.

In some conditions, such as septic shock, adequate O_2 may be delivered to the tissues, but impaired O_2 extraction or diffusion limitation exists at the cellular level. The result is an abnormally high amount of O_2 returning in the venous blood because it is not used at the tissue level. (Chapter 66 discusses shock.) Acid-base alterations (e.g., alkalosis, acidosis) may also interfere with O_2 delivery to peripheral tissues (see Chapter 16).

Clinical Manifestations

Respiratory failure may develop suddenly (minutes or hours) or gradually (several days or longer). A sudden decrease in PaO_2 or a rapid rise in $PaCO_2$ implies a serious condition, which can rapidly become a life-threatening emergency. An example is the patient with asthma who develops severe bronchospasm and a marked decrease in airflow, resulting in rapid respiratory muscle fatigue, acidemia, and acute respiratory failure.

Change in $PaCO_2$ is better tolerated over time because compensation can occur. An example is the patient with COPD who develops a progressive increase in $PaCO_2$ over several days after an acute respiratory tract infection. Because the change occurred over several days, there is time for renal compensation (e.g., retention of bicarbonate). This minimizes the change in arterial pH. (See Chapter 16 for a discussion of renal compensation for acid-base disorders.)

Signs of respiratory failure are related to the extent of change in PaO_2 or $PaCO_2$, the speed of change (acute versus chronic), and the patient's ability to compensate for this change. When the patient's compensatory mechanisms fail, respiratory failure occurs. Because clinical signs vary, it is important to watch trends in ABGs, pulse oximetry, and assessment findings to fully evaluate the extent of change. Frequently, the first sign of respiratory failure is a change in the patient's mental status. Mental status changes often occur early before ABG results are obtained. This is because the brain is very sensitive to variations in O_2 and CO_2 levels and acid-base balance.

Restlessness, confusion, agitation, and combative behavior suggest inadequate O_2 delivery to the brain and should be fully investigated. Conversely, morning headache, a slower respiratory rate, and a decreased level of consciousness may indicate issues with CO_2 removal. Tachycardia, tachypnea, and mild hypertension can be early signs of acute respiratory failure. Such changes can indicate an attempt by the heart and lungs to compensate for decreased O_2 delivery and rising CO_2 levels.

Cyanosis is an unreliable indicator of hypoxemia. It is a late sign of respiratory failure as it often does not occur until hypoxemia is severe (PaO_2 45 mm Hg or less). You must identify the physiologic changes that can occur as a result of hypoxemia or hypercarbia. Your ability to detect the onset of acute respiratory failure and evaluate progression or resolution in response to treatment is essential (Table 67-2).

Consequences of Hypoxemia and Hypoxia. *Hypoxemia* occurs when the amount of O_2 in arterial blood is less than the normal value (normal PaO_2 is 80 to 100 mm Hg). Hypoxia occurs when the PaO_2 falls sufficiently to cause signs and symptoms of inadequate oxygenation (Table 67-2). Hypoxemia can lead to hypoxia if not corrected. If hypoxia or hypoxemia is severe, the cells shift from aerobic to anaerobic metabolism. Anaerobic metabolism uses more fuel, produces less energy, and is less efficient than aerobic metabolism. The waste product of anaerobic metabolism is lactic acid. This is more difficult to remove from the body than CO_2 because it has to be buffered with sodium bicarbonate. When the body does not have enough sodium bicarbonate to buffer the lactic acid produced by anaerobic metabolism, metabolic acidosis, tissue and cellular dysfunction, and cell death may occur. BP and CO can fall. Vasoactive or inotropic drugs may be needed for cardiovascular support. These drugs may be less effective in the presence of a severe acidotic environment.

Permanent brain damage may occur if the hypoxia is severe and prolonged. Renal function may also be impaired. Sodium retention, edema, acute tubular necrosis, and uremia may occur. Gastrointestinal (GI) system alterations include tissue ischemia, increased permeability of the intestinal wall, and possible migration of bacteria from the GI tract into circulation.

TABLE 67-2	**Manifestations of Hypoxemia and Hypercapnia***
Specific	**Nonspecific**
Hypoxemia	
Respiratory	***Central Nervous***
Dyspnea	Agitation
Tachypnea	Disorientation
Prolonged expiration (I:E = 1:3, 1:4)	Restless, combative behavior
	Delirium
Nasal flaring	Confusion
Intercostal muscle retraction	↓ Level of consciousness
Use of accessory muscles in respiration	Coma (late)
↓ SpO_2 (<80%)	***Cardiovascular***
Paradoxic chest or abdominal wall movement with respiratory cycle (late)	Tachycardia
	Hypertension
	Skin cool, clammy, and diaphoretic
Cyanosis (late)	Dysrhythmias (late)
	Hypotension (late)
	Other
	Fatigue
	Inability to speak in complete sentences without pausing to breathe
Hypercapnia	
Respiratory	***Central Nervous***
Dyspnea	Morning headache
Use of tripod position	Disorientation, confusion
Pursed-lip breathing	Agitation
↓ Respiratory rate or rapid rate with shallow respirations	Progressive somnolence
	Elevated intracranial pressure (if monitored)
↓ Tidal volume	Coma (late)
↓ Minute ventilation	***Cardiovascular***
	Dysrhythmias
	Hypertension
	Tachycardia
	Bounding pulse
	Neuromuscular
	Muscle weakness
	↓ Deep tendon reflexes
	Tremors, seizures (late)

I:E, Inspiratory:expiratory ratio.
*List is not all-inclusive.

Specific Clinical Manifestations. The patient in respiratory failure may have a rapid, shallow breathing pattern or a respiratory rate that is slower than normal. Both changes predispose the patient to insufficient CO_2 removal. The patient may increase the respiratory rate in an effort to blow off accumulated CO_2. This breathing pattern requires a substantial amount of work and can lead to respiratory muscle fatigue. A change from a rapid rate to a slower rate in a patient in acute respiratory distress such as that seen with acute asthma suggests extreme progression of respiratory muscle fatigue and increased probability of respiratory arrest.

The patient's position is an indication of the effort associated with the work of breathing (WOB), or the effort used for muscle contraction during inhalation to accomplish lung ventilation. The patient may be able to lie down (mild distress), be able to lie down but prefer to sit (moderate distress), or be unable to breathe unless sitting upright (severe distress). A common position used by patients with moderate to severe COPD is to sit with the arms propped on the overbed table or

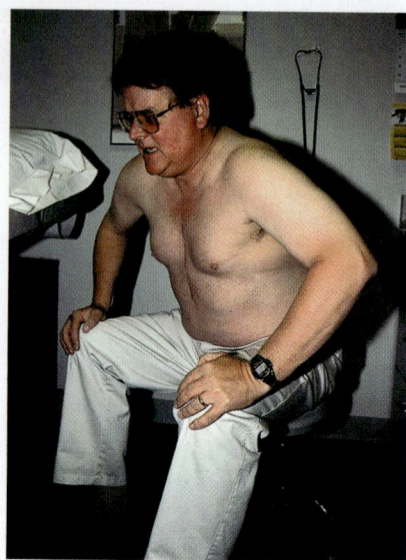

FIG. 67-6 Tripod positioning is used to increase chest and lung expansion and decrease work of breathing for patients with COPD or asthma. (From Wilson SF, Giddens JF: *Health assessment for nursing practice,* ed 4, St Louis, 2009, Mosby.)

on the knees. This so-called *tripod position* helps decrease the WOB, since propping the arms increases the anteroposterior diameter of the chest and changes pressure in the thorax (Fig. 67-6).

The person who is experiencing dyspnea is working hard to breathe. You may see patients using pursed-lip breathing (see Table 28-13). This technique increases SaO_2 by slowing respirations, allowing more time for expiration, and preventing small bronchioles from collapsing. Similarly, the dyspneic patient may be able to speak only a few words at a time between breaths. The patient's ability to speak often indicates the severity of dyspnea. The patient may have "two-word" or "three word" dyspnea. This means that only two or three words can be spoken before pausing to breathe. These are important observations that can help you identify the onset of acute respiratory failure.

You may observe *retraction* (inward movement) of the intercostal spaces or supraclavicular area and use of the accessory muscles (e.g., sternocleidomastoid) during inspiration or expiration. Use of the accessory muscles signifies moderate distress. Paradoxic breathing indicates severe distress. Normally, the thorax and abdomen move outward on inspiration and inward on exhalation.

During *paradoxic breathing,* the abdomen and chest move in the opposite manner—outward during exhalation and inward during inspiration. Paradoxic breathing results from maximal use of the accessory muscles of respiration. The patient may also be diaphoretic from the WOB.

Perform auscultation to assess the patient's baseline breath sounds and any changes from baseline. Note and document the presence and location of any abnormal breath sounds. Crackles (generally heard on inspiration) may indicate pulmonary edema. Loud crackles heard on expiration indicate additional lung secretions and may be symptomatic of pneumonia or COPD. Absent or diminished breath sounds may indicate atelectasis, pleural effusion, or impaired inspiratory effort and hypoventilation. Bronchial breath sounds over the lung

periphery often indicate lung consolidation from pneumonia. A pleural friction rub may also be heard in the presence of pneumonia that involves the pleura.

A thorough assessment may result in early detection of respiratory insufficiency, allowing interventions to be started sooner and preventing respiratory failure. Patients with end-stage chronic lung disease may have low PaO_2 or high $PaCO_2$ levels and crackles as their "normal" baseline. It is important to monitor specific and nonspecific signs of respiratory failure in patients with COPD because a small change can cause significant decompensation (Table 67-2). Immediately report any change in mental status (e.g., agitation, confusion, decreased level of consciousness). This may indicate the onset of rapid deterioration in clinical status and the need for mechanical ventilation. Obtain vital signs as clinically indicated. Changes in vital signs (especially respiratory rate) are often an early sign of respiratory failure.

Diagnostic Studies

After physical assessment, the most common diagnostic studies used to evaluate acute respiratory failure are chest x-ray and ABG analysis. A chest x-ray helps to identify possible causes of respiratory failure (e.g., atelectasis, pneumonia). ABGs determine the levels of $PaCO_2$, PaO_2, bicarbonate, and pH. In respiratory failure, ABGs are used to evaluate oxygenation (PaO_2) and ventilation ($PaCO_2$) status and acid-base balance. Pulse oximetry monitors oxygenation status but reveals little about lung ventilation.

Other diagnostic studies that may be done include a complete blood cell count, serum electrolytes, urinalysis, and ECG. Blood and sputum cultures are obtained as necessary to determine sources of possible infection. If pulmonary embolus is suspected, a CT scan or V/Q lung scan may be done. For the patient in severe respiratory failure requiring endotracheal intubation, end-tidal CO_2 ($ETCO_2$) is used to help confirm correct tube placement within the airway immediately after intubation. (Chapter 65 discusses intubation.) $ETCO_2$ monitoring *(capnography)* and transcutaneous CO_2 monitoring may also be used during ventilator management to assess trends in lung ventilation.[9]

In severe respiratory failure, central venous or PA pressure monitoring or arterial pressure–based CO monitoring is used to measure hemodynamic parameters (e.g., central venous pressure, PA pressures, CO, stroke volume variation, central or mixed venous O_2 saturation [$ScvO_2$ or SvO_2]). These data help to determine the adequacy of tissue perfusion and the patient's response to treatment measures. Hemodynamic monitoring can also determine whether the accumulation of fluid in the lungs is the result of heart or lung problems. It can also provide feedback on the physiologic effects of mechanical ventilation on hemodynamic status.[10] (Chapter 65 discusses hemodynamic monitoring in detail.)

❖ NURSING AND INTERPROFESSIONAL MANAGEMENT: ACUTE RESPIRATORY FAILURE

Because many different problems cause respiratory failure, specific care of these patients varies. This section discusses general assessment and interventions that apply to patients with acute respiratory failure. In acute care settings, collaboration between nursing and other interprofessional care team members (e.g., respiratory therapists) is essential.

Nursing Assessment

Table 67-3 presents subjective and objective data that should be obtained from the patient with acute respiratory failure.

Nursing Diagnoses

Nursing diagnoses for the patient with acute respiratory failure may include, but are not limited to, the following:

- Impaired gas exchange *related to* alveolar hypoventilation, intrapulmonary shunting, V/Q mismatch, and diffusion impairment
- Ineffective airway clearance *related to* excessive secretions, decreased level of consciousness, presence of an artificial airway, neuromuscular dysfunction, and pain
- Ineffective breathing pattern *related to* neuromuscular impairment of respirations, pain, anxiety, decreased level of consciousness, respiratory muscle fatigue, and bronchospasm

Additional information on nursing diagnoses for the patient with acute respiratory failure is presented in eNursing Care Plan 67-1 (available on the website for this chapter).

Planning

The overall goals for the patient with acute respiratory failure include (1) independent maintenance of the airway, (2) effective cough and ability to clear secretions, (3) normal ABG values or values within the patient's baseline, (4) absence of dyspnea or recovery to baseline breathing patterns for patient, and (5) breath sounds within the patient's baseline.

Prevention

As part of the plan of care for any patient who may be at risk for respiratory failure, prevention and early recognition of respiratory distress are important. Prevention involves a thorough history and physical assessment to identify the patient at risk for respiratory failure and then the start of appropriate interventions. These include teaching the patient about deep breathing and coughing, use of incentive spirometry, and ambulation.

Prevention of atelectasis, pneumonia, and complications of immobility, as well as optimizing hydration and nutrition, can potentially decrease the risk of respiratory failure in acutely or critically ill patients. It is also important to consider age-related and acuity-related changes in physiology when assessing risk of acute respiratory failure. Patients at higher risk of acute respiratory failure should be assessed more frequently with additional attention to preventive measures.

Respiratory Therapy

The major goals of care for acute respiratory failure include maintaining adequate oxygenation and ventilation. Interventions include O_2 therapy, mobilization of secretions, and positive pressure ventilation (PPV) (Table 67-4).

Oxygen Therapy. The primary goal of O_2 therapy is to correct hypoxemia. The patient with acute respiratory failure must be able to tolerate the type of O_2 delivery system chosen. For example, a face mask may cause anxiety from feelings of claustrophobia. The anxiety can cause dyspnea, increase O_2 consumption and CO_2 production, and cause the patient to remove the O_2 device. The selected O_2 delivery system must also maintain PaO_2 at 55 to 60 mm Hg or higher and SaO_2 at 90% or higher at the lowest O_2 concentration possible.

Several methods are available to provide O_2 to patients in acute respiratory failure. (Chapter 28 and Table 28-20 discuss

---

TABLE 67-3 Nursing Assessment

Acute Respiratory Failure

Subjective Data

Important Health Information

Past health history: Chronic lung disease, potential occupational exposures to lung toxins, tobacco use (pack-years), alcohol or drug use, previous hospitalizations related to lung disease, thoracic or spinal cord trauma, severe obesity, altered consciousness, age (physiologic and chronologic)

Medications: Use of home O_2, inhalers (bronchodilators), home nebulization, over-the-counter drugs; immunosuppressant (e.g., corticosteroid) therapy, CNS depressants

Surgery or other treatments: Previous intubation and mechanical ventilation, recent thoracic or abdominal surgery

Functional Health Patterns

Health perception–health management: Exercise, self-care activities, immunizations (flu, pneumonia, hepatitis)

Nutritional-metabolic: Eating habits, bloating, indigestion; weight gain or loss, change in appetite. Use of vitamins or herbal supplements

Activity-exercise: Fatigue, dizziness, dyspnea at rest or with activity, wheezing, cough (productive or nonproductive), sputum (volume, color, viscosity), palpitations, swollen feet, change in exercise tolerance

Sleep-rest: Changes in sleep pattern, use of CPAP

Cognitive-perceptual: Headache, chest pain or tightness, chronic pain

Coping–stress tolerance: Anxiety, depression, hopelessness. Risk of drug, alcohol, or nicotine withdrawal

Objective Data

General

Restlessness, agitation

Integumentary

Pale, cool, clammy skin or warm, flushed skin. Peripheral and central cyanosis. Peripheral dependent edema

Respiratory

Shallow, increased respiratory rate progressing to decreased rate. Use of accessory muscles with evidence of retractions, increased diaphragmatic excursion or asymmetric chest expansion, paradoxic chest and abdominal wall movement. Tactile fremitus, crepitus, or deviated trachea on palpation. Absent, diminished, or adventitious breath sounds. Pleural friction rub. Bronchial or bronchovesicular sounds heard in other than normal location, inspiratory stridor

Cardiovascular

Tachycardia progressing to bradycardia, dysrhythmias, extra heart sounds (S_3, S_4). Bounding pulse. Hypertension progressing to hypotension. Pulsus paradoxus, jugular venous distention, pedal edema

Gastrointestinal

Abdominal distention, ascites, epigastric tenderness, hepatojugular reflex

Neurologic

Somnolence, confusion, slurred speech, restlessness, delirium, agitation, tremors, seizures, coma; asterixis, decreased deep tendon reflexes, papilledema

Possible Diagnostic Findings

$\downarrow/\uparrow$ pH, $\uparrow/\downarrow$ $PaCO_2$, $\uparrow/\downarrow$ bicarbonate, $\downarrow$ PaO_2, $\downarrow$ SaO_2, abnormal serum electrolytes, hemoglobin, hematocrit, and white blood cell count. Abnormal findings on chest x-ray. Abnormal central venous or pulmonary artery pressures. Initially cardiac output may be increased due to the stress response. As hypoxemia, hypercapnia, and acidosis become more severe, cardiac output will decrease.

CPAP, Continuous positive airway pressure.

TABLE 67-4   Interprofessional Care
Acute Respiratory Failure

Diagnostic Assessment
- Vital signs
- History and physical examination
- Arterial blood gases
- Pulse oximetry
- Chest x-ray
- CBC
- Serum electrolytes and urinalysis
- ECG
- Blood and sputum cultures (if indicated)
- Hemodynamic parameters: CVP, SVV, PAWP

Management
Respiratory Therapy
- O_2 therapy
- Mobilization of secretions
  - Effective coughing
  - Incentive spirometry
  - Hydration and humidification
  - Chest physiotherapy
  - Airway suctioning
  - Ambulation
  - Positioning: head of bed elevated to assist lung ventilation; tripod positioning for optimal comfort and efficiency during breathing
- Positive pressure ventilation
  - Noninvasive positive pressure ventilation
  - Intubation with positive pressure ventilation

Drug Therapy
- Relief of bronchospasm (e.g., albuterol)
- Reduction of airway inflammation (e.g., corticosteroids)
- Reduction of pulmonary congestion (e.g., furosemide [Lasix], morphine)
- Treatment of pulmonary infections (e.g., antibiotics)
- Reduction of severe anxiety, pain, and agitation (e.g., lorazepam [Ativan], fentanyl [Sublimaze], morphine)

Medical Supportive Therapy
- Management of the underlying cause of respiratory failure
- Maintenance of adequate cardiac output
- Maintenance of adequate hemoglobin concentration

Nutritional Therapy
- Enteral nutrition support
- Parenteral nutrition support

Physical Therapy
- Ambulation
- Muscle conditioning

CVP, Central venous pressure; *PAWP,* pulmonary artery wedge pressure; *SVV,* stroke volume variation.

O_2 delivery devices.) If hypoxemia is secondary to V/Q mismatch, one method is to give supplemental O_2 at 1 to 3 L/minute by nasal cannula. Another method is to give 24% to 32% O_2 by face mask or Venturi mask. This should improve the PaO_2 and SaO_2.

Hypoxemia secondary to an intrapulmonary shunt is usually not responsive to high O_2 concentrations. In this case, the patient usually needs O_2 given by invasive or noninvasive positive pressure ventilation (NIPPV). PPV provides O_2 therapy and humidification, decreases WOB, and reduces respiratory muscle

fatigue. In addition, it assists in opening collapsed airways and decreasing shunt.[11] If respiratory status worsens despite NIPPV, PPV using an endotracheal tube is used and higher O_2 concentrations are given. (Chapter 65 discusses mechanical ventilation.)

High O_2 concentrations replace the nitrogen gas normally present in the alveoli, thus causing instability and atelectasis. In intubated patients, exposure to 60% or higher FIO_2 for longer than 48 hours poses a significant risk for O_2 *toxicity*. In nonintubated patients the risk is less clear. The effects of prolonged exposure to high levels of O_2 include increased pulmonary capillary permeability, decreased surfactant production and surfactant inactivation, and fibrotic changes in the alveoli. (Chapter 28 and Table 28-20 discuss O_2 delivery devices.)

Another possible risk of O_2 therapy is specific to patients with chronic hypercapnia (e.g., patients with COPD). Chronic hypercapnia blunts the response of chemoreceptors to elevated CO_2 levels as a respiratory stimulant. In this case, hypoxia stimulates respiration. Initial O_2 therapy may be provided to patients with chronic hypercapnia through a low-flow device such as a nasal cannula at 1 to 2 L/minute or a Venturi mask at 24% to 28%. O_2 should be given with careful titration and at the lowest possible dose needed to keep SpO_2 and PaO_2 within patient-specific clinical goals. Closely monitor patients for changes in mental status, respiratory rate, and ABGs until their PaO_2 level has reached their baseline normal value.

◆ **Mobilization of Secretions.** Retained pulmonary secretions may cause or exacerbate acute respiratory failure. This occurs because the movement of O_2 into the alveoli and removal of CO_2 are blocked. Secretions can be mobilized by effective coughing, adequate hydration and humidification, chest physiotherapy (physical therapy), airway suctioning, patient positioning, and ambulation when possible.

◆ *Effective Coughing and Positioning.* If secretions are obstructing the airway, encourage the patient to cough. The patient with a neuromuscular weakness from a disease or exhaustion may not be able to generate sufficient airway pressures to produce an effective cough. *Augmented coughing (quad coughing)* may benefit these patients. Perform augmented coughing by placing one or both hands at the anterolateral base of the patient's lungs (Fig. 67-7). As the patient ends a deep inspiration and begins the expiration, move your hands forcefully upward, increasing abdominal pressure and facilitating the cough. This measure helps increase expiratory flow and thereby facilitates secretion clearance.

Some patients may benefit from therapeutic cough techniques. *Huff coughing* is a series of coughs performed while saying the word "huff" (see Table 28-23). This technique prevents the glottis from closing during the cough. Patients with COPD generate higher flow rates with a huff cough than is possible with a normal cough. The huff cough is effective in clearing only the central airways, but it may assist in moving secretions upward.

The staged cough also assists in mobilizing secretions. To perform the *staged cough*, the patient assumes a sitting position, breathes three or four times in and out through the mouth, and coughs while bending forward and pressing a pillow inward against the diaphragm.

Positioning the patient upright, either by elevating the head of the bed at least 30 degrees or by using a reclining chair or chair bed, helps maximize thoracic expansion, thereby decreasing dyspnea and improving secretion mobilization. A sitting

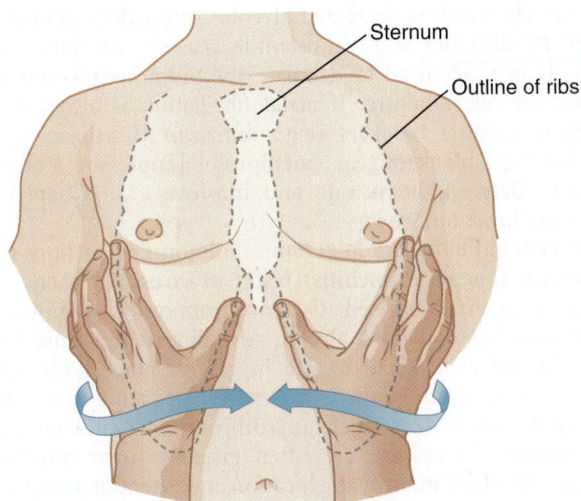

FIG. 67-7 Augmented coughing is performed by placing one or both hands on the anterolateral base of the lungs. After the patient takes a deep inspiration and at the beginning of expiration, move the hand(s) forcefully upward. This increases abdominal pressure and aids in producing a forceful cough. (From American Association of Critical Care Nurses: *AACN advanced critical care nursing,* St Louis, 2009, Mosby.)

position improves pulmonary function and assists in venous pooling in dependent body areas such as the lower extremities. When lungs are upright, ventilation and perfusion are best in the lung bases.

For patients with a unilateral lung disorder such as right-sided pneumonia, lateral or side-lying positioning may be used. This position, termed *good lung down,* allows for improved V/Q matching in the affected lung. Pulmonary blood flow and ventilation are optimal in dependent lung areas. This position also allows secretions to drain out of the affected lung to the point where they may be removed by suctioning. For example, position patients with significant right-sided pneumonia on their left side to maximize ventilation and perfusion in the "good" lung and aid secretion removal from the affected lung (postural drainage). Patients with acute respiratory failure often have pathology affecting both lungs and may require repositioning at intervals on both sides to optimize air movement and drainage of secretions.

All patients should be side lying if there is any possibility that the tongue will obstruct the airway or that aspiration may occur. Airway control with endotracheal intubation and PPV is indicated when patients cannot maintain their airway and lung ventilation.

◆ *Hydration.* Thick and viscous secretions are difficult to expel. Adequate fluid intake (2 to 3 L/day) keeps secretions thin and easier to remove. If the patient is unable to take sufficient fluids orally, IV hydration is used. Thoroughly assess the patient's cardiac and renal status to determine whether he or she can tolerate the IV fluid volume and avoid heart failure and pulmonary edema. Regularly assess for signs of fluid overload by clinical evaluation (e.g., crackles, dyspnea) and invasive monitoring (e.g., increased central venous pressure).

◆ *Humidification.* An appropriate humidification device is an adjunct in secretion management. Aerosols of sterile normal saline, given with a nebulizer, may be used to liquefy secretions. O_2 may also be given by aerosol mask to thin secretions and facilitate their removal. Aerosol therapy may induce

bronchospasm and severe coughing, causing a decreased PaO_2. Frequent assessment of the patient's tolerance to therapy is critical. Mucolytic drugs such as nebulized acetylcysteine mixed with a bronchodilator may be used to thin secretions. A side effect of these drugs is bronchospasm. Therefore during their use, closely monitor the patient's respiratory status.

◆ *Chest Physiotherapy.* Chest physiotherapy is indicated in patients who produce more than 30 mL of sputum per day or have evidence of severe atelectasis or pulmonary infiltrates. Postural drainage, percussion, and vibration to the affected lung segments assist in moving secretions to the larger airways, where they are removed by coughing or suctioning. Positioning affects oxygenation. Patients may not tolerate head-down or lateral positioning because of extreme dyspnea or hypoxemia caused by V/Q mismatch. (Chest physiotherapy is discussed in Chapter 28.)

◆ *Airway Suctioning.* Nasopharyngeal, oropharyngeal, or naso-tracheal suctioning (blind suctioning without a tracheal tube in place) is done if the patient is unable to expectorate secretions. Suctioning through an artificial airway (e.g., endotracheal tube) is also done as needed (see Chapters 26 and 65).

At all times, deep airway suctioning should be done cautiously and the patient should be closely monitored for complications. These could include hypoxia, increased ICP, dysrhythmias, bradycardia, vasovagal response, hypotension from sudden elevation in intrathoracic pressure, and hypertension and tachycardia from noxious stimulation.

❓ CHECK YOUR PRACTICE

You are caring for a 72-yr-old male patient admitted to the critical care unit with a diagnosis of acute respiratory failure. He has a history of COPD. A chest x-ray reveals a left-sided pneumonia. Your patient is awake but mildly confused and has a productive cough.

• What respiratory interventions would you expect to be ordered for this patient?

◆ **Positive Pressure Ventilation.** If initial measures fail to improve ventilation and oxygenation and the patient continues to show signs of acute respiratory failure, ventilatory assistance is needed. Invasive or NIPPV may be considered.[12] NIPPV is used for patients with acute or chronic respiratory failure. During NIPPV, a mask is placed tightly over the patient's nose or nose and mouth and the patient breathes spontaneously while PPV is delivered. With NIPPV, it is possible to decrease the WOB without the need for endotracheal intubation.

Bilevel positive airway pressure (BiPAP) is a form of NIPPV in which different positive pressure levels are set for inspiration and expiration (Fig. 67-8). Continuous positive airway pressure (CPAP) is another form of NIPPV, in which a constant positive pressure is delivered to the airway during inspiration and expiration.[12]

NIPPV is most useful in managing chronic respiratory failure in patients with chest wall and neuromuscular disease (Table 67-1). NIPPV may also be used for patients who refuse endotracheal intubation but still want some palliative ventilatory support (e.g., patients with end-stage COPD).[13] NIPPV is not appropriate for patients who have excessive secretions, decreased level of consciousness, high O_2 requirements, facial trauma, or hemodynamic instability. NIPPV is also used postextubation to avoid reintubation. (Chapter 65 discusses artificial airways, PPV, BiPAP, and CPAP in detail.)

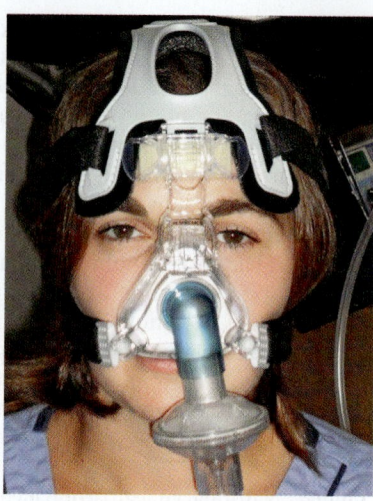

FIG. 67-8 Noninvasive bilevel positive airway pressure ventilation. A mask is placed over the nose or nose and mouth. Positive pressure from a mechanical ventilator assists the patient's breathing efforts, decreasing the work of breathing. (Courtesy Richard Arbour, RN, MSN, CCRN, CNRN, CCNS, FAAN and Anna Kirk, RN, MSN.)

◆ Drug Therapy

Goals of drug therapy for patients in acute respiratory failure include (1) relief of bronchospasm; (2) reduction of airway inflammation and pulmonary congestion; (3) treatment of pulmonary infection; and (4) reduction of severe pain, anxiety, and restlessness.

◆ **Relief of Bronchospasm.** Relief of bronchospasm increases alveolar ventilation. Short-acting bronchodilators, such as metaproterenol and albuterol, reverse bronchospasm. In acute bronchospasm these drugs may be given at 15- to 30-minute intervals until a response occurs. Side effects of these β-adrenergic agonists include tachycardia and hypertension. Prolonged use can increase the risk of dysrhythmias and cardiac ischemia. Monitor ECG and vital signs for any changes when giving these drugs.

The bronchodilator effects of these drugs can sometimes worsen hypoxemia by redistributing the inspired gas to areas of decreased perfusion. Giving the bronchodilator with an O_2-enriched gas mixture usually reduces this effect. (Chapter 28 discusses nursing management related to bronchodilators.) Give these drugs using a hand-held nebulizer or a metered-dose inhaler with a spacer.

◆ **Reduction of Airway Inflammation.** Corticosteroids (e.g., methylprednisolone [Solu-Medrol]) may be used with bronchodilating drugs for bronchospasm and inflammation. When given IV for conditions such as COPD exacerbation or acute asthma, corticosteroids aid resolution of airway inflammation and edema. Clinical effects may require several hours before onset. Inhaled corticosteroids require 4 to 5 days for optimum therapeutic effects and are not used for acute respiratory failure.

> 💊 **DRUG ALERT** IV Corticosteroids
> • Monitor potassium levels, since corticosteroids exacerbate hypokalemia caused by diuretics.
> • Prolonged use causes adrenal insufficiency.

◆ **Reduction of Pulmonary Congestion.** Pulmonary interstitial fluid can accumulate because of direct or indirect injury to the alveolar capillary membrane (e.g., ARDS) or from heart failure. The result is decreased alveolar ventilation and hypoxemia. IV diuretics (e.g., furosemide [Lasix]), morphine, and nitroglycerin are used to decrease the pulmonary congestion caused by heart failure. If atrial fibrillation is also present, calcium channel blockers (e.g., diltiazem [Cardizem]) and β-adrenergic blockers (e.g., metoprolol [Lopressor]) may be used to decrease heart rate and improve CO. (Chapter 34 discusses heart failure.)

◆ **Treatment of Pulmonary Infections.** Pulmonary infections (e.g., pneumonia, acute bronchitis) result in excessive mucus production; fever; increased O_2 consumption; and inflamed, fluid-filled, or collapsed alveoli. Alveoli that are fluid filled or collapsed cannot participate in gas exchange. Pulmonary infections can either cause or exacerbate acute respiratory failure. IV antibiotics, such as azithromycin (Zithromax) or ceftriaxone (Rocephin), are often given to treat infections. Chest x-rays help identify the location and extent of a suspected infection. Sputum cultures help identify the type of organisms causing the infection and their sensitivity to antimicrobial drugs.

◆ **Reduction of Anxiety, Pain, and Agitation.** Anxiety, restlessness, and agitation result from hypoxia. In addition, fear caused by the inability to breathe and a sense of loss of control may increase anxiety. Anxiety, pain, and agitation increase O_2 consumption and CO_2 production from an elevated metabolic rate and increased WOB. This may cause asynchrony with mechanical ventilation and risk unplanned extubation. Several strategies can assist the patient in reducing anxiety and pain.

Sedation and analgesia with drug therapy such as propofol (Diprivan) (used for mechanically ventilated patients), benzodiazepines (e.g., lorazepam [Ativan], midazolam), and opioids (e.g., morphine, fentanyl [Sublimaze]) are used to decrease anxiety, agitation, and pain. Patients receiving these drugs are best managed by following an evidence-based and goal-directed protocol that uses the lowest possible drug dosing and duration of therapy needed to meet patient-specific goals. Some protocols include a regular *"sedation holiday"* (periodically decreasing sedative/hypnotic dosing) for ongoing assessment in patients who are intubated and mechanically ventilated. (Sedation holiday is discussed in Chapter 65.)

> ⚠️ **SAFETY ALERT** Managing Agitation, Pain, and Sedation
> • Agitation is often caused by pain, hypoxemia, electrolyte imbalance, brain injury, and adverse drug reactions.
> • Assess and aggressively treat all reversible causes of agitation.
> • Monitor patients closely for cardiopulmonary depression when giving sedative and/or analgesic drugs.
> • Sedative and analgesic drugs may have a prolonged effect in critically ill patients, delay weaning from mechanical ventilation, and contribute to increased length of stay.

Address treatable causes of agitation (e.g., hypoxemia, pain, hypercapnia) as part of a comprehensive plan of care. Frequently, agitation and mental status changes may be initial consequences of hypoxemia or ventilator asynchrony. You should address these causes and not depend solely on the use of sedatives.

Patients who breathe asynchronously with mechanical ventilation may also benefit from adjustment of ventilator flow rates and other settings. Patients who remain asynchronous with mechanical ventilation despite aggressive sedative and analgesic dosing may require neuromuscular blockade (paralysis) with agents such as vecuronium or cisatracurium (Nimbex). These drugs relax skeletal muscles by interfering with neuromuscular transmission and, ultimately, promote synchrony with mechanical ventilation. Remember that a patient receiving neuromuscular blockade can appear to be asleep but still possibly be awake and in pain. For this reason, deep sedation and analgesia are essential.

> **! SAFETY ALERT   Neuromuscular Blockade**
> - Provide concurrent sedation and analgesia to the point of unconsciousness for patients receiving neuromuscular blockade. This eliminates patient awareness, ensures patient comfort, and avoids the terrifying experience of being awake and in pain while paralyzed.
> - Use neuromuscular blockade for the shortest duration and at the lowest dose possible to avoid complications (e.g., myopathy).

Monitoring levels of sedation in patients receiving neuromuscular blockade is challenging. Noninvasive electroencephalogram (EEG)–based technology may help guide sedative and analgesic therapy in these patients.[14] Levels of drug paralysis are monitored primarily by clinical assessment of ventilation and whether goals of care are being met. A frequent adjunct to monitoring paralysis is the use of a peripheral nerve stimulator (see Fig. 65-19). Clinical assessment is essential to determine the adequacy of sedation, analgesia, and neuromuscular blockade in critically ill patients.

◆ Medical Supportive Therapy

Goals and related interventions to maximize O_2 delivery are essential to improve the patient's oxygenation and ventilation status. The primary goal is to treat the underlying cause of the respiratory failure. Other supportive goals include maintaining an adequate CO and hemoglobin concentration.

◆ **Treating the Underlying Cause.** Interventions are directed toward reversing the disease process that caused the acute respiratory failure. Patients with hypoventilation need to be diagnosed and treated rapidly. Patients with V/Q mismatch, shunting, or diffusion limitation are managed differently depending on the underlying cause. In all patient situations, monitoring treatment effects, including trends in ABGs and changes in respiratory status, is an ongoing process.

◆ **Maintaining Adequate Cardiac Output.** CO reflects the blood flow reaching the tissues. BP and mean arterial pressure (MAP) are important indicators of the adequacy of CO. Always interpret BP and MAP readings within the context of the physical assessment to determine adequacy of CO and tissue perfusion. Usually a systolic BP of 90 mm Hg or more or a MAP greater than 60 mm Hg is adequate to maintain perfusion to the vital organs. At these levels, changes in mental status may be attributed to the level of O_2 and CO_2 rather than decreased cerebral perfusion. In a patient with chronic hypertension, a systolic BP of 90 to 100 mm Hg may be inadequate to maintain systemic and cerebral perfusion. Cerebral perfusion may require a higher BP and MAP to prevent episodes of brain ischemia or hypoperfusion to other organs.

Decreased CO is treated by giving IV fluids, drugs, or both. (Chapter 66 discusses drugs used to treat decreased CO and shock.) CO can also be decreased by changes in intrathoracic or intrapulmonary pressures from PPV. Patients experiencing exacerbation of COPD or asthma and those receiving PPV are at risk of alveolar hyperinflation, increased right ventricular afterload, and excessive intrathoracic pressures. These changes

can limit blood flow from the right side of the heart through the pulmonary vasculature to the left side of the heart and cause hemodynamic compromise (e.g., decreased CO). Blood return from the systemic circulation to the right side of the heart may be impaired, decreasing preload and CO. Closely monitor BP and clinical indicators of adequate CO and tissue perfusion with the start of or changes in mechanical ventilation as these patients are always at risk for hemodynamic compromise.

◆ **Maintaining Adequate Hemoglobin Concentration.** Hemoglobin is the primary carrier of O_2 to the tissues. Delivery of O_2 to the tissues is compromised in anemic patients. A hemoglobin of 7 g/dL (70 g/L) or higher typically ensures adequate O_2 saturation of the hemoglobin for tissue oxygenation.[15] Monitor the patient for signs of blood loss (e.g., hypotension, melena). Transfusion with packed red blood cells may be used if an adequate hemoglobin level is not maintained and the patient is symptomatic.

◆ Nutritional Therapy

Maintenance of protein and energy stores is especially important in patients with acute respiratory failure. The hypermetabolic state in critical illness increases the caloric requirements needed to maintain body weight and muscle mass. Thus nutritional depletion causes a loss of muscle mass, including the respiratory muscles, and may prolong recovery.

The dietitian, in collaboration with the interprofessional care team, determines the optimal method of feeding and optimal caloric and fluid requirements. During the acute manifestations of respiratory failure, the risk of aspiration typically prevents oral intake. Ideally, enteral or parenteral nutrition should be started within 24 to 48 hours. When acute manifestations subside, the patient may resume oral intake as able.

◆ Evaluation

The expected outcomes are that the patient with respiratory failure will
- Maintain a patent airway with effective removal of secretions
- Achieve normal or baseline respiratory rate and rhythm and breath sounds
- Maintain adequate oxygenation as indicated by normal or baseline ABGs
- Experience normal hemodynamic status

Additional outcomes are presented in eNursing Care Plan 67-1 (available on the website for this chapter).

◆ Gerontologic Considerations: Respiratory Failure

Older adults are the fastest-growing age-group in the United States, a trend that is increasingly reflected within the patient populations in acute and critical care settings. Multiple factors contribute to an increased risk of respiratory failure in older adults. The reduction in ventilatory capacity that accompanies aging places the older adult at risk for respiratory failure. Physiologic aging of the lung includes alveolar dilation, larger air spaces, and loss of surface area for gas exchange. Diminished elastic recoil within the airways, decreased chest wall compliance, and decreased respiratory muscle strength also occur.

In older adults, the PaO_2 falls further and the $PaCO_2$ rises to a higher level before the respiratory system is stimulated to alter the rate and depth of breathing. This delayed response can contribute to the development of respiratory failure. In addition, a history of tobacco use is a risk factor that can accelerate age-related respiratory changes. Poor nutritional status and l ess available physiologic reserve in the cardiopulmonary and autonomic nervous systems increase the risk of additional disease states such as pneumonia and heart disease. These may further compromise respiratory function and lead to respiratory failure.

Older adults are more vulnerable to delirium, health care–associated infections (HAIs), and the adverse effects of polypharmacy. Delirium is an independent risk factor for increased mortality and morbidity rates in critically ill patients. It can complicate ventilator management and weaning by interfering with patient cooperation. Delirium associated with agitation increases CO_2 elimination and O_2 consumption, increases the risk for unplanned extubation and device removal, and extends length of hospital stay and ventilator days.[16] (Delirium is discussed in Chapters 59 and 65.)

ACUTE RESPIRATORY DISTRESS SYNDROME

Acute respiratory distress syndrome (ARDS) is a sudden and progressive form of acute respiratory failure in which the alveolar-capillary membrane becomes damaged and more permeable to intravascular fluid (Fig. 67-9). ARDS exists on a continuum. One way to assess the degree of impairment in gas exchange is to measure the PaO_2/FIO_2 (P/F) ratio. Under normal circumstances (e.g., PaO_2 85 to 100 mm Hg; FIO_2 0.21 [room air]), the P/F ratio would be greater than 400 (e.g., 95/0.21 = 452). With the onset and progression of lung injury and impairment in O_2 delivery through the alveolar-capillary membrane, the PaO_2 may remain lower than expected despite increased FIO_2. The PF ratio differentiates between mild, moderate, and severe ARDS[17] (Table 67-5).

The incidence of ARDS in the United States is estimated at more than 150,000 cases annually. Despite supportive therapy, the mortality rate from ARDS is approximately 50%. Patients who have both gram-negative septic shock and ARDS have a mortality rate of 70% to 90%.

Etiology and Pathophysiology

Table 67-6 lists conditions that predispose patients to the development of ARDS. Patients with multiple risk factors are three or four times more likely to develop ARDS.

The most common cause of ARDS is sepsis. Direct lung injury may cause ARDS (Fig. 67-10), or ARDS may develop because of the systemic inflammatory response syndrome (SIRS) (see Fig. 66-1). This is characterized by widespread inflammation or clinical responses to inflammation after a variety of

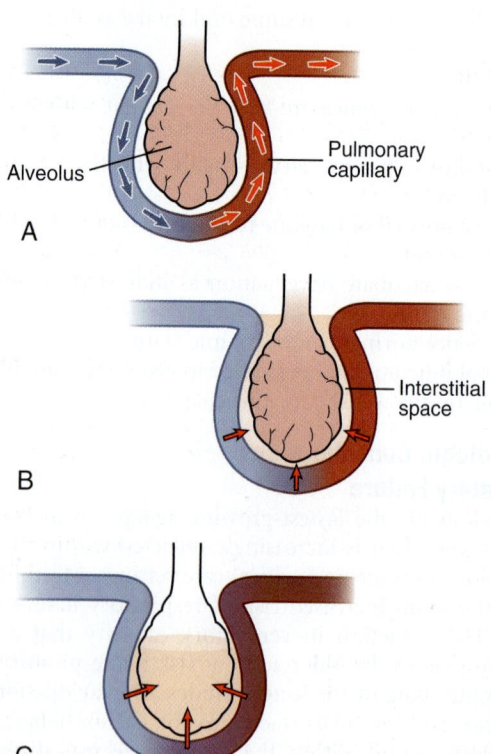

FIG. 67-9 Stages of edema formation in acute respiratory distress syndrome. **A,** Normal alveolus and pulmonary capillary. **B,** Interstitial edema occurs with increased flow of fluid into the interstitial space. **C,** Alveolar edema occurs when the fluid crosses the alveolar-capillary membrane.

TABLE 67-5 Diagnostic Findings in ARDS

Timing

Within 1 week of a known clinical insult or new or worsening respiratory symptoms

Chest X-ray

Bilateral opacities: not fully explained by effusions, lobar/lung collapse, or nodules

Oxygenation

Mild ARDS: PaO_2/FIO_2 ratio >200 to ≤300 with PEEP or CPAP ≥5 cm H_2O

Moderate ARDS: PaO_2/FIO_2 ratio 100 to ≤200 with PEEP or CPAP ≥5 cm H_2O

Severe ARDS: PaO_2/FIO_2 ratio <100 with PEEP or CPAP ≥5 cm H_2O

Modified from Pneumatikos L, Papaloannou VE: The new Berlin definition: what is, finally, the ARDS? *Pneumon* 25(4):365, 2012.

TABLE 67-6 Predisposing Conditions to ARDS

Direct Lung Injury	Indirect Lung Injury
Common Causes	
• Aspiration of gastric contents or other substances	• Sepsis (especially gram-negative infection)
• Viral or bacterial pneumonia	• Severe massive trauma
• Sepsis	
Less Common Causes	
• Chest trauma	• Acute pancreatitis
• Embolism: fat, air, amniotic fluid, thrombus	• Cardiopulmonary bypass
• Inhalation of toxic substances	• Disseminated intravascular coagulation
• Near-drowning	• Opioid drug overdose (e.g., heroin)
• O_2 toxicity	• Severe head injury
• Radiation pneumonitis	• Shock states
	• Transfusion-related acute lung injury (e.g., multiple blood transfusions)

PATHOPHYSIOLOGY MAP

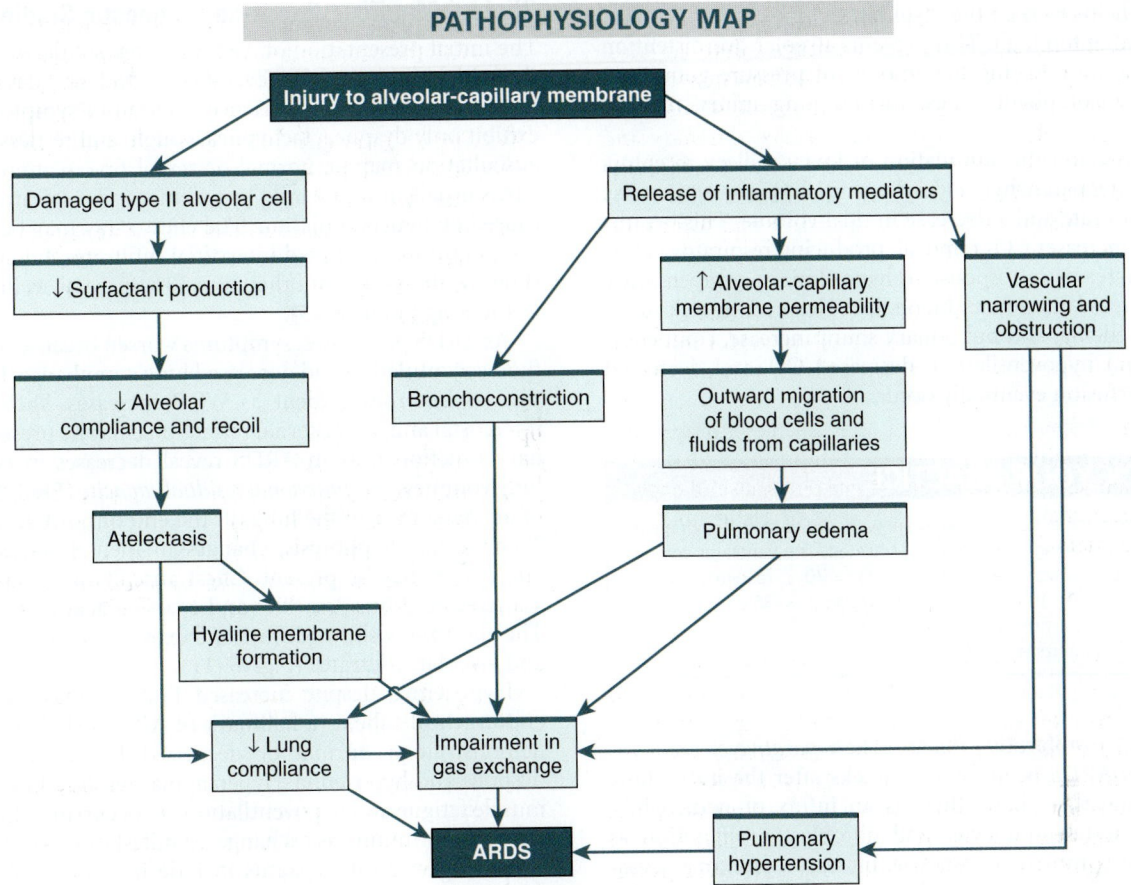

FIG. 67-10   Pathophysiology of acute respiratory distress syndrome (ARDS).

physiologic insults, including severe trauma, gut ischemia, and lung injury. ARDS may also develop as a consequence of multiple organ dysfunction syndrome (MODS). MODS results from organ system dysfunction that progressively increases in severity and ultimately results in failure of one or more body systems. (Chapter 66 discusses SIRS, sepsis, and MODS.)

An exact cause for the damage to the alveolar-capillary membrane is not known. It is thought to be caused by stimulation of the inflammatory and immune systems. This causes an attraction of neutrophils to the pulmonary interstitium. The neutrophils release biochemical, humoral, and cellular mediators that produce changes in the lung. These include increased pulmonary capillary membrane permeability, destruction of elastin and collagen, formation of pulmonary microemboli, and pulmonary artery vasoconstriction (Fig. 67-10). (Chapters 11 and 13 discuss these mediators.)

The pathophysiologic changes in ARDS are divided into three phases: (1) injury or exudative phase, (2) reparative or proliferative phase, and (3) fibrotic phase.

Injury or Exudative Phase.   The *injury or exudative phase* occurs approximately 1 to 7 days (usually 24 to 48 hours) after the initial direct lung injury or host insult. Initially, engorgement of the peribronchial and perivascular interstitial space produces interstitial edema. Next, fluid from the interstitial space crosses the alveolar membrane and enters the alveolar space. Intrapulmonary shunt develops because the alveoli fill with fluid, and blood passing through them cannot be oxygenated (Figs. 67-4 and 67-9).

Alveolar type I and II cells (which produce surfactant) are damaged by the changes caused by ARDS. This damage, in addition to further fluid and protein accumulation, results in surfactant dysfunction. The function of *surfactant* is to maintain alveolar stability by decreasing alveolar surface tension and preventing alveolar collapse. Decreased synthesis of surfactant and inactivation of existing surfactant cause the alveoli to become unstable and collapse (*atelectasis*). Widespread atelectasis further decreases lung compliance, compromises gas exchange, and contributes to hypoxemia.

In addition, during this stage, necrotic cells, protein, and fibrin form hyaline membranes that line the alveoli. Hyaline membranes contribute to the development of fibrosis and atelectasis, leading to a decrease in gas exchange capability and lung compliance.

The primary pathophysiologic changes that describe the *injury or exudative phase* of ARDS are interstitial and alveolar edema and atelectasis. Severe V/Q mismatch and shunting of pulmonary capillary blood result in hypoxemia unresponsive to increasing concentrations of O_2 (termed **refractory hypoxemia**). Diffusion limitation, caused by hyaline membrane formation, worsens the hypoxemia. As the lungs become less compliant because of decreased surfactant, pulmonary edema, and atelectasis, the patient must generate higher airway pressures to inflate "stiff" lungs. Reduced lung compliance greatly increases the patient's WOB.

At this stage, ventilator management often includes a pressure-control type of ventilation. Pressure control ventilation helps to keep the inspiratory and plateau pressures from becoming too high. This prevents alveolar overdistention and rupture. By reducing the amount of pressure going into the stiff, noncompliant lungs, further lung injury may be prevented.[18]

Hypoxemia and the stimulation of juxtacapillary receptors in the stiff lung parenchyma (*J reflex*) initially cause an increase in respiratory rate and a decrease in tidal volume. This breathing pattern increases CO_2 removal, producing respiratory alkalosis. CO increases in response to hypoxemia, a compensatory effort to increase pulmonary blood flow. However, as atelectasis, pulmonary edema, and pulmonary shunt increase, compensation fails and hypoventilation, decreased CO, and decreased tissue O_2 perfusion eventually occur.

? CHECK YOUR PRACTICE

You are caring for a 26-yr-old woman with ARDS who experienced drowning. She is being mechanically ventilated. The ventilator settings are as follows: tidal volume = 350 mL, FIO_2 = 70%, respiratory rate = 10/minute, PEEP = 10 cm H_2O, pressure limit = 35 cm H_2O. The patient's PaO_2 is 83 mm Hg.
• Calculate and interpret the P/F ratio.

Reparative or Proliferative Phase. The *reparative or proliferative phase* of ARDS begins 1 to 2 weeks after the initial lung injury. During this phase, there is an influx of neutrophils, monocytes, and lymphocytes and fibroblast proliferation as part of the inflammatory response. Increased pulmonary vascular resistance and pulmonary hypertension may occur in this stage because fibroblasts and inflammatory cells destroy the pulmonary vasculature. Lung compliance continues to decrease as a result of interstitial fibrosis. Hypoxemia worsens because of the thickened alveolar membrane, causing diffusion limitation and shunting. The proliferative phase is complete when the diseased lung is characterized by dense, fibrous tissue. If the reparative phase persists, widespread fibrosis results. If the reparative phase is stopped, the lesions will resolve.

Fibrotic Phase. The *fibrotic phase* of ARDS occurs approximately 2 to 3 weeks after the initial lung injury. This phase is also called the *chronic* or *late phase* of ARDS. By this time, the lung is completely remodeled by collagenous and fibrous tissues. The diffuse scarring and fibrosis result in decreased lung compliance. In addition, the surface area for gas exchange is significantly reduced because the interstitium is fibrotic, and therefore hypoxemia continues. Pulmonary hypertension results from pulmonary vascular destruction and fibrosis.

Clinical Progression

Progression of ARDS varies among patients. Some survive the acute phase of lung injury. Pulmonary edema resolves, and complete recovery occurs in a few days. The chance for survival is poor in those who enter the fibrotic (chronic or late) stage, which requires long-term mechanical ventilation. It is not known why injured lungs repair and recover in some patients, and in others ARDS progresses. Several factors seem to be important in determining the course of ARDS. These include the nature of the initial injury, extent and severity of comorbidities, and pulmonary complications (e.g., pneumothorax).

Clinical Manifestations and Diagnostic Studies

The initial presentation of ARDS is often subtle. At the time of the initial injury, and for several hours to 1 or 2 days afterward, the patient may not experience respiratory symptoms or may exhibit only dyspnea, tachypnea, cough, and restlessness. Chest auscultation may be normal or reveal fine, scattered crackles. ABGs usually indicate mild hypoxemia and respiratory alkalosis caused by hyperventilation. The chest x-ray may be normal or reveal minimal scattered interstitial infiltrates. Edema may not show on the x-ray until there is a 30% increase in fluid content in the lung (Table 67-5).

As ARDS progresses, symptoms worsen because of increased fluid accumulation and decreased lung compliance. Respiratory distress becomes evident as WOB increases. Tachypnea and intercostal and suprasternal retractions may be present. Pulmonary function tests in ARDS reveal decreases in compliance, lung volumes, and *functional residual capacity* (FRC, the amount of air remaining in the lungs at the end of normal expiration). Tachycardia, diaphoresis, changes in mental status, cyanosis, and pallor may be present. Chest auscultation usually reveals scattered to diffuse crackles and coarse crackles on expiration. The chest x-ray shows diffuse and extensive bilateral interstitial and alveolar infiltrates (Fig. 67-11).

Hypoxemia, despite increased FIO_2 by mask, cannula, or endotracheal tube, is a hallmark of ARDS. ABGs may initially demonstrate a normal or decreased $PaCO_2$ despite severe dyspnea and hypoxemia. Hypercapnia signifies that respiratory muscle fatigue and hypoventilation are occurring, thus interfering with optimum gas exchange. Manifestations of the patient's worsening respiratory status include increasing WOB despite initial findings of normal PaO_2 or SaO_2.

As ARDS progresses, it is associated with profound respiratory distress requiring endotracheal intubation and PPV. The chest x-ray is often termed *whiteout* or *white lung* because consolidation and infiltrates are widespread throughout the lungs, leaving few recognizable air spaces (Fig. 67-11). Pleural effusions may also be present. Severe hypoxemia, hypercapnia,

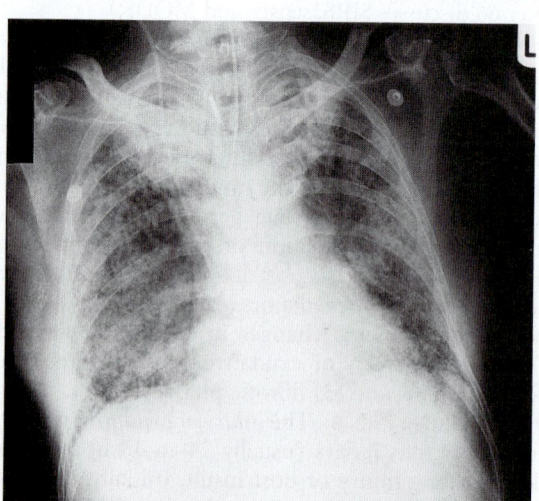

FIG. 67-11 Chest x-ray of a patient with acute respiratory distress syndrome (ARDS). The x-ray shows new, bilateral, diffuse, homogeneous pulmonary infiltrates without cardiac failure, fluid overload, chest infection, or chronic lung disease. (From Cohen J, Powderly WG: *Infectious diseases*, ed 2, St Louis, 2004, Mosby.)

TABLE 67-7 Complications Associated With ARDS

Infection
- Catheter-related infection (e.g., central and peripheral IV catheters, urinary catheters)
- Sepsis

Respiratory
- O₂ toxicity
- Pulmonary barotrauma (e.g., pneumothorax, pneumomediastinum, subcutaneous emphysema)
- Pulmonary emboli
- Pulmonary fibrosis
- Ventilator-associated pneumonia

Gastrointestinal
- Hypermetabolic state, dramatically increased nutrition requirements
- Paralytic ileus
- Pneumoperitoneum
- Stress ulceration and hemorrhage

Renal
- Acute kidney injury

Cardiac
- Decreased cardiac output
- Dysrhythmias

Hematologic
- Anemia
- Disseminated intravascular coagulation
- Thrombocytopenia
- Venous thromboembolism

Endotracheal Tube
- Laryngeal ulceration
- Tracheal malacia
- Tracheal stenosis
- Tracheal ulceration

Central Nervous System and Psychologic
- Delirium
- Posttraumatic stress disorder
- Sleep deprivation

TABLE 67-8 Components of a Ventilator Bundle

- Elevation of head of the bed 30 to 45 degrees
- Daily "sedation holidays" and assessment of readiness for extubation (see Chapter 65)
- Peptic ulcer disease prophylaxis (see Chapter 41)
- Venous thromboembolism prophylaxis (see Chapter 37)
- Daily oral care with chlorhexidine (0.12%) solution (see Table 65-9)

Source: Institute for Healthcare Improvement: How-to guide: prevent ventilator-associated pneumonia. Retrieved from *www.ihi.org/resources/Pages/Tools/HowtoGuidePreventVAP.aspx.*

---

metabolic acidosis, and manifestations of specific organ dysfunction may develop if therapy is not promptly started.

Complications

Complications may develop as a result of ARDS itself or its treatment (Table 67-7). The primary cause of death in ARDS is MODS, often accompanied by sepsis. The vital organs most commonly involved are the kidneys, liver, and heart.

Ventilator-Associated Pneumonia. A frequent complication of ARDS is ventilator-associated pneumonia (VAP). VAP occurs in as many as 68% of patients with ARDS. Risk factors include impaired host defenses, contaminated equipment, invasive monitoring devices, aspiration of GI contents (especially in patients receiving enteral feedings), and prolonged mechanical ventilation. Strategies to prevent VAP include strict infection control measures (e.g., strict hand washing, sterile technique during endotracheal suctioning, frequent mouth care and oral hygiene) and a ventilator bundle protocol[19] (Table 67-8). (Chapter 27 discusses pneumonia, and Chapter 65 discusses VAP.)

Barotrauma. *Barotrauma* may result from rupture of over-distended alveoli during mechanical ventilation. The high peak airway pressures required may predispose patients with ARDS to this complication. Barotrauma results in alveolar air escaping from ruptured alveoli. This can lead to pulmonary interstitial emphysema, pneumothorax, subcutaneous emphysema, pneumoperitoneum, pneumomediastinum, pneumopericardium, and tension pneumothorax.[20] (Chapter 27 discusses pneumothorax.)

To avoid barotrauma and minimize the risk associated with elevated plateau and peak inspiratory pressures, the patient with ARDS is often ventilated with smaller tidal volumes (e.g., 6 mL/kg) and varying amounts of positive end-expiratory pressure (PEEP) to minimize O₂ requirements and intrathoracic pressures. This approach, called the *Acute Respiratory Distress Syndrome Clinical Network (ARDSNet) protocol*, reduces mortality rate and the number of ventilator days for these patients. Unfortunately, one result of this protocol is an elevation in PaCO₂. This is termed *permissive hypercapnia* because the PaCO₂ is allowed to rise slowly above normal limits. It is generally well tolerated as long as the rise in PaCO₂ is gradual to allow systemic and brain circulation to compensate, the pH is 7.2 or higher, and the patient does not have preexisting ICP elevation.[21]

Volutrauma. *Volutrauma* occurs in patients with ARDS or other clinical states requiring mechanical ventilation and large tidal volumes (e.g., 10 to 15 mL/kg) to ventilate noncompliant lungs. Volutrauma results in *alveolar fractures* (damage or tears in the alveoli) and movement of fluids and proteins into the alveolar spaces. To limit this complication, smaller tidal volumes or pressure-control ventilation is now the standard in patients with ARDS (see Chapter 65).

Stress Ulcers. Critically ill patients with acute respiratory failure are at high risk for stress ulcers. Bleeding from stress ulcers occurs in 30% of patients with ARDS who require PPV, a higher incidence than other causes of acute respiratory failure. Management strategies include correction of predisposing conditions such as hypotension, shock, and acidosis. Prophylactic management includes antiulcer drugs such as proton pump inhibitors (e.g., pantoprazole [Protonix]) and mucosal-protecting drugs (e.g., sucralfate [Carafate]). Early initiation of enteral nutrition also helps prevent mucosal damage (see Chapters 39 and 65).

Renal Failure. Renal failure can occur from decreased renal perfusion and subsequent decreased delivery of O₂ to the kidneys. This can result from hypotension, hypoxemia, or hypercapnia. Renal failure may also result from nephrotoxic drugs (e.g., vancomycin [Vancocin]) used to treat ARDS-related infections.

❖ NURSING AND INTERPROFESSIONAL MANAGEMENT: ACUTE RESPIRATORY DISTRESS SYNDROME

The management of a patient with acute respiratory failure (Table 67-4) and the nursing care plan for acute respiratory failure (eNursing Care Plan 67-1, available on the website for this chapter) apply to patients with ARDS. The following section discusses additional interprofessional care for the patient with ARDS (Table 67-9).

TABLE 67-9 Interprofessional Care

Acute Respiratory Distress Syndrome

Diagnostic Assessment

See Table 67-5.

Management

Respiratory Therapy

- O_2 administration
- Positive pressure ventilation with PEEP
- Permissive hypercapnia
- Alternative modes of mechanical ventilation: pressure-control inverse ratio ventilation, airway pressure release ventilation, high-frequency ventilation (see Chapter 65)
- Positioning strategies
  - Prone positioning
  - Lateral rotation therapy
  - Kinetic therapy

Supportive Therapy

- Identification and treatment of underlying cause
- Hemodynamic monitoring
- Nutritional therapy

Drug Therapy

- Inotropic and vasopressor drugs
  - dopamine
  - dobutamine
  - norepinephrine (Levophed)
- Diuretics
- IV fluid administration
- Sedation/analgesia
- Neuromuscular blockade

PEEP, Positive end-expiratory pressure.

◆ Nursing Assessment

Because ARDS causes acute respiratory failure, the subjective and objective data that you should obtain from someone with ARDS are the same as those for acute respiratory failure (Table 67-3). Some patient information may not be possible to obtain initially due to management priorities of oxygenation and ventilation.

◆ Nursing Diagnoses

Nursing diagnoses for the patient with ARDS may include, but are not limited to, those described for acute respiratory failure (see p. 1615).

◆ Planning

Patients with moderate to severe ARDS are cared for in critical care units. With appropriate therapy, overall goals include a PaO_2 of 60 mm Hg or higher and adequate lung ventilation to maintain normal pH. Specific goals for a patient with ARDS include (1) PaO_2 within normal limits for age or at baseline on room air, (2) SaO_2 greater than 90%, (3) resolution of the precipitating factor(s) for ARDS, and (4) clear lungs on auscultation.

◆ Oxygen Administration. The primary goal of O_2 therapy is to correct hypoxemia. Initially use a nasal cannula or face mask with high-flow systems that deliver higher O_2 concentrations to maximize O_2 delivery. Continuously monitor SpO_2 to assess the effectiveness of O_2 therapy. Patients with moderate to severe ARDS and refractory hypoxemia need intubation with mechanical ventilation to maintain the PaO_2 at acceptable levels.

◆ Positive Pressure Ventilation. Endotracheal intubation and PPV provide additional respiratory support. However, even with these interventions it may be necessary to maintain the FIO_2 at 60% or higher to maintain a PaO_2 of at least 60 mm Hg. During PPV, it is common to apply PEEP at 5 cm H_2O to compensate for loss of glottic function caused by the endotracheal tube. In patients with ARDS, higher levels of PEEP (e.g., 10 to 20 cm H_2O) may be used. PEEP increases FRC and opens up collapsed alveoli. PEEP is typically applied in 3- to 5-cm H_2O increments until oxygenation is adequate with FIO_2 less than or equal to 60%. PEEP may improve V/Q in respiratory units that collapse at low airway pressures, thus allowing the FIO_2 to be lowered.

However, PEEP is not a benign therapy. The additional intrathoracic and intrapulmonic pressures can compromise venous return to the right side of the heart, thereby decreasing preload, CO, and BP. High levels of PEEP cause hyperinflation of the alveoli, compression of the pulmonary capillary bed, reduction in blood return to the left side of the heart, and a dramatic reduction in BP. In addition, high levels of PEEP or excessive inspiratory pressures can result in barotrauma and volutrauma.

If hypoxemic respiratory failure persists in spite of high levels of PEEP, alternative modes of mechanical ventilation and respiratory therapies may be used. These include airway pressure release ventilation, pressure-control inverse ratio ventilation, high-frequency ventilation, and permissive hypercapnia (low tidal volumes that allow $PaCO_2$ to increase slowly).[20] (Chapter 65 provides additional information on mechanical ventilation and PEEP.)

Extracorporeal membrane oxygenation (ECMO) and extracorporeal CO_2 removal ($ECCO_2R$) are external devices cannulated within large blood vessels. This allows blood to pass across a gas-exchanging membrane outside the body and then return oxygenated blood back to the body. $ECCO_2R$ with PPV allows the lungs to heal while lung function is inadequate to maintain adequate oxygenation and CO_2 removal.[22]

◆ Positioning Strategies. In the early phases of ARDS, fluid moves freely throughout the lung. Because of gravity, this fluid pools in dependent regions of the lung. As a result, some alveoli are fluid filled (dependent areas), whereas others are air filled (nondependent areas). In addition, when the patient is supine, the heart and mediastinal contents place more pressure on the lungs than in the prone position. Thus the supine position changes pleural pressure and predisposes the patient to atelectasis.

If you turn the patient from supine to prone, air-filled, alveoli in the ventral (anterior) portion of the lung become dependent. Perfusion may be better matched to ventilation.

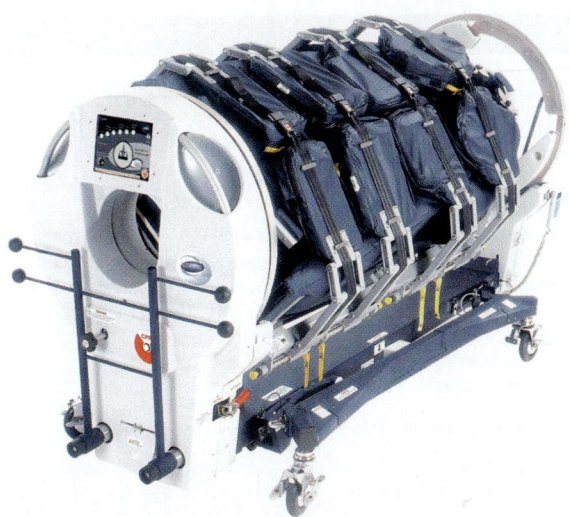

FIG. 67-12 RotoProne bed. (ArjoHuntleigh. Reprinted with permission.) Note: The RotoProne Delta Therapy System allows clinicians to place patients in the prone position, safely and effectively. This product is not specifically indicated for the treatment of ARDS or VAP.

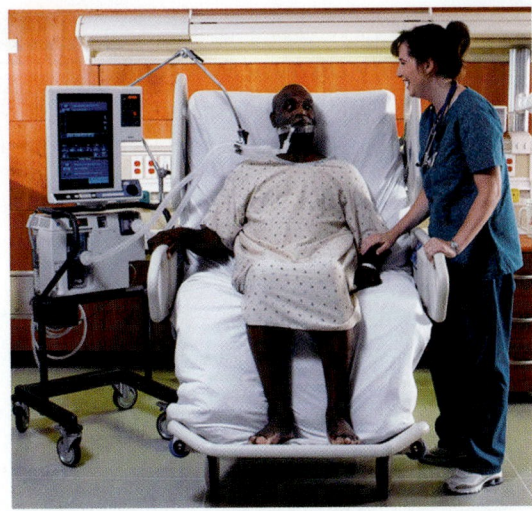

FIG. 67-13 TotalCare SpO2RT Bed System offers continuous lateral rotation therapy and percussion and vibration therapies. Patients can easily and quickly be repositioned. (Copyright 2006 Hill-Rom Services, Inc. Reprinted with permission. All rights reserved.)

Prone positioning may be considered for patients with refractory hypoxemia who do not respond to other strategies to increase PaO_2 (Fig. 67-12). Some patients will have a marked improvement in PaO_2 when prone (e.g., PaO_2 70 mm Hg supine, PaO_2 90 mm Hg prone) with no change in FIO_2.[23]

Prone positioning helps to improve ventilation of better-perfused lung areas. This may be sufficient to allow a reduction in FIO_2 or PEEP. You may observe BP instability owing to fluid shifts and additional need for airway suctioning as secretions are mobilized by gravity.

Currently, there is no reliable way of predicting who will or will not respond to prone positioning.[23] When placing a patient in the prone position, pay special attention to the patient's skin to avoid the development of pressure ulcers.[24]

Other positioning strategies to consider for patients with ARDS include continuous lateral rotation therapy (CLRT) and kinetic therapy. CLRT provides continuous, slow, side-to-side turning of the patient by rotating the actual bed frame less than 40 degrees. The bed's lateral movement is maintained for 18 of every 24 hours to simulate postural drainage and to help mobilize pulmonary secretions. In addition, the bed may also contain a vibrator pack that provides chest physiotherapy. This feature assists with secretion mobilization and removal (Fig. 67-13). Kinetic therapy is similar to CLRT in that patients are rotated side-to-side 40 degrees or more. It is important to obtain baseline assessments of the patient's pulmonary status (e.g., respiratory rate and rhythm, breath sounds, ABGs, SpO_2) and continue to monitor the patient throughout the therapy.

Medical Supportive Therapy

Maintenance of Cardiac Output and Tissue Perfusion. Patients on PPV and PEEP frequently experience decreased CO. One cause is decreased venous return from the PEEP-induced increase in intrathoracic pressure. Impaired contractility and decreased preload can also decrease CO. Hemodynamic monitoring (e.g., CVP, CO, $ScvO_2$, SvO_2) via central venous or pulmonary artery pressure or arterial pressure-based CO monitoring is essential. This allows you to see trends, detect changes, and adjust therapy as needed. An arterial catheter also provides continuous monitoring of BP and sampling of blood for ABGs. If the CO falls, it may be necessary to administer crystalloid fluids or colloid solutions or to lower PEEP. Use of inotropic drugs such as dobutamine or dopamine may also be necessary. (Chapter 65 discusses hemodynamic monitoring.)

Packed red blood cells are used to increase hemoglobin and thus the O_2-carrying capacity of the blood. Controversy exists regarding the optimal hemoglobin level. Some advocate keeping the level around 9 g/dL (90 g/L) with an SpO_2 of 90% or more (when PaO_2 is greater than 60 mm Hg). Others recommend hemoglobin levels greater than 7 g/dL (70 g/L).[15]

Maintenance of Nutrition and Fluid Balance. Maintenance of nutrition and fluid balance is challenging in the patient with ARDS. Consult with a dietitian to determine optimal caloric needs. Enteral or parenteral feedings are started to meet the high energy requirements of these patients.

Increasing pulmonary capillary permeability results in fluid in the lungs and causes pulmonary edema. At the same time, the patient may be volume depleted and thus at risk for hypotension and decreased CO from mechanical ventilation and PEEP. Monitor hemodynamic parameters (e.g., CVP, stroke volume variation), daily weights, and intake and output to assess the patient's fluid status. The patient is often placed on fluid restriction, and diuretics are used as necessary.

Evaluation

The expected outcomes for the patient with ARDS are similar to those for a patient with acute respiratory failure (see p. 1619).

CASE STUDY
Acute Respiratory Distress Syndrome

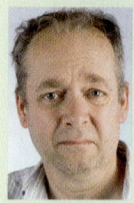

(©Thinkstock)

Patient Profile
J.N. is a 58-yr-old white man who was admitted 12 hr ago to a surgical ICU after emergent surgery for an acute ischemic bowel.

Past Medical History
• Lumbar spine surgery 5 yr ago
• Chronic back pain controlled with oxycodone (OxyContin) 15 mg PO tid

Operative Procedure
• Surgical procedure involved extensive abdominal surgery to repair a perforated colon, irrigate the abdominal cavity, and provide hemostasis
• During surgery his systolic BP dropped to 70 mm Hg
• Six units of packed red blood cells and 4 L of 0.9% saline were infused
• He is receiving 60% O_2 via an aerosol face mask

Postoperative Orders
• Continuous ECG and pulse oximetry monitoring
• Give 0.9% saline at 125 mL/hr via a central venous IV catheter
• Monitor hourly urine output via indwelling bladder catheter
• Pain management via a continuous IV infusion of morphine

Immediate Postoperative Status
• J.N.'s pulmonary status worsens. He requires progressively higher FIO_2 via high-flow face mask and a short trial of noninvasive positive pressure ventilation (NIPPV).
• J.N. continues to experience declining SaO_2 levels and increased WOB as well as worsening hemodynamic status. Emergent endotracheal intubation and PPV are needed.
• Sedation, analgesia, and neuromuscular blockade are started to achieve anxiolysis, pain control, and ventilator synchrony.
• Postintubation chest x-ray reveals 50% right-sided pneumothorax, requiring the emergent chest tube placement. Immediately after chest tube placement, his SpO_2 decreased significantly below baseline to 80% to 82%.
• No significant changes were evident in ventilation or lung compliance, and he remains synchronous with mechanical ventilation.
• ABGs shows $PaCO_2$ increased to 52 mm Hg and PaO_2 decreased to 44 mm Hg.
• J.N. is tachycardic during and immediately after chest tube insertion. A 10-mg bolus of morphine is given followed by an increase in the continuous infusion.
• After 30 min, his O_2 saturation improves to 90% to 91% and ABGs shows improved oxygenation (PaO_2 63 mm Hg) and ventilation ($PaCO_2$ 45 mm Hg).

Postoperative Day 1
• J.N.'s lung function continues to worsen and his hypoxemia is refractory to 100% FIO_2 and high levels of PEEP.
• He experiences kidney and liver failure. There is little hope of weaning him from mechanical ventilation.
• He has an advance directive that indicates he does not want to be kept alive by artificial means.

Subjective Data
• Patient is sedated, paralyzed, and unable to communicate.
• His wife and two adult children are at the bedside and voicing concerns and questions regarding his progress.

Objective Data
Physical Examination
• *General:* Sedated, paralyzed; head of bed elevated 45 degrees; skin cool with moderate diaphoresis
• *Respiratory:* Endotracheal tube in place with PPV. No accessory muscle use, retractions, or paradoxic breathing; respiratory rate 18 breaths/min and in phase with ventilator; SpO_2 85%, bilateral crackles at lung bases. Ventilator settings: tidal volume 350 mL, FIO_2 100%, respiratory rate 10/minute, PEEP 10 cm H_2O, pressure limit 35 cm H_2O.
• *Cardiovascular:* Apical-radial pulse equal, BP 100/60 mm Hg
  • ECG as follows:

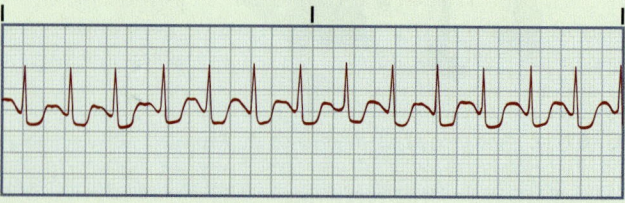

  • Weak peripheral pulses; temperature 101° F (38.3° C) rectally
• *Gastrointestinal:* Surgical dressing dry and intact; colostomy draining serosanguineous drainage
• *Urologic:* Indwelling bladder catheter draining concentrated urine less than 30 mL/hr

Diagnostic Findings
• ABGs obtained 4 hours following intubation and start of PPV: pH 7.15, PaO_2 59 mm Hg, $PaCO_2$ 57 mm Hg, HCO_3 16 mEq/L, O_2 saturation 86%.
• PaO_2/FIO_2 ratio 59
• Chest x-ray: new bilateral, scattered interstitial infiltrates compatible with an ARDS pattern as interpreted by the radiologist

Discussion Questions
1. How does the pathophysiology of ARDS predispose this patient to refractory hypoxemia?
2. What clinical manifestations does J.N. exhibit that support a diagnosis of ARDS?
3. What are the possible causes of ARDS in J.N.?
4. What are the possible complications that J.N. is at risk for developing secondary to ARDS?
5. What are possible reasons for J.N.'s sudden decline in pulmonary status during and immediately after chest tube insertion?
6. ***Evidence-Based Practice:*** You are orienting a new nurse who asks you why you offered J.N.'s family the opportunity to stay at the bedside while the chest tube was placed. How would you respond?
7. What are possible reasons for improved oxygenation and CO_2 levels after administration of additional opioid analgesia?
8. ***Priority Decision:*** What priority interventions should be implemented to improve J.N.'s respiratory status and hypoxemia?
9. ***Priority Decision:*** Based on the assessment data presented, what are the priority nursing diagnoses?
10. ***Teamwork and Collaboration:*** When developing the plan of care for J.N., what tasks can you delegate to unlicensed assistive personnel (UAP)?
11. ***Patient-Centered Care:*** What information should you provide to J.N.'s caregiver(s) given his decline in cardiopulmonary function?
12. ***Patient-Centered Care:*** Given the guidelines in the patient's advance directive, what ethical/legal issues could you encounter in this patient scenario?

Answers available at *http://evolve.elsevier.com/Lewis/medsurg.*

BRIDGE TO NCLEX EXAMINATION

The number of the question corresponds to the same-numbered outcome at the beginning of the chapter.

1. Which signs and symptoms differentiate hypoxemic respiratory failure from hypercapnic respiratory failure (select all that apply)?
   a. Cyanosis
   b. Tachypnea
   c. Morning headache
   d. Paradoxic breathing
   e. Use of pursed-lip breathing

2. The O_2 delivery system chosen for the patient in acute respiratory failure should
   a. always be a low-flow device, such as a nasal cannula or face mask.
   b. administer continuous positive airway pressure ventilation to prevent CO_2 narcosis.
   c. correct the PaO_2 to a normal level as quickly as possible using mechanical ventilation.
   d. maintain the PaO_2 at greater than or equal to 60 mm Hg at the lowest O_2 concentration possible.

3. The most common early clinical manifestations of ARDS that the nurse may observe are
   a. dyspnea and tachypnea.
   b. cyanosis and apprehension.
   c. hypotension and tachycardia.
   d. respiratory distress and frothy sputum.

4. Maintenance of fluid balance in the patient with ARDS involves
   a. hydration using colloids.
   b. administration of surfactant.
   c. fluid restriction and diuretics as necessary.
   d. keeping the hemoglobin at levels above 9 g/dL (90 g/L).

5. Which intervention is most likely to prevent or limit barotrauma in the patient with ARDS who is mechanically ventilated?
   a. Decreasing PEEP
   b. Increasing the tidal volume
   c. Use of permissive hypercapnia
   d. Use of positive pressure ventilation

1. a, b, d, 2. d, 3. a, 4. c, 5. c

For rationales to these answers and even more NCLEX review questions, visit *http://evolve.elsevier.com/Lewis/medsurg.*

ⓔ EVOLVE WEBSITE

http://evolve.elsevier.com/Lewis/medsurg
Review Questions (Online Only)
Key Points
Answer Keys to Questions
• Rationales for Bridge to NCLEX Examination Questions
• Answer Guidelines for Case Study on p. 1626
Student Case Studies
• Patient With Acute Respiratory Failure and Ventilatory Management
• Patient With Pulmonary Embolism and Respiratory Failure
Nursing Care Plans
• eNursing Care Plan 67-1: Patient With Acute Respiratory Failure
Conceptual Care Map Creator
Audio Glossary
Content Updates

REFERENCES

1. Kaynar AM: Respiratory failure: overview. 2015. Retrieved from *http://emedicine.medscape.com/article/167981-overview.*
*2. Chung KF, Wenzel SE, Brozek JL, et al: International ERS/ATS guidelines on definition, evaluation and treatment of severe asthma, *Eur Respir J* 43:343, 2014.
3. Taffet GE, Donahue JF, Altman PR: Considerations for managing chronic obstructive pulmonary disease in the elderly, *Clin Interv Aging* 9:23, 2014.
*4. Barr J, Fraser GL, Puntillo K, et al: Clinical practice guidelines for the management of pain, agitation, and delirium in adult patients in the intensive care unit, *Crit Care Med* 41(1):263, 2013.
5. Ouellette DR: Pulmonary embolism: overview. 2015. Retrieved from *http://emedicine.medscape.com/article/300901-overview.*
6. Cartin-Ceba R, Iyer VN, Krowka MJ: Hepatopulmonary syndrome and portopulmonary hypertension. In Cataldo D, editor: *Contemporary liver transplantation*, Switzerland, 2015, Springer International.
7. Laveneziana P, Webb KA, O'Donnell DE: Static and dynamic hyperinflation in chronic obstructive pulmonary disease. In Aliverti A, Pedotti A, editors: *Mechanics of breathing*, New York, 2014, Springer.
8. Fayyaz J: Hypoventilation syndromes: overview. 2015. Retrieved from *http://emedicine.medscape.com/article/304381-overview.*
9. Huttmann SE, Windisch W, Storre JH: Techniques for the measurement and monitoring of carbon dioxide in the blood, *Ann Am Thorac Soc* 11(4):645, 2014.

10. Terzano C, Romani S, Gaudio C, et al: Right heart functional changes in the acute, hypercapnic exacerbations of COPD, *BioMed Res Int* 2014:596051, 2014.
11. Schnell D, Timsit JF, Darmon M, et al: Noninvasive mechanical ventilation in acute respiratory failure: trends in use and outcomes, *Intens Care Med* 40(4):582, 2014.
12. Kelly CR, Higgins AR, Chandra S: Noninvasive positive-pressure ventilation, *N Engl J Med* 372:e30, 2015.
13. Bumbaeca D, Filip N, Valcu C, et al: Outcome of non-invasive ventilation in acute hypercapnic respiratory failure in the elderly, *Eur Respir J* 44(Suppl 58):P2958, 2014.
*14. Arbour R: Bispectral index monitoring. In Wiegand DL-M, editor: *AACN procedure manual for critical care*, ed 6, St Louis, 2011, Saunders.
*15. Shah A, Stanworth SJ, McKechnie S: Evidence and triggers for the transfusion of blood and blood products, *Anesth* 70(Suppl 1):10, 2015.
16. Inouye SK, Westendorp RGJ, Saczynski JS: Delirium in elderly people, *Lancet* 383(9920):911, 2014.
17. Ferguson ND, Fan E, Camporota L, et al: The Berlin definition of ARDS: an expanded rationale, justification, and supplementary material, *Intens Care Med* 38(10):1573, 2012.
18. Wilson JG, Matthay MA: Mechanical ventilation in acute hypoxemic respiratory failure: a review of new strategies for the practicing hospitalist, *J Hosp Med* 9(7):469, 2014.
19. Kalanuris AA, Zai W, Mirski M: Ventilator-associated pneumonia in the ICU, *Crit Care* 18(208):1, 2014.
20. Terzi E, Zarogoulidis K, Kougioumtzi I, et al: Acute respiratory distress syndrome and pneumothorax, *J Thorac Dis* 6(Suppl 4):S435, 2014.
21. Beitler JR, Schoenfeld DA, Thompson BT: Preventing ARDS: progress, promise and pitfalls, *Chest* 146(4):1102, 2014.
*22. Combes A, Brodie D, Bartlett R, et al: Position paper for the organization of extracorporeal membrane oxygenation programs for acute respiratory failure in adult patients, *Am J Respir Crit Care Med* 190(5):488, 2014.
*23. Beitler JR, Shaefi S, Montesi SB, et al: Prone positioning reduces mortality from acute respiratory distress syndrome in the low tidal volume era: a meta-analysis, *Intens Care Med* 40(3):332, 2014.
*24. Girard R, Baboi L, Ayzac L, et al: The impact of patient positioning on pressure ulcers in patients with severe ARDS: results from a multicentre randomized controlled trial on prone positioning, *Intens Care Med* 40:397, 2014.

*Evidence-based information for clinical practice.

68

Emergency and Disaster Nursing

Linda Bucher

One of the tests of leadership is the ability to recognize a problem before it becomes an emergency.

Arnold H. Glasow

(e) http://evolve.elsevier.com/Lewis/medsurg/

LEARNING OUTCOMES

1. Apply the steps in triage, the primary survey, and the secondary survey to a patient experiencing a medical, surgical, or traumatic emergency.
2. Relate the pathophysiology to the assessment and interprofessional care of select environmental emergencies (e.g., hyperthermia, hypothermia, submersion injury, bites).
3. Relate the pathophysiology to the assessment and interprofessional care of select toxicologic emergencies.
4. Select appropriate nursing interventions for victims of violence.
5. Differentiate among the responsibilities of health care providers, the community, and select federal agencies in emergency and mass casualty incident preparedness.

KEY TERMS

drowning, p. 1639
emergency, p. 1645
family presence (FP), p. 1632
frostbite, p. 1637
heat cramps, p. 1637

heat exhaustion, p. 1637
heatstroke, p. 1637
hypothermia, p. 1638
jaw-thrust maneuver, p. 1630
mass casualty incident (MCI), p. 1645

primary survey, p. 1630
secondary survey, p. 1632
submersion injury, p. 1639
terrorism, p. 1645
triage, p. 1628

This chapter presents an overview of triage and care of select emergency patients. Common emergency situations discussed include heat- and cold-related emergencies, submersion injuries, bites and stings, and various types of poisonings. The chapter concludes with a discussion of terrorism, followed by a description of a mass casualty incident, and the methods of responding to the incident.

The emergency management of various medical, surgical, and traumatic emergencies is discussed throughout the textbook. Tables summarize emergency management of specific problems. Table 68-1 lists the emergency management tables by title, chapter number, and page.

Patients with life-threatening or potentially life-threatening problems as well as less urgent problems come to the hospital through the emergency department (ED). Every year more than 136 million people visit EDs.[1] This number is increasing for a variety of reasons, including (1) the inability to see an HCP, (2) an aging population, (3) shorter hospital stays resulting in frequent readmissions, (4) acute mental health crises, (5) ED closures, and (6) lack of or inadequate health insurance or an HCP. These factors result in chronic overcrowding and long wait times.[2]

Emergency nurses care for patients of all ages and with a variety of problems. However, some EDs specialize in certain patient populations or conditions, such as pediatric ED or trauma ED. The Emergency Nurses Association (ENA) is the specialty organization aimed at advancing emergency nursing practice. The ENA provides standards of care for nurses working in the ED, and a certification process that allows nurses to become certified emergency nurses (CENs).[3]

CARE OF EMERGENCY PATIENT

Recognition of life-threatening illness or injury is one of the most important goals of emergency nursing. Initiation of interventions to reverse or prevent a crisis is often a priority before a medical diagnosis is made. This process begins with your first contact with a patient. Prompt identification of patients requiring immediate treatment and determination of appropriate interventions are essential nurse competencies.

Triage

Triage, a French word meaning "to sort," refers to the process of rapidly determining patient acuity.[4] It is one of the most

Reviewed by Rebecca Personett, RN, PhD, NEA-BC, Professor of Nursing, North Central Texas College, Gainesville, Texas and Brookhaven College, Dallas, Texas; and Matthew Soos, RN, BSN, BA, EMT, Interventional Radiology/Emergency Department Staff Nurse, AtlantiCare Regional Medical Center, Atlantic City, New Jersey.

important assessment skills needed by emergency nurses. Most often you will confront multiple patients who have a variety of problems. The triage process works on the premise that patients who have a threat to life must be treated before other patients.

A *triage system* identifies and categorizes patients so that the most critical are treated first. The ENA and American College of Emergency Physicians support the use of a five-level triage system.[5] The *Emergency Severity Index* (ESI) is a five-level triage system that incorporates concepts of illness severity and resource utilization (e.g., electrocardiogram [ECG], laboratory tests, radiology studies, IV fluids) to determine who should be treated first (Table 68-2). The ESI includes a triage algorithm that directs you to assign an ESI level to patients coming into the ED. The triage algorithm can be found in the ESI Implementation Handbook.[5]

First, assess the patient for any threats to life (ESI-1) (e.g., Is the patient dying?) or presence of a high-risk situation (ESI-2) (e.g., Is this a high-risk patient who should not wait to be seen?). Next, evaluate patients who do not meet the criteria for ESI-1 or ESI-2 for the number of anticipated resources that they may need. Assign patients to ESI-3, ESI-4, or ESI-5 based on this determination. Normal vital signs are required for patients assigned to ESI-3. Patients with abnormal vital signs may be reassigned to ESI-2.[5]

➕ TABLE 68-1 Emergency Management

Emergency Management Tables

Title	Chapter	Page
Abdominal Trauma	42	942
Acute Abdominal Pain	42	939
Acute Soft Tissue Injury	62	1464
Anaphylactic Shock	13	202
Chemical Burns	24	436
Chest Pain	33	723
Chest Trauma	27	519
Depressant Toxicity	10	152
Diabetic Ketoacidosis	48	1144
Dysrhythmias	35	763
Electrical Burns	24	435
Eye Injury	21	371
Fractured Extremity	62	1474
Head Injury	56	1330
Hyperthermia	68	1636
Hypothermia	68	1639
Inhalation Injury	24	435
Sexual Assault	53	1264
Shock	66	1597
Spinal Cord Injury	60	1425
Stimulant Toxicity	10	151
Stroke	57	1354
Submersion Injuries	68	1641
Thermal Burns	24	434
Thoracic Injuries	27	520
Tonic-Clonic Seizures	58	1378

❓ CHECK YOUR PRACTICE

You are working in the ED with your preceptor, who is a triage nurse. A 24-yr-old male arrives and states, "I think I have food poisoning. I've been vomiting all night and now I have diarrhea." The patient reports abdominal cramping that he rates as 6/10. He denies fever or chills. Vital signs: T = 97.8°F (36.6°C), HR = 94, RR = 16, BP = 121/74 mm Hg.

• Assign a triage acuity rating using the ESI (Table 68-2).

After you complete the initial focused assessment to determine the presence of actual or potential threats to life, proceed with a more detailed assessment. A systematic approach to this assessment decreases the time needed to identify potential threats to life and limits the risk of overlooking a life-threatening condition. A primary and secondary survey is the approach used for all trauma patients. For nontrauma patients, the

TABLE 68-2 Five-Level Emergency Severity Index (ESI)

Definition	LEVEL				
	ESI-1	**ESI-2**	**ESI-3**	**ESI-4**	**ESI-5**
Stability of vital functions (ABCs)	Unstable	Threatened	Stable	Stable	Stable
Life threat or organ threat	Obvious	Likely but not always obvious	Unlikely but possible	No	No
How soon patient should be seen by HCP	Immediately	Within 10 min	Up to 1 hr	Could be delayed	Could be delayed
Expected resource intensity	High resource intensity. Staff at bedside continuously. Often mobilization of team response	High resource intensity. Multiple, often complex diagnostic studies. Frequent consultation. Continuous monitoring	Medium to high resource intensity. Multiple diagnostic studies (e.g., multiple laboratory studies, x-rays) or brief observation. Complex procedure (e.g., IV fluids, drugs)	Low resource intensity. One simple diagnostic study (e.g., x-ray) or simple procedure (e.g., sutures)	Low resource intensity. Examination only
Examples	Cardiac arrest, intubated trauma patient, overdose with bradypnea, severe respiratory distress	Chest pain probably resulting from ischemia, multiple trauma unless responsive	Abdominal pain or gynecologic disorders unless in severe distress, hip fracture in older patient	Closed extremity trauma, simple laceration, cystitis	Cold symptoms, minor burn, recheck (e.g., wound), prescription refill

ABCs, Airway, breathing, circulation.
Modified and reprinted with permission. Copyright 1999, Richard C. Wuerz, MD, and David R. Eitel, MD.

primary survey is followed by a focused assessment. (Focused assessments are discussed in Chapter 3.)

Primary Survey

The primary survey (Table 68-3) focuses on airway, breathing, circulation (ABC), disability, exposure, facilitation of adjuncts and family, and other resuscitation aids. If uncontrolled external hemorrhage is noted, the usual ABC assessment format may be reprioritized to <C>ABC for hemorrhage control. The <C> stands for catastrophic hemorrhage and, if present, must be controlled first.[6] Apply direct pressure with a sterile dressing followed by a pressure dressing to any obvious bleeding sites.

The primary survey aims to identify life-threatening conditions so that appropriate interventions can be started. You may identify life-threatening conditions related to ABCs (Table 68-4) at any point during the primary survey. When this occurs, start interventions immediately, before moving to the next step of the survey.

A = Alertness and Airway.
The alertness level of the patient can be an important factor for selecting appropriate airway interventions. Determine level of consciousness (LOC) by assessing the patient's response to verbal and/or painful stimuli. A simple mnemonic to remember is *AVPU: A* = alert, *V* = responsive to voice, *P* = responsive to pain, and *U* = unresponsive.[6]

Nearly all immediate trauma deaths occur because of airway obstruction. Saliva, bloody secretions, vomitus, laryngeal trauma, dentures, facial trauma, fractures, and the tongue can obstruct the airway. Patients at risk for airway compromise include those who drown or have seizures, anaphylaxis, foreign body obstruction, or cardiopulmonary arrest. If an airway is not maintained, obstruction of airflow, hypoxia, and death will result.

Primary signs and symptoms in a patient with a compromised airway include dyspnea, inability to speak, gasping (agonal) breaths, foreign body in the airway, and trauma to the face or neck. Airway maintenance should progress rapidly from the least to the most invasive method. Treatment includes opening the airway using the jaw-thrust maneuver (avoiding hyperextension of the neck) (Fig. 68-1), suctioning and/or removal of foreign body, insertion of a nasopharyngeal or an oropharyngeal airway (in unconscious patients only), and endotracheal intubation. If intubation is impossible because of airway obstruction, an emergency cricothyroidotomy or tracheotomy is performed (see Chapter 26). Ventilate patients with

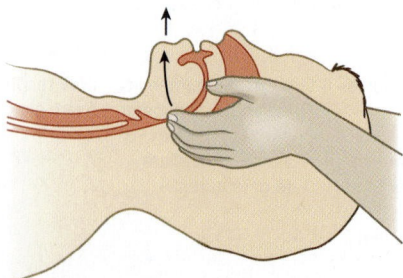

FIG. 68-1 Jaw-thrust maneuver is the recommended procedure for opening the airway of an unconscious patient with a possible neck or spinal injury. With the patient lying supine, kneel at the top of the head. Place one hand on each side of the patient's head, resting your elbows on the surface. Grasp the angles of the patient's lower jaw and lift the jaw forward with both hands without tilting the head.

100% O$_2$ using a bag-valve-mask (BVM) device before intubation or cricothyroidotomy.[7]

Rapid-sequence intubation is the preferred procedure for securing an unprotected airway in the ED. It involves the use of sedation (e.g., midazolam) or anesthesia (e.g., etomidate [Amidate]) and paralysis (e.g., succinylcholine [Anectine]). These drugs aid intubation and reduce the risk of aspiration and airway trauma. (See Chapter 65 for more information on intubation.)

Suspect cervical spine trauma in any patient with face, head, or neck trauma and/or significant upper chest injuries. Stabilize the cervical spine (head maintained in a neutral position) and/or immobilize during assessment of the airway. At the scene of the injury, the cervical spine is immobilized with a rigid *cervical collar* (C-collar) and a *cervical immobilization device* (CID) (also known as "head blocks"). Finally, secure the patient's forehead to the backboard. Do not use sandbags because the weight of the bags could move the head if the patient is logrolled.

B = Breathing.
Adequate airflow through the upper airway does not ensure adequate ventilation. Many conditions cause breathing changes. These include fractured ribs, pneumothorax, penetrating injury, allergic reactions, pulmonary emboli, and asthma attacks. Patients with these conditions may have a variety of signs and symptoms, including dyspnea (e.g., pulmonary emboli), paradoxic or asymmetric chest wall movement (e.g., flail chest), decreased or absent breath sounds on the affected side (e.g., pneumothorax), visible wound to the chest wall (e.g., penetrating injury), cyanosis (e.g., asthma), tachycardia, and hypotension.

Every critically injured or ill patient has an increased metabolic and O$_2$ demand and should have supplemental O$_2$. Give high-flow O$_2$ (100%) via a non-rebreather mask and monitor the patient's response. Life-threatening conditions (e.g., flail chest, tension pneumothorax) can severely and quickly compromise ventilation. Interventions may include BVM ventilation with 100% O$_2$, needle decompression, intubation, and treatment of the underlying cause.

C = Circulation.
An effective circulatory system includes the heart, intact blood vessels, and adequate blood volume. Uncontrolled internal or external bleeding places an individual at risk for hemorrhagic shock (see Chapter 66). Check a central pulse (e.g., carotid) because peripheral pulses may be absent due to direct injury or vasoconstriction. If you feel a pulse, assess the quality and rate. Assess the skin for color, temperature, and moisture. Altered mental status and delayed capillary refill (longer than 3 seconds) are common signs of shock. When evaluating capillary refill in cold environments, remember that a cold temperature delays refill.

Insert IV lines into veins in the upper extremities unless contraindicated, such as in a massive fracture or an injury that affects limb circulation. Insert two large-bore (14- to 16-gauge) IV catheters and start aggressive fluid resuscitation using normal saline or lactated Ringer's solution. Consider intraosseous or central venous access if unable to rapidly obtain venous access. (See Chapter 66 for more information on hypovolemic shock and fluid resuscitation.)

Give type-specific packed red blood cells if needed. In an emergency (life-threatening) situation, give uncrossmatched blood (e.g., O negative) if immediate transfusion is warranted. Pelvic splints or belts for pelvic fracture may be used for bleeding with hypotension.

TABLE 68-3 Emergency Assessment: Primary Survey

Assessment	Interventions
Alertness and Airway With Cervical Spine Stabilization and/or Immobilization	
• Assess for catastrophic external bleeding • Assess alertness (e.g., AVPU) • Assess for respiratory distress • Assess airway for patency • Check for loose teeth or foreign bodies • Assess for bleeding, vomitus, or edema	• Control bleeding with direct pressure and pressure dressings • Open airway • Use jaw-thrust maneuver • Remove or suction any foreign bodies • Insert oropharyngeal or nasopharyngeal airway, cricothyroidotomy • Rapid sequence intubation • Immobilize cervical spine using rigid cervical collar and cervical immobilization device. Secure forehead to backboard
Breathing	
• Assess ventilation • Scan chest for signs of breathing • Look for paradoxic movement of the chest wall during inspiration and expiration • Note use of accessory muscles or abdominal muscles • Observe and count respiratory rate • Note color of nail beds, mucous membranes, skin • Auscultate lungs • Assess for jugular venous distention and position of trachea	• Give supplemental O_2 via appropriate delivery system (e.g., non-rebreather mask) • Ventilate with bag-valve-mask with 100% O_2 if respirations are inadequate or absent • Prepare to intubate if severe respiratory distress (e.g., agonal breaths) or arrest • Have suction available • If absent breath sounds, prepare for needle thoracostomy and chest tube insertion
Circulation	
• Check carotid or femoral pulse • Palpate pulse for quality and rate • Assess skin color, temperature, and moisture • Check capillary refill	• If absent pulse, initiate cardiopulmonary resuscitation and advanced life support measures • If shock symptoms or hypotensive, start two large-bore (14- to 16-gauge) IVs and start infusions of normal saline or lactated Ringer's solution • Consider intraosseous or central venous access if IV access cannot be rapidly obtained • Administer blood products if ordered • Consider autotransfusion if isolated chest trauma • Consider use of pelvic splint or belt in the presence of pelvic fracture with hypotension
Disability	
• Assess level of consciousness by determining response to verbal and/or painful stimuli (e.g., Glasgow Coma Scale) • Assess pupils for size, shape, equality, and reactivity	• Periodically reassess level of consciousness, mental status, and pupil size and reactivity
Exposure and Environmental Control	
• Assess full body for determination of additional or related injuries • Assess environment	• Remove clothing for adequate examination • Stabilize any impaled objects • Keep patient warm with blankets, warmed IV fluids, overhead lights to prevent heat loss, if appropriate • Maintain privacy
Facilitate Adjuncts and Family	
• Assess vital signs including pulse oximetry • Determine caregiver's desire to be present during invasive procedures and/or cardiopulmonary resuscitation	• Obtain bilateral blood pressures if patient has sustained or is suspected of having sustained chest trauma, or if the BP is abnormally high or low • Assign health team member to support caregiver(s)
Get Resuscitation Adjuncts	
• Determine need for additional adjunct measures for monitoring the patient's condition	• Facilitate laboratory tests (e.g., type and crossmatch, complete blood count and metabolic panel, blood alcohol, toxicology screening, arterial blood gases [ABGs], coagulation profile, cardiac biomarkers, pregnancy [urine]) • Continuously monitor ECG for heart rate and rhythm • Insert nasogastric tube; insert orogastric tube in a patient with significant head or facial trauma • Monitor oxygenation and ventilation (e.g., continuous pulse oximetry, capnography) • Manage pain with pharmacologic (e.g., nonsteroidal antiinflammatory drugs, IV opioids) and nonpharmacologic (e.g., distraction, positioning, music) pain management strategies • Provide emotional support to patient and caregiver • Provide additional comfort measures as appropriate (e.g., ice, position of comfort, warm blanket)

AVPU, A = alert, *V* = responsive to voice, *P* = responsive to pain, and *U* = unresponsive.

TABLE 68-4 Potential Life-Threatening Conditions Found During Primary Survey*

Airway
- Inhalation injury (e.g., fire victim)
- Obstruction (partial or complete) from foreign bodies, debris (e.g., vomitus), or tongue
- Penetrating wounds and/or blunt trauma to upper airway structures

Breathing
- Anaphylaxis
- Flail chest with pulmonary contusion
- Hemothorax
- Pneumothorax (e.g., open, tension)

Circulation
- Direct cardiac injury (e.g., myocardial infarction, trauma)
- Pericardial tamponade
- Shock (e.g., massive burns, hypovolemia)
- Uncontrolled external hemorrhage
- Hypothermia

Disability
- Head injury
- Stroke

*List is not all-inclusive.

D = Disability. Conduct a brief neurologic examination as part of the primary survey. The patient's LOC is a measure of the degree of disability. Use the Glasgow Coma Scale (GCS) to determine the LOC (see Table 56-5). Although the GCS is not accurate for intubated or aphasic patients, it is a standardized tool. This allows for consistent communication among the interprofessional care team. Finally, assess the pupils for size, shape, equality, and reactivity.

E = Exposure and Environmental Control. Remove all trauma patients' clothing to perform a thorough physical assessment. This often requires cutting off the patient's clothing. Be careful not to cut through any area that may provide forensic evidence (e.g., bullet hole). Do not remove any impaled objects (e.g., knife). Removing these could result in serious bleeding and further injury. Once the patient is exposed, use warming blankets, overhead warmers, and warmed IV fluids to limit heat loss, prevent hypothermia, and maintain privacy.

F = Facilitate Adjuncts and Family. Obtain a full set of vital signs, including BP, heart rate, respiratory rate, O_2 saturation, and temperature after the patient is exposed. If the patient has sustained or is suspected of having sustained chest trauma, or if the BP is abnormally high or low, obtain the BP in both arms.

Facilitate **family presence (FP)**. Research supports the benefits for patients, caregivers, and staff of allowing FP during resuscitation and invasive procedures.[8] Patients report that caregivers provide comfort, serve as advocates for them, and help remind the interprofessional care team of their "personhood." Caregivers who wish to be present during invasive procedures and resuscitation view themselves as active participants in the care process. They also believe that they comfort the patient and that it is their right to be with the patient.[8] Nurses report that family members serve as "patient helpers" (e.g., provide support) and "staff helpers" (e.g., act as a translator). It is essential to assign a member of the interprofessional care team to explain care delivered and answer questions should a caregiver request FP during resuscitation or invasive procedures.

G = Get Resuscitation Adjuncts. Start additional adjunct measures for monitoring the patient's condition, if not already done. Use the mnemonic "LMNOP" to remember these resuscitation aids:

L: Laboratory tests (e.g., type and crossmatch, complete blood count and metabolic panel, blood alcohol, toxicology screening, arterial blood gases [ABGs], coagulation profile, cardiac biomarkers, pregnancy [urine]).

M: Monitor ECG for heart rate and rhythm.

N: Nasogastric tube to decompress and empty the stomach, reduce the risk of aspiration, and test the contents for blood. Place an orogastric tube in a patient with significant head or facial trauma, since a nasogastric tube could enter the brain.

O: Oxygenation and ventilation assessment. Continuously monitor O_2 saturation and end-tidal CO_2 (if appropriate) (see Chapter 65).

P: Pain assessment and management

Pain is the primary complaint of most patients who come to the ED.[9] Provision of comfort measures is critical when caring for patients in the ED. Many EDs have developed pain management protocols for nurses to treat pain early, beginning at triage.

Pain management strategies should include a combination of pharmacologic (e.g., nonsteroidal antiinflammatory drugs, IV opioids) and nonpharmacologic (e.g., distraction, positioning, music) measures. You play a key role in ongoing pain management because of your frequent contact with patients.

General comfort measures such as providing verbal reassurance, listening, reducing stimuli (e.g., dimming lights, warm blankets), and developing a trusting relationship with the patient and caregiver should be provided to all patients in the ED. Additional measures include splinting, elevating, and icing injured extremities as appropriate.

Secondary Survey

The secondary survey begins after addressing each step of the primary survey and starting any lifesaving interventions. The secondary survey is a brief, systematic process that aims to identify *all* injuries[7] (Table 68-5).

H = History and Head-to-Toe Assessment. The history and mechanism of the injury or illness provides clues to the cause of the crisis (e.g., Were the injuries self-inflicted or a result of abuse?) and suggests specific assessment and interventions. The patient may not be able to give a history. However, caregivers, friends, bystanders, and prehospital personnel can often provide necessary information. Prehospital information focuses on the mechanism and pattern of injury, injuries suspected, vital signs, treatments initiated, and patient responses.

Details of the incident are extremely important because the mechanism of injury and injury patterns can predict specific injuries.[7] For example, a restrained front-seat passenger may have a head injury or knee, femur, or hip fractures from hitting the dashboard and an abdominal injury from the seat belt. If there were deaths at the scene, the patient is at high risk for significant injury.

Patients who jump from buildings or bridges may have bilateral calcaneal (heel) fractures, bilateral wrist fractures, and lumbar spine compression fractures. They are also at risk for aortic tears. Older patients who have fallen may have had a stroke or heart attack that led to the fall.

Prehospital personnel provide a detailed description of the patient's general condition, level of consciousness, and apparent injuries.[7] If the patient is emergently ill, obtain a thorough history from caregivers or friends after the patient is taken to

TABLE 68-5 Emergency Assessment: Secondary Survey

Assessment	Interventions
History and Head-to-Toe Assessment	
History	• Obtain details of the incident/illness, mechanism and pattern of injury, length of time since incident occurred, injuries suspected, treatment provided and patient's response, level of consciousness. • Use the mnemonic **SAMPLE** to determine **S**ymptoms associated with injury or illness; **A**llergies, including tetanus status; **M**edication history; **P**ast health history (e.g., preexisting medical/psychiatric conditions, last menstrual period); **L**ast meal/oral intake; and **E**vents/Environment preceding illness or injury.
Head, Neck, and Face	• Note general appearance, including skin color. • Examine face and scalp for lacerations, bone or soft tissue deformity, tenderness, bleeding, and foreign bodies. • Inspect eyes, ears, nose, and mouth for bleeding, foreign bodies, drainage, pain, deformity, ecchymosis, lacerations. • Palpate head for depressions of cranial or facial bones, contusions, hematomas, areas of softness, bony crepitus. • Examine neck for stiffness, pain in cervical vertebrae, tracheal deviation, distended neck veins, bleeding, edema, difficulty swallowing, bruising, subcutaneous emphysema, bony crepitus.
Chest	• Observe rate, depth, and effort of breathing, including chest wall movement and use of accessory muscles. • Palpate for bony crepitus, subcutaneous emphysema. • Auscultate breath sounds. • Obtain 12-lead ECG and chest x-ray. • Inspect for external signs of injury: petechiae, bleeding, cyanosis, bruises, abrasions, lacerations, old scars.
Abdomen and Flanks	• Look for symmetry of abdominal wall and bony structures. • Inspect for external signs of injury: bruises, abrasions, lacerations, punctures, old scars. • Auscultate for bowel sounds. • Palpate for masses, guarding, femoral pulses. • Note type and location of pain, rigidity, or distention of abdomen.
Pelvis and Perineum	• Gently palpate pelvis. • Assess genitalia for blood at the meatus, priapism, ecchymosis, rectal bleeding, anal sphincter tone. • Determine ability to void.
Extremities	• Inspect for signs of external injury: deformity, ecchymosis, abrasions, lacerations, swelling. • Observe skin color and palpate skin for pain, tenderness, temperature, and crepitus. • Evaluate movement, strength, and sensation in arms and legs. • Assess quality and symmetry of peripheral pulses.
Inspect Posterior Surfaces	• Logroll and inspect and palpate back for deformity, bleeding, lacerations, bruises while maintaining cervical spine immobilization, if appropriate.

the treatment area. The mnemonic *SAMPLE* is a memory aid that prompts you to ask about the following[6]:

S: Symptoms associated with the injury or illness

A: Allergies (e.g., drugs, food, latex, environment) and tetanus status

M: Medication history

P: Past health history (e.g., preexisting medical or psychiatric conditions, previous surgeries, smoking history, recent use of drugs or alcohol, last menstrual period, baseline mental status)

L: Last meal/oral intake

E: Events or environmental factors leading to the illness or injury

Head, Neck, and Face. Assess the patient for general appearance, skin color, and temperature. Check the eyes for extraocular movements. A disconjugate gaze is an indication of neurologic damage. Battle's sign, or bruising directly behind the ear(s), may indicate a fracture of the base of the posterior portion of the skull. "Raccoon eyes," or periorbital ecchymosis, is usually an indication of a fracture of the base of the frontal portion of the skull. Check the ears for blood and cerebrospinal fluid (see Chapter 56 and Fig. 56-13). Do not block clear drainage from the ear or nose.

Assess the airway for foreign bodies, bleeding, edema, and loose or missing teeth. Check for the ability to open the mouth and swallow. Inspect the neck for bruising, edema, bleeding, or distended neck veins. Palpate the trachea to determine whether it is midline. A deviated trachea may signal a life-threatening tension pneumothorax. Subcutaneous emphysema

may indicate laryngotracheal disruption. A stiff or painful neck may signify a fracture of one or more cervical vertebrae. Protect the cervical spine using a C-collar and supine positioning if indicated.

Chest. Inspect the chest for paradoxic chest movements and large sucking chest wounds. Palpate the sternum, clavicles, and ribs for deformity, point tenderness, and crepitus. Auscultate breath sounds and heart sounds. In addition to tension pneumothorax and open pneumothorax, evaluate the patient for rib fractures, pulmonary contusion, blunt cardiac injury, and hemothorax. Obtain a chest x-ray and 12-lead ECG, particularly on patients with known or suspected heart disease. The ECG can help detect dysrhythmias and signs of myocardial ischemia or infarction.

Abdomen and Flanks. The abdomen and flanks are more difficult to assess. Frequent evaluation for subtle changes in the abdomen is essential. Motor vehicle crashes and assaults can cause blunt trauma. Penetrating trauma tends to injure specific, solid organs (e.g., spleen) based on their trajectory. Stabilize any impaled objects. They must be removed in a controlled environment such as an operating room.

Inspect the abdomen for bruising, petechiae, and ecchymosis. Auscultate for bowel sounds. Decreased bowel sounds may indicate a temporary paralytic ileus. Bowel sounds in the chest may indicate a diaphragmatic rupture. Percuss the abdomen for distention (e.g., tympany [excessive air] and dullness [excessive fluid]) and palpate for tenderness.

If you suspect intraabdominal hemorrhage, a *focused abdominal sonography for trauma* (FAST) to identify blood in the peritoneal space (hemoperitoneum) is preferred. This procedure is noninvasive and performed quickly at the bedside. However, a FAST cannot rule out a retroperitoneal bleed. If one is suspected, a CT scan is usually ordered.

Pelvis and Perineum. Gently palpate the pelvis to determine stability. Do not rock the pelvis. Pain may indicate a pelvic fracture and the need for an x-ray. Inspect the genitalia for bleeding, priapism, and obvious injuries. Assess for bladder distention, hematuria, dysuria, or inability to void. The HCP may perform a rectal examination to check for blood, a high-riding prostate gland (e.g., urethral injury), and loss of sphincter tone (e.g., spinal cord injury).

Extremities. Assess the upper and lower extremities for point tenderness, crepitus, and deformities. Splint injured extremities above and below the injury to decrease further soft tissue injury and pain if not done prehospital. Grossly deformed, pulseless extremities should be realigned by the HCP and then splinted. Check pulses before and after movement or splinting of an extremity. A pulseless extremity is a time-critical emergency. Immobilize and elevate injured extremities, and apply ice packs. Prophylactic antibiotics are ordered for open fractures.

Also, assess extremities for *compartment syndrome*. This occurs as pressure and swelling increase inside a section of an extremity (e.g., anterior compartment of lower leg) over several hours. This compromises the viability of the muscles, nerves, and arteries. Potential causes of compartment syndrome include crush injuries, fractures, edema (e.g., burns), and hemorrhage.

I = Inspect Posterior Surfaces. The trauma patient should always be logrolled (while maintaining cervical spine immobilization) to inspect the patient's posterior surfaces and whenever movement is needed. This often needs three to four or more people with one person supporting the head. Inspect the back for ecchymosis, abrasions, puncture wounds, cuts, and obvious deformities. Palpate the entire spine for deformity and pain.

Acute Care and Evaluation

Once the secondary survey is complete, record all findings. Provide tetanus prophylaxis based on vaccination history and the condition of any wounds[10] (Table 68-6).

Regardless of the patient's chief complaint, ongoing monitoring and evaluation of interventions are critical. Provide appropriate care and assess the patient's response. The evaluation of airway patency and the effectiveness of breathing will always be the highest priority. Monitor respiratory rate and rhythm, O_2 saturation, and ABGs (if ordered) to evaluate the patient's respiratory status. Obtain a portable chest x-ray to confirm exact placement of tubes (e.g., endotracheal, gastric).

Closely monitor the LOC; vital signs; quality of peripheral pulses; and skin temperature, color, and moisture for key information about circulation and perfusion. Insert an indwelling catheter to decompress the bladder, monitor urine output, and check for hematuria. Do not insert an indwelling catheter if blood is present at the urinary meatus (e.g., urethral tear) or if scrotal hematoma or perineal ecchymosis is present. Men with a high-riding prostate gland on rectal examination are at risk for a urethral injury. The HCP may order a retrograde urethrogram before inserting a catheter.

Depending on the patient's injuries or illness, the patient may be (1) transported for diagnostic tests (e.g., CT scan, angi-

TABLE 68-6 Tetanus Vaccines and TIG for Wound Management

| Vaccination History | TYPE OF WOUND | |
	Clean, Minor Wounds	All Other Wounds
Age 11 and Older*		
Unknown or <3 doses of tetanus toxoid–containing vaccine	Tdap and recommend catch-up vaccination	Tdap and recommend catch-up vaccination TIG
≥3 doses of tetanus toxoid–containing vaccine *and* <5 yr since last dose	No indication	No indication
≥3 doses of tetanus toxoid–containing vaccine *and* 5–10 yr since last dose	No indication	Tdap preferred (if not yet received) or Td
≥3 doses of tetanus toxoid–containing vaccine *and* >10 yr since last dose	Tdap preferred (if not yet received) or Td	Tdap preferred (if not yet received) or Td

Source: Centers for Disease Control and Prevention: Disaster information: tetanus prevention after a disaster. Retrieved from *www.bt.cdc.gov/disasters/disease/tetanus.asp.*
Td, Tetanus-diphtheria toxoid absorbed; *Tdap,* tetanus toxoid, reduced diphtheria toxoid, and acellular pertussis vaccine; *TIG,* tetanus immune globulin (human).
*Pregnant women: As part of standard wound management care to prevent tetanus, a tetanus toxoid–containing vaccine might be recommended for wound management in a pregnant woman if ≥5 yr have elapsed since previous Td booster. If a Td booster is indicated for a pregnant woman, Tdap should be given.

ography) or to the operating room for immediate surgery; (2) admitted to an intensive care, telemetry, or general unit; or (3) transferred to another facility. You may go with critically ill patients on transports. You are responsible for monitoring the patient during transport, notifying the interprofessional care team should the patient's condition become unstable, and starting basic and advanced life-support measures as needed.

Cardiac Arrest and Therapeutic Hypothermia

Many patients arrive at the ED in cardiac arrest. Patients with nontraumatic, out-of-hospital cardiac arrest benefit from a combination of good chest compressions and rapid defibrillation (see Appendix A), therapeutic hypothermia, and supportive care. Mechanical chest compression devices are often used to provide chest compressions both prehospital and in the ED (Fig. 68-2).

Therapeutic hypothermia for 24 hours after the *return of spontaneous circulation* (ROSC) decreases mortality rates and improves neurologic outcomes in many patients.[11] It is recommended for all patients who are comatose or who do not follow commands after ROSC.[12]

Therapeutic hypothermia, also called *Targeted Temperature Management*, involves three phases: induction, maintenance, and rewarming. The induction phase begins in the ED. The goal core temperature is 89.6° to 93.2°F (32° to 34°C). Recent research has suggested that cooling to a target core temperature of 96.8°F (36°C) results in similar outcomes.[13]

A variety of methods are used to cool patients. These include cold saline infusions and cooling devices (e.g., Arctic Sun). Patients require intubation and mechanical ventilation, invasive monitoring (e.g., arterial and central pressures), and continuous assessment during this therapy. Protocols are used to direct

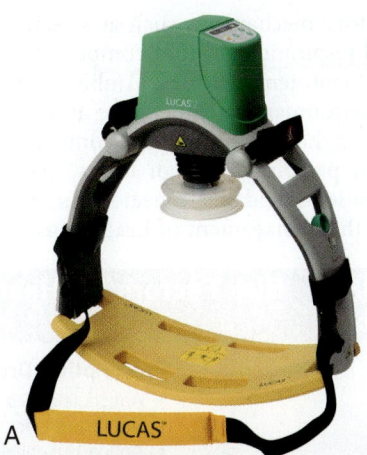

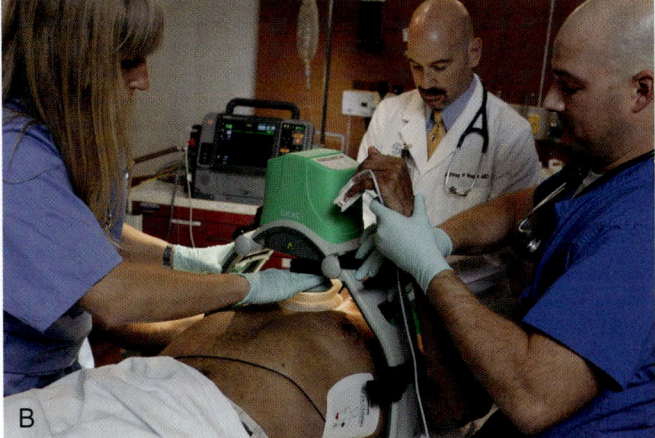

FIG. 68-2 A, LUCAS 2 Mechanical Chest Compression Device. **B,** Application of the LUCAS 2 device on a patient during cardiopulmonary resuscitation. (Reprinted with permission from Physio-Control.)

the care of these patients. (Sample protocols are available at *www.med.upenn.edu/resuscitation/hypothermia/protocols.shtml.*)

Death in the Emergency Department

Unfortunately, a number of patients will not benefit from the skill, expertise, and technology available in the ED. It is important for you to deal with your feelings about sudden death so that you can help caregivers begin the grieving process (see Chapter 9).

Recognize the importance of certain hospital rituals to help caregivers grieve. These can include collecting the personal belongings, viewing the body, and making mortuary arrangements. The death must seem real so that the caregivers can begin to accept the death. You play a significant role in providing comfort to the surviving loved ones after a death in the ED. Whenever possible, provide an area for privacy and, if appropriate, arrange for a visit from a chaplain.[14]

At times, you may need to contact the medical examiner or coroner. Autopsies may have to be arranged at the family's request or in the case of death within 24 hours of ED admission, or from suspected trauma or violence (e.g., gunshot wound).

Many patients who die in the ED could potentially be candidates for *non–heart-beating donation.* Certain tissues and organs (e.g., corneas, heart valves, skin, bone, kidneys) can be harvested from patients after death. *Organ procurement organizations* (OPOs) assist in the process of screening potential donors, counseling donor families, obtaining informed consent,

EVIDENCE-BASED PRACTICE
Translating Research Into Practice

Does Prehospital Therapeutic Hypothermia Improve Outcomes in Cardiac Arrest?

In patients following treatment for cardiac arrest (P), what is the effect of prehospital therapeutic hypothermia (I) versus in-hospital hypothermia or no hypothermia (C) on hospital admission body temperature, survival, and neurologic outcome to hospital discharge and re-arrest (O)?

Synthesis of Best Available Evidence
- Systematic review of randomized controlled trials (RCTs).
- Five RCTs of patients (n = 633) with out-of-hospital cardiac arrest receiving prehospital therapeutic hypothermia, in-hospital hypothermia, or no hypothermia. Outcomes were temperature on hospital admission, survival to hospital discharge, favorable neurologic outcome at hospital discharge, and re-arrest.
- Therapeutic hypothermia helps reduce cerebral metabolism, inhibits excitatory amino acid release, and decreases brain edema and immune response during reperfusion.
- Temperatures on hospital admission for patients with prehospital therapeutic hypothermia were significantly lower compared to out-of-hospital hypothermia or no hypothermia.
- No differences were found related to timing or occurrence of hypothermia for survivor to discharge rates, neurologic outcomes at discharge, or re-arrest.

Conclusion
- After cardiac arrest, prehospital therapeutic hypothermia resulted in decreased patient temperature on hospital admission.

Implications for Nursing Practice
1. What information will you provide to other health team members regarding optimal timing for therapeutic hypothermia?
2. How will you respond to a family member who questions why prehospital therapeutic hypothermia is being done?
3. How would you critically evaluate the strength of evidence for these patients as you consider a change in best practice guidelines?

Reference for Evidence
Diao M, Huang F, Guan J, et al: Prehospital therapeutic hypothermia after cardiac arrest: a systematic review and meta-analysis of randomized controlled trials, *Resuscitation* 84:1021, 2013.

P, Patient population of interest; *I,* intervention or area of interest; *C,* comparison of interest or comparison group; *O,* outcomes of interest; *T,* timing (see p. 15).

and harvesting organs from patients who are on life support or who die in the ED.[15] Approaching caregivers about donation after an unexpected death can be distressing to both the staff and caregivers. However, for many individuals the act of donation may be the first positive step in the grieving process.

Gerontologic Considerations: Emergency Care

The proportion of the population over age 65 is growing, with most leading active lives. Overall, people older than 65 account for 43% of all ED visits.[16] Regardless of a patient's age, aggressive interventions are warranted for all injuries or illnesses unless the patient has a preexisting terminal illness, an extremely low chance of survival, or an advance directive indicating a different course of action.

The older population is at high risk for injury because of many of the anatomic and physiologic changes that occur with aging (e.g., reduced visual acuity, limited neck rotation, slower gait, reduced reaction time). Of the injury-related admissions for people over 65 years old, most are for fractures, with many of these resulting from falls.[16]

The most common causes of falls in older adults are generalized weakness, environmental hazards (e.g., loose mats, furniture), cardiovascular syncope (e.g., dysrhythmias), and orthostatic hypotension (e.g., side effect of drugs, dehydration). When assessing a patient who has fallen, determine whether the physical findings may have caused the fall or may be due to the fall itself. For example, a patient may come to the ED with acute confusion. The confusion may be due to a heart attack or stroke that caused the patient to fall, or the patient may have suffered a head injury as a result of a fall from tripping on a rug.

Understanding the physiologic and psychosocial aspects of aging will improve the care delivered to older adults in the ED (see Chapter 5). Unfortunately, many older adults dismiss their symptoms as simply "normal for their age." It is important to fully explore any complaint by an older adult.

ENVIRONMENTAL EMERGENCIES

Increased interest in outdoor activities such as running, hiking, cycling, skiing, and swimming has increased the number of environmental emergencies seen in the ED. Illness or injury may be caused by the activity, exposure to weather, or attack from various animals or humans. Specific environmental emergencies discussed in this section include heat-related emergencies, cold-related emergencies, submersion injuries, bites, and stings.

HEAT-RELATED EMERGENCIES

Brief exposure to intense heat or prolonged exposure to less intense heat leads to heat stress. This occurs when thermoregulatory mechanisms such as sweating, vasodilation, and increased respirations cannot compensate for exposure to increased ambient temperatures. Ambient temperature is a product of environmental temperature and humidity. Strenuous activities in hot or humid environments, clothing that interferes with perspiration, high fevers, and preexisting illnesses predispose individuals to heat stress (Table 68-7). Table 68-8 presents the management of heat-related emergencies.

TABLE 68-7   Risk Factors for Heat-Related Emergencies

Alcohol

Age
- Infants
- Older adults

Environmental Conditions
- High environmental temperatures
- High relative humidity

Preexisting Illness
- Cardiovascular disease
- Cystic fibrosis
- Dehydration
- Diabetes mellitus
- Obesity
- Previous stroke or other central nervous system lesion
- Skin disorders (e.g., large burn scars)

Prescription Drugs
- Anticholinergics
- Antihistamines
- Antiparkinsonian drugs
- Antispasmodics
- β-Adrenergic blockers
- Butyrophenones
- Diuretics
- Phenothiazines
- Tricyclic antidepressants

Street Drugs
- Amphetamines
- Jimson weed
- Lysergic acid diethylamide (LSD)
- Phencyclidine (PCP)
- 3,4-Methylenedioxymethamphetamine (MDMA, Ecstasy)

Adapted from Howard PK, Steinmann RA, editors: *Sheehy's emergency nursing*, ed 6, St Louis, 2010, Mosby.

TABLE 68-8   Emergency Management

Hyperthermia

Etiology	Assessment Findings	Interventions
Environmental	**Heat Cramps**	**Initial**
• Lack of acclimatization	• Severe muscle contractions in exerted muscles	• Manage and maintain ABCs.
• Physical exertion, especially during hot weather	• Thirst	• Provide high-flow O_2 via non-rebreather mask or BVM.
• Prolonged exposure to extreme temperatures		• Establish IV access and begin fluid replacement for significant heat injury.
Trauma	**Heat Exhaustion**	• Place patient in a cool environment.
• Head injury	• Pale, ashen skin	• For patient with heatstroke, initiate rapid cooling measures: remove patient's clothing, place wet sheets over patient, and place in front of fan; immerse in a cool water bath; administer cool IV fluids or lavage with cool fluids.
• Spinal cord injury	• Fatigue, weakness	
Metabolic	• Profuse sweating	
• Dehydration	• Extreme thirst	
• Diabetes	• Altered mental status (e.g., anxiety)	• Obtain 12-lead ECG.
• Thyrotoxicosis	• Hypotension	• Obtain blood for electrolytes and CBC.
Drugs	• Tachycardia	• Insert urinary catheter.
• Amphetamines	• Weak, thready pulse	
• Antihistamines	• Temperature (99.6° to 105.8°F [37.5° to 41°C])	**Ongoing Monitoring**
• β-Adrenergic blockers		• Monitor ABCs, temperature and vital signs, level of consciousness.
• Diuretics	**Heatstroke**	• Monitor heart rhythm, O_2 saturation, and urine output.
• Phenothiazines	• Hot, dry skin	
• Tricyclic antidepressants	• Altered mental status (e.g., ranging from confusion to coma)	• Replace electrolytes as needed.
Other	• Hypotension	• Monitor urine for development of myoglobinuria.
• Alcohol	• Tachycardia	• Monitor clotting studies for development of disseminated intravascular coagulation.
• Cardiovascular disease	• Weakness	
• CNS disorders	• Temperature >105.8°F (41°C)	

ABCs, Airway, breathing, circulation; *BVM*, bag-valve-mask.

Heat Cramps

Heat cramps are severe cramps in large muscle groups fatigued by heavy work. Cramps are brief and intense and tend to occur during rest after exercise or heavy labor. Nausea, tachycardia, pallor, weakness, and profuse diaphoresis are often present. The condition is seen most often in healthy, acclimated athletes with inadequate fluid intake. Cramps resolve rapidly with rest and oral or parenteral replacement of sodium and water. Elevation, gentle massage, and analgesia minimize pain associated with heat cramps. Instruct the patient to avoid strenuous activity for at least 12 hours. Discharge teaching should emphasize salt replacement during strenuous exercise in hot, humid environments. You can also recommend the use of commercially prepared electrolyte solutions (e.g., sports drinks).

Heat Exhaustion

Prolonged exposure to heat over hours or days leads to heat exhaustion. This is a clinical syndrome characterized by fatigue, nausea, vomiting, extreme thirst, and feelings of anxiety (Table 68-8). Hypotension, tachycardia, elevated body temperature, dilated pupils, mild confusion, ashen color, and profuse diaphoresis are also present. Hypotension and mild to severe temperature elevation (99.6° to 105.8° F [37.5° to 41°C]) are caused by dehydration. Heat exhaustion usually occurs in individuals engaged in strenuous activity in hot, humid weather, but it also occurs in sedentary individuals.

Begin treatment by placing the patient in a cool area and removing constrictive clothing. Monitor the patient for ABCs, including heart dysrhythmias (caused by electrolyte imbalances). Start oral fluid and electrolyte replacement unless the patient is nauseated. Do not use salt tablets because of potential gastric irritation and hypernatremia. Start a 0.9% normal saline IV solution if oral solutions are not tolerated. An initial fluid bolus may be needed to correct hypotension. Always correlate fluid replacement to clinical and laboratory findings. Place a moist sheet over the patient to decrease core temperature through evaporative heat loss. Consider hospital admission for older adults, the chronically ill, or those who do not improve within 3 to 4 hours.

Heatstroke

Heatstroke, the most serious form of heat stress, results from failure of the hypothalamic thermoregulatory processes. It is a medical emergency. Increased sweating, vasodilation, and increased respiratory rate (the body's attempt to lower temperature) deplete fluids and electrolytes, specifically sodium. Eventually, sweat glands stop functioning, and core temperature increases rapidly, within 10 to 15 minutes. The patient has a core temperature greater than 105.8° F (41°C), altered mental status, absence of perspiration, and circulatory collapse. The skin is hot, dry, and ashen. A range of neurologic symptoms occur (e.g., hallucinations, loss of muscle coordination, combativeness) because the brain is extremely sensitive to thermal injuries. Cerebral edema and hemorrhage may occur as a result of direct thermal injury to the brain and decreased cerebral blood flow.

Death from heatstroke is directly related to the amount of time that the patient's body temperature remains elevated.[7] Prognosis is related to age, baseline health status, and length of exposure. Older adults and those with diabetes mellitus, chronic kidney disease, cardiovascular disease, pulmonary disease, or other physiologic compromise are particularly vulnerable.

Interprofessional Care. Treatment of heatstroke focuses on stabilizing the patient's ABCs and rapidly reducing the core temperature. Give 100% O_2 to compensate for the patient's hypermetabolic state. Ventilation with a BVM or intubation and mechanical ventilation may be needed. Correct fluid and electrolyte imbalances and start continuous ECG monitoring for dysrhythmias.

Various cooling methods are available. These include (1) removing clothing, covering with wet sheets, and placing the patient in front of a large fan (evaporative cooling); (2) immersing the patient in a cool water bath (conductive cooling); (3) applying ice packs to the groins and axillae; and, in refractory cases, (4) peritoneal lavaging with iced fluids.

Whatever method is selected, closely monitor the patient's temperature and control shivering. Shivering increases core temperature due to the heat generated by muscle activity. This complicates cooling efforts. Give chlorpromazine IV to control shivering. Antipyretics are not effective in this situation because the elevated temperature is not related to infection.

Monitor the patient for signs of *rhabdomyolysis* (a serious syndrome caused by the breakdown of skeletal muscle). The muscle breakdown leads to myoglobinuria. This places the kidneys at risk for acute kidney injury. Carefully monitor the urine for color (e.g., tea colored), amount, pH, and myoglobin. Finally, obtain clotting studies to monitor the patient for signs of disseminated intravascular coagulation (see Chapter 30).

Patient and caregiver teaching focuses on how to avoid future problems. Provide essential information regarding proper hydration during hot weather and physical exercise. Instruct patients on the early signs of and interventions for heat-related stress.

COLD-RELATED EMERGENCIES

Cold injuries may be localized (frostbite) or systemic (hypothermia). Contributing factors include age, duration of exposure, environmental temperature, homelessness, preexisting conditions (e.g., diabetes mellitus, peripheral vascular disease), drugs that suppress shivering (e.g., opioids, psychotropic agents, antiemetics), and alcohol intoxication. Alcohol causes peripheral vasodilation, increases sensation of warmth, and depresses shivering. Smokers have an increased risk of cold-related injury because of the vasoconstrictive effects of nicotine.

Frostbite

Frostbite is true tissue freezing that results in the formation of ice crystals in the tissues and cells.[7] Peripheral vasoconstriction is the initial response to cold stress and results in a decrease in blood flow and vascular stasis. As cellular temperature decreases and ice crystals form in intracellular spaces, the organelles are damaged and the cell membrane destroyed. This results in edema.

Depth of frostbite depends on ambient temperature, length of exposure, type and condition (wet or dry) of clothing, and contact with metal surfaces. Other factors that affect severity include skin color (dark-skinned people are more prone to frostbite), lack of acclimatization, previous episodes, exhaustion, and poor peripheral vascular status.

Superficial frostbite involves skin and subcutaneous tissue, usually the ears, nose, fingers, and toes. The skin appearance ranges from waxy pale yellow to blue to mottled, and the skin feels crunchy and frozen. The patient may complain of tingling,

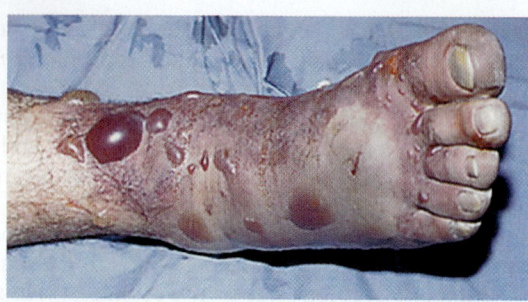

FIG. 68-3 Edema and blister formation 24 hours after frostbite injury occurring in an area covered by a tightly fitted boot. (Courtesy Cameron Bangs, MD. From Auerbach PS, Donner HJ, Weiss EA: *Field guide to wilderness medicine,* ed 2, St Louis, 2003, Mosby.)

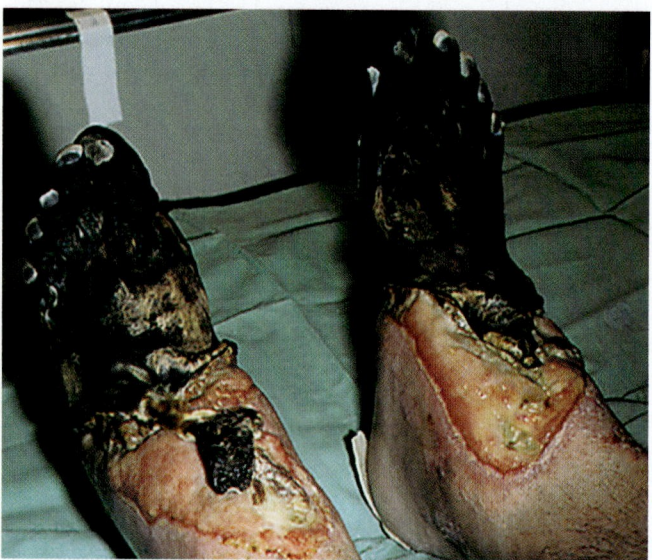

FIG. 68-4 Gangrenous necrosis 6 weeks after the frostbite injury shown in Fig. 68-3. Courtesy Cameron Bangs, MD. (From Auerbach PS, Donner HJ, Weiss EA: *Field guide to wilderness medicine,* ed 2, St Louis, 2003, Mosby.)

numbness, or a burning sensation. Handle the area carefully and never squeeze, massage, or scrub the injured tissue because it is easily damaged. Remove clothing and jewelry because they may constrict the extremity and decrease circulation.

Immerse the affected area in circulating water that is temperature controlled (98.6° to 104°F) [37° to 40°C]). Use warm soaks for the face. The patient often experiences a warm, stinging sensation as tissue thaws. Blisters form within a few hours (Fig. 68-3). The blisters should be debrided and a sterile dressing applied. Avoid heavy blankets and clothing because friction and weight can lead to sloughing of damaged tissue. Rewarming is extremely painful. Residual pain may last weeks or even years. Give analgesia and tetanus prophylaxis as appropriate (Table 68-6). Evaluate the patient with superficial frostbite for systemic hypothermia.

Deep frostbite involves muscle, bone, and tendon. The skin is white, hard, and insensitive to touch. The area has the appearance of deep thermal injury with mottling gradually progressing to gangrene (Fig. 68-4). Immerse the affected extremity in a temperature controlled, circulating water bath (98.6° to 104°F [37° to 40°C]) until flushing occurs distal to the injured area.

After rewarming, the extremity should be elevated to reduce edema. Significant edema may begin within 3 hours, with

blistering in 6 hours to days. IV analgesia is needed in severe frostbite because of the pain associated with tissue thawing. Give tetanus prophylaxis and evaluate the patient for systemic hypothermia.

Amputation may be required if the injured area is untreated or treatment is unsuccessful. It may take as long as 90 days for the final demarcation of the necrotic area.[7] The patient may be admitted to the hospital for observation with bed rest, elevation of the injured part, and prophylactic antibiotics if the wound is at risk for infection.

Hypothermia

Hypothermia, defined as a core temperature below 95°F (35°C), occurs when heat produced by the body cannot compensate for heat lost to the environment.[7] Most body heat is lost as radiant energy, with the greatest loss from the head, thorax, and lungs (with each breath). Wet clothing increases evaporative heat loss to five times greater than normal; immersion in cold water (e.g., drowning) increases evaporative heat loss to 25 times greater than normal. Environmental exposure to freezing temperatures, cold winds, and wet terrain plus physical exhaustion, inadequate clothing, and inexperience predisposes individuals to hypothermia. Older adults are more prone to hypothermia because of decreased body fat, diminished energy reserves, decreased basal metabolic rate, decreased shivering response, decreased sensory perception, chronic medical conditions, and drugs that alter body defenses.[7]

Hypothermia mimics cerebral or metabolic disturbances causing ataxia, confusion, and withdrawal, so the patient may be misdiagnosed. Peripheral vasoconstriction is the body's first attempt to conserve heat. As cold temperatures persist, shivering and movement are the body's only mechanisms for producing heat.

Assessment findings in hypothermia are variable and depend on core temperature (Table 68-9). Patients with *mild hypothermia* (93.2° to 96.8°F [34° to 36°C]) have shivering, lethargy, confusion, rational to irrational behavior, and minor heart rate changes. *Moderate hypothermia* (89.6° to 93.2°F [32° to 34°C]) causes rigidity, bradycardia, slowed respiratory rate, BP obtainable only by Doppler, metabolic and respiratory acidosis, and hypovolemia. Shivering diminishes or disappears at core temperatures of 89.6°F (32°C).[7]

As core temperature drops, metabolic rate decreases two or three times. The cold myocardium is extremely irritable, making it vulnerable to dysrhythmias (e.g., atrial and ventricular fibrillation). Decreased renal blood flow decreases glomerular filtration rate, which impairs water reabsorption and leads to dehydration. The hematocrit increases as intravascular volume decreases. Cold blood becomes thick and acts as a thrombus, placing the patient at risk for stroke, myocardial infarction, pulmonary emboli, and renal failure. Decreased blood flow leads to hypoxia, anaerobic metabolism, lactic acid accumulation, and metabolic acidosis.

Severe hypothermia (below 89.6°F [32°C]) makes the person appear dead and is a potentially life-threatening situation. Metabolic rate, heart rate, and respirations are so slow that they may be difficult to detect. Reflexes are absent, and the pupils fixed and dilated. Profound bradycardia, ventricular fibrillation, or asystole may be present. Every effort is made to warm the patient to at least 86°F (30°C) before the person is pronounced dead. The cause of death is usually refractory ventricular fibrillation.

➕ **TABLE 68-9** **Emergency Management**

Hypothermia

Etiology	Assessment Findings	Interventions
Environmental	• Core body temperature:	**Initial**
• Inadequate clothing for environmental temperature	• *Mild hypothermia:* 93.2°-96.8°F (34°-36°C)	• Remove patient from cold environment.
• Prolonged exposure to cold	• *Moderate hypothermia:* 89.6°-93.2°F (32°-34°C)	• Manage and maintain ABCs.
• Prolonged immersion or drowning	• *Severe hypothermia:* ≤89.6°F (32°C)	• Provide high-flow O₂ via non-rebreather mask or BVM.
Metabolic	• Shivering, diminished or absent at core body temperatures ≤89.6°F (32°C).	• Anticipate intubation for diminished or absent gag reflex.*
• Hypoglycemia	• Hypoventilation	• Establish IV access with two large-bore catheters for fluid resuscitation
• Hypothyroidism	• Hypotension	• Rewarm patient:
Health Care–Associated	• Altered mental status (ranging from confusion to coma)	• *Passive:* Remove wet clothing, apply dry clothing and warm blankets, use radiant lights.
• Administration of neuromuscular blocking agents	• Areflexia (absence of reflexes)	• *Active external:* Apply heating devices (e.g., air or fluid-filled warming blankets), use warm water immersion.
• Blood administration	• Pale, cyanotic skin	• *Active internal:* Provide warmed IV fluids; heated, humidified O₂. Peritoneal lavage with warmed fluids. Extracorporeal circulation (e.g., cardiopulmonary bypass, rapid fluid infuser, hemodialysis).
• Cold IV fluids	• Blue, white, or frozen extremities	• Obtain 12-lead ECG.
• Inadequate warming or rewarming in the ED or operating room	• Dysrhythmias: bradycardia, atrial fibrillation, ventricular fibrillation, asystole	• Anticipate need for defibrillation.*
Other	• Fixed, dilated pupils	• Warm central trunk first in patients with severe hypothermia to limit rewarming shock.
• Alcohol		• Assess for other injuries.
• Barbiturates		• Keep patient's head covered with warm, dry towels or stocking cap to limit loss of heat.
• Phenothiazines		• Treat patient gently to avoid increased cardiac irritability.
• Shock		**Ongoing Monitoring**
• Trauma		• Monitor ABCs, temperature, level of consciousness, vital signs.
		• Monitor O₂ saturation, heart rate and rhythm.
		• Monitor electrolytes, glucose.

ABCs, Airway, breathing, circulation; *BVM,* bag-valve-mask.
*NOTE: Medications and defibrillation may not be effective with core temperatures <86°F (30°C).

Interprofessional Care. Treatment of hypothermia focuses on managing and maintaining ABCs, rewarming the patient, correcting dehydration and acidosis, and treating cardiac dysrhythmias (Table 68-9). Use passive or active external rewarming for mild hypothermia. *Passive* or *spontaneous rewarming* involves moving the patient to a warm, dry place; removing damp clothing; using radiant lights; and placing warm blankets on the patient. *Active external* or *surface rewarming* involves fluid- or air-filled warming blankets, or warm (98.6° to 104°F [37° to 40°C]) water immersion. Closely monitor the patient for marked vasodilation and hypotension during rewarming.

Use *active internal* or *core rewarming* for moderate to severe hypothermia. This refers to the application of heat directly to the core. Techniques include (1) heated (up to 111.2°F [44°C]), humidified O₂; (2) warmed IV fluids (up to 98.6°F [37°C]); (3) peritoneal lavage with warmed fluids (up to 113°F [45°C]); and (4) extracorporeal circulation with cardiopulmonary bypass, rapid fluid infuser, or hemodialysis.

Gentle handling is essential to prevent stimulation of the cold myocardium. Carefully monitor core temperature during rewarming procedures. Rewarming places the patient at risk for *afterdrop,* a further drop in core temperature. This occurs when cold peripheral blood returns to the central circulation. Rewarming shock can produce hypotension and dysrhythmias. Thus patients with moderate to severe hypothermia should have the core warmed before the extremities. Discontinue active rewarming once the core temperature reaches 89.6° to 93.2°F (32° to 34°C).

Patient teaching focuses on how to avoid future cold-related problems. Essential information includes dressing in layers for cold weather, covering the head, carrying high-carbohydrate foods for extra calories, and developing a plan for survival should an injury occur when in an extreme environment.

❓ **CHECK YOUR PRACTICE**

You and your preceptor are working in the ED when the paramedics arrive with a patient who was found lying on the sidewalk outside the downtown bus station. He is wearing only a lightweight shirt and pants. The outdoor temperature is 12°F (-11.1°C). The patient is unresponsive. Initial vital signs are as follows: rectal temperature = 89.5°F (31.9°C), HR = 38, RR = 8, BP (by Doppler) = 86 mm Hg.
• What are your priority interventions for this patient?

SUBMERSION INJURIES

Submersion injury results when a person becomes hypoxic as the result of submersion in a liquid, usually water.[7] More than 50,000 submersion events and approximately 4000 deaths from drowning occur each year in the United States. Most of the victims are children younger than 5 years of age or boys and men between ages 15 and 25. The primary risk factors for submersion injury include inability to swim, use of alcohol or drugs, trauma, seizures, hypothermia, stroke, and child neglect.

Drowning is the process of experiencing respiratory impairment after submersion in water or other fluid. Submersion in cold water (below 32°F [0°C]) may slow the progression of hypoxic brain injury.

Most drowning victims do not aspirate any liquid due to laryngospasm. If liquid is aspirated, it is in small amounts (e.g., 4 mL/kg). Drowning victims who do aspirate water develop

PATHOPHYSIOLOGY MAP

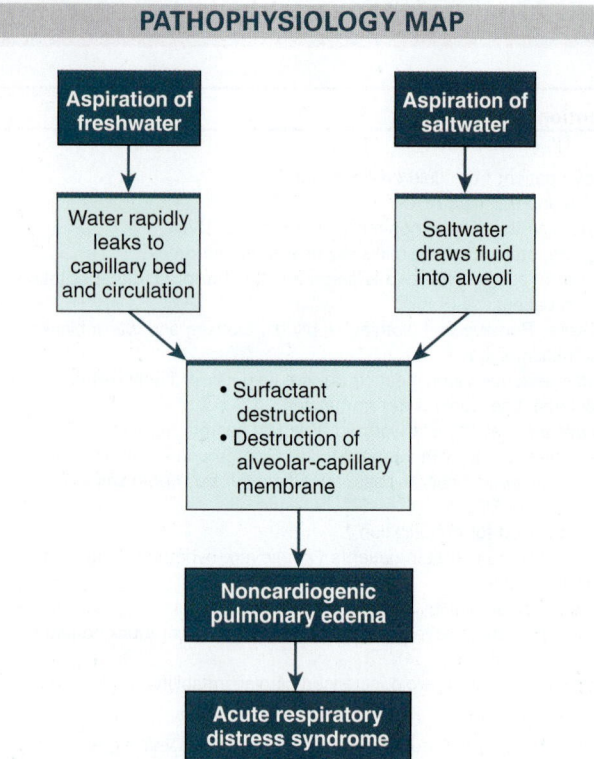

FIG. 68-5 Pathophysiology of submersion injury.

pulmonary edema (Fig. 68-5). Regardless of what type of fluid is aspirated, the end result can be acute respiratory distress syndrome (see Chapter 67).

The osmotic gradient caused by aspirated fluid leads to fluid imbalances in the body. Hypotonic fresh water is rapidly absorbed into the circulatory system through the alveoli. Fresh water is often contaminated with chlorine, mud, or algae. This causes the breakdown of lung surfactant, fluid seepage, and pulmonary edema.

Hypertonic saltwater draws fluid from the vascular space into the alveoli, impairing alveolar ventilation and resulting in hypoxia. The body attempts to compensate for hypoxia by shunting blood to the lungs. This results in increased pulmonary pressures and deteriorating respiratory status. More and more blood is shunted through the alveoli. However, the blood is not adequately oxygenated, and hypoxemia worsens. This can result in cerebral injury, edema, and brain death.

Table 68-10 lists the assessment findings of a patient with a submersion injury. Aggressive resuscitation efforts (e.g., airway and ventilation management), especially in the prehospital phase, improve survival of drowning victims.

Interprofessional Care

Treatment of submersion injuries focuses on correcting hypoxia and fluid imbalances, supporting basic physiologic functions, and rewarming when hypothermia is present. Initial evaluation involves assessment of airway, cervical spine, breathing, and circulation. Table 68-10 lists other interventions.

Mechanical ventilation with positive end-expiratory pressure or continuous positive airway pressure is used to improve gas exchange across the alveolar-capillary membrane when significant pulmonary edema is present. Ventilation and oxygenation are the primary techniques for treating respiratory failure

(see Chapters 65 and 67). Mannitol (Osmitrol) or furosemide (Lasix) is used to treat cerebral edema or decrease free water.

Deterioration in neurologic status suggests cerebral edema, worsening hypoxia, or profound acidosis. Drowning victims may also have head and neck injuries that cause prolonged alterations in the LOC. Complications can develop in patients who are essentially free of symptoms immediately after the drowning episode. Consequently, observe all victims of drowning in a hospital for a minimum of 23 hours.[7] Additional observation is needed for patients who have co-morbidities (e.g., heart disease).

Patient teaching focuses on water safety and how to reduce the risks for drowning. Remind patients and caregivers to lock all swimming pool gates; use life jackets on all watercrafts, including inner tubes and rafts; and learn water survival skills (e.g., swimming lessons). Emphasize the dangers of combining alcohol and drugs with swimming and other water sports.

STINGS AND BITES

Animals, spiders, snakes, and insects cause injury and even death by biting or stinging. Morbidity is a result of either direct tissue damage or lethal toxins. Direct tissue damage is a product of animal size, characteristics of the animal's teeth, and strength of the jaw. Tissue is lacerated, crushed, or chewed, while teeth, fangs, stingers, spines, or tentacles release toxins that have local or systemic effects. Death associated with animal bites is due to blood loss, allergic reactions, or lethal toxins. Injuries caused by select insects, ticks, animals (e.g., dogs, cats), and humans are described here.

Hymenopteran Stings

The *Hymenoptera* family includes bees, yellow jackets, hornets, wasps, and fire ants. Stings can cause mild discomfort or life-threatening anaphylaxis (see Chapter 66). Venom may be cytotoxic, hemolytic, allergenic, or vasoactive. Symptoms may begin immediately or be delayed up to 48 hours. Reactions are more severe with multiple stings. Most hymenopterans sting repeatedly. However, the domestic honey bee stings only once, usually leaving a barbed stinger with an attached venom sac in the skin so that release of venom continues.

African honey bees (killer bees), which look like domestic bees, have migrated into North America. If threatened, these bees aggressively swarm and can repeatedly sting their victims (e.g., humans, animals). These attacks can be fatal.

> **! SAFETY ALERT** **Hymenopteran Stings**
> - Remove the stinger using a scraping motion with a fingernail, knife, or needle.
> - Avoid using tweezers because they may squeeze the stinger and release more venom.
> - Remove rings, watches, or any restrictive clothing around the sting site.

Manifestations vary from stinging, burning, swelling, and itching to edema, headache, fever, syncope, malaise, nausea, vomiting, wheezing, bronchospasm, laryngeal edema, and hypotension. Treatment depends on the severity of the reaction. Treat mild reactions with elevation, cool compresses, antipruritic lotions, and oral antihistamines. More severe reactions require IM or IV antihistamines (e.g., diphenhydramine), subcutaneous epinephrine, and corticosteroids (e.g., dexamethasone). Chapter 13 discusses allergic reactions and related patient teaching.

✚ TABLE 68-10   Emergency Management

Submersion Injuries

Etiology	Assessment Findings	Interventions
• Inability to swim or exhaustion while swimming • Entrapment or entanglement with objects in water • Loss of ability to move secondary to trauma, stroke, hypothermia, myocardial infarction (MI) • Poor judgment due to alcohol or drugs • Seizure while in water	**Respiratory** • Ineffective breathing • Dyspnea • Respiratory distress • Respiratory arrest • Crackles, rhonchi • Cough with pink-frothy sputum • Cyanosis **Cardiac** • Tachycardia • Bradycardia • Dysrhythmia • Hypotension • Cardiac arrest **Other** • Panic • Exhaustion • Coma • Coexisting illness (e.g., MI) or injury (e.g., cervical spine injury) • Core temperature slightly elevated or below normal depending on water temperature and length of submersion	**Initial** • Manage and maintain ABCs. • Assume cervical spine injury in all drowning victims and stabilize or immobilize cervical spine. • Provide 100% O₂ via non-rebreather mask or BVM. • Anticipate need for intubation and mechanical ventilation if airway is compromised (e.g., absent gag reflex). • Establish IV access with two large-bore catheters for fluid resuscitation and infuse warmed fluids if appropriate. • Obtain 12-lead ECG. • Assess for other injuries. • Remove wet clothing and cover with warm blankets. • Obtain temperature and begin rewarming if needed. • Obtain cervical spine and chest x-rays. • Insert gastric tube and urinary catheter. **Ongoing Monitoring** • Monitor ABCs, vital signs, level of consciousness. • Monitor O₂ saturation, heart rate and rhythm. • Monitor temperature and maintain normothermia. • Monitor for signs of acute respiratory failure.

ABCs, Airway, breathing, circulation; *BVM,* bag-valve-mask.

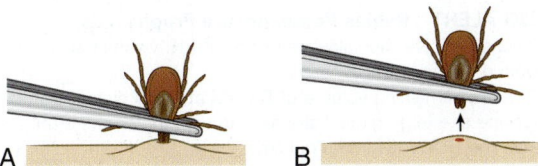

FIG. 68-6 Tick removal. **A,** Use tweezers to grasp the tick close to the skin. **B,** With a steady motion, pull the tick's body up and away from the skin. Do not be alarmed if the tick's mouthparts remain in the skin. Once the mouthparts are removed from the rest of the tick, it can no longer transmit disease.

Tick Bites

Ticks live throughout the United States but are most common in the northwestern, Rocky Mountain, and northeastern regions. Conditions associated with tick bites include Lyme disease, Rocky Mountain spotted fever, and tick paralysis. The infected tick or the release of neurotoxin causes the disease. Ticks release neurotoxic venom as long as the tick head attaches to the body. Therefore safe removal of the tick is essential for effective treatment.

Use forceps or tweezers to grasp the tick close to the point of attachment and pull upward in a steady motion (Fig. 68-6). After you remove the tick, clean the skin with soap and water. Do not use a hot match, petroleum jelly, nail polish, or other products to remove the tick, since these measures may cause a tick to salivate, thus increasing the risk for infection.[17]

Lyme disease is the most common tick-borne disease in the United States. Symptoms appear within days of a bite from the Ixodid (hard) tick that has been attached for at least 48 hours. Exposure to the spirochete *Borrelia burgdorferi* that lives on the tick causes the illness. The first stage of this disease begins with flu-like symptoms (e.g., headache, stiff neck, fatigue). Some patients may develop a characteristic bull's-eye rash (i.e., a circular area of redness 5 cm or more in diameter). Treatment at this stage includes doxycycline (Vibramycin). The rash, if it develops, will disappear even if the patient is not treated.

Monoarticular arthritis, meningitis, and neuropathies occur days or weeks after the initial manifestations. Recommended treatment includes ceftriaxone (Rocephin). Chronic arthritis, peripheral radiculoneuropathy, and heart disease characterize the later stage of the disease. These illnesses can last several months to years after the initial skin lesion. (Chapter 64 discusses Lyme disease.)

Rocky Mountain spotted fever is caused by *Rickettsia rickettsii,* a bacterium that is spread to humans by the Ixodid tick. It has an incubation period of 2 to 14 days. A pink, macular rash appears on the palms, wrists, soles, feet, and ankles within 10 days of exposure. Other symptoms include fever, chills, malaise, myalgias, and headache. Diagnosis is often difficult in the early stages, and without treatment the disease can be fatal. Antibiotic therapy with doxycycline is the treatment of choice.

Tick paralysis occurs 5 to 7 days after exposure to a neurotoxin introduced by a wood tick or dog tick. Classic manifestations are flaccid ascending paralysis, which develops over 1 to 2 days. Without tick removal, the patient dies as respiratory muscles become paralyzed. Tick removal leads to return of muscle movement, usually within 48 to 72 hours.

Animal and Human Bites

Every year more than 5 million animal bites are reported in the United States. Children are at greatest risk. The most significant problems associated with animal bites are infection and mechanical destruction of skin, muscle, tendons, blood vessels, and bone. The bite may cause a simple laceration or be associated with crush injury, puncture wound, or tearing of multiple layers of tissue. The severity of injury depends on animal size, victim size, and anatomic location of the bite. Animal bites from

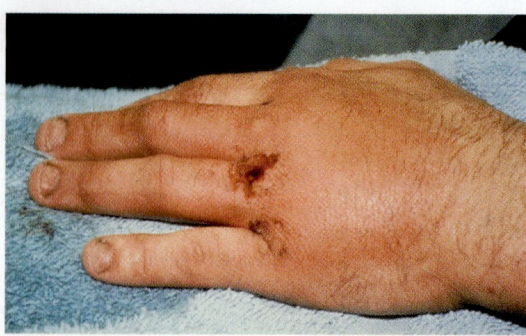

FIG. 68-7 Probable human bite injury, although denied by patient. Human bites cause extensor tendon injuries, fractures, and joint capsule injuries and can harbor foreign bodies. (From Roberts JR, Hedges JR: *Clinical procedures in emergency medicine,* ed 5, Philadelphia, 2009, Saunders.)

dogs and cats are most common, with wild or domestic rodents (e.g., squirrels, hamsters) following as the third most frequently reported offenders.

Dog bites usually occur on the extremities. However, facial bites are common in small children. Most victims own the dogs that bite them. Dog bites may involve significant tissue damage with deaths reported, usually in children. A plastic surgeon should evaluate all disfiguring wounds of the face.

Cat bites cause deep puncture wounds that can involve tendons and joint capsules and result in a greater incidence of infection than with dog bites. Septic arthritis, osteomyelitis, and tenosynovitis can occur as a result of cat bites. The most common causative organisms of infections from dog and cat bites are from the *Pasteurella* species (e.g., *Pasteurella multocida*). Most healthy cats and dogs carry this organism in their mouths.

Human bites also cause puncture wounds or lacerations (Fig. 68-7). These carry a high risk of infection from oral bacterial flora, most commonly *Staphylococcus aureus, Streptococcus* organisms, and hepatitis virus. Hands, fingers, ears, nose, vagina, and penis are the most common sites of human bites and are frequently a result of violence or sexual activity.

Patients with Boxer's fracture (fracture of the fourth or fifth metacarpal) often have concurrent open wounds on the knuckles from striking teeth. The human jaw has great crushing ability, causing laceration, puncture, crush injury, soft tissue tearing, and even amputation. Infection rates are as high as 50% when victims do not seek medical care within 24 hours of injury.

Interprofessional Care. Initial treatment for animal and human bites includes cleaning with copious irrigation, debridement, tetanus prophylaxis, and analgesics as needed. Prophylactic antibiotics are used for animal and human bites at risk for infection, such as wounds over joints, those greater than 6 to 12 hours old, puncture wounds, and bites of the hand or foot. People at greatest risk of infection are infants, older adults, immunosuppressed patients, alcoholics, diabetics, and people taking corticosteroids.

Leave puncture wounds open. Splint wounds over joints. Lacerations are loosely sutured. However, initial closure is used for facial wounds. The patient is admitted for IV antibiotic therapy when an infection is present. These patients have an increased incidence of cellulitis, osteomyelitis, and septic arthritis. Report animal and human bites to the police as required.

Consider *rabies postexposure prophylaxis* in the management of all animal bites. Rabies is generally transmitted via saliva from the bite of an infected animal. It can also be spread by scratches and by contact with infected secretions through mucous membranes. Any warm-blooded mammal (e.g., dogs, raccoons, bats) can carry rabies.

A neurotoxic virus found in the saliva of infected mammals causes rabies. The virus spreads through the CNS via peripheral nerves. After a minimum 2-week incubation period, patients experience flu-like symptoms, pain, paresthesias, or numbness. Rabies prophylaxis must be started before symptoms appear. Otherwise, the disease will progress (e.g., agitation, hypersalivation, dysarthria, hallucinations, nuchal rigidity, seizures, coma) and is fatal. Death results from respiratory and cardiovascular collapse within a few days after the onset of coma.

Consider rabies exposure if an animal attack was not provoked, involves a wild animal, or involves a domestic animal not immunized against rabies. Always provide rabies postexposure prophylaxis when the animal is not found or a wild animal causes the bite. Start the regimen with an initial, weight-based dosage of rabies immune globulin (RIG [HyperRab S/D]) to provide passive immunity. Follow this with a series of four injections of human diploid cell vaccine (HDCV [Imovax Rabies]) on days 0, 3, 7, and 14 to provide active immunity.[18]

Since rabies is nearly always fatal, management efforts are directed at preventing the transmission and onset of the disease. Although death from rabies is significant worldwide, only one to three people die annually in the United States. Rabies vaccine is encouraged for persons who travel globally, since it remains a serious world health concern.

 DRUG ALERT   Rabies Postexposure Prophylaxis

- If possible, give the calculated dose of RIG via infiltration around the wound edges.
- Give any remaining volume of RIG IM at a site distant from the vaccine site (e.g., gluteal site for bite wounds on the arm).
- Give the HDCV IM in the deltoid.

POISONINGS

A poison is any chemical that harms the body. More than 5 million cases of human poisonings occur each year in the United States. Poisonings can be accidental, occupational, recreational, or intentional. Natural or manufactured toxins can be ingested, inhaled, injected, splashed in the eye, or absorbed through the skin. Table 68-11 presents common poisons. Chapter 10 discusses other poisonings related to the use of illegal drugs such as amphetamines, opioids, and hallucinogens. Poisoning may also be due to toxic plants or contaminated foods. (Chapter 41 discusses food poisoning.)

Severity of the poisoning depends on type, concentration, and route of exposure. Toxins can affect every tissue of the body, so symptoms can be seen in any body system. Specific management of toxins involves decreasing absorption, enhancing elimination, and implementing toxin-specific interventions. Consult the local poison control center 24 hours a day (e.g., 800-222-1222) for the most current treatment protocols for specific poisons.[19]

Options for decreasing absorption of poisons include activated charcoal, dermal cleansing, eye irrigation, and gastric lavage. Gastric lavage involves oral insertion of a large-diameter (36F to 42F) gastric tube for irrigation of copious amounts of saline. Elevate the head of the bed or place the patient on the side to prevent aspiration. Patients with an altered LOC or diminished gag reflex are intubated before lavage. Patients who ingest caustic agents, co-ingest sharp objects, or ingest nontoxic

TABLE 68-11 Common Poisons

Poison	Manifestations	Treatment
Acetaminophen (Tylenol)	*Phase 1* (within 24 hr of ingestion): Malaise, diaphoresis, nausea and vomiting *Phase 2* (24-28 hr after ingestion): Right upper quadrant pain, decreased urine output, diminished nausea, increase in LFTs *Phase 3* (72-96 hr after ingestion): Nausea and vomiting, malaise, jaundice, hypoglycemia, enlarged liver, possible coagulopathies, including DIC *Phase 4* (7-8 days after ingestion): Recovery, resolution of symptoms or permanent liver damage, LFT results remain high	Activated charcoal, *N*-acetylcysteine (oral form may cause vomiting, IV form can be used)
Acids and alkalis • *Acids:* Toilet bowl cleaners, antirust compounds • *Alkalis:* Drain cleaners, dishwashing detergents, ammonia	Excess salivation, dysphagia, epigastric pain, pneumonitis; burns of mouth, esophagus, and stomach	Immediate dilution (water, milk), corticosteroids (for alkali burns), induced vomiting is contraindicated
• Aspirin and aspirin-containing drugs	Tachypnea, tachycardia, hyperthermia, seizures, pulmonary edema, occult bleeding or hemorrhage, metabolic acidosis	Activated charcoal, gastric lavage, urine alkalinization, hemodialysis for severe acute ingestion, intubation and mechanical ventilation, supportive care
Bleaches	Irritation of lips, mouth, and eyes, superficial injury to esophagus; chemical pneumonia and pulmonary edema	Washing of exposed skin and eyes, dilution with water and milk, gastric lavage, prevention of vomiting and aspiration
Carbon monoxide	Dyspnea, headache, tachypnea, confusion, impaired judgment, cyanosis, respiratory depression	Removal from source, administration of 100% O_2 via non-rebreather mask, BVM, or intubation and mechanical ventilation; consider hyperbaric O_2 therapy
Cyanide	Almond odor to breath, headache, dizziness, nausea, confusion, hypertension, bradycardia followed by hypotension and tachycardia, tachypnea followed by bradypnea and respiratory arrest	Amyl nitrate (nasally), IV sodium nitrate, IV sodium thiosulfate, supportive care
Ethylene glycol	Sweet aromatic odor to breath, nausea and vomiting, slurred speech, ataxia, lethargy, respiratory depression	Activated charcoal, gastric lavage, supportive care
Iron	Vomiting (often bloody), diarrhea (often bloody), fever, hyperglycemia, lethargy, hypotension, seizures, coma	Gastric lavage, chelation therapy (deferoxamine [Desferal])
Nonsteroidal antiinflammatory drugs	Gastroenteritis, abdominal pain, drowsiness, nystagmus, hepatic and renal damage	Activated charcoal, gastric lavage, supportive care
Tricyclic antidepressants (e.g., amitriptyline)	*In low doses:* Anticholinergic effects, agitation, hypertension, tachycardia *In high doses:* Central nervous system depression, dysrhythmias, hypotension, respiratory depression	Multidose activated charcoal, gastric lavage, serum alkalinization with sodium bicarbonate, intubation and mechanical ventilation, supportive care; never induce vomiting
Alcohol, barbiturates, benzodiazepines, cocaine, hallucinogens, stimulants	See Chapter 10	See Chapter 10

BVM, Bag-valve-mask; *DIC,* disseminated intravascular coagulation; *LFT,* liver function test.

substances should not receive lavage. To be effective, perform gastric lavage within 1 hour of ingestion of most poisons. Problems associated with lavage include esophageal perforation and aspiration.

The most common and effective intervention for management of poisonings is administration of activated charcoal orally or via a gastric tube within 1 hour of poison ingestion. Many toxins adhere to charcoal and pass through the gastrointestinal (GI) tract rather than being absorbed into the circulation. Activated charcoal does not absorb ethanol, hydrocarbons, alkali, iron, boric acid, lithium, methanol, or cyanide.[20] Adults receive 50 to 100 g of charcoal. For some toxins (e.g., phenobarbital, digoxin) multiple-dose charcoal may be needed. Contraindications to charcoal administration include diminished bowel sounds, paralytic ileus, and ingestion of a substance poorly absorbed by charcoal. Charcoal can absorb and neutralize antidotes (e.g., *N*-acetylcysteine for acetamino-

phen toxicity). Do not give these immediately before, with, or shortly after charcoal.

Skin and ocular decontamination involves removal of toxins from skin and eyes using copious amounts of water or saline. Most toxins, with the exception of mustard gas, can be safely removed with water or saline. Water mixes with mustard gas and releases chlorine gas.

As a rule, brush dry substances from the skin and clothing before using water. Do not remove powdered lime with water. It should just be brushed off. Wear *personal protective equipment (PPE)* (e.g., gloves, gowns, goggles, respirators) for decontamination to prevent secondary exposure. Decontamination procedures are usually done by those specially trained in hazardous material decontamination before the patient arrives at the hospital and again at the hospital, if necessary. Decontamination takes priority over all interventions except those needed for basic life support.

Giving cathartics, whole-bowel irrigation, hemodialysis, urine alkalinization, chelating agents, and antidotes increases the elimination of poisons. Cathartics, such as sorbitol, are given together with the first dose of activated charcoal to stimulate intestinal motility and increase elimination.[20] Avoid multiple doses of cathartics because of potentially fatal electrolyte abnormalities. Whole-bowel irrigation is controversial and involves giving a nonabsorbable bowel evacuant solution (e.g., GoLYTELY). Give the solution every 4 to 6 hours until stools are clear. This process can be effective for swallowed objects, such as cocaine-filled balloons or condoms, and heavy metals such as lead and mercury. There is a high risk of electrolyte imbalance caused by fluid and electrolyte losses with this approach.

Hemodialysis is reserved for patients who develop severe acidosis from ingestion of toxic substances (e.g., aspirin). Other interventions include alkalinization and chelation therapy. Sodium bicarbonate administration increases the pH (greater than 7.5), which is particularly effective for phenobarbital and salicylate poisoning. Vitamin C is added to IV fluids to enhance excretion of amphetamines and quinidine. Chelation therapy is considered for heavy metal poisoning (e.g., edetate calcium disodium [calcium EDTA] for lead poisoning). A limited number of true antidotes are available, and many of these agents are themselves toxic.[20]

Focus patient teaching for toxic emergencies on how the poisoning occurred. Arrange for an evaluation and follow-up by a mental health professional for all patients who experience poisoning because of a suicide attempt or substance abuse.

Many health care workers (e.g., nurses, housekeepers) are at risk for exposure to hazardous materials (e.g., antineoplastic drugs, cleaning agents). Always consult the Material Safety Data Sheet (required by the Occupational Health and Safety Administration [OSHA]) for specific information regarding hazardous agents in the workplace. OSHA should evaluate all poisoning related to a workplace hazard.[21]

VIOLENCE

Violence is the acting out of the emotions of fear and/or anger to cause harm to someone or something. It may be the result of organic disease (e.g., temporal lobe epilepsy), psychosis (e.g., schizophrenia), or criminal behavior (e.g., assault, murder). The patient cared for in the ED may be the victim or the perpetrator of violence. Violence can take place in a variety of settings, including the home, community, and workplace.

EDs have been identified as high-risk areas for *workplace violence*.[22] Measures to protect staff include the use of onsite security personnel and police officers, metal detectors, surveillance cameras, self-defense training, and locked access doors. The ENA supports comprehensive workplace violence prevention plans and recommends that they be implemented and evaluated in every ED.[22]

Family and intimate partner violence (IPV) is a pattern of coercive behavior in a relationship that involves fear; humiliation; intimidation; neglect; or intentional physical, emotional, financial, or sexual injury (see Chapter 53 for information on sexual assault). The ENA encourages ED nurses to become certified *sexual assault nurse examiners* (SANEs). These nurses provide expert emergency care, collect and document evidence, participate in staff and community education, and advocate for sexual assault and rape victims.[23]

✳ BECOMING A NURSE LEADER
Patient and Visitor Violence/Abuse

Situation

Since it has always been your desire to be an emergency department (ED) nurse, you are excited when you get to rotate to a busy metropolitan ED during your senior year of nursing school. While in the ED, you witness an intoxicated patient physically attacking and his family verbally abusing the nurses. You are pleased to see the rapid response by the staff and security to deal with the situation. However, you are still frightened and wonder if you should ever work in an ED.

Points for Consideration

- Workplace violence against nurses has become a problem affecting nurses in all settings. It is a serious problem, especially in EDs, mental health facilities, and long-term care facilities.
- Workplace violence can instantly transform nurses from being health care professionals to patients with physical and psychologic trauma caused when patients or visitors attack them.
- You can be a leader in promoting awareness of workplace violence and providing training and education to avoid situations for potential violence. These activities include:[1]
  - Helping to establish policies aimed at preventing workplace violence.
  - Making sure that you are not working alone, especially in certain areas such as the ED.
  - Being aware of your patient's history. Identify in some way the patients' charts if they have past incidents involving violence.
  - Avoiding being physically trapped in a room. Keeping yourself between the patient and the door.
  - Helping to plan work designs that provide for lockable areas for staff only (lounges, lockers rooms, bathrooms) and adequate lighting both inside and outside of the facility.

Discussion Questions

1. What can you do to protect yourself in situations where you are at risk for violence?
2. Describe how the following factors may be related to increased violence in the ED:
   - Prolonged wait times
   - Delays in providing pain medication
   - Influx of patients with mental health issues
   - Workplace design

Reference

1. Emergency Nurses Association: Toolkit—workplace violence. Retrieved from *www.ena.org/practice-research/practice/violencetoolkit/Documents/toolkitpg1.htm*.

IPV is found in all professions, cultures, socioeconomic groups, age groups, and genders. Although men can be victims of family violence and IPV, most victims are women, children, and older adults. Each year, more than 5 million women and 3 million men are treated in EDs for *battery* (assault) by spouses, caregivers, or individuals known to them. Many battered women are pregnant at the time of the assault.[23]

In the ED, you need to screen for family violence and IPV (e.g., Do you feel safe at home? Is anyone hurting you?). Routine screening for this risk factor is required.[23] Barriers to conducting effective screening include limited privacy in the ED, lack of time, and lack of knowledge about how to ask about family violence and IPV. The development and implementation of policies, procedures, and staff education programs improve screening practices.[22]

Start appropriate interventions for patients who you suspect or find are victims of abuse. These include making referrals, notifying appropriate agencies (i.e., as required by law), providing emotional support, and informing victims about their options (e.g., safe house, legal rights).[24]

AGENTS OF TERRORISM

The threat of terrorism is an ongoing concern. Terrorism involves overt actions such as the dispensing of nuclear, biologic, or chemical (NBC) agents as weapons for the express purpose of causing harm. Prompt recognition and identification of potential health hazards are essential in the preparedness of health care professionals.

Biologic agents most commonly used in terrorist attacks include anthrax, smallpox, botulism, plague, tularemia, and hemorrhagic fever. Anthrax, plague, and tularemia are treated effectively with antibiotics if sufficient supplies are available and the organisms are not resistant.

Anthrax vaccine protects against cutaneous and inhalation anthrax. The vaccine is approved by the Food and Drug Administration for at-risk adults (e.g., military personnel) before exposure to anthrax.[25] Smallpox can be prevented or the incidence reduced by vaccination, even when given after exposure. Although botulism is treated with antitoxin, several vaccines are being studied. Vaccines for some hemorrhagic fevers (e.g., yellow fever, Argentine hemorrhagic fever) exist, and others are being investigated (e.g., Ebola).[26]

Chemicals are also used as agents of terrorism and are categorized according to their target organ or effect. For example, sarin is a highly toxic nerve gas that can cause death within minutes of exposure. It enters the body through the eyes and skin and acts by paralyzing the respiratory muscles. Antidotes for nerve agent poisoning include atropine and pralidoxime chloride (2-PAM chloride). Multiple doses may be needed to reverse the effects of the nerve agents.[27]

Phosgene is a colorless gas normally used in chemical manufacturing. If inhaled at high concentrations for a long enough period, it causes severe respiratory distress, pulmonary edema, and death. Mustard gas is yellow to brown and has a garlic-like odor. The gas irritates the eyes and causes skin burns and blisters. Protocols to treat victims of chemical exposure vary and relate to the specific agent.[28]

Radiologic or nuclear agents represent another category of agents of terrorism. *Radiologic dispersal devices* (RDDs), also known as "dirty bombs," consist of a mix of explosives and radioactive material (e.g., pellets). When the device is detonated, the blast scatters radioactive dust, smoke, and other material into the surrounding environment, resulting in radioactive contamination.[29]

The main danger from an RDD results from the explosion, which can cause serious injuries to the victims. The radioactive materials used in an RDD (e.g., uranium, iodine-131) do not usually generate enough radiation to cause immediate serious illness, except to those victims who are in close proximity to the explosion. However, the radioactive dust and smoke can spread and cause illness if inhaled. Since radiation cannot be seen, smelled, felt, or tasted, you should start measures to limit contamination (e.g., covering the patient's nose and mouth) and provide for decontamination (e.g., shower).[29,30]

Ionizing radiation, such as that from a nuclear bomb or damage to a nuclear reactor, represents a serious threat to the safety of victims and the environment. Exposure to ionizing radiation may or may not include skin contamination with radioactive material. Initiate decontamination procedures immediately if external radioactive contaminants are present. *Acute radiation syndrome* (ARS) develops after a substantial exposure to ionizing radiation and follows a predictable pattern.[31] (For additional information on ARS, see *www.bt.cdc.gov/radiation/arsphysicianfactsheet.asp.*)

Explosive devices (e.g., TNT, dynamite) that are used as agents of terrorism result in one or more of the following types of injuries: blast, crush, or penetrating. Blast injuries result from the supersonic overpressurization shock wave caused by the explosion. This shock wave primarily damages the lungs, GI tract, and middle ear. Crush injuries (i.e., blunt trauma) often result from explosions in confined spaces causing structural collapse (e.g., falling debris). Some explosive devices contain materials that are projected during the explosion (e.g., shrapnel), leading to penetrating injuries.

EMERGENCY AND MASS CASUALTY INCIDENT PREPAREDNESS

The term emergency usually refers to any extraordinary event (e.g., multi-vehicle crash) that requires a rapid and skilled response and that the community's existing resources can manage. An emergency is differentiated from a mass casualty incident (MCI) in that an MCI is a man-made (e.g., involving NBC agents) or natural (e.g., hurricane) event or disaster that overwhelms a community's ability to respond with existing resources. MCIs usually involve large numbers of victims, physical and emotional suffering, and permanent changes within a community. In addition, MCIs always require assistance from resources outside the affected community (e.g., American Red Cross, Federal Emergency Management Agency [FEMA]) (Fig. 68-8).

When an emergency or an MCI occurs, first responders (e.g., police, emergency medical personnel) are sent to the scene. Triage of victims of an emergency or an MCI differs from the usual

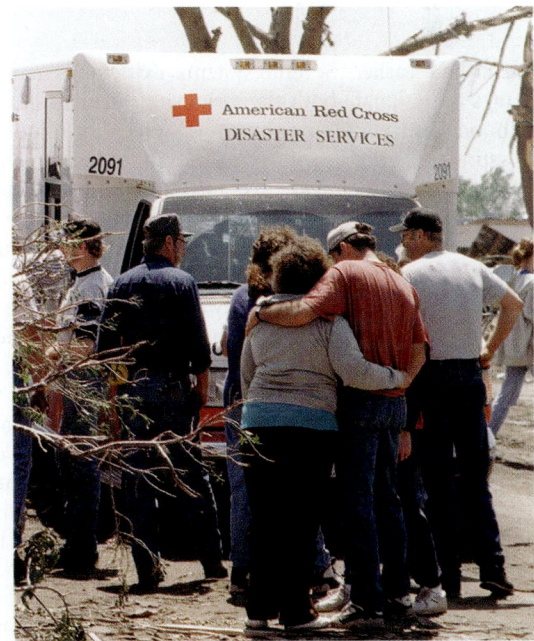

FIG. 68-8 American Red Cross. (Photo used with the permission of the American Red Cross.)

ETHICAL/LEGAL DILEMMAS
Good Samaritan

Situation

You are a registered nurse, employed as a charge nurse at a subacute rehabilitation facility. It is midnight and you are driving home from work when you see a motor vehicle crash with a person at the side of the road waving and yelling for help. You stop and call 911 to report the incident. What do you do next?

Ethical/Legal Points for Consideration

- As a licensed health care professional, you are under no legal obligation to stop and render aid.
- If you do stop, you assume an obligation not to leave the scene until sufficiently trained first responders arrive and assume control.
- Between 50 and 75 yr ago, many states moved to encourage health care professionals to stop and render aid by passing "Good Samaritan" statutes. These statutes, which vary somewhat from state to state, offer immunity from lawsuit for bystanders who offer aid in emergencies except in the case of gross negligence.
- A Good Samaritan must not be in the place of employment or under employment conditions.
- An example of gross negligence may be refusing to assist someone who obviously had a serious hemorrhage in favor of a person with a minor injury because the bleeding person looked old or disheveled.
- Immunity covers only the scene of the accident and not subsequent care under the supervision of HCPs.
- If there is a national disaster, an act of terrorism, or a major emergent need for HCPs, you may be required to go to an assigned site to offer aid. You would not be covered by the Good Samaritan Act under these circumstances.

Discussion Questions

1. What factors do you think contribute to a health care professional's decision whether to stop to provide aid?
2. What basic aid would you feel comfortable providing if you do not have an emergency or trauma background?
3. Would your professional liability (malpractice) insurance cover you if someone claimed that you acted negligently while providing assistance?

triage described earlier. Several systems exist, and many use colored tags to designate both the seriousness of the injury and the likelihood of survival. One system uses green for minor injuries (e.g., sprains) and yellow for urgent, but not life-threatening injuries (e.g., open fractures). Red indicates a life-threatening injury requiring immediate intervention (e.g., shock). Blue indicates those who are expected to die (e.g., massive head trauma), and black identifies the dead.[32]

Triage of victims of an emergency or an MCI must be conducted in less than 15 seconds. In general, two thirds of victims are tagged green or yellow. The remaining are tagged red, blue, or black. Victims need to be treated and stabilized and, if there is known or suspected contamination, decontaminated at the scene. After this, they are moved to hospitals. Many other victims arrive at hospitals on their own (i.e., walking wounded). The total number of victims a hospital can expect is estimated by doubling the number of victims who arrive in the first hour.

Generally, 30% of victims require admission to the hospital, and half of these need surgery within 8 hours.

In addition to the services provided by first responders, many communities have developed *community emergency response teams* (CERTs). CERTs are recognized by FEMA as important partners in emergency preparedness. The CERT training helps citizens understand their personal responsibility in preparing for a natural or man-made disaster. In addition, participants are taught what to expect after a disaster and how to safely help themselves, their family, and their neighbors. Training includes lifesaving skills with emphasis on decision making and rescuer safety. CERTs are an extension of the first responder services. They can offer immediate help to victims and organize untrained volunteers to assist until professional services arrive.[33]

All HCPs have a role in emergency and MCI preparedness. Knowledge of the hospital's *emergency response plan* is essential. This includes individual roles and responsibilities of the members of the response team plus participation in emergency/ MCI preparedness drills on a regular basis. Several types of drills can assess a hospital's level of emergency preparedness. These include hospital disaster drills, computer simulations, and tabletop exercises. Drills allow HCPs to become familiar with the emergency response procedures.[34]

Response to MCIs often requires the aid of a federal agency. The National Incident Management System (NIMS) is a section within the U.S. Department of Homeland Security. NIMS is responsible for coordinating federal, state, and local government efforts to respond to and manage domestic MCIs. One important aspect of NIMS is the development of the *Incident Command System* (ICS). This standardized organizational structure provides for the management of all incidents. NIMS requires that all emergency services–related disciplines (e.g., hospitals, HCPs, emergency response services) wishing to participate in the emergency management of disasters must be NIMS and ICS trained. You can take courses online and at no cost (*http://training.fema.gov/is/nims.aspx*).

The National Disaster Medical System (NDMS) is a part of the U.S. Department of Health and Human Services, Office of Preparedness and Response. The NDMS expands the nation's medical response capability by organizing and training volunteer disaster medical assistance teams (DMATs). Each DMAT consists of members with a variety of health or medical skills and those with specialized support skills (e.g., communications, logistics, security). DMATs are sent to disaster sites with enough supplies and equipment to remain self-sufficient for 72 hours while providing medical care. DMAT personnel are deployed for a period of 2 weeks.[35]

All disasters result in psychologic stress to the individuals involved. This stress can persist for an extended period and is influenced, in part, by the nature of the event, the individual's age, preexisting coping mechanisms, role in the event, and medical and psychologic history. Many hospitals and DMATs have a *critical incident stress management unit*. This unit arranges group discussions to allow participants to share and validate their feelings and emotions about the experience. This is important for emotional recovery.

CASE STUDY

Trauma

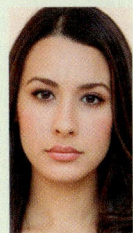

(©Thinkstock)

Patient Profile

D.F., a 20-yr-old Hispanic female trauma victim, is brought to the ED in an ambulance. She was the driver in a motor vehicle crash and was not wearing a seat belt. Two unrestrained children in the car were pronounced dead at the scene. The paramedics stated that there was significant damage to the car on the driver's side.

Subjective Data

• Patient asks, "What happened? Where am I?"
• Complains of shortness of breath and leg pain

Objective Data

Physical Examination

• Vital signs: BP = 85/40 mm Hg, HR = 140 beats/minute, RR = 36 breaths/minute; O$_2$ saturation = 85% with 100% non-rebreather mask
• Decreased breath sounds on left side of chest
• Asymmetric chest wall movement
• Glasgow Coma Score = 14; pupils slightly unequal
• Badly deformed left lower leg with significant swelling and a pedal pulse by Doppler only
• 4-cm head laceration, bleeding controlled

Discussion Questions

1. What are D.F.'s most likely life-threatening injuries?
2. ***Priority Decision:*** What is the priority of care for D.F.?
3. ***Priority Decision:*** What interventions does this patient need immediately?
4. What other interventions should you consider?
5. ***Teamwork and Collaboration:*** What activities could you delegate to unlicensed assistive personnel (UAP)?
6. ***Patient-Centered Care:*** Several family members have arrived in the ED, including the mother of one of the children who died. The second child who died was the patient's child. How should you approach the family?
7. ***Priority Decision:*** Based on assessment data presented, what are the priority nursing diagnoses? Are there any collaborative problems?
8. ***Evidence-Based Practice:*** What are the best practice guidelines for fluid resuscitation in patients who are experiencing hypovolemic shock?

Answers available at *http://evolve.elsevier.com/Lewis/medsurg.*

BRIDGE TO NCLEX EXAMINATION

The number of the question corresponds to the same-numbered outcome at the beginning of the chapter.

1. An older man arrives in triage disoriented and dyspneic. His skin is hot and dry. His wife states that he was fine earlier today. The nurse's next *priority* would be to
   a. assess his vital signs.
   b. obtain a brief medical history from his wife.
   c. start supplemental O$_2$ and have the ED physician see him.
   d. determine the kind of insurance he has before treating him.

2. A patient has a core temperature of 90° F (32.2° C). The *most* appropriate rewarming technique would be
   a. passive rewarming with warm blankets.
   b. active internal rewarming using warmed IV fluids.
   c. passive rewarming using air-filled warming blankets.
   d. active external rewarming by submersing in a warm bath.

3. What are effective interventions to decrease absorption or increase elimination of an ingested poison *(select all that apply)*?
   a. Hemodialysis
   b. Milk dilution
   c. Eye irrigation
   d. Gastric lavage
   e. Activated charcoal

4. An older woman arrives in the ED complaining of severe pain in her right shoulder. The nurse notes that her clothes are soiled with urine and feces. She tells the nurse that she lives with her son and that she "fell." She is tearful and asks you if she can be admitted. What possibility should the nurse consider?
   a. Dementia
   b. Possible cancer
   c. Family violence
   d. Orthostatic hypotension

5. A chemical explosion occurs at a nearby industrial site. The first responders report that victims are being decontaminated at the scene and approximately 125 workers will need medical evaluation and care. The nurse receiving this report should know that this will *first* require activation of
   a. a code blue alert.
   b. a disaster medical assistance team.
   c. the local police and fire departments.
   d. the hospital's emergency response plan.

1. a, 2. b, 3. a, d, e, 4. c, 5. d

For rationales to these answers and even more NCLEX review questions, visit *http://evolve.elsevier.com/Lewis/medsurg.*

⊜ EVOLVE WEBSITE

http://evolve.elsevier.com/Lewis/medsurg
Review Questions (Online Only)
Key Points
Answer Keys for Questions
• Rationales for Bridge to NCLEX Examination Questions
• Answer Guidelines for Case Study on p. 1647
• Answer Guidelines for Managing Care of Multiple Patients Case Study (Section 12) on p. 1649

Student Case Study
• Patient With Musculoskeletal Trauma
Conceptual Care Map Creator
Audio Glossary
Content Updates

REFERENCES

1. Centers for Disease Control and Prevention: Emergency department visits. Retrieved from *www.cdc.gov/nchs/fastats/emergency-department.htm*.

2. American College of Emergency Physicians: Emergency department wait times, crowding and access fact sheet. Retrieved from *http://newsroom.acep.org/index.php?s=20301&item=29937*.

3. Board of Certification for Emergency Nurses: Get certified – CEN. Retrieved from *www.bcencertifications.org/Get-Certified/CEN.aspx*.

4. Rund DA, Rausch TS: *Triage*, St Louis, 1981, Mosby. (Classic)

5. Gilboy N, Tanabe P, Travers DA, et al: Emergency Severity Index (ESI): a triage tool for emergency department, version 4: Implementation handbook 2012 edition, AHRQ Pub No. 12-0014. Retrieved from *www.ahrq.gov/professionals/systems/hospital/esi/esihandbk.pdf*.

6. Emergency Nurses Association: Initial assessment. In *TNCC trauma nursing core course provider manual*, ed 7, Des Plaines, Ill, 2014, Emergency Nurses Association.

7. Hammond BB, Zimmermann PG, editors: *Sheehy's manual of emergency care*, ed 7, St Louis, 2013, Mosby.

*8. Emergency Nurses Association: Clinical practice guideline: family presence during invasive procedures and resuscitation. Retrieved from *www.ena.org/practice-research/research/CPG/Documents/FamilyPresenceCPG.pdf*.

*9. American College of Emergency Physicians: Optimizing the treatment of pain in patients with acute presentations. Retrieved from *www.acep.org/MobileArticle.aspx?id=48089&parentid=*.

10. Centers for Disease Control and Prevention: Tetanus: prevention. Retrieved from *www.cdc.gov/tetanus/about/prevention.html*.

*11. Diao M, Huang F, Guan J, et al: Prehospital therapeutic hypothermia after cardiac arrest: a systematic review and meta-analysis of randomized controlled trials, *Resuscitation* 84:1021, 2013.

*12. O'Gara P, Kushner FG, Ascheim DD, et al: 2013 ACCF/AHA guideline for the management of ST-elevation myocardial infarction, *J Am Coll Cardiol* 61:e78, 2013.

13. Bernard S: Inducing hypothermia after out of hospital cardiac arrest, *BMJ* 348:g2735, 2014.

*14. Emergency Nurses Association: Position statement: palliative and end-of-life care in the emergency department. Retrieved from *www.ena.org/SiteCollectionDocuments/Position%20Statements/PalliativeEndOfLifeCare.pdf*.

15. United Network for Organ Sharing: What every patient needs to know. Retrieved from *www.unos.org/wp-content/uploads/unos/WEPNTK.pdf*.

*16. American College of Emergency Physicians, the American Geriatrics Society, Emergency Nurses Association, and the Society for Academic Emergency Medicine: Geriatric emergency department guidelines. Retrieved from *www.acep.org/geriEDguidelines/*.

17. Centers for Disease Control and Prevention: Tick removal. Retrieved from *www.cdc.gov/ticks/removing_a_tick.html*.

18. Centers for Disease Control and Prevention: Rabies. Retrieved from *www.cdc.gov/rabies/medical_care*.

19. National Capital Poison Control Center: Act fast. Retrieved from *www.poison.org*.

20. Edmunds MW, Mayhew MS: *Pharmacology for the primary care provider*, ed 4, St Louis, 2014, Elsevier.

21. Occupational Health and Safety Administration: Reporting and recording occupational injuries and illness. Retrieved from *www.osha.gov/pls/oshaweb/owastand.display_standard_group?p_toc_level=1&p_part_number=1904*.

*22. Emergency Nurses Association: Position statement: violence in the emergency care setting. Retrieved from *www.ena.org/SiteCollectionDocuments/Position%20Statements/ViolenceintheEmergencyCareSetting.pdf*.

*23. Emergency Nurses Association: Position statement: intimate partner and family violence, maltreatment, and neglect. Retrieved from *http://ncdsv.org/images/ENA_IPVandFamilyViolenceMaltreatmentNeglect_2006.pdf*.

24. Dudgeon A, Evanson TA: Intimate partner violence in rural U.S. areas: what every nurse should know, *AJN* 114:26, 2014.

25. Centers for Disease Control and Prevention: Anthrax. Retrieved from *http://www.cdc.gov/anthrax/medical-care/prevention.html*.

26. Centers for Disease Control and Prevention: Viral hemorrhagic fevers. Retrieved from *www.cdc.gov/ncidod/dvrd/spb/mnpages/dispages/Fact_Sheets/Viral_Hemorrhagic_Fevers_Fact_Sheet.pdf*.

27. Agency for Toxic Substances and Disease Registry: Medical management guidelines for nerve agents: Tabun (GA), Sarin (GB), Soman (GD), and VX. Retrieved from *www.atsdr.cdc.gov/mmg/mmg.asp?id=523&tid=93*.

28. Agency for Toxic Substances and Disease Registry: Medical management guidelines for phosgene. Retrieved from *www.atsdr.cdc.gov/mmg/mmg.asp?id=1201&tid=182*.

29. Centers for Disease Control and Prevention: Frequently asked questions about dirty bombs. Retrieved from *http://emergency.cdc.gov/radiation/dirtybombs.asp*.

*30. Emergency Nurses Association: Position statement: hazardous material exposure. Retrieved from *www.ena.org/SiteCollectionDocuments/Position%20Statements/Archived/Hazardous_Material_Exposure_-_ENA_PS.pdf*.

*31. Military Medical Operations Armed Forces Radiobiology Research Institute: Medical management of radiological casualties. Retrieved from *www.orau.org/PTP/PTP%20Library/library/dod/radiologicalhandbooksp99-2.pdf*.

*32. Lerner EB, Schwartz RB, Coule PL, et al: Mass casualty triage: an evaluation of the data and development of a proposed national guideline, *Disaster Med Public Health Prep* 2:S25, 2008. (Classic)

33. Federal Emergency Management Agency: About community emergency response team. Retrieved from *www.fema.gov/community-emergency-response-teams/about-community-emergency-response-team*.

*34. Agency for Healthcare Research and Quality: Evidence report/technology assessment number 95: training of hospital staff to respond to a mass casualty incident. Retrieved from *http://archive.ahrq.gov/downloads/pub/evidence/pdf/hospmci/hospmci.pdf*.

35. US Department of Health and Human Services: Disaster medical assistance teams. Retrieved from *www.phe.gov/preparedness/responders/ndms/teams/pages/dmat.aspx*.

*Evidence-based information for clinical practice.

CASE STUDY
Managing Care of Multiple Patients

You are working in a 12-bed ICU and have been assigned to care for the following two patients. There is one UAP available to help as needed.

Patients

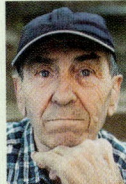
(©Thinkstock)

R.K. is a 72-yr-old white man who was admitted with a massive stroke after collapsing at his home. He is unresponsive, even to painful stimuli. He has an oral endotracheal (ET) tube in place and is receiving mechanical ventilation (assist-control mode, FIO_2 70%, V_T 700 mL, respiratory rate 16 breaths/minute, PEEP 7.5 cm H_2O). His chest x-ray reveals right lower lung consolidation. A subclavian central line was placed to monitor central venous pressure (CVP) and administer fluids and IV antibiotics. His cardiac rhythm on admission was atrial fibrillation with a rapid ventricular response. He is receiving IV diltiazem (Cardizem), and his ventricular response has slowed to 84 bpm. His temperature is elevated despite receiving acetaminophen (Tylenol) q4hr. Additionally, enteral feedings are running at 25 mL/hr via orogastric feeding tube and R.K. has a catheter for urinary drainage.

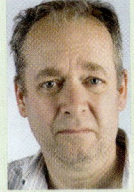
(©Thinkstock)

J.N. is a 58-yr-old white man who was admitted 24 hr ago after emergent surgery for an acutely ischemic bowel. The surgical procedure involved extensive abdominal surgery to repair a perforated colon, irrigate the abdominal cavity, and provide hemostasis. During surgery his systolic BP dropped to 70 mm Hg and remains in the low 90s. He is in sinus tachycardia at a rate of 128 bpm. Six units of packed RBCs and 4 L of 0.9% normal saline were infused. His pulmonary status worsened within 12 hr of admission to the ICU, requiring emergent ET intubation. He developed a right-sided pneumothorax after intubation, and a chest tube was placed at that time. His hypoxemia has rapidly progressed and is now refractory to 100% FIO_2 and high levels of PEEP. His laboratory tests indicate kidney and liver failure. He has an advance directive that indicates he does not want to be kept alive by artificial means, but he currently is full code status. He is sedated, paralyzed, and unable to communicate. His urinary catheter is draining concentrated urine <30 mL/hr and he has a central line in place with 0.9% saline running at 125 mL/hr. His most recent ABGs are as follows: pH 7.12, PaO_2 50 mm Hg, $PaCO_2$ 62 mm Hg, HCO_3^- 17 mEq/L, and O_2 saturation 84%. His PaO_2/FIO_2 ratio is 59, and his chest x-ray shows worsening bilateral interstitial infiltrates compatible with an ARDS pattern.

Discussion Questions

1. ***Priority Decision:*** After receiving report, which patient should you see first? Provide rationale.
2. ***Teamwork and Collaboration:*** Which tasks could you delegate to the UAP *(select all that apply)*?
   a. Record vital signs on R.K. and J.N.
   b. Drain the water from J.N.'s ventilator tubing as needed
   c. Change suction tubing on R.K.'s ET tubes as needed.
   d. Titrate the diltiazem IV drip based on R.K.'s heart rate.
   e. Talk to J.N.'s family regarding his advance directive and current code status.
3. ***Priority Decision and Teamwork and Collaboration:*** As you are assessing J.N., the UAP informs you that R.K. just vomited all over his bed. Which *initial* action would be *most* appropriate?
   a. Ask the UAP to give R.K. a bath while you finish assessing J.N.
   b. Turn off the enteral tube feeding on R.K. and auscultate his lungs.
   c. Ask the UAP to inform the HCP about J.N.'s ABG results while you assess R.K.
   d. Finish assessing R.K. and then suction R.K.'s endotracheal tube to remove any aspirated emesis.

Case Study Progression

R.K.'s lungs are clear to auscultation. Evaluation of his GI status reveals minimal bowel sounds and a gastric residual of 200 mL even after his emesis. You elevate the head of his bed to 60 degrees, hold the tube feeding, and notify his HCP.

4. Which intervention would you expect the HCP to order for R.K.?
   a. Morphine sulfate 2 mg IV stat
   b. Metoclopramide (Reglan) 10 mg IV q6hr
   c. Restart enteral tube feeding while maintaining HOB elevation at 90 degrees
   d. Hold enteral tube feeding for 1 hour and restart with half-strength fluids at same rate
5. J.N.'s ABG results reflect a worsening of his ARDS. You correctly identify that these results demonstrate
   a. uncompensated respiratory acidosis.
   b. uncompensated respiratory alkalosis.
   c. partially compensated respiratory acidosis.
   d. partially compensated respiratory alkalosis.
6. ***Management Decision:*** You walk into J.N.'s room and find his wife whispering in his ear with her hand on the ventilator tubing, appearing to be ready to disconnect him from life support. What is your *best* initial action?
   a. Ask J.N.'s wife to leave the room immediately.
   b. Report the incident to the charge nurse and security immediately.
   c. Ask J.N.'s wife if you could talk to her about her husband's condition.
   d. Report the incident to J.N.'s health care provider to address J.N.'s code status.

Answers and rationales available at *http://evolve.elsevier.com/Lewis/medsurg.*

Basic Life Support for Health Care Professionals

Linda Bucher

Basic life support (BLS) for health care professionals consists of a series of actions and skills performed by the rescuer(s) based on assessment findings. The first action the rescuer performs on finding an adult victim is to assess for responsiveness. This is done by tapping or shaking the victim's shoulder and asking, "Are you all right?" If the victim does not respond, simultaneously scan the victim's chest for signs of breathing and perform a pulse check (described below).

If the rescuer is alone, the rescuer shouts for help. If someone responds, the rescuer asks him or her to activate the *emergency response system* (ERS) (e.g., through the use of a mobile phone) and get an *automatic external defibrillator* (AED) (if available). If no one responds and the rescuer does not have a mobile phone, the rescuer should leave to activate the ERS, get an AED (if available), and return to the victim before beginning *cardiopulmonary resuscitation* (CPR) and defibrillation if necessary.[1]

CARDIOPULMONARY RESUSCITATION

Cardiac arrest is characterized by the absence of a pulse and breathing in an unconscious victim. The current approach for CPR is the chest *compressions-airway-breathing* (CAB) sequence.[1]

The first step in CPR is to perform a pulse check by palpating the carotid pulse for at least 5 but no more than 10 seconds. While maintaining a head-tilt position with one hand on the victim's forehead, locate the victim's trachea using two or three fingers of your other hand. Slide these fingers into the groove between the trachea and neck muscles where the carotid pulse can be felt. The technique is more easily performed on the side nearest you.

If a pulse is felt, give one rescue breath every 5 to 6 seconds (10 to 12 breaths/minute) and recheck the pulse every 2 minutes (Fig. A-1). If no pulse is felt, start CAB.[1,2]

Chest Compressions

The proper technique for providing chest compressions is shown in Fig. A-2. Chest compression technique consists of fast and deep applications of pressure on the lower half of the sternum. The victim must be in the supine position when the compressions are performed. The victim must be lying on a flat, hard surface, such as a CPR board (specially designed for use in CPR), a headboard from a unit bed, or, if necessary, the floor. Position yourself close to the side of the victim's chest. More frequently, mechanical chest compression devices (see Fig. 68-2) are being used to provide chest compressions both prehospital and in the emergency department.

Chest compressions are combined with rescue breathing for an effective resuscitation effort of the adult victim of cardiac arrest. The compression-ventilation ratio for one- or two-rescuer CPR is 30 compressions to 2 breaths (Table A-1). However, if the patient has an advanced airway (e.g.,

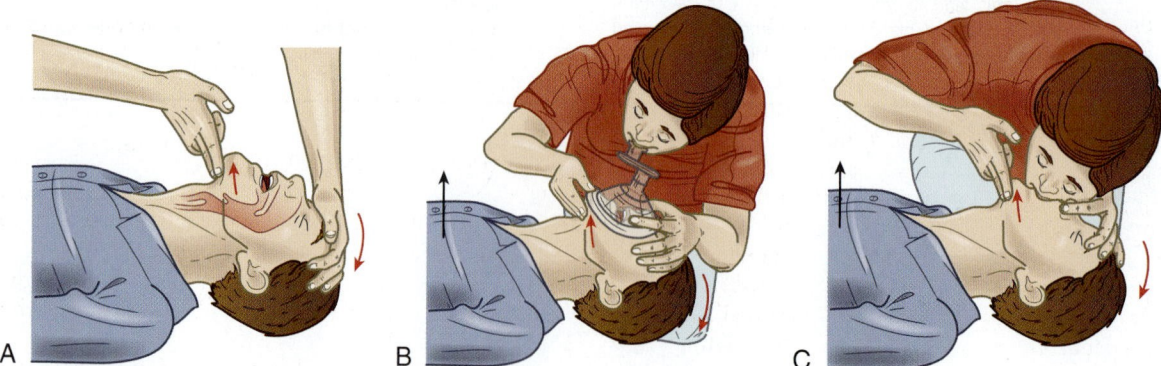

FIG. A-1 The head tilt–chin lift maneuver is used to open the victim's airway to give rescue breaths. **A,** Rescuer places one hand on the victim's forehead and applies firm, backward pressure with the palm to tilt the head back. The chin is lifted and brought forward with the fingers of the other hand. **B,** Mouth-to-barrier device: Rescuer places the device tightly over the victim's mouth and nose and delivers a regular breath. **C,** Mouth-to-mouth technique: Rescuer pinches the victim's nostrils, tightly seals mouth over victim's mouth, and delivers a regular breath. NOTE: Rescuer should observe for a rise in the victim's chest *(black arrows)*.

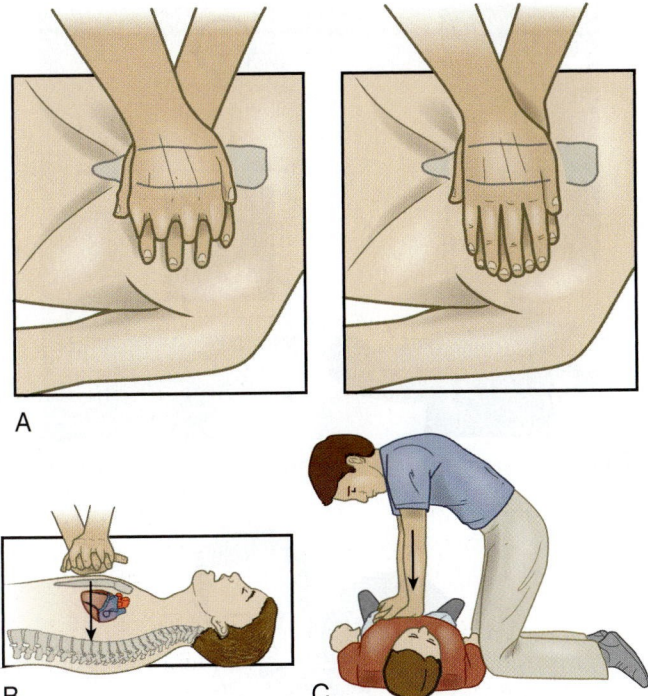

FIG. A-2 Cardiopulmonary resuscitation. **A,** Position of the hands on the lower half of the sternum during chest compressions. **B,** When pressure is applied, the sternum is displaced posteriorly with the heel of the hand. **C,** Arms are kept straight and the rescuer pushes deep (at least 2 in [5 cm]) and fast (a rate of 100-120 compressions per minute).

endotracheal tube, laryngeal mask airway), do not pause between compressions for breaths and deliver 1 breath every 6 seconds (10 breaths/minute).[1]

If a mechanical chest compression device is not used, then it is preferable to have two persons performing CPR. One rescuer, positioned at the victim's side, performs chest compressions while the second rescuer, positioned at the victim's head, maintains an open airway and performs ventilations. To maintain the quality and rate of compressions, rescuers should change roles every 2 minutes.[2] Interruptions in CPR should be limited.

Defibrillation

When the AED or advanced cardiovascular life support (ACLS) team arrives, assess the victim's rhythm. If the victim has a shockable rhythm (e.g., ventricular tachycardia, ventricular fibrillation), deliver one shock and immediately resume CPR for about 2 minutes before checking the rhythm again. If the rhythm is not a shockable rhythm, immediately resume CPR and recheck the rhythm after 2 minutes. CPR should continue between rhythm checks and shocks and until the ACLS team arrives or the victim shows signs of movement.[1]

The American Heart Association includes training in the use of AEDs with instruction of HCPs and laypersons in BLS. Survival from cardiac arrest is the highest when immediate CPR is provided and defibrillation occurs within 3 to 5 minutes.[2] AEDs are found in many out-of-hospital, public settings (Fig. A-3).

Airway and Breathing

If a victim has a pulse but is gasping (e.g., agonal breathing) or not breathing, establish an open airway and begin rescue breathing. Open an adult's airway by hyperextending the head (Fig.

TABLE A-1   Adult One- and Two-Rescuer Basic Life Support With Automatic External Defibrillator (AED)

Assess
- Determine unresponsiveness: tap or shake victim's shoulder; shout, "Are you all right?"
- Check for no breathing or abnormal breathing (e.g., gasping) while simultaneously performing a pulse check (5-10 sec).

Activate Emergency Response System (ERS)
- Activate ERS (e.g., call 911) and get the AED (if available) (outside of hospital).
- Call a code and ask for the AED or crash cart (in hospital).

Begin High-Quality CPR
- If victim has a pulse but is not breathing or not breathing adequately, begin rescue breathing at a rate of 1 breath every 5-6 sec (Fig. A-1) and recheck the pulse every 2 minutes.*
- If there is no pulse, expose the victim's chest and immediately begin chest compressions (Fig. A-2).
- Deliver compressions at a rate of 100-120/minute.
- Compress the chest at least 2 inches (5 cm) but not greater than 2.4 inches (6 cm).
- Allow for complete chest recoil after each compression.
- Deliver a compression-ventilation ratio of 30 compressions to 2 breaths.†
- Minimize interruptions in compressions by delivering the 2 breaths in <10 sec.

Deliver Effective Breaths
- Open airway adequately (Fig. A-1, *A*).
- Deliver breath to produce a visible chest rise (Fig. A-1, *B, C*).
- Avoid excessive ventilation.

Integrate Prompt Use of the AED
- Use AED as soon as possible.
- If rhythm is shockable, deliver one shock and then resume chest compressions immediately after delivery of shock.
- If the rhythm is not shockable, resume CPR and recheck rhythm every five cycles.

Continue CPR
- Continue CPR between rhythm checks and shocks, and until ACLS providers arrive or the victim shows signs of movement.

*If possible opioid overdose, give naloxone if available and per protocol.
†For patients with ongoing CPR and an advanced airway in place, a ventilation rate of 1 breath every 6 seconds (10 breaths per minute) with no interruption in compressions is recommended.
ACLS, Advanced cardiovascular life support; *CPR,* cardiopulmonary resuscitation.
Sources: American Heart Association: *Highlights of the 2015 American Heart Association guidelines update for CPR and ECC,* Dallas, 2015, The Association and American Heart Association: *BLS for healthcare providers—student manual,* Dallas, 2011, The Association.

A-1). Use the *head tilt–chin lift maneuver.* This involves tilting the head back with one hand and lifting the chin forward with the fingers of the other hand. Use the *jaw-thrust maneuver* if you suspect a cervical spine injury (see Fig. 68-1). Attempt to ventilate the victim using a mouth-to-barrier (recommended) device (e.g., face mask or bag-valve-mask) or mouth-to-mouth resuscitation[2] (Fig. A-1, *B, C*).

For mouth-to-mouth resuscitation give ventilations with the victim's nostrils pinched. Take a regular (not deep) breath and tightly seal your lips around the victim's mouth. Give one breath and watch for a rise in the victim's chest. Continue rescue breaths at a rate of 10 to 12 per minute. When the victim has a tracheostomy, give ventilations through the stoma.

TABLE A-2   Management of the Adult Choking Victim

Conscious Adult Choking Victim

Assess Victim for Severe Airway Obstruction

Look for any of the following signs:

- Poor or no air exchange
- Clutching the neck with the hands, making the universal choking sign
- Weak, ineffective cough or no cough at all
- High-pitched noise while inhaling or no noise at all
- Increased respiratory difficulty
- Possible cyanosis

Ask the victim if he or she is choking. If the victim nods yes and cannot talk or has any of the symptoms noted above, severe airway obstruction is present and you must take immediate action.

Abdominal Thrusts (Heimlich Maneuver) With Standing or Sitting Victim (Fig. A-4)

1. Stand or kneel behind victim and wrap arms around the victim's waist.
2. Make fist with one hand.
3. Place thumb side of fist against victim's abdomen. Position fist midline, slightly above navel and well below breastbone.
4. Grasp fist with other hand and press fist into victim's abdomen with a quick, forceful upward thrust.
5. Give each new thrust with a separate, distinct movement to relieve the obstruction. CAUTION: If victim is pregnant or obese, give chest thrusts instead of abdominal thrusts. Position hands (as described) over lower portion of the breastbone and apply quick backward thrusts.
6. Repeat thrusts until object is expelled or victim becomes unresponsive.

Unconscious Adult Choking Victim

If you see a choking victim collapse and become unresponsive:

1. Activate the emergency response system.
2. Lower the victim to the ground and begin CPR, starting with compressions (do not check for a pulse).
3. Open the victim's mouth wide each time you prepare to give breaths. Look for the object. If you see the object and can easily remove it, do so with your fingers. If you do not see the object, continue with CPR using the chest compression–airway–breathing sequence (Table A-1).
4. If efforts to ventilate are unsuccessful, continue with CPR.

Source: American Heart Association: *BLS for healthcare providers—student manual*, Dallas, 2011, The Association.

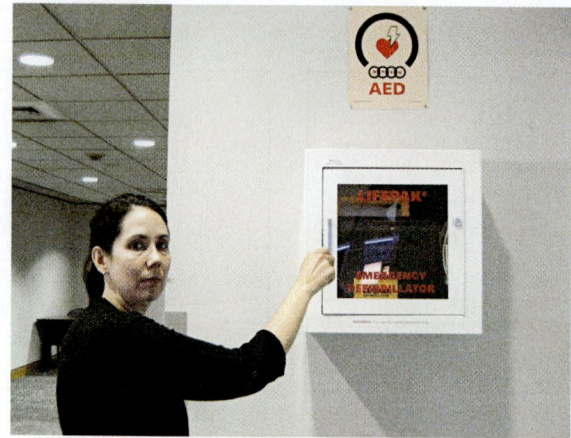

FIG. A-3   Automatic external defibrillator (AED) located in an airport.

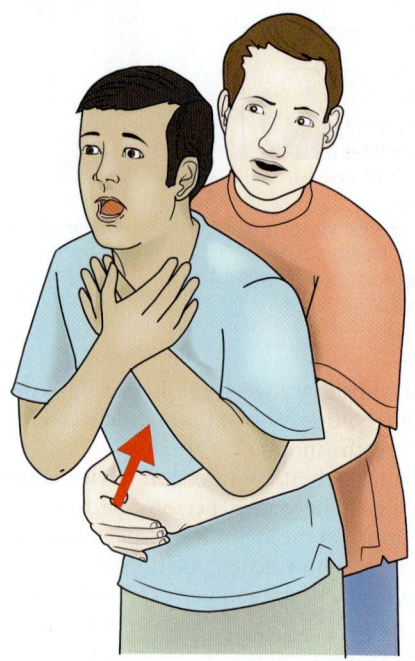

FIG. A-4   Abdominal thrusts (Heimlich maneuver) administered to a conscious (standing) choking victim.

If the victim cannot be ventilated, proceed with CPR. When providing the next rescue breaths, look for any objects in the victim's mouth. If any objects are visible, remove them (Table A-2).

HANDS-ONLY CPR

Hands-only CPR can be used to help adult victims who suddenly collapse from cardiac arrest outside of a health care setting. If you witness this event (as a bystander), you can choose to provide chest compressions only (push fast and deep in the center of the chest) or conventional CPR (described previously). Both methods are effective when done in the first few minutes of an out-of-hospital cardiac arrest.[3]

REFERENCES*

1. American Heart Association: *Highlights of the 2015 American Heart Association guidelines update for CPR and ECC*, Dallas, 2015, The Association.
2. American Heart Association: *BLS for healthcare providers—student manual*, Dallas, 2011, The Association.
3. American Heart Association: Two steps to staying alive with hands-only CPR. Retrieved from *http://www.heart.org/HEARTORG/CPRAndECC/HandsOnlyCPR/Hands-Only-CPR_UCM_440559_SubHomePage.jsp*.

*The CPR guidelines will be updated on an ongoing basis and available at *https://eccguidelines.heart.org/index.php/circulation/cpr-ecc-guidelines-2*.

Activity Intolerance
Activity Intolerance, Risk for
Activity Planning, Ineffective
Activity Planning, Risk for Ineffective
Adaptive Capacity, Decreased Intracranial
Airway Clearance, Ineffective
Allergy Response, Risk for
Anxiety
Aspiration, Risk for
Attachment, Risk for Impaired
Autonomic Dysreflexia
Autonomic Dysreflexia, Risk for
Behavior, Disorganized Infant
Behavior, Readiness for Enhanced Organized Infant
Behavior, Risk for Disorganized Infant
Bleeding, Risk for
Blood Glucose Level, Risk for Unstable
Body Image, Disturbed
Body Temperature, Risk for Imbalanced
Breast Milk, Insufficient
Breastfeeding, Ineffective
Breastfeeding, Interrupted
Breastfeeding, Readiness for Enhanced
Breathing Pattern, Ineffective
Cardiac Output, Decreased
Cardiac Output, Risk for Decreased
Cardiovascular Function, Risk for Impaired
Childbearing Process, Ineffective
Childbearing Process, Readiness for Enhanced
Childbearing Process, Risk for Ineffective
Comfort, Impaired
Comfort, Readiness for Enhanced
Communication, Readiness for Enhanced
Confusion, Acute
Confusion, Chronic
Confusion, Risk for Acute
Constipation
Constipation, Chronic Functional
Constipation, Perceived
Constipation, Risk for
Constipation, Risk for Chronic Functional
Contamination
Contamination, Risk for
Coping, Compromised Family
Coping, Defensive
Coping, Disabled Family
Coping, Ineffective
Coping, Ineffective Community
Coping, Readiness for Enhanced
Coping, Readiness for Enhanced Community
Coping, Readiness for Enhanced Family
Death Anxiety
Decision Making, Readiness for Enhanced
Decisional Conflict

Denial, Ineffective
Dentition, Impaired
Development, Risk for Delayed
Diarrhea
Disuse Syndrome, Risk for
Diversional Activity, Deficient
Dry Eye, Risk for
Electrolyte Imbalance, Risk for
Elimination, Impaired Urinary
Elimination, Readiness for Enhanced Urinary
Emancipated Decision Making, Impaired
Emancipated Decision Making, Readiness for Enhanced
Emancipated Decision Making, Risk for Impaired
Emotional Control, Labile
Falls, Risk for
Family Processes, Dysfunctional
Family Processes, Interrupted
Family Processes, Readiness for Enhanced
Fatigue
Fear
Feeding Pattern, Ineffective Infant
Fluid Balance, Readiness for Enhanced
Fluid Volume, Deficient
Fluid Volume, Excess
Fluid Volume, Risk for Deficient
Fluid Volume, Risk for Imbalanced
Frail Elderly Syndrome
Frail Elderly Syndrome, Risk for
Gas Exchange, Impaired
Gastrointestinal Motility, Dysfunctional
Gastrointestinal Motility, Risk for Dysfunctional
Gastrointestinal Perfusion, Risk for Ineffective
Grieving
Grieving, Complicated
Grieving, Risk for Complicated
Growth, Risk for Disproportionate
Health, Deficient Community
Health Behavior, Risk-Prone
Health Maintenance, Ineffective
Health Management, Ineffective
Health Management, Ineffective Family
Health Management, Readiness for Enhanced
Home Maintenance, Impaired
Hope, Readiness for Enhanced
Hopelessness
Human Dignity, Risk for Compromised
Hyperthermia
Hypothermia
Hypothermia, Risk for
Hypothermia, Risk for Perioperative
Impulse Control, Ineffective
Incontinence, Bowel
Incontinence, Functional Urinary
Incontinence, Overflow Urinary

Incontinence, Reflex Urinary
Incontinence, Risk for Urge Urinary
Incontinence, Stress Urinary
Incontinence, Urge Urinary
Infection, Risk for
Injury, Risk for
Injury, Risk for Corneal
Injury, Risk for Perioperative Positioning
Injury, Risk for Thermal
Injury, Risk for Urinary Tract
Insomnia
Jaundice, Neonatal
Jaundice, Risk for Neonatal
Knowledge, Deficient
Knowledge, Readiness for Enhanced
Latex Allergy Response
Latex Allergy Response, Risk for
Lifestyle, Sedentary
Liver Function, Risk for Impaired
Loneliness, Risk for
Maternal/Fetal Dyad, Risk for Disturbed
Memory, Impaired
Mobility, Impaired Bed
Mobility, Impaired Physical
Mobility, Impaired Wheelchair
Mood Regulation, Impaired
Moral Distress
Nausea
Noncompliance
Nutrition, Imbalanced: Less Than Body Requirements
Nutrition, Readiness for Enhanced
Obesity
Oral Mucous Membrane, Impaired
Oral Mucous Membrane, Risk for Impaired
Other-Directed Violence, Risk for
Overweight
Overweight, Risk for
Pain, Acute
Pain, Chronic
Pain, Labor
Parenting, Impaired
Parenting, Readiness for Enhanced
Parenting, Risk for Impaired
Peripheral Neurovascular Dysfunction, Risk for
Personal Identity, Disturbed
Personal Identity, Risk for Disturbed
Poisoning, Risk for
Post-Trauma Syndrome
Post-Trauma Syndrome, Risk for
Power, Readiness for Enhanced
Powerlessness
Powerlessness, Risk for
Pressure Ulcer, Risk for
Protection, Ineffective
Rape-Trauma Syndrome
Reaction to Iodinated Contrast Media, Risk for
Relationship, Ineffective
Relationship, Readiness for Enhanced
Relationship, Risk for Ineffective
Religiosity, Impaired
Religiosity, Readiness for Enhanced
Religiosity, Risk for Impaired
Relocation Stress Syndrome

Relocation Stress Syndrome, Risk for
Renal Perfusion, Risk for Ineffective
Resilience, Impaired
Resilience, Readiness for Enhanced
Resilience, Risk for Impaired
Role Conflict, Parental
Role Performance, Ineffective
Role Strain, Caregiver
Role Strain, Risk for Caregiver
Self-Care, Readiness for Enhanced
Self-Care Deficit, Bathing
Self-Care Deficit, Dressing
Self-Care Deficit, Feeding
Self-Care Deficit, Toileting
Self-Concept, Readiness for Enhanced
Self-Directed Violence, Risk for
Self-Esteem, Chronic Low
Self-Esteem, Risk for Chronic Low
Self-Esteem, Situational Low
Self-Esteem, Risk for Situational Low
Self-Mutilation
Self-Mutilation, Risk for
Self-Neglect
Sexual Dysfunction
Sexuality Pattern, Ineffective
Shock, Risk for
Sitting, Impaired
Skin Integrity, Impaired
Skin Integrity, Risk for Impaired
Sleep, Readiness for Enhanced
Sleep Deprivation
Sleep Pattern, Disturbed
Social Interaction, Impaired
Social Isolation
Sorrow, Chronic
Spiritual Distress
Spiritual Distress, Risk for
Spiritual Well-Being, Readiness for Enhanced
Spontaneous Ventilation, Impaired
Standing, Impaired
Stress Overload
Sudden Infant Death Syndrome, Risk for
Suffocation, Risk for
Suicide, Risk for
Surgical Recovery, Delayed
Surgical Recovery, Risk for Delayed
Swallowing, Impaired
Thermoregulation, Ineffective
Tissue Integrity, Impaired
Tissue Integrity, Risk for Impaired
Tissue Perfusion, Ineffective Peripheral
Tissue Perfusion, Risk for Decreased Cardiac
Tissue Perfusion, Risk for Ineffective Cerebral
Tissue Perfusion, Risk for Ineffective Peripheral
Transfer Ability, Impaired
Trauma, Risk for
Unilateral Neglect
Urinary Retention
Ventilatory Weaning Response, Dysfunctional
Verbal Communication, Impaired
Walking, Impaired
Wandering

Laboratory Reference Intervals

The tables in this appendix list some of the most common tests, their reference intervals (formally referred to as *normal values*), and possible etiologies of abnormal results. Laboratory results may vary depending on different techniques or different laboratories. Possible etiologies are presented in alphabetic order. Abbreviations appearing in the tables are defined as follows:

mEq = milliequivalent
mm Hg = millimeter of mercury
mm = millimeter
mOsm = milliosmole
L = liter
dL = deciliter (10^{-1} liter)
mL = milliliter (10^{-3} liter)
μL = microliter (10^{-6} liter, 10^{-3} milliliter)
fL = femtoliter (10^{-15} liter, 10^{-12} milliliter)

g = gram
mg = milligram (10^{-3} gram)
mcg = microgram (10^{-6} gram)
ng = nanogram (10^{-9} gram)
pg = picogram (10^{-12} gram)
U = unit
μU = microunit
IU = international unit
mmol = millimole (10^{-3} mole)
μmol = micromole (10^{-6} mole)
nmol = nanomole (10^{-9} mole)
pmol = picomole (10^{-12} mole)
kPa = kilopascal
μkat = microkatal

Source: Burtis CA, Ashwood ER, Bruns DE: *Tietz textbook of clinical chemistry and molecular diagnostics,* ed 5, St Louis, 2013, Elsevier.

TABLE C-1 Serum, Plasma, and Whole Blood Chemistries

| Test | REFERENCE INTERVALS | | POSSIBLE ETIOLOGY | |
	Conventional Units	SI Units	Higher	Lower
Acetone			Diabetic ketoacidosis, high-fat diet, low-carbohydrate diet, starvation	
• Quantitative	<2.0 mg/dL	<344 μmol/L		
• Qualitative	Negative	Negative		
Albumin	3.5-5.0 g/dL	35-50 g/L	Dehydration	Chronic liver disease, malabsorption, malnutrition, nephrotic syndrome
Aldolase	1.5-8.1 U/L	1.5-8.1 U/L	Skeletal muscle disease	Renal disease
α₁-Antitrypsin	78-200 mg/dL	0.78-2.0 g/L	Acute and chronic inflammation, arthritis	Chronic lung disease (early onset), malnutrition, nephrotic syndrome
α₁-Fetoprotein	<10 ng/mL	<10 mcg/L	Cancer of testes, ovaries, and liver	
Ammonia	15-45 mcg N/dL	11-32 μmol N/L	Severe liver disease	
Amylase	30-122 U/L (method dependent)	0.51-2.07 μkat/L	Acute and chronic pancreatitis, mumps (salivary gland disease), perforated ulcers	Acute alcoholism, cirrhosis of liver, extensive destruction of pancreas
Bicarbonate	22-26 mEq/L	22-26 mmol/L	Compensated respiratory acidosis, metabolic alkalosis	Compensated respiratory alkalosis, metabolic acidosis
b-Type natriuretic peptide (BNP)	<100 pg/mL	<100 pmol/L	Heart failure	
Bilirubin			Biliary obstruction, impaired liver function, hemolytic anemia, pernicious anemia	
• Total	0.2-1.2 mg/dL	3-21 μmol/L		
• Indirect	0.1-1.0 mg/dL	1.7-17.0 μmol/L		
• Direct	0.1-0.3 mg/dL	1.7-5.1 μmol/L		

Continued

TABLE C-1   Serum, Plasma, and Whole Blood Chemistries—cont'd

Test	REFERENCE INTERVALS		POSSIBLE ETIOLOGY	
	Conventional Units	SI Units	Higher	Lower
Blood gases*				
• Arterial pH	7.35-7.45	7.35-7.45	Alkalosis	Acidosis
• Venous pH	7.32-7.43	7.32-7.43		
• $PaCO_2$	35-45 mm Hg	4.66-5.98 kPa	Compensated metabolic alkalosis	Compensated metabolic acidosis
• $PvCO_2$	38-55 mm Hg	5.06-7.32 kPa	Respiratory acidosis	Respiratory alkalosis
• PaO_2	80-100 mm Hg	10.6-13.33 kPa	Administration of high concentration of oxygen	Chronic lung disease, decreased cardiac output
• PvO_2	38-42 mm Hg	5.04-5.57 kPa		
Calcium (total)	8.6-10.2 mg/dL	2.15-2.55 mmol/L	Acute osteoporosis, hyperparathyroidism, vitamin D intoxication, multiple myeloma	Acute pancreatitis, hypoparathyroidism, liver disease, malabsorption syndrome, renal failure, vitamin D deficiency
Calcium (ionized)	4.64-5.28 mg/dL	1.16-1.32 mmol/L		
CO_2	23-29 mEq/L	23-29 mmol/L	Same as bicarbonate	
Carotene	10-85 mcg/dL	0.19-1.58 µmol/L	Cystic fibrosis, hypothyroidism, pancreatic insufficiency	Dietary deficiency, malabsorption disorders
Chloride	96-106 mEq/L	96-106 mmol/L	Metabolic acidosis, respiratory alkalosis, corticosteroid therapy, uremia	Addison's disease, diarrhea, metabolic alkalosis, respiratory acidosis, vomiting
Cholesterol	<200 mg/dL	<5.2 mmol/L	Biliary obstruction, hypothyroidism, idiopathic hypercholesterolemia, renal disease, uncontrolled diabetes	Extensive liver disease, hyperthyroidism, malnutrition, corticosteroid therapy
• High-density lipoproteins (HDLs)	Male: >40 mg/dL Female: >50 mg/dL	>1.04 mmol/L >1.3 mmol/L		
• Low-density lipoproteins (LDLs)	Recommended: <100 mg/dL Near optimal: 100-129 mg/dL (2.6-3.34 mmol/L) Moderate risk for CAD: 130-159 mg/dL (3.37-4.12 mmol/L) High risk for CAD: >160 mg/dL (>4.14 mmol/L)	Recommended: <2.6 mmol/L Near optimal: 2.6-3.34 mmol/L Moderate risk for CAD: 3.37-4.12 mmol/L High risk for CAD: >4.14 mmol/L		
Copper	80-155 mcg/dL	12.6-24.3 µmol/L	Cirrhosis	Wilson's disease
Cortisol	8 AM: 5-23 mcg/dL 8 PM: <10 mcg/dL	0.14-0.63 µmol/L <0.28 µmol/L	Cushing syndrome, pancreatitis	Adrenal insufficiency, panhypopituitary states
Creatine	0.2-1.0 mg/dL	15.3-76.3 µmol/L	Active rheumatoid arthritis, biliary obstruction, hyperthyroidism, renal disorders, severe muscle disease	Diabetes mellitus
Creatine kinase (CK)	Male: 20-200 U/L Female: 20-180 U/L	Male: 20-200 U/L Female: 20-180 U/L	Musculoskeletal injury or disease, myocardial infarction, severe myocarditis, exercise, numerous IM injections	
• CK-MB	<4%-6% of total CK	<0.4-0.6	Acute myocardial infarction	
Creatinine	0.6-1.3 mg/dL	53-115 µmol/L	Severe renal disease	
Ferritin	10-250 ng/mL	10-250 mcg/L	Sideroblastic anemia, anemia of chronic disease (infection, inflammation, liver disease)	Iron-deficiency anemia
Folate (folic acid)	3-16 ng/mL	7-36 nmol/L	Hypothyroidism	Alcoholism, hemolytic anemia, inadequate diet, malabsorption syndrome, megaloblastic anemia
Gamma glutamyl transferase (GGT)	0-30 U/L	0-0.5 µkat/L	Liver disease, infectious mononucleosis, pancreatitis, hyperthyroidism	Hypothyroidism
Glucose (fasting)	70-99 mg/dL	3.9-5.5 mmol/L	Acute stress, Cushing disease, diabetes mellitus, hyperthyroidism, pancreatic insufficiency	Addison's disease, hepatic disease, hypothyroidism, insulin overdosage, pancreatic tumor, pituitary hypofunction

PaCO₂, Partial pressure of CO_2 in arterial blood; *PaO₂*, partial pressure of oxygen in arterial blood; *PvCO₂*, partial pressure of CO_2 in venous blood; *PvO₂*, partial pressure of oxygen in venous blood.

*Because arterial blood gases are influenced by altitude, the value for PaO_2 decreases as altitude increases. The lower value is normal for an altitude of 1 mile.

TABLE C-1 Serum, Plasma, and Whole Blood Chemistries—cont'd

| Test | REFERENCE INTERVALS | | POSSIBLE ETIOLOGY | |
	Conventional Units	SI Units	Higher	Lower
Haptoglobin	26-185 mg/dL	260-1850 mg/L	Infectious and inflammatory processes, cancer	Hemolytic anemia, mononucleosis, toxoplasmosis, chronic liver disease
Insulin (fasting)	4-24 μU/mL	29-172 pmol/L	Acromegaly, adenoma of pancreatic islet cells, untreated mild case of type 2 diabetes	Inadequately treated type 1 diabetes mellitus
Iron, total	50-175 mcg/dL	9.0-31.3 μmol/L	Excessive RBC destruction	Iron-deficiency anemia, anemia of chronic disease
Iron-binding capacity	250-425 mcg/dL	44.8-76.1 μmol/L	Iron-deficient state, polycythemia	Cancer, chronic infections, pernicious anemia
Lactic acid (L-Lactate)	6.3-22.5 mcg/dL	0.7-2.5 mmol/L	Acidosis, heart failure, shock	
Lactic dehydrogenase (LDH)	140-280 U/L	0.83-2.5 μkat/L	Heart failure, hemolytic disorders, hepatitis, metastatic cancer of liver, myocardial infarction, pernicious anemia, pulmonary embolus, skeletal muscle damage	
Lactic dehydrogenase isoenzymes				
• LDH$_1$	18%-33%	0.18-0.33	Myocardial infarction, pernicious anemia	
• LDH$_2$	28%-40%	0.28-0.40	Pulmonary embolus, sickle cell crisis	
• LDH$_3$	18%-30%	0.18-0.30	Malignant lymphoma, pulmonary embolus	
• LDH$_4$	6%-16%	0.06-0.16	Systemic lupus erythematosus, pulmonary infarction	
• LDH$_5$	2%-13%	0.02-0.13	Heart failure, hepatitis, pulmonary embolus and infarction, skeletal muscle damage	
Lipase	31-186 U/L	0.5-3.2 μkat/L	Acute pancreatitis, hepatic disorders, perforated peptic ulcer	
Magnesium	1.5-2.5 mEq/L	0.75-1.25 mmol/L	Addison's disease, hypothyroidism, renal failure	Chronic alcoholism, severe malabsorption
Osmolality	275-295 mOsm/kg	275-295 mmol/kg	Chronic renal disease, diabetes mellitus	Addison's disease, diuretic therapy
O$_2$ saturation (arterial) (SaO$_2$)	>95%	>0.95	Polycythemia	Anemia, cardiac decompensation, respiratory disorders
pH	See Blood gases			
Phenylalanine	0.8-1.8 mg/dL	48-109 μmol/L	Phenylketonuria	
Phosphatase, acid	0-0.6 U/L	0-90 μkat/L	Advanced Paget's disease, cancer of prostate, hyperparathyroidism	
Phosphatase, alkaline	38-126 U/L	0.65-2.14 μkat/L	Bone diseases, marked hyperparathyroidism, obstruction of biliary system, rickets	Excessive vitamin D ingestion, hypothyroidism
Phosphorus (phosphate)	2.4-4.4 mg/dL	0.78-1.42 mmol/L	Healing fractures, hypoparathyroidism, renal disease, vitamin D intoxication	Diabetes mellitus, hyperparathyroidism, vitamin D deficiency
Potassium	3.5-5.0 mEq/L	3.5-5.0 mmol/L	Addison's disease, diabetic ketosis, massive tissue destruction, renal failure	Cushing syndrome, diarrhea (severe), diuretic therapy, gastrointestinal fistula, pyloric obstruction, starvation, vomiting
Progesterone (female)				
• Follicular phase	15-70 ng/dL	0.5-2.2 nmol/L	Adrenal hyperplasia, choriocarcinoma of ovary, pregnancy, cysts of ovary	Threatened abortion, hypogonadism, amenorrhea, ovarian tumor
• Luteal phase	200-2500 ng/dL	6.4-79.5 nmol/L		
• Postmenopause	<40 ng/dL	1.28 nmol/L		

RBC, red blood cell; *SaO$_2$,* arterial oxygen saturation.

Continued

TABLE C-1   Serum, Plasma, and Whole Blood Chemistries—cont'd

Test	REFERENCE INTERVALS		POSSIBLE ETIOLOGY	
	Conventional Units	SI Units	Higher	Lower
Prostate-specific antigen (PSA)	<4 ng/mL	<4 mcg/L	Prostate cancer	
Proteins			Burns, cirrhosis (globulin fraction), dehydration	Liver disease, malabsorption
• Total	6.4-8.3 g/dL	64-83 g/L		
• Albumin	3.5-5.0 g/dL	35-50 g/L		
• Globulin	2.0-3.5 g/dL	20-35 g/L		
• Albumin/globulin ratio	1.5:1-2.5:1	1.5:1-2.5:1	Multiple myeloma (globulin fraction), shock, vomiting	Malnutrition, nephrotic syndrome, proteinuria, renal disease, severe burns
Sodium	135-145 mEq/L	135-145 mmol/L	Dehydration, impaired renal function, primary aldosteronism, corticosteroid therapy	Addison's disease, diabetic ketoacidosis, diuretic therapy, excessive loss from GI tract, excessive perspiration, water intoxication
Testosterone	Male: 280-1100 ng/dL	Male: 10.4-38.17 nmol/L		Hypofunction of testes, hypogonadism
	Female: 15-70 ng/dL	Female: 0.52-2.43 nmol/L	Polycystic ovary, virilizing tumors	
T_4 (thyroxine), total	4.6-11.0 mcg/dL	59-142 nmol/L	Hyperthyroidism, thyroiditis	Cretinism, hypothyroidism, myxedema
T_4 (thyroxine), free	0.8-2.7 ng/dL	10-35 pmol/L		
T_3 uptake	24%-34%	0.24-0.34	Hyperthyroidism	Hypothyroidism
T_3 (triiodothyronine), total	Age 20-50: 70-204 ng/dL	1.08-3.14 nmol/L	Hyperthyroidism	Hypothyroidism
	Age >50: 40-181 ng/dL	0.62-2.79 nmol/L		
Thyroid-stimulating hormone (TSH)	0.4-4.2 µU/mL	0.4-4.2 mU/L	Myxedema, primary hypothyroidism, Graves' disease	Secondary hypothyroidism
Transaminases				
• Aspartate aminotransferase (AST)	10-30 U/L	0.17-0.51 µkat/L	Liver disease, myocardial infarction, pulmonary infarction, acute hepatitis	
• Alanine aminotransferase (ALT)	10-40 U/L	0.17-0.68 µkat/L	Liver disease, shock	
Transferrin	190-380 mg/dL	1.9-3.8 g/L		
Transferrin saturation (%)	15%-50%	15%-50%		
Triglycerides	<150 mg/dL	<1.7 mmol/L	Diabetes mellitus, hyperlipidemia, hypothyroidism, liver disease	Malnutrition
Troponins (cardiac)			Myocardial infarction	
• Troponin T (cTnT)	<0.5 ng/mL (<0.5 mcg/L)			
• Troponin I (cTnl)	<0.1 ng/mL (<0.1 mcg/L)			
Urea nitrogen (BUN)	6-20 mg/dL	2.1-7.1 mmol/L	Increase in protein catabolism (fever, stress), renal disease, urinary tract infection	Malnutrition, severe liver damage
Uric acid	Male: 4.4-7.6 mg/dL	Male: 262-452 µmol/L	Gout, gross tissue destruction, high-protein weight reduction diet, leukemia, renal failure	Administration of uricosuric drugs
	Female: 2.3-6.6 mg/dL	Female: 137-393 µmol/L		
Vitamin A (retinol)	30-80 mcg/dL	1.05-2.80 µmol/L	Excess ingestion of vitamin A	Vitamin A deficiency
Vitamin B_{12} (cobalamin)	200-835 pg/mL	148-616 pmol/L	Chronic myeloid leukemia	Strict vegetarianism, malabsorption syndrome, pernicious anemia, total or partial gastrectomy
Vitamin C (ascorbic acid)	0.4-2.0 mg/dL	23-114 µmol/L	Excessive ingestion of vitamin C	Connective tissue disorders, hepatic disease, renal disease, rheumatic fever, vitamin C deficiency
Zinc	70-120 mcg/dL	10.7-120 µmol/L		Alcoholic cirrhosis

TABLE C-2   Hematology

Test	REFERENCE INTERVALS		POSSIBLE ETIOLOGY	
	Conventional Units	**SI Units**	**Higher**	**Lower**
Bleeding time	2-7 min	120-420 sec	Defective platelet function, thrombocytopenia, von Willebrand disease, aspirin ingestion, vascular disease	
Activated partial thromboplastin time (aPTT)	25-35 sec*	25-35 sec*	Deficiency factors I, II, V, VIII; IX, X, XI, XII; hemophilia, liver disease; heparin therapy	
Prothrombin time (Protime, PT)	11-16 sec*	11-16 sec*	Warfarin therapy; deficiency of factors I, II, V, VII, and X; vitamin K deficiency; liver disease	
Fibrinogen	200-400 mg/dL	2-4 g/L	Burns (after first 36 hr), inflammatory disease	Burns (during first 36 hr), DIC, severe liver disease
Fibrin split (degradation) products	<10 mcg/mL	<10 mg/L	Acute DIC, massive hemorrhage, primary fibrinolysis	
D-Dimer	<250 ng/mL	<250 mcg/L	DIC, myocardial infarction, deep vein thrombosis, unstable angina	
Erythrocyte count† (altitude dependent)	*Male:* 4.3-5.7 × 10⁶/μL *Female:* 3.8-5.1 × 10⁶/μL	*Male:* 4.3-5.7 × 10¹²/L *Female:* 3.8-5.1 × 10¹²/L	Dehydration, high altitudes, polycythemia vera	Anemia, leukemia, posthemorrhage
Red blood indices				
• Mean corpuscular volume (MCV)	80-100 fL	80-100 fL	Macrocytic anemia	Microcytic anemia
• Mean corpuscular hemoglobin (MCH)	27-34 pg	27-34 pg	Macrocytic anemia	Microcytic anemia
• Mean corpuscular hemoglobin concentration (MCHC)	32%-37%	0.32-0.37	Spherocytosis	Hypochromic anemia
Erythrocyte sedimentation rate (ESR)	<30 mm/hr (some gender variation)	<30 mm/hr (some gender variation)	*Moderate increase:* acute hepatitis, myocardial infarction; rheumatoid arthritis *Marked increase:* acute and severe bacterial infections, cancer, pelvic inflammatory disease	Malaria, severe liver disease, sickle cell anemia
Hematocrit† (altitude dependent)	*Male:* 39%-50% *Female:* 35%-47%	*Male:* 0.39-0.50 *Female:* 0.35-0.47	Dehydration, high altitudes, polycythemia	Anemia, hemorrhage, overhydration
Hemoglobin† (altitude dependent)	*Male:* 13.2-17.3 g/dL *Female:* 11.7-15.5 g/dL	*Male:* 132-173 g/L *Female:* 117-155 g/L	COPD, high altitudes, polycythemia	Anemia, hemorrhage
Hemoglobin, glycosylated (A1C)	4.0%-6.0%	4.0%-6.0%	Poorly controlled diabetes mellitus	Sickle cell anemia, chronic renal failure, pregnancy
Platelets (thrombocytes)	150-400 × 10³/μL	150-400 × 10⁹/L	Acute infections, chronic granulocytic leukemia, chronic pancreatitis, cirrhosis, collagen disorders, polycythemia, postsplenectomy	Acute leukemia, DIC, thrombocytopenic purpura
Reticulocyte count	0.5%-1.5% of RBC	0.5%-1.5% of RBC	Hemolytic anemia, polycythemia vera	Hypoproliferative anemia, macrocytic anemia, microcytic anemia
White blood cell count†	4.0-11.0 × 10³/μL	4.0-11.0 × 10⁹/L	Inflammatory and infectious processes, leukemia	Aplastic anemia, side effects of chemotherapy and irradiation
WBC differential				
• Segmented neutrophils	50%-70%	0.50-0.70	Bacterial infections, connective tissue diseases, Hodgkin's lymphoma	Aplastic anemia, viral infections
• Band neutrophils	0-8%	0-0.08	Acute infections	
• Lymphocytes	20%-40%	0.20-0.40	Chronic infections, lymphocytic leukemia, mononucleosis, viral infections	Corticosteroid therapy, whole body irradiation
• Monocytes	4%-8%	0.04-0.08	Chronic inflammatory disorders, malaria, monocytic leukemia, acute infections, Hodgkin's lymphoma	
• Eosinophils	0-4%	0-0.04	Allergic reactions, eosinophilic and chronic granulocytic leukemia, parasitic disorders, Hodgkin's lymphoma	Corticosteroid therapy
• Basophils	0-2%	0-0.02	Hypothyroidism, ulcerative colitis, myeloproliferative diseases	Hyperthyroidism, stress

COPD, Chronic obstructive pulmonary disease; *DIC*, disseminated intravascular coagulation.
*Values depend on reagent and instrumentation used.
†Components of complete blood count (CBC).

TABLE C-3   Serology-Immunology

| Test | REFERENCE INTERVALS | | POSSIBLE ETIOLOGY | |
	Conventional Units	SI Units	Higher	Lower
Antinuclear antibody (ANA)	Negative at 1:40 dilution	Negative at 1:40 dilution	Chronic hepatitis, rheumatoid arthritis, scleroderma, systemic lupus erythematosus	
Anti-DNA antibody	<70 IU/mL	<70 IU/mL	Systemic lupus erythematosus	
Anti-Sm (Smith)	Negative	Negative	Systemic lupus erythematosus	
C-reactive protein (CRP)	6.8-820 mcg/dL	68-8200 mcg/L	Acute infections, any inflammatory condition, widespread cancer	
Carcinoembryonic antigen (CEA)	*Nonsmoker:* <3 ng/mL *Smoker:* <5 ng/mL	*Nonsmoker:* <3 mcg/L *Smoker:* <5 mcg/L	Carcinoma of colon, liver, pancreas; chronic cigarette smoking; inflammatory bowel disease; other cancers	
Complement, total hemolytic (CH$_{50}$)	75-160 U/mL	75-160 kU/L		Acute glomerulonephritis, systemic lupus erythematosus, rheumatoid arthritis, subacute bacterial endocarditis
Direct Coombs or direct antihuman globulin test (DAT)	Negative	Negative	Acquired hemolytic anemia, drug reactions, transfusion reactions	
Fluorescent treponemal antibody absorption (FTA-Abs)	Negative or nonreactive	Negative or nonreactive	Syphilis	
Hepatitis A antibody	Negative	Negative	Hepatitis A	
Hepatitis B surface antigen (HB$_s$Ag)	Negative	Negative	Hepatitis B	
Hepatitis C antibody	Negative	Negative	Hepatitis C	
Monospot or monotest	Negative	Negative	Infectious mononucleosis	
Rheumatoid factor (RF)	Negative or titer <1:17	Negative or titer <1:17	Rheumatoid arthritis, Sjögren's syndrome, systemic lupus erythematosus	
RPR	Negative or nonreactive	Negative or nonreactive	Syphilis, systemic lupus erythematosus, rheumatoid arthritis, leprosy, malaria, febrile diseases, IV drug abuse	
VDRL	Negative or nonreactive	Negative or nonreactive	Syphilis	

RPR, Rapid plasma reagin test; *VDRL,* Venereal Disease Research Laboratory.

TABLE C-4 Urine Chemistry

Test	Specimen	REFERENCE INTERVALS Units	REFERENCE INTERVALS SI Units	POSSIBLE ETIOLOGY Higher	POSSIBLE ETIOLOGY Lower
Acetone	Random	Negative	Negative	Diabetes mellitus, high-fat and low-carbohydrate diets, starvation	
Aldosterone	24 hr	3-30 mcg/day (low-sodium diet increases threefold to fivefold)	0.08-0.83 nmol/day	*Primary aldosteronism:* adrenocortical tumors *Secondary aldosteronism:* cardiac failure, cirrhosis, large dose of ACTH, salt depletion	ACTH deficiency, Addison's disease, corticosteroid therapy
Amylase	24 hr	1-17 U/hr	1-17 U/hr	Acute pancreatitis	
Bence Jones protein	Random	Negative	Negative	Multiple myeloma	
Bilirubin	Random	Negative	Negative	Liver disorders	
Calcium	24 hr	100-250 mg/day	2.5-6.3 mmol/day	Bone tumor, hyperparathyroidism	Hypoparathyroidism, malabsorption of calcium and vitamin D
Catecholamines	24 hr			Pheochromocytoma, progressive muscular dystrophy, heart failure	
• Epinephrine		<20 mcg/day	<109 nmol/day		
• Norepinephrine		15-80 mcg/day	89-473 nmol/day		
Creatine	24 hr	<100 mg/day	<763 μmol/day	Liver cancer, hyperthyroidism, diabetes, Addison's disease, infections, burns, muscular dystrophy, skeletal muscle atrophy	Hypothyroidism
Creatinine	24 hr	0.6-2.0 g/day	5.3-17.7 mmol/day	Anemia, leukemia, muscular atrophy	Renal disease
Creatinine clearance	24 hr	59-137 mL/min/1.73 m²	0.59-1.37 mL/sec/m²		Renal disease
Estrogens	24 hr			Gonadal or adrenal tumor	Endocrine disturbance, ovarian dysfunction, menopause
• Female					
• Premenopause		15-80 mcg/day	15-80 mcg/day		
• Postmenopause		<20 mcg/day	<20 mcg/day		
• Male		15-40 mcg/day	15-40 mcg/day		
Glucose	Random	Negative	Negative	Diabetes mellitus, pituitary disorders	
Hemoglobin	Random	Negative	Negative	Extensive burns, glomerulonephritis, hemolytic anemias, hemolytic transfusion reaction	
5-Hydroxyindole acetic acid (5-HIAA)	24 hr	2-7 mg/day	10.5-36.6 μmol/day	Malignant carcinoid syndrome	
Ketone bodies	24 hr	20-50 mg/day	0.34-0.86 mmol/day	Diabetes mellitus, starvation, dehydration	
Metanephrine	24 hr	92-934 mcg/day	500-5100 nmol/day	Pheochromocytoma	
Myoglobin	Random	Negative	Negative	Crushing injuries, electric injuries, extreme physical exertion	
Osmolality	Random	300-1300 mOsm/kg	300-1300 mmol/kg	Dehydration, tubular dysfunction (kidney lost ability to dilute urine)	Tubular dysfunction (kidney lost ability to concentrate urine)
pH	Random	4.0-8.0	4.0-8.0	Urinary tract infection, urine allowed to stand at room temperature	Respiratory or metabolic acidosis
Protein (dipstick)	Random	0-trace	0-trace	Acute and chronic renal disease, especially involving glomeruli; heart failure	
Protein (quantitative)	24 hr	<150 mg/day	<0.15 g/day	Cardiac failure, inflammatory processes of urinary tract, nephritis, nephrosis, strenuous exercise	
Sodium	24 hr	40-220 mEq/day	40-220 mmol/day	Acute tubular necrosis	Hyponatremia
Specific gravity	Random	1.003-1.030	Same as conventional units	Albuminuria, dehydration, glycosuria	Diabetes insipidus
Uric acid	24 hr	250-750 mg/day	1.5-4.5 mmol/day	Gout, leukemia	Nephritis
Urobilinogen	24 hr	0.5-4.0 mg/day	0.8-6.8 μmol/day	Hemolytic disease, hepatic parenchymal cell damage, liver disease	Complete obstruction of bile duct
Vanillylmandelic acid	24 hr	1.4-6.5 mg/day	7-33 μmol/day	Pheochromocytoma	

ACTH, Adrenocorticotropic hormone.

TABLE C-5   Fecal Analysis

Test	REFERENCE INTERVALS Conventional Units	SI Units	POSSIBLE ETIOLOGY Higher
Fecal fat	<6 g/24 hr	Same as conventional units	Chronic pancreatic disease, obstruction of common bile duct, malabsorption syndrome
Mucus	Negative	Negative	Mucous colitis, spastic constipation
Pus	Negative	Negative	Chronic bacillary dysentery, chronic ulcerative colitis, localized abscesses
Blood*	Negative	Negative	Anal fissures, hemorrhoids, malignant tumor, peptic ulcer, inflammatory bowel disease
Color			
• Brown			Various color depending on diet
• Clay			Biliary obstruction or presence of barium sulfate
• Tarry			More than 100 mL of blood in gastrointestinal tract
• Red			Blood in large intestine
• Black			Blood in upper gastrointestinal tract or iron medication

*Ingestion of meat may produce false-positive results. Patient may be placed on a meat-free diet for 3 days before the test.

TABLE C-6   Cerebrospinal Fluid Analysis

Test	REFERENCE INTERVALS Conventional Units	SI Units	POSSIBLE ETIOLOGY Higher	Lower
Pressure	60-150 mm H_2O	60-150 mm H_2O	Hemorrhage, intracranial tumor, meningitis	Head injury, spinal tumor, subdural hematoma
Blood	Negative	Negative	Intracranial hemorrhage	
Cell count (age dependent)			Inflammation or infections of CNS	
• WBC	0-5 cells/μL	$0\text{-}5 \times 10^6$ cells/L		
• RBC	Negative	Negative		
Chloride	118-132 mEq/L	118-132 mmol/L	Uremia	Bacterial infections of CNS (meningitis, encephalitis)
Glucose	40-70 mg/dL	2.2-3.9 mmol/L	Diabetes mellitus, viral infections of CNS	Bacterial infections and tuberculosis of CNS
Protein				
• Lumbar	15-45 mg/dL	0.15-0.45 g/L	Guillain-Barré syndrome, poliomyelitis, trauma	
• Cisternal	15-25 mg/dL	0.15-0.25 g/L	Syphilis of CNS	
• Ventricular	5-15 mg/dL	0.05-0.15 g/L	Acute meningitis, brain tumor, chronic CNS infections, multiple sclerosis	

CNS, Central nervous system.

A

acromegaly   a condition caused by excessive secretion of growth hormone characterized by an overgrowth of the bones and soft tissues.

actinic keratosis   a slowly developing, localized thickening and scaling of the outer layers of the skin consisting of hyperkeratotic papules and plaques as a result of chronic, prolonged exposure to the sun; also known as *solar keratosis.*

acute bronchitis   an inflammation of the lower respiratory tract that is usually due to infection.

acute kidney injury (AKI)   clinical syndrome characterized by a rise in serum creatinine and/ or a reduction in urine output.

acute pancreatitis   an acute inflammatory process of the pancreas caused by autodigestion and marked by symptoms of an acute condition of the abdomen and spillage of pancreatic enzymes into surrounding pancreatic tissues.

acute respiratory distress syndrome (ARDS)   a sudden and progressive form of acute respiratory failure in which the alveolar-capillary membrane becomes damaged and more permeable to intravascular fluid.

acute tubular necrosis (ATN)   a type of intra-renal acute injury of the kidney that affects the renal tubules, caused by renal ischemia and nephrotoxic injury.

adhesion   a band of scar tissue between or around organs.

adventitious sounds   extra breath sounds that are not normally heard, such as crackles, wheezes, and pleural friction rubs.

afterload   the peripheral resistance against which the left ventricle must pump.

allergic rhinitis   the reaction of the nasal mucosa to a specific allergen.

alopecia   partial or complete lack of hair resulting from normal aging, endocrine disorder, drug reaction, chemotherapy, or skin disease.

Alzheimer's disease (AD)   a chronic, progressive, neurodegenerative disease of the brain.

amyotrophic lateral sclerosis (ALS)   a rare progressive neuromuscular disorder characterized by loss of motor neurons and by weakness and atrophy of the muscles of the hands, forearms, and legs, spreading to involve most of the body and face.

anaphylactic shock   an acute and life-threatening hypersensitivity (allergic) reaction to a sensitizing substance, such as a drug, chemical, vaccine, food, or insect venom.

aneurysm   congenital or acquired weakness of the arterial wall resulting in dilation and ballooning of the vessel.

angina   chest pain that is a clinical manifestation of reversible myocardial ischemia.

ankylosing spondylitis   a chronic inflammatory disease that primarily affects the axial skeleton, including the sacroiliac joints, intervertebral disc spaces, and costovertebral articulations.

ankylosis   stiffness or fixation of a joint usually resulting from destruction of articular cartilage and subchondral bone.

aortic dissection   the result of a tear in the intimal (innermost) lining of the arterial wall that allows blood to enter between the intima and media, thus creating a false lumen.

aphasia   an abnormal neurologic condition in which language function is disordered or absent because of an injury to certain areas of the cerebral cortex.

aplastic anemia   a disease with a deficiency of all of the formed elements of blood (specifically red blood cells, white blood cells, and platelets), representing a failure of the cell-generating capacity of bone marrow.

appendicitis   an inflammation of the appendix that, if undiagnosed, leads rapidly to perforation and peritonitis.

arterial blood pressure   a measure of the pressure exerted by blood against the walls of the arterial system.

arteriovenous fistula (AVF)   type of vascular access created most commonly in the forearm with an anastomosis between an artery (usually radial or ulnar) and a vein (usually cephalic).

arteriovenous grafts (AVGs)   fistula made of synthetic materials that forms a "bridge" between the arterial and venous blood supplies.

arthritis   inflammation of a joint; most prevalent types are osteoarthritis, rheumatoid arthritis, and gout.

arthrocentesis   incision or puncture of joint capsule to obtain samples of synovial fluid from within joint cavity or to remove excess fluid.

arthrodesis   the surgical fusion of a joint.

arthroplasty   surgical reconstruction or replacement of a joint.

arthroscopy   insertion of an arthroscope into a joint for visualization or surgery.

ascites   an abnormal intraperitoneal accumulation of a fluid containing large amounts of protein and electrolytes as a result of portal hypertension.

asterixis   flapping tremor commonly affecting the arms and hands that is a manifestation of hepatic encephalopathy.

asthma   a chronic inflammatory lung disease that results in airflow obstruction; characterized by recurring episodes of paroxysmal dyspnea, wheezing on expiration and/or inspiration caused by constriction of the bronchi, coughing, and viscous mucoid bronchial secretions.

asystole   represents the total absence of ventricular electrical activity.

atherosclerosis   formation of focal deposits of cholesterol and lipids known as *atheromas* or *plaque,* primarily within the intimal wall of arteries, that obstruct circulation.

atrial fibrillation   a cardiac dysrhythmia characterized by a total disorganization of atrial electrical activity without effective atrial contraction.

atrial flutter   an atrial tachydysrhythmia identified by recurring, regular, sawtooth-shaped flutter waves.

atrophy   wasting of muscle, characterized by decreased circumference and flabby appearance leading to decreased function and tone.

aura   a sensation of light or warmth or other perception that may be a warning of an attack of a migraine or an epileptic seizure.

auscultation   the act of listening for sounds within the body to evaluate the condition of the heart, blood vessels, lungs, pleura, intestines, or other organs.

autoimmunity   an inappropriate immune reaction to self-proteins.

azotemia   an accumulation of nitrogenous waste products such as blood urea nitrogen (BUN) and creatinine.

B

bariatric surgery   a surgical procedure on the stomach and/or intestines to help a person with extreme obesity lose weight.

Barrett's esophagus   a precancerous esophageal disorder characterized by metaplastic cell changes.

basal cell carcinoma   a malignant epithelial cell tumor arising from epidermal basal cells that begins as a papule and enlarges peripherally, developing a central crater that erodes, crusts, and bleeds.

Bell's palsy   a disorder characterized by a disruption of the motor branches of the facial nerve (cranial nerve [CN] VII) on one side of the face in the absence of any other disease such as a stroke.

benign prostatic hyperplasia (BPH)   a nonmalignant, noninflammatory enlargement of the prostate gland caused by an increase in the number of epithelial cells and stromal tissue.

biologic therapy   treatment using biologic agents such as interferons, interleukins, monoclonal antibodies, and growth factors to modify the relationship between the host and tumor.

borborygmi   audible abdominal sounds produced by hyperactive intestinal peristalsis.

botulism   a rare but serious food poisoning caused by GI absorption of the neurotoxin produced by *Clostridium botulinum,* which results in disturbed muscle innervation.

brachytherapy   radiation delivery system that means "closed" treatment and consists of the implantation or insertion of radioactive materials directly into the tumor or in close proximity to the tumor.

brain attack   a stroke.

bursitis   inflammation of the bursa.

C

calculus   an abnormal stone formed in body tissues by an accumulation of mineral salts.

carcinogens   agents capable of producing cellular alterations leading to the development or increasing the incidence of neoplastic growth.

carcinoma in situ   a lesion with all the histologic features of cancer except invasion.

cardiac index (CI) a measure of the cardiac output of a patient per square meter of body surface area.

cardiac output (CO) the amount of blood pumped by each ventricle in 1 minute.

cardiac pacemaker an electronic device used to increase the heart rate in severe bradycardia by electrically stimulating the heart muscle.

cardiac reserve the ability to respond to demands (exercise, stress, hypovolemia) by altering cardiac output threefold or fourfold.

cardiac tamponade compression of the heart produced by fluid accumulation in the pericardial sac.

cardiogenic shock shock occurring when either systolic or diastolic dysfunction of the myocardium results in compromised cardiac output.

cardiomyopathy a group of diseases that directly affect the structural or functional ability of the myocardium.

carpal tunnel syndrome a condition caused by compression of the median nerve beneath the transverse carpal ligament within the narrow confines of the carpal tunnel located in the wrist.

cataract an abnormal progressive condition of the lens of the eye characterized by an opacity within the lens.

celiac disease an inborn error of metabolism characterized by the inability to hydrolyze peptides contained in gluten.

cell-mediated immunity immunity that is initiated through specific antigen recognition by T lymphocytes, monocytes/macrophages, and natural killer cells.

cellulitis a diffuse, acute bacterial infection of the skin and subcutaneous tissue characterized most commonly by local heat, redness, pain, and swelling.

central cord syndrome damage to the central spinal cord characterized by microscopic hemorrhage, edema of the central spinal cord, and compression on anterior horn cells.

cerebral edema increased accumulation of fluid in the extravascular spaces of brain tissue that can lead to increased intracranial pressure.

cheilosis a disorder of the lips and mouth characterized by bilateral scales and fissures, resulting from a deficiency of riboflavin in the diet.

chemotherapy the treatment of disease with chemical agents.

Cheyne-Stokes respiration an abnormal breathing pattern characterized by alternating periods of apnea and deep, rapid breathing; usually seen as a person nears death.

cholecystitis inflammation of the gallbladder.

cholelithiasis stones in the gallbladder.

chronic kidney disease (CKD) progressive, irreversible loss of kidney function with either the presence of kidney damage or decreased glomerular filtration rate for at least 3 months.

chronic kidney disease (CKD) mineral and bone disorder a systemic disorder of mineral and bone metabolism due to progressive deterioration in kidney function.

chronic pancreatitis progressive destruction of the pancreas with fibrotic replacement of pancreatic tissue.

chronic stable angina chest pain that occurs intermittently over a long period with the same pattern of onset, duration, and intensity of symptoms.

cirrhosis end-stage liver disease characterized by extensive degeneration and destruction of the liver parenchymal cells.

cluster headaches repeated headaches that can occur as clusters, generally at the same time of day or night and followed by periods of remission.

collateral circulation development of arterial branching that occurs within the coronary circulation when occlusion of the coronary arteries occurs slowly over a long period.

coma a profound state of unconsciousness.

community-acquired pneumonia (CAP) a lower respiratory tract infection of the lung parenchyma with onset in the community or during the first 2 days of hospitalization.

compartment syndrome a condition in which elevated intracompartmental pressure within a confined myofascial compartment compromises the neurovascular function of tissues within that space.

complete heart block third-degree atrioventricular heart block in which no impulses from the atria are conducted to the ventricles.

concussion a sudden transient mechanical head injury, such as a blow or explosion, with disruption of neural activity and a change in the level of consciousness.

continuous renal replacement therapy (CRRT) provides a means by which uremic toxins and fluids can be removed slowly and continuously in the hemodynamically unstable patient.

contracture an abnormal, usually permanent condition of a joint, characterized by flexion and fixation.

contusion the bruising of the brain tissue within a focal area without altering the integrity of the pia mater and arachnoid layers.

coronary artery disease (CAD) an abnormal condition that may affect the heart's arteries and produce various pathologic effects, especially the reduced flow of oxygen and nutrients to the myocardium.

cor pulmonale hypertrophy of the right side of the heart, with or without heart failure, resulting from pulmonary hypertension.

crackle short, low-pitched sound consisting of discontinuous bubbling caused by air passing through the airway intermittently occluded by mucus, an unstable bronchial wall, or a fold of mucosa.

crepitation crackling sound or grating sensation as a result of friction between bones.

cryosurgery the use of subfreezing temperatures to perform surgery.

curettage scraping of material from the wall of a cavity or other surface; performed to remove tumors or other abnormal tissue or to obtain tissue.

Cushing syndrome a metabolic disorder resulting from the chronic and excessive production of cortisol by the adrenal cortex or by the administration of glucocorticoids in large doses for several weeks or longer.

cystic fibrosis (CF) an autosomal recessive, multisystem disease characterized by altered function of the exocrine glands involving primarily the lungs, pancreas, and sweat glands.

cystitis an inflammatory condition of the urinary bladder characterized by pain, urgency, frequency of urination, and hematuria.

cystocele herniation or protrusion of the urinary bladder through the wall of the vagina, resulting from weakened connective tissue support between the vagina and bladder.

D

death rattle a sound produced by air moving through mucus that has accumulated in the throat of a dying person who has lost the cough reflex.

debridement removal of dirt, foreign objects, damaged tissue, and cellular debris from a wound or a burn to prevent infection and promote healing.

deep vein thrombosis (DVT) a disorder involving a thrombus in a deep vein; most commonly the iliac and femoral veins.

degenerative disc disease (DDD) progressive degeneration that is a normal process of aging; results in the intervertebral discs losing their elasticity, flexibility, and shock-absorbing capabilities.

dehiscence the separation and disruption of previously joined wound edges, typically an abdominal incision.

delirium a state of temporary but acute mental confusion.

dementia a neurocognitive disorder caused by brain disease, evidenced by chronic personality disintegration, confusion, memory impairment, and deterioration of intellectual capacity and function.

dermatomyositis a disease of the connective tissues characterized by pruritic or eczematous inflammation of the skin and tenderness of the muscles.

diabetes insipidus (DI) a group of conditions associated with deficient production or secretion of antidiuretic hormone (ADH), or a decreased renal response to ADH caused by injury of the neurohypophyseal system.

diabetes mellitus (DM) a multisystem disease related to abnormal insulin production, impaired insulin utilization, or both.

diabetic ketoacidosis (DKA) an acute metabolic complication of diabetes occurring when fats are metabolized in the absence of insulin resulting in formation of acid by-products, such as ketones.

diabetic nephropathy a microvascular complication of diabetes mellitus associated with damage to the small blood vessels that supply the glomeruli of the kidney.

diabetic neuropathy nerve damage caused by the metabolic derangements associated with diabetes mellitus.

dialysis technique in which substances move from the blood through a semipermeable membrane and into a dialysis solution.

dislocation a severe injury of the ligamentous structures that surround a joint resulting in the complete displacement or separation of the articular surfaces of the joint.

disseminated intravascular coagulation (DIC) a grave coagulopathy resulting from the over-stimulation of clotting and anticlotting processes in response to disease or injury.

diverticulitis inflammation of one or more diverticula, resulting in perforation into the peritoneum.

dysarthria a disturbance in the muscular control of speech resulting from interference in the control and execution over the muscles of speech.

dysmenorrhea abdominal cramping pain or discomfort associated with menstrual flow.

dyspareunia abnormal pain during sexual intercourse.

dysphagia difficulty swallowing.

dysphasia difficulty related to the comprehension or use of language.

dysplastic nevi nevi that are larger than usual with irregular borders and various shades of color; also known as *atypical moles*.

dyspnea shortness of breath; difficulty breathing that may be caused by certain heart or lung conditions, strenuous exercise, or anxiety.

E

ecchymoses bruising.

ectopic pregnancy the implantation of a fertilized ovum anywhere outside the uterine cavity.

embolic stroke a stroke that occurs when an embolus lodges in and occludes a cerebral artery, resulting in infarction and edema of the area supplied by the involved vessel.

emergence delirium a neurologic alteration in recovery from anesthesia that can include behaviors such as restlessness, agitation, disorientation, thrashing, and shouting.

empyema an accumulation of purulent exudates in a body cavity, especially the pleural space, that results from bacterial infection, such as pleurisy or tuberculosis.

encephalitis an acute inflammation of the brain that usually caused by a virus.

endometriosis the presence of normal endometrial tissue in sites outside the endometrial cavity.

endotracheal intubation artificial airway created by inserting a tube into the trachea through the mouth or nose, past the larynx, and bypassing the upper airway and laryngeal structures.

enteral nutrition (EN) the administration of a nutritionally balanced, liquefied food or formula through a tube inserted into the stomach, duodenum, or jejunum.

epididymitis acute or chronic inflammation of the epididymis, usually secondary to an infectious process, trauma, or urinary reflux down the vas deferens.

epidural block injection of a local anesthetic into the epidural (extradural) space by either a thoracic or lumbar approach.

epidural hematoma collection of blood between the dura and inner surface of the skull, producing compression of the dura mater and thus of the brain.

epilepsy a condition in which a person has spontaneously recurring seizures caused by a chronic underlying condition.

epistaxis nosebleed.

erectile dysfunction (ED) the inability to attain or maintain an erection that allows satisfactory sexual activity.

erythema redness or inflammation of the skin or mucous membranes that results from dilation and congestion of superficial capillaries.

escharotomy incisions into necrotic tissue from a severe burn performed when eschar formation compromises circulation.

esophageal diverticulum saclike outpouching of one or more layers of the esophagus.

esophageal varices distended, tortuous, fragile veins at the lower end of the esophagus that result from portal hypertension.

evisceration the separation and disruption of previously joined wound edges to the extent that an internal organ, typically intestinal contents, protrudes through the wound.

excision and grafting procedure during which eschar is removed down to the subcutaneous tissue or fascia, depending on the degree of injury; a graft is then placed on clean, viable tissue to achieve good adherence.

exophthalmos protrusion of the eyeballs from the orbits caused by increased fat deposits and fluid in the retroorbital tissues.

external otitis inflammation or infection of the epithelium of the auricle and ear canal.

extreme obesity the classification used to describe individuals with body mass index values >40 kg/m².

F

fat embolism syndrome (FES) embolization of fat globules that occurs in a small percentage of patients with fractures.

fibroadenoma a small, painless, round, well-delineated, mobile benign breast tumor commonly found in young women.

fibrocystic changes a benign condition of the breasts characterized by development of excess fibrous tissue, hyperplasia of the epithelial lining of the mammary ducts, proliferation of mammary ducts, and cyst formation.

fibromyalgia a chronic disorder characterized by widespread, nonarticular musculoskeletal pain and fatigue with multiple tender points.

flail chest instability of the chest wall resulting from multiple rib fractures.

focal seizures seizures that begin in a specific region of the cortex and may be confined to one side of the brain and remain partial or focal in nature, or they may spread to involve the entire brain.

fracture a disruption or break in the continuity of the structure of bone.

fremitus vibration of the chest wall produced by vocalization.

frontotemporal lobar degeneration (FTLD) a rare disorder caused by shrinking frontal and temporal lobes of the brain; characterized by disturbances in behavior, sleep, personality, and eventually memory.

frostbite freezing that results in the formation of ice crystals in the tissues and cells.

full-thickness burn destruction of all skin elements and subcutaneous tissues with possible involvement of muscles, tendons, and bones.

G

galactorrhea a milky secretion from the nipple caused by inappropriate lactation.

gastritis inflammation of the gastric mucosa.

gastroenteritis an inflammation of the mucosa of the stomach and small intestine.

gastroesophageal reflux disease (GERD) any clinically significant symptomatic condition or histopathologic alteration presumed to be secondary to reflux of gastric contents into the lower esophagus.

generalized seizures seizures characterized by bilateral synchronous epileptic discharge in the brain with loss of consciousness for a few seconds to several minutes.

genital herpes a sexually transmitted infection caused by the herpes simplex virus type 2 (HSV-2), resulting in painful genital or anal vesicular lesions.

Glasgow Coma Scale assessment tool for altered states of consciousness that evaluates motor responses, verbal responses, and eye opening.

glaucoma a group of disorders characterized by (1) increased intraocular pressure and the consequences of elevated pressure, (2) optic nerve atrophy, and (3) peripheral visual field loss.

glial cells cells in the central nervous system that provide support, nourishment, and protection to neurons.

glomerular filtration rate (GFR) the amount of blood filtered by the glomeruli in a given time.

glomerulonephritis an immune-related inflammation of the glomeruli characterized by proteinuria, hematuria, decreased urine production, and edema.

goiter enlargement of the thyroid gland that may be associated with hyperthyroidism, hypothyroidism, or normal thyroid function.

gonorrhea infection of the genitalia, the rectum, and/or the oropharynx by *Neisseria gonorrhoeae*, which, if left untreated, leads to the formation of fibrous tissue and adhesions.

Goodpasture syndrome an example of cytotoxic autoimmune disease characterized by the presence of circulating antibodies against the glomerular basement membrane and alveolar basement membrane.

gout recurrent attacks of acute arthritis associated with increased levels of serum uric acid.

Guillain-Barré syndrome an acute, rapidly progressing, and potentially fatal form of polyneuritis possibly caused by a cell-mediated immunologic reaction directed at the peripheral nerves.

gynecomastia a transient enlargement of one or both breasts in men.

H

heat cramps severe cramps in large muscle groups caused by depletion of both water and salt; usually follow vigorous exertion in an extremely hot environment.

heat exhaustion a clinical syndrome characterized by fatigue, light-headedness, nausea, vomiting, diarrhea, and feelings of impending doom precipitated by prolonged exposure to heat over hours or days.

heatstroke the most serious form of heat stress; results from failure of the central thermoregulatory mechanisms and is considered a medical emergency.

heaves sustained lifts of the chest wall in the precordial area that can be seen or palpated.

hematemesis vomiting of blood that indicates bleeding in the upper GI tract.

hemochromatosis an autosomal recessive disease characterized by increased intestinal iron absorption and, as a result, increased tissue iron deposition.

hemodialysis (HD) dialysis that uses an artificial membrane as the semipermeable membrane through which the patient's blood circulates.

hemolytic anemia an anemia caused by destruction of RBCs at a rate that exceeds production.

hemophilia hereditary bleeding disorders caused by defective or deficient clotting factors.

hemorrhagic stroke a stroke that results from bleeding into the brain tissue itself or into the subarachnoid space or ventricles.

hemorrhoids varicosities in the lower rectum or anus caused by congestion in the veins of the hemorrhoidal plexus.

hemothorax accumulation of blood in the pleural space.

hepatic encephalopathy changes in neurologic and mental function resulting from high levels of ammonia in the blood that a damaged liver cannot detoxify.

hepatitis inflammation of the liver.

hepatorenal syndrome type of renal failure in which the kidneys have no structural abnormality and characterized by azotemia, oliguria, and intractable ascites.

hernia a protrusion of a viscus through an abnormal opening or a weakened area in the wall of the cavity in which it is normally contained.

herniated disc herniation of nuclear material from the intervertebral disc that may compress or place tension on a cervical, lumbar, or sacral spinal nerve root.

hiatal hernia herniation of a portion of the stomach into the esophagus through an opening, or hiatus, in the diaphragm.

histologic grading a categorization of tumors in which the appearance of cells and the degree of differentiation are evaluated pathologically.

Hodgkin's lymphoma a malignant condition characterized by proliferation of abnormal giant, multinucleated cells, called *Reed-Sternberg cells*, which are located in lymph nodes.

hordeolum an infection of the sebaceous glands in the eyelid margin; commonly known as a *sty.*

hospice a concept of care that provides compassion, concern, and support for persons in the last phases of a terminal disease.

hospital-acquired pneumonia (HAP) pneumonia occurring 48 hours or longer after hospital admission and not incubating at the time of hospitalization.

human immunodeficiency virus (HIV) a retrovirus that causes HIV infection and acquired immunodeficiency syndrome.

human leukocyte antigens (HLAs) a system consisting of a series of linked genes that occur together on the sixth chromosome in humans and that is used to assess tissue compatibility.

humoral immunity antibody-mediated immunity.

Huntington's disease a genetically transmitted, autosomal dominant disorder that affects both men and women of all races and is characterized by chronic, devastating loss of all neurologic function, resulting in dementia.

hydronephrosis dilation or enlargement of the renal pelvis and calyces resulting from obstruction in the lower urinary tract with backflow of urine to the kidney.

hydroureter dilation of the renal pelvis due to backflow of urine.

hyperaldosteronism excessive aldosterone secretion caused by an adenoma of the adrenal zona glomerulosa or bilateral adrenal hyperplasia.

hypercapnia greater than normal amounts of carbon dioxide in the blood; also called *hypercarbia.*

hypercapnic respiratory failure a condition in which the $PaCO_2$ is above normal in combination with acidemia.

hyperopia farsightedness or the inability of the eye to focus on nearby objects.

hyperosmolar hyperglycemic syndrome (HHS) a life-threatening syndrome that can occur in the patient with diabetes who is able to produce enough insulin to prevent diabetic ketoacidosis but not enough to prevent severe hyperglycemia, osmotic diuresis, and extracellular fluid depletion.

hyperparathyroidism a condition involving increased secretion of parathyroid hormone resulting in increased serum calcium levels.

hypertension a common disorder characterized by sustained elevation of blood pressure.

hypertensive crisis a severe and abrupt elevation in blood pressure.

hyperthyroidism a clinical syndrome in which there is a sustained increase in the synthesis and release of thyroid hormones by the thyroid gland.

hypertrophic scar an inappropriately large, red, raised, and hard scar that occurs when the body produces excess collagen tissue.

hypoparathyroidism a condition of insufficient secretion of the parathyroid glands.

hypopituitarism a rare disorder that involves a decrease in one or more of the pituitary hormones and is marked by excessive deposits of fat and persistence or acquisition of adolescent characteristics.

hypothermia a core temperature <95° F (35° C) that occurs when heat produced by the body cannot compensate for heat lost to the environment.

hypothyroidism insufficient circulation of thyroid hormones resulting in a hypometabolic state.

hypoxemia low oxygen tension in the blood characterized by a variety of nonspecific clinical signs and symptoms.

hypoxemic respiratory failure a condition in which the PaO_2 is 60 mm Hg or less when the patient is receiving an inspired oxygen concentration of 60% or greater.

hypoxia the state in which the PaO_2 has fallen sufficiently to cause signs and symptoms of inadequate oxygenation.

I

ileal conduit urinary diversion procedure in which ureters are implanted into a part of the ileum or colon that has been resected from the intestinal tract and an abdominal stoma is created.

impaired fasting glucose (IFG) an intermediate stage between normal glucose homeostasis and diabetes.

impaired glucose tolerance (IGT) an intermediate stage between normal glucose homeostasis and diabetes in which the blood glucose level is 140 mg/dL (7.8 mmol/L) to 199 mg/dL (11 mmol/L) 2 hours after a meal.

infective endocarditis an infection of the endocardial surface of the heart.

infertility the inability to achieve a pregnancy after at least 1 year of regular intercourse without contraception.

inflammatory bowel disease (IBD) chronic, recurrent inflammatory diseases of the intestinal tract that include ulcerative colitis and Crohn's disease.

insulin resistance a condition in which body tissues do not respond to the action of insulin.

intensive insulin therapy multiple daily insulin injections together with frequent self-monitoring of blood glucose.

intermittent claudication ischemic muscle ache or pain precipitated by a consistent level of exercise, resolves within 10 minutes or less with rest, and is reproducible.

interstitial cystitis chronic, painful inflammatory disease of the bladder probably associated with an autoimmune or allergic response.

intraaortic balloon pump (IABP) a temporary circulatory assist device used to enhance the function of a compromised heart by reducing afterload and augmenting the aortic diastolic pressure.

intracerebral hematoma collection of blood within the parenchyma of the brain, possibly from the rupture of an intracerebral vessel at the time of a head injury.

intracranial pressure the hydrostatic force measured in the brain cerebrospinal fluid compartment.

iron-deficiency anemia a microcytic hypochromic anemia caused by inadequate supplies of iron needed to synthesize hemoglobin; characterized by pallor, fatigue, and weakness.

irritable bowel syndrome (IBS) a disorder characterized by chronic abdominal pain or discomfort and alteration of bowel patterns (diarrhea or constipation).

ischemic stroke a stroke that results from inadequate blood flow to the brain due to partial or complete occlusion of an artery.

isometric contractions muscular contraction that increases tension but does not produce movement.

isotonic contractions muscular contraction with shortening that produces movement.

J

jaundice a symptom of yellowish discoloration of body tissues that results from an increased concentration of bilirubin in the blood.

jaw-thrust maneuver a technique used to maintain an open airway that should be used in emergency situations.

K

keloid an overgrowth of collagenous scar tissue at the site of a skin injury, particularly a wound or a surgical incision; the new tissue is elevated, rounded, and firm.

keratinocytes cells synthesized from epidermal cells in the basal layer; the cells produce a specialized protein (keratin) that is vital to the protective barrier function of the skin.

keratitis an inflammation or infection of the cornea; may be caused by a variety of microorganisms or by other factors.

Korotkoff sounds sounds heard during the taking of a blood pressure reading using a sphygmomanometer and stethoscope.

Kupffer cells a type of macrophage found in the liver that removes bacteria and toxins from the blood.

kyphosis anterior-posterior or forward bending of spine with convexity of curve in posterior direction.

L

leiomyoma a benign smooth muscle tumor that occurs most commonly within the uterus, stomach, esophagus, or small intestine; uterine fibroid.

leukemia a broad term given to a group of malignant diseases characterized by diffuse replacement of bone marrow with proliferating leukocyte precursors.

leukopenia an abnormal decrease in the number of total white blood cells to <4000/μL.

lichenification the thickening of the skin as a result of proliferation of keratinocytes with accentuation of the normal markings of the skin often caused by repeated scratching of a pruritic lesion.

lithotripsy the use of sound waves to break renal stones into small particles that can be eliminated from the urinary tract.

lordosis lumbar spinal deformity resulting in anterior-posterior curvature with concavity in posterior direction.

lumpectomy breast-conserving surgery that involves the removal of the entire tumor along with a margin of normal tissue.

Lyme disease a spirochetal infection caused by *Borrelia burgdorferi* and transmitted by the bite of an infected deer tick; characterized by fever, chills, headache, stiff neck, and migratory joint and muscle pain.

lymphedema accumulation of lymph in soft tissue with swelling resulting from inflammation, obstruction, or removal of lymph channels and nodes.

lymphomas malignant neoplasms originating in the bone marrow and lymphatic structures resulting in the proliferation of lymphocytes.

M

malabsorption syndrome a complex of symptoms resulting from disorders in the intestinal absorption of nutrients, characterized by anorexia, weight loss, abdominal bloating, muscle cramps, bone pain, and steatorrhea.

malignant hyperthermia a rare genetic metabolic disease characterized by hyperthermia with rigidity of skeletal muscles that can result in death.

malignant melanoma a tumor arising in cells producing melanin, usually the melanocytes of the skin.

malignant neoplasm a tumor that tends to grow, invade, and metastasize; usually has an irregular shape and is composed of poorly differentiated cells.

Mallory-Weiss tear a tear that occurs in the esophageal mucosa at the junction of the esophagus and stomach, caused by severe retching and vomiting and results in severe bleeding.

mammoplasty a change in the size or shape of the breast due to surgery.

mass casualty incident a human-caused (e.g., biologic warfare) or natural (e.g., hurricane) event or disaster that overwhelms a community's ability to respond with existing resources.

mastalgia breast pain; can be caused by congestion or "caking" during lactation, an infection, or fibrocystic disease, especially during or before menstruation, or in advanced cancer.

mastitis an inflammatory condition of the breast that occurs most frequently in lactating women, caused by streptococcal or staphylococcal infection.

mean arterial pressure (MAP) a calculated average of systolic and diastolic blood pressures; calculated by adding the diastolic pressure to one third of the pulse pressure.

megaloblastic anemias a group of disorders caused by impaired DNA synthesis and characterized by the presence of large red blood cells.

melena black, tarry stools that indicate slow bleeding from an upper GI source.

menarche the first episode of menstrual bleeding; indicates female has reached puberty.

Ménière's disease a disease characterized by symptoms caused by inner ear disease, including episodic vertigo, tinnitus, fluctuating sensorineural hearing loss, and aural fullness.

meningitis an acute inflammation of the pia mater and the arachnoid membrane surrounding the brain and the spinal cord.

menopause the physiologic cessation of menses associated with declining ovarian function.

metabolic equivalent (MET) a unit of measurement of heat production by the body; used to determine the energy costs of various exercises.

metabolic syndrome a group of metabolic risk factors that increase an individual's chance of developing cardiovascular disease and diabetes mellitus.

metastasis the spread of the cancer from the initial or primary site to a distant site.

migraine headache a recurring headache characterized by unilateral or bilateral throbbing pain and a triggering event or factor; can occur with and without an aura.

mild cognitive impairment (MCI) a state of cognition and functional ability between normal aging and early Alzheimer's disease.

mitral valve prolapse (MVP) a structural abnormality of the mitral valve leaflets and the papillary muscles or chordae that allows the leaflets to prolapse, or buckle, back into the left atrium during ventricular systole.

mixed dementia presentation of two or more types of dementia simultaneously.

multiple myeloma a condition in which malignant neoplastic plasma cells infiltrate the bone marrow and destroy bone.

multiple organ dysfunction syndrome (MODS) the failure of more than one organ system in an acutely ill patient such that homeostasis cannot be maintained without intervention.

multiple sclerosis (MS) a chronic, progressive, degenerative disorder of the central nervous system characterized by disseminated demyelination of nerve fibers of the brain and spinal cord.

murmur a gentle blowing, fluttering, or humming sound heard on auscultation and produced by turbulent blood flow through the heart or the walls of large arteries.

muscular dystrophy (MD) a group of genetically transmitted diseases characterized by progressive symmetric wasting of skeletal muscle without evidence of neurologic involvement.

myasthenia gravis (MG) an autoimmune disease of the neuromuscular junction characterized by the fluctuating weakness of certain skeletal muscle groups.

myasthenic crisis an acute exacerbation of myasthenia gravis triggered by infection, surgery, emotional distress, or overdose or inadequate medication.

myelodysplastic syndrome (MDS) a group of related hematologic disorders characterized by a change in the quantity and quality of bone marrow elements.

myocardial infarction (MI) an irreversible cardiac cellular death caused by sustained myocardial ischemia.

myocarditis a focal or diffuse inflammation of the myocardium.

myopia nearsightedness or the inability of the eye to focus on objects far away.

myxedema the progression of the mental sluggishness, drowsiness, and lethargy of hypothyroidism to a notable impairment of consciousness or coma, which is a medical emergency.

N

nadir the lowest point, such as the blood cell count after it has been depressed by chemotherapy.

nasal polyps benign mucous membrane masses that form slowly in response to repeated inflammation of the sinus or nasal mucosa and project into the nasal cavity.

nephrolithiasis the formation of stones in the urinary tract.

nephrosclerosis a vascular disease of the kidney characterized by sclerosis of the small arteries and arterioles of the kidney, resulting in renal tissue necrosis.

nephrotic syndrome an abnormal condition of the kidney characterized by peripheral edema, massive proteinuria, hyperlipidemia, and hypoalbuminemia.

neurofibrillary tangles tangled bundles of fibers seen in the cytoplasm of abnormal neurons in those areas of the brain most affected by Alzheimer's disease.

neurogenic bladder any type of bladder dysfunction related to abnormal or absent bladder innervation caused by a lesion of the nervous system.

neurogenic bowel loss of voluntary neurologic control over the bowel.

neurogenic shock neurologic syndrome caused by the loss of vasomotor tone caused by spinal cord injury and characterized by hypotension, bradycardia, and warm, dry extremities.

neuropathic pain pain caused by damage to nerve cells or changes in spinal cord processing of nervous system input.

neutropenia an abnormal reduction of the neutrophil count to <1000/μL.

nonalcoholic fatty liver disease (NAFLD) a group of disorders characterized by hepatic *steatosis* (accumulation of fat in the liver) and is not associated with other causes such as hepatitis, autoimmune disease, or consumption of alcohol.

normal pressure hydrocephalus an uncommon disorder characterized by an obstruction in the flow of cerebrospinal fluid; causes a buildup of this fluid in the brain.

nuchal rigidity resistance to flexion of the neck.

nulliparous never having given birth.

nystagmus an abnormal, involuntary, repetitive movement of the eyes.

O

O₂ toxicity a condition of O_2 overdosage caused by prolonged exposure to a high level of O_2.

obese the classification used to describe individuals with body mass index values ≥30 kg/m^2.

obstructive sleep apnea (OSA) a condition characterized by partial or complete upper airway obstruction during sleep.

oliguria producing <400 mL of urine in 24 hours.

oncogenes potentially cancer-inducing genes.

oncotic pressure the osmotic pressure of a colloid in solution.

orchitis an acute inflammation of the testis.

orthostatic hypotension abnormally low blood pressure occurring when an individual suddenly assumes a standing position.

osteoarthritis a slowly progressive, noninflammatory disorder of the diarthrodial (synovial) joints.

osteochondroma primary benign bone tumor characterized by an overgrowth of cartilage and bone near the end of the bone at the growth plate.

osteomalacia a rare condition of adult bones associated with vitamin D deficiency, resulting in decalcification and softening of bone.

osteomyelitis a severe infection of the bone, bone marrow, and surrounding soft tissue.

osteon cylindrical structural units that fit closely together in compact bone, creating a dense bone structure.

osteopenia bone loss that is more than normal (a T-score between −1 and −2.5), but not yet at the level for a diagnosis of osteoporosis.

osteoporosis a metabolic bone disease characterized by low bone mass and structural deterioration of bone tissue, leading to increased bone fragility and pathologic fractures.

osteosarcoma a primary bone tumor that is extremely aggressive and rapidly metastasizes to distant sites; usually occurs in the metaphyseal region of the long bones of the extremities.

osteotomy removing or adding a wedge or slice of bone to change its alignment and shift weight bearing, thereby correcting deformity and relieving pain.

ostomy a surgical procedure in which an opening is made to allow the passage of urine from the bladder or intestinal contents from the bowel through an incision or stoma surgically created in the wall of the abdomen.

otosclerosis a hereditary condition in which irregular ossification occurring on the footplate of the stapes in the oval window results in decreased hearing acuity.

P

Paget's disease of the bone a skeletal bone disorder in which there is excessive bone resorption followed by replacement of normal marrow by vascular, fibrous connective tissue and new bone that is larger, disorganized, and weaker.

Paget's disease of the breast a breast malignancy characterized by a persistent lesion of the nipple and areola with or without a palpable mass.

palliative care an approach that improves the quality of life of patients and their families who face problems associated with serious life-limiting illness.

palpation a physical examination technique in which the examiner feels the texture, size, consistency, and location of certain body parts with the hands.

pancytopenia a marked decrease in the number of red blood cells, white blood cells, and platelets.

paralytic ileus the lack of intestinal peristalsis.

paraplegia paralysis characterized by motor and/or sensory loss in the lower limbs and trunk.

parasomnias unusual and often undesirable behaviors that occur with sleep or during arousal from sleep, such as enuresis (bed-wetting), hallucinations, and eating.

parenteral nutrition (PN) the administration of nutrients by a route (e.g., bloodstream) other than the GI tract.

Parkinson's disease (PD) a disease of the basal ganglia characterized by a slowing down in the initiation and execution of movement, increased muscle tone tremor at rest, and impaired postural reflexes.

paroxysmal nocturnal dyspnea (PND) sudden attacks of respiratory distress that awaken the sleeper, usually after several hours of sleep in a reclining position.

partial-thickness burn varying degrees of epidermal and dermal skin injury in which some skin elements remain viable for regeneration.

pelvic inflammatory disease (PID) an infectious condition of the pelvic cavity that may involve infection of the fallopian tubes, ovaries, and pelvic peritoneum.

peptic ulcer disease (PUD) erosion of the GI mucosa that results from the digestive action of HCl acid and pepsin.

percussion a physical examination technique in which the examiner taps the body with the fingertips or fist.

percutaneous coronary intervention (PCI) a common intervention for coronary artery disease in which a catheter equipped with an inflatable balloon tip is inserted into a narrowed coronary artery and the balloon is inflated.

pericardiocentesis a procedure in which a 16- to 18-gauge needle is inserted into the pericardial space to remove fluid for analysis and to relieve cardiac pressure.

pericarditis a condition caused by inflammation of the pericardial sac.

perimenopause a normal life transition that begins with the first signs of change in menstrual cycles and ends after cessation of menses.

peripheral artery disease (PAD) the progressive narrowing and degeneration of the arteries of the neck, abdomen, and extremities.

peripheral stem cell transplantation the transplantation of stem cells obtained from the peripheral blood in an outpatient procedure; often takes more than one procedure to obtain enough stem cells.

peritoneal dialysis (PD) dialysis using the peritoneal membrane as the semipermeable membrane.

peritonitis the inflammation of the peritoneum.

pernicious anemia a progressive megaloblastic macrocytic anemia resulting from inadequate gastric secretion of intrinsic factor necessary for absorption of cobalamin.

pertussis a highly contagious infection of the lower respiratory tract with a gram-negative bacillus, *Bordetella pertussis*.

petechiae small purplish lesions.

phantom limb sensation the perception of sensations or pain in an amputated limb.

pharmacogenetics the study of variability of responses to drugs due to variations in single genes.

pharmacogenomics the study of variability of responses to drugs due to variations in and interactions of multiple genes.

pheochromocytoma a rare condition characterized by a tumor of the adrenal medulla that produces excessive catecholamines causing persistent or intermittent hypertension.

phimosis a constriction of the uncircumcised foreskin around the head of the penis, making retraction difficult.

pleural effusion an abnormal accumulation of fluid in the intrapleural spaces of the lungs.

pleural friction rub a creaking or grating sound from roughened, inflamed surfaces of the pleura rubbing together, evident during inspiration, expiration, or both.

pleurisy (pleuritis) inflammation of the pleura.

pneumoconiosis a general term for lung diseases caused by inhalation and retention of dust particles.

pneumonia an acute inflammation of the lungs, often caused by inhaled pneumococci of the species *Streptococcus pneumoniae*.

pneumothorax a collection of air or gas in the pleural space causing the lung to collapse.

point of maximal impulse (PMI) the site on the chest wall where the thrust or pulsation of the left ventricle is most prominent.

polycystic kidney disease (PKD) a genetic kidney disorder in which the cortex and medulla are filled with thin-walled cysts that enlarge and destroy surrounding tissue.

polycythemia an abnormal condition with excessive levels of red blood cells.

polymyositis diffuse, idiopathic, inflammatory myopathies of striated muscle, producing bilateral weakness usually most severe in the proximal or limb-girdle muscles; some forms of polymyositis are associated with malignancy.

portal hypertension increased venous pressure in the portal circulation caused by compression and destruction of the portal and hepatic veins and sinusoids.

positive end-expiratory pressure (PEEP) a ventilatory maneuver in which positive pressure is applied to the airway during exhalation.

postural drainage the use of various positions to promote gravity drainage of bronchial secretions.

prediabetes impaired glucose tolerance; occurs when a 2-hour plasma glucose level is higher than normal but lower than that considered diagnostic for diabetes.

prehypertension a disorder characterized by a systolic blood pressure of 120 to 139 mm Hg and a diastolic blood pressure of 80 to 89 mm Hg.

preload the volume of blood in the ventricles at the end of diastole before the next contraction.

premature atrial contraction (PAC) contraction originating from an ectopic focus in the atrium in a location other than the sinus node.

premature ventricular contraction (PVC) a contraction originating in an ectopic focus in the ventricles.

premenstrual syndrome (PMS) a common disorder in women in which a group of physical and psychologic symptoms occur during the last few days of the menstrual cycle and before the onset of menstruation.

presbycusis hearing loss associated with aging.

presbyopia a hyperopic shift to farsightedness resulting from a loss of elasticity of the lens of the eye.

pressure ulcer a localized area of tissue necrosis caused by unrelieved pressure that occludes blood flow to the tissues.

primary hypertension an elevated systemic arterial pressure for which no cause can be found and which is often the only significant clinical finding.

Prinzmetal's angina a variant angina; occurs at rest, usually in response to reversible, severe spasm of a major coronary artery.

prostatitis an acute or chronic inflammation of the prostate gland, usually as a result of infection.

pruritus itching.

psoriasis an autoimmune skin disorder characterized by circumscribed red patches covered by thick, dry, silvery, adherent scales.

pulmonary edema an acute, life-threatening situation in which the lung alveoli become filled with serous or serosanguineous fluid, caused most commonly by heart failure.

pulmonary embolism a thromboembolic occlusion of the pulmonary vasculature resulting from thrombi in the venous circulation or right side of the heart that travel as emboli until lodging in the pulmonary vessels.

pulmonary hypertension elevated pulmonary pressure resulting from an increase in pulmonary vascular resistance to blood flow through small arteries and arterioles.

pulse pressure the difference between the systolic and diastolic pressures.

pursed-lip breathing a technique of exhaling against pursed lips to prolong exhalation, preventing bronchiolar collapse and air trapping.

pyelonephritis a diffuse pyogenic infection of the renal parenchyma and collecting system.

pyrosis a burning sensation in the epigastric or substernal area; heartburn.

R

radical prostatectomy the surgical removal of the entire prostate gland, seminal vesicles, and part of the bladder neck (ampulla).

Raynaud's phenomenon an episodic vasospastic disorder of small cutaneous arteries, most frequently involving the fingers and toes.

refractive error a defect in the ability of the lens of the eye to focus an image accurately on the retina, as occurs in nearsightedness and farsightedness.

renal artery stenosis a partial occlusion of one or both renal arteries and their major branches; is a major cause of abrupt-onset hypertension.

repetitive strain injury (RSI) a cumulative trauma disorder resulting from prolonged, forceful, or awkward movements resulting in strain of tendons, ligaments, and muscles, causing tiny tears that become inflamed.

restless legs syndrome (RLS) the unpleasant sensory and motor abnormalities of one or both legs; characterized by an irritating sensation of uneasiness, tiredness, and itching deep within the muscles of the leg.

retinal detachment a separation of the retina from the retinal pigment epithelium in the back of the eye, allowing the vitreous humor to leak between the two layers.

retinopathy the process of microvascular damage of the retina; may develop slowly or rapidly.

rheumatic fever an inflammatory disease of the heart that potentially involves all layers.

rheumatic heart disease (RHD) the resulting damage to the heart muscle and heart valves from rheumatic fever, a chronic condition characterized by scarring and deformity of the heart valves.

rheumatoid arthritis (RA) a chronic, systemic autoimmune disease characterized by inflammation of connective tissue in the diarthrodial (synovial) joints, typically with periods of remission and exacerbation.

rhinoplasty the surgical reconstruction of the nose.

S

sarcoma a malignant tumor that originates from embryonal mesoderm that becomes connective tissue, muscle, bone, and fat.

scleroderma a disorder of connective tissue characterized by fibrotic, degenerative, and occasionally inflammatory changes in the skin, blood vessels, synovium, skeletal muscle, and internal organs.

scoliosis a lateral S-shaped curvature of the thoracic and lumbar spine.

secondary hypertension elevated blood pressure associated with any of several primary diseases, such as renal, pulmonary, endocrine, and vascular diseases.

seizure a paroxysmal, uncontrolled electrical discharge of neurons in the brain that interrupts normal function leading to a sudden, violent involuntary series of contractions of a group of muscles.

sepsis a systemic inflammatory response to infection.

septic arthritis infectious or bacterial arthritis caused by invasion of the joint cavity with microorganisms; bacterial inflammation of a joint may be caused by the spread of bacteria through the bloodstream from an infection elsewhere in the body or by contamination of a joint during trauma or surgery.

septic shock the presence of sepsis with hypotension despite adequate fluid resuscitation along with the presence of tissue perfusion abnormalities.

sexually transmitted infections (STIs) infectious diseases transmitted most commonly through sexual intercourse or genital contact.

shock a syndrome characterized by decreased tissue perfusion and impaired cellular metabolism resulting in an imbalance between the supply of and demand for oxygen and nutrients.

sickle cell disease (SCD) a group of inherited, autosomal recessive disorders characterized by the presence of an abnormal form of hemoglobin in the erythrocyte.

silent ischemia an asymptomatic ischemia that may damage the heart.

Sjögren's syndrome an autoimmune disease that targets moisture-producing glands, leading to the common symptoms of xerostomia (dry mouth) and keratoconjunctivitis sicca (dry eyes).

Somogyi effect a condition in which an excessive dose of insulin causes blood glucose levels to decline during sleep, triggering the release of counterregulatory hormones that increase the blood glucose levels, resulting in high blood glucose levels at morning testing; indicates a need for reduced dose of insulin.

spermatogenesis the formation of sperm.

spider angiomas small, dilated blood vessels with a bright red center point the size of a pinhead from which small blood vessels radiate.

spinal shock the immediate failure of all spinal cord function at the time of injury below the level of cord damage, resulting in flaccid paralysis, loss of reflexes, and loss of sympathetic innervation.

spondyloarthropathies a group of interrelated multisystem inflammatory disorders that affect the spine, peripheral joints, and periarticular structures.

status epilepticus a state of continuous seizure activity or a condition in which seizures recur in rapid succession without return to consciousness between seizures.

steatorrhea a greater than normal amount of fat in the feces.

stenosis a constriction or narrowing.

stent an expandable meshlike structure designed to maintain vessel patency by compressing the arterial walls and resisting vasoconstriction.

stricture   an abnormal temporary or permanent narrowing of the lumen of a hollow organ.

stroke   the death of brain cells that occurs when there is ischemia to a part of the brain or hemorrhage into the brain.

subarachnoid hemorrhage   a stroke resulting from intracranial bleeding into the cerebrospinal fluid–filled space between the arachnoid and pia mater membranes on the surface of the brain.

subdural hematoma   a collection of blood between the dura mater and the arachnoid layer of the meninges of the brain that is generally of venous origin, usually caused by injury.

sudden cardiac death (SCD)   unexpected death from cardiac causes.

sundowning   a condition in which the individual becomes more confused and agitated in the late afternoon or evening.

surfactant   a lipoprotein that lowers the surface tension in the alveoli, reduces the amount of pressure needed to inflate the alveoli, and decreases the tendency of the alveoli to collapse.

syndrome of inappropriate antidiuretic hormone (SIADH)   a condition associated with overproduction or oversecretion of ADH.

synovectomy   the surgical removal of synovial membrane.

syphilis   the infection of organs and tissues of the body by *Treponema pallidum*.

systemic exertion intolerance disease (SEID)   was formerly called *chronic fatigue syndrome*. Is a serious, complex, multisystem disease in which exertion of any sort (physical, emotional, cognitive) can adversely affect multiple organs.

systemic inflammatory response syndrome (SIRS)   a systemic inflammatory response to a variety of insults, including infection, ischemia, infarct, and injury.

systemic lupus erythematosus (SLE)   a chronic multisystem inflammatory disorder associated with abnormalities of the immune system.

teletherapy   radiation therapy administered by a machine positioned at some distance from the patient; the most common form of radiation therapy treatment.

tenesmus   the painful spasmodic contraction of the anal sphincter and a persistent desire to empty the bowel.

tension pneumothorax   a rapid accumulation of air in the pleural space causing severely high intrapleural pressures with resultant tension on the heart and great vessels.

tension-type headache   a headache characterized by a bilateral feeling of pressure around the head.

tetanus   lockjaw; an extremely severe polyradiculitis and polyneuritis affecting spinal and cranial nerves that results from the effects of a potent neurotoxin released by the anaerobic bacillus *Clostridium tetani*.

tetraplegia   the paralysis of the arms, legs, and trunk occurring with spinal cord damage at C8 or above.

thalassemia   an autosomal recessive genetic disorder of inadequate production of normal hemoglobin.

thoracentesis   a surgical procedure done to remove fluid from the pleural space.

thoracotomy   a surgical opening into the thoracic cavity.

thrombocytopenia   a reduction of the platelet count.

thrombocytosis   a condition marked by excessive platelets; a disorder that occurs with inflammation and some malignant disorders.

thrombotic stroke   a stroke resulting from thrombosis or narrowing of the blood vessel.

thyroiditis   an inflammatory process in the thyroid gland.

thyrotoxicosis   (also called *thyrotoxic crisis* or *thyroid storm*) a hypermetabolic state caused by excessive circulating levels of T_4, T_3, or both.

tinnitus   a subjective noise sensation, often described as ringing, heard in one or both ears.

tonic-clonic seizure   a seizure characterized by loss of consciousness and falling to the ground, followed by stiffening of the body for 10 to 20 seconds and subsequent jerking of the extremities for another 30 to 40 seconds.

tracheostomy   a surgical opening into the trachea through which an indwelling tube may be inserted.

traction   the application of a pulling force to an injured or diseased part of the body or an extremity while countertraction pulls in the opposite direction.

transurethral resection of the prostate (TURP)   a surgical procedure involving the removal of prostate tissue with the use of a resectoscope inserted through the urethra.

triage   a system that identifies and categorizes patients so that the most critical are treated first.

trigeminal neuralgia   a neurologic condition of the trigeminal facial nerve characterized by paroxysms of flashing, stablike pain radiating along the course of a branch of the nerve from the angle of the jaw.

trigger point   a circumscribed hypersensitive area within a tight band of muscle that is caused by acute or chronic muscle strain.

tuberculosis (TB)   an infectious disease caused by *Mycobacterium tuberculosis*; usually involves the lungs but also occurs in the larynx, kidneys, bones, adrenal glands, lymph nodes, and meninges and can be disseminated throughout the body.

tumor angiogenesis   the process of the formation of blood vessels within the tumor itself.

ulcerative colitis   a chronic inflammatory bowel disease that causes ulceration of the colon and rectum.

unstable angina (UA)   an angina that is new in onset, occurs at rest, or has a worsening pattern.

uremia   the presence of excessive amounts of urea and other nitrogenous waste products in the blood; renal function declines to the point that symptoms develop in multiple body systems.

urethritis   inflammation of the urethra.

urinary incontinence (UI)   an uncontrolled leakage of urine; can be caused by anything that interferes with bladder or urethral sphincter control, including confusion or depression, infection, atrophic vaginitis, urinary retention, restricted mobility, fecal impaction, or drugs.

urinary retention   the inability to empty the bladder despite micturition, or the accumulation of urine in the bladder because of an inability to urinate.

urosepsis   a urinary tract infection that has spread into the systemic circulation; life-threatening condition requiring emergency treatment.

uterine prolapse   the downward displacement of the uterus into the vaginal canal as a result of impaired pelvic support.

Valsalva maneuver   a maneuver that involves contraction of the chest muscles on a closed glottis with simultaneous contraction of the abdominal muscles.

varicose veins   the dilated, tortuous subcutaneous veins most frequently found in the saphenous system.

vascular dementia   the loss of cognitive function resulting from ischemic, ischemic-hypoxic, or hemorrhagic brain lesions caused by cardiovascular disease.

vasectomy   the bilateral surgical ligation or resection of the vas deferens performed for the purpose of sterilization.

ventricular assist device (VAD)   a device that is applied externally or internally into the path of flowing blood to augment or replace the action of the ventricle of the heart.

ventricular fibrillation   a severe derangement of the heart rhythm characterized on electrocardiogram (ECG) by irregular undulations of varying contour and amplitude.

ventricular tachycardia (VT)   a condition that occurs when an ectopic focus or foci fire repetitively and the ventricle takes control as the pacemaker.

vertigo   a sensation that a person or objects around the person are moving or spinning; usually stimulated by movement of the head.

vesicants   agents that when accidentally infiltrated into the skin cause severe local tissue breakdown and necrosis.

viral load   the quantity of viral particles in a biologic sample.

Virchow's triad   three important factors in the etiology of venous thrombosis: (1) venous stasis, (2) damage of the endothelium (inner lining of the vein), and (3) hypercoagulability of the blood.

wheezes   a form of rhonchus characterized by a continuous high-pitched squeaking sound caused by rapid vibration of bronchial walls.

window period   a time period of 3 weeks after HIV infection during which an infected individual will not test positive for HIV antibody.

A

AB5000 Circulatory Support System, 754
Abacavir (Ziagen), 187*b*
Abandonment
elder mistreatment, 67*b*
fear of, at end of life, 139
Abatacept (Orencia), 1521*b*-1522*b*, 1529
ABCDE (Awakening and Breathing Trial Coordination, Daily Delirium Monitoring and Management, and Early Exercise and Mobility) bundle, 1582
ABCDE rule, 410, 410*f*
Abciximab (ReoPro), 715*b*-716*b*
Abdomen
abnormalities, 846*b*-847*b*
examination of, 843-844, 1112
auscultation, 843-844
inspection, 843
normal, 846*b*
palpation, 844, 844*f*
percussion, 844, 844*f*
secondary survey, 1633-1634
quadrants of, 843, 843*b*, 843*f*
Abdominal aortic aneurysms, 810, 810*f*-811*f*
clinical manifestations of, 811
interprofessional care for, 811
surgical repair of, 811, 812*f*
Abdominal breathing, 569
relaxation, **83-84**, 84*b*
Abdominal compartment syndrome, 812, 941, 1593
Abdominal distention, 597*b*-598*b*, 846*b*-847*b*
postoperative, 1063
Abdominal pain, 1197*b*
acute, **938-939**, 1013*b*
chronic, **940-941**
Abdominal paradox, 467*b*-468*b*
Abdominal thrusts, 1652*b*, 1652*f*
Abdominal trauma, 941, 942*b*
Abdominal ultrasound, 603*t*, 847*t*-850*t*
focused abdominal sonography for trauma (FAST), 1633-1634
Abdominal wall, in older adults, 840*b*
Abdominal-perineal resection, 956
Abdominoplasty, 890*f*
Abducens nerve, 1305*b*, **1306**
Abduction, 1455*b*
Abiraterone (Zytiga), 1280*b*
Ablation surgery, 1391
ABO blood groups, 600, 601*b*
Abortion, 1243
induced, 1243, **1244**
methods for inducing, 1244*b*
spontaneous, 1243, 1243*b*, **1243-1244**
Abscesses
anorectal, **970**, 970*f*
brain, 1336*b*, **1338-1339**, 1339*b*
lactational breast, **1207**
lung, **512**
peritonsillar, **484**
Absence seizures, 1375-1376
Absent bowel sounds, 846*b*-847*b*
Absent breath sounds, 467*b*-468*b*
Absolute neutrophil count, 632
Absolute refractory phase or period, 761, 762*f*

Abuse
child sexual abuse, 1263
elder abuse, **66-67**, 67*b*, 1414*b*
ACA (Patient Protection and Affordable Care Act), 4
Acanthosis nigricans, 1151
Acapella airway clearance device, 570, 570*f*
Acarbose (Precose), 1131*b*
Accelerated idioventricular rhythm, 764*b*, 770
Acceptance, 728*b*, 1435*b*
Accessory nerve, 1305*b*
Accolate (zafirlukast), 479*b*-480*b*, 547, 548*b*-549*b*
Accountable care organizations (ACOs), 4
Acculturation, 22
AccuNeb (albuterol), 548*b*-549*b*
Accupril (quinapril), 691*b*-693*b*
Accutane (isotretinoin), 417*b*
Aceon (perindopril), 691*b*-693*b*
Acetaminophen (Tylenol), 984*b*
for inflammation, 164, 164*b*
overdose, 1643*b*
for pain, 111-112, 111*b*
Acetazolamide, 381*b*, 1001*b*
Acetylsalicylic acid (aspirin), 1355
Achalasia, 905
Achilles tendon reflex, 1307
Achilles tendonitis, 1456*b*
Acid neutralizers, 903*b*
Acid-base imbalances, **286-297**, 288*b*, 289*f*
in chronic kidney disease, 1077
ROME memory device for, 291*b*
Acid-base regulation, **287-288**
Acid-fast bacteria smear and culture, 469*t*-471*t*
Acidosis, 287
diabetic ketoacidosis, **1142-1145**, 1154*b*
manifestations of, 290*b*
metabolic, 288*b*, **289**
in acute kidney injury, 1072
in chronic kidney disease, 1077
respiratory, 288*b*, **288**
Aciphex (rabeprazole), 903*b*
Aclidinium bromide (Tudorza, Pressair), 548*b*-549*b*
Acne, 403*b*
Acne vulgaris, 417, 417*f*, 419*b*
Acoustic neuroma, 387, 1333*b*
Acquired immunodeficiency syndrome (AIDS), **221**. See also Human immunodeficiency virus (HIV) infection
diagnostic criteria for, 221, 221*b*
Acrochordons, 419*b*
Acromegaly, **1156-1157**
clinical manifestations of, 1157, 1157*f*
dermatologic manifestations of, 399*b*
Acromioplasty, 1466-1467
Acropachy, 1164, 1165*f*
ACS Cancer Survivors Network, 267*b*
Actemra (tocilizumab), 1521*b*-1522*b*, 1529
Actigraphy, **93**
Actinic keratosis, 397, **411**, 412*b*
Action potential, 659, 757-758, 758*b*
Activase (alteplase), 715*b*-716*b*
Activated clotting time, 601*t*, 821*b*
Activated partial thromboplastin time, 601*t*, 821*b*, 1659*b*

Active listening, 49
Active surveillance (watchful waiting), 1278
Active transport, 272
Activity-exercise pattern, 37*b*, 38. See also Physical activity
Actonel (risedronate), 1513
Actos (pioglitazone), 1131*b*
Acupressure, 1080*b*
Acupuncture, **121**, 1523*b*
Acute abdominal pain, **938-939**
emergency management of, 939*b*
etiology and pathophysiology of, 938, 938*f*
Acute abnormal uterine bleeding, 1246
Acute alcohol toxicity, 149
Acute alcoholic hepatitis, 984
Acute angle-closure glaucoma, 380
Acute arterial ischemia, 808
Acute arterial ischemic disorders, **808-809**
Acute blood loss, **614-615**
clinical manifestations of, 615, 615*b*
laboratory results in, 610*b*
Acute bronchitis, **499-500**
Acute care
emergency nursing, 1634
for older adults, 71-74
Acute care nurse practitioners (ACNPs), 1555
Acute chest syndrome, 617
Acute cholecystitis, 1007*b*
Acute coronary syndrome, **718-734**, 718*f*
acute care for, 727-728
ambulatory care for, 730-732
diagnostic studies in, 721-722
drug therapy for, 715*b*-716*b*, 722, **725-726**
ECG changes in, 721, **775-777**, 776*b*
emotional and behavioral reactions to, 728
FITT activity guidelines for, 732, 732*b*
gender differences in, 705*b*
interprofessional care for, 714*f*, **722-726**
monitoring, 727
nursing assessment in, 726*b*
nursing diagnoses for, 726
nursing management of, **726-733**
nutritional therapy for, 726
patient & caregiver teaching for, 730-731, 731*b*
psychosocial responses to, 728*b*
rehabilitation after, 728*b*
sexual activity after, 732-733, 733*b*
Acute coryza, **478-480**
Acute decompensated heart failure
clinical manifestations of, 741-742
clinical mprofile, 742*b*
drug therapy for, 745-746, 745*b*
interprofessional care for, 744-746, 744*b*
Acute diarrhea, 929, 930*b*
Acute disease–related malnutrition, 857
Acute gastritis, 909-910
Acute gastroenteritis, 944
Acute gastrointestinal bleeding, 924, 924*b*
Acute glaucoma, 381*b*
Acute glomerulonephritis, 1041
Acute hemolytic reaction, 650*b*-651*b*
Acute hepatitis, **977-978**
clinical manifestations of, 977, 977*b*
diagnostic findings in, 979, 979*b*
drug therapy for, 975
interprofessional care for, 980-981, 980*b*

NOTE: Disorder names and key terms are in **boldface**. Page numbers in **boldface** indicate main discussions. Page numbers followed by *f*, *t*, or *b* indicate figures, tables, or boxes, respectively.

ABBREVIATIONS

ABG	arterial blood gas	DKA	diabetic ketoacidosis
ACE	angiotensin-converting enzyme	DM	diabetes mellitus; diastolic murmur
ACLS	advanced cardiac life support	DRE	digital rectal examination
ACS	acute coronary syndrome	DVT	deep vein thrombosis
ACTH	adrenocorticotropic hormone	ECF	extracellular fluid
ADH	antidiuretic hormone	ECG	electrocardiogram
AED	automatic external defibrillator	ED	emergency department; erectile dysfunction
AIDS	acquired immunodeficiency syndrome	EEG	electroencephalogram
AKA	above-knee amputation	EMG	electromyogram
AKI	acute kidney injury	EMS	emergency medical services
ALI	acute lung injury	ENT	ear, nose, and throat
ALL	acute lymphocytic leukemia	ERCP	endoscopic retrograde cholangiopancreatography
ALS	amyotrophic lateral sclerosis	ERT	estrogen replacement therapy
AMI	acute myocardial infarction	ESKD	end-stage kidney disease
ANA	antinuclear antibody	ESR	erythrocyte sedimentation rate
ANS	autonomic nervous system	ET	endotracheal
AORN	Association of periOperative Room Nurses	FEV	forced expiratory volume
APD	automated peritoneal dialysis	FRC	functional residual capacity
aPTT	activated partial thromboplastin time	FUO	fever of unknown origin
ARDS	acute respiratory distress syndrome	GCS	Glasgow Coma Scale
ATN	acute tubular necrosis	GERD	gastroesophageal reflux disease
BCLS	basic cardiac life support	GFR	glomerular filtration rate
BKA	below-knee amputation	GH	growth hormone
BMI	body mass index	GI	glycemic index
BMR	basal metabolic rate	GTT	glucose tolerance test
BMT	bone marrow transplantation	GU	genitourinary
BPH	benign prostatic hyperplasia	GYN, Gyn	gynecologic
BSE	breast self-examination	HAI	health care–associated infection
BUN	blood urea nitrogen	HAV	hepatitis A virus
CABG	coronary artery bypass graft	Hb, Hgb	hemoglobin
CAD	coronary artery disease; circulatory assist device	HBV	hepatitis B virus
CAPD	continuous ambulatory peritoneal dialysis	Hct	hematocrit
CAVH	continuous arteriovenous hemofiltration	HCV	hepatitis C virus
CBC	complete blood count	HD	hemodialysis, Huntington's disease
CCU	coronary care unit; critical care unit	HDL	high-density lipoprotein
CDC	Centers for Disease Control and Prevention	HF	heart failure
CIS	carcinoma in situ	HIV	human immunodeficiency virus
CKD	chronic kidney disease	H&P	history and physical examination
CLL	chronic lymphocytic leukemia	HPV	human papillomavirus
CML	chronic myelocytic leukemia	HSCT	hematopoietic stem cell transplantation
CMP	cardiomyopathy	IABP	intraaortic balloon pump
CN	cranial nerve	IBS	irritable bowel syndrome
CNS	central nervous system	ICP	intracranial pressure
CO	cardiac output	I&D	incision and drainage
COPD	chronic obstructive pulmonary disease	IE	infective endocarditis
CPAP	continuous positive airway pressure	IFG	impaired fasting glucose
CPR	cardiopulmonary resuscitation	IGT	impaired glucose tolerance
CRRT	continuous renal replacement therapy	INR	international normalized ratio
CRNA	certified registered nurse anesthetist	IOP	intraocular pressure
CSF	cerebrospinal fluid	IPPB	intermittent positive-pressure breathing
CT	computed tomography	ITP	idiopathic thrombocytopenic purpura
CVA	cerebrovascular accident; costovertebral angle	IUD	intrauterine device
CVAD	central venous access device	IV	intravenous
CVI	chronic venous insufficiency	IVP	intravenous push; intravenous pyelogram
CVP	central venous pressure	JVD	jugular venous distention
D&C	dilation and curettage	KS	Kaposi sarcoma
DDD	degenerative disk disease	KUB	kidney, ureters, and bladder (x-ray)
DI	diabetes insipidus	KVO	keep vein open
DIC	disseminated intravascular coagulation	LAD	left anterior descending
DJD	degenerative joint disease	LDL	low-density lipoprotein